MEDICAL ASSISTING

ADMINISTRATIVE AND CLINICAL COMPETENCIES

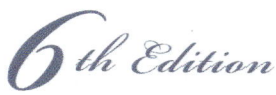
th Edition

MEDICAL ASSISTING

ADMINISTRATIVE AND CLINICAL COMPETENCIES

6th Edition

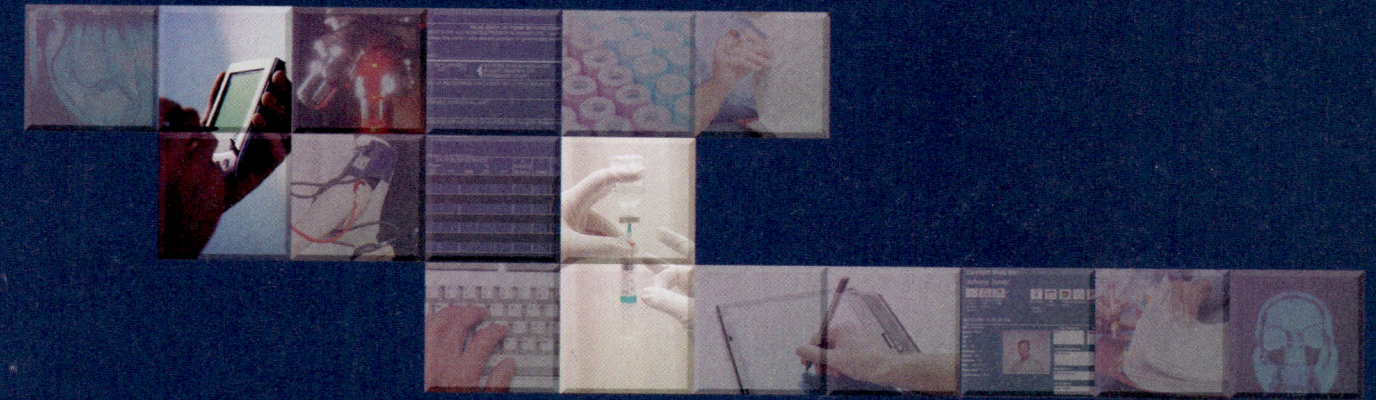

Lucille Keir, CMA-A

Barbara A. Wise, RN, BSN, MA(Ed)

Connie Krebs, CMA-C, BGS

Cathy Kelley-Arney, CMA, RMA, MLTC, BSHS

THOMSON

DELMAR LEARNING

Australia   Canada   Mexico   Singapore   Spain   United Kingdom   United States

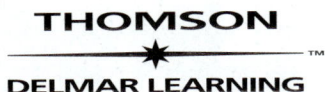

THOMSON

™

DELMAR LEARNING

Medical Assisting: Administrative and Clinical Competencies
Sixth Edition
by Lucille Keir, Barbara A. Wise, Connie Krebs, and Cathy Kelley-Arney

Vice President, Health Care Business Unit:
William Brottmiller

Director of Learning Solutions:
Matthew Kane

Senior Acquisitions Editor:
Rhonda Dearborn

Product Manager:
Sarah Prime

Editorial Assistant:
Laura Pye

Marketing Director:
Jennifer McAvey

Marketing Coordinator:
Andrea Eobstel

Technology Director:
Laurie Davis

Technology Product Manager:
Mary Colleen Liburdi

Technology Project Manager II:
Carolyn Fox

Production Director:
Carolyn Miller

Art Director:
Jack Pendleton

Content Project Manager:
David Buddle

Print Buyer:
Patti Packer

Library of Congress Cataloging-in-Publication Data

Medical assisting : administrative and clinical competencies /
  by Lucille Keir . . . [et al.]. — 6th ed.
    p. ; cm.
  Rev. ed. of: Medical assisting / Lucille Keir, Barbara A. Wise,
    Connie Krebs. 5th ed. c2003.
  Includes bibliographical references and index.
  ISBN-13: 978-1-4180-3266-1
  ISBN-10: 1-4180-3266-2
 1. Medical assistants. I. Keir, Lucille. II. Keir, Lucille. Medical assisting.
  [DNLM: 1. Physician Assistants. 2. Clinical Competence. 3. Practice
Management, Medical. 4. Vocational Guidance. W 21.5 M4896 2007]
  R728.8.K44 2007
  610.73′7—dc22

                                            2007005654

NOTICE TO THE READER

Dedication

I wish to dedicate this edition to my family, for their encouragement and understanding during this revision process, especially for the patience of my three grandchildren, who often had to wait until grandma finished something before they could come stay with me. I also want to remember my two good friends and co-authors, who are no longer with me.

They are truly missed.

Barbara A. Wise, RN, BSN, MA(Ed)

To my husband, Ronnie, who tolerates and loves me no matter what;

To my devoted dog, Tanner, who is always so happy to see me;

To my family of parrots that have been with me so many years and bring me such joy;

And to my brother, Michael, whom I adore and respect more than he can even know.

Cathy Kelley-Arney, CMA, RMA, MLTC, BSHS

CONTENTS

SECTION 3
STRUCTURE AND FUNCTION OF THE BODY   307

CHAPTER 11
Anatomy and Physiology
of the Human Body   308

CHAPTER 15
Specimen Collection and Laboratory Procedures   758

CHAPTER 19
Emergencies, Acute Illness, Accidents, and Recovery   951

SECTION 5
BEHAVIORS AND HEALTH   1003

CHAPTER 20
Behaviors Influencing Health   1004

SECTION 6

EMPLOYABILITY SKILLS   1049

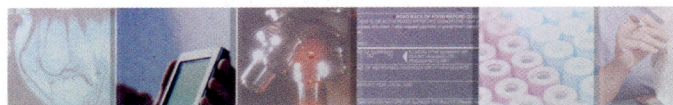

CHAPTER 21
Explore, Enter, and Succeed
in Employment   1050

LIST OF PROCEDURES

FOREWORD

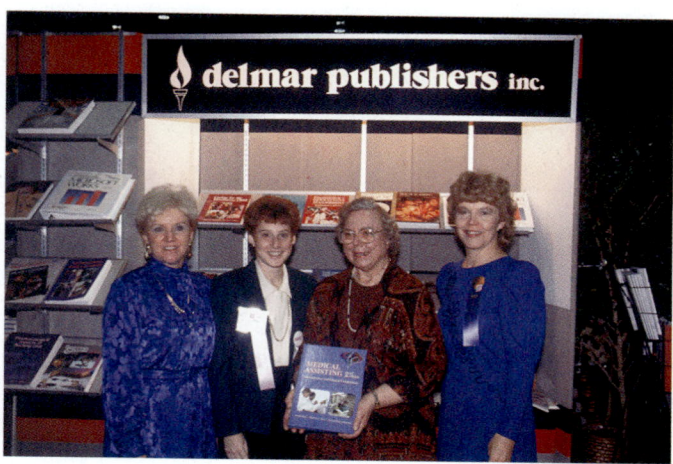

Left to right: Barbara Wise, Marion Waldman (former Delmar editor), Lucille Keir, Connie Krebs

The writing of our book, *Medical Assisting: Administrative and Clinical Competencies*, has been a very rewarding experience, with success that far surpassed our wildest expectations. Initially, the three of us were teaching secondary vocational health occupations in a large city school district. I taught nurse assisting. Lucille Keir and Connie Krebs were teaching medical assisting. They were dissatisfied with having to use three texts, administrative, clinical, and anatomy and physiology, to instruct their program. So, we decided that, among the three of us, we had the ability to write a comprehensive text. Because of this text, we became close friends in addition to educational colleagues.

We submitted our ideas for a text, and on September 23, 1983, we received a letter from the Delmar Editorial Board that our text proposal had been approved! We were going to write a book. Little did we know what a challenge that would be. I have described it as somewhat like giving birth to a first child; it was a new experience, somewhat lengthy and frequently quite painful.

The first edition was published in 1985 and we were ecstatic. When I look at it now, compared to this edition, I wonder why anyone bought it, but apparently a comprehensive text was what other instructors were also looking for. The second revision was much improved and sales were reflecting its acceptance. In the photo above, we are at a Delmar booth at a vocational education conference where the second edition was on display. When we began the third edition, Lucille was gravely ill and was able to contribute very little. She lost her life to cancer before it was published.

Connie and I went on with the third, fourth, and fifth editions. We had physicians, professional colleagues, and subject matter experts contributing to its relevancy and credibility. The text became the leader in its field, growing in all dimensions. Many other texts have replicated our design and format. I truly believe that we are basically responsible for the great improvement in medical assisting educational materials that are available today.

Unfortunately, on February 8, 2005, Connie also lost her life to cancer, and I alone was left to continue this legacy. I have gone on to complete the sixth edition with the help of Michelle Heller, Lyn Veach, Paula Murphy, and Cathy Kelly-Arney. This will be my last edition. After 23 years, I am passing the text responsibility to Cathy. Her years of work experience as a lab tech, medical assistant, and health care education director, in addition to her experience with program curriculum reviews, leaves the text in very capable hands.

I wish to thank all of you who have used this text over the years. I have appreciated your words of kindness and insightful recommendations for revisions. You have given me a sense of achievement that is hard to put into words. I know that Lucille and Connie would be as proud as I am with what we started 23 years ago as I am.

Barbara A. Wise

Barbara A. Wise

PREFACE

Medical Assisting: Administrative and Clinical Competencies, Sixth Edition, is a proven, competency-based learning system with a 23-year history of success. The text is full-color throughout and written in an interesting, easy-to-understand format. The content covers the knowledge, skills, attitudes, and values necessary to prepare you to become a successful, multiskilled medical assistant.

Information is presented in six major sections, which are divided further into 21 chapters and 80 units of instruction. There are hundreds of new color photos, illustrations, charts, and tables to visually supplement and reinforce the written material. New and revised instructor materials and student resources, including a *Workbook, Instructor's Resource Manual, Electronic Classroom Manager, Online Companion,* and *WebTutor,* complete this learning system.

The text and workbook are comprehensive, covering the administrative, clinical, and general areas identified by the current Medical Assisting Role Delineation Study issued by the American Association of Medical Assistants (AAMA) and the National Board of Examiners. The learning and performance competencies are identified at the beginning of each unit of instruction. Performance objectives correlate with each written administrative or clinical procedure.

A clear and concise presentation of human anatomy and physiology is included in the text. The structure and function of each body system is followed by a discussion of the common diagnostic examinations and diseases and disorders of that system. To facilitate learning, an expanded outline format organizes the description, signs and symptoms, etiology, and treatment for each disease.

The entire learning system is designed as an interactive guide for a successful career as a multiskilled medical assistant in today's dynamic health care environment. It can be used in a variety of settings:

- For a structured classroom setting, with the expertise of a qualified instructor
- For individualized instruction of learners in programs of diversified training, because much of the content and format are appropriate for self-study
- For on-the-job training in a physician's office, where the learning package serves as a supplement to employee instruction and as a resource manual
- For review by medical assistants who wish to prepare for the certification exam

Completion of the learning materials, achievement of the learning and performance objectives, and application of the competencies during externship or employment prepare you to successfully complete a national certification exam.

A Student Software CD-ROM accompanies this book and contains interactive software that challenges you to apply content, think critically, develop competency in skills, and improve your knowledge base.

Together the authors have more than 75 years of medical and academic educational preparation and employment experience. In addition, medical assistants, educators, nurse practitioners, physicians from general and specialty practices, a medical laboratory technician, a medical engineer, and a bank manager have reviewed and contributed to this sixth edition.

WHAT'S NEW IN THE SIXTH EDITION?

Many changes were made to reflect the impact of technology, recent legislation, medical advances, and revised accreditation standards. Boxed features and icons highlighting important HIPAA concepts and EHR trends are included throughout each chapter. Other new features have been added, including a Study Checklist, Certification Connection, Activities, and Critical Thinking and StudyWARE Challenges. Limitations on clinical laboratory procedures and the impact of this and other legislation on the operation of a medical office are explained. Other changes involve third-party payments, the shift to managed care, and the communication revolution. The anatomy and physiology content reflects advances in cellular biology applications, new photographs of pathology, and the ever-changing diagnostic and treatment methods. A Spanish Glossary of key terms is found following the English Glossary.

Technology Initiatives

Major new technology initiatives are an integral part of the sixth edition. Highlights include:

- New StudyWARE software with quizzes, activities, and the Competency Challenge is included on the Student Software CD-ROM.

- The Critical Thinking Challenge and a Medical Terminology Audio Library are included on the Student Software CD-ROM.
- Medical Office Simulation Software and case studies accompany the *Workbook*.
- SYNAPSE EHR version 1.0: Electronic Charting Software and task exercises accompany the *Workbook*.

Content Improvements

The major content changes to the text are as follows:

Chapter 1, Health Care Providers, includes a new table format for historical developments and people important to development. Unit 2, The Total Health Care Team, has been revised and streamlined to combine material from fifth edition's Units 2 and 3.

Chapter 2, The Medical Assistant, includes expanded information on the American Medical Technologists (AMT) and National Heathcareer Association (NHA) organizations and provides information about the CMAS, CCMA, and CMAA exams.

Chapter 3, Medical Ethics and Liability, offers a new discussion on HIPAA and the Privacy Rule.

Chapter 4, Professional Communications, reflects the move of material on Career Entry and Employee Evaluation to a more appropriate place in Chapter 21 on employment.

Chapter 5, Medical Terminology, is an entirely new chapter, based on accreditation and certification exam content standards.

Chapter 6, Oral and Written Communications, includes new content on HIPAA guidelines relating to telephone and written communications, and content on computerized appointment scheduling. The latest technology equipment and instructions are provided. The chapter includes new procedures on performing a telephone screening, placing a follow-up call to inform a patient of test results, and responding to written communication.

Chapter 7, Facility and Records Management, starts with a new Unit 1, Preparing for the Day. Unit 2, The Patient's Medical Record, gives an overview of HIPAA relating to the medical record and discusses electronic health records.

Chapter 8, Collecting Fees, has been streamlined. The units have been combined and reorganized.

Chapter 9, Health Care Coverage, offers an updated discussion of Medicare and Medicaid.

Chapter 10, Medical Office Management, starts with a new placement of Unit 1, Safety, Security, and Emergency Plans. Unit 2, The Language of Banking, gives expanded instruction on writing a check and completing a check stub. Unit 5, General Management Duties, includes new content on office liability insurance, equipment inventory and maintenance, and physician's professional meetings. The chapter includes new procedures on establishing and maintaining a petty cash fund, performing an inventory of supplies and equipment, performing routine maintenance of administrative and clinical equipment, and managing a physician's professional schedule and travel.

Chapter 11, Anatomy and Physiology of the Human Body, shows new pathology photographs. In addition, the content was thoroughly reviewed by specialists in each body system.

Chapter 12, Preparing the Clinical Duties, includes a new procedure on performing sterilization through use of an autoclave.

Chapter 13, Beginning the Patient's Record, starts with two brand-new units on in-person screening and the medical history, which include new procedures on performing an in-person screening and taking a medical history. Unit 3, Body Measurements and Vital Signs, added discussion and procedures on body measurements and the temporal artery thermometer and deleted discussion and procedures involving mercury thermometers.

Chapter 14, Physical Examinations and Assessment Procedures, offers new information on the medical assistant's role in the complete physical examination, Pap testing, and prenatal visits. Step-by-step discussion of the physical exam format is presented in outline format. Unit 5, Pediatric Examinations and Procedures, is completely new. This chapter offers several new procedures on preparing and maintaining examination and treatment areas, preparing patients for and assisting with routine physical examinations, and assisting with a gynecologic examination and ThinPrep Pap test.

Chapter 15, Specimen Collection and Laboratory Procedures, has been completely rewritten and reorganized to map to accreditation standards. To this end, all non-CLIA-waived tests have been removed. The chapter includes new procedures on performing an erythrocyte sedimentation rate (ESR), performing a rapid strep screening test for group A strep, instructing a patient in the collection of a clean-catch midstream urine specimen, and performing a wound collection for microbiologic testing.

Chapter 16, Diagnostic Tests, X-Rays, and Procedures, includes new information on RAST testing and a new procedure on performing spirometry testing.

Chapter 17, Minor Surgery in the Medical Office, has been expanded into three distinct units: Unit 1 discusses the care and handling of instruments; Unit 2 informs about preoperative instructions and provides a new procedure on sterile tray set-up; and Unit 3 goes in-depth about assisting with minor surgical procedures, including new information on anesthetics, postoperative instructions, and bandaging.

Chapter 18, Assisting with Medications, gives more information about using the PDR, drug categories and classifications, and controlled substances. New content on principles of IV therapy, vaccinations, and immunizations has been added, along with a new procedure on reconstituting a powdered medication.

Chapter 19, Emergencies, Acute Illness, Accidents, and Recovery, provides new information on recognizing and responding to an emergency, safety and emergencies in children, and CPR for children and adults. It includes a new procedure on performing abdominal thrusts on an adult victim with an obstructed airway.

Chapter 20, Behaviors Influencing Health, discusses the new food pyramid from the U.S. Department of Agriculture and includes a revised discussion of nutrition, calories, and cultural influence on diets. The unit on Habit-Forming Substances was entirely revised by a certified substance abuse nurse.

Chapter 21, Explore, Enter, and Succeed in Employment, has been retitled to reflect revised, more practical chapter content. Unit 1, Externship, is brand new. Unit 3, Career Entry and Success, includes two new procedures on completing a job application and writing an interview follow-up letter.

More Support Materials

This edition marks a drastic improvement in instructor and student support materials:

- A completely revised *Workbook* maps to the text and follows a new unit structure.
- Competency Evaluations include links to ABHES and CAAHEP competencies, with their alphanumeric designations.
- Unit Applications and Procedures are designed to provide Work Products as outlined from CAAHEP.
- The *Workbook* includes case studies that complement Medical Office Simulation Software and SYNAPSE EHR, version 1.0: Electronic Charting Software.
- Microsoft PowerPoint presentations incorporate over 45 minutes of video clips and web links.
- An Image Library includes illustrations and photos from the text.
- A new Online Companion includes content for instructors and students.
- A ready-to-use Curriculum is available on the Online Companion and includes detailed lesson outlines for each unit, suggested activities, and procedures specifically mapping to accreditation competencies.
- WebTutor Advantage on Blackboard or WebCT includes Microsoft PowerPoint, test bank, video clips, animations, quizzes, exams, and static and interactive files for each chapter.

COMPREHENSIVE LEARNING PACKAGE

Student Support

The **Workbook** (ISBN 1-4180-3267-0) has been fully revised to closely map the unit structure of the text. Explore each unit's content through the Words to Know Challenge, Unit Reviews, and Case Studies with critical thinking questions. Following completion of performance objective practice in each chapter, remove the corresponding **Performance Evaluation Checklists** in the *Workbook* and perform the procedures. Each checklist contains columns for multiple attempts, links to both ABHES and CAAHEP competency numbering, appropriate documentation boxes, and work product notations.

SYNAPSE EHR, version 1.0: Electronic Charting Software is packaged free with the *Workbook* and includes four modules to provide experience entering patient information into an electronic chart. Each module assigns specific tasks to the student and concludes with critical thinking questions about the material presented. A Performance Evaluation Checklist follows this section to provide documentation of this competency.

Medical Office Simulation Software is packaged free with the Workbook with six case studies to provide experience using practice management software. Each case study requires the student to register patients, enter and verify insurance information, create appointments, post procedures, and perform billing routines.

The **Online Companion** contains additional games and activities relating to anatomy and physiology, to help reinforce concepts and terminology. To access, go to www.delmarlearning.com/companions, select Allied Health in the drop-down menu, and click on the title of this book.

Instructor Support

The **Instructor's Resource Manual** (ISBN 1-4180-3268-9) provides answer keys for the text and *Workbook*, teaching tips and suggestions, class and individual activities, and lesson outlines for each unit.

The **Electronic Classroom Manager** (ISBN 1-4180-3269-7) is a CD-ROM loaded with content to provide instructors with complete support in the classroom.

- Use the **electronic Instructor's Resource Manual files** to help prepare for class.
- Deliver effective presentations with chapter **Microsoft PowerPoint** presentations, which include visuals and approximately 45 minutes of video clips.
- Create quizzes and tests to monitor student progress with the **Computerized Test Bank** in ExamView, with over 1,700 questions.

- The **Image Library** of over 700 illustrations allows you to pick the important visuals from the text to incorporate into your own class presentations.

The **Online Companion** contains extra content for your classroom. To access, go to www.delmarlearning.com/companions, select Allied Health in the drop-down menu, and click on the title of this book. It includes:

- Password-protected complete **Curriculum,** which includes detailed lesson outlines for each unit
- Updates and additional curriculum, documents, and mapping tools

Check out the **WebTutor** on either Blackboard or WebCT to help manage your course.

- WebTutor Advantage (ISBN 1-4180-3274-3 on Blackboard; ISBN 1-4180-3273-5 on WebCT) provides a course calendar, chat, e-mail, threaded discussions, web links, and a white board and is loaded with content related to each chapter, including quizzes, exams, interactive activities, flash cards, and more.
- WebTutor Toolbox (ISBN 1-4180-3276-X on Blackboard; ISBN 1-4180-3277-8 on WebCT) offers the same course management features and functionality. Chapter content includes objectives, frequently asked questions, and learning links.

ACKNOWLEDGMENTS

A textbook of this nature requires the input and assistance of many friends, professional colleagues and acquaintances, subject matter experts, the publishing team, and the group of reviewers. We owe them all a great deal of appreciation and recognition for their willingness to contribute their time and expertise to assist with this revision.

A special acknowledgment to **National College**, Indianapolis, Indiana, for its participation in the photographing of many figures in this textbook, with special thanks to **Jim Pershing**, Campus Director; **Ted Westlund**, Director of Health Care Education; the staff, faculty, and students at the Indianapolis campus; and **Evie O'Nan**, Director of Health Care Education at the Florence campus and her volunteer students.

Contributors

Special recognition for their contribution to the sixth edition is due to the following:

Michelle Heller, CMA, RMA, program director, Medical Assisting Program at the Ohio Institute of Health Careers, for her guidance, advice, and assistance throughout the revision process.

Lyn Veach, CMA, MLT (ASCP), former medical assistant instructor, Columbus State Community College, for her revision of two units in Chapter 6 and all of Chapters 17 and 18. Lyn also revised several chapters in the *Workbook* and *Instructor's Resource Manual.*

Paula Murphy, MA, reimbursement manager for a large orthoneuro practice, for her expertise in fiscal management and insurance for revising Chapters 8 and 9.

Kent Vedder, BSME, director of engineering for a medical plastics company, for his assistance with electronic communications, computer terminology, and prevention and dealing with computer viruses in Chapter 6.

Cecilia Krebs, CARN (certified addiction RN), for her outstanding in-depth revision of habit-forming substances in Chapter 20, Unit 2.

We continue to acknowledge the following contributors to the fifth edition, whose work remains a part of this text:

Anne Burns, RPh, Clinical Assistant Professor and manager of the Proficiency Practice Laboratory, The Ohio State University College of Pharmacy, for assistance with Chapter 18 on medications.

Holly Herron Meader, RN, MS, Life Flight trauma nurse and critical care outreach manager, for contributions to Chapter 19 on first aid and emergency care.

Susan L. Newell, Key Bank branch manager, for assistance with banking processes and procedures in Chapter 10.

Warner M. Thomas, Jr., attorney at law, for his review and recommendations regarding medical ethics and liability in Chapter 3.

Anatomy and Physiology Chapter

The invaluable contributions from physicians, educators, nurse specialists, and nurse practitioners are truly outstanding. They invested many hours in reviewing, identifying, and recommending content to be added, deleted, or updated in the 13 units of Chapter 11. Words alone are not adequate to express our appreciation. A very special acknowledgment to the following contributors to the sixth and previous editions:

Unit 1 Anatomic Descriptors and Fundamental Body Structure

Carmen Carpenter, RN, MS, CMA, Chair, Allied Health Science and Medical Assisting, South University, West Palm Beach, FL

Stephen D'Ambrosio, PhD, Professor of Radiobiology and Pharmacology, The Ohio State University College of Medicine (fourth and fifth editions)

Unit 2   The Nervous System
Claire V. Wolfe, MD, Physical Medicine and Rehabilitation

Unit 3   The Senses
Janet McOwen, RN, ophthalmology practice
Lawrence Koegel, MD, otorhinolaryngology

Unit 4   The Integumentary System
Kelley Zyniewicz, MD, dermatology practice and Clinical Assistant Professor, Division of Dermatology, The Ohio State University (fifth and sixth editions)

Unit 5   The Skeletal System
John S. Wolfe, MD, orthopedic surgeon

Unit 6   The Muscular System
John S. Wolfe, MD, orthopedic surgeon

Unit 7   The Respiratory System
Karen Bishop, RN, MS, CNP, nurse practitioner, pulmonary medicine practice
Phil Diaz, MD, pulmonary medicine practice and researcher for Ohio State University (fourth and fifth editions)

Unit 8   The Circulatory System
N. Howard Kander, MD, cardiology

Unit 9   The Immune System
Peter Kourlas, MD, oncology
Lisa Smith, RN, MS, AOCN, oncology clinical nurse specialist (fifth edition)
Elaine Glass, RN, MS, OCN, oncology clinical nurse specialist (fourth, fifth editions)

Unit 10   The Digestive System
Thomas Ransbottom, MD, Gastroenterology

Unit 11   The Urinary System
Henry A. Wise, MD, urology (fifth edition)
Michelle Steed, RN, BSN, clinical nurse manager, urology services and dialysis, Riverside Methodist Hospital (fifth edition)

Unit 12   The Endocrine System
Manuel Tzagournis, MD, endocrinology practice and Professor Emeritus, Internal Medicine, Division of Endocrinology, Diabetes and Metabolism, the Ohio State University Hospitals

Unit 13   The Reproductive System
Christine Dombroski, RNC, NP, nurse practitioner in OB/GYN and women's health (fifth and sixth editions)
Henry Wise, MD, urologist (fifth edition)

Pediatric Perspectives content
Cheryl Baxter, RN, MS, pediatric nurse practitioner (fifth edition)

REVIEWERS

The authors are particularly grateful to the reviewers who continue to be a valuable resource in guiding this book as it evolves. Their insights, comments, suggestions, and attention to detail are very important in guiding the development of this textbook.

Jennie Diaz-Ontiveros, CCAM-C
Medical Assisting Instructor
Tri-Cities Regional Occupational Program
Whittier, CA

Brian Dyk
National Academic Director
Heritage Education
Denver, CO

George Fakhoury, MD, DORCP, CMA
Academic Program Manager, Healthcare
Heald College
San Francisco, CA

Dixie Ford, RMA, CMA, AHI
Apollo College
Phoenix, AZ

Sharon Harris-Pelliccia, RPAC
Division Chair, Medical Studies Division
Mildred Elley
Latham, NY

Dayle A. Haworth, MT (ASCP)
Lead Instructor—Medical Assisting Program
Gibbs College
Cranston, RI

Debra Hrisoulas, AA
Medical Assisting Instructor
Platt College
Ontario, CA

Nancy Ingalls, RMA
Medical Assisting Instructor
Apollo College
Mesa, AZ

Shirley Jelmo, CMA, RMA
PIMA Medical Institute
Colorado Springs, CO

Kathryn A. Kalanick
Educational Pathways
Nephi, UT

Claire E. Maday-Travis, MA, MBA, CPHQ
Allied Health Program Director
The Salter School
Worcester, MA

Fred Valdes, MD
Education Consultant, Professor
Florida Metropolitan University
Pompano Beach, FL

Prior Edition Reviewers

Jerri Adler, CMA, CMT
Lane Community College
Eugene, OR

Jennifer Barr
Sinclair Community College
Dayton, OH

Adrienne Lynne Carter-Ward, BA, CMA, NRMA
Skadron College, CSI
San Bernadino, CA

Elizabeth L. Clark, BA, CMA
Everett Community College
Everett, WA

Lisa L. Cook, CMA
Eton Technical Institute
Port Orchard, WA

Cindy Correa
Healthcare Educational Consultant
Denver, CO

Karen Hulse, MT (ASCP)
Lenape Technical Institute
Ford City, PA

Mary Marks, MSN, RNC, PbT (ASCP)
Mitchell Community College
Mooresville, NC

Sharon McCaughrin, CMA
Ross Medical Education Center
Warren, MI

Susan Royce, MS
Design Institute of San Diego
San Diego, CA

Janet Sesser, RMA, CMA
High-Tech Institute
Phoenix, AZ

Melanie Schmidt, RMA, MLT
Arizona College of Allied Health
Phoenix, AZ

Kathy Tozzi, CLPN, RMA, AHI
Cleveland Institute of Dental-Medical Assistants, Inc.
Mentor, OH

How to Use This Book

Unit Objectives list the theoretical and practical objectives at the beginning of each unit.

This edition features new **Performance Objectives** that correlate to the procedures in the chapter, mapping to ABHES and CAAHEP competencies.

UNIT 5
OFFICE MANAGEMENT EQUIPMENT

OBJECTIVES

Upon completion of this unit, you will be able to achieve the following:

LEARNING Objectives

1. Spell and define, using the glossary at th[e] of the text, all the Words to Know in this
2. Explain why a calculator should be used supplies are received.
3. List seven types of material that are oft[en] photocopied.

PERFORMANCE Objectives

NEW

1. Total charges on a calculator.
2. Operate a copy machine.
3. Operate a transcriber.
4. Operate an office computer.

The **Certification Connection** draws a link from unit content to the CMA, RMA, and CMAS exams.

Key terms and ideas are presented in the **Words to Know list** and are highlighted the first time they appear in the unit content.

WORDS TO KNOW

acronym	microfilming
calculator	photocopy
computer	software
dictation	technology
electronic	transcription
hardware	word processor

CERTIFICATION CONNECTION

NEW

CMA
Equipment operation
Computer components

RMA
Transcription and dictation
Computer applications

Within each unit, special content relating to **electronic health records**, **HIPAA**, and **patient education** is highlighted in visual boxes and icons, integrated within the text discussion.

PATIENT EDUCATION

During the patient's office visit, you [may] opportunity to discuss a few of the fo[llowing] which may help the patient better un[derstand] health habits in regard to urinary pro[blems]

1. Remind patients to avoid using p[erfumed] articles (i.e., tissue, tampons, or s[o] irritating to delicate vaginal tissu[e]
2. Advise patients to void when the[y] because delay can cause bladder[
3. Instruct female patients to practi[ce] [incre]ase the sphincter control [ ] urine retention.
[Remind] patient s that they shoul[d] [a]voiding caffeine drinks.
[female] patients that wea[ring] [ti]ght and nylon underwear may be irritating to [vaginal] tissues. Cotton is recommended because it breathes, allowing heat and moisture to escape.

HIPAA

NEW

Maintaining PPI confidentiality, as required by HIPAA, can present a challenge to medical practices establishing paperless office workflows. Confidentiality can be maintained by setting up network security so that only the appropriate users have access to these records. In addition, software applications are commercially available that make it easy for scanned documents to securely become part of an individual's personal records.

EHR CONNECTION

NEW

Appointments, prescriptions, and test results can be easily documented in the patient's electronic record.

ACHIEVE UNIT OBJECTIVES

NEW

- ■ Complete the Workbook activities to meet the learning objectives.
- ■ Practice the procedures in this unit to meet the performance objectives.
- ■ Apply your knowledge at the end of this chapter in completing the Critical Thinking Challenge and Activities, as well as the StudyWARE on your Student CD-ROM.

Achieve Unit Objectives is a checklist at the end of each unit that provides a study plan to review the concepts presented in the unit and helps students get the most out of the entire learning package.

Each **procedure** includes step-by-step instructions with rationales, charting, and log book examples where appropriate.

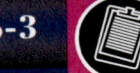

6-3 Telephone a Patient with Test Results

PURPOSE: To telephone a patient with test results, observing HIPAA regulations and following the instructions of the physician.

EQUIPMENT: Patient's chart, telephone, lab results, pen.

PERFORMANCE OBJECTIVE: Using the necessary equipment, follow all the steps in the procedure and inform the patient about laboratory or other test results. Provide patient's chart, with test results attached, to HIPAA the physician. **RATIONALE: The physician must review all test results before they can be released to the patient. Do not release any results that have not been initialed by the physician.**

patient's chart for the signed privacy notice to determine who may receive the information. **NOTE: Be sure to check the signed notice to determine if it is permissible to leave information on an answering machine.**

3. Telephone the patient, identifying an office.

4. Identify the person you are speaking to. **NOTE: Information can only be given to the patient themselves or to persons authorized by the patient to receive PHI.**

5. Inform the patient about test results and any instructions from the physician.

6. Ask the patient to repeat the results to be sure they have the correct information.

7. Instruct the patient to call the office with any questions.

8. Allow the patient to hang up first. **RATIONALE: Allowing the patient to hang up first eliminates the possibility of missing a question or statement from the patient.**

9. Document the call in the patient's chart.

CHARTING EXAMPLE

10-10-xx

Follow-up call to patient with CBC results. Instructed patient to F/U in 6 months for repeat CBC per Dr. Carter.

PERFORMANCE EVALUATION CHECKSHEET

PROCEDURE 15-17   Perform Rapid Strep Screening Te...

TASK	Collect a throat swab from a patient and test the swab for the p... A Strep.
CONDITIONS	In a simulated medical office environment, students will be provided appropriate supplies and equipment to complete the procedure
STANDARD	Student will have a maximum of three attempts to successfully comp... with a minimum score of 35. Any step denoted by an asterisk (*) is a step; if omitted or incorrectly performed, student must repeat the con... The time limit for each attempt is 15 minutes.

PROCEDURE STEPS	POINTS POSSIBLE	FIRST ATTEMPT	SECOND ATTEMPT	THIRD ATTEMPT
Note time began:				
1. Assemble equipment and supplies.	5			
2. Identify patient, introduce yourself and explain procedure.	5			
3. Wash hands and don gloves.	5			
4. *Using the tongue blade and sterile swab, collect specimen from the peritonsillar crypts without touching swab to tongue, cheeks, or lips.	10			
5. *Label the swab with patient's name, date, and health care provider's name.	15			
6. *Properly complete the lab report form with patient's results and report results to health care provider.	15			
Note time ended:				
Points Possible / Points Achieved				

ABHES COMPETENCY: VI.B.1.a.4(bb); VI.B.1.a.4(u); VI.B.1.a.4(j)
CAAHEP COMPETENCY: III.C.3.b(2)(c); III.C.3.b(3)(c)(iv

Evaluator's Signature:
Comments:

The **Workbook** includes **corresponding competency evaluation checklists** with links to ABHES and CAAHEP competency numbering.

StudyWARE™ CHALLENGE   **NEW**

- Study with the flash cards for Chapter 6 to review the key terms in this chapter.
- Solve the crossword puzzle for Chapter 6.
- Complete the multiple choice quiz in test mode for Chapter 6.

At the end of each chapter, reinforce your understanding of the concepts covered through research **Activities.** The **StudyWARE Challenge** provides specific assignments to complete using the Student CD-ROM.

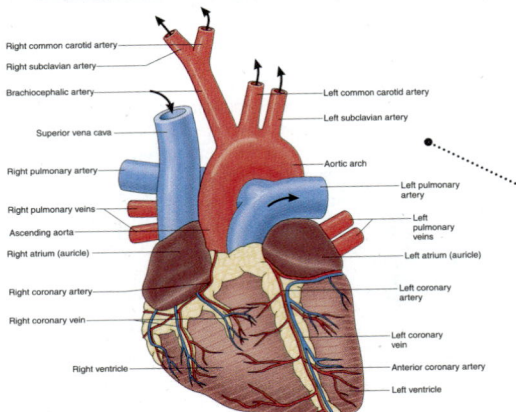

Complete coverage of **Anatomy and Physiology** of the 13 general body systems, including structure and function, diagnostic tests, and diseases and disorders.

NEW

CRITICAL THINKING CHALLENGE

IMPACTING THE PATIENT, THE PRACTICE, AND YOUR CAREER

Jane is the administrative medical assistant who does the office correspondence. The physician had recently dictated some follow-up information to six patients regarding their lab findings following their office visits. As was his practice, he had indicated to her that a copy of the lab reports should be mailed with the short letters. A few days after Jane had completed the letters she received a phone call from one of the patients, Mrs. Turner. It seems Jane had accidentally mixed up the lab reports, and Mrs. Turner had received another patient's reports. She was quite upset primarily because she didn't know who had received her very personal lab findings.

Critical Thinking Challenges conclude each chapter, highlighting students' decisions in relation to the patient, the practice, and their own career.

How to Use the CD-ROM

The Student Software includes **StudyWARE™** with games and activities, the new **Competency Challenge**, the **Critical Thinking Challenge** game simulation, and an **Audio Library**.

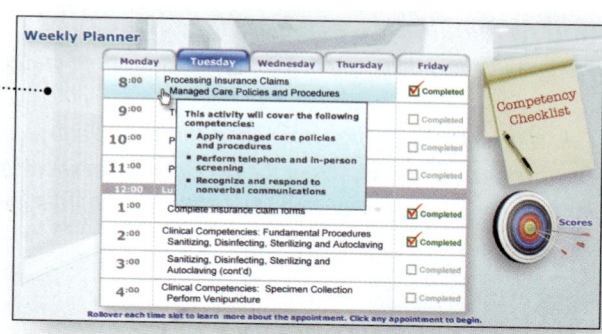

Competency Challenge

Simulating a virtual externship, this challenge includes video-based case studies with interactive exercises that provide an opportunity to test your knowledge and understanding of the educational competencies for the medical assistant.

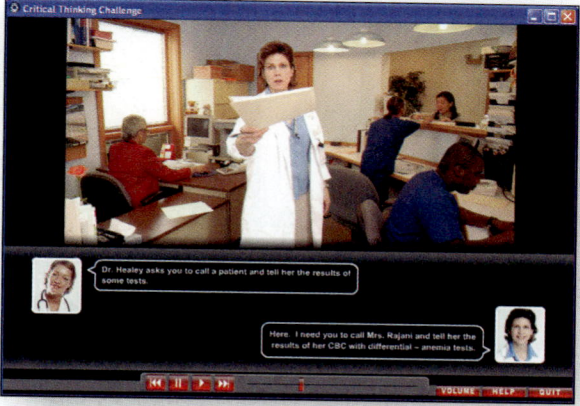

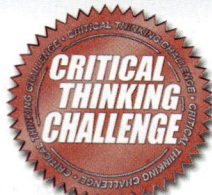

Critical Thinking Challenge

In the Critical Thinking Challenge, you are on a 3-month externship in a medical office. You will be confronted with a series of situations in which you must use your critical thinking skills to choose the most appropriate action in response to the situation.

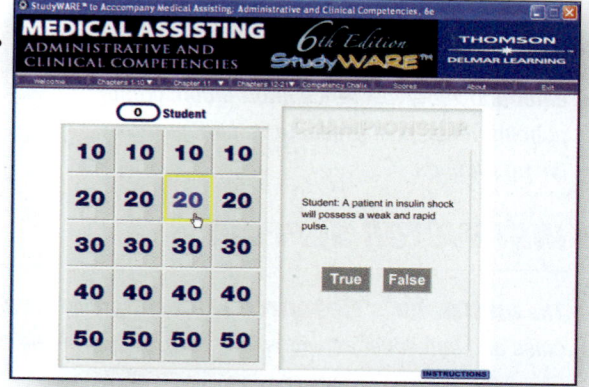

StudyWARE™

StudyWARE™ is interactive software with learning activities and quizzes to help study key concepts and test your comprehension. The activity and quiz content corresponds with each unit in the book.

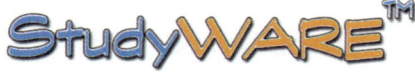

The activities include flash cards, concentration, hangman, crossword puzzles, image labeling, spelling bee, and championship games.

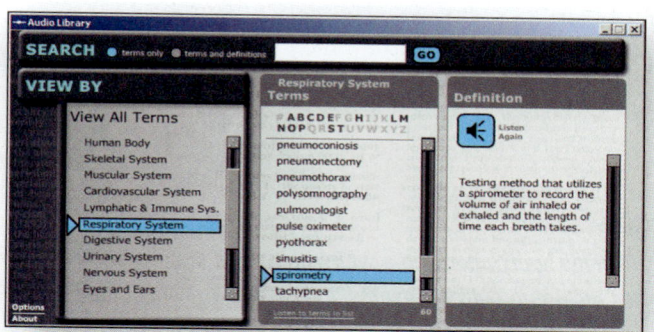

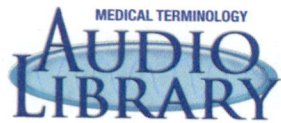

Medical Terminology Audio Library

Practice your pronunciation and recognition of medical terms using the Audio Library. You may search for terms by word or body system. Once you've selected a word, it is pronounced correctly and defined on the screen.

About the Supplements

The **Workbook** has been fully revised to map more closely to the text and follows a new unit structure. Explore each unit's content through the Words to Know Challenge, Unit Reviews, and Case Studies with critical thinking questions.

Unit Applications are designed to provide **Work Products** as outlined by CAAHEP, and Certification and Registration Preparation questions emphasize the importance of credentialing.

Following completion of performance objective practice in each chapter, remove the corresponding **Performance Evaluation Checklists** at the back of the Workbook and perform the procedures. Each checklist contains columns for multiple attempts, links to both ABHES and CAAHEP competency numbering, and documentation boxes.

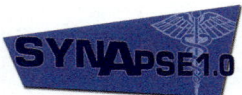

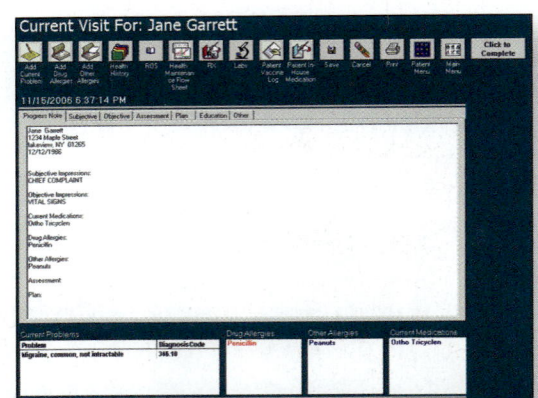

SYNAPSE, version 1.0: An Electronic Charting Simulation is packaged free with the Workbook and includes five modules to provide experience entering patient information into an electronic chart. Each module assigns specific tasks to the student and concludes with critical thinking questions about the material presented.

Medical Office Simulation Software is packaged free with the Workbook with six case studies to provide experience using practice management software. Each case study requires the student to register patients, enter and verify insurance information, create appointments, post procedures, and perform billing routines.

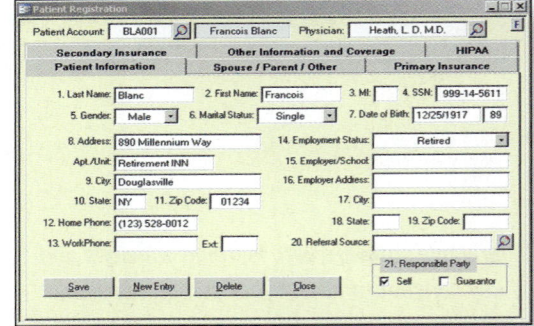

INSTRUCTOR SUPPORT

The **Instructor's Resource Manual** provides answer keys for the text and Workbook, teaching tips and suggestions, class and individual activities, and sample syllabi and course outlines.

The **Electronic Classroom Manager** is a CD-ROM loaded with content to provide instructors with complete support in the classroom, including electronic Instructor's Manual files, Microsoft PowerPoint presentations, a **Computerized Test Bank**, and an **Image Library**.

The **Online Companion** contains extra content for the classroom.
- Password-protected complete **Curriculum**, which includes detailed lesson outlines for each unit
- Updates and additional curriculum documents and mapping tools
- Additional games and activities for students

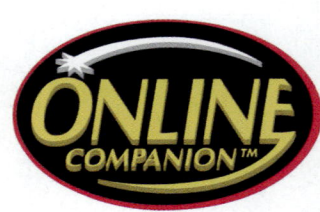

WebTutor on either Blackboard or WebCT to help manage your course.
- WebTutor provides a course calendar, chat, e-mail, threaded discussions, web links, and a white board.
- WebTutor Advantage is loaded with content related to each chapter, including quizzes, exams, interactive activities, flash cards, and more.

SECTION 1
Medical Health Care Roles and Responsibilities

1

Health Care Providers

Health care providers have held prominent positions in society since the beginning of time. A look into the history of medicine reveals that for thousands of years, disease was thought to be the result of evil spirits and demons, brought on by disobedience to the gods. Therefore, early medical practitioners were primarily religious leaders. Eventually, scientific interest led to the discovery of microorganisms and understanding of the human body. Unit 1 of this chapter highlights ancient, medieval, and modern health care practitioners. It also discusses the great advancements in medicine that came with the modern era of "super" surgery, the installation of artificial parts, and the ethical and moral questions of stem cell and DNA capabilities. In recent years the government and health consumers have intervened in many ways to affect the delivery of health care in the United States.

Because of the complexity of health care, many different health care practitioners and specialists are needed to provide complete patient care. They work in a variety of settings providing specialized care or services related to their education or training.

Due to the vast amounts of accumulated knowledge and clinical procedures, it is also impossible for a physician to provide competent care in all areas of medicine. In order to meet the needs of patients, some physicians become medical specialists, spending additional years in the study of one particular field of medicine. Unit 2 identifies members of the total health care team and gives brief descriptions of their roles in health care.

Because of the great technologic advances in health care that have controlled plagues, increased survival rates, and extended the years of life, another major problem has developed: overpopulation. Unless controlled, the masses of people will outstrip the world's capacity to support their existence. The current presence of air, water, and land pollution and the destruction of vital resources are evidence of impending problems. Once again disease, famine, and epidemics of viruses yet unknown and uncontrolled may affect the people of the world.

UNIT 1
A BRIEF HISTORY OF MEDICINE

OBJECTIVES

Upon completion of this unit, you will be able to achieve the following:

LEARNING Objectives

1. **Spell and define, using the glossary at the back of the text, all the Words to Know in this unit.**
2. **Explain how the caduceus may have been acquired as the medical symbol.**
3. **Explain the reason Hippocrates is known as the Father of Medicine.**
4. **State why many of Galen's findings were invalid.**
5. **Explain the differences in the role of the physician, the surgeon, and the barber-surgeon.**
6. **Identify the contributions of Jenner, Pasteur, Lister, Roentgen, Reed, Barton, Blackwell, Nightingale, Curie, Papanicolaou, Domagk, Banting, Fleming, Salk, Sabin, and DeBakey.**

WORDS TO KNOW

acupuncture	epidemics	practitioners
anesthesia	exorcism	Roentgen
apothecaries	guilds	scientific
apprenticeship	Hippocratic oath	surgeons
asepsis	infectious	surgery
caduceus	pandemic	trephining
cautery	physicians	vaccination
disease	plague	

ANCIENT HISTORY

To fully understand the high technical level of current health care and the responsibilities of those who provide it, we must look back at its history and learn how it has developed. Ancient times were filled with **infectious disease** and **epidemics** as well as illnesses and injuries caused by dietary deficiencies and unhealthy or hostile environments. Eighty percent of primitive human beings died by the age of 30 as a result of a hunting accident or violence. Primitive individuals lived primarily alone, so there was little risk of widespread diseases or **plagues**. However, when they began settling in communities, farming, and domesticating animals, epidemic diseases resulted from overcrowding, filth, and the natural presence of microorganisms. Initially, tuberculosis, tetanus, malaria, smallpox, typhus, typhoid, and, later, leprosy ravaged early civilizations.

Because these ancient people did not understand the concept of microorganisms or the function of the human body, the presence of disease was credited to evil spirits and demons brought on as punishment for disobedience to the gods. Therefore, medical practice became the role of priests or medicine men. "Treatments" involved rituals to drive out demons. At times, a surgical procedure called **trephining** was performed. This remarkable operation involved cutting a hole in the skull with a flint knife presumably to treat migraines, epilepsy, paralysis, or insanity. Later, it was used to treat head injuries incurred in battle or from accidents. Archaeologists have examined hundreds of skulls and have determined that some trephining ended in death, but surprisingly, the majority showed healing and several years of survival.

Early Egypt

Evidence has been found in Egyptian tombs and on papyri that indicates that the people of the area around the Nile River had developed a level of medical practice as early as 3000 BC. Egyptian **physicians** were priests who studied medicine and **surgery** in the temple medical schools. They too tried to drive out evil spirits with spells. If this failed, they used concocted repellents to fight the demons. These were made from the excretions of the lion, panther, gazelle, and ostrich. Insects, either crushed or alive, were swallowed along with the backbones of ravens and fat from black snakes. In addition to the "black magic," they also used about one third of the medicinal plants still used in pharmacies today.

Egyptians believed that blood in the body flowed through canals like those constructed along the Nile for irrigation. When it was thought that the body's canals were "clogged," they were opened by bloodletting or the application of leeches. The leech not only removed blood and disease toxins but also produced hirudin in the process, which prevented coagulation. The use of leeches continued until the 19th century and is being reintroduced today in specific traumas where a large amount of blood is present within the tissues. Egyptian physicians (priests) were very conservative in treating patients. They adhered to rules of the Sacred Books so they would be free from blame if a patient died. If the physician tried a different treatment and the patient did not survive, the physician was executed; therefore, medical progress was impossible. The conservative physicians became famous and were in high demand. An Egyptian named Imhotep was considered outstanding and became the physician for the royal family. As a reward, he was given deity and named the Egyptian God of Medicine.

People from surrounding regions had medical problems similar to those of the Egyptians. The average person lived in squalor, drank filthy water, and had very poor personal hygiene. By the year 2000 BC, the ruler of Babylon established a legal code for medical practice that set fees for services and established rules of conduct. It provided that the physician's hands be cut off if the physician killed a patient or destroyed the patient's sight. It is worth noting that these stiff penalties applied only to patients from nobility—a slave just had to be replaced.

India's Contribution

The Sacred Books tell of priest-doctors in India around 1500 BC and listed their deadly diseases as malaria, dysentery, typhoid, cholera, the plague, leprosy, and smallpox. The Hindus had the world's first nurses and hospitals. There was extensive use of drugs, including those for **anesthesia** that undoubtedly assisted with the main Hindu contribution to the art of healing: surgery. Their knowledge of anatomy was limited, but their **surgeons** performed a fairly technical form of cataract and plastic surgery. Early writings reveal that they used approximately 120 surgical instruments in many different operations. The Hindu environment was greatly improved with walled sewer drains and underground water pipes. Their level of

medical knowledge and drugs spread to other lands through trade and migration and by conquerors.

China's Contribution

The Chinese, India's neighbor, had a highly developed center of early medical learning. Their belief in evil spirits as the cause of illness gradually changed; they began searching for medical reasons for illness. About 3000 BC, the emperor, who was known as the Father of Chinese Medicine, followed a document called *Great Herbal* (a translation), which contained over a thousand drugs; some are still in use today. The art of **acupuncture** was originally used as a means to drive out demons. Today, the ancient procedure has become a respected alternative form of treatment. Acupuncture consists of the insertion of needles of various metals, shapes, and sizes into one or several of the 365 specified spots on the head, trunk, and extremities. It is believed to relieve internal congestion and restore the equilibrium of the bodily functions.

Greek Influence

The Greeks also played a large role in the development of medicine. Beginning about 2000 BC, they invaded many lands and established a remarkable civilization. They acquired knowledge from their conquered but still practiced the religious/healing rituals. They believed Apollo, the Sun God, taught the art of medicine to a centaur who in turn taught others, including Asklepios, the Greek God of Healing, who lived around 1250 BC. The priests in the temples of Asklepios (also called Aesculapius) used massage, bathing, and exercise in treating patients. They also depended on the magical power of large, yellow, nonpoisonous snakes. After patients purified themselves by bathing and made offerings to the god, they were given tablets to read that described cures of former patients. Then they were put into a drug-induced sleep in the temple. During the night, the snakes licked the wounds and Asklepios applied salves. The god was usually depicted holding a staff with a serpent coiled around its shaft. This is probably the origin of the medical symbol known as a **caduceus** (Figure 1-1), even though it shows two instead of one coiled serpents, as did the staff of Aesculapius. Both are accepted as symbols of medical practice.

The Greeks absorbed ideas, drugs, and earlier methods of treatment from their predecessors. Their great interest in the unknown led them to question the accepted knowledge and seek information themselves. They began to investigate the causes of and reasons for illness in nature, which started the tradition of medical inquiry. About 500 BC, Alcmaeon dissected animals to study sight and hearing. Another Greek named Empedocles believed that blood gave life and the heart dis-

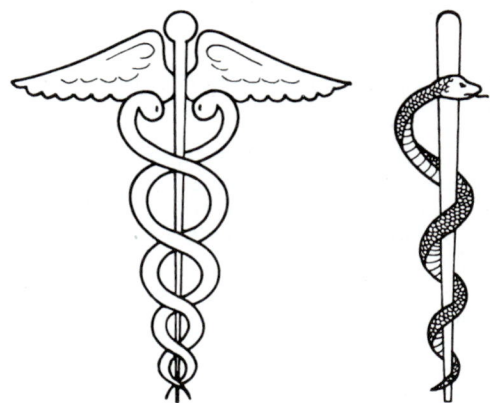

FIGURE 1-1   A caduceus (left) and the staff of Aesculapius (right)

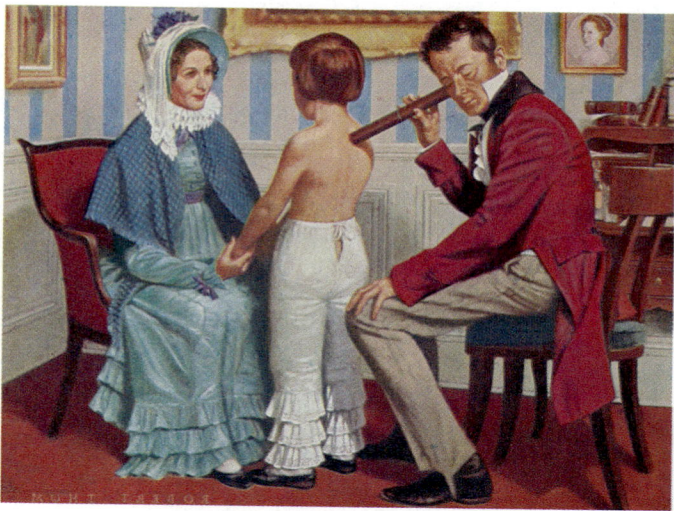

FIGURE 1-2   Laennec and the stethoscope *(Courtesy of Parke-Davis and Company, © 1957)*

tributed it around the body. Medical schools began to observe what happened in illness rather than accept the teachings of the past.

Hippocrates

Hippocrates, the founder of **scientific** medicine, was born in about 460 BC on the Island of Cos. During his 99 years of life, he took medicine out of the realm of priests and philosophers and produced an organized method of gaining knowledge through the means of observation. He taught that illness was the result of natural causes and not punishment for sin. He advocated examining a patient's environment, home, and place of work. He stressed the importance of diet and cleanliness. He felt medical knowledge could only be acquired through accurate clinical observation of the sick. He discovered that the course of certain diseases could be traced by listening to the chest of a patient. Over 2,000 years passed before a French physician named Laennec invented the stethoscope to improve this method of observation (Figure 1-2).

Hippocrates studied with the most distinguished teachers of the day. He practiced in many parts of the Greek world and was admired for his cures. He wrote many detailed studies, among which are ones on prognostics, fractures, and surgery. He is best known for his code of behavior known as the **Hippocratic oath**, which medical schools still teach and physicians repeat as they enter practice (Figure 1-3). For all his accomplishments, Hippocrates became known as the Father of Medicine.

Aristotle

Aristotle, a contemporary of Hippocrates, was a philosopher and scientific genius and became the tutor of Alexander the Great. He brought together medicine,

biology, botany, and anatomy. His findings were based upon animal dissection because human dissection was illegal where he lived. However, in Alexandria, Egypt, human dissection was legal. Students throughout the ancient world went there to study and use its library of 700,000 books. Alexandria became the center of learning and the home of a famous medical school. However, it declined with the rise of the Roman Empire, and medicine reverted to supernatural theories of disease.

Roman Influence

Medicine was held in very low esteem in the Roman Empire. The Romans distrusted and despised the wandering Greek physicians who came to Italy about 200 BC, many as slaves. Roman men treated their own families with early, primitive methods. In 46 BC, Julius Caesar gave physicians citizenship rights and they began to achieve status. But the great demand for physicians opened medicine to anyone, and little clinical teaching took place. The teachings of Hippocrates were largely ignored, and rival schools of medicine argued about his ideas.

About this time Claudius Galen, a physician from Asia Minor, emerged, professing to following the teachings of Hippocrates. He was born in 129 AD and became a surgeon for a gladiatorial school after minimal medical training. He received much experience treating the severe wounds the gladiators received in the arenas. He later went to Rome and quickly became famous, but his arrogance caused hostility from other physicians and he was forced to return home. He was called back to Rome by Marcus Aurelius, the emperor. Galen successfully cured the emperor's stomachache, and he remained in Rome until his death in 199 AD. Galen produced over

---

OATH OF HIPPOCRATES

I swear by Apollo, the physician, and Aesculapius and health and all-heal and all the Gods and Goddesses that, according to my ability and judgment, I will keep this oath and stipulation:

TO RECKON him who taught me this art equally dear to me as my parents, to share my substance with him and relieve his necessities if required; to regard his offspring as on the same footing with my own brothers, and to teach them this art if they should wish to learn it, without fee or stipulation, and that by precept, lecture, and every other mode of instruction, I will impart a knowledge of the art to my own sons and to those of my teachers, and to disciples bound by a stipulation and oath, according to the law of medicine, but to none others.

I WILL FOLLOW that method of treatment which, according to my ability and judgment, I consider for the benefit of my patients, and abstain from whatever is deleterious and mischievous. I will give no deadly medicine to anyone if asked, nor suggest any such counsel; furthermore, I will not give to a woman an instrument to produce abortion.

WITH PURITY AND WITH HOLINESS I will pass my life and practice my art. I will not cut a person who is suffering from a stone, but will leave this to be done by practitioners of this work. Into whatever houses I enter I will go into them for the benefit of the sick and will abstain from every voluntary act of mischief and corruption; and further from the seduction of females or males, bond or free.

WHATEVER, in connection with my professional practice, or not in connection with it, I may see or hear in the lives of men which ought not to be spoken abroad I will not divulge, as reckoning that all such should be kept secret.

WHILE I CONTINUE to keep this oath unviolated may it be granted to me to enjoy life and the practice of the art, respected by all men at all times but should I trespass and violate this oath, may the reverse be my lot.

FIGURE 1-3   The Oath of Hippocrates

500 books during this time. His theories were accepted for the next 1,300 years because he claimed they had the authority of Hippocrates (Figure 1-4). However, he had ignored observation and explained diseases as unbalanced "humors." The body was believed to be composed of and regulated by the four fluids (humors) of life, namely the blood, phlegm, black bile, and yellow bile. An imbalance or disturbance of the humors was

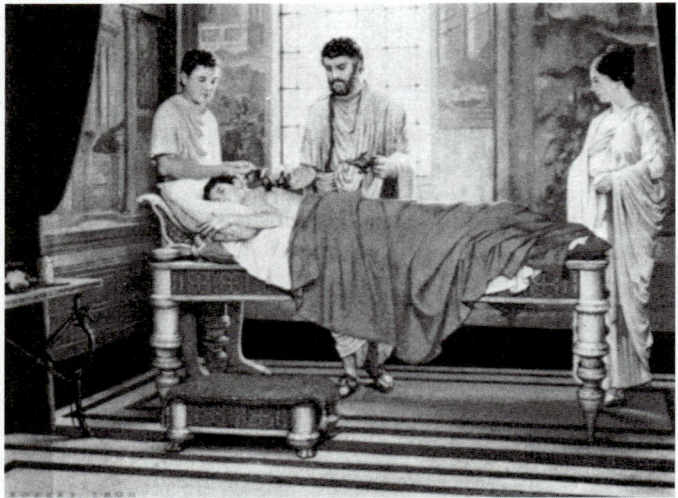

FIGURE 1-4   Galen: An influence for 45 generations *(Courtesy of Parke-Davis and Company, © 1957)*

thought to result in illness. He prescribed diets, massage, exercise, and drugs to cool, heat, dry, or moisten the body as needed. His beliefs regarding blood and circulation set back medical progress. He did believe that knowledge of anatomy was necessary, so he dissected pigs and apes and related his findings to humans because human dissection was still illegal. His viewpoints went unchallenged until the 16th century.

The Romans made almost no contribution to medicine but established superior methods of sanitation and water supply. They realized disease was connected to filth and overcrowding. They drained the marshes to reduce the incidence of malaria. There were laws to maintain public health and clean streets. They built an extensive underground sewer system and pure water aqueducts capable of bringing an estimated 300 million gallons of drinking water a day into the city. Medical officers and surgeons, usually Greek, served in the army. A private hospital system was also developed, first for the wealthy and slaves, then for the campaign armies. Later, public hospitals were founded, and the hospital movement expanded with the growth of Christianity and its tradition of caring for the sick.

Despite Rome's advances, the empire began to fall as political, social, and economic factors collapsed. The real cause, however, was the spread of disease that resulted from the disuse of the drainage system and the return of the swamps that followed invasions by other empires. The resulting malaria and smallpox killed thousands. In 542 AD, the remnants of the eastern Roman Empire were destroyed by the first major historically known **pandemic** (a disease occurring at the same time in different places) of the bubonic plague. It had come from China and had spread through trade routes to Egypt along the coast of North Africa to Palestine, Syria, and into Europe. It affected all the known world.

MEDIEVAL HISTORY

The great Roman Empire was overrun by barbarians. Europe was controlled by Teutonic tribal groups. The people were agricultural, and established health standards vanished. The centers of learning and medicine decayed. From the 5th to the 16th centuries, there was no progress in medical knowledge or practice. There was a blend of pagan magic, superstition, and herbalism. According to Hastings in *Medicine, An International History,* the Anglo-Saxon settlers in Britain believed illness was caused by "nine venoms, the nine diseases, or of 'worms,' elves, and witches." It was treated with charms and incantations or with herbs, some of which were effective. However, the settlers lived in filth and had a total absence of sanitation and personal hygiene. Writings from the 6th to the 10th centuries tell of epidemics of smallpox, dysentery, typhus, and plague. In addition, there was widespread famine.

The Role of the Church

Eventually, medicine passed into the hands of the Christian Church and Arab scholars. The church did not foster medical science. They recommended prayer and fasting because they believed that illness was a punishment for sin. In 391 AD, a religious fanatic mob burned the great library at Alexandria. Christianity forbade human dissection, so anatomy and physiology died except for the erroneous pages of Galen. Priests again became healers, using **exorcism** and holy relics to cure the sick. Parts of the body were assigned a patron saint who could cure and inflict disease. The church did care for the sick and established religious orders that provided care. Most monasteries had rooms and herb gardens to care for their own sick and members of the general public. The monasteries also took on the task of translation and transcription of the ancient manuscripts of the classical physicians, a task that preserved and circulated information before the invention of the printing press.

Arab Influence

A second storehouse of medical knowledge was in the Moslem Arab Empire, which, by 1000 AD, extended from Spain to India. The Arabs were eager for knowledge, and the classical learning was translated into Arabic. Medicine began a revival. Arab physicians learned much about epidemics, but their great knowledge of chemistry resulted in their major medical contribution in pharmacology. They also continued the Roman system of hospitals, including at least four major teaching centers. One had specialized wards for specific conditions. All patients were admitted regardless of race, creed, or social status. Upon departure, patients were given sufficient money to cover their convalescence.

One of the greatest physicians was known as Rhazes, the Arab Hippocrates. He was 40 before beginning medical study and was responsible for the construction of a hospital. He produced about 150 books, including a medical encyclopedia weighing 22 pounds. He based his diagnosis upon observation of disease, and his major contribution was distinguishing smallpox from measles. Anatomy was still based upon Galen. Because it was considered unclean to touch the human body with the hands, the Arabs were not good surgeons. This was left to inferior practitioners; however, Rhazes is credited with the use of animal gut sutures to sew wounds. The major surgical instrument was the **cautery** (a red-hot iron) applied to wounds and infected ulcers to "burn out the poison," always very painful and disfiguring and often fatal.

Medical Schools

The union of medical knowledge from both the East and West produced an outstanding medical school at Salerno, Italy, around 850 AD. It was believed to be founded by a Jew, a Roman, a Greek, and an Arab and was open to both men and women of all nationalities. Because it was not a church school, it could teach medicine using a sound basis. It became the convalescent center for wounded Crusaders. By the 12th century it had a highly organized curriculum upon which students were examined and issued degrees to become the first "true" doctors. Both anatomy and surgery were taught, but it was still based upon animal dissection. Other medical centers followed, including ones in Paris, Oxford, and Cambridge. Despite earlier beliefs, however, religious and scholarly factions prohibited advancement. Hippocrates and Galen remained the unquestioned authorities. Medical teaching was predominately oral since books were scarce (for example, the medical school in Paris had only 12 books at the end of the 14th century). Dissection was rare. One university did secure the right to dissect one executed criminal every 3 years, but it allowed only a superficial examination of the chest and abdomen.

Barber Surgeons

Medieval European surgeons' practice was limited to nobility, the high clergy, and wealthy merchants. Other patients and minor surgeries were treated by ignorant barber-surgeons. They cut hair, practiced bloodletting, opened abscesses, and occasionally did amputations—all with the same razor. Their trademark became the white poles around which they wrapped their blood-stained bandages. The red and white pole has descended to barbers today.

The Great Diseases

The Roman tradition of hospitals continued, but public health and personal hygiene was gone. The environment was overrun with disease. Famine and population movement due to wars increased the problems. Typhus was flourishing due to the custom of wearing the same underclothing, which was often infested with fleas. Tuberculosis was endemic due to poverty and food shortage. Tuberculosis of the neck was common, and its principal remedy was "the king's touch." In one month in 1277 AD, Edward I touched 543 persons attempting to effect a cure. Smallpox was returned to Europe by the Crusaders in the 13th century, causing at least 20 epidemics. Danish ships even spread the disease to Iceland.

Two of the greatest medieval diseases, however, were leprosy and the bubonic plague. Leprosy was present in the early centuries, brought perhaps by the Roman soldiers. It was one of the few diseases recognized as being contagious but was believed to be a result of sins against God. The afflicted were herded into leper houses outside the towns, forbidden to marry, proclaimed dead citizens, and ordered to wear a black cloak with white patches. In 1313, King Philip the Fair wanted to burn them all but was forbidden by the church. Incidences of leprosy decreased with the coming of the "Black Death" (the bubonic plague), which killed many lepers. Black Death was a term used to describe the dark, mottled appearance of the corpse due to hemorrhages beneath the skin. (In 1905, it was determined that this disease was caused by a bacillus that grew in fleas of infected black rats.) The disease was devastating. Symptoms included sudden shivering, headache, vomiting, and pains in the abdomen and limbs, followed by delirium. Large, painful boils appeared at the body joints, and, unless treated, it proved fatal in 5 days. Other variations included the pneumonic plague, which affected the lungs and caused death in 3 days, and the septicemic plague, caused by direct bacillus injection into the blood by the flea, which caused death within 24 hours.

The plagues probably began after flooding drove rodents inflicted with fleas from their habitats. China reported 13 million deaths. The plague traveled to India, Asia Minor, Egypt, and North Africa. One army fighting for a trading port realized they were becoming infected, catapulted their infected corpses into the port, and fled homeward to Sicily. This same sequence occurred in other areas, thereby carrying the plague into other ports. By 1352, all of Europe, Iceland, Greenland, and Russia were infected. The plague was blamed on a corrupt atmosphere: foul vapors created by Jupiter, infection from decomposing bodies of a plague of locusts, and, the most favored, invisible arrows shot by Christ. All were attributed to the wrath of God. Finally, the Jews were blamed. All Jews living in Switzerland and Germany, approximately 28,000 people, were put in wooden buildings and burned alive. Before it subsided, it is estimated that 30% of the total European population died. There were four additional outbreaks before the end of the 14th century. In *Medicine, An International History,* Hastings states, "infectious disease has been a more deadly enemy to man than war—hence the ghastliness of the modern concept of bacteriological warfare." The Black Death was not forgotten, and fear of the plague was an important motivation to stimulate a return to medical learning.

EARLY MEDICAL PIONEERS

Beginning in Italy in the 14th century, there was a revival of culture and concern for life. Gradually, people began to escape the limitations of the church. There was a new attitude toward the human body. The classical artists, Michelangelo, Dürer, and da Vinci, began to practice dissection in order to draw the human body—especially the bones, muscles, and internal organs—accurately.

Vesalius

An anatomist named Vesalius was from a medical family in Brussels. Vesalius did his own dissections on corpses that he took from the gallows or bought from grave robbers. He determined that the structures he dissected were not as Galen had described. In 1537 he became a professor of surgery and anatomy, and four years later, while dissecting a monkey, he discovered that Galen's descriptions had been the result of animal dissection, not human. He published a book on the human body that contained over 300 illustrations proving Galen's errors; however, he made little attempt to discuss physiology or the function of organisms.

William Harvey

In 1578, an Englishman named William Harvey observed that blood in the arteries always flowed away from the heart while blood in the veins flowed toward it, with valves that prevented it from changing direction. He also realized that the same blood had to be pumped repeatedly. He knew blood passed through the lungs to be purified, but he died without discovering the capillaries between the arteries and veins.

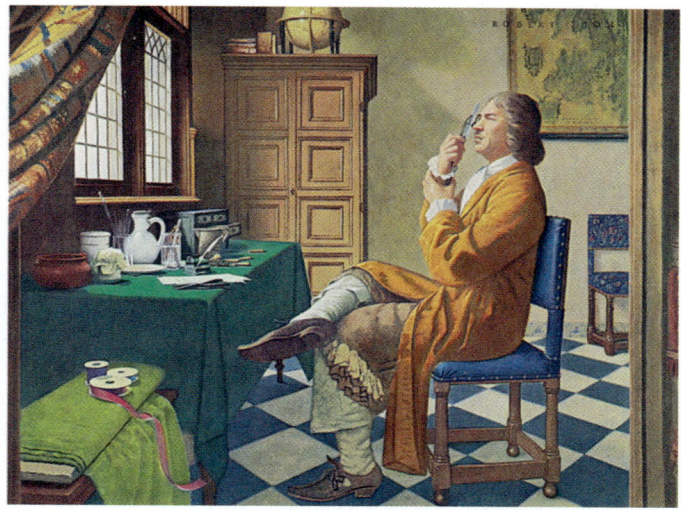

FIGURE 1-5   van Leeuwenhoek and his microscope *(Courtesy of Parke-Davis and Company, © 1957)*

The First Microscope

The microscope was the invention of an Italian named Malpighi and a Dutchman named van Leeuwenhoek (Figure 1-5). Malpighi first saw capillaries in 1661. van Leeuwenhoek was a wealthy merchant and in his leisure built over 200 microscopes (some of which magnified up to 270 times), allowing him to see, for the first time, red blood cells.

Ligatures and Forceps

An outstanding surgeon of this era was a Frenchman named Pare. He studied 4 years at the Paris hospital and earned his Diploma of Barber-Surgeon. For the next 30 years, he accompanied the army in its many battles, making discoveries first-hand. He discovered it was possible and much more successful to tie bleeding vessels with a ligature, rather than to burn them with a cautery. He invented special forceps to grasp arteries and developed new techniques for treating fractures and dislocations.

The Guilds

The practice of medicine in the beginning of the 17th century was divided among the members of three **guilds** (an association of persons engaged in a common trade or calling for mutual advantage and protection): the physicians, the surgeons, and the **apothecaries**. The physicians were the most prestigious because they usually possessed a university degree. They preferred studying, teaching, and debating the theories of disease to actually dealing directly with the sick. They limited their practice to the upper classes. The surgeons were

considered inferior to the physicians. They were divided into two classifications: Surgeons of the Long Robe and the more humble barber-surgeons. Only a few surgeons held university degrees. They were trained largely in hospitals or through **apprenticeships** (a period of time when one is bound by agreement to learn some trade or craft). Barber-surgeons used their razors for opening veins as well as barbering. The apothecaries were tradesmen and were permitted to treat people with the drugs they made, prescribed, and sold. They were the general **practitioners** for the masses and also learned through apprenticeships.

MODERN MEDICAL PIONEERS

The discovery and conquest of the Americas had far-reaching medical impact. Colonists from Spain, Portugal, Holland, and France who landed in South, North, and Central America brought the diseases from the Old World and infected the Native Indians who had no built-up resistance. Entire native tribes were destroyed, making it easy to occupy their lands. However, the Indians were infected with syphilis and "sent" it back to Europe with sailors. Syphilis flourished and spread throughout Europe. Reportedly, one third of all the people in Paris alone were infected.

There were only three or four trained physicians in all of Virginia before 1700. The Virginia Company offered free passage to apothecaries and their families to increase medical immigration. It was necessary for the settlers to practice self-medication using herbs and old practices. Bleeding was still practiced for fevers, infections, and even toothaches. One French surgeon reportedly bled his patient 64 times in 8 months. To aid in digestion, some physicians recommended swallowing grit. Queen Anne's physician prescribed drinking 50 live millipedes in water twice daily. The preparations in the medicines still contained ingredients recommended in ancient Egypt.

Humans had been "practicing" medicine for thousands of years, but only since the development of the microscope and the discovery of microbes has it progressed.

With the emphasis on scientific inquiry, medicine changed rapidly. Many people made contributions that changed medical practice. Table 1-1 lists the more familiar persons and their contributions.

Polio

In 1949 there were 43,000 cases of polio in the United States alone. Dr. Jonas Salk and a group of researchers at the Harvard Medical School successfully isolated the polio virus after discovering that it grew in human intestines and was carried in water and food to other contacts. In April of 1954, Dr. Salk began massive trials of

TABLE 1-1   Contributions of Medical Pioneers

Name/Date	Country of Residence	Contribution
Trotula Platearius 1100 AD	Italy	Earliest known female physician. She specialized in obstetrics and gynecology and wrote a textbook, *Diseases of Women,* which was used for 700 years.
Gabriel Fahrenheit 1688–1736	Germany	A physicist who introduced the thermometric scale and developed the mercury thermometer.
Edward Jenner 1749–1823	England	Gave the first vaccination to an 8-year-old boy using the exudate from a cowpox lesion of a dairymaid. He injected the boy with smallpox 2 months later, but it did not develop.
Rene Laennec 1781–1826	France	Invented the stethoscope because he could not hear the heart and lungs of an obese patient with his ear. It was originally a rolled-up piece of paper but became a wooden tube.
WTG Morton 1819–1868	United States	Introduced the use of ether to make his patients more comfortable during surgery.
Florence Nightingale 1820–1910	England (primarily)	Founder of modern nursing. She was sent with 38 nurses to care for Crimean War casualties. She established a formal school of nursing at St. Thomas Hospital in London in 1860.
Clara Barton 1821–1912	United States	A civil war nurse; recognized the need for support services for soldiers. She established the American Red Cross in 1881 and served as its first president.
Elizabeth Blackwell 1821–1910 (Figure 1-6)	United States	First woman physician in the United States. She was rejected by 17 schools before being accepted. In 1853 she and two women physicians opened a medical college for women in New York, and in 1857, a hospital exclusively for women.
Louis Pasteur 1822–1895 (Figure 1-7)	France	A chemist who discovered microorganisms could be destroyed by heating. The treatment of milk with heat to destroy organisms carries his name, pasteurization. He also discovered a vaccine to prevent and treat rabies.
Joseph Lister 1827–1912 (Figure 1-8)	England	A surgeon who realized microbes in the air caused infections after surgery. He used diluted carbolic acid to disinfect the skin, his hands, and instruments and developed a pump to spray the air. This was the foundation for medical **asepsis.**

(continues)

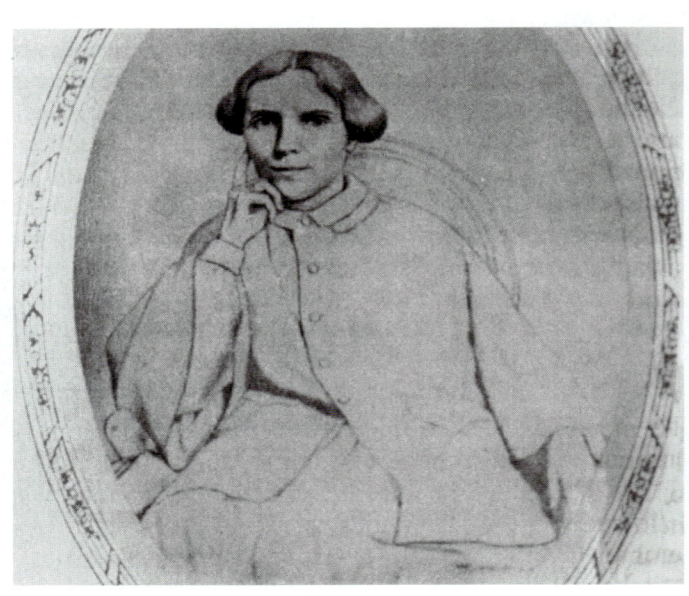

FIGURE 1-6 Elizabeth Blackwell, the first woman in the United States to qualify as a doctor *(Courtesy of Hobart and William Smith Colleges)*

TABLE 1-1   Contributions of Medical Pioneers (Continued)

Name/Date	Country of Residence	Contribution
Wilhelm von Roentgen 1845–1923	Germany	Discovered x-rays, which were later called **Roentgen** rays in his honor. This gave physicians the ability to see inside the body without surgery.
Elias Metchnikoff 1845–1916	Russia	Worked at Pasteur's Institute and became director after Pasteur died. He discovered how white blood cells protect the body from disease.
Walter Reed 1851–1902	United States	An army major serving in Cuba he discovered the cause of yellow fever as a virus carried by a mosquito. By preventing bites, the disease was curtailed and the Panama Canal was built.
Marie Curie 1867–1934	Poland	First world-famous woman scientist. She discovered radium, and her work led to the use of radium in the treatment of cancer.
Alexis Carrel 1873–1944	France	Came to the United States and discovered severed arteries could be joined and again be functional. Also did animal research transplanting bones, blood vessels, and organs.
Elsie Strang L'Esperance 1878–1959	United States	Graduated from medical school established by Elizabeth Blackwell. She had a concern for early cancer detection and established the Strang Clinic.
George Papanicolaou 1883–1962	United States	Dr. Papanicolaou worked at the Strang Clinic on diagnosing cervical cancer. His discovery, the Pap test, has become routine and has saved the lives of thousands of women.
Frederic Banting 1891–1941	Canada	Discovered and isolated insulin in 1921, giving diabetics a more normal life.
Gerhard Domagk 1895–1964	Germany	A bacteriologist experimenting with mice, he discovered a red dye called prontosil killed coccus-family organisms. This led to the development of sulfa drugs that cure 90% of coccal infections.
Sir Alexander Fleming 1881–1964	Scotland	While experimenting with bacteria, a mold accidentally got on a culture and prevented the bacteria from growing. Later this mold was studied and became the beginnings of penicillin.

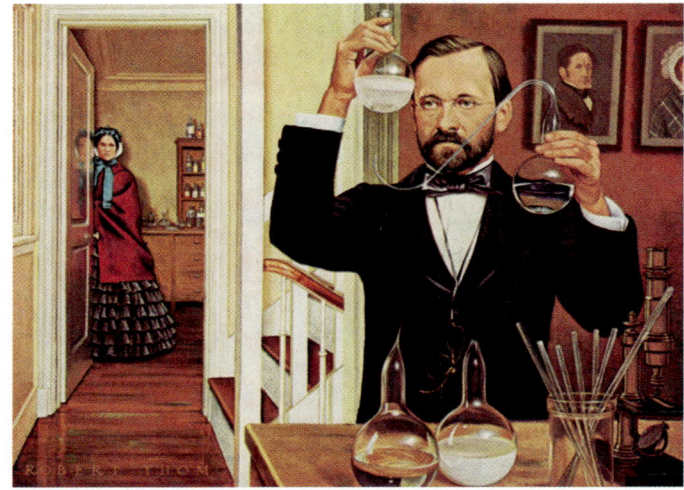

FIGURE 1-7   Pasteur: The chemist who transformed medicine *(Courtesy of Parke-Davis and Company, © 1957)*

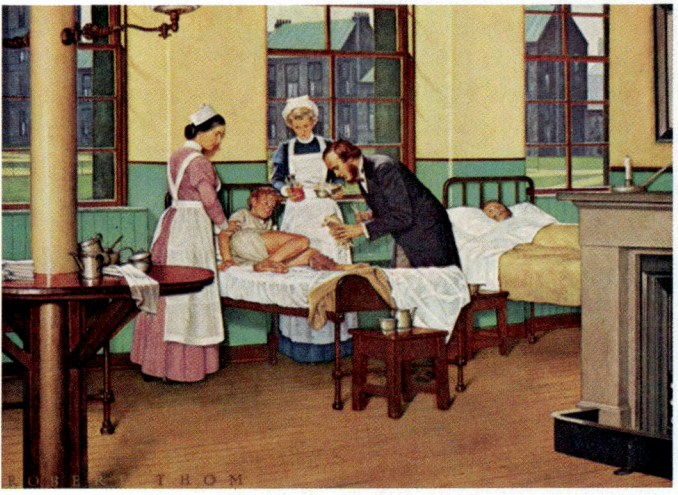

FIGURE 1-8   Lister introduces antisepsis *(Courtesy of Parke-Davis and Company, © 1957)*

a vaccine. By the end of that summer, 1,830,000 children in America had been successfully protected.

Following **vaccination**, some of the children developed polio, and there was a lot of discussion regarding the use of the vaccine. In 1953, after a time of trial and testing, Dr. A. B. Sabin developed an attenuated oral vaccine composed of dead viruses. It stimulated production of antibodies in the human body and was 90% effective in preventing polio. The vaccine has been called one of the miracles of modern medicine. In 1961 the U.S. Public Health Department licensed Sabin's vaccine, saying it produced immunity quicker, involved no injection, and lasted longer.

New Equipment

In Holland in 1938, William J. Kolff tried to develop an artificial kidney device after helplessly watching his young patient die from kidney failure. A short time later, a colleague introduced him to a new product called cellophane, and he was able to use it to perfect his machine. After World War II, he brought it to the United States and joined the staff at the Cleveland Clinic in Ohio. The early treatments required long periods of time, 3 to 4 days each week, being attached to the machine. In 1966, with the help of colleagues at The Engineering Science Group, Kolff developed a dialyzing unit that encircled one arm and a fluid reservoir with activated charcoal that could be worn around the waist. This mechanism provided continuous dialysis and allowed for freedom from the machine.

A gigantic leap in diagnostic capabilities came about during the 1950s, with the use of radioisotopes. Before then, only x-rays could see inside the body, and that image was a still, flat picture. Doctors had to rely on palpation and tests for additional information. With the use of isotopes, however, organs could be visualized clearly with a scanner and observed for function as they absorbed, retained, or disposed of the isotope. Isotopes can be composed of iodine, fluorine, mercury, gold, copper, arsenic, or technetium. The type used depends on the organ being studied.

Replacement Parts

Many things have been developed to take the place of the body's natural parts, such as sea coral for bone, artificial metallic joints, plastic eye lenses, and lifelike limb prostheses. However, some artificial parts have truly been lifesavers. Late in 1950, Dr. Michael DeBakey of Baylor University in Waco, Texas, successfully replaced arteries with Dacron tubing, and patients did not experience immune reactions. Later Teflon tubing was also used. Dr. Charles Hufnagel of Georgetown University Medical Center in Washington, D.C., re-

placed a heart valve with the first artificial one in 1953. In 1957, Dr. C. Walton Lillehei and two electronic engineers perfected a pacemaker with silver-plated wires going through the chest and attaching to the surface of the heart.

A Swedish doctor, Ake Senning, was the first to implant a pacemaker, but the short battery life made it impractical. In May of 1970, the first pacemaker with a 10-year battery was implanted in a French woman. By July 1972, two U.S. surgeons had implanted the first nuclear-powered pacemaker, which had an extended period of use.

By 1960, Dr. DeBakey and his team developed the first auxiliary heart pump and attached it to a patient experiencing heart failure. The patient died 3 days later from pneumonia. In April 1966, an improved model was used; however, the patient died after 5 days, even though the pump was still working. Research has continued on the perfection of artificial organs, but it has not been particularly successful. In July 2001, the first totally implantable artificial heart, developed by the AbioCor company, was placed in a patient who had only a few days to live. The heart battery was powered externally through the skin. The expectation was that the patient would only live for about 60 days. He survived 151 days, dying on November 30, 2001, because of a stroke and internal bleeding.

There have been a total of 14 patients who have received the artificial heart in its initial experimental phase. All patients were in end stages of heart failure, were not suitable for a transplant, and had no other options to live. Their life expectancy was less than 30 days. The "heart's" original 60-day goal for life was at least twice the patient's anticipated life. One patient lived a total of 512 days and was able to return to many of his former activities; he died in February of 2003 when the artificial heart, designed to function no more than 1 year, wore out. At present, the heart is being redesigned to make it smaller. In its original size, only those with large chest cavities could accommodate the 2-pound heart. The FDA has temporarily withdrawn approval for additional trials because all participants have died, some during surgery or soon thereafter. Other mechanical hearts are available to support people while waiting for a transplant but are not implantable devices.

Presently many body parts can be replaced with artificial substitutes and in some cases, such as heart valves, with matching parts from animals. But replacing the vital functioning organs, like the heart, lungs, kidney, or pancreas, can be relatively successful only with transplants from a compatible donor. Efforts are being focused on the importance of designating oneself as a donor to meet the needs of thousands who are enrolled on waiting lists, anticipating their lifesaving gift.

Electronic Clothing

A newly developed device allows continuous monitoring of a person by sensors imbedded into a self-contained, vestlike garment that only weighs 10 ounces. It is called SmartShirt, Life Shirt, or the Health Buddy Appliance, depending on the manufacturer. The vest is capable of measuring 30 physiologic signs, such as cardiac and respiratory function, measuring oxygen levels through an attached finger clip, identifying the location of a bullet hole in the chest, and measuring vital signs. The data is stored on a memory card of a hand-held computer that clips on a belt. The device has applications for hospitalized patients, law enforcement, racecar drivers, and the chronically ill, whose data can be assessed over the web with the proper connections.

CONTROVERSIAL DISCOVERIES

Stem Cells

A huge step in modern medicine is the ability to use stem cells to correct many problems within the body. Stem cells are extracted from an embryo when it has developed about 150 cells. They are grown in a culture and can develop into all of the body's tissues. Many researchers see stem cells as a way to treat many diseases. Healthy stem cells can replace diseased ones to cure patients with incurable diseases. To date, the most promising early research is in diabetes. Stem cells can develop into pancreatic tissue to replace that which is nonfunctioning. The use of stem cells is a highly controversial process that is filled with ethical, moral, and legal implications. Reportedly, stem cells will be able to:

- Repair brain cells damaged by Alzheimer's disease
- Replace corneas
- Provide muscle or bone for any body part
- Replace heart valves
- Repair or replace damaged liver cells
- Repair spinal nerves
- Repair or replace skin after burns
- Repair bone cartilage in joints

The cells themselves will be capable of multiplying indefinitely to make more stem cells. This scientific discovery may be one of the most significant of the century if scientists can "grow" new body parts on demand and insert healthy cells where damaged ones are developing.

DNA

Another very significant scientific discovery also is changing the practice of medicine. An international effort has resulted in the defining of the human genome, the identification of the genes in the DNA of cells. The ability to know which gene certain characteristics come from or which gene is responsible for certain diseases and disorders opens the possibility for scientific intervention into an unknown number of areas. As with stem cell technology, manipulating genes is also filled with ethical, legal, and moral issues. On the positive side, DNA determination is an asset in identifying risk of disease, criminal activity, and identification of casualties. Chapter 11, Unit 1, discusses the Genome Project and its applications.

NEW TECHNOLOGY

New computer-driven technology is making incredible medical breakthroughs. A micro-miniaturization technique permits visualization inside the digestive system. A tiny camera-radio-LED mechanism is enclosed in a small capsule that is swallowed, thereby eliminating endoscopies. The device sends images twice per second to an outside recording device. After 8 hours the capsule is eliminated naturally from the body.

Other artificial organs are also being developed, as are artificial skin and blood. In Europe, an internal mechanical pancreas is being perfected to produce insulin. An artificial liver is being studied at the University of Michigan. In Portugal, eight blind patients can now experience limited vision with a video camera after having electrodes and a tiny computer implanted in their brains. The development of cochlear implants has allowed over 40,000 people who were once deaf to hear.

It is anticipated that by 2010, you will be able to have a home monitoring device that will check your heart, kidneys, and circulatory system at home and send the information to your doctor. There is also a tiny chip that can monitor and transmit your temperature. Scientists believe that within 50 years we may be able to replace most of our worn-out parts.

Many modern-day miracles of medicine are being performed nearly every day, but only after time is it possible to determine which ones will truly make a difference. Innovations are apparently limited only by the imagination and perseverance of scientists and researchers.

THE IMPACT OF GOVERNMENT ON HEALTH CARE

In 1946, Congress passed the Hill Burton Act that provided for the improvement and construction of hospitals. Big cities renovated existing buildings and established ICU units, trauma centers, and outpatient services. Small towns and rural areas were provided with regional health centers. Professional administrators began to manage hospital operations.

Private clinics sprung up to care for specific diseases. Hospitals that once cared for tuberculosis (TB) patients are now closed because of the success of antibiotics. Large mental institutions are also gone as a result of the efforts to assimilate these persons into society.

TABLE 1-2   Organization And Legislation Affecting Health Care

Date	Organization/ Legislation	Description
1930	National Institutes of Health (NIH)	Had its beginnings in 1887 as a laboratory researching the causes of cholera and tuberculosis. There was no treatment for either disease. In 1930 the NIH was established under the U.S. Department of Health and Human Services (DHHS). There are 13 research institutes (e.g., National Cancer Institute) that work to improve health and provide information to health care professionals. They support biomedical research in the cause and prevention of disease at the institutes and at universities and hospitals.
1948	World Health Organization (WHO)	A specialized agency of the United Nations that cooperates to control and eradicate disease worldwide. They share information and technology and deliver medical supplies and drugs where needed.
1965	Medicaid	A Title under the Social Security Amendments that provides government funding to the states to help pay for the medical care of indigents. States establish criteria for qualification and set fee schedules to reimburse physicians who provide services.
1966	Medicare	National health insurance for persons over 65, or those who are blind, disabled, or have certain kidney conditions. It is administered by the Centers for Medicare and Medicaid Services (CMS) through the DHHS. Medicare has Part A, which covers hospitalization, and Part B, which covers physicians and other medical providers.
1967	Clinical Laboratory Improvement Act (CLIA)	Established guidelines for operating laboratories. A congressional investigation into physician's office labs (POL) resulted in the 1988 amendments. The labs were found deficient in both quality of service and results mainly due to lack of accredited technologists. The new law set standards for laboratories and listed tests which were exempt from CLIA that could be performed in a POL with a certificate of waiver.

(continues)

Custodial nursing homes and the hospice movement were developed to meet society's needs.

Following World War II, big medical centers with schools of medicine, nursing, pharmacy, dentistry, and allied and public health began accelerating research. Research was also being carried out by pharmaceutical firms, independent institutes, the armed forces, and health departments. New equipment (such as the electron microscope), new techniques using nuclear and molecular biology, biophysics, and the recent breaking of the genetic code have revolutionized research.

The federal government has provided much impetus and influence in the growth of medicine through funding, grants, and regulations. Legislation gave status to Public Health Services and the Food and Drug Administration. In 1953, the two became part of the Department of Health, Education, and Welfare, which has since become the Department of Health and Human Services.

Building on the successful organizations of the National Cancer Institute (1937) and the old Hygenic Lab of the Public Health Services, Congress passed acts that ultimately led to the creation of the National Institutes of Health (NIH), which are clusters of research institutes that focus on major diseases.

Congress also enacted legislation in 1965 in an effort to establish an effective and comprehensive federal health care program in the form of national health insurance with Medicare for the aged and Medicaid for the poor. Now there is an effort to try to control the massive costs of these programs.

Table 1-2 lists organizations or legislation that has affected the delivery of health care. A review of the information will give you some insight as to why certain policies and procedures are followed in the medical office.

THE IMPACT OF CONSUMERS ON HEALTH CARE

Group Involvement

In the 1960s, many critics of mainline medicine became organized. There were organized efforts to stop vaccinations programs, the fluoridation of water, and the use of animals in research. A more subtle criticism was voiced against modern therapeutic practices. There were complaints about unnecessary surgery, excessive use of drugs, over-medicalization of childbirth, intimidating and painful procedures, and the use of heroic measures for prolonging life.

A more informed society began to question the previously unquestioned medical authority. Grievances

TABLE 1-2   Organization And Legislation Affecting Health Care (Continued)

Date	Organization/ Legislation	Description
1968	Uniform Anatomical Gift Act	Allows living individuals to indicate their desire for their body or organs to be gifted to research, transplant services, or a tissue/organ bank at the time of their death.
1970	Occupational Safety and Health Administration (OSHA)	Originally an act to reduce the incidence of injury, illness, and deaths in the workplace. It is under the U.S. Department of Labor and since the end of the 1980s has been extended to the health care industry. The threat of HIV and AIDS brought about guidelines to protect workers from bloodborne organisms by requiring compliance to standards covering body fluids, needles, sharps, spills, personal protective equipment, and other hazards.
1970	Controlled Substance Act	The Drug Enforcement Administration (DEA), which is part of the U.S. Department of Justice, works with all levels of government to address the serious use and abuse of drugs. Physicians must apply for registration and receive a DEA number in order to administer, prescribe, or dispense drugs. The act also specifies the proper storage or disposal of controlled drugs.
1996	Health Insurance Portability and Accountability Act (HIPAA)	HIPAA legislation is intended to limit health administration costs, provide for patient information privacy, and prevent fraud and abuse. The regulations deal with many areas, such as electronic transmission of data, release of personal information, security of records, establishing individuals as HIPAA officers, etc.
2006	Medicare D	Everyone who receives Medicare was eligible to join a prescription drug plan to assist in payment of medication costs. Multiple insurance companies provide plans from which to choose coverage based on drugs covered, drug costs, monthly premiums, co-payments, and deductible costs.

from organized consumers, senior citizens, churches, and feminists groups began opposing specific medical practices and demanded more humane environments and treatments. Because of the lack of confidence in the medical establishment and the authoritarian manner of practice, many people defected to alternative health therapies (refer to Chapter 20, Unit 4).

Recognizing problems, medical schools began addressing the issues of philosophy, social concerns, and ethics and incorporated these courses in their curriculum. Other forms of medical care, such as osteopathy and optometry, flourished and became accepted by mainline medicine. Chiropractic medicine was without orthodox approval but flourished. Other alternatives to medicine were Christian Science and faith healing among fundamentalist churches.

Individual Changes

There was a great search for humane treatment by literate lay people. There was a revival of homeopathy and consideration of the whole person in holistic medicine. There was a renewed interest in herbal medicine and folk remedies.

Contacts made overseas by military and traveling Americans exposed them to Asian medical and health

concepts. It generated interest in Zen, yoga, and martial arts. Acupuncture gained a measure of official acceptance following President Nixon's visit to China, and it is prominent in Asian-American communities today.

The promotion of physical exercise, sports, and recreation is directed toward promoting and maintaining good health. This is evident in the popularity of activities such as body building, aerobics, and running, as well as the proliferation of gyms and health clubs.

A sizeable portion of the population is now vegetarian. Health food stores have proliferated. There is a growing feeling of nonestablishment: a "heal thyself" attitude. There are "fat farms," multiple fad diets, liposuction, television and video exercise enthusiasts, and a mountain of health-related books. Pressure from activists forced the development of food labels to identify the nutritional content of foods. The relationship between food and the major illnesses of heart disease, diabetes, and stroke are being studied.

The sexual revolution in the past four decades fostered the idea that more frequent, less inhibited sex was healthy. Accommodation to homosexuality occurred. The liberation of women and the freedom of sexual behavior brought a new role to the physician. Sexually transmitted diseases (STDs), antibiotic therapy, birth control, sex-change surgery, breast enhancement, sterilization, and abortion all created new areas of counseling and treatment.

A new era developed. Sexual hygiene and education and birth control devices became common topics of discussion. Studies of sexual habits were conducted by two famous teams: Alfred Kinsey and colleagues from 1948 through 1953 and William Masters and Virginia Johnson from the 1960s through 1980.

In 1980, rigorous campaigns were begun to encourage the use of condoms in an effort to control the spread of STDs, especially the newest one, acquired immune deficiency syndrome (AIDS). There was a great deal of public exposure to sexual behavior.

Physicians are now faced with a new problem to solve. Because of people's lack of physical activity and the convenience of prepackaged food, fast food, junk food, and eating out, the population has become obese and is displaying a number of medical conditions relating to obesity. This is a problem not only for the adult population, but also for children who are becoming obese at alarming rates. In addition to treating diseases, physicians now find themselves dealing with dietary problems and prescribing preventive and curative therapies in an attempt to get at the real cause of health problems. Unfortunately, no magic pill has yet been discovered, and human nature being what it is, the problem of obesity will not be an easy one to solve.

ACHIEVE UNIT OBJECTIVES

- Complete the Workbook activities to meet the learning objectives.
- Apply your knowledge at the end of this chapter in completing the Critical Thinking Challenge and Activities, as well as the StudyWARE on your Student CD-ROM.

UNIT 2
THE TOTAL HEALTH CARE TEAM

OBJECTIVES

Upon completion of this unit, you will be able to achieve the following:

LEARNING Objectives

1. Spell and define, using the glossary at the back of the text, all of the Words to Know in this unit.

2. Discuss the role of the health care professionals listed in this unit.

3. Explain why it is necessary to have a basic understanding of other health care team members.

4. Identify four types of medical practice.

5. Explain the titles of the seven types of doctors, identifying their designating initials.

6. Properly pronounce and define the area of expertise for each physician specialist.

7. Properly pronounce and define the area of expertise for each nonphysician specialist.

WORDS TO KNOW

admission clerk
allergist
anesthesiologist
cardiologist
chiropractor
cytologist
dental assistant
dental hygienist
dentist (DDS)
dermatologist
dietitian
doctorate
electrocardiogram
 technician
 (ECG tech)
emergency
 medical
 technician
 (EMT)
endocrinologist
gastroenterologist
gerontologist
gynecologist
hematologist
histologist
internist

laboratory
 technician
licensed practical
 nurse (LPN)
nephrologist
neurologist
nurse assistant
 (NA)
nurse midwife
nurse practitioner
nutritionist
obstetrician
occupational
 therapist (OT)
occupational
 therapy
 assistant (OTA)
oncologist
ophthalmic
 technician (OT)
ophthalmologist
optometrist
orthopedist
osteopathy
otorhinolaryng-
 ologist

paramedic
pathologist
pediatrician
pharmacist (RPH)
pharmacy
 technician
phlebotomist
physical therapist
 (PT)
physician's
 assistant (PA)
podiatrist
psychiatrist
psychologist
radiologist
radiology
 technician
registered nurse
 (RN)
respiratory
 therapy
 technician
surgeon
unit clerk
urologist
x-ray technician

 CERTIFICATION CONNECTION

CMA
Working as a team member
 to achieve goals

HIPAA

Health Insurance Portability and Accountability Act (HIPAA) regulations do not interfere with the exchange of personal health information among team members. The Privacy Rule permits freedom to share personal health information among health care providers who are involved in the direct treatment of a patient without further authorization. Broad permission includes any and all services provided by one or more health care providers. Doctors may share information concerning treatment and care of a patient when referred to another physician. The only exception relates to psychotherapy, which requires authorization and special treatment to disclose information.

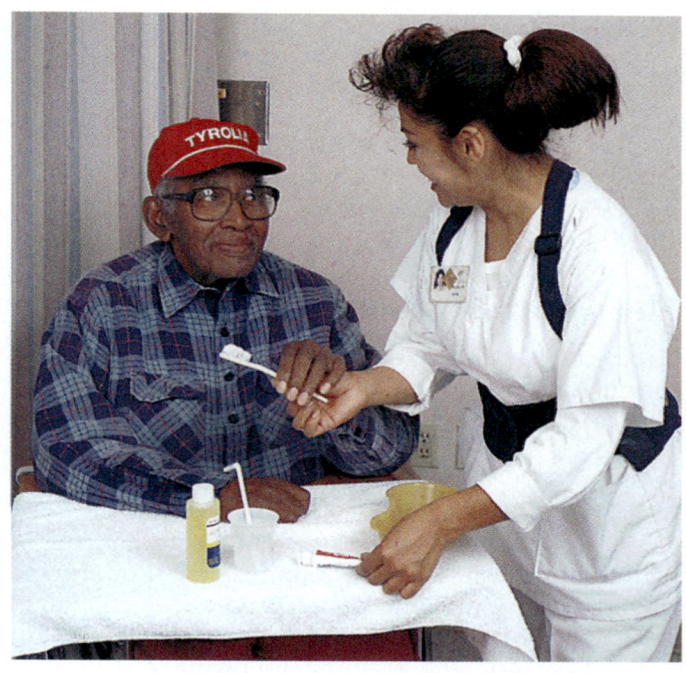

FIGURE 1-9   The nursing assistant assists with daily living skills.

ALLIED HEALTH CARE TEAM MEMBERS

There are many health professionals who provide specific care to patients. They work in a variety of settings such as hospitals, laboratories, municipal safety divisions, provider offices, pharmacies, convalescent and extended care facilities, and for home health care agencies. It is important for you to have some understanding of the specific duties for which they have been trained and their role in total patient care. Unless you work in a group practice or clinic you probably will not work directly with most of these team members, but you may have contact with them by telephone or by written communication. Often patients can have several health problems at the same time, and cooperation with other members of the health care team to accommodate the patient is vital. Knowing the role each professional plays in the total health care of patients will enable you to speak more intelligently with others in the medical field and become more efficient in your role as the medical assistant.

The following pages briefly discuss the various team member roles, their educational preparation, and the certification or licensure credentials.

Admissions Clerk

An **admissions clerk** in the hospital or medical center has basic medical terminology and administrative medical office skills. Obtaining a basic medical history and other important information from patients when they are admitted is the primary duty of this person. A college degree is desirable, but not essential.

Certified Ophthalmic Technician

Certified **ophthalmic technicians (COTs)** are valuable members in the field of ophthalmology. Often they are initially medical assistants with a versatile background

in both administrative and clinical office procedures and a basic understanding of medical terminology. Additional training is necessary, and certification is required to perform delicate ophthalmic tests and procedures for patients. All COTs must also keep current with the latest treatments, medications, and equipment in assisting patients and physicians.

Certified Nurse Assistant

The certified **nurse assistant (CNA)** provides basic nursing skills and patient care to those in nursing homes, retirement and adult day care facilities, and home health care under the supervision of the registered or licensed nurse (Figure 1-9). CNAs may be employed by some hospitals and are also referred to as nurse aides, nurse technicians, and orderlies.

Cytologist

A **cytologist** is a laboratory technician who specializes in the study of the formation, structure, and function of cells.

Dental Assistant

A **dental assistant** helps a dentist in the performance of generalized tasks, including chairside assistance, clerical work, reception, and some radiography and dental laboratory work. The person learns duties in school or on the job and becomes certified by taking the national certification examination to become a CDA, Certified Dental Assistant.

Dental Hygienist

A **dental hygienist** is a person with special training to provide dental services under the supervision of the dentist. Services supplied by a dental hygienist include dental prophylaxis, radiography, application of medications, and provision of dental education chairside and in the community.

Electrocardiogram Technician

Electrocardiogram (ECG) technicians are skilled in performing electrocardiograms and may be employed in medical clinics and hospitals.

Emergency Medical Technician

Emergency medical technicians (EMTs) are trained in and are responsible for the administration of specialized emergency care and the transportation to a medical facility of victims of acute illness or injury. All EMTs have ongoing training following certification and must be recertified every 2 years.

Histologist

A **histologist** is a medical scientist who specializes in histology, which is the science dealing with the microscopic identification of cells and tissues. Histologists are employed in private laboratories, clinics, and hospitals.

Laboratory Technician

A medical technologist or **laboratory technician** is one who, under the direction of a pathologist or other physician or medical scientist, performs specialized chemical, microscopic, and bacteriologic tests of blood, tissue, and bodily fluids. Those who have successfully completed the examination by the Board of Registry of the American Society of Clinical Pathologists, or a similar professional body, are designated as certified medical technologists (CMTs).

Medical Assistant

A medical assistant is a professional trained to work under the direction of a physician in offices and a variety of health care settings. They provide a wide range of administrative and clinical skills in patient care and office operations. Training is available from public vocational high schools and adult education, community, and technical schools; private career training institutes; and colleges. Graduates of programs accredited by the Commission on Accreditation of Allied Health Education Programs (CAAHEP) or Accrediting Bureau of Health Education Schools (ABHES) are eligible to take a certification examination given by the American Association of Medical Assistants (AAMA). Successful candidates become certified medical assistants and use the initials CMA following their name. Medical assistants can also obtain a registration credential, which is given by the American Medical Technologists (AMT) organization. Candidates must be high school graduates or have a GED, complete an ABHES accredited program or one that is regionally approved, or have armed forces training or 5 years medical assistant work experience. Successful completion of the examination provides the registration credential and the use of the initials RMA following their name.

Multi-Skilled Health Care Assistants

Multi-skilled health care assistants are coming of age as a result of health care reform. In the efforts to hold down the cost of health care, many medical facilities have become more and more interested in the health care worker who offers a variety of skills in the area of patient care. There is a vast array of titles for this multi-skilled person that seems to vary from one facility to another, as do the expectations of the job. Some medical centers refer to this employee as a patient care technician (PCT). A background in medical assisting or nurse assisting is most helpful, and most often required. Additional training is provided by the nursing staff, with certification exams that follow. Under the supervision of registered nurses, the duties of this position range from performing vital signs and ECGs to turning patients, drawing blood, and changing dressings, as well as many other responsibilities.

Nurses

Nursing is the practice of those activities contributing to health or recovery from illness. The following are areas of nursing:

Registered Nurse   In the United States a **registered nurse (RN)** is defined as a professional nurse who has completed a course of study at a state-approved school of nursing and passed the National Council Licensure Examination (NCLEX-RN). RNs are licensed to practice by individual states. Employment settings for RNs include hospitals, convalescent facilities, clinics, and home health care, to name a few.

Nurse Midwife   A **nurse midwife** is a professional RN who has had extensive training and experience in labor and delivery. Most states require a certification in addition to the state nurse license. The midwife assists the birthing mother throughout her pregnancy, the delivery of her infant at home or in a medical facility, and the postpartum period. Nurse midwives manage normal pregnancies and deliveries that potentially have no risks of developing complications.

Nurse Practitioner   A **nurse practitioner** is an RN who, by advanced training and clinical experience in a branch of nursing (they hold a Master's degree), has acquired expert knowledge in that branch of practice. Nurse practitioners are employed by physicians in private practice or in clinics. Some states permit independent practice.

Practical Nurse   Sometimes referred to as licensed vocational nurses, **licensed practical nurses (LPNs)** are trained in basic nursing techniques and direct patient care. They practice under the direct supervision of an RN or a physician and are employed in hospitals, convalescent centers, nursing homes, and home health care.

Nutritionist

A **nutritionist** studies and applies the principles and science of nutrition (the study of food and drink as related to the growth and maintenance of living organisms).

Dietitian   A **dietitian** has specialized training in the nutritional care of groups and individuals and has successfully completed an examination and maintains continuing education requirements of the Commission on Dietetic Registration. This member of the health care team assists patients in regulating their diets. Dietitians are employed in hospitals and clinics. One of the duties of a nutritionist or dietitian is to instruct patients to select a daily well-balanced special or regular diet.

Occupational Therapist

An **occupational therapist** practices occupational therapy most often in the hospital setting. An occupational therapist may be licensed, registered, certified, or otherwise regulated by law. Occupational therapy is defined by the American Occupational Therapy Association as: "the use of purposeful activity with individuals who are limited by physical injury or illness, psychosocial dysfunction, developmental or learning disabilities, poverty and cultural differences, or the aging process to maximize independence, prevent disability, and maintain health. The practice encompasses evaluation, treatment, and consultation."

Occupational Therapy Assistant

The **occupational therapy assistant (OTA)** is an important member of the health care team. The certified occupational therapy assistant, or COTA, generally has achieved an associate's degree in applied sciences and works under the direction of a registered occupational therapist. The duties include assisting patients in learning (or relearning) self-care, functional duties of their employment, and recreational activities according to their individual needs.

Office Manager/Business Office Manager

An office manager or business office manager has managerial skills in the business operations of the medical office, clinic, or hospital. A degree in business administration is most desirable.

Paramedic

Paramedics act as assistants to physicians or in place of a physician, especially in the military. They are trained in emergency medical procedures and supportive health care tasks. They are employed as municipal safety personnel and by private emergency services providers.

Pharmacist

A **pharmacist** is a specialist in formulating and dispensing medications, licensed by individual states to practice pharmacy (the study of preparing and dispensing drugs). Pharmacists are employed in hospitals, medical centers, and pharmacies. A bachelor's degree and 2 years of postgraduate study in pharmacology are required.

Pharmacy Technician

Pharmacy technicians assist licensed pharmacists in preparing medications for patients and, in certain cases, administering the medicine. They also assist in clerical duties such as telephone communication, typing, and filing and often in patient education regarding medicines. Requirements and duties may vary in different states; however, professional certification can be obtained through individual state pharmacy boards.

Phlebotomist

Skilled **phlebotomists** are extensively trained in the art of drawing blood for diagnostic laboratory testing. Most often they are also lab technicians. They must be nationally certified and are employed in medical clinics, hospitals, and laboratories. (Under the supervision of a physician, the medical assistant who has had instruction, practice on a training arm, and evaluation proving competency in this skill may perform this procedure to obtain blood specimens for analysis.)

Physical Therapist

A **physical therapist** is licensed to assist in the examination, testing, and treatment of physically disabled or handicapped people and those patients who are going

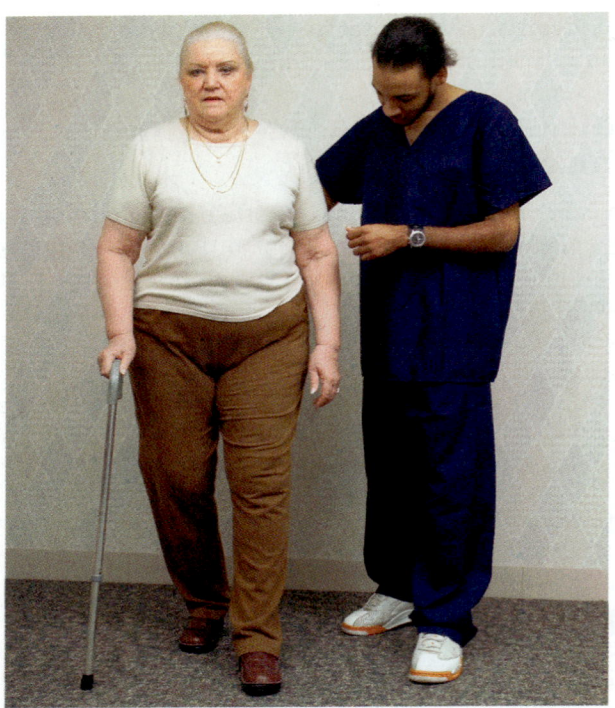

FIGURE 1-10 A physical therapist explains to a patient the correct way to use ambulatory equipment.

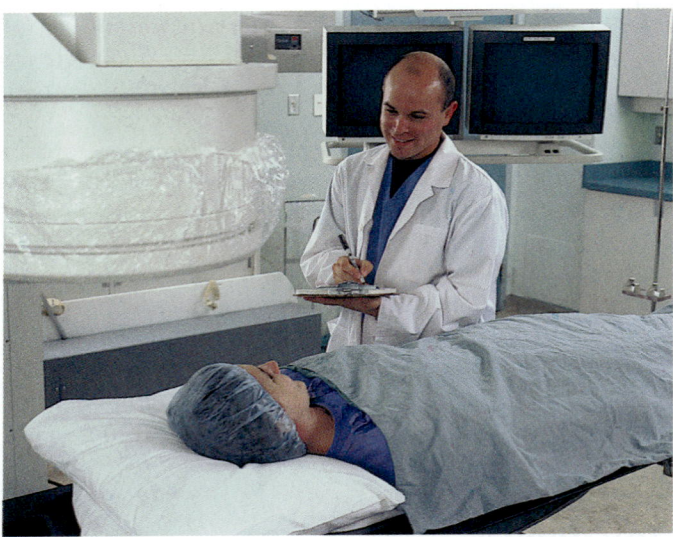

FIGURE 1-11 An x-ray technician explains the x-ray procedure to a patient.

through a physical rehabilitation program following accident, injury, or serious illness. They use special exercises, the application of heat or cold, ultrasound therapy, and other techniques (Figure 1-10). They qualify by earning a Bachelor's of Science degree in physical therapy or completing a special 12-month certificate course after obtaining a Bachelor's of Science degree in a related field.

Physician Assistant

A **physician assistant (PA)** is a person trained in certain aspects of the practice of medicine or osteopathy to provide assistance to the physician. These individuals are trained by physicians and practice under their direct supervision, within the legal license of a physician, according to the laws of each state. Students who have successfully completed pre-med requirements can apply for the required 2-year physician assistant program.

Radiology Technician, Radiologic Technologist, X-Ray Technician

An **x-ray technician**, **radiology technician**, or radiologic technologist (Figure 1-11) is one who has had specialized training in the various techniques of visualization of the tissues and organs of the body and who, under the supervision of a physician radiologist, operates radiologic equipment and assists radiologists and other health professionals. Competence must be proved by the American Registry of Radiologic Technologists.

Respiratory Therapy Technician

Respiratory therapy technicians are graduates of an AMA-approved school designed to qualify persons for the technician certification examination of the National Board for Respiratory Care. These members of the health care team perform procedures of treatment that maintain or improve the ventilatory function of the respiratory tract in patients. The training period for this field is usually a 1-year program in a hospital setting.

Unit Clerk

A **unit clerk** performs routine clerical and reception tasks in a patient care unit of a hospital. This position requires a self-motivated, mature individual to handle the stress of the hectic pace of coordinating personnel and their duties at the nurses' station. This position is also called unit coordinator, unit secretary, administrative specialist, ward clerk, or ward secretary. Training is on the job or possibly included in a health care program such as medical assisting.

Because medical assistants are versatile health care workers, it is reasonable for them to seek employment in many of the previously mentioned areas of the medical field. Once they have gained basic entry-level skills in medical assisting, they are able to adapt easily to a specialty practice with additional training.

PHYSICIAN TEAM MEMBERS

Physicians invest a minimum of 9 years in learning how to practice medicine, which is the art and science of the diagnosis, treatment, and prevention of disease and the maintenance of good health. Until recently, their training, education, and practical experience included a 4-year college degree in pre-med, 4 years in medical school, and 1 year of internship. Following this and successful completion of the state board examination for licensure, the person was then considered a general practitioner and was ready to begin a private practice. This license to practice medicine is renewed periodically throughout the physician's life. Today the phrase "post-graduate year following medical school" (PGY-1) denotes the internship stage of training.

General or Family Practice

The field of general practice covers perhaps the broadest spectrum. The general practitioner sees all kinds of patients with all kinds of problems. Most can be handled by the general practitioner. If, however, the symptoms of a case suggest a serious or perhaps unknown cause, the patient may be referred to a specialist for further diagnosis or treatment (Figure 1-12). When the patient's specific need or problem has been remedied or the recovery plan has been established, the patient returns to the "family doctor" for continued care.

Physician Specialties   The advances in modern medicine have made it impossible for physicians to study every aspect of medicine. Because of this some have become medical specialists. Specialty areas require

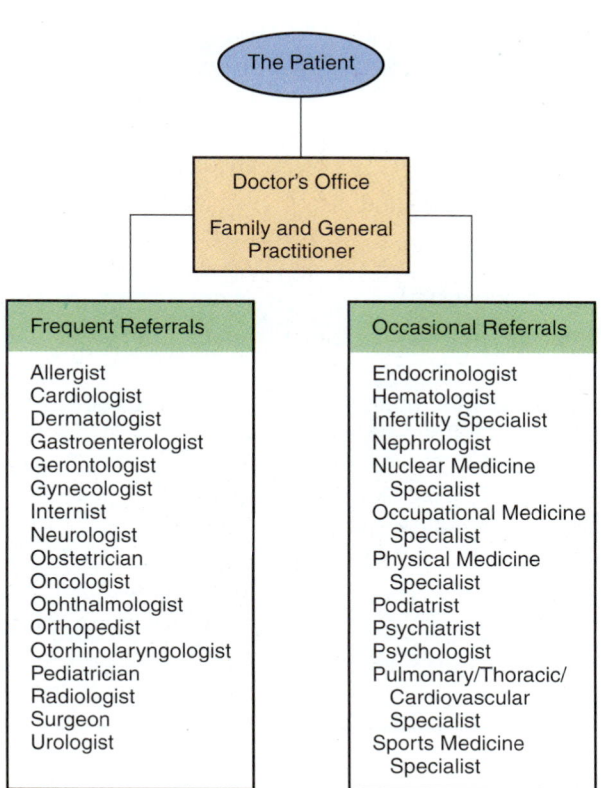

FIGURE 1-12   Frequency of referrals

additional years of study in the particular area of choice. It usually requires a minimum of 2 to as much as 6 years of additional study known as residency or PGY-2, 3, 4, and so on. After satisfactorily accomplishing all requirements, the physician is awarded a certificate of competency in the specialty area and is recognized as a diplomat or fellow of that specialty.

In addition to specialty areas, some physicians have a particular interest that is not a specialty but is an area they believe worthy of their time and effort to help their patients toward better health. These areas are viewed as subspecialties or areas of special interest.

Because medical assistants generally are employed by physicians in their offices, they need a basic understanding of the various medical specialties and special interests. The medical assistant who works for a general practitioner may need to initiate contacts with specialists through referrals and be knowledgeable about these areas to help reinforce or clarify the physician's directions to the patient. Knowing about these various practices will also help the medical assistant decide in which area to seek employment. Most specialists maintain office practices and have a need for medical assistants just as general and family practitioners do. Adapting to these special areas after acquiring basic skills and knowledge should be relatively easy. A medical assistant interested in advancement must be willing to put forth the necessary effort.

To help you become familiar with these specialties, Table 1-3 contains basic information concerning each area. Note that a few specialty practices are not listed in the table. The specialty practices of emergency or trauma medicine, anesthesiology, and pathology are usually hospital-based; rarely do they have private practice offices where patients are seen. These specialists work as members of the health care team contributing their expert skills and knowledge in serving patients. More precise knowledge of all these practices will come with experience and further study.

SUBSPECIALTY OR SPECIAL INTEREST AREAS

In the following sections you will be introduced to the subspecialty (S) or special interest (SI) areas that branch off from a particular specialty practice. A brief description and definition of each area will give you a basic idea of the roles they play in the health care team. As you learn and study the duties and responsibilities of the medical assistant, you may discover a particular area of interest of your own. When the time comes for your internship and then later for you to begin the job search for gainful employment, you will have a basic understanding of the variety of practices so that you will be better prepared to make a decision regarding where to apply.

TABLE 1-3   Physician Specialties

Specialty	Title of Practitioner	Area of Specialization	Types of Patients Seen
Allergy	**Allergist**	Diagnosing and treating conditions of altered immunologic reactivity (allergic reactions)	Adults of all ages, children, both sexes
Anesthesiology	**Anesthesiologist**	Administering anesthetic agents before and during surgery	Adults of all ages, children, both sexes
Cardiology	**Cardiologist**	Diagnosing and treating abnormalities, diseases, and disorders of the heart	Adults of all ages, children, both sexes
Dermatology	**Dermatologist**	Diagnosing and treating disorders of the skin	Adults of all ages, children, both sexes
Endocrinology	**Endocrinologist**	Diagnosing and treating diseases and malfunctions of the glands of internal secretion	Adults of all ages, children, both sexes
Family practice	Family practitioner	Similar to general practice in nature, but centering around the family unit	Adults of all ages, infants and children of all ages, both sexes
Gastroenterology	**Gastroenterologist**	Diagnosing and treating diseases and disorders of the stomach and intestines	Adults of all ages, children, both sexes
Geriatrics	**Gerontologist** or geriatrician	Diagnosing and treating diseases, disorders, and problems associated with aging	Older adults, both sexes
Gynecology	**Gynecologist**	Diagnosing and treating diseases and disorders of the female reproductive tract; strong emphasis on preventive measures	Female adolescents and adults
Hematology	**Hematologist**	Diagnosing and treating diseases and disorders of the blood and blood-forming tissues	Adults of all ages, infants and children, both sexes
Infertility	Infertility specialist	Diagnosing and treating problems in conceiving and maintaining pregnancy	Couples who desire to have children but cannot
Internal medicine	**Internist**	Diagnosing and treating diseases and disorders of the internal organs	Adults of all ages, children, both sexes
Nephrology	**Nephrologist**	Diagnosing and treating diseases and disorders of the kidney	Adults, children, both sexes
Neurology	**Neurologist**	Diagnosing and treating diseases and disorders of the central nervous system	Adults, children, both sexes
Nuclear medicine	Nuclear medicine specialist	Diagnosing and treating diseases with the use of radionuclides	Adults, both sexes
Obstetrics	**Obstetrician**	Providing direct care to women during pregnancy, childbirth, and immediately thereafter	Pregnant women
Occupational Medicine	Occupational medicine specialist	Diagnosing and treating diseases or conditions arising from occupational circumstances (e.g., chemicals, dust, or gases)	Adults of all ages, both sexes
Oncology	**Oncologist**	Diagnosing and treating tumors and cancer	Adults of all ages, children, both sexes
Ophthalmology	**Ophthalmologist**	Diagnosing and treating diseases and disorders of the eye	Adults of all ages, children, both sexes

(continues)

TABLE 1-3   Physician Specialties (Continued)

Specialty	Title of Practitioner	Area of Specialization	Types of Patients Seen
Orthopedics	**Orthopedist**	Diagnosing and treating disorders and diseases of the bones, muscles, ligaments, and tendons and fractures of the bones	Adults of all ages, children, both sexes
Otorhinolaryngology	**Otorhinolaryngologist**, commonly referred to as an ENT (ear, nose, and throat) specialist	Diagnosing and treating disorders and diseases of the ear, nose, and throat	Adults of all ages, children, both sexes
Pathology	**Pathologist**	Analysis of tissue samples to confirm diagnosis	Usually has no direct contact with patients
Pediatrics	**Pediatrician**	Diagnosing and treating diseases and disorders of children; strong emphasis on preventive measures	Infants, children, and adolescents
Physical medicine	Physical medicine specialist	Diagnosing and treating diseases and disorders with physical agents (physical therapy)	Adults, children, both sexes
Plastic surgery	Plastic surgeon	Evaluates and improves appearance of scars, deformities, and birth defects; also provides elective procedures that patients desire for aesthetic purposes	Adults of all ages, children, both sexes
Psychiatry	**Psychiatrist**	Diagnosing and treating pronounced manifestations of emotional problems or mental illness that may have an organic causative factor	Adults of all ages, children, both sexes. (Note: Child psychiatry is a further specialized field dealing exclusively with children and adolescents.)
Pulmonary specialties	Pulmonary, thoracic, or cardiovascular specialist	Diagnosing and treating diseases and disorders of the chest, lungs, heart, and blood vessels	Adults, both sexes
Radiology	**Radiologist**	Diagnosing and treating diseases and disorders with Roentgen rays (x-rays) and other forms of radiant energy	Adults of all ages, children, both sexes
Sports medicine	Sports medicine specialist	Diagnosing and treating injuries sustained in athletic events	Adults, especially young adults (athletes), both sexes
Surgery	**Surgeon**	Diagnosing and treating diseases, injuries, and deformities by manual or operative methods	Adults of all ages, infants, children, both sexes
Trauma medicine	Emergency physician (commonly referred to as ER or trauma physician since most work in hospital emergency rooms)	Diagnosing and treating acute illnesses and traumatic injuries	Adults of all ages, infants, children, both sexes
Urology	**Urologist**	Diagnosing and treating diseases and disorders of the urinary system of females and genitourinary system of males	Adults of all ages, infants, children, both sexes

Acupuncture

This method of treatment originated in the Far East and has been gaining in popularity in western countries since the 1970s. This procedure involves the insertion of fine thin needles into specific sites of the body to alleviate pain or to treat a specific body system or area (its use is still controversial). (SI)

Adolescent Medicine

This area branches from pediatrics and specifically deals with youngsters aged 11 to 20 years, or the years of puberty to maturity. (S)

Aerospace Medicine

Physicians who extend their practice of medicine to this area do research in the effects of the environment in space on people. The areas of greatest concern are pathology, physiology, and psychology. (SI)

Alcoholism (Chemical Dependency)

These physicians treat patients who have addiction to alcohol and drugs. (SI)

Allergy and Immunology

An allergy is an acquired hypersensitivity a person exhibits to a substance that normally does not cause a reaction. Physicians interested in allergies sometimes combine these areas because they are closely related. Immunology is the study of how the body deals with immunity to disease (it is a subspecialty sometimes practiced alone). (S)

Diabetes

As implied, these physicians have a special interest in treating only patients who have been diagnosed with diabetes. (SI)

Emergency Medicine

Physicians practicing this subspecialty are concerned with the diagnosis and treatment of patients with conditions that have resulted from injury or trauma or from sudden illness. (S)

Gynecologic Oncology

The subspecialty of gynecology that deals with the diagnosis and treatment of cancer of the reproductive tract of women of all ages is called gynecologic oncology. (S)

Hypertension

A physician who subspecializes in this area treats patients who have high blood pressure (hypertension). (SI)

Hypnosis

This method of treatment is becoming more popular with physicians. This procedure is used mainly in psychotherapy in which the patient is induced into a trancelike sleep to help change the memory or the perception of something in that person (such as weight control or an unwanted behavior like smoking). Its use in medicine is to help patients deal with pain and stress, which affect their overall health. (SI)

Nutrition

This area of special interest includes patients with disorders or diseases related to how the body uses food and drink for growth and maintenance. (SI)

Pediatric Allergists

These physicians deal only with treating children who have allergies. (S)

Preventive Medicine

This branch of medicine deals with the prevention of both mental and physical illness and disease. It is sometimes referred to as general preventive medicine (GPM). (S)

Rheumatology

Physicians in this subspecialty treat inflammatory disorders of the connective tissues and related structures. (S)

Sleep Disorder

As the name implies, physicians who deal with these patients are interested in the various stages of sleep and the effects of sleep deprivation. (SI)

Surgery

Most of the subspecialty areas of this branch of medicine and **osteopathy** are listed below:

- Cardiovascular
- Colon (and rectal)
- Cosmetic (plastic and reconstructive)
- Hand
- Head and neck
- Neurologic
- Orthopedic
- Pediatric
- Spine
- Thoracic
- Urologic
- Vascular

With the great strides that medical science achieves, the field of medicine continues to evolve with remark-

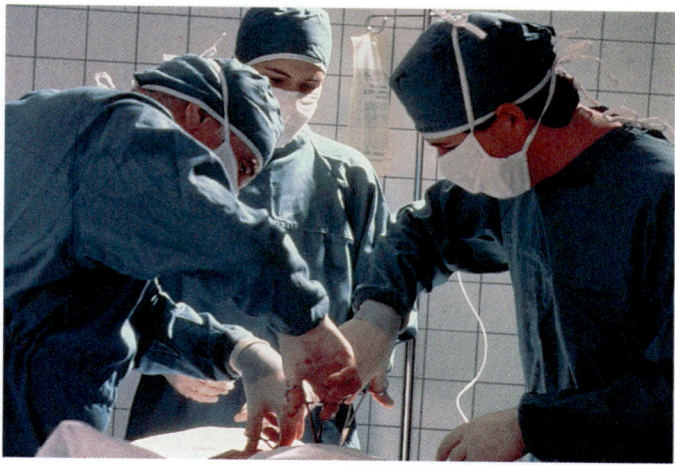

FIGURE 1-13   A successful operation requires the cooperation and expertise of the surgeon and the entire surgical team.

able new treatments, medications, and discoveries. Being an integral part of the health care team is exciting (Figure 1-13). New areas of special interest and subspecialties are ever-changing with the latest findings. Keeping abreast of these changes by attending ongoing educational programs to increase your knowledge will help you to become not only more confident in your work, but a valuable medical assistant as well.

A NOTE REGARDING DOCTORS

A basic understanding of the term *doctor* will be helpful. The term comes from Latin; it means *to teach*. Persons who hold doctoral degrees (**doctorates**) are entitled to be addressed as "Doctor" and to write the initials that stand for their doctorate after their name. A doctorate requires specific study in a field of knowledge after a Baccalaureate and a Master's degree have been earned. It generally involves a set amount of course work followed by extensive research into a topic of interest and the development and publication of a dissertation about the findings. Doctorates are attainable in most disciplines such as nursing, mathematics, education, chemistry, philosophy, and so on. This "doctor" title uses the initials PhD. The abbreviation "Dr." is the proper way to address a physician or any other type of doctor who has earned this title. In the medical field, the abbreviation "Dr." denotes that the person is qualified to practice medicine. In other fields, it means that the person has achieved the highest academic degree awarded by a college in the particular discipline.

Nonphysician Specialties

There are many other health care professionals with the title "doctor" who are not physicians but provide services to patients. Table 1-4 lists the ones with whom you are most likely to have contact.

Doctor of Medicine (MD) and Doctor of Osteopathy (DO)

One of the areas of greatest confusion is the differentiation between MDs and DOs. Holders of either degree are licensed physicians. The degrees themselves originate from somewhat different schools of thought. (Interestingly enough, it was an MD who founded the osteopathic movement that now produces DOs.) Physicians of both schools must satisfactorily complete board examinations in the state where they wish to practice medicine.

The development of osteopathy has become an accepted medical treatment because of the efforts of a physician named Dr. Andrew T. Still. In 1874, Dr. Still began to practice the philosophy of osteopathy (the practice of being concerned with the patient as a whole person) and to use an alternative method to treat them. He was concerned with the overuse of drugs and medicines and feared that surgery was used too quickly to relieve patients' suffering. Because there was no college that taught the practices of osteopathy, Dr. Still traveled the country giving demonstrations to those who were interested about how to alleviate illness with manipulation therapy. His sons later joined him in giving instruction to students in the first school of osteopathy. The premise of osteopathy is that relieving structural stress increases the body's functional capabilities and allows the body to heal itself.

The charter for the American School of Osteopathy was obtained in 1892 in Kirksville, Missouri. This later became the Associated Colleges of Osteopathy and the degree of Doctor of Osteopathy (DO) was accepted. During World War II, osteopathic physicians became respected and appreciated for their services to both soldiers and the general public. Today, there is a mutual respect among physicians of MD and DO degrees.

In the United States today, medical licensing boards permit DOs to perform the same duties as MDs. Should you find employment working for either a DO or MD, you will be able to apply the same administrative and clinical knowledge and skills.

Although you are training primarily to assist physicians, with a little adaptation you could also move into assisting chiropractors, psychologists, or podiatrists. To move into the dental or optometric field would require additional training.

Types of Practices

The actual business of practicing medicine may be conducted in several ways. Many physicians prefer to have a solo practice, or sole proprietorship, meaning that the individual alone makes all decisions regarding the practice. Being employed as a medical assistant in this type of office requires that you have both administrative and clinical skills essential for the smooth operation of that practice, especially if you are the only employee.

TABLE 1-4   Nonphysician Specialties

Specialty	Title of Practitioner	Degree	Area of Specialization	Types of Patients Seen
Chiropractic	**Chiropractor**	DC, or Doctor of Chiropractic	Manipulative treatment of disorders originating from misalignment of the spinal vertebrae	Adults of all ages, children, both sexes
Dentistry	**Dentist**	DDS, or Doctor of Dental Surgery	Diagnosing and treating diseases and disorders of the teeth and gums	Adults of all ages, children, both sexes
Optometry	**Optometrist**	OD, or Doctor of Optometry	Measuring the accuracy of vision to determine whether corrective lenses are needed	Adults of all ages, children, both sexes
Podiatry	**Podiatrist**	DPM, or Doctor of Podiatric Medicine	Diagnosing and treating diseases and disorders of the feet	Adults of all ages, children, both sexes
Psychology	**Psychologist**	PhD, or Doctor of Philosophy	Evaluating and treating emotional problems; these professionals give counseling to individuals, families, and groups	Adults of all ages, children, both sexes

In a partnership, two or more physicians have a legal agreement to share in the total business operation of the practice. In this case, usually two to several medical assistants (or other members of the health care team) are employed to care for patients and conduct business.

A group practice consists of three or more physicians who share a facility for the purpose of practicing medicine. In this legal contract the doctors share expenses, income, equipment, records, and personnel. Many times these practices are a health maintenance organization (HMO) or an independent practice association (IPA) type of practice. You will learn more about these in Chapter 9. Usually, several professionals make up the health care team in this setting. Medical assistants, lab technicians, radiology technicians, nurses, physician assistants, and the physicians work together in providing health care.

ACHIEVE UNIT OBJECTIVES

- Complete the Workbook activities to meet the learning objectives.
- Apply your knowledge at the end of this chapter in completing the Critical Thinking Challenge and Activities, as well as the StudyWARE on your Student CD-ROM.

CRITICAL THINKING CHALLENGE

IMPACTING THE PATIENT, THE PRACTICE, AND YOUR CAREER

Lisa had been employed by Dr. Slack for only about 1 month. Today, Janet Small was being seen for low back pain. As Lisa was interviewing her to determine the history of her complaint and what she had done about it, Janet remarked she had been seeing a chiropractor for 2 months but she still was having problems. Lisa told Janet, "You know they aren't really doctors, don't you? I've heard about people who have gone to them and had all kinds of problems afterward. In fact, my grandmother was having some back problems and she went to a chiropractor. She still has numbness in her left leg."

QUESTIONS

1. How might Lisa's remarks affect the patient?
2. How would this discussion reflect on the practice?
3. How might Lisa's career be affected?

ACTIVITIES

1. If you enjoy history, go online and search for some of the persons identified in Unit 1. You can either enter the name in the search space or click on the Research icon at the top of your screen and choose a reference book. Microsoft Internet Explorer has the *Encarta Encyclopedia,* which will give you many interesting facts.

2. You can try the same exercise with the different allied health careers. Enter a career title in the search space and you will get thousands of choices.

3. Look in the yellow pages of your phone book under physicians (or however it may be listed). Observe that they are listed alphabetically both individually and by the practice name. Directories will also list physicians by specialty and sometimes by geographic location. Observe the number of physicians in some of the more common specialty areas.

StudyWARE™ CHALLENGE

- Study with the flash cards for Chapter 1 to review the key terms in this chapter.
- Complete the true/false quiz in test mode for Chapter 1.

RESOURCES

AbioCor™ Replacement heart. Retrieved June 19, 2006, from *www.mos.org/cst-archive/article/3737.*

American Medical Association. (1999). Health Professions Education Directory (27th ed.). Chicago: Author.

Clayman, C. B. (Ed.). (1989). *Encyclopedia of medicine.* New York: Random House.

Hastings, R. P. (1974). *Medicine: An international history.* New York: Praeger.

Jones, B. E. (1978). The difference a D.O. makes. Oklahoma City, OK: Times-Journal Publishing Company.

Lippincott's textbook for medical assistants. (1997). Philadelphia: Lippincott-Raven Publishers.

Louderback, J. (2003). *Medical miracles.* McLean, VA: Gannett Satellite Information Network, Inc.

Marks, G., & Beatty, W. K. (1973). *The story of medicine in America.* New York: Scribners.

Mosby. (2002). *Mosby's medical, nursing, and allied health dictionary* (6th ed.). St. Louis, MO: Author.

Raven, S., and Weir, A. (1981). *Women of achievement.* New York: Harmony.

Sicherman, B., & Green, C. H. (1980). *Notable American women: The modern period.* Cambridge, MA: Belknap.

Venes, T. (2001). *Taber's cyclopedic medical dictionary* (19th ed.). Philadelphia: F.A. Davis.

WEB LINKS

www.abms.org (American Board of Medical Specialties) *This web site provides information on specialization and certification in medicine.*

www.ama-assn.org (American Medical Association) *A voluntary organization of physicians in the United States that sets standards for the medical profession and advocates on behalf of physicians and patients.*

www.aoa-net.org (American Osteopathic Association) *The main representation organization of osteopathic physicians in the United States. Serves as the primary certifying body of DOs and is the accrediting agency for all osteopathic medical colleges and health care facilities.*

www.cdc.gov (Centers for Disease Control and Prevention) *One of 13 major operating components of the Department of Health and Human Services. It is charged with prevention and control of infections and chronic diseases, injuries, workplace hazards, disabilities, and environmental threats.*

www.hhs.gov (Department of Health and Human Services) *U.S. government's principal agency, consisting of over 300 programs, for protecting the health of all Americans and providing essential human services, especially for those who are least able to help themselves.*

www.nih.gov (National Institutes of Health) *Part of the U.S. Department of Health and Human Services; the primary federal agency for conducting and supporting medical research.*

www.who.int (World Health Organization) *WHO is the United Nations specialized agency for health with the objective of attaining the highest possible level of health for all peoples.*

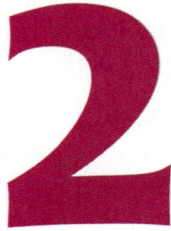

CHAPTER 2

The Medical Assistant

UNIT 1
Training, Job
Responsibilities,
and Employment
Opportunities

UNIT 2
Personal Characteristics

UNIT 3
Professionalism

The American Association of Medical Assistants (AAMA) describes the medical assistant profession as follows: "The medical assistant is a professional, multi-skilled person dedicated to assisting in patient care management. This practitioner performs administrative and clinical duties and may manage emergency situations, facilities, and/or personnel. Competence in the field also requires that a medical assistant display professionalism, communicate effectively, and provide instruction to patients."

During the evolvement of the practice of medicine, physicians have come to realize the value of medical assistants. Many years ago, physicians could treat patients alone. There was no need for appointments, filing of insurance forms, or extensive recordkeeping. There was rarely any thought of a lawsuit.

Times have changed dramatically. It is now necessary to document every transaction between the physician or the office staff and the patient to validate appropriate and responsible care. Accurate and comprehensive records are vital. Attention to every office management detail is essential as well.

This chapter discusses the training opportunities and job responsibilities of a medical assistant. It also describes highly desirable personal characteristics that will help make you a valuable asset to the physician. In addition, it identifies those attributes of professionalism that elevate your working experience to a higher level and provide you with personal satisfaction.

UNIT 1
TRAINING, JOB RESPONSIBILITIES, AND EMPLOYMENT OPPORTUNITIES

OBJECTIVES

Upon completion of this unit, you will be able to achieve the following:

LEARNING Objectives

1. Spell and define, using the glossary at the back of the text, all the Words to Know in this unit.
2. Name the two factors that are causing increased employment opportunities in the health care field.
3. Identify three types of schools that offer programs in medical assisting.
4. Explain the purpose of the Role Delineation Study.
5. List the 10 areas of competence identified by the Role Delineation Study.
6. Explain the term "career laddering."
7. Identify the 14 fastest-growing health occupations, according to the United States Department of Labor.

WORDS TO KNOW

administrative	hygienist	rehabilitation
associate's	license	centers
degree	methodical	rehabilitative
bookkeeper	nuclear medicine	therapy
certificate of	technologist	Role Delineation
completion	professional	Study
clinical	proprietary	secretary
competency	radioactive	therapeutic
compliance	agents	therapist
confidential	receptionist	ultrasound
curriculum		technologist

CERTIFICATION CONNECTION

CMA
Professionalism
- Displaying professional attitude
- Job readiness and seeking employment
- Working as a team member to achieve goals

Communication
- Professional communication and behavior

RMA
Interpersonal relations

CMAS
Professionalism

You have chosen to become a medical assistant. The following questions can help interested individuals decide whether to pursue the career:

- Do you like people?
- Do you want variety in your work?
- Can you "take hold" and get things done?
- Are you **methodical** and accurate in what you do?
- Can you be trusted with **confidential** information?

If you can answer yes to these questions, you may have the appropriate characteristics of a medical assistant. You will be pleased to learn that, according to the United States Department of Labor, this occupation is one of the health care areas identified to experience significant growth in the near future. Health occupations make up 47%, nearly half, of the total 30 identified fastest-growing occupations. Specifically, medical assisting is expected to be one of the fastest-growing occupations through the year 2014.

In this unit, you will learn about the training and responsibilities of a medical assistant. You will also read about opportunities for employment in medical assisting as well as how experience, together with additional training, can qualify you for other health care jobs in the future.

Health care occupations have developed from the physician's need to enlist the help of other persons to provide technical and efficient care for greater numbers of patients. In addition to medical assistants who work directly with the physician, a large number of highly technical and **professional** people perform a great number of diagnostic and supporting functions. In the 1998–2008 Employment Occupational Outlook Bulletin, the United States Department of Labor data indicated that 14 health care related occupations would be growing faster than the average overall workforce through the year 2008. Opportunities would be plentiful in these broad occupational groups, with a predicted average growth rate of 29.6%.

TABLE 2-1 Projected Percentages of Growth in the Fastest-Growing Health Occupations, 2004–2014

Occupation	Projected Growth
Home health aides	56%
Medical assistants	54.6%
Physician assistants	52.1%
Physical therapist assistants	44.2%
Dental assistants	42.7%
Personal and home care aides	41%
Physical therapists	36.7%
Diagnostic medical sonographers	34.8%
Physical therapist aides	34.4%
Occupational therapist assistants	34.1%
Occupational therapists	33.6%

Source: The Bureau of Labor Statistics, Monthly Labor Review, November 2005

Table 2-1 lists the projected percentages of growth in the fastest growing health occupations. Table 2-2 also lists data available from the United States Department of Labor. The first two columns show the 2004 and the 2014 projected employment figures of representative health care occupations. The third and fourth columns show the increase in percentage of employment and the total number of new employees needed within the 10 years.

The health occupations boom is the result of two factors: extended lifetimes of Americans and rapidly evolving medical technology. Data have shown that the population over age 85 is growing at a rate of four times the total population. As people age, they develop more health problems and therefore require more services. With the development of new diagnostic tests and methods of treatment, someone must be trained to operate the equipment and provide the service. Occasionally, it means that a completely new field of employment is needed, such as has occurred with **nuclear medicine technologists**.

TABLE 2-2 Current and Projected Employment in Health Occupations

Occupation	Number Employed in 2004	Number Projected to be Employed in 2014	Percent Increase	Total Job Openings, 2004–2014
Cardiovascular technologists	45,000	60,000	32.6%	23,000
Clinical lab technologists and technicians	302,000	371,000	22.7%	150,000
Dental assistants	267,000	382,000	42.7%	189,000
Emergency medical technicians	192,000	244,000	27.3%	74,000
Home health aides	624,000	974,000	56%	431,000
Licensed practical nurses	726,000	850,000	17.1%	282,000
Massage therapists	97,000	120,000	23.6%	42,000
Medical assistants	387,000	589,000	52.1%	273,000
Medical records and health information technicians	159,000	205,000	28.9%	69,000
Occupational therapy assistants and aides	27,000	35,000	32.5%	12,000
Pharmacy technicians	258,000	332,000	28.6%	107,000
Physician assistants	62,000	93,000	49.6%	40,000
Radiologic technologists and technicians	182,000	224,000	23.2%	76,000
Registered nurses	2,394,000	3,096,000	29.4%	1,203,000
Surgical technologists	84,000	109,000	29.5%	36,000

Source: The Bureau of Labor Statistics, Monthly Labor Review, November 2005

Another shift has resulted from the changing nature of how health care services are being delivered. A good example of this is the explosion of home health care. Employment in this area is expected to increase 56%. This reflects the growing population of the elderly and the disabled who will need assistance, but the trend will be toward providing it in their homes instead of within a more expensive health care facility.

TRAINING

Since you are reading this text, you are probably enrolled in a formal training program to acquire the knowledge and skills needed to become a medical assistant. Thirty years ago it was relatively easy to be hired and trained on the job. This may still take place in some offices, usually where there are multiple employees so work can continue while a new person learns. But today, with the fast-paced, complex level of skills required to provide medical care and conduct the business affairs of the practice, the value of a trained employee is recognized as a real asset by the physician.

Degree Programs

Training programs vary in length and design. In many states, vocational education offers medical assisting programs. It can be an educational option in public high schools, usually for junior and senior students. Vocational programs may also be offered at the adult level to meet the needs of post-high school individuals. Many technical and community colleges offer training as well. Programs leading to a **certificate of completion** or diploma are usually 1 year in length. An **associate's degree** program would require 2 years of course work and include subject areas that complement the **curriculum**. Another major source of training is available from private **proprietary** schools. This training may also vary in length and content depending upon the school's philosophy, affiliation, and educational goals. Regardless of the type of school, the *basic* medical assistant curriculum should be similar.

From 1979 through 1996, the AAMA maintained a document called the DACUM (*Developing a Curriculum*). This publication identified the areas of practice and the **competencies** required for the occupation of medical assistant. This document was updated in 1984 and 1990. In 1997, the DACUM was replaced by the **Role Delineation Study**. Two groups of practicing certified medical assistants (CMAs) were surveyed by the National Board of Medical Examiners and AAMA. Based upon the groups' practical experiences, they listed all current competencies essential for medical assistants. The lists of competencies were combined with the 1990 DACUM to form a survey instrument that was sent to a random sample of CMAs who represented many areas

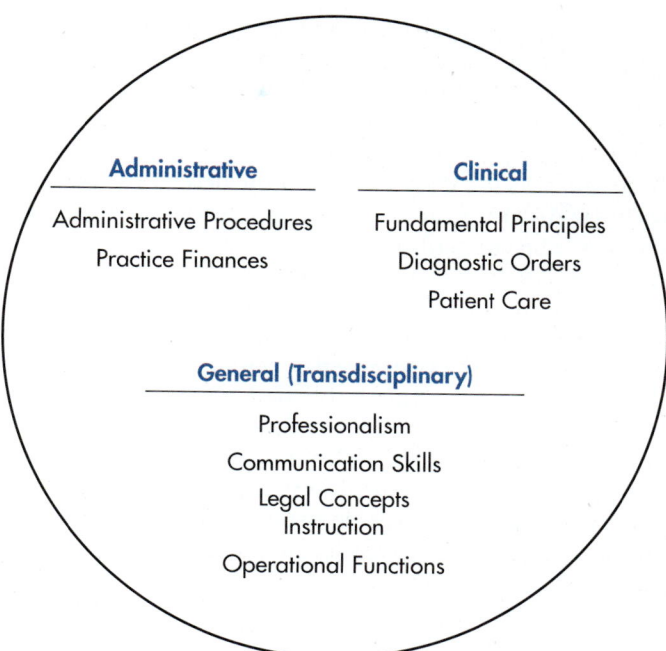

FIGURE 2-1 Areas of competence for the entry-level medical assistant, from the Role Delineation Study and Chart

of practice and geographic locations and a variety of backgrounds. The responses were evaluated and became the content for the areas of competence for entry-level medical assistants found in the Role Delineation Study. The AAMA Curriculum Review Board finalized the list of competencies, which became the *Standards and Guidelines of an Accredited Educational Program for the Medical Assistant* and replaced the previous *Essentials*.

The Role Delineation Study identifies three broad areas of practice: **Administrative**, **Clinical**, and General. These are further divided into 10 areas of competence as listed in Figure 2-1. The complete Medical Assistant Role Delineation Chart illustrating all skills (standard and advanced) within each area of competence is shown in detail in Appendix A. These competencies are deemed necessary by the AAMA for the entry-level practice of medical assisting. Mastery of the competencies will prepare you to successfully complete national certification examinations administered by the AAMA or AMT and acquire credentials as evidence of your qualifications. (This is more fully discussed in Chapter 2, Unit 3.)

Accrediting Organizations

An organization that governs programs of educational preparation of medical assistants is the Commission on Accreditation of Allied Health Education Programs (CAAHEP), an autonomous accrediting body sanctioned by the Council for Higher Education Accreditation

(CHEA). CHEA is a private, nonprofit national organization that coordinates accreditation activity in the United States. General educational requirements cover the program length, the facility, the administration and faculty, library access, finances, and other areas of operation. In addition, specific criteria are established in cooperation with the AAMA regarding the preparation of medical assistants. The curriculum must cover content in nine specific areas, including an externship with a minimum 160 contact hours of practical experience. Educational programs desiring to acquire this accreditation standard participate in an on-site review process that measures their compliance to the established standards.

Another accrediting agency of medical assistant programs is the Accrediting Bureau of Health Education Schools (ABHES). Medical assisting programs accredited by ABHES comply with program standards, course requirements, facility requirements, and other areas of operation. The curriculum must cover content in 11 areas and must include an externship of a minimum of 160 contact hours. Programs who wish to be accredited by ABHES participate in accreditation workshops, as well as internal and on-site review processes.

Graduates from programs certified by CAAHEP and/or ABHES are eligible to sit for national exams to become credentialed or registered medical assistants. Credentialing agencies include the American Association of Medical Assistants (AAMA) and the American Medical Technologists (AMT). Refer to Chapter 2, Unit 3, for more information.

In 2005, there were more than 520 programs accredited by CAAHEP. Additionally, ABHES accredited more than 107 programs institutionally and 55 programmatically.

JOB RESPONSIBILITIES

The role of the medical assistant is to provide skillful execution of administrative, clinical, and general duties as an integral and supportive part of the physician's practice. Performing clinical skills is an extension of the physician's role of assessment, examination, diagnosis, and treatment. Performing administrative skills helps manage the business affairs of the practice. The performance of general skills is concerned with legal, ethical, moral, and professional conduct in the execution of your duties. Table 2-3 lists examples of the variety of skills to be acquired in administrative, clinical, and general areas.

Many other tasks are performed regularly. A particularly important one is patient education. It is a task that requires special attention to the patient's response to ensure there will be **compliance** with the instruction. The assistant must carefully explain and/or demonstrate the procedure or activity and follow up with questioning to confirm understanding. The assistant

TABLE 2-3 Medical Assistant Skills in Administrative, Clinical, and General Areas	
Administrative	Schedule appointments
	Prepare correspondence
	Handle telephone calls
	Complete insurance forms
	Obtain initial patient data
Clinical	Take medical histories
	Take vital signs
	Assist with medical procedures
	Prepare patients for examinations
	Prepare medications
General	Demonstrate initiative and responsibility
	Treat all patients with compassion and empathy
	Use medical terminology appropriately
	Teach methods of health promotion
	Work as a team member
	Maintain confidentiality
	Document accurately
	Follow federal, state, and local legal guidelines

should not assume something has been learned until the patient can explain or perform it.

It is also important for medical assistants to have a basic understanding of the anatomy and physiology of the human body. This knowledge helps in the comprehension of the need for diagnostic and treatment procedures ordered by the physician. A working knowledge of medical terminology is also essential to communicate with other health care professionals and to assist patients in understanding information or instructions given to them.

Other major responsibilities of a medical assistant are the legal, moral, and ethical issues confronted on a daily basis. The medical assistant must be constantly aware of these concerns in order to respect the values of others and to eliminate the chance for personal or employer liability. This subject matter is more fully discussed in Chapter 3. To get an overview of all the tasks a medical assistant will be expected to perform, look through the "Procedures" list in the front pages of this book (page 11). Job responsibility, however, goes beyond just the execution of procedures; it includes a personal commitment to assist the physician in every way possible in order to provide total quality patient care.

EMPLOYMENT OPPORTUNITIES

The practice of medicine has changed dramatically. Today, medical assistants work in physicians' offices, clinics, hospitals, and other facilities, performing both administrative and clinical duties, under the supervision of the physician. The efficient medical practice requires much attention to detail to provide the best care possible to patients. It is essential to keep thorough records. The need for a **receptionist**, **secretary**, **bookkeeper**, and technician, in addition to a medical assistant or nurse, may be required. Some small individual practices may still be able to operate with only one support person, who will handle all the administrative, clinical, and operational duties alone.

Some physicians like to manage their office operations themselves, but most prefer to concentrate on patient care and give office management responsibilities to a professional member of their staff. This person can discuss fees, arrange collection of accounts, order supplies, perform banking activities, schedule staff hours, pay office expenses, and do many other operational duties. Medical assistants who have office experience and administrative ability are often given the responsibility of performing the duties of the office manager.

Medical assistants who specialize in certain fields may have other responsibilities. A podiatry assistant may make castings of feet, take x-rays, and assist in surgery. Ophthalmic assistants administer diagnostic tests, measure eye muscle function, explain proper care and use of safety glasses and eye shields, and demonstrate the care and insertion of contact lenses.

According to the latest statistics released by the Department of Labor Bureau, the health service industry employed 12.9 million individuals in 2002. Approximately 16% of all new wage and salary jobs created between 2002 and 2012 will be in health services, for a total of nearly 3.5 million new jobs. Medical assisting is projected to be the fastest growing occupation among the health service industry for this period, with an anticipated increase of 59%. In 2002, there were 330,000 employed medical assistants in various facilities.

Salaries vary depending upon experience, skill level, geographic location, and nationally recognized credentials. The median annual earnings reported in 2002 for medical assistants was $23,940. The following groups varied from this annual median as follows:

General medical and surgical hospitals	$24,460
Offices of physicians	$24,260
Outpatient care centers	$23,980
Other ambulatory health care services	$23,440
Offices of other health care practitioners	$21,620

CAREER LADDERING

You may be completely satisfied as a medical assistant and find great pleasure in your work. This is very admirable—you are providing a valuable service. But perhaps, after a period of time, you decide you would like to pursue another occupation for personal reasons, achievement needs, or financial gain. The term *career laddering* refers to other occupations in which you might be employed based upon your interest, training, and experience. The "ladder" can be lateral or vertical. In addition to the advancement to a medical office manager, there is hospital-based employment that medical assistants can fulfill. Examples of lateral jobs are unit secretaries, admissions clerks, medical records clerks, medical secretaries, phlebotomists, and ECG technicians.

Other job opportunities may be possible with some additional instruction, and you may already possess a portion of the skills. Patient care technician, a developing job category, is seen as an alternative position for a medical assistant. It is also hospital based and incorporates skills from medical, nursing, and medical laboratory assisting. The job tends to be defined by the employing facility, who also is currently providing the training. At this time, there are no recognized criteria or standards of practice.

The following brief descriptions of other health careers will provide you with some information about the type of employment, the training required, and an average salary amount. Each of these positions would require additional training but would also provide you with a personal challenge and reward your efforts. *Note:* Salary scales may vary widely according to geographic area.

Additional information is available from the web sites of state and federal governments, educational organizations, and professional associations. Refer to suggested web links at the end of this chapter.

Licensed Practical Nurses (LPNs)

Where Employed   LPNs work under the supervision of registered nurses and physicians. They work in hospitals, nursing homes, private home care, and physicians' offices and clinics. The growing elderly population will increase the need for LPNs in nursing homes, group homes, and residential care facilities (Figure 2-2).

Training   Training is usually a 1-year program of classroom and clinical practice. All LPNs must pass a state licensing examination to begin practice. Training is available at approved schools of practical nursing operated by vocational-technical schools and community colleges. A current **license** is required in order to work

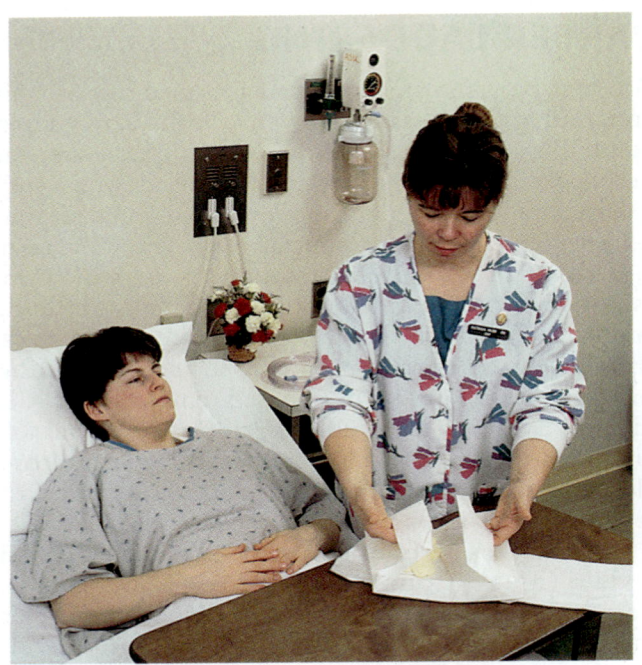

FIGURE 2-2   Licensed practical nurse

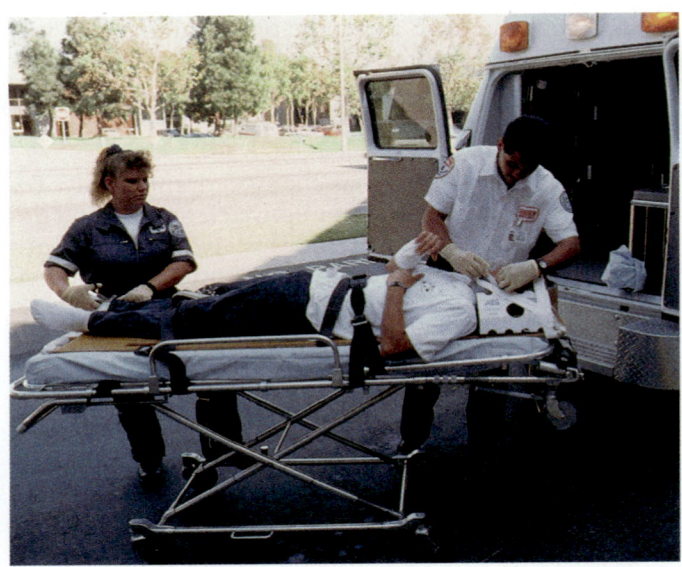

FIGURE 2-3   Emergency medical technicians

as an LPN. Renewal is subject to continuing education credits in most states.

Salary   Average annual salary is approximately $31,440 for a 40-hour week, excluding shift differentials.

Emergency Medical Technicians (EMTs)

Where Employed   EMTs work for private ambulance services or municipal fire, police, or rescue squads. EMTs provide immediate, on-site care in cases such as auto accidents, heart attacks, drownings, injuries, and shootings. EMTs transport patients to a medical facility (Figure 2-3). They work in teams under the direction of a dispatcher. There are three levels of practice: basic, advanced, and paramedic. The growing population and an increase in the total number of elderly people will increase the need. There is a high turnover rate for EMTs because of the stressful nature of the job.

Training   The basic training course is from 100 to 120 hours of classroom instruction plus 10 internship hours in a hospital emergency room. Training is provided by vocation-technical schools and community colleges in conjunction with hospitals, police, fire, and health departments. There are certification exams for each level that must be passed to work in that capacity.

Salary   Salaries vary according to the level of expertise and the employer. The average paramedic or EMT earns $24,030.

Recreational Therapists

Where Employed   Recreational **therapists** work in hospitals, **rehabilitation centers**, nursing homes, senior citizen facilities, and community recreational departments. They may assess a patient's condition by consulting medical records, the family, and the patient. A **therapeutic** program of individual or group activities can be developed by a recreational therapist and may contain sports, arts, crafts, music, or outings. With advances in medical technology, more people survive illness and trauma and require **rehabilitative therapy**. Again, the increased number of elderly individuals will require a larger amount of services.

Training   A bachelor's degree is the usual requirement, but an associate's degree program may be sufficient for some positions, such as a nursing home director of activities (Figure 2-4). Certification by the National Council for Therapeutic Recreation requires a bachelor's degree.

Salary   A recreational therapist earns approximately $30,540 annually. Nursing care facilities pay a median annual income of $25,010.

Respiratory Therapists

Where Employed   Respiratory therapists normally work 40 hours per week but may work irregular night and weekend hours. Almost all work is in either respiratory care, anesthesiology, or pulmonary care departments of a hospital. Some may be employed by medical rental companies, home health care providers,

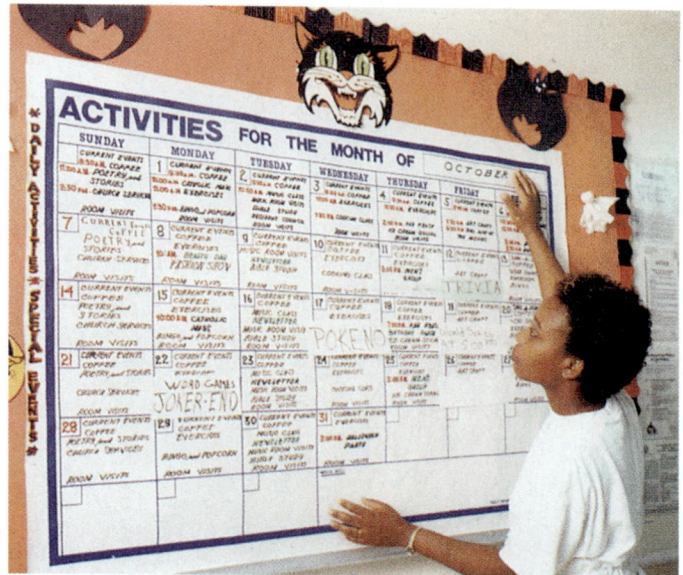

FIGURE 2-4   Recreational therapist/activity director

and nursing homes. The increasing elderly population and the rapid rise in the number of patients with acquired immune deficiency syndrome (AIDS) will increase the need for therapists.

Training   Most programs are 2 years in length. There are 4-year and advanced 2-year programs that are helpful for acquiring a supervisory position. In addition, there is a 1-year technician program that permits employment in some settings. Most employers require all levels to obtain the Certified Respiratory Therapist (CRT). An advanced level certification is a Registered Respiratory Therapist (RRT).

Salary   The respiratory therapist's average annual salary is approximately $40,220.

Dental Hygienists

Where Employed   Almost all dental **hygienists** work in private dental offices. Some may work in public health agencies, schools, hospitals, or clinics. They regularly work 40 hours per week but may often work part-time in more than one office. Dental hygienists provide preventive dental care by examining, cleaning, and taking x-rays of the teeth. They also remove sutures, teach oral hygiene, and provide restorative work. Population growth, higher incomes, and more elderly individuals with natural teeth will increase the demand for dental services.

Training   Training is obtained at accredited dental hygiene programs of 2 or 4 years in length. All hygienists must pass the American Dental Association's Na-

tional Dental Examination in order to be licensed in their state of practice.

Salary   The median hourly earnings are approximately $26.59, but this varies greatly in relation to the number of hours worked.

Nuclear Medicine Technologists

Where Employed   About 90% of nuclear medicine technologists work in hospitals, with the remaining 10% working in clinics and physicians' offices. Hospital employees usually work irregular hours and on-call rotations. Technologists locate and track **radioactive agents** that have been introduced into a patient's body as part of a diagnostic examination. The radioactive material, absorbed by a specific organ, produces images that are recorded on the photographic film of high-tech cameras. Technologic advances will increase nuclear medicine practice and the number of procedures, therefore requiring more technicians.

Training   There are different levels of training, varying from 1 to 4 years in length, that permit performance of various functions. **Ultrasound** and radiologic **technologists** complete 1-year certificate programs (Figure 2-5). Advanced practice in nuclear medicine technology requires a 2-year certificate or associate's degree. Many states require licensure. Federal standards covering administration and operation of radiation detection equipment must be met.

Salary   The average technologist salary for a 40-hour week, excluding shift differentials, is approximately $48,750 annually.

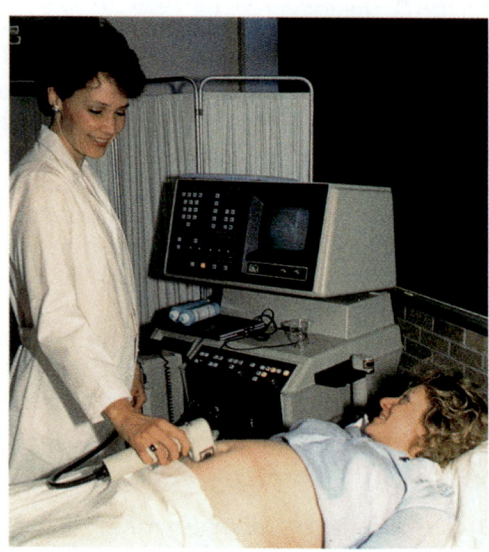

FIGURE 2-5   Registered diagnostic medical sonographer performing fetal ultrasound examination

Physician Assistants (PAs)

Where Employed PAs are employed primarily in physicians' offices and clinics and work about 40 hours per week. Some hospitals employ PAs in their emergency department, on two 24-hour or three 12-hour shifts per week. Approximately 30% work in smaller communities where physicians are scarce. Depending on the state where they are licensed, PAs can treat injuries, suture wounds, apply splints and casts, examine patients, order and interpret lab and x-ray procedures, make diagnoses, treat, and prescribe most medications.

Training The average PA program is 2 years in length and is offered by medical schools, vocational-technical schools, and 4-year colleges. Graduates from accredited programs who become certified by an examination can use the letters PA-C following their name. Almost all states require certification. Recertification every 6 years, plus 100 hours of continuing education every 2 years, is required to maintain the certificate.

Salary The average annual salary is approximately $64,670, with surgeons paying a slightly higher wage.

Pharmacy Technicians

Where Employed Pharmacy technicians work in pharmacies in hospitals, grocery stores, and retail pharmacies. Opportunities also exist with pharmaceutical firms and wholesale pharmaceutical distributors. Duties include the preparation of prescriptions under the direct supervision of the pharmacist (Figure 2-6). Pharmacy technicians may also work in the retail side of the business. In some hospitals, pharmacy technicians dispense routine medications to patients under the supervision of registered nurses (RNs).

Training The length of preparation varies and can occur during on-the-job training or by completing a certificate program or a 2-year associate's degree college program. A National Pharmacy Technician Certification Examination is available through the Pharmacy Technician Certification Board. It offers the title of certified pharmacy technician (CPhT).

Salary The average pharmacy technician salary is $22,256 per year for a 40-hour week, but the job may require hours outside the regular 8-to-5 time frame.

Occupational Therapy Assistants

Where Employed Employment is under the supervision of a registered occupational therapist. Hospitals, rehabilitation facilities, retirement homes,

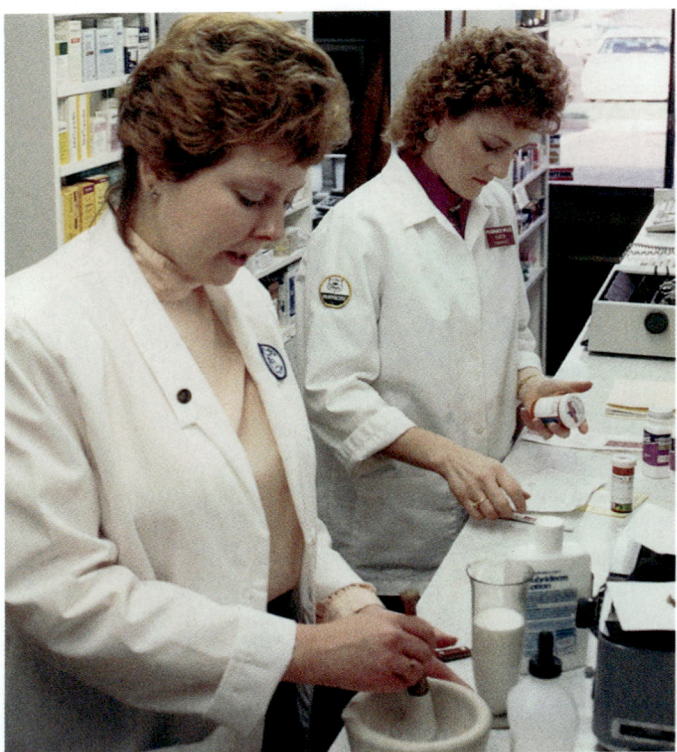

FIGURE 2-6 Pharmacy technicians prepare medications to be dispensed by pharmacists *(Courtesy of the Michigan Pharmacists Association and the Michigan Society of Pharmacy Technicians)*

psychiatric institutions, and nursing homes employ occupational therapy assistants (OTAs). Their duties involve helping individuals with mental or physical disabilities to learn or regain their highest level of functioning. This is achieved through activities that teach fine motor skills, day-to-day life skills, and the arts. OTAs prepare activity materials; maintain supplies, equipment, and tools; and document an individual's progress.

Training OTAs must obtain an associate's degree and pass a national certification examination.

Salary The average OTA working a 40-hour week earns $36,660 annually.

Obviously, there is much opportunity within the health care field. Regardless of whether you remain a medical assistant or choose to practice in another field, you must be prepared to continue with life-long learning to maintain competency in your area of practice. At the present time, it appears that your efforts will be rewarded with the security of employment opportunities in the future. You are fortunate—this is not true in many fields of work.

ACHIEVE UNIT OBJECTIVES

- Complete the Workbook activities to meet the learning objectives.
- Apply your knowledge at the end of this chapter in completing the Critical Thinking Challenge and Activities, as well as the StudyWARE on your Student CD-ROM.

UNIT 2
PERSONAL CHARACTERISTICS

OBJECTIVES

Upon completion of this unit, you will be able to achieve the following:

LEARNING Objectives

1. Spell and define, using the glossary at the back of the text, all the Words to Know in this unit.
2. List the 17 highly desired character traits of health care workers.
3. Identify five personality qualities desired.
4. Name the four voice characteristics desired.
5. Give two reasons why health care workers need to be concerned about their appearances.
6. List the nine things that contribute to a professional appearance.

WORDS TO KNOW

accurate	enthusiasm	perseverance
adapt	flexible	personality
appearance	honesty	posture
attitude	initiative	punctuality
confidential	innate	reliable
cooperate	intelligence	respectful
courteous	monotone	self-control
dependable	patience	tact
empathy	perceive	trait

CERTIFICATION CONNECTION

CMA
Professionalism
- Displaying professional attitude
- Working as a team member to achieve goals

RMA
Interpersonal relationships

CMAS
Professionalism

HIGHLY DESIRABLE CHARACTERISTICS OF HEALTH CARE WORKERS

There are many personal character **traits** that are highly desirable for health care workers. Some characteristics seem to be almost **innate**, while others must be learned. All traits can be enhanced by consciously making an effort to improve them. Your ability to work well with your employer, supervisors, and coworkers and your effectiveness in dealing with patients is greatly influenced by your personal characteristics.

First, let us examine some character traits as they relate to the manner in which job responsibilities are performed. As you read and consider the content, try to *honestly* examine your own character traits. Then we'll look at a few **personality** qualities and consider the messages they send when there is either verbal or nonverbal interaction with others.

Character Traits

For each of the following character traits, rate yourself on a scale of 1, 2, or 3: 1 = not usually, 2 = usually, and 3 = always. Can you score at least 30?

Accurate (detailed correctness, exactness). Performing procedures in the correct manner is extremely important. Findings may be inaccurate or the process unsafe if you are careless. The **accurate** recording of patients' remarks and findings from vital signs or other assessments is critical, as is the preparation of medications and injections. Thus, you must always be conscious of accuracy (Figure 2-7).

Adaptable (the ability to adjust, to make fit). In employment, it will often be necessary to **adapt** to a change in a situation to benefit the operation of the office, such as changing your schedule to work for someone or performing duties not usually your responsibility. Your willingness to be **flexible** and to "**cooperate** will be noticed by your employer or supervisor and, in the future,

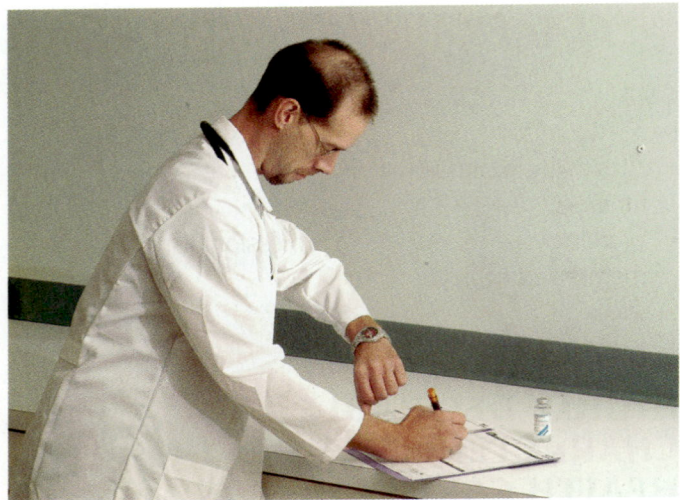

FIGURE 2-7 Accuracy is crucial when recording information.

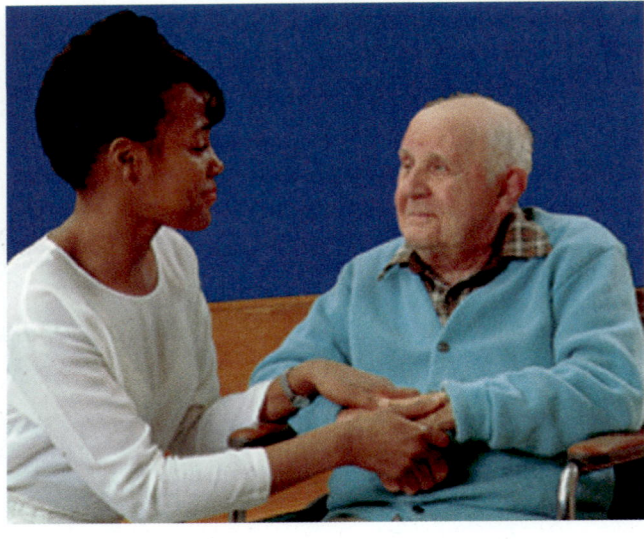

FIGURE 2-8 Have empathy for others.

if you should need someone to adapt to your situation, that individual will be more willing to work it out with you.

Conservative (to be cautious, prudent, to handle with care, not wasteful). You will be handling equipment, materials, and supplies daily. It is important that you conserve office equipment usefulness and not carelessly waste products. Treat the things in the office as if they were your own. Waste is lost profit.

Courteous (to be polite, well-mannered). You will be a representative of your employer and are expected to be **courteous** to coworkers, patients, and office visitors. This will not always be easy. It is never easy to be nice to someone who has been making it difficult for you. But, be courteous despite difficulties, and you will know you acted properly—it might even change the situation for the better.

Dependable (can be relied upon, responsible). Can people depend on you to carry out your responsibilities without the need of constant supervision? When you agree to do something, do you always follow through? If you are **dependable**, you are at work, organized, and ready to start the day when the first patient arrives. When you are dependable, the physician and the office staff know you are reliable and can direct their attention to other matters.

Confidential (prudent, cautious—especially in speech). You must use good judgment in any discussion regarding a patient. You have access to **confidential** information that is not for discussion outside the office. The only exception is when there is a need to share information with other health professionals to whom you are making a referral for therapy or treatment. Always observe confidentiality—never give out information about a patient over the phone or in writing without the patient's written permission. Even the completion of the patient's insurance claims requires the patient's authorization.

Empathetic (trying to identify one's feelings with those of another). Empathy is not the same as sympathy. Most patients do not want you to feel sorry for them; they just want you to try to understand how they feel. **Empathy** is the ability to put yourself in another person's place. Imagine you are wheelchair-bound with a condition that requires you to depend upon others for all your needs (Figure 2-8). Everyone feeling sorry for you will not be of any benefit, but if everyone could see the situation from your viewpoint, they would realize that you just need physical assistance and their support.

Enthusiastic (zeal, intense interest). **Enthusiasm** shows in your facial expressions and the general manner in which you carry out your responsibilities. Your **posture**, voice, and mannerisms should all indicate that you like what you are doing. You usually will look your best and do your best when you are enthusiastic, and people will enjoy being around you. Enthusiasm must be genuine, however, or it becomes an effort for you and it won't convince anyone else.

Honest (trustworthy, the quality of being truthful). You know the saying "Honesty is the best policy." In health care this is extremely important. You cannot lie about something you did or did not do for a patient, because you are dealing with a living human being. You cannot use correction fluid to correct a mistake, but you can admit to the mistake so that it can be amended or counteracted. **Honesty** also refers to being trustworthy. You will have access to office equipment and supplies, coworkers' personal belongings, and perhaps money; you *must* be trustworthy. No business can tolerate or afford a thief or a liar.

Initiative (ambition, hustle, setting something in motion). A person with **initiative** is a self-starter and a valuable member of a health care team. This member recognizes work to be done—even though it may not be an assigned job—and will either do the work or offer assistance. A self-starter does not have to be told or reminded of routine tasks. A person with initiative will also volunteer to take on a task or project to learn something new.

Patient (calmness in waiting, tolerant). It is very hard to be "patient" with a patient when you have many tasks to do. The elderly, especially, require **patience** because they are often slow to move and need assistance. If they are also lonely, they may take advantage of having someone to talk to. You are sure to have a "chronic complainer" who goes on and on about symptoms or the need for treatment until it begins to bother you. In your haste to stay on schedule and keep ahead of the physician, you will have to learn how to *politely* explain to patients that another person or duty needs your attention now and you must move on. The physician cannot afford for you to be impolite or impatient.

Perseverance (persistent, continued, or prolonged effort). **Perseverance** means to stick with a task until it is completed. Posting financial information, completing insurance forms, or filing may be postponed at times until it becomes a real task to accomplish and requires self-discipline to persevere until it is done. You may also need this quality when having difficulty getting a piece of equipment to function properly or when performing a certain procedure. In this manner, perseverance and patience go hand in hand.

Punctual (in exact agreement with appointed time). You are expected to be at work and on time every day. **Punctuality** is a part of being dependable. When you arrive at the established time and are ready to assume your responsibilities, the entire office will operate more smoothly. In contrast, when you are late, it often seems that you never get "caught up," and your whole day goes poorly. This is a trait you definitely can acquire with self-discipline.

Reliable (trustworthy, dependable, responsible). This trait is similar to being dependable. If you are **reliable**, the physician knows you can be expected to perform in the same consistent manner as you have in the past. In both your personal and professional life, you know how important it is to have someone who is reliable and who will always be there should you have the need.

Respectful (showing regard for, considerate, courteous). Being friends with everyone with whom you work will probably not happen. You will have differences of opinion at work and at home about how people act or what they say. You don't have to agree with them, but realize they have a right to their actions and respect that right. Even if you do not care for someone personally, it is important to be courteous and **respectful**. That is the mark of a mature, civil person. There will be patients with whom you'll have difficulty, but you must always be tolerant and considerate. The trait of being respectful is necessary for good human relations.

Self-Control (show restraint, in check). Being in control of your actions is very important. There will be times when you may be tempted to blurt out remarks or display some negative action, but it is not appropriate in the workplace. **Self-control** is also very important when there is something trying that has to be done. Then, you must concentrate even harder on not losing your composure. Losing self-control usually makes matters worse, because then you must apologize for your actions. Lack of self-control could also result in the termination of your employment.

Tact (delicate skill in saying or doing the right thing). **Tact** is a trait that may not be easy to acquire. Often, we respond to actions and statements *before* we think. Tact is being able to perceive a situation and knowing the right thing to say or do when dealing with people in a difficult situation. Tact is especially difficult and important when dealing with ill people. You must be very careful about what you say when responding to their questions.

This is the end of the discussion of highly desirable character traits. How do you rate?

PERSONALITY QUALITIES

In addition to the character traits discussed, there are other personality qualities that affect the way character traits are **perceived** by others. An individual could show initiative, dependability, honesty, and other traits, but if they are not likeable, they will not get along well with their coworkers. These qualities might be more difficult to acquire since they seem to be connected to one's personality. *New World Concise Webster's Dictionary,* 10th edition, defines personality as "existence as a person; the assemblage of qualities, physical, mental, and moral, that set one apart from others." Let's look at some of these qualities that we like in people.

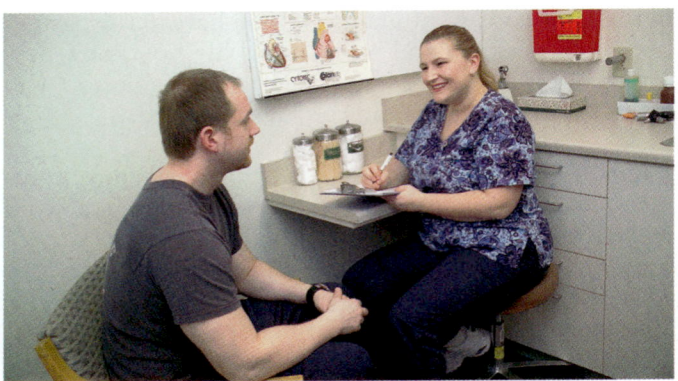

FIGURE 2-9   Maintain a friendly, professional relationship with patients.

Friendly Attitude and Genuine Liking of People

(real, concerned, caring viewpoint): A friendly **attitude** will be recognized by the persons you deal with in the office. You should know and use the names of your patients while carrying on conversations with them. Be friendly, but at the same time maintain a professional relationship (Figure 2-9). You can show a true concern for their welfare without becoming personally involved. For example, if an elderly person needs assistance but has no family support, you cannot take this on personally but you can contact community resources to arrange for the assistance. Good interpersonal relations require dealing with people so that your self-image and theirs remain positive and intact. Courtesy is never out of style. A simple "please" and "thank you" is appropriate with all ages.

Intelligence

(ability to apply the mind effectively to any situation, clear thinking plus good judgment): **Intelligence** is not just a high IQ or a college degree, for neither of these is of value if the owner can't appropriately apply knowledge to life situations. You can acquire knowledge from study and experience. There is no end to what you can learn; that information, effectively applied, is intelligence. Everything you learn affects you and, in turn, the people with whom you interact. Use every opportunity to expand your knowledge—not only of health care, but also of the world of information that is available (Figure 2-10). You will find that a willingness to learn advances your professional status. You will also find that your professional skills will improve with experience and new technology. Your knowledge can be expanded by observing, reading, and attending seminars. Physicians will often sponsor your attendance at workshops and educational seminars if you show an interest in learning.

Another good source of information is the Internet. Once you learn to "surf the net" you can bring up information on almost any topic. You should, however, be cautious of any information you read or download. There are no standards by which web sites are held or

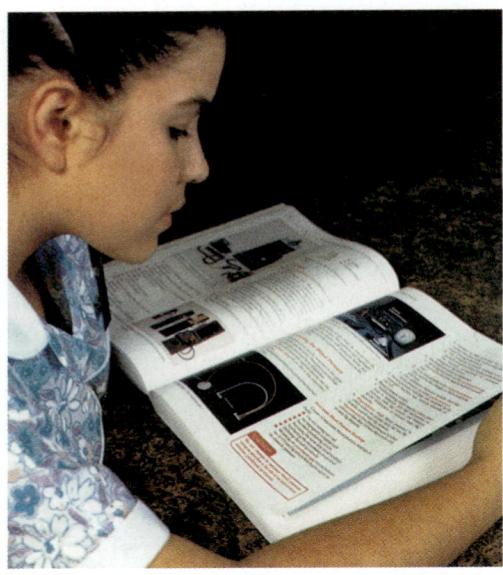

FIGURE 2-10   Do not let opportunities to learn pass you by.

judged, and the person providing the information may be without qualifications. Remember also that any research, wonderful discovery, or cure may not be worth the time it takes to read it. Be very cautious. Consider the source of the information. If it is from a known educational institution, the national or state government, or a recognized organization, it is probably reliable.

Pleasant Personality

(cheerful, agreeable personal qualities): A pleasant personality is tremendously important because of the continuous stream of persons with whom you will come into contact. Because of their illnesses, the situation will not always be the best, but if your contact with them is cheerful and pleasant, it will make their time in your office a little easier to bear. Your interaction with the physician and other team members will be much more enjoyable if you are pleasant. No one enjoys being around someone who is always complaining or is negative about everything. It has been said that success is 90% personality. Impressions about people are, at least initially, formed from the way we perceive their personality. A chance at success may not occur if the perception is negative.

Pleasant Voice

(pleasing to hear): A voice has four characteristics: pitch, force, quality, and rate. The pitch of your voice refers to its highness or lowness. If you have a medium pitch, you are fortunate because it is considered the most pleasing to hear. If you are told your voice sounds high, consider exercises to lower its pitch. Record your voice and listen to it. You can also determine your pitch by using a piano. Sing "ah" to find the lowest note you can sing, then sing up the scale four whole notes. This will be your best speaking voice pitch. If you currently speak above it, practice reading aloud at the new note pitch. This will also allow you to develop variety in the range of your pitch. Without variation, your speech will be **monotone**, which is unpleasant to hear. The force of your voice makes it possible for you to be heard. You generally need little force in office communications; in fact, you must guard against being overheard by patients. If you do find it necessary to increase the intensity of your voice, be careful it does not become irritating. The quality of your voice is reflected in the manner in which you pronounce vowels. Relaxation exercises will improve vocal quality. A good exercise for the jaw muscles is a yawn. The rate of your speech is determined by how long you hold sounds and by the pauses between words and phrases. Most of us speak too rapidly. Communication requires understanding, and it is extremely hard to understand someone who runs their words together and does not enunciate clearly. Again, you can improve your rate of speech by listening to your recorded voice as you read aloud. With practice, you can adjust your rate and improve your communication skills. Practice is also needed to eliminate using "uh," "er," and "you know" when you speak. A simple pause, while you think of what to say, is much more pleasant for the listener.

Genuine Smile   (real expression): A genuine smile is a welcome sight to patients and visitors entering a physician's office. It conveys that you acknowledge them and are interested in being of service. You may be surprised by how many smiles you receive in return. Besides, it's hard to be unpleasant with someone who is smiling at you.

Positive Attitude   Your attitude shows everyone who sees you or speaks to you, by telephone or in person, how you feel about your work, others, and yourself. You display your attitude in the way you get along with others and interact with them. The importance of a positive attitude cannot be overemphasized. The many hassles and conflicts that arise with patients and colleagues during everyday activity in the busy medical office can be handled much more effectively if you possess and project a positive attitude. Having a good outlook on life carries over into every area and promotes well-being.

PERCEPTION AS A PROFESSIONAL

There are two other observations about you that speak very loudly, yet do not require a word to be spoken. Since you are a health care worker and consider yourself to be a professional, you are expected to "look the part."

Good Health   (state of wellness): The patients and visitors coming into a physician's office gain the first impression of the practice from the medical assistant or receptionist who greets them. A neat, attractive person has a good psychological effect on everyone. To look your best, you must be in good health. This re-

quires a routine of rest, well-balanced meals, exercise, and recreation. As a health care professional, you are perceived as an example. What message are you sending? If you need medical attention, you should see your personal physician without delay. No patient wants to receive medical attention from someone who appears unhealthy. Patients may resent, and rightly so, any exposure to illness. Many people are in a rather fragile state of health. They come to the physician to get assistance with their own illness or injury; they do not need to be exposed to additional problems.

Personal Appearance   (individual image, a look, visible): Your **appearance** says volumes about you. Neat, well-groomed professionals look self-confident, display pride in themselves, and give an impression of being capable of performing whatever duties need to be done (Figure 2-11). Not only does the patient feel the provider is competent, but the provider also feels good. We have all experienced days when we didn't feel good about the way we looked that, in turn, affected our performance. In order to present yourself in the best possible light, you must adhere to some general guidelines for a professional appearance:

1. *Cleanliness* is the first essential for good grooming. Take a daily bath or shower. Use a deodorant or antiperspirant. Shampoo your hair often. Brush and floss your teeth daily.

2. *Hand care* is critical. Take special care of your hands. Keep hand cream or lotion in convenient places to use after washing your hands. Because this is done frequently, hands tend to chap and crack, which can allow organisms entry into your body—a risk

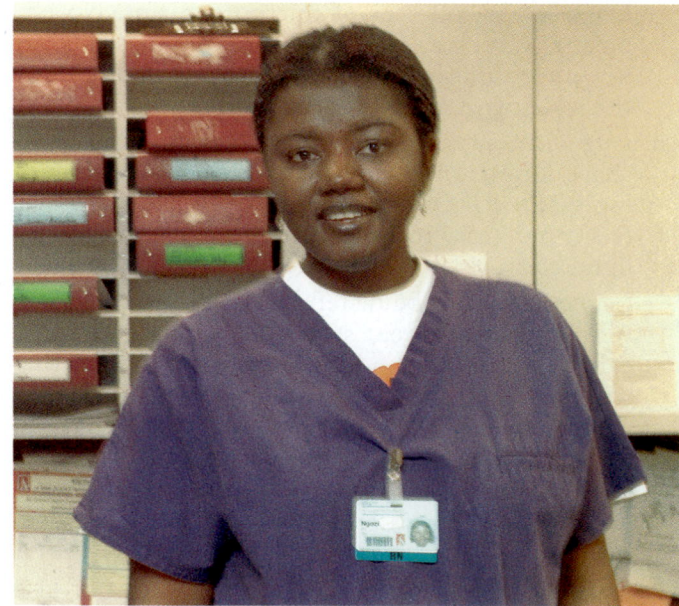

FIGURE 2-11   Present a professional appearance.

you cannot afford. Also, keep your fingernails manicured at a moderate length. If you work in a uniform and want to use nail polish, choose clear or light shades. Even in street clothes, bright or trendy colors are not appropriate for the office.

3. *Hair* must be clean and away from your face. Long hair should be worn up or at least fastened back. It is not a good idea to have to keep pushing your hair out of the way while working with patients. You only add their organisms to your environment, and perhaps take them home with you. Patients may also be susceptible to "receiving" something from your hair if you touch them after arranging your hair.

4. *Proper attire* may vary with medical specialty. For instance, many pediatric practices prefer that medical assistants wear colorful prints with patterns of cartoon characters that children will recognize to help them feel more at ease. Psychiatry and psychology medical office assistants may not be required to wear uniforms, as their clinical duties would be limited. Looking like a professional will not only encourage the respect of others for your profession, but it will help you to feel an integral part of the health care team. When uniforms are required, they must be clean, fit well, and be free from wrinkles. Uniform shoes should be kept clean and have clean shoestrings; hose must not have runs. Pay attention to the undergarments that you wear beneath the uniform so that they do not show through the fabric of your uniform.

5. *Jewelry,* except for a watch or wedding ring, is not appropriate with a uniform. Small earrings may be worn but still may get in the way when you use the telephone. Not only does jewelry look out of place, it is a great collector of microorganisms. Novelty piercings, such as nose rings and tongue studs, are not appropriate for professional grooming. Save the wearing of these for after work hours.

6. *Fragrances,* such as perfumes, colognes, and aftershave lotions, may be offensive to some patients, especially if they are suffering from nausea. If you feel it necessary to wear something, use one with a light, clean-smelling fragrance.

7. *Cosmetics* should be tasteful and skillfully applied. All major department stores have salespeople who can help you select and learn to apply products that will enhance your appearance.

8. *Gum* chewing is very unprofessional. A large piece of gum interferes with speech, and cracking gum is totally unacceptable. If you feel you need gum for a breath concern, use a breath mint or mouthwash instead.

9. *Posture* affects not only your appearance but also the amount of fatigue you experience. The ease at which you move around reflects your poise and confidence. To check your posture, back up to a wall, place your feet apart (straight down from your hips), and try to insert your hand through the space between your lower back and the wall. If you can, you need to improve your posture. Pull your stomach in, tuck under your buttocks, and try to place your spine against the wall. Your shoulders should be relaxed with your head held erect. This will probably feel very unnatural, but practice keeping your body straight and head erect when you walk and you will see how much better you look and feel.

Remember that your personal hygiene must be impeccable, because setting a good example for others is a part of your responsibility in the care of others. Although it seems redundant, daily showering, clean attractive hair, and neatly manicured nails show others that you take pride in yourself and give them a model by which to pattern themselves.

A lot of different elements make up our personal characteristics and have a definite effect upon how we feel about ourselves and how others perceive us. This discussion should help you to evaluate yourself and help identify things you can do to improve your effectiveness when interacting with people.

ACHIEVE UNIT OBJECTIVES

- ☐ Complete the Workbook activities to meet the learning objectives.
- ☐ Apply your knowledge at the end of this chapter in completing the Critical Thinking Challenge and Activities, as well as the StudyWARE on your Student CD-ROM.

UNIT 3
PROFESSIONALISM

OBJECTIVES

Upon completion of this unit, you will be able to achieve the following:

LEARNING Objectives

1. Spell and define, using the glossary in the back of this text, all the Words to Know in this unit.
2. Describe the origin of the medical assistant profession.

3. **Describe the history and purpose of the AAMA and the AMT.**

4. **Explain the definition of medical assisting according to the AAMA and the AMT.**

5. **Describe and discuss the original and current AAMA logos.**

6. **Describe the three levels of membership with the AAMA and the value of each level.**

7. **Define and discuss the meaning of professionalism.**

8. **Explain the *Standards of Practice* set by the AMT.**

9. **Explain the purpose of continuing education and how to acquire it.**

10. **Identify the qualifications for and methods of acquiring medical assistant certification from the AAMA and AMT.**

11. **Describe methods for revalidation of medical assistant certification from the AAMA and AMT.**

12. **Explain advantages of membership in one or more of the professional organizations contained in this unit.**

13. **List additional purposes of the AAMA and the AMT besides membership.**

WORDS TO KNOW

accredited	competent	pro tem
barter	professionalism	revalidation
certification		

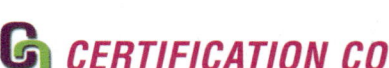

CERTIFICATION CONNECTION

CMA
Professionalism

CMAS
Professionalism

RMA
Professionalism

HOW MEDICAL ASSISTING BEGAN

In Chapter 1, you learned about the many pioneers in this field. These leaders in the practice of medicine obviously had the best interest of their patients in mind as they treated them as efficiently as they could with what little was available. The sick went to be treated without an appointment and they waited as long as necessary to be seen by the physician. Payment for medical care was a **barter**-type, often with food or whatever the patient or the family had of value. If one had no means of payment, the doctor treated the person anyway. No medical records were kept because they were not even thought to be necessary in those days. Because the physician was considered to be a valuable close family friend whose knowledge and life-saving skills were well respected by the entire community, it was very rare for a lawsuit to be filed against the physician.

Since those days, the practice of medicine has changed dramatically. Accurate and comprehensive records are vital in the managed care of patients. Documentation of every transaction between physician and patient is a must. The efficiently run medical practice requires absolute attention to every detail to protect the reputation of the physician and to make it possible to render the best care possible to the patient. Because medical school offers little or no background in managing the "business of medicine," the physician must entrust this responsibility to a competent individual. Even today, the common term "my office nurse" is often used by physicians in reference to a member of their office personnel. This can often be misleading, as there may in actuality be no nurses employed in the facility. Using this term casually is not a wise practice, because it is deceiving to the public. The art and skill of nursing is for the most part aimed toward the critically ill and those patients requiring bedside care. Obviously, in an ambulatory setting such as an office or clinic, and in some departments in medical centers and hospitals, medical assistants can be and are employed in a wide variety of positions. This person, who works under the supervision of the physician, performs a wide variety of administrative and clinical duties and is given the title of medical assistant. During the evolvement of the practice of medicine, physicians have realized the value of both administrative and clinical medical assistants to run their offices and assist in many other roles with appropriate instruction and evaluation. Unit 1 of this chapter discusses the many roles and responsibilities that await the medical assistant in the wealth of opportunities in the medical field.

HISTORY OF PROFESSIONAL ORGANIZATIONS

The American Association of Medical Assistants

In 1955, medical assistants from 15 states met in Kansas City, Kansas, and adopted the name American Association of Medical Assistants (AAMA). The representatives elected **pro tem** officers and made plans for

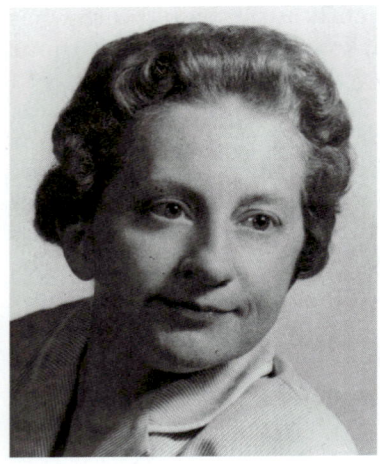

FIGURE 2-12 Maxine Williams, founder and first national president of the AAMA *(Courtesy of the American Association of Medical Assistants)*

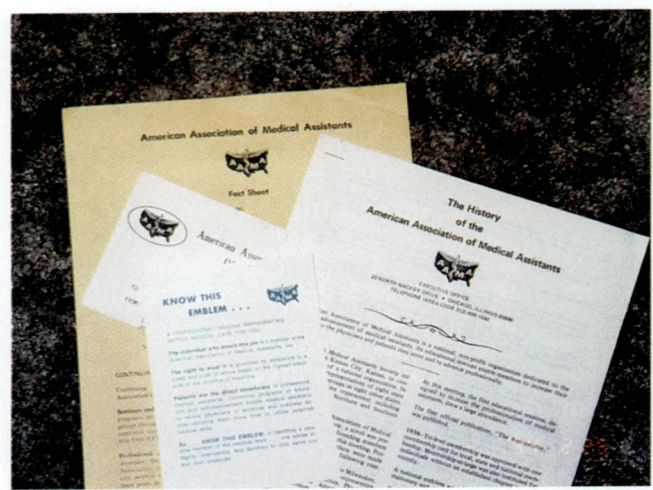

FIGURE 2-13 Original logo of the AAMA *(Courtesy of the American Association of Medical Assistants)*

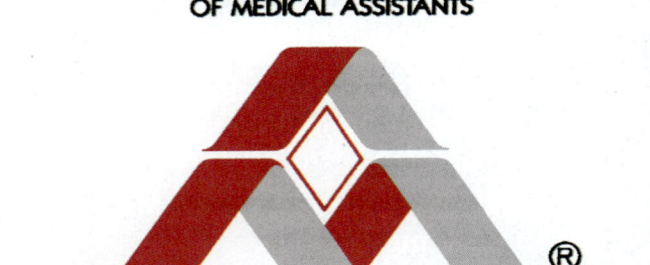

FIGURE 2-14 Logo of the AAMA *(Courtesy of the American Association of Medical Assistants)*

an organizational meeting to be held the following year. In October of 1956, physicians and advisors of the American Medical Association (AMA) met with 250 members of medical assistant societies from 16 states. At this meeting, the AAMA was officially founded with advice, assistance, and moral support from the AMA. The founder and first national president of the AMA was Maxine Williams (Figure 2-12). The primary purpose of the AAMA was to raise the standards of the medical assistant to a professional level. Physicians realized then, as they do now, that health care professionals were needed to assist them in a multitude of office duties for which nurses had not been trained. They also needed help in the physician-patient relationship. Another concern was that of instilling in young people a desire to carry the profession of medical assisting into the future. The *Maxine Williams Scholarship Fund* was established to award several $500 scholarships annually to students who were seriously interested in pursuing a career as a medical assistant. (*Note:* The scholarships are awarded on the basis of interest, need, and aptitude. Applications are available from the AAMA executive office. Applicants must have the completed form postmarked no later than May 1 of the year in which the scholarship will be used.)

In 1958, a national emblem was selected for use on AAMA stationery and official publications (Figure 2-13). The current logo for AAMA, introduced in 1978, is shown in Figure 2-14. The AMA received word from the United States Department of Health, Education, and Welfare that medical assisting had been formally recognized as an allied health profession and that its educational programs were eligible for federal funding by the Bureau of Health Manpower.

The AAMA Board of Trustees approved the current definition of medical assisting in February 1991: "Medical assisting is a multi-skilled allied health profession whose practitioners work primarily in ambulatory settings, such as medical offices or clinics. Medical assistants function as members of the health care delivery team and perform administrative and clinical procedures."

The American Academy of Professional Coders

The American Academy of Professional Coders (AAPC) was founded in 1988 to promote professionalism and encourage and support education, networking, and certification. Setting high ethical standards for its 22,000 members is a top priority. The AAPC offers training through their *Independent Study Program* and the *Professional Medical Coding Curriculum* and two distinct types of

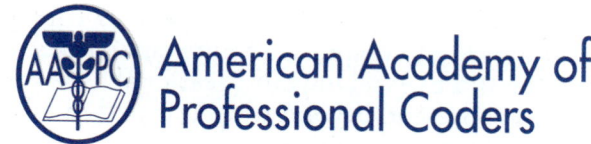

FIGURE 2-15 Logo of the AAPC (Courtesy of the American Academy of Professional Coders)

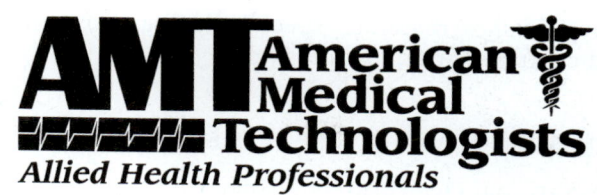

FIGURE 2-16 Logo of the American Medical Technologists (AMT) (Courtesy of the American Medical Technologists)

certification examinations. The Certified Professional Coder (CPC) is one who codes for professional services. The Certified Professional Coder-Hospital (CPC-H) is one who codes for the outpatient facility. *Specialty Proficiencies* provide further indication of a qualified professional in the coding field. In order to remain in good standing, credentialed members are required to submit continuing education units (CEUs) annually. The AAPC offers continuing education through its annual national conference, workshops, and the *AAPC Coding Edge,* the bimonthly news magazine that contains educational news for coding professionals. For further information, contact the AAPC at 800-626-2633 or at the web site www.aapc.com. The current logo for AAPC is shown in Figure 2-15.

American Medical Technologists

In 1976 the American Medical Technologists (AMT) association organized a nationally recognized body to address the needs of medical assistants and award the title of Registered Medical Assistant (RMA) following the successful completion of an Accrediting Bureau of Health Education School's (ABHES) accredited medical assisting program and after passing the national registry examination. Other criteria for registry through the AMT are that one must have graduated from a nonspecific accredited medical assistant program and have been employed full-time in the medical field for 1 year or part-time for 2 years. The current AMT logo is shown in Figure 2-16. The RMA must complete continuing education credits to stay current in the field.

A national board of directors is elected to conduct the business of the organization, such as educational programs, legal concerns, certification, and other national issues. The national board appoints state and local members to council positions. This leadership group works directly with the needs of the membership. Members receive a professional publication, *AMT Events,* which provides timely information regarding educational seminars, the annual meeting held in late June, test sites for certification, and home education programs. The AMT registers other health care professionals, including phlebotomists, medical lab assis-

tants, and medical lab technicians, which the medical assistant could become with additional study and training. Those who desire to become RMAs through the AMT must send the application form to the AMT Registry Office by the deadline date with the application fee, a copy of their high school diploma or GED certificate, a copy of the notarized cardiopulmonary resuscitation (CPR) current certification, and any other pertinent documentation. All information sent to this office must be in English.

Professional organizations for continuing education and membership are listed at the end of this chapter.

American Association for Medical Transcription (AAMT)

One who interprets and transcribes patient information from oral to printed form with the use of a typewriter or word processor is known as a medical transcriptionist. These professionals are medical language specialists who must possess excellent skills in the areas of listening, English grammar and punctuation, spelling, and transcription technology. Additionally, the medical transcriptionist must have a solid foundation in anatomy and physiology, disease processes, medical-legal and ethical areas, and professionalism.

The AAMT is the professional organization for the advancement of medical transcription and for the education and development of medical transcriptionists as medical language specialists. This organization was incorporated in 1978 in Modesto, California. The AAMT publishes a bimonthly journal to inform association leaders of important relevant information. State or regional component associations offer members delegate representation at the national convention, and local chapters offer educational opportunities. Voluntary certification by examination is offered by the AAMT. This certification is valid for 3 years. The certified medical transcriptionist must achieve 30 continuing education credits (CEU) in each 3-year cycle for recertification or successful reexamination. The AAMT offers a national convention, continuing education programs, workshops, and seminars for members. This organization also publishes materials specifically for those in the medical transcription profession.

National Healthcareer Association

The National Healthcareer Association (NHA) was established in 1989 as a certification agency. Today, the NHA provides products and services to health care professionals, including continuing education, program development, career and networking services, as well as 14 certification exams, including Certified Clinical Medical Assistant (CCMA) and Certified Medical Administrative Assistant (CMAA). More than 150,000 certifications have been issued to health care professionals since testing began. To qualify to sit for a certification exam, you must be a graduate of a health care training program, or have 1 or more years of full-time job experience. Exams are given in 950 locations, both online and in traditional paper-and-pencil testing format. For more information, visit the NHA's Web site, www.nhanow.com.

PROFESSIONALISM

On your journey of study to become a medical assistant you must also become aware of just what a professional is and what that means to you. "One who is trained and skilled in the methods of the profession" is the coined definition that can apply to *any* profession regarding technical and ethical standards of the particular skill area. In an article in the January/February 1987 issue of the AAMA's *Professional Medical Assistant (PMA)* magazine, Barbara Smith defined **professionalism** as "a state of mind. It is a particular blend of self-esteem, self-confidence, enjoyment of life, respect for the feelings of others, as well as specific knowledge and skills."

The AMT outlines the requirements of professionalism in the *Standards of Practice* (Figure 2-17). All AMT members, RMAs, and every member of the health care delivery team are urged to follow these standards.

True professionalism goes well beyond a mere definition. Standards of conduct are certainly a noble consideration, especially in the revered field of medicine. The physician and the field of medicine, in general, have always been highly respected and admired by society. And, rightfully so, those who seek the services of professionals in the health care field have expectations of being treated with respect and dignity. It takes a certain type of person to work with the sick and injured day in and day out. You have been introduced to the personal characteristics that health care professionals should possess. Those necessary attributes are used perpetually in patient care. It is all part of being a professional.

Professionalism is a complex issue. It is your personal standard of conduct, morality, and ethics. It is having the will to excel in your vocational aspirations and to go above and beyond what is expected of you. Professionalism is seen in those who aspire to become certified and **revalidate** when the time comes. The professional is one who seeks out the ways and means to grow personally as well as professionally and encourages others to do the same. The leaders of these organizations, the pacesetters of the AAMA and AMT, have paved the way of the professional medical assistant. You are learning a fine tradition of the example they set for the future of the profession of medical assisting and in the establishment of continuing education programs. You have a great opportunity because of the efforts of a few medical assistants who saw the vision of the profession and had the desire to do something about it. That is what professionalism is all about. They did something above and beyond their 9-to-5 job. The seeds they planted have taken root and have bloomed into a formally recognized profession.

AAMA AND AMT EXAMINATIONS

The AAMA and AMT are national certifying bodies for health professionals. The AAMA administers an exam for individuals to become credentialed as a certified medical assistant (CMA), and the AMT offers exams for individuals to become credentialed as a registered medical assistant (RMA) or certified medical administrative specialist (CMAS).

Credentialing is a way to distinguish yourself and show employers proficiency in entry-level medical assisting skills. In addition, the AAMA and AMT certification and recertification exams cover content on professionalism, including:

- Professional organization
- Accepting responsibility for actions
- Performing within ethical boundaries
- Code of ethics
- Patients' rights
- Current issues in bioethics
- Maintaining confidentiality
- Releasing patient information
- Intentional tort
- Invasion of privacy
- Slander and libel
- Promoting competent patient care
- Working as a team member to achieve goals
- Team member responsibility

Keeping these professional components in mind as you learn skills and procedures will help you toward your goal of becoming a concerned and **competent** medical assistant.

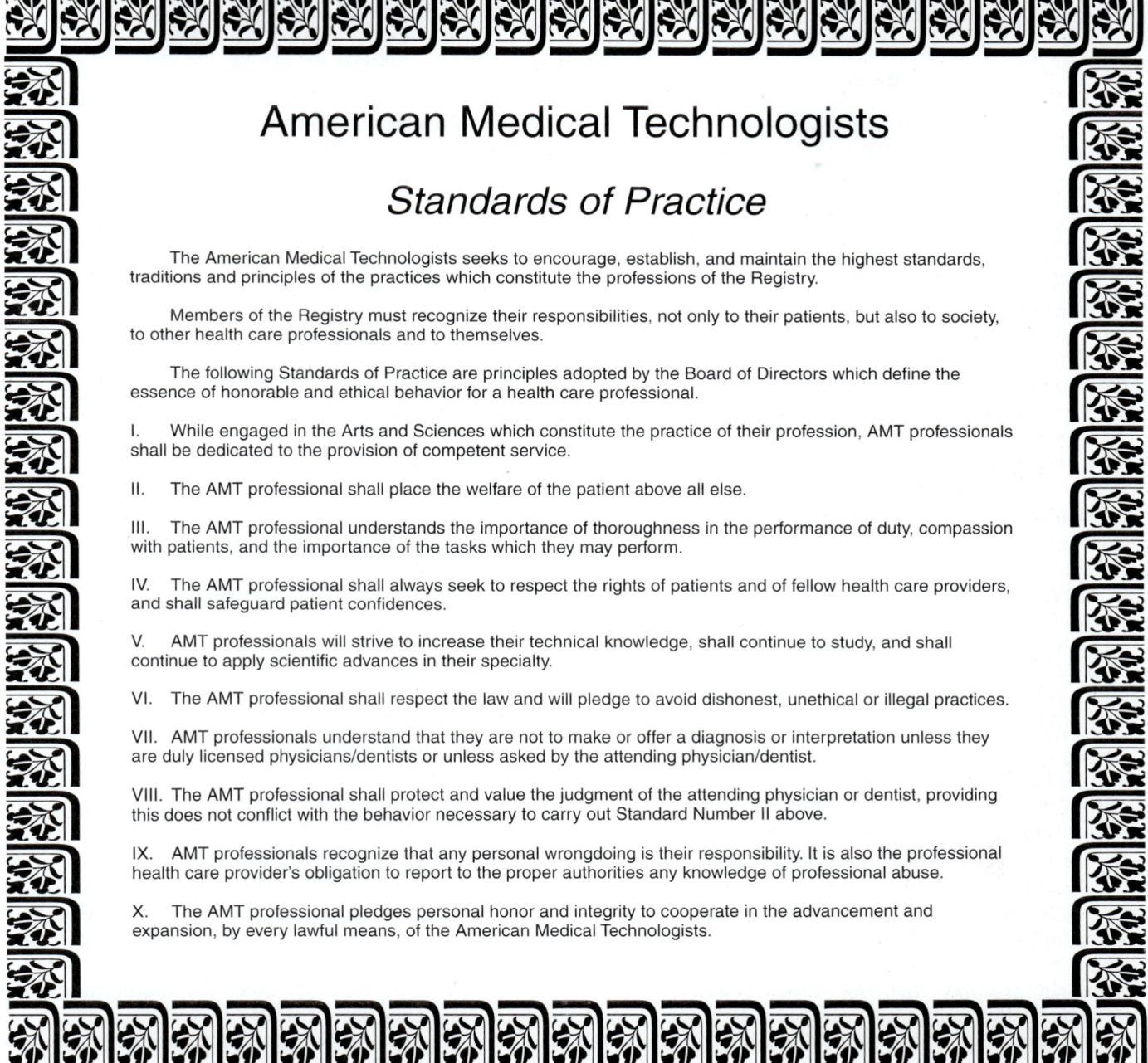

American Medical Technologists

Standards of Practice

The American Medical Technologists seeks to encourage, establish, and maintain the highest standards, traditions and principles of the practices which constitute the professions of the Registry.

Members of the Registry must recognize their responsibilities, not only to their patients, but also to society, to other health care professionals and to themselves.

The following Standards of Practice are principles adopted by the Board of Directors which define the essence of honorable and ethical behavior for a health care professional.

I.   While engaged in the Arts and Sciences which constitute the practice of their profession, AMT professionals shall be dedicated to the provision of competent service.

II.   The AMT professional shall place the welfare of the patient above all else.

III.   The AMT professional understands the importance of thoroughness in the performance of duty, compassion with patients, and the importance of the tasks which they may perform.

IV.   The AMT professional shall always seek to respect the rights of patients and of fellow health care providers, and shall safeguard patient confidences.

V.   AMT professionals will strive to increase their technical knowledge, shall continue to study, and shall continue to apply scientific advances in their specialty.

VI.   The AMT professional shall respect the law and will pledge to avoid dishonest, unethical or illegal practices.

VII.   AMT professionals understand that they are not to make or offer a diagnosis or interpretation unless they are duly licensed physicians/dentists or unless asked by the attending physician/dentist.

VIII. The AMT professional shall protect and value the judgment of the attending physician or dentist, providing this does not conflict with the behavior necessary to carry out Standard Number II above.

IX.   AMT professionals recognize that any personal wrongdoing is their responsibility. It is also the professional health care provider's obligation to report to the proper authorities any knowledge of professional abuse.

X.   The AMT professional pledges personal honor and integrity to cooperate in the advancement and expansion, by every lawful means, of the American Medical Technologists.

FIGURE 2-17   AMT *Standards of Practice (Courtesy of the American Medical Technologists)*

Becoming Certified

At the 1995 AAMA convention in San Antonio, Texas, the certification board voted that as of February 1, 1998, only those individuals who have successfully completed an accredited medical assistant program may sit for the national certification examination. The AAMA (**certification**) exam is designed to evaluate entry-level competency in medical assisting. Administrative and clinical skills, anatomy and physiology, human relations, medical terminology, professionalism, communication, and medical-legal issues are included in this exam. It is offered three times each year at over 100 test centers nationwide. The National Board of Medical Examiners serves as an educational test consultant and works with the AAMA in preparing the examination. To be eligible for the certification exam you must be a graduate of a CAAHEP (**accredited**) medical assistant program or a graduate of an ABHES-accredited program with 1 year of documented work experience.

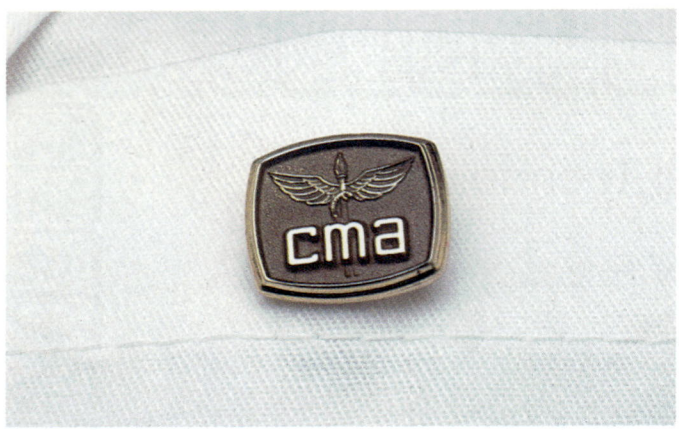

FIGURE 2-18   Certified medical assistant (CMA) pin *(Courtesy of the American Association of Medical Assistants)*

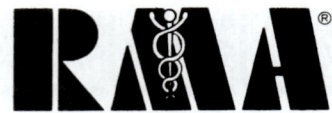

FIGURE 2-19   Logo of the Registered Medical Assistant (RMA), representing a credential awarded by the AMT *(Courtesy of the American Medical Technologists)*

As of 1998, certified medical assistants (CMAs) must recertify every 5 years to demonstrate current knowledge of administrative, clinical, and general medical information. A CMA remains current through December 31 of the fifth year following certification or recertification. Recertification reinforces the validity of the CMA credentials and helps maintain continued acceptance by physicians, patients, and other health care professionals. This requirement may be met in one of two ways:

1. By earning 60 recertification points through continuing education courses or academic or other formal credit that has relevancy to medical assisting, with the points distributed equally among the three areas covered in the examination.
2. By retaking the certification examination.

Those who sit for the exam and are successful in achieving a passing score are entitled to the CMA designation following their names. Figure 2-18 shows a photo of the official CMA pin from the AAMA. NOTE: There are also attractive pins sold in uniform shops around the country that say "medical assistant" or "certified medical assistant" as accessory items. Even though these pins inform the onlooker that one is a medical assistant, they are not authorized by the AAMA and do not reflect the wearer's credibility regarding AAMA certification.

Becoming Registered

The RMA exam is designed to evaluate the competence of the entry-level medical assistant (Figure 2-19). The format and questions on the exam are developed by the Education, Qualifications, and Standards Committee of the AMT and then approved by the AMT Board of Directors.

The RMA exam consists of 210 four-option multiple-choice questions in Administrative, Clinical, and General content areas.

General Medical Assisting Knowledge:
- Anatomy and physiology
- Medical terminology
- Medical law
- Medical ethics
- Human relations
- Patient education

Administrative Medical Assisting Knowledge:
- Insurance
- Financial bookkeeping
- Medical receptionist, secretarial, clerical

Clinical Medical Assisting Knowledge:
- Asepsis
- Sterilization
- Instruments
- Vital signs and measurements
- Physical examinations
- Clinical pharmacology
- Minor surgery
- Therapeutic modalities
- Laboratory procedures
- Electrocardiography (ECG)
- First aid and emergency response

To be eligible for the RMA exam, you must be a graduate of an ABHES– or CAAHEP–accredited program or a formal medical services training program of the U.S. Armed Forces or meet the requirements for medical assisting experience.

The RMA exam can be taken at a computerized testing center or as a pencil-and-paper test. Computerized testing can be scheduled daily, except Sundays and holidays. Applications can be downloaded from the AMT web site, www.amt1.com.

Medical Administrative Specialist

The AMT also offers the Certified Medical Administrative Specialist (CMAS) exam, which includes 210 four-option multiple-choice questions covering front office medical assisting skills.

Medical Assisting Foundations:
- Medical terminology
- Anatomy and physiology

- Legal and ethical considerations
- Professionalism

Basic Clinical Medical Office Assisting:
- Basic health history interview
- Basic charting
- Vital signs and measurements
- Asepsis in the medical office
- Examination preparation
- Medical office emergencies
- Pharmacology

Medical Office Clerical Assisting:
- Appointment management and scheduling
- Reception
- Communication
- Patient information and community resources

Medical Records Management:
- Systems
- Procedures
- Confidentiality

Health Care Insurance Processing, Coding, and Billing:
- Insurance processing
- Coding
- Insurance billing and finances

Medical Office Financial Management:
- Fundamental financial management
- Patient accounts
- Banking
- Payroll

Medical Office Information Processing:
- Fundamentals of computing
- Medical office computer applications

Medical Office Management:
- Office communications
- Business organization management
- Human resources
- Safety
- Supplies and equipment
- Physical office plant
- Risk management and quality assurance

To be eligible to sit for the CMAS exam, you must be a graduate of a medical administrative program accredited by the ABHES or another regionally or nationally accredited institution approved by the U.S. Department of Education or possess acceptable experiencer requirements as outlined on the AMT website, www.amt1.com. The CMAS exam is also administered in computerized and paper-and-pencil formats.

CONTINUING EDUCATION

In addition to sitting for a national exam after completing studies in medical assisting, you should carefully consider the many benefits of joining a professional organization such as the AAMA. An *active member* must be a CMA or an individual who was an active member on December 31, 1987, and who maintains continuous active membership. An *associate member* is one who is not eligible for another category of membership but who is interested in the profession of medical assisting. Those enrolled in a medical assistant program may become student members at a reasonable cost. Student membership may be retained for dues 1 year after graduation if active or associate membership is not chosen.

One of the best and most appropriate ways for you to continue your education is through AAMA tri-level membership (local, state, and national levels). Hundreds of educational programs offering CEUs are conducted throughout the year. Physician advisors are among the professionals who speak at the monthly meetings and other educational activities. Many physician employers and office managers offer financial assistance to employees to encourage attendance and participation in seminars, workshops, and conventions where important current topics are shared. Members are entitled to special rates for all educational pursuits offered by the organization as well as many other financial advantages (such as group rates). Soon after joining, members automatically begin receiving AAMA's bimonthly magazine, *CMA Today,* which is devoted to educational articles that are written by experts in allied health and related fields. This magazine contains current medical research reports, the latest state and federal health legislative news, education program announcements, and articles offering CEU credit. Most organizations at the state level keep members informed with a news publication containing educational articles as well as dates for programs, meetings, and other activities relevant to the medical assistant. Many local chapters send notices to their members about meeting times and other important information.

The AAMA and the AMT additionally provide guided study programs at a reasonable cost in a wide range of areas such as Human Relations, Medical Law, and Communication Skills, among others. These professionally designed courses allow medical assistants to learn and study at home at their own pace. CEUs are awarded for the successful completion of the examinations accompanying each home study course.

Employers are impressed with applicants who take the initiative in belonging to one or more such organizations. Membership not only shows your interest in self-improvement, but also shows your initiative in improving your skills for the welfare of the patients you serve. Most employers encourage their employees to attend seminars, workshops, and courses that offer education that relates to the medical office practice, both clinical and administrative. Some employers even pay for the costs of membership and for educational program fees. Well-informed personnel provide competent care to patients and assist in quality management of administrative tasks.

Additional information may be obtained by writing, faxing your request, retrieving information from web sites, or calling the professional organizations listed at the end of this unit.

ACHIEVE UNIT OBJECTIVES

- Complete the Workbook activities to meet the learning objectives.
- Apply your knowledge at the end of this chapter in completing the Critical Thinking Challenge and Activities, as well as the StudyWARE on your Student CD-ROM.

CRITICAL THINKING CHALLENGE

IMPACTING THE PATIENT, THE PRACTICE, AND YOUR CAREER

Janet and Rebecca are medical assistants working in a busy clinic that employs five physicians, two physician assistants, and two nurse practitioners. Both are recent graduates from different institutions; these are their first positions in their chosen profession. Janet reports to work the first week promptly each day with her hair pulled away from her face, her uniform clean and pressed, her make-up appropriately applied, and impeccable personal hygiene. Rebecca, on the other hand, reports to work that first week an average of 15 minutes late; her hair hangs in her face and is dirty, her uniform is wrinkled with stains, she has multiple obvious piercings and uncovered tattoos, she wears excessive jewelry, and her personal hygiene leaves a lot to be desired. During that first week, the health care providers and patients prefer working with Janet, and Rebecca is scheduled to work in medical records away from the patients.

QUESTIONS

1. Is there any impact on patients if Rebecca is scheduled to work with them?
2. If you feel that there could be a negative impact if Rebecca works with patients, what impact (if any) do you think that could have on the practice?
3. Given the scenario, contrast the career impacts for both Janet and Rebecca.

ACTIVITIES

1. Go to the Internet to research the differences between the registered medical assistant (RMA), certified medical assistant (CMA), and the certified medical administrative specialist (CMAS). Write a short paper outlining the differences in the credentials and the organizations awarding the credentials.
2. Go to the Internet to look up the American Association of Medical Assistants (AAMA) and the Accrediting Bureau of Health Education Schools (ABHES) and write a short paper describing the differences in these accrediting bodies.
3. Interview a certified medical assistant, registered medical assistant, and certified medical administrative specialist regarding continuing education requirements for their credentials.

StudyWARE™ CHALLENGE

- Study with the flash cards for Chapter 2 to review the key terms in this chapter.
- Solve the crossword puzzle for Chapter 2.
- Complete the multiple choice quiz in test mode for Chapter 2.

RESOURCES

American Association of Medical Assistants. (2002). *AAMA role delineation study: Occupational analysis of the medical assisting profession*. Chicago: Author.

American Medical Technologists, Telephone 847-823-5169.

Gillyatt, P. (1996, July). How to answer your own medical questions. *Harvard Health Letter, xii*(2), 9–12.

Lindh, W. Q., Pooler, M. S., Tamparo, C. D., & Dahl, B. (2006). *Delmar's comprehensive medical assisting: Administrative and clinical competencies* (3rd ed.). Clifton Park, NY: Thomson Delmar Learning.

U.S. Department of Labor. (2005). *Occupational outlook handbook* (2002–12 ed.). Washington, DC: Bureau of Labor Statistics.

WEB LINKS

www.aama-ntl.org (American Association of Medical Assistants)
Provides information about career opportunities, CAAHEP-accredited programs, and the CMA exam.

www.abhes.org (Accrediting Bureau of Health Education Schools)
Provides a list of ABHES-accredited programs.

http://stats.bls.gov (U.S. Department of Labor, Bureau of Labor Statistics)
Provides employment statistics.

CHAPTER

3

Medical Ethics and Liability

During the past 20 years the number of patients bringing lawsuits against physicians has increased dramatically. Medical liability insurance rates have increased so much that physicians have difficulty affording liability insurance. Laws may vary in different states, but ethical standards are the same in every state. **Ethics** deals with moral choices and rules of conduct. All members of professional organizations that deal with patient health care and have a high regard for morality and competence follow a code of ethics specific to their profession.

UNIT 1
Ethical and Legal Responsibilities

UNIT 2
Professional Liability

UNIT 1
ETHICAL AND LEGAL RESPONSIBILITIES

OBJECTIVES

Upon completion of this unit, you will be able to achieve the following:

LEARNING Objectives

1. Spell and define, using the glossary at the back of the text, all the Words to Know in this unit.
2. List licensure requirements for physicians.
3. Describe methods of licensure.
4. List exceptions to the need for licensure.
5. Define the components of public and private law.
6. Recognize the differences between ethics and law.
7. Identify areas of medical ethics of particular concern to medical assistants.
8. List the five primary elements of the American Association of Medical Assistants Code of Ethics.
9. Describe the reason diagnostic related groups are causing an ethical issue for physicians.
10. Name one societal group being denied health insurance.
11. List ethical considerations surrounding the life of a fetus.
12. List and define the three categories of medical transplants.
13. Name the most common type of transplant.
14. Describe a living will.
15. Name four examples of tort law.
16. Define the term *emancipated minor* and give examples.
17. Describe the three parts of the physician-patient contract.
18. Define the terms *implied consent* and *express consent.*
19. Prepare common consent forms used in medical offices.
20. Define the term *privileged communication.*
21. List instances of legally required disclosure.
22. Explain the terms *defamation of character, libel,* and *slander.*
23. Describe the conditions for revocation or suspension of a medical license.

WORDS TO KNOW

agent	enact	*non compos*
artificial	endorsement	*mentis*
insemination	ethics	peer review
assault	explicit	proxy
battery	expressed	prudent
biennially	forged	quackery
civil law	fraudulent	rational
coercion	genetic	reciprocity
confidentiality	implied	revoke
criminal law	incompetent	statutes
defamation	intimidation	surrogate
emancipated	liability	tort
minor	moral	

CERTIFICATION CONNECTION

CMA
Medicolegal guidelines and
  requirements

CMAS
Legal and ethical
  considerations

RMA
Documentation
Understand and utilize
  proper documentation
  of patient encounters

Our founding fathers saw a need for regulation of the practice of medicine, and in colonial days medical practice acts were in effect for the protection of citizens. These acts were gradually repealed because it was believed the Constitution gave everyone the right to practice medicine. This resulted in a period of time in the nineteenth century when **quackery** was common. After a Supreme Court decision in 1899 upheld a state's right to establish qualifications for people wishing to practice medicine, all states soon had once again established medical practice acts. Most state **statutes** define two basic elements that constitute the practice of medicine. One is diagnosis and the other is the prescribing of treatment. Only a licensed physician (and some mid-level practitioners) can engage in the diagnosis and prescribing of treatment for the physical condition of human beings. In general terms, medical practice acts define the practice of medicine and establish requirements for licensure and grounds for suspending or **revoking** a license.

LICENSURE REQUIREMENTS

Licensure requirements are established by each state. A physician is usually required to:

- Be of legal age
- Be of good moral character
- Have graduated from an approved medical school
- Have completed an approved residency program or its equivalent
- Be a resident of the state where the physician is practicing
- Have passed the oral and written examinations administered by the National Board of Medical Examiners and the state where the physician is practicing

Physicians who have all the necessary requirements for licensure may also be licensed by **reciprocity** or **endorsement**. A physician who has been licensed in one state and wishes to move to another state may be granted a license by reciprocity if it is determined that the original licensure requirements are equal to the requirements in the new state. Many physicians take the test administered by the National Board of Medical Examiners at the same time they take their first state test. The high standards of the national board make it possible to obtain a state license by endorsement when the national board examinations have been successfully passed.

Physicians are required to renew their license annually or **biennially**. You should be sure the physician has a record of all continuing medical education credits (CMEs) earned since the previous renewal, as this is a requirement in many states. Physicians earn CMEs by attending seminars and scientific meetings as well as university courses. The renewal notice will notify the physician of the number of CMEs necessary to renew the license.

There are some exceptions to the rule requiring a current state license to practice medicine. Any physician is free to administer first aid outside the state of residence.

Physicians in military service must be licensed to practice medicine in their home states. They do not need to be licensed in the state where they are stationed as long as they practice only on the military base.

Each state's Board of Medical Examiners provides procedures for revocation or suspension of licensure. In some states the board has the power to revoke a license, and in other states a special review committee has this authority.

A physician may lose the license to practice medicine if convicted of a crime such as murder, rape, violation of narcotic laws, or income tax evasion. A medical license may also be revoked for unprofessional conduct. The most usual offenses in this category are betrayal of patient-physician confidence, illegal use of drugs and alcohol, and inappropriate sexual conduct with patients.

A license may be revoked because of proven fraud in the application for a license. In some cases **fraudulent** diplomas are used. Fraud in the filing of claims for services that were not rendered and fraud in the use of unproven treatments are also grounds for revocation of a license.

Physicians who are found to be incompetent to practice because of mental incapacity also may have their license revoked.

ETHICAL CONSIDERATIONS

Whereas laws concern matters enforced through the court system, ethics deals with what is morally right and wrong. The ethical standards established by a profession are administered by **peer review**, and violation of the standards may result in suspension of membership.

Physician's Code

The American Medical Association (AMA) Principles of Medical Ethics defines the standards of conduct and behavior for physicians. These nine principles are the basis of the AMA's Code of Medical Ethics, which is a comprehensive ethics guide for physicians. Refer to www.ama-assn.org to view the principles in their entirety.

Medical Assistant's Code

As an agent of the physician, you, the medical assistant, are also governed by ethical standards: The American Association of Medical Assistants (AAMA) Code of Ethics is, in many respects, similar to that of the American Medical Association (AMA).

A code of ethics is made up of statements regarding how individuals affiliated with an organization should conduct themselves. The AAMA's Code of Ethics indicates that medical assistants will abide by ethical and **moral** principles as they relate to the profession (Figure 3-1). It also states that medical assistants should strive to deserve the high regard of the medical profession and the general public. It continues with five specific pledge statements concerning how medical assistants will conduct themselves in the performance of their profession. In addition, the Medical Assistants' Creed contains eight statements that medical assistants agree to accept as evidence of their desire to practice their profession to the best of their ability (Figure 3-2). By adhering to these two ethical

---

CODE OF ETHICS
of the American Association of Medical Assistants

The Code of Ethics of AAMA shall set forth principles of ethical and moral conduct as they relate to the medical profession and the particular practice of medical assisting.

Members of AAMA dedicated to the conscientious pursuit of their profession, and thus desiring to merit the high regard of the entire medical profession and the respect of the general public which they do serve, do pledge themselves to strive always to:

A. render service with full respect for the dignity of humanity;

B. respect confidential information obtained through employment unless legally authorized or required by responsible performance of duty to divulge such information;

C. uphold the honor and high principles of the profession and accept its disciplines;

D. seek to continually improve the knowledge and skills of medical assistants for the benefit of patients and professional colleagues;

E. participate in additional service activities aimed toward improving the health and well-being of the community.

FIGURE 3-1 Code of Ethics of the American Association of Medical Assistants *(Courtesy of the American Association of Medical Assistants)*

MEDICAL ASSISTANT'S CREED

The creed of the American Association of Medical Assistants reads as follows:

I believe in the principles and purposes of the profession of medical assisting.

I endeavor to be more effective.

I aspire to render greater service.

I protect the confidence entrusted to me.

I am dedicated to the care and well-being of all people.

I am loyal to my employer.

I am true to the ethics of my profession.

I am strengthened by compassion, courage, and faith.

FIGURE 3-2 Medical Assistant's Creed *(Courtesy of the American Association of Medical Assistants)*

---

standards (Medical Assistant's Code of Ethics and Medical Assistant's Creed), you will uphold the professional quality of medical assisting.

STATE AND FEDERAL LAWS

The physician must release patient information when the patient authorizes the release or if the release is required by law. State laws vary regarding release of information. Information that must be reported includes:

- Births and deaths
- Cases of violence such as gunshot wounds, knifings, and poisonings
- Sexually transmitted diseases
- Suspected cases of abuse (child, spousal, or elders)
- Cases of contagious, infectious, or communicable diseases

Medical assistants should check with local authorities for the procedures to be followed in making these reports. They need to be aware also of other required local reports. When a physician moves or retires, it is important that the original records be kept until the period for filing of liability suits has expired. A copy of the records is provided to a new physician if one takes over the practice.

You will often find it necessary to make decisions based on the professional nature of your employment. Patients can be extremely insistent at times, but you must be firm in carrying out the expectations of your employer and your profession. A patient may, for instance, demand that you call in a prescription for medication when the physician is not immediately available. Be firm and say that only the physician can give you the orders to do this. Carefully record on the chart the request of the patient and how it was taken care of. *Never put yourself in the position of practicing medicine.*

The Federal Drug Administration has established five categories, or "schedules," that classify chemical substances with specific regulations as to their use. The states also have laws that further define the use of drugs. It is important for the medical assistant to understand that only the physician (and some midlevel providers) can legally prescribe medications. The medical assistant must understand that certain medications cannot be refilled and that restrictions limit the number of times some medications can be refilled. Some medication orders must be accompanied by a written prescription before they can be filled, while others can be called in by telephone. It is important to remember that all patients should be scheduled to see the physician at regular intervals to check all medications they are currently taking.

The United States Department of Justice Drug Enforcement Administration publishes a physician's manual that gives all the information necessary for office personnel to understand the provisions of the Controlled Substances Act. This booklet is free and is furnished on request.

The Drug Enforcement Administration also publishes a *Physician's Manual,* which includes recommendations for physicians about the care and security of prescription pads to help reduce the number of **forged** prescription orders:

1. Prescription pads should be stored in a safe place (locked cabinet) to discourage theft. There should be a minimum number of prescription pads used.

2. Schedule II controlled substances are to be written in ink or typed and signed by the physician.

3. The prescription should contain the amount of the medication in Arabic or Roman numerals as well as the written number to deter changing the amount.

4. Unless absolutely necessary, the amount (number) of a controlled substance should be limited when writing prescriptions.

5. The amount of controlled substances carried in the doctor's medical bag should be kept at a minimum.

6. If the physician keeps a medical bag in the car, it must be locked in the trunk.

7. Use caution when prescribing controlled substances to a patient who has disclosed that another doctor has prescribed a controlled drug. Check with the doctor at the patient's medical facility, or examine the patient to make a decision regarding a prescription for a controlled drug.

8. Prescription blanks should never be signed in advance.

9. Controlled substances must be accurately recorded and maintained to comply with the regulations of the Controlled Substance Act.

10. Verify prescription orders with the pharmacist to assist with the dispensing of the correct medication.

11. To report or obtain information regarding prescription medications, contact the nearest DEA field office.

LEGAL AND ETHICAL ISSUES

In the practice of medicine it can be difficult to distinguish between legal and ethical issues. The trend in the United States is to demand good health care as a right for everyone. However, not all citizens are willing to finance such a program. The use of diagnosis related groups (DRGs) in determining the payment hospitals will receive for Medicare patients raises both ethical and legal questions. The problem with the system arises when patients may be discharged too early simply because the hospital will not be paid for more than the DRG-allowed number of days. The physician knows the legal responsibility is to the well-being of the patient, but the hospital must have money to stay in business, and the physician wants to stay in good standing with the hospital. In a case in California, Wickline v. State of California, 1986, a physician was held liable for releasing a patient too early. In fact, the physician had failed to protest the third party's decision to shorten the patient's recommended hospital stay. In this case, the third party payer was a California Medicare agency called MediCal.

Insurance companies are presenting more ethical questions to medical care providers when they refuse insurance to individuals who have acquired immune deficiency syndrome (AIDS) and human immunodeficiency virus (HIV).

Many ethical considerations surround the life of a fetus, an infant's birth, and the newborn: New technologies allow us to have more control over birth by detecting *in utero* abnormalities. The improved techniques of **artificial insemination** bring before the court system the problems associated with **surrogate** motherhood and paternal responsibility. Many advances have been made in the use of fetal tissue in transplants. Our society must study the ethical and emotional considerations of ending a pregnancy if a serious **genetic** deficiency is found before birth or allowing the infant to be born handicapped.

The use of transplants has added another series of ethical problems. Medical transplants are divided into three categories:

- Autograft: transplantation of a person's own tissue from one body site to another (can also be used to describe transplant between identical twins)
- Homograft: transplantation of tissue from one person to another
- Heterograft: transplantation of animal tissue to a human being

The blood transfusion is the most common transplant. Nearly all the major organs of the body may be transplanted, and research continues to improve these possibilities.

THE UNIFORM ANATOMICAL GIFT ACT

The Uniform Anatomical Gift Act was passed in 1968. By 1978 it was reported that all 50 states had established some system of organ and tissue donor identification so that individuals can ensure that when they die they will be identified as a donor. Any person of sound mind and legal age may donate any body part after death for research or transplant. The family may make this decision for the donor if the donor has not done so while living. The time of death must be determined by a physician who will not be involved in the transplant in any way. No money can be exchanged for making an anatomical donation. Many states allow residents to mark and sign a donor card on the back of their driver's license.

Different ethical problems affect the use of organs from living donors. As the technology of transplantation becomes more readily available, the demand for organs will grow. One source estimated that since the year 2000, most of the poor in India are surviving with only one kidney as the result of the common practice of selling their kidneys to wealthy foreigners.

Another ethical issue of concern is the ability to *grow* tissue and organs from manipulated stem cells or cultivated *donor* tissue. This research is highly controversial yet highly motivated by the need for replacement organs to sustain life, and the experimentation continues.

LIVING WILL

The health care team will provide a larger percentage of care to geriatric patients as the quality of care extends life expectancy. It is important that everyone in the office listen to older patients and allow them to make decisions regarding a living will. A majority of the states now have laws that define policies on withholding life-sustaining procedures from hopelessly ill patients. The living will is signed when the patient is competent and must be witnessed by two individuals. The effect of this living will is to protect the wishes of the patient who may become incompetent and thus unable to make **rational** decisions. The patient and all family members should discuss these issues while the patient is still rational and can fully comprehend the implications. A chosen family member should then be made aware of the responsibility of carrying out the patient's wishes as it becomes necessary. Copies of the living will should be filed with the family, the primary physician, and the family's attorney.

DURABLE POWER OF ATTORNEY

Choice in Dying, Inc., now stresses the importance of also completing a durable power of attorney for health care form, authorized by either your state's statute or some other legal authority. This allows you to appoint another person (known as your **agent**) to make health care decisions for you if at any time you become unable to make them yourself. It is strongly advised that you appoint an agent, assuming there is someone who can be trusted to make the decisions you would make if you could, and who is willing to act for you in this way. The appointed **proxy** (agent) must be aware of your wishes and understand the complete document before giving consent to carry out the agreement. It may be helpful to record the wishes of a living will and power of attorney on a videotape so there could be no doubt that you made the statements regarding care. It is also recommended that a copy of the video be kept by the appointed attorney. The video dialogue should state the date it is made, who has copies, and the living will/advanced directives of the patient.

ACCEPTING OR REFUSING TREATMENT

A medical "Miranda warning" law approved by Congress and signed by President George Herbert Walker Bush gives patients legal options for refusing or accepting treatment if they are incapacitated. The law, which took effect in November 1991, applies to hospitals, hospices, nursing homes, health maintenance organizations (HMOs), and other health care facilities that receive money from Medicare and Medicaid programs. Under the law, patients must receive written information explaining their right-to-die options according to their state laws. The law stipulates that hospitals and other providers must note on medical records whether patients have legal directives on treatment. Providers also must have procedures to ensure that they comply with a patient's wishes.

Every member of the medical care team must be current in cardiopulmonary resuscitation (CPR) certification. An ethical question arises when the older or terminally ill patient does not wish to be resuscitated in the event of a cardiopulmonary arrest. The courts have held that individuals have the right to make decisions that affect their own deaths.

LEGAL MATTERS

In the United States the laws are divided into the categories of public law and private law. The various branches of public law include **criminal law**, constitutional law, administrative law, and international law. Criminal law deals with offenses against all citizens. The practice of medicine without a license is an offense under the criminal law. Constitutional law defines the powers of the government and the rights of its citizens. Each state has a constitution that defines its powers over matters not covered by the federal government, which are spelled out in the United States Constitution. Administrative law is concerned with the powers of government agencies. International law is concerned with agreements and treaties between countries.

The practice of medicine is primarily affected by private law or **civil law**, specifically by contract law and tort law. The patient-physician relationship is considered a contractual one. A **tort** is defined as any of a number of actions done by one person or group of persons that causes injury to another. Violations of tort law may be intentional or negligent. Negligence is an act or failure to act as a reasonably **prudent** physician under the same or similar circumstances that directly or proximately causes injury to a patient. The negligent causing of an injury, when committed by a physician in the course of professional duties, is commonly referred to as *malpractice*. Intentional torts also result in professional **liability** suits. Libel and slander are two forms of **defamation**. Libel refers to written statements; slander refers to oral remarks. **Assault** is defined as a deliberate attempt or threat to touch without consent. Another intentional wrong is **battery**, which is the unauthorized touching of another person. A patient has a right to refuse treatment. If any treatment is provided without consent, a charge of battery may be filed by the patient. Other civil laws govern property ownership, corporations, and inheritance.

Patient-Physician Contract

The contract between a patient and a physician has three parts (Figure 3-3). They are the offer, the acceptance, and the consideration. The offer takes place when a competent individual indicates a desire to become a patient. The acceptance takes place when an appointment is given and the physician examines the patient. The consideration is the payment given in exchange for services. When a child is a patient, the par-

1. The offer—desire to become patient

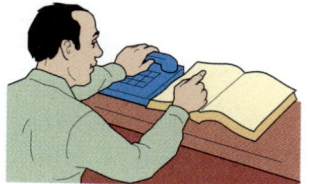

2. Acceptance

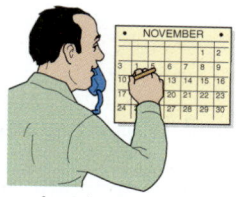

a. Appointment is given

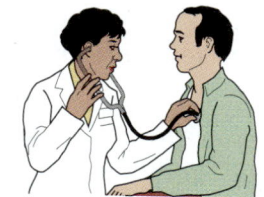

b. Physician examines patient

3. Consideration—payment made for services

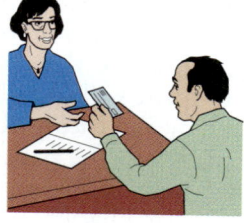

FIGURE 3-3   The three parts of the patient-physician contract

ent is expected to pay. A young person is considered to be a minor until reaching full legal age, known as the age of majority. The statutes defining the age of majority vary from state to state. The medical assistant needs to be aware that the rights of minors in medical treatment are changing. More than half of the states allow minors the right to consent to treatment or consultation for pregnancy, contraception, venereal disease, drug abuse, or alcoholism.

An **emancipated minor** is an individual who is no longer under the care, custody, or supervision of parents. The emancipated minor may be married, in the armed forces, or self-supporting and living apart from parents. An emancipated minor can legally consent to medical care.

An individual who has been judged by the courts to be mentally **incompetent** must have an appointed guardian. The general legal term for all varieties of mental illness is ***non compos mentis***. The guardian is responsible for both the payment of bills and the care of the patient. In this case the parents are not responsible for payment. When a patient-physician contract is entered into, the physician is responsible for the care of that patient until the physician officially withdraws from the case or the patient discharges the physician.

Consent for Treatment

The contract between the patient and the physician may be either **implied** or **expressed**. An express, or written, contract must be entered into if a third party is to be responsible for payment. If this agreement is not in writing, it is not possible to press for payment. The fact that the patient has come to see the physician implies consent for treatment. The instances when express consent is required are:

- Proposed surgery or other invasive treatments such as lumbar punctures, sigmoidoscopies, and biopsies
- Use of experimental drugs
- Use of unusual procedures that may involve high risk

There are exceptions to the rule for surgery. Minor procedures generally involve only an explanation by the physician and oral consent of the patient. Notes regarding this conversation, however, need to be entered by the physician in the patient's medical record.

Figure 3-4 shows an example of a consent form. Remember that it is your responsibility to know what consent forms your employer uses. The physician may wish to develop consent forms individualized for the practice. It is important that these be **explicit** as to what is to be done. Experiments have been conducted using a tape recorder to keep a record of the information given the patient before a consent form is signed. These were discussions with patients who had to be told they

CONSENT TO OPERATION, ANESTHETICS, AND OTHER MEDICAL SERVICES

I authorize the performance upon _____ the following operation:

_____

to be performed under the direction of Dr. _____.

- The nature of the operation is as follows:

_____

- The purpose of the operation is as follows:

_____

- The possible alternative methods to treatment are:

_____

- The possible consequences of this operation are:

_____

- The risks involved are as follows:

_____

- The possible complications are as follows:

_____

I have been advised of the serious nature of this operation, and have been advised that if I desire more information about any of the above items, including risks and complications, that it will be given to me.

I do not request further information about any of the above items in this consent form.

_____   _____

Signature of Patient   Witness

_____   _____

Date   Date

FIGURE 3-4   Sample consent to treatment form

had cancer. The results showed that most of these patients had little or no memory of what had been discussed because they were extremely upset by the diagnosis. In some of these cases the patients were certain they had not been fully informed, but replay of the tape proved they had been. The medical assistant should understand that the physician must be legally responsible for obtaining informed consent from a patient. You should not be given that responsibility. Informed consent is necessary to avoid a claim of assault and battery. The law describes this as a threat to make a physical attack on someone and carrying out the attack. You will be expected to prepare consent forms and ideally be present to listen so that you may help determine whether the patient understood before signing the consent form.

If an all-purpose form is used, it is important to cross out the paragraphs that do not apply. You may be asked to sign as a witness. What you say when you ask a patient to sign after the physician has explained the risks is important. A suggested statement is: "If you have no further questions for the doctor and you understand the consent form, will you please sign it?" You can help the patient by indicating the line where the signature is required, or ask the patient to sign on the line you have marked with an "X."

If a physician is to treat a patient with unusual or experimental medication, it is best to use a consent to treatment form. When a physician is to perform a sterilization procedure, it is preferable to have both husband and wife sign a request for sterilization form.

RIGHT TO PRIVACY

Patients have the right to privacy when they are being examined and treated. Even though many physicians have arrangements with medical facilities to offer training opportunities for medical students or residents, the patient always has the right to refuse to have observers present. Patients must first be asked if it is acceptable for observers to be present during the examination. If the patient refuses, no **intimidation** or **coercion** should be expressed to make the patient change the decision. Physicians may protect themselves by having an authority to admit observers form signed.

Information contained in a patient medical record and information exchanged between a physician and a patient are considered privileged communications. Every patient has a legal right to privacy and **confidentiality**. Information disclosed to the health care team must be kept in the strictest confidence, and you must be ever mindful of the legal implications of handling patients' records. Information concerning patients may be given to another member of the health care team, such as a laboratory technician or referring physician, only when it pertains directly to the course of treatment. For example, another medical office may telephone you to inquire about a patient's medical history for diagnostic purposes, to confirm symptoms, or to verify birth date. In complying with referral appointments or scheduled tests, patients will have given *implied consent* for necessary information to be transmitted concerning their condition. Implied consent means that the patient has expressed a desire to become a patient by making an appointment, being examined by the physician, and making payment for services rendered.

Medical information may be given to parties not concerned in the patient's treatment only when the patient has signed a release of information form.

A large number of states have **enacted** privileged communication statutes to offer additional protection to the patient. You will find that curious and well-meaning friends and relatives will ask about patients, yet you must remember to give only information that has been authorized by the patient. Each time a patient authorizes release of information, the form must state specifically who is to receive what information covering what time period. This authorization must be kept in the medical record.

All health care providers must be aware of any state regulations governing the reporting of HIV-positive tests. At issue is the right of the patient to confidentiality and the rights of citizens to be protected from accidental exposure to the HIV virus. Such exposure might occur when police, fire, emergency medical service, or other medical personnel come into direct contact with the blood or body fluids of a patient.

In all fifty states, confirmed cases of HIV/AIDS constitute a reportable condition either by statute or administrative regulation.

ACHIEVE UNIT OBJECTIVES

- ☐ Complete the Workbook activities to meet the learning objectives.
- ☐ Apply your knowledge at the end of this chapter in completing the Critical Thinking Challenge and Activities, as well as the StudyWARE on your Student CD-ROM.

UNIT 2
PROFESSIONAL LIABILITY

OBJECTIVES

Upon completion of this unit, you will be able to achieve the following:

LEARNING Objectives

1. Spell and define, using the glossary at the back of the text, all the Words to Know in this unit.
2. List rights of the physician in providing medical care.
3. List rights of the patient in receiving medical care.
4. Describe the correct procedure for terminating the physician-patient contract.
5. Define and give examples of abandonment.
6. Define and give examples of professional negligence.
7. Give an example of an implied agreement.
8. Describe the precaution that should be observed in giving written instructions to a patient.
9. List the reasons for keeping medical records.

10. Describe who owns medical office records and who has a right to the information in them.

11. List the recordkeeping necessary to provide legally adequate records.

12. Describe the kinds of notes that are not appropriate in a patient chart.

13. Name the six basic principles for preventing unauthorized disclosure of patient information.

14. List six office procedures that can cause problems when the physician is involved in a lawsuit.

15. Describe the acceptable method for making changes in medical records.

WORDS TO KNOW

abandonment	doctrine	*res ipsa loquitur*
breach	encompass	*respondeat*
chronologic	harmonious	*superior*
competent	liability	*subpoena duces*
confrontation	obligate	*tecum*
defamation	procrastination	venereal
deposition	rapport	

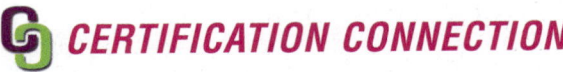

CERTIFICATION CONNECTION

CMA
Medicolegal guidelines and requirements
• Licenses and accreditation
• Legislation
• Physician-patient relationship

RMA
Documentation
Understand and utilize proper documentation of patient encounters

CMAS
Legal and ethical considerations

PHYSICIAN AND PATIENT RIGHTS

Physicians have the right to determine whom they will accept as patients. Physicians who have been in practice for a long time may also build up a patient load that is as large as one person can care for adequately. Because a physician must care for all patients accepted, it is not unusual for a physician to decide to see no new patients. A physician may not, on the other hand, refuse to provide emergency service if assigned to an emergency, and most physicians will provide emergency service whenever the need exists. Because they do not have to continue the patient's treatment once the emergency services have been provided, the patient is stabilized and the patient's regular physician takes over the case.

Physicians have the right to decide what types of medicine they wish to practice and where. They have the right to establish their own working hours, to charge for their services, and to take a vacation if they provide names of qualified substitutes to care for their patients while they are unavailable. Physicians have the right to change the location of their office but must notify patients in advance to give them adequate time to make alternative plans for medical care.

Patients have the right to receive care equal to the standards of care in the community as a whole. Patients have the right to choose the physician from whom they wish to receive treatment from the listing of physicians who are enrolled in their particular insurance plan. Of course, a patient may always see any physician desired as long as they take full responsibility for payment of services rendered; this means that the patient pays cash at the time of service if the patient's insurance plan will not cover the services of that particular physician. If a patient becomes a member of an HMO, the right to choose a physician may be restricted to physicians who are members of the chosen HMO. A patient has the right to accept or reject treatment and to know whether the prescribed treatment has side effects, what the prognosis is, what effect the treatment will have on the body, and any treatment alternatives.

A physician may choose to withdraw from the care of a patient who does not follow instructions for treatment or keep follow-up appointments or who leaves a hospital against medical advice. Withdrawal must be by means of a letter sent by certified mail with return receipt requested as proof the letter was received (Figure 3-5). The return receipt should be filed in the patient record. The letter should state the reason for the withdrawal and needs to state the date the withdrawal will become effective. If the patient needs follow-up, the letter should recommend that the patient make an appointment with another physician. It is appropriate to indicate that a copy of the medical records will be sent to the new physician if the patient will send written authorization to do so. The letter should be signed by the physician.

A patient has a choice and a right to change physicians. The patient should notify the physician, but if this does not take place in a written form the physician may send a letter confirming the dismissal. This letter should also be sent by certified mail, return receipt re-

Inner City Health Care
222 S. First Avenue
Carlton, MI 11666

December 5, 20XX

CERTIFIED MAIL

Rhoda Au
41 Academy Road
Carlton, MI 11666

Dear Ms. Au:

I find it necessary to inform you that I am withdrawing further professional medical service to you because of your persistent refusal to follow my medical advice and treatment.

Since your condition requires medical attention, I suggest that you place yourself under the care of another physician without delay. If you so desire, I shall be available to attend you for a reasonable time after you have received this letter, but in no event later than January 7, 20XX. This should give you sufficient time to select a physician from the many competent practitioners in this area.

You may be assured that, upon receiving your written request, I will make available to the physician of your choice your case history and information regarding the diagnosis and treatment which you have received from me.

Very truly yours,

Mark Woo

Mark Woo, MD
MW:kr

FIGURE 3-5   Sample letter notifying the patient of the physician's withdrawal from the case

quested, and a copy of the letter and the receipt should be filed in the patient chart.

A physician who has begun care of a patient must carry through until the patient no longer needs treatment or decides to see a different physician, or the physician has withdrawn from care. A physician who has undertaken care of a patient and is then not available to continue that care may be sued for **abandonment**, unless coverage for the patient by some equally qualified physician is provided. If a patient is admitted to the hospital and the physician does not see the patient right away to check on the patient's condition and order treatment, the physician may risk being accused of abandonment by the patient or by a family member of the patient. If a physician is ill, the office staff must refer patients who need care to other qualified physicians who will care for them.

Physicians are not **obligated** to provide follow-up care when they see a patient for preemployment or in-surance examinations, or on other occasions when the request comes from someone other than the patient (e.g., when a school athletic department requests assessment of a potential athlete).

MEDICAL ASSISTANT RIGHTS

The medical assistant has the right to be free from sexual discrimination. This may involve a man or woman being refused employment because the job is usually filled by someone of the opposite sex. It can involve not receiving promotions, being paid less for the same work, or being treated as inferior in any way.

Title VII of the Civil Rights Act of 1964 defines sexual harassment as "Unwelcome sexual advances, requests for sexual favors, and other verbal or physical conduct of a sexual nature when submission or rejection of this conduct explicitly or implicitly affects an individual's employment, unreasonably interferes with an individual's work performance or creates an intimidating, hostile or offensive work environment." Sexual harassment can occur in a variety of circumstances:

- The victim as well as the harasser may be a woman or a man. The victim does not have to be of the opposite sex.
- The harasser can be the victim's supervisor, an agent of the employer, a supervisor in another area, a co-worker, or a nonemployee.
- The victim does not have to be the person harassed but could be anyone affected by the offensive conduct.
- Unlawful sexual harassment may occur without economic injury to or discharge of the victim.
- The victim has a responsibility to establish that the harasser's conduct is unwelcome.
- A written account of each incident of sexual harassment should be documented with the names of witnesses, date, time, and place of occurrence.

It is in the victim's best interest to directly inform the harasser that the conduct is unwelcome and must stop. Each instance reported to authorities is handled on a case-by-case basis and involves a thorough investigation.

NEGLIGENCE

Torts is the branch of private law that deals with **breach** of legal duty. Torts **encompass** such wrongs as invasion of privacy, personal injury, malpractice, and slander or libel. The tort of negligence is a primary cause of malpractice suits.

Physicians are expected to be as well trained and to exercise the same degree of skill with the same degree of judgment as other physicians in similar circumstances. These criteria are used in determining the standard of care. In lawsuits involving specialists, the standard of care is that practiced nationally rather than that in a given community.

In a case of negligence the patient must establish that he or she was examined by the physician, that the physician did or did not do something another physician under similar circumstances would or would not have done, whichever the case may be, and that the negligence injured the patient. Testimony of a physician as an expert medical witness is almost always necessary in a case of negligence. In some cases the testimony of an expert witness is not required. In these instances the **doctrine** is *res ipsa loquitur*, or *the thing speaks for itself.* These cases involve such situations as a sponge or instrument left in the patient during surgery, an injury done to the bladder while performing a hysterectomy, or an infection caused by the use of unsterilized instruments. The doctrine has different interpretations in different states.

Physicians are responsible for the actions of their employees. This **liability** is expressed in the doctrine of *respondeat superior* (let the master answer). This is the law of agency, and you are an agent for the physician. Any individual entering the profession of medical assisting is considered to be accepting a position as a health care professional. If you violate the standard of care, you create the basis for a medical malpractice lawsuit. The physician is responsible for the acts of the medical assistant in the care of patients, and it is reasonable to expect the care to be as professional as the care given by the physician. A medical assistant is not licensed to practice medicine and cannot decide for a patient what care should be given.

Negligence is doing or not doing something that a *reasonable* person would do or not do in a given situation. Malpractice is a *professional's* negligence. Under ordinary circumstances, a medical assistant performing the administrative duties of a receptionist or secretary would be considered a person who could be charged with negligence. A medical assistant performing clinical procedures such as drawing blood or administering injections would be considered a professional and could be charged with malpractice.

Medical assistants who have had special training are expected to perform at a higher standard of care than those with no special knowledge or training. The medical assistant is not always covered by the physician's insurance, but insurance is available for the protection of medical assistants if they want to purchase their own coverage (or have the employer purchase it for them).

The Good Samaritan Act

The Good Samaritan Act originated in California in 1959 to protect the physician who gives emergency care from liability for any civil damages. The physician can help in an emergency without fear of being charged with neglect or abandonment for follow-up care. Now all states have Good Samaritan statutes. The statute requires that emergency care be given to the best ability of the person providing the care. In some states, the statute includes coverage for any health professional or citizen with first aid skills. The Good Samaritan law does not cover physicians if they receive compensation for the emergency care, however.

An implied agreement is considered to be a legal contract in a medical office. The medical assistant should never make a promise of a cure. You should be certain the patient understands that the instructions you give come directly from the physician or from written instruction sheets. When you hand a patient a written instruction sheet you need to be certain that the patient can read the instructions. Illiterate people are often reluctant to let anyone know that they cannot follow the directions for use of medications or preparation for a diagnostic test. One indicator of illiteracy might be the patient who becomes a "pest" by asking over and over for office staff to explain the instructions given by the physician. This patient might also ask you to explain a printed instruction sheet as a means of getting you to read it aloud. Informative videos that present detailed instructions regarding procedures, tests, and examinations for patient education are available from many pharmaceutical companies (or you can make them yourself) for patients to view while they are waiting to see the physician. Their questions and any further explanation can then follow at the end of their office visit.

The importance of doing everything possible to avoid a medical malpractice suit cannot be overemphasized. Simply being accused can have severe effects and repercussions on the physician, the physician's practice, and family. Those physicians who are wrongly accused of serious charges of neglect or malpractice can have ongoing problems with public mistrust and other issues depending on the extent of publicity. This misfortune can affect the livelihood of the physician and ruin the physician's medical practice. A physician can be ethical, honest, and **competent**, and still be sued for medical malpractice by a single patient who for some reason did not realize the expected result of treatment. This is another reason why the medical assistant is vital in providing patient education to supplement the physician's orders. The great increase in malpractice cases has caused physicians to order more tests and x-rays than are really necessary because they may feel the need to protect themselves from the possibility of missing a diagnosis and therefore being sued by the patient. The medical assistant is an extremely important person in the practice of preventive medicine in the medical office. When a friendly, **harmonious** interpersonal relationship is found in the office (known as **rapport**), the patient is much less likely to feel angry about anything associated with the care received. The well-trained medical assistant will understand the basic skills in good human relations and will then avoid **confrontations** that could lead to lawsuits against the office.

The patient who suffers nerve damage as the result of a medical assistant giving an improperly administered injection may sue both medical assistant and physician under this doctrine. You should always inform the physician immediately of any mistakes you have made in the care of a patient so that corrective measures may be taken. You should never attempt to perform a procedure for which you have not been trained. Finally, you should be sure you understand your job responsibilities as outlined in a written procedures manual, which should be periodically updated.

You must be especially careful what you say about a patient within hearing distance of anyone but the physician or other office personnel. Statements regarding patients may be considered **defamation** of character and a breach of confidentiality. If you should make public the fact that a patient has a **venereal** disease, for example, this could be damaging to the patient.

You play an important role in preventing negligence by scheduling appointments for careful follow-up, knowing how and where to reach the physician at all times during the day, and making sure that the telephone is adequately covered at all times. The patient who feels well cared for will not be anxious to sue the physician. The patient who can never reach the physician for advice or who has difficulty obtaining an appointment will be much more apt to sue on the grounds of negligence.

The medical assistant should investigate the use of an arbitration agreement procedure by contacting the local or state medical society. Not all states have an arbitration statute at the present time, but it is well worth investigating as a possible way to settle legal problems without going to court.

Because the incidence of malpractice suits has increased, the medical assistant may need to be involved in preparing materials for court. This may include the professional training and experience of the physician as well as the patient medical record.

The attorney may agree to taking the testimony of the physician by **deposition**. A deposition is oral testimony and may be taken in the attorney's office or the physician's office in the presence of a court reporter. Some depositions are also videotaped.

A medical assistant may also receive a **subpoena duces tecum** to appear in court with patient records. This occurs when the physician is not available at the time needed in court.

Statute of Limitations

A statute of limitations is a law that designates a specific limit of time during which a claim may be filed in malpractice suits or in the collection of bills. Each state

is obligated to protect individuals by establishing the statutes that regulate the time period. It is important to research the current law by contacting your state medical association.

MEDICAL RECORDS

The medical office staff must understand the importance of maintaining complete, accurate, up-to-date records on all patients. You must have complete records to give adequate care to patients. Your records may be used in research into certain illnesses or forms of treatment, and your records must be complete for protection in case of a lawsuit. A patient record that would meet this criterion would include: (1) personal information such as full name, address, occupation, marital status, and insurance carrier; (2) patient's personal family, sociocultural, and medical history; (3) all details of physical examinations, laboratory and x-ray findings, diagnoses, and treatments; and (4) consent forms for procedures done and authorization forms for release of medical information. **Procrastination** cannot be tolerated in handling medical records. As legal documents, they are subject to critical inspection at any time.

You should always take a medical history in a private room or ask the patient to personally complete the information. Make entries on the patient medical record only as requested by the physician. All entries should be factual. All results of findings on a patient should be recorded, even if they are normal or negative. Errors on a medical record must be corrected by drawing a single line through incorrect material and adding your initials, the date, and the reason for the change. All prescription refills should be recorded, along with missed appointments, the reason for the missed appointment, and follow-up. Requests for medical information should be recorded along with the information given. Any failure to follow the treatment or advice of the physician should be noted. All notations should be in black ink, as pencil is too easily erased. Blue ink, as well as other colors, and pencil do not copy well. This is a concern for duplicating reports and records for referrals. Standard abbreviations should be used. Upon the death of a patient, a copy of the death certificate should be filed in case of subsequent requests for information. A quality medical record indicates quality medical care.

Medical records are considered the property of the physician who treats the patient. No record should be shown to a patient without the knowledge of the physician, as there may be some reason the patient should not see all of the record.

Each office should have a written policy regarding releasing information from a medical record. This policy must take into consideration local or state statutes.

In some states, the legislature has given the patient, the physician, or an authorized agent the right to examine or copy the medical record. The requirement of confidentiality regarding the medical record is no longer recognized when the patient initiates a malpractice claim against a physician.

Any review of the chart by the patient should be done when the physician is present to interpret medical terms or abbreviations. Some physicians give patients a copy of their medical records and believe this reduces any anxiety regarding their health.

For legal and practical purposes, it is a wise choice to ask the patient at the initial office visit who in their family should receive medical information regarding the patient's health status; then have the patient sign the appropriate form and list all of the names provided. This directive protects the patient's confidentiality and will also protect the practice from potential problems if the staff pays attention to this important information.

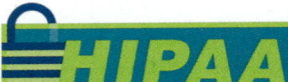

Prevention of unauthorized release of medical information regarding a patient requires that the following are practiced:

- Confidentiality applies to every patient regardless of their personal characteristics or lifestyle.
- Be aware of laws (federal, state, and local), ordinances, regulations, and rules, as well as public health programs.
- All requests from third parties require the patient's signature for medical information to be released. Keep a current "signature on file" form in the front of the patient's chart.
- Never give out medical information about a patient when you are not certain that a signed permission form exists.
- Patients should be provided with medical information regarding their diagnosis and treatment, and it is their decision to release or not to release that information. Documentation should be obtained with the patient's signature before disclosing medical information to anyone.
- If you are legally required to release medical information regarding a patient because of the seriousness or risk of the disease spreading to others, it should first be discussed with the patient.

It is a good policy to refuse to answer a telephone question as to whether an individual is a patient; a person coming to the office for information regarding a patient should produce an authorization to disclose information before any is given. It is important to check the specific details authorized to be released and to ask for photo identification of the individual or organization requesting the information. The signed authorization should be placed in the patient chart with a copy of the information released.

The complete, unaltered medical record is a legal document and is the best defense for a physician who is charged with malpractice. The first step a lawyer will take in a malpractice case against a physician is to obtain a copy of the patient's records and have them examined by an independent physician.

The following office procedures have caused problems in malpractice suits:

1. Procrastination or delay in filing lab test results or reporting them to the physicians.
2. Incomplete medical records.
3. Illegible records.
4. Unexplained altered medical records.
5. Faking or forging a document or signature.
6. Loss of records.

Correcting Medical Records

There are acceptable methods of making changes in medical records. A single line should be drawn through an incorrect entry. The initials of the person making the correction should be written in the margin along with the date the error was discovered. The corrections should appear in the record in **chronologic** order.

Records Retention

In addition to having complete, up-to-date records, you must be aware of the need for keeping these records even after care has ceased or the patient has died. Records should be kept as long as the statute of limitations is in effect on a case history. A few states designate the length of time records must be kept. Federal law dictates that you and your office have a responsibility to see that necessary records are kept for any narcotics used in the office. You also may be responsible for keeping accurate financial records. Within the following pages of this book, whenever appropriate, points will further remind you of the medicolegal importance of the subject matter.

HEALTH INSURANCE PORTABILITY AND ACCOUNTABILITY ACT OF 1996

One of the most recent developments in patient confidentiality has been addressed through the Health Insurance Portability and Accountability Act of 1996 (HIPAA), which was put into place in August 1996. Because the privacy of personal information is such an important issue for everyone, the Department of Health and Human Services (DHHS) wrote the Privacy rule to ensure nationwide standards were mandated to protect private health information.

Although the law was enacted in 1996, the privacy standards did not go in effect until April 2003, which served to standardize how all patient information would be handled throughout the country. Every health care provider must have specific policies in effect in order to comply with HIPAA, and staff in each provider's office must be trained to adhere to HIPAA. There will be at least one person in each provider's office that is the designated HIPAA officer to oversee the compliance; this helps to ensure that patient confidentiality is not compromised in any way.

Additionally, the Privacy Rule required providers to distribute to every patient a Notice of Privacy Practices; this document informs the patient of the following six components:

- How a patient's protected health information is used and disclosed

- The provider's duties to protect the patient's privacy
- Written notice of the provider's practices to ensure each patient's privacy
- The terms of the provider's notice
- The patient's individual rights concerning protected health information
- How to contact the office to obtain further information or to file a complaint

Because of the extent of the ruling, one must be exceptionally careful with regard to releasing patient information without specific authorization and consent. For instance, a patient has the right to block access of their protected health information if they so choose. Noncompliance with the Privacy Rule has civil penalties associated with it, and if the noncompliance is severe enough, criminal penalties may apply. If in doubt when releasing patient information, check with the designated HIPAA officer at your facility to prevent any violation of the ruling.

ACHIEVE UNIT OBJECTIVES

- ■ Complete the Workbook activities to meet the learning objectives.
- ■ Apply your knowledge at the end of this chapter in completing the Critical Thinking Challenge and Activities, as well as the StudyWARE on your Student CD-ROM.

CRITICAL THINKING CHALLENGE

IMPACTING THE PATIENT, THE PRACTICE, AND YOUR CAREER

Natalie Jones, CMA, has been charged with the responsibility of filing medical charts all morning. During a break, Ashleigh Miller, CMA, charted a prescription refill phoned in to a pharmacy for a patient; however, she spilled coffee on the chart. Ashleigh returned the chart to Natalie and asked her to file it back and started to walk away. Natalie calls to Ashleigh and tells her that she cannot put a wet, soiled chart into the shelf. Ashleigh proceeds to replace several pages of progress notes, including the file jacket. She hurriedly scribbled information, some of it recorded erroneously, throws the soiled pages away, and hands the chart back to Natalie for filing.

QUESTIONS

1. What impact could these actions have on the patient?
2. What impact could these actions have on the practice (think about if that chart is subpoenaed or audited)?
3. What impact could this have on Natalie's career?
4. What impact could this have on Ashleigh's career?

ACTIVITIES

1. Go to the Internet and research the statute of limitations for collection of professional medical bills in your state.

StudyWARE™ CHALLENGE

- Study with the flash cards for Chapter 3 to review the key terms in this chapter.
- Solve the crossword puzzle for Chapter 3.
- Complete the true/false quiz in test mode for Chapter 3.

RESOURCES

Flight, M. (2002). *Law, liability, and ethics for medical office professionals* (4th ed.). Clifton Park, NY: Thomson Delmar Learning.

Krager, C., & Krager, D. (2004). HIPAA for medical office personnel. Clifton Park, NY: Thomson Delmar Learning.

WEB LINKS

www.aama-ntl.org (American Association of Medical Assistants)
The home page for the American Association of Medical Assistants.

www.ama-assn.org (American Medical Association)
The home page for the American Medical Association.

CHAPTER 4

Professional Communications

One of the most important skills a medical assistant can possess is the art of communicating effectively with others. Both clinical and administrative duties require a constant exchange of written, oral, and nonverbal information.

You must be able to convey messages to many different people and receive vital information in the same manner. You will have daily contact with patients, colleagues, and other professionals, by phone, face to face, or by letter. Telephone and written communications and office mail will be discussed later in this text. This chapter deals with both verbal and nonverbal messages. Understanding how one gives and receives these is vital in the exchange of communication.

In dealing with patients and their families, learning to listen and to offer advice in a calm, professional manner will help to reduce unnecessary stress for all concerned. Times of sadness and pain can be extremely difficult for those closely involved. You can be instrumental in providing comfort and compassion to those in need.

Because the medical office is usually a very active place with many people coming and going, asking questions, and making payments or appointments, intraoffice communication can become hurried and ineffective. A harmonious team effort makes for an efficient and pleasant work environment. If an atmosphere of accord and cooperation exists among the staff, patients will sense this during their visits. If an uneasy situation exists, with friction evident, this may add to a patient's apprehensions and anxieties. Working together for the single purpose of providing quality health care to patients in a relaxed and friendly manner will help ease the daily pressures for the members of the medical office team and contribute greatly to their collective effectiveness.

UNIT 1
VERBAL AND NONVERBAL MESSAGES

OBJECTIVES

Upon completion of this unit, you will be able to achieve the following:

LEARNING Objectives

1. **Spell and define, using the glossary at the back of the text, all the Words to Know in this unit.**
2. **Describe the basic pattern of communication.**
3. **Give examples of nonverbal communication.**
4. **Explain how verbal and nonverbal communication can sometimes be misinterpreted.**
5. **Describe ways that tone and speed of speech can affect the message.**
6. **Discuss the importance of dress in nonverbal communication.**
7. **Explain *perception* and state its importance in communication.**
8. **List and explain the three types of listening and how they affect communication**

WORDS TO KNOW

active listening	convey	interpret
articulate	distort	intuition
conceptualize	empirically	perception
contradict	incongruous	scrupulously

CERTIFICATION CONNECTION

CMA
Adapting communication to an individual's ability to understand
Recognizing and responding to verbal and nonverbal communication
Professional communication and behavior

Evaluating and understanding communication
Interviewing techniques

RMA
Interpersonal relations

CMAS
Medical office clerical assisting–communication

To become effective in the art of communication, it may help to **conceptualize** the communication process (Figure 4-1). The message originates with the sender. The encoded message takes form based upon the sender's reference points. The message is picked up by the intended receiver, who immediately begins to decode it based on reference points. In responding (or providing feedback), the whole process is reversed: the original receiver becomes the sender, and the original sender becomes the receiver. In receiving this feedback, the original sender (now the receiver) can assess and evaluate how well the original message was received and **interpreted** and make any necessary adjustments or clarification.

The whole process seems simple enough, and generally it works well. However, many things can happen to affect the quality of the message or even **distort** it. You must be aware of these potential problems.

Foremost is the issue of reference points. For example, the spoken messages may include terminology familiar to you but unknown to the patient. Therefore, though the message will be heard, it may not be understood. Talking to patients on a level that they can easily understand is a skill requiring quick judgment. You will have to adapt to a vast number of different personalities in **conveying** information.

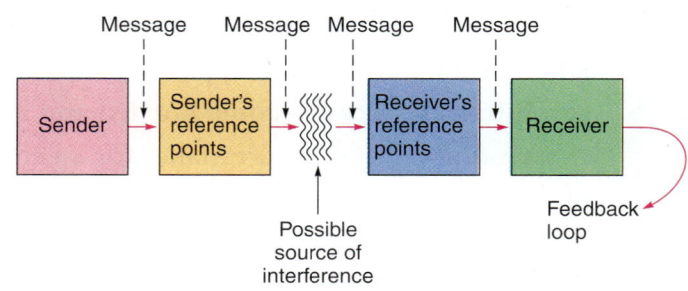

FIGURE 4-1 A model of the communication process

Some patients may be hearing- or sight-impaired, developmentally disabled, or non-English speaking, and will therefore require extra understanding. If a patient is in some way disabled, a family member or friend usually accompanies the person, thereby helping with your task of transmitting necessary information. It is important, however, that you speak to all patients directly and acknowledge their presence. It is rude and impolite to discuss their health care with another person and ignore the patients as if they were not even present.

There are many sources of interference or distractions, such as others talking, phones ringing, phone conversations, coworkers, pagers, interruptions, music, and, more often in pediatrics and family/general practice, little ones crying. The patient could also be preoccupied with what the doctor has just said or have a personal problem. It is best to speak one-on-one with the patient in an area where there will not likely be any distractions or interference. The following gives an example of a conversation in which the medical assistant is using active listening skills with the patient during triage:

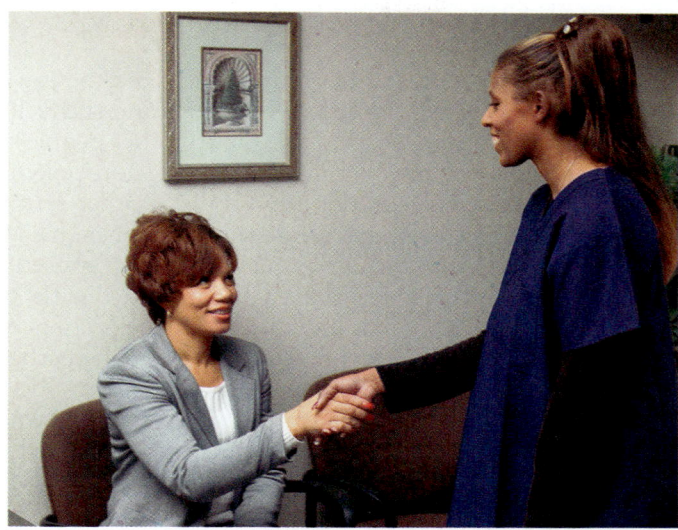

FIGURE 4-2 Make eye contact with patients when communicating verbal messages.

Medical assistant: "Now Mrs. Owen, tell me what problems you have been having."

Mrs. Owen: "Well, I've been having a lot of indigestion lately, about a month or so, and I take antacids for it but it isn't going away. It bothers me a lot in the evening."

Medical assistant: "Okay, Mrs. Owen, you say that you've been having what you think might be indigestion for approximately a month and it seems worse at night, and you take antacids for this problem. Does it help?"

Mrs. Owen: "It seems to a little but this indigestion never goes away completely."

Medical assistant: "Could you tell me what other kinds of medication you are taking?"

Mrs. Owen: "I only take aspirin sometimes for arthritis pain."

Medical assistant: "So you are taking aspirin. How much and how often?"

Mrs. Owen: "Come to think of it, I have been taking aspirin about 3 or 4 times a day for the past 2 months."

Medical assistant: "I wrote all of this down for the doctor to talk to you about in just a little while. Is there anything else that you need to see Doctor Lang about today?"

Mrs. Owen: "No, thanks. I just want my stomach to feel better."

The spoken word must be delivered in an **articulate**, clear manner if the intended message is to be received. Correct pronunciation and proper grammar help to convey meaning. You must also be aware of the rate of the spoken word. Patients need to be spoken to in an unrushed manner so that the information has a chance to register and questions can be asked. Speaking in a pleasant tone of voice is necessary to keep the listener's interest in what you are saying. You must also remember to look the person in the eye while you are conversing. Eye contact makes people pay attention to the words you are saying because it gives them a feeling of importance and expresses a sincere interest in their well-being (Figure 4-2).

Listening involves giving attention to the persons trying to communicate with you. **Active listening** is the participation in a conversation with another by means of repeating words and phrases or giving approving or disapproving nods. This signals to the message sender that you are hearing and following what is being said. This method of conversation is highly recommended for health care providers and patients in communicating needs, because it requires both parties to interact. The listener must make an effort to pay attention and follow the speaker. Distractions can create problems and interfere with what is being said; it takes concentration and self-control to keep focused on a topic when there are many activities and interruptions going on, as often happens in a medical facility. Taking a patient into an exam room or to a quiet space away from noise is the most practical way to communicate important information.

Common courtesy is an art that seems to have been lost to some degree. In a professional setting it is essential to be **scrupulously** polite. *Please, Thank you, Excuse me,* and *May I help you?* should be words in frequent use. In this way the entire health care staff will show respect for others and a sense of caring.

PERCEPTION

Perception in the context of communication may be considered as being aware of one's own feelings and the feelings of others. The feelings you have about other people's moods and the way they act are perceptual, nonspoken communication between you. **Intuition** is another term for perception in this sense. While they cannot be measured **empirically**, these feelings may be strong indeed. Therefore, they must be recognized and reckoned with.

Being perceptive is a skill acquired with experience and practice. Keeping your eyes and ears open to the needs of others and what is going on will help you develop it. Developing the ability to perceive your own needs is a part of perception that will enhance your effectiveness. Planning and thinking ahead will help you develop in this area.

BODY LANGUAGE

The image you project is of utmost importance. Your overall appearance sends out messages to anyone who looks at you. Appropriate dress, uniform, or businesslike attire should be worn. Your professional appearance sends a nonverbal message that you have authority and confidence and are in charge.

Body language is a complex communication process. It involves unconscious use of posture, gestures, and other forms of nonverbal communication. It is possible to **contradict** a verbal message by an inappropriate or **incongruous** facial expression. Even when a person says nothing and thinks that the message being sent is positive, body language will send the true message. When a person says, for instance, "I'm OK," and you see the person grimacing with pain, the conflicting message shows through.

Facial Expression

Part of perception is being aware of how others think you feel, or see you. You create this impression partly by your facial expression. The most common example of a positive, happy facial expression is a smile (Figure 4-3). This nonverbal signal conveys a positive attitude. Frowning and looking glum only add to other people's troubles. It is especially important to be pleasant and friendly to those seeking medical attention, because their worries concerning their condition are already on their minds. Adding your troubles to theirs is highly inappropriate. A positive attitude and a receptive awareness will show in your facial expression.

Eye contact shows that you are interested in giving and receiving messages of mutual concern and interest. It has been said that the eyes are the windows of the soul. Looking into another's eyes while engaging in conversation permits an open, honest transmission of thoughts and ideas. Looking away while people are talk-

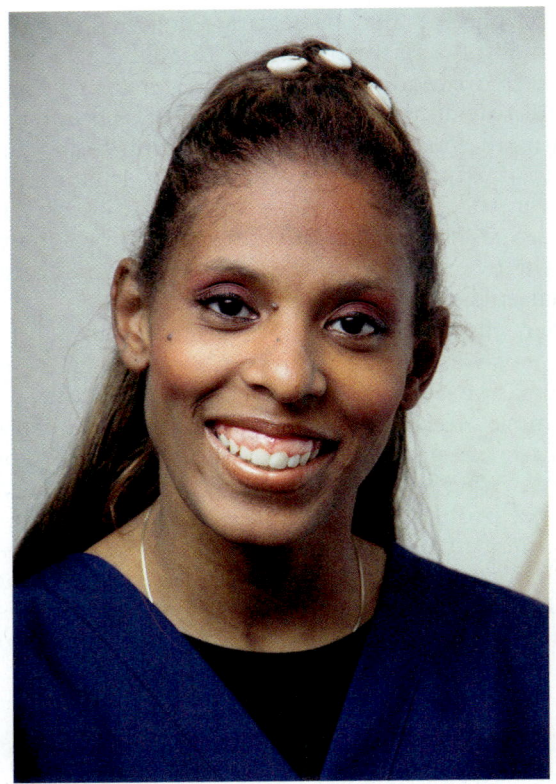

FIGURE 4-3 Smiling conveys a positive attitude.

ing to you makes them feel that what they are saying is not important. Interest and attention soon disappear and the intent of your message may be distorted or lost.

Gestures

Still another way of transmitting nonverbal messages is by gesturing. Gestures are body movements that enhance what is being said. You may know people who seemingly could not talk if they had to sit on their hands. Try to follow their example. Using hand and body gestures to accentuate a point can help the receiver understand your meaning. To emphasize the subject matter in conversation, gestures help to convey the message (Figure 4-4).

In your dealings with patients you will encounter many people who are from different cultures, countries, and social backgrounds. Some gestures, facial expressions, or remarks may be offensive to them. Use caution when you are not sure of a remark or gesture; it may be taken the wrong way. It is a good practice to have an interpreter for patients who do not speak the same language that you do. You can ask the interpreter to explain those things that you are not sure of and to alert you to those things you should be careful of in dealing with patients in the future.

There are many gestures that we use daily that have become such a part of our personalities that we do not

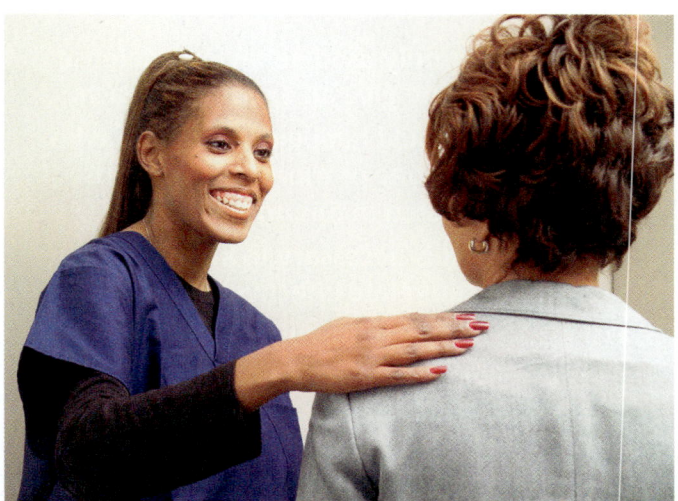

FIGURE 4-4 Gestures are a way to transmit nonverbal messages.

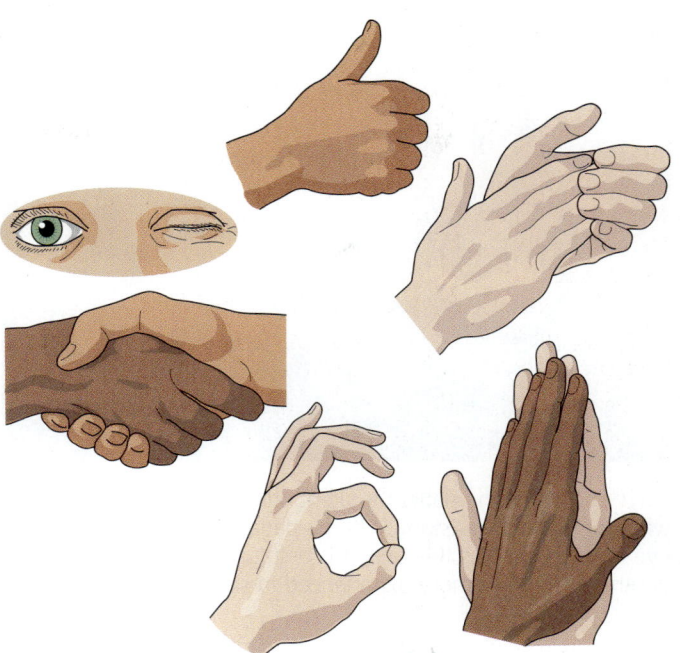

FIGURE 4-5 Common positive gestures (clockwise, from top): thumbs up, applause, high-five, okay, handshake, and winking. Note that some gestures may not be perceived as positive to persons from other cultures or backgrounds.

even realize we do them anymore. Some of them are positive and some are not. Some that are positive and very popular are thumbs up, okay, high-five, applause, winking, and a handshake. These are all ways of showing signs of acceptance, encouragement, appreciation, and friendliness (Figure 4-5). If you pay attention, the intended message is clearly understood without saying anything at all. Some of the ways of telling if a person is upset or not interested (negative body language) are crossed arms, looking at one's watch, rolling of the eyes, tapping of the foot or fingers, sighing, and talking under one's breath. And there are still other gestures that are very rude and socially unacceptable. Usually it helps to ignore the patient who seeks attention by using this type of behavior. If this is not effective, it may be necessary to call for assistance from a supervisor, security, or the police if nothing else works. It should not be a part of your job description to put up with verbal or physical abuse of any kind. If the patient is mentally ill or is under the influence of drugs or alcohol, a certain amount of understanding and tolerance must be employed by all. However, seeking assistance in these situations before a problem escalates is always recommended.

A handshake is a sign of friendship. Another meaningful body movement is a hug to convey feelings of warmth and affection. A comforting touch helps patients feel that you care and gives them a sense of security and acceptance. Studies have shown that patients who have been touched, by a hand on the shoulder or a hand held, respond significantly better in treatment than those not touched. Patting someone on the back and saying "Good for you" is a positive reinforcer. You might do that in praise of a patient who followed the prescribed treatment of the physician and lost 10 pounds and who needs positive recognition of these achievements to encourage con-

tinued compliance. There are, however, patients who may be offended by your touching them or whose religious beliefs, culture, or ethnic origin do not allow this. When touching patients in the office to offer comfort or praise, do so in the presence of other professionals for your protection against possible misunderstandings. This will safeguard you from being unfairly accused of touching someone inappropriately.

There is also a proper distance you should maintain when speaking to others. If you are engaged in a personal conversation, the accepted space between two people is from 1.5 to 4 feet. For social conversation among people, the distance between people is from 4 to 12 feet, which is about the distance at which you and your patients will be communicating. In a public setting the space can be 12 to 25 feet. Keep in mind that touch, gestures, and language barriers are important considerations when communicating with patients.

In reinforcing a patient's actions, you should display a positive attitude, facial expression, gestures, and eye contact—all the communication skills so far mentioned. In addition, your tone of voice should be happy and sincere. Patients who believe you are pleased with their progress are more willing to strive to follow future treatment because of the resulting positive feelings.

Another powerful nonverbal communication tool is silence. This method can indeed be most frustrating for the person to whom it is directed. In dealing with

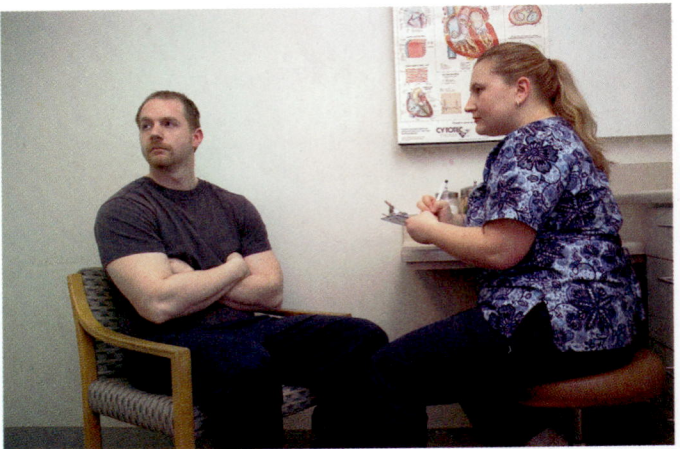

FIGURE 4-6   The patient is silent and is avoiding eye contact with the medical assistant. When a patient is silent and avoids eye contact, such as this one, it is helpful to solicit help from another individual more experienced in such situations.

patients who exhibit this nonverbal way of communicating, it is best if the inexperienced medical assistant asks for help from a supervisor, a physician, or another staff member who has skill in dealing with this type of situation (Figure 4-6). Patients who exhibit behavior such as this may have serious underlying problems.

ACHIEVE UNIT OBJECTIVES

■ Complete the Workbook activities to meet the learning objectives.

■ Apply your knowledge at the end of this chapter in completing the Critical Thinking Challenge and Activities, as well as the StudyWARE on your Student CD-ROM.

UNIT 2
BEHAVIORAL ADJUSTMENTS

OBJECTIVES

Upon completion of this unit, you will be able to achieve the following:

LEARNING Objectives

1. Spell and define, using the glossary at the back of the text, all the Words to Know in this unit.

2. List the commonly used behavioral defense mechanisms and give an example of each.

3. Explain what could happen to a person who habitually uses one or more of the defense mechanisms listed in this unit.

4. Explain why it is necessary to know yourself before you can relate effectively to others.

5. List problem-solving steps, and apply them to a particular problem you may have.

6. Explain the importance of mental and emotional status in regard to overall health.

WORDS TO KNOW

adjustment	intellectualization	repression
analytical	malinger	strategem
ardently	projection	sublimation
compensation	rationalization	suppression
denial	regression	unobtrusive
displacement		

CERTIFICATION CONNECTION

CMA
Adapting communication to an individual's ability to understand
Recognizing and responding to verbal and nonverbal communication
Professional communication and behavior

Evaluating and understanding communication
Interviewing techniques

RMA
Interpersonal relations

CMAS
Medical office clerical assisting—communication

We discussed in Unit 1 of this chapter how keeping a positive attitude is of primary importance in our interactions with others. Even though we strive for a good rapport with coworkers, patients, family, and friends, we must realize that we are human beings. Perfection in any relationship, even the best one, is certainly a desirable goal but is rather unrealistic. Understanding ourselves and others is essential in meaningful communications. Often in our daily transactions of conveying and receiving messages, we use certain coping skills to keep ourselves from getting hurt or to protect our image. These complex **strategems** are called defense mechanisms.

DEFENSE MECHANISMS

These defenses are largely unconscious acts we use to help us deal with unpleasant and socially unacceptable circumstances or behaviors. They help us make an emotional **adjustment** in everyday situations. Surely we all use various defense mechanisms from time to time. However, habitual use can cause one to become somewhat out of touch with reality.

Repression

The most commonly used defense mechanism is **repression**, which is the forcing of unacceptable or painful ideas, feelings, and impulses into the unconscious mind without being aware of it. Certainly, we have all wished something unpleasant would happen to another person when we have experienced feelings of hostility, jealousy, or intense anger from interacting with that person. These feelings do not vanish but are placed in our unconscious and may surface in dreams or subtle **unobtrusive** behaviors.

Repression, like all of the defense mechanisms, tends to protect us from unwanted messages about ourselves that make us feel bad.

Suppression

Suppression is a term to describe a condition in which the person becomes purposely involved in a project, hobby, or work so that a painful situation can be avoided. There are those who, rather than face a difficult problem within a relationship, for instance, throw themselves into their work so much that there is little or no time for the relationship. This is a good way to avoid communication because the legitimate "work" has to be done. However, people only fool themselves until something has to be done to relieve the stress this kind of behavior causes.

Displacement

Displacement is the transfer of emotions about one person or situation to another. A typical example of displacement for the medical assistant might be as follows: In the course of the day, a medical assistant has many duties to perform for many others, and one patient in particular becomes overly demanding and rude. The medical assistant holds back the strong feelings that arise and deals with the situation professionally. Later in the evening at home, the medical assistant feels all the pent-up anger surface and explodes at a family member. Although this is done unconsciously, after the fact the medical assistant realizes that actions have been displaced from where they originated to an innocent, unsuspecting target.

Projection

In **projection**, you might unconsciously blame another person for your own inadequacies. An extreme form of projection can lead to hostile, even aggressive behavior if you perceive another person to be the cause of the painful feelings. For example, an obese patient who has gained a few pounds may blame the medical assistant by saying that the scales were set up or read incorrectly.

Rationalization

With **rationalization**, you justify behavior with socially acceptable reasons and tend to ignore the real reasons underlying the behavior. This self-disciplined, unconscious act is relatively harmless. However, habitual use of this defense mechanism, as well as all the others discussed in this unit, can become nonproductive or even destructive because they distort reality. A typical rationalization might be, "I dieted strictly all day; therefore, it's okay to eat a couple of candy bars later in the evening after supper."

Intellectualization

Intellectualization is still another means of denying socially unacceptable feelings or strong feelings that cannot be easily expressed. With this mechanism, you use reasoning to avoid confronting emotional conflicts and stressful situations. For example, you might discuss all the facts and provide endless information about how to begin caring for an elderly relative, elaborating on special diets and home health care to avoid dealing with the true feelings of sadness that may accompany the person's illness.

Sublimation

Sublimation is used unconsciously to express socially unacceptable instinctive drives or impulses in approved and acceptable ways. An example of sublimation might be a 30-year-old father who is a frustrated athlete forcing his child to excel in a sport. Or, an artist may unconsciously direct sexual impulses in the form of constructive writing, sculpture, painting, or photography.

Compensation

Compensation is somewhat similar to sublimation in that it is positive. When you use this defense mechanism, you use a talent or an attribute to the fullest to compensate for a realized personal shortcoming. For example, a person who can no longer participate in sports because of illness or injury may find satisfaction in writing about the game, helping with coaching, or becoming an ardent fan of a well-known team.

Temporary Withdrawal

Temporary withdrawal is a defense mechanism that is a retreat from facing a painful or difficult situation. This avoidance of something that is unpleasant is another way of protecting ourselves from disagreeable feelings. Watching TV or reading excessively to avoid dealing with an issue are common types of withdrawal.

Putting off issues only makes the situation worse. As withdrawal goes on, it produces anxiety and makes the problem more difficult to face.

Daydreaming

A healthy type of temporary withdrawal that all of us do from time to time is daydreaming. This is a way to momentarily escape from reality and relax. At times, you can become very creative and return refreshed from daydreams. If, however, this form of escape is done too often and for too long, it becomes unhealthy and should be of concern.

Malingering

Another common defense mechanism is **malingering**. When you malinger, you deliberately pretend to be sick to avoid dealing with situations that are unpleasant or cause anxiety. A malingering individual might stay home sick on a day when he or she was to give a presentation, when in fact that person is not sick and is actually enjoying the time at home.

Denial

Denial seems to be a commonly used defense mechanism. It is the refusal to admit or acknowledge something so that you do not have to deal with a problem or situation. When you are not accepting the phases of life that may produce anxiety, you sometimes use denial as an emotional defense. Denial is usually seen only in psychosis in adults who have reacted to a traumatic situation of extreme stress.

When one who has been given the diagnosis of a terminal illness does not accept the reality of it and believes that a recovery is certain, that person is going through the denial stage.

Regression

Regression is behaving in ways that are typically characteristic of an earlier developmental level. This usually happens in times of high stress.

For example, a college student consoles herself during final exam week with eating hot fudge sundaes as she did as a child with her mother whenever problems at school piled up. Occasionally we may see someone regress to sucking their thumbs or twirling their hair when they are stressed or very tired.

Indeed, we all use many and perhaps all of these defense mechanisms from time to time. Because they are mostly used without conscious awareness, they may be relatively harmless. However, habitual use of defense mechanisms can veil reality and interfere with facing personal issues and crises, as well as with open and honest communication with others.

Procrastination

This defense mechanism is a threat to us all. It robs us of time and energy if we let it become a habit. Procrastination is defined as "always putting off until tomorrow what you could do today." This is surely familiar to you. There is nothing wrong with doing as much as you can within reason and ability in a day and leaving some things to do the next day. The problem with procrastination is that it becomes easier to put off more tasks. This creates stress on the job for you and coworkers because there is so much to do the next day, and catching up is difficult. Occasional procrastination is understandable, but if it becomes a habit, it is detrimental to your character and your workload. Coworkers will not be pleased to always bail you out because you never complete your work on time. You must be aware of this and not give in to a habit of procrastinating so that you will be more productive.

PROBLEM SOLVING

In our complex daily lives, we use many coping skills to deal with our difficulties. Defense mechanisms have already been discussed. Another approach to handling interpersonal problems and concerns is to develop problem-solving skills. Taking a step-by-step approach helps one look realistically and logically at a problem. This method encourages **analytical** thinking and confident decision making.

The basic steps in problem solving are:

1. Determine just what the problem is and write it down. Ask if there is a problem chain or a series of events that is a contributor.
2. Gather facts and ideas to help you decide what to do about it.
3. Use analytical and creative thinking. (List your decisions and what you think their outcome will be.)
4. Prioritize your decisions and begin testing them one by one until results are satisfactory to you and others concerned.

If results are not pleasing, begin again with step one. Often, step one alone triggers an answer to a problem. Sitting down and writing out what the problem actually is can be most therapeutic. Once you begin to use this skill to think logically about major problems, such as changing employment, relocating geographically, or locating a suitable day care facility, you will begin to think more logically in all matters. Making a habit of this skill will increase your peace of mind and reduce stress because you will deal with problems more efficiently and spend less time and energy worrying about what to do. This skill can be a great stride toward eliminating procrastination.

The medical assistant who concentrates on patient education may want to pass this helpful skill on to patients.

MENTAL AND EMOTIONAL STATUS INFLUENCING BEHAVIORS

Medical assistants, in both administrative and clinical capacities, have many opportunities daily to observe patients' mental and emotional states. These observations have a direct influence on the medical assistants' behaviors, which in turn directly influence their overall health. We must keep in mind that all medical personnel are patients too. Therefore, all of the information we learn about patients applies to us as well.

Stress in life can lead to ill health. A true understanding of one's self is the primary key to understanding others.

Learning about yourself requires you to take a good hard look at who and what you really are. When assessing your "self," your individual presence may come to mind first. This presence comprises both your physical self (your body) and your self-image (how you view yourself). Another aspect of self, as termed by psychologists, is the "self-as-process." This refers to the ongoing process inside each of us that deals with constant changes, or adjustments, in our lives.

Your response to others is dealt with by your social self. You have many different roles with which you identify **ardently**. Finally, you have an "ideal self." This is what you picture yourself to be—the perfect model you have of yourself.

We are, indeed, complex beings, capable of doing just about anything we choose. Unfortunately, many of us never come close to realizing our true potential. This may be due to never having to look at ourselves squarely. Sometimes it can be quite difficult and even unpleasant to be honest about ourselves.

A good way to begin a basic assessment of yourself is by making a list of all the strengths you have, as well as all your weaknesses. This technique can help point out your abilities and qualities and identify areas that need to be changed. Keeping a journal or a diary, even if only temporarily, is another way to vent feelings, look at problems, and realize and assess your behavior patterns to better know your true self.

An ideal time to reevaluate yourself and renew your goals and aspirations is annually on your birthday. Many people prefer the traditional New Year's resolution. Knowing yourself will help you become a more complete person and will help you relate to others more effectively.

COMMUNICATING EMOTIONAL STATES

In Unit 1 of this chapter, we discussed verbal and nonverbal messages. Communication is a complex process, and one must be aware of all of its facets so that complete information exchange may occur.

The perceptive medical assistant should be able to decide what "feeder questions" to ask a patient to determine whether the look on the patient's face matches the patient's emotional demeanor. The following are feeder questions the medical assistant may use to find out the emotional states of the patients they interview. After greeting the patient with a kind "hello," the medical assistant may want to ask "What seems to be the problem today?" or "What brings you here to see the doctor today?" or "Can you tell me about the problem you seem to be having?" or "Can we talk about what has been giving you concern that brings you in to see the doctor?"

For a follow-up visit, ask "Are you feeling any better since you were in to see the doctor last?" or "You don't seem to be feeling too well; do you feel any better?" or "Can you tell me how you've been doing since you were here last?"

Hearing patients' answers can provide a general idea of how they feel emotionally. Of course, one can only accomplish this by taking time to find out. That means giving the patients your undivided attention, if only for a few minutes. Unfortunately, many health care professionals lack the skills and perhaps even the concern to establish this rapport, and therefore fail to develop this skill. Remember that the manner in which you speak, your tone of voice, and your body language convey your attitude. Make sure that you show professionalism and compassion when you serve all patients. The medical assistant can be instrumental in pointing out factors that can interfere with a particular treatment approach planned by the physician (Figure 4-7). Patients will likely respond to and comply with the doctor's orders far more readily if the medical assistant imparts a genuine concern for their well-being with each contact.

If a patient seems quieter than usual, you may determine after talking to the patient (with eye contact, of course) that the patient is preoccupied by some problem or matter that he or she will reveal if you show interest and take time to listen. Often a statement that begins with "I" can open up a conversation with another

1. Travel (business or pleasure)
2. Work schedule (irregular hours)
3. Relocating/moving
4. Lifestyle/cultural influences
5. Economic concerns
6. Comprehension of physician's orders
7. Disability/mental incompetence
8. Being unclear about the directions or the importance of the treatment plan

FIGURE 4-7 Factors that can interfere with patient compliance in treatment plans

person. For instance, you may say to a patient, "I noticed as you were walking in today that you don't seem to be as lively as usual. Is anything in particular bothering you?" This gives patients a feeling that you really pay attention to them, that you care about how they are, and that you are showing it. This can make the patient feel more at ease and may gain better compliance with the physician's orders. If the patient is not allowed to express certain feelings, he or she may not be attentive enough to listen to the physician's orders, which need to be followed for optimal health benefits. The medical assistant plays an important role in assisting both physician and patient in providing quality health care.

Using the statements that begin with "I" can be of help to the health care team as well. You can also use an "I" statement with a coworker, such as, "I noticed that the filing is getting piled up; need some help?" This way of offering help is much easier to answer with a positive response because the person is not being accused of doing a poor job of filing. The blame falls on the volume of filing, not the coworker. When conversing with coworkers it is important to speak sincerely and to communicate your feelings as professionally as you do with patients. This can prevent a serious situation because the habit of giving and expecting respect and courtesy has been established.

UNIT 3
PATIENTS AND THEIR FAMILIES

OBJECTIVES

Upon completion of this unit, you will be able to achieve the following:

LEARNING Objectives

1. Spell and define, using the glossary at the back of the text, all the Words to Know in this unit.
2. Explain why it is important to develop rapport with patients and their families.
3. Describe means of safeguarding the patient's right to confidentiality.
4. Describe the patient's options in relation to the physician's treatment plan.
5. Describe the stages that follow diagnosis of a terminal illness.
6. Describe your role in dealing with the terminally ill patient.
7. Explain the purpose of the living will.
8. State the purpose of the hospice movement.
9. List the services of the hospice movement.

WORDS TO KNOW

absurd	holistic	living will
advance directives	hospice movement	marginal nonchalant
commiserate	hostility	solace
devastate	incomprehensible	terminal
fortitude	inevitable	

ACHIEVE UNIT OBJECTIVES

- Complete the Workbook activities to meet the learning objectives.
- Apply your knowledge at the end of this chapter in completing the Critical Thinking Challenge and Activities, as well as the StudyWARE on your Student CD-ROM.

CERTIFICATION CONNECTION

CMA
Adapting communication to an individual's ability to understand
Recognizing and responding to verbal and nonverbal communication

Patient instruction
Professional communication and behavior
Evaluating and understanding communication
Interviewing techniques

RMA	**CMAS**
Interpersonal relations	Medical office clerical assisting—communication

The medical profession's first responsibility is to the patient. Thus you must be able to relate to people of all ages, from tiny infants to senior citizens. The development and growth of your own personality and interests will help you do so.

The ability to converse about a variety of subjects shows an interest in people and makes you interesting to be with. Conversation with patients helps to ease their anxieties and encourage a sense of friendship and trust. At times a patient needs to express pent-up feelings, and you will often be the one who provides this necessary listening service. Sincere empathy will often begin to relieve the inner fears and anxieties of a patient who is experiencing an illness for the first time.

Patients and family members may need to discuss again the treatment plan the physician has already discussed with them. Often patients do not hear all of what has been said by the physician because they have been preoccupied with worry about their illness. Their questions may sometimes seem trivial, but to the patient they are real and pressing issues that need immediate attention. Be mindful of those patients who are disabled, are from another culture, or speak another language. Offer compassion as best as possible when conversing with them about patient care. An interpreter should be scheduled to translate for the patient and family members if no family member speaks English. Provide translators with printed patient education materials that they can review with the patient.

This is the reason that giving printed instructions to patients is so important. If the patient is preoccupied when the instructions are given, printed material is also given to the patient, who can read the information later. Usually a phone call will be initiated by the patient at a later time to have questions answered or for clarification or reassurance about something.

Many patients have never before experienced sickness or injury. They may never have set foot in a health care facility. Having to face strange new surroundings, unfamiliar medical language, and possibly puzzling procedures will add to a patient's apprehensions. The way the patient is treated in these new situations will determine how the patient and members of the family accept the diagnosis and prognosis of the patient's condition. Tact and good communication skills will help to promote rapport with all patients and their family members.

RIGHT TO PRIVACY

Refer to Chapter 3 for a review of privacy practices. Medical information may be given to parties not concerned in the patient's treatment *only* when the patient has signed a release of information form. Medical insurance forms, for instance, have a section patients must sign to authorize the release of information to insurance companies (Figure 4-8). Only those persons specified in writing by the patient may receive information concerning the patient's condition. Usually the medical facility has a patient information release form, which is completed during the initial visit. Persons to contact in case of emergency are listed by the patient; this is when you should inquire about who may be informed about the patient's condition. This document should be filed in the patient's chart for future reference.

Many patients have answering machines and e-mail. You must have a signed permission form on file to leave a message on an answering machine (or voice mail) or e-mail concerning the patient. There may be others listening to or reading your message(s) before the patient retrieves the message(s), and the patient may not want the information known to others. Even a reminder of an appointment should have signed permission before a message is left. The privacy of each patient must always be protected. Those of legal age have the right to privacy in all matters of treatment, and even parents may not be given information about a family member's condition unless specific written permission accompanied by the patient's signature is secured.

RELEASE AND ASSIGNMENT

Date ______________

To ____
INSURANCE COMPANY

____

Group No. ______________ Certificate No. ______________

I hereby authorize Dr. ______________________________

to release to your company or its representative, any information including the diagnosis and the records of any treatment or examination rendered to me during the period of such Medical or Surgical care.

I also authorize and request your company to pay directly to the above named doctor the amount due me in my pending claim for Basic Medical, Major Medical and/or Surgical treatment or services, by reason of such treatment or services rendered to:

____
PATIENT

____
SIGNATURE OF INSURED

______________________ ______________________
WITNESS ADDRESS

FIGURE 4-8 Release of information form

In the normal course of conversation with a patient, you may be told personal information that should be kept to yourself, unless doing so would be harmful to the patient. The patient will usually tell you how far the information should go, or whom to tell or not to tell. Emotional stress and other critical data should be relayed to the physician, for it may have some bearing on the condition of the patient. You must use judgment in this important area. A patient who is experiencing domestic problems, for instance, may be asking for help by telling you about the situation.

There also will be patients who have no medical insurance to cover the cost of treatments or other diagnostic procedures; you should guide them to seek public assistance, if possible. Patients usually realize that professionals can put them in touch with assistance and sometimes expect that it will be forthcoming if they merely suggest that help is needed. Tact is required in handling delicate matters of this nature. Patients trust the medical profession to safeguard matters discussed in the privacy of the medical office. Directly asking each patient who may receive this confidential information and having appropriate release forms signed will ensure that the patient is aware of what has been done and will also protect you from liability.

CHOICE OF TREATMENT

Advising patients of the choices they have in the treatment of their illnesses is often part of your responsibilities. A full explanation of the diagnosis, prognosis, and options in treating the condition are given to the patient by the physician. However, some patients have a difficult time making up their minds and may need additional information and further discussion before deciding to accept a treatment plan (especially when it involves a major event such as elective surgery). There are life-threatening situations in which patients must make these decisions quickly. Often family members must help patients with these difficult decisions.

You play an integral part in reinforcing the physician's orders. You should become proficient in identifying those patients who still seem confused after leaving their conference with the physician. Restating what the physician has already said may be all you need to say to some patients to initiate their compliance. Some patients may have had trouble with the wording used by the physician and look to you to interpret. It is difficult at times to make clear to patients all that is involved in the course of treatment. Great skill in perception is essential for all health care team members to ascertain if the treatment approach is fully understood by the patient. Perception is a valuable skill that takes time and experience to master.

It is prudent to advise patients to seek a second opinion if they harbor any doubts concerning their condition. It may be that patients disbelieve the diagnosis.

Having a second, or even a third, opinion will help them to accept their illness. Many insurance companies encourage patients to seek other opinions before treatment is initiated. This is wise, especially if the patient is troubled about the possible outcome.

Patients still may have difficulty in complying with physicians' orders (e.g., regarding weight reduction, exercising, or taking prescribed medicine). Patients must be given sound reasons for following the advice of the physician even though they already know that it is for their own good. The prescribed treatment plan will most likely change the patient's lifestyle. The patient who has just been diagnosed as hypertensive may have to cope with several lifestyle changes, such as losing weight, following a special diet, and giving up cigarettes. If reinforcement and encouragement are not sufficiently provided to the patient by members of the health care team, cooperation may be **marginal**. The risks of not following the physician's advice should be outlined in the simplest terms. Acting **nonchalant** or showing no interest in the patient will not be much help in prompting a patient to follow orders.

The final choice whether to accept and follow the outlined plan of treatment is always the patient's. Knowing what is best does not always dictate compliance. Motivation is the key. Giving patients realistic suggestions can help them accept a treatment plan that may initially have seemed impossible to follow. Changing behavior will probably be resisted. The patient who experiences setbacks, who does not remember to take medication, or who breaks away from the prescribed diet will need additional encouragement to get back on track. You can be of particular value in this type of situation. You must always be reinforcing with your remarks made to patients concerning the intended goals of treatment. Furthermore, by being a good role model, you subtly reinforce the physician's advice. An assistant who should be but is not following a weight-reduction plan will give a negative impression to a patient who has just been told to do so by the physician. A patient who has been instructed by the physician in personal hygiene will be less likely to follow advice if the medical assistant does not also heed the advice.

In conversing with patients you will find that their areas of interest will prompt ideas for encouraging compliance with treatment. One good motivator is the physician's fee for services. Many patients quickly realize that they should follow the physician's advice, for it will certainly be more costly in the long run if they do not.

Approach-Avoidance Conflict

Approach-avoidance behavior protects one from reaching a set goal that seems too difficult to complete. This is a personal conflict and can cause one considerable stress. The person wants to reach a goal, but keeps avoiding the final step of the plan. Think of the patient who makes an appointment for the removal of a mass in the colon. The patient schedules the appointment, yet when the time comes for it, the patient cancels because he or she fears that the surgical biopsy will reveal cancerous tissue. Every time a person who has approach-avoidance conflict sets a goal or makes a plan of some magnitude, the outcome is that the person does not follow through because of fear of the end result.

TERMINAL ILLNESS

Dealing with patients who have been diagnosed as having a **terminal** illness is a challenging and rewarding experience: challenging because of its difficulty and rewarding because of the knowledge that you are giving supportive care when patients and their families need it most.

Many patients have a hard time accepting the diagnosis. Their initial reaction is to deny it. Indeed, knowing that one's life is about to end is an almost **incomprehensible** fact. Patients wrestling with this new reality claim that the diagnosis is **absurd**, but ignoring the problem cannot provide **solace**.

As frustration mounts and anger becomes apparent, patients may feel isolated, for they see others as the picture of health. Feelings of **hostility** are natural and **inevitable**. Patients in this plight may lash out at anyone with whom they come in contact. Blaming themselves and others becomes a means of dealing with their anger for a time. Questioning becomes a way of venting anger for some. "Why does this have to be?" is the most troublesome question. Following this stage of anger is a period of depression. This is the reaction to the final realization of the course of their illness. Patients in this stage are usually ready to talk about their illness, hoping someone will understand. It is a difficult subject to talk about, but you may be influential in helping them to respond and talk about their fears. Eventually patients attempt to accept the terminal illness by bargaining, or seeking ways of "buying" more time. This sometimes gives them inner strength to live a while longer: they are holding on to see someone be married, wanting to hold the new grandchild, or waiting for someone to return from the service. In this stage of bargaining, patients may look for spiritual inspiration. The zest for life is strong, and the fight is one not easily given up.

In the final stages of terminal disease, patients come closer to accepting the course of their disease. This is truly a sad time for patients and their families. To know that one may not see the next spring, or to know that one will no longer experience the joys and pleasures of loved ones, can be **devastating** to the patient. Empathy and genuine compassion may be offered to a patient who is reaching out for comfort. You will be touched deeply, and your **fortitude** will be challenged to the maximum in interacting with the patient and family members during this most stressful time (Figure 4-9).

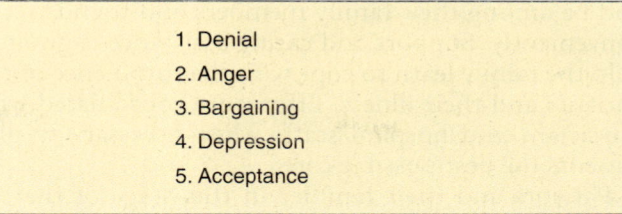

1. Denial
2. Anger
3. Bargaining
4. Depression
5. Acceptance

FIGURE 4-9   The stages of terminal illness

Finally, patients resign themselves to impending death. An inner peace is often evident in patients in this final stage of their illness, and they are more willing to make plans for their final days.

Some patients prefer to spare family members the ordeal of prolonging treatment when their physicians reach the decision that death is likely to occur in the near future. Late in 1991 a law was passed in the United States that requires all health care providers to inform and advise patients and their families of **advance directives**. The **living will** is a legal document that allows patients to terminate medical procedures that would sustain their lives if they became unconscious or unable to make further decisions. This document is not recognized in all states in the United States, but it is fast becoming a more acceptable way for patients to let others know when they want to have their life support discontinued. Advance directives also refers to the living will because it gives direction to those who will be following the wishes of the patient who prepared the legal document. With this legal form, the patient can state exactly how far lifesaving efforts should go or can establish a do not resuscitate (DNR) order. This documentation helps the patient and family avoid an agonizingly long period in waiting for the inevitable.

When the patient signs this document, a copy should be filed with the physician, the attorney, and the family. In assisting patients with this procedure, it is helpful if you remind them to make sure that all details have been worked out and that the family has been properly informed about who is responsible for honoring the document. Patients now know that they have a right to die with dignity and that they have a choice in making their last days of life more meaningful.

For many years a concerned group of individuals has recognized and **commiserated** with grief-stricken, terminally ill people. This concerned group has formed the **hospice movement** to provide some health care to those with terminal illness. In recent years the hospice movement has gained strength. Instead of the tiring and impersonal surroundings that are sometimes associated with hospital care, hospice helps the family provide care so that patients can remain in their comfortable, familiar home surroundings during the last days of their lives and be among their family members and friends more conveniently. Support and caring assistance is given to help the family learn to cope with the turbulence of the patients and their illness. Efforts are coordinated with physicians and hospital staffs when necessary to give patients the best possible care.

Patients and their families in this stage of the patient's illness may need more spiritual guidance. The counsel of a minister, priest, or rabbi may also be found through hospice, because **holistic** care is the purpose of the hospice movement. Once the patient has been informed by the physician that he or she has a terminal illness, you should refer patients to the local hospice movement for consultation.

Society is returning to the idea that there is a human need to share the experiences of birth and death with loved ones. These natural parts of life have been largely removed from our experience for some time now. We have even become uneasy in talking about them. The need for human love during significant times is evident in the return to the practice of entering and leaving this world at home.

ACHIEVE UNIT OBJECTIVES

- ☐ Complete the Workbook activities to meet the learning objectives.
- ☐ Apply your knowledge at the end of this chapter in completing the Critical Thinking Challenge and Activities, as well as the StudyWARE on your Student CD-ROM.

UNIT 4
OFFICE INTERPERSONAL RELATIONSHIPS

OBJECTIVES

Upon completion of this unit, you will be able to achieve the following:

LEARNING Objectives

1. Spell and define, using the glossary at the end of the text, all the Words to Know in this unit.
2. Describe relationships between the medical assistant, the employer, and coworkers.

3. List positive methods for dealing with stress.
4. Describe the reasons for staff meetings.
5. Explain methods of intraoffice communication.
6. State the purpose of an employee evaluation.
7. Describe the obligations of the employer and the new employee in providing a smooth transition in the workplace.

WORDS TO KNOW

description	obligation	petty
evaluation	perplexing	transition
externship		

CERTIFICATION CONNECTION

CMA
Professional communication and behavior
Evaluating and understanding communication
Maintaining the physical plant—personnel
Office policies and procedures

RMA
Interpersonal relations

CMAS
Medical office clerical assisting—communication

The medical assistant employed in a medical office or clinic must learn to positively relate not only to patients but to other members of the health care team as well. Dealing with the needs of patients on a day-to-day basis can sometimes become an overwhelming task. Schedules in most medical practices can easily become overbooked; sometimes it seems everyone has an emergency and must be seen by the physician today! Health care employees should be able to shift gears and handle these situations gracefully and efficiently. The essential ingredient in running a medical office smoothly is cooperation. When each employee contributes, the result is a good team that works together for quality patient care.

The field of medicine is by its nature stress-filled. Patients are troubled by an abnormal state of health and are naturally anxious and on edge. They may exhibit their feelings by acting irritable and uncooperative at times. They not only expect but demand patience and understanding from medical personnel.

STAFF ARRANGEMENTS

Picture the ideal medical office where patients and medical staff are going about the business at hand in a pleasant, efficient manner. Everyone gets along well with everyone else, patients are smiling and friendly, and every interchange is courteous. The schedule is kept down to the minute, all the filing is caught up, the phone rings only when there is nothing else pressing at the moment, referral reports are all back, and everything runs like clockwork. This picture is unreal. This ideal situation is what every medical practice hopes to achieve, but to bring this model practice into existence would require the perfection of all persons involved. This is, of course, impossible. Nevertheless, each member of the staff has a unique set of values, principles, and standards, and each must respect the others to ensure compatible relationships.

The number of employees varies in each type of medical practice. Some physicians in private practice employ only one medical assistant to perform both administrative and clinical duties. This is a tremendous responsibility and requires a highly motivated and mature personality. A medical assistant's compensation may sometimes seem minimal when the job includes long hours and limited benefits. A good rapport with the employer is necessary to accomplish the objectives of daily patient care. Usually a good friendship develops between the physician and medical assistant over time, and working together is an enjoyable learning experience for both. Interest in each patient is easy to cultivate since individual contact is made at each office visit. You may get to know patients even better than the physician because of frequent phone conversations with patients. You will soon become the physician's right hand by supplying important patient information obtained in this manner.

Communication lines must remain open with this one-to-one relationship, as in all employer-employee relationships. If misunderstandings occur, they must be rectified as soon as possible. More complex problems can mushroom if incidental misunderstandings are not cleared up. Solutions to these problems must be worked out together. You will have to be assertive in decisions concerning administrative, clinical, and personal employment matters. Being on one's own as a medical assistant in a private practice has its rewards as well as its disadvantages.

Many physicians in both private and group practices find it necessary to employ several medical assistants. Although this can be an enjoyable experience for all members of the staff, a great deal of cooperation and respect for one another is necessary for a harmonious relationship among the staff members to be maintained. Specific job **descriptions** encourage each employee to remain in a particular area to promote efficiency. Overstepping boundaries may cause friction and misunderstandings; at the same time, all staff members must be willing to pitch in where help is needed. Again, a positive attitude is needed to create a pleasant work environment.

The physician usually delegates responsibility for office management to one of the employees, most often the one with greatest seniority, qualifications, or both. This frees the physician to attend to patients and also relieves the physician of personnel management. This is a major area of importance, especially in large clinics with many employees, and, as a rule, it is an area physicians are not trained to handle. Often these supervisory or personnel management positions are filled by registered nurses, but they also have little or no specific training in medical office management. Their training centers primarily around the hospital model and direct patient care. Since a trained medical assistant can, in most states, perform most of the procedures that a nurse can, under the supervision of a physician, resentment may arise. You must come to grips with this reality before accepting a position where it may be a source of irritation and discontent.

Physicians and office managers appreciate the versatility of the medical assistant, respect their initiative and industriousness, and employ them with pride and satisfaction (Figure 4-10). However, each medical practice has its own unique office policy regarding employees. There are some physicians who would rather take charge of their own office business affairs.

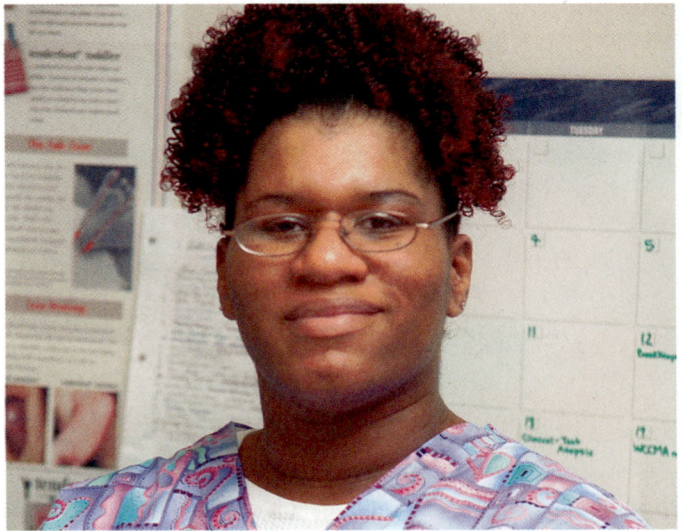

FIGURE 4-10 The medical assistant is a versatile member of the office staff.

Working closely with others can have both positive and negative effects. In a large office practice or clinic, when there are many employees, a certain amount of give and take must prevail. Completing assigned tasks is expected so that the work is shared equitably. **Petty** differences should be settled with tact. Sharing enlightening experiences and significant events with other employees is a natural inclination. This is fine if it does not interfere with patient care. A certain amount of self-discipline and self-control is necessary in a professional setting. Remaining aware of the situation at hand will help you perceive what is appropriate.

INTRAOFFICE COMMUNICATION

Many physicians hold regular staff meetings that all employees are expected to attend. They are usually held in the medical office either before or after patients have been seen and are announced far enough in advance so that arrangements can be made to attend. Many staff meetings are scheduled at regular times (e.g., the second Friday of each month, a meet-and-eat meeting at noon every other Wednesday). At these meetings decisions concerning office policy changes are reached and problems are discussed (Figure 4-11). This is a time for new ideas to be expressed and exchanged. It also allows all members of the staff to get to know each other.

Some situations between employees may be impossible to iron out. These are usually personality conflicts, and the usual course of action, if the situation does not improve, is termination of one of the employees (usually the one who is more troublesome or less valuable to the practice). This kind of **perplexing** problem may be discussed during a staff meeting. Personnel managers are often aware of these problems before they are reported, and they are usually handled privately.

Employers sometimes use office meeting time for inservice programs, such as training in cardiopulmonary resuscitation. Some employers encourage holiday celebrations on occasion to promote better working relationships.

An intraoffice memo is a means of communicating important information to members of the staff, especially between regularly scheduled staff meetings. Each employee is instructed to read the memo and initial it, indicating that the information has been received, and then pass it on to another employee. This helps ensure that all employees are informed. Word of mouth is not a sure way to relay an important announcement, for it may get distorted en route.

Some offices and clinics use a bulletin board as a means of intraoffice communication. Notices of educational programs, seminars, or meetings are posted for all members of the staff to read, in an area such as the staff room or eating area.

CAREER ENTRY

According to recent statistics, there is an increasing need for qualified medical assistants across the nation. Employers in the health care field are recognizing the benefits of employing medical assistants who have had specific training in this most versatile field. This, of course, eliminates the need for extensive and expensive additional training on the job. **Externship** plans are very successful in cooperative programs because they provide soon-to-graduate medical assistant students experience in different offices. The supervisor agrees to allow the instructor to periodically visit the facility and observe the student's performance. Other training programs not accredited by the AAMA require only that students observe for a certain number of hours to fulfill the program's standards. In either case, the trend is most welcomed following the past practice of hiring assistants without any training in the field, who sought either full-time or part-time employment in the physicians' offices or clinics.

The **transition** from student to medical assistant, at any age, poses certain adjustment considerations to all concerned in the health care setting. Employers have an **obligation** to assist the new employee in feeling accepted in the profession and to give helpful advice with patience. The new employee is obligated to strive to perform skills with both proficiency and efficiency. An effort to get along with others is required of each member of the health care team. A smooth transition with a new member of the team is possible

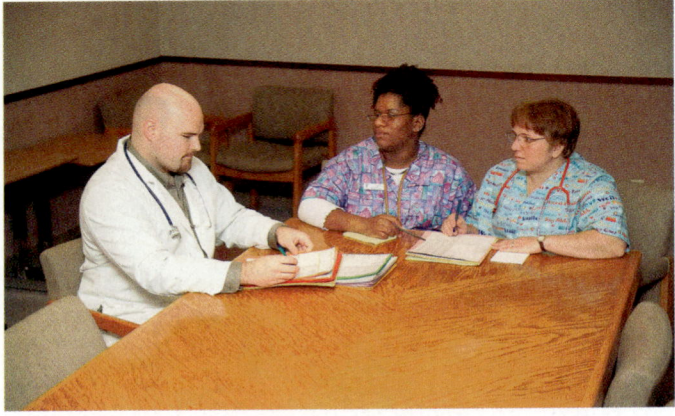

FIGURE 4-11 Physicians hold regular meetings in the office to communicate important information to the members of the staff.

if each employee recognizes the individual worth of each person and the value of each position in fulfilling the health care needs of the patients.

EMPLOYEE EVALUATION

In most employment situations, an **evaluation** of work performance is made on an annual basis. This is filed in your record. The initial employment review is usually held after a probationary period of 30, 60, or 90 days. In this meeting, you and your employer will discuss your job performance. Evaluation forms outline the most important qualities and abilities needed for the job and include a section for strengths and weaknesses to be listed. An example of an employee evaluation form can be found in Chapter 21, Unit 2, with further discussion on securing employment. Employers are always aware of an employee's behavior. Little goes unnoticed when you share a daily routine. Your attitude shows at all times. Even though the word *attitude* may not be a part of the evaluation, the other categories cover it comprehensively.

Initiative is an important factor. Demonstrating resourcefulness will help you advance in your career. Following office policy is also important. Being on time and being dependable on the job are always pleasing to employers. Absences and tardiness are difficult to tolerate from employees who make it a habit. Another area of extreme importance to employers is the quality and quantity of your work. Performing assigned tasks in a reasonable amount of time, without needing to be reminded, is a valuable trait.

The employee evaluation need not be a threat to the conscientious medical assistant. It is a time when questions about advancement and salary may be openly discussed. If you have lived up to the standards of the job, your performance should receive a favorable review.

Some employers find that annual evaluations motivate employees and keep communication lines open. Others choose not to have official evaluations, but wish employees to discuss whatever is on their mind at any time. For some office personnel this works quite well. For the private practice physician with one or two medical assistants this is usually the case.

ACHIEVE UNIT OBJECTIVES

■ Complete the Workbook activities to meet the learning objectives.

■ Apply your knowledge at the end of this chapter in completing the Critical Thinking Challenge and Activities, as well as the StudyWARE on your Student CD-ROM.

CRITICAL THINKING CHALLENGE

IMPACTING THE PATIENT, THE PRACTICE, AND YOUR CAREER

Two medical assistants are working in the same office with a family practitioner. On this particular day, they are overbooked and understaffed, and as a consequence, both medical assistants have worked through their lunch hour. Connie does not cope as well with the stressful situation as does Sammie and is short with and rude to the patients. Sammie has been pleasantly answering the phone, courteously rooming the patients, and assessing their conditions for priority. However, Sammie runs out of patience when she finds Connie in the break room, reading a magazine. When Sammie asks Connie to assist her, Connie becomes angry and tells her that she needs a break and to leave her alone.

QUESTIONS
1. What impact do Connie's actions have on the patients?
2. What impact do Connie's actions have on the practice?
3. What impact do Connie's actions have on her career?
4. What impact do Sammie's actions have on her career?

CRITICAL THINKING CHALLENGE

IMPACTING THE PATIENT, THE PRACTICE, AND YOUR CAREER

Jennifer and Brenda have just returned from lunch, laughing about a funny story they heard earlier. Jennifer, still smiling and chuckling about the funny story, brings the first patient back to an examination room. However, the patient thinks that she is laughing at him and asks her what is so funny in a sarcastic tone. Brenda hears the man's tone and comes into the room to explain about the funny story and why they have been laughing.

QUESTIONS

1. Had the patient not received an explanation of why the girls were laughing, what impact might that have had on him?
2. Had the girls not explained to the patient about the funny story, what impact could that have on the practice?
3. If the girls had not explained the circumstances to the patient, what impact, if any, would that have on their careers?

ACTIVITIES

1. Write an essay on your view of professionalism as a medical assistant. Think about how you would like to be treated as a patient and approach this from that point of view.

StudyWARE™ CHALLENGE

- Study with the flash cards for Chapter 4 to review the key terms in this chapter.
- Solve the hangman activities for Chapter 4.
- Complete the multiple choice quiz in test mode for Chapter 4.

RESOURCES

Milliken, M. E. (2004). *Understanding human behavior* (7th ed.). Clifton Park, NY: Thomson Delmar Learning.
Physicians' desk reference. (Updated annually). Oradell, NJ: Thomson Medical Economics.

WEB LINKS

www.epic.org (Electronic Privacy Information Center)
This is the web site of a public interest research center in Washington, D.C., established to focus public attention on emerging civil liberties issues and to protect privacy, the First Amendment, and constitutional values.

www.mentalhelp.net (Mental Help Net)
This web site, maintained by a psychologist, provides information on mental health, including defense mechanisms.

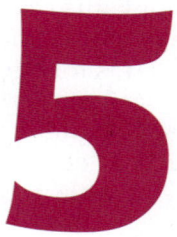

CHAPTER

5

Medical Terminology

Working in the medical field, whether administratively or clinically, demands that you have a good working knowledge of medical terminology. Medical terminology is the language dealing with health care, and as a medical assistant, you need to be able to define medical terms, build medical terms, spell correctly, and use proper application of medical terms when working with patients and other health care professionals. What seems to be a minor error on your part can adversely affect a patient's care, so developing a working relationship with this new language is essential for the success of your career.

UNIT 1
INTRODUCTION TO MEDICAL TERMINOLOGY

OBJECTIVES

Upon completion of this unit, you will be able to achieve the following:

LEARNING Objectives

1. **Spell and define, using the glossary at the back of the text, all the Words to Know in this unit.**

2. **Understand the basic principles behind medical terminology and its applications.**

3. **Gain an understanding of how to properly break medical terms apart to aid in defining their meaning.**

4. **Understand how to build medical terms using word roots or combining forms as well as modifying their meanings by adding prefixes and/or suffixes.**

5. **Receive an introduction to Greek and Latin origins of medical terms.**

WORDS TO KNOW

combining forms	suffix
prefix	word root

 ## CERTIFICATION CONNECTION

CMA
Medical terminology
- Word building and definitions
- Uses of terminology

RMA
Medical terminology
- Word parts
- Definitions
- Common abbreviations
- Spelling

CMAS
Medical terminology
- Use and spell basic medical terms appropriately
- Identify root words, prefixes, and suffixes
- Define basic medical terms

One of the most common complaints that students in medical assisting often have is that medical terminology is a new language, one that is foreign and difficult to understand. That is actually true. Most medical terms derive from Greek or Latin origins, and the Latin language is classified as a "dead" language. So, it is no wonder that students wrestle with medical terminology.

The Romans of ancient times recorded their teachings in Latin; the Romans were one of the first people to develop medical procedures, diagnoses, and treatments. About the same time, the Greek physicians were also developing medical studies and recording their findings. Thus even today, you will find that a great majority of the medical terms you encounter have either Latin or Greek foundations. For example, the Romans believed that a woman's uterus was what caused her to be moody and unpredictable, hence placing the combining form of *hyster/o* to denote that part of a woman's anatomy. They weren't that far off the mark if you carefully consider their findings—think about moods and emotions associated with the menstrual cycle (premenstrual syndrome or PMS) as well as menopause. Some terms are associated with the physician who discovered a particular part of the anatomy or a disease—the Fallopian tubes are names after Fallopius, the physician who discovered them and named them after himself. The surgical term designated for delivering a baby by other than natural means—the Cesarean section—is supposedly the manner in which Julius Ceasar was delivered into this world.

There are other cultures that have influenced medical terminology as well, but by and large, these two languages have had the greatest impact on the "language of health care." Through memorization and constant review of the **word roots**, **combining forms**, **prefixes**, and **suffixes**, you can learn this new language, but it will take some effort on your part. As you will find as you read through and practice in this chapter, there are distinct differences in the various components of medical terms. Word roots and combining forms are the part of the word that identify the structure to which the prefix and/or the suffix may be added. The difference between the word root and the combining form is that a vowel is added to the word root when necessary to make the terms easier to pronounce and more logical. The prefix is the component that goes at the *beginning* of the word to modify its meaning, and the suffix is the component that is added to the *end* of the medical term. A suffix can change a word from a noun to an adjective when added to either the word root or the combining form.

One of the best learning tools for a student is to make flash cards and refer to them often. Remember being in elementary school and using flash cards for the multiplication table? It may seem very basic for a post-secondary level, but using this type of review is very effective in imprinting medical terminology in your memory. The StudyWARE software on the CD accompanying this book offers electronic flash cards of many of these terms, but it is still a very useful tool for you as the student to make your own flash cards and concentrate on the word roots, prefixes, and suffixes that give you the most problems.

This chapter is an introduction to the world of medical terminology, meant to give you a basis on which to build your knowledge. Accept the challenge of learning this new language and talking the talk of health care!

BREAKING A MEDICAL TERM APART

When you are breaking a medical term apart in an attempt to define it, you should start with the suffix. Look at the suffix to determine its meaning. Next look to see if there is a prefix; if there is, identify the meaning of the prefix. The last step is to determine the word roots or combining forms and define them. Put all of the word components together, and you will have a very rudimentary definition of the medical term.

- Example: Define the term **hypogastric.**

You have not learned any of the components, but do not despair—just follow the example to get an idea of how the process works. First, the suffix is -*ic*, which means "pertaining to." Next, there is a prefix, *hypo-*, which means "below" or "underneath." The word root is *gastr* (the combining form would be *gastr/o*), which means stomach.

Refer to Figure 5-1, which illustrates how to put all of this together for a definition: pertaining to below the stomach. That is exactly what the term means. See how easy that was! It is just a process of learning the components and remembering the "rules."

Now try a harder one.

- Example: Define the term **otorhinolaryngologist.**

That is a long term, but do not let it intimidate you. Remember, first identify the definition of the suffix,

which is -*logist*, meaning "one who studies." This particular term does not have any prefixes, although it does contain three combining forms. *Ot/o* refers to the ears, *rhin/o* refers to the nose (think of a rhinoceros's nose with its big horn), and *laryng/o* refers to the throat; put all of this together, and you have "one who studies the ear, nose, and throat," more commonly known as an ENT specialist (ear, nose, and throat). You have probably heard of one of these specialists.

Another thing to remember is that there are several suffixes that mean the same thing, several prefixes that mean the same, and combining forms and word roots that are alike. Learning the most appropriate application of each takes time and practice. Now you are ready to try building a medical term. Once again, remember that although you have not seen or memorized the various parts that make up medical terms, the earlier you are exposed to this process, hopefully, the easier it will be for you.

> Remember the rules:
>
> - A prefix always goes to the left (front of the word) and is denoted with a hyphen to the right.
> - A suffix always goes to the right (back of the word) and is denoted with a hyphen to the left.
> - The word root or combining form is the part of the word that applies to a part of the anatomy, and there can be more than one of these in a medical term.

Use the following definition to build a medical term:

- A condition of painful urine

Remembering that you define a medical term by first identifying the suffix, start with the suffix for "condition," which is -*ia*. The next step is the prefix, as it modifies the medical term, so "painful" would be *dys-*. The final step is to identify the word root or the combining form for "urine"; since the suffix begins with a vowel, we'll choose to use the word root—it does not make sense to put two vowels together when building medical

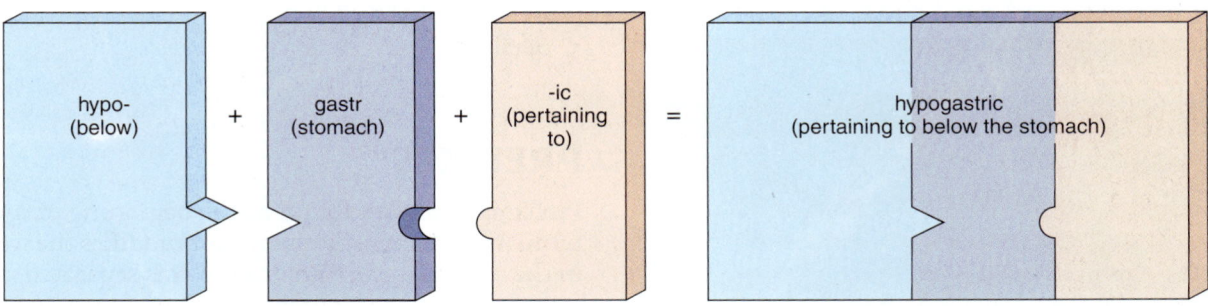

FIGURE 5-1   A medical term may be taken apart to determine its meaning. Hypogastric means "pertaining to below the stomach."

terms. The word root for "urine" is *ur*. Here is what happens when all of the various components are combined:

$$\text{dys-} + \text{ur} + \text{-ia} = \text{dysuria}$$

Now, build one that uses a combining form instead of just the word root and note the difference in how the terms are constructed. Use this definition to build the medical term:

● An inflammation of the muscle of the heart

First, identify the suffix for "inflammation," which is *-itis*. The combining form for "muscle" is *my/o*, and the combining form for "heart" is *cardi/o*. Looking at the combining forms for muscle and heart, it does not make sense to put the two combining forms together without the combining form vowel *o*; however, it is hard to pronounce and appears illogical if the combining vowel *o* is used when adding the suffix, since it begins with a vowel itself. Look at each possibility; you can see how strange one of the terms seems as opposed to the other:

$$\text{my/o} + \text{cardi/o} + \text{-itis} = \text{myocardioitis (\textbf{incorrect})}$$

or

$$\text{my/o} + \text{cardi} + \text{-itis} = \text{myocarditis (\textbf{correct})}$$

SPELLING MEDICAL TERMINOLOGY

Spelling is *very* important; misspelling a term can mean the difference in a diagnosis or treatment. Some medical terms are pronounced the same, so you need to know the application of the medical term in each of those instances in order to properly spell it in a patient's medical record. For example, *ilium* and *ileum* are pronounced identically although they are two entirely different structures. If a health care provider asks you to obtain pre-authorization for a patient to have a portion of the small intestine removed, and when completing the form, you type the term *iliectomy*, instead of the patient having a portion of the small intestine removed, this medical term would be requesting pre-authorization for the patient to have a portion of a hip bone removed! So, be very careful and attentive to your spelling.

ACHIEVE UNIT OBJECTIVES

- ■ Complete the Workbook activities to meet the learning objectives.
- ■ Apply your knowledge at the end of this chapter in completing the Critical Thinking Challenge and Activities, as well as the StudyWARE on your Student CD-ROM.

UNIT 2
PREFIXES, SUFFIXES, WORD ROOTS, AND COMBINING FORMS

OBJECTIVES

Upon completion of this unit, you will be able to achieve the following:

LEARNING Objectives

1. **Understand how prefixes alter the meaning of a medical term and be able to appropriately use prefixes with combining forms.**
2. **Understand how suffixes change a medical term and be able to appropriately use suffixes with combining forms.**
3. **Define the difference between a combining form and a word root.**
4. **Demonstrate a basic knowledge in building medical terms.**

CERTIFICATION CONNECTION

CMA
Medical Terminology
- Word building and definitions
- Uses of terminology

RMA
Medical Terminology
- Word parts
- Definitions
- Common abbreviations
- Spelling

CMAS
Medical Terminology
- Use and spell basic medical terms appropriately
- Identify root words, prefixes, and suffixes
- Define basic medical terms

PREFIXES

Prefixes are always found at the beginning of a medical term. A prefix actually changes or modifies the word root in the medical term. When a prefix is separated from the term, most often the prefix is followed by a hyphen.

To see how a prefix can change the meaning of a term when added to the beginning of a term, for instance, look at the medical term *gastric*, which means "pertaining to the stomach." If we add the prefix *hypo-* to the term, it becomes *hypogastric*; *hypo-* means "below or underneath." Thus, the term now has a definition of "pertaining to below the stomach," which is quite different than the original term with which we started. Often you will find that prefixes will indicate a location, presence or absence, quantity, size, frequency, or position. In this particular case, location is identified with the prefix *hypo-*.

Exceptions

Usually, prefixes are not altered when added to a combining form or word root; however, there are exceptions to this. A basic rule of thumb is that if the combining form/word root begins with a vowel, you would select the most appropriate prefix that is applicable that ends in a consonant. Remember, though, these are only guidelines; you will often find exceptions as you work with medical terms. Look at the following examples for a better understanding: *Uria* would be a condition of urine, and we want to build a medical term that means a condition of "no urine." The two choices for a prefix that relate to "no/without" are *a-* and *an-*. Looking at the basic guideline, the best selection for the prefix would be *an-*, making the medical term *anuria*. If the prefix of *a-* had been selected, the term would have been *auria*—doesn't that look strange? One example of changing the prefix to make the medical term easier to pronounce would be *antacid*, meaning "against acid"; it's doubtful that you have ever seen or will see the term *antiacid*, although according to the "rules" of prefixes, that is really the way the term should be written. Learning the prefixes and their meanings and using your common sense is the most effective way to apply your knowledge for building medical terms.

Common prefixes are listed in Table 5-1.

TABLE 5-1   Common Prefixes

Prefix	Meaning	Example
a-, an-	Without	*Arrhythmia* is without a rhythm; *anuria* is a condition without urine.
ante-, pre-, pro-	Before	*Antenatal* or *prenatal* vitamins are vitamins taken before the baby is born. *Prophylactic* medications are used before a disease might occur.
anti-, contra–	Against	*Anticoagulants* are chemicals that work against the blood's clotting ability. Many medications are *contraindicated* when using other medications, meaning that they are against being used together.
bi-, diplo-	Two	*Bilateral* means "pertaining to two sides"; *diplococci* are bacteria appearing in pairs (twos).
brady-	Slow	*Bradycardia* is a condition of a slow heart (rate).
circum-	Around	*Circumference* is the measurement around an object.
de-	Away from	*Dehydration* is the process of taking water away from the body.
dia-, trans-	Through	*Diathermy* is a treatment modality of passing heat through the skin to the underlying tissues. *Transcutaneous* medications are absorbed through the skin.
dys-	Abnormal, painful, difficult	*Dysuria* is a condition of painful urination.
ecto-	Outside	*Ectopic* pregnancies occur when the ovum becomes fertilized outside of the uterus.
endo-	Within	*Endoscopies* are procedures in which an instrument is placed within the body for viewing structures.
epi-	Upon, over	The *epidermis* is the outermost layer of skin over the dermis.
eu-	Normal, good	*Euthyroid* indicates that that thyroid function is normal.
ex-, exo-, extra-	Out of, away from, outside	*Exophthalmos* is an abnormal condition of the eyeballs in which they appear to be out of the sockets, *exoskeleton* is a skeleton on the outside of the body, and *extracurricular* refers to activities outside of the classroom.
hemi-, semi-	Half	*Hemiplegia* is paralysis occurring on one side of the body; semiconscious is being half conscious and half unconscious.

(continues)

TABLE 5-1   Common Prefixes (Continued)

Prefix	Meaning	Example
hyper-, poly-	Above normal, excessive	*Hyperthermia* is an abnormal body temperature that is above normal; *polyuria* is a condition of excessive urination, often occurring in diabetic patients.
hypo-, sub-	Below normal, below, underneath, inferior	*Hypodermic* injections are administered below the dermis of the skin. *Substernal* chest pain would be underneath the breastbone of the rib cage.
inter-	Between	*Intercostal* spaces are located between the ribs.
intra-	Within	*Intracellular* fluid is the fluid found within the cells.
iso-	Same	*Isotonic* saline has the same pH as blood.
mal-	Bad, not adequate	*Malabsorption* occurs when the body has bad or inadequate absorption through the gastrointestinal tract.
megalo-, mega-, macro-	Large, big	*Megalocytes* are large cells.
micro-	Small, tiny	A *microscope* is an instrument used for viewing tiny things.
mono-	One	A *monocyte* is a cell that contains only one nucleus.
multi-, pluri-	Many	*Multipara* indicates that a woman has had more than one pregnancy (many pregnancies).
oligo-	Few, scanty, sparse	*Oliguria* is a condition in which scanty urine is produced.
pan-	All	*Pancytopenia* is an abnormal decrease in the number of all cells.
peri-	Around	*Perianal* pertains to the area around the anus.
post-	After, following	*Postmortem* is after death.
quadra-, quadri-	Four	*Quadrants* are imaginary divisions of four sections; *quadriplegia* is the paralysis of all four extremities.
re-	Again, backward	*Reproduce* is to produce again.
super-, supra-	Above, superior, more	*Superman* has powers above the normal mortal man; *suprapubic* is the area immediately above the pubis.
tachy-	Fast, abnormally fast	*Tachycardia* is a condition of an abnormally fast heartbeat.
ultra-	Beyond	An *ultrasound* is a radiologic procedure that goes beyond the speed of sound.
uni-	One, single	*Unilateral* pertains to one side only.

SUFFIXES

When suffixes are written as separate components, they begin with a hyphen, followed by the suffix. Some suffixes are actually stand-alone nouns that can be added to combining forms for more specificity of a particular term. Suffixes can change a medical term to an adjective as well. For example, *pyr/o* is the combining form that means "fire." *Mania* is a stand-alone term that can also be used as a suffix and means "an unusual preoccupation or obsession." To build a term that means an obsession with fire, these words combine to form *pyromania*, a term that you have probably heard in the past.

Dissecting a term is a good exercise for learning about suffixes.

Hydrophobic: -ic + phob/o + hydr/o

Remember that to take a medical term apart to define it, you should start with the suffix, followed by the prefix (if there is one), and finally the combining forms. As you learn the meanings of combining forms, breaking medical terms apart to define them will become more logical for you. In this term (Figure 5-2), *-ic* means "pertaining to," *phob/o* means "abnormal fear," and *hydr/o* means "water"; thus our term means "pertaining to an abnormal fear of water" (an adjective). *Hydrophobia*, "an abnormal fear of water," is another term for rabies. Animals infected with rabies avoid water because they cannot swallow—the rabies paralyzes the throat muscles, which is also why affected animals froth at the mouth and drool.

A list of common suffixes and their meanings can be found in Table 5-2.

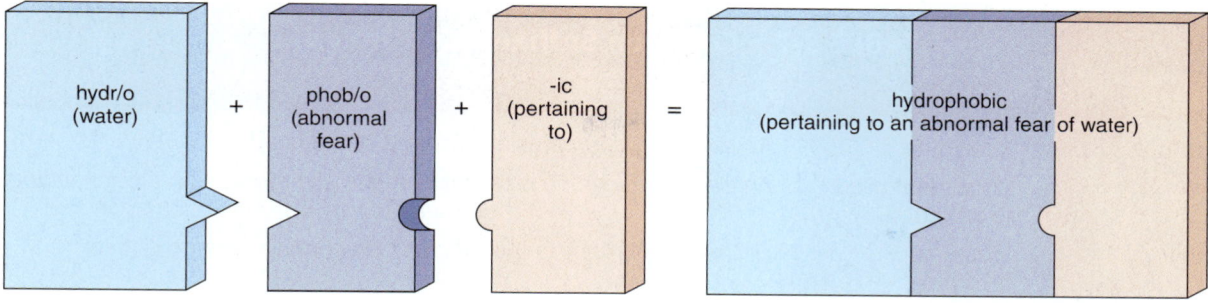

FIGURE 5-2   Hydrophobic means "pertaining to an abnormal fear of water."

TABLE 5-2	Common Suffixes	
Prefix	**Meaning**	**Example**
-ac, -al, -ar, -ary, -eal, -ia, -ic, -ory, -ous -tic	Pertaining to	*Ventricular* is pertaining to the ventricles.
-ad	Toward	*Caudad* is toward the tail.
-algia, -dynia	Pain	*Arthralgia* is pain in the joint(s). *Cephalodynia* is pain in the head or a headache.
-ase	Enzyme	*Amylase* is an enzyme that breaks down starches.
-asthenia	Weakness	*Myasthenia gravis* is great muscle weakness.
-blast	Baby, immature	*Erythroblasts* are immature red blood cells most often found in the bone marrow.
-cele	Hernia, abnormal protrusion	A *rectocele* is an abnormal protrusion from the rectum.
-cide, -cidal	Killing, destroying	*Bacteriocidal* solutions kill bacteria.
-crine	To secrete	The *endocrine* system secretes hormones.
-cyte	Cell	A *leukocyte* is a white blood cell.
-derma	Skin	*Scleroderma* is "hard" skin.
-ectasia, -ectasis	Stretching, dilating	*Bronchiectasis* is a lung condition in which the bronchioles are stretched out permanently.
-ectomy	Surgical removal	A *hysterectomy* is the removal of the uterus.
-edema	Swelling, fluid accumulation	*Lymphedema* is fluid accumulation and swelling when the lymph nodes cannot circulate lymph back through the vascular system, usually due to an obstruction.
-ema, -iasis, -ism, -lepsy, osis	Condition, abnormal condition	*Erythema* is a condition with redness; *hyperthyroidism* is a condition of above-normal thyroid function; *candidiasis* is a condition of a yeast infection; *hidrosis* is a condition of abnormal sweating. *Narcolepsy* is an abnormal condition of sleep.
-emesis	Vomiting	*Hyperemesis* is excessive vomiting.
-emia	Blood	*Anemia* is a condition of low (no) blood.
-esthesia	Sensation, feeling	*Anesthesia* produces a lack of feeling or sensation.
-gen, -genesis, -genic	Producing, production, production of, formation	A *carcinogen* is something that produces cancer, *carcinogenesis* is the formation of cancer, and *carcinogenic* is a substance capable of producing cancer.
-globin, -globulin	Protein	*Hemoglobin* is the protein in red blood cells that transports oxygen; an *immunoglobin* is a protein that helps to protect us against infections.

(continues)

TABLE 5-2   Common Suffixes (Continued)

Prefix	Meaning	Example
-gram	Recording	An *electrocardiogram* is a recording of the heart.
-graph	Instrument used to record	An *electrocardiograph* is the instrument used to make an electrocardiogram.
-graphy	Process of recording	*Electrocardiography* is the process of recording the heart's beat.
-itis	Inflammation	*Gastritis* is inflammation of the stomach.
-kinesia, -kinesis	Movement	*Dyskinesia* is painful movement of the body.
-logist	One who studies	A *cardiologist* is one who studies the heart.
-logy	The study of	*Cardiology* is the study of the heart.
-lysis, -lytic	Destruction	*Hemolysis* occurs when red blood cells are destroyed.
-malacia	Softening	*Nephromalacia* is a condition occurring when the kidney(s) soften.
-mania, -manic	Abnormal preoccupation or obsession	*Pyromania* is an abnormal obsession with fire, and a *pyromaniac* is a person with this preoccupation.
-megaly	Enlargement	*Acromegaly* is enlargement of the extremities.
-meter, -metry	Measuring device, process of measuring	A *spirometer* measures the amount of air inhaled and exhaled through the respiratory system. *Pelvimetry* is the process of measuring a pregnant woman's pelvis.
-oid	Resembling	*Osteoid* is resembling bone.
-oma	Tumor	A *lipoma* is a fatty tumor.
-opia	Vision	*Diplopia* is double vision.
-ose	Sugar	*Lactose* is the sugar found in milk.
-ostomy	Formation of a new opening	A *gastrostomy* is a new opening in the stomach to provide nutrients to patients who are unable to swallow.
-para, -parous	Bearing, producing child	*Unipara* refers to a woman who has given birth to one child.
-pathy	Disease	*Lymphadenopathy* is a disease of the lymph glands.
-penia	Deficiency	*Thrombocytopenia* is a deficiency of clotting cells (platelets).
-pepsia	Digestion	*Eupepsia* is normal digestion.
-pexy	Surgical fixation	*Mastopexy* is surgical fixation of the breasts.
-phage, -phagy, -phagia	To eat or digest	*Macrophages* are large cells that ingest foreign matter. *Dysphagia* is difficult or painful digestion.
-phasia	Speaking	*Dysphasia* is difficult speaking, as in laryngitis.
-phil, -philia	To love	An *eosinophil* loves the red dye found in Wright's and Giemsa stains.
-phobia	Abnormal fear	*Necrophobia* is an abnormal fear of death.
-phonia	Sound	*Aphonia* is the lack of sound (or not being able to hear sound).
-phrenia, -phrenic	Mind, diaphragm	*Schizophrenia* is a split personality; the *phrenic* nerve enervates the diaphragm.
-plasty	Surgical repair	*Rhinoplasty* is surgical repair of one's nose.
-plegia, -plegic	Paralysis	*Quadriplegia* is paralysis of four limbs; a *quadriplegic* is a person that has this condition.
-pnea	Breath or breathing	*Dyspnea* is difficult breathing.
-poiesis	Formation	*Hematopoiesis* is the formation of blood.

(continues)

TABLE 5-2   Common Suffixes (Continued)

Prefix	Meaning	Example
-ptosis	Sagging or drooping	*Blepharoptosis* is a drooping eyelid.
-rrhage, -rrhagia	Heavy discharge	*Hemorrhage* is a heavy discharge of blood.
-rrhaphy	Suturing	*Cardiorrhaphy* is a suturing of the heart.
-rrhea	Discharge, flowing	*Diarrhea* is flowing of feces through the anus.
-rrhexis	Rupture	*Cardiorrhexis* is a rupture of the heart.
-scope, -scopy	Instrument, process of using the instrument	*Microscopes* are instruments used to view tiny objects; *microscopy* is the process of examining the tiny objects.
-somnia	Sleep	*Polysomnia* is much sleep.
-stasis	Stopping	*Homeostasis* is the process of stopping processes in the body to maintain an equilibrium.
-stenosis	Narrowing	*Esophagostenosis* is the narrowing of the esophagus.
-stomy	Opening	*Gastrostomy* is making a new opening into the stomach.
-tome	Instrument used for cutting	A *gastrotome* is an instrument used for cutting into the stomach.
-tomy	The process of cutting	*Nephrotomy* is the process of cutting into a kidney.
-trophic, -trophy	Nutrition	*Atrophic* pertains to a lack of nutrition, commonly found in limbs that have been bound by casts.
-uria	Urine	*Dysuria* is painful or difficult urination.
-version	Turning	*Cardioversion* is turning or converting the heart to a normal rhythm.

WORD ROOTS AND COMBINING FORMS

Combining forms are the word roots that have a vowel added to the end of the root to make it easier to combine with suffixes or other word roots. Usually, the combining form vowel is not used if the suffix begins with a vowel, but once again, there are exceptions to this rule. Most often the combining form vowel is an *o*, but other vowels may be used depending on the word root; the other two most common vowels seen in combining forms are *a* and *i*.

Some examples of the differences in combining forms and word roots are listed in Table 5-3.

Remember, the difference between combining forms and word roots is simply that a combining form has a vowel added to the basic part of the word to which suffixes or other word roots/combining forms may be added. The combining form vowels make the medical term easier to pronounce and more sensible. Different books identify combining forms in various manners, so do not be dismayed if you come across a different way of identifying combining forms—the principle is the same regardless of the designation.

TABLE 5-3   Common Combining Forms and Word Roots

Combining Form	Word Root	Meaning
cardi/o	cardi	Heart
carp/o	carp	Wrist
cyan/o	cyan	Blue
hemat/o, hem/o	hemat, hem	Blood
lip/o	lip	Fat
muscul/o	muscul	Muscle
neur/o	neur	Nerve
ren/o	ren	Kidney

Unit 4 presents multiple tables identifying combining forms as they pertain to individual body systems. You have already seen some examples of combining forms as an introduction, and as the chapter progresses, you will see many more.

ACHIEVE UNIT OBJECTIVES

- Complete the Workbook activities to meet the learning objectives.
- Apply your knowledge at the end of this chapter in completing the Critical Thinking Challenge and Activities, as well as the StudyWARE on your Student CD-ROM.

UNIT 3
FORMING PLURALS FROM SINGULARS

OBJECTIVES

Upon completion of this unit, you will be able to achieve the following:

LEARNING Objectives

1. Spell and define, using the glossary at the back of the text, all the Words to Know in this unit.
2. Determine whether a term is singular or plural.
3. Demonstrate knowledge of converting medical terms from singular to plural and vice versa.

WORDS TO KNOW

plural
singular

 ## CERTIFICATION CONNECTION

CMA
Medical Terminology
- Word building and definitions
- Uses of terminology

RMA
Medical Terminology
- Word parts
- Definitions
- Common abbreviations
- Spelling

CMAS
Medical Terminology
- Use and spell basic medical terms appropriately
- Identify root words, prefixes, and suffixes
- Define basic medical terms

FORMING PLURALS

In our everyday English language, it is relatively simple to make a **plural** form of a **singular** term; we simply add an s—*runner* becomes *runners*, *car* becomes *cars*. In other cases, adding "es" will change a singular term to a plural—*business* changes to *businesses*. However, because many of the medical terms derive from Latin, Greek, or other foreign origins, the rules are more complex. It is important that you learn the proper conversions for changing a singular medical term to a plural one. It is also vital that you can recognize the differences in plural and singular medical terms for the most appropriate application and definition of such terms. For instance, it is not uncommon to hear lay people say "appendixes" rather than "appendices," but the rule for changing appendix to plural form is to drop the *x* and add *ces*. When you hear someone make an erroneous reference such as this, you can smile because you know the basic rules of properly changing singular terms to plural ones. Practice makes perfect, so when you are unsure about the proper conversion from singular to plural and vice versa, consult a reference rather than make an error.

Table 5-4 lists the basic rules for changing singular medical terms to plurals.

TABLE 5-4	Singular to Plural	
Singular Ending	**Plural Ending**	**Example**
-a	-ae	*Vertebra* (singular) becomes *vertebrae* (plural).
-ex, -ix	-ices	*Apex* changes to *apices*; *appendix* in plural form is *appendices*.
-is	-es	*Diagnosis* (singular) becomes *diagnoses* (plural).
-nx	-nges	*Phalanx* (digit such a finger or toe), when counting more than one, changes to *phalanges*.
-um	-a	*Atrium* changes to *atria*.
-us	-i	*Bacillus* becomes *bacilli* in plural form.

ACHIEVE UNIT OBJECTIVES

- Complete the Workbook activities to meet the learning objectives.
- Apply your knowledge at the end of this chapter in completing the Critical Thinking Challenge and Activities, as well as the StudyWARE on your Student CD-ROM.

UNIT 4
UNDERSTANDING AND BUILDING MEDICAL TERMS OF BODY SYSTEMS

OBJECTIVES

Upon completion of this unit, you will be able to achieve the following:

LEARNING Objectives

1. **Spell and define, using the glossary at the back of the text, all the Words to Know in this unit.**
2. **Demonstrate the ability to select and define combining forms for each body system.**
3. **Demonstrate the ability to appropriately add prefixes to combining forms for each body system.**
4. **Demonstrate the ability to appropriately add suffixes to combining forms for each body system.**
5. **Have the ability to break medical terms apart to define their meanings.**
6. **Appropriately use medical terms in applications.**

WORDS TO KNOW

abduction	cryptorchidism	human organism
acne vulgaris	cusp	hyperglycemia
adduction	dermatology	inferior
alimentary canal	dialysis	inferior vena
alopecia	diaphragm	cava
anatomical	digestive	integumentary
position	dorsal	system
anterior	erythrocyte	internal
ascites	eversion	inversion
atria	extend	jaundice
atrium	external	lateral
bicuspid	feces	leukocyte
bolus	femoral	medial
cell	femur	micturition
cervicitis	flex	mitral
cholecystolithiasis	gastrointestinal	myocardium
chyme	(GI) system	nephron
circumversion	histologist	

neuron	pyelonephritis	thorax
ophthalmologist	septum	tissue
phlebotomist	superficial	tricuspid
pneumonitis	superior	ventral
polyneuralgia	superior vena	ventricle
posterior	cava	viscera
prone	supine	

CERTIFICATION CONNECTION

CMA
Medical Terminology
- Word building and definitions
- Uses of terminology

RMA
Medical Terminology
- Word parts
- Definitions
- Common abbreviations
- Spelling

CMAS
Medical Terminology
- Use and spell basic medical terms appropriately
- Identify root words, prefixes, and suffixes
- Define basic medical terms

ANATOMICAL POSITION, DIRECTIONAL TERMS, AND BODY PLANES

The first point of reference is the **anatomical position** when discussing directional terms and body planes. The anatomical position is always the same no matter where you reference it: the body is upright, arms at the side, with the palms facing forward. From the anatomical position, you can then view the body for the **anterior** or **ventral** (front) and the **posterior** or **dorsal** (back) areas (Figure 5-3). As body systems are discussed later in this chapter, references will be made to their locations with respect to these directional terms.

Terms may also relate to positioning of the body and directions related to those positions (see Figure 5-3). For instance, **inferior** would relate to a part of the body that is below another part of the body: The knees are *inferior* to the hips. **Superior** tells us that the position would be above: The head is *superior* to the chest. Some other directional terms are:

- **Lateral**—the arms are *lateral* (to the side) of the chest.
- **Medial**—the sternum is *medial* (middle) to the chest.
- **Internal**—the digestive organs are *internal* (deep) in the abdomen.
- **Superficial**—the wound was *superficial* (on the surface) to the calf.

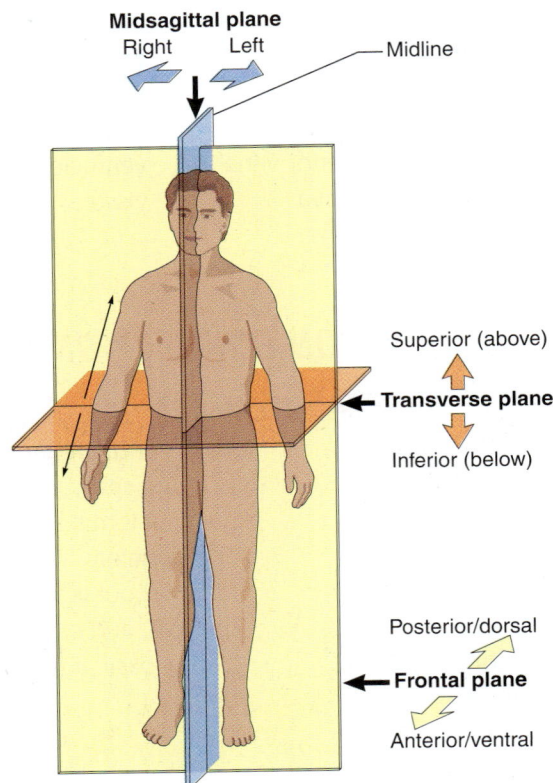

FIGURE 5-3   Body directions and positions

There are also terms that are relative to the body when it is not in the anatomical position; **prone** would tell you that the person is lying face down, and **supine** is when the person is lying on his or her back.

There are also imaginary planes of the body that are envisioned to "dissect" it for identifying certain structures. These imaginary lines divide the body into front and back, left and right, top and bottom.

Also found in medical terminology are references to movement of certain parts of the body; for instance, **abduction** means to move something away from the midline, such as in moving the arm away from the trunk. A tip to remember this is to think about a child abduction—the child is "taken away" from the home (midline); using word associations such as this will help in your recall of terms. **Adduction** is to bring something back to the midline, such as moving the arm back to the trunk of the body. To remember this term look at the first three letters of the term itself— "add." If you are taking the arm back to the midline, you are "adding" it back to the trunk. **Circumversion** is to move a limb in a circle; word association to help you remember this is to think back to your high school days when you measured the *circumference* of a circle. There are lots of little tricks to help you remember these terms. When one wants to leave a building, which door is taken? The *exit* door, right? Using that

TABLE 5-5 Directional Terms		
Combining Form and Word Root	**Meaning**	**Example**
anter/o, anter	Anterior, front	*Anteroposterior* refers to from the front to the back.
coron/o, coron	Crown	The *coronal* plane from the crown of the head divides the body into anterior (front) and posterior (back) sections.
dist/o, dist	Distant, far (usually from point of attachment)	The foot is *distal* to the hip as compared with the knee.
dors/o, dors	Back	The *dorsal* fin of a shark is the fin that can be seen above the surface of the water.
later/o, later	To the side	The arms are *lateral* to the trunk of the body.
lumb/o, lumb	Lower back	The *lumbar* spine is located below the thoracic spine, in the small of the back.
medi/o, medi	Toward the middle	The location of the human heart can be described as *medial*.
poster/o, poster	Back, rear, posterior	When an x-ray is requested as *posteroanterior*, the beam goes from the back of the body to the front.
proxim/o, proxim	Near, proximal (usually when describing points of attachment)	The elbow is *proximal* to the shoulder.
somat/o	Body	*Somatic* tremors are involuntary movements of the body, often caused by Parkinson's disease.
ventr/o, ventr	Toward the front or belly	The digestive organs are located in the *ventral* cavity.

| TABLE 5-6 Body Planes, Cavities, and Sections ||
Description	Definition
Abdominal cavity	Houses the digestive and accessory organs.
Abduction	Taking away from the midline
Adduction	Bringing toward the midline
Coronal, frontal plane	Divides the body into front and back sections (anterior and posterior)
Cranial cavity	Contains the brain
Dorsal cavity	Contains the spine
Medial, midsagittal plane	Divides the body into left and right sections
Pelvic cavity	Contains the reproductive organs, portions of the large intestine, bladder and urethra
Prone position	Face down, lying on the belly
Supine position	Face up, lying on the back
Thoracic cavity	Houses the heart and lungs as well as some other organs
Transverse plane, horizontal plane	Divides the body in half at the waist

premise, **eversion** is turning an appendage out, while **inversion** is moving an appendage in toward the center. When a man wants to show off his deltoid muscles in his upper arms, he **flexes** his arm to make the muscle more pronounced; he brings the extremity up to make the degree in the joint as small as possible. When the man has shown off his muscles for you, he will **extend** his arm, meaning that he makes the angle of the joint larger by straightening the joint out.

More directional terms and planes of the body are listed and defined in Tables 5-5 and 5-6.

STRUCTURE OF THE HUMAN BODY

A comprehensive exposure to the anatomy and physiology of the body appears in Chapter 11, but a brief introduction to help you understand the organization of the body is essential in this chapter.

The basic unit of the human body is the **cell**, and of course, the cell is composed of many smaller units. The combining form for cell is *cyt*/o, and the suffix for the same word is *-cyte*. In subsequent parts of the chapter, you will see more references to cells that are specific to tissues and organs. For instance, **erythrocytes** are red

blood cells that will be discussed in the circulatory system; **leukocytes** are white blood cells that are essential to our immune systems in that they help to protect us from infections in various ways. Cells organize to become **tissue**, and tissues become organized to form *organs*. The combining form for tissue is *hist*/o, so when you come across the word **histologist**, you will be able to identify that this is someone who studies or specializes in tissues. Organs work together to be organized into *organ systems*, which ultimately are organized into the **human organism**, a very highly structured living being. The organ systems that compose the living human body will be referenced in this chapter as related to medical terminology.

THE INTEGUMENTARY SYSTEM

The skin, or the **integumentary system**, is the most external and visualized organ in the human body, as well as the largest organ of the human body. The study of the skin is called **dermatology**, so usually patients will not have any idea of the reference to the integumentary system. Most people do not fully realize or appreciate the complexity of the skin and its structures, nor the important role the skin plays in keeping us healthy and protected from external dangers. Technically, the skin is composed of three layers: the outermost or the *epidermis*; the "true" skin or *dermis*; and the anchoring layer, which is actually below the skin, the *hypodermis*. There are several layers that make up the epidermis; they are discussed in Chapter 11. The integumentary system includes not only the skin, but the nails of the hands and feet, hair on various areas of the body, sweat glands, oil glands, the specialized glands of the ear that produce wax, and the associated structures for each of these. The skin is our first line of defense against foreign invaders, so protecting the skin is of utmost importance in remaining healthy. Some terms related to the integumentary system need to be memorized as they will not break down into components. An example of one of these terms is **alopecia**, the medical term meaning "baldness." Another example is **acne vulgaris**, an unfortunately common affliction with teenagers; *vulgaris* literally means "vulgar," and extreme cases of acne can be quite disconcerting to see. As you are reading through Chapter 11, acquaint yourself with these various diseases and disorders to be proficient in problems associated with the skin as well as diagnosis and treatments for such problems.

Thinking back to directional terms, the skin is the most **external** or superficial organ that we have. Injuries that occur beneath this structure would be considered **internal** or deep injuries.

Table 5-7 lists and defines the most common combining forms related to the integumentary system.

TABLE 5-7   Integumentary System

Combining Form	Definition	Example
adip/o, lip/o	Fat	*Adipose* tissue is the layer just below the skin, consisting primarily of fat cells. A *lipoma* is a benign, fatty tumor.
albin/o, leuk/o	White, without color	*Albinism* is a condition in which there are no melanocytes to provide color to the skin, giving the person a white appearance. *Leukoderma* is abnormal patches of white skin.
cutane/o, derm/o, dermat/o, integument/o	Skin	A *subcutaneous* injection is given beneath the skin's layers; a *dermatologist* is one who specializes in disorders of the skin.
cyan/o	Blue	*Cyanosis* of the nail beds or lips is a bluish tint due to the lack of oxygen.
erythem/o	Red	*Systemic lupus erythematosus* is an autoimmune disease often characterized by a red butterfly rash on the face.
melan/o	Black	*Malignant melanoma* is a black tumor of the skin.
onych/o	Nail	*Onychomycosis* is an abnormal fungal infection of the nails.
scler/o	Hard, hardening	*Scleroderma* is a condition of hardened skin.
xanth/o, icter/o	Yellow	*Xanthoderma* is yellowish appearing skin. A patient described as being *icteric* has a yellow discoloration of the skin from a liver disorder. Sometimes the word "jaundice" is used for the same condition.
xer/o	Dry	*Xeroderma* is a condition of extremely dry skin.

THE MUSCULOSKELETAL SYSTEM

Beneath the integumentary system, the musculoskeletal system forms the structural support that allows us to stand upright. Within this system you will find the bones of the skeletal system as well as the muscles that move the bones. There are 206 bones in the human body; by learning the name of each of the bones, you will have a good basis for knowing the combining forms for each of them. Additionally, when you learn the combining forms for the names of the bones, it will be easier to identify other structures. For instance, the combining form for **femur** (the thighbone) is *femor/o*. While that may not seem significant now, later when you hear a reference to the **femoral** artery, based on your working knowledge of the bones of the body, you will know that this artery is located in the upper leg (thigh). The human body also has 646 muscles, but you won't need to know as many of those for combining forms as you will for bones. Classifications of the muscle types, such as smooth muscle or striated muscle, and terms pertaining to the membrane separating the muscles and attaching the muscles will be your most common usage. One of the most common combining forms for muscle is *my/o*; this fact should help you in defining terms you encounter with other body systems. An example of one of these terms not associated with the musculoskeletal system but utilizing this combining form is **myocardium**; try breaking this term apart to define it.

- Step 1: Identify and define the suffix: *-ium*, membrane
- Step 2: Identify and define the combining form(s): *my/o*, muscle; *cardi/o*, heart
- Step 3: Add the component definitions together: "membrane of muscle of the heart"

The meaning, although a little distorted in this example, is the muscular layer of the heart, which is defined by a membrane that separates the muscle portion of the heart from the outer and inner membranes. Sometimes you will have to adapt your literal definition of the terms to the structure of the specific body system.

Table 5-8 identifies and defines the most common combining forms for the musculoskeletal system.

THE CARDIOVASCULAR SYSTEM

The cardiovascular system is composed of the heart and its associated structures; there are vessels that carry blood rich in oxygen and nutrients throughout our bodies all the way to the cellular level, and there are ves-

TABLE 5-8   The Musculoskeletal System

Combining Form	Definition	Example
ankylos/o	Stiffening	*Ankylosing spondylitis* is an abnormal stiffening of the spine that results in a lack of mobility.
arthr/o	Joint	*Arthritis* is inflammation of a joint.
carp/o	Wrist (bones)	*Carpal tunnel syndrome* affects the nerves in the wrist.
cervic/o	Neck	The *cervical* spine is the vertebrae that compose the neck.
chondr/o	Cartilage	*Costochondritis* is an inflammation of the cartilage around the ribs that often mimics the pain of a heart attack.
cost/o	Ribs	When performing an electrocardiogram, the medical assistant needs to locate the *intercostal* spaces for proper electrode placement.
crani/o	Skull, head	The *cranial* cavity is located within the skull.
dactyl/o	Digit	*Dactylography* is the process of taking someone's fingerprints.
femor/o	Femur (thighbone)	The *femoral* artery is located near the femur in the upper part of the leg.
fibul/o	Fibula (smaller bone in the calf)	A *fibular* fracture would be a break of the fibula.
humer/o	Humerus (upper bone in the arm)	When one hits the *humeral* nerve, it is often described as hitting the "funny" bone.
ili/o	Ilium (pelvic bones)	The *iliac* crest of the pelvis is used as a landmark for administering intramuscular injections.
lamin/o	Lamina of a vertebra	A *laminectomy*, removing a portion of the vertebra, may be performed by a surgeon to relieve back pain.
mandibul/o	Mandible (lower jaw, only movable bone in the skull)	*Temporomandibular joint* (TMJ) pain occurs when the bone of the mandible does not align correctly with the temporal bone to which it is attached.
maxill/o	Maxilla (upper jaw)	*Maxillary* sinuses are located just above the maxilla of the face.
muscul/o, my/o	Muscle	*Muscular* pertains to muscles; the *myocardium* is the muscular portion of the heart.
orth/o	Straight, straighten	An *orthopedist* is one that specializes in straightening bones.
oste/o	Bone	*Osteitis* is inflammation of a bone.
patell/o	Patella (knee cap)	The *patellar* reflex is solicited when striking a patient's leg just below the knee cap.
pelv/i	Pelvis	The *pelvic* cavity is housed within the bony structure of the pelvis.
phalang/o	Fingers or toes	*Phalangitis* is inflammation of a finger or a toe.
rachi/o, spondyl/o, vertebr/o	Vertebra(e), spine	*Rachitis* and *spondylitis* are both inflammation of the vertebrae/spine. The *vertebral* column is composed of bones of the spine.
stern/o	Sternum (breastbone)	*Substernal* chest pain is pain described as being just below the breastbone, often indicating a heart attack.
ten/o, tend/o, tendin/o	Tendon	*Tendonitis* is inflammation of a tendon.
tibi/o	Tibia (shin)	A *tibial* contusion, caused by striking the shin, is quite painful.

sels that transport the used by-products for disposal by the body.

The heart is composed of three layers of muscle and divided into right and left sections with chambers in each of these sections. The left side of the heart is responsible for pumping the oxygen and nutrient-rich blood out through the aorta and ultimately to the cellular level. The right side of the heart receives the oxygen-poor, waste-rich blood, which is pumped back through the lungs for reoxygenation. Directionally, the heart is usually described as being **medial**, or located mostly in the middle of the chest or **thorax**. Other directional terms that will help with understanding of the venous structures that return oxygen-poor blood to the lungs include the **superior vena cava**, the large vein that collects blood from the upper (superior) structures such as the head and neck, and the **inferior vena cava**, the corresponding large vein that collects blood from the lower (inferior) structures such as the legs, abdomen, and pelvic regions.

The heart is also divided into right and left sections by tissue called the **septum**. As mentioned, the left side of the heart is responsible for routing the oxygen-rich blood through the aorta, arteries, and arterioles to supply the cells with necessary oxygen and nutrients; the right side of the heart receives the oxygen-poor blood from the cells for routing to the lungs for an exchange of carbon dioxide and oxygen. The heart is futher divided into four chambers: The two **superior** structures are called the **atria** (plural for **atrium** since there is a right and left), and the two inferior structures called the **ventricles** (plural for ventricle). Aiding the proper flow of blood through the heart are valves that prevent regurgitation of the blood back into chambers of the heart. By learning the prefixes for numbers, you can more easily identify the structure of the valves; between the left atrium and left ventricule is the **bicuspid** or **mitral** valve. The prefix of *bi-* refers to the number two, so you would know the valve has two sections or **cusps**; the reference to mitral goes back to Roman times and the head covering that priests wore for Roman Catholic services. These "hats" were composed of two pieces of material, thus the reference to two. The valve that maintains proper blood flow through the right side of the heart between the atrium and ventricle is the **tricuspid** valve—of course, the prefix of *tri-* refers to the number three.

The aorta, arteries, and arterioles are the vessels that transport the oxygen-rich blood throughout the body. The exchange between the oxygen and carbon dioxide (this is the blood that has waste products) occurs at the capillary level, and the blood is then routed through the venules, veins, and vena cavae before being returned to the right side of the heart. The vessels transporting the blood from the left side of the heart

are more muscular and thicker-walled than the vessels returning the blood to the right side of the heart because they are under great pressure. Chapter 11 provides a more in-depth discussion of the structural differences in arteries and veins and the reasons for these differences.

Also included with the cardiovascular system are the blood system, lymphatic system, and immune system. The vascular part of the system routes the blood cells throughout the body, helps to protect the body by providing immunity and responses to pathogenic invaders, and transports lymph fluid.

Try defining a couple of practice words to build a better understanding of medical terms associated with this system.

Define **phlebotomist.**

- Step 1: Identify and define the suffix: -ist, one who
- Step 2: Identify and define any prefix: (in this word, there is no prefix)
- Step 3: Identify and define combining forms or word roots: *phleb/o*, vein; *tom/o*, (surgical) incision
- Step 4: Combine the definitions: "One who [makes a surgical] incision into a vein." Isn't that exactly what a phlebotomist does when taking your blood? Those trained in phlebotomy use needles to make a small incision into a **superficial** vein to aspirate blood for diagnostic testing.

Build a word for "pertaining to the atrium and ventricle."

- Step 1: Select the most appropriate suffix for "pertaining to": in this case, it is *-ar*. Sometimes selecting the most commonly used and most appropriate suffix for "pertaining to" can be quite a challenge.
- Step 2: Select the combining form for "atrium": *atri/o*
- Step 3: Select the combining form for "ventricle": *ventricul/o.*
- Step 4: Place the word components together and review to see if you will need the combining form vowels to build your word.

atri/o + ventricul/o + -ar = atrioventricular

Note the use of the combining form vowel for ventricle and absence of the one for atrium. Remember your basic rules: if you are adding combining forms together and the second word component begins with a consonant, the combining form vowel will be used with the first. However, if adding a component that begins with a vowel, the combining form vowel is usually dropped, as it was in *ventricul/o.*

You need to be familiar with the combining forms relating to the cardiovascular system identified and defined in Table 5-9.

TABLE 5-9   The Cardiovascular System

Combining Form	Definition	Example
aden/o	Gland	*Lymphadenopathy* is often found with viral illnesses such as infectious mononucleosis.
angi/o, vas/o	Vessel	*Angioplasty* may be performed when a blockage is found in a blood vessel to repair or remove the blockage.
aort/o	Aorta	An *aortic* aneurysm is a ballooning out of this major vessel and is frequently life-threatening.
arteri/o	Artery	*Temporal arteritis* is an inflammation of the temporal artery.
ather/o	Yellow, fatty plaque	*Atherosclerosis* is hardening of the arteries due to deposits of yellow, fatty plaque.
atri/o	Atrium (atria), upper chambers of the heart	The *atrioventricular* node is located between the atrium and ventricle of the heart and provides stimulation for the heart's beat.
cardi/o	Heart	*Cardiac* surgery pertains to surgery on the heart.
erythr/o	Red	*Erythrocytes* are the red blood cells, which are responsible for transporting oxygen.
hem/o, hemat/o	Blood	*Hemodialysis* is cleansing of the blood by a machine; a *hematologist* is one who specializes in blood disorders.
leuc/o, leuk/o	White	*Leukocytes* are the white cells that help to protect the body from infections.
lymph/o	Lymph	*Lymphoma* is a tumor found in the lymph system.
phleb/o, ven/o	Vein	A *phlebotomist* or *venipuncturist* is a person that draws a patient's blood for diagnostic testing.
splen/o	Spleen	When a person's spleen becomes overactive and removes too many blood cells, a *splenectomy*, removal of the spleen, may have to be performed.
thromb/o	Clot	*Thrombophlebitis* is an inflammation of a vein due to a blood clot.
ventricul/o	Ventricle, lower chambers of the heart	*Ventricular* bigeminy is an abnormal heart rhythm involving the ventricles of the heart.

THE RESPIRATORY SYSTEM

When you think of breathing, you likely think only of the lungs; however, there is much more to the respiratory system than the lungs. One must envision the pathway of air into the body to realize all of the structures that compose the respiratory system. Air first enters the body through the mouth or the nose, moves down through the throat (*pharynx*), then the voice box (*larynx*), the airway (*trachea*), the bronchi, the bronchioles, and ending at the *alveoli*, the microscopic air sacs that exchange oxygen and carbon dioxide through the processes of inspiration (breathing in) and expiration (breathing out).

The lungs are located superior to the abdominal organs, positioned just above the **diaphragm**, which is the muscle that literally divides the body's thoracic cavity from the abdominal cavity. You may find it surprising that the right and left lungs are not identical to one another as is the case with the kidneys. Both lungs are composed of lobes; the right lung has two lobes that are wider than the three lobes found in the left lung, but the right lung is shorter than the left lung to provide enough room for the liver to be positioned beneath the diaphragm. The left lung is more narrow to provide room for the heart. Therefore, having a lobectomy is different from having a pneumonectomy. Remember that the suffix *-ectomy* means "surgical removal," so the difference in these two operations is that the lobectomy is the removal of only a lobe of the lung while the pneumonectomy is the removal of an entire lung. Another important set of terms in relation to the respiratory system includes those that refer to air or oxygen, which keep our organs, tissues, and cells healthy. Probably one of the more common combining forms that you already know is aer/o; think about the terms *aerobic* and *aerodynamic*. Another common combining form for air or oxygen is ox/o; an example is pulse oximeter, which is a device usually clipped to a

TABLE 5-10   Common Combining Forms and Suffixes Related to the Respiratory System

Combining Form	Definition	Example
aer/o	Air	*Anaerobic* microorganisms prefer a lack of air for growth.
atel/o	Imperfect	*Atelectasis*, when taking the literal definition, means imperfect stretching. In premature infants, atelectasis indicates that the lungs cannot fully expand.
bronch/o, bronchi/o	Bronchus (bronchi)	*Bronchitis* is an inflammation of the bronchi found in upper respiratory tract infections; *bronchiectasis* is an abnormal stretching of the bronchi.
bronchiol/o	Bronchioles (little bronchi)	Toddlers are often diagnosed with *bronchiolitis*, an inflammation of the bronchioles.
laryng/o	Larynx (voice box)	A *laryngectomy* is the surgical removal of the larynx, usually due to cancer.
lob/o	Lobes	*Lobar* pneumonia indicates an infection in only one lobe of a lung. A *lobectomy* is the surgical removal of a lobe of a lung.
muc/o	Mucus	The *mucous* membranes are responsible for secreting mucus in the respiratory tract.
nas/o, rhin/o	Nose	*Nasal* sprays are used in the nose to alleviate symptoms of *rhinitis*, an inflammation of the nose and nasal passages.
ox/o	Oxygen	*Hypoxia* is a condition of below-normal oxygen levels.
pharyng/o	Pharynx (throat)	The *pharyngeal* tonsils are the lymph glands found in the back of the throat.
pleur/o	Pleura (membrane surrounding each lung)	*Pleurisy* is an inflammation of the pleura around one of the lungs.
pneum/o, pnemon/o	Lung, air	A *pneumothorax* is a collapsed lung from air rushing in; *pneumonitis* is an inflammation of a lung, more commonly known as *pneumonia*.
pulmon/o	Lung	Chronic obstructive *pulmonary* disease (COPD) is a disease that affects the lungs and the oxygen levels.
sinus/o	Sinus(es)	*Sinusitis* is an inflammation of the sinuses, often from an allergic reaction.
spir/o	To breathe	A *spirometer* is a device used to measure the amount of air a patient breathes in and out. *Respiratory* literally means "pertaining to repeat(ed) breathing."
tonsill/o	Tonsil(s)	In repeated cases of strep throat, a *tonsillectomy*, surgical removal of the tonsils, may be performed.
trache/o	Trachea (windpipe)	A *tracheotomy* is performed when a person is unable to breathe through the mouth or nose; this involves creating a new opening for air to pass.
Suffix		
-ptysis	To spit	*Hemoptysis* is spitting up blood.

finger to measure the oxygen content in the blood without actually taking any blood from the patient.

Practice building and defining terms relating to the respiratory system.

Define the term **pneumonitis**.

- Step 1: Identify and define the suffix: *-itis,* inflammation (of)
- Step 2: Identify and define combining forms or word roots: *-pneumon/o,* lung(s)
- Step 3: Combine the definitions: "inflammation of the lungs," more commonly, and erroneously, referred to as *pneumonia,* which in its literal definition means "an abnormal condition of the lungs."

Build a word that means "a condition of difficult (painful) voice or speaking."

- Step 1: Select the most appropriate suffix that means "pertaining to," which in this case is *-ia.*
- Step 2: Select the most appropriate prefix that means "painful"; the prefix is *dys-.*
- Step 3: Select the combining form for "voice/speaking"; for this term, we need to use "phon/o."
- Step 4: Put the word parts together to make a term, remembering that prefixes are always at the beginning of the word and suffixes go at the end of the terms.

dys- + phon/o + -ia = dysphonia

Remember that if the suffix begins with a vowel, the combining form vowel is dropped.

You will need to learn the terms associated with the structures of the respiratory system as well as the process of breathing. A listing and definitions of the combining forms, and suffixes related to the respiratory system are provided in Table 5-10.

THE GASTROINTESTINAL (DIGESTIVE) SYSTEM

Often when one thinks about the **gastrointestinal (GI) system**, the stomach is what comes to mind. Just as with the respiratory system, there are many structures that compose the gastrointestinal or **digestive** system, as well as accessory structures that assist with the digestion of nutrients that are taken into the body.

When nutrients are taken into the body, the first place the food enters is through the mouth. Within the mouth are several digestive structures, such as the tongue, teeth, and salivary glands. As food is chewed, the tongue and teeth help to break it into smaller parts; the tongue mixes saliva with the smaller parts and pushes the food back to the throat as a **bolus**. This bolus makes its way through the pharynx to the esophagus and is deposited in the stomach. The stomach secretes enzymes and gastric juices to further liquefy the bolus. The bolus is then transformed into **chyme** and moved into the first portion of the small intestine, the duodenum. The small intestine is divided into three sections: the duodenum, the jejunum, and the ileum. Most of digestion occurs within the small intestine.

The next structure in the journey is the large intestine, which is also divided into parts. The first part of the large intestine is the cecum, the part of the large intestine from which the appendix projects; this is followed by the *ascending* colon (ascending refers to going up), the *transverse* colon (transverse means across), the *descending* colon (going down), the *sigmoid* colon (sigmoid means "resembling an *s*"), then the *rectum* and the *anus*. The large intestine's responsibility is primarily to reabsorb water and package the waste for disposal as **feces**. Thus, the digestive system, or **alimentary canal**, begins at the mouth and terminates at the anus, making it quite a complex system indeed. (*Aliment/o* is the combining form for "nutrition," and the suffix *-ary* refers to "pertaining to"; that is certainly the function of the alimentary canal.) Within the digestive system are accessory organs that assist in the processing of nutrients; these include the teeth, tongue, liver, pancreas, and gallbladder. The proper medical term for the appendix is *vermiform appendix*; the word vermiform loosely means "shaped or appearing like a worm" (*verm/i*). Refer to Chapter 11 for figures illustrating the digestive system—the appendix does look a lot like a worm!

There are some terms that you simply need to memorize, as they are not constructed like other medical terms

in this chapter. For instance, **viscera** is a collective term that means the internal organs, and **ascites** is an abnormal fluid accumulation in the abdominal cavity. The abdominal cavity is lined and protected by a membrane known as the peritoneum (you might identify the suffix *-eum*, which means membrane). Look at the term cirrhosis. Literally defined, this word means "a condition of yellow," but that does not make much sense medically. However, if you know anything about this disease, many times the patient will present with a yellow discoloration of the skin (**jaundice**), because the liver is no longer functioning normally. The problem with this generality is that not all patients with cirrhosis have a yellowish skin color. When the condition was first diagnosed in Greek medicine, because physicians at that time did not have the medical technologies that we have, the patient was diagnosed based on the yellowish color caused by the failing liver; hence, the term as we know it. The term *jaundice* is derived from the French term for yellow; once again, it is probably easier if you memorize the term as meaning "a yellowish discoloration of the skin."

To reinforce, define a medical term and then build one. Define the term **cholecystolithiasis**.

- Step 1: Identify and define the suffix: *-iasis,* an abnormal condition
- Step 2: Identify and define the first combining form: *chol/e,* bile (gall)
- Step 3: Identify and define the second combining form: *cyst/o,* bladder
- Step 4: Identify and define the last combining form: *lith/o,* stone
- Step 5: Combine the definitions to define the entire term: "an abnormal condition of gallbladder stone(s)," or more commonly, gallstones.

Build a term that means "surgical removal of half of the stomach."

- Step 1: Select the suffix that means surgical removal: *-ectomy*
- Step 2: Select the prefix that means half: There are two prefixes that mean this, *hemi-* and *semi-*. In this case, we will use *hemi-*.
- Step 3: Select the combining form that pertains to the stomach: *-gastr/o.*
- Step 4: Combine the word components to make the medical term, reviewing to see if a combining form vowel will have to be dropped to make the correct medical term.

hemi + gastr/o + -ectomy = hemigastrectomy

Once again, the combining form vowel is not used when combining with the suffix since the suffix begins with a vowel.

Table 5-11 identifies and defines the most common combining forms and suffixes associated with the gastrointestinal system.

TABLE 5-11 **Common Combining Forms and Suffixes Related to the Gastrointestinal System**

Combining Form	Definition	Example
abdomin/o	Abdomen	*Abdominal* pain is pain felt pertaining to the abdomen.
aden/o	Gland	*Sialadenitis* is inflammation of the salivary glands.
aliment/o	Nourishment, food	*Hyperalimentation* is the process of providing more or additional nourishment.
amyl/o	Starch	*Amylase* is an enzyme secreted by the pancreas that breaks down starches into simple sugars.
an/o	Anus	An *anal* fissure is a tear in the anus, the terminal portion of the digestive (GI) tract.
append/o, appendic/o	Appendix	An *appendectomy* is the surgical removal of the appendix, a small projection off the cecum; *appendicitis* is the condition that most frequently leads to this operation.
bucc/o	Cheek	Dentists frequently administer local anesthetic into the *buccal* (cheek) area.
cec/o	Cecum (first segment of the large intestine)	The ileocecal junction is where the small intestine merges with the large intestine.
cheil/o	Lip(s)	*Cheilitis* is an inflammation of the lip.
cholecyst/o	Gallbladder	*Cholecystolithiasis* is the condition most commonly referred to as gallstones.
choled/o	Common bile duct	*Choledolithotomy* is the process of removing stones from the common bile duct.
col/o, colon/o	(Large) intestine, colon	A *colostomy* is the formation of a new opening into the colon; a *colonoscopy* is the process of using a lighted instrument to visualize the colon.
dent/i, dent/o odont/o	Tooth (teeth)	A *dentist* is a tooth specialist.
duoden/o	Duodenum (first section of the small intestine)	*Duodenal* ulcers develop as a result of too much stomach acid passing from the stomach into the duodenum.
enter/o	(Small) intestine	*Enteral* stasis is a condition that occurs when digestion fails to take place in the small intestine.
epiglott/o	Epiglottis	*Epiglottitis* is an inflammation of the epiglottis, the structure that closes over the trachea to prevent food from passing into the respiratory system.
esophag/o	Esophagus (food tube)	*Esophageal* ulcers can occur when a patient has gastroesophageal reflux disease (GERD) and acid backs up into the esophagus.
gastr/o	Stomach	A *gastrectomy* is partial surgical removal of the stomach.
gloss/o, lingu/o	Tongue	*Ankyloglossia* is a condition of being "tongue tied."
hepat/o	Liver	*Hepatitis* is a viral inflammation of the liver; there are at least five different viruses cause hepatitis.
ile/o	Ileum (last section of the small intestine)	The *ileocecal* junction is where the ileum joins with the first section of the large intestine, the cecum.
intestin/o	Intestine	*Gastrointestinal* pertains to the stomach and intestines.
jejun/o	Jejunum (second section of the small intestine)	A *jejunectomy* is the surgical removal of the jejunum.
lith/o	Stone, calculus	*Sialolithectomy* is the surgical removal of salivary stones.
or/o, stomat/o	Mouth	*Oral* means pertaining to the mouth.
pancreat/o	Pancreas	*Pancreatitis* is an inflammation of the pancreas that causes the patient a good deal of pain; *pancreatic* secretions include amylase, lipase, and insulin.

(continues)

TABLE 5-11   Common Combining Forms and Suffixes Related to the Gastrointestinal System (Continued)

Combining Form	Definition	Example
periton/o	Peritoneum	The *peritoneal* cavity is lined by the peritoneum and houses the viscera.
pharyng/o	Pharynx (throat)	*Oropharyngeal* means "pertaining to the mouth and the throat."
proct/o, rect/o	Rectum	A *rectal* examination involves digital examination of the rectum; a *proctologist* is a specialist in rectal diseases.
sial/o	Saliva	*Sialolithiasis* is a condition of having stones in a salivary (gland).
sigmoid/o	Sigmoid colon	A *sigmoidectomy* is the surgical removal of the sigmoid colon, part of the large intestine.
Suffix	**Meaning**	**Example**
-ase	Enzyme	*Amylase, protease,* and *lipase* are all enzymes that break down food products for assimilation into the body.

THE URINARY SYSTEM

The urinary system is instrumental in ridding the human body of waste products that build up in the bloodstream and excreting that waste in the form of urine. The urinary system is composed of two kidneys, two ureters, one bladder, and one urethra. The body filters the blood in the **nephrons** of the kidneys; the nephrons are the microscopic functional cells of the kidney. Think about to whom you would be referred if you were having problems with your kidneys—a nephrologist, not a "kidneyologist." Ultimately the process of secreting urine for transport out of the body begins in the kidney in the nephrons; once the blood has been filtered and waste products removed, the urine is sent through the ureters to the bladder. The filtration process that occurs within the nephron and its complicated microscopic structure is a highly complex procedure that is explained in detail in Chapter 11. The bladder is responsible for housing the urine until there is a sufficient quantity to be transported out of the body by voiding, or **micturition**. There are many medical terms that relate to the urinary system, so an introduction to the terminology is necessary here.

The most common combining form on which many of the urinary system medical terms are based is *ur/o*, so learning this word component will help you interpret many of the terms associated with this system. *Ur/o* refers to the urine; a urologist is a specialist who is consulted when a patient is having problems with micturition (voiding). One common problem associated with the urinary system is formation of kidney stones, which are commonly referenced in that manner; however, the terms renal calculi and nephrolithiasis are also appropriate for this abnormal condition. When the kidneys fail to function properly, the waste products that would normally be transported out of the body in the urine will build up in

the bloodstream; patients experiencing this condition often must have their blood artificially cleansed by **dialysis**. Otherwise, a condition known as uremia will occur, a term that literally means "urine in the blood."

To reinforce these concepts, define and build the following medical terms.

Define the term **pyelonephritis.**

- Step 1: Identify and define the suffix: *-itis,* inflammation (of)
- Step 2: Identify and define the first combining form: *pyel/o,* (renal) pelvis
- Step 3: Identify and define the second combining form: *nephr/o,* kidney
- Step 4: Combine the definitions to identify the meaning of the term: "inflammation of the pelvis of the kidney." In this particular term, kidney is a bit redundant, as the combining form *pyel/o* refers to the renal pelvis, which is contained within the kidney.

Build a medical term that means "the process of viewing the bladder with a lighted instrument."

- Step 1: Select the suffix that means the process of viewing with a lighted instrument: *-scopy*
- Step 2: Select the combining form that means bladder: *cyst/o.*
- Step 3: Combine the word components, remembering that the suffix always goes at the end of the word.

Cyst/o + -scopy = cystoscopy

Remember that the process of viewing is different from the instrument that is used for the examination. A "scope" is the instrument, but "scopy" is the process of using that scope.

Table 5-12 lists and defines the most common combining forms associated with the urinary system.

TABLE 5-12   Common Combining Forms Related to the Urinary System

Combining Form	Definition	Example
bacteri/o	Bacteria	*Bacteriuria* indicates the presence of bacteria in the urine, usually from a urinary tract infection (UTI).
cyst/o	Bladder, sac	A *cystoscopy* is viewing the interior of the bladder with a lighted instrument.
glomerul/o	Glomerulus, filtering unit of a nephron	*Glomerulonephritis* is an inflammation of the glomerulus of the nephrons.
hemat/o	Blood	In some cases of nephrolithiasis, *hematuria*, or blood in the urine, is present.
lith/o	Stone, calculus	*Nephrolithiasis* is a condition of having kidney stones.
nephr/o, ren/o	Nephron, functional cell of the kidney, kidney	A *nephrectomy* is the removal of a kidney; the *renal* artery supplies blood to the kidney.
noct/o	Night	Older patients frequently complain of *nocturia*, a condition of having to get up during the night to void.
py/o	Pus	*Pyuria* is the presence of pus in the urine.
pyel/o	Renal pelvis	*Pyelolithotomy* is the surgical removal of kidney stones from the renal pelvis.
ur/o, urin/o	Urine	*Pyuria* is an abnormal condition of pus in the urine; a *urinometer* is an antiquated device that was used to measure the specific gravity of urine.
ureter/o	Ureter	An *ureteroscopy* is the procedure that is used to view the ureter(s) with a scope.
urethr/o	Urethra	A voiding *cystourethrogram* is an examination that is done while a patient is voiding that allows visualization of the bladder and the urethra.

THE NERVOUS SYSTEM

There are two major divisions to the nervous system: the central nervous system, consisting of the brain and spinal cord, and the peripheral nervous system, the portion that allows for awareness of surroundings through various receptors and communications with the brain. The brain is protected by the bony covering of the skull or cranium, while the fragile and delicate spinal cord is protected by the vertebrae of the spinal column. Without proper functioning of the nerve impulse centers in the brain as well as an intact spinal cord, voluntary movement of the extremities would be difficult if not impossible. The functional cells of the nervous system are **neurons**, so many of the medical terms related to the nervous system are based around this term. Not also that there are various parts of the brain and its protective covering, known collectively as the meninges.

Practice defining and building medical terms associated with this system.

Define **polyneuralgia**.

- Step 1: Identify and define the suffix: *-algia*, pain
- Step 2: Identify and define the prefix: *poly-*, many
- Step 3: Identify and define the combining form: *neur/o*, nerve

- Step 4: Combine the word component definitions to define the term: "pain in many nerves"

Build a medical term that means "pertaining to the nerves and muscles."

- Step 1: Select a suffix that means "pertaining to": in this case, *-ar*
- Step 2: Select the combining form that means "nerves": *neur/o*
- Step 3: Select the combining form that means "muscles": in this case, *muscul/o*
- Step 4: Combine the word components to make the medical term, dropping combining form vowels where indicated and remembering that a suffix is always at the end of the word.

    neur/o + muscul/o + -ar = neuromuscular

Look carefully at how the term is constructed: The second combining form began with a consonant, so the combining form vowel was maintained, but the suffix began with a vowel, so the combining form vowel was dropped.

For this system of the body, you need to learn the combining forms associated with the parts of the brain and the membranes lining the brain for protection, as

TABLE 5-13   Common Combining Forms Related to the Nervous System

Combining Form	Definition	Example
cerebell/o	Cerebellum	If there is an interruption in *cerebellar* nerve impulses, voluntary movements of the body become difficult.
electr/o	Electricity	An *electroencephalogram (EEG)* is a recording of the electrical impulses transmitted by the brain.
encephal/o, cerebr/o	Brain, cerebrum	Viral *encephalitis* is an inflammation of the brain by a virus; the *cerebral* part of the brain is what gives each individual unique personalities and thought processes.
mening/o	Meninges	*Meningococcal encephalitis* is an infection of the meninges resulting in inflammation of the brain.
neur/o	Nerve	*Neuralgia* is a generalized term meaning pain in a nerve.
phas/o	Speech	Occasionally when a patient has a stroke, *aphasia*, or inability to speak, may occur.

well as some of the pathologic conditions that affect the nervous system.

Table 5-13 lists and defines the common combining forms associated with the nervous system.

THE ENDOCRINE SYSTEM

The endocrine system is a unique system within the human body; the word endocrine, when broken down into its components (*endo-* and *crin/o*), literally means to "secrete within." Although each gland produces a secretion, it is not visible externally because the product—a hormone—is released directly into the bloodstream—hence to "secrete within." Laboratory tests can measure the level of hormones in the bloodstream to determine whether they are adequate; these are quite common blood tests drawn in health care providers' offices.

The organs of the endocrine system also are very specific in the way they operate; each hormone secreted by an endocrine organ targets a specific organ. The same hormone will not affect any other organ within the body. For instance, when the pituitary gland releases thyroid stimulating hormone (TSH), the hormone travels straight to the thyroid gland to stimulate it to produce more hormones for increasing the metabolism. But if your body needed more insulin, TSH would have absolutely no effect on your blood sugar (insulin's job is to lower blood sugar levels). Often the endocrine system and its secretion of hormones is likened to a lock and key; only one key will fit a lock, and only one hormone affects a particular organ.

The terms that you will encounter related to this system will most often refer to specific endocrine glands. Practice defining and building medical terms related to this system.

Define **hyperglycemia.**

- Step 1: Identify and define the suffix: *-emia*, blood
- Step 2: Identify and define the prefix: *hyper-*, above normal
- Step 3: Identify and define the combining form: *glyc/o*, sugar or glucose
- Step 4: Combine the word component definitions: "blood above normal glucose." This is an example of a term that requires you to change the order of adding the definitions together to make the word make sense. Rearranging the literal definition yields "above-normal blood sugar/glucose," which is correct.

Build a medical term that means "an abnormal condition of below-normal parathyroid (function)."

- Step 1: Select a suffix that means abnormal condition: in this case, *-ism*
- Step 2: Select a prefix that means below normal: for this word, choose *hypo-*
- Step 3: Select the combining form for parathyroid: *parathyroid/o*.
- Step 4: Put the word components together to make the term, remembering that the suffix always goes at the end of the word and the prefix goes at the beginning and watching the combining form vowels.

hypo- + parathyroid/o + -ism =
hypoparathyroidism

Another prefix that also means "below normal" is *sub-*, but this prefix is less common. It may be confusing to build medical terms before you have learned the most common terms. Also note that the combining form vowel was dropped when adding the suffix because the suffix began with a vowel.

Table 5-14 lists and defines the endocrine glands' combining forms and suffixes.

TABLE 5-14   Common Combining Forms and Suffixes Related to the Endocrine System

Combining Form	Definition	Example
gluc/o, glyc/o	Sugar, sweet	*Glucosuria* and *glycosuria* both mean "sugar in the urine."
parathyroid/o	Parathyroid glands	*Hyperparathyroidism* is a condition of excessive parathyroid activity.
thym/o	Thymus gland	*Thymosin* is a hormone secreted by the thymus gland.
thyr/o	Thyroid gland, shield	*Thyrotoxicosis* is a serious condition of the thyroid being "poisoned."
toxic/o	Poison, toxin	See previous example.
Suffix		
-oid	Resembling	*Thyroid* means "resembling a shield."
-ose	Sugar	*Sucrose* and *lactose* are different types of sugars than *glucose*.

THE SPECIAL SENSES

The special senses include those organs that provide vision, hearing, balance and upright stature, smell, and taste. Also included are the receptors of the skin that allow for the sense of touch, pain, and temperature (although there are few medical terms specifically associated with these senses). Most of the word components that you need to learn are associated with the various organs in the special senses. The organs associated with the senses include the *eye, ear, tongue,* and receptors embedded in the skin. The receptors in the skin associated with the sense of touch are varied in that some receptors differentiate between heat and cold *(thermoreceptors),* while others help in the sensation of pain *(nociceptors).* In some cases, there will be more than one combining form associated with an organ, so learning the most appropriate word component is essential to success with this section. For instance, both *ophthalm/o* and *opt/i* are combining forms for the eye, and *ot/o* and *aur/o* are combining forms for the ears. *Gloss/o* and *lingu/o* both refer to the tongue. Follow the examples to define and build medical terms.

Define **ophthalmologist**.

- Step 1: Identify and define the suffix: *-logist,* one who studies (or specializes)
- Step 2: Identify and define the combining form: *ophthalm/o,* eyes
- Step 3: Combine the word component definitions to define the term: "one who studies or specializes in the eyes," a term given to a medical doctor for this field

Build a medical term that means "a condition of tiny/small ear."

- Step 1: Choose a suffix that means "condition": for this word it will be *-ia*
- Step 2: Choose a prefix that means "tiny or small": *micro-*
- Step 3: Choose the most appropriate combining form for ear: in this case, it is *ot/o*
- Step 4: Put the word components together in their proper order, dropping combining form vowels where indicated.

$$micro- + ot/o + -ia = microtia$$

Let's review how this word was constructed since it is slightly different from some of the other examples presented in this chapter. First, take note that an exception was made when the prefix was added in that the *o* at the end of *micro-* was dropped, because the combining form begins with a vowel. Remember that this is unusual, and it is not common practice to change prefixes in such a manner. Also, because the suffix begins with a vowel, the combining form vowel was dropped. Without these changes, the resulting word would have been "microootia."

Table 5-15 lists and defines the combining forms, prefixes, and suffixes related to the special senses.

THE REPRODUCTIVE SYSTEM

There are two separate reproductive systems for the male and female. Each system has its own associated terms.

The reproductive system is responsible for allowing the human race to reproduce and perpetuate the species through new birth. Thus, this section introduces terms not just specific to the reproductive system, but also to human development from fertilization through birth.

The primary structure associated with the female reproductive tract is the ovary (of which there are two); the remaining structures are accessory organs. Included in these accessory organs are the uterus, the fallopian or

TABLE 5-15   Common Combining Forms Related to the Special Senses

Combining Form	Definition	Example
audi/o	Sound, hearing	An *audiogram* is a record of how well a patient is able to hear various pitches of sound.
aur/o, ot/o	Ear	*Aural* and *otic* drops are used in the ear to soften ear wax. *Microtia* is a condition of very small ears.
blephar/o	Eyelid	*Blepharoptosis* is a sagging (drooping) eyelid.
conjunctiv/o	Conjunctiva(e)	*Conjunctivitis* is an inflammation of the mucous membrane lining of the eye, commonly referred to as "pink-eye."
corne/o	Cornea	A *corneal* abrasion is a scratch on the cornea of the eye.
myring/o, tympan/o	Ear drum	A *myringotomy* is often performed on children to relieve pressure on the ear drum; *a tympanic* thermometer is one inserted into the ear canal to measure temperature.
ocul/o, ophthalm/o	Eye	*Ocular* implants are placed in the eye; an *ophthalmologist* is a specialist in the eye and associated diseases.
olfact/o	Smell	The *olfactory* nerve endings in the nose provide the sense of smell.
retin/o	Retina	*Retinal* surgery would be performed to repair a detached retina.
Prefix		
presby-	Aging, elderly	*Presbyopia* and *presbycusis* are medical terms given to diminished vision and hearing associated with the aging process.
Suffix		
-cusis	Hearing	*Presbycusis* is the medical term given to hearing loss that occurs as a result of the aging process.
-ptosis	Sagging or drooping	*Blepharoptosis* is a sagging (drooping) eyelid.

uterine tubes, the vagina, and external accessory organs. Combining forms associated with this system are deeply rooted in Greek and Latin terms, making it more difficult to remember and memorize the terms. Also keep in mind that the female breasts are accessory organs for the reproductive system.

The primary structure in the male reproductive system is the testis (of which there are two); the remaining structures are accessory organs and include the internal structures such as the epididymis, the vas deferens, the seminal vesicle, the prostate gland, and the bulbourethral or Cowper's glands. The remaining structures are categorized as external reproductive organs.

The cycle of development of an embryo until it becomes a neonate or infant is also pertinent. At fertilization, the result of the combining of the sperm and the ovum is termed a zygote; the zygote will not implant itself into the uterine wall for about 3 days. Once the zygote implants, it is called an embryo until the end of the eighth week of development, after which it is called fetus. While the embryo/fetus is developing and growing, it is enclosed in a protective sac known as the pla-

centa or amniotic sac. Once the fetus has been delivered outside of the mother's body, it is referred to as a neonate or newborn until the fourth week of life, at which time it is called an infant. This term applies until the child is a year old.

Practice defining and building medical terms for each reproductive system.

Define **cervicitis.**

- Step 1: Identify and define the suffix: *-itis*, inflammation
- Step 2: Identify and define the combining form: *cervic/o*, neck (of the cervix in this case)
- Step 3: Add the definitions together to define the word: "inflammation of the neck (of the uterus)"

Define **cryptorchidism.**

- Step 1: Identify and define the suffix: *-ism*, condition
- Step 2: Identify and define the first combining form: *crypt/o*, hidden
- Step 3: Identify and define the second combining form: *orchid/o*, testes

Step 4: Add the word component definitions together to define the word: "a condition of hidden testes." When one of the testes fails to descend as it should, it remains in the abdominal cavity rather than in the scrotum, and thus the testis is "hidden." Hence, the definition "a condition of an undescended testis" may be more appropriate.

Build a medical term that means "surgical removal of an ovary, fallopian tube, and uterus."

- Step 1: Select the suffix that "means surgical removal": *-ectomy*
- Step 2: Select the combining form that refers to ovary: *oophor/o*
- Step 3: Select the combining form that means "fallopian tube": *salping/o*
- Step 4: Select the combining form that refers to the uterus: *hyster/o*
- Step 5: Combine the word components in their proper order, paying attention to the combining form vowels and dropping those indicated.

oophor/o + salping/o + hyster/o + -ectomy = oophorosalpingohysterectomy

The first combining form vowel was retained because the next combining form begins with a consonant. The same is true when the third combining form is added; however, the combining form vowel for

TABLE 5-16	Common Combining Forms Related to the Reproductive System	
Combining Form	**Definition**	**Example**
amni/o	Amnion	*Amniocentesis* is a surgical puncture of the amnion (amniotic sac) for diagnostic testing for birth defects.
cervic/o	Neck, cervix (neck) of the uterus	*Cervical* cancer may be revealed with the use of a Pap smear.
colp/o, vagin/o	Vagina	A *colposcopy* is examination of the vagina with a lighted instrument; *vaginitis* is inflammation of the vagina, usually bacterial or fungal.
embry/o	Embryo	*Embryology* is the study of human development through the eighth week after conception.
gravida	Pregnancy	The terms *nulli gravida* indicates a woman has never been pregnant.
gyn/o, gynec/o	Female, woman	A *gynecologist* is a specialist in the anatomy of the female reproductive system.
hyster/o, metr/o, uter/o	Uterus	A *hysterectomy* is the surgical removal of the uterus; a *uteroscopy* may be performed prior to the surgery. *Metrorrhagia* is uterine bleeding at a time other than the monthly cycle.
lact/o	Milk	*Prolactin* is a hormone secreted by the pituitary gland so a mother can nurse her baby by producing milk.
mamm/o, mast/o	Breast	A *mammogram* is a common radiologic test for detection of breast cancer; a *mastopexy* may be done to correct sagging breasts.
men/o	Month, menstruation	*Menopause* is when a woman no longer has monthly periods.
nat/o	Birth	A *neonate* is a newborn; the *prenatal* period pertains to the months prior to the baby's birth.
oophor/o, ovari/o	Ovary	An *oophorectomy*, surgical removal of an ovary, may be performed in the case of an *ovarian* cyst.
orch/o, orchi/o, orchid/o, test/o	Testes	*Cryptorchidism* is a condition in which one or both testes (testicles) have not descended in the male and may require an *orchiopexy* to correct. *Testosterone* is the hormone produced by the testes in the male.
ov/o	Egg	*Oval* means "pertaining to an egg"; an oval is shaped like an egg.
prostat/o	Prostate	A *prostatectomy* is the surgical removal of the prostate.
salping/o	Tube (fallopian)	*Salpingitis* is an inflammation of the fallopian tube that may impede pregnancy.
sperm/o, spermat/o	Sperm	A *spermaticide* is used to kill sperm and prevent pregnancy.

TABLE 5-17   Common Medical Abbreviations

Abbreviation	Meaning	Abbreviation	Meaning
ASHD	Arteriosclerotic heart disease	GU	Genitourinary
CA, ca	Cancer, carcinoma	GYN	Gynecology
COPD	Chronic obstructive pulmonary disease	IV	Intravenous
CVA	Cerebrovascular accident (stroke)	MI	Myocardial infarction
ECG, EKG	Electrocardiogram	MS	Musculoskeletal
EEG	Electroencephalogram	UA	Urinalysis
EGD	Esophagogastroduodenoscopy	UGI	Upper GI (series)
GERD	Gastroesophageal reflux disease	URI	Upper respiratory infection
GI	Gastrointestinal	UTI	Urinary tract infection

uterus was dropped because the suffix begins with a vowel.

Build a medical term that means "the process of producing or originating sperm cells."

- Step 1: Select the suffix that means "originating or beginning": -genesis
- Step 2: Select the combining form that relates to sperm: spermat/o
- Step 3: Add the word components together to make the medical term

Spermat/o + -genesis = spermatogenesis

Once you have the opportunity to learn more about the anatomy of the reproductive systems for both the male and female, come back to this chapter and refresh your knowledge of the medical terms; they will likely make more sense to you then. Table 5-16 lists and defines the combining forms associated with the reproductive system and human development through birth.

COMMON ABBREVIATIONS

In the anatomy and physiology section of the book, you will be introduced to many abbreviations as they relate to diagnostic tests, diseases, and treatment modalities. However, Table 5-17 offers a brief introduction to some of these.

ACHIEVE UNIT OBJECTIVES

- Complete the Workbook activities to meet the learning objectives.
- Apply your knowledge at the end of this chapter in completing the Critical Thinking Challenge and Activities, as well as the StudyWARE on your Student CD-ROM.

CRITICAL THINKING CHALLENGE

IMPACTING THE PATIENT, THE PRACTICE, AND YOUR CAREER

Jennifer Hooper is a competent medical assistant; however, Jenni has dyslexia, which is of constant concern to her. She is working with Dr. Betty Shrader, a surgeon, scheduling patients for operations and procedures. Dr. Shrader tells Jenni that she would like for Ms. Debbie Jones to be scheduled for a nephrectomy as soon as possible. When Jenni writes down the procedure, she records the operation as a phrenectomy and calls the hospital later in the afternoon to schedule Ms. Jones for the operation.

QUESTIONS

1. What impact will this have on the patient?
2. What impact could this have on the practice of Dr. Shrader?
3. What could this do to Jenni's career?

ACTIVITIES

1. Select a body system from the chapter and write a short story appropriately using as many of the medical terms as possible.
2. Ask your instructor for a medical transcription reference that has a patient's chart notes and compare the application of the medical terms in the body of the transcription.

StudyWARE™ CHALLENGE

- Study with the flash cards for Chapter 5 to review the key terms in this chapter.
- Solve the crossword puzzle for Chapter 5.
- Complete the true/false quiz in test mode for Chapter 5.

RESOURCES

Ehrlich, A. (2005). *Medical terminology for health professions* (5th ed.). Clifton Park, NY: Thomson Delmar Learning.

WEB LINKS

www.medterms.com (MedTerms Medical Dicionary) *Online medical dictionary and glossary with medical definitions.*

SECTION 2

The Administrative Medical Assistant

The office assistant must have sufficient knowledge of medical terminology to deal efficiently with the unending variety of telephone calls received daily. A pleasant voice and good listening skills are essential. Practicing patience and demonstrating compassion to those in need of such attention are important. The medical assistant needs to have legible handwriting for recording appointments and messages. Typing or keyboarding skills are necessary if appointments are to be made on a computer. You will have an opportunity to demonstrate your knowledge of anatomy, medical terminology, spelling, grammar, and punctuation when you answer the office phone and as you complete progress notes on charts. You will also use these skills in the completion of correspondence. You may have the responsibility of processing incoming and outgoing mail. Written communication skills must be as flawless as possible. A number of people may view the letters or forms you send out, and each will receive a mental picture of you and your office—good if the work is neat and correct, and definitely questionable if it is inaccurate or messy.

UNIT 1
TELEPHONE COMMUNICATIONS

OBJECTIVES

Upon completion of this unit, you will be able to achieve the following:

LEARNING Objectives

1. Spell and define, using the glossary at the back of the text, all the Words to Know in this unit.

2. Describe methods of screening incoming calls.

3. Explain the proper protocol for answering the telephone in the medical office.

4. Explain the procedure for handling nonemergency calls.

5. List the information that should be included in all telephone messages.

6. Describe the different types of phone calls that a medical assistant may have to answer in the medical office, and explain how each should be handled.

7. Explain the protocol for handling callers who refuse to identify themselves.

PERFORMANCE Objectives

1. Perform a telephone screening.

2. Obtain a telephone message from a recording device.

3. Obtain a telephone message from an outside answering service.

4. Place a follow-up call to inform the patient of test results.

WORDS TO KNOW

confirmed	expressed	personality
empathy	fax	screening
etiquette		

 CERTIFICATION CONNECTION

CMA

Adapting communications to an individual's ability to understand

Recognize and respond to verbal communication

Professional communication and behavior

Evaluating and understanding communications

Interviewing techniques

Telephone techniques

CMAS

Communications

RMA

Employ appropriate telephone etiquette

Perform appropriate telephone screenings

Instruct patient via telephone

Inform patient of test results per physician's instructions

Record, process, and document results received from outside provider

Employ active listening skills

ANSWERING THE TELEPHONE

The telephone is the center of all activity in the medical office just as it is with any business. The professional attitude conveyed is critical to the success of the business of practicing medicine. The medical assistant who handles phone calls must be courteous, articulate, and a careful and active listener. The rapport established by the medical assistant will contribute to successful communication with patients. Most medical facilities have telephones with multiple lines. Someone should answer each line as soon as possible—at least by the third ring. Sometimes all lines ring continually. Some basic guidelines for handling several ringing lines include the following:

- Excuse yourself and ask the patient you are speaking to if they can hold.
- Answer the second call, determine the nature of the call (be sure it is not an emergency), and ask if they can hold.
- Return to the first call and thank them for holding.
- Resolve the first call and return to the second call.

An automated answering device can also be utilized to answer calls more efficiently. A recording asks the caller to hold and informs them that their call will be answered in the order in which it was received. Some recordings offer a menu of options to properly route calls to the correct person or department.

Phone Menus

Most business phone systems have a menu for the caller to be connected to the proper person or department. By pushing the correct number as directed by the recorded message (e.g., "Press one to reach the billing department, press two to speak to the scheduling department, press three for prescription refills,"), the caller can be connected to the desired party. The system is designed to be more efficient and to not only keep the caller from being on hold for too long, but to help avoid being disconnected. The caller should be instructed at the beginning of the recorded message to hang up immediately and call EMS or 911 (as applicable to the caller's geographic area) if there is a medical emergency. Each call should be answered as soon as possible no matter what the nature of the call is. Courteous and expedient return of a call not only is most efficient, but it promotes a positive atmosphere.

Telephone Screening

An established phone screening manual should be kept near the phone for reference so that each assistant who answers the phone will ask standard questions and give the standard advice that has been pre-authorized by the physician. The assistant must learn how to logically proceed through a set of questions that will reveal the caller's condition and help to determine, if necessary, how soon the patient should be seen by a physician. This process is called telephone screening. If the assistant does not know how to handle a patient, or if the questions have not been addressed in the manual, referring the problem to one who is more experienced is necessary and appropriate. Never guess in response to a patient's questions and do not treat any question lightly. If there is a serious telephone emergency that cannot be handled in the facility, it is best to refer the patient to an emergency medical service and explain that they will send someone as soon as possible to help. It may be best to direct the person to an emergency room of the nearest hospital. It is important to have all emergency phone numbers listed by each phone in the office. In stressful times, this will be helpful in giving the patient phone numbers they might need quickly or in calling an emergency service for the patient. The assistant must ask questions of coworkers and supervisors as they learn how to best deal with problems. If you are speaking to a patient face-to-face at the office and you must answer the phone, say to the patient, "Excuse me for a moment, please," answer the phone call, and then continue with what you were doing. All emergency calls must be handled immediately.

Nonemergency Calls

If the person on the phone needs additional information, or if the call is going to take a while, excuse yourself from the phone call by saying, "May I put you on hold for a moment?" However, if it will be more than one minute, the caller should not be placed on hold; in this case say, "May I call you back with that information?" Be sure to check the patient's phone number before hanging up, because it may have changed since the patient's last appointment. Find out a good time to call back. There may be times when the patient has to wait to speak to the physician. In this case, you should check back frequently until the doctor answers to let the patient know that he has not been forgotten. During the hold time, many medical facilities provide the caller with helpful information that contains reminders of immunization updates, services and procedures offered by the staff, routine office hours, what to do and whom to call in an emergency, and other relevant information. The assistant must beware of leaving callers on hold for too long. You can be sure that callers will let you know how long they had to wait and how many times they heard the entire recording.

Transferring Telephone Calls

If you need to transfer a patient's call to another department or office, first give the caller the phone number, extension number, and the person's name to whom you are transferring them in case there is a disconnection. You should signal (or page) the person, and when the person answers, explain who is waiting to speak to her and give a brief summary of what it is regarding. If a patient is calling for information, pull the chart and have it ready for the physician along with any test or lab reports associated with the call. If using a public address system, be very careful with confidentiality and state only the person's name and that they have a call on line 1. Make sure you inform the caller that the person they wish to speak with has been paged and will be with them as soon as possible. There may be times when the physician is close to the phone; simply ask the doctor to take the call and tell him who is calling and what the call is regarding. Always use common courtesy when handling any telephone call. Establishing good communication, especially over the phone, is essential to building good rapport. A telephone log should be maintained that lists all calls received, along with the name and telephone number of the person you should call back. The log may also contain information on the best time to return the call and what the call is regarding. Telephoning a person at an appropriate time can eliminate playing "phone tag."

Refer to Procedure 6-1 for the steps to follow when performing telephone screening.

DOCUMENTING TELEPHONE MESSAGES

 Documenting telephone messages is of vital importance and should be treated likewise. Of primary concern is the issue of confidentiality due

PROCEDURE PROCEDURE PROCEDURE PROCEDURE PROCEDURE PROCEDURE PROCEDURE

6-1  Perform a Telephone Screening

PURPOSE: Answer the office telephone promptly and efficiently in a professional manner.

EQUIPMENT AND SUPPLIES: Telephone, paper, pen, computer—if available.

PERFORMANCE OBJECTIVE: In a simulated situation, answer the telephone by the third ring, identifying yourself and the office.

1. Answer the phone promptly (by the third ring) in a polite and pleasant manner.

2. Identify the office and yourself by name. **NOTE: Your voice must be clear and distinct. Speak at a moderate rate, expressing consideration for the needs of the caller.**

3. Listen to and record the name and phone number of the caller, the reason for the call, and the date and time of the call. **NOTE: Obtain the correct spelling and pronunciation of the caller's name.**

4. Before placing a caller on hold, determine whether the call is an emergency situation, and if so, process the call immediately.

5. If a caller must be placed on hold, try to check with him periodically to let him know you haven't forgotten about him.

6. Complete all calls placed on hold in a timely manner.

7. Screen and complete as many calls as possible before adding names to the physician's call back list.

8. Respond to an untimely request to speak to the physician by taking a message for the physician to return the call or having advice relayed by you.

---

to HIPAA regulations. Data regarding patients may not be given out over the telephone to anyone unless the patient has given written permission for the release of specific information with a signature. It is equally important that the date, time, a brief message regarding the call, and the initials of the person who responded to the call be recorded. Then any questions concerning a call may be further explained by the person whose initials are on the message. All calls should be documented in the same manner. All messages that are urgent should be given priority and handled as soon as possible to prevent further discomfort, pain, and anxiety for patients.

Many offices now utilize an outside answering service to answer calls during lunch breaks, after office hours, and on weekends. The caller often appreciates talking with a real person rather than a recording, especially in an emergency situation.

MESSAGING DEVICES

Voice mail, pagers, and other answering devices make communications much more accessible than ever before. Answering machines are especially useful for short time blocks such as during lunch time. If the standard in your medical office is an answering machine that records messages whenever the physician is not in the office, it should tell the caller how to contact the physician or how to leave a message. This must be done day and night, 365 days a year. Messages need to be played back and recorded as soon as possible. Then, all of the

calls need to be returned in the order of their importance within an appropriate and reasonable time period. Remember to check the **fax** machine, because messages and other patient-related information can be faxed to the office at any time. Returning phone- or fax-requested patient information should also be done promptly.

Confidentiality is a primary concern. All documents with information regarding patients should be kept out of reach of others who are not part of the medical office staff. Some physicians prefer to have patients call them at their home, while others employ an answering service to screen calls and take only urgent cases at home. In this instance, the one who screens the calls will contact the doctor at home (or by pager) and have the doctor return the patient's call. Refer to Procedure 6-2 for the steps to follow when obtaining telephone messages from a phone recording device or answering service.

A telephone message pad and pen should be placed by each office telephone. You cannot rely on memory in a busy office where there are constant interruptions. Individual offices have a variety of methods for recording telephone messages. You may use a preprinted duplicate message pad; the top sheet is removed and the carbon remains as a permanent record of calls received. The office may use a secretarial notebook that is dated each day; calls are recorded and checked off when returned. You need to develop a follow-up method to be sure calls

PROCEDURE PROCEDURE PROCEDURE PROCEDURE PROCEDURE PROCEDURE PROCEDURE

6-2   Obtain a Telephone Message from a Phone Recording Device

PURPOSE: To obtain accurate message(s) from a recording device or answering service, obtaining all necessary information from the caller to correctly process requests.

EQUIPMENT AND SUPPLIES: Telephone message device, pen, paper/phone message log or computer, appropriate patients' charts.

PERFORMANCE OBJECTIVE: In a simulated situation, obtain a telephone message from a recording device or answering service.

1. Assemble all necessary items in an area away from noise and distractions.

2. Check the recording device or answering service and write out each message accurately. **NOTE: You may have to listen to the recording more than one time in order to obtain complete information, as some voices may be difficult to understand. It is a good practice to ask another staff member to listen if you have difficulty.**

3. If obtaining messages from an answering service, call the service and obtain all messages from a representative of the service.

4. Sometimes, answering services will send you an e-mail message or a fax, which provides you with a hard copy that can be filed in the patient's chart.

5. Always clarify any discrepancies in e-mails or faxes with the service.

6. Sign your initials after the message. The date and time of the message must also be written.

7. List all patients who leave messages so you can pull their charts.

8. Prioritize messages according to the nature of their seriousness and distribute to the appropriate staff member or department to be processed.

have been returned. The call pad or messages should not be filed until the requests have been given a response. Some offices have a stamp made up to indicate in the patient chart a telephone communication and a brief note with the date the patient was contacted. It is not advisable to have loose slips of paper in the file, as they are easily lost. If these are kept in the chart, they should be filed shingle fashion on a sheet of paper with the most recent call on top.

Self-stick telephone message forms are helpful in establishing effective control of patient calls. One form comes in a single looseleaf style with a stub (like that of a checkbook or loan payment book) that remains in a binder for future reference. Another style has a duplicate copy that remains in a spiral binder and provides a master reference for future review. When a call is received from a patient, the message form is completed. After completing the form, tear it at the perforation and attach the form to the patient's chart. If a patient call requires a return call from the physician, the form is attached to the front of the patient's chart and given to the physician. When the physician completes the call and records the message, the form is simply removed from the front of the chart and placed in the proper location on the inside of the chart for future reference. Another telephone message form is a log sheet and message slip with carbon. The benefits of this system are that you do not have to rewrite the message in the patient's chart,

use a telephone stamp, or be concerned about loose slips of paper falling out of the chart. The carbon copy is a permanent record of calls for reference. Examples of telephone message forms are shown in Figures 6-1 and 6-2A. Figure 6-2B illustrates the recording of a message from a patient on a chart.

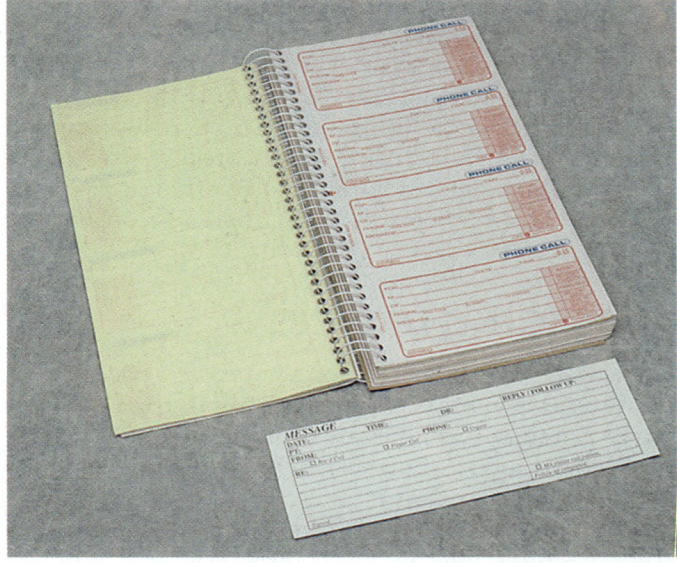

FIGURE 6-1 These telephone message forms have a carbon copy that stays intact for a permanent record of each call.

PHONE MESSAGE

For _____ Date ____ Time _____ AM/PM

Mr/Ms _____

Of _____

Phone _____ Page # _____ Fax _____

☐ Phoned   ☐ Please call—urgent
☐ Returned call   ☐ Stopped in
☐ Will call again   ☐ Wants appointment
☐ Personal   ☐ See me for message

Message

_____

_____

_____

_____

_____

Call taken by _____ Date ____ Time ____

FIGURE 6-2A   A telephone message form

Date/time

Mr. Silvers called to let Dr. Lang know that his dentist, Dr. Edwin Blair, gave him an antibiotic, penicillin 500 mg, #32, 4x da, for 8 days, for an abscessed tooth.

FIGURE 6-2B   Example of recording a phone message on the patient's chart

Important elements included in a telephone message are:

- Caller's full name, spelled correctly
- Brief note indicating the nature of the call
- Action required
- Date, time of call, initials of person receiving call
- Phone number of caller; include the area code if this is a long distance call

If the telephone has a speaker phone or a headset, your hands will be free to use a pen to either write a message or use the keyboard to log in the patient's call, retrieve the patient's file, or schedule an appointment. Figure 6-3 shows a medical assistant using a headset in a phone conversation. The proper position of a phone with a receiver is shown in Figure 6-4. When you hold the receiver of the telephone, it should be 2 to 3 inches

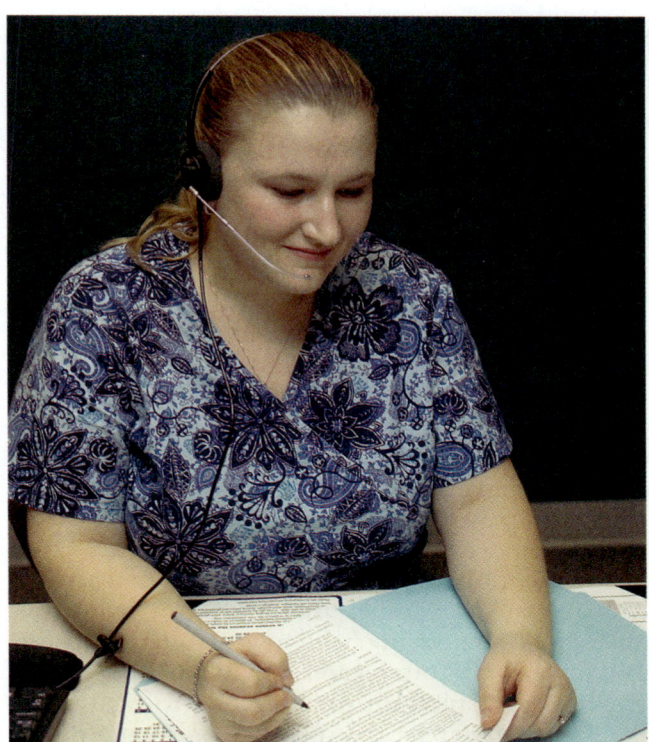

FIGURE 6-3   This medical assistant is using a headset to answer calls to free her hands to use the keyboard, take messages, open mail, and so on.

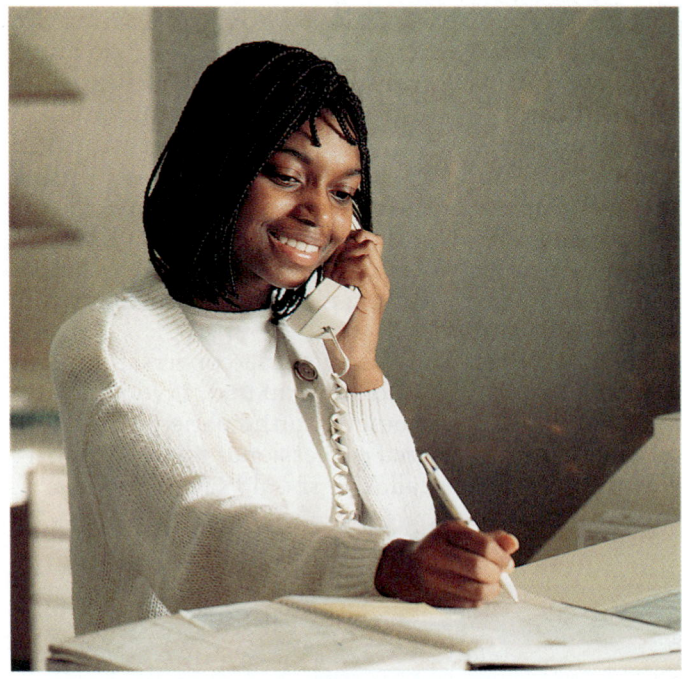

FIGURE 6-4   This medical assistant is holding the phone receiver at a proper distance. Even though the caller cannot see the receptionist, her pleasant attitude is evident.

in front of your mouth so that the caller may clearly hear your voice. Many professional offices have cordless phones, with long cords on the receiver for ease in accessing files as needed. The hold button, transfer extension dialing, conference calling, and other features may vary from office to office. You should be honest about your knowledge and experience with phone systems. You must ask to have a certain feature explained and demonstrated to you if you do not know how to use it. You must use proper technique with a telephone system or the caller may be rudely interrupted or accidentally disconnected during a call. Since you never know who is on the other end of the phone, always answer as promptly as possible in a professional manner. Emergencies can happen at any time, and your efficiency on the phone could affect the outcome.

The following example highlights the proper manner of a polite and efficient way to answer a call: "Good morning, Central Medical Center, Ellen speaking, how may I help you?" The caller usually is prompted to give you her name after saying hello to you and explains the reason for the call. Your response should be appropriate and spoken in a pleasant tone of voice to each caller. Make sure that you get the complete name and phone number of the patient in case your call is interrupted. This is a safe practice to follow in case the call is an emergency and you get cut off. If the information that the patient gives you is not clear, you must say, for example, "Could you please repeat that for me?" or "Would you spell your name for me again, please?" It is better to ask someone to repeat what was said initially than to have to go back over the whole conversation and redo all of it—the patient may wonder if you paid attention to *anything* that was said. You should convey confidence rather than insecurity. If you cannot understand someone because their voice is too soft, ask them to speak a little louder. If the person talks too loud, ask if they could speak a little softer, faster, slower, and so on. It is also a good practice to ask patients each time you speak to them (over the phone or in person) if there is any change in their address, phone numbers, and so on, to keep files current.

When you are finished with the conversation, it is best to allow the caller to hang up first. If you hang up first you might miss something the patient wanted to add. It is not considered professional to say "Bye-bye" when you finish the call. You should say "Good-bye."

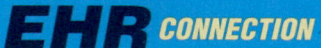

EHR *CONNECTION*

Appointments, prescriptions, and test results can be easily documented in the patient's electronic record.

When you have more than one telephone line coming in to the office, never answer the second line with "Hold the line, please," and then go back to your first call. You need to place the first call on hold properly and find out who is on the second line. Then you can determine whether or not it is an emergency and, if it is not, ask the second caller to hold while you finish the first call. Keep all calls as brief as possible. Personal calls and personal business should be kept to a minimum.

Your voice is part of your **personality**, but over the telephone, your voice *is* you. Callers form a picture of you as they listen to your voice. Does your telephone personality reveal a confident, courteous, friendly, and efficient medical assistant? It is equally easy to be heard as uncertain, irritated, abrupt, or inefficient.

Since the phone call is often the first contact a patient has with the office, your manner of speaking and the **empathy** you convey are a part of establishing an appropriate image of the practice.

COMMON TYPES OF PHONE CALLS

The process of **screening** calls requires you to be aware of the most frequent types of phone calls that will be received in the medical office. They are:

- Referrals
- Patients who are calling for appointments, prescriptions, or the results of tests
- Emergency calls
- Other physicians, hospitals, or laboratories
- Personal calls and general business calls

Table 6-1 lists examples of calls received in the medical office and where they should be routed. Knowing where to send a call when it comes in can save time and frustration.

Appointments, Prescriptions, and Test Results

Patients who phone for appointments should be given a choice of two appointment times. Usually one of the times will be satisfactory, and this will eliminate the patient asking for multiple dates and times that are not available. Do not say "When would you like to come in?" It is better to say "Do you prefer mornings or afternoons?" Do not say "Are you a patient here?" It is better to say "When did we last see you?" Do not say "What's the problem?" It is better to say "What is the reason for your visit?" The appointment should be **confirmed** by reading the scheduled time back to the patient after it has been recorded in the appointment book.

You will find that patients will frequently ask to speak with the physician. Never say "The doctor is busy," as this may give the impression that the doctor does not want to be bothered by the caller. Be aware of

TABLE 6-1 Routing Calls in the Medical Office				
Type of Call	**Immediately Routed to Physician**	**Record Message for the Physician**	**Routed to Clinical Medical Assistant**	**Routed to Administrative Medical Assistant**
Any situation deemed to be an emergency by the physician	X			
Critical lab results	X	X — Route to the physician immediately after recording the results.		
Progress report from a patient		X		
Patient requesting test results	X (abnormal results)		X (if results are normal)	
Billing or insurance calls				X
Prescription refills			X	
Referrals			X	
Scheduling appointment				X
Another physician	X			
Hospital calling for orders	X			
Patient complaints		X		
Patient requesting medical advice	X			
Third party request for information about a patient	X			

the statements you make in reporting why the physician cannot speak on the telephone. It would be much better to state "The doctor is with a patient now. May I take a message and we will return the call as soon as possible?" The caller will usually respect the right of others to have the full attention of the physician and will not expect to interrupt the doctor except for an emergency.

Prescriptions

Each office will have its own rules for calling pharmacies for prescription refills. It is important that you learn the rules for the office in which you work and follow them without exception. The general rule is that a medical assistant does not give out information or call in a prescription without the **expressed** direction of the physician.

Write messages requesting prescriptions or test results in legible handwriting. If a patient requests a prescription refill, you need to know the name and phone number of the pharmacy as well as the name of the medication, strength, and prescription number. You also should record a telephone number where the patient can be reached in case the physician needs to talk

with the patient before prescribing the medication. The physician may need to examine the patient first, in which case you would need to call and schedule an appointment.

Many physicians prefer to have prescriptions and refills faxed to the patient's pharmacy. This practice is very efficient because it usually requires only one phone call, the one initiated by the patient for the medication refill. The fax document provides a paper trail for the patient's chart and should be filed as soon as possible. The medical assistant needs to ask the patient a few questions to note on the fax form, such as birth date, social security number, medical insurance number, and current phone number. It is vital that all information be kept in strict confidence.

A brief entry should be entered on the progress notes of the chart regarding the date and the name of the medication that was faxed to the pharmacy (with: "See fax"). Add your initials to indicate that you completed the procedure.

Another expedient and efficient method of dealing with medications may be available in certain instances. Patient information and the prescription can be entered into the computer and sent directly to the pharmacist. The patients can then go to the pharmacy and pick up their medications.

Test Results

Patients will call the office on a daily basis to request test results. Always observe your office's policy for releasing results. Most physicians will want to speak with the patient themselves if the test results are abnormal, while some will allow the medical assistant to give normal results over the telephone. The physician will usually want to examine the results and initial them before releasing the chart to the medical assistant. Refer to Procedure 6-3 for the steps to follow when telephoning a patient with test results.

Professional Calls

When a physician telephones to speak to your employer, politely ask the caller for his name and inform the physician. Professional **etiquette** dictates that a physician will not keep a colleague waiting unless the physician is involved with an emergency or a surgical procedure.

Calls received in your office regarding x-ray or laboratory results need to be recorded accurately. Always record the name of the person giving the report. It is best to read back everything you have written down to be sure it is correct and complete before allowing the caller to leave the line.

Business, Personal, and Legal Calls

Your employer should let you know how to handle calls from family members, business associates, and salespeople. Calls from attorneys requesting information about a patient must be handled with great caution. Attorneys know the patient must give written permission to divulge information to anyone regarding their health, yet attorneys will call and ask for information. Pull the patient chart and look for authorization listing the name of the attorney and the signature of the patient. If you find it, you may answer questions about the patient. Some physicians may still want you to check with them before releasing information. If you do not find authorization listing the name of the attorney, you must tell the caller to send an authorization signed by the patient and then you will be able to release information. It is ad-

---

PROCEDURE PROCEDURE PROCEDURE PROCEDURE PROCEDURE PROCEDURE PROCEDURE

6-3  Telephone a Patient with Test Results

PURPOSE: To telephone a patient with test results, observing HIPAA regulations and following the instructions of the physician.

EQUIPMENT: Patient's chart, telephone, lab results, pen.

PERFORMANCE OBJECTIVE: Using the necessary equipment, follow all the steps in the procedure and inform the patient about laboratory or other test results. Protect PHI (protected health information) according to HIPAA and document the call.

1. Obtain patient's chart, with test results attached, from the physician. **RATIONALE: The physician must review all test results before they can be released to the patient. Do not release any results that have not been initialed by the physician.**

2. Check the patient's chart for the signed privacy notice to determine who may receive the information. **NOTE: Be sure to check the signed notice to determine if it is permissible to leave information on an answering machine.**

3. Telephone the patient, identifying yourself and the office.

4. Identify the person you are speaking to. **NOTE: Information can only be given to the patient themselves or to persons authorized by the patient to receive PHI.**

5. Inform the patient about test results and any instructions from the physician.

6. Ask the patient to repeat the results to be sure they have the correct information.

7. Instruct the patient to call the office with any questions.

8. Allow the patient to hang up first. **RATIONALE: Allowing the patient to hang up first eliminates the possibility of missing a question or statement from the patient.**

9. Document the call in the patient's chart.

CHARTING EXAMPLE

10-10-xx

Follow-up call to patient with CBC results. Instructed patient to F/U in 6 months for repeat CBC per Dr. Carter.

L. Leonard, CMA

HIPAA

When relaying information to or regarding a patient by telephone, the following HIPAA guidelines should be observed to protect the privacy of individual health information.

1. Some patients request that any communications with them by the medical office be confidential. The patient will usually give an alternate telephone number to contact them, other than their home number. Careful attention must be paid to ensure that the patient's request is being granted.
2. It is permissible to call the patient at their home number if they have not requested confidential communications.
3. When calling a patient, identify yourself and the office.
4. A message may be left on a recording device or with another individual for the patient to return the call. Be sure to leave the appropriate telephone number. No medical information or test results may be left on a recording device or with another individual.
5. Confidential information may be discussed with the patient over the telephone, taking special care not to divulge information where it can be overheard by a third party.
6. The patient may designate another individual or individuals that may receive protected health information about them.

PHI (protected health information) must be kept in secure areas so that unauthorized individuals may not obtain it. The following are considered to be PHI and must be protected:

- Information on a computer monitor
- Medical records or patient charts
- Verbal conversations
- Patient financial records

visable to return a call from an attorney even if you have authorization so you can be sure to whom you are talking. Anyone can call and claim to be a patient's attorney. Unless you know the caller, you cannot be sure you are talking to the correct individual.

Only information that has been authorized by the patient in writing, with the patient's signature, may be given to another party. Otherwise, the patient record is considered confidential information, and you may be liable for your actions.

Difficult Calls

There are a few calls that will be a challenge to you no matter when they are received. These can include a call from an angry patient, a prank call, an obscene call, and

"bogus" business calls. These types of calls should be reported to the police department if they persist. As with any phone call you receive, you should be as tactful, professional, and courteous as possible.

When an angry patient phones you and begins to rant and rave about something that you know nothing about, you should first, as calmly as possible and in a soft tone, ask the person to please start from the beginning and tell you his concerns. In this way, you can either answer the patient's needs or direct him to the proper person or department so that the problem can be resolved. If the patient is speaking so loudly that you have to hold the receiver away from your ear, ask the person to please hold for a few seconds while you pull his chart. This will allow for a little time for the patient to calm down. If the caller uses profanity, you should remind the caller that you will not continue the call unless you can be spoken to in a courteous manner. There are times when the only way to sensibly handle a situation like this is to ask the office manager, your supervisor, or the physician to speak to the patient. Another way that may be helpful is to take the complaint and phone number and ask if you may call the patient back after you determine the extent of the problem. Explain that you need to discuss the issue with the proper person and that you will call back with an answer. Let the patient know when to expect your call so they don't get even angrier unnecessarily waiting for an answer. Whatever the case may be, it should be noted on the patient's chart regarding the nature of the problem and the outcome.

Prank calls are not common, but if you need to deal with this, you should alert all office personnel so that no one will be caught off guard. Usually the prank is childish and not harmful. The best way to handle this type of call is to simply hang up. Being disconnected will discourage the prankster from repeating this call. Simply hanging up may be sufficient to stop obscene calls. Alert all other office staff of the call. As stated earlier, if the calls persist, they should be reported to the police.

The phone company should be contacted to trace calls of this nature, and criminal charges may be brought against the offender. You should keep a record of the date and time of the calls until the phone company becomes involved. Most phone directories have a section that outlines the steps that should be taken in situations such as bothersome and harassing calls. Simply telling the caller that you have reported the problem may be enough to make them stop calling. Taking action as soon as the situation occurs is the most sensible course.

Another type of call that you should be aware of is the "bogus" business call. Occasionally you may receive a call from a fake business owner who claims to have a special deal on office or medical equipment or supplies. Beware of this type of practice when the party demands payment before goods are received, because likely no goods are ever delivered. Do not make any business deal with any new company without checking them out first. All business should be conducted with well-established, reputable companies with good references to ensure solid business practices.

Follow-up Calls

Often physicians advise patients to call the next day to report their progress. You should determine whether you are to take the call and relay the message to the doctor (and record the patient's report on her chart), or if the physician wishes to speak directly to the patient when she calls. It is also a good practice to check with the physician to see if you should contact the patient if you do not receive the follow-up call from her by a predetermined time. Make sure that you have the current home, cell phone, pager, or work number(s) before the patient leaves your office so that you will be able to call her if necessary. It is also a good practice to make sure that the patient's chart has a current phone number of a relative or friend in the event that the patient cannot be contacted.

Physician Visits Outside the Office

When a patient calls and requests a house call, be sure you check with your physician employer before you schedule one. If your employer makes house calls, you should have a city map or county map to help locate any new patient scheduled.

Many physicians visit patients in hospitals and nursing homes on a regular basis. You need to establish a method of recording these visits and hospital calls. The physician should have a list of calls to be made each day along with a checklist of needed follow-up and charges for services.

Long Distance Calls

You may need to place long distance calls. If you are calling an area outside of your time zone, you should consult the telephone directory for the map of time zones (Figure 6-5) so you can establish the appropriate time to call. Take into consideration when it is lunch break in a different time zone so that you will not waste time trying to phone an office when the staff is not available to take your call. Be sure you know the code needed to dial for your long distance service, in addition to the telephone numbers of the persons you need to call. A record book should be kept on all long distance calls made.

Call Monitoring

Your employer may ask you to monitor a call either by an extension phone or speakerphone. Listen quietly and take notes of the conversation. It is important to make certain the caller agrees to your listening and tak-

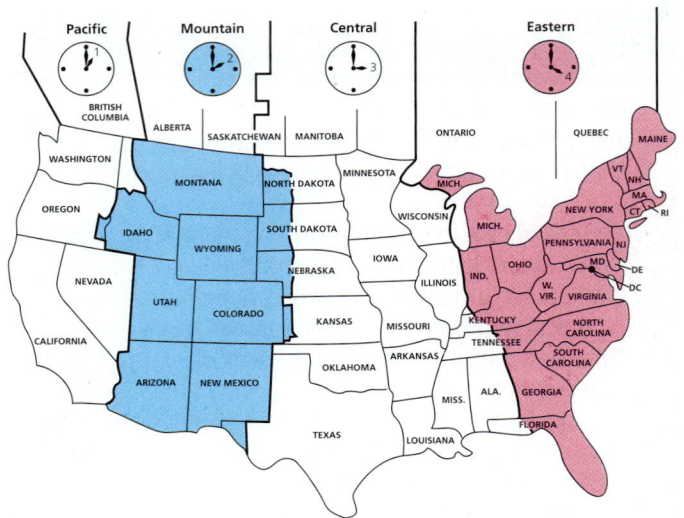

FIGURE 6-5 Make sure you place long distance calls within regular business hours by referring to a time zone map such as this.

ing notes. It is illegal for you to do this without the consent of the caller. Another type of monitoring is to record the phone call so that it may be played back if necessary at a later time. This, also, is illegal without the party's written consent.

Refusal or Inability to Identify

Your office may have a specific method of handling individuals who call and refuse to identify themselves. A good general rule is to suggest that the individual write a letter to the physician and mark it *personal,* in which case the physician will receive it unopened. Most physicians do not wish to talk to unidentified callers during busy office hours.

The guidelines for handling the physician's telephone can be summarized as follows:

1. Answer the telephone as promptly as possible.
2. Keep a pad and pen next to the telephone at all times.
3. Verify the caller's name and correct spelling. If an adult calls about a child, make sure you have the correct last name. Do not assume the child's last name is the same as the caller's name.
4. Determine the reason for the call.
5. Handle as many telephone calls as you possibly can without disturbing the physician.
6. If the physician prefers to speak to a patient, call the physician to the telephone after asking who is calling. Pull the patient's chart and give it to the physician.
7. Whenever possible, if you cannot handle the call alone, take a message for the physician. The physician will tell you what to do or call the patient back as time allows.

8. Make a memorandum for the physician of every telephone call. Use printed telephone memorandum pads that show date of call, time of call, name of caller, telephone number, and message.

9. Always know where to reach the physician. If the message is urgent and the physician is not in the office, page or telephone at once and relay the message.

10. If the physician cannot be reached, have the message by your phone. When your employer checks in, you may relay the message.

11. Learn how much medical information the physician wishes you to give over the telephone. Patients frequently call the office because they have forgotten the physician's instructions about treatments or medications. If these instructions are clearly stated in the chart, or in a preapproved triage manual, it may be possible for the assistant to repeat them to the patient.

12. When answering a second line, determine whether it is an emergency or another physician before placing the caller on hold and returning to finish the first call.

13. Allow the caller to say "Good-bye" and to hang up first.

If you have answered the phone and no one responds after you try twice to converse, simply hang up. Some phone systems may have caller ID, which may help in this type of situation. Immediately returning the call in this case may link you to a person in distress. **CAUTION:** Never tell anyone over the phone (or in person) that you are alone (even if you are), as this could be an invitation for undesirable behaviors. For your safety, it is not wise to work alone when there is no one near for assistance. If you must, and only if it is absolutely necessary for you to complete your responsibilities, a neighboring office staff or someone you trust should be informed of your being alone.

FINDING PHONE NUMBERS

You can save a great deal of time by keeping an up-to-date index of your most frequently called numbers by the telephone. It is a good idea to keep a back-up list of all e-mail addresses in case they are lost on the computer. In addition, when you need to use the telephone directory, it is helpful to know how it is organized.

The introductory section usually contains:

- Emergency numbers
- Community service numbers
- General telephone information
- Directory assistance information
- Rates for telephone calls
- Out-of-city area codes and time zones
- Money-saving tips on use of the telephone
- Directions for making international calls
- Rights and responsibilities
- Directory listings

You will find an alphabetic listing of individuals in the white pages. There may be separate listings of business and professional organizations in a second section of the white pages. An index of city, county, state, and United States government offices may be found in a separate section. Local zip code numbers by street address are usually in the introduction or a separate section of the telephone book. This section can be taken out of the large phone book and kept on the top of the desk in a stand-up organizer for easy access. This makes your job less taxing and eliminates the need to lift a heavy book many times each day. There are also books of complete listings of all zip codes in the country available. This is a necessary reference to have in the office, as it saves you from making frequent calls to the post office for information. Within the "rights and responsibilities" section of a telephone directory, you will find very helpful information regarding phone service and safety.

The contents section should be reviewed with each new updated directory as it will contain information that may have changed from the last edition. Another feature most telephone companies now have are specialized services and equipment for the deaf known as TTY (teletypewriter) or TDD (telecommunications device for the deaf). These devices allow the medical assistant to communicate with the hearing impaired patient by typing messages regarding prescriptions, test results, etc. You may have an opportunity to pass this information on to patients who may need these services and not be aware of them. The yellow pages (or classified directory) list the name, address, and phone number of every business subscriber, grouped under product and service headings. The classified directory also contains an index that can help you determine the headings under which a specific type of product or service may be listed.

ACHIEVE UNIT OBJECTIVES

■ **Complete the Workbook activities to meet the learning objectives.**

■ **Practice the procedures in this unit to meet the performance objectives.**

■ **Apply your knowledge at the end of this chapter in completing the Critical Thinking Challenge and Activities, as well as the StudyWARE on your Student CD-ROM.**

UNIT 2
SCHEDULE APPOINTMENTS

OBJECTIVES

Upon completion of this unit, you will be able to achieve the following:

LEARNING Objectives

1. Spell and define, using the glossary in the back of this text, all the Words to Know in this unit.

2. List and discuss ways that an office staff can establish the most desirable method of scheduling for their individual needs.

3. Explain what is meant by "establishing a matrix," and explain why it is important.

4. List and explain the various methods of scheduling.

5. Describe the advantages and disadvantages of each method of scheduling.

6. List and discuss the most important points to consider in determining appointment scheduling when someone calls the office.

7. Describe the importance of a triage manual for handling telephone calls.

8. Explain the most practical way to schedule a patient who is always late.

9. Explain and discuss the purpose of the rules for handling a canceled appointment.

10. List and discuss the goals of the physician, the medical assistant, and the patient regarding the appointment schedule.

11. List common abbreviations and their meanings used in making appointments.

12. Describe various ways of recording appointment schedules and give advantages and disadvantages of each.

13. State what information should be included in a procedure manual to help the medical assistant with making referral appointments.

14. Explain the procedures for making various appointments.

PERFORMANCE Objectives

1. Schedule an appointment.
2. Arrange a referral appointment.

WORDS TO KNOW

downtime	obliterate
flex time	ramification
gatekeeper	unstructured
guarantor	utilization
matrix	

CERTIFICATION CONNECTION

CMA
Utilizing appointment
  schedules/types
Appointment guidelines
Appointment protocol

CMAS
Appointment management
  and scheduling

RMA
Scheduling

EHR CONNECTION

Electronic scheduling saves time. Many programs automatically locate the next available appointment. Follow-up appointments can even be scheduled from the exam room, eliminating the need for the patient to stop at the window to schedule the next appointment.

APPOINTMENT STRATEGIES

One of the most primary and vital functions in the course of managed care is the scheduling of appointments (see Procedure 6-4). Managing time well for the physician and support staff will help keep patient flow at a satisfactory pace and promote a good professional working relationship. This may seem like an ideal situation that is unattainable. However, if there is genuine cooperation among all staff members, the schedule should flow well, with some understandable exceptions due to emergencies and other unpredictable situations from time to time. Office hours may be scheduled with appointments made during specific times, or left as an open, **unstructured** block of time.

PROCEDURE PROCEDURE PROCEDURE PROCEDURE PROCEDURE PROCEDURE PROCEDURE PROCEDURE

6-4  Schedule Appointments

PURPOSE: Schedule appointments according to office rules, by appointment book or computer.

EQUIPMENT AND SUPPLIES: Appointment book and pen, computer and scheduling program, monitor, printer, and appointment cards.

PERFORMANCE OBJECTIVE: In a simulated situation, schedule an appointment for a patient by either appointment book or computer, remembering to follow HIPAA guidelines for protecting PHI.

1. Determine the means of scheduling: appointment book or computer entry.

2. Mark off the hours when the physician will be unable to see patients. Include daily hospital rounds, lunch hour, meetings, and vacation.

3. Attempt to give patients two choices of times for the appointment. **NOTE: In black ink, record patients'** names as well as phone number(s) so that you can easily and quickly get in touch with them if necessary.

4. Ask patients to schedule their next appointment before leaving the office.

5. Write patients' names in the schedule book, or enter the patient's name in the appropriate space on the appointment screen.

6. Complete an appointment card and give it to the patient. Be sure to record the appointment first in the appointment book and then on the appointment card.

7. Avoid over-scheduling and leave sufficient time for same-day appointments.

8. Allow time for the doctor to return phone calls. **NOTE: Patient charts should be pulled and given to the doctor for these calls.**

First, the entire staff must be made aware of the intended schedule of the physician(s) in the medical facility. An inservice or an orientation is a practical way to inform employees about the schedule and enforce the established guidelines for "office hours." An organized routine helps the office staff as well as the patients with intended goals. In addition to providing the public with the routine hours when services are provided in printed form, the information should be posted at the entrance of the medical facility, on appointment cards, and on other printed materials. This information should also be placed in phone directories and wherever may be applicable. This way, everyone will know when the doctor is in and at what time business calls and appointments are taken. More discussion about an office policy manual is provided in Chapter 10.

After the office hours have been determined, the appointment schedule must be fashioned to meet the specific goals of the physician(s) and staff. Figure 6-6 outlines the goals that must continually be considered when scheduling.

Several styles of appointment books are available to schedule an entire year or more. A standard type of appointment book contains each day of the year printed with hours ranging from 8:00 AM to 5:00 PM, as shown in Figure 6-7. Individual medical facilities can have appointment books custom-made for their needs. Where several physicians' schedules are kept, the computer is the most desirable log of appointments, as it eliminates the awkward use of several appointment books.

The goals of the patient, the physician, and the medical assistant need to be considered. In general, the *goals of patients* are:

1. A minimum wait for an appointment
2. A minimum wait in the office
3. Maximum time with the physician

The general *goals of physicians* are:

1. Cost-effective use of time
2. Adequate time with the patients
3. Uninterrupted time
4. Time for referrals, emergencies, and so on

The general *goals of the medical assistant* are:

1. A smooth-running office
2. To close the office on time
3. A lunch hour and breaks
4. Patient and physician goals

FIGURE 6-6 Goals of the patient, the medical assistant, and the physician must be considered when preparing an appointment schedule.

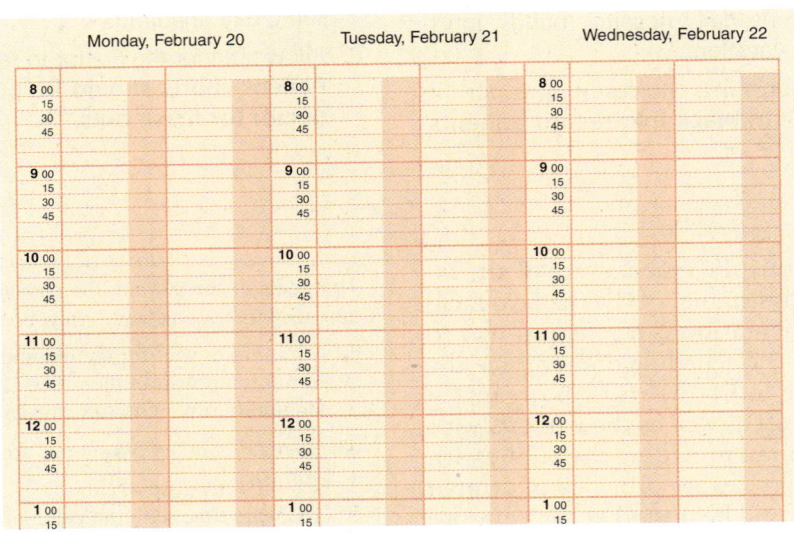

FIGURE 6-7 Appointment scheduling styles

When you use computerized appointment scheduling, you totally replace the paper appointment book (Figure 6-8). You should certainly have an accounts receivable system well established before converting to appointment scheduling. This feature should not be added if you have a single terminal but can be effective if you have several terminals. You also must consider how you would handle **downtime**, when, for whatever reason, the computer is not functional. This is a reality you need to plan for before it takes place so the office will run as smoothly as possible through the downtime. Downtime in this context refers to the time when the computer is basically not working and you are unable to enter or obtain information.

A computerized appointment system automatically locates the next available time, gives you a record of all appointments already made, allows you to locate a specific date and time, and prints copies of the daily schedule. These printed copies should be filed with the accounting records of the day as a legal document that you could be called on to produce in the event of an IRS audit of the office practice. Figure 6-9 shows part of a daily schedule from a computerized appointment scheduling system. Most computer systems can be used to print charge slips for the patients as they are seen. The patient's next scheduled appointment can be printed at the bottom of the charge slip, which is also a receipt of payment of the services of that day's office visit.

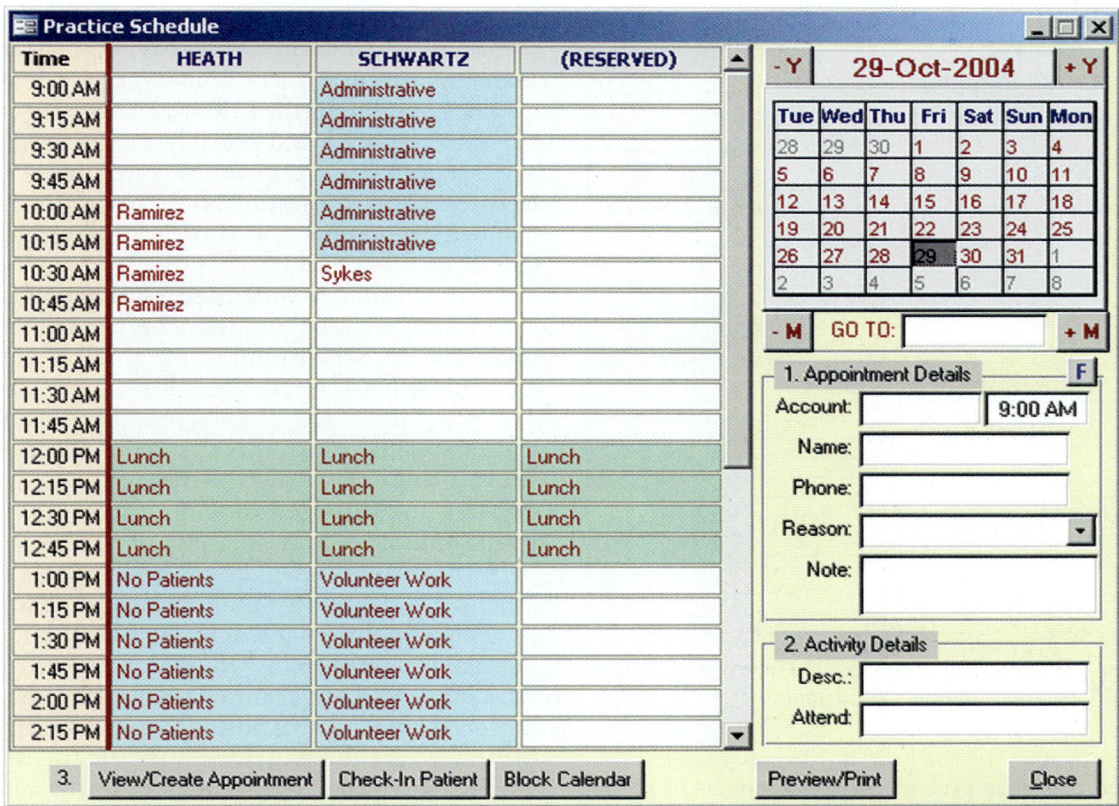

FIGURE 6-8 Computerized appointment schedule

Schedule For Friday, October 29, 20XX

Time	HEATH	Reason	SCHWARTZ	Reason	(RESERVED)	Reason
9:00 AM			Administrative			
9:15 AM			Administrative			
9:30 AM			Administrative			
9:45 AM			Administrative			
10:00 AM	Manuel Ramirez Colonoscopy		Administrative			
10:15 AM	Manuel Ramirez Colonoscopy		Administrative			
10:30 AM	Manuel Ramirez Colonoscopy		Eugene Sykes	Severe sore throat		
10:45 AM	Manuel Ramirez Colonoscopy					
11:00 AM						
11:15 AM						
11:30 AM						
11:45 AM						
12:00 PM	Lunch		Lunch		Lunch	
12:15 PM	Lunch		Lunch		Lunch	
12:30 PM	Lunch		Lunch		Lunch	

FIGURE 6-9 Daily schedules can be printed out from a computerized appointment scheduling system and filed.

ESTABLISHING A MATRIX

The appointment book or computer program schedule must have a fixed **matrix**. Establishing the matrix refers to the practice of blocking off time slots with an "X" as shown in Figure 6-10. Spaces blocked by an "X" indi-cate that the physician or other health care professional will not be available during those times to treat pa-tients. For instance, nothing should be scheduled be-tween the hours of 8:00 AM and noon on Thursdays, and nothing scheduled before 9:00 AM and after 4:45 PM

Tuesday, March 10, 20xx

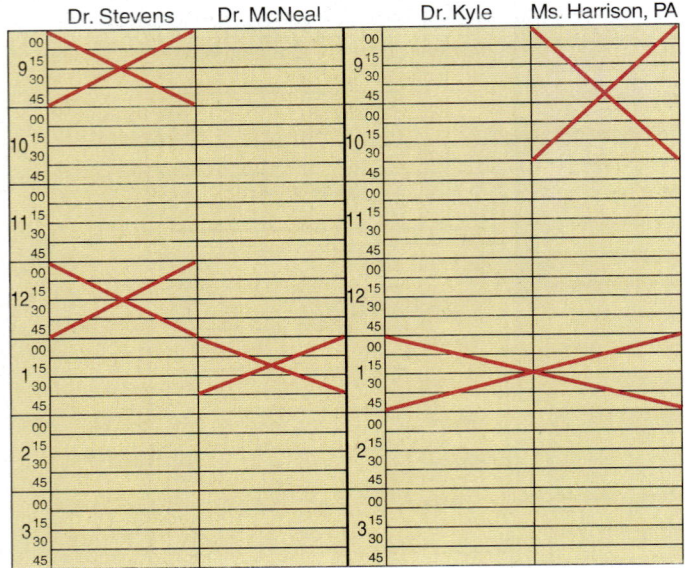

FIGURE 6-10 Appointment schedule with matrix established for three physicians and a physician assistant.

on Fridays because the physician(s) will not be in to see patients. It can also mean simply that no one should be scheduled in this time slot because it is reserved specifically for urgent conditions and same-day appointments. All staff members need to be aware of the exact meaning of the matrix. An entire day with an X through it means that the doctor is out, an X through the afternoon time slots means that the doctor is out only in the afternoon, and an X from 11:00 AM to 11:45 AM or 2:45 PM to 3:15 PM usually means that this time is reserved for catch-up. Time slots that are blocked off may be referred to as **flex time**, which can be used to return patient phone calls. If there is an established "lunch" time each day from 12:00 PM to 1:00 PM, it should be crossed out also. The matrix should be established for the entire year as soon as dates of activities are known.

Another practice that may be helpful is to highlight in a color (or several) for specific types of appointments (e.g., yellow is urgent, green is recheck, blue is injection, and so on). A separate schedule or section of the master schedule for those professionals in your facility (physician assistant, medical assistant, insurance secretary, and so on) who take appointments for various services, apart from the physician's appointment schedule, should also be kept. Figure 6-10 gives an example of a multiple appointment schedule. Patients who only need to be given immunizations, have weight and blood pressure checked, urinalysis rechecks, and so on, do not need to be seen by the doctor unless there is a problem. Appointment times should be scheduled to avoid having all patients show up at the same time. This can save the physician valuable time that may be spent in providing managed care to others. This type of schedule should also have an established matrix. This is a sensible practice that helps to avoid possibly having to reschedule patients because of unplanned meetings, vacations, or lectures. Clear communication among the entire staff will help to prevent confusion, mistakes, and misunderstandings.

Once the matrix has been established, the style of scheduling must be decided. There are several different methods of scheduling. The preferred method of scheduling that is adopted for a particular medical practice is up to the physician and the staff. The medical assistant must have excellent communication skills, a solid knowledge of the signs and symptoms of diseases and disorders, and an understanding of medical terminology and anatomy in order to proficiently perform telephone screening and prepare an efficient schedule. Obtaining the most precise assessment of a patient's condition and actively listening to what is being said is referred to as telephone screening. Using this type of assessment technique should result in obtaining accurate information and yield appropriate and complete care. When patients phone the medical facility with a request to see the doctor, the medical assistant must find out who the caller is (ask the correct spelling of the caller's name) and determine whether the person has previously seen the doctor.

Patients who either stop at the desk after seeing the doctor or who stop in to make an appointment should be given the same courtesy that patients receive over the phone. Offer the person a choice between two dates and times, allow sufficient time for the person to decide, and then confirm it by repeating it to the person before writing (printing) it in the appointment book or entering it in the computer. Remember to write the phone number(s) of the patient in the schedule book next to the name (so that you can call the patient quickly, if necessary, without pulling the chart) and note briefly (using abbreviations) the nature of the office visit. Write the time and date on an appointment card and politely hand it to the patient. Figure 6-11 shows an example of an appointment card that is given to the patient that indicates the date, day, and time of the patient's next appointment. At this time you should also provide the patient with any appropriate printed instructions or educational materials regarding the patient's condition, further treatment, or scheduled studies. Keep in mind that all appointment cards or forms that are used for this purpose should have the full name of the physician, complete address, phone number, and type of practice printed clearly on them. If the practice is new or in a new location, it is a convenience to the patient to have a small map or instructions of how to get to the office. If there are other office locations, they should also be listed with

Appointment for _Linda Parker_

On _Thurs. 4/5_   at   _9:30_   (AM/PM)

With Dr. Catherine Lang—Baldwin Family Practice Center
712 Central Parkway
Central City, XX   Zip Code

Telephone # 000/555-5000   Fax # 000/555-5001

If unable to keep this appointment, please give 24-hours notice or a charge will be made for the reserved time.

FIGURE 6-11 An example of a typical appointment card to give the patient that has the date (and day) and time of the next scheduled appointment.

complete information. Many appointment cards for professional services state that the patient must give the staff a 24-hour notice if a change in the scheduled appointment must be made. A verbal reminder to patients also helps to reinforce this policy. This can be very helpful in maintaining a smooth schedule. Many practices also provide patients with a telephone reminder of their appointment the day before. Remember to always protect PHI.

A new patient must provide you with complete information not only so that you can prepare a chart for the initial appointment, but also in case it becomes necessary to reach the patient before the scheduled appointment. If data is on the computer, the needed information can also be called up immediately.

Many medical facilities are now utilizing computerized scheduling instead of a paper appointment book. Software is available that will establish the matrix for a particular type of practice, as well as automatically locate the next available appointment.

Programs are available that allot the necessary amount of time for a specific procedure, along with alloting customized time slots for routine visits. Some software programs will automatically document no-shows and cancellations and make them a part of the patient's medical record.

A hard copy of the day's schedule can be easily produced and placed in designated areas of the office for easy reference by all staff members.

APPOINTMENT SCHEDULING STRATEGIES

As you gain experience in listening to patients' complaints over the phone, you will become more proficient in assessing problems. Using a preapproved telephone screening manual or a medical office handbook is a wise practice, as it reinforces continuity among staff members. All employees must be in-

structed to use the same format and ask the same questions every time of every patient who complains of similar symptoms. Following these screening guidelines that have been approved by the physician will help uncover serious conditions and lead to more efficient care of patients. Overlooking any of the questions or leaving out any part of a patient's symptoms is potentially a serious risk to both the patient and the medical practice. You must be careful not to put words in the caller's mouth. Asking precise questions and waiting for a response from the patient is recommended. The caller must inform you of what has been done to relieve the problem, and if it has been successful. When writing down information, be exact in how much and how often regarding medications, home remedies, and other treatments. Never leave out information that the patient tells you no matter how minor it may seem to you. The information disclosed to you by the patient should provide you with sufficient information to determine how soon the appointment should be made.

A patient's health maintenance organization (HMO) often determines which physicians the insured may see. Those physicians who contract with a specific company are designated as "in network." Many times a patient is calling to schedule an appointment because the physician is on a list of "in network" providers. If the physician can no longer accept new patients at this time, the patient must be informed. It is a courtesy to suggest one or two other physicians who may be currently accepting new patients.

Scheduling Methods

All staff members must be willing to work cooperatively and efficiently in order to provide quality care to patients. Included in the many choices for scheduling appointments are the following methods: clustering, double-booking, open hours, single-booking, streaming, wave, and modified wave. Table 6-2 lists these methods of scheduling with a description of the purpose of each. Any one of these methods can be used exclusively or in combination with one or more others to fit the specific individual needs of the practice. Even when appointment times have been assigned to patients, it is a good policy to have the patients sign in when they arrive in the office. This helps to identify new patients who need to complete initial forms for their chart. This way, current patient information is obtained, as well as the order in which the patient should be taken back. A sign should be posted giving instructions for patients to "sign in" as they arrive. Leaving the sign-in sheet out for all to read is a risk, because it allows all patients to read everyone's name. You know that you would not leave the appointment book open for the general public to read because it would break the confidentiality of patients. The ideal way to keep

TABLE 6-2 Methods of Scheduling	
Method	**Description**
Clustering	Patients with similar complaints or diagnoses are scheduled every 10 minutes throughout a particular segment of the day or a particular day of the week.
Double-booking	The same appointment time is given to two or more patients.
Open hours	No scheduled appointments. Patients sign in upon arrival and are seen by the physician in that order.
Single-booking	Used when an appointment for a patient will take a longer period of time. Single-booking means a single patient is booked for a specific amount of time.
Streaming	Appointments are scheduled for a particular amount of time based on patient need. This type of scheduling is designed to keep a continuous flow of patients coming through the office.
Wave	Patients are scheduled during the first 30 minutes of each hour, leaving the last 30 minutes for same-day appointments.
Modified wave	Scheduled the same as wave, with the exception of scheduling patients in the last 30 minutes at 10–20 minute intervals.

this from being a potential problem is to write the information down yourself as patients arrive, or enter it into the computer, keeping the screen from the view of others. Figure 6-12 shows an example of a patient sign-in sheet.

MAINTAINING THE SCHEDULE

After a period of time, through trial and error, each medical practice staff arrives at a schedule that works best for them. An assessment should be made of the efficiency of the schedule, and appropriate changes should be made to create better patient flow. Management consultants suggest an evaluation of old appointment sheets for a 12- to 15-week period. The number of work-ins, cancellations, and no shows and the time spent with specific exams and complaints of patients will help determine the course for revising the scheduling techniques. The time slots needed for various procedures, exams, and consultations can then be handled in short, medium, long, and extended appointment times. Often, a patient needs to have several procedures performed or must see one or more doctors in an office or a medical center. Coordinating all of these appointments for the patient on the same day will save the person from having to repeat unnecessary visits. The medical assistant may be expected to provide an explanation of different medical specialties, medical terms, instructions for procedures, exams, or treatments for patients who are unfamiliar with such matters. Sending the patient printed instructions regarding procedures and exams along with an appointment card prior to the scheduled appointment helps get them prepared and reduces their anxiety. Further discussion and helpful information about diagnostic examinations is provided in Chapters 15 and 16.

Patients with a scheduled appointment may become angry if they have to wait for a long time. Understandably, this patient may wonder why an appointment was even made. Surveys have shown that patients usually do not mind as much as a half-hour wait but tend to become angry if it is any longer. This could lead to medical-legal **ramifications** if it is not handled properly. Time is as valuable to patients as it is to you and the physician. Delays should be made known to patients tactfully as soon as they are realized. Patients need to be given the choice of waiting for as long as it may be or rescheduling for another appointment time altogether. Announcing that there will be a delay as soon as you have been given the information (e.g., that the doctor is caring for a patient with an emergency at the hospital) is something that patients will understand and appreciate. Patients appreciate your letting them know so that they can make a choice about waiting or returning at another time.

Handling Patients without Appointments

There may be a time when a patient who has an appointment brings along a family member or a friend to be seen. When a patient arrives who has no appointment, you need to explain that an appointment is necessary. It is advisable to have a sign near the reception window that indicates the office hours and that patients are seen by appointment *only*. Cooperation is usually attained when the patient realizes appointments must be scheduled. Patients who are persistent should be referred to the office manager or physician. Depending on the patient's complaint, the physician will sometimes make an exception. However, the patient must be informed of the importance of schedul-

Patient Sign-In   Date: _____

Please sign in and notify us if:
you are a new patient, your insurance, telephone number or address have changed.

NO.	Please Print Name Sign-in on next available #	Appt. Time	Time Seen	Appointment with	Note if first visit, new phone, address or insurance change
24	24				
25	25				
26	26				
27	27				
28	28				
29	29				
30	30				
31	31				
32	32				
33	33				
34	34				
35	35				
36	36				
37	37				
38	38				
39	39				
40	40				
41	41				
42	42				
43	43				
44	44				
45	45				
46	46				

FIGURE 6-12   An example of a patient sign-in sheet. *(Courtesy of Bibbero Systems, Inc., Peteluma, CA. (800) 242-2376; www.bibbero.com)*

ing an appointment ahead of time. If the patient's complaint is a serious emergency, you should automatically call for emergency medical service. In some cases, the physician may agree to take care of the emergency and then refer the patient to another physician for continuous managed care.

Canceled or Missed Appointments (No Shows)

If a patient cancels or does not show up for the scheduled appointment, it should be noted in the person's chart and the appointment time given to another patient as soon as possible. The physician should be notified about the patient's cancellation or "no show." The physician will advise you about further action as war-

ranted by the patient's condition. For example, if a patient is being treated for a wound that requires follow-up care and a dressing change, the patient may cancel (or just not come) and the wound area could become infected. The patient might decide to sue the doctor for inadequate care. The record of the canceled appointment or no show is important in proving that the patient had an appointment but failed to follow the physician's instructions. The patient's name should be left in the appointment book with a single line drawn through it. It is also wise to phone the patient at home and leave a message about the missed appointment. If patients cannot be reached by phone, a letter should be mailed regarding the missed appointment with a request that another appointment be arranged by calling the office. This provides legal protection if a lawsuit is filed against the physician for failure to provide care for the patient. Negligence is difficult to prove when efforts to offer medical help have been made.

Appointment Book Maintenance

You should never erase a name or use correction fluid to obliterate a name in the book. Do not use pencil. There are those who, even though it is not a suggested practice, use pencil in their appointment books. If this is the case, the entries should be written over at the end of the day in black ink. Having used pencil and possibly erasing from time to time during the course of the day may raise questions as to what names were erased, and why it was done. Having a patient's name in the schedule book even though the appointment may not have been kept will help defend efforts of providing the patient with the opportunity for medical care if ever the need arises. If there is no name on the appointment schedule because it has been erased, it is very difficult to prove that care was offered to the person. Management consultants advise that no altering of the schedule be done, as it may look as if one was trying to conceal information or fraudulently add it in at a later date. The appointment schedule is an official legal document and must be legible. For a cancellation, place a large letter "C" at the beginning of the person's name to indicate a cancellation, or "C&C" to indicate that the patient did call to tell you the reason the appointment had to be canceled. Some office personnel find it helpful to use a stamp to record in the chart the fact that the patient did not keep the appointment. The date, time, and reason for the missed appointment along with your initials should be noted. All staff members should be given a copy of the abbreviations common to your facility so that there is consistency with their use and the meanings are clear. A list of some common abbreviations that can be used in the appointment schedule is shown in Figure 6-13. A more extensive list of abbreviations is in the appendix of this text.

For legal reasons, all appointment schedule books must be kept for 3 years.

SCHEDULING BUSINESS APPOINTMENTS

In addition to routine scheduled appointments, emergency situations, and unexpected disruptions, there are other ancillary health professionals who may stop in to give the physician new information regarding medications, office equipment, medical supplies, and so on. A better way to deal with this before it becomes a routine disruption is to offer a regular appointment to the salesperson or pharmaceutical representative. A standing appointment will give the physician the opportunity to acquire the most current information on products and

BP✓	blood pressure check
C&C	called and canceled
C	canceled
Cons	consultation
CP	chest pain
CPE (CPX)	complete physical examination
ECG	electrocardiogram
FU	follow-up examination
Inj	injection
Lab	laboratory studies
NP	new patient
NS	no show
P&P	pap and pelvic
PT	physical therapy
Re✓	re-check
Ref	referral
RS	reschedule
Sig	sigmoidoscopy
S/R	suture removal
Surg	surgery

FIGURE 6-13 The entire staff must know abbreviations specific to the practice and their meanings and use them consistently. Here is a sample list.

have any questions answered immediately by the professional salesperson. Many reps bring in a variety of complimentary items, including lunch and other treats for the office staff. Leaving brochures and sample medications is another common practice of sales reps. You will have to organize and file or store all of the items that are left after the physician sees them. There is no need to schedule an extended amount of time for these individuals. Often the doctor chats briefly in the hallway, and only a portion of the time blocked out for the appointment is actually used. Many physicians prefer not to see these salespeople and ask that they talk to the office manager or medical assistant or just send information by mail. If another doctor or a family member stops in to see the physician, you should politely interrupt and let the physician know so that the guest does not have to wait. A reminder to the physician-employer of how many patients are waiting in the reception room is a good idea before the meeting ensues.

The medical assistant should note trouble spots in the schedule and report them to the physician or office manager periodically. This subject can be presented at staff meetings so that, by sharing ideas and suggestions, a better schedule may result. If the problem is that patients have had to wait far too long to see the doctor over a period of time (that is, more often than not), then it is possible that there are more appointments made than the doctor can see in the set "office hours," and the simple remedy is that fewer appointments should be scheduled. It is vital to the success of a schedule that the medical assistant maintain open communication with the physician and staff regarding patient flow.

If all efforts to improve scheduling problems have failed, an efficiency expert may be consulted for an objective viewpoint. Those not involved in the daily schedule of the office are better able to provide objective solutions. An efficiency expert's expertise can make all staff members more aware of how the schedule affects everyone throughout the office. The ideal schedule should provide a comfortable pace for the staff without making the patients feel rushed or slighted. *The importance of building good rapport with patients is invaluable; scheduling is where it begins.*

ADHERING TO A REALISTIC SCHEDULE

Since the physician generally expects the medical assistant to schedule appointments in time slots that are realistic for presenting complaints of the patients, a sample guideline for some typical office visits is presented in Figure 6-14. The actual amount of time spent with patients will depend on the speed of the staff, the patient, and the physician, as well as how talkative all concerned are before, during, and after the service rendered. A good rapport is built with patients when the service is achieved, pleasantries are ex-

changed, and the time seems to pass quickly. Variations and rearranging of appointments may be necessary according to the way the course of events unfolds during any given day in the medical practice. Experience will be the best teacher in arriving at a successful schedule. Adding the patient's phone number next to his name on the appointment schedule makes it easy to contact the patient if it becomes necessary to alter the office schedule.

Maintaining the Physician's Schedule

In addition to scheduling patients, the medical assistant has the responsibility to help the physician stay on schedule. Sometimes there is an obvious slowing down on the part of the physician or other staff members, and the schedule backs up. If the physician agrees that catching up is nearly impossible, the medical assistant may call patients and delay their arrival time or reschedule them for another day. It is a necessary courtesy for you to explain tactfully to all patients who are waiting to see the physician when the schedule is getting behind because of an emergency. Remember that each patient has the right to feel that her time is just as important as anyone else's time, and therefore you should offer to reschedule the appointment if the patient so chooses. A notation should be made in the patient's chart that because of an emergency the appointment was rescheduled and how long the patient had waited. The medical assistant may also want to work out a signal with the physician for those times when the patient gets too talkative and is taking more time than was allotted for the appointment. A suggestion is to interrupt by a signal over the speaker, such as "Excuse me, Doctor, you have a call on line five" (and there are only four phone lines). You may decide that a simple knock on the door or a particular signal on his or her pager can help the physician stay on task to avoid getting further behind.

Handling Late Patients

There are occasional patients who seem to be late for every appointment. In this situation, you may schedule them just after you come back from lunch and work them in when they arrive, or you may decide to schedule them at the end of the day. If the person does not arrive for the appointment at the time it was scheduled, a reasonable time of waiting is documented, and attempts are made to reach the patient by phone to determine if she is still coming. Late arrivals can be told that they need to reschedule their appointment if it is impossible to work them in. Late and missed appointments should be documented in the chart. After the first offense, established office policy

12	Lunch	
12.15		
12.30	Carol Wang - Sig 555-0050	
12.45	↓	
1	Kenneth Franks BP ✓ Lab	
1.15	↓	555-8846
1.30	Susan Steele - ECG	
1.45	↓	555-4495
2	Arnold Wing - CPE	
2.15		
2.30		555-6483
2.45	↓	
3	Work-ins	
3.15	Peggy Watters Inj	555-9913
3.30	Walter Matthews PT	
3.45	↓	555-2237
4	Latasha Peters Cons	
4.15	↓	555-7702
4.30	Work-ins	
4.45	Robert James BP ✓ 555-4951	

FIGURE 6-14 Sample time blocks for commonly scheduled appointments in a medical office

regarding late or missed appointments should be explained. If the appointment was at the end of the day, the patient should be advised regarding the length of waiting time established. With documentation in the chart, a pattern of late arrivals or missed appointments can be verified to discuss with the patient. If there are some extenuating circumstances such as transportation, child care, or work-associated problems, then a solution must be found to solve the problem. Late arrival problems may be alleviated if a printed sign posted in the reception area and a statement in the office information brochure states that patients who are late past a specific period must reschedule their appointment. Providing printed information regarding office hours as well as posting them will help to prevent such situations.

At certain times of the year there seem to be expected conditions that wreak havoc with a schedule, such as colds and flu in the winter months, injuries during winter and spring breaks from school, rashes and other ailments related to summer, and so on. These problems must be taken into account when preparing the daily schedule, especially the types of problems specific to the particular practice where you are employed. Figure 6-15 offers a list of some helpful points to keep in mind when scheduling appoint-

1. Have the full name spelled correctly.
2. Make the appointment for the next hour available.
3. Be sure the date and time are clearly understood.
4. Allow enough time for each appointment.
5. Check to see that no one else is scheduled at the same time for the same service.
6. Ask the time of day each patient prefers for an appointment: AM or PM?
7. When scheduling a series of appointments for the same patient, try to use the same day and time to make it easier for the patient to remember.
8. Offer a choice: "Would you like to come today at 3:00 or tomorrow at 9:00?"
9. If you have to refuse a request for an appointment at a certain time, explain why this is necessary and try to find another time that is convenient for the patient.
10. Enter the appointment in your appointment book or computer.
11. Complete an appointment card and hand it to the patient.
12. Try to allow extra time for emergencies each day.

FIGURE 6-15 Main points to remember when making appointments

ments. The saying "Time is money" is a good thought to consider. It should remind us to use time well and for the purpose intended. Efficient use of the physician's time and that of the entire staff in treating patients is the main purpose of a schedule.

REFERRAL APPOINTMENTS

When a patient develops a condition or requires an examination that your office cannot perform, your employer will refer the patient to an appropriate colleague or facility. The office should have a list of names, addresses, and phone numbers of physicians your employer wishes to refer patients to in different specialty areas. The patient should be provided with at least two names from which to choose for a referral. Keep a list of the name, address, and phone number of facilities where you might refer patients (e.g., laboratories, x-ray facilities, and community clinics). Keep in mind that certain managed care plans require referrals (see Procedure 6-5) to specialists within the plan with the approval of the primary care physician (**gatekeeper**). A list of these plans and participating physicians is an excellent time saver.

When a patient is to be admitted to the hospital, it is important to know what admission information the hospital will require. Be prepared when you call to give the necessary information regarding the patient.

When scheduling a hospital admission, you may be asked to identify the attending physician for the admission, the service admitting under (i.e., whether medical, surgical, or obstetric), the admission date requested, and the type of reservation. The type of reservation might be inpatient, admitting day surgery (ADS), ambulatory surgery (AS; patients who walk in, have surgery, and go home), or outpatient. Other information needed is listed here:

1. Full name of the patient (include birth name of married female patient if the woman has changed her name)
2. Age and date of birth
3. Sex of patient
4. Marital status
5. Social Security number
6. Address (including zip code)
7. Telephone numbers (home, pager or cell phone, and work) of patient and closest relative
8. Primary insurance of **guarantor** and Social Security number of this individual
9. Employer of guarantor and work telephone number
10. Hospital insurance coverage along with verification if prior authorization is granted
11. Name, address, and phone number of referring physician

PROCEDURE PROCEDURE PROCEDURE PROCEDURE PROCEDURE PROCEDURE PROCEDURE

6-5  Arrange a Referral Appointment

PURPOSE: Schedule a referral appointment for a patient in a professional manner.

EQUIPMENT AND SUPPLIES: Patient's chart with referral request, phone directory, phone, pen, and paper.

PERFORMANCE OBJECTIVE: In a simulated situation, schedule a referral appointment for a patient by phoning the appropriate medical facility.

1. Obtain patient's chart with request for referral to other facility.

2. Use the phone directory to obtain phone number and address of the referral office.

3. Place the call to the referral office and provide the receptionist with:

   - Your name and physician's name, address, and phone

   - Patient's name, address, and so on and reason for the appointment. **NOTE: It is a courtesy to also write down the name of the person who schedules the referral appointment for the patient for any** further questions the patient may have and for directions on how to get there.

   - Indicate if you will send a confirmation letter of the referral request by mail or fax.

   - Record the appointment information on the patient's chart; also write the time, day and date, name, address, and so on on paper for the patient to keep. **NOTE: If the patient is standing before you while you make the referral appointment call, be sure to ask if the date is okay before you finalize the conversation. (If the patient is not present, you must phone the patient to confirm the appointment.)**

4. Give the patient printed instructions regarding the appointment, as appropriate, and directions to the facility.

5. Initial the patient's chart, signifying the completion of the request.

---

12. The physician needs to furnish the diagnosis and plan of care for the **utilization** committee review.

13. If surgery is to be scheduled, you need to give the date of surgery, expected length of procedure in hours, name of procedure, type of anesthesia, units of blood needed, and whether x-rays will be taken.

14. When preadmission testing is to be carried out, you need to know the date, time, and names of tests, x-rays, ECG, and patient prep. If a generally required test is not ordered, you need to explain why it was not ordered.

The following conditions will generally justify inpatient hospital care for an otherwise outpatient procedure if the severity of the illness or intensity of service needed warrants it:

1. Severe myocardial insufficiency (with or without angina)
2. Chronic congestive heart failure
3. Chronic obstructive lung disease
4. Bronchial asthma
5. Diabetes
6. Thyroid disease
7. Hypertension

FOLLOW-UP APPOINTMENTS

It is the medical assistant's responsibility to assist patients with their payments and any necessary follow-up or referral appointments after the physician has seen them.

The need for a follow-up appointment may be marked by the physician on the charge slip, or the patient may be told to inform you of this need. The patient should be given the choice of two appointment times, and only after the entry is made in the appointment book should an appointment card be prepared and given to the patient. This practice will prevent the possibility of forgetting to enter the patient's name in the book.

Physicians who treat patients who need regular follow-up but do not make appointments a year in advance may choose to send a recall notice. This notice could be a preprinted card sent to the patient as a reminder to call or write for an appointment. An example would be a reminder for an annual Pap test. Some offices find it helpful to send a reminder notice of appointments that were made far in advance. You might even ask the patient to address such a card at the time the appointment is made. The patient is handed an appointment card, which he may lose, and at the same time addresses a card with the appointment time marked on it. You place this in a file under the date when it should be mailed.

ACHIEVE UNIT OBJECTIVES

- ■ Complete the Workbook activities to meet the learning objectives.
- ■ Practice the procedures in this unit to meet the performance objectives.
- ■ Apply your knowledge at the end of this chapter in completing the Critical Thinking Challenge and Activities, as well as the StudyWARE on your Student CD-ROM.

UNIT 3
WRITTEN COMMUNICATIONS

OBJECTIVES

Upon completion of this unit, you will be able to achieve the following:

LEARNING Objectives

1. Spell and define, using the glossary at the back of the text, all the Words to Know in this unit.
2. List seven types of correspondence medical assistants may need to prepare.
3. Name instances when form letters may be indicated.
4. Explain how HIPAA affects correspondence.
5. Explain the purpose of information sheets.
6. Name six specific criteria for written communications.
7. Name and give examples of the eight parts of speech.
8. Identify the nine standards for producing a mailable business letter.
9. Name the 12 components of a business letter.
10. Use standard proofreading marks.
11. Identify 11 common errors in written communications.

PERFORMANCE Objectives

1. Respond to and initiate written communications.
2. Compose a business letter.

WORDS TO KNOW

adjective	interjection
adverb	mailable
apostrophe	misspelled
clause	modifies
communication	noun
compose	postscript
congratulations	preposition
conjunction	pronoun
context	proofread
contraction	punctuation
correspondence	signature
critique	stationery
denote	thesaurus
ellipses	verb
galley proofs	watermark
hyphen	

CERTIFICATION CONNECTION

CMA
Recognizing and responding to verbal and nonverbal communication
Professional communication and behavior
Fundamental writing skills

CMAS
Employ effective written and oral communication

Medical office information processing

RMA
Compose correspondence employing acceptable business format
Employ effective written communication skills, adhering to ethics and laws of confidentiality

WRITTEN COMMUNICATION

What is **communication**? One dictionary defines it as "the giving or receiving of information; a system for sending and receiving messages." You can communicate in many ways, such as talking, gesturing, or writing.

Written communication is often called **correspondence**. Again, the dictionary says correspondence is "communication by the exchange of letters." An individual who is hired by a newspaper or magazine to furnish news regularly from a certain place is called a correspondent. There are schools from which you can receive instruction in a particular subject by mail. They are known as correspondence schools. But in its broader sense, correspondence can be thought of as any exchange of information between persons. With this interpretation, correspondence or written communication could include the sending of notes; inneroffice communications (IOCs); form letters; information sheets; and business, professional, and personal letters.

In a physician's office, written communication is often necessary:

- To officially inform the staff of a policy or decision
- To contact professional colleagues
- To correspond with professional associations
- To request or respond to a medical consultation
- To engage in business communications with medical suppliers, financial consultants, attorneys, and insurance companies
- To send personal messages

Communication and HIPAA Regulations

Communications that include personal information about patients require specific handling. With the enactment of HIPAA, rules about the security of patients' personal information (PPI) as contained in medical records were identified. Care must be taken to prevent disclosure to entities that are not directly involved with the provision of health care. Most physicians have developed specific Release of Information forms that follow the HIPAA guidelines. Patients are requested to sign these forms giving permission for physicians to communicate personal information when it is necessary for the provision of their care. Some examples of instances would be:

- To request a consultation from a specialist
- To provide results to the referring physician from a specialist
- To provide information to a hospital or nursing care facility
- To assure third-party approval of a procedure

The patient is provided with a written statement from the physician's practice that explains their adherence to the HIPAA regulations in regards to their personal information. Patients are asked to sign a form indicating they have received a copy of this document.

Access to the patient's record may be limited within an office to only those people who have a need to view the chart. Therefore, preparing written communication may be limited to those approved individuals. Others would be prohibited from access to patient information by the security officer as directed by the HIPAA regulations.

Inneroffice Communication

IOC is an informal, memo-style communication that is usually specific to one concern. It is an effective way of being certain that everyone is aware of some event, policy, concern, and so on. If you want to ensure that everyone reads the memo, a copy must be given to each person, or a copy can be posted or circulated with an attached list of all people involved, who then must enter their initials next to their names to indicate they have read the IOC. An example might look something like Figures 6-16A and B.

Informal Notes

Informal notes would be indicated for times when "thank you's," **congratulations**, or similar expressions are desired. Usually, these are personal and informal in nature. Often they are written on a first-name basis.

Personal Letters

The physician may ask for assistance with personal correspondence. It is common for medical assistants to correspond with travel agencies, mail order catalogs, perhaps clothing suppliers, and specialty shops. A competent medical assistant should be able to **compose** (write) the necessary letter after receiving the specific information desired, so all the physician has to do is provide a **signature**.

Professional Letters

Physicians may need to write to their professional associations, licensing boards, and other physicians regarding some issue or concern affecting personal medical activities or their professional practice. Perhaps your employer holds an office in a medical society that requires communicating with the members or issuing the group's opinion on a particular subject to the community or media. Some physicians hold office on a hospital medical board, which might necessitate issuing of written communication. Physicians who participate in research do a great deal of professional correspondence in regard to the experimental studies being conducted. Some physicians enjoy writing professional journal articles about a unique patient or explaining a procedure they have developed. Obviously, these specific writings require detailed dictating and perfect transcription.

But some professional letters may not be that critical. Suppose your employer wrote a medical journal

SAMUEL E. MATTHEWS, MD
100 EAST MAIN STREET, SUITE 120
YOURTOWN, US 98765-4321

DATE: April 3, 20--
TO: Office staff
FROM: Doctor Sam
SUBJECT: New office computer system

Representatives from ABC Electronics will be at our office on April 10 and 11 to provide instruction on the use of our new equipment. Please see Joyce and schedule yourself into one of the four orientation sessions. After you have selected your time, enter your initials next to your name on the sheet at her desk to verify you have responded to this memo.

Thank you for your cooperation in this matter.

FIGURE 6-16A Inneroffice communication (IOC)

SAMUEL E. MATTHEWS, MD
100 EAST MAIN STREET, SUITE 120
YOURTOWN, US 98765-4321

After you have read the memo and selected a time for your orientation, please initial below on the line by your name. Your initials verify your response to the memo to attend one session presented by ABC Electronics on April 10 or 11.

_____ Amy Adornio	_____ Gerri Gore
_____ Betty Barry	_____ Harry Hecht
_____ Chuck Cukovich	_____ Inez Immel
_____ Diane Delong	_____ Jacki James
_____ Emily Everett	_____ Kelly Kendzierski
_____ Frank Flaherty	_____ Lisa Long

FIGURE 6-16B Inneroffice communication (IOC) circulation sheet

article about a new method of treatment he has developed that has proved very successful. The medical association planning committee is scheduling presenters for their next convention. Your employer has received a request to make a presentation about his new treatment at the convention. He asks you to write a response for his signature. In preparation for this task, you and the physician refer to the office calendar and his personal schedule. He discovers that he and his family have scheduled a vacation to begin the day after the conference closes, but he could make the presentation at the beginning of the meeting. You confer with the office scheduler to block off the additional days until the presentation is confirmed. Refer to Procedure 6-6 for guidelines to compose a response to a communication.

Business Correspondence

The greatest amount of correspondence, however, is of the business type, required to manage the affairs of the practice. This would include the referrals, consulting, annual examination reminders, collection letters, school and work releases, suppliers of equipment and materials, and other correspondence necessary to the office operation. These types of letters can be individually composed, or a form letter may be used. Prewritten form letters can be developed and stored electronically on computers. When needed, the letter is pulled up; the appropriate date, name, address, amount due, and so on is added; and it is printed without the need to prepare the total letter. Form letters are especially well suited for:

- Return to work or school approvals (following surgery or illness)
- Annual diagnostic examination reminders (eye examinations, Pap tests, mammogram, sigmoidoscopy)
- Delinquent account reminders, usually in about three increasing levels of request intensity
- Office visit verifications (for work or school absence)
- Athletic participation approvals
- Providing information to referred patients, such as appointment confirmation, office location, information needed, and examination preparation.

 Be sure to check the patient's chart for a signed form to release information and be certain there are not restrictions as to whom or where information can be sent.

Several businesses offer prepared medical forms both in hard copy for completion or as software packages for computer use.

The *master* of each hard-copy form letter is stored in a file, and copies are made as needed. Specific information appropriate to the recipient is entered in the blank areas. In the past, such letters were common, and the specific information was added by using a typewriter. Of course, this was less than desirable, because it was difficult to "line up" the type so the added words looked like they were part of the original document. With the advent of the computer, hard-copy form letters are seldom used. Today, any such form of correspondence

6-6  Respond to Written Communication

PURPOSE: Compose a response to received correspondence.

EQUIPMENT AND SUPPLIES: Computer, received correspondence, and letterhead paper

PERFORMANCE OBJECTIVE: With access to equipment and supplies and information from physician, draft a letter to respond to a received correspondence. The letter must meet mailable standards as identified in this text.

1. Position the cursor at least three lines below the letterhead.
2. Enter the date using the selected letter style.
3. Move the cursor down about five lines.
4. Enter the inside address as identified on the received correspondence.
5. Double space after the address.
6. Enter an appropriate salutation using the name of the writer of the received letter.
7. Double space.
8. Enter the reference line (e.g., reference the conference presentation).
9. Double space.
10. Type the body of the letter:
    a) Re-iterate the question asked.
    b) State the answer.
    c) Express appreciation and anticipation of an answer.
11. Enter a complimentary closing.
12. Enter four lines.
13. Enter the physician's name.
14. Double space.
15. Enter the typist's initials.
16. Print a draft copy and proofread.
17. Make corrections to the document and print on letterhead.
18. Prepare an envelope.
19. Give the letter and envelope to the physician for a signature.
20. Make a copy for the physician's personal use and one for the office file or save in appropriate folder in the computer.

---

would be limited to very informal and routine messages that are filled in with handwritten information.

Software form letters are very efficient and convenient. The appropriate form letter can be pulled up from the file, and the necessary specific information can be added and the form printed out. When the same form letter will be sent to several people, specific information for each person such as name, address, and salutation can be added in a data format and then merged to produce individualized letters.

Information Sheets

Specific written instructions regarding the examinations and diagnostic tests performed in your office are very beneficial to patients. They help to reinforce what you have explained and serve as a reminder after they leave the office. They typically explain to patients how to prepare themselves for a particular test or what to expect when the test is performed. Usually there is a place on the form to enter the date and time the examination is scheduled. These information sheets can be prepared

and stored in the files to be used as needed. They are an excellent example of patient education material.

PREPARING WRITTEN COMMUNICATION

Almost every day, when the mail carrier arrives, there will be something received that requires a response. Your employer may want to review all the mail personally and request that you only open the envelopes and arrange everything neatly on the desk. Some physicians allow the mail to be opened and sorted, referring to only professional or personal material that requires their response; anything pertaining to the practice operation is handled by the office manager.

After a few days, the physician will need to devote some time to drafting responses to inquiries or responding to referrals. Some may use a dictating machine, while others may prefer to dictate in person. Surgeons and other specialists who have a large number of referral patients will have the greatest amount of responses to compose. Usually a type of form letter is developed with the opening and closing paragraphs being a standard format and the middle of the letter specific to the patient. This format only requires minimal dictation, after the opening "Thank you for referring . . ." and the closing "If I can be of any additional assistance . . ." Of course, occasionally, written communication is required that is specific to a request or concern so the total correspondence is individualized.

Probably the most important criteria about any communication is that it be written using proper grammar and punctuation and have no **misspelled** words. It also must be spaced on the page properly and be neat and clean. Try not to use the same major word twice in the same or even consecutive sentence. The following information will assist you in producing attractive, error-free communications.

Spelling

Spelling is difficult for some people. If you are one of them, you will have to try exceptionally hard until you master certain rules and habits. There are 14 rules about spelling that are very helpful once you understand how to use them. Refer to Figure 6-17. Here are some ideas that might help.

- If you have certain words that you cannot seem to spell correctly, try making an alphabetical list of them to use as a quick reference.
- Make a mental picture of the word correctly spelled.
- Pronounce the word correctly several times.
- Write the word, dividing it into syllables and inserting accent marks.
- Write or type the word several times.
- Learn to use a general and medical dictionary when you are in doubt.
- When you use a word processor or computer software to compose correspondence, be sure to run your document on the spell checker. It will catch most errors. (Unfortunately you cannot rely on the checker completely, because it is possible that the word is spelled correctly but you have entered the wrong word, a word "out of **context**." Examples of this are using "their" for "there," "cite" for "sight," "rite" for "right," "your" for "you're," and several others.)

If you are using Microsoft Word as your software, you may not have to perform a spell check. Misspelled words are almost immediately underlined in red to alert you. Words that the software thinks you have misused, such as "which" instead of "that," or thinks you perhaps left off an *s* or *d*, will be underlined in green. At times the software will make changes to formatting that you are applying, and you will need to re-enter your content so it will stay. This, for example, occurs when doing a list of bulleted items in which you don't want the first letter capitalized. Also, when you have been entering information in a certain format for a while and you want to change back to the default format, you may have to pull down Format and go into Styles and Formatting to turn it off. Even though the software at times can cause irritation, its capabilities are almost unlimited. Make every attempt to learn to utilize it so that you can create a variety of interesting and professional documents.

Parts of Speech

To compose effective, well-written communications, you need to be aware of the eight parts of speech and how they are used (Table 6-3).

Once you have the spelling and the parts of speech under control, it is time to put the words together in sentences. Written material should be composed of sentences of differing lengths and complexity to appropriately match the written matter being prepared. Patient referral or business letters require concise material, while personal correspondence or medical articles can contain more variety. Be careful not to make run-on sentences containing too many clauses. The following information outlines sentence construction.

Sentence Structure

When writing letters, write in complete thoughts. A *simple sentence* consists of only one complete thought, that is, one independent clause with a subject and a verb.

> **EXAMPLES:**
> Physicians examine patients.
> Physicians prescribe medication.
> The receptionist scheduled appointments.

A *compound sentence* contains two or more independent clauses, separated by a comma.

> **EXAMPLES:**
> The physician dictates letters, and the medical assistant transcribes them.
> Administrative medical assistants perform clerical duties, and clinical medical assistants perform clinical duties.
> Laboratory technicians analyze specimens, and medical assistants assist with physical examinations.

A *complex sentence* contains one independent clause and one or more dependent clauses. A dependent clause cannot stand alone as a sentence.

> **EXAMPLES:**
> The doctor, who is off on Thursdays, sees allergy patients in the morning. (An adjective clause)
> Patients are sometimes quite apprehensive when they come to the office for diagnostic examination. (An adverb clause)
> Physicians require that patients receive proper instructions for diagnostic procedures. (Noun clause)

Rule 1. Write *ie* when the sound is *ee*, as in:

achieve	piece
field	shield
grief	yield

EXCEPT after *c*, as in:

conceive	perceive
deceive	receive

OTHER EXCEPTIONS:

leisure	seize
neither	weird

Rule 2. Write *ei* when the sound is not long *e*, especially when the sound is long *a*, as in:

freight	veil
height	vein
sleigh	weigh

EXCEPTIONS:
friend
mischief

Rule 3. The prefixes *mis, il, in, im,* and *dis* do not change the spelling of the root word:

mis + spell = misspell
il + legal = illegal
il + literate = illiterate
in + audible = inaudible
im + mature = immature
dis + appear = disappear

Rule 4. Only one word in English ends in *sede: supersede.* Only three words end in *ceed:* exceed, proceed, and succeed. All other words of similar sound end in *cede,* as in:

concede
recede
precede

Rule 5. The suffixes *ly* and *ness* do not change the spelling of the root word:

sudden + ness = suddenness
final + ly = finally
truthful + ly = truthfully
lean + ness = leanness

EXCEPTIONS: Words ending in *y* preceded by a consonant change *y* to *i* before any suffix not beginning with *i:*
kindly + ness = kindliness
happy + ly = happily
happy + ness = happiness

Words ending in *y* preceded by a vowel also follow this rule.

Rule 6. Drop the *e* from the end of a word before adding the suffixes *al, ed, ing,* and *able:*

complete—completed—completing
care—caring
fine—final
love—lovable
observe—observable

EXCEPTIONS: Words ending in *ce* and *ge* usually keep the silent *e* when the suffix begins with *a* or *o* in order to preserve the soft sound of the final consonant:
notice + able = noticeable
change + able = changeable

Rule 7. Keep the final *e* before a suffix beginning with a consonant:

large + ly = largely
care + ful = careful
care + less = careless
state + ment = statement

EXCEPTIONS:
argue + ment = argument
true + ly = truly

Rule 8. With words of one syllable ending in a single consonant preceded by a single vowel, double the consonant before adding *ing, ed,* or *er:*

sit + ing = sitting
hop + ed = hopped
dip + er = dipper
run + ing = running
swim + ing = swimming

Rule 9. If a one-syllable word ends in a single consonant not preceded by a single vowel, do not double the consonant before adding *ing, ed,* or *er:*

reap + ed = reaped
heat + ing = heating

Rule 10. To make a word ending in *y* plural, check the letter before the *y.* If it is a vowel, just add *s:*

birthday—birthdays
day—days
ray—rays
toy—toys

If it is any other letter, change the *y* to *i* and add *es:*

city—cities
lady—ladies
study—studies
guppy—guppies
fly—flies

Rule 11. Most nouns (names of people, places, things, ideas) become plural by adding *s:*

boy—boys	desk—desks
dog—dogs	window—windows

Rule 12. The plural of nouns ending in *s, x, z, ch,* or *sh* is formed by adding *es:*

wax—waxes
dish—dishes
waltz—waltzes

Rule 13. The plural of most nouns ending in *f* is formed by adding *s.* The plural of some nouns ending in *fo* or *fe* is formed by changing the *f* to *v* and adding *s* or *es:*

gulf—gulfs	knifes—knives
belief—beliefs	life—lives

Rule 14. The plural of nouns ending in *o* preceded by a vowel is formed by adding *s.* The plural of nouns ending in *o* preceded by a consonant is formed by adding *es:*

patio—patios
ratio—ratios
tornado—tornadoes
hero—heroes

EXCEPTIONS:
eskimo—eskimos
silo—silos

FIGURE 6-17   Spelling rules

TABLE 6-3   The Eight Parts of Speech

Speech Part	Description	Word Examples	Example of Use
Noun	The name of anything, such as a person, a place, an object, an occurrence, or a state	assistant, office, attention, laboratory, Texas, computer	The *assistant* draws *blood* and takes it to the *laboratory*.
Pronoun	A substitute for a noun	she, her, he, him, his, which, some, everyone, it, their, they, nobody	*He* called *her* to see if *she* knew if *anyone* else was going to the inservice program.
Verb	A word or word group that expresses action or a state of being	write, perform, cut, assist, attend, run, jump, enter	The assistant *measured* the patient's blood pressure and *entered* the findings on the chart.
		am, is, are, will be, have been, feel, seem, appear	
Adjective	Describes, limits, or restricts a noun or pronoun	efficient, dedicated, tall, thin, dependable, irregular	Joyce is an *efficient* and *dependable* medical assistant.
Adverb	**Modifies** a verb, adjective, or another adverb. Adverbs commonly end in "-ly" and are used to answer questions.	How? What? When? Where? How often?	*Frequently* Jane arrives *early* for work and often stays *late*.
Preposition	Shows the relationship of an object to some other word in the sentence	of, with, without, for, above, below, on, from, between	*Between* you and me, Dr. Morrison's handwriting is, *without* a doubt, the most difficult *to* read.
Conjunction	Connects words, phrases, and clauses	and, but, or, for, because, if	We can work Jane in *if* she can be here by 1:00 *but* not at 3:00 as she requested.
Interjection	Used to express strong feeling or emotion. These words are usually followed by an exclamation point or a comma.	oh, hurray, ouch, wow	*Hurray*! We received the research grant.

A *compound–complex sentence* contains two or more independent clauses plus one or more dependent clauses.

EXAMPLE:

Medical assistants should seek continuing education because medical technology is constantly changing, and the medical assistant must keep current with new procedures.

Punctuation Marks

To make sentences easier to read and to tell a reader when you come to the end of a thought, a variety of markings called **punctuation** are used. The most common are the comma, period, apostrophe, hyphen, and ellipsis. The following information describes the correct usage of these marks.

- A *period* is placed at the end of each sentence.
- A *comma* or period should appear before an ending quotation mark: "or."

There are four general rules for the use of a comma:

1. Use between main **clauses** connected by *and, but, so, for, or, nor,* and *yet.* If main clauses are short, no comma is needed.
2. Use following long introductory phrases or clauses that may begin with words such as *after, whenever, if, until, since,* and *once.*
3. Use to separate items in a series.
4. Use to set off nonrestrictive modifiers. A *nonrestrictive phrase* or clause is a nonessential phrase or clause. It just adds descriptive or explanatory detail. A *restrictive modifier* restricts or limits the noun it modifies.

EXAMPLES:

The medical assistant, being dedicated to his profession, helps the doctor in countless ways.

The medical assistant, who is a part of the medical team, needs to be especially careful in attending to details.

An **apostrophe** is used in **contractions** to signify that one or more letters have been left out. Be sure if you use *it's* that you mean *it is. Who's,* meaning *who is,* should not be confused with *whose; there's,* meaning *there is,* is not to be confused with *theirs.*

An apostrophe is also used to signify possession in a noun.

EXAMPLES:

The medical assistant's pen, pencil, and notepad are always beside the office telephone.

The assistant's stethoscope hangs in the examination room.

Carefully check all **hyphens** at the end of a line to be sure the word is divided correctly. Check your dictionary if you are in doubt about the end of a syllable.

Two forms of **ellipses** may be used—three and four dots. The three-dot ellipsis is used with spaces at each end and between the dots to signify an omission of words.

EXAMPLE:

"They come in two varieties—the three-dot variety . . . and the four-dot variety."

The four-dot ellipsis signifies an omission of words and the end of a sentence with no space between the last letter and the first dot.

EXAMPLE:

"The four-dot. . . ."

Use a *semicolon* between two clauses of a compound sentence when they are not joined by a conjunction, unless they are very short and are used informally. Samples of conjunctions are therefore, however, then, and nevertheless. The semicolon can also be used for clarity.

A *colon* is used to formally introduce a word, a list, a statement or question, a series of statements, or a long quotation. It is used after the salutation of a business letter and between numbers denoting time.

Quotation marks are used to enclose a direct quote. They are also used with titles of articles, chapters of books, and titles of short poems and stories. Spoken words in written narrative are also placed in quotes. A *question mark* or an *exclamation mark* is placed inside the quotation marks *if it is a part of the quotation* and outside if it applies to the main clause. Question marks are placed after every direct question. The exclamation mark is used after words, expressions, or sentences to show strong feeling.

Parentheses may be used to enclose matter apart from the main thought. Even though it may contain a complete sentence, it does not have to start with a capital or end with a period; however, if it is an interrogative statement (question), it ends with a question mark.

Capitalization

Capitalize names of persons and places, the first word in a sentence, names of holidays, principal words in titles of major works, and any product or title that might be trademarked. Many medical terms begin with a capital letter because they are names of the physicians who named them. Medications are usually trademarked. Again, use your dictionary when in doubt.

Be especially careful to check every word in a heading or title for correct spelling. Use your medical dictionary or a good general dictionary. Always have these reference books in the office.

Numbers

The use of numbers must be consistent. If you follow a specific reference style book (e.g., *The Chicago Manual of Style, CBE Style Manual, AMA Manual of Style*), you should follow its instructions for using numerals or spelling out the numbers. Also, follow the rules your employer wishes to be used for your office.

In the absence of other references and if the physician's preference is unknown, usually any number under 10 is spelled out, while those above are used in numeric form. A partially contradicting general rule says to spell out the number if it can be done in one or two words. A number at the beginning of a sentence must be spelled out. A person's age and the time of day are also usually written out. Dates, street numbers, and page numbers are written in figures. When several numbers are mentioned within a short space, figures should be used for all of them.

COMPOSING A BUSINESS LETTER

A business letter has several distinct components. The following identifies and provides a description of each part. Refer to the sample letters in Figure 6-18.

- The letterhead: Preprinted name, complete address, and phone number (optional)
- Dateline: Date letter is dictated or composed, if not dictated
- Inside address: Address of person to whom the letter is being sent
- Salutation: The greeting to the recipient
- Reference: To identify what or about whom the letter is concerning
- Body: The content of the letter
- Complimentary closing: Expressing the closing of the letter
- Sender's signature: Signature of the writer
- Title: Writer's title, if appropriate (e.g., Vice President, Director)
- Reference initials: Initials of the letter typist

- Enclosures: Any identified materials to be sent with the letter
- Copies: "cc," meaning "carbon copy," identifies another person or persons to whom a copy of the letter is sent

With all the previous information, you are now ready to compose a business letter. The word processing software default formatting is usually appropriate for composing letters. In fact, in some version of Microsoft Word, once you begin entering information in a letter format, an icon will appear asking you, "It looks like a letter, do you need help?" If you require different margins, learn how to change the settings and explore other formats. With Word, for example, try using Tools, click on Letters and Mailings, then the Letter Wizard. This will allow you to select a letter style and a page design that will accommodate your letterhead, among other things. As mentioned before, the capabilities of software are very helpful if you can learn to use them. There are certain steps in the process to consider in order to produce a final copy without errors.

- Determine what information needs to be included (a) to answer a letter, (b) to respond to a verbal request, (c) to request information, and (d) to obtain a specific response.
- Determine the style for the letter, and set margins for appropriate placement on the page.
- Select the type of font and size.
- Compose a rough draft using concise, easy to understand sentences. Use the words "I" and "we" as infrequently as possible, especially to begin sentences. Remember it is awkward to use the same word twice in one sentence or even in two consecutive sentences. The use of a **thesaurus** to increase the usage of different words makes the content more interesting.
- Proofread the draft and edit the content. Eliminate redundant (extra, unnecessary) phrases.
- Compose the final copy, and prepare the envelope.
- Sign it or give it to the sender to sign.

In a specialist's office, one of the most common letters received is a request from another physician for a consultation of a patient (Figure 6-18). You will often find it necessary to correspond with the patient if you need to send any special instructions, directions to your office, and other information. Be certain the material has ample time to arrive at the patient's home before the date of the examination. The content of the correspondence usually covers:

- The reason for the appointment
- The date and time of the appointment (it should request notification if the appointment cannot be kept)
- A statement saying that if there are any questions, please feel free to call your office. Be sure to include your office's phone number.

Samuel E. Matthews, MD
100 East Main Street, Suite 120
Yourtown, US 98765-4321

October 7, 20--

Robert Smith, M.D.
50 North Broad Street
Mytown, US 43200

Dear Dr. Smith:

I am referring Susan B. James to your office for evaluation of severe headaches of approximately six months duration. She was treated initially at a pain clinic in Yourtown. Susan will be calling your office for an appointment. I am sure you will find her to be a most cooperative patient.

I would appreciate a report of your diagnosis and recommended course of treatment.

Sincerely,

Samuel E. Matthews, M.D.

lk

FIGURE 6-18 Sample referral letter

The sample letter in Figure 6-18 from Dr. Matthews fails to give Dr. Smith's office the address or telephone number for Susan James, whom he is referring. In this case, Susan has been instructed to phone Dr. Smith for an appointment. It will be important for the medical assistant who schedules the appointment to get the personal information so that instruction for the consultation can be sent.

The office visit will require a follow-up letter from the specialist to the referring physician, identifying the findings, diagnosis, and recommended course of treatment.

MAILABLE STANDARDS

All communications leaving your office should meet the standards for a **mailable** letter. These include:

- Appropriate letter placement on page (Figure 6-19A)
- The right margin is fairly even; top and bottom margins are generous.
- Punctuation and spacing that follow acceptable business practice
- Divided words at end of line are done correctly.
- Letter content is accurate as dictated.
- All parts ("enclosures") of the letter are included.
- No spelling errors

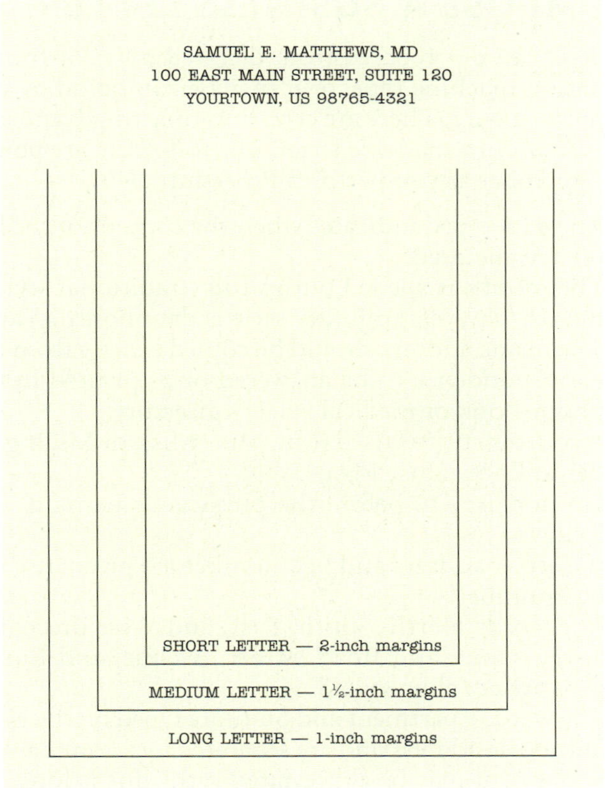

SAMUEL E. MATTHEWS, MD
100 EAST MAIN STREET, SUITE 120
YOURTOWN, US 98765-4321

SHORT LETTER — 2-inch margins

MEDIUM LETTER — 1½-inch margins

LONG LETTER — 1-inch margins

FIGURE 6-19A　Placement of letter

Samuel E. Matthews, MD
100 East Main Street-Suite 120
Yourtown, US 98765-4321

August 15, 20--　　　　　　　**(DATELINE)**

Robert Smith, M.D.
50 North Broad Street
Mytown, US 43200　　　　　　　**(INSIDE ADDRESS)**

Dear Dr. Smith:　　　　　　　**(SALUTATION)**

RE: Amy D. James　　　　　　　**(REFERENCE)**

I am referring Amy James to your office for an eye
examination. She is complaining of some difficulty with
reading. She will be returning to school soon, and her parents
wish to ensure that her vision is properly corrected.

Mrs. James will call your office for an appointment. I would
appreciate a report of your findings.

Sincerely yours,　　　　　　　**(COMPLIMENTARY CLOSE)**

　　　　　　　　　　　　　　(SIGNATURE OF SENDER)

Samuel E. Matthews, MD　　　**(NAME TYPED)**

lk　　　　　　　　　　　　　**(REFERENCE INITIALS)**

(ENCLOSURE, IF ANY)

FIGURE 6-19B　Sample full block letter

Samuel E. Matthews, MD
100 East Main Street-Suite 120
Yourtown, US 98765-4321

　　　　　　　August 15, 20--　**(DATELINE)**

Robert Smith, M.D.
50 North Broad Street
Mytown, US 43200　　　　**(INSIDE ADDRESS)**

　　　　　RE: Amy D. James　**(REFERENCE)**

Dear Dr. Smith:　　　　**(SALUTATION)**

I am referring Amy James to your office for an eye examination. She is complaining of some difficulty with reading. She
will be returning to school soon, and her parents wish to ensure that her vision is properly corrected.

Mrs. James will call your office for an appointment. I would appreciate a report of your findings.

(COMPLIMENTARY CLOSE)　Sincerely yours,
　　　　　　　　　　　　(SIGNATURE OF SENDER)

(NAME TYPED)　　　Samuel E. Matthews, MD
(TITLE IF NEEDED)

lk
(ENCLOSURE, IF ANY)　　**(REFERENCE INITIALS)**

FIGURE 6-19C　Sample modified block letter

Samuel E. Matthews, MD
100 East Main Street, Suite 120
Yourtown, US 98765-4321

　　　　　　　August 15, 20--　**(DATELINE)**

Robert Smith, M.D.
50 North Broad Street
Mytown, US 43200　　　　**(INSIDE ADDRESS)**

　　　　　RE: Amy D. James　**(REFERENCE)**

Dear Dr. Smith:　　　　**(SALUTATION)**

　　I am referring Amy James to your office for an eye examination. She is complaining of some difficulty with reading. She
will be returning to school soon, and her parents wish to ensure that her vision is properly corrected.

　　Mrs. James will call your office for an appointment. I would
appreciate a report of your findings.

(COMPLIMENTARY CLOSE)　Sincerely yours,
　　　　　　　　　　　　(SIGNATURE OF SENDER)

(NAME TYPED)　　　Samuel E. Matthews, MD
(TITLE IF NEEDED)

lk　　　　　　　　　**(REFERENCE INITIALS)**
(ENCLOSURE, IF ANY)

FIGURE 6-19D　Sample modified block letter with indented
paragraphs

SELECTING A LETTER STYLE

Letter styles vary in the location of some of the parts. Compare Figures 6-19B, C, and D. They are samples of the full block letter, the modified block letter, and the modified block letter with indented paragraphs. Notice the different placement of the parts of the letter with each style. Your employer may have a preference, so be sure you know which one is to be used. In full block style, the dateline, address, salutation, body of letter, complimentary close, typed signature, and the initials of the typist are flush with the left margin. This is a popular style because no tab stops are needed. Another popular style is the modified block with the dateline, complimentary close, and typed signature beginning a bit right of center. This style is compatible with most letterheads. The dateline sets the style. If you place the date at the right, you must follow with modified block style, lining up the complimentary close and typed signature with the date. The least popular of the three styles customarily used in the medical office is the modified block with indented paragraphs.

Stationery

The type and quality of **stationery** makes a statement about the physician's office. If it becomes your responsibility to select the stationery, be sure to inspect any anticipated choice carefully. The letterhead style and content is usually the choice of the physician. Letterhead stationery and matching envelopes are usually 16-, 20-, or 24-pound weight. The larger the number, the heavier the paper. It is usually ordered by the ream, which consists of 500 sheets of paper. Continuation pages are plain bond and should match the weight, texture, and brightness of the letterhead.

A **watermark** appears on bond paper and should read across the paper in the same direction as the typing. You can determine the correct watermark side by holding the paper to the light.

Be certain to make a copy of every business letter or report to be sent from the office. Copies of correspondence regarding patients need to be filed in their charts. Correspondence in answer to business letters need to be copied and placed in the appropriate file.

EHR CONNECTION

Offices with EHR will file patient correspondence in their respective personal electronic file and the business correspondence in the appropriate office correspondence file folder.

COMPOSE A BUSINESS LETTER

A letter can be prepared from dictated notes or from a dictation machine tape, or it may be composed by you at the keyboard. There are certain formatting standards that result in a mailable letter. The following are points to remember as you perform Procedure 6-7:

- The date typed indicates when the content of the letter was dictated.
- The month is spelled out in full (traditional style is month/day/year; military style is day/month/year).
- The inside address should be copied exactly from the correspondence to be answered or as printed in the phone book or medical society directory.
- A courtesy title is used (Mr., Mrs., Miss, or Ms. If gender unknown, use Mr.).
- Do not use Dr. before the physician's name if MD follows.
- If a street address and box number are given, use the box number.
- The words North, South, East, and West preceding street names and Road, Street, Avenue, and Boulevard are *not* abbreviated.
- The words Apartment and Suite are typed on the same line as the address and are separated by a comma.
- Apartment may be abbreviated if the line is long.
- The name of the city is spelled out and is separated from the state by a comma.
- The state name can be spelled out or abbreviated (see Unit 4 for a list of abbreviations) and is separated from the zip code by one space; there is no punctuation between the state and the zip code.
- A proper salutation is Dear, followed by the title and the person's last name. If the correspondence is to a colleague or friend, a first name is appropriate (ask the physician). When writing to a business, use "Dear Sir" or "Dear Madam."
- To use a reference line, type "RE:," then the person's full name. This line goes two spaces *below* the salutation, flush with the left margin in block style. It may be lined up with the date and follow the address in the modified block style. It is a common error to type the reference line prior to the salutation, because that is where most physicians who dictate correspondence name the person.
- Always double space between paragraphs, flush left with block style and indented five spaces with modified block.
- If a second page will be necessary, stop the first page at the end of a paragraph, if possible. If not, include at least two lines from the broken paragraph on the bottom of the first page.
- The bottom margin must measure at least one inch.
- The last word on a page cannot be divided.
- Capitalize only the first word of a complimentary closing; follow with a comma.

PROCEDURE PROCEDURE PROCEDURE PROCEDURE PROCEDURE PROCEDURE PROCEDURE

6-7  Compose a Business Letter

PURPOSE: To prepare a mailable business letter.

EQUIPMENT AND SUPPLIES: Computer, paper, dictation machine or dictation tape, and transcriber.

PERFORMANCE OBJECTIVE: Given access to equipment and supplies, complete a mailable letter following the steps in the procedure within the number of attempts and time frame specified by the instructor. The final copy must meet the mailable standards described in this text.

NOTE: In order to transcribe a dictated letter from a machine or tape, it will be necessary to activate the equipment to listen to the dictation. It is a good idea to listen to the entire letter before beginning to type in order to judge its length and be aware of its content. Start and stop the tape as necessary throughout the procedure to produce the letter.

1. Move the cursor down at least three lines below the letterhead.

2. Enter the date. **NOTE: Be sure that the location is appropriate for the chosen style.**

3. Move to the fifth line below the date.

4. Enter the inside address. **NOTE: Be sure the address is in the appropriate location for the style of letter. Use the appropriate courtesy title and enter the name exactly as printed on the received letterhead or as is in the phone or medical society directory.**

5. Double space after the last line of the address.

6. Enter the appropriate salutation, followed by a colon.

7. Double space.

8. Enter the reference line in the location appropriate for letter style. Type RE: Enter the name of the patient or person about whom the letter is written.

9. Double space.

10. Enter the body (content) of the letter.
    - Be sure the paragraph style is appropriate to the style of the letter.
    - Always double space between paragraphs.

- If a second page is needed, end the first page at the end of a paragraph. If this is not possible, place at least two lines of the paragraph on the first page. Do not divide the last word on the first page.

11. When a second page is necessary, enter the second page heading in vertical or horizontal format. **NOTE: Includes name, page number, and date.**

12. Continue body of letter.

13. Enter a complimentary closing in letter style format.

14. Go down four lines.

15. Enter the sender's name in letter style format exactly as printed on letterhead. **NOTE: An official title follows the name on the same line separated by a comma, or it is placed directly below, with no comma required.**

16. Double space.

17. Enter reference initials to indicate the typist.

18. Single or double space if enclosing materials.

19. Enter the preferred style enclosure. **NOTE: Number and identify if there is more than one enclosure.**

20. Single or double space if copies will be sent.

21. Enter cc and the recipient(s) name(s). **NOTE: Enter bcc on file copy if sending a blind copy.**

22. Double space.

23. Enter PS for postscript, if desired.

24. Print a draft copy.

25. Proofread the letter.

26. Print the letter on letterhead.

27. Prepare an envelope.

28. Present the letter with envelope to the person who dictated it for signature.

29. File a copy in the chart if it concerns a patient or in the appropriate business folder.

30. If the office has EHR, file it in the appropriate folder or the patient's file.

- The formality of the letter determines the closing: "Cordially" or "Sincerely" is considered informal, whereas "Very truly yours" is more formal.
- The sender's name is entered four spaces below the closing, exactly as on the letterhead; an official title follows on the same line, separated by a comma, or it can be typed on the next line with no comma.
- The typist's initials, in lower case, are placed two spaces below the sender's name. When the sender

will not be signing the letter, both dictator's (in upper case) and typist's initials are used. Typists do not use their reference initials on letters they sign.

- When items will be enclosed with the letter, enter "Enclosure" or "Enc." one or two lines below reference initials; number and identify if more than one enclosure is included.
- If copies are sent to others, enter "cc" (for carbon copy) and the other receiver's name one or two spaces below the initials or last notation. When more than one individual is carbon copied, list their names alphabetically or by rank. When a copy is sent to another person without the knowledge of the recipient, it is known as a *blind carbon copy* (bcc). No notation is placed on the recipient's letter, but *bcc* is placed on the file copy to **denote** it was sent.
- A **postscript** (PS) is entered two spaces below the last notation.
- When using a second page, a heading of the patient's name, page number, and date, is entered either vertically or horizontally, one inch from the top. If the letter does not concern a patient, the receiver is listed.
- The letter continues on the third line after the heading; the page should contain at least two lines of a paragraph.
- Print a draft copy and proof it. Proofing on screen is difficult because you cannot view the entire letter at one time. Correct and save the copy. Print the letter on a letterhead.
- Prepare an envelope and give with letter to the writer for a signature.

paragraph indents, spacing on the page, etc. Then they read for content, to make certain correct words, punctuation, and grammar are used. Last, they do a check of spelling. Because we can be fooled by what we think we see when we read normally, spelling is checked by reading the content *backward,* checking each word, one word at a time. Going through these steps should ensure an error-free communication. If possible, as a final precaution, have someone else **critique** the letter.

When you proofread a draft copy, you should use standard proofreader's marks to indicate changes that need to be made. Knowledge of these marks is very helpful if your employer writes for professional journals or other publications. Materials that are submitted may be returned by the publisher with these markings and any other clarifications or changes the publisher may desire. The final draft of copy to be published is called **galley proofs**. It will require very careful proofreading for any remaining errors before the material goes to print. The most common proofreading marks are shown in Figure 6-20.

Good transcription and composing skills and the ability to produce error-free communications are very desirable traits. They can make you an asset to the physician's practice. If you enjoy this type of work, it will probably be possible for you to specialize in communication preparation.

Medical assistants can be self-employed by establishing arrangements with physicians to pick up dictation tapes and return accurately completed correspondence within a short time frame.

Proofreading

All written communication must be **proofread** before it is sent. This is a process of carefully reading printed material and marking errors for correction. The spell checker and immediate feedback of composition errors from word processing software will identify most common errors. However, it will still miss the correctly spelled wrong word and out-of-context words. Watch for certain things that seem to be problems, such as:

words ending in "s"	periods
combinations of punctuation	commas
capital letters	two-letter words
numbers	dashes
apostrophes	double letters in words
hyphens	

Proofreading requires concentration and attention to details in a step-by-step process. Career proofreaders use at least a three-read system. First they read through the material to make sure it makes sense and to check for errors in composition such as a misaligned margin,

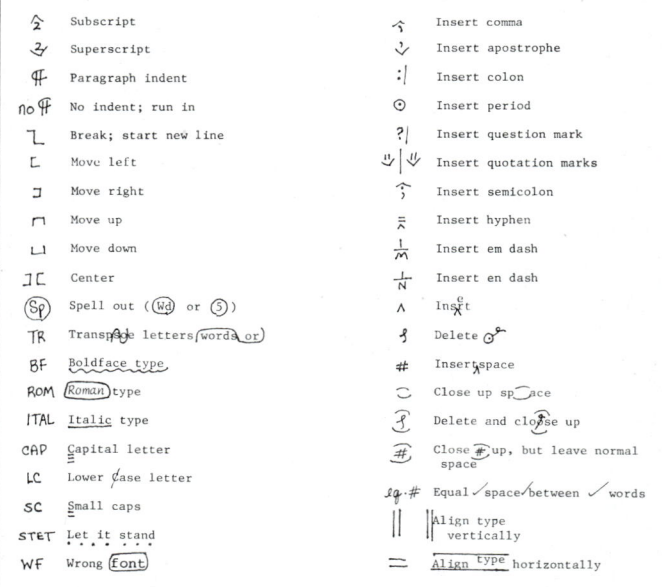

FIGURE 6-20 Proofreader's marks

ACHIEVE UNIT OBJECTIVES

- ☐ Complete the Workbook activities to meet the learning objectives.
- ☐ Practice the procedures in this unit to meet the performance objectives.
- ☐ Apply your knowledge at the end of this chapter in completing the Critical Thinking Challenge and Activities, as well as the StudyWARE on your Student CD-ROM.

UNIT 4
RECEIVING AND SENDING OFFICE COMMUNICATIONS

OBJECTIVES

Upon completion of this unit, you will be able to achieve the following:

LEARNING Objectives

1. Spell and define, using the glossary at the back of the text, all the Words to Know in this unit.
2. Explain how to sort, open, and annotate incoming mail.
3. Describe how vacation mail might be handled.
4. Identify postal services that may be required by an office.
5. List points to remember in processing metered mail.
6. List six classifications of mail.
7. Describe two reasons to use a certificate of mailing.
8. Explain why you might use certified mail.
9. Describe the purpose of use of registered mail.
10. Explain what restricted delivery means.
11. Explain the purpose of a return receipt.
12. Name six means of communication other than by mail.
13. Name six uses for a fax machine.
14. Describe the characteristics of an electronic address.
15. Define the term "computer virus."
16. List four guidelines to avoid acquiring a virus through e-mail.

WORDS TO KNOW

abbreviations	polling
annotating	postmark
cancellation	priority
certified	receipt
consecutively	recipient
domestic	registered
envelope	restricted
facsimile	standard
foreign	teleconference
guaranteed	thermally
judgment	transmitted
periodical	

CERTIFICATION CONNECTION

CMA
Receiving, organizing, prioritizing, and transmitting information
Computer applications, electronic mail
Internet services
Screening and processing mail

CMAS
Processing incoming and outgoing mail
Employ e-mail applications

RMA
Employ procedures for integrity of information and compliance with HIPAA Security and Privacy regulations (Firewall software and hardware)

INCOMING MAIL

The amount of mail coming into physicians' offices depends on the number of physicians. In smaller offices the task of handling the mail is manageable, but in large clinics it may be necessary to have a mail clerk who is responsible for sorting and delivering the mail within the clinic.

The office policy manual should give instructions regarding the handling of mail. If no manual is available, the office manager or the physician should be consulted. Following are some generally accepted practices.

SORTING MAIL

Incoming mail should first be sorted. Any mail marked *personal* should be placed on the physician's or office manager's desk unopened. Special delivery mail, Mailgrams, or special messenger mail should be opened immediately. (The Mailgram is a postal service offered jointly by the United States Postal Service [USPS] and Western Union.) Mailgrams are transmitted over Western Union's communication network to printers located in over 140 post offices, placed in special envelopes carrying the postal service emblem, and delivered the next day by regular carrier.

There are many different types of mail that come into a physician's office. Office policy will determine whether it is sorted and placed on the physician's desk or the office manager's desk or whether a combination of both occurs in relation to the type of mail received. The process will depend upon the number of physicians, the office management design, and the assignment of personnel. The actual processing of the mail may be done by the manager, the receptionist, or an administrative medical assistant. The following are some examples of mail that will be received:

Special delivery mail
Mailgrams
Special messenger mail
Correspondence from patients
Payments from patients
Payments from insurance companies
Requests for information from insurance companies
Referral letters or reports from physicians
Laboratory reports
Hospital reports
Professional organization mail
Professional journals
Magazines
Newspapers
Advertisements
Promotional literature and samples from pharmaceutical companies

Mail may be sorted into categories, such as mail from patients, physicians, insurance companies, and miscellaneous sources. Other classes of mail, such as magazines, professional journals, and newspapers, should be separated from drug samples and advertisements.

OPENING MAIL

When opening mail, you will need a letter opener, paper clips, a stapler, and a date stamp. It is more efficient to stack all envelopes so that they are facing in the same direction. A quick tap on the desk will move contents away from the flap side of the **envelope**. Open each letter along the flap edge, being careful to remove all contents from each envelope. As the mail is removed, be sure the contents contain the same name and return address shown on the envelope. Some offices want you to keep the envelope with the mail received, and certainly you should if it is needed to help identify the contents. Otherwise you may discard the envelopes.

Date-stamp the correspondence and attach any enclosures. If an enclosure is indicated on the letter but is missing, it is necessary to write "None" after the "Encl." notation and circle it to indicate need for follow-up.

A word of caution regarding mail: From time to time someone may use the mail to send material that is explosive, contaminated, or otherwise dangerous. It is possible that a disgruntled patient could seek to harm or at least frighten the physician or the office staff. Although this is probably highly unlikely, for your own safety and that of the office, you should be aware of what is considered to be a suspicious letter or package. The USPS has suggested that certain things would make a letter seem suspicious:

- It is unexpected or from someone you do not know.
- It is addressed to someone no longer at your address.
- It is handwritten and has no return address or bears one that you cannot confirm is legitimate.
- It is lopsided or lumpy in appearance.
- It is sealed with an excessive amount of tape.
- It is marked with restrictive endorsements such as *Personal* or *Confidential*.
- It has excessive postage.

Other suggestions regarding packaging that could make it seem suspicious are:

- A package wrapped with string (against postal regulations, could have been delivered by other means)
- Any sound coming from a package

If such a letter or package should arrive, what should you do?

- Don't handle a letter or package that you suspect is contaminated.
- Don't shake it, bump it, or sniff it.
- Wash your hands thoroughly with soap and water.
- Notify local law enforcement authorities.

PROCESSING INCOMING MAIL

Exercise your best **judgment** to determine which mail can be handled without the aid of the physician. This type of mail would include routine office expense bills, insurance forms, and checks for deposit. If cash is received in the mail, you should always seek a witness to verify the amount of money and have that person sign a receipt along with you to be sent to the patient. This helps avoid the possibility of the patient saying that more was sent than was actually found in the envelope. This can happen quite innocently by human error.

If you are employed by a surgeon, the mail will contain copies of hospital summaries and dictated operative notes. These can be filed directly in the patients' charts. Often copies are sent to the referring physician. Other hospital, laboratory, or special examination reports received should be seen by the physician and initialed before they are filed. Requests regarding patients or other office matters should be placed in a designated area for the physician to see and respond to each day.

The medical assistant can perform a valuable, time-saving service for the physician by **annotating** the incoming mail, or identifying important points to be noticed. If any correspondence or a patient's chart will be needed to answer mail, it should be pulled and placed with the mail to facilitate the response.

Notifications of meetings, miscellaneous correspondence, and professional journals are placed under the stack of mail. Some physicians want to see all supply catalogs and pharmaceutical company descriptions of products. In other offices, many of these items are disposed of immediately, especially if they concern areas of practice the office does not provide. Items that may be needed for future reference should be placed in a designated file.

Drug samples that may be used should be placed in a designated area for future use. Samples that will not be used should never be placed in the trash, because they could cause harm to individuals taking them without medical evaluation and advice. Often, community clinics and service organizations can make good, safe use of donated samples. The office should have a box to collect samples for this purpose.

VACATION MAIL

When the physician is away from the office for professional meetings or on vacation, the medical assistant may be asked to carefully read all mail and decide how each piece will be handled. You should discuss what to do with urgent mail before the physician leaves. The physician may want you to call to discuss or, in some cases, to copy and forward the mail. Never send the original. If the physician will be away for a long time, you may need to send mail more than once. If so, be sure to number the envelopes **consecutively** and keep track of what you send so that you can be sure all the mail is received. When responding to the person who sent urgent mail, you may also wish to send a brief note explaining the reason for the delay in answering. If the office will be closed temporarily or permanently, be sure to go to the post office and complete a form to have mail held or forwarded to another address. Never send the form by mail, because it may be delayed. The USPS cannot take verbal orders for this purpose. Allowing mail to accumulate invites theft.

FIGURE 6-21   Example of a bar code *(Courtesy of United States Postal Service.)*

MACHINABLE MAIL

The United States Postal Service (USPS) uses optical character readers (OCRs) and bar code sorters (BCSs) to read the addresses on envelopes you mail. The BCS equipment is capable of sorting over 36,000 pieces of mail per hour, but only if envelopes are properly addressed.

Each piece of mail passes by the computer's scanner for a quick read of the delivery address. Then, it goes to the OCR's printer, which sprays on a bar code representing the zip code or ZIP + 4 code for the address. The bar code is a series of little lines seen at the bottom of letters from utility companies, banks, retailers, and other businesses (Figure 6-21). Next, the mail piece goes to one of the OCR's sorting channels reserved for the proper delivery area. From there, the bar coded mail is fed to BCSs for the final separations. The BCS processes mail just as quickly and in much the same way as the OCR reads addresses, except its scanner recognizes only one thing—the bar code. As the bar code on your mail piece passes the BCS lens, it is quickly read and sent to the appropriate channel for delivery.

ADDRESSING ENVELOPES

Addresses must be typed or machine printed in order to be processed by automatic equipment. A standard type font is also required. Script or executive type cannot be used because the letters run together. The OCR must be able to see a clear space between each character and word, or it won't know where one word ends and the next begins. Capitalize everything, using plain block letters. Omit all punctuation, except the hyphen in the ZIP + 4 code. Use approved abbreviations whenever possible. Lines of the address should be formatted with a uniform left margin. Also, be sure your toner is producing good quality print so that there is adequate contrast to be scanned.

The letter envelope must also be of a proper size. Envelopes smaller than $3\frac{1}{2} \times 5$ inches are not mailable. Envelopes larger than $6\frac{1}{8} \times 11\frac{1}{2}$ inches are mailable but must be processed by hand and will require additional postage.

ADDRESS BLOCK LOCATION

The shaded area in Figure 6-22 illustrates the area on the face of the mail piece where address information should be located to be read by the OCRs. The OCRs and BCSs register mail pieces on the bottom edge;

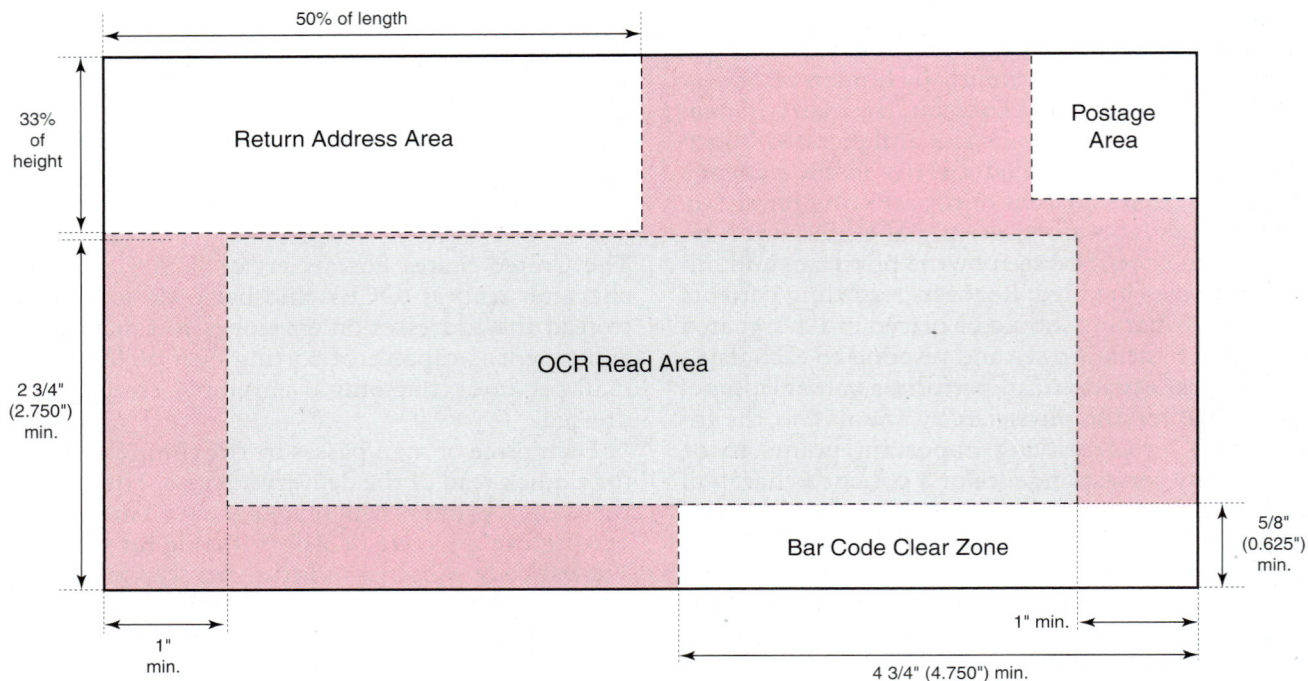

FIGURE 6-22 Designated zones for accurate reading of envelopes by optical character reader (OCR) and bar code scanner (BCS) *(Courtesy of United States Postal Service)*

therefore, all vertical measurements are relative to the bottom edge.

Where possible, the entire address (exclusive of the optional lines above the name of recipient line) should be contained in an imaginary rectangle that extends from ⅝ inch to 2¾ inches from the bottom of the mail piece, with 1-inch margins on each side. At a minimum, all characters of the last line of the address block—the post office (city), state, and zip code or ZIP + 4—should be located within an imaginary rectangle that extends from ⅝ inch to 2¼ inches from the bottom of the mail piece, with 1-inch margins on each side. Make sure the address is as complete as possible, including all apartment or suite numbers.

Care must be taken to make the lines straight, as slanted lines cannot be read by the OCR process. The only **abbreviations** permitted in the name of the city are those found in the "Abbreviations" section of the *National Zip Code Directory*. The OCR cannot read a non-standard abbreviation.

No portion of the return address should appear in the OCR read area. Special notations for the recipient such as *PERSONAL* or *CONFIDENTIAL* should be typed in all capitals aligned with and two lines below the return address.

The zip code is critical to the rapid delivery of mail. The first number of the zip code refers to a region of the United States, from 0 for the East Coast to 9 for the West Coast and Hawaii. The next two numbers refer to

the major post office in the region, and the final two identify the local delivery post offices. The ZIP + 4 coding allows even better use of automated processing in that the first two additional numbers denote a delivery sector, which may be several blocks, a group of streets, several office buildings, or another small geographic area. The last two numbers denote a delivery segment, which might be one floor of an office building, one side of a street, specific departments in a firm, or a group of post office boxes.

The USPS will offer assistance in converting to ZIP + 4, but the confidential nature of medical office records means that patient interests would best be served by converting your own records. The customer service representative at the post office can answer your questions on the use of the *ZIP + 4 National State Directory*.

Now that you know how to address an envelope correctly, it is time to put it all together. The name of the intended **recipient** (business or individual) should appear on the first line. The line above the name of recipient line is an optional line for additional address information. When needed, it should be used to direct mail to the attention of a specific person when a business name has been placed on the name of the recipient line or to provide other information that will facilitate delivery (e.g., the name of a department within a company).

The line immediately below the recipient line is designated the *delivery address line*. The street address, post office box number, rural route number and box number, or highway contract number and box number should appear on this line. Figure 6-23 lists examples of USPS approved address abbreviations that can be used. Mail addressed to multiunit buildings should include the apartment number, suite, room, or other unit designation immediately after the street address of the building, on the same line. When the length of the delivery address is such that it prevents the placement of the unit number or other designation on the same line, the number or designator should be placed on the line immediately above the delivery address line. When use of the building name in the address is necessary, it should also be placed on the line above the delivery address line.

For **domestic** mail, the post office (city), state, and zip code or ZIP + 4 should appear, in that order, on the bottom line of the address. However, if all three elements will not fit on that line, the zip code or ZIP + 4 may be placed on the line immediately below the post office and state, aligned with the left edge of the address block. The standard two-letter state abbreviations should also be used (Figure 6-24). The ZIP + 4 codes should always be printed as five digits, a hyphen, and four digits. The hyphen should be treated as any other character as far as spacing and stroke width are concerned. Figure 6-25 shows a properly addressed envelope with all components in the correct format and location. This address can easily be read by the OCR equipment.

Mail addressed to **foreign** countries should include the country name printed in capital letters (no abbreviations) as the only information on the bottom line.

EXAMPLE:

MR THOMAS CLARK
117 RUSSELL DRIVE
LONDON WIP6HQ
ENGLAND

Mail addressed to Canada may use either of the following formats when the postal delivery zone number is included in the address:

MRS HELEN SAUNDERS	MRS HELEN SAUNDERS
1010 CLEAR STREET	1010 CLEAR STREET
OTTAWA ON K1AOB1	OTTAWA ON CANADA
CANADA	K1AOB1

The post office will furnish additional information on mailing to foreign countries if assistance is needed.

COMPLETING MAILING

When you are satisfied that your letter and envelope are complete, place the flap of the envelope over the top of the letter and secure it with a paper clip. If enclosures are indicated, be sure these are included. It is a good idea to have a signature folder in which finished mail waiting to be signed is placed.

When the mail has been signed, fold it and place it in the envelope. A letter for a standard-size business

Annex	ANX	Parkway	PKY
Apartment	APT	Pike	PIKE
Attention	ATTN	Place	PL
Avenue	AVE	Plaza	PLZ
Boulevard	BLVD	Post Office	PO
Canyon	CYN	President	PRES
Causeway	CSWY	Ridge	RDG
Circle	CIR	River	RIV
Court	CT	Road	RD
Department	DEPT	Room	RM
East	E	Route	RT
Expressway	EXPY	Rural	R
Freeway	FWY	Rural Route	RR
Heights	HTS	Secretary	SECY
Highway	HWY	Shore	SHR
Hospital	HOSP	South	S
Institute	INST	Southeast	SE
Junction	JCT	Southwest	SW
Knolls	KNLS	Square	SQ
Lake	LK	Station	STA
Lakes	LKS	Street	ST
Lane	LN	Suite	STE
Meadows	MDWS	Terrace	TER
North	N	Treasurer	TREAS
Northeast	NE	Turnpike	TPKE
Northwest	NW	Union	UN
Palms	PLMS	Vice President	VP
Park	PK	View	VW

FIGURE 6-23 Examples of USPS-approved address abbreviations (Courtesy of United States Postal Service)

Alabama	AL	Montana	MT
Alaska	AK	Nebraska	NE
Arizona	AZ	Nevada	NV
Arkansas	AR	New Hampshire	NH
California	CA	New Jersey	NJ
Canal Zone	CZ	New Mexico	NM
Colorado	CO	New York	NY
Connecticut	CT	North Carolina	NC
Delaware	DE	North Dakota	ND
District of Columbia	DC	Ohio	OH
Florida	FL	Oklahoma	OK
Georgia	GA	Oregon	OR
Guam	GU	Pennsylvania	PA
Hawaii	HI	Puerto Rico	PR
Idaho	ID	Rhode Island	RI
Illinois	IL	South Carolina	SC
Indiana	IN	South Dakota	SD
Iowa	IA	Tennessee	TN
Kansas	KS	Texas	TX
Kentucky	KY	Utah	UT
Louisiana	LA	Vermont	VT
Maine	ME	Virginia	VA
Maryland	MD	Virgin Islands	VI
Massachusetts	MA	Washington	WA
Michigan	MI	West Virginia	WV
Minnesota	MN	Wisconsin	WI
Mississippi	MS	Wyoming	WY
Missouri	MO		

FIGURE 6-24 Two-letter state abbreviations (Courtesy of United States Postal Service)

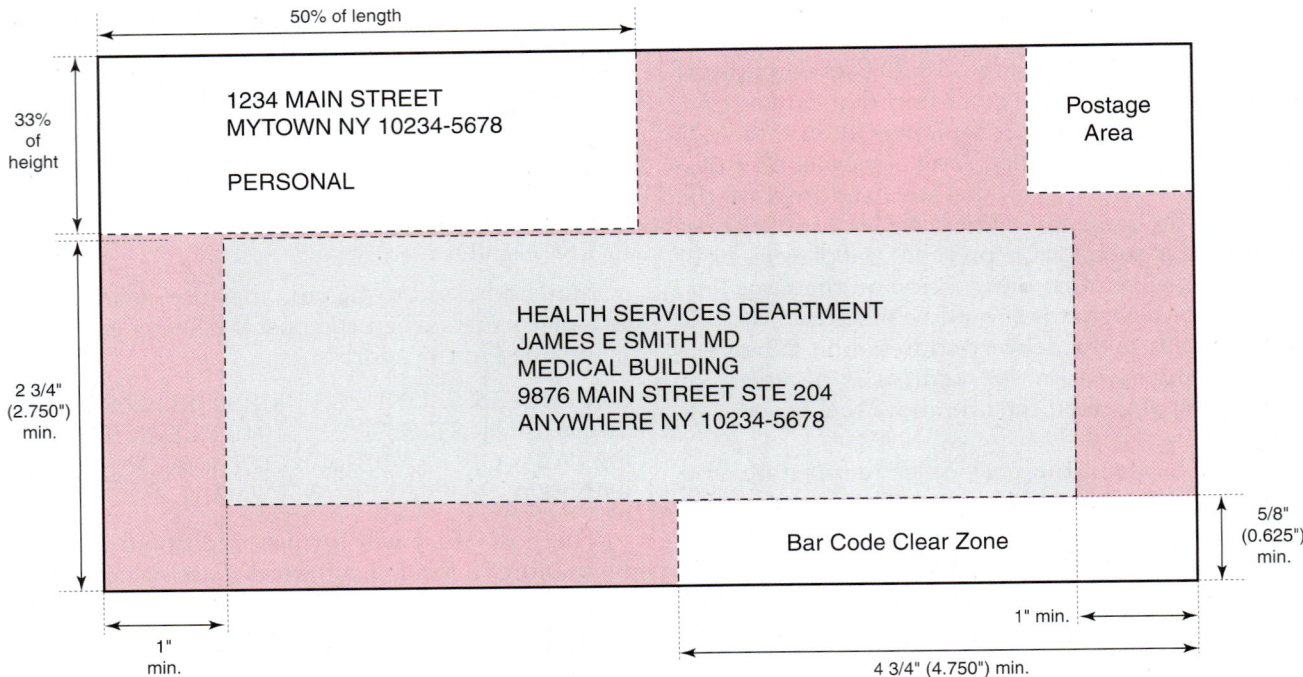

FIGURE 6-25 Properly addressed envelope

envelope should be folded by bringing the lower third of the letter up and making a crease, then folding the top third of the letter down to about half an inch from the creased edge and making a second crease (Figure 6-26A). The second crease goes into the envelope first. To fold a standard-size letter for a 6¾″ envelope, bring the bottom edge to within half an inch of the top edge and crease. Fold from the right side about one third the width of the sheet and crease. Fold from the left edge to within half an inch of the second crease. Insert the left-edge crease into the envelope first (Figure 6-26B).

An alternative folding method places the top third of the letter at the front (Figure 6-26C). This allows immediate identification of the recipient upon opening the envelope. It also might be appropriate if your envelopes have an address window that would match the location of the inside address, thereby eliminating the need to address the envelope.

If you have a large number of envelopes to seal, you can speed up the process by placing eight or ten envelopes address side down with flaps open in a shingle fashion. Use a damp sponge to wet all the flaps at once and then, starting with the one on top, turn down each flap and seal (Figure 6-26D). Be sure that the sponge is not too wet, as it will wet the envelopes and may spread the glue so that the letters stick together before you can seal them.

STAMP OR METER MAIL

The cost of sending mail is an expenditure that must be examined to be sure you obtain the most for your money. Your local post office can furnish you with current information. Postage rates, categories, and regulations are changeable, so you need to be current.

Mail may be either stamped or metered. Stamps may be purchased at a post office or obtained through the mail by using a specially printed envelope available through the post office. If you have a large volume of mail, it is preferable to use a postage meter. This machine can be leased from several authorized dealers, but the license to use it must be obtained from the USPS. A medical office can obtain a license by submitting an application to the post office where the metered mail will be deposited.

Postage meters contain a sealed unit that houses the printing die and two recording counters. One counter adds up all postage printed by the meter. The other counter subtracts and shows the balance of postage remaining in the meter. When you purchase an amount of postage, the post office will open the meter with a key, set the counter for the amount of postage purchased, and relock the meter. When the prepaid amount has been spent, the meter will lock automatically. The postage meter prints prepaid postage either directly on the mail or on adhesive strips that are then affixed to the mail. The metered mail imprint, or me-

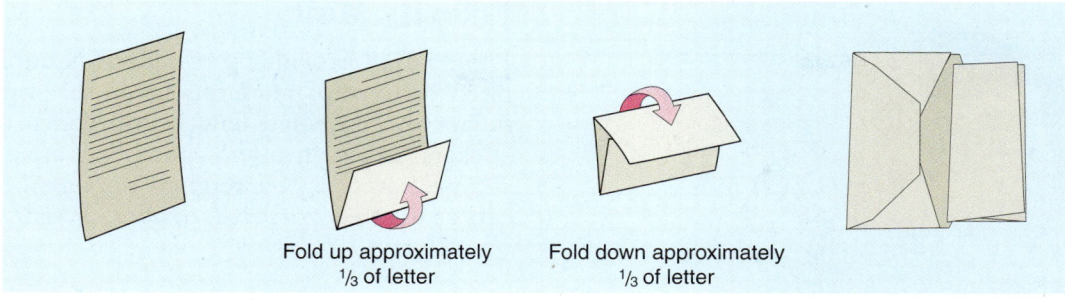

FIGURE 6-26A   Folding of a letter for a standard-size business envelope

Fold up approximately ⅓ of letter

Fold down approximately ⅓ of letter

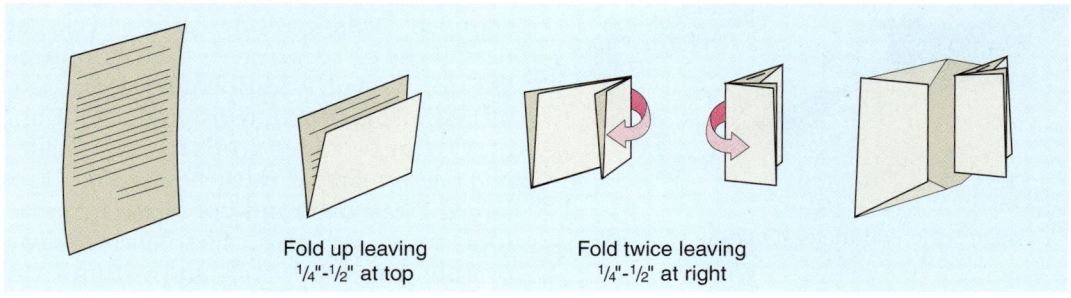

FIGURE 6-26B   Folding of a letter for a 6¾″ envelope

Fold up leaving ¼″–½″ at top

Fold twice leaving ¼″–½″ at right

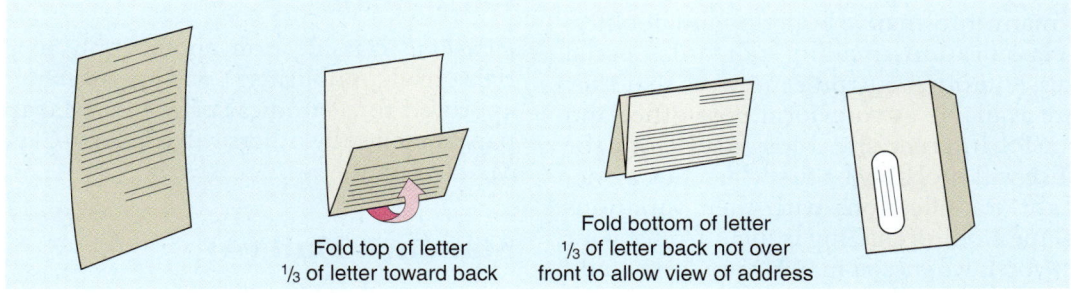

FIGURE 6-26C   Alternative fold for business envelope

Fold top of letter ⅓ of letter toward back

Fold bottom of letter ⅓ of letter back not over front to allow view of address

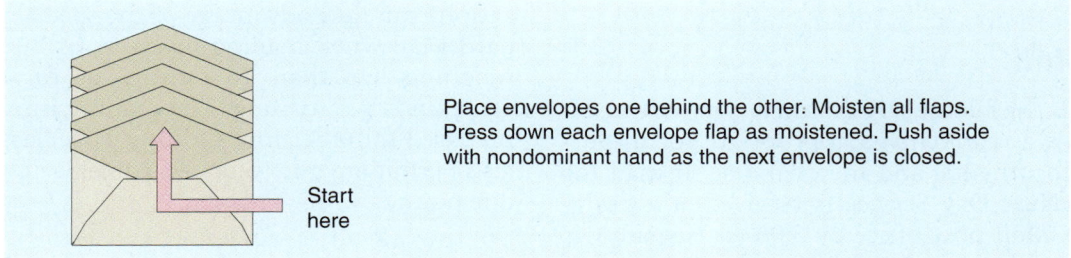

FIGURE 6-26D   Sealing envelopes in shingle fashion

Start here

Place envelopes one behind the other. Moisten all flaps. Press down each envelope flap as moistened. Push aside with nondominant hand as the next envelope is closed.

tered stamp, serves as postage payment, **postmark**, and **cancellation** mark. All mail classes, amounts of postage, and quantity of mail may be metered. Metered mail, when bundled, can provide faster service than stamped mail because it is already postmarked and will bypass postal cancellation equipment.

To expedite the processing of metered mail, remember to: (1) change the date on the meter daily, (2) apply the correct amount of postage by weighing the mail before affixing postage, (3) check the imprint to be sure it is clear and readable, and (4) use fluorescent ink in the meter (Figure 6-27).

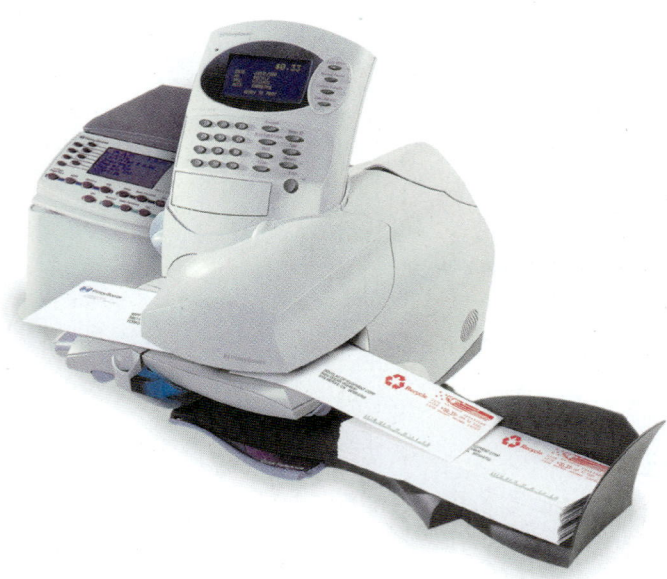

FIGURE 6-27 Postage scale and meter *(Courtesy of Pitney Bowes, Inc.)*

MAIL CLASSIFICATIONS

The USPS has many informative bulletins and booklets regarding the classifications, mailing standards, special mailing services, and other customer services that they offer. These are available at your local post office and through the USPS Internet site. Most mail from the physician's office will probably be first class, but a brief discussion of the classifications with their variations and additional methods of mailing is included for your information. If you have special mailing needs, it would be advisable to consult with your local post office for advice and up-to-date regulations, because they tend to change periodically.

Express Mail

Express Mail is the fastest service and is **guaranteed** delivery 365 days a year. This is appropriate for important letters, documents, and merchandise. If mail for Express Mail Next Day Service is received at a designated Express Mail post office by 5:00 PM (usually), it will be delivered by noon or 3:00 PM the next day. If overnight is not possible to the destination, then a guaranteed second-day delivery service is available. Merchandise is automatically insured up to $500, and up to $5000 for a fee. If you wish, you can waive the recipient's signature requirement so that the delivery can be left if the recipient is not there (unless it is insured above $500). Special envelopes, boxes, and tubes are provided free of charge. The rates vary by the amount of material mailed.

Priority Mail

Priority Mail provides preferential handling and expedited delivery of materials up to 70 pounds and 108 inches in combined length and width. Priority Mail stickers, labels, envelopes, and boxes are provided at no charge. Rates vary by weight. This classification of mail can be insured, *registered*, *certified*, or sent COD (collect on delivery).

First-Class Mail

First-Class mail is for sending letters, postcards, stamped cards, greeting cards, checks, and money orders. If the piece is heavier than 11 ounces, it is handled as Priority Mail. Additional services, such as certificates of mailing, certified, registered, COD, and *restricted* delivery, can be added to First-Class Mail. If the piece is NOT letter-size, it must be marked "First Class," or a large, green-diamond-bordered first-class mail envelope must be used. First-Class delivery is usually overnight in local cities and within two days to most states.

Periodicals

Periodicals classification applies only to printed materials from publishers and registered news agents approved for Periodical privileges. Magazines or newspapers mailed by others will use First-Class or Standard Mail (A) rates.

Standard Mail (A)

Standard Mail (A) is a classification used by retailers, catalogers, and other advertisers to promote products and services. Churches and other eligible nonprofit organizations can take advantage of the special rates of Standard Mail when mailing in excess of 200 pieces, each weighing less than 16 ounces, or for sending over 50 pounds per mailing. The mailing must be specially prepared for efficient handling. This classification will also permit anyone to mail a parcel weighing less than one pound.

Standard Mail (B)

Standard Mail (B) is for parcels weighing one pound or more. If a First-Class Mail piece is attached or enclosed, you will pay for it in addition to the Standard Mail (B) parcel charge. Insurance to cover the value of articles mailed can be purchased. Parcels mailed under this classification can weigh up to 70 pounds. There are special rates for books or catalogs. The delivery time is slower, perhaps taking up to 9 days.

SPECIAL MAILING SERVICES

There are other special mailing services you may want to use when mailing personal or confidential patient information. These are in addition to the various classifications discussed.

Certificate of Mailing

A certificate of mailing is a *receipt* showing evidence that the piece was mailed. It is purchased at the time of mailing. This is helpful when you want to prove that something was mailed or a deadline was met. There is no proof of delivery, and no insurance against loss is provided with the certificate.

Certified Mail

Certified mail provides proof of mailing and delivery of the mail. The sender receives a mailing receipt when the item is mailed, and a receipt of delivery is kept at the recipient's post office. If the sender wishes, a proof-of-delivery return slip can be purchased. This service is available only for First-Class or Priority Mail. It does not carry insurance protection. This is appropriate to use if the physician is terminating services to a patient for some reason. A signed return receipt should be purchased to provide evidence to be placed in the discharged patient's chart.

Collect on Delivery (COD)

Collect on delivery (COD) is used when you wish to collect payment for merchandise and/or postage when the item is delivered. It can be used with First-Class, *registered*, Express, Priority, or Standard Mail. The receiver must have ordered the material. Fees include insurance coverage limited to $600.

Insurance

Insurance can be purchased for up to $5000 for regular Standard Mail and for mail sent at Priority or First-Class Mail rates. A *restricted* delivery, return *receipt*, or special handling service can be purchased for items insured over $50.

Registered Mail

Registered mail is the most secure option offered. It provides protection for valuables and important mail. Registered articles are placed under tight security from the point of mailing to the point of delivery. First-Class Mail or Priority Mail postage is required. Return receipt

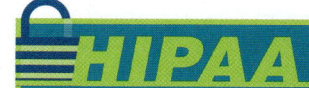

The restrictive delivery method of sending correspondence could work well to maintain compliance with HIPAA rules. It is always advisable to check the patient's chart to see whether there are restrictions for sending sensitive personal information. With restricted delivery, you would be certain only the patient receives the correspondence. For example, a wife could be assured her husband would not open a lab report that has an abnormal finding before she had a chance to read it. Or, if mail is sent to a place of business, a secretary would not open and read personal communication.

and restricted delivery is available. Insurance up to $25,000 can be purchased.

Restricted Delivery

Restricted delivery means that the mail is delivered only to a specific addressee or someone authorized to receive mail for the addressee. This can be used to be certain that only the patient receives specific communication, such as lab reports, a copy of a consultant examination, or any other personal material.

Return Receipt

Return receipt is the sender's proof of delivery. It can be purchased at the time of mailing for mail sent COD; Express Mail insured for more than $50; or registered, certified, or restricted mail. The receipt shows who signed for the item and the date it was delivered.

Other services are available should there be a need. Depending upon what you want to send, FedEx and UPS offer other alternatives.

If you have deposited mail and find you want it back, you will need to file a written application at the local post office, with an envelope addressed exactly as the one you wish returned. If the post office finds that the letter has left the local post office, the postmaster will telephone or telegraph the destination post office, at your expense, to have the letter returned to you.

If you have mail returned because the patient has moved and left no forwarding address, you can try contacting the patient's employer for a new address or talking with the individual who referred the patient. When a letter is returned after an attempt has been made to deliver it, you must prepare a new envelope and put on new postage before remailing it. A letter is sometimes returned because you have made an error, such as transposing numbers in an address.

ALTERNATIVE WAYS TO COMMUNICATE

There are many ways to receive and send information in today's technological society. Some common methods are fax, pager, cellular phone, voice mail, conference call, teleconferencing, e-mail, and the Internet.

Fax Machines

Facsimile (fax) machines (Figure 6-28) can be used by hospitals, physicians' offices, and clinics to send and receive information regarding patients over telephone lines. The machine makes it possible to send and receive letters, medical reports, laboratory reports, and insurance claims. Physicians may use the fax machine to send prescription orders to pharmacies. The office may also use it for ordering office or medical supplies.

A fax machine is connected to a telephone line. The machine scans a document and converts the image to *electronic* impulses that are **transmitted** over the telephone lines. The receiving fax machine converts the impulse to make an identical copy of the original. Fax machines may print on **thermally** treated or plain paper. The thermally treated paper eventually fades when exposed to sunlight; therefore, you would usually photocopy an important document onto bond paper.

The fax machine is available with many special features. Certainly a concern in the medical office is the transmission of confidential material. It is possible to have a secret code that will lock out unauthorized **polling**. The fax machine may also be able to store multiple documents in memory and have automatic dialing, with redialing when a busy signal is detected. The fax machine can be a *plain-paper* type using standard

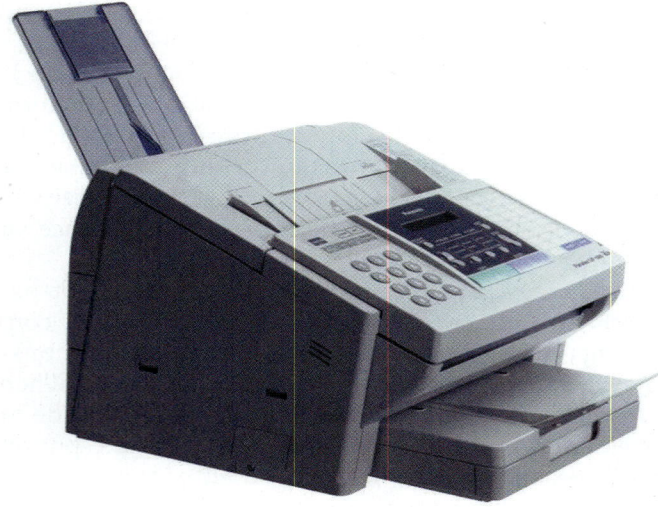

FIGURE 6-28 Fax machine *(Courtesy of Panasonic Document Imaging Co.)*

8½ × 11-inch copy paper or a type that uses a paper roll that is automatically cut to the length of each page of received message. If the recording paper runs out, the message is stored in memory and will be automatically printed out when new paper is loaded. A battery safeguards the document memory in case of power failure. The machine may be equipped with a white-line skip function that automatically skips over horizontal blank spaces on a document. This feature allows a standard document to be transmitted in as little as 12 seconds.

You will need to learn the specific procedure for operating the fax machine you will be using. However, there are general rules that are important to the use of any fax machine.

1. Always remove paper clips and staples from material to be scanned so you will not damage the fax machine.
2. Make a test copy if the document has color. Dark colors may block copy and can slow transmission.
3. Do not use correction tape or fluid on documents to be transmitted.
4. Do consider using typed words for numbers to avoid problems with interpretation.
5. If the material you are faxing is confidential, before sending it, call to alert the recipient to be watching for the material.
6. The first sheet of any transmission is called the fax page. It includes the date, name of recipient, recipient's address and fax number, and the number of pages being sent (including the fax page). The name and fax number of the sender will also be included. Any other special information required for routing instructions should be added.
7. Be familiar with error messages the fax machine may display and learn how to correct these problems. The machine may be equipped with built-in service diagnostic codes that can be automatically transmitted over telephone lines to a service provider. Most service calls can be resolved by telephone, therefore reducing costly equipment downtime and labor costs.
8. You may need to resend a message if noise or interference on the telephone line resulted in an unclear transmission.
9. Check to be sure the transmission is completed. The display will indicate that the message was sent, identifying the date and time of transmission. Remove the original from the machine.

 With all the emphasis on protection of patient personal information, sending of this type of information by fax should be carefully weighed against the use of other methods. An article published in *The Doctor's Office* discusses many of the things we

DON'T FAX YOUR WAY INTO A LAWSUIT

One of the cornerstones of the doctor/patient relationship is professional confidentiality. But quality care often depends on sharing patient information, swiftly and accurately, with other medical professionals.

About the fastest and most accurate way to transmit medical information is by fax. But faxed records can all too easily fall into the wrong person's hands.

In this lawsuit-driven age, all of us know why we must never fax confidential records, but in our convenience-driven culture, we also know that confidential records are being faxed every day, all across America. So the question becomes: How can we keep faxed records as confidential as mailed, messengered, or verbally-summarized-over-the-phone records?

The answer is to set up a Fax Security System, as follows:

Fax Security System

1. Make sure you have an Authorization To Release Records form, dated and signed by the patient or legal guardian, before you fax any information (just as you'd make sure you had a signed release if you wanted to send records any other way).
2. Never fax financial information. You can justify (in court) the faxing of medical information on the basis of medical necessity; but you cannot justify (anywhere) the faxing of financial data that the patient deems confidential.
3. Before you fax, ask yourself: "Is this really necessary? Or are we better off mailing or messengering these records?"
4. After you answer yourself, ask your office manager: "Will you sign an approval to fax these records? You will? I'll do it right away. You won't? Thanks for taking the decision off my back."
5. Only fax to telecopiers located in physician offices, nursing stations, or other secure areas. Do not fax to machines in mail rooms, office lobbies, or other open areas unless they are secured with passwords. When in doubt about the machine's exact location, "Hold your fax 'til you see the whites of their thermal paper."
6. Use a cover sheet that contains the warning: "The following material is strictly confidential; all persons are advised that they may be prosecuted under federal and state law for sharing this information with unauthorized individuals."
7. If your fax has a display showing the phone number being faxed to, make sure the displayed number corresponds to the number you want to fax to.
8. After faxing, call the faxee and confirm that the fax was received. If not, use your "recall" to find the last number dialed (your manual should show you how). Fax an urgent alert to that number and ask "all persons of goodwill to immediately and effectively destroy all documents received in the previous transmission."

Photocopy this Fax Security System and post it right above your fax machine. Make sure every staff member reads and understands it.

Oh? You say you can't be bothered with all this "security stuff"? That's all right; there's a much easier item to post for practices that aren't all that security-conscious: Your lawyer's telephone number.

FIGURE 6-29 Don't fax your way into a lawsuit. *(Copyright © 1994 The Doctor's Office. Reprinted with permission.)*

should consider before sending information by fax (Figure 6-29).

Pagers

Physicians commonly wear pagers so they can be contacted regardless of where they are or what they are involved in. A pager is a small electronic device that is activated by a telephone signal. When you wish to contact the physician, you simply dial the number. After it rings, a series of beeps will be heard, and you then enter the phone number from which you are calling. Meanwhile, the pager being worn by the physician will be activated and will produce a beeping sound or, if the sound is turned off, will vibrate to alert the wearer of a call. The phone number of the caller will be displayed in the pager's small viewing area, and the physician can go to a phone and make the call. Newer models have the ability to receive small messages, which print out on the pager viewing area. An additional feature provided by some paging services allows voice messages to be left, which can be retrieved by the receiver from any phone. Pagers are very beneficial and allow people to stay in contact even when they are not near a phone.

Voice Mail

Voice mail is another way to communicate. It is similar to a telephone answering machine, except voice mail can receive messages and place them in your "mailbox" even if your phone is busy. Basically, if you call and the individual is either not there to answer or is talking on the line, a recording comes on. The message is usually spoken by the individual and typically changes daily. It may tell you the date and explain where the person may be. It may also give you the individual's schedule for the next couple of days. It will then typically request that you leave a message. When the individual checks the phone, an audible cue, such as an intermittent dial tone, alerts the individual to a message in the voice mailbox, or the phone may be equipped with a message light. Another advantage of voice mail is that the sender, with the proper software, can record a message and then direct it to several mailboxes. This is especially helpful within a company or association to notify several people of an event or a meeting. These messages can also be retrieved from any phone by accessing the voice mailbox using a personal identification number.

Cellular Phones

The ease and portability of cellular phones make them another option for communication. As phone technology makes them smaller and lighter, they have become an easily carried device. Slim, pocket-sized phones and some slightly larger than a credit card are available. Of course their greatest advantage is the familiarity of use and the ability to give and receive information instantly. Perhaps their only disadvantage may be difficulty of reception within certain environments and within certain locations. The inconvenience of ringing at inappropriate times can be solved, for the most part, by adjustment of the ringer's volume or activation of the signaling mode. Technology has rapidly changed the cellular phone into a multitasking device that can photograph and send pictures, text message information, download and play music, and display television programming. Future capabilities will undoubtedly be developed.

Conference Calls

The telephone can be used to simultaneously conduct conversations with several people in various locations at the same time. This allows business to be conducted, meetings to occur, and professional or personal communication to be carried out. Conference calling saves time, travel, and money—all important in managing practice expenses. If your phone system is not equipped to allow multiple connections, conference calls may be arranged with your local phone service provider.

Teleconferencing

This means of exchanging information is like a conference call, except everyone can see and hear each other at the same time. All are linked together by way of telecommunications equipment. There are cameras, speaker phones, connection devices, and television monitors in each location. The phone company for the meeting originator will contact all other sites and network the phones together. With the aid of the phone, camera, and television, participants can see and talk to each other. A **teleconference** can involve several people in many different locations. Ideas can be presented, concerns expressed, and new techniques shown; teleconfer-

encing is the next best thing to actually being together in a meeting, yet it conserves travel time and expense.

Telemedicine

As early as January 1997, *The Harvard Health Letter* reported that an exciting long-distance medical care was happening and may become more routine. It enabled physicians to "see" patients at other sites miles away from the physician's home base or office. It involves the use of electronic stethoscopes, digitized x-ray transmissions, and interactive video to examine, diagnose, and treat patients. In Kansas, nurses who make home visits to chronically ill patients began using interactive video to enable them to "see" more people. The home-care agency sets up a camera and a 13-inch TV in a participant's home. The nurse sends a "buzzer" sound to alert the patient that the call will occur in two minutes. The patient sits in front of the camera and talks with the nurse as together they perform a series of tasks by using digital equipment attached to the TV. The electronic stethoscope is placed on the chest to check the patient's heart; a blood pressure cuff gets a reading; a finger stick and the blood sugar level is measured; and the finger oximeter measures the amount of oxygen in the blood. Patients seem to like the approach, and it has greatly boosted efficiency. When driving from patient to patient, only five people could be seen in a day; now the nurses are able to "see" three times as many patients.

Telemedicine enables primary care physicians to immediately consult with a faraway specialist while the patient is still in their office. For example, the cardiologist can listen to a patient's heart with the electronic stethoscope and assist the primary physician in diagnosing a murmur or irregularity. It has been adapted to permit "house calls" to people who find it physically difficult to visit care facilities or for those who live or are stranded by weather in remote areas. Health care reform may encourage this form of practice as a more efficient use of resources (e.g., skilled specialists). A California pilot program links physicians at Stanford University with patients at a nursing home, an urban clinic, and a multispecialty medical practice. This allows experts from the university to participate in the examination of high-risk or problem cases. Through the use of high-resolution computerized images, it is possible for the specialist to view a skin rash, a fetal ultrasound, or the retina of the eye. The capabilities are endless. By 1996, doctors at the New England Medical Center in Boston conducted about 1,500 consultations with regional and overseas patients—one as far away as South America.

A new technology being used by cardiac surgeons at The Ohio State University Hospital sounds like science fiction. With the use of computers, an operative console, and a robot, a surgeon is able to perform surgery through very small incisions in the chest. The surgeon sits at the console in an adjoining room and manipulates the hand controls. The computer translates the motions into a language the robot can understand. The robot's thin *arms and hands* are fitted with very small instruments and actually perform the surgery. One procedure that can be done in this fashion is a coronary bypass. The robot can harvest a vein from the inside of the chest wall and transplant it to the heart surface.

The most immediate advantage of this type of surgery is a great reduction in recovery time and patient discomfort, because the opening is very small compared with when the hands of the surgeon must actually get inside the chest. Often, these patients are not good operative risks, and reducing the invasiveness of the procedure is very beneficial. It has been suggested that, with the proper technical equipment in place, it would be possible to perform procedures at great distances from the surgeon through the use of communication technology. Someday a surgical specialist in the United States could perform a procedure in the outback of Australia while sitting at a console dressed in jeans and a sweatshirt.

There are some issues to be settled regarding these forms of medical practice. Items such as costs to initiate the technique and legal, ethical, and professional concerns need to be addressed. Some physicians see it as threatening since they would have to compete with many more physicians than just those in their local area. And, of course, there is the issue of malpractice liability. If the consult is out of state, whose state laws apply? Another factor is privacy when sending personal medical records through telecommunication systems. Congress passed legislation requiring federal health officials to develop specifications for a national computer network to enable doctors, hospitals, insurers, and others to transfer patient records electronically.

Another big question is medical licensure, since physicians are licensed only in the state in which they practice. Currently, 10 states are requiring that doctors who practice within their boundaries hold a state license, even if their presence is purely electronic. The AMA went on record recommending full licensure for each state except in emergencies and physician-to-physician consultation. Some states feel a limited telemedicine credential would be sufficient. Telemedicine physicians feel it is time for a national licensure to be established for physicians to solve the problem completely. This new form of medical practice will be interesting to watch develop.

E-Mail

E-mail, or "electronic mail," is possible with a computer, appropriate software, and the Internet. Before you can send or receive messages, you need to have an e-mail "address." E-mail can be exchanged within a company or clinic, or outside to anyone with a phone and an e-mail address. Electronic addresses have certain common characteristics. They begin with the person's name, some abbreviated form of it, or any other combination of words or numbers the individual desires. Next may come the name or abbreviation of a business or company when it is a business address. Then the "@" symbol follows, which denotes the beginning of the individual's server's address. The name of the Internet service provider (ISP) is next, which is then followed with a "dot" and an abbreviation such as "com," "org," "gov," or "net" to designate commerce, organization, government, or the Internet.

It is desirable to pay for the registration of your e-mail address to ensure no one else can choose the same one. A registered name is known as a *domain name* and usually needs to be renewed every year. To communicate by e-mail, you will need some form of communication software on your computer and an electronic service provider to connect your computer to the Internet. When you send a message, the software converts the typed words into standard digital language and sends it via the phone line to your e-mail server's computers. There the server checks the "domain name" (that part that follows the "@" in the address) and forwards the message over the Internet to the recipient's e-mail server. The recipient's server files the message until the recipient's computer checks for e-mail messages and then delivers the message to the computer. Once again, the digital message is translated back into words that can be read. This all occurs in a matter of a few seconds.

E-mail allows for the almost instant exchange of information without the costs associated with long-distance phone calls. In addition, the advantage of transmitting written material makes it appropriate for transferring reports, documents, correspondence, and all forms of written communication. Not only can material from one computer be sent to another, but material can also be scanned from other sources and sent over the Internet. When you receive communication, you can "open" your e-mail and read the information. If you wish to save it, it can be printed out or sent to your hard disk and stored.

The Internet/World Wide Web

This communication link allows you access to information from all over the world. It can be a great source of data from health organizations such as the American Cancer Society and the Centers for Disease Control and Prevention. Another capability through the Internet, which your physician may wish you to use, is the ability to schedule airline, hotel, and other services directly without going through various agents. Again, to access the "information superhighway," as the Internet is called, you will need a computer, the appropriate software, and a modem. If you learn how to identify what you are looking for, you probably can find it. All you have to do is give the ISP computer your subject matter. You enter the appropriate key words into a "search engine" such as Yahoo or Google. In return, you receive a listing from which you can select a more specific entry. When this is viewed, it may be further definable until you are able to pinpoint the topic you want. You can access a source's "home page" to obtain the source's general information. By identifying your topic more specifically, you can bring the appropriate information to your screen to view. You can read it there, produce a hard copy with your printer, or store it on your disk.

The Internet contains a wealth of information, but there can be serious problems associated with some online sources. Patients should be warned especially about going to web sites for medications. Some sites may be tempting with lower prices and the ability to obtain drugs upon request, often with a minimum of medical inquiry. Self-medication could cause serious problems from drug interactions with the prescribed medications ordered by the physician.

You need to take certain precautions when reading and evaluating web sites. Remember, there is no official agency that reviews or evaluates the information. The controls over legitimate sites come from the sponsoring organizations or governmental agencies. You may want to follow some simple web site guidelines such as:

1. Check the source. Are there links to professional affiliations or are there professional credentials?

2. Be cautious about personal testimonies from "users"; they often are just receiving monetary compensation for making statements.

3. Watch for dates of the information; the information may be very old and no longer valid.

4. Use your analytic skills to interpret *scientific* studies or reports. Who did the research? How many people were included in the study? Is the amount of time spent appropriate to arrive at the stated conclusions? Is there more than one study on the subject to give its results credibility?

As you become more familiar with technical reading and practice analyzing information, you will be able to make good decisions.

It is possible to enter, obtain, and exchange information, as well as conduct business transactions such as banking, all electronically. The amount of material available is mind boggling. It is possible to look at books, museums, association's publications, the world's encyclopedias, and on and on. However, there is some concern about the lack of security. With all the providers and information routing involved, interception of information is possible. Because of this and the nature of medical records and the need to provide for privacy of information, electronic communication may not be advisable in a medical office.

This new technology has made great changes in the way we access and exchange information. The storehouse of historical data is unbelievable; the ability to have instant connection with virtually every person, business, university, organization, and even government is possible. It is important that you learn to use new technologies. When things change, you must change with it or be left behind and unable to compete in the new workplace.

According to information released by the Pew Internet & American Life Project, in December 2004, 63% of the adults in the United States had Internet access. Use among adults older than 65 years represented only 22% of the total number, but that percentage had increased 44% during the four preceding years. At the other end of the adult age group, the 18 to 29 year olds, 77% are Internet users. The Computer Industry Almanac reported that in 1998 in the United States, there were 76.5 million people with access to the Internet, but that number was anticipated to grow to 207 million by 2005. Worldwide, 147 million users were reported in 1998, with a projected growth of 720 million by 2005. This form of communication is definitely becoming a preferred method of information exchange.

Computer Viruses

With the increased use and dependence on the Internet for communication and information gathering, you need to be aware of the very real threat that computer viruses pose. A virus is information that is sent electronically to interfere with or destroy your electronic files. There are standard methods of protection offered by employing firewalls and antivirus software (with the virus database kept up-to-date) to protect your computer while browsing and downloading files. You must be especially careful with respect to the use of e-mail. The following rules of thumb can help keep your computer virus-free:

1. Before opening an e-mail, look at the subject and who sent it. If you receive an e-mail from an unfamiliar source or with a suspicious subject (e.g., the subject is out of character with what you would expect to receive from the sender), do not open it! Delete and purge the suspicious e-mail immediately.

2. Never open an executable or script file (files with a "exe." or ".vbs" suffix) unless you are expecting to receive such a file from the sender. Opening these types of files is particularly dangerous because they can cause any number of actions, ranging from sending an e-mail to everyone in your address book to completely erasing the contents of your hard drive.

3. Use antivirus software to scan e-mails before opening them (either through your e-mail server or from your local mail application). Keep in mind that this is not entirely effective, because new viruses are being created and deployed continuously and may

not be detectable even if you have the most up-to-date virus database.

4. Last but not least, be aware that operating systems and the services and programs they run can be inherently open to attack. If you are computer-savvy, keep abreast of the latest patches and software upgrades that address security. Otherwise, consult with the administrator of your computer network to be sure you are protected.

ACHIEVE UNIT OBJECTIVES

- ☐ **Complete the Workbook activities to meet the learning objectives.**

- ☐ **Apply your knowledge at the end of this chapter in completing the Critical Thinking Challenge and Activities, as well as the StudyWARE on your Student CD-ROM.**

UNIT 5
OFFICE MANAGEMENT EQUIPMENT

OBJECTIVES

Upon completion of this unit, you will be able to achieve the following:

LEARNING Objectives

1. **Spell and define, using the glossary at the back of the text, all the Words to Know in this unit.**

2. **Explain why a calculator should be used when supplies are received.**

3. **List seven types of material that are often photocopied.**

4. **Give two reasons why records are microfilmed.**

5. **Explain when dictation on a tape should be saved.**

6. **Define all the computer terms listed in the unit.**

7. **List four items known as computer hardware.**

8. **Explain why the backing up of computer data is necessary.**

PERFORMANCE Objectives

1. **Total charges on a calculator.**

2. **Operate a copy machine.**

3. **Operate a transcriber.**

4. **Operate an office computer.**

WORDS TO KNOW

acronym	microfilming
calculator	photocopy
computer	software
dictation	technology
electronic	transcription
hardware	word processor

CERTIFICATION CONNECTION

CMA
Equipment operation
Computer components

RMA
Transcription and dictation
Computer applications

CMAS
Fundamentals of computing

The medical assistant may be responsible for the operation of many pieces of business equipment while performing administrative duties. A variety of office machines contribute to the efficiency of an office. Some are rather simple, whereas others can be quite complicated, requiring specialized training and practice to master. This unit identifies a variety of office equipment that could be found in a medical practice.

A variety of machines and equipment is required to manage the business operation of a medical office. Large multi-physician offices and clinics have more patients and employees and therefore require a greater number and larger capacity of equipment. Smaller offices and single-physician practices will likely have less-specialized equipment and will concentrate on the essentials, primarily because of costs and limited operating personnel. The following material discusses the types of common office management equipment found in a medical practice.

CALCULATOR

There are many occasions when an accurate calculation of figures is necessary. Some examples are:

- Determining total charges when preparing a patient's statement
- Submitting an insurance claim for services rendered
- Preparing bank deposits
- Reconciling a bank statement

The summation of the daily log of receipts and charges is easier and more accurate when calculating equipment is used. Of course, care must be taken to enter the figures accurately, or the results will be incorrect.

With the increasing use of office management software, manual totaling is less common. Performing the proper keystrokes will supply the total of charges and receipts on a daily, weekly, monthly, or even annual basis, as desired. However, once again the accuracy depends upon the correct entry of charge data and receipts.

A calculator can be very useful when checking shipments or deliveries from various office suppliers. Often not all items ordered are shipped, but you may have been charged for the total order. Also, there could be errors when ordering a quantity of the same item. Items are usually listed as a "per item" charge and then multiplied times the number ordered and/or shipped. A simple calculation with the calculator assures you have been charged correctly.

If the **calculator** produces a hard copy, the entries can be easily reviewed. If it displays the amount digitally in the display window, each entry can be viewed for accu-rate keying when entered, but it would be wise to also repeat the calculation to see if you get the same answer twice. A simple 10-key calculator with a few additional function keys is usually adequate for general office management (Figure 6-30). Calculators are powered by various sized batteries, electricity, or even light from the sun or a lightbulb. Some models can use either electricity or a battery. Printing calculators use a roll of narrow paper upon which the numbers are printed, similar to what you receive from the grocery store. Having a printed copy of your entries makes it possible to compare and recheck entries. It is much easier to find an error of omission or an inaccurate entry when you can see the figures. Perform Procedure 6-8 to total a list of charges on a calculator.

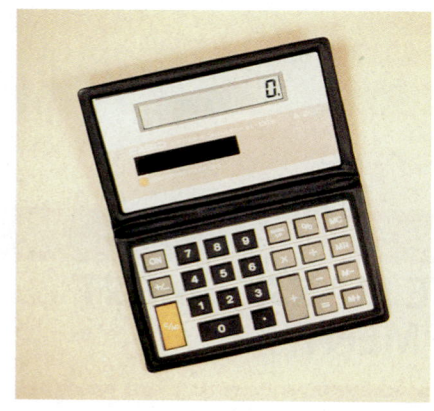

FIGURE 6-30 Ten-key calculator

PROCEDURE PROCEDURE PROCEDURE PROCEDURE PROCEDURE PROCEDURE PROCEDURE PROCEDURE

6-8 Total Charges on a Calculator

PURPOSE: To accurately total a list of numbers using a calculator.

EQUIPMENT: Calculator, a list of 20 charges to be calculated, and pen or pencil.

PERFORMANCE OBJECTIVE: Provided with necessary equipment and materials, calculate a list of 20 charges, performing any necessary mathematical functions, and correctly determine the total amount. The total must agree with the instructor's results.

1. Turn on the calculator.

2. Check the paper supply if it is a printing model.

3. Clear the machine. **RATIONALE: The digital display window or printed tape gives visual evidence that the machine is cleared.**

4. Perform the necessary mathematical functions and enter the figures to be calculated.

5. Total the entries and record the displayed total.

6. Double-check the tape or refigure on the digital display to be sure you get the same answer twice.

7. Record the total from the digital display or circle the total on the tape.

COPY MACHINE

The copy machine is extremely important to the efficiency of the office (Figure 6-31). A **photocopy** of correspondence, an insurance form, a patient's record, laboratory reports, or account information is often needed (Procedure 6-9). Most machines can be set to use either letter- or legal-sized paper. Frequently, prepared literature, information sheets, and initial information forms will require copying. Many machine models can produce color copies, which greatly enhances information materials. Some offices may use the copier for monthly billing. The accounting record is copied, folded, and inserted into an envelope and mailed, thereby eliminating preparation of a separate statement. Remember, the copier is not for your personal use. Generally, if the equipment is owned by the practice, you will be permitted to make a few copies if necessary. Some machines are leased and have attached counters that record the number of times the camera flashes making copies. Offices are charged a rate reflective of their usage. With this arrangement, use of the copier is restricted. NOTE: Care should be taken to avoid copying material that carries a copyright protec-

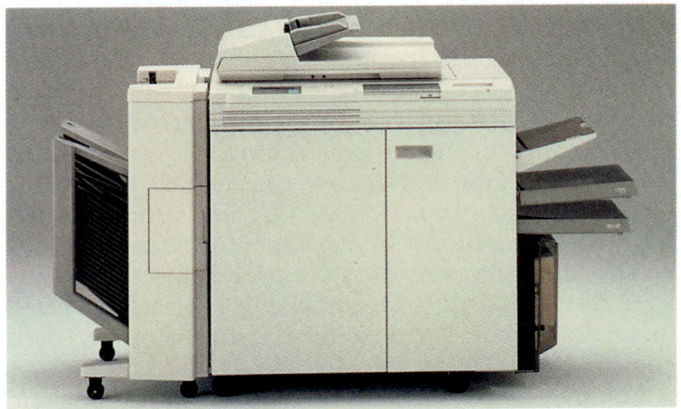

FIGURE 6-31   Photocopy machine

PROCEDURE PROCEDURE PROCEDURE PROCEDURE PROCEDURE PROCEDURE PROCEDURE PROCEDURE

6-9   Operate a Copy Machine

PURPOSE: To accurately prepare settings on a copy machine in order to produce a duplicate of the original in the size, number, and order desired.

EQUIPMENT: Copy machine, paper, and material to be copied.

PERFORMANCE OBJECTIVE: Given access to a copy machine and supplies, demonstrate adjustment of settings to produce the specified copy or copies following the steps in the procedure.

1. Assemble the material to be copied.
2. Determine the number of copies needed.
   RATIONALE:
   a. **You usually make one file copy of every letter you send. If copies are to be sent with the letter, you need additional copies.**
   b. **Two copies of most medical legal reports are needed.**
   c. **If you are making copies of instruction sheets for patients, copy enough for a month's use at one time.**
3. Turn on the copy machine. **NOTE: Some offices leave the machine on all day because it requires a warm-up period before it can be used. If this is not your office policy, turn the machine off when finished.**

4. Adjust the settings for what you want to copy.
   NOTE:
   a. **Legal- or letter-size paper**
   b. **Regular copy/lighter/darker (can be adjusted as needed to produce acceptable copy)**
   c. **Regular, reduced, or enlarged copy**
   d. **Number of copies**
5. Check the paper supply. **RATIONALE: Assure adequate supply. Some machines may jam when supply becomes too low. Also, check paper in the appropriate size supply tray. The last person using the copier may have used colored paper, a different size, or letterhead paper.**
6. Raise the lid and place the material to be copied, one sheet at a time, face down on the glass. **NOTE: On self-feeding models, place material on feeder tray. If there is more than one page, arrange them in proper order.**
7. Close the lid.
8. Press the button or key pad to activate the copier.
9. Remove the original(s) and copy/copies. Remove special paper, if used, from supply.
10. Return the machine to "standard" settings if you changed them.
11. Turn off the machine (if policy dictates).

tion, as this is considered illegal unless permission to copy is obtained from the writer or publisher.

Routine maintenance will improve the quality of copies made. Offices should have service arrangements with suppliers of equipment and copy materials. Service representatives can demonstrate cleaning of the glass, feed rollers, and surfaces and show you how to maintain the toner. Large copiers can be programmed to perform several functions such as enlarging or reducing copy size, stapling, sorting, off-set stacking, one- or two-sided copying, and insertion of cover sheets. You should ask for additional instruction before attempting to perform these functions. If you happen to cause a paper jam or in some way render the copier inoperable, it may be necessary to call the technician for service. This will invariably occur when some urgent materials need copied!

You may be assigned to provide routine cleaning and maintenance of the copier. Usually each morning the glass and rollers should be cleaned and the exterior wiped of dust or smudges. Pick up any discarded paper clips or staples that might get into the copier. The paper supply should be filled and the toner checked and replaced as needed. Depending on the model, some toner cartridges can be refilled by a service provider at reduced costs. Be sure to have at least one replacement cartridge in reserve, depending upon the amount of copying done in your office.

Newer models of office copy machines are capable of serving as printers and scanners and are connected directly to the office computer network. Instead of a document being sent to a printer and then using a copier to make copies, the printer is built into the copier, thereby eliminating one paper copy and one peripheral piece of equipment. A copy machine can produce copies at a much lower cost than a printer, and the features of speed, collating, off-set stacking, and others can be very time saving. Smaller combination machines have been in use in homes and small offices for several years. The all-in-one, printer, fax, scanner, and copy machine is attached to the computer and replaces four individual pieces of equipment.

MICROFILM

The medical assistant may need to be familiar with the microfilming process (Figure 6-32). Microfilming is a method of preserving material by reducing it to minute film images. **Microfilming** of office records can provide the necessary record security while using a minimum of storage space. The machine is easy to operate. Documents are placed on the scanner's feed tray. The machine automatically detects the size of the document and produces image data on the microfilm in the correct proportions. The film is contained on a reel that the machine automatically monitors to determine the amount of film remaining.

The digital microfilm scanner connected to the file printer (Figure 6-33) displays the image on the screen and converts film images to letter- or ledger-sized laser-quality printouts. With the appropriate interface board, the scanner can be connected to a computer that would allow the scanned images to be converted electronically over fax, e-mail, or the Internet or stored on disks.

Medical record archiving is changing with the increased use of electronic equipment. As more physicians move toward electronic health records and the paperless office, all information will be entered and stored in files on the computer. These electronic files will in turn be backed up and stored on large-capacity CDs, DVDs, or tapes. Physicians may utilize a combination of storage devices. Perhaps records beyond a certain age, 10 years for example, may already be placed on microfilm, while

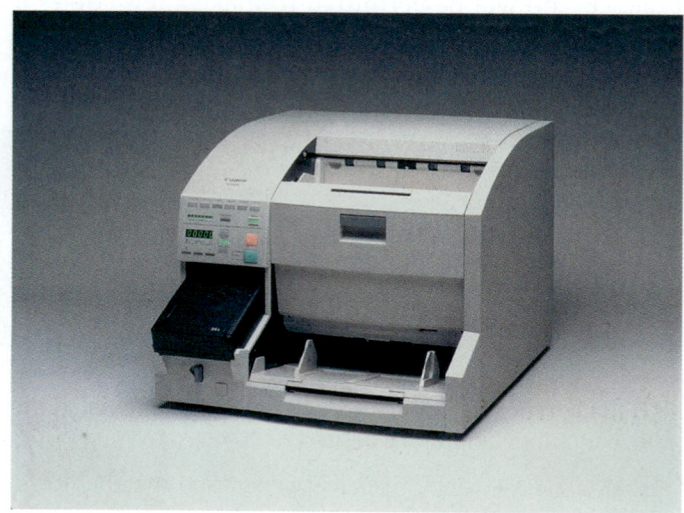

FIGURE 6-32 Microfilm machine *(Photo courtesy of CanonUSA, Inc.)*

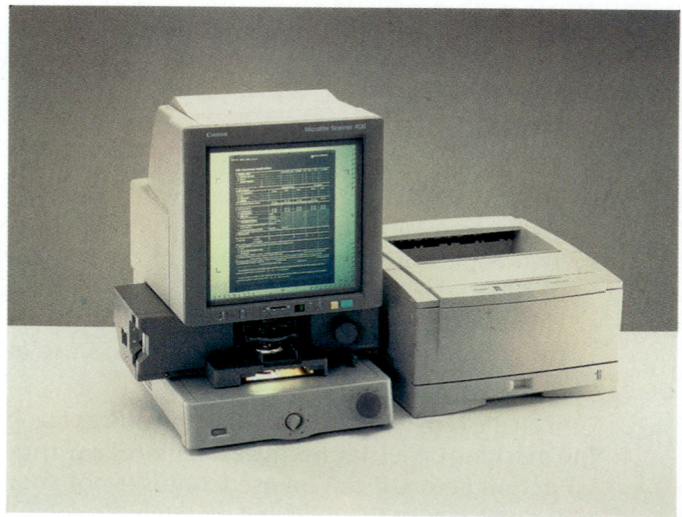

FIGURE 6-33 Microfilm reader-printer machine *(Photo courtesy of CanonUSA, Inc.)*

HIPAA

Maintaining PPI confidentiality, as required by HIPAA, can present a challenge to Medical practices establishing paperless office workflows. Confidentiality can be maintained by setting up network security so that only the appropriate users have access to these records. In addition, software applications are commercially available that make it easy for scanned documents to securely become part of an individual's personal records.

more recent records will be scanned onto electronic storage for easier access. The decision will depend upon time, ease of use, cost, and personal preference.

DICTATION-TRANSCRIPTION MACHINE

The most common forms of dictation-transcription equipment used in the physician's office are the desktop machines (Figure 6-34). Several kinds of machines are available: a unit for **dictation** only, a unit for **transcription** only, or a combination unit that can be used for both purposes. Many physicians use portable dictating equipment that can be operated by battery or electricity. The physician may use it in the office, in the car, at home, or while attending meetings. Some physicians will dictate their notes following each patient's appointment. When office hours are over, they will give you the tape so their observations, comments, and findings can be entered on the respective patient's EMR or chart.

The medical assistant can help the physician use the equipment more efficiently by tactfully dis-

cussing any problems encountered while transcribing. Tell the physician when the dictation is good. If you are experiencing difficulties due to dictation or mechanical reasons, explain precisely the problem and offer specific solutions. Sometimes a list of helpful hints to improve dictation and reduce the chance of error can be used to help the physician and therefore the transcriptionist. The list of suggestions might include the following:

1. Check the machine to be sure it is recording.
2. Indicate the date and what is being dictated (chart note, letter, research paper, report, and so on).
3. Remember that he is talking to a person through the machine.
4. Dictate the name of the patient and/or the name of the person or firm who will be the recipient of the message.
5. Dictate the street address, city, state, and zip code to which correspondence is to be sent and the number of copies needed.
6. Dictate punctuation such as "period," "comma," or "paragraph."
7. Refrain from eating, drinking, or listening to loud music or television while the dictation is being done.
8. Speak in a normal, clear voice.
9. End with an appropriate message to indicate the dictation is completed.

The dictation machine that is taken out of the office must be kept in operating order at all times—you never know when the physician will put it to use. When it is in the office, check to be certain it is ready for use. Replace the batteries as needed and maintain a supply of erased tapes for reuse.

When preparing to do transcription, keep in mind some helpful guidelines. If you know a certain transcription is a priority, do it first. It is also best to do the oldest dictation first so you can get caught up to date. Hopefully you can work where it is quiet and not be interrupted. Once you select the tape, insert it in the machine, and you are ready to begin.

The transcription machine is operated by using a foot control that starts the machine. When the pedal is released, the machine stops. It also has a backup pedal that allows you to relisten to the transcription if you need to hear it again before you transcribe. You will learn how to press the pedal, listen, and then begin typing the sentences with a minimum of time. With practice and speed, you may be able to type and listen almost simultaneously. The machine has controls for automatic rewind and fast forward. The speed control can be adjusted to either slow down or speed up the voice message. The speed control should generally be adjusted for the normal voice quality for the physician making the dictation. Refer to Procedure 6-10 to transcribe a dictated document.

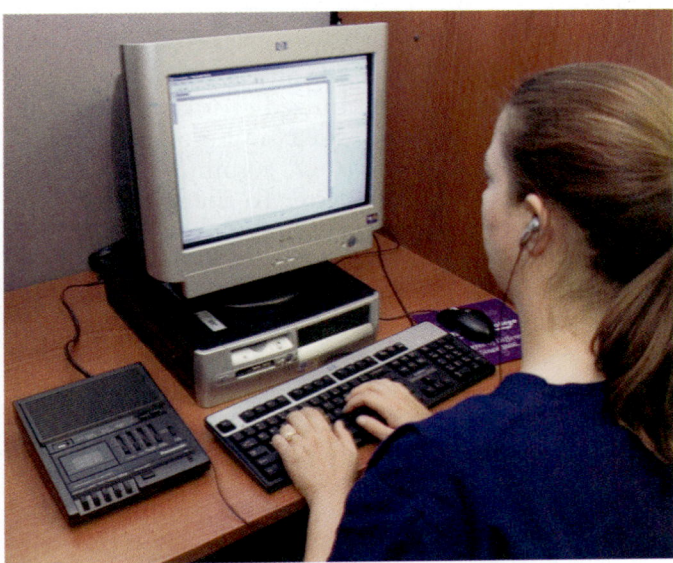

FIGURE 6-34 Dictation-transcription machine

6-10  Operate a Transcriber

PURPOSE: To operate a transcriber to produce a printed copy from recorded material.

EQUIPMENT: Transcriber, dictation tape, headset, foot control, computer, and paper.

PERFORMANCE OBJECTIVES: Given access to equipment and supplies, operate the transcriber, following all steps in the procedure to complete an accurate transcription within a specified time period.

1. Turn on the transcriber.
2. Verify that a headset with earphones and the foot control are attached to the unit.
3. Select a dictation tape. **RATIONALE: Type rush reports or oldest dictation first.**
4. Adjust the headset with earphones. **NOTE: Earphones should not be shared. RATIONALE: Prevents the spread of organisms.**
5. Insert the tape. Press the play tab or the pedal to listen for the beginning of the dictation.
6. Listen for the physician's instructions. **NOTE: The material to be typed will guide you in selecting the appropriate paper. It may be a chart note, a report, or a letter requiring letterhead paper.**
7. Adjust the volume, tone, and speed controls for clearest communication reception.
8. Bring up the word processing screen, and set margins and tabulator stops as needed.
9. Enter the recorded information.
10. Alternately press and release the foot pedal to listen and transcribe the recorded material. **NOTE: Consult a dictionary if a word is unfamiliar. If you are unable to understand a word or words, leave a blank, note the place on the tape, and ask someone else to listen. If necessary, ask the dictating physician for assistance so you can complete the work.**
11. Turn off the machine and place accessory items in their proper storage space.
12. Save the dictation tape. **RATIONALE: In case questions should arise before the physician will approve the report or sign the letter.**
13. Erase the tape following the approval of the material or physician's signature on the letter, so the tape can be used again.

Word Processing

The term word processing came into being with the development of electronic features for typewriters and the computer. First the typewriter was combined with electricity enabling the typist to increase typing speed as well as greatly reducing the amount of force necessary to strike the keys. It even returned the carriage automatically. Then a correction tape was added, which allowed you to back up to your mistake and then enter the correct letters. Some models would allow editing changes on the whole current line being written, which showed in a window, before it was actually typed when you advanced to the next line. A unique feature allowed you to insert different wheels of type styles called daisy wheels, so you could add variety to your work. Soon small screens were added so you could view your work before it was actually typed. These advanced machines were known as **word processors** and could store text on a small floppy disk and print copies from an add-on sheet or tractor feed paper supply.

With the innovation of computer language, instructions could be installed in a machine enabling it to do many functional operations, and the computer was born. In order for the computer "machine" with its built-in functions to work, instructional programs for producing text documents, bookkeeping, graphic designs, medical office operations, and a vast number of other applications, known as software, were developed. The computer has revolutionized the way information is produced, transmitted, used, and stored in today's world. The field of written communications has changed from the simple letter to the combined text and graphics of professional printers.

Word processing software is available for all computers (Figure 6-35). These programs provide almost limitless composition of written and graphic materials. You have the ability to select from a number of print font styles and sizes, which can be bolded, italicized, underlined, superscripted or subscripted, printed with shadows, and more. You can vary line spacing and margins and set columns, borders, bullets, and tabs. You can rearrange content by highlighting, cutting, and then pasting it in the new location. It is possible to insert page breaks, use auto shapes that allow you to add

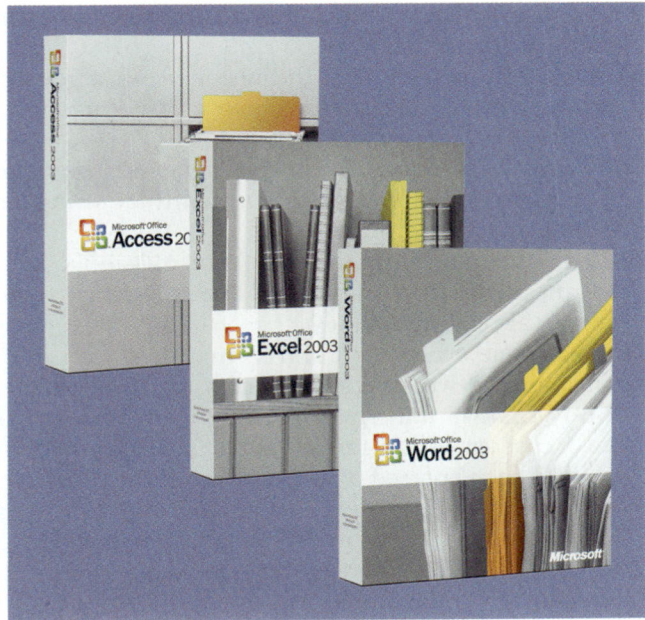

FIGURE 6-35   Word processing and other application software commonly used in medical offices

text boxes, draw lines, input clip art or content from files, draw and insert tables, and much more. With practice you can not only create quality standard correspondence but also outstanding reports, articles, and presentations for your employer.

The ability to view the document while it's being developed is very helpful. By selecting the print preview screen, you can visualize the whole finished product for page placement and balance before actually printing it. This is especially important before printing a letter on letterhead paper.

THE COMPUTER

In a text titled *Computer Fundamentals for an Information Age,* authors Shelly and Cashman define a computer as follows:

A **computer** is an **electronic** device, operating under the control of instructions stored in its own memory unit, which can accept and store data, perform mathematical and logical operations on that data without human intervention, and produce output from the processing.

Computers come in a variety of makes, styles, sizes, capacities, and price ranges. However, they all perform about the same way. Some can be carried like a small notebook; others are large, designated primary network machines. Many have the capacity to convey sound, and some are capable of responding to voice commands. A recent development is a wireless mouse and keyboard using "Blue Tooth Technology." It operates

by radio frequencies. Clicking the mouse or inputting from the keyboard transmits signals to receivers in the computer ports, thereby eliminating the need for cumbersome cables. In reality, you could sit across the room in an easy chair with the keyboard in your lap and operate your computer, provided the screen was large enough to be seen.

The computer has changed the way information is processed and stored. An individual with computer skills can be a valuable employee. With **technology** constantly changing, it is necessary to update and learn new applications almost continuously. It would be wise to take every opportunity possible to acquire additional skills.

Physicians are aware of the advantages of using computers in the office. The office can have direct-line insurance reporting by computer: the necessary information is entered into the office computer and travels to the insurance company computers. This eliminates paperwork, and the speed of processing claims is enhanced considerably. The insurance company, in turn, sends confirmation of payment back to the office and issues the check for payment.

Written communication is much more efficient with the use of computer software. Office management software can help eliminate human error in totaling charges and receipts while quickly providing financial status figures. Some physicians are going to electronic health records using computers to enter all patient information and office visit progress notes instead of writing on charts. Information now contained in file cabinet after file cabinet can be stored on high-density disks in a fraction of the space and can be called up with a few keystrokes. Maintaining the privacy of personal information stored in computers is addressed by HIPAA.

HIPAA

A system is to be established in an office to limit access to computer information in relation to the requirements of the job. Employees with computer access should have a password to safeguard the information. Even protecting the display on a monitor from being viewed by others is to be achieved by the positioning of a flat screen monitor or using a screen blocker.

The exchange of information over the Internet allows for almost instant communication. A physician requesting consultation can send patient information to a colleague and receive immediate feedback. All this information traveling through cyberspace has caused another problem of protection. HIPAA has directed that firewalls and encrypted data be used to prohibit unauthorized access to electronically transmitted data.

Computer Terms

With the development of the computer came a whole new vocabulary of technical terms, as well as new meanings for old words. In order to communicate with other users, it is important to understand and use computer language. The following are some of the most commonly used terms relating to the computer and its components. Become familiar with them quickly.

- **@**—the symbol that represents the word "at" that is used in e-mail addresses. It separates the user name from the name of the mail server.
- **attachment**—a file such as a letter or document that you send along with an e-mail message.
- **backup**—duplicate of data files made to protect information. Records should be backed up daily. Some experts recommend twice daily.
- **batch**—an accumulation of data to be processed.
- **boot**—to start up a computer.
- **bug**—an error in a program.
- **catalog**—a list of files on the storage media.
- **CD-ROM**—compact disk read-only memory. A type of optical disk capable of storing large amounts of data, typically 650–700 MB.
- **CPU**—central processing unit, or the "brain" of the system. The memory is made up of **bits.** A bit is a single **BI**nary digi**T.** *Binary* refers to a situation in which there are only two choices: for example, yes/no, on/off, pass/fail. *Digit* refers to a single number. A bit is either 0 or 1. A **byte** is the fundamental group of bits that a computer will treat as a word. A byte consists of 8 bits. A 16-bit processor is twice as fast as an 8-bit processor. One **K** (kilobyte) is equal to 1,024 bytes. A 64-K computer can handle 65,536 bytes. The greater the number of bytes, the greater the memory. Present-day computers will usually have 512 MB (one megabyte is one million bytes) of memory and a hard-drive storage capacity of 80 GB (one gigabyte is one billion bytes).
- **cursor**—a marker on the screen that shows where the next letter, number, or symbol will be placed (may be an underline dash or a blinking rectangle or square).
- **data**—information that can be processed or produced by a computer.
- **debugging**—finding errors and correcting them in computer programs.
- **disk**—a round plate on which data can be encoded. There are two basic types of disks: *magnetic disks* and *optical disks.*
- **disk drive**—the device used to get information on and off a disk.
- **domain**—a group of computers and devices on a network that are administered as a unit with common rules or procedures. Within the Internet, domains are defined by IP addresses. All devices sharing a common part of the IP address are said to be in the same domain.

- **dot-matrix printer**—printer that uses dots to form letters and numbers.
- **download**—to retrieve information from a source, such as a computer, the Internet, or an e-mail, and transfer it to another computer.
- **downtime**—a period of lost work time during which a computer is not operating or is malfunctioning because of machine failure.
- **electronic mail (e-mail)**—the transmission of letters, messages, or memos from one computer to another over telephone lines.
- **file**—a single, stored unit of information that is given a file name by which it can be accessed from storage.
- **floppy disk**—a flat, rigid, plastic square that looks like a coaster with a metal center. It stores content that has been entered into a computer. The disk permits taking information from one computer and transferring it to another. When the disk is inserted into the disk drive of another computer, the information can be transfered and used.
- **font**—a family or assortment of characters of a given size or style.
- **GB (gigabyte)**—approximately one billion (1,000,000,000) bytes (1,073,741,824 bytes to be more exact).
- **hard copy**—the readable paper copy or printout of information.
- **hardware**—the electronic, magnetic, and electromechanical equipment of a computer system (such as keyboard, disk drive, monitor, CPU, and printer).
- **home page**—the first page of a web site.
- **HTTP**—Hyper Text Transport Protocol; retrieves hypertext documents (web pages).
- **input**—data or commands entered into the computer.
- **interface**—the hardware and software that enable individual computers and components to interact.
- **Internet**—a global network that allows computers to connect to each other.
- **ISP**—Internet Service Provider, a company that provides users with Internet access.
- **K**—computer-shorthand for 1,024 bytes; a term used to measure computer memory capacity.
- **KB (kilobyte)**—about one thousand (1,000) bytes.
- **keyboard**—an input device resembling a typewriter keyboard that converts keystrokes into electrical signals that are displayed on the screen as words or symbols.
- **MB (megabyte)**—approximately one million (1,000,000) bytes (1,048,576 bytes to be more exact).
- **memory**—internal storage areas on the computer.
- **menu**—a display of available machine functions for selection by the operator.
- **microprocessor**—a silicon chip that contains a CPU.
- **modem (MO**dulator/**DEM**odulator)—a device or program that enables a computer to transmit data over telephone or cable lines.

- **monitor**—visual display unit with a screen called a cathode-ray tube (CRT) or flat panel LCD screen.
- **mouse**—a handheld computer input device, separate from a keyboard, used to control cursor position on a video display terminal (VDT).
- **output**—what the computer produces after recorded information is processed, revised, and printed out.
- **peripheral**—anything you plug into a computer; for example, a printer, disk drive, CRT terminal, or printer.
- **printer**—a device that produces hard copy. It may be dot-matrix, ink-jet, thermal, or laser.
- **program**—a set of instructions written in computer language.
- **prompting**—messages issued to a user requesting information necessary to continue processing.
- **RAM**—**acronym** for **R**andom **A**ccess **M**emory. This is a temporary, or volatile, memory. RAM is synonymous with main memory—the memory that is available for programs to use. When you turn off the computer, this memory is gone, unless it is saved.
- **ROM**—acronym for **R**ead **O**nly **M**emory. This is permanent special memory used to store programs to boot the computer or store diagnostics.
- **scanner**—a device that can read text or illustrations printed on paper and translate them into electronic files that can be stored, displayed on a screen, or used by other programs.
- **scrolling**—moving the cursor up, down, right, or left through information on a computer display to view information otherwise not visible.
- **search engine**—a program that searches documents for specified keywords and returns a list of the documents where the keywords were found.
- **security code**—user name and password. Used to prevent unauthorized access to data in a system.
- **server**—a computer or device on a network that manages network resources. Examples would be file servers (storage devices), print servers (manage one or more printers), network servers (manage network traffic), database servers (process database queries), and web servers (serve up web pages).
- **software**—computer programs necessary to direct the hardware of a computer system to perform specific tasks.
- **terminal**—in networking, a terminal is a personal computer or workstation connected to a mainframe. The personal computer usually runs terminal emulation software that makes the mainframe think it is like any other mainframe terminal.
- **URL**—the global address of documents and other resources on the World Wide Web.
- **Web browser**—software application used to locate and display web pages.
- **write-protect**—process or code that prevents overwriting of data or programs on a disk.

Input into a computer is by means of a keyboard very much like that on a typewriter. There are added keys to give you expanded capability. You do not need to be an expert on computer technology or programming to make good use of a computer.

When discussing computers, reference is made to hardware and software. The **hardware** refers to the hard disk drive, the CPU, the monitor, and the keyboard. **Software** is the programs containing instructions to the computer that enable it to perform tasks. You interact with the software to produce correspondence, maintain records, calculate financial statements, and perform many other tasks. Software is available on disks and is downloadable from the Internet to be installed onto the computer's hard drive. Software disks are available on floppy disk, CD-ROM (Figure 6-36A),

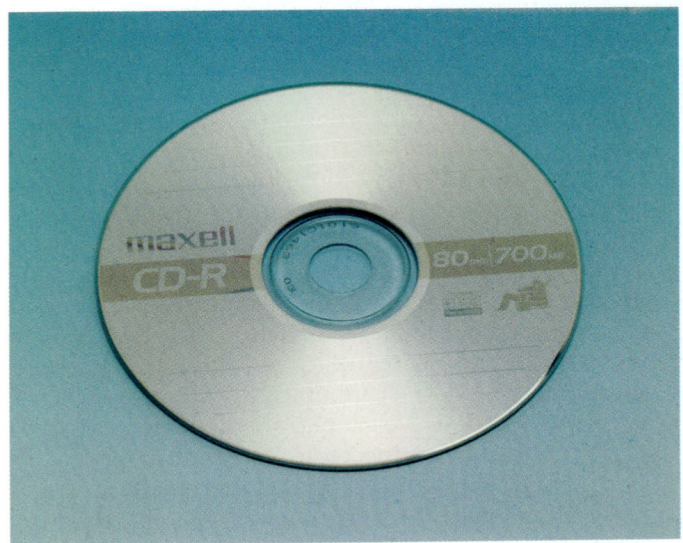

FIGURE 6-36A   CD-ROM

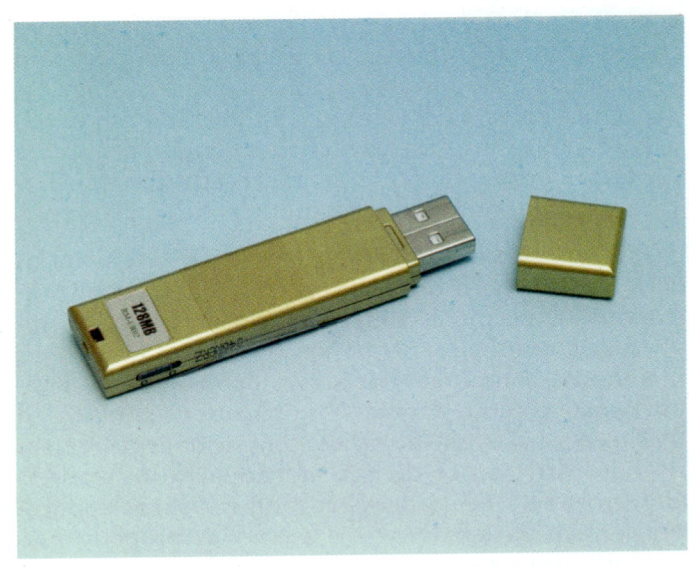

FIGURE 6-36B   USB flash drive

or DVD-ROM, depending on the size of the program. When you input data with a software program, the data resides in main memory until it is saved in a file on the hard drive or other storage device.

The information stored on a disk is called a *file*. It is necessary to assign a name to information to be saved so that it may be *called up* from the storage disk. Computer manufacturers usually provide basic software programs that are compatible with their hardware. A computer is useless without the software instructions for accessing and inputting data.

The main storage component for a computer is its hard drive, an oxide-coated metal platter that is sealed inside a housing to ensure dust-free operation. The hard drive can store enormous amounts of information, which can be retrieved almost immediately.

Various types and capacities of storage devices are available to supplement internal hard drive storage capacity. Examples are:

- **CD-R**—can be burned using computers that have a CD burner onto a recordable (CD-R) disk. Storage capacity is typically 640–700 MB.
- **CD-RW**—short for CD-ReWriteable disk. This type of disk enables you to write onto it in multiple sessions. Storage capacity is the same as CD-R.
- **DVD+R** and **DVD-R**—short for DVD Recordable disk. A DVD-R disk can only record data once, and then the data becomes permanent on the disc. Single-layer disks can store up to 4.7 GB of data, and dual-layer disks can store up to 8.5 GB of data.
- **external hard drive**—a peripheral (external) hard drive that can be connected to a computer via a USB port or Firewire (IEEE 1394). External hard drives are available with capacities up to 400 GB. External hard drives are useful for backing up or storing large amounts of data beyond the capacity of the computer's internal hard drive.
- **USB Flash Drives**—a small, portable flash memory card that plugs into a computer's USB port and functions as a portable hard drive with storage capacities up to 2 GB (Figure 6-36B). USB flash drives have less storage capacity than external hard drives but are extremely portable and useful for transferring data to or from any computer with a USB port.

PCs store their software programs as well as input data on their hard drive. In offices with several workstations or personal computers, the individual computers or terminals can be networked to a server or mainframe computer. The server or mainframe computer may contain databases, applications, and stored files to be shared in the office. This arrangement frees up hard drive space on the individual work stations and provides a centralized location for client applications, such as e-mail, to be served. A properly networked system permits input and updating of records from all stations and allows the information to be accessed from all stations.

Electrical surges and power outages can destroy information currently being used by the computer if it has not yet been saved by the operator or automatically by the program. This is most likely to occur during a severe storm. Loss of data due to electrical surges and power outages can be prevented by the installation of a protective device known as an Uninterrupted Power Supply (UPS), which contains a battery backup system. A UPS is capable of sensing a surge or outage and automatically switches to a backup battery to preserve the data. The size of the battery determines the length of time the equipment can be sustained. The primary purpose is to allow you time to save your document, exit the program, and shut down your system until the power is again stable.

It is very important to establish a "backup policy" to make copies of office programs and data. Often this is performed each night. Computer hard drives can "crash," causing the loss of all programs and stored data. Programs and extensive data can be copied by a tape backup device that is a peripheral to the computer, thereby providing a durable copy of information. All central computer data should be backed up on tape daily. Some offices may even contract to have materials backed up in an off-site facility in order to protect against loss of files from fire or natural disaster.

PRINTERS

To produce hard copy from computer files, you must have a printer. Three types of printers are appropriate for a medical office: dot-matrix, ink-jet, or laser. The dot-matrix produces print made up of pin-head dots and can produce "near letter quality" printing. Depending on the type of printer you have, you may set "draft mode," and the printer will print more than twice as fast as it will on letter quality. Printer speed is expressed in terms of the number of pages printed per minute. An ink-jet printer might print in three different modes. In draft, when less dots or less ink is used, the page can be printed faster. When printing in letter quality, when a professional looking finish is desired, all the dots or maximum ink coverage is used, and therefore the process is slowed. For example, the printer may print five pages a minute in draft, three pages a minute in "normal," and only one page a minute in best or letter-quality mode. The purpose of the draft setting is to conserve printer toner or ink when printing a large number of pages of a document that is not in its final stages.

The letter-quality printers may have many print styles built in, and more can be loaded into the printer. Ink-jet printers produce letter-quality copy by "spraying" letters onto the paper. A variety of type fonts allow great varia-

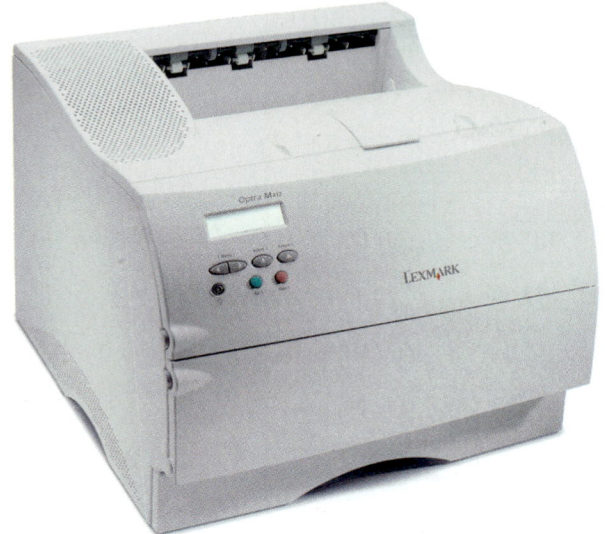

FIGURE 6-37   Laser printer *(Courtesy of Lexmark, Inc.)*

tion of print styles, and many interesting features can be added to your office's print communications.

Laser printers are more expensive, but the print quality is comparable to typeset material. A toner cartridge inside the printer contains the printer's powered "ink" material that produces the type or graphic images. The cartridge will last for approximately 5000 pages of text. The laser printer can also have postscript capability, which takes advantage of the high-resolution output capabilities of this type of device (Figure 6-37).

COMPUTER SOFTWARE

Computer software capabilities are virtually limitless. Software companies are continually designing programs that make it possible to direct a computer to produce different prescribed outcomes. It takes many months to research, write, and test a comprehensive software program. When the project is begun, the newest technology is used. By the time the project is completed and fully tested, the newest technology may be almost outdated. It is important to keep this in mind if you are in a position to recommend use of specific software.

Medical management software is available from many different companies. The software programs make it possible to keep patient information with no limit to the number of patients, except as limited by the capacity of the computer memory. It provides information needed for billing, such as primary and secondary insurance. It is easy to look up patient treatment or payment history, print patient mailing labels, find phone listings, or set up a recall/reminder system.

The procedure and diagnosis codes are built into the program. (Figure 6-38). The codes may be searched by number or by description.

The computer program allows for posting charges and payments. The program allows the medical assistant to input the necessary information and then push one key to print a completed insurance form. The information in the computer may be retrieved at any time.

Reports can be prepared with a minimum of effort when data is regularly put into the computer. Accounts receivable may be printed by date or age or alphabetically. Accounts receivable may be broken down between insurance company and patient. A detailed summary of income between two given dates may be easily prepared. The report of charges between any two dates may be accessed in detail or summary. A day sheet can be easily prepared. Physicians may find a need for a statistical report of diagnosis and procedure code usage, which can be retrieved from the stored data. Reports can also be sorted and output by individual patient, physician, or insurance company.

The patient entry screen provides for the entry of account information for each patient (Figure 6-39). All the data needed to properly bill the account is included.

The transactions entry screen is where all charge entries are done, including the entries for payments made at the time of service. During charge entry, a running total of the account is displayed at all times. When you have finished making entries for the patient, the account updates immediately. When you have finished your entries for each patient, you will be given the option of printing a patient statement. Prompt billing of patients means faster payment, and efficient, accurate submission of claims means a higher percentage of payment.

The medical office daily register report shows charges and receipts for daily records.

The utility menu screen gives you access to all the functions that let you set up and maintain the custom files to be used by the system, establish the format for your custom forms, and do the maintenance work to keep your system running efficiently. Once these files are established, the data in them is a keystroke away when the system is in use. See Chapter 8, Unit 4, on computer billing.

These illustrations of computer screens are only a sampling of the many office procedures possible with computers. It is important to note that many of the software manufacturers make programs that are compatible with more than one brand of computer.

Some believe that in the future it will be common practice to use a hand-held scanner (like those used in department stores) to scan the bar code on the patient charge slip and thus automatically enter the code number of the procedure or illness and the charge for service. This would eliminate the possibility of error in typing the figures into the computer.

The computer should be useful for inventory control of office supplies, to personalize form-letter mailings

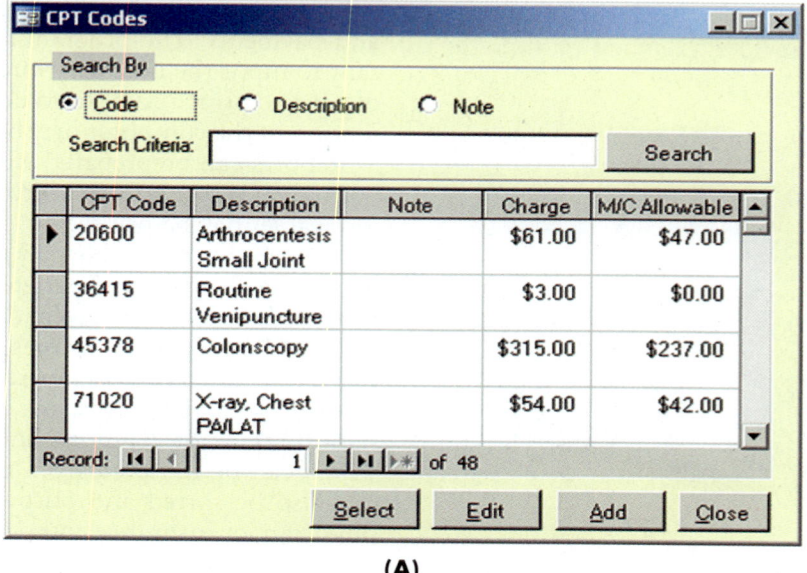

FIGURE 6-38 (A) CPT procedure codes and (B) ICD-9-CM diagnosis codes may be quickly called up alphabetically or numerically using medical practice management software. *(Current Procedural Terminology © 2005 American Medical Association. All rights reserved.)*

for collections, to reschedule annual checkups, and to gather research data.

Some physicians find the computer essential if they are engaged in research and need to quickly identify all patients with a specific diagnosis. It is also valuable in the quick identification of patients taking a particular drug if the manufacturer should issue a warning about side effects.

You may be involved in the use of a computer for patient education. This is similar to the television programs used by some offices. The medical assistant may load the programs into the computer, discuss with patients what they will see, and ascertain whether patients

have further concerns after they complete the viewing. Information programs have been developed for diabetes, cancer, pregnancy, health hazards of smoking, and many other subjects.

You have learned in this unit that using computers in medical offices can be extremely important in helping to complete your work. You should use any opportunity you have to practice with the computer. You should learn the vocabulary and how to read and understand an instruction manual. You need to practice on a typewriter if an extra computer is not available so that you will have accurate keyboarding skills.

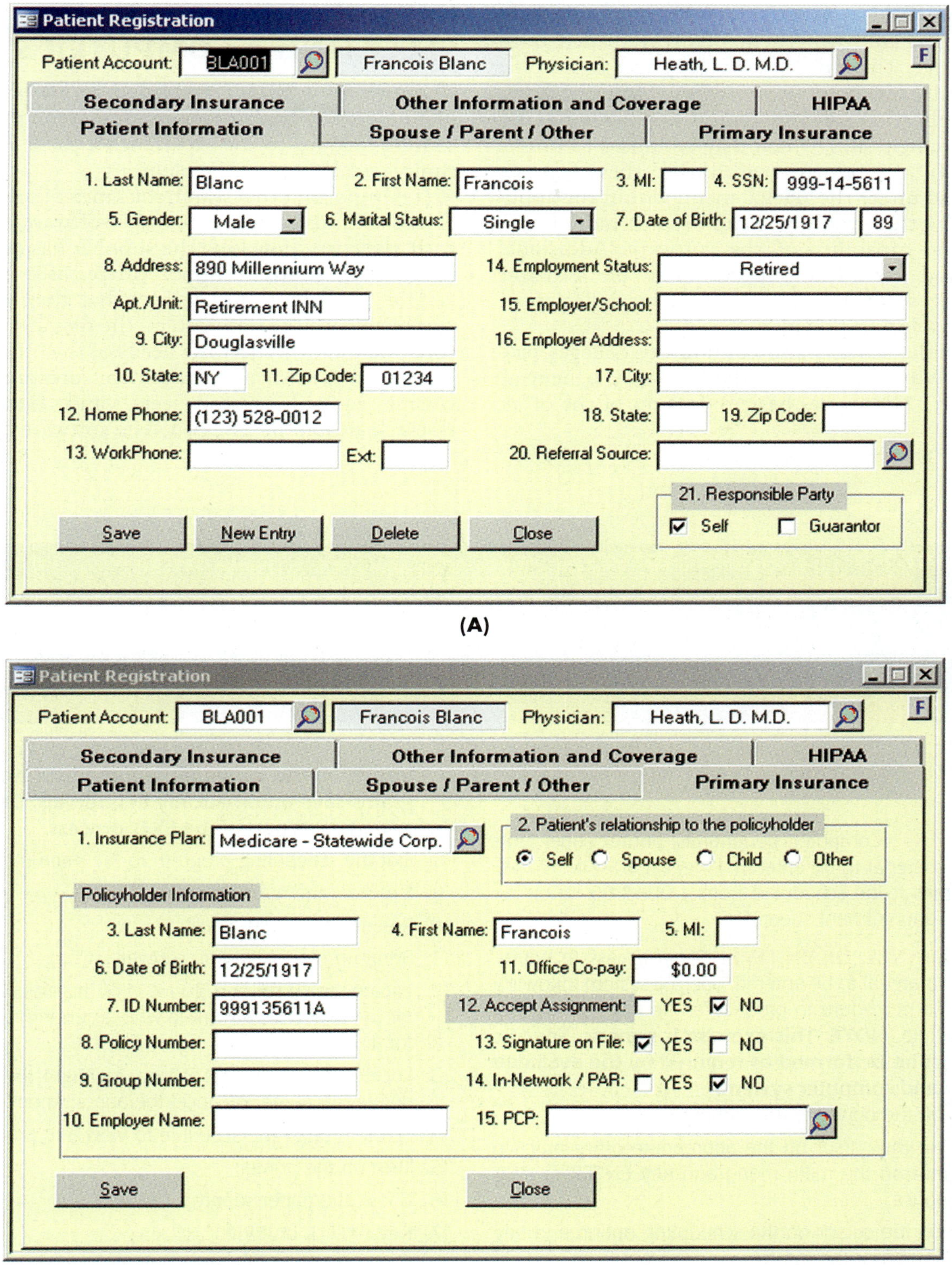

Patient Registration

Patient Account: BLA001 🔍   Francois Blanc   Physician: Heath, L. D. M.D. 🔍   **F**

| Secondary Insurance | Other Information and Coverage | HIPAA |
| Patient Information | Spouse / Parent / Other | Primary Insurance |

1. Last Name: Blanc   2. First Name: Francois   3. MI: [ ]   4. SSN: 999-14-5611

5. Gender: Male ▼   6. Marital Status: Single ▼   7. Date of Birth: 12/25/1917   89

8. Address: 890 Millennium Way   14. Employment Status: Retired ▼

Apt./Unit: Retirement INN   15. Employer/School: [ ]

9. City: Douglasville   16. Employer Address: [ ]

10. State: NY   11. Zip Code: 01234   17. City: [ ]

12. Home Phone: (123) 528-0012   18. State: [ ]   19. Zip Code: [ ]

13. WorkPhone: [ ]   Ext: [ ]   20. Referral Source: [ ] 🔍

21. Responsible Party
☑ Self   ☐ Guarantor

[Save]   [New Entry]   [Delete]   [Close]

(A)

Patient Registration

Patient Account: BLA001 🔍   Francois Blanc   Physician: Heath, L. D. M.D. 🔍   **F**

| Secondary Insurance | Other Information and Coverage | HIPAA |
| Patient Information | Spouse / Parent / Other | Primary Insurance |

1. Insurance Plan: Medicare - Statewide Corp. 🔍

2. Patient's relationship to the policyholder
● Self   ○ Spouse   ○ Child   ○ Other

Policyholder Information

3. Last Name: Blanc   4. First Name: Francois   5. MI: [ ]

6. Date of Birth: 12/25/1917   11. Office Co-pay: $0.00

7. ID Number: 999135611A   12. Accept Assignment: ☐ YES ☑ NO

8. Policy Number: [ ]   13. Signature on File: ☑ YES ☐ NO

9. Group Number: [ ]   14. In-Network / PAR: ☐ YES ☑ NO

10. Employer Name: [ ]   15. PCP: [ ] 🔍

[Save]   [Close]

(B)

FIGURE 6-39   The patient information screen contains areas to input (A) demographic information and (B) insurance information.

Most computer systems ship with electronic help files, tutorials, and owner's manuals preloaded onto the hard drive. These documents help you to become familiar with your computer hardware and operating system. Application software typically comes with CDs or electronic help files, which may be linked to online assistance. In a Windows environment, these features can be found under the "Help" menu within the application. Using these tools, you can become more familiar with the capability of the software. Additional training and technical support may be available through the software manufacturer, local dealer, or third-party solution provider.

Many public schools and community colleges provide adult education classes that are very beneficial. Procedure 6-11 discusses basic operation of the office computer.

IMPORTANT FACTORS IN SELECTING A COMPUTER SYSTEM

The medical assistant employed in an office that is planning to upgrade the computer system will be able to look forward to the experience if there is an opportunity to take part in the planning.

It is important to research the kinds of software available, the kinds of computers the software can be used with, the costs, how long the supplier has been in business, and the kinds of support offered after installation.

After the physicians decide what they want to accomplish with the new system, the first step is to select software that will meet the needs of the office. Applications such as medical management software, word processing, e-mail, spreadsheets, and databases for research should be assessed. The software can then be

---

PROCEDURE PROCEDURE PROCEDURE PROCEDURE PROCEDURE PROCEDURE PROCEDURE

6-11 Operate an Office Computer

PURPOSE: To operate a computer system to enter, revise, delete, and save data and print a hard copy of a document.

EQUIPMENT: Computer, peripherals, printer paper, and prepared material to be entered. (Suggest a list of 12 "patient" names to be scheduled from 1:00–3:00 PM on an electronic appointment sheet.)

PERFORMANCE OBJECTIVE: Given access to equipment and material to be entered, operate system following steps in the procedure to produce an accurate print copy of a schedule. **NOTE: This exercise is generic. Specific steps must be performed as required by the available software and computer system.**

1. Turn on the power to the computer.
2. Position the cursor on the appropriate office practice program on the main menu and key ENTER or click the mouse.
3. Position the cursor on the scheduling option and key ENTER or click the mouse.
4. Locate the cursor in or click on the first cell to be completed.
5. Enter a 1:00 PM appointment for the first patient on the list.
6. Enter the remaining names at 15-minute intervals.

7. SAVE the data. **NOTE: If input is not saved, it will be lost when the computer is turned off. Some programs save automatically at intervals. Others will save data as part of the EXIT process.**
8. Exit the scheduling program to the main menu.
9. Exit from the main menu.
10. Re-enter the main menu.
11. Bring up the scheduling software.
12. Locate the cursor at 2:30 PM, click the mouse, and enter the patient as a work-in who is currently scheduled for 1:30 PM.
13. Locate the cursor at 1:30 PM, highlight the cell, and delete the name to cancel the appointment.
14. Scroll through the schedule to view and proofread.
15. Turn on the printer.
16. Check the paper supply.
17. Key or click on PRINT.
18. Select from the available options (current page, number of copies).
19. Print the document.
20. Exit the program.
21. Exit the main menu and the system.
22. Turn off the power to the printer and the computer according to office policy.

matched with compatible computer hardware. Items to consider are:

- Operating system
- Hard drive capacity
- Memory requirements
- Processor speed
- Networking requirements

There are hidden costs to consider. Maintenance agreements for hardware and software should be reviewed and the costs weighed against the services provided. Technical support (online or by phone), accidental damage coverage, on-site service, and software updates should be evaluated. Review existing office insurance policies to determine whether they are adequate to cover the cost of the computer system. If not, determine the cost of additional insurance to cover loss due to theft, fire or flood damage, and natural disasters. Costs to train the office staff on the new applications should also be determined.

When considering a major software purchase (such as Medical Management Software), companies should refer you to current users to help determine the reliability and usability of the software. It is always important to obtain cost estimates from at least three companies.

The appropriate software matched with an efficient computer makes for an effective system to meet the current and future needs of the practice.

ACHIEVE UNIT OBJECTIVES

- Complete the Workbook activities to meet the learning objectives.
- Practice the procedures in this unit to meet the performance objectives.
- Apply your knowledge at the end of this chapter in completing the Critical Thinking Challenge and Activities, as well as the StudyWARE on your Student CD-ROM.

CRITICAL THINKING CHALLENGE

IMPACTING THE PATIENT, THE PRACTICE, AND YOUR CAREER

Jane is the administrative medical assistant who does the office correspondence. The physician had recently dictated some follow-up information to six patients regarding their lab findings following their office visits. As was his practice, he had indicated to her that a copy of the lab reports should be mailed with the short letters. A few days after Jane had completed the letters she received a phone call from one of the patients, Mrs. Turner. It seems Jane had accidentally mixed up the lab reports, and Mrs. Turner had received another patient's reports. She was quite upset primarily because she didn't know who had received her very personal lab findings. Mrs. Turner talked with Jane and asked her how this could have happened. She felt her privacy had been violated. She demanded Jane immediately contact the other patients and retrieve her copy of the lab report.

QUESTIONS

1. How does Jane's error affect the patient?
2. How could the HIPAA rules affect the practice?
3. How can the error affect Jane's employment?

ACTIVITIES

1. Suppose your employer is going to move the office to a new location. There have been notices posted in the office and printed handouts to alert those patients who have been in. However, the physician feels that all the patients should receive a written notice, since some have not been in lately. You have been given the task of preparing a letter containing the necessary information: the date of the move, new address and phone number, directions, and an appropriate statement concerning the change.

2. After you have prepared the notice, you are to decide which would be the best way to address all the letters: either directly on the envelope or onto mailing labels and then onto the envelopes.

3. Inquire at the post office about bulk mailing costs and the process. Based upon 2,500 pieces of mail, determine the amount that could be saved with the office preparing the mailing.

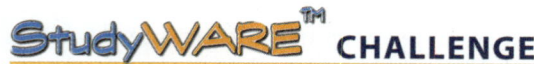 **CHALLENGE**

- Study with the flash cards for Chapter 6 to review the key terms in this chapter.
- Solve the crossword puzzle for Chapter 6.
- Complete the multiple choice quiz in test mode for Chapter 6.

RESOURCES

Battenberg, E. (2001, February 26). *Traffic control: Taking the mystery out of e-mail.* Columbus, OH: The Columbus Dispatch Co.

Lindh, W., Pooler, M., Tamparo, C., & Dahl, B. (2006). *Thomson Delmar Learning's comprehensive medical assisting: Administrative and clinical competencies* (3rd ed.). Clifton Park, NY: Thomson Delmar Learning.

Steinbacher, R. (2000). *Computer Friendly.* Erie, PA: Green Tree Press, Inc.

United States Postal Service. (1995). *Addressing for success.* Washington, DC: Author.

United States Postal Service. (1998, March). *Consumer's guide to postal services and products.* Washington, DC: Author.

United States Postal Service. (2001, January). *Quick service guide.* Washington, DC: Author.

WEB LINKS

www.cc.nih.gov/ccc/ceg/info.html (Confidentiality Education Group [CEG])
  This web site provides guidelines for faxing and e-mailing medical information.

www.usps.com (United States Postal Service)
  This web site provides postal information.

www.webopedia.com (Webopedia)
  An online computer terminology dictionary

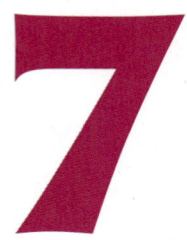

CHAPTER 7

Facility and Records Management

The medical assistant is often the first person into the medical office each day. Some of the responsibilities included with facility management are opening and closing the office, having patients' charts pulled and ready for the day, ensuring the waiting area is straightened, preparing charge slips either on paper or electronically, and organizing new patient data to establish the chart.

Medical records consist of a complete and detailed patient information form, health history, physical examination, diagnostic reports, and treatment notes that allow the physician to provide necessary care for patients. The records must be accurate, complete, and filed so that they may be quickly found when needed.

HIPAA mandates the confidentiality of the records must be maintained by careful management as they are used. Efficiency is essential to a well-run medical facility. Filing needs to be current at all times.

UNIT 1
PREPARING FOR THE DAY

OBJECTIVES

Upon completion of this unit, you will be able to achieve the following:

LEARNING Objectives

1. Spell and define, using the glossary at the back of the text, all the Words to Know in this unit.

2. List five things to check in a reception room environment.

3. List four tasks to do before opening the office, in addition to the reception room check.

4. Explain why the receptionist is an important position.

5. List at least five responsibilities of the receptionist.

6. Identify five pieces of information found on a completed charge slip.

7. List four things you will find inside a new patient's chart folder.

8. List two reasons to use a "checklist."

PERFORMANCE Objectives

1. Open the office.
2. Obtain new patient information.
3. Close the office.

WORDS TO KNOW

appointment	communication	intervention
atmosphere	confidentiality	receptionist
brochure	environment	schedule

CERTIFICATION CONNECTION

CMA
Maintaining the physical plant
• Office environment

RMA
Medical receptionist/ secretarial/clerical
• Reception

CMAS
Reception

PREPARING FOR THE DAY

There is no set list of things to do in order to prepare for the day. Preparation procedures vary according to the type of practice, number of physicians, weekly schedules, and many other variables. Some doctors may not see patients every day. Surgeons frequently reserve a day or two a week for surgery and have office hours on the other days. Physicians who are affiliated with university schools of medicine will teach and work with medical students and may see personal patients only one or two days a week. The following content discusses general things that need to be considered when preparing to receive patients in the office.

Opening the Office

The staff should arrive at the office in time to make preparations for receiving patients. If adequate time is not available, it seems like you can never get organized or "caught up." There are several things that need attention before the first patient arrives. Procedure 7-1 addresses many of these tasks.

1. *Unlock the reception room door.* This refers to the door to the outside hallway or building exterior. The door between the reception room and the interior of the office should probably be locked from the reception room side for safety reasons. Be certain that the lock is set on the outside door so that it does not relock itself when it is closed. Check any open/closed sign for proper reading.

2. *Observe the physical environment of the reception room.* Studies have shown that the reception room **atmosphere** can be an **intervention**, or, in other words, a "go between" or mediation to the outcome of the office visit. Atmosphere affects how people experience their environment and may have a relationship to their response to treatment:

   • *Check the temperature.* The room temperature should ensure the patient's comfort.
   • *Look at the room's appearance.* The room should appear pleasant and well maintained. The arrangement of chairs can "say" secluded or sociable, which affects **communication** in the room. The presence of large plants and attractive paintings soften the office **environment**. The choice of color and lighting affects behavior. Soft colors and subdued light tend to calm the hostile person. The use of relaxing background music has become commonplace in medical and dental offices. Aquariums can provide diversion and have an enjoyable bubbling sound. Try standing in the reception

PROCEDURE PROCEDURE PROCEDURE PROCEDURE PROCEDURE PROCEDURE PROCEDURE

7-1　　Open the Office

PURPOSE: To prepare the office to see patients.

MATERIALS: A simulated office, if available; otherwise, role-play, explaining the procedure.

PERFORMANCE OBJECTIVE: Following all the steps in the procedure, role-play the actions necessary to prepare a medical office to see patients. Actions must be verbally described while performing.

1. Unlock the reception room door.
2. Adjust heat or air-conditioning for the comfort of the patients.
3. Check for safety hazards in the office. **NOTE: Check for frayed electric wires, damaged furniture, or objects on the carpet that might cause patients to fall.**
4. Check magazines for condition and date. **NOTE: Be sure magazines are current. Torn or damaged magazines should be removed from the waiting room.**
5. Check the telephone answering device or call the answering service for any messages.
6. Pull the charts of patients to be seen. **NOTE: Write or stamp with today's date. Check the patient's previous visit to see whether any studies were ordered. RATIONALE: Results must be filed in the chart before the patient is seen.**
7. Check examination rooms to be sure they are clean and stocked with supplies. **NOTE: This is necessary in case the physician saw a patient after office hours and did not put things away.**
8. Fill and turn on sterilizer.
9. Prepare hazardous waste disposal containers.
10. If it is the policy of the office, prepare a list of the patients to be seen and the times of their appointments and place copies in designated areas.

room and looking around. Be conscious of the sights, sounds, and even smells you perceive.

- *Perform a safety check.* Remember to make a daily visual check of electrical devices, furniture, floors, and lighting before any patients arrive. Care should be taken to make the whole office "accident-proof." An incident in the office can result in a patient filing a suit for alleged pain and injury. If anyone should be injured, no matter how insignificant it may seem, the medical assistant must have the individual examined by the physician. If the patient should claim they were not injured and refuse examination, the incident must still be carefully recorded on their chart and the refusal of care noted. Some physicians may require a signed release of responsibility in order to protect against a later claim of injury.

- *Check the reading material.* Neatly arrange magazines. Make them accessible in several seating areas. Remove torn and very outdated material. Encourage the physician(s) to subscribe to a variety of reading materials appropriate to both males and females of all ages. Many physicians have a prepared **brochure** that describes their practice, discusses the office policies, and provides information regarding appointments, office hours, and other useful details. An as-

sortment of informative health-related pamphlets may also be found in a display rack (Figure 7-1). Copies of professional medical journals or similar technical material is not appropriate for general display.

- *Check the toys and books.* If children's toys or books are provided, they require constant monitoring. All toys should be washable and of a safe design and material with no sharp edges or parts small enough for a child to swallow. The toys should be cleaned regularly. During daily inspection, remove any broken or visibly soiled toys or books. If at all possible, the children's play area should be situated in a corner or within a half-walled space to contain things within a controlled area to reduce the possibility of adults falling over objects on the floor. In some offices, it may be necessary for the medical assistant to keep children entertained while adults are being examined (Figure 7-2). In pediatricians' offices, there are usually two reception rooms, or at least a room with a separate section, each with its own play area. One is considered the well area, while the other is the "sick" area. This allows for the separation of children with fevers, coughs, nausea and vomiting, diarrhea, and other disease conditions from the well children.

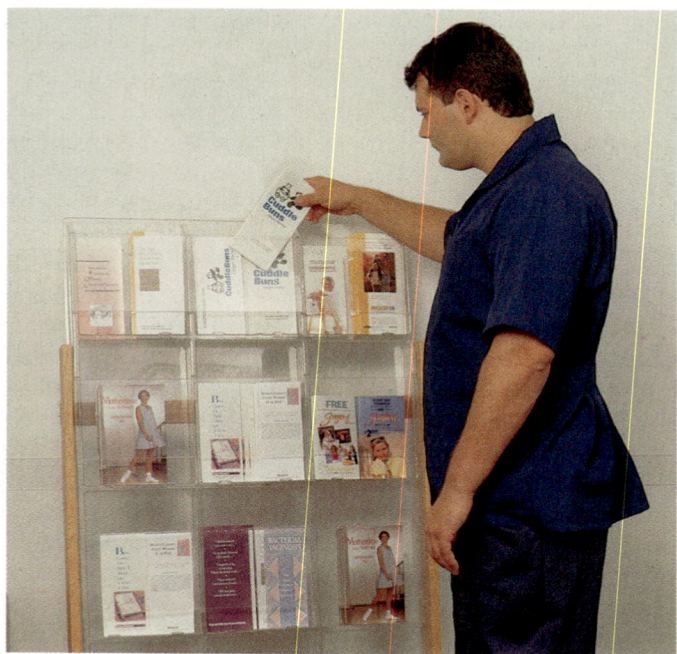

FIGURE 7-1 Office practice brochures and other handouts should be accessible to patients and visitors.

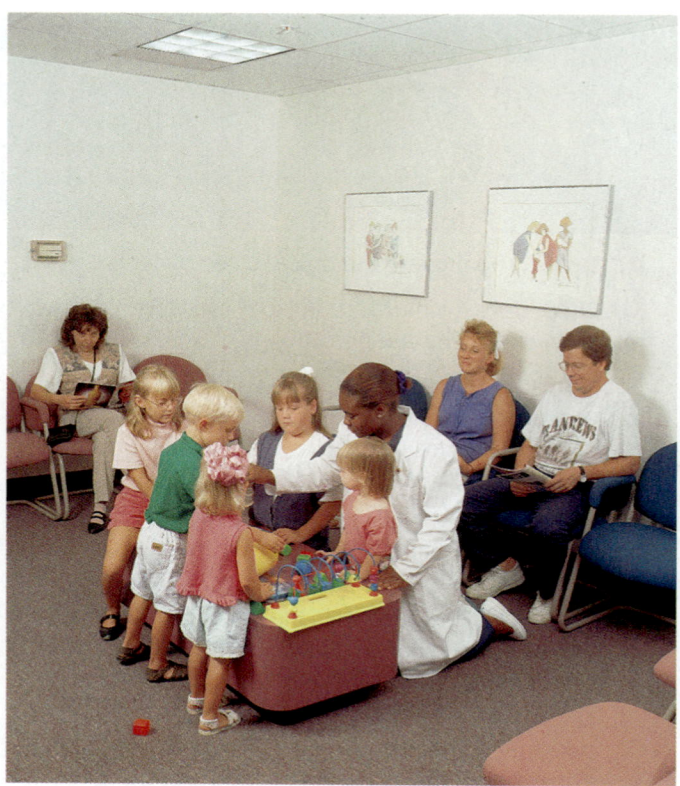

FIGURE 7-2 The medical assistant may need to entertain children while parents are in the examination room or physician's office.

- *Display the smoking policy.* In view of regulations against the use of smoking materials in public areas and the overwhelming evidence of the effects of secondhand smoke, a medical office probably does not permit smoking. Be certain the "No Smoking" sign is displayed and that it is enforced. There should be no ashtrays accessible.

3. *Retrieve telephone messages.* Retrieve and record all messages on the answering machine. If an outside service is used, call and obtain the messages.

4. *Pull charts.* Look at the appointment book or run a hard copy from the computer of all patients who have appointments that day. Pull the charts of previously seen patients. Be certain to attach reports of any previously ordered studies to the chart. Have materials ready for initiating charts for scheduled new patients. This process can often be done the night before to reduce morning preparation duties. Many offices like to post a copy of the day's **schedule** in a common area for reference. Some physicians want a list of patients and appointment times on their desk for their personal use.

5. *Inspect examination rooms.* Visually inspect all rooms for cleanliness. Even if they were cleaned when closed the previous office day, the physician may have seen a patient after hours. Replace examining paper and be certain waste receptacles are emptied. Observe room temperature and plug in any discon-

nected electrical equipment. Be certain everything is in working condition. Restock supplies so that needed materials are available.

6. *Check common work areas.* Check for cleanliness and be certain everything is in order. Check the water level in the autoclave and turn it on. Be sure hazardous waste disposal containers are available for use in all areas where needed.

THE RECEPTIONIST

The medical assistant may fulfill the role of the **receptionist**, whose responsibility it is to greet and receive patients. This is a very significant role. The receptionist is usually the first person a patient encounters in the office. It is extremely important that this initial experience be very positive:

- Greet patients promptly and courteously (Figure 7-3).
- Maintain eye contact when talking to patients.
- Call patients by their full names.
- Actively listen to patient remarks and show that you care about their concerns.
- Explain patient instructions thoroughly.

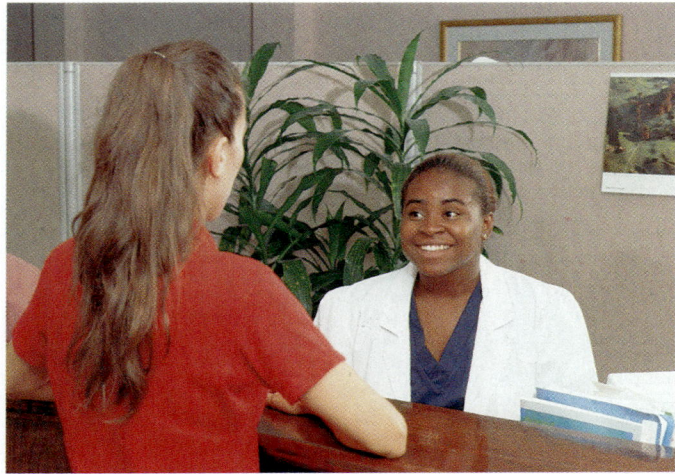

FIGURE 7-3   The receptionist should greet each patient with a warm and friendly smile.

- Do not question or discuss personal matters with patients in the reception room.
- Respect the patient's right to **confidentiality**.

The receptionist is usually charged with answering the phone, making routine calls, and scheduling **appointments**. This responsibility requires an understanding of common diseases and disorders and the basic office operational procedures. It often demands tactful dealings with patients. The receptionist must determine when to enlist the assistance of other professionals in dealing with patients' concerns and requests.

The receptionist should be positioned within the office in such a way as to have a clear view of the reception room. If the space is behind a wall with a glass window partition, the reception room may not be easily seen. The area must be observed frequently to monitor the activity and to check for new arrivals who may fail to come to the window. A separated physical arrangement does have the advantage of providing privacy for engaging in telephone conversations, talking with patients, or performing duties.

It is important to monitor the social climate of the reception area. Be alert to any behavior that may cause an unfavorable impression of the office. Remember: People are affected by their environment.

Be especially alert if a very ill patient enters the office. The ill patient should not have to sit and wait in a reception room. As soon as possible, assist the patient into an examination room where the patient can be made comfortable until the physician can see him or her. Remember to ensure the patient's safety. Warn the patient (and advise any companions) to be careful while lying on the narrow examination table.

Charge Slips

The receptionist may also be given the responsibility of preparing the charge slip that accompanies the patient's chart. This form is often called the encounter form. Medical offices usually have a slip that lists the procedures, with the respective codes, that are performed in the office. The charge slip has a space for the patient's name and date and may request additional information. Some large clinics prepare "charge cards" that are used to stamp the patient's name and account number on the charge slip. When the physician completes the examination or treatment, the charges are entered on the slip, and it is given to the patient with instructions to take it to a designated person on the way out of the office (Figure 7-4).

Forms will vary from one type of practice to another. Where computers are used, the form will be designed to be compatible with the software program being used.

New Patients

The receptionist is usually responsible for the completion of the new patient information form (Figure 7-5). If this is to be done in an interview format, be sure that others cannot overhear the questioning process. Usually, a new patient is given the form and a clipboard and requested to complete the information. A pen or pencil should be provided. It is important to give clear instructions and ask if there are any questions. Be observant. If the patient seems reluctant to accept the form, appears confused, or is not making progress, it may indicate a reading problem. Quickly offer to assist. Check to be sure this form is complete and signed by the responsible party.

At this time, it is normally routine to request insurance cards from the patient so that they may be copied, on both sides, for the necessary billing information. If necessary, verification of coverage can be obtained by phoning the insurance company. The copy of the card and the preliminary form are placed in a folder along with chart sheets and any other referral materials received. If the filing method is numeric, the patient's name or number is typed onto a label, which is attached to the tab of the folder. Refer to Chapter 7, Unit 3, for more information regarding filing procedures.

Before the patient is seen, the charge slip is completed and attached to the chart. The chart is then placed in a designated area until the patient is taken to an examination room. Then it is placed in a holder outside the room, ready for the physician when the patient is seen. Procedure 7-2 discusses the steps in obtaining new patient information.

PLEASE RETURN THIS FORM TO RECEPTIONIST

NAME _____

2330

PLACE OF SERVICE:
( ) OFFICE
( ) NEW YORK COUNTY HOSPITAL
( ) COMMUNITY GENERAL HOSPITAL
( ) RETIREMENT INN NURSING HOME
( ) _____

DATE OF SERVICE _____

A. OFFICE VISITS - New Patient

Code	History	Exam	Dec.	Time	
___ 99201	Prob. Foc.	Prob. Foc.	Straight	10 min.	_____
___ 99202	Ex. Prob. Foc.	Ex. Prob. Foc.	Straight	20 min.	_____
___ 99203	Detail	Detail	Low	30 min.	_____
___ 99204	Comp.	Comp.	Mod.	45 min.	_____
___ 99205	Comp.	Comp.	High	60 min.	_____

B. OFFICE VISIT - Established Patient

Code	History	Exam	Dec.	Time	
___ 99211				5 min.	_____
___ 99212	Prob. Foc.	Prob. Foc.	Straight	10min.	_____
___ 99213	Ex. Prob. Foc.	Ex. Prob. Foc.	Low	15 min.	_____
___ 99214	Detail	Detail	Mod.	25 min.	_____
___ 99215	Comp.	Comp.	High	40 min.	_____

C. HOSPITAL CARE   Dx Units

1. Detailed (30 min) ___ ___ 99221 _____
2. Subsequent Care ___ ___ 99231 _____
3. Critical Care (300-74 min) ___ ___ 99291 _____
4. each 30 min. ___ ___ 99292 _____
5. Discharge Services ___ ___ 99238 _____
6. Emergency Room ___ ___ 99282 _____

D. NURSING HOME CARE

Dx Units

Initial Care - New Pt.
1. Expanded ___ ___ 99322 _____
2. Detailed ___ ___ 99323 _____

Subsequent Care - Estab. Pt.
3. Problem Focused ___ ___ 99311 _____
4. Expanded ___ ___ 99312 _____
5. Detailed ___ ___ 99313 _____

E. PROCEDURES

1. EKG w/interpretation ___ 93000 _____
2. Colonoscopy ___ 45378 _____
3. Arthrocentesis, Small Jt. ___ 20600 _____
4. X-Ray Chest PA/LAT ___ 71020 _____

F. LAB

1. Preg. Test, Quantitative ___ 84702 _____
2. VDRL ___ 86592 _____
3. Blood Sugar ___ 82947 _____
4. UA, Routine w/Micro ___ 81000 _____
5. UA, Routine w/o Micro ___ 81002 _____
6. Pap Smear ___ 88150 _____
7. CBC w/differential ___ 85031 _____
8. Strep Screen ___ 87081 _____
9. Mono Screen ___ 86308 _____
10. Hematocrit ___ 85014 _____
11. ESR ___ 85651 _____
12. Uric Acid ___ 84550 _____

F. Cont'd   Dx Units

13. Potassium ___ 84132 _____
14. Comprehensive Metabolic Panel ___ 80053 _____
15. Routine Venipuncture ___ 36415 _____
16. Wet Prep ___ 82710 _____
17. Cholesterol ___ 82465 _____
18. ___ ___ _____

G. INJECTIONS

1. Influenza Virus Vaccine ___ 90659 _____
2. Tetanus Toxoids ___ 90703 _____
3. Pneumoccoccal Vaccine ___ 90732 _____

H. MISCELLANEOUS

1. _____ ___ _____
2. _____ ___ _____

AMOUNT PAID $ _____

DIAGNOSIS NOT LISTED BELOW _____

Mark diagnosis with	
(1=Primary, 2=Secondary, 3=Tertiary)	

DIAGNOSIS	ICD-9-CM 1, 2, 3	DIAGNOSIS	ICD-9-CM 1, 2, 3	DIAGNOSIS	ICD-9-CM 1, 2, 3
Abdominal Pain	780.0_ _____	Depression, NOS	311 _____	Peptic Ulcer Disease	536.9 _____
Allergic Rhinitis, Unspec.	477.9 _____	Diabetes Mellitus,		Peripheral Edema	782.3 _____
Angina Pectoris, Unspec.	413.9 _____	Non Insulin Dependent	250.00 _____	Peripheral Vascular Insufficiency, Unsp.	443.9 _____
Atypical Chest Pain, Unspec.	786.50 _____	Insulin Dep.	250.02 _____	Pharyngitis, Acute	462 _____
Asthma w/ Exacerbation	493.92 _____	Drug Reaction	995.2 _____	Pharyngitis, Strep	034.0 _____
Asthmatic Bronchitis	493.90 _____	Dysuria	788.1 _____	Pneumonia	486 _____
Atrial Fibrillation	427.31 _____	Eczema	692.2 _____	Prostatitis, NOS	601.9 _____
Anemia, Iron Deficiency, Unspec.	280.9 _____	Fever, Unknown Origin	780.6 _____	PVC	427.69 _____
Anemia, Pernicious	281.0 _____	Gastritis	535.0_ _____	Rash, Non Specific	782.1 _____
Anemia, NOS	285.9 _____	Gastroenteritis, NOS	558.9 _____	Seizure Disorder	780.3_ _____
Bronchitis, NOS	490 _____	Gastroesophageal Reflux	530.81 _____	Serous otitis Media, Chronic	381.10 _____
Bronchiolitis	466.1_ _____	Hypertension, Unspec.	401.9 _____	Sinusitis, Unspec.	461.9 _____
Cellulitis, NOS	682.9 _____	Hepatitis A, Infectious	070.1 _____	Tonsillitis, Purulent	463. _____
Cardiac Arrest	427.5 _____	Hypokalemia	276.8 _____	Bronchitis, Acute	466.0 _____
Congestive Heart Failure	428.0 _____	Hypercholesterolemia, Pure	272.0 _____	Upper Respiratory Infection, Acute	465.9 _____
Contact Dermatitis	692 _____	Hypoglycemia	251.2 _____	Urinary Tract Infection	599.0 _____
COPD	496 _____	Impetigo	684 _____	Urticaria	708.9 _____
Cardiac Pulmonary Disease	416.9 _____	Lymphadenitis, Unspec.	289.3 _____	Vertigo, Acute	780.4 _____
CVA, Acute, NOS	436 _____	Mononucleosis	075 _____	Viral Syndrome	079.99 _____
CVA, Old or Healed	438 _____	Myocardial Infarction, Acute, NOS	410.9 _____	Weakness, Generalized	780.79 _____
Degenerative Arthritis		Otitis Externa, Acute	380.10 _____	Weight Loss	783.21 _____
(Specify Site) _____	715.9 _____	Otitis Media	381.4 _____		
Dehydration	276.5 _____	Organic Brain Syndrome	310.9 _____		

ABN: I UNDERSTAND THAT MEDICARE PROBABLY WILL NOT COVER THE SERVICES LISTED BELOW

A. _____ B. _____ C. _____
Patient
Date _____ Signature _____
Doctor's Signature _____
RETURN: _____ Days _____ Weeks _____ Months

DOUGLASVILLE MEDICINE ASSOCIATES
5076 BRAND BLVD.
DOUGLASVILLE, NY 01234
PHONE No. (123) 456-7890
❐ L.D. HEATH, M.D.   ❐ D.J. SCHWARTZ, M.D.
SS# 999-00-1111   SS# 999-00-1235
EIN# 00-1234560

REF# 122949-SB 11.24.03   TO REORDER CALL INHEALTH RECORD SYSTEMS 800-477-7374

FIGURE 7-4 A charge slip, or encounter form *(Used with permission. InHealth Record Systems, Inc., 5076 Winters Chapel Road, Atlanta, GA 30360, 800-477-7374, www.inhealthrecords.com)*

PATIENT INFORMATION   DATE:

PATIENT'S NAME		MARITAL STATUS		DATE OF BIRTH		SOCIAL SECURITY NO.
		S | M | W | DIV | SEP				

STREET ADDRESS ☐ PERMANENT ☐ TEMPORARY	CITY AND STATE		ZIP CODE	HOME PHONE NO.

PATIENT'S EMPLOYER	OCCUPATION (INDICATE IF STUDENT)	HOW LONG EMPLOYED?	BUSINESS PHONE NO.

EMPLOYER'S STREET ADDRESS	CITY AND STATE		ZIP CODE

IN CASE OF EMERGENCY CONTACT:			DRIVERS LIC. NO.

SPOUSE'S NAME

SPOUSE'S EMPLOYER	OCCUPATION (INDICATE IF STUDENT)	HOW LONG EMPLOYED?	BUSINESS PHONE NO.

EMPLOYER'S STREET ADDRESS	CITY AND STATE		ZIP CODE

WHO REFERRED YOU TO THIS PRACTICE?

IF THE PATIENT IS A MINOR OR STUDENT

MOTHER'S NAME	STREET ADDRESS, CITY, STATE AND ZIP CODE		HOME PHONE NO.
MOTHER'S EMPLOYER	OCCUPATION	HOW LONG EMPLOYED?	BUSINESS PHONE NO.
EMPLOYER'S STREET ADDRESS	CITY AND STATE		ZIP CODE
FATHER'S NAME	STREET ADDRESS, CITY, STATE AND ZIP CODE		HOME PHONE NO.
FATHER'S EMPLOYER	OCCUPATION	HOW LONG EMPLOYED?	BUSINESS PHONE NO.
EMPLOYER'S STREET ADDRESS	CITY AND STATE		ZIP CODE

INSURANCE INFORMATION

PERSON RESPONSIBLE FOR PAYMENT, IF NOT ABOVE	STREET ADDRESS, CITY, STATE AND ZIP CODE		HOME PHONE NO.
☐ COMPANY NAME & ADDRESS	NAME OF POLICYHOLDER	CERTIFICATE NO.	GROUP NO.
☐ COMPANY NAME & ADDRESS	NAME OF POLICYHOLDER	POLICY NO.	
☐ COMPANY NAME & ADDRESS	NAME OF POLICYHOLDER	POLICY NO.	

☐ MEDICARE	MEDICARE NO.	☐ MEDICAID	PROGRAM NO.	COUNTY NO.	ACCOUNT NO.

In order to control our cost of billing, we request that office visits be paid at the time service is rendered. We would rather control our billing costs than be forced to raise our fees.

AUTHORIZATION: I hereby authorize the physician indicated above to furnish information to insurance carriers concerning this illness/accident, and I hereby irrevocably assign to the doctor all payments for medical services rendered. I understand that I am financially responsible for all charges whether or not covered by insurance.

_____
Responsible Party Signature

FIGURE 7-5   New patient information form *(Courtesy of Bibbero Systems, Inc., Petaluma, CA, 800-242-2376; www.bibbero.com)*

PROCEDURE PROCEDURE PROCEDURE PROCEDURE PROCEDURE PROCEDURE PROCEDURE

7-2  Obtain New Patient Information

PURPOSE: To obtain initial information from a new patient.

MATERIALS: An assigned "patient," a patient initial information form, a clipboard, a pen, a mock insurance card, a charge slip, chart folder, tabs, and computer.

PERFORMANCE OBJECTIVE: In a simulated situation, clearly communicate instructions and complete the steps in the procedure to obtain patient information and assemble all required materials.

1. Take the new patient to a private area to ask preliminary questions, or ask the new patient to complete a data sheet. **NOTE: Give the patient a clipboard and pen and offer assistance, if needed. Ask the patient to return the form when it is completed. A medical history is a potential legal document. Check to be sure the form is completed accurately and legibly, and signed where appropriate.**

2. Prepare a patient folder by typing the patient's name on a label and attaching it to the tab of the folder.

3. Transfer information from the form to the chart sheet.

4. Copy the insurance card (both sides).

5. Insert the chart, sheets, information form, and insurance card copy in the folder.

6. Prepare a charge slip.

7. Place the folder in the area reserved for charts of patients to be seen. **NOTE: If you have received any referral material on a new patient, be sure to place it with the chart.**

CLOSING THE OFFICE

At the end of the day, the examination rooms should be restocked and cleaned, and discarded material should be placed for pick-up. This saves time the next morning.

Charts must be collected, checked for completeness, and filed in a locked cabinet. If there is not time to file, place charts in a separate folder of "charts to be filed" and place in the cabinet to be filed the next day. (Some

---

PROCEDURE PROCEDURE PROCEDURE PROCEDURE PROCEDURE PROCEDURE PROCEDURE

7-3 Close the Office

PURPOSE: To prepare the office to be closed.

MATERIALS: A simulated office, if available; otherwise, role-play, explaining the procedure.

PERFORMANCE OBJECTIVE: Following all the steps in the procedure, role-play the actions required to close the office. Actions must be verbally described while performing the procedure.

1. Check to see that records are collected and filed in locked cabinets.

2. Place any money received in the safe or take to the bank to be deposited.

3. Turn off all electrical appliances. **NOTE: Many offices ask that you unplug electrical appliances. RATIONALE: Eliminates the chance of electrical fire.**

4. Check that rooms are cleaned and supplied for the next day.

5. Straighten reception room if time allows.

6. Pull charts for the next day if time allows.

7. Activate the answering device on the phone or notify the answering service and indicate when you will be back in the office.

8. Turn off lights.

9. **NOTE: Activate alarm system, if available.**

10. Set the lock and close the door.

11. Check to ensure that it is locked.

doctors may dictate their notes, which must first be typed onto the chart before it can be filed.) All electrical appliances and the autoclave must be turned off. Receipts collected during the day can be taken to the bank for deposit or locked in the office safe. If there is time, tidy the reception area and pull the next day's records. Always take a walk through the office to complete your checklist of things to do. Activate your answering system and turn off the lights. Activate the alarm system, if available, and securely lock the door. See Procedure 7-3.

ACHIEVE UNIT OBJECTIVES

- Complete the Workbook activities to meet the learning objectives.
- Practice the procedures in this unit to meet the performance objectives.
- Apply your knowledge at the end of this chapter in completing the Critical Thinking Challenge and Activities, as well as the StudyWARE on your Student CD-ROM.

UNIT 2
THE PATIENT'S MEDICAL RECORD

OBJECTIVES

Upon completion of this unit, you will be able to achieve the following:

LEARNING Objectives

1. Spell and define, using the glossary at the back of the text, all the Words to Know in this unit.
2. Describe the importance of the medical record as a legal document.
3. List examples of subjective information.
4. List examples of objective information.
5. Describe methods of recording progress notes.
6. Describe the correct procedure for making corrections to progress notes.
7. List the differences between a conventional record and the problem-oriented medical record.
8. Explain the History Physical Impression Plan (HPIP) method of recording patients' medical information.
9. Describe the major sections of a medical record.
10. Explain the reason for a tickler file.
11. Explain the purpose of chart audits and their importance.

WORDS TO KNOW

audit	objective	progress notes
charting	procrastinator	subjective
jeopardize		

CERTIFICATION CONNECTION

CMA
Medicolegal guidelines and
  requirements
Records management

RMA
Medical law
Administrative medical
  assisting: records and
  chart management

CMAS
Legal and ethical
  considerations
Medical records
  management

The patient history is the most important record kept in the medical office. The dates of any injuries, dates of treatment, and all notes regarding the condition of the patient must be accurate in every detail. In a lawsuit resulting from an injury, the patient chart information could win or lose the case.

Each office has its own method of **charting** patient information during visits. Some physicians ask the medical assistant to record the findings of a physical examination as it is being completed. Some physicians take the time to write all physical findings and **progress notes** for each visit. Many physicians prefer to dictate progress notes; then it becomes the duty of the medical assistant to type them or process the data using a word processor or computer. If dictating and transcribing the information is the preferred method, the printed document must be dated and placed in the patient's chart with a notation: for example, *"As dictated by Dr. H.G. Brown."* Keep in mind that confidentiality is vitally important, especially where many staff members have access to patient files and when the patients and their families may have a clear view of the monitor screen at times. Safeguarding personal and private patient information is always necessary.

Computer-generated patient records begin with entering the patient's general information for billing and scheduling. Computerized patient records also include the medical history appropriate for each particular type of medical practice. The extent of computer use in patient records is a decision made by the employer and the office manager.

Software packages are available to fit the needs of the practice according to the types of functions desired. Computerized medical records and examination formats, as well as billing and insurance with Current Procedural Terminology (CPT) and International Classification of Diseases (ICD) codes and other helpful and time-saving programs, are designed to make processing and retrieving information easy and efficient in the daily practice of managed care of patients.

HIPAA AND THE MEDICAL RECORD

The Health Insurance Portability and Accountability Act of 1996, or HIPAA as it is commonly called, required many changes for health providers as well as health insurance carriers. While the act has a larger scope than just privacy of health records, this is the area of concentration we will discuss in this unit. The areas that pertain primarily to records management include:

1. Maintaining the privacy of health information
2. Establishing standards for any electronic transmission of health information and related claims
3. Ensuring the security of all electronic health information

In April 2003, the privacy standards for all medical data became effective, resulting from many patients' feeling that their confidential, personal information was too open to others. Medical facilities realized that they needed to limit what information was released and to whom it was released. HIPAA is more lenient than most people realize, and the Privacy Rule allows each organization to do what it feels is reasonable within the mandated guidelines, but it does not specify how organizations must comply with the rule. All health care providers will have certain policies and procedures in place to document compliance, and it is essential that each employee follows those policies for all health information that is released as related to their responsibilities. Each office now has a HIPAA officer that understands the ruling, trains the staff in aspects of the ruling, and is charged with the responsibility of keeping up-to-date on any changes. The ruling also has designated that a Privacy Officer must be assigned to track who has access to protected health information within an office.

With the trend in many medical offices to go to electronic medical records instead of paper records, there are additional considerations regarding records management and HIPAA compliance. There is a Security Rule within HIPAA that mandates not only the privacy of medical records, but the security of those records, too. Actually, the focus of the Security Rule is on electronic information and ways to protect it from invasion, accidental disclosure, or loss of the records. Within the Security Rule, providers must demonstrate compliance in these four core areas:

1. Ensure confidentiality, integrity, and availability of all electronic Protected Health Information that the providers compose, receive, maintain, or send out.
2. Have policies and procedures in place that will protect against use or disclosures of the electronic information that is not required or permitted under the Privacy Ruling.
3. Have policies and procedures in place to protect against threats or hazards to the Protected Health Information records.
4. Demonstrate compliance with the Security Ruling within the workplace.

There are varying detailed categories within the rule that will serve to show compliance. If an office is audited, the Centers for Medicare and Medicaid Services (CMS) will ask for documentation to see how an office is living up to the expectations of the Security Rule. The categories that are reviewed during an audit include:

- Administrative safeguards
- Physical safeguards
- Technical safeguards
- Organizational requirements
- Documentation

Understanding the rationale for many of the security policies you will find within a health care provider's office will help you work with the office for the security of such records. Part of your training within an office setting will be to orient you to that specific office's requirements for compliance.

HIPAA

You may wonder what all of this has to do with you, both as a student and later as an employee. When you go to your externship, you will have access to Protected Health Information in patients' files, whether they are paper or electronic medical records. It is essential that you understand how important it is to protect privacy of the patients' information. In offices where an advanced electronic medical records system is in place, you may not be permitted access to the database for the security of those records, in accordance with HIPAA. As an employee, you will most likely have access to medical records, and understanding all of the implications associated with the privacy and security of those records is crucial to the health care provider. Taking the necessary safeguards with releasing information from medical records must be in the forefront of your mind while in the office setting.

THE PURPOSE OF RECORDS

The complete medical record has several important purposes:

1. It serves as a basis for planning patient care and for continuity in evaluating the patient's condition and treatment. The personal and family history and the findings of the physician must be combined with the results of laboratory studies, x-rays, and any indicated special tests. The review of all of these facts together help the physician determine the diagnosis and course of treatment. This would not be possible without a well-documented, accurate record. The patient history or family history may alert the physician to certain conditions such as a family history of diabetes or exposure to hazardous substances.

2. The medical record furnishes documentary evidence of the course of the patient's medical evaluation, treatment, and change in condition. The charting of progress notes is extremely important and should give an indication of the patient comments, physician's evaluation, prescribed treatment, and need for further follow-up.

3. The record furnishes evidence of communication between the physician and any other health professional contributing to the patient's care. The chart should include a record of reports from other physicians asked to evaluate the patient with special laboratory, x-ray, or diagnostic procedures.

4. It affords protection of the legal interests of the patient and the physician. The complete accurate record would be necessary if the patient wished the physician to testify in an injury case. The complete accurate record is also necessary if the patient sues

the physician for malpractice. The patient must always sign an authorization form before any information may be released. An authorization must indicate who is to be allowed to receive the information.

5. The medical record helps to establish a database for use in continuing education and research. The accurate record of patients is a useful resource for research concerning response to medications or procedures in every phase of medical treatment.

6. Insurance companies routinely send a representative to perform chart **audits** (inspections) of medical records of patients insured through their company. Medical offices receive an overall grade that reflects the thoroughness and quality of their recordkeeping. Offices that consistently score low **jeopardize** future contracts with those insurance companies.

The information in the medical record is classified as subjective or objective. The **subjective** information is supplied by the patient and includes routine information about the patient, past personal and medical history, family history, and chief complaint. The physician and various members of the health care team provide **objective** information (e.g., vital signs, exam findings, diagnostic tests, etc). The objective information includes examination, results of any laboratory studies, special procedures, x-rays, the diagnosis, treatment prescribed, and progress notes.

PARTS OF THE MEDICAL RECORD

The medical record is generally divided into the following sections:

- Administrative data
- Financial and insurance information
- Correspondence
- Referral
- Past medical records
- Clinical data
- Progress notes
- Diagnostic information
- Lab information
- Medications

Administrative Data and Financial and Insurance Information

Prioritizing matters of importance is the logical thing to do. Being prioritized and completing one task at a time will help reduce stress and help you be efficient. Each patient should be asked to fill out demographic information on a patient data form during the first office visit. Ask the patient to complete all blanks, such as full name, Social Security number (SS#), birth date, spouse's name, address, work and home phone numbers, insurance information, emergency contact information, etc.

Your Practice Name Here

Authorization for Disclosure of Health Information

Patient Name:_____

Date of Birth:_____ Phone:_____

Address:_____

City:_____ State:_____ Zip:_____

1. *I authorize the use or disclosure of the above named individual's health information as described below.*

2. *The following individual or organization is authorized to make the disclosure:*

Name:_____

Address:_____

City:_____ State:_____ Zip:_____

3. The type and amount of information to be used or disclosed is as follows: (include dates where appropriate)

_____ Complete health records   _____ Lab results/X-ray reports

_____ Physical exam   _____ Consultation reports

_____ Immunization record

_____ Other (please specify):_____

4. I understand that the information in my health record may include information relating to sexually transmitted disease, acquired immunodeficiency syndrome (AIDS) or human immunodeficiency virus (HIV). It may also include information about behavioral or mental health services and treatment for alcohol and drug abuse.

5. *This information may be disclosed to and used by the following individual or organization.*

Name:_____

Address:_____

City:_____ State:_____ Zip:_____

For the purpose of _____

6. I understand that I have a right to revoke this authorization at any time. I understand that if I revoke this authorization I must do so in writing and present my written revocation to the health information management department. I understand that the revocation will not apply to my insurance company when the law provides my insurer with the right to contest a claim under my policy. Unless otherwise revoked, this authorization will expire on the following date, event, or condition: _____ .

7. If I fail to specify an expiration date, event, or condition, this authorization will expire in sixty days. I understand that authorizing the disclosure of this health information is voluntary. I can refuse to sign this authorization. I need not sign this form in order to ensure treatment. I understand that I may inspect or copy the information to be used or disclosed, as provided in CFR 164.524. I understand that any disclosure of information carries with it the potential for an unauthorized redisclosure and the information may not be protected by federal confidentiality rules. If I have questions about disclosure of my health information, I can contact:

_____ ,

Privacy Officer for_____ .

_____   _____

Signature of patient or legal representative   Signature of witness

Date:_____   Date:_____

PLEASE NOTE: This information has been disclosed to you from confidential records protected from disclosure by state and federal law. No further disclosure of this information should be done without specific, written, and informed release of the individual to whom it pertains or as permitted by state law and federal law 42 CFR, part II.

FIGURE 7-6   Example of a new patient information form, including HIPAA disclosure(s).

Demographic information should be updated at every visit. Make sure that the information is updated on the patient's chart and in the computer. Refer to Figure 7-6 for an example of a patient information sheet. Place an attractive sign in the reception area and at the checkout window that directs a simple question to patients such as, "Do we have your current address and phone number?" Another example of a sign to post is, "Please let us know if there are any changes we should know about your address, phone, workplace, etc." Some offices post a sign or notice on the back of the exam room door. This way a patient can read the reminder and let the medical assistant know of any changes. This information must be obtained from patients at the reception window.

Correspondence

This section of the medical record includes all correspondence received concerning the patient. Referral or follow-up letters from specialists, informational or request-of-information letters from insurance companies, and any correspondence from the patient should be filed in the patient's chart as soon as possible when it is received.

Referral

Frequently, patients need to be sent to other facilities for specified diagnostic testing and to specialists for conditions beyond the expertise of the preferred provider. In order for the insurance company to pay for these visits, the preferred provider generally will need to submit a referral to the hospital, specialist, or other provider. It is imperative that the referring physician sends the patient to a participating provider listed on the patient's insurance plan. Often explaining this to the patient is one of the most important duties of the medical assistant. Failure to comply with these conditions could make the referring physician responsible for the cost of the diagnostic tests, which could result in a costly mistake of thousands of dollars.

Past Medical Records

Physicians usually request medical records from prior physicians for reference purposes. Knowing the patient's medical history is quite helpful in providing quality health care.

Progress Notes

Progress notes are the chronologic listing of visits, prescription refills, all calls that pertain to the patient, and all calls that the patient has had with any member of the health care team. Any time a patient has an interaction with anyone in the medical office, it should be recorded in the patient's progress notes.

The progress notes should be arranged in chronologic order, with the most recent date on top. If several notes are recorded on a page, the last on the page should be the most recent. The chart should be carefully dated for each visit. As discussed in Chapter 3, each no show, cancellation, telephone call, or prescription needs to be recorded as a progress note in the record of the patient, along with the date each took place, and signed by the individual making the entry.

The initial visit for any condition is usually written as a chief complaint on the progress note. It is a brief description of what is wrong with the patient. A history of the present illness and any remedies taken by the patient are usually included. Over-the-counter (OTC) medications should also be included. The patient's medication and drug allergies should be recorded and updated during each subsequent visit. Use standard abbreviations whenever possible when charting information. Using a + (plus) sign to indicate that the patient has the symptom and a − (minus) sign to indicate that the patient does not have that symptom provides valuable information for the physician (Figure 7-7). The level of pain that the patient experiences must also be

---

Example 1:

Ms. Sabrina K. Lane, DOB 12/23/1977
01/15/XX Pt C/O urinary sx × 3 d +frequency, +burning, +pain/urination, +N/−E, +chills, −fever, −pus or blood in urine, −back or abdominal pain, −vag sx, LMP
01/05/XX − OTC meds, current prescribed meds: Ortho-Novum 7-7-7 and tetracycline. NKDA.

          D. Brown, CMA

Example 2:

01/18/XX TC [telephone call]: pt called to tell Dr. Smith that the Macrobid makes her sick. Her sx are worse. Called in new Rx for Cipro 500 mg, BID to XYZ pharmacy per Dr. Smith.

          D. Brown, CMA (KL)

Example 3:

01/20/XX TC: pt called and said that sx are better and that Cipro does not make her sick. Pt encouraged to continue Cipro and to follow up with an appointment in 1 wk per Dr. Smith.

          D. Brown, CMA (KL)

Example 4:

01/27/XX Pt here for a F/U [follow-up] for UTI. Pt states that she took all of the Cipro and is presently asymptomatic.

          D. Brown, CMA (KL)

FIGURE 7-7 Examples of charting entries on progress notes. Remember, you should only use the designation of CMA if you are a certified medical assistant holding current status.

recorded on the chart. Use the standard scale of 1 to 10, with 10 being the worst. The physician will complete the progress notes by listing all objective findings and assessment and plan for further treatment and by signing the chart once the patient's examination is completed.

Diagnostic Information

All x-rays and non-lab-related testing should be placed in chronologic order in this section of the patient's chart.

Lab Information

All lab reports should be placed in chronologic order in this section of the chart. Notice in the charting examples that follow in this unit that the medical assistant signs her name and credentials after recording the procedure that she completed. In the parentheses are the physician's initials that signify that the physician has approved the orders that were completed.

Medications

Copies of prescriptions and documentation of any medications that are administered in the office are usually placed in this section of the chart. Administrative data are usually placed on one side of the chart and clinical data on the other side of the chart. This makes it easier and more expedient to locate each of the sections for information about a patient.

DATING, CORRECTING, AND MAINTAINING THE CHART

It is extremely important to record the date when documenting the patient's chief complaint or additional information on progress notes. In pertinent cases, such as car or industrial accidents, the time should also be recorded. You should make sure that you indicate AM or PM when noting the time unless you are recording in military time. The date may be written in ink or stamped. Every time a patient is given a prescription over the phone or is given a report or advice should also be recorded with the date and time. Failure of a patient to keep an appointment should always be recorded by the date stamp on the chart. When it is necessary to start a new page, the patient's name and birth date should be written at the top of each new page. If office staff other than the physician are making notes on the chart, these should be signed by the person making the notation.

In making a correction on progress notes, a handwritten entry should have a single line drawn through it and the correction written above or following it. An indication of correction should be made in the margin and should bear the initials of the person making the correction. Using correction fluid or erasing the error is never done because it looks as if one were trying to cover up or completely eliminate what was written. This could raise suspicion if there were ever a legal question regarding a patient and treatment. Write or print in a neat and legi-

ble manner. Be careful to spell the patient's name correctly and learn how to pronounce it accurately. (If necessary, you should ask the person to give you a phonetic spelling with accent symbols to show how to pronounce the name correctly. Some examples of difficult names to pronounce, followed by their phonetic spelling, are: Gnomic, gno′-mic [no′-mic]; Coughlin, cog′-lin; Chappelle, cha-pell′; Skowronski, Sko′-ron-ski; Zielachowski, zi-la-chow′-ski.) Charting becomes a part of the permanent record, and one should respect this fact. Using black ink will make much better photocopies of the record. When you finish with a patient's chart, always try to straighten up the forms and make the chart neat before filing it. Forms and other documents tend to shift with handling, and they sometimes become folded or tattered, which eventually makes them difficult to read. After you have completed recording or filing additional information in a patient's chart, you should return it to the files as soon as possible. Having stacks of files pulled too far in advance of the patients' appointments is not necessary and is not practical. Patient charts should be filed when not in use for a specific purpose.

For many years, the typewriter was a staple piece of equipment in the medical office; today, however, with computers in offices, you will find that typewriters are seldom used for transcription of medical records' content. The common practice is that dictated notes are transcribed using a computer; the transcriptionist will type the office notes and proofread prior to printing to catch any errors before the document is printed. However, if an error is found within the body of the progress/chart note, a single line should be drawn through the error with a correction made, the date of the correction, and identification of who has made the change.

In each medical specialty there will be unique terms and phrases; a working knowledge of these terms and phrases will make your job easier. Most medical offices have installed software packages on their computers that will perform spelling checks of anatomical terms, surgical terms, and medications as the text is typed within the program. This streamlines the process and makes the work easier, as you don't have to continually refer to a medical dictionary. Many physicians also use abbreviations in handwritten notes and dictation, so having a knowledge of these is useful. See Figure 7-8 for steps to follow in managing records.

TRACKING MEDICAL RECORDS

Every office or clinic has a system to track outstanding work that must be completed before releasing the chart to be filed. Many medical practice offices separate the charts at the physician's station or desk into specific stacks. Divisions may include:

- Charts to be filed
- Prescription refills
- Lab results
- Coding/financial corrections

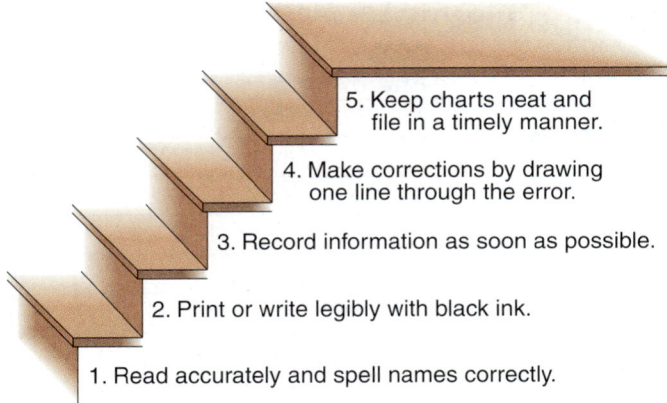

5. Keep charts neat and file in a timely manner.

4. Make corrections by drawing one line through the error.

3. Record information as soon as possible.

2. Print or write legibly with black ink.

1. Read accurately and spell names correctly.

FIGURE 7-8   Follow these steps for proper records management.

- Charts awaiting dictation
- Referrals

The physician will work on these stacks throughout the day, generally in the order of the most urgent to the least. It is the medical assistant's responsibility to track the stacks and complete any assigned work such as prescription call-ins, phoning patients with lab results, and sending completed charts to the central filing area. Time management is essential when working on these tasks. The assistant who works throughout the day to eliminate these stacks is the assistant who will get to leave at the usual closing time each day.

Many fine physicians are **procrastinators** when it comes to completing paperwork in the office. It is the duty of the medical assistant to see that it gets done, even if this requires daily reminders.

CALL-BACKS

As mentioned earlier in this unit, the medical assistant will make calls to patients, pharmacies, and labs. These are frequently referred to as *call-backs*. There will be some occasions when the medical assistant will be unable to complete all calls that need to be made. The following list categorizes calls that should take precedence.

1. All abnormal lab results, especially prothrombin time levels and other medication levels
2. Prescription refills
3. Patient concerns that were not handled at the time of the initial call

None of the above issues should ever be left until the following day without the direct approval of the physician.

Calling a patient with lab results is part of a process known as *following up test results*. It is common for a health care provider to assign the responsibility of screening test results to the medical assistant; this is a process in which you review laboratory results for any abnormal

values. The normal values are reviewed by the provider, but the abnormal values take priority over these so that immediate action can be taken on these results. It is very important that you fully understand the instructions to be given to the patient when following up, and even more critical is being certain that you document the call to the patient. Be sure when documenting any call that you include the date and times of the call; if not using military time, don't overlook designating AM or PM in the record. When making calls of this nature, you must also be sure that the patient understands the message that you are conveying. When calling patients about normal lab results, it is still imperative that you document the call in the medical record for future reference. If you are unable to reach the patient, a note of this must be made in the medical record.

A helpful practice for keeping track of referral appointments, follow-ups, and re-checks is to use a small, recipe card-sized filing unit called a tickler file. A more in-depth discussion of tickler files will be presented at the end of the chapter.

THE PROBLEM-ORIENTED MEDICAL RECORD

In the early 1970s Lawrence L. Weed, M.D., a professor of medicine at the University of Vermont's College of Medicine, originated a system of recordkeeping for patients that he named the problem-oriented medical record (POMR). In the traditional medical record, the progress notes are recorded according to the source they come from—the physician, laboratory, or physician's assistant—with no special attempt to record a relationship between them. The POMR record begins with the standard database, which includes patient profile, chief complaint, review of systems, physical examination, and laboratory reports. The chart usually contains a page near the front cover that lists and dates chronic problems. The page may also contain such information as a medication list, a preventive care list, and an education section that dates when patient education was given to the patient (Figure 7-9). This allows the physician to review at a glance the patient's past history without having to read through each individual entry of the progress notes. Using this system, the physician can make an assessment of the patient's health status to date. It works especially well in group practice settings because it promotes the continuity of patient care among the group members. The physician will first record findings on the progress notes of the chart using the subjective objective assessment plan (SOAP) method that follows (Figure 7-10):

S—Subjective impressions
O—Objective clinical evidence
A—Assessment or diagnosis
P—Plans for further studies, treatment, or management

This process makes the chart easier to review and helps in follow-up of all problems the patient may have.

Problem and Medication List

Patient Name: **DOB:**

Allergies: **Pharmacy #**

Date	Dx #	Chronic Problems	Dx #	Chronic Medications	Date		Refills					
					Start	Date						
					Stop	Initials						
					Start	Date						
					Stop	Initials						
					Start	Date						
					Stop	Initials						
					Start	Date						
					Stop	Initials						
					Start	Date						
					Stop	Initials						
					Start	Date						
					Stop	Initials						
					Start	Date						
					Stop	Initials						
					Start	Date						
					Stop	Initials						
					Start	Date						
					Stop	Initials						

Preventive	Date	Date	Date	Date	Date	Date
History Update Every 2 Years						
Breast Exam (plus Self-Exam)						
Mammogram						
DEXA						
Diabetic Blood Sugar Monitoring						
Diabetic Foot Care						
Diabetic HbA1c						
Diabetic LDL						
Diabetic Retinal Exam						
Diabetic Proteinuria						
Fasting Glucose						
Lipid Panel						
Pap/Pelvic						
Prostate Exam, PSA						
Rectal Exam						
Sigmoid/Colonos						
Stool for Occult Blood						
Testicular Exam (plus Self-Exam)						

Immunizations

Vaccination	Schedule	Date	Date	Date	Date
Hepatitis	As appropriate				
Influenza	At risk—q1y				
Pneumovax	At risk X 1				
Td Booster	PRN—q10y				

Education

	Date	Date	Date	Date
Advanced Directives/ Power of Attorney				
Alcohol/Drug Use				
Birth Control/Menopause				
Diabetes				
Diet				
Exercise				
Smoking				
Stress				

FIGURE 7-9   A sample patient problem and medication list that also provides space for dates and details of preventive actions, patient education, and immunizations, as well as the patient's pharmacy phone number.

OUTLINE FORMAT PROGRESS NOTES

Patient Name ___Yvette Garcia___

Page ___4___

Prob. No. or Letter	DATE	**S** Subjective	**O** Objective	**A** Assess	**P** Plans
5	9/6/01	Patient complains of two days of severe high epigastric pain and burning, radiating through the back. Pain accentuated after eating.			
			On examination there is extreme guarding and tenderness, high epigastric region no rebound. Bowel sounds normal. BP 110/70		
				R/O gastric ulcer, pylorospasm	
					To have upper gastrointestinal series. Start on Ametidine 300 mg daily Eliminate coffee, alcohol & aspirin Return two days.

Start each Progress Note (Subjective, Objective, form. Write through the intervening columns to the   Assessment and Plans) at the appropriate right margin of the page.   shaded column to create an outline

FIGURE 7-10   Example of Subjective objective assessment plan (SOAP) progress note page *(Courtesy of Bibbero Systems, Inc., Petaluma, CA, 800-242-2376; www.bibbero.com)*

EHR CONNECTION

In 2004, President George W. Bush addressed the American Association of Community Colleges annual convention in Minneapolis, Minnesota. One comment he made was based on conclusions drawn by researchers and leaders in the medical informatics field regarding electronic health records. In his speech to the group, President Bush made reference to how far behind the times the United States is with regard to patients' records. Specific mention was made that the current health care system utilizes paper files for tracking patients; there are multiple problems associated with paper files. For instance, charts get misplaced, information may not be consistently in the same place within the record, and handwritten notes can be illegible. President Bush also added that the antiquated method of maintaining paper files on patients is a real threat to patients and their safety. To this end, President Bush has added the incentive for medical practices to convert to electronic health records by approving projects that will encourage the implementation of such technology in medical practices.

Basically, the electronic health record (EHR) is a computer-based record for each individual patient. You will find reference to the EHR in several terms such as electronic medical records, computer health records, and electronic charts. However, they all mean virtually the same thing, and for this text, the term "electronic health record" is used in a generic sense. Some of the advantages of EHRs include:

- Having a set database for recording the patient's demographics, allergies, lab results, and improved accessibility of the record to health care providers.
- Many testing facilities such as radiology and laboratory departments record the patients' results in an electronic database; with the implementation of electronic health records, the results of such testing may be directly transmitted to the provider, reducing the time in receiving the results and establishing a regimen of care for the patient. In most cases, there is an alert for abnormalities when transmitting results in this manner.
- Prescriptions can be entered in the EHR, minimizing the possibility of misinterpretation from unreadable handwriting; additionally, the prescription orders can be sent to the pharmacy reducing the time for filling prescriptions. Software associated with EHR is usually designed to screen medications for possible interactions and patient allergies to lessen the change of an adverse reaction.

- The EHR aids in reminding the health care provider for routine testing such as mammography, vaccinations, and cardiovascular procedures.
- In a multi-physician practice, the EHR helps to coordinate care plans among those physicians, provides diagnosis and plans in place, and helps to eliminate duplicate testing.
- Chart notes are immediately available in cases in which a patient requires a referral or consultation with another provider. Software is available that takes notes made in the electronic database and converts them into full sentences. Also, software is available that has voice recognition for transcribing the dictated notes.
- Some EHR software is designed to assign CPT and ICD codes derived from the data entered into the patient's record during the visit, decreasing the time for filing insurance claims and increasing reimbursement.
- EHR software manufacturers also have recognized the need for ensuring the correct patient is being treated; many of the databases have a built-in feature that includes a photograph of the patient to ensure the correct patient's record has been selected for entering information during the visit.
- The more sophisticated EHR software programs are designed to detect trends in the patient's health history and map lab results and/or radiographic interpretations for better health care management.

An executive order executed in April 2004 by President Bush established the Office of National Coordinator for Health Information Technology. Dr. David Brailer, the national coordinator, is responsible for implementing health information technology in the public and private sectors for the reduction of medical errors, quality improvement of health care, and providing a greater value for the expenses associated with health care. In July 2004, Dr. Brailer, presented a framework for such strategic action that would expedite the adoption of such implementation.

Many individuals think that using the EHR system means that there will no longer be paper copies of medical records; however, that is not necessarily true. The EHR system is another way to keep accurate and accessible records that may be shared across the health care field for better access by clinicians as well improved patient care.

Ms. Sabrina Katherine Lake   DOB 12/23/1977
01/29/XX

Subjective   Pt states, "I've been feeling very tired and weak for the
              past month," LMP 01-15-XX very heavy flow. Exam: 6 #
              Wt loss since last visit 12/19/XX.
Objective   BP 112/70, Hb 10.4, Hct 31%. Decrease in muscle
              strength, pale.
Assessment   R/O anemia.
Plan   CBC with diff sent to lab, return in 1 week.

FIGURE 7-11A   A labeled sample of the subjective objective assessment plan (SOAP) method of charting.

Mr. Dennis J. Roberts   DOB 8/25/XX
3/4/XX

(H) Hx   C/O severe H/A Rt side of his head lasting several
               hours to up to 3 days; has had 4 in the past 6 wks,
               pain is increasing each time; takes ASA for pain.
(P) PX   Neurologic exam shows slight tremor in both hands.
(I) Impression R/O encephaloma.
(P) Plan   CAT scan of cranium. Refer to Clearbrook Neurological
               Associates.

FIGURE 7-11B   A sample of the history physical impression plan (HPIP) method of charting as related to the subjective objective assessment plan (SOAP).

Figures 7-11A and B are two methods of charting patients' medical information. Notice how similar they are. Following these formats in recording findings of patients yields better point-of-care service because there is a logical sequence to follow. There is less chance of overlooking a problem or a plan to treat patients.

Another similar system of recording medical information about patients is the history physical impression plan (HPIP) method:

H—History (subjective findings)
P—Physical exam (objective findings)
I—Impression (assessment/diagnosis)
P—Plan (treatment)

ACHIEVE UNIT OBJECTIVES

- Complete the Workbook activities to meet the learning objectives.

- Apply your knowledge at the end of this chapter in completing the Critical Thinking Challenge and Activities, as well as the StudyWARE on your Student CD-ROM.

UNIT 3
FILING

OBJECTIVES

Upon completion of this unit, you will be able to achieve the following:

LEARNING Objectives

1. Spell and define, using the glossary at the back of the text, all the Words to Know in this unit.
2. Explain basic filing methods.
3. List the steps used in filing.
4. Describe methods of removing and replacing patient files.
5. List the storage media used for "paperless" filing systems.
6. List and discuss the sections of a medical chart.
7. Describe purging files.
8. Explain ways to locate a missing chart.
9. Explain the pros and cons of alphabetical and numeric (digital) filing systems.

PERFORMANCE Objectives

1. File items alphabetically.
2. Pull a file folder from alphabetic files.
3. File items numerically.
4. Pull a file folder from numeric files.

WORDS TO KNOW

accumulated	expedite	subsequent
caption	illuminating	supplemented
chronologic	purge	systematically
data	sequence	unproductive

CERTIFICATION CONNECTION

CMA
Records management

RMA
Records and chart
  management

CMAS
Medical records
  management

IMPORTANCE OF FILING

Assembling and filing the patient's medical record are necessary to good patient care. Records must be filed accurately and **systematically**. Accuracy in assembling and filing the patient's medical record is necessary in providing quality managed care. Carelessly filed records produce chaos in the office. Reports that are lost or filed in the wrong chart or hidden in stacks of unfiled material will result in many hours of **unproductive** time spent searching for them. An efficient office requires accurate filing daily. Not only does this maintain efficiency, it also reduces the chance of accidental loss of correspondence and reports.

FILING STEPS

Folders or cards are easily filed alphabetically or numerically, but the procedure for filing reports and letters requires several steps (Figure 7-12).

Step One: Inspect

Generally, the medical assistant is the first to *inspect* reports. The reports are divided into negative/normal and positive/abnormal for the physician to read. It is the practice of some physicians to have the medical assistant send reports or phone patients about diagnostic reports if the reports are normal or negative. Many physicians prefer to review all reports regardless of the findings. After the physician reads a report, a check mark in the right upper corner of the document or a circle around the abnormal finding is made in red, and a notation is made about the follow-up (e.g., "Repeat mammography in 3 months," "Schedule an appointment for consultation," "Needs chest x-ray," etc.). A letter may be dictated, or a referral may be necessary (Figure 7-13).

Patient: Carol Sue Lamp   ✓

City Hospital
Troy, Ohio

ROENTGEN FINDINGS

Examination of the pelvis. AP supine including the upper third of the femora bilaterally visualizes advanced degenerative arthritis of the right hip with narrowing almost to obliteration of the hip joint space and with degenerative changes and cystic formation affecting the articulating surfaces of the head of the femur as well as the acetabulum. The remaining pelvis and left hip appears essentially normal.

Impression: Advanced degenerative arthritis right hip, otherwise normal pelvis and left hip.

FIGURE 7-13   The check mark in the upper right-hand corner of this report shows that the physician has read the report and notified the patient, and it is ready to be released to file in the patient's chart. Most physicians will make a notation referencing their review of the document.

Step Two: Indexing

The second step is *indexing*. This requires that you make a decision as to the name, subject, or other **caption** under which you will file the material. Materials for patients should be filed under the patient name. Research papers can be filed under illness, procedure, treatment, medication, or author. A cross-reference may be helpful in finding things later (Figure 7-14). For example, a research paper might be filed under the title, *Diabetes*, and a cross-reference to the article placed under the author's name, *Allen, John*.

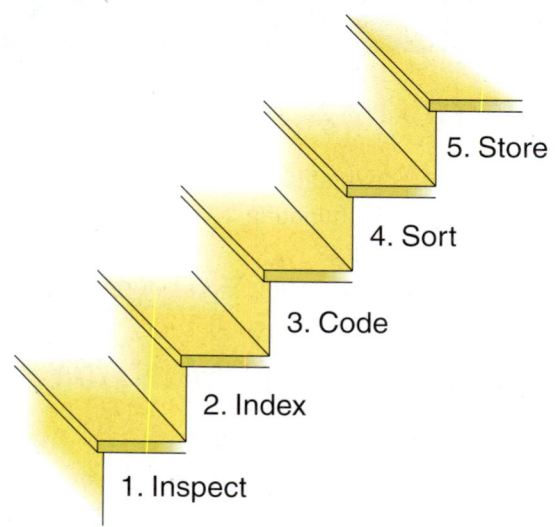

FIGURE 7-12   Follow these steps in order when filing.

5. Store
4. Sort
3. Code
2. Index
1. Inspect

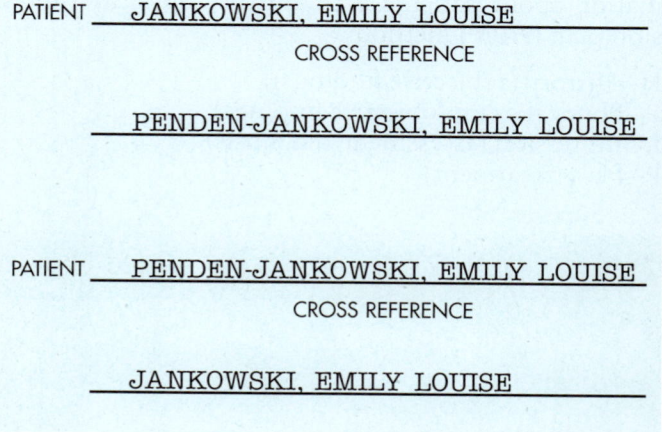

PATIENT   JANKOWSKI, EMILY LOUISE
CROSS REFERENCE

PENDEN-JANKOWSKI, EMILY LOUISE

PATIENT   PENDEN-JANKOWSKI, EMILY LOUISE
CROSS REFERENCE

JANKOWSKI, EMILY LOUISE

FIGURE 7-14   Example of a cross-reference card for effective and efficient filing.

Step Three: Coding

Coding is the third step and is done by marking the index caption on the papers to be filed. If the name, subject, or a number appears on the paper, you can underline or circle it, preferably with a colored pencil or a color highlighter (Figure 7-15). (Your employer may have a preference as to the color to be used for the coding process.) If the name, subject, or other caption does not appear on the material to be filed, write the caption in the upper right-hand corner. The medical assistant (or whoever is reviewing the chart or report) should sign the chart (with first-name initial and full last name, e.g., J. Williams) or report signifying that the patient has been contacted. The physician should review all charts and place his or her initials in parentheses after the medical assistant's signature to signify that the physician is aware that orders were carried out. As soon as the recommendations have been completed and the patient has been informed, the chart is ready for sorting to be filed.

Step Four: Sort

The fourth step is to *sort* the material. A desk sorter may be used to put papers in alphabetic order after they have been coded. This speeds up the process of filing (Figure 7-16). This sorter or an expanding alphabetic file for sorting reports, mail, and other items can provide a temporary file of these records until they can be placed in the patient's permanent chart. On days when it is especially hectic and all the filing has not yet been

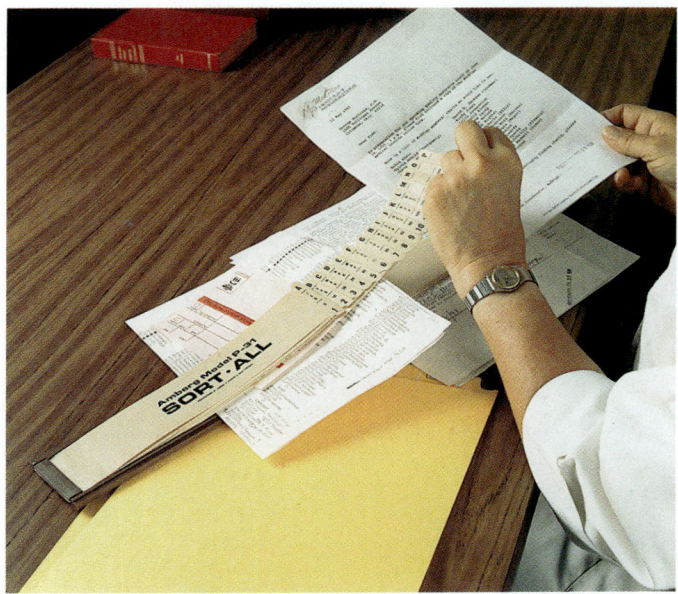

FIGURE 7-16   A desk sorter to alphabetize reports makes filing more streamlined and efficient.

completed, this means of sorting can help you locate a particular report quickly. This can be a practical answer to more efficient filing because each letter of the alphabet is in groups and thus filing goes much more quickly. Also, there are times when the patient's chart is in another department, and mail, for example, can be placed in this temporary file for ease in obtaining information to answer a phone call without having to take time out to go and get the entire chart.

Step Five: Storing

The final step is *storing*. You must first locate the file drawer or shelf with the appropriate caption. Then find the folder in which the reports will be stored. Lift the folder and place it on a flat surface before adding any material. This procedure makes it easier for you to make sure the caption on the folder agrees with the caption on the paper to be filed. Place the papers with the heading to the left and the most recent material on top. Some offices attach laboratory reports to the folder in a "shingle" fashion (Figure 7-17). The first is attached at the bottom of the page, and each **subsequent** report partially overlaps the previous ones.

FINDING A MISSING CHART

There are times when a chart seems nowhere to be found. There are a few steps to consider in locating the missing chart. First, go to the files where the chart you need should be, and look through several of the charts in front of and after this location. The chart may have

---

Patient: <u>Marsha Leonard</u>

Tri-County Hospital
Miami, Ohio

ROENTGEN FINDINGS

Films of 8/31/XX. Review of the PA and lateral chest film of 8/31/XX shows the traches to be shifted slightly to the left by a soft tissue mass in the right thoracic inlet in the superior mediastinal area. This probably represents tumor and is again seen on the lateral view lying in the anterior portion of the thoracic inlet on the right. Heart is otherwise normal. Lungs are otherwise clear.

FIGURE 7-15   Underlining the patient's name on a report, usually in a colored ink or highlighter, is one way of signifying that the patient has been notified and that the report has been released to be filed in the patient's chart.

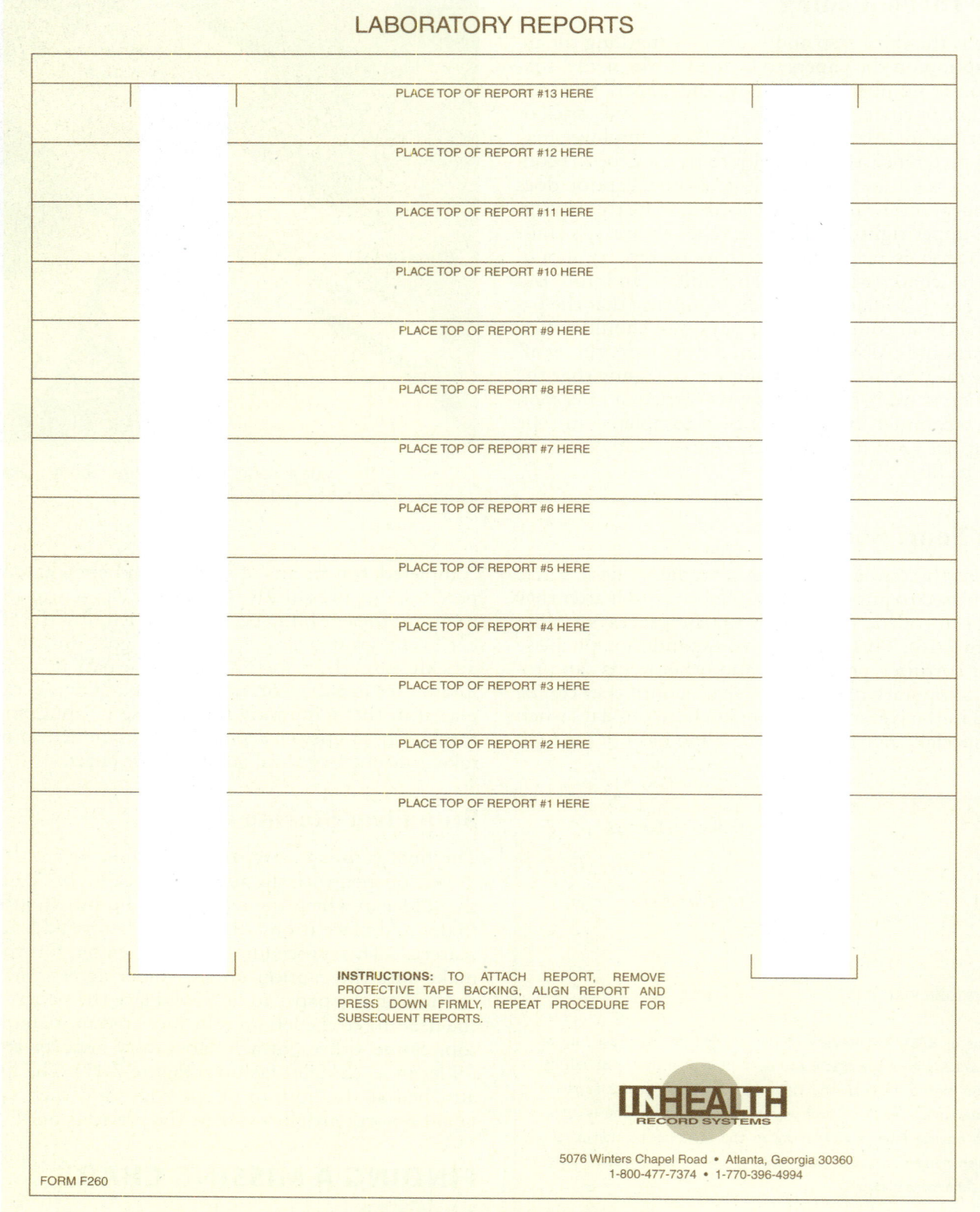

FIGURE 7-17 This type of report is filed by shingle fashion, with the most recent report on the top. *(Used with permission. InHealth Record Systems, Inc., 5076 Winters Chapel Road, Atlanta, GA 30360, 800-477-7374; www.inhealthrecords.com)*

been accidentally placed within one of the other charts near where it belongs. Second, check the name of the chart you need, and see if the chart was filed alphabetically by the person's first name. Next, check the day's schedule, and see if the chart is out for the patient to be seen. If you know the person was seen earlier in the day or week and you cannot locate the chart, look on the day's schedule when the patient was last seen, and check in several of the charts of those seen before and after the patient. It could have been placed within one of those charts by mistake. If you still cannot find the chart, the other logical places to look are on the desk of the physician, in the insurance or billing department, with the lab technician or office manager, or on the cart of the charts being pulled for the day or charts to be filed.

FILING STORAGE

Every office that requires you to file paper records will have storage units for this purpose. Files come in many different styles, shapes, and sizes. There are vertical or lateral file cabinets, card index files, open shelf files, and tub files (Figures 7-18 and 7-19). To save space, many offices are using movable shelving systems (Figure 7-20). Automation has made its way to the medical office.

Automated shelving units not only save space but also provide extra security for the medical records. The carriers rotate automatically, bringing requested files to your fingertips so that you avoid reaching, bending, or

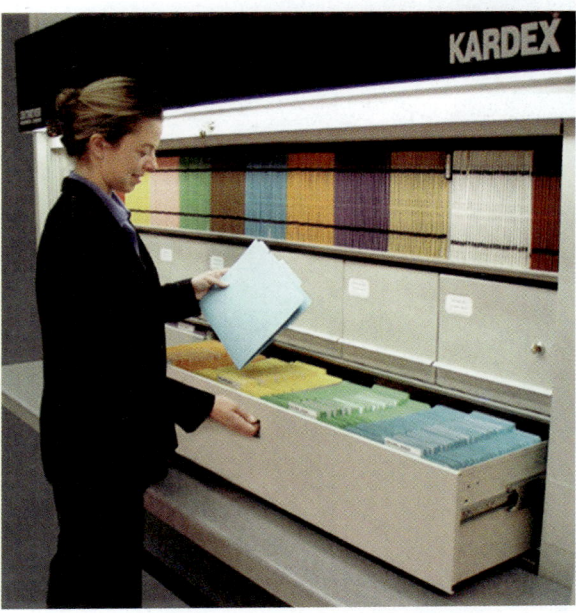

FIGURE 7-19   An example of filing a patient's record in pull-out drawer files *(Courtesy of Kardex. Kardex Systems Inc. PO Box 171, Marietta OH 45740, 800-234-3654 Kardex.com)*

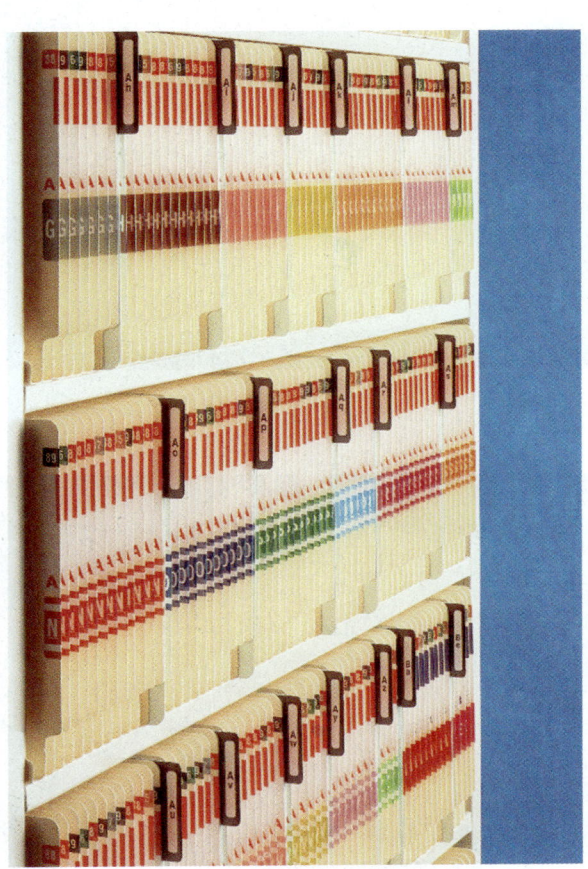

FIGURE 7-18   Retrieval of a chart from lateral shelf files *(Courtesy of Smead Manufacturing Company)*

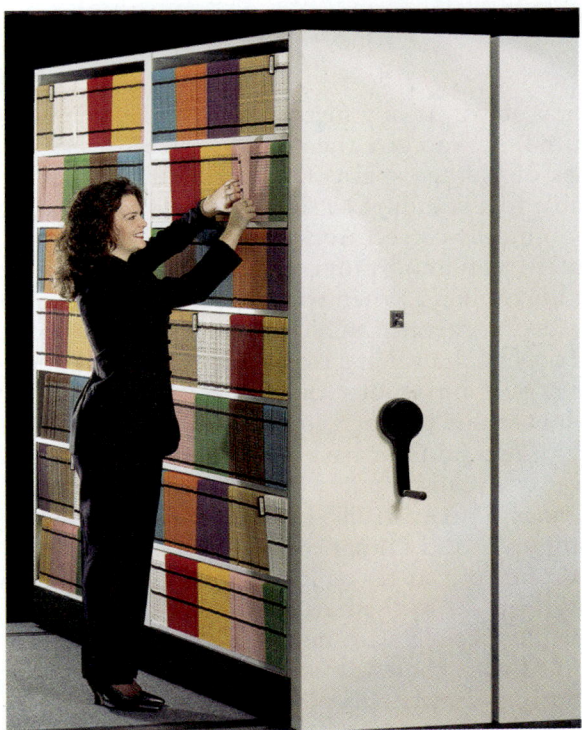

FIGURE 7-20   The Kompakt movable shelving provides maximum file space while taking up a minimum of floor space. *(Courtesy of Kardex)*

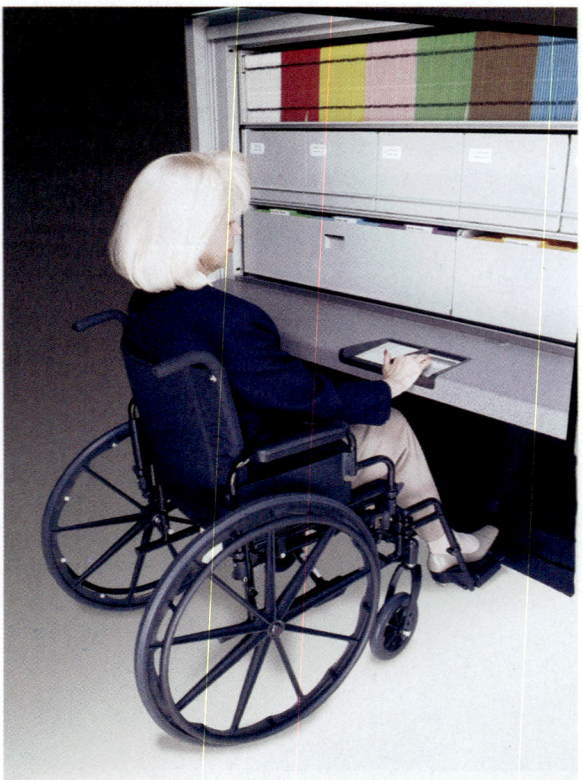

FIGURE 7-21 With the Lektriever 2000, the work surface is adjustable to a standing or sitting position; its design is ergonomically correct for all employees, including those with disabilities. *(Courtesy of Kardex.)*

FILING SUPPLIES

Filing supplies include guides, OUTguides or OUT-folders, folders, vertical pockets, index tabs, and various colored self-stick number and letter labels, as well as the standard office equipment such as stapler, staple remover, tape, etc. (Figures 7-22 and 7-23). A properly organized filing system will have many dividers or guides that identify sections within the file. The guides should be constructed of heavy material to stand up under continual wear. They reduce the area to be searched and allow you to locate a folder more quickly. The number of guides used is a matter of personal preference and will be determined by each office.

An OUTguide or folder is used to temporarily replace a folder that has been removed. It is thick and may be of a distinctive size and color for easier detection. The use of OUTguides makes refiling much easier and also alerts the medical assistant to missing files. The OUTguide may also have lines for recording information, such as where the missing folder may be located, or it may have a plastic pocket for inserting an information card. In a large office with several physicians and employees, it is

wasting steps. At any given time, the Lektriever 2000 (Figure 7-21) can give the operator access to 350 linear inches of storage space. The work surface area is adjustable to a standing or sitting position, providing an ergonomically-correct work height for all workers.

Safety is an important consideration when you work with file cabinets. When you leave a file drawer open at floor level, someone can fall over it. If you pull out more than one file drawer at a time in a vertical file cabinet, it can tip over and injure you. Be careful when pulling a file drawer out to reach material in the back, because some drawers do not have a stop to prevent the entire drawer from falling out.

Caution: There can also be the danger of a file cabinet tipping over and falling on you if you pull the entire top drawer out as far as it can open and do not have enough weight in the bottom drawer(s). This can be a problem especially with new file drawers as they are being filled with charts. It is best to start placing files in the bottom drawers first to avoid the possibility of injury a potential mess of papers and forms if a drawer were to fall. Always be mindful to keep all drawers, cabinet doors, step stools, or any other source of a possible accident closed or out of the path of others.

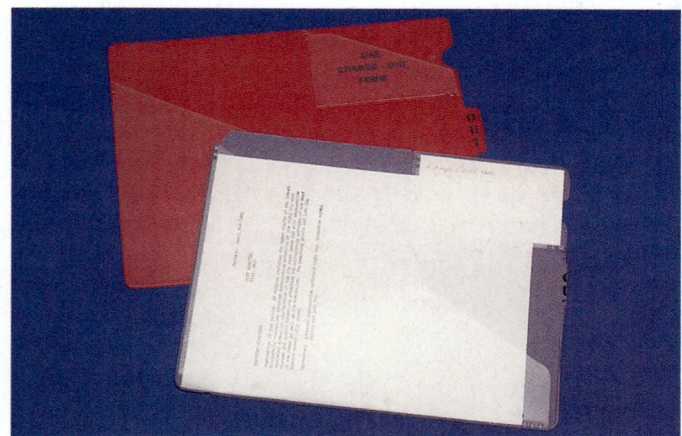

FIGURE 7-22 Example of OUTguide cards

FIGURE 7-23 Examples of top-cut and end-cut file folders

essential to know who has the folder when it is out of the file. Occasionally, a record may be sent to another physician or treatment facility, and it is extremely important that this information be recorded. The OUTfolder is also useful in providing a place to file material until the original folder is returned. Make sure you check with the physician before allowing a patient to take an entire chart. This is not an accepted practice and requires written permission and signatures with an expected date of return. It is only allowed in exceptional cases. A copy of, or a written summary of, a patient's health records is the usual procedure in sending information regarding a patient to another physician or health care facility.

A color coding system may be used to **expedite** both filing and finding of folders. Ordinary manila folders may be coded with colored strips or dots along the edge of the folder. The coding may be used to identify portions of the alphabet or patients of different physicians within an office. Color coding is also useful in identifying different types of insured patients. Everyone should have a key to the color coding through use of a procedure manual or posted chart.

A more sophisticated and efficient way of creating color-coded labels can be achieved by using your printer. Software programs are now available that can create color-coded indexing, text, bar codes, graphics, and full color images directly onto label paper or printable folders using your desktop color printer.

Offices that bar code their files can eliminate the need for OUTguides by scanning files prior to leaving the file area (Figure 7-24). The file clerk not only scans records when they leave the file area but also scans records in each department at least once or twice a day. This provides a great tracking system when the file leaves one area and is

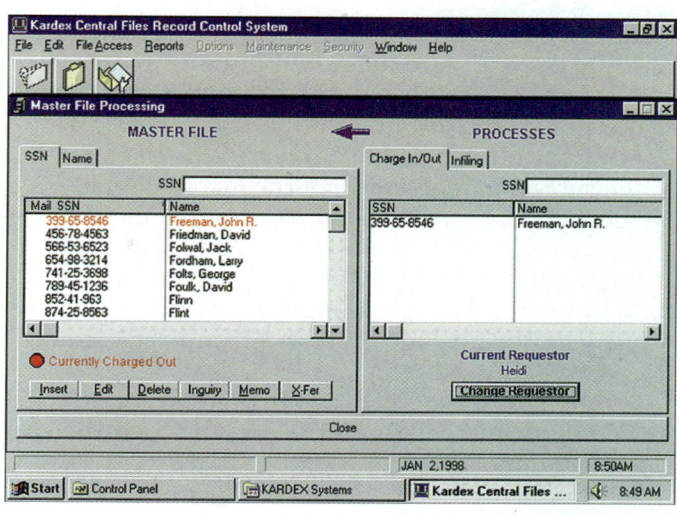

FIGURE 7-25   Charts that have been scanned can be viewed on a computer monitor to easily locate them. *(Courtesy of Kardex.)*

moved to another area. When the clerk inserts the file name into the computer, the file name pops up and identifies in chronologic order each department that has had the file since its initial removal. A list of files is shown in Figure 7-25. This system not only reduces the search time but also greatly decreases the number of lost files.

PAPERLESS FILES

Storage units used to house paperless media are either card files, drawers, open shelves, or racks. Shelves or drawers are used to store boxed rolls of microfilm. Card files are used for microfiche and aperture cards. (Aperture cards are one tiny negative mounted on a data processing card.) These types of records require an **illuminating** and magnifying viewing device to read the stored information.

If you are hired to work with a paperless filing system, you will be taught how to use the special filing equipment on the job. You will be using computers to handle **data.** There will be automatic storage and retrieval units to master. Storage of a vast array of information regarding patient records, employee information and payroll, scheduling, statistics regarding medical conditions, office management, taxes, inventory, and a host of other records can be filed and stored on a computer system with easy retrieval whenever necessary. This eliminates clutter and the need for filing space. Software companies provide advice for practical use to fit particular needs of the practice.

FILING SYSTEMS

Most filing systems are based directly or indirectly on an alphabetic arrangement. In alphabetic filing, the names of persons, firms, or organizations are arranged as in the telephone directory. This is the simplest and most commonly used method of filing. In numeric filing, the material is arranged in numeric order in the

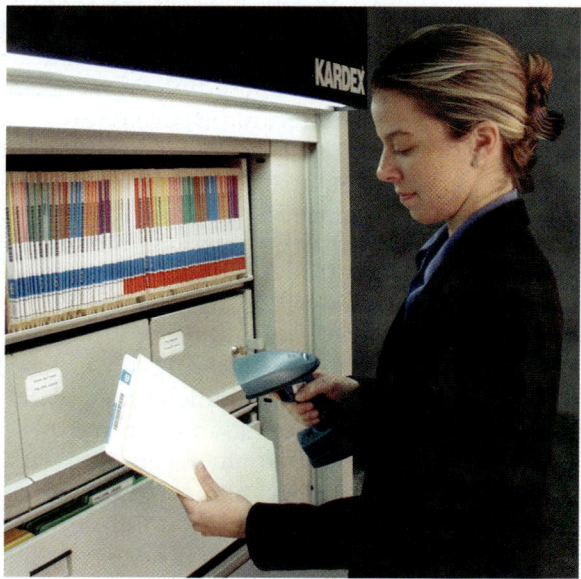

FIGURE 7-24   A scanner can be used to track where charts are located in the office. *(Courtesy of Kardex.)*

main file. The main file is **supplemented** by an alphabetically arranged card index. The number under which a given item is to be filed can be determined by referring to the alphabetic card index file.

A subject file is based on an outline or classification of the subject matter to which the material refers. In a physician's office, it is customary to maintain files of reference materials **accumulated** by subject matter.

In geographic filing, material is arranged alphabetically by political or geographic subdivisions such as country, state, city, and even street, and each subdivision is alphabetized.

Chronologic filing refers to filing according to date. Arranging documents with the most current date on top is recommended.

When you are filing additional documents in a patient's chart, place them in order of dates with the most current date on top. Patient files are generally arranged in an orderly fashion in sections as follows (with the chart opened flat): progress notes are on the right with physical exam form under them; imaging reports and lab reports are shingled on the inside (right) back cover of the chart; and on the inside cover (left) are immunization records, medication list, and patient data. This is one way to organize a chart. Follow the office policy of your place of employment.

Files are also arranged by color-coding them in either alphabetic or numeric order or by category. Figure 7-26 shows movable file shelving that is color-coded. Each cat-

egory (e.g., allergy patients, workers' compensation, charts of patients who are delinquent in payments, etc.) is assigned a different color. This is done to expedite patient care and processing of payment of services. This type of indexing also helps to reduce the time that it takes to file and retrieve patient charts. Misfiles are quickly spotted with this system. Also, the colors of the charts are very bright and attractive. The office manager is generally the one who makes the decision about filing systems.

FILING ALPHABETICALLY

The most common method of filing is alphabetic. Patient charts are filed in alphabetic order. They are also labeled with colorful numeric codes. Procedure 7-4 explains the steps necessary in filing alphabetically. The rules for filing material alphabetically must be learned. They are as follows.

RULE 1. In filing the names of persons, the surname or last name is considered first, the first name or initial second, and the middle name or initial third.

EXAMPLE: John E. Brown is filed as Brown, John E.

RULE 2. Names are filed alphabetically in an A-to-Z **sequence** from the first to the last letter, considering each letter in the name separately and each unit separately. The following names are listed in correct filing order:

Allard, Wm.
Allen, E. S.
Allen, Edna
Allen, Wm. A.
Allen, William C.
Allens, M. R.

- When the surnames of two persons are spelled differently, the first and middle names or initials need not be considered. See the first two names in the preceding list. The order of these two names is determined by the fourth letter in the surname.
- When a shorter surname is identical with the first part of a longer surname, the shorter name is listed first. The rule is sometimes stated as "nothing before something." See the fifth and sixth names in the preceding list.
- When the surnames are alike, the order in filing is determined by the first names or initials. When the surname and first names or initials are alike, the filing order is determined by the middle names or initials. See the fourth and fifth names in the preceding list.
- An initial is listed before a name beginning with the same letter. See the second and third names in the preceding list. This again is the example of "nothing before something."
- An abbreviated first or middle name is treated as if it were spelled out in full. See the fourth and fifth names in the preceding list.

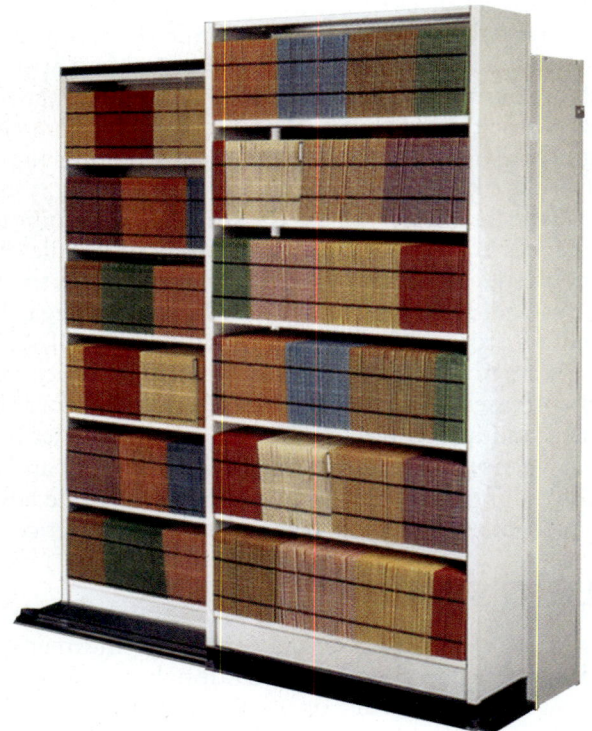

FIGURE 7-26 These movable shelving units are attractive space savers. *(Courtesy of Kardex.)*

7-4    File Item(s) Alphabetically

PURPOSE: To file and store patient file(s) or other items accurately in alphabetic order.

EQUIPMENT AND SUPPLIES: Items to be filed, cabinet for files.

PERFORMANCE OBJECTIVE: In a simulated situation, given patients' files or other items, accurately file and store the file(s) or other items within 10 minutes.

1. Use the rules for filing items alphabetically. **NOTE: Double check the spelling of the name for accuracy when using the cross-reference file. (Refer to Figure 7-27.)**

2. Determine the appropriate storage file.

3. If you are filing new material, scan the guides for the area nearest to the letters of the name(s) on the items that you have to file. **NOTE: When filing items such as lab reports or letters, be extremely careful to** place them in the correct chart. **Remove the chart, open it, and place the item in the chart with the top of the item toward the top of the inside of the chart on the appropriate left or right side. Be sure to place dated items in chronologic order with the most recent date on top.**

4. Place the folder in the correct alphabetic order between two files. **NOTE: Be sure to insert the new file *between* two other folders and NOT within another folder where it could be lost.**

5. If you are filing material previously in the file, scan for the OUTguide. Remove the OUTguide after you have replaced the materials. **NOTE: Check to be sure it was marking the space for the file you just returned and not another.**

(Procedure 7-5 discusses pulling a file folder from alphabetic files.)

RULE 3. A prefix (also called a surname particle), such as Mc, Mac, De, Le, and von, is considered as part of the surname.

EXAMPLES:
MacAdams, Bruce
McAdams, Helen
VonBergen, T. R.

RULE 4. In filing the name of a married woman, her legal name is used. The title Mrs. is disregarded in filing but is placed in parentheses after the name.

EXAMPLE: Mrs. R. A. (Betty A.) Smith is filed as Smith, Betty A. (Mrs. R. A.).

RULE 5. Most firm names are filed as they are written. The apostrophe is disregarded in filing.

EXAMPLES:
Herb's Auto Service
Walters Printing Company

RULE 6. Firm names that include the full name of an individual are filed with the name of the individual transposed.

EXAMPLE: Edward Wenger Company is filed as Wenger, Edward Company.

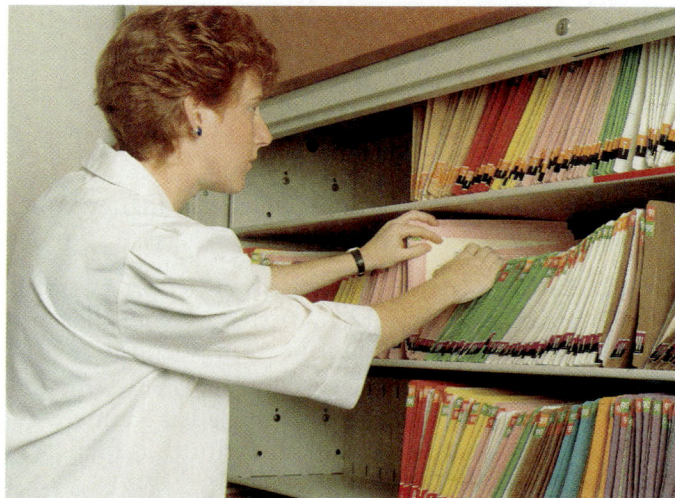

FIGURE 7-27 These charts are filed alphabetically; note that they also have numerical codes.

RULE 7. When the article *the* is part of a title, it is placed in parentheses and disregarded in filing.

EXAMPLES: Sam the Barber is filed as Sam (the) Barber; The Family Steak House is filed as Family Steak House (The).

PROCEDURE PROCEDURE PROCEDURE PROCEDURE PROCEDURE PROCEDURE PROCEDURE

7-5 Pull File Folder from Alphabetic Files

PURPOSE: To obtain the correct patient file(s) from the file cabinet.

EQUIPMENT AND SUPPLIES: Name of patient file to be pulled, OUTguide (card), pen, cabinet of patient files.

PERFORMANCE OBJECTIVE: In a simulated situation, given the patient's name, accurately prepare the OUTguide and pull the file, replacing the file with the OUTguide within 10 minutes.

1. Find the name of the patient in the alphabetic file. Double check the spelling of the name for accuracy.

2. Complete the OUTguide with the date and your name. **NOTE: If you are pulling files for the day, OUT-guides may not be necessary. When pulling files for another person, write that person's name and your initials.**

3. Pull the file(s) needed and replace with the OUTguide(s).

RULE 8. *And, for, of,* etc., are disregarded in filing but are not omitted.

EXAMPLE: Adams & Smith Pharmacy is filed as Adams (&) Smith Pharmacy.

RULE 9. Abbreviations such as *Co., Inc.,* or *Ltd* in a firm name are indexed as though spelled out.

EXAMPLE: Frank Smith Co. is filed as Smith, Frank Company.

RULE 10. Hyphenated surnames and hyphenated firm names are indexed as one unit.

EXAMPLES: Dunning-Lathrop & Assoc. Inc. is filed as Dunning-Lathrop (&) Associates, Incorporated; Lester Smith-Mayes is filed as Smith-Mayes, Lester.

RULE 11. Numbers are usually filed as though spelled out.

EXAMPLE: 5th Avenue Store is filed as Fifth Avenue Store.

RULE 12. Professional or honorary titles are not considered in filing but should be written in parentheses at the end of the name for identification purposes.

EXAMPLES: Dr. Anne Lewis is filed as Lewis, Anne (Dr.); President John Kennedy is filed as Kennedy, John (President); Prof. William S. Smith is filed as Smith, William S. (Prof.).

- Titles are filed as written when they are part of a firm name. Foreign or religious titles followed by one name are also filed as they are written.

EXAMPLES:

Dr. Scholl's Foot Powder

Prince Phillip

RULE 13. Terms of seniority, such as *Junior, Senior, Second,* or *Third,* are not considered in filing. If two names

are otherwise identical, the address is used to make the filing decision in the order: state, city, street.

EXAMPLES:

Willard Keir, Sr.

Willard Keir, Jr.

Filed as:

Keir, Willard, Sr. (Cleveland, Ohio)

Keir, Willard, Jr. (Columbus, Ohio)

RULE 14. File the names of federal, state, or local government departments first by political division and then by name of department.

EXAMPLE: Drug Enforcement Administration, Cincinnati, Ohio is filed as Cincinnati, City, Drug Enforcement Administration, Cincinnati, Ohio.

FILING NUMERICALLY

The second filing method used, especially in very large clinics, is the numerical system (Procedure 7-6). This system provides the most patient privacy, as all that is visible on the folder is the patient number. As mentioned before, a cross-index or cross-reference is required in the form of an alphabetic card file, and a number is assigned to each patient. First locate the alphabetic card to determine the patient's number, and then locate the numbered file.

Most offices use the same number of digits for each number assigned, and the numbers are always filed in order from smallest to largest. If the zero (0) falls before another number, it is disregarded when filing. A system using six digits would begin 000001, 000002, 000003, and so on.

Some systems use the same terminal digit or digits to designate shelves or drawers. The patients are assigned numbers, which are separated into twos (2s) or threes (3s). The numbers are then read from the right hand group of numbers to the left hand group. After

PROCEDURE PROCEDURE PROCEDURE PROCEDURE PROCEDURE PROCEDURE PROCEDURE

7-6  File Item(s) Numerically

PURPOSE: To file and store patient file(s) or other items accurately in numerical order.

EQUIPMENT AND SUPPLIES: Items to be filed, cabinet for files.

PERFORMANCE OBJECTIVE: In a simulated situation, given the patient's file or other items, accurately store the file(s) or other items within 10 minutes.
1. Use the rules for numerical filing. **NOTE: Double check the spelling of the name for accuracy when using the cross-reference file.**

2. Determine the appropriate storage file.
3. Match the first two or three numbers with those already in the file. If using terminal digits, match the last two numbers.
4. Match the remaining numbers with those in the file. **NOTE: If you have assigned a number to a new patient, it should probably be at the very end of the file.**

(Procedure 7-7 discusses pulling a file folder from numerical files.)

PROCEDURE PROCEDURE PROCEDURE PROCEDURE PROCEDURE PROCEDURE PROCEDURE

7-7  Pull File Folder from Numeric Files

PURPOSE: To obtain the correct patient file(s) from the file cabinet.

EQUIPMENT AND SUPPLIES: Name of patient file to be pulled, OUTguide (card), pen, cabinet of patient files.

PERFORMANCE OBJECTIVE: In a simulated situation, given the patient's name or account number, accurately prepare the OUTguide and pull the file, replacing the file with the OUTguide, within 10 minutes.
1. Find the name of the patient in the card file to obtain the account number. Double check the spelling of the name for accuracy.

2. Complete the OUTguide with the date and your name. **NOTE: If you are pulling files for the day, OUTguides may not be necessary. When pulling files for another person, write that person's name and your initials.**
3. Locate the corresponding section of the numeric file.
4. Scan the files for the number.
5. Pull the requested file and replace with the prepared OUTguide.

the last two or three digits are sorted together in numeric order, you next consider the middle digits and sort them in order. Finally, you consider the first group of digits and sort them in order.

For example, the numbers of charts in one series might end in 25 and another series might end in 35. Charts labeled 10-07-25 and 02-17-25 would then be filed separately from charts labeled 08-17-35 and 12-25-35. The order of the charts numbered above would be:

02-17-25
10-07-25
08-17-35
12-25-35

FILING BY SUBJECT

In a medical office it is necessary to have files for business information. You must file financial records, copies of inventory, copies of orders, and records of supplies and equipment received. You should have a file for tax records, insurance policies, and canceled checks. The subject headings of these files would be relatively easy to determine, but it is more difficult to determine where to file some general correspondence or reprints of medical research publications.

Very often reprints are filed with a cross-index, one file for the subject and one for the author with a listing of reprint subjects available. The miscellaneous folder is an important subject file. When you have one letter on a subject it should go into the miscellaneous file indexed by subject or names. The material in each subject file is filed in chronologic order with the most recent entry on top. When five papers are assembled in the miscellaneous file on one subject or person, a separate folder should be prepared and the material removed from the miscellaneous file.

USING A CHRONOLOGIC (TICKLER) FILE

A chronologic file is commonly called a "tickler file" and is used as a follow-up method for a particular date (Figure 7-28). The file may be an expanding file, a card file, or even a portion of a file drawer. It consists of dividers with the names of all the months and dividers numbered from 1 to 31 for the days of the month. Some offices have patients fill out a card to be sent as a reminder to return for examination, testing, or injections. The patient addresses the card, and the office retains it in the tickler file to be mailed at the appropriate time. Place the month card in the front of the file each month and check each day to see if anything needs to be done. Reminders for equipment servicing, carpet cleaning, completing monthly orders, making an appointment for a patient to have elective surgery, sending a reminder to a patient who needs to be seen for follow-up, and scheduling a speaker for an in-service are among the many types of reminders that can be included in this file. These 5 × 7-inch cards should have the party's name and phone number, the date and reason for the reminder, the referral facility phone number, etc. There should also be a line for the person who completes the task to sign and date that it was completed. The tickler file should be the responsibility of the administrative medical assistant, who is generally the person who handles the reception of and check out duties for patients. This file should be checked every day at the same time. Once the reminder is sent, the card should be kept for a period of weeks, months, or however long your employer/office manager requires. This is a smart practice because it serves as a reference in case of a misunderstanding or a question about the way the patient or a referral was notified, when it was made, and who was responsible.

Many software companies now manufacture programs that can be installed on office computers that serve as electronic tickler files. The programs are automated to "pop up" on the screen to remind an individual of the task needing to be completed.

DESKTOP FILES

A convenient desktop file such as the one shown in Figure 7-29 makes it easy to flip to the phone number or address you need quickly. Other helpful materials that will fit neatly on the desktop are a list of frequently called referral facilities, pharmacies, labs, and hospitals. Using supplies that make your job easier is most practical. Being efficient in recordkeeping is a key factor in helping the workday go smoothly.

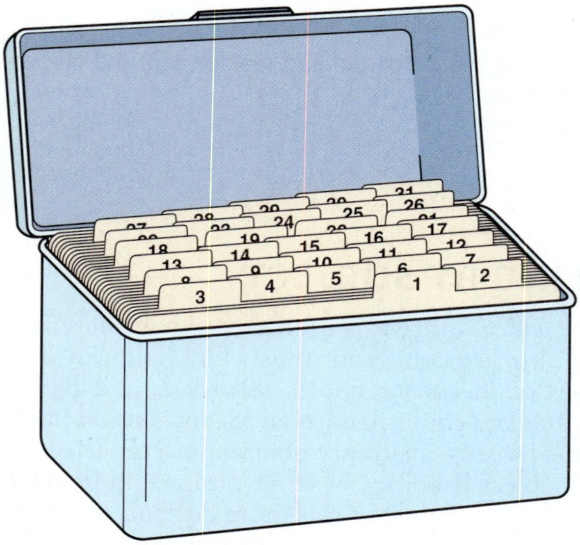

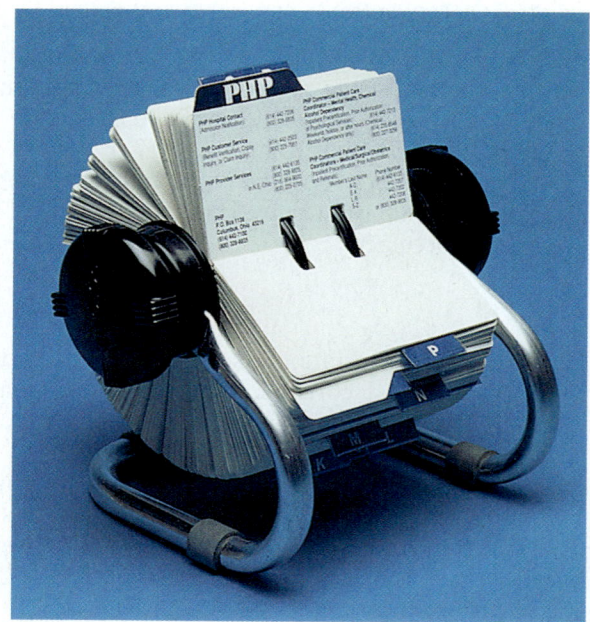

FIGURE 7-28 Using a tickler file such as this will help to plan and keep track of important dates, events, and responsibilities.

FIGURE 7-29 This desktop Rolodex file takes up little space but still provides fingertip access to important phone numbers.

PURGING FILES

In all medical practices, at some point the shelves holding the files become full, and there is no room for any more charts. Periodically you must purge files of those patients who are no longer being seen by the physician(s). **Purge** means to clean out. You simply take out the inactive charts to make room on the file shelves or in drawers for new and active patients. Basically, you are moving files into other file cabinets or storage boxes. Files are generally purged when the shelves become too full, at the end of each quarter, or biannually. Purging can also be done routinely with charts that have been inactive 2 years or more (depending on the office policy). If you use year tab stickers to make new charts, those files that are to be purged can be easily spotted. Purging can be time-consuming and should be accomplished over a given period of time. When you purge files, it must be accomplished in a systematic manner. There has to be a plan and a place to accommodate the inactive files. If inactive files are boxed, it is critical to label them accurately. Some practices have inactive patient charts on microfilm to be stored. Caution should be taken by those involved in moving volumes of files and charts to lift only a small amount at a time to prevent back strain and other injuries. Those who lift any heavy object should practice proper body mechanics, lift carefully, and lift only a reasonable

number of charts at a time. Figures 7-30A and B show correct movement when lifting to prevent injury. A helpful means in moving great numbers of charts from one file-shelving unit to another is shown in Figure 7-31. This way you can easily transport a large number of files with the wheeled cart and eliminate making so many trips to the inactive file cabinet or room.

Inactive files must be available because the patient may return. Transferring records of deceased patients should be delayed until all requests for forms have been completed. At that time, the files can be closed and may be placed in the deceased storage area. The transport file cart may also be used daily for charts that are ready to be filed, keeping them separated from those charts out for patient care and phone call-backs. The charts can be placed in alphabetic or numeric order for convenience for filing and if another team member needs one of the patient charts.

Security is necessary in keeping this stored information regarding patients confidential. The files should be locked when there is no one monitoring them. Frequently, records of patients are kept in medical practices no matter how far back the date goes. You can see that putting this information on disk or on microfilm

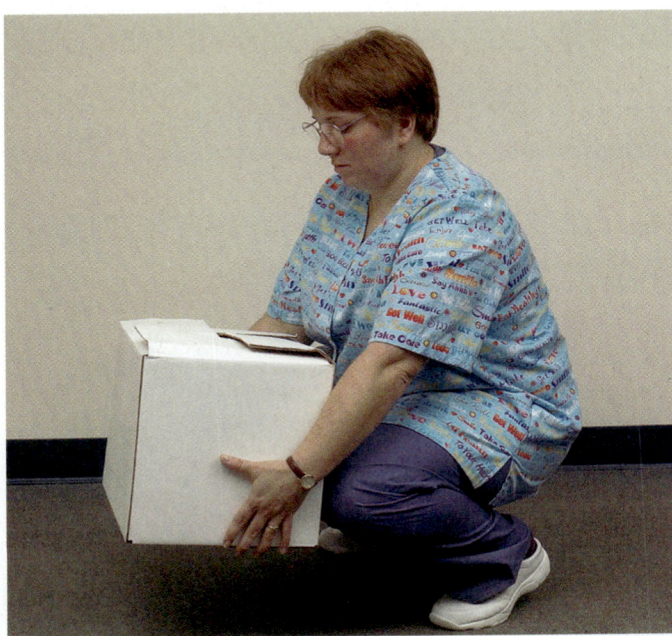

FIGURE 7-30A The steps to proper lifting: 1. Bend at the knees and hips, and stand close to the object. Keep your back straight and lift using the muscles in your arms and legs, not your back.

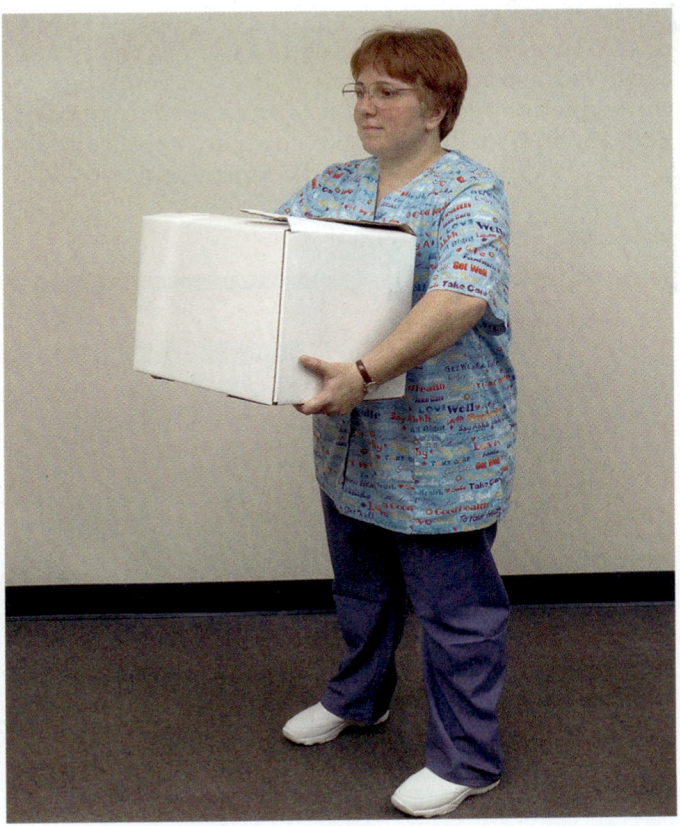

FIGURE 7-30B 2. Once lifted, keep the object close to your body.

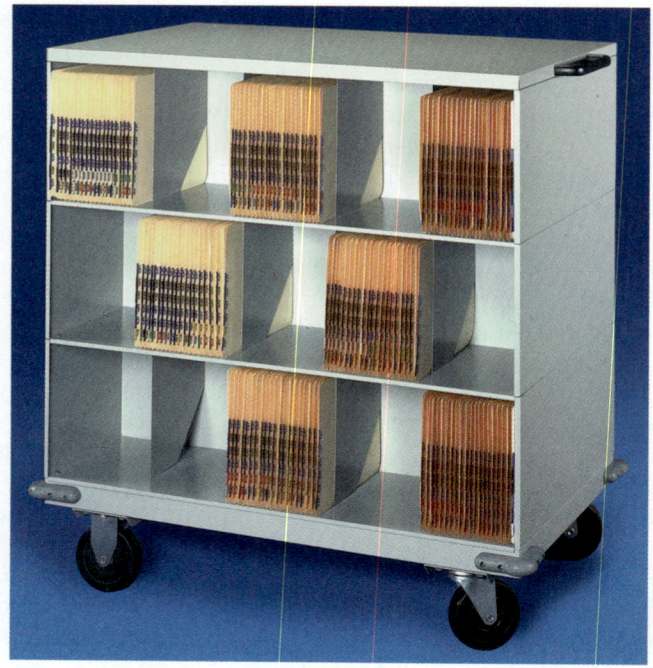

FIGURE 7-31 This filing cart is an easy way to transport large numbers of patient charts at one time or to designate charts that need to be filed. *(Courtesy of Colwell, a division of Patterson Dental Supply, Inc., 800-637-1140)*

to save space is often necessary to save the cost of additional storage space. You must check in your state for the regulations concerning files and the time you must keep them. Usually medical records are kept from 3 to 7 years. In different states and countries this may vary.

It is vital to ascertain the necessary time limit in keeping these documents in your state or country.

In addition to purging and storing files, all appointment books, laboratory logs, telephone message books, the facility's triage manual, and any other records pertaining to patient care should be kept and stored for future reference because patient information is valuable and could possibly be necessary in a medical-legal case.

All office records should be in closed files when not in use. Professional liability insurance policies, life insurance policies, canceled checks, wills, licenses, deeds, stocks, and bonds should be kept in a safe or in a fireproof box. Receipts for business and medical equipment and any warranties should also be kept in fireproof storage until you no longer have the equipment.

ACHIEVE UNIT OBJECTIVES

- ☐ Complete the Workbook activities to meet the learning objectives.
- ☐ Practice the procedures in this unit to meet the performance objectives.
- ☐ Apply your knowledge at the end of this chapter in completing the Critical Thinking Challenge and Activities, as well as the StudyWARE on your Student CD-ROM.

CRITICAL THINKING CHALLENGE

IMPACTING THE PATIENT, THE PRACTICE, AND YOUR CAREER

As an extern student, you have been placed in a busy family practice office. One of your first assigned responsibilities is to file outside reports in the charts after the physician has released them for filing. The office uses a numeric filing system; there is a cross-reference file for assigning the numeric codes to the appropriate patient. You complete your filing assignments for the day and return to the office the next week. The office manager asks you to come into her office in the afternoon and shows you the chart of Mathew George, which has George Mathews' lab results in it. Mr. Mathews has insulin-dependent diabetes.

QUESTIONS

1. What impact could this have on the patient?
2. What impact could this have on the practice?
3. What impact could this have on your career?

ACTIVITIES

1. Describe how you would respond to the following scenario:

   Manfred Hager was seen in the physician's office earlier today with acute respiratory failure from COPD; Mr. Hager was admitted to ICU in serious condition, which was documented in his medical record. This afternoon, you receive a phone call from an individual who inquires about Mr. Hager's condition. You inform the caller that Mr. Hager has been admitted to the ICU. The caller demands more information specific to his illness, which you cannot provide, but the individual does not understand why you cannot provide the information.

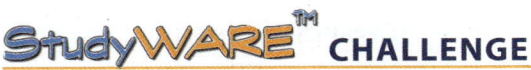 **CHALLENGE**

- Study with the flash cards for Chapter 7 to review the key terms in this chapter.
- Solve the hangman activities for Chapter 7.
- Complete the true/false quiz in test mode for Chapter 7.

RESOURCES

Lindh, W. Q., Pooler, M. S., Tamparo, C. D., & Dahl, B. M. (2006). *Thomson Delmar Learning's comprehensive medical assisting: Administrative and clinical competencies* (3rd ed.). Clifton Park, NY: Thomson Delmar Learning.

Kardex Systems, Inc., Marietta, OH 45750.

Krager, C., & Krager, C. (2004). *HIPAA for medical office personnel*. Clifton Park, NY: Thomson Delmar Learning.

Merriam-Webster, Inc. (Ed.). (1994). *Merriam-Webster's collegiate dictionary* (10th ed.). Springfield, MA: author.

Smead Manufacturing Co., Hastings, MN 55033.

White House Press Office, Washington, DC.

U.S. Department of Health and Human Services, Washington, DC.

WEB LINKS

www.kardex.com (Kardex® Information and Materials Management Systems)
   Provides information on office products.

www.smeadsoftware.com (Smead Software Solutions)
   Provides information on products that provide record management software.

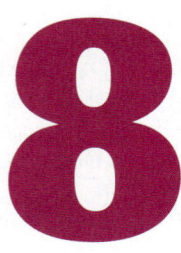

CHAPTER

8

Collecting Fees

The medical assistant has a great deal of responsibility in relation to ensuring his or her practitioner is paid for the services provided to all patients. Ultimately all charges incurred by the patient are the responsibility of the patient. There may be third parties such as insurance companies, employers, etc., who will play a role in the payment process; but this never removes the patients' responsibility for services they have received. The medical assistant should be equipped with information to refer **indigent** patients or those on limited incomes to local clinics that will treat the patients and charge them on a sliding scale according to their ability to pay. The medical assistant is involved in explaining fees and payment policies and virtually every aspect of collecting for the services the physician has provided.

UNIT 1
PAYING FOR MEDICAL SERVICES

OBJECTIVES

Upon completion of this unit, you will be able to achieve the following:

LEARNING Objectives

1. Spell and define, using the glossary at the back of the text, all the Words to Know in this unit.
2. Name the factors in determining fees for patient care.
3. List the information that should be obtained for every new patient.
4. List some circumstances when you may need to discuss payment planning with a patient.
5. Describe credit arrangements that can be used to finance medical care.
6. Describe the reason for accepting credit cards as payment for services rendered.

WORDS TO KNOW

complexity	indigent	substantial
date of birth (DOB)	Social Security number (SSN)	

 ## CERTIFICATION CONNECTION

CMA
Patient instruction
Releasing medical information
Physician-patient relationship
Computer applications
Bookkeeping systems
Third-party billing
Accounting and banking procedures

CMAS
Communication
Procedures
Confidentiality
Insurance billing and finances
Patient accounts

RMA
Terminology
Patient billing
Reception
Records and chart management

Most physicians have traditionally been reluctant to discuss fees with patients. It is fairly common for the medical assistant to be the one who must answer these questions. When a patient is unhappy about medical costs, it is important to listen and try to explain why the charges are as stated. The physician should be told when a patient is unhappy with the cost of treatment, and it may be necessary for the physician to talk with the patient about the concern regarding cost of care.

Physicians must set their fees based on their professional financial profile and the fees appropriate for similar specialists in the community. In considering the fee for services to the patient, the physician considers the time spent with the patient, the **complexity** of the diagnosis, and the treatment. In addition, the cost of maintaining an office and staff is considered. The physician can also obtain usual and customary fee schedules from the local medical society or a medical practice management firm.

In some instances, you will find that insurance companies and government agencies establish a fee profile for the physician based on charges averaged over a period of time. This is one of the reasons it is so critical to learn to code patient visits accurately. When such a profile is established, it represents the highest payment the insurance company or government agency will make for the services listed in the profile.

PERSONAL DATA SHEET

The patient should complete a personal data sheet at the initial office visit (Figure 8-1). This information form can be custom-designed and purchased from a printing company, or you may design one specifically for your office practice by using the office computer.

At each subsequent office visit, it is important to verify and update the patient's current phone, address, employment, and insurance information. Often patients may forget to inform you of a change because the nature of their visit is stressful. If you approach the patient in a polite and friendly manner to ask for the update, the patient is generally cooperative. The following information should always be obtained:

- Patient's full name, correctly spelled
- **Date of birth (DOB).** This is especially useful if your office treats two people with the same or similar names.
- **Social Security number (SSN)**
- Marital status
- Current address and length of time at that address (A person who moves frequently may lack stability in payment of bills.)
- Telephone numbers at home and at work or pager, cell phone, e-mail, and fax numbers
- Name and relationship of person legally responsible for charges. Under normal circumstances parents are

PATIENT DATA SHEET

Patient's Name _____

            Last   First   Middle

Address _____

City _____ State _____ Zip+4 _____

Date of Birth _____ Social Security Number _____

Home Phone _____ Pager/Cell Phone _____

Employer _____ Work Phone _____

Occupation _____

Address _____

INSURANCE INFORMATION

Subscriber's Name _____

Insurance Company _____

Policy Number _____ Group Number ____ Union/Local ____

If Group Insurance, Name of Policy Holder (e.g., employer, union)

_____

Insured's ID or Medicare Number (include any letters) _____

Effective Date of Insurance _____ Coverage _____

Exclusions or Exceptions _____

ADDITIONAL COVERAGE

Other Health Insurance? Yes _____ No _____

Copy of Insurance Card(s)? Yes _____ No _____

If Yes, Name of Policy Holder _____ Company _____

Plan Name and Address _____

Policy or Medical Assistance Number _____

Patient's Signature _____ Date _____

Subscriber's Signature _____ Date _____

(if patient is a minor)

FIGURE 8-1 Patient data sheet

Jason E. Jackson, MD
8247 Central Avenue
Stockdale, NY 23456-7890
345-678-9100

Date: 6-17-XX   Patient: <u>Julia Renee Price</u>

Party Responsible for Payment: <u>Martina J. Burnette</u>

I, <u>*Martina J. Burnette*</u>, agree to pay for all examinations and treatments for Julia Renee Price.

Margo Little   *6-17-XX*
Witness   Date

FIGURE 8-2 Example of third-party liability statement

MEDICAL RECORDS RELEASE   Date _____

I, Kendra Leigh Forest, 4406 Slate Run Drive, Bluestone MI,

request that all of my medical records be released from:

    Catherine R. Lang, MD
    431 S. Water Street
    Bluestone, MI 12345-6789
    123/789-0123

To: Jason E. Jackson, MD
    8247 Central Avenue
    Stockdale NY 23456-7890
    345/678-7890

Sonia D Philips *3-7-xx*   *Kendra Leigh Forest* *3-7-xx*
Witness   Date   Patient   Date

FIGURE 8-3 Records release form

---

considered responsible for the charges of their children. However, if a third party is involved, an oral agreement is not binding, and the individual who will pay the bill needs to sign a simple statement before care is given. This statement may be a form you have prepared or it may be a handwritten statement (Figure 8-2).

- Patient's occupation, with name, address, and phone number of employer. If a patient has a spouse, you should also obtain the spouse's occupation and name, address, and phone number of employer.
- The name of the person who referred the patient to your clinic. This information can be valuable if the patient later moves without leaving a forwarding address.
- Health insurance information. Ask to see the patient's identification card (or cards, if they are covered by more than one plan). You need to make a copy of both sides of the card(s) on your copy machine to be sure you have all the information. Some states require a consent for release of information separate from the printed one on insurance forms. If this is the case in your state, be sure that this form also is completed at the time of the first visit (Figure 8-3). Be sure you have complete information regarding all insurance carried.

- A copy of the patient's driver's license, if legal in your state, or the driver's license number. Patients who know that you have this information in their chart are more likely to take responsibility for their bills.

HIPAA

Most insurance carriers have begun to use numbers *other than* the insured's Social Security number for the policy number. This is another step at ensuring the protection of protected health information. You will see many different variations of combinations of letters and numbers as policy (identification) numbers.

PAYMENT PLANNING

The medical assistant can assist patients who are going to have a baby, elective surgery, or extensive therapy by helping them develop a payment plan. When the patient knows in advance that there will be costly medical expenses, the medical assistant should review the patient's health insurance coverage. Some physicians use a cost estimate sheet to give the patient an idea of the cost for surgery or long-term treatment (Figure 8-4). The estimate may include the approximate cost of the anesthetist, any consultants, and hospital charges. It is important the patient understand that the anticipated costs provided on the estimate are just that—an estimate. In the event of unforeseen complications or additional problems, expenses are likely to be higher than the estimate provided. Covering this topic thoroughly prior to the care being provided will aid the medical assistant in the collection efforts.

If it appears that the patient will need to pay a **substantial** sum out-of-pocket, the medical assistant should discuss with the patient the manner in which payments will be made. Even if patients have medical insurance, there could be a substantial amount that their particular insurance company does not pay, or the copay is a sizable amount. Often the costs accumulate over a long period of time, as with physical therapy, and the amount the patient owes is quite significant. Assisting the patient in planning a reasonable payment schedule for these expenses will help the patient to be more at ease and have less worry about financial matters. The patient can concentrate on getting well. If the patient does not have current resources to pay the full amount in one payment, the medical assistant should offer the option of a fixed sum as a down payment and regular payments of a fixed amount on specified dates. The Truth in Lending Act, which is enforced by the Federal Trade Commission, specifies that when there is an agreement between the physician and a patient to accept payment in more than four installments, the physician is required to provide disclosure of finance charges (Figure 8-5). The patient must sign this form in your presence, and the disclosure statement must be kept on file for 2 years. If

SURGERY COST ESTIMATE

Catherine R. Lang
123-789-0123

Patient _____ Date _____

Scheduled surgery time: _____

At _____ Hospital/Medical Center

On the day of your scheduled surgery you should arrive at _____ am/pm and go to the _____ floor.

Check with your insurance company for the cost that you are expected to pay (your co-pay) unless your insurance covers the total cost. Plan for budgeting payments or coinsurance for this service.

For your information, in addition to the hospital costs for your surgery without complications, you will be charged for the following:

• Operating Surgeon _____ $_____ to $_____
• Assisting Surgeon _____ $_____ to $_____
• Anesthetist _____ $_____ to $_____

The total cost of the surgery and related charges are based on the length of time for the procedure. Your costs also will vary with the procedure's complexity and length of time of your hospital stay. For the surgical procedure that you are having, the average length of stay in the hospital is _____ days. The hospital room charges depend on your preference of a semi-private or private room. Be sure to bring your insurance information with you the day of your surgery. You will be telephoned ahead of time by a hospital admissions clerk to discuss specific information and to give you a confirmed time for your surgery. This person may also ask you to come to the hospital a few days or a week before your surgery to do a series of blood tests and a preadmission exam.

If you have any questions or concerns, please call us at the number at the top of this estimate.

FIGURE 8-4 Example of a surgery cost estimate and information sheet

Catherine R. Lang, MD
431 S. Water Street
Bluestone, MI 12345-6789
123-789-0123

FEDERAL TRUTH IN LENDING STATEMENT
For Professional Services Provided

Patient _____ Date _____

Address _____
_____

Parent/Guardian _____
1. Fee for Service .... $_____
2. Down Payment .... $_____
3. Unpaid Balance .... $_____
4. Amount Financed .... $_____
5. Finance Charge .... $_____
6. Annual Percentage Rate
   of Finance Charge .... _____
7. Total Amount of Payments (#s 4 + 5) $_____
8. Deferred Payment Price (#s 1 + 5) $_____

Total payment due (#7) is payable to Dr. Catherine R. Lang at the above address in monthly payments of $_____, the first of which is payable on _____, 20XX. Each subsequent payment is due on the 15th of each month until paid in full.

_____ _____
Date   Signature of Patient/Parent/Guardian

FIGURE 8-5 A federal Truth in Lending form

the physician makes no specific arrangement for more than four payments and bills each month for the full amount, rather than installment amounts, there is no need for the signed statement.

CREDIT CARD USAGE

Our society enjoys convenience. This remains true even in paying for our medical expenses. Credit and debit cards are used in almost every facet of personal business, including paying copays, deductibles, and co-insurances. The credit card offers convenience in several ways. A checkbook is much bulkier and cannot be carried by two people at one time, whereas multiple cards can be issued for a credit card account; therefore each spouse can carry a card. Carrying cash to pay for services puts one at some risk in the event it is lost or stolen, whereas a credit card that is lost or stolen can be put on hold with a telephone call and another one re-issued. Many people do not even carry checkbooks any longer because they know "plastic" is accepted almost everywhere. Your office should display a sign indicating the methods of payment your practice accepts. Signs can be obtained from the bank the practice does business with reflecting the logos of the different types of cards you accept.

Acceptance of credit and debit card payments is especially helpful when placing a call to a patient who owes a balance on a delinquent account. The medical assistant can inform the patient that a credit card payment can be taken over the telephone to take care of the balance at the time of the call. A receipt can be mailed to the patient, and there is no need to continue to send statements and letters requesting payment.

Another advantage of credit card use for paying for medical services is that the monies are generally available to the physician within 24 hours of depositing. This service does not come without cost to the physician, however. Generally, a fee of 1% to 3% is assessed to the physicians, based upon either the revenue collected or the volume of credit card transactions. Many physicians feel this is to their advantage because office time is not used for collection of any delinquent accounts.

Some banks have set up financing programs in which the bank sends the money directly to the physician after deducting a handling charge. It is important for the physician to be sure that any outside financing arranged for patients is managed in a professional manner and that no unreasonable pressure tactics are used. In larger cities the physician may want to check credit references before extending credit for a large surgical fee. Some large medical societies have Bureaus of Medical Economics that perform a collection service and also provide credit information.

If you should receive a request from a credit bureau, you can say when a patient's account was opened, the current balance, and the largest amount of the account at any time. **However, you will be in violation of the law if you make any statements regarding paying habits of the patient or the character of the patient.**

ACHIEVE UNIT OBJECTIVES

- ☐ Complete the Workbook activities to meet the learning objectives.
- ☐ Apply your knowledge at the end of this chapter in completing the Critical Thinking Challenge and Activities, as well as the StudyWARE on your Student CD-ROM.

UNIT 2
BOOKKEEPING PROCEDURES

OBJECTIVES

Upon completion of this unit, you will be able to achieve the following:

LEARNING Objectives

1. Spell and define, using the glossary at the back of the text, all the Words to Know in this unit.
2. Describe exceptions to usual billing procedures.
3. Describe the advantages of a one-write bookkeeping system.

PERFORMANCE Objectives

1. Transfer charges from a charge slip to the daily log.
2. Post charges from the daily log to a patient ledger card.
3. Type an itemized statement.
4. Process a credit balance and refunds.

WORDS TO KNOW

assets	business	journalizing
bankruptcy	associate	ledgers
bookkeeper	agreement	petition
	(BAA)	posted

practice   protected health   trial balance
   management   information
   system (PMS)   (PHI)

CERTIFICATION CONNECTION

CMA   Fundamentals of
Legislation   computing
Formats
Equipment operation   **RMA**
Computer applications   Finance/bookkeeping
Bookkeeping systems   (terminology)
Accounting and banking   Patient billing
   procedures   Collections
                             Fundamental medical
CMAS   office accounting
Fundamental financial   procedures
   management   Financial mathematics
Patient accounts

BOOKKEEPING TERMS

Some of the basic terminology used in recording office business transactions includes:

- *Daily journal* or day sheet. All patient charges and receipts are recorded here each day.
- *Account.* A record for each patient, which will show charges, payments, and balance due.
- *Accounts receivable.* All of the outstanding accounts (amounts due).
- *Posting.* Transfer of information from one record to another.
- *Debit.* A charge, added to existing balance.
- *Credit.* A payment, subtracted from existing balance.
- *Balance.* Difference between debit and credit.
- *Adjustment.* Professional courtesy discounts, write-offs, or amounts not paid by insurance. If no adjustment column is included, discounts are listed in red in the debit column.
- *Debit balance.* Reflects the amount paid is less than the total due.
- *Credit balance.* Reflects the amount paid is greater than was due or the account is being paid in advance of service provided. A credit balance is written in red ink, circled, or noted in parentheses.

Daily Log

The medical assistant should record the charges, or no-charge visits, for each patient on the daily log sheet (Figure 8-6). They should be itemized, and a total should be put in the charge column. Payments should be placed in the credit (paid) column. Payment types should be noted in the paid column for ease of balancing the daily log. Note the check or money order number, type of credit card used, or whether cash was paid. When a patient pays in any form, a receipt should be given so the patient has a record of the payment. In particular, a receipt must be given to the patient after a cash payment, and patients should be informed that it is not safe to pay accounts by mailing cash payments. The daily log sheet will reflect the names of all patients treated in the office each day and any payments received in the mail or from patients who come to the office just to pay the bill. Unassigned columns on the daily log may be used to distribute charges or receipts among partners or to distribute charges by departments, such as laboratory, x-ray, or physical therapy, or by medication type in cases such as chemotherapy.

Patient Accounts

Many health care providers use computerized billing systems that allow for timely filing of encounters and itemized statements, with immediate access to patient demographic information and account status. Often these systems can also generate reports that are used to improve the efficiency of the practice.

Some health care providers use ledger cards. The medical assistant who must transfer the charges from the day sheet to the patient account card should do this when there will be a minimum of interruptions (Procedures 8-1 and 8-2). The variety of ledger cards available makes it possible to increase efficiency by using the one that best suits your needs. It is a good policy to place a small check mark on the day sheet after each entry has been **posted** to the account card. Then if you are interrupted you will know where to begin again in your posting job.

Statements

Statements (Procedure 8-3) must be accurate in every detail, from the name of the patient to the figures for charges and payments (Figure 8-7). If your office uses monthly billing, send out bills on the last day of the month. Your patients are more likely to pay if statements are received on a regular basis. If you have a large number of statements to send, cycle billing should be used. With this system, account cards are divided into groups to correspond to the number of times you will be billing. You then maintain the same cycle each month so that patients learn when to expect your statement. You might send A through F on the tenth of each month, G through M on the twentieth, and N through Z at the end of the month.

Statements can also be generated through your **practice management system (PMS)**. You may choose to

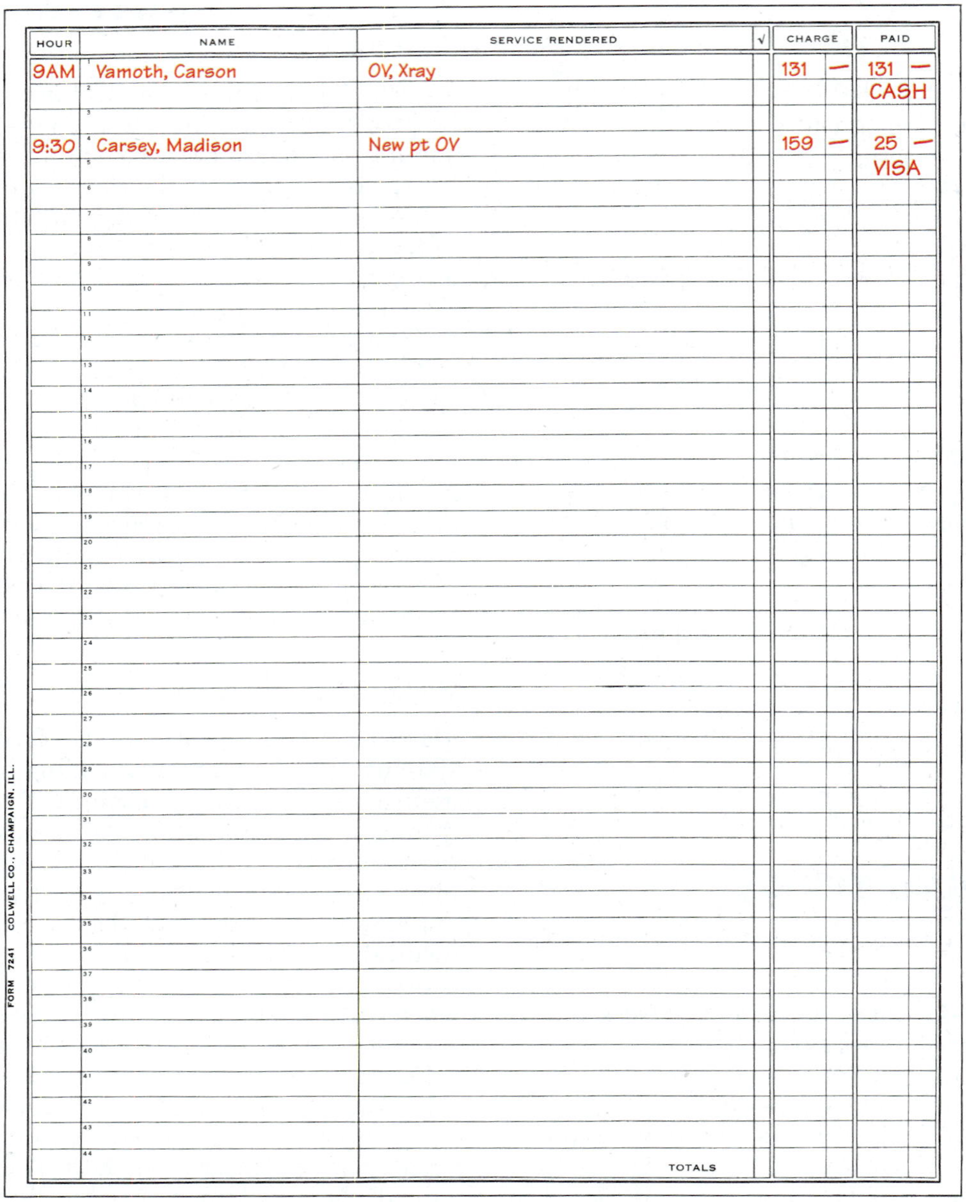

HOUR	NAME	SERVICE RENDERED	√	CHARGE	PAID
9AM	Vamoth, Carson	OV, Xray		131 —	131 — CASH
9:30	Carsey, Madison	New pt OV		159 —	25 — VISA
		TOTALS			

FIGURE 8-6 Daily log sheet

print and process them for mailing in house, or your practice may send the statements electronically to a billing service that may print, sort, stuff, add postage to, and mail the statements for you. It may be cost effective to handle statements in this fashion. Check around for the best pricing and service available in your area. Another service the outside company may offer is updated address information for your patients. This saves your practice valuable time and money by not having to deal with skip trace efforts. If your practice processes statements in house, check into renting or leasing envelope-stuffing machinery. The machinery folds, stuffs, and inserts statements quickly.

The medical assistant's role may be that of a bookkeeper. A **bookkeeper** is one who records information. You may be required to keep a record of accounts receiv-

able and payable. The office accountant or Chief Financial Officer (CFO) in larger organizations, will inform you of any records you need to provide to prepare summary reports of financial information, which are as important in the practice of medicine as in any well-run business. The accountant will analyze the figures and prepare reports that not only tell the present status of accounts receivable and payable, but compare current reports with other years or periods of time. A breakdown of the most cost-efficient procedures and least cost-efficient procedures may be revealed in such a summary. The accountant may be the person designated to prepare payroll checks and pay the quarterly amounts due to government agencies for taxes withheld.

The medical assistant who is going to do bookkeeping must be accurate in every detail. There is no "al-

8-1      Prepare a Patient Ledger Card

PURPOSE: Accurately prepare a patient ledger card.

EQUIPMENT: Blank ledger card(s), typewriter or pen with black ink, patient information sheet, or a computer.

PERFORMANCE OBJECTIVE: In a simulated medical office situation, prepare a patient ledger card following the steps in the procedure. The instructor will observe each step.

1. Type the name of the patient, last name first.
2. Type the complete address with zip code. **NOTE: On a ledger card to be photocopied, the name and address are completed in the same manner as an ad-** dress on an envelope, because the copy of the card is folded and mailed in a window envelope.
3. Type the name and address of the person responsible for charges, if different from the patient.
4. Type the telephone number of the patient.
5. Type the name of the insurance company.
6. Type the name of the referring individual.
7. If this is a continuation of a previous card, carry forward any balance due.

8-2      Record Charges and Credits

PURPOSE: Accurately record charges, payments, and adjustments on patient ledger cards/computerized account day sheets.

EQUIPMENT: Ledger cards, typewriter or pen with black ink, daily log, or a computer.

PERFORMANCE OBJECTIVE: In a simulated medical office situation, record charges, credits, and adjustments following the steps of the procedure. The instructor will observe each step.

1. Pull the ledger card for the patient.

   NOTE:

   - **If you can record charges near your ledger file it will be efficient to do one at a time. Tilt up the card behind the one you are posting to use as a marker.**

   - **If you must post away from your ledger file, pull all the cards you need at one time, then return all to the file when done.**

2. Post all charges and credits (payments and adjustments) for a patient and check them off on the day sheet before you go on to the next patient.

   NOTE:

   - **Use small, neat figures.**

   - **Note the dividing line between dollars and cents. In some cases this is a darker line.**

   - **Never use dollar signs on account cards.**

3. Charges are posted in the debit column. **RATIONALE: If a balance is shown on the card, add the new debit to get a new balance.**

4. Payments and adjustments are posted in the credit column and are subtracted from the balance due. **NOTE: If the credit is greater than the balance due, the difference is a credit balance and is shown in red.**

5. The balance column should always reflect the current status of the account.

most right" in bookkeeping. The work either is 100% correct, or it is incorrect and must be corrected. The bookkeeper must enjoy detail work and must make clear, legible figures using a fine-point, black ink pen. Care must be taken to record figures in correct columns as debit or credit and always in straight columns. Care must also be taken to place the decimal point correctly and always double check figures on a calculator or adding machine. An adding machine tape is helpful in that you can double check figures easily.

PROCEDURE PROCEDURE PROCEDURE PROCEDURE PROCEDURE PROCEDURE PROCEDURE

8-3  Generate an Itemized Statement

PURPOSE: Accurately prepare an itemized statement.

EQUIPMENT: Ledger cards, typewriter (or computer and printer), appropriate stationery for statement.

PERFORMANCE OBJECTIVE: In a simulated medical office situation, generate itemized statements with 100% accuracy following the steps in the procedure. The instructor will observe each step.

1. Stack ledger cards beside the computer or typewriter.
2. Assemble statement forms and window envelopes.
3. Stamp the ledger card on the line below the last entry with a date stamp.
4. Type the name and complete address in an area that will show in the window envelope.
5. If there is a balance from the previous month, list that first under services.

6. Type each service charge and payment for the current month.
7. The last line should show the current balance due.
   a. Generate an itemized patient account statement from the computerized billing system.
8. Fold and place the statement in an envelope with the address showing through the window.
   NOTE:
   - **You may want to stuff all the envelopes after you have typed all the statements.**
   - **Be careful to place only one statement in each envelope.**
9. Fan out several envelopes with flaps exposed.
10. Dampen a sponge and wipe over all the flaps at once.
    NOTE: Be careful not to overwet.
11. Fold down the flaps and seal.

Employees have been fired from their jobs because of carelessness with figures in simple math. You should practice adding and subtracting numbers without the use of paper and pen or computer. The bookkeeper who can independently compute numbers quickly and accurately is considered an asset to any office.

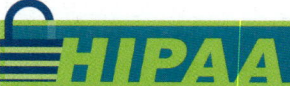

If it is decided that an outside company will be used to print and process your statements, you should have them sign a **Business Associate Agreement (BAA)**, thereby ensuring the company understands your expectations as to what they will do with the privileged information they will have access to. The BAA will also establish guidelines regarding what will occur if an inappropriate disclosure of **protected health information (PHI)** takes place.

Catherine R. Lang, MD
431 S. Water Street
Bluestone, MI 12345-6789
123-789-0123

Ms. Glenda Page
145 Central Avenue
Bluestone, MI 12349-6784
123-786-9876

| DATE | | DESCRIPTION | CHARGE | CREDITS | | CURRENT BALANCE |
				PAYMENTS	ADJ.	
		BALANCE FORWARD →				
4/12/XX	Sara	Allergy Injection	18.00			18.00
5/02/XX	Glenda	Exam	65.00	65.00		18.00
		UA	20.00			38.00
5/15/XX		Allergy Injection	18.00	20.00		36.00
5/18/XX	Sara	Exam	25.00	20.00		41.00
		Ace Wrap	10.00			51.00

276L   PLEASE PAY LAST AMOUNT IN THIS COLUMN ▲

FIGURE 8-7 An example of an itemized statement of a patient's account

THIS IS A COPY OF YOUR ACCOUNT AS IT APPEARS ON YOUR LEDGER CARD

BOOKKEEPING

As a bookkeeper, the medical assistant prepares the daily log or journal and posts charges and payments on the patient **ledger** card or enters the payment into the computer. The patient ledger card is a record of all charges or services rendered, any payments made by the patient or the insurance carrier, and any adjustments. If your office has a computer system that has software that includes a bookkeeping program, all charges and other information are entered into the computer. Make sure that you double check your entries to proofread for errors. Note that it is easy to transpose numbers as well as letters. The entries on the daily log are called **journalizing**. The entries should be kept in chronologic order. The total amount of cash and checks, including credit/debit card payments, should be recorded on a cash control sheet. This may be a daily record sheet or a monthly record showing an entire month with a line used each day to show income in cash and checks, any deposits made, and any amounts not deposited and therefore carried over to the next day.

When the balance is carried forward it is important to record it under "previous balance" for the next day, where it will be added to the total received to calculate "total on hand." This kind of record is also helpful in double checking your bank deposit slips. The cash and checks should equal the amount shown on the cash control sheet (Figure 8-8). This amount should also equal the amount of the bank deposit for the day.

An accounts receivable record should be kept daily. This record represents the total amount owed to the physician for services rendered. The total should be the same as the total of balances on all the active patient ledger records. The process of running such a total is called a **trial balance**. The accounts receivable balance is carried forward from month to month and added to the daily charges. The payments made by patients and any adjustments are subtracted to determine the true account receivable each day.

This single-entry method of bookkeeping records all increases and decreases in the **assets** of the practice. As-

sets are anything that have value that are owned by a business. Examples of assets are office furniture, equipment, the building itself, and the land on which the building stands.

EXCEPTIONS TO USUAL PROCEDURES

There are a number of exceptions to the usual billing procedures. Some physicians complete physical examinations for individuals applying for insurance coverage. In this case the bill is sent to the insurance company. Physicians who specialize in sports medicine and examine athletes may be paid by the school or team referring the patient.

When it is necessary to collect a bill owed by a deceased patient, the statement is sent to the estate of the deceased in care of any known next of kin at the patient's last known address. Do not address the statement to a relative unless you have a signed agreement that that person will be responsible for the bills. You may need to contact the probate court to obtain the name of the administrator of the estate if the patient expired in a nursing home and had no known next of kin.

When your office receives an official notice that a patient has filed for **bankruptcy**, you may send no more statements and can make no attempt to collect the account. The patient who has filed a wage earner's bankruptcy will pay a fixed amount to the court to be divided among the creditors. Your office may receive only a dollar at a time. Accept this and credit the account. You will be notified of a creditors' meeting in a straight **petition** for bankruptcy, but it is usually best just to be sure they have a copy of the statement and wait to see if you will receive any money. Sometimes the patient wishes to continue seeing the physician and will make payments on the account independently on a cash basis.

The physician may examine a patient in consultation in a legal claim, and in this case the person or agency requesting the consultation is responsible for

CASH CONTROL SHEET								
Day	Total Rec'd	Total Cash	Total Charges	Total Checks	Previous Balance	Total Available	Deposit	Balance Carried Forward
2	$2820.00	260.00	2820.00	2560.00	–0–	2820.00	2820.00	–0–
3	$ 600.00	–0–	600.00	600.00	–0–	600.00	–0–	500.00
4	$4750.00	650.00	4750.00	4100.00	500.00	6000.00	6000.00	–0–

FIGURE 8-8　Example of a cash control sheet

the charges. The statement is sent with the consultation report. Other examples of third-party billing are auto accidents, workers' compensation, and Medicaid.

Some offices use outside billing services to handle all aspects of their accounts receivable, insurance and patient billing, as well as collections. In this case you need to be sure all charges and payments are sent so that the statements will be accurate and complete. The disadvantage of this system is that you do not have records in your office of current balances for your patients. In this case, if patients ask you a question about their account, refer them to contact the outside billing service directly.

PEGBOARD SYSTEM

The pegboard system is referred to as the *write-it-once* system. Although pegboard systems are used less today than in the past, it is a very efficient system. This system shows that you can make an entry on the ledger, the daysheet, and the charge slip simultaneously. The base or board has pegs, which you should place up and to the left. This log holds all of your daily entries; it becomes a listing of patients seen, as well as a complete financial record of charges made and payments received. You position a shingle of receipt/charge slips on top of the daily log, with the notches fitted over the pegs. Working downward from the top of the daily log, the shingle must be placed so that the charge/receipt slip nearest the top of the pegboard has its posting line directly over the first available line on the daily log. At the beginning of each day this will be at the top of the daily log. These forms are prenumbered in the lower right

corner; be sure to use them in numeric sequence to preserve the strong audit trail designed into the system. The receipt/charge slip serves several functions. It is the charge slip for current fees; a receipt for any payment received either by check or cash; and a statement of account showing previous balance, today's charges, today's payments, and the new balance. It also shows the next appointment if there is one. After the pegboard system is completed you are ready for your first patient of the day (Figures 8-9A and B).

When you check in a patient, pull the appropriate ledger card from your file tray. If the patient is new to your practice, prepare a ledger card. Post to the first available charge/receipt slip the existing balance (if zero, write —0—), and the patient's name. What you are writing on the charge/receipt slip is being written simultaneously on the daily log sheet. You then detach the charge slip portion at the perforation and forward it to the doctor with the patient's clinical record. The doctor will check the services received by the patient and give the slip to the receptionist. The medical assistant will then position the ledger card so that the posting line of the receipt slip is directly over the first available line on the ledger card and post the receipt number, date, and professional services rendered, using the codes preprinted on the form. The total charges are figured from the charge slip and entered in the charge space on the receipt slip. This is the time to ask for payment. If there is no charge, the entry is written *n/c.*

Post any payment received in the paid space on the receipt slip. If there is no payment, record as —0—. Post the new balance in the appropriate space (again, if zero, write —0—). In one writing you have created for

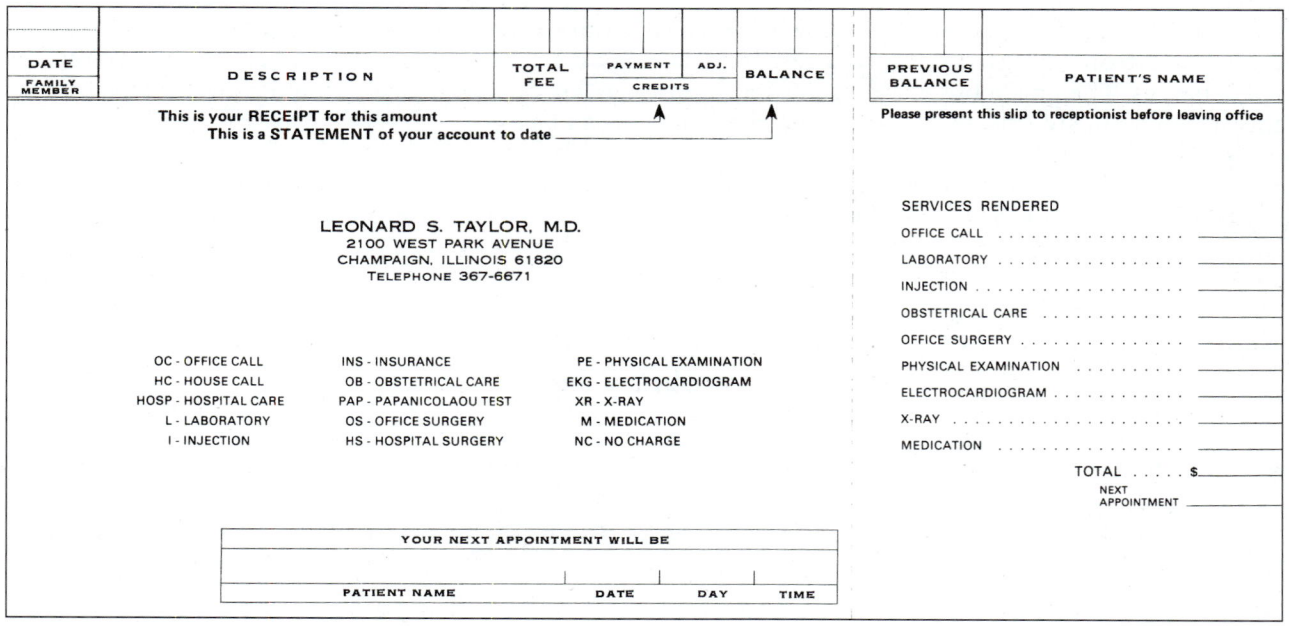

FIGURE 8-9A Pegboard charge, receipt, and appointment slip *(Courtesy of Colwell, a division of Patterson Dental Supply, Inc., 800-637-1140)*

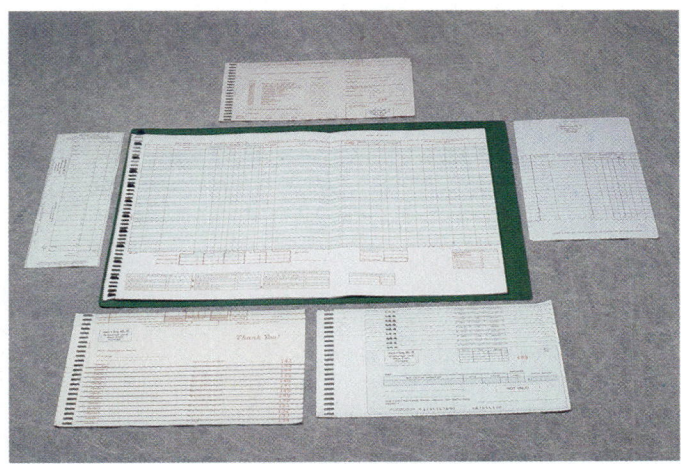

FIGURE 8-9B Pegboard, ledger card, and charge slip, ready to be assembled *(Courtesy of Colwell, a division of Patterson Dental Supply, Inc., 800-637-1140)*

the patient a combination receipt and statement. With the same one-write system, you have recorded the financial data you need on both the patient's ledger card and the daily log sheet. You are now ready to detach the receipt slip from the shingle at the perforation and remove it from the pegboard.

Arrange the patient's next appointment, if necessary, and record the date and time in the appropriate spot on the receipt slip. Also be sure to record the appointment in the appointment book before handing the receipt to the patient. Never write in the appointment space while the receipt is still attached to the shingle. The last step is to return the patient ledger card to its proper position in the file tray.

If payment is made other than when service is rendered, the receipt slip is used if the payment is made in person. If the payment is received in the mail, it is written directly on the ledger card and through it to the

---

PROCEDURE PROCEDURE PROCEDURE PROCEDURE PROCEDURE PROCEDURE PROCEDURE PROCEDURE

8-4  Process a Credit Balance and Refund

PURPOSE: Accurately process a credit balance and refund on patient ledger cards or a computerized account.

EQUIPMENT: Ledger cards, company check, envelope, typewriter or pen with black ink, or a computer.

PERFORMANCE OBJECTIVE: In a simulated medical office situation, process a credit balance for refund following the steps of the procedure. The instructor will observe each step.

1. Pull the ledger card for the patient. **NOTE: Review the credit on the ledger card to determine which date of service the credit is from. Be certain the credit is from an actual overpayment and not an adjustment taken incorrectly before proceeding to refund any money.**

2. Post the amount of the overpayment in the credit column with a negative (−) sign preceding it. This indicates the amount that will be refunded and the amount added back onto the account, bringing the balance to a zero status instead of a negative status.

3. Indicate on the ledger card the date the refund is being processed and to whom the refund is being issued. **NOTE:**

   ■ **If the refund is due to the patient, verify that you have the current address before mailing a check. Sometimes addresses are updated in the charts and not on the ledger cards/computer accounts.**

   ■ **If the refund is due to an insurance company, verify where the refund is to be mailed. Often the claims address and refund address differ from one another.**

4. Insert the company check into the typewriter.

5. Type the date the check is being issued in the appropriate field on the check.

6. Type the name of the person or company and their address in the Pay to the Order of section of the check.

7. Type the dollar amount to be refunded in the appropriate field of the check. Example: $32.75

8. Type that same dollar figure, spelling out the number values. Example: $32.75 would be reflected as Thirty Two and 75/100.

9. Remove the check from the typewriter. Check all typing for accuracy and compare the refund amount with the amount indicated on the ledger.

10. Obtain the proper signature(s) on the check. **NOTE: Checks may only be signed once a week, two times each month, etc. Keep the refund check in a safe or under lock and key until you are able to obtain the necessary signature(s).**

11. Copy the check for your accounts payable records.

12. Address an envelope to the payee.

13. Mail the check.

14. Return the ledger card to the ledger card file.

daily log sheet. The new balance is then posted on the ledger card after it is removed from the daily log sheet.

At the close of the day, remove remaining charge/receipt slips from the pegboard and verify that all receipt numbers are listed on the daily log. You will usually have several blank lines at the bottom of the sheet; on the last line write "End of (date)." Use a new log sheet each day. Add each column and post totals in spaces provided. Save your tapes and double check the figures. It is a simple matter to have an up-to-date account of accounts receivable at all times with this system. The total owed to the physician by all patients is increased by the day's charges and reduced by the day's receipts. The total of the receipts should be the amount of the bank deposit each day. To protect the employees of the office against a possible bank error, the daily cash summary and the bank deposit slip should be initialed by at least two persons.

ACHIEVE UNIT OBJECTIVES

- ■ **Complete the Workbook activities to meet the learning objectives.**
- ■ **Practice the procedures in this unit to meet the performance objectives.**
- ■ **Apply your knowledge at the end of this chapter in completing the Critical Thinking Challenge and Activities, as well as the StudyWARE on your Student CD-ROM.**

UNIT 3
BILLING AND COLLECTIONS

OBJECTIVES

Upon completion of this unit, you will be able to achieve the following:

LEARNING Objectives

1. **Spell and define, using the glossary at the back of the text, all the Words to Know in this unit.**
2. **Describe the advantages of computerized billing.**
3. **Describe different ways to locate an account in a computer system.**

4. **Describe an account history.**
5. **List reasons why billing statements would/should be withheld.**
6. **Define "aging of accounts."**
7. **Define the statute of limitations.**

PERFORMANCE Objectives

1. **Demonstrate use of the telephone for collection of accounts.**
2. **Compose collection letters suitable for a variety of situations.**
3. **Post NSF checks and collection agency payments.**

WORDS TO KNOW

account history	antagonize	idle
accounts receivable (A/R)	at the time of service (ATOS)	reputable
		skip
aging of accounts	date of service (DOS)	termination
alpha search	expended	year to date (YTD)

CERTIFICATION CONNECTION

CMA
Formats
Equipment operation
Computer applications
Bookkeeping systems
Coding systems
Accounting and banking procedures

CMAS
Medical records management
Medical office financial management
Medical office information processing

RMA
Finance/bookkeeping (terminology)
Patient billing
Collections
Fundamental medical office accounting procedures
Financial mathematics
Oral and written communication
Computer applications

Billing is the most common use for a computer in the medical office. Many different computer systems and software packages are available. It is important to determine the needs of the office prior to purchasing. You may also:

- Visit medical offices in similar practice to discuss advantages and disadvantages of their system and software packages
- Ask personnel in other medical practices about their equipment, software, and service
- Attend trade shows and demonstrations of medical practice software
- Have representatives from various companies present hands-on in-service presentations of their medical practice systems and software for all medical office personnel, including the physician(s)

Practice management software offers a variety of services, such as posting electronic claims, providing statistics on the number of patients seen per day (week, year), the diagnoses, and monthly and year-to-date billing information. Software should also provide Current Procedural Terminology (CPT) and International Classification of Diseases (ICD) codes for processing insurance claims efficiently. Although the system may provide CPT and ICD codes, care must be taken to ensure that the most current codes are used, because these are updated annually. Careful and thoughtful consideration must be given before a new system is purchased. Cost is the primary concern. Often the existing hardware may need to be upgraded, thereby eliminating the additional expense of a complete new system. If the billing system software is self-contained for the practice, patients' questions may be answered by the administrative assistant who handles the billing. Making a back-up file disk of all transactions daily is necessary to keep billing records secure. Patients can have more personalized service if all transactions are done on site. If the billing is sent out to a billing service, patients must deal with yet another person for any billing questions or problems. With planning, each method can be equally efficient.

The computer terminology for a patient ledger is **account history**. This is simply a record of the information that should be obtained for every new patient. You need to know the name and address of the person responsible for payment of the account, all data regarding insurance, and all necessary information regarding family members under the same insurance. All of this information can be obtained by viewing the Patient Data Sheet (see Figure 8-1). Generally, account histories follow the same organized plan used for ledger records of patients. You may have a choice in determining how you will find an account entered in the computer system. When the system will accept a number only, you must maintain a cross-reference file of an alphabetical listing of patients along with their account numbers. The easiest

and fastest method is called an **alpha search**. You type in the first few letters of the name, and the screen will automatically list all names of patients starting with those letters. You select the name you wish to make an entry for and type in the appropriate entry. The account history automatically shows the balance of the account and the number of days the account has been due. The entire account activity is available to view on the screen or to make a printout for the patient.

Your system should allow you to remove inactive accounts from the computer just as you remove inactive ledger cards. When a physician's office converts to a computerized system, it is important to choose the CPT codes commonly used in the practice. They are then programmed into the computer along with the descriptions of the codes and the fees to be charged for each. The ICD diagnostic codes may be programmed into the computer for insurance claims use. The computer can be coded to indicate the source of the payment: insurance, cash, check, money order, or credit/debit cards. Adjustment codes can be used for returned checks, contractual adjustments, and any cancelled account balances.

Some computers can be programmed to create charge slips. When the patient hands a computer-generated or handwritten charge slip (also referred to as a "walk out" slip, or superbill) to the receptionist, the charge and payments may be entered on the patient account history. In some offices, the receptionist would check to be sure that the services rendered were indicated on the charge slips and then send the slip to the business office for processing in the computer. All charge slips must be accounted for each day. The computer can create a statement or receipt to be handed to the patient before he or she leaves the office.

Computers can be programmed to lead you through the entry of every transaction by means of questions flashed on the screen or statements telling you what to do next. A medical assistant should be an accurate typist to operate a computer efficiently. If an error is posted on a transaction, there are ways to delete the transaction and start over again with a correct entry.

Computerized insurance claims can greatly improve cash flow. A claim can be completed in a matter of seconds for every patient visit.

Prior to sending any claims to a third party to acquire reimbursement, whether on behalf of the patient or for the practitioner, you need to have permission from the patient to file the claim on their behalf. This can be accomplished by having the patient sign and date a Centers for Medicare and Medicaid Services (CMS) form, or you may have specific language reflected in your new patient paperwork asking for this permission. It is a good idea to get the patient's signature annually for filing purposes. This is known as "signature on file." You should retain the paperwork reflecting the signature in the patient medical record.

The computer can speed up monthly billing and can be programmed to withhold statements on accounts for which you do not need or wish to send statements. Some examples are government-assisted patients, workers' compensation claims, or families of patients who have recently passed. The computer statement is considered to be an efficient collection method for the office because it not only shows an itemized account of all transactions, but the age of the account can also be listed. The statement should show the portion of the amount due that is current, over 30 days, over 60 days, and over 90 days.

The computer can furnish you with a daily journal report. This report can be a record of cash control also, as a listing of checks and cash can be shown separately. All computer systems should be set up to record deleted transactions as a printed safeguard against anyone tempted to steal money by entering a transaction and then deleting it.

The computer can be used to print out monthly summaries of charges, payments, and accounts receivable. **Year-to-date (YTD)** reports can be easily produced. You may print out a record of all outstanding accounts with an analysis of account aging.

The computer can provide a detailed list of patients seen by each physician in a large clinic and the services rendered. It can be used to determine the number of patients seen with a specific diagnosis or for a particular procedure for research summaries.

The medical assistant can also program the computer to print a list of hospital and nursing home patients to be seen. Such a list improves the accuracy in recording all out-of-office patient charges.

When you have a computer system with many of the printout possibilities detailed here, you will find the business management of the office much more efficient. You will also find you can complete all of these procedures in a fraction of the time required to do them by more conventional methods.

COLLECTING OVERDUE PAYMENTS

Computers can help in analyzing accounts receivable for accounts past due. This process is known as **aging of accounts**. It is basically a means of dividing accounts into categories according to the amount of time since the first billing date. Accounts are considered current if within 30 days of the billing date.

In order to stay on top of your **accounts receivable (A/R)** due from your patients, you will need some type of reporting system to see who has not paid on their account. Your practice management software should have the capability of allowing you to request reports by different parameters: accounts older than 60 days without any patient payment, accounts that have not had any patient payments posted in the last 30 days, etc. Each practice will have their own set of guidelines for when they consider an account to be delinquent. No account should be referred to a collection agency unless the physician has given approval for this to be done. However, federal law requires that when you have stated you will turn the account over for collection you must follow through and do so if the bill is not paid. You cannot make **idle** threats.

ADVANTAGEOUS COLLECTION OPPORTUNITIES

The patient's gratitude for the services received is highest at the time of service; that is why you should collect any amount of money that is appropriate at that time. If you are participating with the patient's insurance plan and they owe a copay **at the time of service (ATOS)**, collect only the copay. If they are uninsured (self-pay), collect in full ATOS. As soon as the patient leaves your office suite, the gratitude begins to fall, and so do your chances of collecting.

The best opportunity for collecting is when you have the patient in the office. This is true for balances due ATOS and for past due balances. The next opportunity you have to collect is by sending a statement, a collection letter, or over the telephone. The least effective means of collecting past due amounts is through written communication, whether by statement or letter. The best collection opportunity after face-to-face contact is by telephone.

The challenge with telephone collection is getting the patient to the phone. With technology advances such as caller identification and call blocking it can be difficult to even reach the patient by telephone. When a person other than the patient answers the telephone and asks who is calling, the patient may refuse to take the call once they realize it is the physician's office they owe money to calling.

Prior to making collection calls for your practice, obtain permission to do so from your office/business manager or the physician. Check the laws in your state for appropriate calling hours. Several states allow calls from 8:00 am until 9:00 pm. Do not call before or after stated times or you can be liable for harassment. Calls should be made from an area of the office where there is no chance that other patients or visitors to the office can overhear what you are saying. This is also a requirement of HIPAA.

MAKING THE COLLECTION CALL

Prior to making the collection call you should review the account to verify whether any payments have been posted since the collection report was run from your practice management system. Review the notes on the account. If notes are made in more than one area of an account, review the notes in each area. Know where the patient balance is coming from—which **date(s) of service(s) (DOS)**.

Verify that the insurance has been billed and has responded to any DOS in question. Have an idea of what you are going to say to the patient before placing the call. Attempt to reach the patient at the home number first. Try the cell and work number next. If the patient requests that you do not call them at work again, you must honor the request. Ask for the patient by full name when placing your call. "May I speak with Jane Ann Jones, please?" would be an appropriate way to begin your call. Once you are certain you are speaking with the correct person, identify yourself and where you are calling from: "This is Juanita Gomez calling from the business office of Dr. Pamela Martin." Get right to the point of your call: "I am calling today regarding your past due balance with Dr. Martin." You want to answer any questions the patient may have. If the patient indicates dissatisfaction with the results of medical care, be sure to convey this information to the physician. On occasion patients do not pay their bills because they have questions about the service or how it was billed. Once you have answered their questions they may be willing to pay the bill with a credit/debit card while you are on the phone. If the patient is unable to pay the entire bill all at once, offer them a payment plan following the guidelines that have been provided to you. Ten percent of the balance on a monthly basis is usually the lowest amount a practice will agree to. Once you agree on an amount you need to agree upon a specific date each month that the patient is going to *mail* the payment. If their balance is $250 and they agree to pay $25 a month on the 12th of each month, it will take them 10 months to pay the bill in full.

Balance of account $250
Monthly payment $25
250 ÷ 25 = 10 months

Typically payment plans are set up to have the account paid in full within 12 months. Extremely large balances from costly surgeries may take much longer than 12 months to pay. Follow your practice's guidelines when setting up payment plans with patients. At the end of the call repeat everything the patient has agreed upon: "Ms. Jones, you agree to pay $25 each month, on the 12th of the month, for the next 10 months to pay your balance in full." Note the account to reflect the agreement and any other pertinent information from the call. You should also discreetly note on the inside of the patient medical record about the payment plan. This will inform the receptionist about the agreement in case the patient questions something at their next visit, and the receptionist will know not to attempt to collect on the old balance when the patient is in the office.

Each month run the report that reflects accounts with delinquent balances. You can check the report for payments that have been received on the accounts where payment plans have been established. Your software might offer a report specifically for accounts that have been set to "budget payment plan." A specific field in the demographic or collection screen might be available to notate when an account has been set up for budget payments.

COLLECTION LETTERS

Some physicians feel that collection cards or stickers are a sufficient reminder, but others prefer the use of collection letters (Procedure 8-5). Consult the office procedure manual or your employer regarding preferences for follow-up on the collection of accounts. You may want to compose a series of standardized letters that you can personalize as needed (Figure 8-10). When

    Since your last office visit in May we haven't received any word
of how you are feeling or any payments on your account.

    If arrangements can't be made to pay the full amount of $____ by
June 12, please let us know so that the office can help you make arrangements
for your payments.

    You have always paid promptly on your account in the past, so you
must have accidentally overlooked the statements we've sent. If that is
the case, please accept this as a friendly note to remind you of your
account due in the amount of $_____.

    We can no longer carry your account on our books. The balance of $_____
must be paid within 10 days.

    Our collection agency receives all delinquent accounts on the 25th of
each month.

FIGURE 8-10   Three different samples of possible wording for collection letters

8-5  Compose a Collection Letter

PURPOSE: Compose collection letters appropriate for the aged accounts.

EQUIPMENT: Personal computer or typewriter, stationery, patient ledgers, envelopes.

PERFORMANCE OBJECTIVE: Using a typewriter or a personal computer, compose appropriate mailable collection letters for assigned accounts to be collected according to the procedure that follows.

1. Identify patients to whom an initial collection letter should be sent. **NOTE: If you categorize your collection accounts you will be more efficient. Complete all #1 letters before proceeding to all #2 letters, etc.**

2. Compose a rough draft, with the first paragraph indicating why you are writing.

3. The second paragraph should indicate what response or reaction you expect.

4. Reread the rough draft to be sure you have written clearly, correctly spelled words (if using a spell checker, be careful to proofread the letter to make sure you have not missed an error before you print from the computer or before you take the letter out of the typewriter), and correctly punctuated sentences.

5. Type the letter.

   Note:

   - **Follow standard letter form (block or modified block).**

   - **Proofread the letter.**

   - **Sign the letter with your name unless the physician wishes to sign. Remember to type your position below your name and your title (Mr., Mrs., Miss, or Ms.) before your name.**

   - **Do not use identification initials if you sign the letter.**

6. If using a computer software program that prints address labels, print those needed and affix to the envelopes.

7. Fold the letter, place it in the envelope, seal it, affix appropriate postage, and mail.

---

composing collection letters, avoid words that tend to **antagonize**, such as *neglected, ignored,* and *failure*. Words such as *missed, overlooked,* and *forgotten* are not quite so negative and seem more human. Decide whether you are going to use a series of two or three letters. The last letter in the series will usually inform the patient that you must resort to a collection agency if you do not receive payment by a *specified* date. Use your knowledge of the patient to decide what type of letter to use. You would use a stronger-sounding first letter for someone with a poor payment record. For a patient who has an excellent payment record, your first letter would be a gentle reminder. Every effort must be **expended** to collect as many accounts as possible without resorting to a collection agency, which charges a percentage of everything collected. Most offices avoid collection agencies if at all possible.

An example of a form letter that can be used to obtain an answer in writing of reasons for nonpayment of an account is shown in Figure 8-11. If you can get this kind of letter signed by patients, you not only know the reasons for nonpayment, but you have a signed paper acknowledging the amounts they owe the physician. If you know the reason for nonpayment, it is easier to help work out a solution for payment. If the payment is not made within the prescribed period used by your office, the fact that you have a signed statement from the patient acknowledging the amount owed is helpful in a collection situation. The patient cannot deny the debt.

Each state has laws (called *statutes of limitations*) that establish the number of years during which legal collection procedures may be filed against a patient. If a patient is being treated for a chronic illness, there is no **termination** of the illness or treatment unless the patient dies or changes physicians. The last date of debit or credit on the patient account card is the starting date for that particular debt. If the last date was June 2006, a 2-year statute could be collected through June 2008. In written contracts the statute of limitations starts from the date due. Some states have a shorter time limit on the statute of limitations on single entry (single charge) accounts.

When statements you have mailed are returned marked *moved, no forwarding address,* you have to consider the possibility that the patient is a **skip** (collection agency slang), or has moved to avoid payment of bills. The first step is to check your records to make sure you mailed to the correct name, address, and zip code. If

Catherine R. Lang, MD
431 S. Water Street
Bluestone, MI 12345-6789
123-789-0123

May 23, 20XX

Ms Glenda Page
145 Central Avenue
Bluestone, MI 12349-6784
123-786-9876

Dear Ms. Page:

Our policy is giving our patients the best medical services possible. We also expect that payments for our services be made in a timely manner. Because your account is past due, and before it is turned over to a collection agency, we would like to hear from you about what can be done to settle your account. Please select your choice of how you would like to take care of your obligation by checking one of the following, sign and return to us within 3 days from its receipt. Your account balance is $_____.

☐ I would prefer to settle this account. Payment in full is enclosed.

☐ I would like to make regular payments of $_____/month until the account is paid in full. My first payment is enclosed.

☐ I would prefer that you assign this account to a collection agency. (Failure to return this letter will automatically result in this action.)

☐ I don't believe I owe this amount for the following reasons(s):

_____
Signature of patient   Date

Please indicate your preference above and sign and return this letter.

Thank you for your cooperation.

Sincerely,

Catherine R. Lang, MD

Catherine R. Lang, MD

FIGURE 8-11   Sample collection letter requesting statement from patient explaining how account will be settled

these are all correct, place a telephone call to see if the old phone number was transferred to a new address. You may call referring individuals to try to obtain a new address for the patient, although you must not indicate your reason for needing the new address other than that you need to verify it. You may call the patient's employer for information regarding address change, identifying yourself by name only and asking that the patient return your call. You may find the patient simply forgot to inform the post office of an address change. You may also find the patient has left his or her place of employment, in which case you should check with your employer about referring the account for collection. The longer you wait, the less chance you have to collect.

Your employer should have arrangements with a **reputable** collection agency. The office reputation can be severely damaged if the agency you work with uses unethical collection methods. When the decision to refer an account for collection has been made by your employer or the business/office manager, send the collection agency the full name of the patient, name of spouse or person responsible for the bill, last known address, full amount of debt, date of last entry on ledger card or computerized account, occupation of debtor, and business address. Send no further statements, and refer any calls regarding the account to the collection agency. If you should receive any information regarding the account or any payments, you should forward them to the collection agency.

PROCEDURE PROCEDURE PROCEDURE PROCEDURE PROCEDURE PROCEDURE PROCEDURE PROCEDURE

8-6  Post Non-Sufficient Funds (NSF) Checks and Collection Agency Payments

PURPOSE: Post NSF checks and collection agency payments on ledger cards or a computerized account.

EQUIPMENT: Ledger cards, returned NSF checks from the bank, checks from the collection agency, typewriter or pen with black ink, or a computer.

PERFORMANCE OBJECTIVE: In a simulated medical office situation, accurately post NSF checks and collection agency payments following the steps of the procedure. The instructor will observe each step.

SCENARIO: Your office recently placed several accounts with an outside collection agency the practice uses for collection efforts when the practice has been unsuccessful in collecting the debt from the patient. One of the accounts was turned over to the agency because the patient had a habit of presenting checks that bounced due to lack of funds in their account to cover the amount the checks were issued for. Today you received another NSF check written for payment on this patient's account. You also received the first collection agency payment on this same account.

1. Pull the ledger card for the patient.

2. Post the NSF check under the debit/charges column, adding back onto the account, the amount the check was originally issued for. **NOTE: Debit the account the amount that was originally credited to the account. You originally *de*creased the account balance for** the amount the check was written for. Now you want to *in*crease the account balance for this same amount since the check did not clear the bank.

3. Date your entry, noting NSF on the description portion of the ledger card. **NOTE: The balance that was created by adding back in the NSF check amount will need to be placed with the collection agency.**

4. Review the check sent from the collection agency..

5. Post the amount of the check received from the collection agency in the credit column on the ledger card. Compute the new balance.

NOTE:

■ **If your practice's protocol is to adjust all balances from the accounts with an adjustment indicating "placed with outside collections" at the time you turn the account over to the agency, you may need to make an additional adjustment to the account. Make certain you do not reflect a credit on the account by posting the collection agency payment.**

■ **If your practice's protocol is to reflect the amount of the payment the collection agency withheld as their fee for collecting on outstanding balances, an additional adjustment may be required.**

ACHIEVE UNIT OBJECTIVES

■ **Complete the Workbook activities to meet the learning objectives.**

■ **Practice the procedures in this unit to meet the performance objectives.**

■ **Apply your knowledge at the end of this chapter in completing the Critical Thinking Challenge and Activities, as well as the StudyWARE on your Student CD-ROM.**

ACTIVITIES

1. Select two solo practitioner web sites and two group web sites to perform this activity. Compare the type of information reflected on each web site. Look for the following:

   ● Are their hours listed?
   ● Methods of payment accepted
   ● Biography of the physician(s)
   ● Health plans physician(s) are participating in
   ● Collection policies

   Considering only the information posted on the web site, which of the four practices would you select to

CRITICAL THINKING CHALLENGE

IMPACTING THE PATIENT, THE PRACTICE, AND YOUR CAREER

It was Clara's second day at the office. A coworker, Yvonne, was helping Clara get settled and showed her how to obtain a completed data sheet for each patient. After lunch Yvonne noticed that one of the charts of the patients seen in the morning did not have a patient data form. When asked why, Clara said that the patient could not understand her, so Clara had let it go. Taking a closer look at the chart, they realized the patient was new to the area and spoke very little English. Yvonne asked the physician about this, who said that the patient was only in for some medicine for a rash on her hands and that a data sheet was not necessary. Looking up the charges and posting of accounts, Yvonne found that the patient had paid cash for the visit.

HOW MIGHT THE PATIENT BE AFFECTED IN THIS SITUATION?

1. Is it possible that due to the language barrier that the patient could not clearly convey a chief complaint about the rash on her hands?
2. What if the patient had allergies that she was unable to clearly communicate to the physician and support staff?
3. Was she able to understand the directions provided to her at the time of service regarding use of the medication for the rash?

WHAT IMPACT MIGHT THIS SITUATION HAVE ON THE PRACTICE?

1. How would the practice reach the patient if there were a problem with the medication that was provided or prescribed ATOS?
2. If upon a closer look at the cash that was presented for payment, after the patient left, it was realized to be counterfeit, how would the practice recover the lost funds?
3. Should a new employee be shown a task one time and then left alone to perform the task without any guided supervision? Should someone witness the new employee performing each task at least once during his or her orientation?

COULD THERE BE ANY POSSIBLE EFFECTS ON YVONNE'S OR CLARA'S CAREERS?

1. How could Clara have handled the situation differently?
2. Is there reason to be concerned about Clara's judgment in this situation?
3. Did Yvonne respond appropriately?

go to and why? What similarities do all four sites reflect? Are there specific similarities on the solo practitioner web sites versus the group practices?

2. Role-play with a classmate in a collection call scenario. One student will be the patient and the other will be the medical assistant placing the collection call. Work through the following scenario:

Erika Baker has been asked by her office manager to call patients today who have a patient balance between $100 and $500 that is past due. Her manager has told her that she expects her to collect on at least 25% of the accounts she calls on today. It is getting late in the afternoon, with only one hour left in the business day. Erika is behind meeting the 25% goal her leader established for her. The next person on the list is a patient Erika remembers from working at the front desk during the maternity leave of another coworker. This patient was routinely late for her appointments, was rather loud, and always brought food into the waiting room, leaving her trash behind when she was called to the exam room. When anyone attempted to collect her copays ATOS, the patient had every excuse imaginable and would become even louder if anyone continued to pursue her for the day's payment. It is time to place the call.

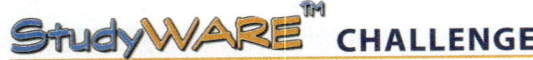 **CHALLENGE**

- Study with the flash cards for Chapter 8 to review the key terms in this chapter.
- Solve the crossword puzzle for Chapter 8.
- Complete the multiple choice quiz in test mode for Chapter 8.

RESOURCES

Lindh, W. Q., Pooler, M. S., Tamparo, C. D., & Dahl, B. M. (2006). *Thomson Delmar Learning's comprehensive medical assisting: Administrative and clinical competencies* (3rd ed.). Clifton Park, NY: Thomson Delmar Learning.

Simmers, L. (2004). *Diversified health occupations* (6th ed.). Clifton Park, NY: Thomson Delmar Learning.

WEB LINKS

www.ftc.gov/os/statutes/fdcpa/fdcpact.htm (Fair Debt Collection Practices Act)
Provides guidelines for fairly collecting on debts.

www.nclc.com (National Consumer Law Center)
Provides information pertaining to medical debt and how to get out of it. Click on the Action Agenda link and then the Older Consumers link. This page contains links to additional topics, including consumer information for seniors, which leads to specific articles, such as "Medical Debt and Seniors: How Consumer Law Can Help."

www.nlm.nih.gov/services/freemedcare_int.html. (United States National Library of Medicine)
Reflects links to web pages relating to discounted or free medical care.

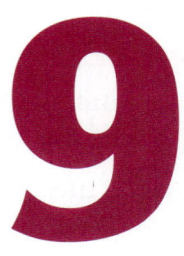

Health Care Coverage

The largest industry in the United States is insurance. The purpose of insurance is to protect us or compensate us from losses we may incur. We are able to insure our homes, automobiles, health, life, and valuables; however, this protection from loss comes at a cost. Premiums for insurance coverage of any type bear expense. The amount of coverage one selects and the amount of deductible associated with the policy will determine the expenses the insured will encounter.

In the medical field you will come across many different types of insurance coverage; health maintenance organization plans (HMOs), preferred provider health organizations (PPOs), health savings accounts (HSAs), health reimbursement arrangements (HRAs), and traditional style-health plans. People like to have choices. Employers like to be able to offer choices. Selecting the plan that best fits the employer's or the employee's wallet or that of the self-insured can require a bit of shopping around to determine the best product for the best price.

While the costs associated with medical care continue to escalate, insurance agencies continue to look for ways to cut costs. The U.S. government continues to spend thousands of dollars searching for a better way to cover and contain medical expenses. Yet the focus should not only be on the expenses associated with medical care but also on patients and their needs. Patients (consumers) should not have to worry if the latest and greatest diagnostic test available for their condition will be covered by their insurance; or should they?

UNIT 1
Fundamentals of Managed Care

UNIT 2
Health Care Plans

UNIT 3
Preparing Claims

The debate continues regarding just how much of our medical expenses insurance should cover. One belief is that if you keep patients involved in paying for portions of their health care, they will make wiser spending choices than they would if insurance paid 100% of all health care expenses.

What is certain is that the traditional type of insurance that once covered the cost of our medical care is fast becoming extinct. Even though traditional private insurance is fading, there are still individuals who choose to pay high premiums so that they may have the flexibility to seek medical care from health care professionals of their choice. This is referred to as fee-for-service care. The different types of plans are briefly explained in Unit 1 and are discussed further in Unit 2 of this chapter.

Health care reform has, in many cases, changed the way individuals select a physician. Often members of health insurance plans are required to select a physician from a published directory of participating physicians. The directory lists the physicians who have signed agreements with the insurance plan to provide care for their members. The physicians are listed by their specialty and the county of location. Many large insurance companies publish their provider directories online on the company's web site. The web site should reflect the most accurate listing of participating physicians. Patients should call the office of their selected provider (physician) to determine whether they are accepting new patients and to be certain the provider is currently participating with their health care plan. (The printed directory may not have the latest additions or deletions of providers.)

Both administrative and clinical medical assistants will find it necessary to keep abreast of changes in insurance billing and coding procedures and learn to **implement** them in a timely manner to guarantee the income of the practice. A discussion of the language of insurance, managed care, various medical care plans, and preparing claims for payment is offered in this chapter.

UNIT 1
FUNDAMENTALS OF MANAGED CARE

OBJECTIVES

Upon completion of this unit, you will be able to achieve the following:

LEARNING Objectives

1. Spell and define, using the glossary at the back of this text, all the Words to Know in this unit.
2. Describe the changes in health care coverage in the last two decades and the reasons for the change.
3. Explain the purpose of HMOs.
4. Explain the concept of managed care.
5. Distinguish the two major classes of health insurance.
6. Explain the reason for keeping patient insurance information confidential.
7. Define the terms listed in this unit.
8. List the different types of health insurance discussed in this unit.
9. Explain the birthday rule.

WORDS TO KNOW

birthday rule	direct payment	primary
cessation	encompass	reimbursement
coordination of benefits	implement	secondary
	premium	

CERTIFICATION CONNECTION

CMA
Patient instruction
Legislation
Releasing medical
  information
Physician-patient
  relationship

CMAS
Insurance processing
Fundamental financial
  management

RMA
Records and chart
  management

HEALTH MAINTENANCE ORGANIZATIONS

Managed care is a phrase regarding health insurance that became popular in the late 1980s in the United States. Initially, it was used in the early 1970s to convey the concept of promoting good health and preventive medicine. The contracts of these plans, which were negotiated between the insurance company and the employer, grew in popularity. This medical insurance coverage is a great employee benefit and has created much competition over the years. These insurance plans are referred to as health maintenance organizations (HMOs). The contracts offer people affordable health care plans because they are provided through their place of employment at a reasonable cost. The employer pays a large amount of the cost for the plan. The employee's cost is a reasonable group **premium** rate for health insurance coverage (a part of their employee benefits) that requires only a copayment at the time of the medical service. This is a good arrangement for individuals and families. These organizations employ physicians and other providers of medical care, and patients visit them for their needs. Today, managed care is an organized system of medical team members and groups who provide quality and cost-effective care that **encompasses** both the delivery of health care and the payment of these services.

The primary purpose of HMOs is the containment of health care costs. Promoting wellness by offering members counseling about nutrition, exercise programs, stress management, weight control, low-fat diet, smoking **cessation**, drug rehabilitation, and the like are efforts to keep people well and thereby cut the costs of medical care. Encouragement of annual physicals and PAP tests, breast self-exams, testicular self-exams, mammographies, prenatal programs, well-baby check-ups, and immunizations, and, in general, requesting that people see their physician as soon as any problems are noticed, all help to reduce medical care costs.

The two major types of health insurance are individual and group. Any individual may buy individual health insurance by paying the required premium. Group health insurance generally costs less and is more comprehensive. The group may be employees, a union, or any other party. Complete coverage may or may not be paid by the employer. The employee may have to pay an additional premium to include other family members in the coverage. Most people have some form of health and accident insurance coverage because they realize that a serious illness or injury can be devastating to family or individual finances. Insurance seldom pays all medical costs.

There are many different types of medical care coverage plans (third-party payers). They will be discussed further in this chapter. A brief definition of each type can be found in the list of important terms in Table 9-1 that are used in working with patients and their various plans. Those you will be in contact with are Medicare, Medicaid, TRICARE (CHAMPUS), CHAMPVA, workers' compensation, HMOs, preferred provider organizations (PPOs), and private insurance companies.

One of the most helpful points that the medical assistant can stress to patients is to have them check their insurance policy regarding their coverage. Many times there is a misunderstanding or a lack of comprehension on the patient's part as to the type of coverage their insurance allows. If the patient seems to be confused, it is a good idea to suggest that he phone the insurance company and speak to someone in customer service. This is helpful to the patient because he receives answers to his questions. Even though it would be a kind gesture on the medical assistant's part to go over the policy with the patient, there is not sufficient time for this activity in a professional setting where other patients need attention. It is fair to let patients know that not all physicians are members of all plans. Each insurance company sends members a packet of information when the contract is issued. Periodic supplemental information should also be received by the patient in the mail. You can ask the patient to gather this together and look for a *provider of services* booklet. This will help the patient to find the names of the physicians who are participating members of the patient's HMO.

Primary and Secondary Insurance Coverage

When greeting the patient in the office upon arrival for an appointment, ask the patient for a current insurance card(s). Make a copy of both sides of the card(s); it will be needed to complete forms or to request information regarding that patient and her coverage

TABLE 9-1 Terms Used in Health Insurance

Accounts payable—The total amount owed by the practice to suppliers and other service providers.

Accounts receivable—The total amount of all charges for services rendered to patients that have not been paid to the physician.

Admitting physician—The physician who admits a patient to the hospital (not necessarily the patient's attending physician).

Advance directives—A printed and signed statement to direct those who will take care of medical decisions for a patient when the patient becomes unable to make decisions. (Also known as a living will.)

Assignment of benefits—The authorized signature of the patient for payment to be paid directly to the physician for services.

Attending physician—The physician who cares for a patient in the hospital (not necessarily the physician who admitted the patient).

Authorization to release medical information (release of medical information form)—A form that must be signed by the patient before any information may be given to an insurance company.

Balance billing—The amount of the charges to the patient for medical services that the insurance company did not pay.

Capitation—The health care provider is automatically paid a fixed amount per month regardless of provided services for each patient who is a member of a particular insurance organization.

Civilian Health and Medical Program of the Veterans' Administration (CHAMPVA)—Established in 1973 for the spouses and dependent children of veterans who have total, permanent, service-connected disabilities.

Claim—A request for payment under an insurance organization made by either the physician (medical assistant) or the patient.

Coding—Transference of words into numbers to facilitate the use of computers in claim processing.

Coordination of benefits (COB)—Procedures used by insurers to avoid duplication of payment on claims when the patient has more than one policy. One insurance becomes the primary payer, and no more than 100% of the costs are covered.

Copayment or coinsurance—A specified amount that the insured must pay toward the charge for professional services rendered.

Current Procedural Terminology code (CPT)—Coding system published by the American Medical Association that translates services received by a patient into a numeric value for convenience and continuity of reporting these services to third parties for payment. The system is recognized by governmental payers and private insurance companies.

Deductible—A predetermined amount that the insured must pay each year before the insurance company will pay for an accident or illness.

Diagnosis related group (DRG)—A system developed by Yale University to group together major diagnostic categories, organized by body systems, from which the 470 DRGs are drawn.

Effective date—The date when the insurance policy goes into effect.

Electronic claims—Also referred to as electronic media claims, electronic data interchange, and electronic claims processing.

Encounter form—See "Superbill."

Endorser—The one who writes his/her signature on the back of a check that is made out to another person.

Early and periodic screening, diagnosis, and treatment (EPSDT)—This program requires screening and diagnostic services to determine any diseases or disorders, as well as complete health care, in children from birth through 21 years. (Also called Healthchek.)

Explanation of benefits (EOB)—A printed description of the benefits provided by the insurer to the beneficiary.

Fee disclosure—The action of health care providers informing patients of charges before the services are performed.

Fee schedule—A list of approved professional services for which the insurance company will pay with the maximum fee paid for each service.

Fee slip—A printed (computer) form with the patient's information, listing the services and code numbers with the charges.

Gatekeeper—A term given to a primary care physician for coordinating the patient's care to specialists, hospital admissions, and so on.

Group insurance—Insurance offered to all employees by an employer.

CMS 1500—The standard claim form of the Centers for Medicare and Medicaid Services to submit physician services for third-party (insurance companies) payment.

Health Care Procedural Coding System (HCPCS Code)—An alphanumeric coding system devised by the federal Centers for Medicare and Medicaid Services (CMS) as a supplement to the CPT code and distributed by the regional fiscal agents of Medicare, TRICARE (CHAMPUS), and Medicaid.

Health maintenance organization (HMO)—A prepaid group practice serving a specific geographic area with a wide range of comprehensive health care at a fixed fee schedule; HMOs are interested in promoting wellness and good health, thus containing the cost of health care. These can be sponsored and operated by the government, medical schools, clinics, foundations, hospitals, employers, labor unions, hospital medical plans, or the Veterans' Administration.

Indemnity plan—A commercial plan in which the company (insurance) or group reimburses physician or beneficiaries for services.

(continues)

TABLE 9-1   Terms Used in Health Insurance (continued)

Independent practice association (IPA)—A group of independent physicians who provide health care to a group of patients who pay an annual fee in advance.

Individual insurance—Insurance purchased by an individual for self and any eligible dependents.

International Classification of Diseases (current number), Revision, Clinical Modification (ICD-9-CM)—The coding system used to document diseases, injuries, illnesses, and mortalities.

Loss-of-income benefits—Payments made to an insured person to help replace income lost through inability to work because of an insured disability.

Managed care—A system of medical team members organized into groups to provide quality and cost-effective care that encompasses both the delivery of health care and payment of the services.

Medicaid—A joint funding program by federal and state governments (excluding Arizona) for low-income patients on public assistance for their medical care.

Medicare fee schedule—A list of approved professional services that Medicare will pay for with the maximum fee that it pays for each service.

Medigap (Medifill)—Private insurance to supplement Medicare benefits for noncovered services.

Member physician—A physician who has contracted to participate with an insurance company to be reimbursed for services according to the company's plan.

National Committee for Quality Assurance (NCQA)—A nonprofit organization created to improve patient care quality and health plan performance in partnership with managed care plans, purchasers, consumers, and the public sector.

Out-of-area—HMO members are generally covered for emergency services out of their geographic area, but other coverages may not always be provided.

Patient status—Refers to patient's eligibility for benefits. Insurance companies frequently have stipulations that services be provided on an inpatient or outpatient basis; there are also requirements for prior authorization from the insurance company for certain services or procedures to be performed.

Point-of-service (POS) plan—An open-ended HMO, POS encourages their members to choose a primary care physician.

Preadmission testing (PAT)—Routine tests required for all patients before hospital admission to screen for abnormal findings that could interfere with the patients' hospital stay or scheduled procedure.

Precertification—Prior authorization must be obtained before the patient is admitted to the hospital or some specified outpatient or in-office procedures.

Preexisting condition—A condition that existed before the insured's policy was issued.

Preferred provider organization (PPO)—This plan offers different insurance coverage depending on whether the patient receives services from a contracting network or non-network physician. The benefits are higher if the physician provider is a member of the PPO (or is a network physician).

Premium—Monies paid for an insurance contract.

Release of medical information form (authorization to release medical information)—A form that must be signed by the patient before any information may be given to an insurance company.

Resource-based relative value scale (RBRVS)—Fee schedule based on relative value of resources that physicians spend to provide services for Medicare patients.

Service area—The geographic area served by an insurance carrier.

Skilled nursing facility—A medical facility that is licensed (as defined by Medicare) to primarily provide skilled nursing care to patients.

Subscriber—The person who has been insured; an insurance policy holder.

Superbill—A printed form containing a list of the services with corresponding codes (encounter form).

Third-party check—A check from one person that is made out to a second person for payment of a third person.

Third-party payer—An insurance carrier, who is not the doctor or patient, who intervenes to pay the hospital or medical bills per contract with one of the first two parties.

TRICARE—Civilian Health and Medical Program of the Uniformed Services (CHAMPUS)—Established to aid dependents of active service personnel, retired service personnel and their dependents, and dependents of service personnel who died on active duty, with a supplement for medical care in military or Public Health Service facilities.

Usual and customary fee—The usual fee is the charge physicians make to their patients; the customary fee is one within the range of usual fees charged by physicians in a given geographic and socioeconomic area who have similar training and experience.

Utilization management—A panel that tracks what their members receive and checks if their medical care meets the standards of the organization.

Utilization review—A review carried out by allied health professionals at predetermined times to assess the necessity of the particular patient to remain in an acute care facility.

Walkout statement—A printed form with the patient's charges and the amount paid for the services rendered, which the patient takes with her.

Workers' compensation—Government program that provides insurance coverage for those who are injured on the job or who have developed work-related disorders, disabilities, or illnesses.

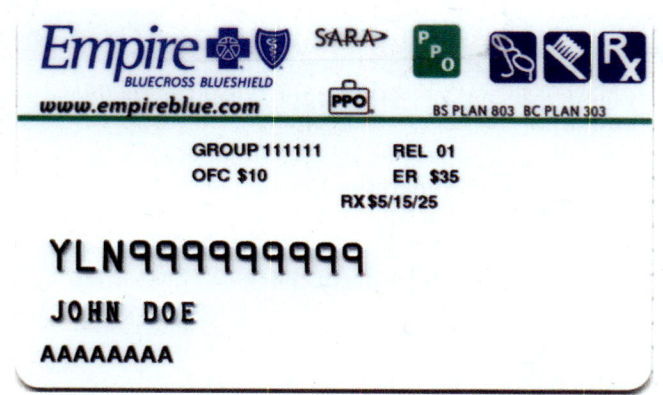

FIGURE 9-1 Empire Blue Cross/Blue Shield insurance card *(Courtesy of Empire Blue Cross/Blue Shield)*

Please present your insurance card to the receptionist when you arrive for your appointment.
Thank you!

FIGURE 9-2 Sample of a sign that could be posted at the receptionist's window to help keep records current

(Figure 9-1). It may be necessary to change the copy ratio or brightness quality on your copier prior to copying the insurance card. Font size on the cards and colored backgrounds sometimes make it difficult to read copies of the cards.

It is a good idea to write the date at the bottom of each card copy when the copy is made. The date will alert the medical assistant as to the last time a copy of the card was obtained. Keeping up-to-date with patient's current insurance coverage can be a challenge. Patients may have more than one insurance plan. Often families have coverage from each spouse's place of work. Many insurance companies include a "nonduplication of benefits" or "**coordination of benefits**" clause in the policy. If a child is covered by both parents' insurance, it will be necessary to determine who is considered the **primary** carrier (responsible for payment first) and who is the **secondary** carrier (responsible for payment after primary coverage). The charges are filed first with the primary carrier. After the claim has been processed and an explanation of benefits is received, the balance is submitted to the secondary carrier for payment. The charges are usually covered, or nearly so, with both plans. Responsibility for primary coverage will be based upon the language contained in the policies. For example, one spouse may have a good plan as a fringe benefit; then the other may decide to refuse the option to contribute to a plan and instead participate in a supplemental coverage that will become the secondary coverage. There can be many variables.

Covering dependent children is another variable. The primary coverage is usually responsible, but if both parents have equal coverage, another variable may be the determining factor. In this situation the **birthday rule** will apply. This rule states that:

- The plan of the parent whose birthday occurs first in the calendar year is primary, and the other parent's plan is secondary.

- If both parents have the same birthdate, the plan in effect the longest is primary.
- If the parents divorce and retain their plans, the parent with custody is primary.
- If a court order exists that dictates which parent is responsible for medical expenses, the court order supersedes the birthday rule.

More information regarding primary and secondary insurance coverage will follow later in this chapter.

Those who have Medicare may also have additional insurance coverage to supplement their insurance costs. Remember to ask for their current information and insurance card(s), because changes may occur from one visit to another. Keep in mind that Medicare patients tend to continue to carry their traditional red-white-and-blue insurance card even if they have opted into a Medicare HMO. A patient may present to you his traditional Medicare card when he is actually insured by one of the HMOs. A patient cannot be covered by traditional Medicare and a Medicare HMO simultaneously; they either have one or the other. Posting a sign that says, "Please give your insurance card to the receptionist when you arrive—thank you" (Figure 9-2) will help with obtaining current information from all patients served. Current insurance information is imperative to correctly bill for services rendered.

THE INSURANCE PAPER TRAIL

An example of how the paper trail for services rendered to patients is initiated and progresses is provided in Unit 3. The importance of accuracy and completeness is made evident by this series of forms and billing statements generated by only one patient for a relatively minor procedure. The medical assistant must be careful in documenting all information. Legible writing or printing as well as exactness is critical in successful **reimbursement** for services. Another sign that will help in collecting fees for services is one that states clearly, "Payment for services is appreciated at the time of service" (Figure 9-3). Even if this pay-

> We appreciate payment at the time of service.   Thank you!

FIGURE 9-3   Sample of a sign to inform patients that payment at time of service is expected

ment is the copay amount, it can save time and work in ending the potential future paper trail. Submitting a claim form for the services to the patient's insurance provider will speed up the cash flow of the practice. Patients will comply with requests if they are made in a pleasant manner. It is the usual custom to have insurance payments and reimbursements sent directly (**direct payment**) to the physician. In cases in which the patient is reimbursed for medical services (indirect payment), the payment may be delayed because the patient may put off sending in the payment for one reason or another.

Table 9-1 listed many of the terms (with brief definitions) used in dealing with insurance claims. As medical terminology and anatomy are necessary for dealing with patients and procedures, so too is the terminology used in preparing insurance claims. You should familiarize yourself with these important words and their meanings to communicate needs and expectations of both patients and insurance companies. Your knowledge will help to expedite the processing of claims accurately and efficiently, thereby bringing payment for medical services to the practice in a timely manner. For those who prepare claims, it is necessary to keep current with any changes in policy, terminology, and procedures. There are newsletters, periodicals, and workshops offered to help in providing data to keep up with the latest information. It is to your advantage and that of the practice where you are employed to participate in these informative offerings. Knowledge in the important task of processing claims will decrease the frustration that is often associated with the complications of preparing and processing claims for patient services.

When filing claims for reimbursement of services rendered, be certain that you have the proper forms signed with authorization to release information regarding the patient. The authorization forms should be updated periodically. Dependent upon the wording on the form, this may be necessary each time the patient's insurance coverage changes. Always retain copies of signed and dated authorizations in the pa-

tient's medical record. If information is given to a third party without the signed authorization of the patient, the one who gave the information may be charged with breach of confidentiality. A contract is legally binding. Those who enter into a contract have certain expectations. A contract is an agreement between two (or more) parties for certain services or obligations to be fulfilled. Where there is a concern as to the competence of the patient, or if the patient is a minor, a guardian must sign for any information to be released as well as for any service to be completed. Refer to Chapter 3 regarding legal terms.

ACHIEVE UNIT OBJECTIVES

- ☐ Complete the Workbook activities to meet the learning objectives.
- ☐ Apply your knowledge at the end of this chapter in completing the Critical Thinking Challenge and Activities, as well as the StudyWARE on your Student CD-ROM.

UNIT 2
HEALTH CARE PLANS

OBJECTIVES

Upon completion of this unit, you will be able to achieve the following:

LEARNING Objectives

1. Spell and define, using the glossary at the back of the text, all the Words to Know in this unit.
2. Identify the original purpose of an indemnity-type insurance plan.
3. Identify the health care philosophy of an HMO.
4. Name the types of HMOs and explain their differences.
5. Explain how a PPO differs from an HMO.
6. List five federal health care plans.
7. Name the three centers that were established by the changes in 2001.

WORDS TO KNOW

accreditation
annuity
capitation
comprehensive
connotations
deductible
flexible spending
    account
health
    maintenance
    organization
    (HMO)

health
    reimbursement
    arrangement
    (HRA)
health savings
    account (HSA)
indemnity
Medicaid
Medicare
Medigap
periodic

preauthorization
preferred
    provider
    organization
    (PPO)
premiums
quality assurance
restricted
statutory
supplement
utilization

CERTIFICATION CONNECTION

CMA

Legislation
Documentation/reporting
Physician-patient
    relationship
Computer applications
Internet services
Resource information and
    community services—
    services available
Third-party billing

CMAS

Patient information and
    community resources
Insurance processing

RMA

Finance/bookkeeping—
    terminology
Patient billing
Financial mathematics
Medical receptionist/
    secretarial/clerical—
    terminology

COMMERCIAL HEALTH INSURANCE

A large segment of the population is covered by commercial insurance policies. These private, commercial insurance companies control the price of **premiums** paid and specify the benefits they will provide.

Blue Cross and Blue Shield health insurance plans are generally well known. Physicians helped originate them. Blue Cross was originally set up to pay for hospital expenses but now covers outpatient services as well. Blue Shield was originally used to pay for physicians' services. In the early years, Blue Cross and Blue Shield was an **indemnity**-type plan with an annual **deductible** and copayment. They have changed with today's health care demands and now also offer a variety of HMO, PPO, point of service (POS), HSA, HRA and indemnity-type plans.

Indemnity-type insurance has the least amount of structural guidelines for patients to follow. Patients are able to see the physician of their choice without having to deal with listings of participating physicians and other managed care guidelines. The patients are also able to see specialists without having to obtain referrals from another physician. However, this freedom of choice comes at a higher cost to the patient. Patients are required to pay for their services in full at the time service is provided. The plan has an annual deductible that must be satisfied before the insurance company will cover any of the patient's expenses. Traditional indemnity coverage is sometimes referred to as an "80/20 plan." The carrier will pay 80% of the expenses, and the insured will pick up the other 20%. This is after the deductible has been satisfied. An encounter form or an itemized statement will be provided to the patient to file for reimbursement from the insurance carrier. Some practices will file the claim to the insurance company as a courtesy to the patient.

HMOs are plans set up to provide **comprehensive** health care with an emphasis on wellness and preventive medicine. The patient is encouraged to have annual physicals to identify health problems early. Some HMOs have the subscribers choose a primary care physician (PCP) to oversee their medical care. The PCP is responsible for referring the patient to a specialist if needed. Another cost containment measure with HMOs is preauthorization for all inpatient hospital stays, some outpatient surgeries, costly services such as magnetic resonance imaging (MRI) services, and referrals to physicians outside the panel of providers.

Determining Carrier Coverage

The terms *precertification, preauthorization,* and *predetermination* refer to a patient's eligibility for services. Many times these terms are used interchangeably, but there are technical differences, and they do not all mean the same thing.

- *Precertification* refers to the discovery as to whether a treatment (surgery, hospitalization, diagnostic test) is covered under the patient's insurance contract.
- **Preauthorization** relates not only to whether the services are covered, but also whether the proposed treatment is medically necessary.
- *Predetermination* refers to the discovery of the maximum amount of money that the carrier will pay for primary surgery, consultation service, postoperative care, etc.

Atlhough these conditions are all similar because they affect the patient's ability to receive services, they are also specific and different in their application and effect on the patient's coverage.

Most HMOs require the patient to pay a copayment at the time service is rendered, usually $10 to $25. The physician's office staff then files the claim with the insurance carrier for the balance due. In addition to physicians, the HMO also contracts with hospitals, laboratories, and other ancillary services, such as pharmacies. There are at least four different types of HMOs.

Types of HMOs

- **Staff model HMO** is a plan in which all services (physical therapy, radiology, and so on) are provided at the same location. The PCP is responsible for routine care and referrals. True emergency (life-threatening) care does not require preauthorization. If the patient is traveling outside the HMO geographic service area, she must call and preauthorize any nonemergency care. Failure to do so will result in the HMO refusing payment of the services.
- **Group model HMOs** are multispecialty practices contracted to provide health care services to members. The physicians are reimbursed on a capitated basis. **Capitation** means that physicians are paid a set fee per patient on their patient listing each month, whether the patient is seen one or more times or not at all.
- **Open-ended HMOs** allow members greater freedom in their choice of care. They do not have a PCP and can self-refer to specialists. If they choose to use a nonpanel provider, the benefit is more like an indemnity plan with a deductible and coinsurance. If they choose a panel provider they receive the HMO benefit.
- **Point-of-service (POS)** is another type of HMO and has gained in popularity in recent years. The organization consists of a network of physicians and hospitals that contract to provide an insurance company or an employer with services for their members or employees at a discount rate. This benefits the insurance company by reducing the cost of care, which in turn should reduce the cost of the insurance for the employer. The physicians benefit by gaining a group of patients from whom they can receive payments.

HMO Accreditation

To qualify as an HMO, an organization must present proof of its ability to provide comprehensive health care. To retain eligibility, the HMO must submit **periodic** performance reports to the Department of Human Services. The National Committee for Quality Assurance (NCQA) is responsible for assessing, measuring, and reporting outcomes of HMOs. They also provide the **accreditation** for HMOs after reviewing the HMOs' performance and procedures. It is important for the physician's office to keep complete and accurate records for their patients, maintenance records on all equipment, and records of medications dispensed from their offices; office safety procedures, office cleanliness and appearance, and accessibility are all components to the NCQA standards. There are four levels of accreditation:

1. Full accreditation is given for 3 years, indicating excellent performance.
2. HMOs that are well equipped to make recommended improvements are given a 1-year accreditation.
3. Provisional accreditation for 1 year is given if it appears that the potential for improving the HMO is there.
4. Accreditation is denied if the HMO does not meet the NCQA standards.

Independent Practice Associations

Independent practice associations (IPAs) are individual health care providers who join together to provide prepaid health care to groups and individuals who purchase coverage. This is a **restricted** health plan, as only panel providers, hospitals, laboratories, and other ancillary services can be utilized for benefits to be paid. The IPA physicians can hire their own staff and maintain private offices. Primary care physicians are usually paid on a capitated basis while the specialists are paid on a fee-for-service basis.

Preferred Provider Organization

A **preferred provider organization (PPO)** is not an HMO. The PPO affords the patient the option of using network or non-network physicians and hospitals. Benefits are greater if a network physician or hospital is utilized. The patient assumes a greater financial responsibility if non-network physicians or hospitals are used. PPO members do not have a PCP, but they do have more patient care management than an indemnity-type plan because of the limitations of the provider panel. A PPO usually has deductibles and copayment requirements, and some plans even have coinsurance amounts due from the insured. The physician's office generally files the claim for services rendered.

Many physicians belong to multiple HMOs, PPOs, and IPAs, unless restricted by specific terms of an insurance carrier contract or because of certain regulations in their area.

MANAGED CARE DELIVERY SYSTEMS

With the advent of health care reform, managed care delivery systems are gaining prominence in the types of plans employers are offering employees. Managed care plans integrate the financing and appropriate delivery of services to covered persons by contracting with selected providers for comprehensive health care services, with specific standards for the specialty of the provider and programs for **quality assurance** and **utilization** review. The PCP or gatekeeper is responsible for coordinating all care for the patient. The patient must first consult with his PCP for a referral before seeking the services of a specialist. The PCP is encouraged to use the specialists listed with the HMO/IPA panel of physicians. There may be circumstances when a referral is necessary outside the panel as the specialty may not be part of the panel. Some managed care plans will allow a woman only one visit a year to her gynecologist for her annual well-woman exam and Pap smear. If there are any gynecologic problems prior to the next well-woman exam, she will need a referral from the PCP to see the gynecologist again. Managed care also encourages mammograms for women based on the American Cancer Society guideline.

Well-child care is also promoted by HMOs. This includes periodic visits for screenings of height, weight, vision, and hearing; neurologic exams; immunizations at appropriate intervals; and tuberculosis (TB) Mantoux tests. Most managed care plans require that the patient pay a copayment, usually between $10 and $25, at the time of service. The administrative medical assistant in the physician's office files the claim for reimbursement of charges for services rendered for the visit.

Managed care plans employ a large staff of provider/professional relations representatives. These representatives periodically personally call on physicians' offices to provide new information, distribute new policy manuals, offer assistance in navigating through their web sites, and answer questions that the staff or physicians may have regarding their particular company. Also, monthly newsletters are either mailed or available on the company's web site to providers' offices to keep them apprised of changes between representative's visits. Some managed care plans also offer periodic seminars on their policies and claim-filing procedures.

CONSUMER-DRIVEN HEALTH PLANS (CDHPs)

Insurance companies and employers like to see consumers making informed choices regarding use of their health care dollars. The Federal government created CDHPs, specifically health savings accounts, in 2003. Insurance companies responded to the demands for additional options beyond HMOs, PPOs, and traditional coverage by developing CDHPs. The plans typically have high deductibles and lower monthly premiums. Some fear that health care services are overutilized because consumers think, "I do not know what my doctor charges, I just know I pay a copay." When patients have CDHP-type coverage, they no longer think of going to the physician's office and just paying a copay; instead they want to know how much the service is going to cost before it is provided, because a set amount of money is available to pay for their health care through the high-deductible plans described in the following sections. Several plans are now available that offer different options to meet the needs of the public.

Health Savings Account (HSA)

A **health saving account (HSA)** is a tax-sheltered savings account, similar to an IRA, that can be used to pay for medical expenses. Any amount not used in a given year remains in the account and continues to gain interest. An HSA has a high deductible and must be paired with a qualified health plan. Preventive care is not subject to the deductible. Contributions to the plan can be made by the employee or employer. The maximum contributions for 2006 are $2,650 for an individual and $5,250 for a family. Small medical expenses can be paid for through the HSA, up to the deductible amount, as long as they are considered a qualified medical expense. Some examples of qualified medical expenses are ambulance service, braces, home improvements to assist a disabled person, and telephone or TV equipment to assist the hearing and visually impaired. Examples of nonqualified expenses include babysitting and child care for a healthy individual, funeral expenses, and diaper service. Usually PPO type coverage kicks in to pay for medical expenses after the deductible is met.

Health Reimbursement Account (HRA)

Like an HSA, a **health reimbursement account (HRA)** is used to pay for medical expenses. It can be paired with a standard or high-deductible health plan. An employer can contribute to an HRA, but an employee cannot. In 2006 there were no restrictions to the amount of money that could be deposited into an HRA. The employer owns the money in this account, and it may not be portable when the employee leaves the company.

Flexible Spending Account (FSA)

A **flexible spending account (FSA)** is referred to as a cafeteria plan. There are three components to the plan:

1. Health insurance premiums
2. Qualified medical expenses
3. Dependent care expenses

The plan is usually funded by the employee. In some instances an employer may be able to contribute small amounts. This is a "use it or lose it"-type plan. The money belongs to the employee; however, any unused amounts at the end of the year are returned to the employer. An employee should give careful consideration to how much money she wants to put in the plan, knowing that if she does not use it she loses it. Qualified medical expenses are the same for the HSA, HRA, and FSA. Employees are not required to pay any Federal, Social Security, or state (in most cases) taxes on contributions.

GOVERNMENT HEALTH PLANS

Workers' Compensation

Employees in the United States have the benefit of being covered by workers' compensation laws. For many years the name of the coverage was known as workman's compensation, but it was changed to avoid **connotations** of gender bias. Every state has these laws to cover employees who are injured while working or become ill as a result of their work. In addition to state statutes, there are federal statutes covering federal employees injured on the job—United States Longshoremen and Harbor Workers Compensation, Federal Coal Mine Health and Safety Compensation, and special benefits for workers in the District of Columbia. The state compensation laws cover those workers not protected by federal statutes. The employer pays the premium for workers' compensation insurance, with the premium based on the risk involved in performance of the job.

Physicians who treat patients under workers' compensation plans are usually required to register with the state Workers' Compensation Board on an annual basis. The code assigned to each physician will limit care to a particular medical specialty.

There are four principal types of state benefits: (1) the patient may have medical treatment in or out of a hospital; (2) if there is determined to be a temporary disability, the patient may receive weekly cash benefits in addition to medical care; (3) when a percentage of permanent disability is found, the patient is given weekly or monthly benefits, and in some cases a lump-sum settlement; or (4) payments are made to dependents of employees who are fatally injured. Benefits also include comprehensive vocational rehabilitation for severely disabled employees.

In most states the report of an industrial injury is initiated by the employer and sent to the physician, who reports to the insurance company responsible for paying the claims (Figure 9-4). A few states have their own state fund for workers' compensation, and in these states the forms must be forwarded to the state office responsible. Time requirements for filing a claim vary. When the physician receives the form, it is considered authorization for treatment.

A patient who has an industrial injury should have a separate file set up for that injury and a separate account card. If the patient's record is required in a court case for settlement of the claim, there is no chance of violating the patient's confidentiality if other medical records are in a separate file. The patient is never billed in these cases unless treatment was given without authorization or was considered excessive by the Workers' Compensation Commission, in which case you may bill the patient's private insurance and then the patient for the portion denied by the commission. Patients who have a continuing partial or permanent disability are reevaluated at intervals, and the physician must furnish a supplemental report.

The medical assistant must keep current files of procedures to be followed and forms to be used, as these are frequently changed. The public affairs section or office services section of your state workers' compensation carrier will furnish any needed information. Visiting the web site of the Bureau of Workers' Compensation for your state on a frequent basis is also a good way of stay abreast of updates and changes.

The complete and accurate preparation of forms will ensure prompt payment of services. The following details are necessary for reimbursement:

- An accurate claim number appears on all forms and bills.
- The patient's complete name, the date, and the nature of the treatments is included.
- The payee name, address, and number are listed on the form.
- Fees for laboratory or x-ray examinations with interpretations are attached.
- If a surgical billing, a copy of the operative report is attached.
- Fee totals are accurate.
- Forms and bills must be legible.
- The form is signed by the physician.

A bill may be disallowed if it is not filed within the **statutory** time limit. If the claim is rejected for late filing and your records prove your original billing was filed within the statutory time limit, that information should be submitted for reconsideration of the claim. Always retain a copy of your billing. A code number should identify each patient.

Medicaid

Medicaid is health care coverage for individuals of limited or low income. It is a government program that came into being in 1965 and is funded by both the federal and state governments. The federal government sets minimum standards for Medicaid coverage. Each individual state has the ability to enhance the benefits to a higher level if they wish. Any enhancements to the federal standards are paid for by the state government of that individual state.

There are different categories of eligible recipients, including pregnant women and aged, blind, or disabled

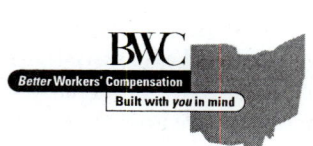

First Report of an Injury, Occupational Disease or Death

WARNING:
Any person who obtains compensation from BWC or self-insuring employers by knowingly misrepresenting or concealing facts, making false statements or accepting compensation to which he or she is not entitled, is subject to felony criminal prosecution for fraud.
(R.C. 2913.48)

Injured worker and injury/disease/death info.

| Last name, first name, middle initial | Social Security number | Marital status ☐ Single | Date of birth |

Home mailing address | Sex ☐ Male ☐ Female | ☐ Married ☐ Divorced | Number of dependents

City | State | 9-digit ZIP code | Country if different from USA | ☐ Separated ☐ Widowed | Department name

Wage rate $ _____ Per: ☐ Hour ☐ Month ☐ Week ☐ Year ☐ Other | What days of the week do you usually work? ☐ Sun ☐ Mon ☐ Tues ☐ Wed ☐ Thur ☐ Fri ☐ Sat | Regular work hours From _____ To _____

Have you been offered or do you expect to receive payment or wages for this claim from anyone other than the Ohio Bureau of Workers' Compensation? ☐ Yes ☐ No If yes, please explain. | Occupation or job title

Employer name

Mailing address (number and street, city or town, state, ZIP code and county)

Location, if different from mailing address

Was the place of accident or exposure on employer's premises? ☐ Yes ☐ No
(If no, give accident location, street address, city, state and ZIP code)

| Date of injury/disease | Time of injury _____ ☐ a.m. ☐ p.m. | If fatal, give date of death | Time employee began work _____ ☐ a.m. ☐ p.m. | Date last worked | Date returned to work |

Date hired | State where hired | Date employer notified

Description of accident (Describe the sequence of events that directly injured the employee, or caused the disease or death.) | Type of injury/disease and part(s) of body affected (For example: sprain of lower left back)

Benefit application/medical release – I am applying for recognition of my claim under the Ohio Workers' Compensation Act for work-related injuries that I did not purposely inflict. I request payment for compensation and/or medical expenses as allowable. Direct payment(s) to the providers of any medical services are authorized. I understand that I am allowing any provider who attends to, treats or examines me to release all medical, psychological and/or psychiatric information that is causally or historically related to physical or mental injuries relevant to issues necessary to the administration of my workers' compensation claim to the Ohio Bureau of Workers' Compensation, the Industrial Commission of Ohio, the employer listed in this claim, that employer's managed care organization and any authorized representatives. I further authorize the Ohio Rehabilitation Services Commission to release information about my physical, mental, vocational and social conditions that is causally or historically related to physical or mental injuries relevant to issues necessary for the administration of my workers' compensation claim to the aforementioned parties.

| Injured worker signature | Date | E-mail address | Telephone number ( ) | Work number ( ) |

Treatment info.

| Health-care provider name | Telephone number ( ) | Fax number ( ) | Initial treatment date |

Street address | City | State | 9-digit ZIP code

Diagnosis(es): Include ICD code(s)

Will the incident cause the injured worker to miss eight or more days of work? ☐ Yes ☐ No | Is the injury causally related to the industrial incident? ☐ Yes ☐ No

Health-care provider signature | 11-digit BWC provider number | Date

Employer info.

Employer policy number | **Check if** ☐ Employer is self-insuring ☐ Injured worker is owner/partner/member of firm

| Telephone number ( ) | Fax number ( ) | E-mail address | Federal ID number | Manual number |

Was employee treated in an emergency room? ☐ Yes ☐ No | Was employee hospitalized overnight as an inpatient? ☐ Yes ☐ No

If treatment was given away from work site, provide the facility name, street address, city, state and ZIP code

☐ **Certification** - The employer certifies that the facts in this application are correct and valid. | ☐ **Rejection** - The employer rejects the validity of this claim for the reason(s) listed below: | **For self-insuring employers only** ☐ **Clarification** - The employer clarifies and allows the claim for the condition(s) below: ☐ **Medical only** ☐ **Lost time**

Employer signature and title | Date | OSHA case number

BWC-1101 (Rev. 8/2005) | This form meets OSHA 301 requirements
FROI-1 (Combines C-1, C-2, C-3, C-6, C-50, OD-1, OD-1-22)

FIGURE 9-4 First report form for workers' compensation

individuals, to name a few. Eligibility requirements can differ from state to state. Medicaid cards are issued to recipients on a monthly basis. Always verify current coverage before rendering services in order to ensure that your physician will be paid. There are time limits for filing claims for reimbursement.

Patients need to seek care from a participating provider. Not all physicians are Medicaid providers. Physicians are not required to accept Medicaid patients, nor are they required to apply to participate. If a physician is not participating and renders treatment to a Medicaid patient, it is very unlikely that they will receive any payment from Medicaid. A physician must be participating in order to receive reimbursement for services provided. Medicaid HMO plans are offered within some state's programs. Participation in traditional Medicaid does not mean a physician is automatically participating in the HMO; typically there is a separate contract that must be signed.

Medicaid patients should be treated medically, personally, and professionally in the same manner as any other patient.

Medicare

Medicare is a program of health insurance administered under the Social Security Administration for people over the age of 65 who meet the eligibility requirements and have filed for coverage. In addition, those who are disabled, receiving Social Security benefits, or in end-stage renal disease, regardless of their age, are also eligible. Patients are issued a red-white-and-blue membership card to verify their coverage (Figure 9-5).

Part A Medicare is for hospital coverage, and any person who is receiving monthly Social Security benefits is automatically enrolled. Along with health care costs in general, the annual deductible increases each year. Most patients now carry additional coverage to supplement their Medicare coverage to help offset the expenses of the annual deductible and coinsurance due after Medicare has paid its portion. The term **Medigap** is sometimes used to describe this type of supplemental insurance.

Part B of Medicare is for payment of other medical expenses, including office visits, x-ray and laboratory services, and the services of a physician in or out of the hospital. The premiums are automatically deducted for those who wish the coverage and are on Social Security, railroad retirement, or civil service **annuity**. Other individuals who are eligible pay premiums directly to the Social Security Administration.

Medicare HMOs are in operation in many states. The HMOs usually offer the patient additional services outside of what traditional Medicare covers. A patient can be insured with a Medicare HMO and also carry supplemental insurance. HMO benefits vary from plan to plan. You must keep abreast of the plans offered in your area. It is not uncommon for patients to ask questions about their HMO coverage while they are in the office. It is helpful if you are able to offer them telephone numbers of the HMO so the HMO can address their coverage and other related questions.

Medicare uses Social Security numbers along with an alpha character to define the beneficiary's health insurance claim (HIC) number. This is the number used to identify the patient when submitting claims. A Social Security number followed by the letter "A" indicates the Social Security number belongs to the card holder. If the number is followed by the letter "B," it indicates the Social Security number belongs to the card holder's spouse.

Medicare Administration and Claims Processing   Physician providers and medical assistants need to keep current with the regulations governing health care and processing of claims. Professional orga-

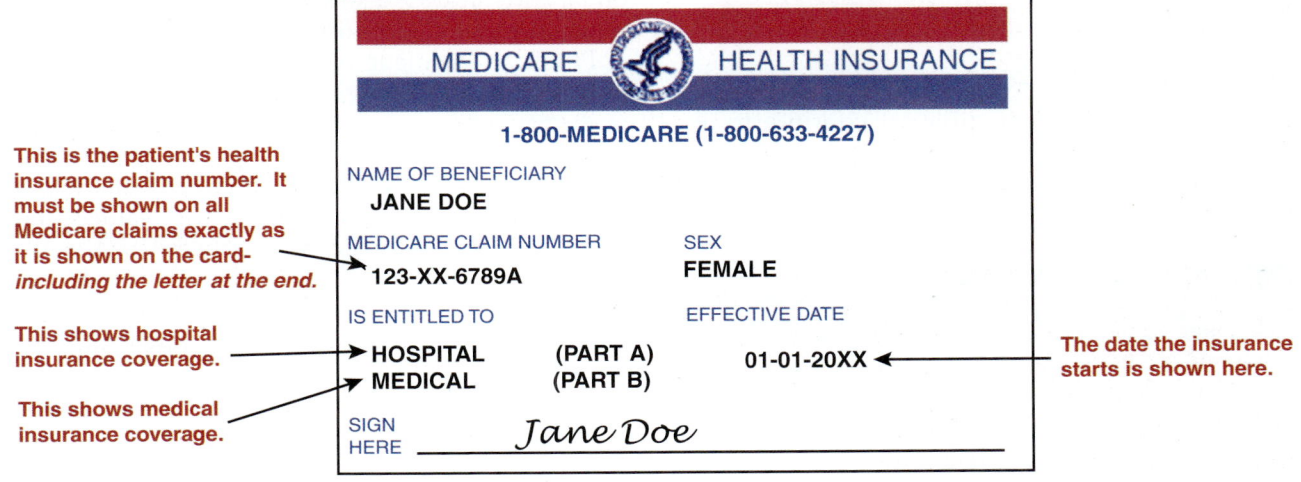

FIGURE 9-5   Medicare identification card

nizations, inservice education providers, and insurance companies offer periodic training sessions and seminars to inform the medical community of changes. When Medicare and Medicaid were enacted originally in 1965 as part of the Social Security Act, they came under the Social Security Administration. In 1977, they were transferred to the Department of Health and Human Services and to the Health Care Financing Administration (HCFA). This name was later changed to Centers for Medicare and Medicaid Services (CMS). Changes occurred in attempts to improve the health care delivery system.

Beginning in September 1990, The Omnibus Budget Reconciliation Act (OBRA) of 1989 required that all physicians and suppliers submit Medicare claims for their patients. Physicians and suppliers are not responsible for filing the Medicare claim if the service is not covered by Medicare or for filing other health insurance claims. Claims must be filed within a year of the time the service is received by the patient. In some cases the Medicare insurance carrier will automatically send the amount not covered on to the private insurance carrier, which may pay the deductible and the 20% not covered, eliminating the need to fill out additional forms.

Physicians who sign a contract with Medicare to be a participating provider will receive payment directly from Medicare for services rendered. Physicians who choose not to be a participating provider can collect only the Medicare-approved amount for the service rendered. They cannot balance bill the patient for the difference between what Medicare approves and what the physician charges. The maximum amount a nonparticipating provider can collect is 115% of the Medicare fee schedule.

Patients insured with Medicare Part B have an annual deductible to satisfy (pay) before any portion of their medical expenses will be paid by Medicare. The deductible is paid to the provider of services. The deductible amounts for previous years were as follows:

2004	$100
2005	$110
2006	$124

It is expected that the deductible will continue to rise due to the continued increase in costs associated with medical care. Medicare pays 80% of the approved amount once the deductible is satisfied. The remaining 20% is paid by either the patient's supplemental insurance, once their deductible is satisfied with the supplemental plan, or by the patient. Medically necessary lab services are paid at 100%, and the patient is never billed for associated costs.

Most Medicare patients will have some form of supplemental or Medigap insurance to cover the deductible and the 20% copayment. Medigap is health insurance offered by private companies to persons eligible for Medicare benefits and is specifically designed to supplement Medicare benefits. Medicare generally forwards the claim information directly to the Medigap carrier, thus saving the office staff time. It is important to ask the patient about any supplemental insurance at the time of service. Make a copy of both sides of the Medicare and supplemental insurance cards for your records. (A copy of both sides of *all* insurance cards should be made at each visit.) If the patient does not have a commercial supplemental insurance and is unable to pay the deductible or co-insurance, their 20%, the patient may be eligible for Medicaid. In this case, Medicare would be the primary insurance and Medicaid would be secondary and balance billed for the deductible and co-insurance.

Another variable with primary and secondary coverage occurs when a person qualifies for Medicare by virtue of age but remains employed. If the employee continues to work and is employed by a company with 20 or more employees, the group plan is billed as primary and Medicare is billed as secondary. Health insurance coverage provided through employment group plans terminates when the employee retires, and Medicare becomes the primary coverage. Supplemental coverage is often available through the company's retirement plan. However, if a Medicare beneficiary is retired but has a working spouse with health insurance, and the beneficiary is an eligible dependent on the spouse's policy, then the spouse's plan becomes primary and Medicare is secondary. Medicare is also secondary when patients are receiving Veterans Administration benefits.

Physician payment reform (PPR) is another part of OBRA passed by Congress that made sweeping changes in the payment of physician services by Medicare Part B.

- The PPR payment is based on a fee schedule, which is based on a resource-based relative value system referred to as the Medicare fee schedule (MFS).
- Medicare volume performance standards (MVPS) have been established to track annual increases in Medicare Part B payments for physicians' services and levels for future years.
- Various financial protections for the beneficiary have been developed.
- Payment and medical policies used by Medicare carriers have been standardized.

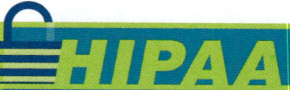

In order to be in HIPAA compliance, providers are required to submit all Medicare claims electronically as of October 1, 2005. This requirement applies whether Medicare is the primary or secondary coverage for the patient.

Patient's Name: _____   Medicare # (HICN): _____

ADVANCE BENEFICIARY NOTICE (ABN)

NOTE: You need to make a choice about receiving these health care items or services.

We expect that Medicare will not pay for the item(s) or service(s) that are described below. Medicare does not pay for all of your health care costs. Medicare only pays for covered items and services when Medicare rules are met. The fact that Medicare may not pay for a particular item or service does not mean that you should not receive it. There may be a good reason your doctor recommended it. Right now, in your case, **Medicare probably will not pay for –**

| **Items or Services:** |
| |
| |

| **Because:** |
| |
| |

The purpose of this form is to help you make an informed choice about whether or not you want to receive these items or services, knowing that you might have to pay for them yourself. Before you make a decision about your options, you should **read this entire notice carefully.**

- Ask us to explain if you don't understand why Medicare probably won't pay.
- Ask us how much these items or services will cost you (**Estimated Cost: $ _____**), in case you have to pay for them yourself or through other insurance.

PLEASE CHOOSE **ONE** OPTION. CHECK **ONE** BOX. **SIGN & DATE** YOUR CHOICE.

☐ **Option 1. YES. I want to receive these items or services.**

I understand that Medicare will not decide whether to pay unless I receive these items or services. Please submit my claim to Medicare. I understand that you may bill me for items or services and that I may have to pay the bill while Medicare is making its decision. If Medicare does pay, you will refund to me any payments I made to you that are due to me. If Medicare denies payment, I agree to be personally and fully responsible for payment. That is, I will pay personally, either out of pocket or through any other insurance that I have. I understand I can appeal Medicare's decision.

☐ **Option 2. NO. I have decided not to receive these items or services.**

I will not receive these items or services. I understand that you will not be able to submit a claim to Medicare and that I will not be able to appeal your opinion that Medicare won't pay.

_____   _____
Date   Signature of patient or person acting on patient's behalf

NOTE: Your health information will be kept confidential. Any information that we collect about you on this form will be kept confidential in our offices. If a claim is submitted to Medicare, your health information on this form may be shared with Medicare. Your health information, which Medicare sees, be will kept confidential by Medicare.

OMB Approval No. 0938-0566   Form No. CMS-R-131-G   (June 2002)

FIGURE 9-6 Advance beneficiary notice *(Reprinted according to http://www.cms.hhs.gov web site content reuse policy)*

Medicare is only permitted to pay for services or supplies that are considered medically reasonable and necessary for the diagnosis given. Medicare will not pay for cosmetic surgery or experimental, unproved, or investigational services. Beginning in 2005, *new* Medicare beneficiaries were provided coverage for one routine physical exam. There are other preventive screenings and tests that Medicare offers limited benefits for. If the physician does provide a noncovered service, the patient must be informed in advance and an Advance Beneficiary Notice (ABN; Figure 9-6) must be signed by the patient. The notice must state the specific service, the date of service, the anticipated amount of cost that Medicare is not going to cover, and the specific reason the service is not covered. The following are some examples of advanced notice statements which can be used:

- Medicare usually does not pay for this service.
- Medicare usually does not pay for this injection.
- Medicare does not pay for this service as it is considered experimental.

In addition to using the ABN when you know that a service is statutorily not covered, it should also be used when you anticipate that a service may not be covered. The same information should be supplied to the patient. This information must be shared with the patient and the form completed in advance of the services being rendered or it is not considered to be valid and you cannot hold the patient responsible for the bill associated with the service.

If the patient is not informed in advance of a noncovered service, the patient will not be responsible for payment, and any money collected will need to be refunded.

Current Medicare requirements specify that nonparticipating surgeons must notify all patients in writing of their estimated charge, the estimated Medicare approved charge, and the difference between the two in advance of elective operations that involve charges over $500.

Another change occurred when CMS designated a uniform health insurance claim form to standardize information requested and the method in which it was submitted. This form is known as the CMS-1500, formerly the HCFA-1500 (Figure 9-7). Regulations were established requiring that all claims submitted by Medicare contractors after May 1, 1992, had to be on an original CMS-1500 claim form. Photocopied forms would not be acceptable and would be returned regardless of whether the provider accepted assignment. The only practitioners who can currently bill Medicare with the hard copy CMS-1500 forms are businesses with less than 10 full-time employees, including physicians.

In 1997 the State Children's Health Insurance Program (SCHIP) was included as part of the Balanced Budget Act. The program was an attempt to respond to the growing problem of families without health insurance coverage, which in reality means that many children do not receive even basic medical care.

A major change in health care administration occurred in October 2001. A massive restructuring took place "to better serve the needs of Medicare/Medicaid beneficiaries and health care providers." The Health Care Financing Administration was renamed the Centers for Medicare and Medicaid Services (CMS). This change was part of a package of reforms to "change the agency and drive it to be responsive and effective." The CMS is "organized around three centers to clearly reflect the agency's major line of business: traditional fee-for-service Medicare, Medicare+Choice, and state-administered programs such as Medicaid and SCHIP." One center is known as the Center for Medicare Management and focuses on the traditional fee-for-service program. It is charged with responding to Medicare and Medicaid beneficiaries and health care providers to strengthen health care services and information availability.

The second center, The Center for Beneficiary Choices, focuses on providing beneficiaries with information on Medicare, Medicare Select, Medicare+Choice, and Medigap. It is also responsible for managing the Medicare+Choice plan, consumer research and demonstration, and grievance and appeals functions.

The third center is The Center for Medicaid and State Operations, which focuses on programs administered by states, which include Medicaid, SCHIP, insurance regulation functions, survey and certification, and the Clinical Laboratory Improvements Act (CLIA).

The following services are available to help Medicare beneficiaries and caregivers understand Medicare costs, coverage, and options available (such as Medigap and Medicare+Choice):

- Customer service representatives at the CMS call center provide information 24 hours a day, 7 days a week. They can be reached at 800-Medicare (800-633-4227) to ask questions and to request written information through the mail.
- A web-based information site is available at www.medicare.gov.
- Information for physicians and their staff is accessible at www.cms.gov.

TRICARE (CHAMPUS)

As part of the United States Department of Defense, the Civilian Health and Medical Program of the Uniformed Services TRICARE (CHAMPUS) was established to aid dependents of active service personnel, retired service personnel and their dependents, and dependents of service personnel who died on active duty, with a **supplement** for medical care in military or Public Health Service facilities. The word *dependents* refers to spouses and dependent children. All members of TRICARE (CHAMPUS) over the age of 10 are issued an identification card. A patient who lives within 40 miles of a uniformed services hospital will need a *nonavailability statement* to be cared for in a civilian or physician's office. This simply means that the necessary services are not available at the service hospital or that for medical reasons it would be better to continue care under the civilian physician who has been treating the patient. Authorization is not necessary if the patient lives more than 40 miles from a military medical facility that could furnish the necessary care.

The Civilian Health and Medical Program of the Veterans' Administration (CHAMPVA) was established in 1973 for the spouses and dependent children of veterans who have total, permanent, service-connected disabilities. This service is also available for the surviving spouses and dependent children of veterans who have died as a result of service-connected disabilities. The local VA hospital determines eligibility and then issues identification cards. The insured members can then choose their own private physicians. There are deductibles and cost-sharing requirements your office needs to be aware of.

If your office needs additional information on military benefit programs, you can contact your local health

1500

HEALTH INSURANCE CLAIM FORM

APPROVED BY NATIONAL UNIFORM CLAIM COMMITTEE 08/05

| | PICA | | | | | | | | | PICA | |

CARRIER

1. MEDICARE   MEDICAID   TRICARE CHAMPUS   CHAMPVA   GROUP HEALTH PLAN   FECA BLK LUNG   OTHER   1a. INSURED'S I.D. NUMBER   (For Program in Item 1)
(Medicare #)   (Medicaid #)   (Sponsor's SSN)   (Member ID#)   (SSN or ID)   (SSN)   (ID)

2. PATIENT'S NAME (Last Name, First Name, Middle Initial)

3. PATIENT'S BIRTH DATE   MM   DD   YY   SEX   M   F

4. INSURED'S NAME (Last Name, First Name, Middle Initial)

5. PATIENT'S ADDRESS (No., Street)

6. PATIENT RELATIONSHIP TO INSURED
Self   Spouse   Child   Other

7. INSURED'S ADDRESS (No., Street)

CITY   STATE

8. PATIENT STATUS
Single   Married   Other

CITY   STATE

ZIP CODE   TELEPHONE (Include Area Code)
(   )

Employed   Full-Time Student   Part-Time Student

ZIP CODE   TELEPHONE (Include Area Code)
(   )

9. OTHER INSURED'S NAME (Last Name, First Name, Middle Initial)

10. IS PATIENT'S CONDITION RELATED TO:

11. INSURED'S POLICY GROUP OR FECA NUMBER

a. OTHER INSURED'S POLICY OR GROUP NUMBER

a. EMPLOYMENT? (Current or Previous)
YES   NO

a. INSURED'S DATE OF BIRTH   MM   DD   YY   SEX   M   F

b. OTHER INSURED'S DATE OF BIRTH   MM   DD   YY   SEX   M   F

b. AUTO ACCIDENT?   PLACE (State)
YES   NO

b. EMPLOYER'S NAME OR SCHOOL NAME

c. EMPLOYER'S NAME OR SCHOOL NAME

c. OTHER ACCIDENT?
YES   NO

c. INSURANCE PLAN NAME OR PROGRAM NAME

d. INSURANCE PLAN NAME OR PROGRAM NAME

10d. RESERVED FOR LOCAL USE

d. IS THERE ANOTHER HEALTH BENEFIT PLAN?
YES   NO   **If yes**, return to and complete item 9 a-d.

PATIENT AND INSURED INFORMATION

READ BACK OF FORM BEFORE COMPLETING & SIGNING THIS FORM.
12. PATIENT'S OR AUTHORIZED PERSON'S SIGNATURE I authorize the release of any medical or other information necessary to process this claim. I also request payment of government benefits either to myself or to the party who accepts assignment below.

SIGNED _____ DATE _____

13. INSURED'S OR AUTHORIZED PERSON'S SIGNATURE I authorize payment of medical benefits to the undersigned physician or supplier for services described below.

SIGNED _____

14. DATE OF CURRENT: ILLNESS (First symptom) OR   MM   DD   YY   INJURY (Accident) OR   PREGNANCY(LMP)

15. IF PATIENT HAS HAD SAME OR SIMILAR ILLNESS. GIVE FIRST DATE   MM   DD   YY

16. DATES PATIENT UNABLE TO WORK IN CURRENT OCCUPATION   MM   DD   YY   FROM   TO   MM   DD   YY

17. NAME OF REFERRING PROVIDER OR OTHER SOURCE

17a.
17b. NPI

18. HOSPITALIZATION DATES RELATED TO CURRENT SERVICES   MM   DD   YY   FROM   TO   MM   DD   YY

19. RESERVED FOR LOCAL USE

20. OUTSIDE LAB? $ CHARGES
YES   NO

21. DIAGNOSIS OR NATURE OF ILLNESS OR INJURY (Relate Items 1, 2, 3 or 4 to Item 24E by Line)
1. ____.____   3. ____.____
2. ____.____   4. ____.____

22. MEDICAID RESUBMISSION CODE   ORIGINAL REF. NO.

23. PRIOR AUTHORIZATION NUMBER

24. A. DATE(S) OF SERVICE From To MM DD YY MM DD YY	B. PLACE OF SERVICE	C. EMG	D. PROCEDURES, SERVICES, OR SUPPLIES (Explain Unusual Circumstances) CPT/HCPCS MODIFIER	E. DIAGNOSIS POINTER	F. $ CHARGES	G. DAYS OR UNITS	H. EPSDT Family Plan	I. ID. QUAL.	J. RENDERING PROVIDER ID. #
1									NPI
2									NPI
3									NPI
4									NPI
5									NPI
6									NPI

25. FEDERAL TAX I.D. NUMBER   SSN   EIN

26. PATIENT'S ACCOUNT NO.

27. ACCEPT ASSIGNMENT?   (For govt. claims, see back)
YES   NO

28. TOTAL CHARGE
$

29. AMOUNT PAID
$

30. BALANCE DUE
$

31. SIGNATURE OF PHYSICIAN OR SUPPLIER INCLUDING DEGREES OR CREDENTIALS (I certify that the statements on the reverse apply to this bill and are made a part thereof.)

SIGNED _____ DATE _____

32. SERVICE FACILITY LOCATION INFORMATION

a. NPI   b.

33. BILLING PROVIDER INFO & PH # (   )

a. NPI   b.

PHYSICIAN OR SUPPLIER INFORMATION

APPROVED OMB-0938-0999 FORM CMS-1500 (08/05)

FIGURE 9-7   Health insurance claim form, CMS-1500

benefits advisor (HBA) at the nearest military hospital or clinic or the office of TRICARE (CHAMPUS) in Aurora, Colorado. Check out TRICARE's web site at www.tricare.osd.mil for contact information via the web or telephone.

Easter Seal/Crippled Children

All states operate Crippled Children's Services with federal support under Title V of the Social Security Act. The intent of this service is to locate disabled children under 21 or those who have potentially crippling conditions to see that appropriate health care is furnished. Part or all of this treatment may be paid for if the family's resources are not adequate. Some Crippled Children's Services are being changed to Easter Seal rehabilitation centers because of the stigma attached to the words *crippled children*. Some Easter Seal rehabilitation centers are now operated as private nonprofit organizations.

ACHIEVE UNIT OBJECTIVES

- Complete the Workbook activities to meet the learning objectives.
- Apply your knowledge at the end of this chapter in completing the Critical Thinking Challenge and Activities, as well as the StudyWARE on your Student CD-ROM.

UNIT 3
PREPARING CLAIMS

OBJECTIVES

Upon completion of this unit, you will be able to achieve the following:

LEARNING Objectives

1. Spell and define, using the glossary at the back of the text, all the Words to Know in this unit.
2. Explain why claim forms were developed.

3. Explain the meaning of primary and secondary coverage and how it affects coverage.
4. Name the two main classifications of codes and explain their basic difference.
5. Explain the meanings of both the "reason rule" and sequencing.
6. List four general coding rules.
7. Identify two things to be done before completing a patient's claim form.
8. List six common errors made when filing claims.
9. Explain the purpose of an insurance log, listing six of the items to enter.
10. Name four pieces of information to have before calling to follow up on a delinquent insurance claim.
11. Explain the phrase "accept assignment."
12. Describe what action should be taken when a procedure is not covered by insurance.
13. Name five of the seven items necessary for adequate documentation on a patient's record.
14. Identify three ways to stay current with Medicare and other insurance company regulations.

PERFORMANCE Objectives

1. Properly identify CPT and ICD coding applications.
2. Demonstrate completion of a claim form.

WORDS TO KNOW

bundle	International	reason rule
carrier	Classification	reimbursement
contributory	of Diseases	secondary
Current	modifier	sequenced
Procedural	nomenclature	specificity
Terminology	numeric	third-party
encounter	preferred	reimbursement
fee schedule	primary	truncated

CERTIFICATION CONNECTION

CMA

Releasing medical
   information

Equipment operation

Computer components

Computer applications

Internet services

Process for filing
   documents

Coding systems

Third-party billing

CMAS

Insurance processing

Insurance coding

Insurance billing and
   finances

Fundamental financial
   management

Fundamentals of computing

Medical office computer
   applications

RMA

Finance/bookkeeping–
   terminology

Patient billing

Medical
   receptionist/secretarial/
   clerical–terminology

THE BEGINNING OF CLAIM FORMS

The preparation of claims for the purpose of receiving payment for medical services is a fairly recent development in the history of health care. For centuries, providers were paid directly with some form of money, bartered goods, or the exchange of services. With industrialization and the scientific advancement of medicine, this was no longer appropriate. At the same time, people began receiving employment benefits such as vacations and pensions. Soon, other benefits such as health care were added and the new industry of health insurance exploded. The phrase "**third-party reimbursement**" was coined to indicate payment of services rendered by someone other than the patient. With this intermediate step came the need for some form of paperwork to serve as the means of reporting the health care provided to the source of payment: the claim form was developed. Today, the most common third-party reimbursers are federal and state agencies, insurance companies, and worker's compensation.

Originally, patients would provide the physician with forms obtained from their employer's benefits office for their insurance coverage. The patient completed his portion of the form and either signed or did not sign the section that authorized payment for services to be made directly to the physician. If it was not signed, the patient paid the charges and then the insurance company sent the payment to the patient. It was customary for physicians to charge a small fee to complete forms after the first one was done. Patients often had multiple coverage and could even "make money" with covered conditions. Medical findings, diagnoses, and treatments were described verbally in medical terminology, and fees were paid as requested if they were reasonable. Third-party reimbursement was simple and fairly easy. The contract for services was primarily between the physician and the patient; controls were minimal. As time went by, medicine evolved into a very sophisticated science. Medical care became extremely complicated and technologic advances caused a rapid rise in medical costs. Premiums for insurance coverage skyrocketed. Unemployed and retired persons had to resort to community clinics in order to obtain health care.

THE HISTORY OF CODING

While medical care was evolving into a highly technical service, another need was surfacing: some method of collecting health data so that physicians, scientists, and government agencies could assess the incidences and treatments of diseases. As early as the 1890s, a physician developed a classification of causes of death. From this beginning, the American Public Health Association recommended that this classification system be adopted by those responsible for recording deaths in Canada, Mexico, and the United States. It was decided that the classification should be revised every 10 years. In 1938, the fifth revision had evolved into the **International Classification of Diseases** (ICD). A few years later hospitals began trying to classify diseases and their medical records departments used a modified ICD version to code and index records.

The initial reason for classifying deaths was to provide a means of assessing statistically the prevalence of certain diseases or disorders or the incidences of fatal injuries. Later, codes were used in order to retrieve medical records by diagnosis or surgical procedure to be useful in medical research and education. As other applications became evident, the system provided a method of identifying the incidence of diseases and disorders being treated throughout the world. Reported prevalence provides statistics for assessing the status of people within and among various countries. As the need for greater **specificity** of medical conditions became desirable, the codes were revised, expanded, and refined.

By 1978, the World Health Organization published the ninth version of the ICD (ICD-9), and in the United States the *International Classification of Diseases, 9th Revision, Clinical Modification (ICD-9-CM)* was issued and will remain in effect until the 10th revision is released. The 10th revision contains ICD changes made by the World Health Organization and the clinical modifications (CM) changes made by the National Center for Health

Statistics in the United States. The new code book will serve every field of health care. Its full title will be *International Statistical Classification of Diseases and Related Health Problems*. The book will go beyond classification of disease and injuries to the coding of ambulatory care and risk factors encountered in primary care. It will also include additional clinical details about current diseases as well as those diseases discovered since the last revision. However, for the most part it will retain the same format. Some change will occur in the Injury and Poisoning chapter, where injuries will be catalogued by the anatomic site instead of by type of injury. Another change involves the E codes that were used for external causes of disease. E codes will be used for endocrine system diseases, while the external causes will be listed under V codes. The new code book will be published in three volumes and include the following:

Volume 1—The tabular listing of alpha-numeric codes as in ICD-9

Volume 2—An instructional manual that provides rules and guidelines of coding

Volume 3—An alphabetic index of the codes in the tabular list

The codes now allow for the expression of extensive verbal descriptions into a numeric system. Coding is, in reality, the transferal of verbal or written descriptions of disease or injury into numeric designations to achieve uniform data that can be easily entered into electronic processing and storage systems.

USE OF CURRENT ICD CODES

The ICD codes became useful for reporting all medical care on claim forms for Medicare, Medicaid, and other third-party payers of medical services. Later, the impact of the Catastrophic Coverage Act of 1988 on the physician's office changed the way physicians manage their practices. Since April 1, 1989, ICD coding is no longer an option; it is required on all Medicare and other government health care claims. The act mandates submission of an appropriate diagnostic code or codes for each service provided under Medicare B, or other coverage, for which payment is requested. Specific coding guidelines have been developed for physicians' offices. It is very important that coding be done properly. The physician's **reimbursement** is based upon the codes that are submitted.

The ICD codes are descriptive of the *disease* or *condition* presented by the patient. The ICD code selected by the physician must be as specific to the patient's diagnosed condition as possible. Another coding system based on the *procedures* and *services* the physician or the office staff provides for the patient are known as the Current Procedural Terminology (CPT) codes. These codes must be appropriate for the ICD code of the dis-

ease or payment will not be approved by the **carrier**. Accurate and precise coding not only helps to optimize reimbursement, it is essential for carrier acceptance. Mistakes not only cost the physician, but patients are also affected when services are not covered.

The coding systems established a way to communicate numerically with carriers and at the same time provided a means to collect numeric data for national and international purposes. It is a complex system, but with experience it becomes more manageable. One of the most important factors to remember is that the codes have to be **sequenced** in relation to the intensity and level of service provided. Basically this involves listing the primary reason for the office visit first and other reasons next in order of their importance. The staff person who processes claim forms needs to be a detail-oriented individual. This is a very important role in the medical practice and is not suitable for a beginning employee.

PERFORMING CODING FUNCTIONS

To become an accurate and efficient coder, three things are necessary: a working knowledge of medical terminology, an understanding of anatomy and physiology, and comprehension of ICD characteristics and terminology. Coding requires attention to detail. Work experience and a period of learning with the help of an experienced coder can be very beneficial. In this unit, only a brief introduction to the process is presented. This responsibility can best be learned by actual performance using the coding materials provided by your employer. Because various companies produce manuals with the ICD codes, with different methods of organization of the information, specific directions are not practical. Excellent resources for obtaining coding books or instructional manuals are the American Medical Association (AMA), Ingenix, or PMIC. There are hundreds of book titles published annually to assist with the coding process.

The standard codes were taken from the federal government's official Centers for Medicare and Medicaid Services (CMS) material. Some coding books arrange diseases and injuries in two volumes.

Volume I—A tabular list, organized into 17 chapters, with conditions listed by body systems in one chapter and by conditions according to their causes in another chapter. Other information in Volume I includes supplementary classifications such as:

- V-codes—Factors influencing health status and contact with health service
- E-codes—External causes of injury and poisoning

Volume I also contains appendices of:

- M-codes—Morphology of Neoplasms
- Classification of Drugs by the American Hospital Formulary
- Classification of Industrial Accidents According to Agency
- List of Three-Digit Categories

Volume II—An alphabetic index organized into three main sections:

- Section 1—Alphabetic Index to Diseases and Injuries
- Section 2—Table of Drugs and Chemicals
- Section 3—Index to External Causes of Injuries and Poisonings (for assigning E-codes)

Some references have a Section 4—Index to Procedures, while others have a Volume III, which is used by hospital coders to code procedures (physicians' offices use the CPT coding for their procedures, so this section or volume is *not* used for coding in the medical office).

In addition, many code books have enhancement variations. Some are loose-leafed, and some highlight codes to be avoided or ones that require additional information. Some carry additional explanations of diseases or disorders, while others are color-coded to identify cautions, signs, symptoms, external causes, and so on.

ICD-9-CM 2007

One example of an ICD code book is published by Ingenix. It contains both Volumes I and II. The tabular section with disease classifications and increasing specific codes is arranged numerically from 001, Infectious and Parasitic Diseases, to 999.9, Other and unspecified complications of medical care, not elsewhere classified. A partial page is shown in Figure 9-8. This book has some features that help ensure accurate coding:

- Boxes preceding the ICD indicate that a fourth and/or fifth digit are available for greater specificity.
- Code descriptions have colored backgrounds to indicate the type of code and bring attention and unspecified or other specified codes.
- At the bottom of each page a key indicates what the different symbols represent.

The diagnosis with a proper code is easily recognized. Note the description of the conditions in 240.0 and 240.9. In addition to the codes, notice the black boxed *excludes* feature that indicates other code numbers used for these conditions. New lines of information are identified with a solid black diamond, while a revised line is an outlined black diamond. This code book also includes anatomic illustrations of various body structures to aid in selecting codes.

Coding Rules

The general coding rules are:

1. Code correctly and completely any diagnosis or procedure that affects the care, influences the health status, or is a reason for treatment on that visit.
2. Code the minimum number of diagnoses that fully describe the patient's care received on that visit. The diagnosis must reflect the patient's need for treatment, x-rays, diagnostic procedures, or medications.
3. Code each problem to the highest level of specificity (3rd, 4th, or 5th digit) available in the classification (see Figure 9-8).
4. Sequence codes correctly so that it is possible to understand the chronology of events (e.g., the reason for the visit and care).

The *main rule* to remember is the "**reason rule**," which says that the reason for the patient visit (encounter) is coded *first*.

This is **primary**; other "side" issues are coded next, in order of importance. There is a situation when the main rule will not apply. Sometimes, after the patient has been examined, another condition is discovered that differs from the condition for which the patient had originally sought treatment. In this situation, the diagnosis that required the greatest amount of effort would be coded first. At first, coding is confusing and difficult, but with experience, it will become easier.

IDENTIFYING THE DIAGNOSIS

Identifying the diagnosis may be a difficult task for the beginning coder. Remember to follow the rules and suggestions mentioned previously. Physicians usually help by marking indications on the patient's encounter form or superbill as well as recording diagnoses on the chart. However, it is necessary for the coder to read the chart, or if employed by a surgeon, the operative report, in order to determine any other codes that might apply. Remember, this affects your rate of payment. Some code books provide cues in their listings. Claims with codes that should be carried to the 4th or 5th digit to make the diagnosis more specific, but are not, *will be rejected and returned*. To complicate matters further, the rules are always changing. In 1996, Medicare had made five "changes" by July 1 that affected how claims are filed. One referred to rebundling of codes when multiple procedures are performed and said that generally reimbursement would be given only for the *major* procedure. To **bundle** refers to the process of considering several parts as a whole. At other times, Medicare will unbundle a multilevel procedure and allow billing on each portion. The **truncated** (cutoff) ICD coding rul-

Chapter heading

3. ENDOCRINE, NUTRITIONAL AND METABOLIC DISEASES, AND IMMUNITY DISORDERS (240-279)

Excludes statement

EXCLUDES *endocrine and metabolic disturbances specific to the fetus and newborn (775.0-775.9)*

Instructional note

Note: All neoplasms, whether functionally active or not, are classified in Chapter 2. Codes in Chapter 3 (i.e., 242.8, 246.0, 251-253, 2555-259) may be used to identify such functional activity associated with any neoplasm, or by ectopic endocrine tissue.

Major topic heading

DISORDERS OF THYROID GLAND (240-246)

Category code

✓4th **240 Simple and unspecified goiter**
DEF: An enlarged thyroid gland often caused by an inadequate dietary intake of iodine.

Subcategory code

240.0 Goiter, specified as simple
Any condition classifiable to 240.9, specified as simple

240.9 Goiter, unspecified

Description statements

Enlargement of thyroid	Goiter or struma:
Goiter or struma:	hyperplastic
NOS	nontoxic (diffuse)
diffuse colloid	parenchymatous
endemic	sporadic

EXCLUDES *congenital (dyshormonogenic) goiter (246.1)*

DISEASES OF OTHER ENDOCRINE GLANDS (250-259)

✓4th **250 Diabetes mellitus**
EXCLUDES *gestational diabetes (648.8)*
hyperglycemia NOS (790.6)
neonatal diabetes mellitus (775.1)
nonclinical diabetes (790.29)

Subclassification codes for 5th digit assignment

> The following fifth-digit subclassification is for use with category 250:
> ▲ **0 type II or unspecified type, not stated as uncontrolled**
> Fifth-digit 0 is for use for type II patients, even if the patient requires insulin
> ▶ Use additional code, if applicable, for associated long-term (current) insulin use V58.67 ◀
> ▲ **1 type I (juvenile type), not stated as uncontrolled**
> ▲ **2 type II or unspecified type, uncontrolled**
> Fifth-digit 2 is for use for type II patients, even if the patient requires insulin
> ▶ Use additional code, if applicable, for associated long-term (current) insulin use V58.67 ◀
> ▲ **3 type I (juvenile type), uncontrolled**

AHA: 2Q, '02, 13; 2Q, '01, 16; 2Q, '98, 15; 4Q, '97, 32; 2Q, '97, 14; 3Q, '96, 5; 4Q, '93, 19; 2Q, '92, 5; 3Q, '91, 3; 2Q, '90, 22; N-D, '85, 11

DEF: Diabetes mellitus: Inability to metabolize carbohydrates, proteins, and fats with insufficient secretion of insulin. Symptoms may be unremarkable, with long-term complications, involving kidneys, nerves, blood vessels, and eyes.
DEF: Uncontrolled diabetes: A nonspecific term indicating that the current treatment regimen does not keep the blood sugar level of a patient within acceptable levels.

✓5th **250.0 Diabetes mellitus without mention of complication**
Diabetes mellitus without mention of complication or manifestation classifiable to 250.1-250.9
Diabetes (mellitus) NOS
CC Excl: For code 250.01-250.03: 250.00-250.93, 251.0-251.3, 259.8-259.9

AHA: 4Q, '97, 32; 3Q, '91, 3, 12; N-D, '85, 11;
For Code 250.00;
4Q, '03, 105, 108; 2Q, '03, 16 1Q, '02, 7, 11;
For Code 250.01:
4Q, '03, 110; 2Q, '03, 6 **For Code 250.02:** 1Q, '03, 5

FIGURE 9-8 ICD-9-CM diseases tabular list *(From ICD-9-CM for Hospitals—Volumes 1, 2 & 3, 2005 Professional. Reprinted with permission of Ingenix.)*

ing, which became effective July 1, 1996, stated that claims must be coded to the highest level of specificity or they will be rejected and the provider will be required to file a new claim.

The standardized *required* form will accept up to four diagnostic codes (see Figure 9-7, line 21). Remember: you only receive reimbursement for procedures or services that relate to the identified diagnostic codes. Again, refer to Figure 9-7 line 21. The form asks you to relate the diagnosis code to the procedure and enter that in line 24 D and E. There must be a reason for the procedure to be done. For example, if a patient just wanted to know her blood type, but there was no *reason* (diagnosis) that the information was necessary, the procedure code would probably be rejected.

While the government was busy publishing the ICD code books, the American Medical Association developed and published *The Physicians' Current Procedural Terminology (CPT)* code book. This is a descriptive listing of codes for reporting medical services and procedures performed by physicians. NOTE: These two standard **nomenclature** code books (ICD, CPT) are published *annually* and are absolutely essential to the function of the medical office. Each year codes are added, deleted, changed, or modified for the new editions. Books can be ordered in advance and are released in the fall. Some governmental and commercial payers require that you begin to use the next year's codes as of October 1 of the current year. Check with payers to see what their requirements are. There are payers that wait to begin to use the new codes as of January 1 of the following year and others will wait until as late as April 1 of that year.

Healthcare Common Procedure Coding System (HCPCS) Level II Code Set

An additional set of codes used to identify products and supplies, which are not identified in CPT, are the Healthcare Common Procedure Coding System (HCPCS) codes. The CMS maintains and distributes HCPCS codes. The codes are composed of one alpha and four numeric characters. *J* codes identify injectables. *L* codes identify orthotics. HCPCS codes are used in outpatient settings only. Like the CPT and ICD books, HCPCS codes are published annually. Not all insurance companies recognize HCPCS codes. Verify with the companies you send claims to whether or not they will accept HCPCS codes.

CURRENT PROCEDURAL TERMINOLOGY CODES

The **Current Procedural Terminology (CPT)** codebook has a systematic listing and coding of procedures and services performed by physicians. Each procedure or service is identified with a five-digit code, which is used to report services. The main body of the material is listed in six sections:

1. Evaluation and Management (E/M)
2. Anesthesiology
3. Surgery
4. Radiology (including Nuclear Medicine and Diagnostic Ultrasound)
5. Pathology and Laboratory
6. Medicine (except Anesthesiology)

Within each section are subsections with anatomic, procedure, condition, or descriptor subheadings. The procedures and services with their identifying codes are presented in **numeric** order with one exception: the entire Evaluation and Management section is placed at the beginning of the listed procedures. These items are used by most physicians in reporting a significant portion of their services. At the end of the book are the appendix and the index. Following the index is a page listing instructions for the use of the CPT index. The index has four general categories. Each category has examples to assist the user in understanding the category.

Using the CPT Book

To determine a code, the name of the procedure or service that most accurately identifies the service performed is selected. This could be a diagnostic procedure, radiologic examination, or surgery. Other additional procedures performed or pertinent services may be listed, including any modifying or extenuating circumstances. Any service or procedure that is coded *must be* adequately documented in the medical record. As with ICD codes, you can rely on the physician for assistance. Generally, services performed in the office are marked on the patient's encounter form. Care must be taken not to miss items like injections, urinalysis, or blood samples, or the need to use a **modifier** for prolonged E/M services. If you must code from operative reports, it will be necessary to review the description the surgeon dictated to be certain all pertinent codes have been identified.

The introduction in the CPT code book gives excellent instructions on the use of CPT terminology and coding. The book is divided into specialty sections, but codes from any section may be used to give an adequate description of a treatment or procedure rendered by a qualified physician. In reading the introduction, you will find guidelines are presented at the beginning of each section to define items that are necessary to interpret and report the procedure and services to be found in that section. In some instances a specific procedure or service may need to be slightly altered. Instructions and the appendix explain the use of modifiers. Some examples of when these would be used are if unusual events occurred, if a service was performed by more than one physician, or if only the professional or technical component of a radiologic procedure were to be billed for.

If you cannot find a code listed for a procedure or service your employer has performed, a provision has been made for the use of specific code numbers for reporting unlisted procedures. In these instances a description of the service must also be provided.

It is important to use the current year's code book to check the codes you are using to be sure they have not been changed. A special appendix in the book provides a complete list of the codes deleted, revised, and added to the book. Another detail requiring attention is the superbill or encounter form. Usually they are preprinted with the most frequently used ICD and CPT codes listed to facilitate coding by the physician and insurance coder. When new books are issued, these frequently used codes especially need to be checked to ensure they remain accurate and valid. If changes have occurred, the slip may need reprinting.

Software companies have made it possible for physicians' offices to design their own superbills in whatever format they choose. The software contains all the ICD and CPT codes, and the practice chooses the ones appropriate to their services. Once the superbill is designed, it can be printed out from a computer. Errors and fraudulent billing codes are reduced when completing a claim form. The software even warns the user when fourth and fifth digits are required. Updating the software when codes are revised will also allow the program to scan the designed superbill to identify code changes.

Features of the CPT Book

The CPT 2007 book uses symbols to indicate specific information about code numbers, much like those found in the ICD publications. Figure 9-9 is a sample of breast incision and excision codes that illustrates

one of the symbols. In addition, notice the descriptive language and symbols that explain the specificity of the procedure:

+ Add-on code
▲ Revised code
● New code
►◄ New or revised text

The AMA also offers versions of the CPT book in CD format, and the CPT book's contents can be downloaded to a computer. Other coding publications are avilable for immediate download as well. You can veiw these publications by visiting their web site at www. ama-assn.org.

Evaluation and Management Services Guidelines

The E/M section codes are divided into 17 categories of provider services beginning with *Office and Other Outpatient Services* and ending with *Other Procedures*. The E/M codes are related to medical services as opposed to surgical services. Figure 9-10 illustrates two of the five coding areas for a new patient office visit. The codes are important because they describe the nature of the physician's actions, such as:

- Place of service
- Level of history and examination required
- Degree of decision making involved
- Extent of the patient's problem
- Amount of time the physician spent

Another classification that affects coding is whether the patient is new or established.

Within each category or subcategory of E/M services, three to five levels are available for reporting purposes. The levels include examinations, evaluations, treatments, conferences with or concerning patients, preventive pediatric and adult health supervision, and

---

BREAST

Incision

19000	Puncture aspiration of cyst of breast
+19001	each additional cyst (List separately in addition to code for primary procedure)
	(Use 19001 in conjunction with 19000)
	(If imaging guidance is performed, see 76095, 76096, 76393, 76942)
19020	Mastotomy with exploration or drainage of abscess, deep
19030	Injection procedure only for mammary ductogram or galactogram
	(For radiological supervision and interpretation, see 76086, 76088)
	(For catheter lavage of mammary ducts for collection of cytology specimens, use Category III codes 0046T, 0047T)

FIGURE 9-9 Sample CPT codes showing procedures and symbols to denote new, revised, add-on, and surgical procedures only (Current Procedural Terminology ©2006 American Medical Association. All rights reserved.)

NEW PATIENT

99201   **Office or other outpatient visit** for the evaluation and management of a new patient, which requires these three key components:

- **a problem focused history;**
- **a problem focused examination;**
- **straightforward medical decision making.**

Counseling and/or coordination of care with other providers or agencies are provided consistent with the nature of the problem(s) and the patients and/or family's needs.

Usually, the presenting problem(s) are self limited or minor. Physicians typically spend 10 minutes face-to-face with the patient and/or family.

99202   **Office or other outpatient visit** for the evaluation and management of a new patient, which requires these three key components:

- **an expanded problem focused history;**
- **an expanded problem focused examination;**
- **straightforward medical decision making.**

Counseling and/or coordination of care with other providers or agencies are provided consistent with the nature of the problem(s) and the patient's and/or family's needs.

Usually, the presenting problem(s) are of low to moderate severity. Physicians typically spend 20 minutes face-to-face with the patient and/or family.

FIGURE 9-10   Sample CPT-E/M codes for new patient office or other outpatient services (Current Procedural Terminology ©2006 American Medical Association. All rights reserved.)

similar medical services. The levels encompass wide variations in skill, effort, time, responsibility, and medical knowledge required for the prevention or diagnosis and treatment of illness or injury.

In addition to the levels are descriptors that recognize seven components that are used in defining the levels of E/M services:

1. History
2. Examination
3. Medical decision making
4. Counseling
5. Coordination of care
6. Nature of presenting problem
7. Time

The first three are considered key components in selecting a level of E/M services. The next three and the nature of the presenting problem are considered **contributory** factors in the majority of **encounters** (contacts). It is *not* required that these services be provided at every patient encounter. The actual performance of any diagnostic test or study requires separate specific coding in *addition* to the appropriate E/M code. Several other items unique to the section are described in the E/M guidelines, which are fairly easy to read and understand. If you refer to the first page of the E/M section of the CPT code book, you will see codes for a new patient that show four levels of history and examina-

tion. Selecting the appropriate E/M and CPT codes is a complex clinical decision that is ultimately the responsibility of the physician. Completion of Procedure 9-1, "Perform Procedural and Diagnostic Coding," will provide you with practice in locating and applying CPT and ICD codes.

COMPLETING THE CLAIM FORM

Be certain that you have a copy of the patient's insurance coverage card and have secured his or her signature on a form to permit release of information before processing claims. This form will also have an "assignment of benefits" clause that authorizes benefits be paid directly to the provider.

Obtaining the appropriate signatures for releasing patient information to any third-party payer should be a priority when the patient completes her initial new patient information paperwork. The paperwork could include a statement similar to the following:

> I request that payment of authorized Medicare benefits be made on my behalf to Dr. _____ for any service furnished to me by that physician. I authorize release of medical information about me needed to determine these benefits or benefits payable for related services.

The form should be signed by the patient and dated.

PROCEDURE PROCEDURE PROCEDURE PROCEDURE PROCEDURE PROCEDURE PROCEDURE

9-1  Perform Procedural and Diagnostic Coding

PURPOSE: To accurately locate and apply a procedure code and diagnosis code.

EQUIPMENT: Encounter form and current year's CPT and ICD books.

PERFORMANCE OBJECTIVE: Accurately identify the correct CPT code in the CPT book to describe the service indicated on the encounter form in narrative form. Locate the diagnosis code that describes the narrative diagnosis listed on the encounter form. Indicate the correct CPT and ICD on the form once it is identified by using the coding manuals. Follow the procedural steps listed here to accomplish this task.

1. Identify the narrative procedure listed. **NOTE: It may be difficult to read the handwriting of the practitioner. Seek clarification of a word or spelling if you are unsure; *never* guess or assume. If no one is able to assist you in determining what the narrative reflects, go to the author of the narrative description to seek clarification.**

2. Determine the main term(s) listed in the narrative.

3. Turn to the alphabetic index in the CPT book. **NOTE: The index is located at the *back* of the CPT book. Main terms are listed alphabetically.**

4. Locate the main term by viewing all of the listings. **NOTE: If you cannot locate a term where you think it would be, consider a synonym of that term. What type of service or procedure was performed? Maybe it can be located by anatomic site, by abbreviation, or by condition or disease.**

5. Locate the appropriate subterm under the main term that best describes the services the practitioner provided.

6. There might be one code listed to the right of the description, several codes separated by commas, or a range of codes indicated by a hyphens. **NOTE: Locating the main and subterms in the index is only part of the process of identifying the correct code. *Never code* directly from the index, even if only one code is listed when you locate the main and subterms.**

7. Turn to the CPT code(s) (five-digit number) in the main part of the CPT manual. Does the description mirror the services your practitioner provided? If so, apply this code to the encounter form. **NOTE: Remember that if a range of codes or a series of codes separated by commas was listed in the index, you must** look at all of these codes before making your CPT code selection.

8. Review the narrative diagnosis finding indicated on the encounter form.

9. Locate the index of the ICD manual. **NOTE: The alphabetic index of ICD is located at the *front* of the manual. This is identified as Volume II.**

10. Identify the main term(s). **NOTE: Keep in mind that terms such as "broken" may be located by looking under "fracture," and "collar bone" may be found under the term "clavicle." If you cannot locate a term where you think it would be, consider a synonym of that term.**

11. Locate the appropriate subterm under the main term that best describes the practitioner's finding. **NOTE: If a patient has a broken collar bone, locate the main term *fracture* (which will be in bold font and flush with the left margin of the column it is listed in) and then *clavicle* as the subterm. The subterm will not be bolded and will be indented under the main term.**

12. A three-to-five digit ICD will be listed at the end of the subterm. **NOTE: Coding ICDs to the highest level of specificity is extremely important. An ICD code will have a minimum of three digits and could have an additional one to two digits following a decimal point after the third digit. If a 4th or 5th digit is available to describe the diagnosis, it must be used. Payers are very particular about specificity in diagnosis coding.**

13. Locate the ICD in the tabular list of the ICD book. This is also known as Volume 1. **NOTE: The tabular list reflects all ICDs that are located in the alphabetic index; however in the tabular list the codes are listed numerically beginning with category 001 and ending with category 999. Watch for coding conventions such as *Includes and Excludes, Use Additional Code, and And and With.* These are helpful tools in identifying whether you are selecting the appropriate code(s).**

14. Indicate the correct ICD on the encounter form. **NOTE: Correct coding takes a great deal of practice. The more the medical assistant codes, the better he will become. Just like practice at clinical skills refines a medical assistant's ability to perform clinically, the same holds true with the administrative function of applying CPT and ICD coding skills.**

HIPAA

HIPAA guidelines require that the patient be informed regarding the medical practice's intentions on why, how, and what it plans to do with the patient's protected health information (PHI). The medical assistant can accomplish this by providing the patient with a copy of the practice's Notice of Privacy Policies.

The CMS has developed codes for Medicare that allow for uniformity throughout the country. The two levels of codes range as follows:

1. The CPT codes are established and updated by the American Medical Association. These are five-digit numeric codes ranging from 00000 to 99999 for physicians' services, such as examinations, surgeries, radiology, and pathology.

2. HCPCS codes were developed by the Center for Medicare and Medicaid Services. The Alpha-Numeric Workgroup with in CMS, the Health Insurance Association of America, the Blue Cross and Blue Shield Association work collaboratively to maintain the codes. These alpha-numeric codes range from A0000 to V9999 and are used for physician and nonphysician services not listed in the CPT.

Another important number necessary for completion of Medicare claims is the physician's National Provider Identification (NPI) number. In 2007, the NPI replaced the PIN, or physician's identifying number, and the UPIN, or unique physician's identifying number, previously used. The NPI is a ten-digit number; the first seven digits are unique to the physician, the eighth digit is a check digit, and the last two have to do with location. The NPI will be used in blocks 24 and 33 of the approved form to identify who provided the service. When the physician refers a patient to another practice for services, the referring physician's NPI will appear in block 17b of the form. If this number is missing from the claim, the claim will be returned.

Medicare provides annual updated policy manuals, seminars, and monthly newsletters to keep physicians and their staffs current on Medicare policy. The best way to keep up-to-date on Medicare's constant changes is to visit the CMS web site often and sign up for their listserv. Every time there is a news release an announcement will be sent to your e-mail address. You can click on the link to view the release.

In processing Medicare insurance forms, you must use ICD codes for diagnosis, CPT codes for treatment, and HCPCS codes for any supplies or appliances used.

Today the patient has little or no responsibility for filing claims. The physician is *required* to file Medicare claims, and it is normally an obligation when contracting as a provider with other carriers. Once the physician has billed the primary coverage and the primary carrier has responded, either the carrier will automatically forward the claim to a secondary carrier, or the physician as a courtesy may choose to file for the secondary coverage. Often this is to the physicians' advantage, as the supplemental amount is usually paid directly to them. After primary and secondary carriers have responded, the remaining approved balance can be billed to the patient for payment.

As stated previously, government-sponsored health care claims must be filed on the approved insurance claim form (refer to Figure 9-7). Regulations also require that the form be an original; copies are not acceptable. Procedure 9-2 "Complete a Claim Form," will give you some practice in preparing a form. CMS forms can be obtained from many office supply companies, as well as the AMA. The forms are designed for use with computer printers. In addition to government mandatory use, all other insurance companies will accept the form. This is helpful, especially with patients who have **secondary** coverage; it eliminates the need to complete two forms. Even if the secondary carrier has its own claim form, a copy of the approved form can be attached and will be acceptable.

MAINTAINING AN INSURANCE LOG

A method for monitoring the status and payment of insurance claims should be established. It is easy to forget about filed claims, and soon a sizeable amount of money is owed to the physician. Some practices use an insurance log (a book in which a list of insurance claims is kept). When a claim is filed, it is noted on a log. The log should have columns for recording pertinent information. Tracking the following is helpful in monitoring claim status:

- The date the claim is filed
- The insurance company's name
- The patient's name
- The amount of the claim
- The amount paid
- The secondary company's name
- The date filed
- The amount billed
- The amount paid
- The date the patient was billed
- The follow-up date

Today, most offices use computer software designed for monitoring insurance claims. The information can be entered on the grid and brought up on the screen for review or printed out so it is possible to see the total file at once.

By looking at the log or the computer file, you can quickly see the status of each claim. If claims become

PROCEDURE PROCEDURE PROCEDURE PROCEDURE PROCEDURE PROCEDURE PROCEDURE

9-2   Complete a Claim Form

PURPOSE: To accurately complete a claim form for processing.

EQUIPMENT: CMS-1500 form, patient record, account ledger or information, computer, and software.

PERFORMANCE OBJECTIVE: Given access to all necessary equipment and information, follow the procedure to complete an approved claim form without error within the instructor's prescribed time limit.

1. Check for a photocopy of the patient's insurance card.

2. Check the chart to see whether the patient signature is on file for release of information and assignment of benefits. **NOTE: If one is not on file, the patient must sign the form. It is best to have it signed before the form is completed. If the completed form is forwarded to the patient to be signed and sent to the insurance company, it is best to send a stamped and addressed envelope to avoid a delay in forwarding the form to the insurance company.**

3. Using Figure 9-7 as a guide, complete the following entries:

   A. Check the appropriate box at the top of the form.

   B. Enter the name of the patient (be certain the name used on the form is the same as that on the identification card).

   C. Enter the birth date and check the box for male or female. **NOTE: Use eight digits to write the birth date (e.g., 08/23/1929).**

   D. Fill in the rest of the numbered boxes on CMS-1500 using these steps, which correspond to the box numbers.

4. Enter the insured's name.

5. Enter the patient's full address and telephone number.

6. Enter the patient's relationship to the insured.

7. Enter the insured's full address and telephone number.

8. Enter the patient's status.

9. Enter the other insured's name and necessary information:

   - Other insured's policy or group number
   - Other insured's birth date, and check box for male or female
   - Employer's name or school name
   - Insurance plan name or program name

(Fill in "none" or N/A, for not applicable, so there is no doubt you have observed this section.)

10. Check the appropriate box regarding employment and accident. (Do not leave all these boxes blank.)

11. Enter the insured's policy number and other necessary information:

    - Insured's birth date, and check box for male or female
    - Employer or school name
    - Insurance plan name or program name
    - Is there another health benefit plan?

12. Obtain the patient's or authorized person's signature.

13. Obtain the insured's signature, or stamp "signature on file" if you have the record to prove it.

14. Record the date the current illness began.

15. Record the date the patient was first treated for the same or similar illness.

16. Enter the dates the patient is unable to work or leave blank.

17. Complete with the name of the referring physician or leave blank.

17a. Enter the non-NPI number of the referring physician.

17b. Insert the NPI number of the referring physician.

18. Complete with dates of hospitalization or leave blank.

19. Leave blank.

20. Mark the appropriate box regarding lab services.

21. Enter an ICD code on a separate line for each diagnosis.

22. Complete if Medicaid.

23. Complete if applicable with medical authorization code.

24. Complete A through H with appropriate CPT or HCPCS codes for services. **NOTE: List each service separately with the most important listed first.**

24a. Enter the rendering provider's non-NPI (legacy) number in the shaded area. Enter the provider's NPI number in the nonshaded area. **NOTE: Certain type of providers will not have an NPI number. Another type of identifying number might be required. The shaded area in 24J is provided in order to report this number.**

25. Add the physician's Social Security number or practice tax identification number and mark the appropriate box.

(continues)

9-2  Complete a Claim Form (Continued)

26. Add the patient's account number if applicable.

27. Check one box regarding assignment. **NOTE: Must be marked "yes" to accept assignment.**

28. Enter the total charged.

29. Enter the amount paid.

30. Enter any balance due. **NOTE: Form will be rejected if this not completed.**

31. Obtain physician's signature and date. **NOTE: Medicare will accept a stamped signature. All carriers will accept physicians' typed name and credentials as indication of their signature.**

32. Enter the name and address of the facility where services were rendered, if other than home or office.

32a. Enter the NPI number of the facility.

32b. Enter the non-NPI number of the facility. **NOTE: Certain types of facilities may not have an NPI number. Another type of identifying number might be required.**

33. Enter the physician's name, address, and telephone number. **NOTE: Do not use punctuation in the address. If you supply a 9-digit zip code, it is acceptable to use a hyphen to separate the last 4-digits.**

33a. Enter the NPI number of the provider.

33b. Enter the non-NPI number of the provider. **NOTE: Certain types of providers will not have an NPI number. Another type of identifying number might be required.**

delinquent, a carrier can be easily identified and contacted. As a general rule, claims are paid in a timely fashion after billing, usually within 30 to 60 days for a paper claim and as little as 10 to 14 for a claim that is filed electronically. At times, a carrier will deny ever receiving a claim. If your office manually completes claims, it is wise to make copies prior to sending them out. In the event the carrier states they never received the claim, a copy of the original will come in handy. If you are using a practice management (PM) system to generate claims, you will be able to regenerate the claim to send a second time. When claims are *not* approved or are rejected because of errors, you will be able to refile upon submitting additional information or correcting the errors. When a claim is returned after being denied, it may not be eligible for refiling.

DELINQUENT CLAIMS

If an electronically submitted claim has not been paid 3 weeks after submission (6 weeks for a paper claim), and you have not received a denial, it is time to follow up. Most carriers provide a toll-free number on the insurance card provided to the patient. Before you make the call, be sure you have the following information available: your practice's tax identification number; patient's name; identification number; group name or number; and, if the patient *is not* the insured, the insured's (e.g., spouse's) name. Once the account is identified, they will request the date(s) of service and

the total amount submitted. The carrier will then give you the status of the claim. If it is still in process, request an anticipated date of payment. If the claim is delayed pending additional information, be sure to follow up quickly and return the material requested. If the company has no record of receiving a claim, ask if you may submit a *copy* of the claim previously submitted and verify the mailing address. Also ask if you could direct the claim to a specific person to accelerate the process. It is helpful to have a specific contact person in case further discussion is necessary. In the event the claim is close to the filing statute date, inquire if you can fax the claim. If the carrier indicates that the claim has been paid, ask when the payment was made and to whom it was sent. If it was sent to the patient, you will need to send the patient a statement.

COMMON CLAIM ERRORS

In a recent survey of insurance companies, the following common errors were listed as causes of claim payment delays:

1. The patient's—not the policyholder's—Social Security number or identification number is used as the certificate number. The claim would be rejected for lack of membership.

2. The "Coordination of Benefits" section is not completed, thereby suspending the claim for additional information.

3. Use of incorrect ICD codes.

4. Use of an incorrect or deleted CPT code could result in a decreased payment or a rejection.

5. Use of an incorrect provider identification number could result in misdirection of payment.

6. Superbills attached to a claim form are sometimes illegible.

7. Member does not respond to the request for clarification of insurances covering injury or illness when another party might have responsibility.

8. Lack of operative report if procedure is unusual or complicated or fee is unusual.

9. Incorrect spelling of patient's name.

10. Inconsistent use of patient's name; for example, middle name is used as first, nicknames are used instead of correct first name (i.e., Bill instead of William).

11. An incorrect patient birth date is reported.

12. Use of an incorrect place of service code will suspend a claim.

ELECTRONIC CLAIM FILING

Many offices electronically process claim forms to the insurance carrier. The turn-around time is shortened, and there is a reduction in preparation time. Your PM system must have the software required for filing claims electronically. A program is run on your system to flag claims that need to be billed to the carriers. The claims are put into batches. Batches of claims are sent electronically to a clearinghouse. The clearinghouse runs a claims scrubber on all of the claims to check for missing or invalid data. Any claims that are not "clean" are returned to you via a status report. These claims need to be reviewed and any errors will need to be corrected in order for you to submit the claims again. Clean claims are forwarded to the appropriate payer for processing. The cost of the service is considered money well spent, because the claims are "clean" when submitted and reimbursement is received within a few weeks.

ACCEPTING ASSIGNMENT

Medicare and other carriers enlist physicians to "sign up" as approved or **preferred** providers. Usually, the physician agrees to treat people enrolled in the program for an "agreed" rate for services. This rate is referred to as a **fee schedule**. In return for being willing to participate and accept a reduction in charges, the physician is ensured a supply of patients enrolled in the health care program. Physicians often contract with many carriers in order to be able to provide services for a large group of current as well as future patients. (This concept was covered earlier in this chapter when carriers and managed care were discussed.)

Particularly with Medicare patients, the contracted provider agrees to accept the "approved amount" as their fee; this agreement is known as "accepting assignment." The difference between the amount charged and the payment received is "written off" by the physician as a provider adjustment. The physician or any other provider can charge the patient only for the part of the deductible that has not been met and the small leftover balance from the approved charge. The provider can also charge for any service *not* covered by Medicare. If your physician is making a charge for a noncovered service, be certain the patient understands that the charges will be his or her responsibility. It is a good idea to have a statement signed by the patient that states the fee is *not* covered so that the patient cannot later refuse to pay and claim noncoverage was unknown.

All physicians, whether they choose to participate or not, must abide by Medicare laws. When the doctor does *not* accept assignment, he must be paid directly by the patient, who is responsible for the entire bill, even if it is higher than the Medicare-approved amount. However, even when a doctor does not accept assignment, the most that can be charged is 115% of what Medicare approves. Doctors and other providers who exceed limits can be fined.

MEDICARE AUDIT

The importance of complete records and documentation is never as critical as when the office is involved in a Medicare audit. Audits may be conducted if there is any question as to the amount of service rendered in exchange for the claims paid. Records are essential to provide evidence that diagnoses and treatments were appropriate and that the services paid for were actually provided. The level of service must also be documented. Failure to adequately document the level of service could cause a downcoding by Medicare and can result in the charge of "fraud." Anyone knowingly submitting a false claim or creating a false record or statement in order to receive payment from the federal government will be fined a civil penalty of not less than $5,500 and not more than $11,000. Documentation is essential. Remember: When records are reviewed by third-party payers, "If it is not documented, it was never done." Office staffs should monitor physicians' records and inform them of what is needed if necessary. Not only does it ensure adequate documentation but it also ensures that the physician receives the maximum reimbursement due. Of the following seven items, at least five must be documented in the office medical records:

- Complaints and symptoms
- Duration and course of illness
- Details of illness
- Examination and findings
- Laboratory and x-ray values and findings
- Diagnosis or problem
- Treatment, injection, or advice

REIMBURSEMENT

Remember that Medicare reimburses the approved fee at the rate of 80% after the year's annual deductible amount has been paid by the patient. Secondary payment is then sought to cover the 20% not covered. Many secondary carriers likewise will pay 80% of the 20% not covered of the approved amount, after the deductible is met. The remaining small percentage and the initial annual deductible is the responsibility of the patient. Figure 9-11 is a summary of the Medicare and secondary insurance "explanation of benefits" reports, resulting from an actual minor medical situation, in the approximate order they were received. In this example, the patient is a 65-year-old female who had a suspicious mammogram that resulted in an incisional biopsy of two areas of microcalcification in the same breast. The procedure was performed in the same-day surgery department of a hospital.

The importance of detailed descriptions, procedure codes, and accurate records is very evident. With insurance payment of medical charges, there are several factors to be considered: annual deductibles, approved fee schedules, and percentages of approval rates, which all influence the amount paid. Review the summary. Notice how much of the charges are approved and how much is the patient's responsibility. Follow the initial charges through deductibles, Medicare, secondary coverage, sometimes refiling, and finally, the patient's responsibility. This excessive amount of paperwork is a good example of why patients become so confused with insurance coverage and payment, and why medical assistants seem to never finish filing claims.

THE FUTURE OF INSURANCE CLAIMS

As long as there are third-party payers, the filing of some sort of claim will continue. Probably the greatest change will come in how the filing is done. Providers will take advantage of the electronic process. With the capability of computer programs, it is possible to use software that, given a diagnosis, automatically identifies coding, sequences it, and compares it to the treatment codes. An annual update for the software program is required to screen for any changed, added, or deleted codes. This eliminates much of the rejection and refiling problems. A built-in fee by the carriers for the physician's filing expenses would also be a helpful update.

MAINTAINING CURRENCY

Staying informed and up-to-date with Medicare is a never-ending process. Ideally, in each practice someone is designated the claims filer and is expected to maintain currency. This can be done in various ways. Medicare updates are discussed in bulletins available monthly to the practice. Many practice specialty organizations will have newsletters, specific to their needs, to keep members informed. Other insurance carriers will send newsletters to their participating physicians describing any changes in their coverage or processing.

Seminars are conducted frequently. The annual major update seminar sponsored by your state medical association is practically a requirement in order for any practice to survive. Other seminars are conducted by private companies and can prove very informative. The content, of course, depends upon the amount of time and the expertise or focus of the presenting organization.

It is very important that you closely review any in-service advertisement. It should identify the content, perhaps include an outline, and if objectives are listed, give you a good idea of expected outcomes. Another assurance of its value is the approval for CEUs by the AAMA or the ARMA. If not preapproved, however, remember that you can submit information and request CEUs for educational seminars you attend, but approval is not ensured. Make certain you understand what is being offered and to what extent it will be presented so that your investment of time and money will be worthwhile.

ACHIEVE UNIT OBJECTIVES

- Complete the Workbook activities to meet the learning objectives.
- Practice the procedures in this unit to meet the performance objectives.
- Apply your knowledge at the end of this chapter in completing the Critical Thinking Challenge and Activities, as well as the StudyWARE on your Student CD-ROM.

DATE OF FORM	DATE OF SERVICE	SOURCE OF FORM	PROVIDER OF SERVICE	SERVICE PROVIDED—CODE	CHARGE	MEDICARE APPROVED	MEDICARE PAID	SECONDARY INSURANCE PAID	PATIENT RESPONSIBILITY	COMMENTS
2005 10/9	9/27	Medicare	Radiologist #1	Mammogram—7609L XA Both Breasts	$135.00	$65.91	-0-	-0-	$65.91	$65.91 applied to '05 deductible
11/2	10/3	Medicare	Surgeon	Office Consult—99242	$105.00	$89.56	$36.38	-0-	$53.18	$44.09 applied to '05 deductible
11/10	10/11	Medicare	Primary physician	Office Consult—99243 ECG—93000 Chest x-ray—71020-XA Blood draw—36415	$130.00 54.00 69.00 7.00 $260.00	$119.40 25.68 34.71 3.00 $182.79	$95.52 20.55 27.77 2.40 $146.24	-0- -0- -0- -0-		$36.55 to be billed to insurance
11/30	10/17	Medicare	Radiologist #2	Place needlewire—19290 X-ray needlewire placement in breast—76096-26 X-ray specimen—76098-26	$275.00 140.00 22.00 $437.00	$152.40 28.73 8.21 $189.34	$121.92 22.99 6.57 $151.48	-0- -0- -0-	$30.48 $5.74 $1.64 $37.86	
11/30	10/17	Medicare	Surgeon	Excision breast lesion—19125	$800.00	$428.42	$342.74	-0-		$85.68 to be billed to insurance
11/20	10/17	Medicare	Anesthesia #1	4.3 Anesthesia—00400 Chest skin surgery QKQS	$350.40	-0-	-0-	-0-	-0-	Requested information had not been received.
11/20	10/17	Medicare	Pathologist	1 Tissue exam—88305-26 1 Tissue exam—88307-26 1 Consult in surgery—88329	$165.00 230.00 70.00 $465.00	$41.26 86.65 49.61 $177.52	$41.26 86.65 49.61 $177.52	-0- -0- -0-	-0- -0- -0-	Lab services are paid at 100% of the Medicare allowable. Patient does not owe any copay or coinsureace on lab work.
11/20	10/17	Medicare	Anesthesia #2	4.3 Anesthesia—00400 Chest skin surgery QKQS	$111.25	-0-	-0-	-0-	$111.25	Charges denied, other insurance may pay.
11/20	10/17	Insurance	Surgeon	Procedure—excision				$68.55	$17.13	Insurance paid 80% of $68.55
12/2	10/11	Insurance	Prmy Phys	Medical x-ray, testing	$260.00			$29.24	$7.31	Insurance paid 80% of $36.55
12/14	10/3	Insurance	Surgeon	Medical	$105.00	$89.56	$36.38	$42.55	$10.63	Insurance paid 80% of $53.18
12/15	10/17	Medicare	Hospital	Laboratory Radiology Pharmacy Surgical service	$155.00 399.00 182.88 2,317.92 $3,054.80	$1,527.40	$916.44	-0-	$610.96	Deductible met.
2006 1/5	10/3 and 10/17	Statement	Surgeon	Balance after insurance payments		—	—		$24.44	Pt bal after Medicare and insur.
1/16	10/11	Statement	Prmy Phys	Balance after insurance payments					$7.31	Pt bal after Medicare and insur.
1/27	10/17	Insurance	Hospital	Surgical services	$3,054.80	$1,527.40	$916.44	$610.96	-0-	Paid in full by insurance.
1/26	10/17	Insurance	Radiologist #2	X-ray services balance after insurance payments	$437.00	$189.34	$151.48	$30.29	$7.57	
2/12	10/17	Statement	Radiologist #2	X-ray services balance after insurance payments	$437.00	$189.34	$151.48		$7.57	Remaining balance due.

FIGURE 9-11 Summary of insurance explanation of benefits form and medical statements received in connection with one routine breast incisional biopsy procedure

CRITICAL THINKING CHALLENGE

IMPACTING THE PATIENT, THE PRACTICE, AND YOUR CAREER

Maria was employed by Dr. Grey 6 months ago to process all insurance-related business. She had 2 years of experience with another physician and has attended updating seminars sponsored by her medical assistant association. Accepting the position with Dr. Grey seemed almost too good to be true. She is allowed to work a flexible, hourly schedule, which helps her manage her responsibilities as a single parent of two children. In addition, she was able to increase her salary and will be eligible to participate in the practice's profit-sharing plan after 1 year. She enjoys working with the three other office employees and often receives praise from them and the physician for her management of the insurance affairs.

About 3 months ago, Maria began to wonder about some charges listed on occasional encounter forms but dismissed the thought. Lately, however, after more careful observation, she is almost certain the physician is identifying charges that are not actually being done. For instance, he listed two hospital visits she is almost certain he did not make. She can also think of at least four instances last week when an office urinalysis was charged and not done. And 2 weeks ago, she knew an ECG was falsely charged. Subtler charge irregularities involved the listing of some office visits as comprehensive when in reality they were only focused. She was certain this occurred this week with Mrs. Lopez and Mr. Lee, because neither one of them was in the office more than 10 minutes each. She likes her job very much and knows she is considered a valued employee, but she is concerned about this issue.

WHAT IMPACT MIGHT THIS SCENARIO HAVE ON THE PATIENTS INVOLVED?

1. Could the patient's insurance premiums be affected by false or altered claims submitted?
2. Would patients question the urinalysis charges that would be reflected on their explanation of benefits from their insurance carrier?
3. Do you think patients would question the level of visit charged in the case of a focused exam versus a comprehensive exam, or do you think they would just pay their copay and not question the level of care charged?

WHAT IMPACT WOULD THE PHYSICIAN'S ACTIONS IN THIS SCENARIO HAVE ON THE PRACTICE?

1. How would an insurance company become aware that the physician may be altering or falsifying claims?
2. How would upcoding and charging for services not provided affect collections for the practice?
3. Do you think the physician is putting his participation status with the health plans at risk? If so, in what way?

WHAT IMPACT COULD THIS SITUATION HAVE ON THE MEDICAL ASSISTANT'S CAREER?

1. If the practice was audited and the physician was found guilty of submitting false or altered claims, would Maria be at fault also?
2. If Maria voiced her concerns to her manager or the physician, as well as documented on her own her suspicions and when she discussed them with the manager or physician, would she still be at fault?
3. Should Maria inform the patients involved of her suspicions? Why or why not?
4. There is a phone number to report suspected Medicare fraud (800-477-8477). Should she call and report her suspicions?

CRITICAL THINKING CHALLENGE

IMPACTING THE PATIENT, THE PRACTICE, AND YOUR CAREER

A patient presents at your office for treatment for what appears to be a work-related injury. You determine through obtaining the chief complaint from the patient and from the information reflected in the chart regarding where she is employed and a brief listing of her job responsibilities that the injury very likely could be work related. When you inquire a little further and specifically question whether the visit is related to an injury that occurred at work, the patient responds, "Well, yes, this did happen at work but I want my private insurance billed. I do not want this turned in as a workers' compensation claim." The patient was very clear in voicing where she wanted the claim for the service to be billed.

WHAT IMPACT COULD THIS SCENARIO HAVE ON THE PATIENT?

1. Do you think the patient is fearful of losing their job if a workers' compensation claim is filed for this injury?
2. Do you think the patient will follow the medical advice offered to her today if it involves seeing another physician and therefore greater expenses?
3. Could the patient be withholding details of the event that led to the injury? Is she possibly intoxicated or on illegal drugs?

WHAT IMPACT COULD THIS SCENARIO HAVE ON THE PRACTICE?

1. Can patients choose which insurance company or third party they want their claims billed to?
2. Do you need to be concerned with possibly losing this patient from the practice if you do not follow her wishes and file the claim only with her private insurance?
3. Where could you refer this patient for care in the event your physician is not participating as a Bureau of Workers' Compensation provider?

WHAT IMPACT COULD THIS SCENARIO HAVE ON THE CAREER OF THE MEDICAL ASSISTANT?

1. What action will you take?
2. Are you obligated to follow the patient's wishes?
3. Who should you make aware of the patient's request in relation to where the claim is to be filed?
4. If you file this claim with the commercial carrier, instead of BWC, and they see it is an injury, how do you think the claim will be processed?
5. If the carrier asks the patient for details that led to the injury, do you think the patient will respond to the request?

ACTIVITIES

1. Go to CMS's web site at www.cms.gov and type "electronic claims" in the search box. How many entries are there for this topic? What happens when you narrow the search by typing "how to file electronic claims"? Did the number of entries on the topic increase or decrease?

2. Ask the following questions to your friends or relatives and share the answers with your classmates. You may be surprised by the answers you receive. Be sure to let your subjects know that this is for a class assignment to put them at ease in answering the questions.

   - Do you know what type of insurance coverage you have? Is it an HMO, PPO, or traditional insurance?
   - In relation to medical insurance, does the term "birthday rule" mean anything to you?
   - What does coordination of benefits mean?
   - Does your physician's office have a sign at the front desk that implies you will need to show your insurance card at every visit?
   - Do they ask to see your card and do they make a copy of it?

   Questions to answer before you perform this activity:

   - Do you think patients know what kind of coverage they have?
   - Do you think patients pay attention to signs that are posted?

StudyWARE™ CHALLENGE

- Study with the flash cards for Chapter 9 to review the key terms in this chapter.
- Solve the hangman activities for Chapter 9.
- Complete the true/false quiz in test mode for Chapter 9.

RESOURCES

American Medical Association. (2000). *Current procedural terminology, CPT™ 2006 standard edition*. Chicago, IL: Author.

Connecting Consumer Choice to Healthcare. Retrieved July 5, 2006, from www.connectyourcare.com/cyc2/glossary.html

Health Savings Accounts vs. Health Reimbursement Accounts vs. Medical Saving Accounts vs. Flexible Spending Accounts. Retrieved July 5, 2006, from www.wsma.org/memresources/hsa_compare_chart.pdf

Medicode (2006). *Physician ICD-9-CM volumes 1 & 2*. Los Angeles, CA: Practice Management Information Corp.

Mosio, M. A. (2006). *A guide to health insurance billing* (2nd ed.). Clifton Park, NY: Thomson Delmar Learning.

Rowell, J., & Green, M. A. (2006) *Understanding health insurance* (8th ed.). Clifton Park, NY: Thomson Delmar Learning.

Thompson, T. G. (2001, June 22). *Renaming and restructuring of Health Care Financing Administration (HCFA) to Centers for Medicare and Medicaid Services (CMMS)* (Press Release). Washington, DC: U.S. Department of Health and Human Services.

WEB LINKS

www.ama-assn.org (American Medical Association)
   Provides information on CPT coding.

www.cms.hhs.gov (Centers for Medicare and Medicaid Services—formerly the Health Care Financing Administration [HCFA])
   Provides information on Medicare and Medicaid programs and services.

www.palmettogba.com (Palmetto Government Benefits Administrators)
   Provides helpful information to physicians and patients regarding Medicare programs.

www.wsma.org (Washington State Medical Association)
   Upon entering the web site, type "HRA comparison chart" in the search box. Click on "Washington State Medical Association—ReferenceFour." Under Practice Operations click on "HSA Comparison Chart." Select "Health Savings Accounts/Medical Savings Accounts," and select "HSA Comparison Chart." Provides comparative information regarding health savings accounts, flexible spending accounts, and health reimbursement accounts.

www.connectyourcare.com (Connect Your Care)
   To access the glossary, select "Individuals and Employees" after entering the web site. Select "Glossary." Provides a glossary of terms relating to the insurance industry.

10 Medical Office Management

Many factors affect the overall operation of the medical office and often become the responsibility of an office manager. First, the office should be a safe, secure, and environmentally friendly workplace. Safety involves not only the use or condition of the physical equipment and furnishings in the office, but also the human activities of the office personnel, patients, and visitors. Modifications for individuals who are physically challenged are necessary to make the environment a friendlier and safer place for them. The working environment must allow for a focus on the provision of care rather than concern about personal safety.

Second, the office needs a manager who is responsible for the efficient day-to-day operation of the practice. In addition to the physical characteristics of the office, there must be a method to manage the office staff, the finances, and the general operational duties. Individual or small group practices may assign an individual to deal with these duties. Medical assistants who have adequate office experience and possess management abilities are often selected to be office managers. Large group practices, clinics, and physician corporations, who have multiple physicians and many employees, however, may choose an individual with a business background or a management company to oversee the operation.

Third, the fiscal operation of the office also requires someone to manage the daily receipts, expenditures, and other financial matters of the practice. Many physicians find that even with an efficient manager, a professional accounting firm is still necessary for the preparation of tax forms, financial statements, and maintenance of salary records, but the manager is still responsible for providing the necessary data for the firm.

Because individual physician preferences result in a wide array of management possibilities, this chapter discusses general administrative duties and responsibilities and also includes information regarding the role of an office manager. Physicians place great confidence in their manager's ability to efficiently and effectively handle the administrative affairs of the office. The following units outline the skills and duties related to the fiscal and physical operation of a medical office, such as:

- Banking transactions
- Office expenditures
- Accounting records
- Employer records
- Office environment and equipment responsibilities
- Hiring, training, evaluating, and dismissing personnel
- Providing essential reference materials
- Attending office management seminars

UNIT 1
SAFETY, SECURITY, AND EMERGENCY PLANS IN THE MEDICAL OFFICE

OBJECTIVES

Upon completion of this unit, you will be able to achieve the following:

LEARNING Objectives

1. Spell and define, using the glossary at the back of the text, all the Words to Know in this unit.

2. Name four things to check to ensure safety in a reception room.
3. List four hazards in a reception/business office area.
4. Name three things in an examination room that might be unsafe.
5. Name the three elements necessary for fire.
6. List four ways a fire might start.
7. Name six items that are considered to be protective barriers to prevent skin and mucous membrane exposure to pathogens.

WORDS TO KNOW

assault	extinguisher	safety
barrier	hazard	security
biohazardous	irrational	universal
emergency	precautions	precautions
environment	prevention	ventilation
evacuated	reception	volatile

CERTIFICATION CONNECTION

CMA
Maintain the physical plant

RMA
Office safety

CMAS
Medical office management (safety, physical office plant)

A SAFE, HEALTHY ENVIRONMENT THROUGHOUT THE MEDICAL OFFICE

The medical office, like the home, is a place where you should feel safe and secure. But just like a home, it takes conscious effort to ensure that the office has a protective, healthy **environment**. The medical assistant is part of the team responsible for recognizing any **safety**, security, or operational **hazard**; helping to eliminate it; and warning coworkers and patients of any dangers.

Safety in the Working Environment

The physician's office environment must ensure the health and safety of the physician and staff and all persons being treated, as well as those accompanying them. This refers not only to the physical surroundings in the office but also the general maintenance of the facility, the mechanical condition of the equipment, and the procedures used to control the presence of harmful microorganisms. The effort to reduce or eliminate exposure to harmful organisms is known as *infection control*.

All types of health care settings must maintain procedures to control the transmission of organisms. By the very nature of the services provided, health care workers are constantly coming into contact with patients who are ill or who may have contagious diseases. The patients in this setting are also exposed to organisms from other patients. It is extremely important for the health and safety of all concerned that the spread of these organisms be prevented. Awareness has been heightened by the ever-present possibility of the spread of hepatitis and HIV viruses.

For the protection of employers and employees, federal and state agencies have established legislation dealing with policies, procedures, and guidelines to reduce disease transmission. The United States Department of Labor established regulations through the Occupational Safety and Health Administration (OSHA). These guidelines deal primarily with requirements of employers to provide employees with safe working conditions to protect them from harmful exposure and substances. An example of this regulation is the provision of latex and vinyl gloves to protect employees during patient contact.

The United States Public Health Department has the Centers for Disease Control and Prevention (CDC) in Atlanta, Georgia. It is the CDC's responsibility to collect data on pathogens and diseases and establish guidelines to prevent their spread. The CDC has developed a system of classifications or categories of infectious diseases related to their method of spread. It was this agency that established guidelines concerning contact with blood and body fluids referred to as **universal precautions**. These guidelines were developed to control the spread of hepatitis and AIDS. Universal precautions have since been incorporated into guidelines called Standard Precautions. These expanded **precautions** are set infection control guidelines to be used by all health care professionals when caring for all patients. The new guidelines combine the basic principles of the universal precautions with the recommendations of personal protective equipment used to provide protection from all body fluids regardless of whether blood is present or not.

A third governmental agency also establishes regulations for the safety of patients and health care workers. The Clinical Laboratory Improvement Amendments (CLIA) legislation is governed by the United States Department of Health and Human Services. It is their responsibility to ensure the public is safeguarded by regulating all testing of specimens coming from the human body. All clinical laboratories must adhere to the strict regulations set forth by the legislation. The original standards were strengthened in response to the public's complaints regarding misread Pap smears that resulted in unnecessary deaths. Laboratory tests are now categorized in relation to their complexity, and laboratories are only approved to perform testing in relation to their level of certification.

This discussion is only an introduction to the regulations. They are more thoroughly discussed in Chapter 12.

Safety in the Reception Room

A safe environment begins at the front door. The **reception** room requires a safety check every morning to ensure it presents no hazards for patients and visitors. Observe the condition of the furniture carefully. Pay attention to chair and table legs—they must be stable and able to support appropriate weight. Lamps and electrical cords should be examined. Bulbs should not dim or flicker, and cords should be in good condition with no evidence of fraying. Be sure lighting is adequate so that even people with impaired vision can see well. Check the floor to be certain there are neither carpet wrinkles nor anything lying on the floor that might cause someone to fall. Avoid the use of decorative or throw rugs.

Safety in the Receptionist/Business Office

In the receptionist/business office area, pay special attention to file drawers and cupboard doors. NEVER open more than one file drawer in a vertical file at a time, because the unbalanced weight could cause the cabinet to tip forward. Many people have sustained back and extremity injuries from the automatic reaction to "catch" a cabinet. Also, be careful with opened bottom drawers. You can easily trip over an open drawer. Wall cupboards pose another safety hazard. If the door is left open, you could strike your head quite forcefully when you stand up or rise up from underneath. All electrical cords must be kept behind desks and other office furnishings so that they will not be tripped over. All equipment should operate properly and show no evidence of electrical shorts or damage.

Safety in the Examination Room

The examination table must be cleaned after each patient. The table must operate properly, and the medical assistant must be thoroughly competent in its use.

Assist patients as necessary to sit or lie on the table. If the use of a stool is necessary, be exceptionally cautious to guard against the patient stepping on the edges, which could cause it to tip. Very ill patients, elderly patients, and children should not be left alone on an examination table where they could fall. Small children accompanying a parent are best left with another office staff member while the parent is in the examination room.

Children, and some adults, also have a natural curiosity about "things" in the examination room cabinets or on counters. Anything that might be hazardous or could become contaminated should be kept out of sight. Prescription pads should not be left lying around where they could be stolen and possibly used to obtain controlled substances. In an examination room, there is a lot of equipment with electrical cords that must be positioned so that they will not interfere with movement or walking in the room.

Safety Rails and Floor Coverings

The installation of handrails in hallways and bathrooms within the office assists elderly patients and weak or motor-impaired people in moving throughout the office with greater stability and less chance of falling. Be certain the floors are clear of any materials and that carpets are smooth and secured—loose rugs are very dangerous, especially over tile or vinyl flooring. The medical assistant must always be on guard to be certain no one falls.

Safety in the Laboratory Area

Chemicals kept in the office for laboratory work must be properly labeled and stored. Chemicals that could become **volatile** when kept beyond their expiration date must be monitored carefully. The testing of patients' urine, blood, and other specimens requires special procedures. Containers for the disposal of used equipment and **biohazardous** waste must be readily accessible. A strict adherence to standard precautions is essential to the maintenance of a safe and healthy lab environment.

Personal Safety

All health care workers must practice standard precautions to protect themselves against acquiring HIV, hepatitis B, or other infectious diseases. *Caution:* All patients should be considered infected, because medical history and examination cannot reliably identify all patients infected with HIV or other blood-borne pathogens. Protection involves the use of appropriate **barrier** precautions to prevent skin and mucous membrane exposure when there is contact with blood or

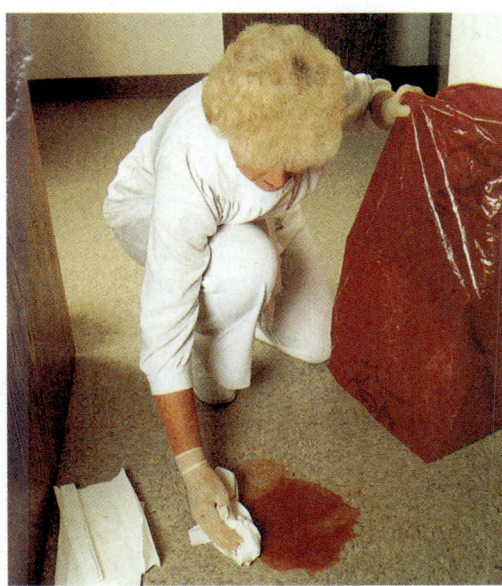

FIGURE 10-1   Clean up spills immediately. When blood or other body fluids are involved, universal precautions must be observed.

other body fluids of any patient. This means the appropriate use of and gloves, face shields, masks, protective eyewear, aprons, and gowns as needed. Persons likely to be in an emergency situation also need to make use of mouthpieces, **ventilation** bags, and other ventilating devices in order to avoid direct contact with saliva or possible blood due to an injury. Precautions are identified later in this text as they become necessary within procedures. Look for the glove icon at the top of a procedure instruction.

Spills and Dropped Objects

It is very important to clean up spilled liquids immediately. When the spill involves bodily fluids such as blood or urine, universal precautions must be observed by using gloves and placing materials in a biohazardous waste bag (Figure 10-1). The area must be thoroughly cleaned with an effective disinfectant or a 10% solution of household bleach. The used paper towels or cloths should also be discarded into the hazardous waste container.

Objects dropped on the floor must also be picked up immediately in order to prevent falls. Glass fragments are best picked up using a brush or broom and dust pan. Glass must be discarded in such a way that it will not puncture the plastic bag liner of the waste receptacle—this could accidentally cut someone's hands when it is removed. Fragments could be carefully wrapped in layers of newspaper or placed inside empty cardboard or plastic containers before being deposited into the receptacle.

GENERAL OFFICE SAFETY

Fire

Fire **prevention** is very important to everyone's safety. Only three elements need to be present for a fire to start: heat, fuel, and oxygen (Figure 10-2). Today, there are rare exceptions to the "no smoking" regulations in medical and public facilities. Yet, there is still a possibility of a carelessly discarded match or cigarette ash dropping onto furniture or being discarded into a trash container. Some facilities provide floor model ashtrays just outside their entrance for disposal of smoking materials. If the ashtrays contain sand in which materials can be placed, they are relatively safe. However, types with metal tops that open can be an ideal place for a fire to start, because people tend to use the ashtray as a receptacle for their trash. Any regular ashtray may contain smoldering, smoking materials

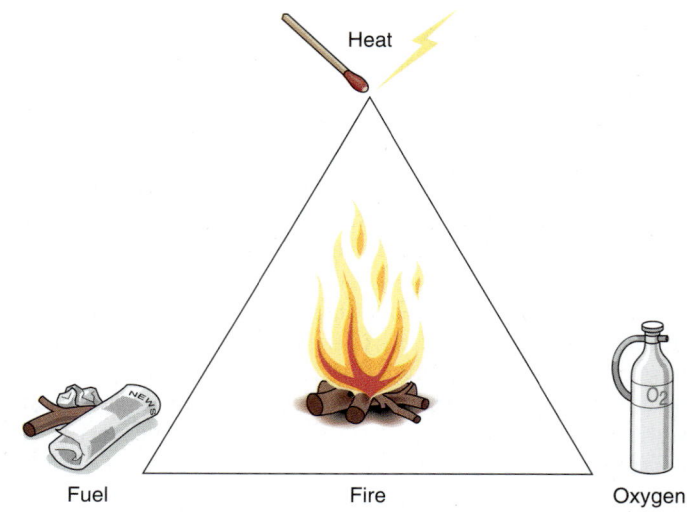

FIGURE 10-2 The fire triangle—elements needed for combustion (burning)

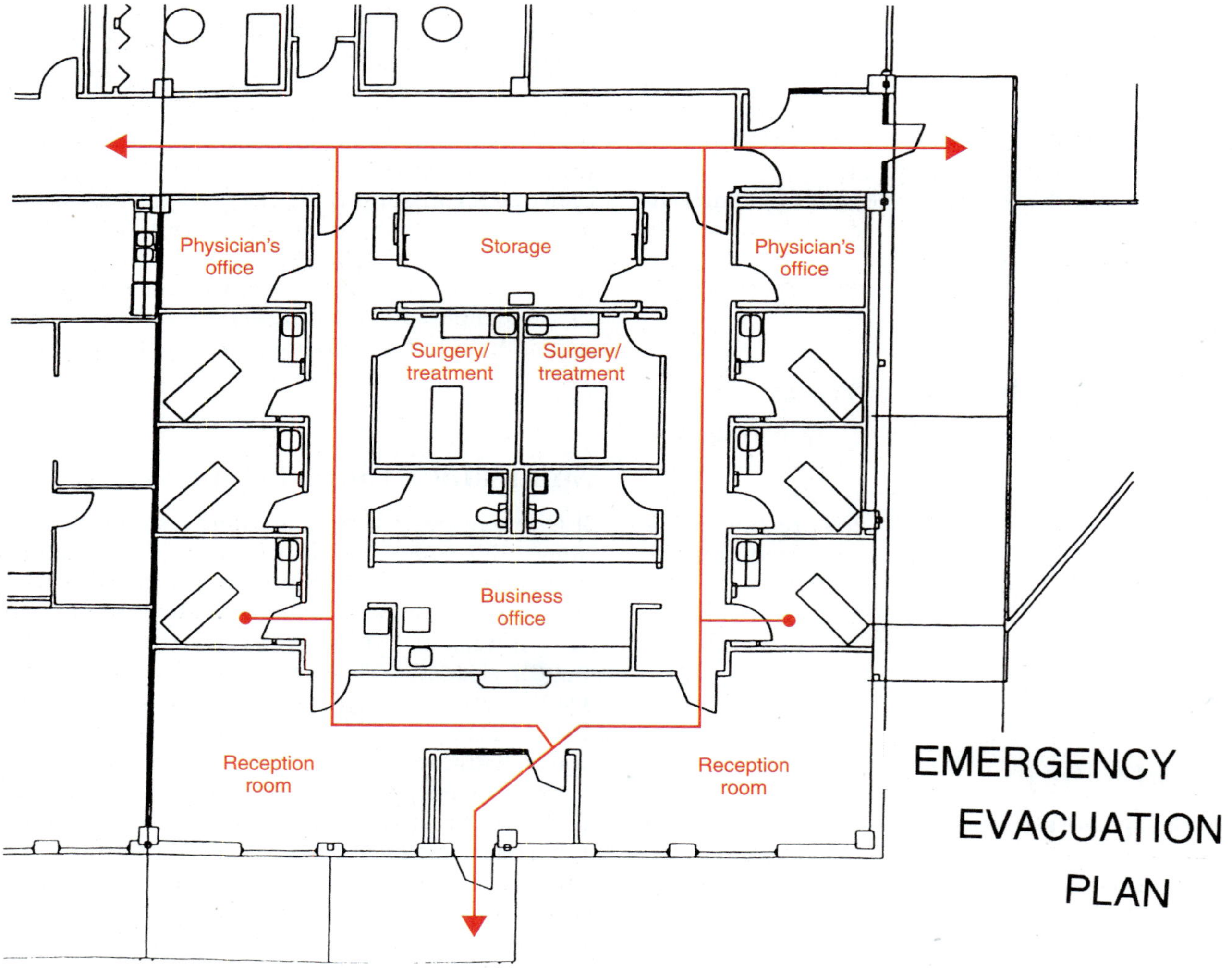

FIGURE 10-3 Know the quickest route to exit the building.

that are best emptied into a toilet and flushed rather than into a wastebasket, which could later burst into flame.

Fires can also be started by other causes. A defective outlet or frayed wires on any electrical appliance or office equipment could short out and start a fire. Coffee pots and water sterilizers can also boil dry and cause a fire. It is a good policy to unplug all electrical appliances whenever the office is closed.

The office should have an established policy regarding the procedure to follow in case of fire. There should be a planned route of escape prominently posted (Figure 10-3). All patients and office staff must be **evacuated** from the building, and the fire department must be notified. Exit signs should be clearly posted. All stairways and hallways should be free from clutter to allow quick, safe passage. When appropriate, knowing the location of the fire **extinguisher** and using it properly could prevent a fire from spreading. This knowledge should be everyone's responsibility (Figures 10-4A, B, and C).

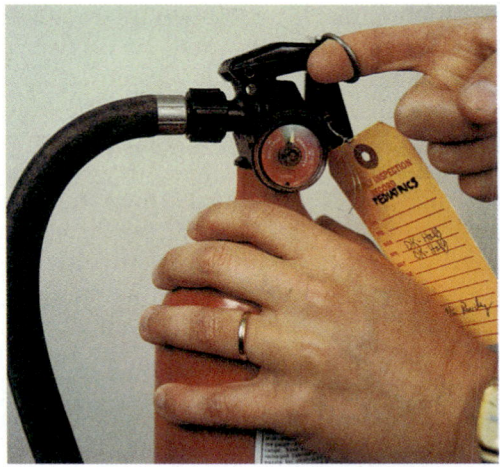

FIGURE 10-4B   Pull the ring.

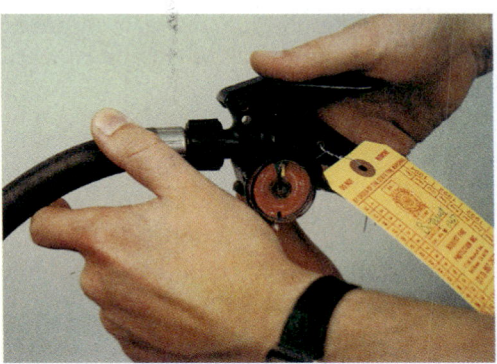

FIGURE 10-4C   Squeeze the handle and point the hose at the base of the fire.

Natural Disasters

A severe weather warning is another event that requires an established policy as to what to do in case it occurs. Natural disasters such as strong electrical storms and tornados are unpredictable and can claim lives if necessary steps are not taken. In these instances, people must remain inside and take shelter in the predetermined safest area. In areas where there is danger from earthquakes, it is wise to stand in doorframes or beneath a sturdy structure. It may be dangerous to go outside where you could be struck by falling trees and buildings or come into contact with downed power lines. Yet, remaining in a multistory building may not be the safest policy, either. People living in high-risk areas generally know the appropriate action to take.

Electrical power is sometimes disrupted during such an **emergency**. Never use an elevator during a threaten-

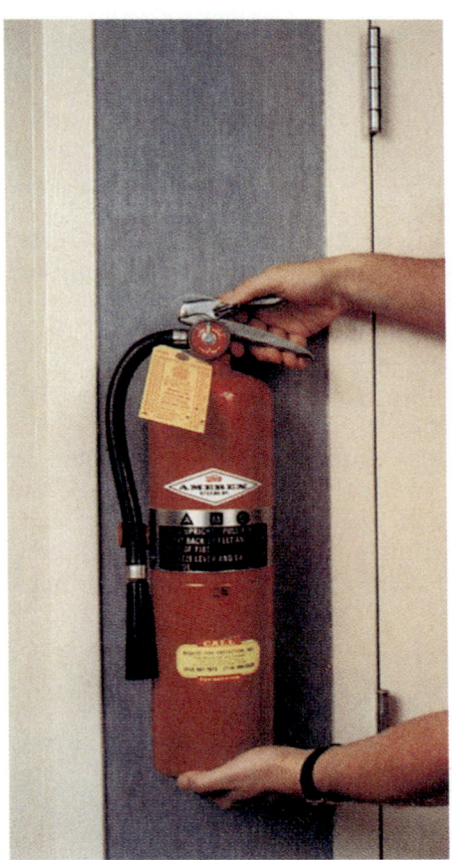

FIGURE 10-4A   Know the location of the fire extinguisher and how to use it.

ing situation, because the power could go off, trapping you inside until power is restored or you are rescued. Large medical facilities may have electrical generators to provide emergency lighting during emergency situations. Battery-powered lights should always be available and accessible.

Routine fire and weather drills prepare people psychologically to act in a safe and responsible manner. A practical time to review drill procedures is at a staff meeting or during new employee orientation. Those who are prepared have a greater chance of surviving a crisis than those who do not know what to do or how to act. Keeping calm and confident in times of emergency helps to reduce panic and **irrational** behavior in oneself and others. It is not practical to decide at the time of such an emergency what to do with the patients and the staff. Each member of the office team should be assigned specific duties and know how to carry them out safely and efficiently.

Development of emergency plans, assignment of duties, and practice drills are usually the responsibility of the office manager.

Emergency Phone Numbers

A list of emergency phone numbers should be posted by the phone for quick access. Such numbers may include, but are not limited to, police, fire department, emergency service, poison control center, building security, utility companies, hospital emergency room, and a hospital admissions office. When an urgent situation arises, you don't want to have to search for phone numbers.

SECURITY IN THE MEDICAL OFFICE

The increased incidences of crime makes security a prime concern. A criminal may think a physician's office has cash from daily receipts or could be taken from people in the office, such as employees or patients, and decide to commit a robbery. There is also the misconception that large amounts of drugs are kept on site and could be easily attained. Unfortunately, sexual **assault** can also occur when the interior office is accessible from the reception area. In order to provide a degree of **security**, police recommend that doors between these areas be equipped with snap locks to prevent unwanted entry. Also, any opening between the two areas, such as a window, should be covered with a grill if it is possible to climb through it. (This author knows of an incident when an intruder crawled through the reception room window and assaulted a nurse who was working alone in an office.) If there are private entry doors, be certain they are kept

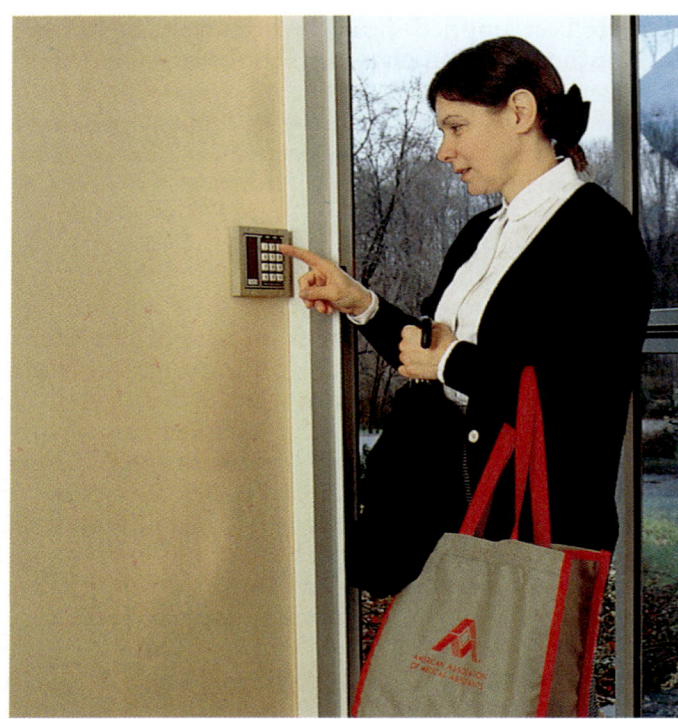

FIGURE 10-5   Enter the security code when opening the door.

locked at all times. If you must enter or leave the office after dark, be especially alert. The outside area should be well lit. If building security people are available, ask for an escort.

Many offices today are equipped with electronic security systems. If you are the first staff member to arrive at work, it will be necessary to enter the code before opening the door or enter the code on an internal key pad before the entrance delay period expires (Figure 10-5). Both these systems lend a feeling of safety and security, but be aware, it only takes a few seconds for someone to grab your purse or wallet or force you to hand over office money or drugs. Never enter the office if there is evidence of forced entry or if it appears that someone might either be inside or has been inside. Leave at once and call building security or the police.

ACHIEVE UNIT OBJECTIVES

- Complete the Workbook activities to meet the learning objectives.
- Apply your knowledge at the end of this chapter in completing the Critical Thinking Challenge and Activities, as well as the StudyWARE on your Student CD-ROM.

UNIT 2
THE LANGUAGE OF BANKING

OBJECTIVES

Upon completion of this unit, you will be able to achieve the following:

LEARNING Objectives

1. **Spell and define, using the glossary at the back of the text, all the Words to Know in this unit.**

2. **Differentiate between savings and checking accounts.**

3. **Explain the significance of the ABA and MICR codes.**

4. **Define the banking terms listed in this unit.**

5. **Differentiate among cashier's, certified, limited, postdated, stale, traveler's, and voucher checks.**

6. **Explain the difference between overdraft and overdrawn.**

7. **Explain the "stop payment" process.**

WORDS TO KNOW

agent	insufficient	promissory
certified	limited check	transaction
collateral	negotiable	voucher
currency	overdraft	warrant
debit	payee	withdrawal
deposit	power of	
endorsement	attorney	

CERTIFICATION CONNECTION

CMA
Banking procedures

CMAS
Banking

RMA
Understand check processing procedures and requirements

This unit presents the most common banking terms and their definitions to help you understand financial transactions. The medical assistant who works as the office manager must have a good working knowledge of banking and basic accounting procedures. These skills are not only important in the physician's office but also in the management of your own personal finances.

As the manager, knowledge of banking terms will help you communicate with the bank officials where the office has its account as well as the accounting firm personnel who prepare the office financial forms.

BANKING TERMS

- *Agent*. An agent is a person authorized to act for another person. You are the agent for your employer in the office. Bank officials are agents for the bank.

- *American Bankers Association (ABA) number*. A code number found in the right upper corner of a printed check. It may be above the check number on a business check or below the check number on a personal check.

- *ATM*. An automated teller machine (ATM) is a banking machine operated by inserting a credit or bank card and entering a personal identification number (PIN) code. Deposits, transfers, withdrawals, and other banking functions can be performed at the ATM location.

- *Bank statement*. A record of a checking account sent to the customer, usually on a monthly basis, showing the beginning balance, all deposits made, all checks drawn, all bank charges, and the closing balance. The customer's canceled checks are returned with the statement. With the increased use of electronic banking, statements and cancelled checks are available online and do not have to be sent.

- *Bankbook*. In the case of a savings account it is called a savings passbook and contains a record of deposits, withdrawals, and interest earned, with the dates of all the transactions. This book must be presented with each deposit or withdrawal. At regular intervals, usually quarterly, interest earnings are credited to an account. These earnings should be entered in the passbook by the bank. Some banks indicate the passbook should be presented for interest entry at least once in a 3-year period.

- *Cashier's check*. The purchaser pays the bank the full amount of the check. The bank then writes a check on its own account payable to the party specified. This type of check "guarantees" the recipient that the full amount of money indicated on the check will be paid on processing.

- *Certified check*. The bank stamps the customer's own check *certified* and then holds the certified amount in reserve in the customer's account until the check is cashed. This is a guaranteed check and so is always acceptable when a personal check is not.

- *Check register*. Also referred to as a check stub. It is a record showing the check number, person to whom the check is paid, amount of the check, date, and balance. It is kept by the person writing the check as a record of the transaction.

- *Checking account.* A bank account against which checks may be written. The bank will issue the checks and deposit slips.
- **Currency**. Paper money issued by the government.
- **Debit**. An entry in an account of an amount owed that has been charged to the account.
- *Debit card.* A card similar to a credit card that withdraws money from the account to pay for the debit. Another type of debit card is used specifically to make purchases, in effect replacing a check. These are called check cards.
- **Deposit**. An amount of money (cash or checks) placed in a bank account.
- *Deposit record.* A record of a deposit that is given to the customer at the time of the deposit. It is important to keep the deposit record as proof of the deposit in case the bank fails to list the deposit on the bank statement.
- *Deposit slip.* An itemized list of cash and checks deposited in a checking account. It is important to keep a copy of all deposit slips to verify deposits.
- *Direct deposit.* When an amount is sent electronically by the payer directly into a savings or checking account of the payee.
- *Electronic check.* A check paid directly from a checking account via the Internet. The account owner establishes a list of recurring payees, their corresponding account numbers, and the electronic or actual addresses. To pay a bill, the list is called up, the payee identified, the amount of payment entered, and the payment command given. The bank electronically completes the transaction within a day or two without the need for a paper check, envelope, or stamp.

- *Electronic fund transfer (EFT).* A method of crediting or debiting accounts by computer without checks or deposit slips.
- **Endorsement**. The payee's signature on the back of a check. It is a transfer of title on the check to the bank in exchange for the amount of money on the face of the check.
- *Endorser.* The payee on a check. If the name is spelled incorrectly on the face of the check, it should be endorsed in the same way and then endorsed correctly.
- **Insufficient** *funds.* A bank term used to indicate that the writer of the check did not have enough money in the account to cover the check. An office usually has a policy regarding returned checks, which normally involves contacting the patient immediately and asking the person to pick up the check and bring a cash payment. These checks are sometimes described as *bounced,* and the account is called *overdrawn.*
- **Limited check**. A check that will be marked void if written over a certain amount. These checks are often used for payroll or for insurance payments. A check may also list a time limit during which it must be cashed. It must be cashed within the time limit or you will find it is not **negotiable**.
- *Magnetic ink character recognition (MICR).* This technique consists of characters and numbers printed in magnetic ink at the bottom left side of checks and deposit slips (Figures 10-6 and 10-7).
- *Maker.* The individual who signs a check or the corporation that pays it.
- *Money order.* Negotiable instrument often used by individuals who do not have checking accounts or to meet the requirement for purchasing an item or service. Money orders may be purchased for a fee from banks, credit unions, post offices, and many other money order service locations.

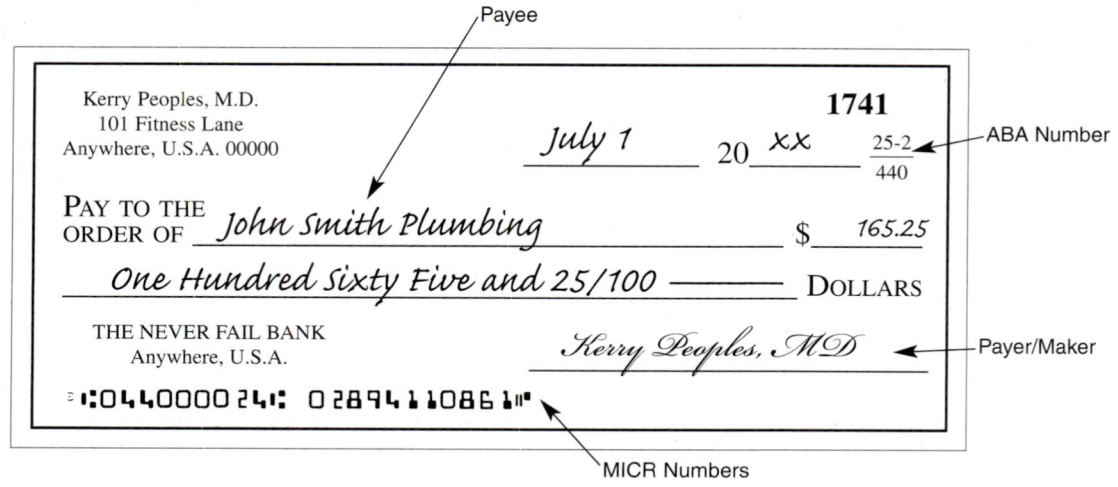

FIGURE 10-6 Check with MICR numbers

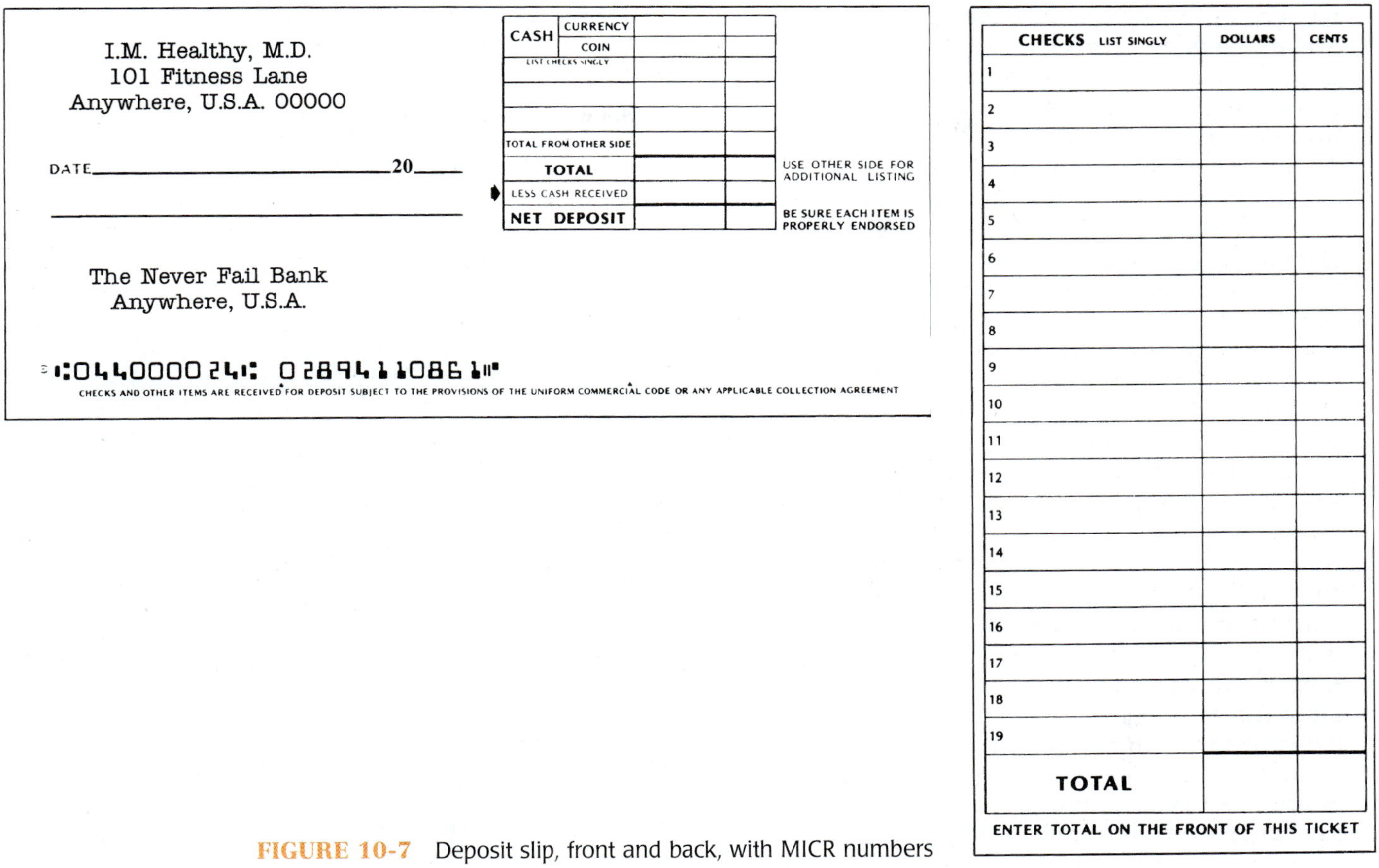

I.M. Healthy, M.D.
101 Fitness Lane
Anywhere, U.S.A. 00000

DATE________________________20____

CASH	CURRENCY		
	COIN		
LIST CHECKS SINGLY			
TOTAL FROM OTHER SIDE			
TOTAL			
LESS CASH RECEIVED			
NET DEPOSIT			

USE OTHER SIDE FOR ADDITIONAL LISTING

BE SURE EACH ITEM IS PROPERLY ENDORSED

The Never Fail Bank
Anywhere, U.S.A.

⑆044000024⑆ 0289411086 1⑈

CHECKS AND OTHER ITEMS ARE RECEIVED FOR DEPOSIT SUBJECT TO THE PROVISIONS OF THE UNIFORM COMMERCIAL CODE OR ANY APPLICABLE COLLECTION AGREEMENT

CHECKS LIST SINGLY	DOLLARS	CENTS
1		
2		
3		
4		
5		
6		
7		
8		
9		
10		
11		
12		
13		
14		
15		
16		
17		
18		
19		
TOTAL		

ENTER TOTAL ON THE FRONT OF THIS TICKET

FIGURE 10-7 Deposit slip, front and back, with MICR numbers

- *Negotiable.* Refers to the fact that something is able to be transferred or exchanged. On a check the words "Pay to the order of" are considered to make the check negotiable. In other words, the amount written can be transferred from the account of the payer to the payee.
- *Note.* Legal evidence of a debt. A **promissory** note is a written promise to pay. A **collateral** note is a written promise to pay with the additional requirement that the maker of the note must list marketable securities that may be sold by the creditor if the maker does not pay the note within the time limit promised.
- *One-write check writing.* System that makes it possible to make a record on a check register as you write a check. This is excellent for payroll because you can record deductions for the employee and office records in one writing.
- *Online banking.* Banking on the bank's Internet web site is called online banking. It is possible to check account information, transfer money, and pay bills over the Internet.
- *Overdraft checking accounts.* Accounts that allow checks to be written for a larger amount than is currently in the account. The **overdraft** is covered by the bank in the form of a loan for which interest is charged.
- ***Payee***. The person to whom a check is written. The name of the payee is listed on the check after the words "Pay to the order of."
- *Payer.* The person who signs the check.
- *Postdated check.* A check made out with a future date. You may have patients who wish to pay while they are in the office but will not have the money in their account until next pay day, which is the date they will put on the check. Never deposit these checks until the date for which they are made out. The practice of writing a postdated check is illegal in some states; be sure you know the law in your state.
- ***Power of attorney***. A legal procedure that authorizes one person to act as an agent for another. This is often necessary when patients are not physically or mentally capable of taking care of their own financial affairs.
- *Savings account.* A bank account upon which the depositor can earn interest. The amounts deposited may be recorded in a passbook. (Note that many banks now also give interest on checking accounts if a minimum balance is maintained.)
- *Service charge.* Fee charged by the bank on a monthly basis for services rendered. If a specified minimum balance is maintained in the account, the bank may

not charge because it has the use of that money. Some banks charge for every **transaction**, whether depositing money or writing checks.

- *Special checking account.* Many different names and definitions apply, depending on the area of the country. It may be an account on which interest is paid if an established minimum balance is maintained in the account; an account for senior citizens for which no handling charges are made; or an account that charges fee for checks only. Banks are continually offering new plans to attract depositors.

- *Stale check.* A check presented too long after it was written to be honored by the bank. Some checks specify that they must be cashed within 90 days, and if presented after that date the bank will not honor payment. A period of 6 months is generally considered enough time for a check to be presented for payment.

- *Stop payment.* A method by which the maker of a check may stop payment. The bank charges a sizable fee for this service. Some banks will accept a stop order by phone if it is promptly followed by completion of a form, which the bank furnishes. The payer must furnish the number of the check, date issued, name of payee, amount of check, and the reason for stopping payment. The bank will then refuse to honor the check. A stop payment order is used when a check is lost or if there is a disagreement regarding a product or service received.

- *Teller.* The bank employee who is the main contact between the customer and the bank.

- *Traveler's check.* A special check used by individuals who are traveling and do not wish to carry a large amount of cash. Personal checks are sometimes not accepted outside of the area of the bank upon which they are drawn. Therefore, in exchange for cash, banks will issue traveler's checks. These must be signed individually at the time of purchase and again when they are used. They are usually considered the same as cash, but some merchants still require some identification before they accept a traveler's check. Lost traveler's checks can usually be replaced if you can produce a list of their serial numbers. Traveler's checks are listed as checks on a deposit slip.

- **Voucher** *check.* A check with a detachable voucher form that is used to show the reason for which the check was drawn. This kind of check is often used by insurance companies. The voucher form is removed before the check is endorsed and deposited.

- **Warrant**. This is evidence of a debt due but is not negotiable. It can be converted into a negotiable instrument or cash. An insurance adjustor may issue a warrant as evidence that a claim should be paid. The warrant authorizes the insurance company to issue a check to settle the claim.

- *Wire transfer.* Money can be transferred electronically from the payer's account to another account overnight if the name and number of the receiving account and the name and identification number of the receiving bank are given. There is usually a fee of about $20 charged for the service.

- **Withdrawal**. Removal of funds from a depositor's account. This may be done by means of a passbook, a withdrawal slip, a check, or electronic fund transfer.

ACHIEVE UNIT OBJECTIVES

- ☐ **Complete the Workbook activities to meet the learning objectives.**

- ☐ **Apply your knowledge at the end of this chapter in completing the Critical Thinking Challenge and Activities, as well as the StudyWARE on your Student CD-ROM.**

UNIT 3
CURRENCY, CHECKS, AND PETTY CASH

OBJECTIVES

Upon completion of this unit, you will be able to achieve the following:

LEARNING Objectives

1. **Spell and define, using the glossary at the back of the text, all the Words to Know in this unit.**

2. **Explain the handling of currency in the office.**

3. **Identify the seven features of a check that make it negotiable.**

4. **List the five features of a check that banking institutions look for to guard against fraud.**

5. **Describe precautions with checks received from patients.**

6. **Explain blank and restrictive endorsement.**

7. **Explain special concerns with mail deposits.**

8. **Describe establishing and maintaining a petty cash fund.**

PERFORMANCE Objectives

1. **Prepare a check.**
2. **Prepare a deposit slip.**
3. **Reconcile a bank statement.**
4. **Establish and maintain a petty cash fund.**

WORDS TO KNOW

authorization	negotiable	third party
currency	reconcile	transaction
denomination	register	void
depleted	signature	voucher

 ## CERTIFICATION CONNECTION

CMA
Accounting and banking
procedures

RMA
Banking procedures

CMAS
Medical office financial
management

CURRENCY

Currency is the name given to the cash money we use in our society. It is made up of paper bills in $1, $2, $5, $10, $20, $50, $100, and other larger denominations. Cash money also comes in the form of coins in denominations of 1, 5, 10, 25, 50, and 100 cents. *Note:* Fifty-cent pieces are no longer made and are disappearing from circulation.

The presence of cash in the office presents an area of concern. Because currency and coin are instantly expendable, care must be taken to keep it secured. All cash money should be placed out of sight as soon as received, in a cash box, file drawer, or some other secure location. Care should be taken that your *place* is not in view of patients in the reception area. Usually, all daily proceeds are either locked in a safe or deposited at the close of the day.

FEATURES OF A CHECK

Checks have a long history. The first recorded use of a check was in 1374. They were rare before 1700 but became common after World War II. It is believed about 63 billion checks are processed in the United States every year, and that number is growing. With this great amount it is understandable why coding to make machine processing possible and electronic transfer of funds are increasingly necessary. With this increase in checks also comes the increase in the number of bad checks and fraud.

There are seven features you must examine to ensure a check is valid. You should question any missing or contradicting feature (Figure 10-8):

1. The date: Watch for a stale date (6 months or older), a postdate (a future date), or a preprinted date requirement such as *void after 60 days*. A check with these features is not valid before or after a specific period of time.

2. Words of *negotiability:* A check must say "Pay to the order of" or "Pay to the bearer" to be **negotiable**.

3. The payee: The check must identify to whom the check is written. In the office, this will be the physi-

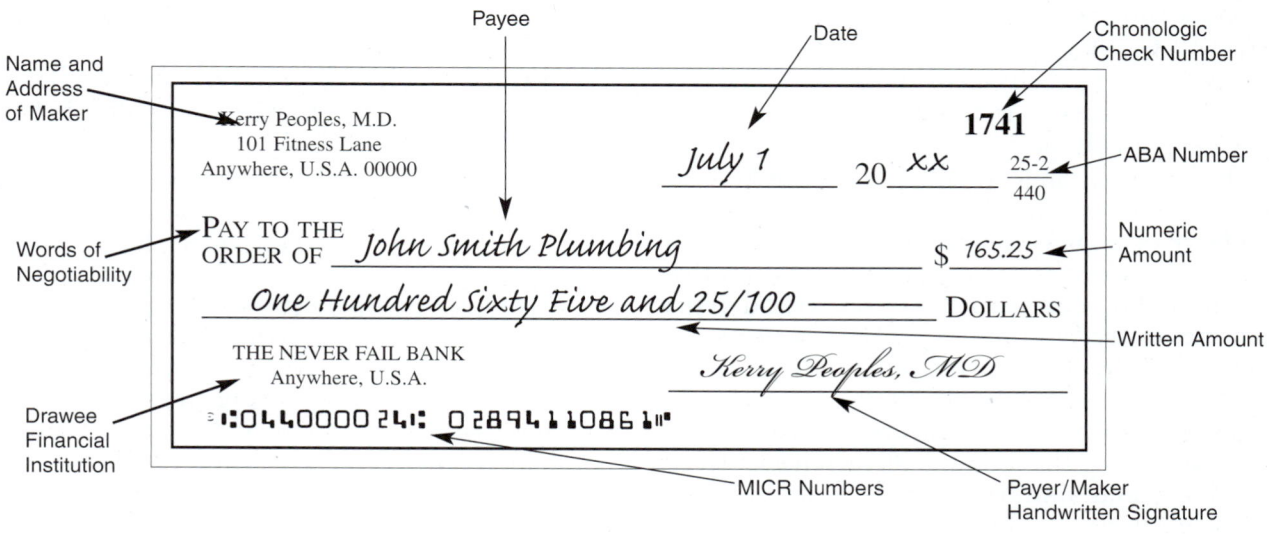

FIGURE 10-8 Features of a check

cian who receives checks as payment for care provided. A payee can also be a person or company that has rendered the practice a service for which a check is written.

4. The numeric amount: This is the amount in numbers that the check is written for.

5. The written amount: This is the amount written in words. It must agree with the numeric amount.

6. The drawee financial institution: This identifies where the check is payable. Checks issued by the government, traveler's checks, corporate checks, and money orders do *not* have a drawee institution printed on them because they are the drawee.

7. The signature: The signature is usually handwritten but can also be a reproduced facsimile.

There are five other features that banks have instituted to guard against fraud, but they are not necessary for validity. If they are missing, it is best to scrutinize the check very carefully.

1. The name and address of the maker: This is usually preprinted by the check printer.

2. A chronologic check number: This is printed at the right upper corner of the check.

3. The check routing symbol (ABA number): It is in fractional form and identifies the institution involved in the clearing process. This number was originated by the American Bankers Association. The purpose is to have a method of identifying the area where the bank on which the check is written is located, and to identify the bank within the area. It may be written as a fraction ($\frac{51-44}{119}$) on a business check, or hyphenated (25-2/440) on a personal check.

4. Magnetic ink character recognition (MICR) numbers: These are numbers that aid in the clearing process. The numbers are printed with special magnetic ink and identify:
   - The Federal Reserve district and branch
   - The drawee financial institution
   - The maker's account number
   - Usually the check number

   This information is specific to each checking account and is imprinted on each check and deposit slip by the company printing the checks. The first series of numbers is the routing information that identifies the bank and area. The second series identifies the account numbers. The last series corresponds to the check number.

   When the bank processes the check, additional magnetic ink numbers are printed across the bottom identifying the amount of the check. These characters and numbers can be read by high-speed machinery, which greatly enhances the bookkeeping procedures in the bank by simplifying the sorting of checks and the printing of individual monthly statements.

5. One rough or perforated edge: This is where the check is separated from a book or sheet of checks. This will not be found in government or traveler's checks.

WRITING CHECKS

The office manager may be required to write checks to pay for equipment, supplies, or wages. It is very important to perform this task with complete accuracy. The office will receive statements from utility companies, medical suppliers, periodical publishers, perhaps a rental agency or mortgage company, and various other businesses. Each statement must be checked to be certain it is for services or materials you receive. Checks may also be written for employee salaries, tax payments, physician's expenses, the office petty cash fund, and other needs. Checks can be processed traditionally, like your own personal account, or be computer written in the office, in which case you will need to learn how to use the software. You will bring up the check form on the screen and complete the entries. With software, your balance is automatically adjusted for you each time you add a deposit or write a check. With either method, the same entries are required.

There are five essential factors that you must include when writing a check:

1. The date: The month can be written or numerical

2. The payee: The person or business that the check is written to

3. The numeric amount: The amount of the check in numbers. Keep the numbers close to the dollar sign so other numbers cannot be inserted to increase the amount of the check.

4. The written amount: The amount of the check written in terms of dollars and fractions of dollars. For example, a check for $25.89 is written Twenty-five and 89/100. Fill in the remainder of the space with a line to prevent insertion of words to increase the amount.

5. The payer signature: Signature of the person owning the account or other designated individuals.

In addition to the traditional check, the corresponding check stub or **register** must also be accurately completed (Figure 10-9). (When using computer software, the check is recorded electronically) This supplies a record of the expenditure as well as a running balance of the account. It is a good practice to complete the stub or register before writing the check in order to avoid accidental overdraft or forgetting and then mailing the check and not knowing the payee or the amount to deduct from the balance. Some traditional checkbooks have a duplicate feature

1741 $ 165.25

Date: July 1   20xx

To: John Smith Plumbing

For: Repair faucet leak

Balance Forward	$ 8,645.89
Deposits	—
Total	$ 8,645.89
This Check	$ 165.25
Balance Forward	$ 8,480.64

FIGURE 10-9   Check stub

that imprints a copy of each check when it is written, therefore preventing this situation.

To properly complete the stub or register:

1. Use black or blue ink.
2. Enter the check number if it is not preprinted.
3. Enter the date.
4. Identify the payee.

5. Bring forward the balance from the previous stub.
6. List any deposits.
7. Enter the amount of the check being written.
8. Enter the new balance.

When the check is finished, it is attached to the billing statement and given to the physician for signature prior to mailing.

Physicians may give check-signature power to an office manager to eliminate the need for their personal **signature**. A signature **authorization** card obtained from the bank must be completed to allow someone other than the recorded owner of the account to execute checks. Some offices, as a means of monitoring expenditures and preventing employee embezzlement, require two signatures on a check or have a policy that the individual writing the check (e.g., bookkeeper) must have another authorized person (often the office manager) sign the check. This also provides an opportunity to question expenditures and maintain a sense of cash flow. If a mistake is made in writing a check, it is necessary to write "**VOID**" across the check and stub and write a new one. Practice preparing checks by following Procedure 10-1, and using the workbook samples.

Payment of Invoices

One area of expenditure that must be carefully monitored is payment of invoices for office equipment and supplies. When a statement is received from a supplier, it is essential to know that everything on the invoice and the amount or number of each item has in fact been received.

PROCEDURE PROCEDURE PROCEDURE PROCEDURE PROCEDURE PROCEDURE PROCEDURE PROCEDURE

10-1  Prepare a Check

PURPOSE: Accurately prepare a check and stub or register.

EQUIPMENT: Checkbook, pen with black or blue ink, computer, and computer checks.

PERFORMANCE OBJECTIVE: In a simulated medical office situation, given the necessary equipment, a payee, the amount due, a signature name, and a previous balance, prepare a check and stub following the steps of the procedure. The check must be without error and contain the five essential factors, and the stub entries must agree with the check information with the balance be accurately figured.

1. Complete the check stub:
   - Enter the check number if it is not preprinted.
   - Enter the date.
   - Enter the payee name.
   - Bring forward the balance.
   - Add any deposits.
   - List the amount of the check.
   - Compute the new balance.
2. Complete the check:
   - Enter the date.
   - Enter the payee.
   - Enter the correct numeric amount.
   - Enter the correct written amount.
3. Obtain a signature.

The shipment must be compared with packing slips or invoices at the time it is received and notification of any discrepancy made to the supplier. Frequently, partial shipments are sent and some items are on back order. Payment of the total amount of the invoice would represent payment for goods not received. Some difficulty may also arise in trying to obtain materials not sent once you have paid in full for the shipment. The provider assumes everything was shipped as stated on the invoice because no questions were raised when the shipment was received.

PATIENTS' CHECKS

Certain precautions need to be observed when accepting checks from patients:

- Be sure the check has the seven features that make a check valid and that no corrections have been made.
- Do not accept a **third-party** check unless the check is from an insurance company. A third-party check is generally one made out to the patient by someone unknown to you. Because you do not know how credit-worthy the check writer is or have any personal information about the individual, it is unwise to accept a third-party check that another person has written.
- You might have patients who want to write a check for more than the amount due so they can have some cash in hand. This is generally not a good policy, and it would be advisable to refuse such a check. When you accept the check as payment and give out an additional amount in office cash, you risk not only the check not being honored by the bank, but also your office will lose the cash that was given to the patient.
- Do not accept a check marked "paid in full" or "payment in full" unless it does pay the account in full, including charges incurred on the day the check is written. If there is still a balance, you will be unable to collect if you accept and deposit such a check. People often write "paid in full" or "payment in full" on the memo line on the front of a check. Be sure to check this line because it is easy to overlook. When you receive a check, stamp it with the deposit endorsement (see the next section) to protect against theft.
- Do not accept a postal money order with more than one endorsement, because two is the limit honored.

ENDORSEMENT

An endorsement is a signature or a signature plus other information on the back of a check. The endorsement of a check transfers all rights in the check to another party. Endorsements should always be made in ink and may be made with a pen or rubber stamp. The end of the check to be endorsed can be identified by holding the check on the right end as you look at it, turning it over, and endorsing the opposite or left end. All checks received in the office, whether in person or through the mail, should be protected by endorsement at the time received.

The two kinds of endorsement commonly used are blank endorsement and restrictive endorsement. A *blank endorsement* is a signature only. It should not be used until the check is to be cashed, because if the check is stolen with such an endorsement, someone else could endorse the check below your name and cash the check. A *restrictive endorsement* is used to endorse checks when they are received. It is a stamp or written information that states, "PAY TO THE ORDER OF (name of bank where check is to be deposited)" followed by the name of the physician. If such a check is stolen it could not be used in any way.

If the name of the payee is misspelled, it should be endorsed the same way followed by the correct signature directly below.

Effective September 1, 1988, federal regulations required all endorsements to be within 1½" of the "trail-

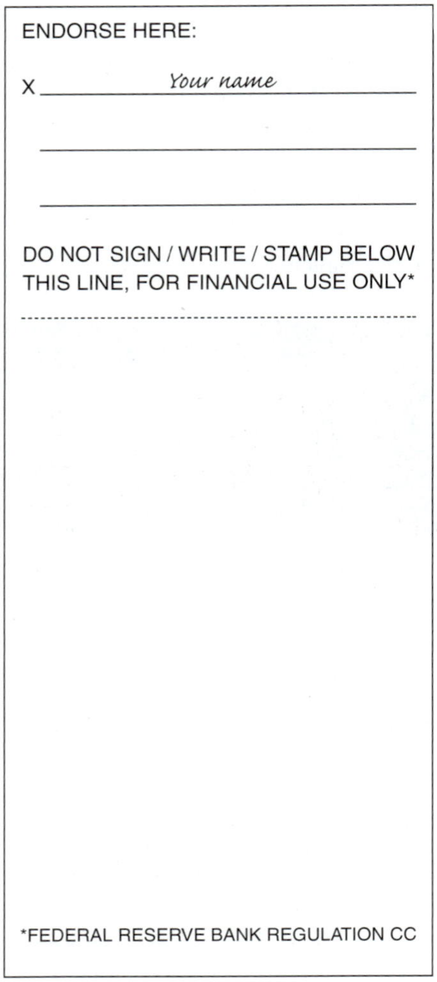

ENDORSE HERE:

X _____ *Your name*

_____

_____

DO NOT SIGN / WRITE / STAMP BELOW THIS LINE, FOR FINANCIAL USE ONLY*

\- -

*FEDERAL RESERVE BANK REGULATION CC

FIGURE 10-10 Proper placement of signature endorsement

ing edge" of all checks. Checks on which the endorsement extends beyond the 1½" area may be refused by the financial institution for improper endorsement. To avoid processing delays, be sure to endorse all checks as described (Figure 10-10).

MAKING DEPOSITS

The manager is also expected to deposit cash and checks received in the office. This may be a daily task, or it may be as infrequent as once a week for a physician with a limited practice. Deposits should be prepared in a secure place out of people's view. Currency should be sorted:

- Put all bills of the same **denomination** together.
- Face bills the same direction, portrait side up.
- Stack in order from highest to lowest denomination (for example, 50s, 20s, 10s, 5s, then 1s).

Count and enter the total amount of the bills on the currency line of the deposit slip (see Figure 10-7). Next, count and enter the total amount of coins on the coin line. If there is a large amount of coin, it should be placed in wrappers.

Check to be sure all the checks have been endorsed. Arrange them facing up from the largest amount to the least. List checks by number, last name of maker, and amount on deposit slip. A computer-generated list or an additional sheet of check listings is acceptable if a deposit slip is attached. If a money order is received,

identify it as MO and the payee's name. If there are more checks than can be listed on the deposit slip front, use the back, total the amount, and bring it forward to the correct line. Total the amount of the checks and enter it on the slip. To avoid errors, total the actual checks and compare with the total listed amount. Total the deposits and enter the amount on the deposit slip. Make a copy of both sides of a deposit slip in case any question about the deposit should arise. When the deposit slip is finished, enter the amount in the checkbook and add it to the existing balance, enter it on the daily log sheet, or post it on the appropriate computer screen.

Deposit slips are imprinted with the account number in MICR numbers that match those on the checks. These numbers make it possible for checks and deposit slips to be sorted and recorded by computer. Banks will accept a list of deposited items on something other than the bank-provided deposit slip as long as the bank deposit slip is attached (see Figure 10-7).

Following the steps in Procedure 10-2, complete a deposit slip correctly. The workbook has a page of checks with stubs for you to practice.

Deposits are usually placed in a zippered bank bag to be taken to the bank. They can be taken inside and given to a teller or deposited in the night depository. Care should always be taken when transporting money. Be aware of your surroundings and do not put yourself in a questionable situation. If there is any chance you are being watched, do not leave your car. It

---

PROCEDURE PROCEDURE PROCEDURE PROCEDURE PROCEDURE PROCEDURE PROCEDURE

10-2   Prepare a Deposit Slip

PURPOSE: Accurately prepare a deposit slip.

EQUIPMENT: Deposit slip, pen with black or blue ink, and cash and checks to be deposited.

PERFORMANCE OBJECTIVE: Prepare a bank deposit slip, following the steps in the procedure. All cash, checks, and coin must be entered without error and the deposit accurately totaled within the time established by the instructor.

1. Separate money to be deposited by check, currency, and coin.
2. Arrange currency by denomination, portrait, and direction.
3. Total the currency and record it on the deposit slip.
4. Count the coins; wrap large amounts.
5. Enter the amount of coins on the deposit slip.
6. Check to ensure all checks are endorsed.
7. Arrange checks face up from greatest to least.
8. Enter checks by number, maker, and amount on the deposit slip.
9. Total all checks listed on the back and enter the total; bring it forward.
10. Total the currency, coin, and checks and enter it on the slip.
11. Make a copy of the deposit slip for your office files.
12. Enter the deposit total in the checkbook.
13. Deposit at the bank
14. File a record of the deposit.

probably is a good idea to vary the deposit day and time if possible so you do not become predictable.

You should receive a record of the deposit when it is made or by mail if night deposited. This should be filed to prove a deposit was made if the bank fails to credit the account on the monthly statement.

DEPOSIT BY MAIL

Checks may be deposited by mail. You should avoid sending cash or currency by mail, but if you must, then send it registered. The deposit slip and money are prepared as for any deposit. The checks should be endorsed by restrictive endorsement only. If no stamp is available, the handwritten notation "for deposit only to the account of (name of your employer)" or "to the account number" will suffice. You should request a receipt, as this record is necessary to prove a deposit was made. It is extremely important that you have an accurate record of all checks deposited with the check number, whom the check is from, and the amount of check so that you can follow up if necessary. It is a good idea to neatly arrange the checks on the photocopier glass and then photocopy them. If checks become lost in the mail, it will be necessary to notify all payees to stop payment and issue you new checks.

RECONCILING BANK STATEMENTS

An important part of banking is the reconciliation each month of the bank statement with the office records. You need to be sure that you and the bank agree as to the amount of money in the account. You will receive a statement that shows all banking **transactions** concerning the account along with the checks that the bank has received and processed. Most statements contain a section similar to Figure 10-11 that allows you to list outstanding checks and do other calculations to **reconcile** the amounts.

An outstanding check is one you have written that does not appear on your bank statement because the payee has not yet cashed the check. Look at the statement and put a check mark on each stub or register entry that matches a bank statement entry. A check stub or registry entry not checked indicates an outstanding check. The total of the outstanding checks is entered on the worksheet.

Items withdrawn from the account by the bank for charges, automatic payments, and such that appear on the statement but are not in your checkbook must be totaled and entered on the appropriate line on the worksheet. Check the statement for deposits and compare the statement with your checkbook record. If you made a deposit since the statement was printed, it will not appear. Be sure make certain an earlier deposit was not omitted from the statement.

```
RECONCILING THE BANK STATEMENT

Bank Statement Balance        $_____

Less Outstanding Checks

  #_____ $_____

  #_____ $_____

  #_____ $_____

  #_____ $_____

  #_____ $_____

  #_____ $_____

  #_____ $_____

Total      _____          $_____

Plus deposits not shown      $_____

CORRECTED BANK STATEMENT              $_____

Checkbook balance            $_____

Less bank charges            $_____

CORRECTED CHECKBOOK BALANCE           $_____
```

FIGURE 10-11 Reconciliation form

Finally, the account may earn interest that you have not recorded in the checkbook. Enter that on the form. Once you have all the amounts, and do the math, the corrected checkbook amount should reconcile (be consistent with) the bank statement.

With the convenience of online banking, some recurring expenses may be paid by electronic check. Unless a record is made in the traditional checkbook, there will be a difference in the balance. Be certain to check for these expenditures when you are reconciling the monthly statement. The statement will list the transaction as a "bill pay" and identify the payee. Other funds could be added or withdrawn by electronic transfer to and from other accounts or as automatic deposits or withdrawals. These will also be listed and will affect your reconciling balances. Follow Procedure 10-3 and the workbook exercises to practice reconciling a bank statement.

PETTY CASH AND OTHER ACCOUNTS

Since it is not reasonable to write checks for small office transactions, most physicians have a petty cash fund. The physician will determine the amount of the fund and for what it will be used. The fund is estab-

PROCEDURE PROCEDURE PROCEDURE PROCEDURE PROCEDURE PROCEDURE PROCEDURE

10-3  Reconcile a Bank Statement

PURPOSE: Accurately reconcile a bank statement.

EQUIPMENT: Bank statement and canceled checks or photocopies, reconciliation worksheet, pen or pencil, calculator or adding machine.

PERFORMANCE OBJECTIVE: Given all necessary equipment, follow the procedure steps to reconcile a bank statement so that the checkbook balance equals the bank statement balance.

1. Compare the opening balance on the new statement with the closing balance on the previous statement. **NOTE: If they do not agree, contact the bank.**

2. List the bank balance in the appropriate space on the reconciliation worksheet.

3. Compare the check entries on the statement with the returned checks. **NOTE: The bank may have your checks in numeric order; if not, you should place them in order.**

4. Determine whether you have any outstanding checks.

5. Total the outstanding checks.

6. Subtract from your checkbook balance items such as withdrawals, automatic payments, or service charges that appear on the statement but not in the checkbook. **NOTE: These items are indicated by a code such as *AP* for automatic payment or *SC* for service charge.**

7. Add to your checkbook balance any interest earned as indicated on your statement. **NOTE: Some banks pay interest if a specified minimum amount is maintained in the account.**

8. Add to the bank statement balance any deposits not shown on the bank statement (e.g., amounts deposited since the statement was prepared).

9. The balance in your checkbook and the bank statement should agree. **NOTE: If they do not agree, subtract the lesser figure from the greater for a possible clue to the error and recheck all figures.**

---

lished by writing a check payable to "cash" or "petty cash." The check is then cashed and the money kept in a separate locked cash box. The money is often used for postage due letters, inexpensive office supplies, and small charitable donations.

A **voucher** form or expenditure list should be completed each time payment is made from this fund. When the amount in the fund is nearly **depleted**, another check is written for the difference between the established original fund amount and the remaining amount. The expense records are kept in a file to verify the use of the petty cash fund. Figure 10-12 shows a petty cash fund ledger form to monitor expenditures.

Practice completing a petty cash form by referring to Procedure 10-4 and using the following amounts. Assume the physician has said that when the balance goes below $5.00, it should be brought back up to the $25.00 level. For what amount should the check be written?

$25 beginning cash
#1 voucher: $5.00 donation
#2 voucher: $1.50 parking
Bill: $3.80 package shipping
#3 voucher: $4.75 Girl Scout cookies
Bill: $1.39 mailing envelope
#4 voucher: $3.75 gift card

DATE	DESCRIPTION	VOUCHER NUMBER	TOTAL AMOUNT	OFFICE EXPENSE	DONA-TIONS	MISC.	BALANCE
10/1	Fund established						25.00
10/5	Postage due	1	.40	.40			24.60
10/8	Parking fee	2	1.60			1.60	23.00
10/10	Coffee	3	2.98				20.02

FIGURE 10-12 Petty cash form

ACHIEVE UNIT OBJECTIVES

- ■ **Complete the Workbook activities to meet the learning objectives.**

- ■ **Practice the procedures in this unit to meet the performance objectives.**

- ■ **Apply your knowledge at the end of this chapter in completing the Critical Thinking Challenge and Activities, as well as the StudyWARE on your Student CD-ROM.**

PROCEDURE PROCEDURE PROCEDURE PROCEDURE PROCEDURE PROCEDURE PROCEDURE

10-4  Establish and Maintain a Petty Cash Fund

PURPOSE: Establish and accurately maintain a petty cash fund.

EQUIPMENT: Petty cash form, pen.

PERFORMANCE OBJECTIVE: Given an initial amount of cash, a petty cash form, vouchers, bills, and a pen, correctly enter the items and compute the balance accurately.

1. Enter the opening balance on the petty cash form.
2. Refer to a voucher and enter the description, number, and amount dispersed and compute the balance.
3. Refer to a bill and enter the description and amount dispersed and compute the balance.
4. Continue until all items are listed and the remaining balance is computed.
5. Notify the physician or manager to write a new check for the difference between the balance and the established fund amount when it reaches the agreed-upon level.

UNIT 4
EMPLOYEE, SALARY, BENEFITS, AND TAX RECORDS

OBJECTIVES

Upon completion of this unit, you will be able to achieve the following:

LEARNING Objectives

1. **Spell and define, using the glossary at the back of the text, all the Words to Know in this unit.**
2. **Explain the W-4, W-2, and I-9 forms.**
3. **Identify nine items that may be needed for payroll records and a personnel file.**
4. **Differentiate between hourly wage and a salary.**
5. **Identify the information required for payroll records.**
6. **List the four factors that affect the amount of federal tax withheld.**
7. **Differentiate between gross and net salary.**
8. **Describe salary benefits, identifying six examples.**

WORDS TO KNOW

accountant
benefits
bereavement
   time
complimentary
deductions
disability
exemption
fringe benefits
gross
Internal Revenue
   Service
longevity
net
productivity
profit sharing
unemployment
vested

CERTIFICATION CONNECTION

CMA
Office policies and
   procedures
Employee payroll

CMAS
Medical office financial
   management (payroll)

Medical office
   management (human
   resources)

RMA
Employee payroll

EMPLOYEE REQUIREMENTS AND RECORDS

All employees in a physician's office must have a Social Security number. This is a nine-digit number that is obtained from the Social Security Administration. Forms to apply for a Social Security number can be obtained from the local Social Security office, **Internal Revenue Service** office, and post offices. Each employee must also complete an Employee's Withholding Allowance Certificate (W-4 form) indicating the number of **exemptions** claimed (Figure 10-13). Any employee who fails to complete a

Form W-4 (2005)

Purpose. Complete Form W-4 so that your employer can withhold the correct federal income tax from your pay. Because your tax situation may change, you may want to refigure your withholding each year.

Exemption from withholding. If you are exempt, complete only lines 1, 2, 3, 4, and 7 and sign the form to validate it. Your exemption for 2005 expires February 16, 2006. See Pub. 505, Tax Withholding and Estimated Tax.

Note. You cannot claim exemption from withholding if (a) your income exceeds $800 and includes more than $250 of unearned income (for example, interest and dividends) and (b) another person can claim you as a dependent on their tax return.

Basic instructions. If you are not exempt, complete the **Personal Allowances Worksheet** below. The worksheets on page 2 adjust your withholding allowances based on itemized deductions, certain credits, adjustments to income, or two-earner/two-job situations. Complete all worksheets that apply. However, you may claim fewer (or zero) allowances.

Head of household. Generally, you may claim head of household filing status on your tax return only if you are unmarried and pay more than 50% of the costs of keeping up a home for yourself and your dependent(s) or other qualifying individuals. See line **E** below.

Tax credits. You can take projected tax credits into account in figuring your allowable number of withholding allowances. Credits for child or dependent care expenses and the child tax credit may be claimed using the **Personal Allowances Worksheet** below. See Pub. 919, How Do I Adjust My Tax Withholding? for information on converting your other credits into withholding allowances.

Nonwage income. If you have a large amount of nonwage income, such as interest or dividends, consider making estimated tax payments using Form 1040-ES, Estimated Tax for Individuals. Otherwise, you may owe additional tax.

Two earners/two jobs. If you have a working spouse or more than one job, figure the total number of allowances you are entitled to claim on all jobs using worksheets from only one Form W-4. Your withholding usually will be most accurate when all allowances are claimed on the Form W-4 for the highest paying job and zero allowances are claimed on the others.

Nonresident alien. If you are a nonresident alien, see the Instructions for Form 8233 before completing this Form W-4.

Check your withholding. After your Form W-4 takes effect, use Pub. 919 to see how the dollar amount you are having withheld compares to your projected total tax for 2005. See Pub. 919, especially if your earnings exceed $125,000 (Single) or $175,000 (Married).

Recent name change? If your name on line 1 differs from that shown on your social security card, call 1-800-772-1213 to initiate a name change and obtain a social security card showing your correct name.

Personal Allowances Worksheet (Keep for your records.)

A Enter "1" for **yourself** if no one else can claim you as a dependent . . . . A ____

B Enter "1" if: { • You are single and have only one job; or • You are married, have only one job, and your spouse does not work; or • Your wages from a second job or your spouse's wages (or the total of both) are $1,000 or less. } . B ____

C Enter "1" for your **spouse.** But, you may choose to enter "-0-" if you are married and have either a working spouse or more than one job. (Entering "-0-" may help you avoid having too little tax withheld.) . . . . C ____

D Enter number of **dependents** (other than your spouse or yourself) you will claim on your tax return . . . . D ____

E Enter "1" if you will file as **head of household** on your tax return (see conditions under **Head of household** above) . E ____

F Enter "1" if you have at least $1,500 of **child or dependent care expenses** for which you plan to claim a credit . F ____

(**Note.** Do **not** include child support payments. See **Pub. 503,** Child and Dependent Care Expenses, for details.)

G **Child Tax Credit** (including additional child tax credit):

- If your total income will be less than $54,000 ($79,000 if married), enter "2" for each eligible child.
- If your total income will be between $54,000 and $84,000 ($79,000 and $119,000 if married), enter "1" for each eligible child plus "1" **additional** if you have four or more eligible children. G ____

H Add lines A through G and enter total here. (**Note.** This may be different from the number of exemptions you claim on your tax return.) ▶ H ____

For accuracy, complete all worksheets that apply. { • If you plan to **itemize or claim adjustments to income** and want to reduce your withholding, see the **Deductions and Adjustments Worksheet** on page 2. • If you have **more than one job** or are **married and you and your spouse both work** and the combined earnings from all jobs exceed $35,000 ($25,000 if married) see the **Two-Earner/Two-Job Worksheet** on page 2 to avoid having too little tax withheld. • If **neither** of the above situations applies, **stop here** and enter the number from line H on line 5 of Form W-4 below. }

- - - - - - - - **Cut here and give Form W-4 to your employer. Keep the top part for your records.** - - - - - - - -

Form **W-4**

Department of the Treasury
Internal Revenue Service

Employee's Withholding Allowance Certificate

▶ **Whether you are entitled to claim a certain number of allowances or exemption from withholding is subject to review by the IRS. Your employer may be required to send a copy of this form to the IRS.**

OMB No. 1545-0010

2005

1 Type or print your first name and middle initial | Last name | 2 Your social security number

Home address (number and street or rural route) | 3 ☐ Single ☐ Married ☐ Married, but withhold at higher Single rate.
Note. If married, but legally separated, or spouse is a nonresident alien, check the "Single" box.

City or town, state, and ZIP code | 4 **If your last name differs from that shown on your social security card, check here. You must call 1-800-772-1213 for a new card.** ▶ ☐

5 Total number of allowances you are claiming (from line **H** above **or** from the applicable worksheet on page 2) 5 ____

6 Additional amount, if any, you want withheld from each paycheck . . . . 6 $ ____

7 I claim exemption from withholding for 2005, and I certify that I meet **both** of the following conditions for exemption.

- Last year I had a right to a refund of **all** federal income tax withheld because I had **no** tax liability **and**
- This year I expect a refund of **all** federal income tax withheld because I expect to have **no** tax liability.

If you meet both conditions, write "Exempt" here . . . . ▶ 7 ____

Under penalties of perjury, I declare that I have examined this certificate and to the best of my knowledge and belief, it is true, correct, and complete.

Employee's signature
(Form is not valid
unless you sign it.) ▶ Date ▶

8 Employer's name and address (Employer: Complete lines 8 and 10 only if sending to the IRS.) | 9 Office code (optional) | 10 Employer identification number (EIN)

For Privacy Act and Paperwork Reduction Act Notice, see page 2. Cat. No. 10220Q Form **W-4** (2005)

Form W-4 (2005) Page **2**

Deductions and Adjustments Worksheet

Note. Use this worksheet *only* if you plan to itemize deductions, claim certain credits, or claim adjustments to income on your 2005 tax return.

1 Enter an estimate of your 2005 itemized deductions. These include qualifying home mortgage interest, charitable contributions, state and local taxes, medical expenses in excess of 7.5% of your income, and miscellaneous deductions. (For 2005, you may have to reduce your itemized deductions if your income is over $145,950 ($72,975 if married filing separately). See *Worksheet 3* in Pub. 919 for details.) . . 1 $ ____

2 Enter: { $10,000 if married filing jointly or qualifying widow(er); $ 7,300 if head of household; $ 5,000 if single or married filing separately } . . . . 2 $ ____

3 **Subtract** line 2 from line 1. If line 2 is greater than line 1, enter "-0-" . . . . 3 $ ____

4 Enter an estimate of your 2005 adjustments to income, including alimony, deductible IRA contributions, and student loan interest 4 $ ____

5 **Add** lines 3 and 4 and enter the total. (Include any amount for credits from *Worksheet 7* in Pub. 919) . 5 $ ____

6 Enter an estimate of your 2005 nonwage income (such as dividends or interest) . . . . . 6 $ ____

7 **Subtract** line 6 from line 5. Enter the result, but not less than "-0-" . . . . 7 $ ____

8 **Divide** the amount on line 7 by $3,200 and enter the result here. Drop any fraction . . . . 8 ____

9 Enter the number from the **Personal Allowances Worksheet,** line H, page 1 . . . . . . 9 ____

10 **Add** lines 8 and 9 and enter the total here. If you plan to use the **Two-Earner/Two-Job Worksheet,** also enter this total on line 1 below. Otherwise, **stop here** and enter this total on Form W-4, line 5, page 1 . 10 ____

Two-Earner/Two-Job Worksheet (See *Two earners/two jobs* on page 1.)

Note. Use this worksheet *only* if the instructions under line H on page 1 direct you here.

1 Enter the number from line H, page 1 (or from line 10 above if you used the **Deductions and Adjustments Worksheet**) 1 ____

2 Find the number in **Table 1** below that applies to the **LOWEST** paying job and enter it here . . 2 ____

3 If line 1 is **more than or equal to** line 2, subtract line 2 from line 1. Enter the result here (if zero, enter "-0-") and on Form W-4, line 5, page 1. **Do not** use the rest of this worksheet . . . . . . 3 ____

Note. If line 1 is *less than* line 2, enter "-0-" on Form W-4, line 5, page 1. Complete lines 4–9 below to calculate the additional withholding amount necessary to avoid a year-end tax bill.

4 Enter the number from line 2 of this worksheet . . . . . . 4 ____

5 Enter the number from line 1 of this worksheet . . . . . . 5 ____

6 **Subtract** line 5 from line 4 . . . . 6 ____

7 Find the amount in **Table 2** below that applies to the **HIGHEST** paying job and enter it here . . 7 $ ____

8 **Multiply** line 7 by line 6 and enter the result here. This is the additional annual withholding needed . 8 $ ____

9 Divide line 8 by the number of pay periods remaining in 2005. For example, divide by 26 if you are paid every two weeks and you complete this form in December 2004. Enter the result here and on Form W-4, line 6, page 1. This is the additional amount to be withheld from each paycheck . . . . . 9 $ ____

Table 1: Two-Earner/Two-Job Worksheet

Married Filing Jointly						All Others	
If wages from **HIGHEST** paying job are—	AND, wages from **LOWEST** paying job are—	Enter on line 2 above	If wages from **HIGHEST** paying job are—	AND, wages from **LOWEST** paying job are—	Enter on line 2 above	If wages from **LOWEST** paying job are—	Enter on line 2 above
$0 - $40,000	$0 - $4,000	0	$40,001 and over	30,001 - 36,000	6	$0 - $6,000	0
	4,001 - 8,000	1		36,001 - 45,000	7	6,001 - 12,000	1
	8,001 - 18,000	2		45,001 - 50,000	8	12,001 - 18,000	2
	18,001 and over	3		50,001 - 60,000	9	18,001 - 24,000	3
$40,001 and over	$0 - $4,000	0		60,001 - 65,000	10	24,001 - 31,000	4
	4,001 - 8,000	1		65,001 - 75,000	11	31,001 - 45,000	5
	8,001 - 18,000	2		75,001 - 90,000	12	45,001 - 60,000	6
	18,001 - 22,000	3		90,001 - 100,000	13	60,001 - 75,000	7
	22,001 - 25,000	4		100,001 - 115,000	14	75,001 - 80,000	8
	25,001 - 30,000	5		115,001 and over	15	80,001 - 100,000	9
						100,001 and over	10

Table 2: Two-Earner/Two-Job Worksheet

Married Filing Jointly		All Others	
If wages from **HIGHEST** paying job are—	Enter on line 7 above	If wages from **HIGHEST** paying job are—	Enter on line 7 above
$0 - $60,000	$480	$0 - $30,000	$480
60,001 - 110,000	800	30,001 - 70,000	800
110,001 - 160,000	900	70,001 - 140,000	900
160,001 - 280,000	1,060	140,001 - 320,000	1,060
280,001 and over	1,120	320,001 and over	1,120

Privacy Act and Paperwork Reduction Act Notice. We ask for the information on this form to carry out the Internal Revenue laws of the United States. The Internal Revenue Code requires this information under sections 3402(f)(2)(A) and 6109 and their regulations. Failure to provide a properly completed form will result in your being treated as a single person who claims no withholding allowances; providing fraudulent information may also subject you to penalties. Routine uses of this information include giving it to the Department of Justice for civil and criminal litigation, to cities, states, and the District of Columbia for use in administering their tax laws, and using it in the National Directory of New Hires. We may also disclose this information to other countries under a tax treaty, to federal and state agencies to enforce federal nontax criminal laws, or to federal law enforcement and intelligence agencies to combat terrorism.

You are not required to provide the information requested on a form that is subject to the Paperwork Reduction Act unless the form displays a valid OMB control number. Books or records relating to a form or its instructions must be retained as long as their contents may become material in the administration of any Internal Revenue law. Generally, tax returns and return information are confidential, as required by Code section 6103.

The time needed to complete this form will vary depending on individual circumstances. The estimated average time is: Recordkeeping, 45 min.; Learning about the law or the form, 12 min.; Preparing the form, 58 min. If you have comments concerning the accuracy of these time estimates or suggestions for making this form simpler, we would be happy to hear from you. You can write to: Internal Revenue Service, Tax Products Coordinating Committee, SE:W:CAR:MP:T:T:SP, 1111 Constitution Ave. NW, IR-6406, Washington, DC 20224. **Do not** send Form W-4 to this address. Instead, give it to your employer.

FIGURE 10-13 Form W-4, Employee's Withholding Allowance Certificate

W-4 form will have withholding figured on the basis of being single with no exemptions. A new W-4 form must be completed if there is a change in marital status or a change in the number of exemptions.

Recent federal legislation requires employees to complete an Employment Eligibility Verification, Form I-9 (Figure 10-14). The form is issued by the Department of Justice, Immigration and Naturalization Service. Its purpose is to ensure all persons employed are either United States citizens, lawfully admitted aliens, or aliens authorized to work in the United States. By law, this form must be completed before an individual can be officially hired. **Accountants** will not permit salary to be paid to individuals who do not have a form I-9 on file.

In addition to these federal requirements, forms must also be processed for state and local tax records. Local government tax is paid to the city where employment occurs regardless of where the employee lives.

All employees should have the following documents or information available when filling out initial payroll forms:

- Driver's license or other state picture identification
- Social Security card and a copy of Social Security numbers of all dependents
- If not a United States citizen, a green card or equivalent

Other documentation needed for your personnel file include:

- Immunization record
- Copies of any professional license, registration, or certification
- Evidence of pertinent diplomas, degrees, or certificates
- Evidence of professional liability insurance (if applicable)
- Verification of Occupational Safety and Health Administration/Clinical Laboratory Improvement Amendments (OSHA/CLIA) training
- Exposure classification record

The very nature of work in a physician's office brings you into contact with pathogens. Because of the chance of exposure to hepatitis B in blood and other body fluids, OSHA regulations require that you have a series of vaccinations, provided by your employer, for your protection. If your particular office responsibilities make it unlikely that you will come in contact with the virus, you may be permitted to decline the vaccine. You may need to sign a form stating that you have declined and that should you come upon a spill of blood or body fluids, you will avoid contact and notify a properly trained person to handle the material. At any time should your job responsibilities change, you may need to receive the vaccine. Figure 10-15 is a sample of a form that would become part of your personnel file.

MEDICAL OFFICE REQUIREMENTS AND RECORDS

The physician's office must have a federal tax reporting number, which is obtained from the Internal Revenue Service. In states that require employer reports, a state employer number must also be obtained.

When payroll checks are prepared, a record must be kept showing Social Security, federal taxes, any state and city taxes, and insurance amounts deducted from earnings. Employees may be paid an hourly wage or a salary (a fixed amount paid on a regular basis for a prescribed period of time). The Federal Fair Labor Standards Act regulates the minimum wage and requires that overtime be paid to hourly wage earners at a minimum rate of one and one-half times the regular rate for hours above 40 hours per week. It is necessary to keep records of hours worked, total pay, and all **deductions** withheld for all employees.

All employees are expected to work the assigned number of hours per day, week, and month. Any time off must be reconciled on the payroll records and the salary adjusted according to office policy.

Several office supply businesses furnish forms for payroll recordkeeping. Office management software also provides screens for recording payroll data. There should be a page for each employee's payroll record. The heading should give the following:

- Name
- Address
- Telephone
- Social Security number
- Date of employment

There are columns in which the following information can be recorded:

- Date of check
- Hours worked (regular and overtime)
- **Gross** salary
- Individual deductions: federal income tax, Social Security tax, state tax, local tax, insurance, and perhaps uniforms
- **Net** pay (the actual amount of the paycheck after deductions).

When an accountant or management firm is employed to prepare payroll, office records must be given to them by a designated date(s) each month so that payroll can be prepared and records maintained.

The amount of federal tax withheld is based on the amount earned, marital status, number of exemptions claimed, and length of the pay period. The Internal Revenue Service will provide the charts used to figure deductions for federal income tax and Society Security tax. State and local taxes are usually a percentage of gross earnings. The net pay (pay actually given to the employee) is the

Department of Homeland Security
U.S. Citizenship and Immigration Services

OMB No. 1615-0047; Expires 03/31/07

Employment Eligibility Verification

Please read instructions carefully before completing this form. The instructions must be available during completion of this form. ANTI-DISCRIMINATION NOTICE: It is illegal to discriminate against work eligible individuals. Employers CANNOT specify which document(s) they will accept from an employee. The refusal to hire an individual because of a future expiration date may also constitute illegal discrimination.

Section 1. Employee Information and Verification. To be completed and signed by employee at the time employment begins.

Print Name: Last	First	Middle Initial	Maiden Name
Address (Street Name and Number)		Apt. #	Date of Birth (month/day/year)
City	State	Zip Code	Social Security #

I am aware that federal law provides for imprisonment and/or fines for false statements or use of false documents in connection with the completion of this form.

I attest, under penalty of perjury, that I am (check one of the following):

☐ A citizen or national of the United States
☐ A Lawful Permanent Resident (Alien #) A _____
☐ An alien authorized to work until _____

(Alien # or Admission #) _____

Employee's Signature	Date (month/day/year)

Preparer and/or Translator Certification. *(To be completed and signed if Section 1 is prepared by a person other than the employee.) I attest, under penalty of perjury, that I have assisted in the completion of this form and that to the best of my knowledge the information is true and correct.*

Preparer's/Translator's Signature	Print Name
Address (Street Name and Number, City, State, Zip Code)	Date (month/day/year)

Section 2. Employer Review and Verification. **To be completed and signed by employer. Examine one document from List A OR examine one document from List B and one from List C, as listed on the reverse of this form, and record the title, number and expiration date, if any, of the document(s).**

List A	OR	List B	AND	List C
Document title: _____		_____		_____
Issuing authority: _____		_____		_____
Document #: _____		_____		_____
Expiration Date (if any): _____		_____		_____
Document #: _____				
Expiration Date (if any): _____				

CERTIFICATION - I attest, under penalty of perjury, that I have examined the document(s) presented by the above-named employee, that the above-listed document(s) appear to be genuine and to relate to the employee named, that the employee began employment on *(month/day/year)* _____ **and that to the best of my knowledge the employee is eligible to work in the United States. (State employment agencies may omit the date the employee began employment.)**

Signature of Employer or Authorized Representative	Print Name	Title
Business or Organization Name	Address (Street Name and Number, City, State, Zip Code)	Date (month/day/year)

Section 3. Updating and Reverification. To be completed and signed by employer.

A. New Name (if applicable)	B. Date of Rehire (month/day/year) (if applicable)

C. If employee's previous grant of work authorization has expired, provide the information below for the document that establishes current employment eligibility.

Document Title: _____   Document #: _____   Expiration Date (if any): _____

I attest, under penalty of perjury, that to the best of my knowledge, this employee is eligible to work in the United States, and if the employee presented document(s), the document(s) I have examined appear to be genuine and to relate to the individual.

Signature of Employer or Authorized Representative	Date (month/day/year)

NOTE: This is the 1991 edition of the Form I-9 that has been rebranded with a current printing date to reflect the recent transition from the INS to DHS and its components.

Form I-9 (Rev. 05/31/05)Y Page 2

FIGURE 10-14 Employment Eligibility Verification, Form 1-9

SAMPLE

Exposure Classification Record of Employee

The following employee was classified according to work task exposure to certain body fluids as required by the current OSHA infection control standard on (Date) _____ as follows:

Employee Name: _____ SS# _____

_____ Category 1. "All procedures or other job related tasks that involve an inherent potential for mucous membrane or skin contact with blood, body fluids, or tissues, or a potential for spill or splashes of (blood or body fluids)."

_____ Category 2. Tasks in which "The normal work routine involves no exposure to blood, body fluids, or tissues, but exposure or potential exposure may be required as a condition of employment." For example, receptionists, accounting, or insurance staff or others who may, as a part of their duties, be asked to help in clean up, instrument recirculation, laboratory, or other similar procedures where exposure may result.

_____ Category 3. Tasks in which "The normal work routine involves no exposure to blood, body fluids, or tissues. Persons who perform these duties are not called upon as part of their employment to perform or assist in emergency medical care or first aid or to be potentially exposed in some other way."

Employer Signature _____

Because of a change of job assignment, the above employee was reclassified according to tasks exposure on (Date) _____ as follows:

_____ Category 1

_____ Category 2

_____ Category 3

Employer's Signature _____

Because of a change of assignment, the above employee was reclassified according to task exposure on (Date) _____ as follows:

_____ Category 1

_____ Category 2

_____ Category 3

Employer's Signature _____

NOTE: This record should be retained for length of employment plus thirty years.

FIGURE 10-15 Sample Exposure Classification Record, which shows exposure categories into which employee's tasks fall. This record is kept for 30 years. *(Courtesy POL Consultants, 2 Russ Farm Way, Delanco, NJ 08075, 856-824-0800)*

gross earnings minus taxes and other deductions. The physician must provide the employee with a statement of gross pay and deductions along with the check each pay period. The tax deductions withheld must be sent on a quarterly basis to the federal, state, and local government offices along with the reporting forms provided by the tax offices. The local, state, and federal governments supply the guidelines necessary to complete these reports.

A W-2 form (Figure 10-16), which is a summary of all earnings for the year and all deductions withheld for federal, state, and local taxes, must be provided to each employee by January 31st of each year. The Social Security Administration must also receive a report of W-2 forms each year. The physician who has several employees may also need to submit reports to the state and federal government for **unemployment** taxes. This tax is not deducted from the employee's earnings for federal tax but may be deducted in some cases for state unemployment tax.

BENEFITS

Full-time employed medical assistants and other medical office employees can expect **benefits** in addition to their salary. These are sometimes known as **fringe benefits**. Benefits will vary according to the situation of the employee and the generosity of the physician(s). The following are examples of benefits that may be offered.

- Vacation: Usually a minimum of 2 weeks with pay after completing a year of full-time employment; increases with **longevity**.
- Holidays: A minimum of six paid holidays per year—New Year's, Memorial Day, Fourth of July, Labor Day, Thanksgiving, and Christmas.
- Sick time: Some physicians will pay employees when they need to be out of the office because of illness. Most will pay for 3 to 5 sick days per year.
- Personal time: This is time that an employee can take off for physician or dental appointments and other personal matters without having to use vacation or sick time. Three days per year is the usual amount.
- **Bereavement time**: This is the time that an employee can take off when a family member or very close friend dies. The amount of time is usually based on the relationship of the employee with the deceased.
- Jury duty: Some physicians will pay employees when they are summoned to appear in court. The amount of time granted is based on the court order. It may be possible to get excused from duty if your position is considered critical to your employer.
- Paid time off (PTO): Some practices group holidays, personal days, and vacation time into one category called PTO benefits. Using a mathematical equation based upon the employee's date of hire, a percentage of PTO is accrued each pay period.

a Control number				Safe, accurate, FAST! Use	IRS e~file	Visit the IRS website at www.irs.gov/efile.
		OMB No. 1545-0008				

b Employer identification number (EIN)	1 Wages, tips, other compensation	2 Federal income tax withheld
c Employer's name, address, and ZIP code	3 Social security wages	4 Social security tax withheld
	5 Medicare wages and tips	6 Medicare tax withheld
	7 Social security tips	8 Allocated tips
d Employee's social security number	9 Advance EIC payment	10 Dependent care benefits
e Employee's first name and initial Last name	11 Nonqualified plans	12a See instructions for box 12

13 Statutory employee ☐ Retirement plan ☐ Third-party sick pay ☐	12b
14 Other	12c
	12d

f Employee's address and ZIP code						
15 State Employer's state ID number	16 State wages, tips, etc.	17 State income tax	18 Local wages, tips, etc.	19 Local income tax	20 Locality name	

Form **W-2** **Wage and Tax Statement**   **2005**   Department of the Treasury—Internal Revenue Service

Copy B—To Be Filed With Employee's FEDERAL Tax Return.
This information is being furnished to the Internal Revenue Service.

FIGURE 10-16   Form W-2 summarizes all earnings and deductions for the year and must be prepared for each employee by January 31.

● Health insurance: Available; may require some copayment and may not be provided if employee is covered by insurance with spouse's employment.
● **Disability** insurance: Will cover a percentage of the salary if the employee is unable to work because of a disabling condition.
● Life insurance: Usually for a set amount, for example, equal to a year's salary.
● **Profit sharing**: A form of pension plan to employees who meet certain requirements, such as being at least 21 years old, working a minimum of 1,000 hours in a year, and remaining employed for at least a year to establish eligibility. Each plan will have its own requirements. For example, an amount equal to a certain percentage of the employee's salary is deposited annually into the plan by the employer. This amount accumulates interest and grows tax free until it is withdrawn. The employee is normally responsible for the taxes due. There is usually a period of time, 5 years for example, before an employee becomes **vested** in the plan. This means the person must be employed at least 5 years before being eligible to receive the money in the account should employment be terminated. This type of benefit can add up to a

nice sum. As an example, a person earns $10 per hour, $20,800 per year. If 10% of the salary ($2080) is placed into the plan for 10 years, it would be valued at $20,800 plus the interest earned. Even if there were no increase in salary and therefore no increase in annual contributions, with an interest rate of only 5%, the amount would be approximately $23,000 at the end of 10 years—a very impressive fringe benefit.

Another benefit, which is often overlooked, is the medical care you may receive as an employee. Depending on the type of practice in which you work, you may realize a considerable amount of **complimentary** health care. It is also of benefit to be a physician's employee when you need referral to another physician or medical specialist.

Another nice benefit that some physicians may permit is complimentary lunches that are sponsored by drug companies to have an opportunity to present their products to the physician and staff.

Medical practices that offer a good benefit package in addition to a competitive salary usually have a much more stable staff. This, in turn, results in reduced expense and maintenance of a high level of **productivity** because training time for new employees is not needed.

UNIT 5
GENERAL MANAGEMENT DUTIES

OBJECTIVES

Upon completion of this unit, you will be able to achieve the following:

LEARNING Objectives

1. Spell and define, using the glossary at the back of the text, all the Words to Know in this unit.
2. Discuss refunds to patients.
3. Explain why no shows are a concern.
4. Describe a method to ensure inventory supplies.
5. Identify office equipment requiring frequent attention.
6. Identify six organizations that might inspect a physician's office.
7. Describe a manager's responsibility to the employees.
8. Describe a manager's responsibility to the physicians.
9. List general facility responsibilities.

PERFORMANCE Objectives

1. Perform an inventory of supplies and equipment.
2. Perform routine maintenance of administrative and clinical equipment.
3. Manage the physician's professional schedule and travel.

WORDS TO KNOW

delegation	fiscal	management
expenditure	inventory	negligent
extensive	maintenance	reimbursement

CERTIFICATION CONNECTION

CMA
Maintaining the physical plant
Equipment and supply inventory
Office policies and procedures
Managing physician's professional schedule and travel
Maintaining liability coverage

CMAS
Medical office management (human resources, supplies and equipment, physical office, plant)

RMA
Supplies and equipment management
Employ procedures in compliance with OSHA guidelines and regulations (employee training program)

Many duties performed in a medical office can be categorized under the broad classification of general **management** duties. These are activities that coordinate and maintain the functions within an office. This unit identifies a wide range of miscellaneous duties to acquaint you with those "behind the scenes" activities needed to efficiently operate a successful medical practice.

DAILY AND MONTHLY ACCOUNT RECORDS

Medical offices use a variety of bookkeeping and accounting systems. Regardless of the system used, some method will be needed to maintain a sense for **fiscal** status. It is essential to identify expenditures and income totals to ensure the practice is earning sufficient income to meet office expenses, employee salaries, taxes, insurance premiums, and benefits payments and to provide an income for the physician. In addition, it is necessary to build assets for equipment purchases, investments, and perhaps the hiring of additional employees when needed.

In a medical practice, a percentage of patients may be **negligent** in paying for services. This can represent a sizeable amount of lost income. If it is allowed to continue or increase in percentage, it can present a serious problem and must be dealt with by the manager. Because of this fact, many physicians now require payment when services are delivered. In long-term care situations, such as with obstetric patients, a standard fee to cover the anticipated form of delivery is established, and the patient makes periodic payments prior to the delivery.

It is necessary to keep a record of accounts receivable. You can do this with a record page that allows you to begin the month with the amount carried over from the preceding month. Then each day you list charges and receipts and increase or decrease your total accounts receivable balance depending on whether your receipts or charges were greater. A trial balance, or total of all outstanding accounts, should be calculated each month. The total should agree with the accounts receivable balance.

The accounts payable records include all invoices for purchases, the checkbook, and the disbursement record. All **expenditures** must be carefully entered. Office expenses must be separated from the physician's personal expenses. Office expenses are tax deductible, but not all personal expenses are.

The practice management software should allow calculations of daily, weekly, and year-to-date figures to provide reports for analyzing income sources. It should also provide lists of outstanding receivables and have the capability of generating a list of delinquent accounts.

Many offices send their billing and invoices to an accounting service through a telephone-linked terminal. Still other offices prepare all accounting records in a batch and take them to an accounting service computer center to be processed.

When a personal accountant is employed, the records will be maintained and a report provided to the medical practice each month that indicates the expenditures, balances, and accounts receivable.

In addition to those already mentioned, the 1099 payment reporting forms issued by third-party payers, which indicate the total amount paid directly to the physician during the year, must be saved and given to the accountant for inclusion with the tax forms.

MISSED APPOINTMENTS

Another related area that a manager may need to address is missed appointments. A missed appointment policy should be distributed in new-patient packets either prior to or during the first office visit. If a patient does not show, no payment is received for that scheduled time of the day. In addition, another patient who needed to schedule an appointment was either scheduled at another time or referred if necessary. As an example, say there is one no show, for an average charge of $50. If this occurs 3 days in a week for 48 weeks during a year, $7,200 of income is lost. A policy of calling to remind patients of upcoming appointments can be estab-

lished or a fee assessed for additional missed appointments after the patient has been notified in writing.

Any time a patient calls to cancel an appointment, it is critical that it is recorded in the patient's chart or entered into the computer system. This will document that the patient failed to keep an appointment and eliminate accidental billing.

OFFICE POLICY MANUAL

The office manager is responsible for developing and maintaining the policy and procedure manuals for the office. An office manual may include policy on such topics as:

- Absenteeism
- Paid time off (PTO)
- Harassment
- Confidentiality
- Continuing education
- Chain of command
- Expected performance
- Employment evaluation

OFFICE PROCEDURE MANUAL

An office procedure manual will identify the common procedures performed in the office. The manual may include such procedures as:

- Opening and closing the office
- Laboratory tests
- Documentation requirements
- OSHA/CLIA requirements
- Basic clinical procedures
- Basic administrative procedures
- Emergency procedures

The office manager should address these manuals during the employee's orientation. Employees should always sign a statement that they have read and fully understand the information included in the manuals.

The office manager will usually be responsible for maintaining and updating the policy manual. When a new operational policy is adopted, it must be put into writing and added to the manual. As new procedures become necessary, the manager should also develop the written procedure guidelines and add them to the procedure manual.

HIPAA AND OFFICE POLICY

When the HIPAA rulings began in 1996, policy manuals required updating to include the new directives for protecting patient information and providing security measures and specific instruction for electronically transmitting patient data. Office managers had to attend meetings to learn the requirements of the law and then provide training for their office personnel, including the physicians. Dealing with patient information to families, other health care entities, insurance companies, and business associate contacts required following strict guidelines. It was a challenge to an office to continue business while changing procedures to comply with HIPAA.

The legislation also created three separate roles to be established. A person must be designated the HIPAA Officer to coordinate and oversee compliance with the rules. A person must also be designated Security Officer and is responsible for the security of the patients' records. A third position is a Privacy Officer, who is to keep track of who has access to the protected information. The three positions may be filled by as few as two people, with a third as backup, or several people can be designated in large practices. The office manager most often fills the role of at least one of these positions.

OFFICE LIABILITY INSURANCE

The individual physician or the physicians within a group practice will purchase insurance to protect their personal and professional assets in the event they are found liable for some action or lack of action. Cost of such coverage varies greatly in relation to the type of practice. Lately some specialty physicians have closed their practices because the excessive premiums charged for liability coverage would require them to see more patients and work longer hours to maintain their level of income. A few have decided to practice without any coverage, often providing care at a lesser cost, and informing their patients that they have no liability coverage. If they should be found negligent, they would have to pay the amount awarded from their personal assets.

Many physicians will also provide coverage for their employees, because they frequently are named in a lawsuit. The names of the covered persons are identified with the policy, and the manager may be required to maintain an up-to-date list of employees in order to ensure everyone is covered. Depending upon the wording of the policy, it may state that all persons receiving wages from the practice are covered, and the listing of individuals would therefore not be necessary. All employees should be informed of their exposure to suit when they are hired.

It is also important to see that premiums are paid when due in order to keep the policy in effect; a lapsed policy is of no benefit. If liability is not offered by the practice, medical assistants should purchase their own policy to protect their personal assets. Practicing medical assistants have the option to purchase coverage at special rates through the American Association of Medical Assistants.

STAFF MEETINGS

The office manager is also responsible for conducting staff meetings. The meetings should last from 30 minutes to 1 hour. Many times they are associated with lunch or a continental breakfast to use time more effectively. Employees should receive pay for staff meeting time.

To have a successful meeting, it is necessary to have an agenda or order of business so that it will be organized and the topics to be covered will be known in advance. If decisions are made that will affect office operation, be sure a written record in the form of minutes is kept so that there will be a reference for any necessary changes in the policy and procedure manual. The meetings should be informative and beneficial and should concern the operation of the office. The meeting should never be allowed to turn into a "gripe session." Discussing personal issues associated with individual employees should be avoided when the total staff is present. If an employee wants to discuss an issue that may be considered controversial, the manager will need to schedule a private meeting to determine the appropriateness of how the issue may affect the practice.

In large practices with several physicians, perhaps a physician's assistant, and nurse practitioners in addition to medical assistants, technicians, and a support staff of secretaries and clerks, it may be more beneficial to hold separate meetings. The manager and physicians have different concerns and business to discuss than do the rest of the staff. Depending upon the agenda, it would be up to the manager to differentiate the group and coordinate the information between them.

It is important that all employees attend staff meetings in order to learn about any new procedures, policies, or decisions that will affect them. A memo requiring sign-off by each person validates notification. Noting attendance at meetings will identify anyone who did not receive the information.

PRACTICE INFORMATION BROCHURE

The office manager may be asked to compose an information brochure. It should be printed on a good quality paper. If the practice has a logo, this could be placed on the cover of the brochure. The brochure can be as simple as a single sheet neatly folded or as complex as a booklet. An added touch would be a picture of the physician(s) and a map showing the office location. A brochure can be sent to a new patient as confirmation of an appointment or given to the patient at the initial appointment. The brochure will need to be updated as physicians or services are added or deleted from the practice.

The brochure may also contain some of the following information:

- Brief explanation of office policies
- Brief description of physician's education and practice interests
- Hospital affiliation
- Office hours
- After-hours policy
- Phone number and extensions
- Appointment policy (missed and cancellation)
- Payment policies

PATIENT REFUNDS

Managers usually assume the responsibility of verifying overpayment to a patient's account before approving **reimbursement** to the patient. This situation occurs when both the patient and the insurance company pay the physician or an error in the amount due is made (see Chapter 8).

EQUIPMENT MAINTENANCE AND SUPPLY INVENTORY

The manager or the medical assistant is expected to keep track of equipment **maintenance** and maintain an **inventory** of clinical and administrative supplies. An office that has been in operation for several years will have an established list of companies that supply its needs. You should not change to another company without consulting the physician. You should be alert to the best quality for the best price, however. You will be a valuable member of the health care team if you are able to control costs without sacrificing the quality of the products and supplies you use.

A card system or electronic file of suppliers and equipment maintenance companies is absolutely necessary. A list of all the suppliers of goods and services might be compiled by category, such as administrative, laboratory, clinical, and general. The entries of these businesses should name the company, the address and phone number, and a contact person if possible. A list of what products or services they provide should be entered for each company. General office supplies, for example, may be purchased from the local office supply store, but printer and copier cartridges may be supplied by an electronics store or ordered from the manufacturer. There are many variables, but knowing who and where to call saves valuable time. Individual physicians' offices may join to form a business organization. Together, they have some advantages such as lower pricing because of large quantity purchasing. In this situation, supplies are obtained through the organization.

Office supplies need to be properly stored in clean, dry areas near where they will be used. For example, supplies for administrative use need to be in that area of the office, while materials used in the examination rooms should be stored there. Some items require special storage, such as a locked cabinet for narcotics or refrigeration for some laboratory items. All items need to be inventoried or counted on a regular basis to be sure there is adequate supply on hand to operate the office. If items are time sensitive (date expirations), store in order of expiration, with the first to expire in front. Discard expired items properly.

One area that might need special attention may be linen supply. When actual cloth material that requires laundering is used, there may be a time factor involved with getting fresh linens delivered, so supplies cannot be allowed to get too low.

A minimum amount of supplies to be maintained should be determined and would depend upon the type of office practice and the number of patients seen on an average day. It would be better to err on excess than not have adequate supply. An example of a small practice inventory sheet to be used to check supplies for two examination rooms might look something like Figure 10-17. It could include the date and initials of the person performing the inventory. By noting the items on hand, it is easy to see what needs to be ordered. After completing the form, give it to the person responsible for ordering supplies. Procedure 10-5 describes performing a basic inventory of supplies.

Office equipment represents another large investment. It is important to keep files of equipment manuals and purchase records in order to validate warranties. It is also important to have an inventory of equipment owned by the practice. It should name the items and the date purchased and may include identifying numbers either in the form of applied inventory tags or model numbers from the manufacturer. Periodically, it is a good practice to take inventory to review equipment age and determine whether equipment is still on site. The inventory needs to be updated whenever a new piece of equipment is purchased or an old piece is discarded.

It is also important to keep equipment in proper operating order by providing good office maintenance. It is not possible to give quality care to patients with faulty office equipment. The office may have contracted for routine service that occurs on a regular basis for some pieces of equipment. When equipment is not working properly, go through a troubleshooting checklist, usually included in the manual, to see if you can correct a problem before requesting a service call. Remember, repair personnel charge the same for plugging in a machine as for doing repairs.

A record of regularly scheduled maintenance is necessary. There are daily, weekly, monthly, quarterly, and

Examination Room Supply Inventory

Date: _6-28-20XX_   Taken by: _G Stone, MA_

	Item	Supply minimum	Amount on hand	Place order
1.	Table paper	2 Rolls	1	✓
2.	Cover sheets	1 Box	2	
3.	Pillow covers	2 Boxes	2	
4.	Examination vests	1 Box	1 1/2	
5.	Examination gowns	1 Box	0	✓
6.	Tissues	6 Boxes	10	
7.	Examination gloves	2 Boxes	4	
8.	Alcohol wipes	2 Boxes	1	✓
9.	Otoscope covers	2 Boxes	3	

FIGURE 10-17   Sample supply inventory checklist

PROCEDURE

10-5   Perform an Inventory of Supplies and Equipment

PURPOSE: To obtain the current status of supplies.

EQUIPMENT: Clipboard, supply inventory checklist, and pen.

PERFORMANCE OBJECTIVE: Given a clipboard, supply list, and pen, arrange any items that are time sensitive in front. Count the number of items in storage and accurately record on the list.

1. Enter the date on the form.

2. Check the package dates on time-sensitive materials.

3. Arrange the supplies with the first to expire dates in front.

4. Count each category of items on the inventory list.

5. Enter the number of items left in storage in the appropriate place.

6. Note on the form the supplies below the minimum amount.

7. Sign the form.

8. Give the completed form to the appropriate person to order supplies.

annual inspections to make. When equipment is examined, serviced, or repaired, it should be recorded. When the office is going through an on-site review process by a governing agency or insurance company, evidence of equipment maintenance is one area that is evaluated. The inventory list of equipment combined with records of maintenance and repair should satisfy the requirement. Examples of some of the items checked under the review guidelines are listed in Figure 10-18.

Performing routine maintenance is a frequent activity involving checking electric cords, batteries, equipment cleaning, equipment condition, and the like in both the administrative and clinical areas. This is a day-to-day inspection to ensure equipment is in operable condition. A sample of a partial checklist is shown in Figure 10-19. Refer to Procedure 10-6 to perform a routine maintenance activity.

RESPONSIBILITY FOR DECISION MAKING

In large practices, clinics, and corporations, it is advisable to divide the decision-making responsibilities among the physicians according to their area of interest or expertise. When decisions need to be made, the manager has to confer with only that physician or two instead of the total partnership. An example of division of responsibility is:

- Employment/personnel concerns
- Purchasing and office facility concerns
- Lab and radiology issues
- Fees, investments, and other financial matters

Decisions made by designated physicians are then usually discussed at a general meeting.

From time to time, the manager may also be involved in the review and the eventual negotiations required for agreement to a managed care contract. Managers can provide insight and make inquiries from a different viewpoint than the physicians. When managers have been promoted from medical assistant administrative or clinical positions, they have a valuable understanding of the patient care requirements specified in the managed care contract.

Groups of physicians who form a business partnership to buy supplies in larger quantities may also work together to negotiate for higher reimbursement from insurance providers in exchange for more physician choices for the managed care clients. The manager's input may well affect people in other offices.

The office manager may also be asked to contribute to the determination of fee schedules for patient care. The manager will have a continuing awareness of the costs involved for the physician to perform certain diagnostic studies or the cost of disposable products and supplies involved in certain procedures. When the costs

Type	Frequency
Housekeeping schedule	Daily
Refrigerator and freezer temperatures	Daily
Cold sterilization to check the efficacy of the solution	Daily
Autoclave controls such as Steri-Strips	Daily in most states
Calibration of equipment	Daily or each shift in applicable cases
Quality control for lab procedures	Daily
Inventory of controlled substances	Daily
Spore checks	Weekly or monthly depending on the state
Checking for outdated sterilized instruments	Monthly
Checking for outdated samples in the drug sample closet, refrigerator, freezer, and drug cabinets	Monthly
Infectious waste logs	Monthly
Changing X-ray processing chemicals	According to manufacturer's instructions
Fire extinguisher gauge and pin inspections	Monthly
Eyewash station	Monthly
Emergency/crash kits	Monthly
Automated external defibrillator (AED) or defibrillator units	Monthly
Lab proficiency testing	Quarterly
Evacuation drills	One or two times annually
Hazard communication training	Annually
Blood-borne pathogen training	Annually
Exposure control plan	Annually
Review of safety manual	Annually
OSHA form 200 posted (if more than 10 employees)	Annually
Laboratory policy and procedure manual updated/reviewed	Annually
Emergency preparedness drills	Annually
Radiology policy and procedure drills updated and reviewed	Annually or according to state guidelines
X-ray certificate current	Annually, depending on the state guidelines
Federal CLIA certificate updated	Every two years
CPR certification	Every two years
Equipment maintenance	Every one to three years

FIGURE 10-18   Documentation schedule

Equipment Maintenance Checklist

Date: 4/10/20XX

Taken by: S. White, MA

	Item	Perform maintenance	Inspected	Repairs needed
1.	Copier	Clean glass, rollers, check toner	✓	—
2.	Printer	Clean, check cartridge/toner	✓	Noisy, call service
3.	Computer	Clean glass, check power cord, cables	✓	—
4.	Exam table 1	Clean, check cover	✓	Cover worn
5.	Electric exam table 2	Clean, check cover, power cord, operable	✓	—
6.	Sphygmomanometer 1	Check cuff, tubing, valve, bulb	✓	Bulb soft
7.	Sphygmomanometer 2	Check cuff, tubing, valve, bulb	✓	—
8.	Ophthalmoscope 1	Power supply, cord, bulb	✓	—
9.	Ophthalmoscope 2	Power supply, cord, bulb	✓	Replaced bulb
10.	Exam light 1	Clean, power cord, bulb	✓	—

FIGURE 10-19 Sample routine maintenance checklist

of the products and supplies increase, the fees may have to be adjusted to accommodate the increased expense.

RESPONSIBILITIES TO EMPLOYEES

The manager in large practices often has the following responsibilities related to the support staff employees:

- Interview, hire, and terminate employees in concert with physicians if desired
- Supervise or personally train employees. This applies to new personnel as well as updating current staff.
- Conduct staff meetings to inform, discuss, and exchange information
- Make out work schedules
- Arrange vacations and coverage
- Conduct performance evaluations, establishing probationary periods as deemed necessary
- Consult physicians concerning salary increases and benefit changes

RESPONSIBILITY FOR THE FACILITY

The physical structure of the office must be observed and maintained. The manager assumes responsibility for:

- Maintenance of office services such as cleaning and laundry
- Subscriptions to magazines and health-related literature
- Monitoring and paying utilities
- Suggesting improvements: repairs, decorating, and organization of rooms

A manager who has served successfully in the position may also be given the responsibility to handle renewals of business and professional insurance policies. This could also involve researching different providers and making comparisons of coverage and benefits to obtain the most coverage for the amount spent. Another area that is often the responsibility of the man-

10-6  Perform Routine Maintenance of Administrative and Clinical Equipment

PURPOSE: To perform activities to ensure the operability of equipment.

EQUIPMENT: Equipment list, clipboard, pen, and access to any necessary maintenance supplies.

PERFORMANCE OBJECTIVE: Given an equipment list, clipboard, and pen, inspect each item for cleanliness and safe condition and ensure operability. Provide routine maintenance. Note and report any equipment requiring repair.

1. Date the maintenance sheet.
2. Inspect each item on the list for cleanliness.
3. Clean the item appropriately.
4. Check equipment for safety factors:
   a. Electric cord and plugs
   b. Tighten loose screws/bolts.

5. Check for operability:
   a. Test any light source; replace burned out bulbs.
   b. Inspect items for wear; order replacement parts.
6. Check required operational standards:
   a. Freezer temperature
   b. Refrigerator temperature
   c. Autoclave test strip
7. Briefly operate seldom used equipment. **RATIONALE: To ensure in working condition if needed**
8. Report equipment requiring repairs.
9. Sign the maintenance sheet.

---

ager is the negotiation of leases and prices for equipment and supply contracts. Careful comparisons of equipment features, supply packaging amounts, and price will determine the best purchase option.

RESPONSIBILITIES TO PHYSICIANS

Physicians also need to be kept informed and aware of conditions affecting the practice. The manager has a great deal of obligation to the physicians. Some areas the manager must consider are:

- Assisting in creating or updating business policies to increase efficiency
- Attending meetings pertaining to office management such as those sponsored by the medical association and other professional organizations
- Updating physicians on Medicare, health plans, and insurance company policy changes, fee schedules, and reimbursement rates (for example, changes in Current Procedural Terminology [CPT] and International Classification of Diseases [ICD] codes or descriptors or the reduction in Medicare coverage affecting reimbursement when accepting consignment). Approximately 85% of a physician's income is from third-party payers, either directly or indirectly. It is critical that physicians learn to code their services correctly to obtain the full amount allowed for their care.

- Ordering CPT and ICD books annually and reviewing for deleted or added numbers
- Holding physician meetings to discuss practice concerns

PHYSICIAN'S PROFESSIONAL MEETINGS

The physician may ask the manager for assistance with office scheduling and travel arrangements in order to attend or make a presentation at a professional meeting. The schedule can be marked so that no patients are booked if it is known far enough in advance. If patients have already been scheduled, they will have to be contacted and offered alternative times. Physicians may also want another physician contacted to cover during their absence. When physicians practice within a group, it is usually possible to schedule patients with another group member.

Sponsors of a medical meeting, like the AMA, will send conference information flyers, have a special section in their professional publications, or provide information on their web sites to identify meeting dates, location, major presenters, session topics, and many other features of the conference. They will also identify the hotel or hotels where rooms have been blocked for the attendees. Conference headquarters and meeting rooms may be held in one of the hotels or at a nearby convention center. It is usually convenient to be as close to the meetings as possible. Other activities are sometimes arranged for family members to enjoy during the meetings. Registration for the conference will probably consist of completing the form, selecting a lodging preference, indicating any additional activities, and submitting the registration fee.

There are many things to be considered before you make travel plans. Once you have all the details you can proceed with making arrangements. Have the practice credit card available on which to charge the reservation and tickets.

- Dates:
  - Will the physician combine the conference with personal time off before or after the meetings? (This is very possible when meetings are held in areas near special attractions such as Disney World, Las Vegas, or Washington, D.C.)
  - Will the physician attend all or part of conference?
- Attending alone or with family
- Hotel and room style preference
  - Compare prices among identified hotels.
- Airline reservations
  - Is the physician a frequent flyer member with one or more airlines?
  - Air transportation to the conference is often contracted at a special rate with one or two airlines and is available by using a special code identifier when booking.
  - Compare flight times and prices.

- Use a travel agent instead of the association's arrangements. Note that it is not always possible to get room reservations if associations have all the rooms blocked.
- Make your own arrangements online.

There are many variables possible when making travel plans. Follow the steps in Procedure 10-7 as one way to manage a physician's professional schedule and travel.

Once arrangements have been completed, prepare an itinerary sheet that lists dates, airline, flight numbers and times, hotel name, phone numbers, and any other pertinent information for the physician's quick reference. Tickets obtained online list all the flight numbers, departure times, connecting flights, arrival times, and meal information and can be printed out. This becomes an e-ticket, and no paper tickets will be mailed or need to be picked up. Give the itinerary, reservation information, and e-tickets to the physician. Maintain a copy for office reference.

RESPONSIBILITY FOR PREPARING FOR A SITE VISIT

Many different organizations inspect physicians' offices from time to time, including:

- Insurance companies
- CLIA

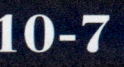 

PROCEDURE PROCEDURE PROCEDURE PROCEDURE PROCEDURE PROCEDURE PROCEDURE PROCEDURE

10-7 Manage a Physician's Professional Schedule and Travel

PURPOSE: To arrange for a physician's absence and travel to a professional event.

EQUIPMENT: Computer, practice credit card, event information, and physician's preferences.

PERFORMANCE OBJECTIVE: Given all necessary equipment and information, arrange an office schedule, send an event registration, make a lodging reservation, and schedule travel to meet a physician's specifications.

1. Obtain all event, lodging, and travel details from the physician.
2. Arrange the office schedule for the absence:
   a. Block appointments.
   b. Arrange coverage as instructed.
3. Complete the event registration information.
4. Make a lodging selection on the registration form.

5. Register for any additional activities.
6. Total the registration costs and prepare a check or enter the charge information.
7. Copy the registration form.
8. Go online to contact the preferred conference airline.
9. Select the most convenient flight schedule.
10. Process a ticket request using the identifying code and credit card payment.
11. Print out the e-ticket.
12. Record the itinerary specifics for quick reference and make a copy.
13. Give the physician the itinerary, a copy of the registration, and e-tickets.
14. Ensure the arrangements meet the physician's needs.

- Commission on Office Laboratory Accreditation (COLA)
- OSHA
- Local or state board of health
- Drug Enforcement Agency (DEA)

Many insurance companies will announce their visits in advance. Other organizations such as CLIA, OSHA, and boards of health do not always give advance notification. It is imperative that office managers familiarize themselves with the latest guidelines from each of these organizations.

PREPARING FOR AN INSURANCE SITE REVIEW

It is the responsibility of the office manager to prepare the office for the site visits. Responsibilities need to be delegated to the office staff. Good teamwork is essential when preparing for site visits. Many different areas are examined during the review. They can be divided into categories such as:

- Site guidelines
- Building/facility
- Service accessibility
- Pharmaceuticals
- Laboratory
- Equipment
- Medical records, general
- Medical records, content and structure
- Staffing issues
- Radiology
- Patients' rights
- Medical records, preventive medicine items

These tables would be extremely useful to managers who are preparing for an insurance site visit.

PREPARING FOR DISASTER

The manager may need to receive instruction related to national disasters. After the discovery of anthrax in government buildings in Washington, D.C., the Centers for Disease Control and Prevention issued bulletins with instructions for care of exposed individuals should it occur elsewhere. After the attacks on September 11, 2001, communities have been charged with developing strategies and procedures to care for catastrophic events and the massive amount of injures that could occur. In Ohio, public health nursing personnel have been making presentations to medical assistant students regarding their possible involvement. It is believed they could be used as assistants to disaster-trained professionals to record and document information. As of yet, physician's offices have not been contacted, and the primary responsibility rests with hospital and public safety personnel.

MOVING THE OFFICE

Medical offices change locations for many different reasons. Some offices outgrow their space. Others find a facility that is more economical or in a better and more convenient location. The office manager is usually the one who coordinates the move. Prior to the change, communication with the practice owner is essential. Goals need to be clearly defined. The following content represents many of the responsibilities that arise as a result of an office move.

Responsibilities at Existing Facility

Responsibilities at the existing facility may include:

- Purging medical records
- Purging x-rays
- Arranging for storage of purged records
- Discarding or cleaning and storing items that are no longer relevant
- Obtaining a minimum of three written estimates from moving companies

Movers can have many hidden costs. Do not accept an estimate that reveals only one price. Have the company itemize what you are being charged. At the time of the move, the moving representative might indicate that additional services can be provided. Determine what the additional services are and how much they will cost. If you decide to accept more services, get the new price in writing before allowing the movers to perform the services.

You will need to notify many businesses of your move. This is a good time to carefully evaluate which businesses you wish to continue to work with and which you want to replace. The following is a partial list of businesses you will need to notify several weeks prior to your move:

- Gas company
- Electric company
- Telephone company
- Waste management
- Vending machine company
- Carpet runners supplier
- Security company
- Landscaping/snow removal services
- Background music provider
- Equipment leasing companies
- Post office
- Directory assistance
- White business and yellow pages
- Biohazardous waste removal
- Medical bureau
- Cleaning company
- Periodicals companies

If there is more than one physician in the practice, each one will need to be listed with the post office, phone company, medical bureau, and so forth. If the practice has a name, information for that too will need to be changed. All companies that provide services will need to be notified and work together to make certain that the office has uninterrupted service throughout the entire move.

Other businesses that need to be notified of your move include the hospitals and insurance companies with which the practice has current contracts, state medical boards, laboratories, CLIA, COLA, x-ray board, and all physicians who send referrals or to whom the practice sends referrals.

The patients are the biggest group to be notified. This is most effectively done by sending a form letter to each one. The database in the computer should be able to produce names and addresses to merge with the form letter's text to make it seem more personal. Names and addresses can be printed directly on the envelope or onto mailing labels, which can be affixed to the envelope. The move should be announced to patients coming to the office as soon as it is known because of the need to make follow-up appointments. The move also can become part of the office's recorded phone message. An announcement in the local newspaper would also be beneficial.

Responsibilities at the New Facility

Many things will need to be taken care of at the new facility prior to the move. If the facility is new or requires some remodeling, it may be necessary to work with construction contractors. Interior designers can take care of the decorating. Furniture, window coverings, and other items for the new facility will need to be ordered. Equipment and supplies will need to be stocked, utilities turned on, and the phone system installed to operate properly. Moving an office is a very involved task that must be organized to be as efficient and smooth as possible. Moving also requires things to be up and running almost the same day.

The Day of the Move

The staff should be divided on the day of the move; part of the staff will remain at the old location, and part will go to the new location. Organization is imperative. Each team member will have specific responsibilities. Once everything has been moved from the old facility and all areas have been checked for any missed items and completely cleaned, they can join the other staff members at the new facility.

MANAGER'S REWARDS

The role of office manager can be as limited or **extensive** as the physician(s) feels comfortable in the **delegation** of authority. A trusted employee who performs well in the role of office manager becomes a tremendous asset to the practice. This role in large medical offices carries a great amount of authority and responsibility, but the rewards are worthwhile both financially and personally. It is a challenge you should look forward to accepting should the opportunity arise.

ACHIEVE UNIT OBJECTIVES

- ☐ **Complete the Workbook activities to meet the learning objectives.**
- ☐ **Practice the procedures in this unit to meet the performance objectives.**
- ☐ **Apply your knowledge at the end of this Chapter in completing the Critical Thinking Challenge and Activities, as well as the StudyWARE on your Student CD-ROM.**

ACTIVITIES

1. Search "Medical Office Management" on the web. Look for entries that offer certificates or associate degrees. Look at the curriculum and costs.
2. Search "Internal Revenue Service" on the web; click on the first entry, go to "Individual" information, and look for "Events in Life that Impact Your Tax." Identify the events that might change your tax status. Publication #505 explains how your taxes are figured.
3. Contact a few banks regarding opening a business account. Determine which one has the best offer. Compare items such as monthly charges, per-check charge, per-deposit charge, minimum balance required, and interest paid.

StudyWARE™ CHALLENGE

- Study with the flash cards for Chapter 10 to review the key terms in this chapter.
- Solve the hangman activities for Chapter 10.
- Complete the multiple choice quiz in test mode for Chapter 10.

CRITICAL THINKING CHALLENGE

IMPACTING THE PATIENT, THE PRACTICE, AND YOUR CAREER

Michelle has been the office manager for a three-physician practice for the past 2 years. Rosie, one of five medical assistants, has worked for the practice for 5 years. She is very professional, can be depended on to perform her responsibilities, and is well liked by the patients. Recently, a friend of hers who works in a surgeon's office has been trying to encourage her to come work with her. Michelle does not want to lose a good employee, yet she realizes Rosie's dilemma because she could earn another $100 a month if she were to leave. Michelle talked with the physicians about giving Rosie a raise, but they feel they do not want to set a precedent of counter-offering a salary. In addition, the pay scales are established in the policy manual, and increases are tied to longevity and performance, as well as figured on a percentage of the current salary. They were concerned that the other staff members might resent Rosie receiving "special" treatment. Still, Michelle wants to keep Rosie on the staff and realizes she must figure out another way to do so.

Following are two ideas often used in business as a means to provide additional compensation. The third comment is for you to consider in relation to what makes someone happy in their job. Think about each of these statements and try to determine how they might or might not affect the patients, the practice, and the careers of both Michelle and Rosie.

QUESTIONS

1. What do you think about establishing a different job description with perhaps a little more responsibility in order to justify a salary increase?
2. Could additional fringe benefits be established for employees such as Rosie who have been employed for 5 years?
3. How would being given more responsibility, a *title,* and a sense of control over some portion of the operation provide an incentive for Rosie?

RESOURCES

Krager, D., & Krager, C. (2005). *HIPAA for medical office personnel.* Clifton Park, NY: Thomson Delmar Learning.

Lindh, W., Pooler, M., Tamparo, C., & Dahl, B. (2006). *Comprehensive medical assisting: Administrative and clinical competencies* (3rd ed.). Clifton Park, NY: Thomson Delmar Learning.

Simmers, L. (2001). *Diversified health occupations* (5th ed.). Clifton Park, NY: Thomson Delmar Learning.

WEB LINKS

www.epracticemanagement.org (American Academy of Medical Management)
   Web site for the American College of Medical Management.

www.btcc.com (Bankers Training and Consulting Company)
   Provides financial news and several links to other web sites.

SECTION 3

Structure and Function of the Body

Anatomy and Physiology of the Human Body

The human body is a fantastic combination of parts that function in an organized manner, far more efficiently and effectively than any machine ever developed. This chapter describes the body's fundamental structure and the body systems and discusses how all the parts work together.

The diseases and disorders affecting the human body are a result of impairment, deterioration, or malfunction of one or more of its component parts. This chapter presents the anatomy of each body system and how that system physiologically functions within itself and with the other body systems. Following the presentation of each system will be a discussion of characteristic pathophysiologic conditions and disorders, many of which result from the body's inability to adapt or defend itself. A basic discussion of the critical role of the immune system in maintaining a healthy state will help you to correlate your knowledge of the body's complex interrelationships. With this understanding, you will be able to see how the patient's concerns and complaints, the physician's examination, and the clinical findings fit together to indicate the diagnosis and the plan of treatment the physician prescribes.

The preparation of material relating to the structure and function of the human body is exciting yet at times quite technical. The inclusion of diagnostic examinations, diseases and disorders, and usual methods of treatment further complicates the content. In order to obtain the most recent information available, many medical newsletters and health-related association publications have been reviewed. Many professional colleagues revised the content and provided new information. Almost daily, the print and electronic media releases information on new research findings and results of studies that are rapidly changing the manner in which health care is provided. All these data are beyond the capability of any one individual to fully acquire or use. The speed at which scientific discovery occurs can be explosive once a specific "piece of the puzzle" is found. Before this material is published, another discovery may cause the information to be inaccurate or obsolete. You must be alert to information about new findings. Evaluate it carefully. Look for *fact*, not "seems-to-be" results. Observe the persons studied in any research to see if it makes a reported finding seem valid for the total population. It is hardly significant when the findings are shown to be in a small group of people who are living in the same area or are all about the same age and sex. You live in a time when scientific capability is raising many ethical, moral, and legal questions. The possibility of altering our very cellular structure is at hand. Be inquisitive, be excited, be informed, and you will be knowledgeable.

UNIT 1
ANATOMIC DESCRIPTORS AND FUNDAMENTAL BODY STRUCTURE

OBJECTIVES

Upon completion of this unit, you will be able to achieve the following:

LEARNING Objectives

1. Spell and define, using the glossary at the back of the text, all the Words to Know in this unit.

2. Describe the anatomical position.

3. Apply the appropriate terminology to anatomical directional references on the human body.

4. Locate the eight body cavities on an illustration.

5. Name the major organ(s) located within each body cavity.

6. Identify the regions of the abdomen.

7. Describe the basic characteristics of the cell.

8. Explain what happens when a mutation occurs.

9. Name the patterns of inheritance, and explain how they affect a trait.

10. Describe the six ways molecules pass through cell membranes.

11. Describe the identifying characteristics of the following genetic conditions: cleft lip, cleft palate, Down syndrome, spina bifida, Klinefelter's syndrome, talipes, and Turner's syndrome.

12. Explain DNA "fingerprinting."

13. Describe the four main types of body tissues.

14. Name the 10 systems of the body.

WORDS TO KNOW

abdominal	cytology	exocytosis
abdominopelvic	cytoplasm	extremities
anatomic	cytotechnologist	filtration
anatomy	dehydration	frontal
anterior	diaphragm	gene
biochemistry	diffusion	Golgi apparatus
buccal	distal	gross anatomy
cardiac	DNA	histology
carriers	dominant gene	histotechnologist
caudal	dorsal	homeostasis
cavities	edema	horizontal
cell membrane	elements	hypertonic
centrioles	endocytosis	hypochondriac
chromosomes	endoplasmic	hypogastric
congenital	reticulum	hypotonic
connective	epigastric	iliac
coronal	epithelial	inferior
cranial	etiology	inguinal

involuntary	neuron	retroperitoneal
isotonic	normal saline	ribosome
keloid	nucleolus	skeletal
lateral	nucleus	smooth
lumbar	orbital	spinal
lysosomes	organ	striated
medial	organelles	superior
membrane	osmosis	syndrome
microscopic	osseous	system
anatomy	pathophysiology	thoracic
midline	pelvic	tissue
midsagittal	peritoneum	trait
mitochondria	phagocytosis	transverse
mitosis	physiology	umbilical
muscle	pinocytosis	ventral
mutation	posterior	voluntary
myelin	proximal	X-linked
nasal	pubic	
nerve	quadrant	
neurilemma	recessive gene	

CERTIFICATION CONNECTION

CMA
Diagnostic procedures
Common diseases and
  pathology
Anatomy and physiology

CMAS
Anatomy and physiology

RMA
Anatomy and physiology

ANATOMY AND PHYSIOLOGY DEFINED

Two terms are used in discussing the study of the human body: **anatomy**, which is the study of the physical structure of the body and its organs, and **physiology**, which is the science of the function of cells, tissues, and organs of the body. In other words, anatomy describes the framework and physical characteristics, whereas physiology explains how everything works together to support life.

Anatomy can be subdivided into various areas of study. For instance, the term **gross anatomy** refers to the study of those features that can be observed with the naked eye by inspection and dissection. As an example, the pathologist, when examining a tissue specimen, will describe its gross **anatomic** surface appearance and then proceed with the dissection and its description.

An area of study known as **microscopic anatomy** deals with features that can be observed only with the use of a microscope. Referring again to the pathologist, a fragment of a specimen can be properly prepared on a slide and observed with a microscope to complete the de-

scription of the specimen's characteristics and formulate an opinion as to its identity or state of condition.

There are two related areas of microscopic anatomy, **cytology**, the study of cell life and formation, and **histology**, the study of the microscopic structure of tissue. **Cytotechnologists** and **histotechnologists** are laboratory specialists who precisely prepare cells and tissue for microscopic examination and diagnosis by the pathologists.

Physiology is the study of the interrelationships of all the functioning structures of the body. When everything is in harmony and all biological indicators are within acceptable limits, the individual is referred to as being in a "steady state" or "normal." This state is also known as **homeostasis**. When the normal physiology is disrupted to the point of instability and begins to deteriorate, pathophysiologic mechanisms are likely to occur and may result in the development of a disease condition. **Pathophysiology** is the study of mechanisms by which disease occurs, the responses of the body to the disease process, and the effects of both on normal function.

Pathophysiology attempts to bring together the clinical signs and symptoms present with the knowledge of the effects of the disease processes on the body, from the cellular level to the total human being. Often close observation of the clinical signs of a disease state has led to the discovery of physiologic functions previously unknown. This is currently apparent in the great effort to understand the immune system to find a way to effectively control and eventually eliminate acquired immunodeficiency syndrome (AIDS) and cancer.

Fortunately, the healthy body has an enormous capacity to protect itself by compensating, defending, and adapting to the pathophysiologic effects of disease. However, when this fails, appropriate medical intervention can often correct or at least control the disease process.

LANGUAGE OF MEDICINE

The members of the health care team must be able to accurately communicate information, findings, and instructions among themselves. Much of the language of medicine is precise and is specific to the field of health care. For instance, it is necessary to not only know about the human body but also to be able to physically and verbally locate body structures and be able to describe the site of a patient's complaint or injury. The following fundamental descriptive terminology will be essential to the understanding of body references.

ANATOMIC DIRECTIONAL TERMS

Certain directional terms are universally used in describing anatomic structures. A body is said to be in the anatomic position when standing erect, with arms

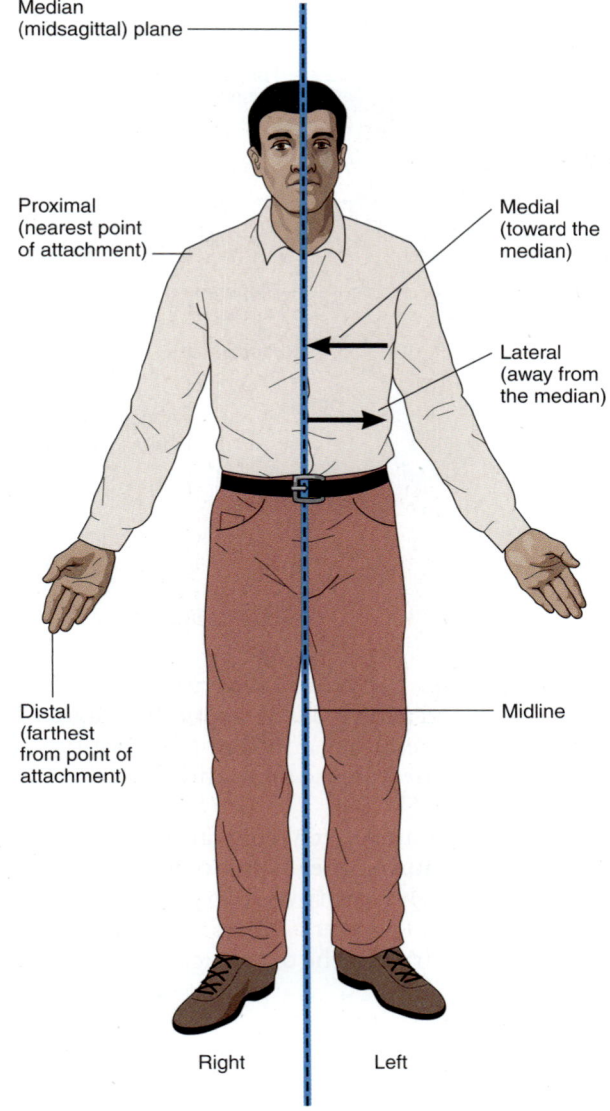

Median (midsagittal) plane

Proximal (nearest point of attachment)

Medial (toward the median)

Lateral (away from the median)

Distal (farthest from point of attachment)

Midline

Right   Left

FIGURE 11-1   Anatomic position with directional references

down at the sides, and the palms of the hands facing forward (Figure 11-1). This means that when the person is facing you, his right side is on your left, as if you were looking in a mirror. When reference is made to a body structure or a specific area, it is in relationship to this anatomical position. The same is true when you are studying illustrations in this textbook or labeling a drawing in the workbook.

Dividing the body vertically down the front will result in a right and left half. This imaginary line is known as the median or **midsagittal** plane. The right and left designations always refer to right and left in anatomic position. Anything located toward the **midline** is said to be **medial**, whereas anything away from the midline is said to be **lateral**.

Two other terms are used to describe the relationship of the **extremities** or ends of the body, such as the arms and legs, to the trunk of the body. **Proximal** indicates nearness to the point of attachment, whereas **distal** indicates distance away from the point of attachment. These terms are also applicable when describing parts of the arms, legs, fingers, or toes. For example, the thumb and great toe have proximal and distal sections, whereas the other fingers and toes have proximal, middle, and distal sections (Figure 11-2).

If you draw a line vertically through the side of the body from the top of the head to the feet, you will make a front and back section (Figure 11-3). This line is known as the **frontal** or **coronal** plane. The front is known as the **anterior** or **ventral** section; the back is called the **posterior** or **dorsal** section.

Finally, drawing an imaginary line **horizontally** (across) the body creates a **transverse** plane. The portion of the body above the line is known as **superior** or **cranial**. The portion below the line is called **inferior** or **caudal**. It is not necessary that the body be divided into equal parts. The terms superior and inferior refer to any relationship of structures above or below a "line" and de-

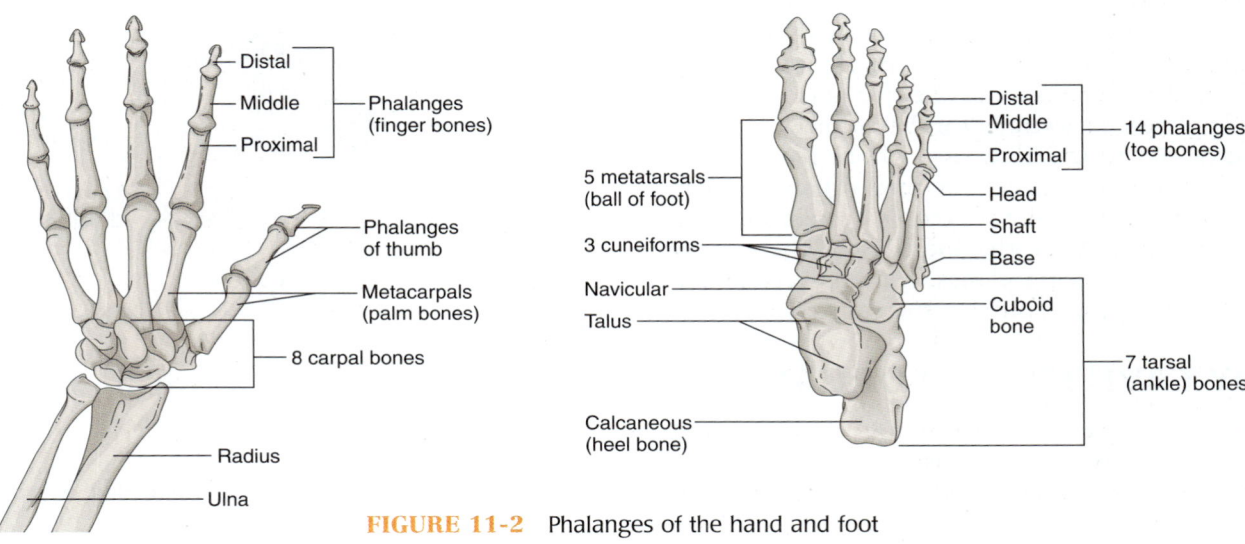

Distal
Middle — Phalanges (finger bones)
Proximal

Phalanges of thumb

Metacarpals (palm bones)

8 carpal bones

Radius

Ulna

5 metatarsals (ball of foot)

3 cuneiforms

Navicular

Talus

Calcaneous (heel bone)

Distal
Middle — 14 phalanges (toe bones)
Proximal

Head

Shaft

Base

Cuboid bone

7 tarsal (ankle) bones

FIGURE 11-2   Phalanges of the hand and foot

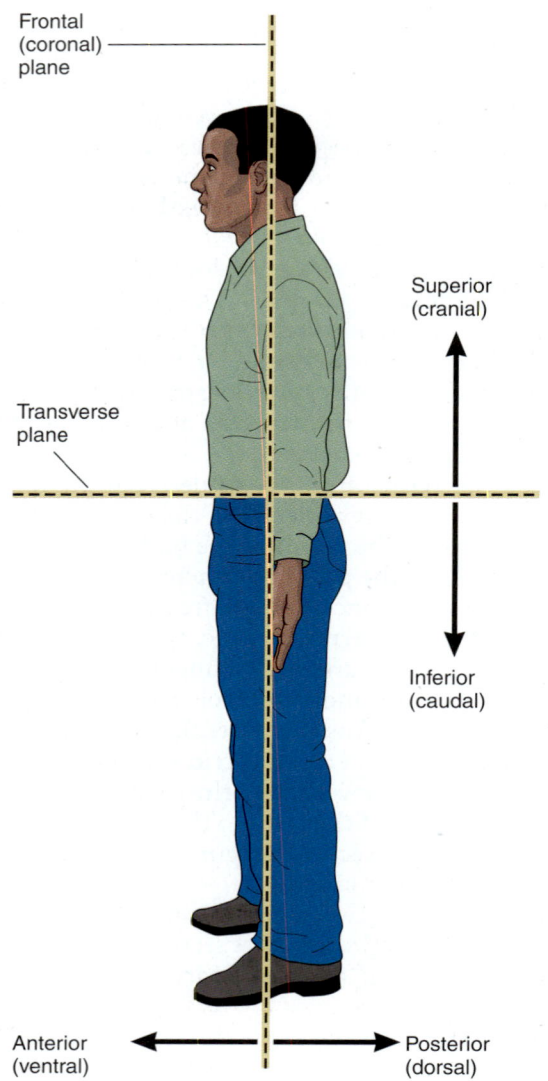

FIGURE 11-3 Anatomic directional references

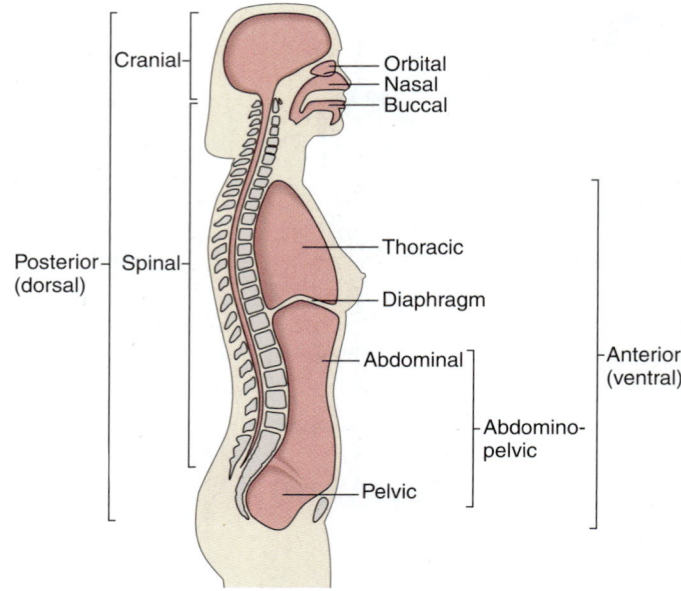

FIGURE 11-4 Body cavities

diaphragm divides the anterior cavity into an upper thoracic cavity and a lower abdominopelvic cavity. The thoracic cavity (chest) has a wall of ribs that protects its vital organs—the heart, lungs, and the great blood vessels (Figure 11-5).

The diaphragm alternately contracts and relaxes to move the lungs, causing breathing to occur.

The abdominopelvic cavity has two parts, an upper abdominal portion and a lower pelvic portion. The abdominal portion extends from the diaphragm to the top edge

pend on where it is drawn. For example, with a transverse line at the waist, the chest is superior to the abdomen, but if at the neck, the chest is inferior to the head. All anatomic directional terms are appropriate only when describing the relationship of one structure to another.

These planes or sections can be applied to internal structures and to the body as a whole. *Incisions* (cuts) made on the body surface or into organs are often made along a plane. The surgeon's description of the operation will identify the location of the incisions made using referencing planes. A tissue specimen cut along the transverse plane is known as a *cross section*.

BODY CAVITIES AND ORGANS

The body is divided into two main cavities, an anterior or ventral cavity and a posterior or dorsal cavity (Figure 11-4). A dome-shaped muscle known as the

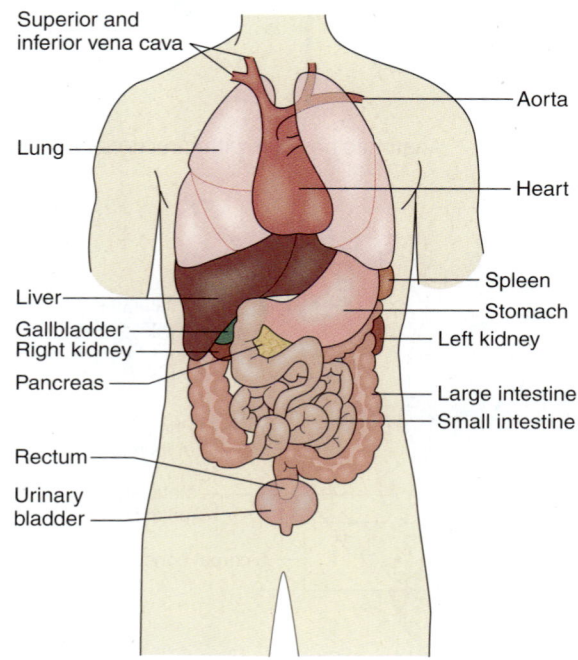

FIGURE 11-5 Thoracic and abdominal organs

of the pelvic girdle (bones). The organs found in the abdomen are the stomach, small intestines, most of the large intestine, the liver, spleen, pancreas, and gallbladder. The kidneys are located in the dorsal abdominal area but are behind the peritoneal **membrane** that lines the cavity and thus are technically outside the abdominal cavity. This space is referred to as **retroperitoneal**, behind the **peritoneum**. The pelvic cavity is surrounded by the pelvic girdle, which provides protection for the urinary bladder, the last portion of the large intestine, and the internal reproductive organs. Since organs of the digestive system are found in both cavities, frequently the term abdominopelvic is used to describe this area.

The posterior dorsal body cavity includes a cranial and a spinal section. The cranial cavity is totally encased by the bones of the skull, which provides protection for the brain. The cranial cavity is joined at its base by the **spinal** cavity, which extends through the center of the column of vertebrae (bones). This bony structure contains the spinal cord and protects it from injury.

There are three other small cavities, the **orbital** for the eyes, the **nasal** for the structures of the nose, and the **buccal** or mouth.

Abdominal Regions

The abdomen is such a large area of the body that it is necessary to divide it into quadrants or regions for purposes of identification or reference. There are two recognized methods. One creates **quadrants** known as the right and left upper quadrants (RUQ and LUQ) and the right and left lower quadrants (RLQ and LLQ) (Figure 11-6).

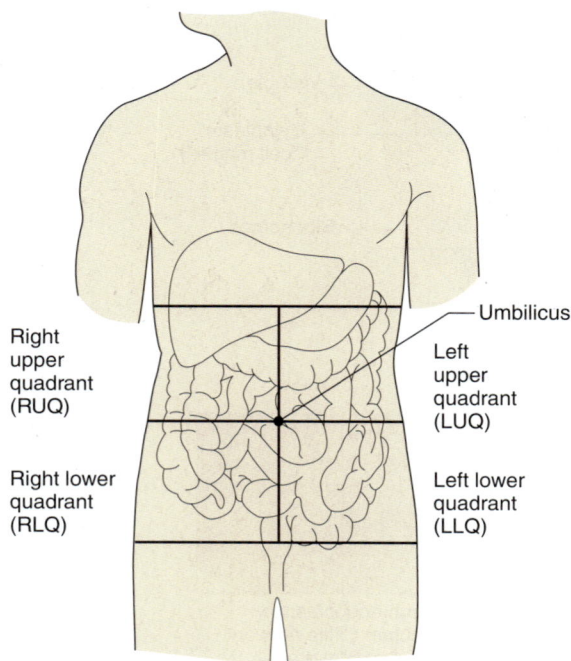

FIGURE 11-6   The four abdominal quadrants

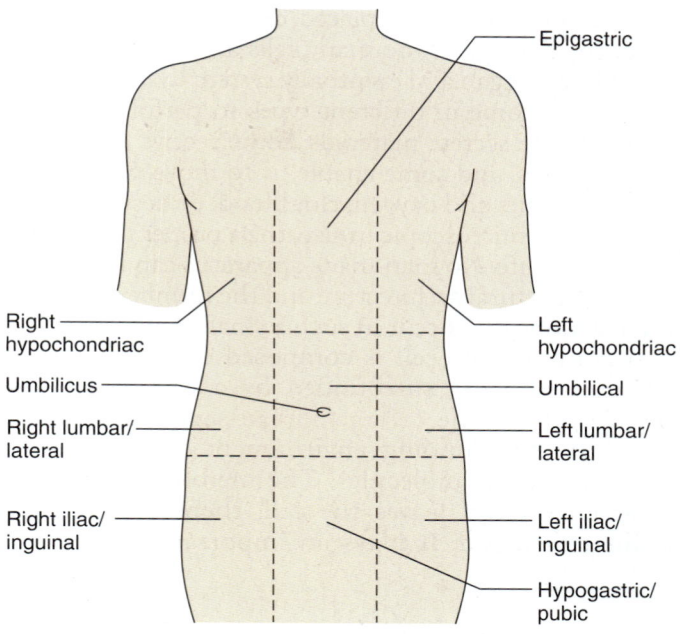

FIGURE 11-7   Nine regions of the abdomen

A more exacting division results in nine regions identifiable by location and an anatomical reference point. The divisions create three central areas:

- **Epigastric** (over the stomach)
- **Umbilical** (around the umbilicus)
- **Hypogastric** (below the stomach; also known as **pubic**)

These are surrounded by six side areas:

- Right and left **hypochondriac** (below the cartilage, referring to the ribs)
- Right and left **lumbar** (loin or side region; also called lateral)
- Right and left **iliac** (referring to the ileum portion of the pelvic bone; also known as the **inguinal**, meaning groin, region)

Figure 11-7 shows these nine regions of the abdomen.

THE CELL

To understand the structure of the body, you must first learn about its basic building block, the cell. This fascinating wonder is a living, working, microscopic image of the body. It requires nutrients and oxygen to survive, performs specific functions, produces heat and energy, and gives off waste products. Many cells can reproduce themselves to replace missing cells.

Cells vary greatly in size and shape. The body contains about 75 trillion cells. Some cells, such as those of the skin or in the intestines, are lost as part of a natural process. These cells are replaced by new cells in line behind them within the tissue structure. Cells lost by injury may or may not be replaced, depending on the severity of the damage. If too many cells are lost and cannot be replaced, organ and eventually system dysfunction results. Cells come in different types to perform specific duties. Some secrete materials, some receive and transmit impulses, and some enable us to move. Still others carry nutrients and oxygen, clot blood, or destroy bacteria. Though microscopic in size, their proper function is essential to life. No man-made apparatus can match the cell for structural architecture and the number of chemical reactions that occur in such a small space.

A conventional cell is composed of a fluid called **cytoplasm** and is surrounded by a cell membrane (Figure 11-8). The **cell membrane** separates the cell from the surrounding environment. It consists of protein and fat molecules. The membrane controls what enters and leaves the cell, thereby regulating cellular function. It plays an important role in the

health and welfare of the cell. Enclosed within the membrane is the sticky semifluid material known as cytoplasm. It is a combination of protein, lipids (fat), carbohydrates, minerals, salts, and water (over 70%). Chemical reactions such as cellular respiration and protein synthesis occur in the cytoplasm.

The Organelles

Within the cytoplasm of the cell are many minute bodies called **organelles** that perform amazing tasks. The organelles are the **nucleus**, **mitochondria**, **ribosomes**, **centriole**, **endoplasmic reticulum**, **Golgi apparatus**, and **lysosomes**. Refer to Table 11-1 for a summary of the organelles' functions. Scientists still do not understand how some functions are carried out, but they do know some organelles physically separate the chemical reactions occurring in the cytoplasm because many reac-

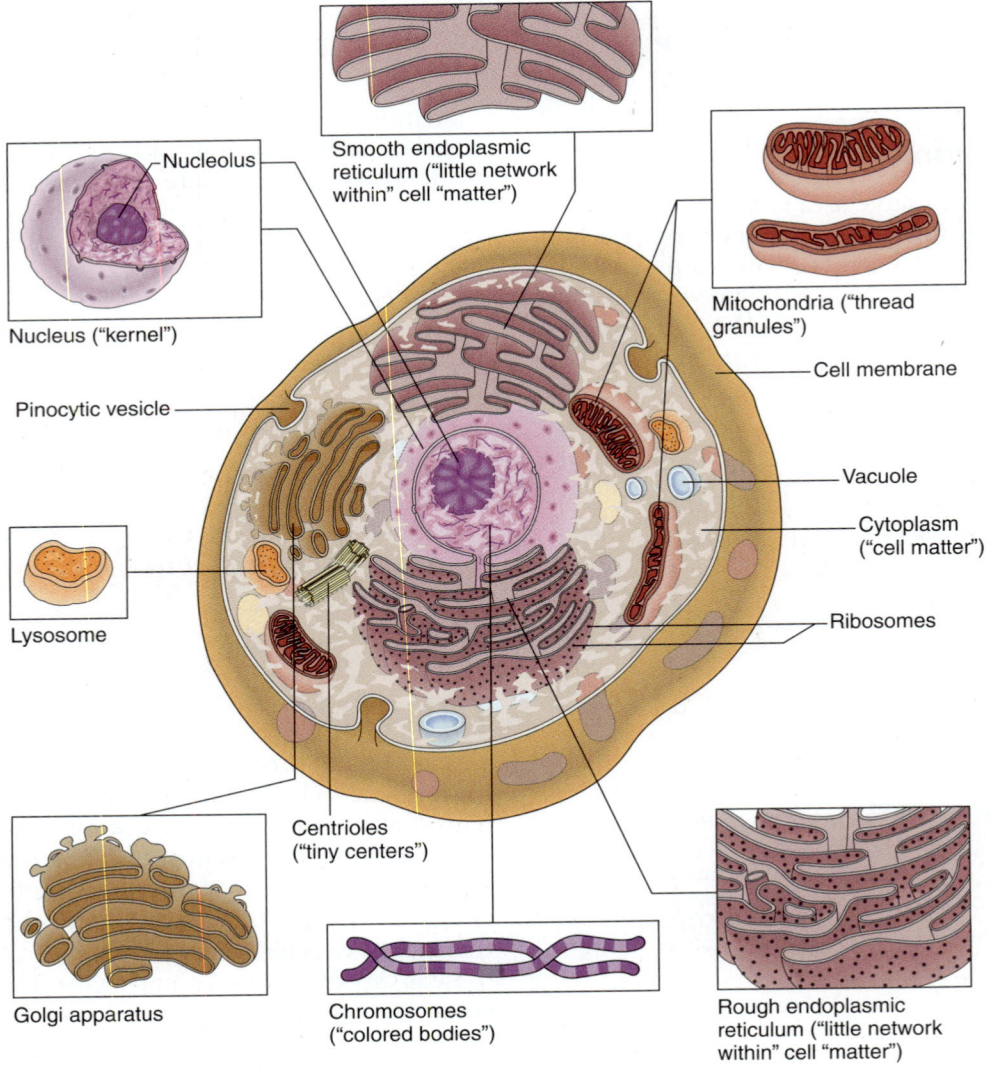

FIGURE 11-8 Structure of a basic cell

TABLE 11-1   Cell Organelles

Organelle	Function
Cell membrane	Regulates transport of substances into and out of the cell.
Cytoplasm	Provides an organized watery environment in which life functions take place by the activities of the organelles contained in the cytoplasm.
Nucleus	Serves as the "brain" for the control of the cell's metabolic activities and cell division; has DNA and genes.
Nuclear membrane	Regulates transport of substances into and out of the nucleus.
Nucleoplasm	A clear, semifluid medium that fills the spaces around the chromatin and the nucleoli.
Nucleolus	Functions as a site for RNA synthesis.
Ribosomes	Serve as sites for protein synthesis.
Endoplasmic reticulum	Provides passages through which transport of substances occurs in cytoplasm.
Mitochondria	Serve as sites of cellular respiration and energy production; the "powerhouse" of the cell.
Golgi apparatus	Manufactures carbohydrates and packages secretions for discharge from the cell.
Lysosomes	Serve as centers of cellular digestion.
Pinocytic vesicles	Transport large particles into a cell.
Centrosome	Contains two centrioles that are functional during animal cell division.
Centrioles	Provide spindle fibers for attaching chromosomes during cellular division.

Adapted from Scott & Fong, Body Structures and Functions, 10th ed. Copyright 2004. Thomson Delmar Learning.

tions are not compatible. Organelles also control the time when reactions take place, such as producing or processing a molecule in one organelle and then later using the molecule in another reaction.

Organelle Structure and Function

The *nucleus* is a dense mass within the cytoplasm and is the control center of the cell. It is surrounded by its own nuclear membrane. Materials pass in and out of the nucleus from the cytoplasm through pores in the membrane. The membrane is continuous with the endoplasmic reticulum, which often has ribosomes attached. It regulates the chemical reactions and controls the process of mitosis (cell division) for reproduction.

Within the nucleus are the structures called **chromosomes**. Each member of a species has a specific number of chromosomes. Human beings have 46 individual or 23 pairs of chromosomes that store the hereditary material passed on from one generation to the next. Twenty-two pairs of chromosomes are autosome (same in number and kind), and one pair are sex chromosomes, either both X if female or an X and a Y if male. One chromosome from each of the 23 pairs is contributed by the mother and one by the father. When the egg and sperm unite at fertilization, their chromosomes are united so that the new cell, a zygote, will also contain 23 pairs. The sex of the child is determined by whether it is combined with a father's cell carrying an X or a Y chromosome.

Chromosomes are rod-shaped structures composed of long strands of molecules known as deoxyribonucleic acid (**DNA**). DNA is the material within the chromosome that encodes the **genes** that are located at specific sites on the chromosome. The DNA carries all of the genetic information necessary for cellular functions. DNA is composed of sugar, phosphate, and four bases: adenine, cytosine, guanine, and thymine. The genetic coding makes it possible for the exact duplication of the cell.

Genes

Every individual has a different DNA code, but the code in all cells of the same individual are identical. It is the arrangement of the base pairs of the DNA code that makes for the differences. The genes are the units of instruction that produce or influence particular characteristics or traits and the capabilities of an organism. Genes are specific segments of DNA molecules that are located on the chromosomes in the cell nucleus. They act in pairs to dictate traits from eye color to the chemical reactions that determine not only cell structure but also function and, therefore, heredity. A gene consists of sequences of thousands of DNA base pairs. Originally scientists estimated there were over 100,000 pairs or more of genes, but we now know there appears to be 35,000 to 45,000 genes that compose the DNA of a cell. This great number of genes helps explain why there is so much variety in the human race, and yet each individual's structure is uniquely and identifiably their own. Consider that during meiosis, each parent's chromosomes are halved, "shuffled," and then combined at fertilization. The father and mother each contribute half of the child's total number of genes to their offspring. The new being now has a unique combination of genes and, consequently, traits.

The nucleus itself will have at least one **nucleolus**. In a nucleolus, portions of ribonucleic acid (RNA) are assembled with proteins to make subunits of the ribosomes, which then pass through the nuclear pores of the nuclear membrane into the cytoplasm, to become a complete two-part ribosome to synthesize protein. Ribosomes are found circulating in the cytoplasm or attached to the endoplasmic reticulum.

Centrioles are the two cylinder-shaped organelles near the nucleus. During mitosis, the centrioles separate and form spindle fibers that attach to the chromosomes to ensure their equal distribution to the two new daughter cells.

Endoplasmic reticulum crisscrosses the cytoplasm in a network fashion. When attached to the nuclear membrane, it serves as a passageway for the transportation of materials in and out of the nucleus. If grouped together, they can store large amounts of protein. The difference between rough and smooth endoplasmic reticulum is the presence of *ribosomes* on the membrane. Ribosome sites of protein synthesis give the membrane a rough appearance.

Mitochondria are round or rod-shaped organelles that supply the cell's energy. There may be one to over a thousand in each cell depending on how much energy that type of cell requires. Mitochondria have a double-membraned structure with the inner membrane folding into ridges. The cell is capable of cellular respiration because the enzymes located in the ridges break down nutrient molecules and oxygen to provide carbon dioxide, ATP (adenosine triphosphate; energy for the cell), and water.

The *Golgi apparatus* is a stack of membrane layers that synthesize carbohydrates and combine them with molecules of proteins. The organelle appears to store and prepare secretions to excrete from the cell. Therefore, the cells of the gastric, salivary, and pancreatic glands have large numbers of Golgi apparatus.

Lysosomes are round or oval structures. They have a strong digestive enzyme that consumes protein molecules such as those found in old worn cells, bacteria, or foreign matter. This is a very important function of the body's natural immune system.

Pinocytic vesicles are pocket-like formations in the cell's membrane. These structures permit large molecules like protein and fat, which cannot pass through the pores of the cell membrane, to enter with the extracellular fluid into the vesicle. Then the "pocket" closes, forming a vacuole (bubble) in the cytoplasm. This process is called **endocytosis**. When liquid droplets, instead of protein or fat molecules, are enclosed, the process is known as **pinocytosis**, which means "cell drinking." A related term, **exocytosis**, refers to a similar process whereby substances are moved from the cell to the outside. On entering the cytoplasm, most vesicles fuse with lysosomes, and their contents are digested. Special white blood cells known as phagocytes rely on endocytosis to destroy harmful bacteria in the body. As you learn more about your body, you will begin to appreciate what a magnificent piece of "equipment" it is and how important it is that you care for it properly. You have the physical and mental power to have a great impact on your health and your life.

Table 11-1 summarizes the organelles and their role in the function of the cell.

PASSING MOLECULES THROUGH CELL MEMBRANES

As stated before, the cell membrane controls materials entering and leaving the cell. This is necessary for the cell to acquire substances from its environment to be processed for its use, for secretion, and for excretion of waste materials. There are six processes by which materials pass through a cell membrane: **diffusion**, **osmosis**, **filtration**, active transport, **phagocytosis**, and pinocytosis.

Diffusion is a process whereby gas, liquid, or solid molecules distribute themselves evenly through a medium. When the medium is a fluid and the molecules are solid, they are called solutes (Figure 11-9). When solutes and water pass across a membrane to distribute themselves, they will move from an area of higher concentration to an area of lesser concentration. Diffusion plays a vital role in the body. For example, higher concentrations of oxygen in the alveolus (air sac) of the lung cross the membrane into the lesser concentrated area of the red blood cell in the capillary (see Figure 11-9). The blood cell, now with a high concentration of oxygen, circulates in the blood to a body cell with lower oxygen concentration and exchanges its oxygen for the cell's higher concentration of waste products. Hence, the body's cells "breathe" in a process called *internal respiration*.

Osmosis is a process of diffusion of water or another solvent through a selective permeable membrane, one through which some solutes can pass but others cannot (Figure 11-10). In the illustration, the membrane will only allow the salt and water to pass through; therefore, the salt leaves the greater concentrated area within the membrane to go to the lesser concentrated water. At the same time, the water leaves its higher concentrated area to enter the lesser concentrated area within the membrane. When the water molecules are equal on both sides, the diffusion will stop. The pressure of the water molecules inside the membrane is then said to be at *equilibrium*, a state known as the *osmotic pressure*.

The osmotic characteristics of solutions are classified by their effect on red blood cells (Figure 11-11). If

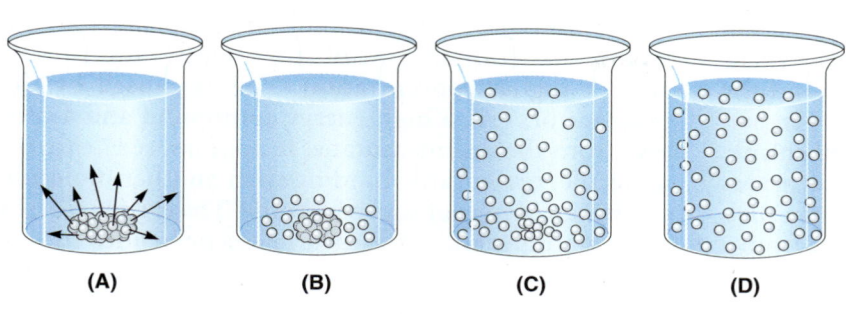

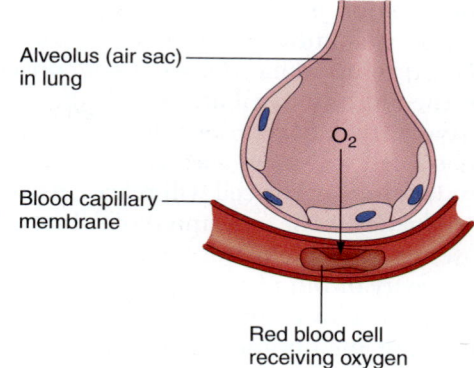

Diffusion:

(A) A small lump of sugar is placed into a beaker of water, and its molecules dissolve and begin to diffuse outward. **(B and C)** The sugar molecules continue to diffuse through the water from an area of greater concentration to an area of lesser concentration.
(D) Over a long period, the sugar molecules are evenly distributed throughout the water, reaching a state of equilibrium.

Example of diffusion in the human body: Oxygen diffuses from an alveolus in a lung where it is in greater concentration, across the blood capillary membrane, and into a red blood cell where it is in lesser concentration.

FIGURE 11-9   The process of diffusion

Initial stage

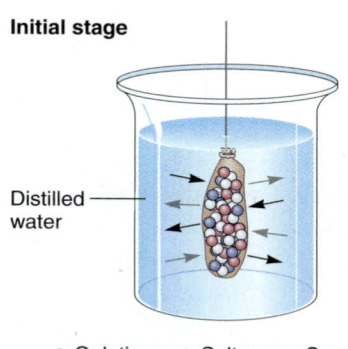

Distilled water

(A) Initially, the sausage casing contains a solution of gelatin, salt and sucrose. The casing is permeable to water and salt molecules only. Since the concentration of water molecules is greater outside the casing, water molecules will diffuse into the casing. The opposite situation exists for the salt.

10–12 hours later

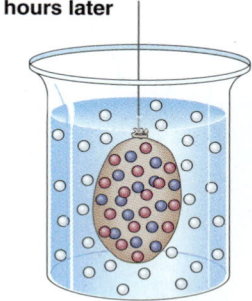

(B) The sausage casing swells because of the net movement of water molecules inward. However, the volume of distilled water in the beaker remains constant.

● Gelatin   ○ Salt   ● Sucrose

FIGURE 11-10   Osmosis is the diffusion of water through a selective permeable membrane. A sausage casing is an example of a selective permeable membrane.

Hypertonic solution

Hypotonic solution

Isotonic solution

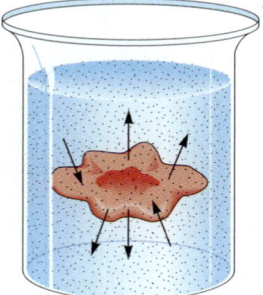

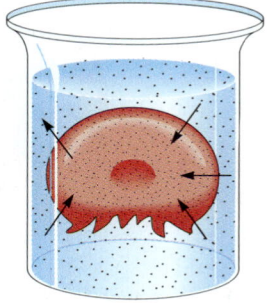

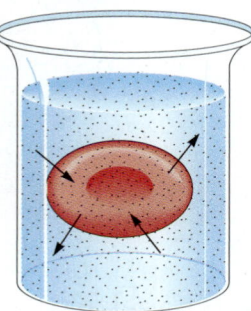

⸫ Water molecules

Hypertonic solution (seawater)
a red blood cell will shrink and wrinkle up because water molecules are moving out of the cell.

Hypotonic solution (freshwater)
a red blood cell will swell and burst because water molecules are moving into the cell.

Isotonic solution (human blood serum)
a red blood cell remains unchanged because the movement of water molecules into and out of the cell are the same.

FIGURE 11-11   Movement of water molecules in solutions of different osmolalities

the solution is of the same osmotic pressure as blood serum, it is known as an **isotonic** solution. A 0.9% salt (NaCl) solution has the same salt concentration as that of the red blood cell and is called **normal saline**. If the osmolality is lower, the solution is **hypotonic**, and the blood cell will swell with water and burst. In a **hypertonic** solution, the cell will release its water and shrink.

Filtration is the movement of solutes and water across a semipermeable membrane as a result of a force such as gravity or blood pressure. The particles move from a higher to a lower area of pressure. The size of the pores of some membranes allow only small molecules to leave. This process occurs in the kidneys where small molecules of water and waste products are filtered from the blood in the capillaries, whereas the large protein molecules and red blood cells are retained (Figure 11-12).

A good example of filtration can be observed with a drip coffee maker.

Active transport refers to molecules moving across a membrane from an area of low concentration to an area of higher concentration. This is caused by the presence of ATP, a high-energy compound and a protein from the cell membrane. It appears as a "carrier" molecule, temporarily binding with another molecule on the outer edge of the membrane. The carrier crosses the membrane and releases its "passenger" into the cytoplasm. The carrier then receives more energy from the membrane and returns to the outer surface to transport another molecule. The carrier can also reverse the process and carry molecules from the inside to the outside.

Phagocytosis is known as "cell eating." White blood cells become phagocytes and engulf bacteria, cell fragments, or damaged cells (Figure 11-13). The white cell forms a vacuole by enfolding its membrane and enclosing the particle. When it is completely enclosed, digestive enzymes enter from the cytoplasm and destroy the trapped material. This process is extremely important to the body's ability to maintain a healthy state.

Pinocytosis, as discussed earlier, is called "cell drinking" and involves the engulfing of large molecules of liquid material. Once inside the cytoplasm, the fluid is digested by the cell.

Another area of great importance to the welfare of the human body is its chemistry. The study of chemical

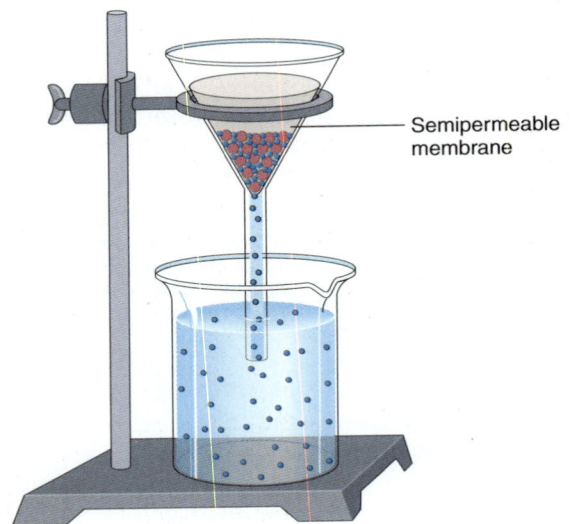

Filtration: Small molecules are filtered through the semipermeable membrane, whereas the large molecules remain in the funnel.

Semipermeable membrane

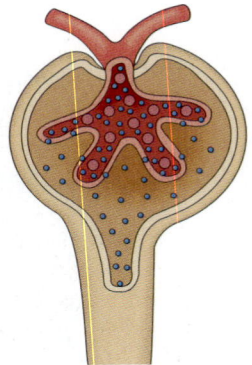

Example of filtration in the human body: Glomerulus of kidney; large particles like red blood cells and proteins remain in the blood, and small molecules like urea and water are excreted as a metabolic excretory product—urine.

FIGURE 11-12   Filtration is a passive transport process.

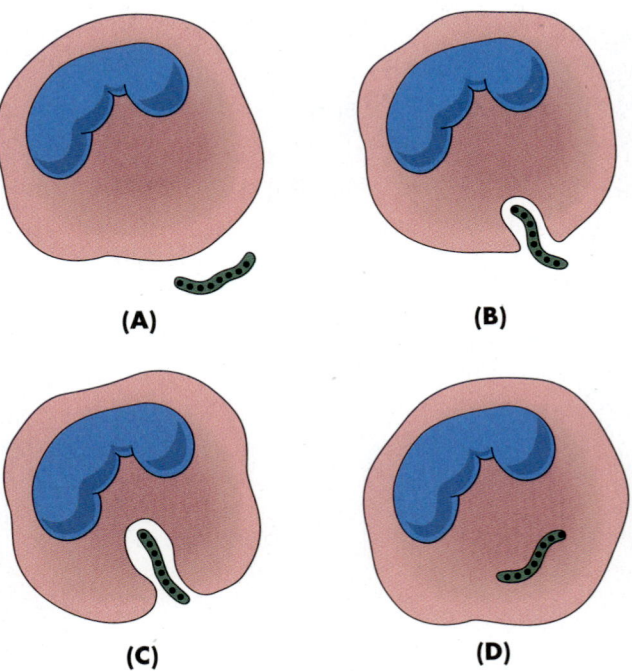

(A)   (B)

(C)   (D)

FIGURE 11-13   Phagocytosis of bacteria by a white blood cell. Phagocytosis can occur in the bloodstream, or white cells may squeeze through capillary walls and destroy bacteria in the tissues.

TABLE 11-2   Names, Location, or Use of Some Common Acids and Bases

Name of Acid	Where Found or Used	Name of Base	Where Found or Used
Acetic acid	Vinegar	Ammonium hydroxide	Household liquid cleaners
Boric acid	Weak eyewash	Magnesium hydroxide	Milk of Magnesia
Carbonic acid	Carbonated beverages	Potassium hydroxide	Caustic potash
Hydrochloric acid	Stomach	Sodium hydroxide	Lye
Nitric acid	Industrial oxidizing acid		
Sulfuric acid	Batteries and industrial mineral acid		

reactions within the body is called **biochemistry**. The basic building blocks of all matter are the **elements**, substances in their simplest form. There are 92 natural and at least 13 man-made elements. Of these, about 20 are in all living things. Four of these 20 elements make up 97% of all living matter. They are carbon, oxygen, hydrogen, and nitrogen. The remaining 16 elements are sodium, chlorine, magnesium, phosphorus, sulfur, calcium, potassium, iron, copper, manganese, zinc, boron, tin, vanadium, cobalt, and molybdenum. Because the last four elements occur in the body in such minute amounts, they are known as *trace elements*.

Many elements combine together in specific amounts to form new substances known as *compounds*. Some common compounds are water (hydrogen and oxygen), carbon dioxide (carbon and oxygen), salt (sodium and chloride), hydrochloric acid (hydrogen and chlorine), and sodium bicarbonate (sodium, hydrogen, carbon, and oxygen). Compounds can be classified in one of three groups: acids, bases, or salts. An acid compound will have positively charged ions of hydrogen and negatively charged ions of some other element. They have a sour taste such as is found in some citrus fruits (limes and lemons). However, an unknown substance should not be tasted to determine its acidity; it should be tested by the special dyes contained in litmus paper. If acid is present, blue litmus paper will turn red.

A base compound is also called an alkali. A base substance will have negatively charged hydroxide ions and positively charged ions of a metal. Bases have a bitter taste and will turn red litmus paper blue. Table 11-2 lists some common acids and bases and identifies where they are found.

When an acid and a base are combined, they form a salt and water. A common example is sodium chloride (table salt), which is the result of combining hydrochloric acid with sodium hydroxide. When the water evaporates, the salt remains.

Frequently the determination of acidity or alkalinity of a body fluid or solution is desired. This measurement is referred to as the pH. A pH value of 7.0 on the pH scale indicates the solution has the same amount of hydrogen ions as hydroxide ions and therefore is neutral. An example of a neutral solution is water. A pH value between 0 and 6.9 indicates an acidic solution. The lower the number, the stronger the acid or hydrogen ion concentration. A pH value of 7.1 to 14.0 indicates the solution is basic or alkaline. The higher the number is above 7.0, the stronger the base or hydroxide ion concentration. The pH inside most cells is maintained between 7.2 and 7.4. The pH values of some common acids, bases, and human body fluids and their effect on a pH testing strip are shown in Figure 11-14.

CELLULAR DIVISION

The division of cells is known as mitosis and is controlled by the nucleus of the cell (Figure 11-15). When a cell is preparing to divide, the two pairs of centrioles, just outside the nucleus, move to opposite sides of the cell (A). Spindle fibers form and attach to the chromosomes, which "line up" in the center (B). The chromosomes divide and move toward the centrioles at different ends of the cell (C). The spindles then dissolve, and a nuclear membrane develops around each new set of chromosomes (D). For unknown reasons, the cell then pinches itself in two, thereby making two new cells (E) called daughter cells. Mitosis results in the formation of two daughter nuclei with the exact same genes as the mother cell nucleus. The purpose of cell division is to provide exact duplication of cells for growth and repair of the body. In the unit on immunity, you will discover what happens when an antigen (foreign matter) interferes with this copying process.

All cells do not reproduce at the same rate. The bloodforming cells of the bone marrow, the cells of the skin, and the cells of the intestinal lining reproduce continuously. Muscle cells only reproduce every few years; however, muscle tissue formed of voluntary muscle cells may be hypertrophied (enlarged) with exercise. This is apparent from the great increase in muscle size produced by body builders who use weights and repeti-

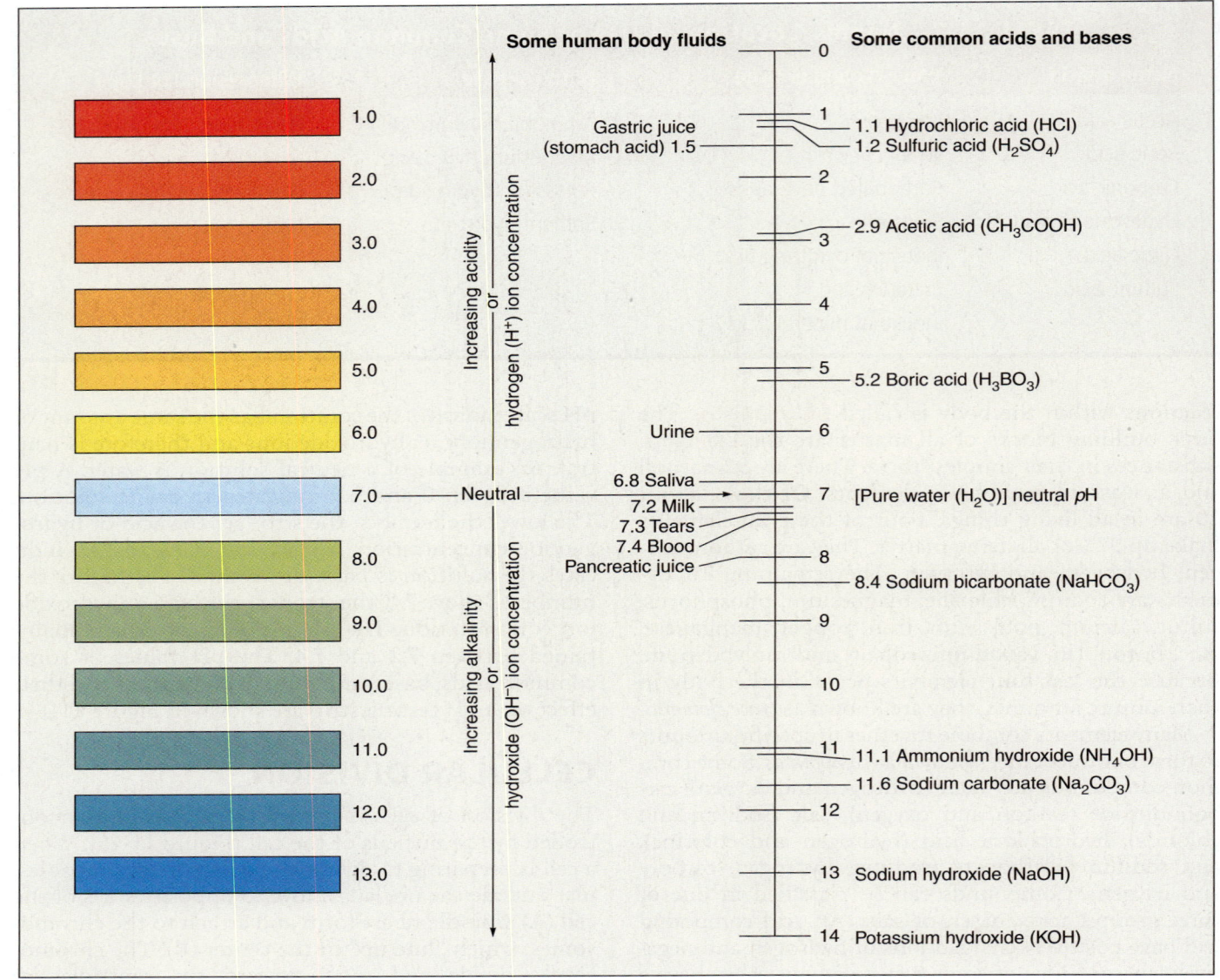

FIGURE 11-14 pH values of some common acids, bases, and human body fluids and the collar changes that can occur to a pH strip when tested.

tions of routines to achieve muscle definition and enlargement. Cells of the **nerve** tissue, or **neurons**, do not increase in number after birth, and some cannot be regenerated if damaged or destroyed.

There are many kinds of cells with different shapes and sizes. The characteristics shown previously in Figure 11-8 are common to most cells. However, cells like those in the blood (red, white, and platelets) and the nerve cells are very different and perform specialized functions. With this specialization, some of the other cell functions may be lost, such as the ability of some nerve cells to reproduce. Specialization also results in an interdependence among cells to enable them to

carry out their activities. One type of cell that is very different is the sex cell (gamete), which is responsible for reproduction. During a process known as meiosis, the ovum from the female and the spermatozoon from the male each reduce their respective 46 chromosomes to 23, one half the normal amount. When fertilization occurs, the two cells combine to form a single cell called a zygote, which will then have the full set of 46 chromosomes, 23 from each parent. The zygote will subsequently, by mitosis, divide again and again until the new being is fully developed. This cellular activity will be more fully discussed in the unit on the reproductive system.

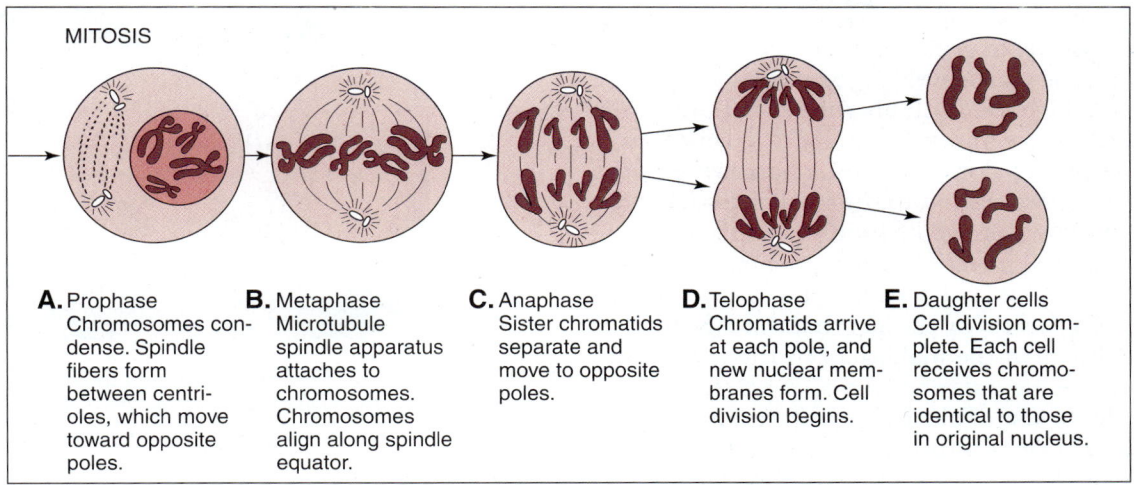

MITOSIS

A. Prophase
Chromosomes condense. Spindle fibers form between centrioles, which move toward opposite poles.

B. Metaphase
Microtubule spindle apparatus attaches to chromosomes. Chromosomes align along spindle equator.

C. Anaphase
Sister chromatids separate and move to opposite poles.

D. Telophase
Chromatids arrive at each pole, and new nuclear membranes form. Cell division begins.

E. Daughter cells
Cell division complete. Each cell receives chromosomes that are identical to those in original nucleus.

FIGURE 11-15   Stages of mitosis in cells

HOMEOSTASIS

The body has many control systems, some of which operate within the cell. It is important that the fluid within the cell (*intracellular fluid*) maintains the proper chemical and pH balance for the cell to maintain life. The fluid surrounding the cells (*extracellular fluid*) mixes with the fluid of the blood to supply the cell with food and other substances. When the internal environment is functioning properly and all the organs and tissues of the body are performing their appropriate tasks, a condition of *homeostasis* exists. This is a stable condition of the internal environment. This condition continues until one or more of the control systems loses the ability to maintain it. When this occurs, all cells of the body suffer. A moderate dysfunction causes illness; a severe dysfunction leads to death.

MUTATIONS AND TRAITS

Remember that the DNA is a code that provides information to the cell. It has been compared with the dots and dashes of the Morse code or the "0s" and "1s" of the computer binary code. When these symbols are arranged in different sequences, they form different words. The same is true of DNA. When DNA is being replicated, if some is lost, rearranged, or paired in error, the resulting change in instruction of the genetic code could lead to an improperly functioning or missing protein when the DNA's code is translated. This is known as **mutation**. Genetic mutations can be caused by internal or external factors. Internal factors are those that occur during replication and abnormal metabolism. External causes include chemicals, x-rays, sunlight, and other radiations. A mutation is a change in a cell resulting from a chemical change in the structure of the gene. It is first reflected in the RNA copy, then in the enzyme or protein, and finally in the appearance of new **trait**. A trait is the recognizable result of the effect of a gene or group of genes. Mutations may be either dominant or recessive. They may result in no change or can produce minimal or drastic alterations. They can be beneficial or lethal. Mutations provide an essential key for evolutionary change, even among humans.

Single genes may be involved in one of three patterns of inheritance as they produce recognizable traits. These are known as dominant, recessive, and X-linked. A **dominant gene** can produce a trait without regard to the nature of its pair member (Remember: There are two genes, one each from the mother and father). Dominant disorders are usually milder and result in structural defects rather than abnormalities in function. A **recessive gene** is one whose presence within the pair does not result in a recognizable trait *unless* both members of the gene pair are of a similar mutation; in this case, a recessive disorder would occur. People who have one dominant and one recessive gene are known as **carriers**. The third pattern of inheritance is sex- or **X-linked** because the defective gene is carried on the X chromosome. In some instances, the pattern is dominant with direct inheritance, and in others it is recessive, depending primarily upon which parent has the defect and whether the child is male or female.

Another classification of traits deals with results caused by two mechanisms: multifactorial inheritance and chromosomal aberrations. Multifactorial inheritance refers to the combined influence of a number of genes and environmental factors causing a trait to be expressed. The environment can be within the uterus before birth or in general following birth. The trait appears as a result of the accumulation of sufficient factors to raise the level of genes above a certain threshold, beyond which the trait develops. Examples of this are height and intelligence. Both are influenced prenatally by parental influence and postnatally by environment. Another example is pyloric stenosis, a narrowing of the opening from the stomach into the small intestines that interferes with the passage of food. It is linked to the possibility of a viral infection during pregnancy, and it is known that the child's sex is a factor. Development of the disorder is *influenced* by the fact that the threshold of the factor is lower in the male than in the female. Examples of environmental exposures that are classified as toxins include the use of alcohol (which results in small birth weights), liver dysfunction, and the condition known as fetal alcohol syndrome. Another toxin is the drug diethylstilbesterol (DES), which can adversely affect sex organ development.

Chromosomal abnormalities are the result of either a group of genes occurring in excess or as a deficit of genetic materials. There is a difference in the general effects depending on whether the abnormality affects pairs numbered 1-22, called autosomes, or the X and Y chromosomes of the 23rd pair. Autosome genetic imbalance is invariably associated with mental retardation and exerts influence on the development of the physical structure of the early embryo and fetus. Incorrect numbers of X and Y chromosomes are among the most common chromosomal abnormalities. Chromosomal abnormality can occur as the result of abnormal cell division and from exposure to toxins.

GENETIC AND CONGENITAL DISORDERS

As we have learned, genetic and **congenital** disorders can result from improper sex cell division at the time of fertilization, from the inheritance of an altered gene or genes, from environmental factors, or from toxins. They cause structural defects, retardation, and physiologic disorders. These are collectively called genetic or congenital disorders.

There is a difference between the two. The word congenital is defined as "occurring during fetal life; not hereditary." In other words, it is a "born with" condition. Genetic disorders result from initial cellular structure at conception. The more common disorders are discussed in the following content.

Cleft Lip

Description—The presence of a structural defect of the upper lip.
Signs and symptoms—It is characterized by a vertical split in the upper lip that often continues into the nostril. A cleft lip can be unilateral (one side) or bilateral (both sides) (Figure 11-16A).

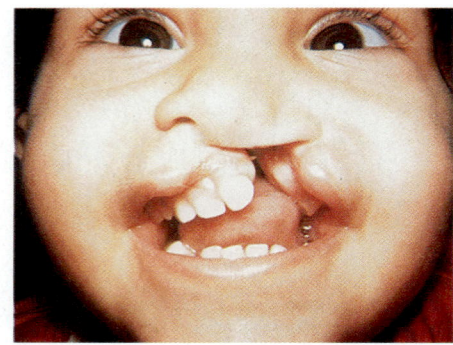

FIGURE 11-16A Cleft lip *(Courtesy of Dr. Joseph Konzelman, School of Dentistry, Medical College of Georgia)*

Etiology—It is caused by the failure of the soft or bony tissues to unite during the 8th to 12th week of gestation.
Treatment—Modern plastic surgery is very successful at closing the clefts and normalizing the infant's appearance.

Cleft Palate

Description—The presence of a structural defect in the roof of the mouth.
Signs and symptoms—It is characterized by an opening or hole to a total split of the palate. It is often associated with a cleft lip (Figure 11-16B).
Etiology—It is caused by the failure of the soft and bony tissues to unite during the 8th to 12th week of gestation.
Treatment—Surgical intervention is necessary. The cleft can cause feeding problems for an infant because liquid is able to get into the nose and breathing passages. A temporary solution to the problem involves the use of various types of nipples or an inverted "spoon-like" feeder with a nursing nipple, which provides an artificial roof in the mouth. This allows the infant to suck milk until surgical repair can be done.

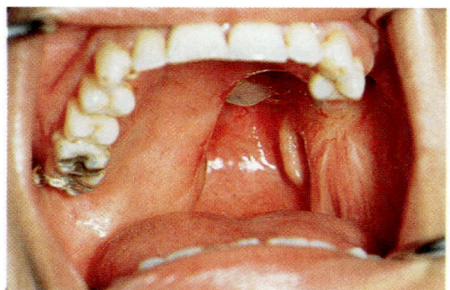

FIGURE 11-16B Cleft palate *(Courtesy of Dr. Joseph Konzelman, School of Dentistry, Medical College of Georgia)*

Color Vision Deficiency

Description—An inherited trait that makes perception of colors inaccurate. It is erroneously called "color blindness" because most people see some color; rarely do people see only black, white, and gray (monochromatism).

Signs and symptoms—Most affected people see colors and do not realize they have a deficiency until they have a color vision test. The most common problem is distinguishing reds and greens, which can be a problem when driving an automobile. (See Ishihara color vision acuity color plates, Chapter 14, Unit 1.)

Etiology—The deficiency is caused by a defective gene carried on the X chromosome and occurs most frequently among men. Because men have only one X chromosome, it is more likely to be expressed. Women have two X chromosomes and are likely to have a normal gene that will dominate the defective one. Rarely the condition is caused by a severe lack of vitamin A or by retinal disease or cataracts.

Treatment—There is no treatment to correct the problem. Individuals with the deficiency must learn to compensate. It is estimated that seven million drivers in North America have the condition. The difficulty in recognizing traffic light colors and red taillights on cars accounts for some accidents. Studies have shown color defective drivers take much longer to respond to color signals. Traffic lights have been redesigned so red is at the top, amber in the middle, and green at the bottom. Experts suggest that adding a distinctive shape for each color would also be beneficial. White borders have been added to red stop signs to make them more visible. It has also been suggested that taillights be changed to green because it is the least sensitive color. Drivers must learn to compensate for their deficiency by allowing more distance from the car ahead and approaching intersections with extra caution.

Cystic Fibrosis (Sis'-tic Fi-bro'-sis)

Description—A generalized dysfunction of the exocrine glands, affecting multiple organ systems. It is the most common fatal genetic disease of Caucasian children, affecting 1 in every 2,000 live births. About 50% die by age 16; the rest survive up to age 30.

Signs and symptoms—They may take years to develop and include sweat gland dysfunction resulting in salty tasting skin; wheezing; dry, nonproductive cough; dyspnea; clubbed fingers; bulky, foul-smelling stools; and excessive appetite but poor weight gain.

Etiology—An autosomal recessive trait that probably causes an alteration in a protein or an enzyme.

Treatment—Treatment is aimed at helping the child lead as normal a life as possible. Salt is prescribed generously, and pancreatic enzymes and vitamins A, D, E, and K are added to food. Breathing exercises, aerosol therapy, postural drainage, and oxygen assist with breathing. Antibiotics are used aggressively when episodes of acute pulmonary infection occur. There is no cure.

PEDIATRIC PERSPECTIVE

Research by Dr. Jeffrey Bartlett at Children's Hospital in Columbus, Ohio, may lead to a strategy to permit delivery of a normal copy of a gene to replace a defective one. He has been able to modify a nonpathogenic virus so that it will carry a "treated" gene to the epithelium of the airway cells. Patients with cystic fibrosis have defective fibrocystic genes that result in the development of the disease. This discovery will not only benefit these patients but will affect many other gene therapy processes.

Down Syndrome (Sin'-drom)

Description—A well-known genetic **syndrome** (group of features) caused by improper cell division. Incidence in North America is about 1 in every 1,000 live births, depending on the mother's age.

Signs and symptoms—It is characterized by slanting eyes, a fold at the inner eye, a large tongue, pug nose, and microcephaly (small head). Other distinguishing features are a simian crease (a single transverse palmer crease), slow dental development, small external ears, and a short neck. Mental retardation occurs in all cases, and there is some degree of growth restriction (Figure 11-17).

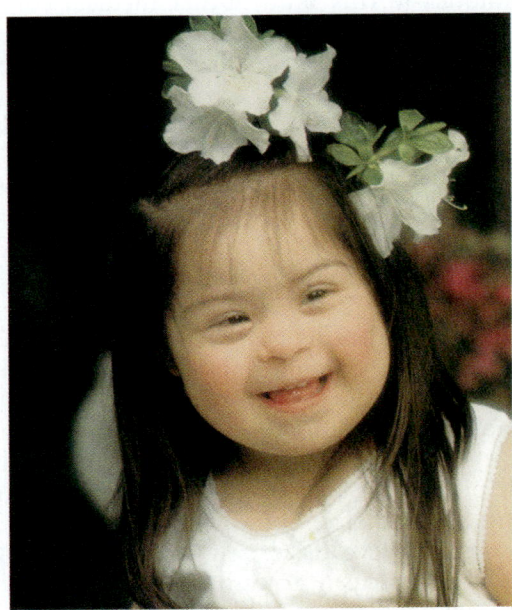

FIGURE 11-17   Child with Down syndrome features *(Copyright Marijane Scott, Marijane's Designer Portraits, Down Right Beautiful 1996 Calendar)*

Etiology—Improper cell division results in the number 21 chromosome occurring in triplicate rather than as a pair, so the individual has 47 instead of 46 chromosomes per cell. Another form occurs when the long arm of chromosome number 21 breaks and attaches to another chromosome.

Treatment—There is no treatment to correct the disorder. Amniocentesis, a diagnostic test, is recommended when prenatal interviews indicate the possibility of a genetic problem. (See Unit 13.) It is also indicated in pregnancies of women older than age of 35. At 20 years of age, a woman has about 1 chance in 2,500 of having a child with Down syndrome, but by age 45, the risk rises to 1 in 40. Amniocentesis requires a small amount of amniotic fluid, which surrounds the fetus, to be withdrawn from the pregnant uterus. Skin cells from the fetus can be found floating in the amniotic fluid and can be grown in a culture for examination. The test can either relieve parental anxiety or can allow them time to prepare for managing a Down syndrome child. Early pregnancy termination can be achieved if findings are a cause of great concern for the parents.

Within a few years another option may be open to parents. In May of 2000, one of the scientific groups of the consortium working to decode the human genome completed the DNA sequence of the 21st chromosome. They learned it has only 225 genes and an approximate 33,827,477 decodable units of DNA. When scientists can identify the location and function of each gene on the chromosome, perhaps gene therapy could be devised to correct the abnormality. (See Discoveries in Human Genetics and New Genetic Techniques in this unit.) Other medical conditions have also been traced to this chromosome, such as acute myeloid leukemia, Alzheimer's disease, epilepsy, Lou Gehrig's disease, and schizophrenia. This widely diverse group of seemingly unrelated diseases demonstrates the complexity of the human body.

Dwarfism

Description—Dwarfism is a condition that causes an abnormally short or undersized person. There are about 200 conditions that result in dwarfism, most of which are genetic in origin. Dwarfism can also result from an endocrine dysfunction (lack of growth hormone), a deficiency disease, or from renal insufficiency. People with this condition prefer the term "little person" or "person of short stature" when referring to their size. Some will accept "dwarf," but the term "midget" is mostly unacceptable. Achondroplastic dwarfism accounts for about 70% of all cases of short stature. This genetic type results from an autosomal dominant gene. It affects 1 in every 26,000 to 40,000 births.

Signs and symptoms—Achondroplastic dwarfism is characterized by a normal-sized trunk but shortened extremities, particularly shortened upper arms and thighs; an enlarged head; bowed legs; shortened hands and fingers; and prominent buttocks. The average height for adult males is 52 inches (4 feet, 4 inches) and adult females is 49 inches (4 feet, 1 inch).

Etiology—Achondroplastic dwarfism results from a newly mutated *FGFR3* gene. It is random and unpreventable. In fact, 85% of children with the condition are born to parents of average size. One copy of the altered gene in each cell is sufficient to cause the disorder. Other cases are the result of an inherited *FGFR3* gene from a parent with the condition. No environmental or other factors have been identified. Depending on the cause of short stature, little people can have average-sized children.

Treatment—Supplemental growth hormone and other treatments that are indicated with some forms of dwarfism are not effective with achondroplastic dwarfism. Because the etiology is genetic, no form of drug therapy would be beneficial. A degree of additional height can be achieved through a surgical procedure known as limb-lengthening, which is usually performed on the lower extremities. Upper arm lengthening can also be performed in situations in which shortness causes difficulty with performing personal care or if desired for a more balanced appearance.

Figure 11-18 shows extremely rare 13-year-old identical twin achondroplastic dwarfs with a 13-year-old average-size friend. The twins were born to average-size parents and have two older average-size siblings. Neither parent could identify any family history of either dwarfism or the occurrence of twins. At age 9 the boys decided they wanted leg-lengthening surgery after seeing a program on television. At this time they were only 38 inches tall. They were experiencing difficulty in managing routine things at school such as climbing stairs and using the drinking fountains and bathroom facilities. Boarding the school bus presented an additional challenge.

Limb lengthening involves cutting the femur, tibia, and fibula of both legs. The bones are held in line with an external fixator (a scaffold-like frame) with metal pins or wires into the bone (Figure 11-19). The frame allows for tension and "distraction" by slowly turning attached mechanisms a few times each day to pull apart the cut bone. The tension on the bone stimulates it to grow gradually, filling in the gap as it is widened. The surrounding muscles, nerves, skin, and blood vessels also grow. Periodic x-rays measure the degree of growth of new bone and determines the rate at which lengthening can be achieved. The maximum rate for children is 1 mm per day, or an inch per month. After the bone is lengthened, it must heal completely in the length-

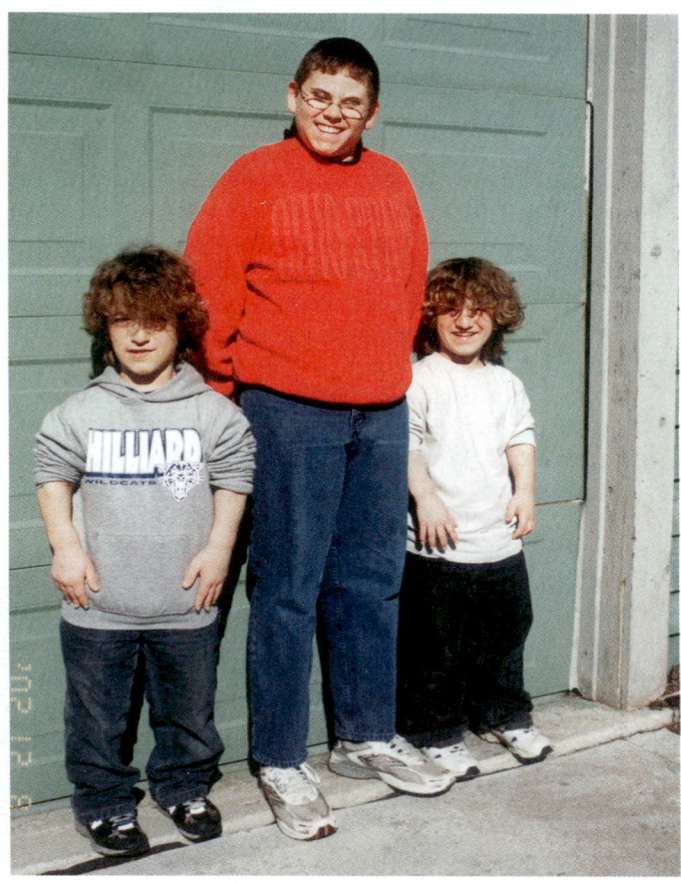

FIGURE 11-18   Thirteen-year-old identical twin male achondroplastic dwarfs with an average-size thirteen-year-old male friend. The twins have had limb-lengthening surgery, which added 4 inches to their leg length.

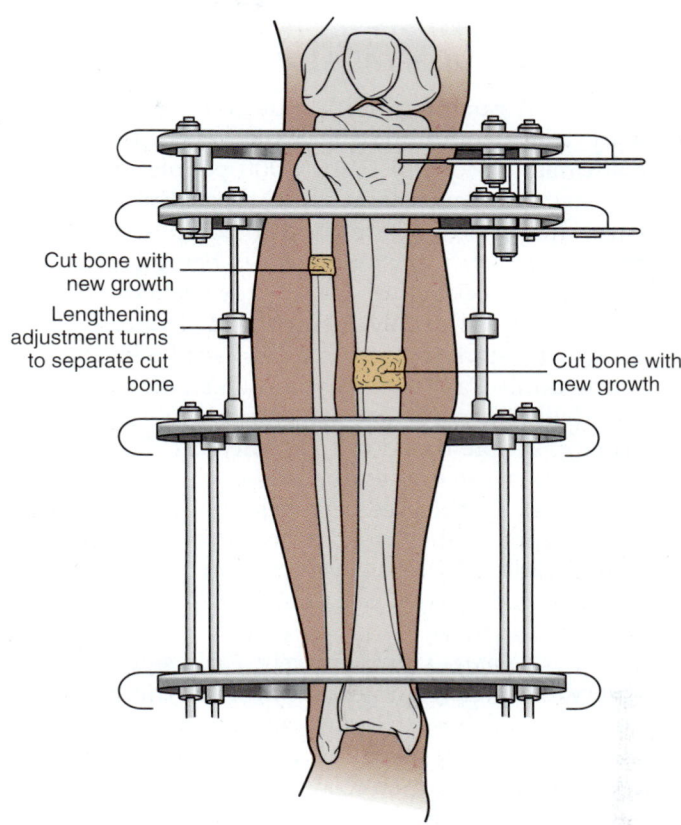

Cut bone with new growth

Lengthening adjustment turns to separate cut bone

Cut bone with new growth

FIGURE 11-19   External fixator attached to tibia and fibula after limb lengthening surgery

ened position before the frame can be removed. The process usually takes between 2½ to 3 months per inch depending upon age, general health, and rehabilitation success. A cast may be applied after the frame is removed to give temporary support if necessary. An additional lengthening procedure can be performed after several years if desired.

The procedure is not without discomfort and is prone to infection at the pin sites. The twins' mother turned 8 fasteners ¼ turn, three times per day per child for 2 months to separate the bones. They achieved a 2-inch lengthening at the femur and another 2 inches at the tibia and fibula for a total of 4 inches in leg length. After the maximum length was achieved, it took 2 months for their bones to harden and another 2 months in rehabilitation to regain leg strength and usage. The prolonged recovery period presents many challenges not only for the children but also for the parents. The procedure is available at only a few sites in the United States, thereby necessitating an extended period of time at a distant health care facility for most patients. At this time the twins are not planning to have an additional procedure. At 13 years old, they are now 47 inches tall, having grown an additional 5 inches during the 4 years since surgery.

Galactosemia (Ga-lakto-se'-me-a)

Description—An inherited metabolic disorder involving the digestion of milk and milk products. It occurs in about 1 in every 50,000 births.

Signs and symptoms—Usual signs are the failure to thrive, diarrhea, jaundice from liver damage, and severe vomiting. Other symptoms include enlargement of the spleen, cataracts, and a pseudo (false) brain tumor. Continued ingestion of galactose or lactose foods may cause mental retardation, progressive liver damage, and death.

Etiology—A recessive gene causes an inability to normally metabolize the sugar galactose, which is formed by the digestion of lactose in milk.

Treatment—Elimination of galactose and lactose from the diet will cause the side effects to subside. Infants must have breast or cow's milk replaced with a soybean-based formula. A galactose-free diet must be maintained throughout life. Screening of newborns is required in some states.

Hemochromatosis (He-mo-kro-ma-to'-sis)

Description—A genetic condition of iron overload in the body. It is a common genetic disorder, affecting approximately 5 out of every 1,000 people. It is most prevalent in Caucasians of northern European descent. It has been overlooked in the past by physicians, but now more attention is being paid to its presence. Screening for the disorder is being recommended for all family members of diagnosed persons, but a team researching the disorder believes all young adult Caucasians should be screened at least once before age 40. The screening involves an inexpensive, simple blood test that detects the presence of a marker for iron status. Researchers found 70% to 80% of first-degree relatives (siblings, children, and parents) of diagnosed individuals were affected. Complications of cirrhosis of the liver, arthritis, diabetes, and congestive heart failure can be avoided by early intervention.

Signs and symptoms—Unfortunately, early signs are not observable. When complications arise, the signs and symptoms of those disorders are recognizable. Other signs may include increased skin pigmentation, usually bronze from increased melanin accumulation, but a metallic gray may also be visible from iron deposits in the skin. Other common abnormalities include depressed secretions from the pituitary gland, calcium deposits in cartilage, and iron deposits in the synovial fluid of the joints. Males may also have testicular atrophy and loss of libido.

Etiology—Complications arise because the body absorbs too much iron from foods as a result of a faulty metabolism. The absorbed iron is deposited in the tissues of the body. The slow accumulation of iron deposits in the cells causes tissue damage and the typical clinical features.

Treatment—The primary treatment is the removal of excess iron by withdrawing blood frequently until serum iron levels drop within normal range. It may take up to 3 years to obtain acceptable results. A drug, deferoxamine, mobilizes iron stores and promotes their excretion, but it is only about half as effective as blood withdrawal. Other systemic diseases that have developed must also be treated.

Hemophilia (Hemō-fil'e-a)

Description—A sex-linked bleeding disorder carried by females but occurring only in males. Incidence is approximately 5 in every 40,000 live births.

Signs and symptoms—It is characterized by abnormal bleeding, which may be mild to severe, depending upon the degree of clotting deficiency. Typically there is easy bruising, hematomas, a tendency for nose-bleeds, bleeding gums, and prolonged bleeding after injury or dental or surgical procedures. In severe cases, internal bleeding into joints, organs, and from major blood vessels is a cause for great concern. It is very dangerous when bleeding occurs within the brain, throat, or heart; this can lead to shock and death.

Etiology—An inherited X-linked recessive trait with known transferral percentages. Female carriers have a 50% chance of transmitting the gene to each daughter, who then becomes a carrier, and a 50% chance of transmitting the gene to each son, who would develop hemophilia. The trait causes abnormal bleeding through the absence or deficiency of a clotting factor. A diagnosis is made following evidence from a clotting factor profile and a positive family history.

Treatment—The disorder is not curable but can be controlled to prevent anemia and severe deformities. Bleeding must be quickly stopped by administering the deficient clotting factors to raise the plasma levels so that the individual can form clots. Fresh, frozen plasma may be used if factors are not immediately available.

Klinefelter's Syndrome (Kline'-fel-ters)

Description—A sex-linked disorder caused by chromosome abnormality affecting, in varying degrees, approximately 1 in every 600 males.

Signs and symptoms—Mild cases probably go undetected. It usually becomes apparent at puberty when the penis and testicles fail to mature fully, often leading to sterility. Other symptoms are breast enlargement, mental retardation, sparse body hair, abnormal body build (long legs with a short, obese trunk), a tendency toward alcoholism, and often personality disorders.

Etiology—One or more extra X chromosomes resulting from abnormal meiosis. The severity depends on the number of extra X chromosomes—the more extra chromosomes, the more severe the disorder.

Treatment—If begun early, treatment with testosterone (the male hormone) may help reverse the feminine characteristics but will not reverse the sterility or mental retardation. Psychotherapy is indicated when sexual dysfunction causes emotional maladjustment.

Phenylketonuria (Fenil-keto-nure-a) (PKU)

Description—A devastating, genetic metabolic disease, requiring early intervention to prevent its development and progress.

Signs and symptoms—The warning symptoms are not readily observable, so early detection and prevention are necessary. PKU disorders can be diagnosed from blood and urine tests. Newborns' blood is routinely checked at birth, but because enzyme levels may be normal at that time, a follow-up urine test is done at about the second week of life.

Etiology—The inability of the newborn's body to act upon an amino acid called phenylalanine. The newborn lacks the necessary liver enzyme, so the amino acid builds up in the blood and tissues, causing brain damage, which results in profound retardation, seizures, and stunted growth.

Treatment—A restrictive diet is indicated to keep levels of phenylalanine low. This requires elimination of natural proteins from the diet and a milk substitute that has a normal amount of other amino acids, carbohydrates, and fat until at least age 5 or 6. The child must avoid breads, cheese, eggs, meat, poultry, fish, nuts, flour, and legumes. This must be carefully monitored to avoid brain damage.

Spina Bifida (Spi'-na Bi'-fid-a)

Description—A structural malformation of the spine in which the posterior portion of the spinal tissues fails to close during the first 3 months of pregnancy. These malformations occur in three forms: spinal bifida occulta, meningocele, and myelomeningocele. (See Spinal Cord Defects, Chapter 11, Unit 2, for more information. See also Figure 11-45.)

Talipes (Tal'i-pez)

Description—A structural malformation of the feet, commonly called clubfoot (Figure 11-20).

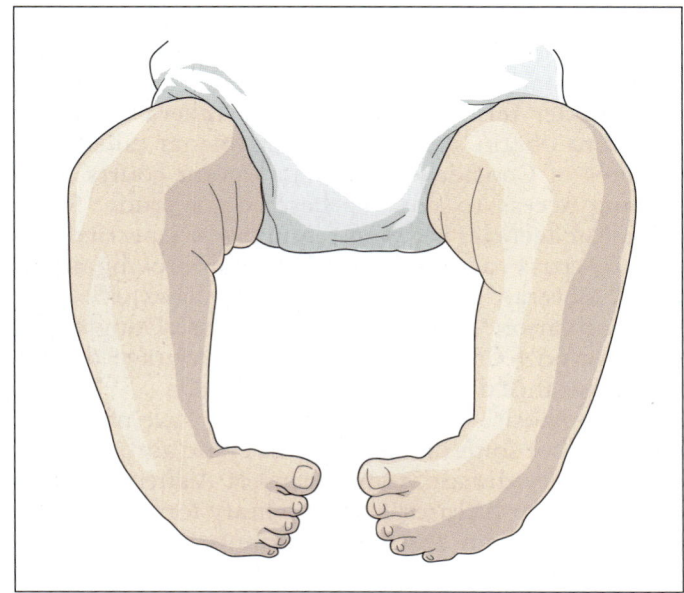

FIGURE 11-20 Talipes

Signs and symptoms—It is characterized by varying degrees of inward, outward, downward, or upward turning of one or both feet.

Etiology—The result of a deformed talus (foot bone) and a shortened Achilles tendon, apparently caused by a combination of genetic and in utero environmental factors. There is a strong heredity factor in some instances and an apparent arrestment of development during the 9th and 10th weeks of life when the feet are formed.

Treatment—A distinction needs to be made between true and apparent clubfoot. X-ray reveals whether the talus and calcaneus bones of the foot are superimposed. Correction involves three stages: correcting the deformity, maintaining the correction, and long-term observation. Surgical correction is done shortly after birth. Repositioning is maintained by a cast. After correction, proper alignment must be maintained through exercise, night splints, and special shoes. A deformity that resists manual correction or a neglected clubfoot will require surgical adjustment of the bone and tendons.

Turner's Syndrome (Turn-ers Sin'-drom)

Description—A sex-linked disorder with a group of structural defects that affects about 1 in 10,000 newborn females.

Signs and symptoms—It is characterized by short stature, webbing of the neck, a low hairline, a wide chest with broadly spaced nipples, poor breast development, and underdevelopment of the genitalia. The ovaries fail to develop, making the female sterile. Often it is not recognizable until lack of menses and developing genitalia become apparent. The disorder also causes an abnormality of the aorta and edema of the legs and feet.

Etiology—The affected individual has only 45 chromosomes because the sex cells fail to divide correctly in meiosis, causing only one sex chromosome to be present in the cells.

Treatment—The use of estrogen (female hormone) after age 13, to prevent growth from stopping, will induce sexual maturation but doesn't reverse the sterility. Psychotherapy is indicated to deal with the emotional adjustment required to deal with the disorder.

DISCOVERIES IN HUMAN GENETICS

An article titled "Vital Data" appeared in the March 1996 publication of *Scientific American*. It reports that in 1990 a 15-year, $3 billion, federally funded study called "The Human Genome Project" was formed to analyze human genetics at the molecular level. The project was launched because it seemed to promise the best hope for ultimately defeating not only diseases long known to be inherited but also those with more subtle links, like cancer. The planners estimated it would take several tens of thousands of technician years to find the sequence of all the DNA bases and the human genes and 390,000 pages to list them. The sequencing, it was believed, would reveal the possible functions and location of the estimated 100,000 human genes. But first it was necessary to devise "a genetic map," or diagram, which describes how thousands of known marker sequences in the chromosomes separate and recombine. They also needed physical maps to show the order along a chromosome of recognizable sequence sites. Using the maps, a researcher could compare a given condition's pattern of inheritance with that of the marker sequences. This makes it possible to determine where a gene that causes the condition might be located. Computers can then "match" the reams of data coming from sequencing machines onto the sites on a physical map. By comparing the two maps, it is possible to quickly find genes associated with an illness.

In February of 2001, two different scientific groups published the first drafts of the human genome in two leading scientific journals, *Science* and *Nature*. This accomplishment has revolutionized the understanding and treatment of disease. The genome is the approximate 3 billion letter code of the human DNA that is the chemical sequence containing the basic information for building and running a human body. This chemical sequence determines every characteristic in the human body, from eye color to vulnerability to disease.

The number of genes discovered was surprisingly lower than expected, 20,000 to 25,000 genes, not much greater than the number found in other species, such as the fruit fly. The sequencing of the human genome was completed 5 years earlier than expected because of the significant development of new technologies. These same technologies are now being used to help diagnose human diseases, design custom treatments, and even identify criminals.

Although the newly discovered maps of the genome are considered to be just drafts, they are already providing breakthroughs in medicine. It is predicted that science will be able to zero in on the genetic factors involved in diabetes, heart disease, and other common disorders within the next 5 to 10 years. Cancer drugs are already being targeted at the molecular level of the disease. Companies have been formed that are taking blood samples from volunteers with known diseases to compare the codes and to identify the responsible genes.

In the course of this project, many other genetic technologies have been developed, such as gene therapy and gene transplantation. When genetic mutations are isolated, tests can be developed to identify their presence. Diagnostic technology has been developed that can simultaneously analyze DNA from patients for the presence of many different mutations on multiple genes. When the effects of mutations are known, test results can be a medical bonanza. It will be possible to indicate how likely a person is to develop a disease and, hopefully, determine a treatment or at least a method of control. In the course of the genome project, other genetic technologies like gene therapy and gene transplantation have been developed that will hopefully permit treatment of faulty genes in the future. Although science is much closer to understanding defects in genes and the diseases that result, cures based upon changes in the genetic code may be years away while new drugs and ways to deliver corrected genes into defective cells are developed.

The exciting new technology is not without its critics. Abuses of the new science have already begun. Commercial value of certain DNA sequences are enormous. Scientific companies have "gene-based patents," which are certain to lead to vicious legal battles. Drug companies are spending hundreds of millions of dollars to identify genes connected to diseases because it will lead to molecules that are good targets for drugs and diagnostic reagents.

There is a potential problem with protecting against the misuse of individual genetic information. Discrimination in employment and life and health insurance has already surfaced. People with a genetic condition, or who are at risk for one, are often turned down for employment or insurance, and some have lost their current jobs and coverage. They are declining the opportunity to have their children tested, even when it would be medically valuable, for fear of "labeling" them and therefore making their insurability or future employment questionable. There is concern that insurers might even classify the mutations as a pre-existing condition and refuse to cover any treatments related to that condition. Some testing is being done under false names, and researchers are being forced to obtain special legal documents called Certificates of Confidentiality that prevent courts from gaining access to data gathered in a study. Some adoption agencies are even requiring prospective parents to "pass" a genetic test before approving adoptions. Several states have enacted laws to limit descrimination based on genetic data. Congress is working on federal legislation to discourage or prevent insurance discrimination nationally.

On the positive side, mutated genes have now been identified for some diseases such as cystic fibrosis, polycystic kidney disease, some forms of Alzheimer's and cardiovascular diseases, and hereditary forms of breast and colon cancers. Tests are becoming more commonplace. If someone is identified as having the mutated gene, the known percentages for its disease probability can be provided. With the near certainty for contracting specific inherited malignancies, some people have gone so far as to elect surgical removal of both breasts and entire colons in order to save their lives. Until unique new therapies can be developed, little else can be done.

Some researchers worry about uncontrolled testing and the interpretation of results. Many physicians are not well enough informed to be giving genetic advice. The psychologic harm from DNA testing is also receiving growing attention. The fear of consequences and of discrimination overshadows the benefits. Genetic counselors believe that because of the potential for harm, children should not be tested for mutation-predicting diseases that will not develop until adulthood *unless* there is a possible medical intervention available. Yet the tests have gone on. One incident occurred reportedly because parents wished to avoid paying for a college education if their child was likely to develop a hereditary disease for which there is no cure. Truly, standards are needed. Leaders of the genome project acknowledged from the beginning that human genetics can be used to harm as well as to help. They have devoted millions of dollars to studying ethical, legal, and social questions. Yet, technical gains are outrunning the attempts of professional societies and government regulators to guide the use of the technology. Governments around the world are working on legislation to protect individual rights and confidentiality. On October 13, 2003, the President's Council on Bioethics presented their research on this area in a document entitled "Beyond Therapy: Biotechnology and the Pursuit of Happiness." This 300+ page document summarizes the reflections of the Council on a wide range of ethical issues "from gene therapy for fetuses to the development of psychotropic and 'age retarding' drugs." Just how far should scientific technology go to alter the human? Where does relieving human suffering end and manipulation for personal desire begin? This area of science will be a topic for discussion for years to come.

NEW GENETIC TECHNIQUES

Polymerase Chain Reaction

Polymerase chain reaction is a technique being used in molecular biology to allow scientists to isolate, characterize, and produce large quantities of specific pieces of DNA from very small amounts of starting material that would otherwise be undetectable. Practical applications are applied to prenatal and postnatal diagnosis of genetic diseases, infectious disease (such as AIDS), and cancer. It assists in the matching of transplant recipients with donors, in the study of human genetic history and evolution, and in DNA fingerprinting by forensic scientists.

DNA Fingerprinting

DNA fingerprinting is a detection and identification method that was first announced by a British geneticist in 1985. Except for identical twins, the DNA code for each individual is unique. Examination of blood, semen, and other body fluids at a crime scene can render positive identification when compared with the DNA molecules of the suspect. The evidence of a DNA match, in view of the great variance among the population, is considered to be a positive identification.

Genetic Counseling

Genetic counseling provides information to a couple regarding their risks of having a child with a genetic disorder. Even "normal" couples face some risk with any pregnancy. About 3% of all live-born infants have a significant birth defect. Counseling is available to those couples who perceive their risk to be greater than the population in general. Information provided should include known risk statistics and offer available alternatives such as amniocentesis, pregnancy termination, adoption, artificial insemination (if the male has the risk factor), or information to permit understanding and acceptance of a pregnancy situation for which the parents agree no termination action will be taken.

Gene Therapy

Gene therapy is a new frontier in medicine. Persons who are born with a congenital disorder resulting from a defective gene could have a perfect gene inserted into their cells, preventing the development of or correcting the effects of the disease. This therapy began in 1990 when genetically engineered cells were infused into a 4-year-old girl with a life-threatening immune deficiency. The infused cells were from her own blood into which researchers had inserted copies of a missing gene that produces the missing immune product. Again in 1991, gene therapy was used to treat cancer. Two patients who had advanced skin cancer were infused with their own white blood cells after they had been genetically altered to produce a tumor-killing protein. These early experimental attempts were the front-runners to the new exacting technology that will result from the genome project.

Genetic Engineering

Genetic engineering is being used in the prenatal diagnosis of inherited diseases. The DNA pattern of cells from the parents, who may carry a gene for a congenital disorder, and the pattern of the fetus are compared. The disease status of the fetus can currently be determined in the following instances: thalassemia, Huntington's disease, cystic fibrosis, and Duchennes' muscular dystrophy.

Genetic engineering has allowed discoveries that could not otherwise have been made. An example is the discovery of oncogenes and tumor suppressor genes that play a role in causing some cancers. Scientists were able to cut the cancer-causing DNA into segments and identify the specific segments that were responsible for transforming normal cells into cancer cells. Much research remains to be done to achieve the promise of gene therapy and genetic engineering, but its value could be enormous.

There is always controversy when new techniques are introduced, but manipulating human cellular structure appears to have many ethical and moral issues to be resolved. On one hand is the opportunity to eliminate the devastating physical and mental conditions resulting from defective genes, and few people would deny the social and economic advantages of this capability. On the other hand, there are those who say man is playing "God," and that is not right. There is also the criticism that if you have enough money, you could "buy" perfect children of the sex, color, intelligence, and projected size you desired. When technology is known, regardless of ethical controls (which have yet to be developed), someone will always be operating outside the accepted practice for a price.

The reality of genetic identification discrimination hangs in the balance. Only the future will determine that outcome. As the director of the National Center for Human Genome Research said in *Scientific American,* "as the number of genetic tests grow, we are going to see it [genetic identification discrimination] happen on a larger scale, since we're all at risk for something."

Stem Cell Research

Two great areas of scientific inquiry have generated hope for medical breakthroughs, the Human Genome Project and stem cell research. Both have had their share of controversy as to moral and ethical implications. Scientists believe that offered the possibility of stem cell research, they could regenerate any tissue in the human body and therefore cure many medical conditions such as Parkinson's disease, diabetes, paralysis, and heart failure.

Stem cells can be embryonic or adult. The embryonic cells are obtained from the inner cell mass of a week-old embryo. Usually these are excess cells created during infertility treatment in standard in vitro fertilization practices. The participants donate the excess cells for research purposes rather than have them destroyed. Embryonic stem cells have the potential to de-

velop into all or nearly all of the tissues of the body. The cells are cultured and can grow and divide indefinitely. The cells develop into a stem cell line, descended from the original. Batches of cells are then separated and distributed to researchers in the United States, Australia, India, Israel, and Sweden. Private research has developed more than 60 genetically diverse stem cell lines.

Adult stem cells are unspecialized, can renew themselves, and become specialized to yield cells from the tissue from which they originated. However, no adult cells have been able to develop into different tissues.

The use of federal money to fund stem cell research became a topic of debate. Scientists wanted unlimited support to find cures for many diseases. Religious leaders condemned the research because it involves prohibiting the development of the embryo, thereby violating the sanctity of human life. In August of 2001, the Bush Administration announced that federal funds could be used only on the existing stem cell lines because those embryos were already destroyed and no longer had the possibility of further human development. This decision allowed for the scientists to explore the potential of this research to benefit people who suffer from life destroying diseases and yet preserved the value and sanctity of human life by prohibiting additional embryos for federally funded research.

Other decisions were also made regarding the research criteria, the denying of funds for additional cells, embryos, or cloning. A President's Council of Bioethics was created to "study the human and moral ramifications of developments in biomedical and behavioral science and technology." They are looking at issues such as "stem cells and embryo research, assisted reproduction, cloning, genetic screening, gene therapy, euthanasia, psychoactive drugs, and brain implants." It will be very interesting to watch how these very important medical, legal, ethical, and moral concerns shape our future scientific policy.

TISSUES

As you are already aware, not all cells are alike. They may be transparent, as in the eye, or transmit electrical impulses or nutrients. Some have long, thin fibers, and others produce secretions. When cells of the same type group together for a common purpose, they form a **tissue**. Tissues are composed of 60% to 99% water. The essential substances needed by the body are either dissolved or suspended in the tissue fluids. Therefore, water is indispensable to cell life, and lack of it causes death more rapidly than lack of any other substance, except oxygen.

Two common medical terms describe the opposites of tissue fluid balance. When there is too little fluid, the condition is known as **dehydration**. An abnormal accumulation of excess fluid, causing puffiness of the affected tissues, is known as **edema**.

Tissue Classifications

Tissues can be classified into four main types: **epithelial**, **connective**, nerve, and muscle.

Epithelial   Epithelial tissues form the body's glands, cover the surface of the body, and line the cavities. Epithelium is the main tissue of the skin, which serves as a protective covering for the body. Epithelium also covers all the organs and lines the intestinal, respiratory, and urinary tract and uterus. Some epithelial tissues secrete fluids, such as mucus and digestive juices. Others selectively absorb nutrients, chemical elements, and water. The epithelium of the urinary bladder is uniquely arranged in folds to allow for expansion as the bladder fills.

Epithelial tissues in glands specialize to provide specific secretions for the body. Glands that secrete directly into the blood in the capillaries are known as *endocrine* or ductless glands.

Glands that produce secretions through ducts within the body are classified as *exocrine* (Figure 11-21). Two glands, the liver and pancreas, produce both endocrine and exocrine secretions.

Connective   Connective tissue forms the supporting structure of the body, connecting other tissues together to form the organs and body parts.

There are three categories of connective tissue: (1) connective tissue proper, (2) supportive connective, and (3) fluid connective tissue. Connective tissue in the form of adipose or fat tissue, stores the body's reserve of food, fills the area between tissue fibers, insulates against heat and cold, and pads the body structures (Figure 11-22). Supportive connective tissue is stretchable and forms the subcutaneous layer of the skin. A dense supportive connective tissue in the form of tendons, ligaments, and organ capsules serves to support and protect organs and lend elasticity to the walls of arteries (Figure 11-23).

Blood and lymphatic vessels, lymph, the blood, and blood cells are forms of fluid connective tissue. Cells in the blood carry nutrients and oxygen to the cells and

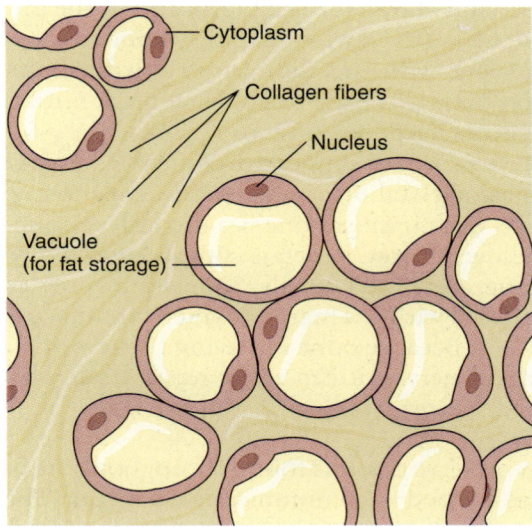

FIGURE 11-22   Connective (adipose) tissue throughout the body

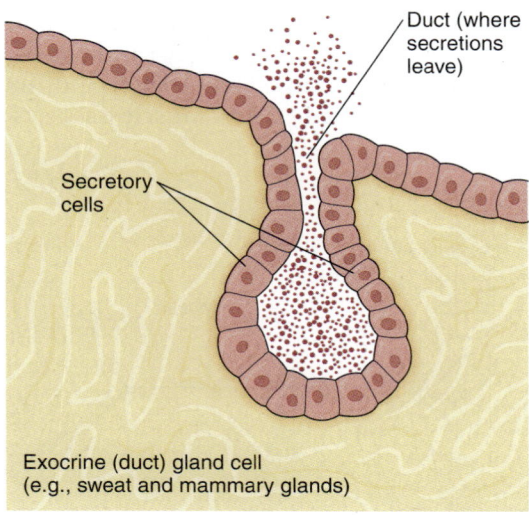

FIGURE 11-21   Epithelial cell tissue of an exocrine gland

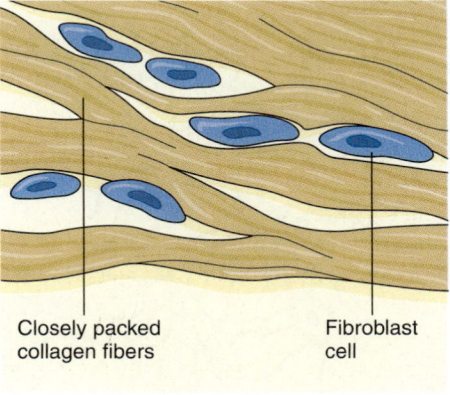

FIGURE 11-23   Dense supportive connective tissue in ligaments and tendons

pick up metabolic wastes for elimination. Lymph fluid consists of water, glucose, fats, and salt and is present in the spaces between the cells of the tissues and within the lymph vessels. Connective tissue plays a major role in the repair of damaged body tissue. The repair process involves new blood vessel formation and the growth of new connective tissue known as scar tissue. Excessive blood vessel development in the early stages may result in a condition called "proud flesh." In instances of surgery or suturing (sewing) of a clean wound, the need for tissue regrowth and therefore the resulting scar are reduced because the cut edges are brought together closely by the surgical process. An excessive growth of scar tissue is called a **keloid**.

Supportive connective tissue can be found in the cartilage and bones of the body. Cartilage is located between the bones of the spine (where it acts as a shock absorber and allows for flexibility) and in the ear, nose, and voice box (to provide shaping). Bone tissue is actually cartilage with the addition of calcium salts. This addition takes place gradually from birth until the tissue becomes hardened (Figure 11-24).

Bone is a form of supportive connective tissue that is also called skeletal or **osseous** tissue. It is not a lifeless material. Within most bone is a medullary cavity filled with yellow marrow, which is composed of fat, connective tissue, and blood vessels. Some long bones contain cavities filled with red marrow, which manufactures red blood cells. Because bone is a living tissue with a blood supply and nerves, it can easily repair itself when it is damaged.

Nerve Nerve tissue is found throughout the body. It serves as the body's communication network. The basic structural unit of the tissue is the neuron, which con-

sists of a nerve cell body and fibers that resemble tree branches (Figure 11-25). The dendrites bring impulses to the cell body; the axon conducts impulses away. Neurons range from a fraction of an inch up to 3 feet in length.

There are three types of nerve cells or neurons. A *sensory neuron* in the skin or sense organs picks up a stimulus and sends it toward the spinal cord and brain. An *interneuron,* or *connecting neuron,* carries the impulse to another neuron. A *motor neuron* receives an impulse and sends a message, which causes a reaction.

Clusters of neurons form the nerve tissue. Nerves throughout the body join together to form the spinal cord, which in turn transmits electrical impulses to and from the brain. Nerves outside the brain and spinal cord are called *peripheral nerves*. Most of the fibers of these nerves are covered with a fatty insulating material called a **myelin** sheath, which is then covered with a thin membrane called **neurilemma**. If a sheathed nerve fiber is damaged or cut, it can be surgically repaired, and a new fiber may form within the sheath, but nerve tissue recovers very slowly. Unfortunately, fibers of the brain and spinal cord lack sheaths and cannot be restored by surgery when damaged or cut.

Muscle Muscle tissue is designed to contract on stimulation. Tissue that can be controlled at will with impulses from the brain is called **voluntary** muscle tissue. This type is found connected to the bones of the body and is called **skeletal** or **striated** muscle (Figure 11-26A). It gives us the ability to move our bodies.

Involuntary muscle action occurs without control or conscious awareness. There are two types of involuntary muscle tissue. One type, called **smooth** muscle tissue, is found within the walls of all the organs of the body except the heart. This type of tissue moves food and waste material through the digestive tract and changes the size of the iris of the eye and the diameter of arteries (Figure 11-26B). The other type of involuntary muscle tissue, called **cardiac** muscle tissue, is found

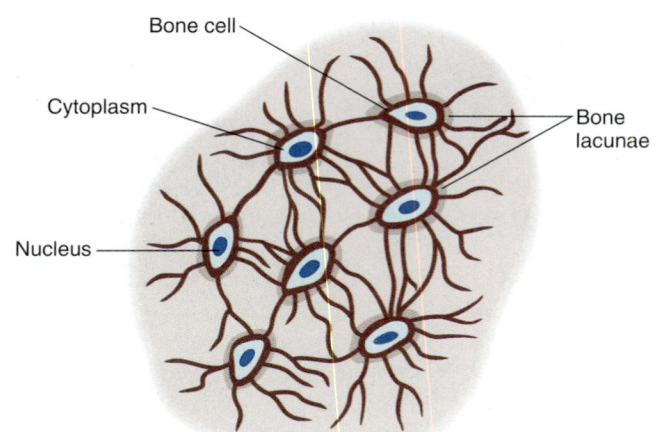

FIGURE 11-24 Supportive connective tissue found in bone

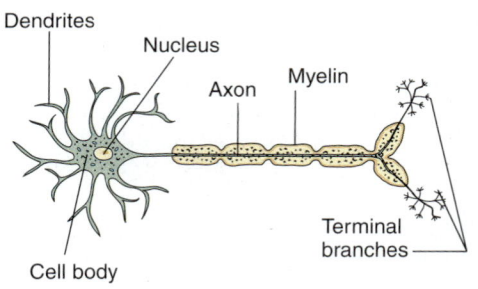

FIGURE 11-25 A motor neuron

only in the heart. Cardiac muscle fibers are joined in a continuous network and must contract together in a forceful, rhythmic action to pump blood throughout the body (Figure 11-26C).

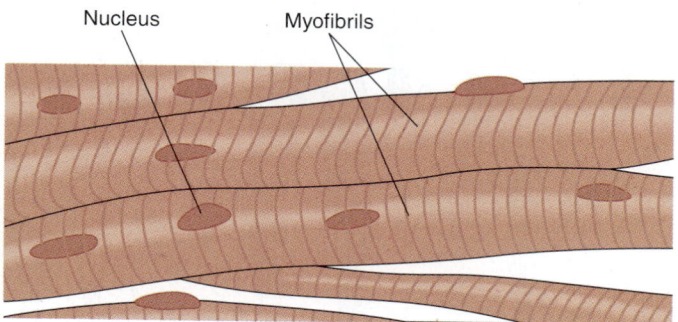

FIGURE 11-26A Skeletal muscle tissue (striated voluntary) attached to bone

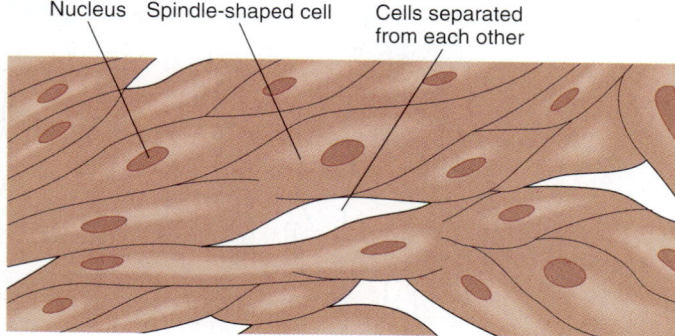

FIGURE 11-26B Smooth muscle tissue in the walls of organs and blood vessels

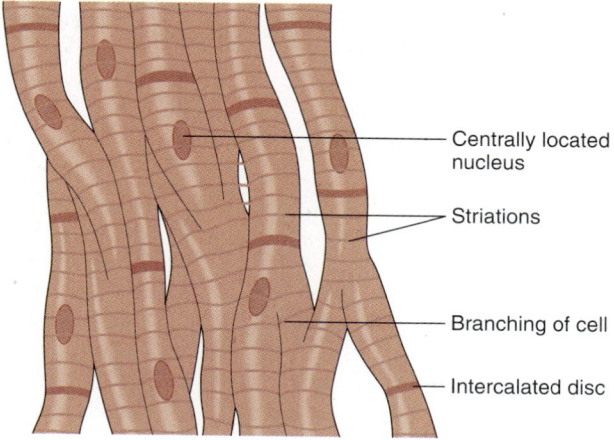

FIGURE 11-26C Cardiac muscle tissue of the heart

ORGANS

The **organs** of the body are made of two or more types of tissue that work together to perform a specific body function. For example, the stomach is constructed with walls of smooth muscle tissue to "churn" the food; it is lined with one type of epithelial tissue, which secretes gastric juices, and covered with another type, which protects the organ; connective tissue fills the spaces between the other tissue fibers; nerve tissue controls the rate at which material is emptied from the stomach. (The roles of the organs will be discussed in more detail in the remaining units of this chapter.)

SYSTEMS

Organs of the body that perform similar functions are organized into a body **system**. Again as an example, the stomach joins with the mouth, throat, esophagus, and small and large intestines to make up the alimentary tract of the digestive system. The alimentary tract combines with the teeth, tongue, salivary glands, liver, pancreas, and gallbladder to form the total digestive system. The other systems of the body, which will be discussed individually, are the integumentary, skeletal, muscular, respiratory, circulatory, urinary, nervous, endocrine, and reproductive systems.

One additional "system" will also be discussed later in this chapter. The immune system is not considered to be a system. However, because the body's health and well-being directly depend on an intact and effective immune response, you should have a basic knowledge of its role in disease response. As scientists begin to better understand how it functions and what can be done to correct its malfunction, perhaps we can solve the mysteries of cancer, AIDS, and many other immunologically based disorders. The basics of the complex subject of immunology are discussed in Unit 9.

Even a body system cannot function alone. All systems must combine their individual contributions for the health and well-being of the total human body. Figure 11-27 illustrates the systems of the body.

The following is a summary of the fundamental structure of the human body: it is composed of billions of cells, which are grouped together to form tissues that bind together to form organs to perform the functions of a system that cooperates with other systems to become the human body (Figure 11-28).

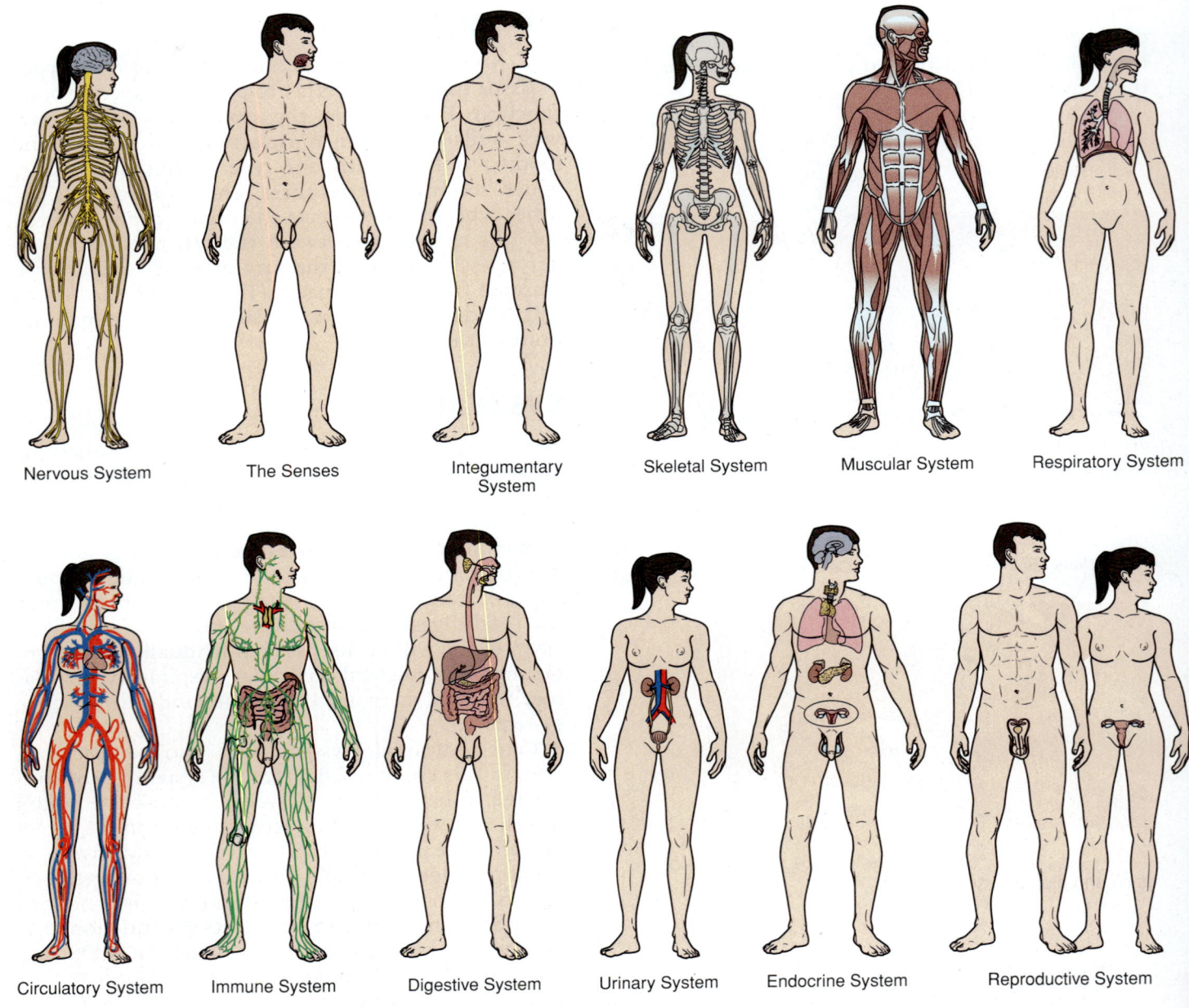

Nervous System   The Senses   Integumentary System   Skeletal System   Muscular System   Respiratory System

Circulatory System   Immune System   Digestive System   Urinary System   Endocrine System   Reproductive System

FIGURE 11-27   The body systems

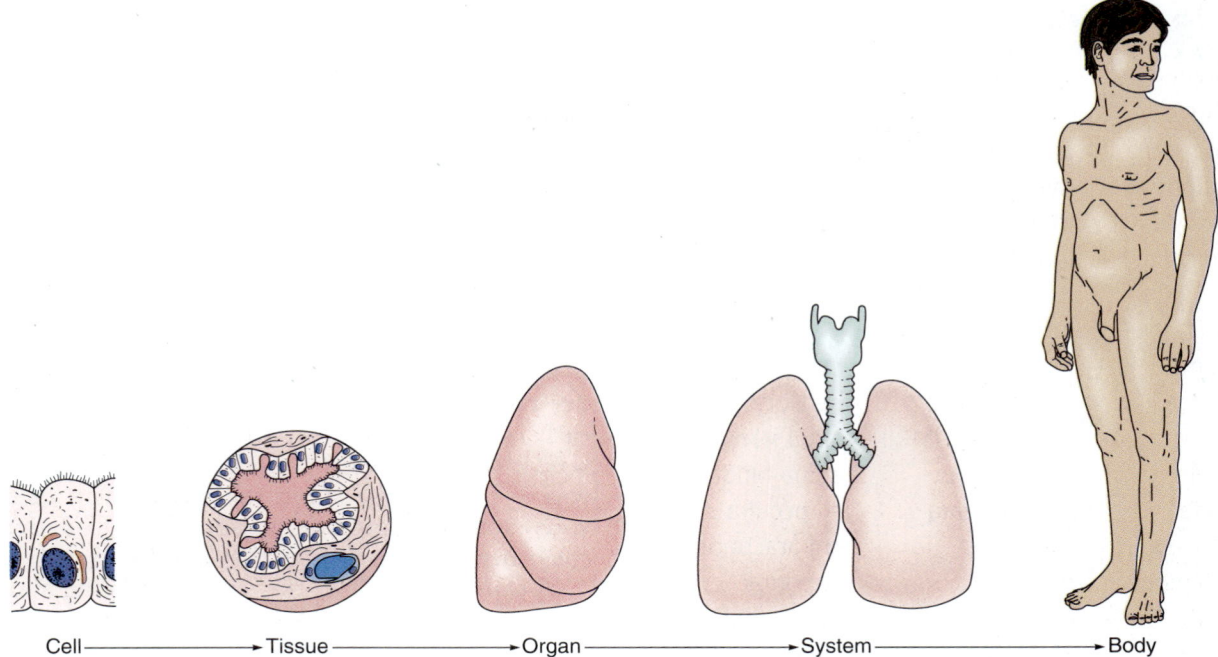

Cell　———————→ Tissue　———————→ Organ　———————→ System　———————→ Body

FIGURE 11-28　　Fundamental cell-to-human-body-structures sequence

ACHIEVE UNIT OBJECTIVES

- ☐ Complete the Workbook activities to meet the learning objectives.
- ☐ Apply your knowledge at the end of this chapter in completing the Critical Thinking Challenge and Activities, as well as the StudyWARE on your Student CD-ROM.

UNIT 2
THE NERVOUS SYSTEM

OBJECTIVES

Upon completion of this unit, you will be able to achieve the following:

LEARNING Objectives

1. Spell and define, using the glossary at the back of the text, all the Words to Know in this unit.

2. Name the two main divisions of the nervous system.

3. Identify the two types of peripheral nerves and explain the function of the spinal nerves.

4. Describe simple and complex reflex actions.

5. Describe a synapse and the effects of various substances on its action.

6. Describe the purpose of the automatic nervous system, and explain the action of its two divisions.

7. Identify the main parts of the brain and their functions.

8. Name the coverings of the brain and spinal cord, and describe their purpose.

9. Describe the function of cerebrospinal fluid.

10. Name common diagnostic tests used to identify neurologic disorders and possible reasons for their use.

11. List the functions of the hypothalamus.

12. Describe 25 diseases or disorders of the nervous system.

WORDS TO KNOW

action potential
angiography
arachnoid
arteriography
auditory
autonomic
axon
central
cerebellum
cerebrospinal
    fluid
cerebrum
coma scale
computerized
    axial tomog-
    raphy (CAT or
    CT scan)
cranium
dendrite
dura mater
electroencepha-
    lography (EEG)

electromyography
frontal
ganglion
hypothalamus
interneurons
longitudinal
    fissure
lumbar puncture
magnetic
    resonance
    imaging (MRI)
medulla
    oblongata
meninges
midbrain
migraine
motor
myelography
occipital
olfactory
optic
parasympathetic

parietal
peripheral
pia mater
plexuses
pons
positron emission
    tomography
    (PET scan)
sciatica
sensory
skull x-ray
spina bifida
    occulta
subarachnoid
subdural
sympathetic
synapse
syndrome
temporal
thalamus
thorax
ventricle

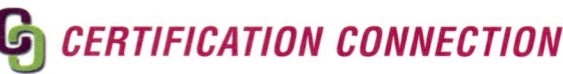

CERTIFICATION CONNECTION

CMA
Diagnostic procedures
Common diseases and
    pathology
Anatomy and physiology

CMAS
Anatomy and physiology

RMA
Anatomy and physiology

The nervous system is the communication network that organizes and coordinates all the body's functions. It is a complex and somewhat difficult system to understand, and in most texts, it is not usually discussed early in the study of the body systems. However, in this text, it is being presented first. Hopefully, this will help you to better understand the involvement of the nervous system's regulatory action in the functioning of the other body systems as they are discussed.

You might think of the system as being something like your telephone system. You can make local, instate, national, and international calls. You can easily call next door, but the further away you wish to call, the more number messages and the more "routing" of signals you need to complete your call. The phone picks up your voice (stimulus), converts it to impulses, and sends it along a charged line to a bundle of lines and on to phone company switching equipment. Every so of-

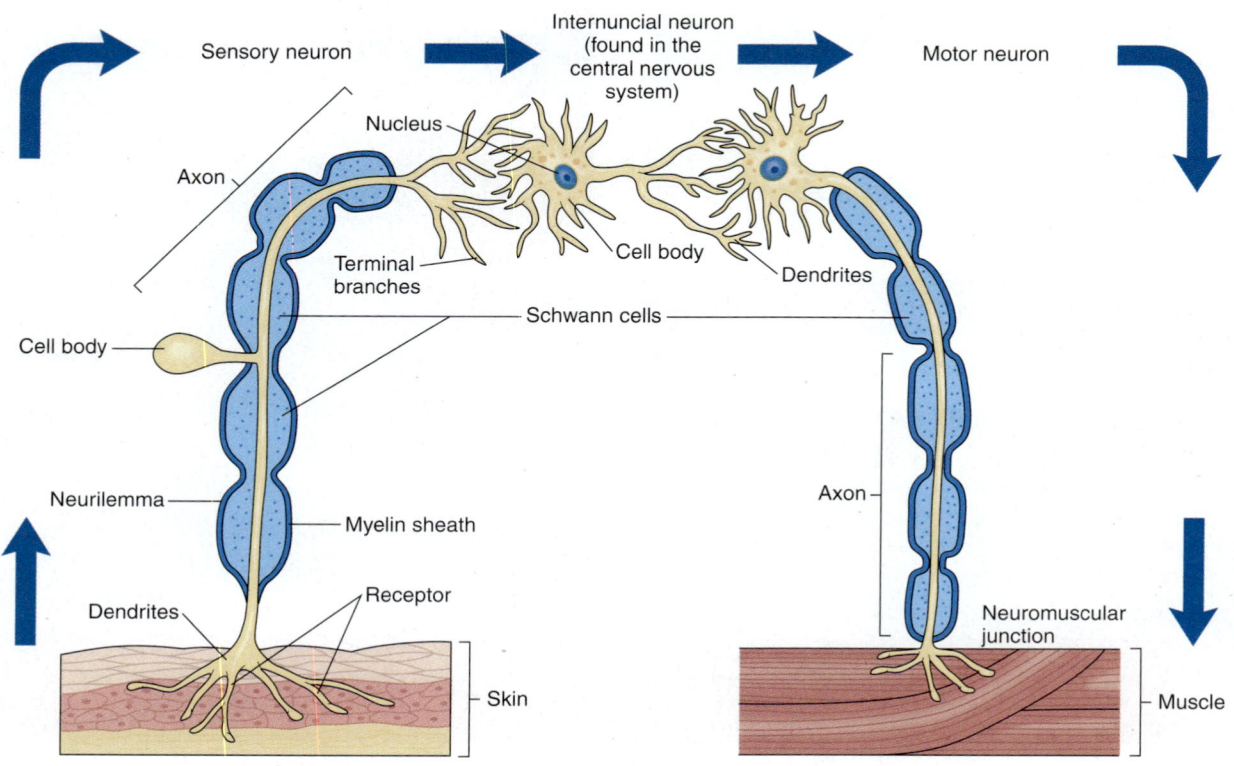

FIGURE 11-29   Types of neurons

ten, the impulse is "boosted" to maintain your "voice." It may even be given special treatment and sent through space and bounced off a satellite, but the message is forwarded to its destination. Your nervous system operates in a similar but much more complicated manner. The system has two main divisions: the **central** nervous system (CNS), which consists of the brain and the spinal cord, and the **peripheral** nervous system, which includes all the nerves that connect the CNS to every organ and area of the body. The **autonomic** nervous system is a specialized part of the peripheral system and controls internal organs and other self-regulating body functions.

Like in all systems, the basic functioning unit is the cell; in this system the unit is a nerve cell or neuron. As described in Unit 1, there are three types of neurons in nerve tissue: **sensory**, connecting, and **motor**. They receive stimuli or impulses, transmit impulses to other neurons, and deliver response actions to the muscles and glands. Connecting neurons are also called *associative* or *internuncial neurons*. Figure 11-29 illustrates the three types of neurons.

All nerve cells have a nucleus, cytoplasm, and a cell membrane. Scattered throughout the cytoplasm are little microscopic granular "dots" called Nissl bodies. They are involved in protein synthesis and metabolism. The cell body has processes that are extensions of cytoplasm called **dendrites** and **axons**. A neuron may have many dendrites but only one axon. These extensions are also called *fibers*. Around the long, thin axons of peripheral nerves are the Schwann cells. They form a tight protective covering called the myelin sheath and also play a part in the transmission of messages. The myelin is then surrounded by the neurilemma, an elastic sheath covering.

A nerve is composed of bundles of nerve fibers bound together by connective tissue. If a nerve is composed of fibers going from the sense organs to the spinal cord or brain, it is a *sensory* or *afferent nerve*. If it is carrying impulses from the brain or spinal cord to a muscle, organ, or gland, it is known as a *motor* or *efferent nerve*. Some nerves have both kinds of fibers and are known as *mixed nerves*.

MEMBRANE EXCITABILITY

Nerves carry impulses by creating electric charges in a process known as membrane excitability. Neurons have a membrane that separates the cytoplasm inside from the extracellular fluids outside the cell, thereby creating two chemically different areas. Each area has differing amounts of potassium and sodium ions and negative charged ions (anions) and positive charged ions (cations), with the inside being the more negatively charged. When a neuron is stimulated, ions move across the membrane, creating a current that, if large enough, will briefly change the area inside of the neuron to be more positive than the outside area. This state is known as **action potential**. Neurons and other cells that produce action potentials are said to have membrane excitability.

To understand how impulses are carried along nerves or throughout a muscle when it contracts, we need to learn a little more about membrane excitability. Ions cross a membrane through channels, some of which are open and allow ions to "leak" (diffuse) continuously. Other channels are called "gated" and open only during action potential. Another membrane opening is called a sodium-potassium pump. By active transport, it maintains the flow of sodium and potassium ions from higher to lower concentration levels across the membrane and restores the cytoplasm and extracellular fluid to their original value after an action potential occurs. This action is in response to an imbalance between the cytoplasm and the extracellular fluid. When diffusion takes place, particles move from an area of greater concentration to an area of lesser concentration.

The following simplified description explains how this whole process works.

1. A neuron membrane is "at rest." There are larger amounts of potassium and negative ions inside the cell and a greater concentration of sodium and positive ions outide in the cytoplasm. The reverse is true outside the cell in the extracellular fluid. Most of the open channels are for potassium to pass through, so it leaks out of the cell.

2. As the K+ ions leave, the inside becomes relatively more negative until some K+ ions are attracted back in, the electrical force balances the diffusion force, and movement stops. The inside is still more negative, and the amount of energy between the two differently charged areas is ready to work (carry an impulse). This state is called *resting membrane potential* (Figure 11-30A). The membrane is now polarized. The sodium ions are not able to move in because their channels are closed during the resting state; however, if a few leak in, the membrane pump sends an equal number out.

3. Now suppose a sensory neuron receptor is stimulated by something, such as a sound. This will cause a change in the membrane potential. The stimulus energy is converted to an electrical signal, and, if it is strong enough, it will depolarize a portion of the membrane and allow the gated sodium ion channels to open (Figure 11-30B).

4. The sodium and positive ions move through the gated channels into the cytoplasm, and the inside becomes more positive until the membrane potential is reversed and the gates close to sodium ions.

5. Next, the potassium gates open, and large amounts of potassium and negative ions reenter the cell, resulting in the repolarization of the membrane (Figure 11-30C). After repolarization, the sodium-

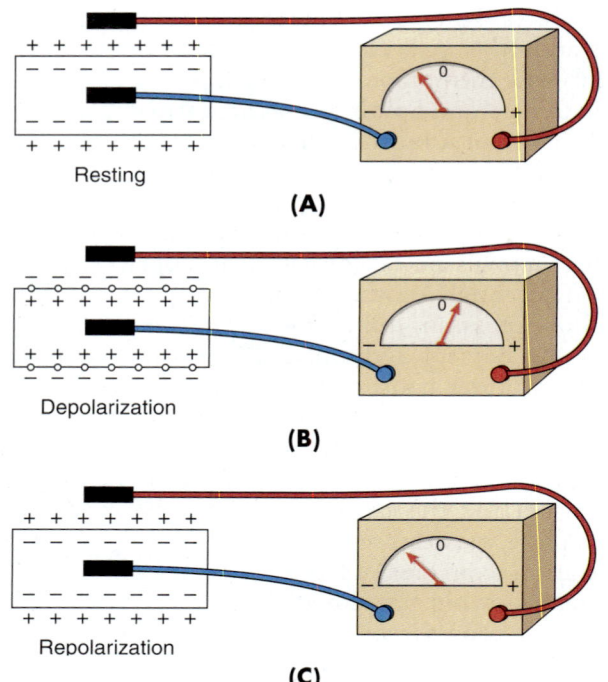

FIGURE 11-30   Sequence of events in membrane potential and relative positive and negative states: (A) Normal resting potential—negative inside, positive outside. (B) Depolarization—positive inside, negative outside. (C) Repolarization—negative inside, positive outside.

potassium pump restores the initial concentrations of sodium and potassium ions inside and outside the neuron.

This whole process occurs in a few milliseconds. When this action occurs in one part of the cell membrane, it spreads to adjacent membrane regions, continuing away from the original site of stimulation, sending "messages" over the nerve. This cycle is completed millions of times a minute throughout the body, day after day, year after year.

But what happens when the impulse reaches the end of the neuron? You will recall that impulses travel across a neuron from the dendrites to the cell body and then to the axon. Here there is a minute space between the dendrites of the next neuron called a **synapse**, which the impulse must "jump" chemically. This space is technically called a *synaptic cleft*. Impulses from the sending cell release chemical messengers called neurotransmitters into the cleft. These substances are signaling molecules that can cause a rapid change in the membrane potential of the receiving cell. These chemicals can either speed up or slow down the transmission. Normally nerve impulses travel about 200 miles per hour. The intake of alcohol, for instance, seems to aid the chemical that causes impulses to be blocked, and our reactions are therefore slowed down. Other chemicals, such as stimulant drugs and wartime nerve gases,

cause the release of a chemical that allows the transmission of impulses to speed up, even to the point of causing a flood of impulses to the brain resulting in the possible breakdown of the body's ability to function.

Scientists have discovered that a number of mental disorders are the result of imbalances in brain chemistry. This has resulted in the design of new medications for treating specific mental disorders and behavior problems. The best known of the new drugs is probably Prozac. It inhibits the sending cell from reabsorbing the chemical serotonin. Research indicated that depressed people had less serotonin than people who were not depressed, so by blocking its reuptake, the effect of a small amount of serotonin on the receiving cell is boosted (Figure 11-31).

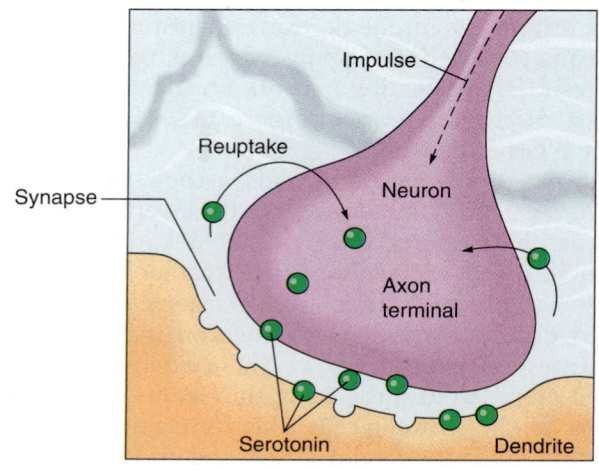

Before medication

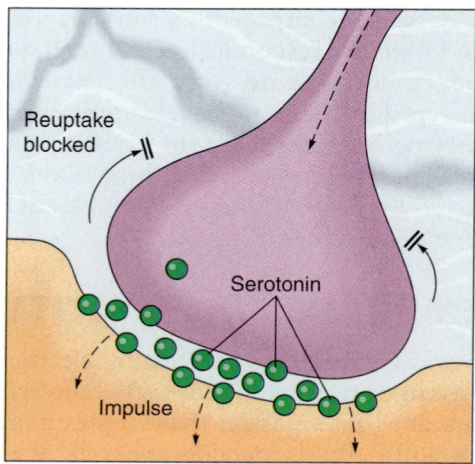

After medication

FIGURE 11-31   Transmission of a nerve impulse across a synapse is chemical. People who are depressed have less of the neurotransmitter serotonin. *Note:* The serotonin is released from the axon before the medication is reabsorbed by the sending cell. With the presence of a serotonin uptake inhibitor, such as Prozac, the reabsorption is blocked or slowed to increase the effect of serotonin of the receiving call.

A disease condition called tetanus results from the effects of the bacterium *Clostridium tetani* on the nervous and muscular systems. Bacteria invade the body through a puncture wound from a contaminated object or an animal bite. The tissues deep in the puncture do not receive oxygen, so they die off and the bacteria multiply. A substance is released by the bacteria that is toxic to the motor neurons that innervate the muscles. A neuron normally stimulates muscle tissue through *balanced chemical messages,* which alternately contract and relax the muscle tissue. This balance is essential to our ability to maintain erect stature and movement. However, with the release of the neurotoxin from the bacteria, excitation is unbalanced, and the inhibitory synapses of the motor neurons of the brain and spinal cord are affected, thereby allowing excessive contraction of the muscles. (Without the control of the "inhibitor," the message goes on full permission to contract.) The muscles cannot relax, and there is a prolonged, spastic paralysis of the muscles, which can result in death.

With these examples, it is apparent how the function of the nervous system affects the total welfare of the body. It is now important to learn how the nerves are organized in the communication network.

PERIPHERAL NERVOUS SYSTEM AND SPINAL CORD

The peripheral nervous system includes 12 pairs of cranial nerves that connect the brain directly to the sense organs (eye, ear, tongue, nose, and skin), the heart, the lungs, and other internal organs. Some cranial nerves, like the optic nerve from the eye, have only sensory fibers, whereas others, like those to the heart and lungs, are mixed nerves containing both sensory and motor fibers. The peripheral system also includes 31 pairs of spinal nerves. The spinal nerves are both motor, to provide a function or movement, and sensory, to perceive stimuli; therefore, they are also mixed nerves (Figure 11-32).

All spinal nerves enter and leave the spinal cord, which is located within the canal created by an opening in each of the bones (vertebrae) of the spinal column. A cross section of the cord would reveal a rounded white mass of myelinated nerve fibers with a notched area on the anterior surface (Figure 11-33). The white matter is mainly axons of **interneurons**. Some axons are grouped together into major sensory nerves going to a specific section of the brain. Others are grouped into major motor nerves going to their muscle or organ destination. Still others connect with each other up, down, and within the gray matter to provide control over activities that occur within the cord itself. In the center of the white area is a gray area in the shape of an H, which is the nerve cell bodies and their fibers without the myelin covering. The gray matter is involved mainly with reflex connections in the spinal cord that deal with the reflexes involved in such things as walking or blinking.

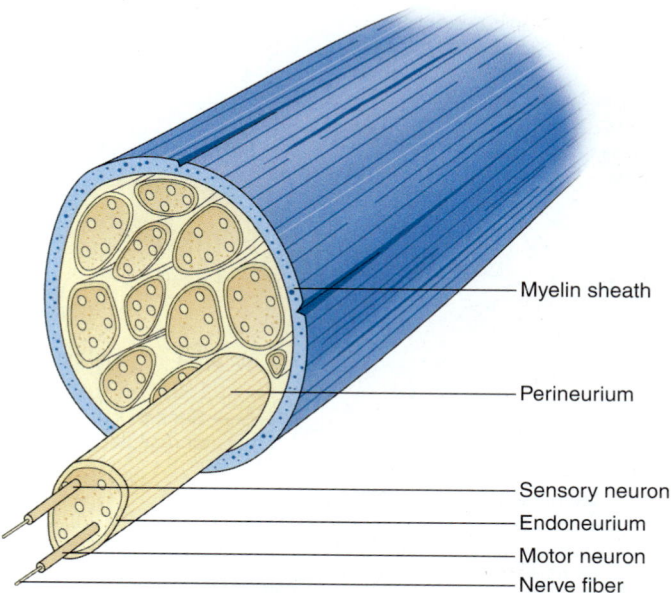

FIGURE 11-32　Cross section of a spinal nerve showing both sensory and motor nerves (greatly enlarged)

- Myelin sheath
- Perineurium
- Sensory neuron
- Endoneurium
- Motor neuron
- Nerve fiber

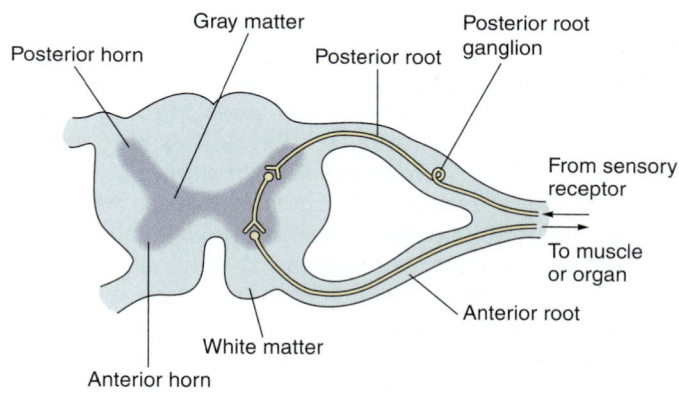

Gray matter
Posterior horn
Posterior root
Posterior root ganglion
From sensory receptor
To muscle or organ
Anterior root
White matter
Anterior horn

FIGURE 11-33　Cross section of the spinal cord

A spinal nerve splits into two roots as it enters the cord. The posterior root carrying sensory fibers to the cord enters at the posterior horn of the H. The bulge on the posterior root contains the sensory nerve cell bodies and is called a **ganglion**. The anterior root of the nerve leaves at the anterior horn of the H, carrying motor nerve fibers that have their cell bodies inside the gray matter of the cord. Neurons within the cord connect sensory to motor nerves.

Sensory neurons transmit messages from millions of special receptor cells to the spinal cord and on to the brain for interpretation and decisions. If a reaction is needed, impulses from the CNS are transmitted to the appropriate muscle or organ over the motor neurons. Connecting interneurons route impulses throughout the body, permitting any nerve to communicate with any other nerve.

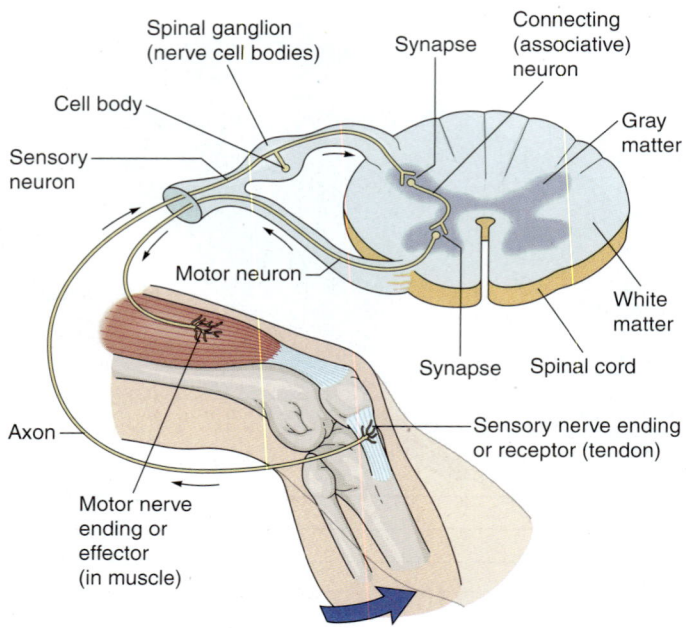

FIGURE 11-34 Reflex action. In this example, tapping the patellar tendon of the knee results in extension of the leg, producing the knee jerk reflex.

In very simple reflex actions in which no interpretation or decision is required, the nerve impulse travels only to the spinal cord and back. The knee jerk test often used by physicians illustrates such a simple reflex and provides an evaluation of the nervous system. When the knee is hanging completely relaxed, the leg should kick up sharply when the tendon below the kneecap is lightly tapped (Figure 11-34). If there is no response, a nervous system disease or disorder can be suspected.

In more complicated reflex actions, such as the body coming into contact with something harmful, the sensory impulse is relayed through nerve cells to the spinal cord and up to the brain (Figure 11-35). There the impulse is interpreted, and the motor neurons carry the message back down the spinal cord and out the appropriate motor nerves to the muscles and the legs move the body away.

Autonomic Nervous System

The autonomic nervous system is part of the peripheral nervous system. These nerves are involuntary and unconsciously regulate functions such as breathing, heartbeat, and digestion. The system consists of nerves, ganglia, and **plexuses** (networks of nerves). There are two divisions of the autonomic system. The **sympathetic** division accelerates activity in the smooth, involuntary muscles of the body's organs, and the **parasympathetic** division reverses the action and slows down activity. For example, the sympathetic nerves

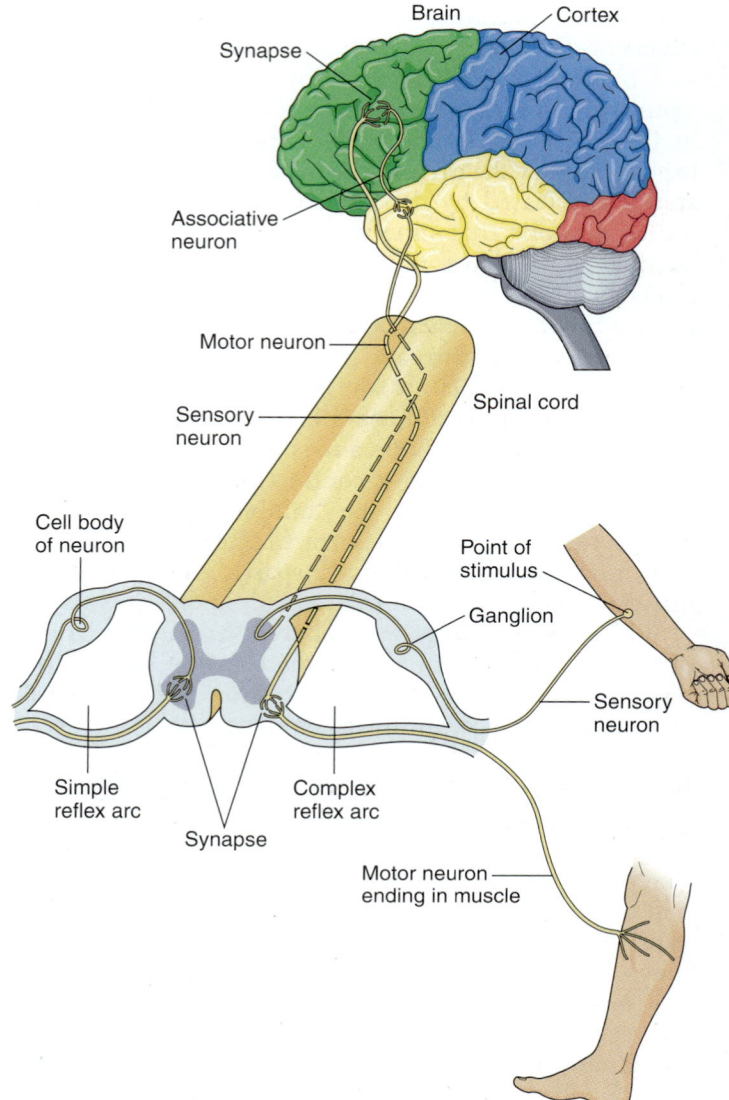

FIGURE 11-35 Complex reflex action

constrict blood vessels and speed up the heartbeat; the parasympathetic nerves dilate the blood vessels and slow down the heartbeat. These activities continuously balance each other to maintain homeostasis in the body. However, this on and off mechanism does not apply to all organs, because some do not have a dual nerve supply. Also, nerves in both divisions can have excitatory or inhibitory effects. At any given time, the actual effect depends on the net outcome of the two opposing signals.

The *sympathetic nervous system* begins at the base of the brain and runs down both sides of the spinal column in two tracts. These consist of nerve fibers and ganglia. The sympathetic nerves extend to all the vital internal organs, the blood vessels, the iris of the eye, and even to the sweat glands (Figure 11-36).

Sympathetic Outflow   **Parasympathetic Outflow**

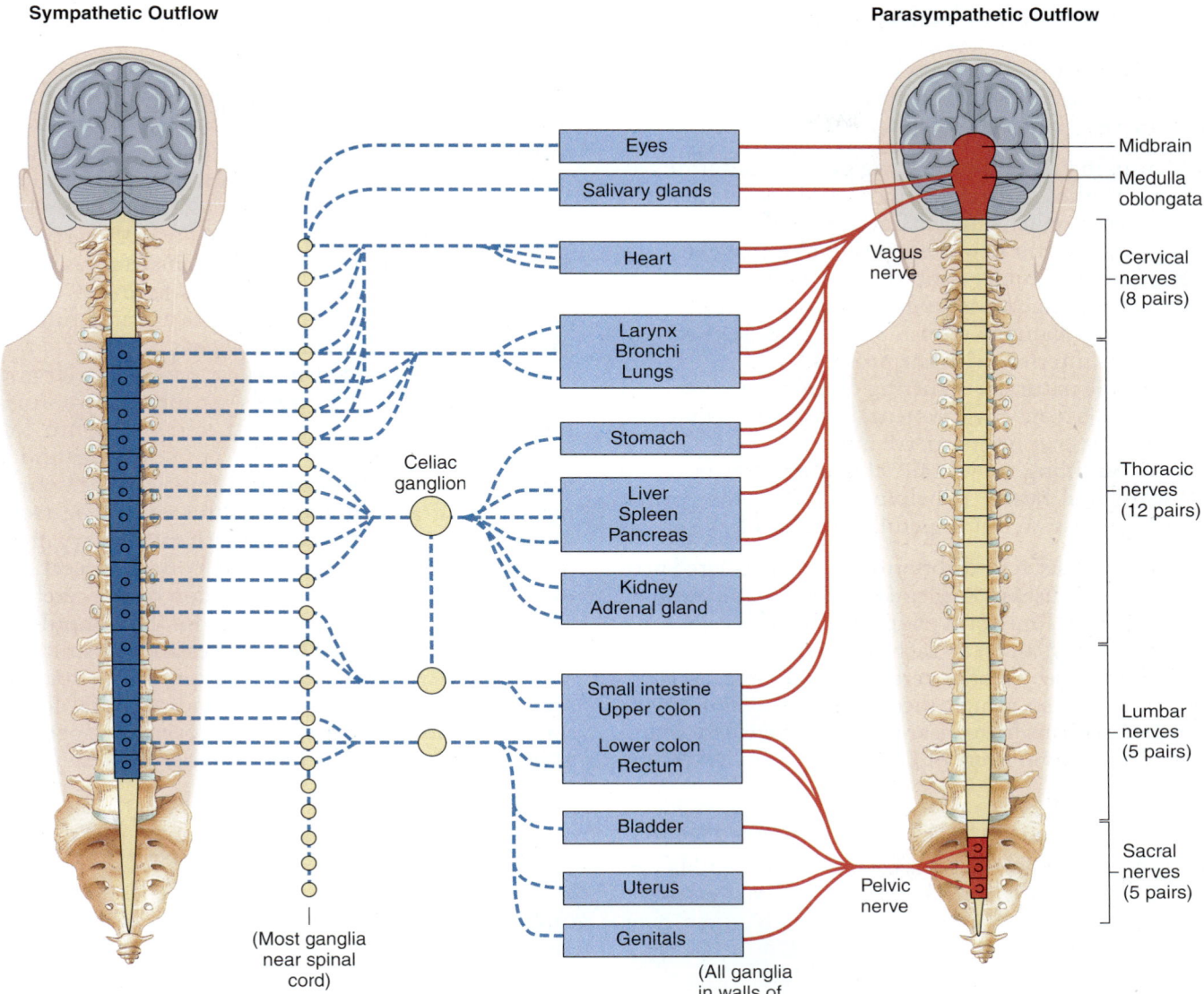

FIGURE 11-36 Autonomic nervous system. Shown here are the main sympathetic and parasympathetic pathways leading out from the central nervous system to some major organs. As the lists of examples suggest, in some cases, the sympathetic and parasympathetic nerves operate antagonistically in their efforts on the organ. Keep in mind that both systems have paired nerves leading out from the brain and spinal cord.

The *parasympathetic system* has two important nerves, the vagus and the pelvic nerve. The vagus extends from the medulla oblongata of the brain and branches to the neck, chest, and upper abdominal organs. The pelvic nerve exits the spinal cord around the hip area and branches into the lower abdominal and pelvic organs. Both systems are strongly affected by emotions such as fear, anger, and stress.

The action of the autonomic system is extremely important to our ability to react in an emergency. It is frequently called our "flight-fright mechanism" because it accelerates our body functions to permit escaping or otherwise dealing with danger.

CENTRAL NERVOUS SYSTEM

The Brain

The brain is a large mass of nerve tissue with about 100 billion neurons. Scientists call it the most complex and challenging structure ever studied. This small organ, weighing only about 3 pounds, is a mass of interconnecting nerve cells that "talk" to each other continuously in both chemical and electrical language. The new discoveries in genetics and the ability to view its structure with new sophisticated equipment is allowing scientists to begin to understand how the brain functions. They are learning how groups of specialized cells produce memory, language, emotion, perception, and other complex activities. Understanding how a healthy brain operates allows them to determine what goes wrong when disease strikes. The following discoveries are very exciting:

- Identifying disease-producing genetic mutations allows diagnosis of some inherited disorders and the ability to predict who will develop them. This knowledge will permit new therapies to alter the genes.
- Beginning to understand the programmed death of nerve cells that leads to degenerative diseases or expands the damage after a stroke may lead to new drugs to interfere with the process.
- Using the naturally occurring chemicals that protect nerve cells from environmental destruction may prevent disease or reverse nerve injury.
- Understanding how brain chemistry affects mood and mental health is helping not only the patient with depression but hopefully others as well.

Scientists have found abnormal genes associated with Huntington's disease, Alzheimer's disease, amyotrophic lateral sclerosis, one form of epilepsy, two types of muscular dystrophy, and Tay-Sachs disease, which *primarily* affects Jewish people of eastern European descent. However, there is also a high incidence among non-Jewish French Canadians living near the St. Lawrence River and in the Cajun community of Louisiana.

The Structure and Function of the Brain

The brain is protected and supported by surrounding membranes known as **meninges** (Figure 11-37). It is further protected by the **cranium** (skull). The brain surface has extensive deep furrows and folds and is divided into two hemispheres by a **longitudinal fissure**. The hemispheres are connected internally with nerve fibers and share information. The cerebral surface is covered with ridges and furrows known as *fissures* if they are deep or *sulci* if they are shallow. The elevated ridges between the sulci are called *convolutions*.

The brain is divided into five parts. The largest is the **cerebrum**, which controls sensory and motor activities. The cerebrum is further divided into lobes (Figure 11-38 A and B). The **frontal** lobe behind the forehead seems to be related to emotions, personality, moral traits, and intellectual functions. The frontal lobe is also the motor area for active voluntary muscle movements and two areas that control speech. The **occipital** lobe is the far back portion of the cerebrum. This area is associated with vision. The impulses of color and light received by the eyes are transmitted by the **optic** nerve fibers to the occipital lobe for interpretation. Between the frontal and occipital lobes is the **parietal** lobe; the motor area governing speech lies at its junction with the frontal lobe. It is the parietal

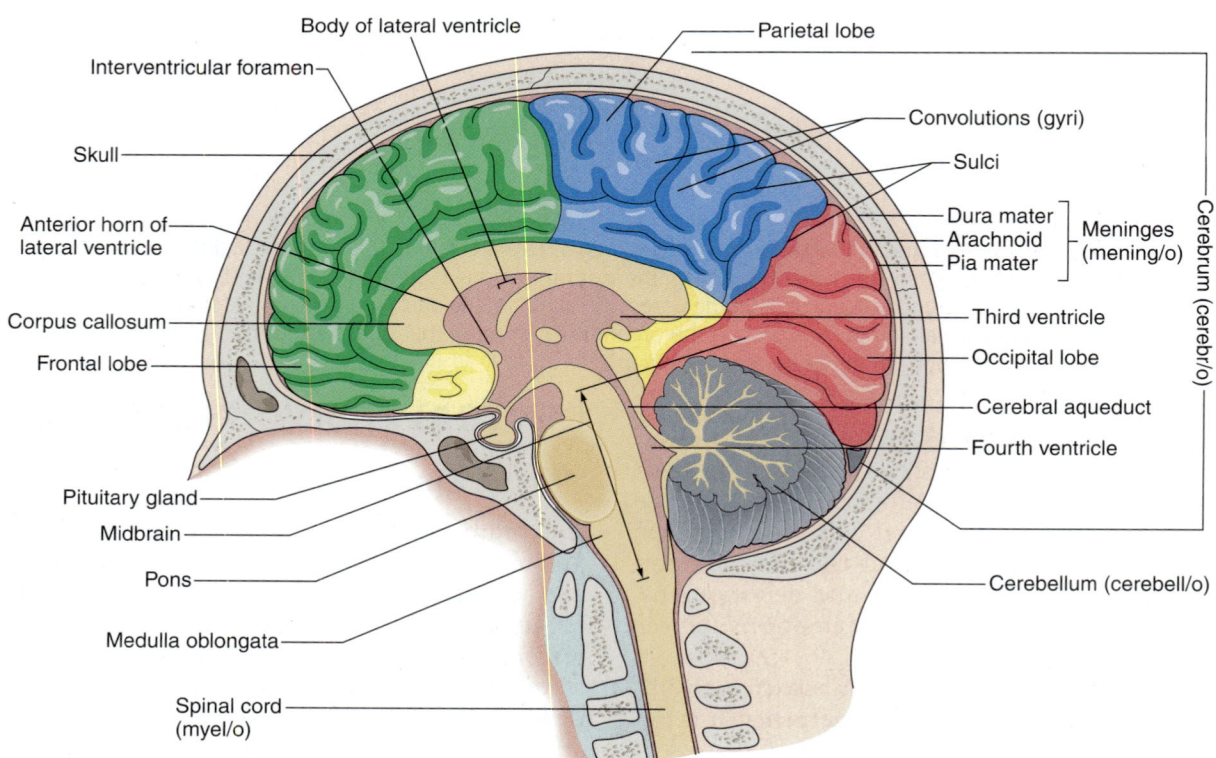

FIGURE 11-37   Cross-section of the brain

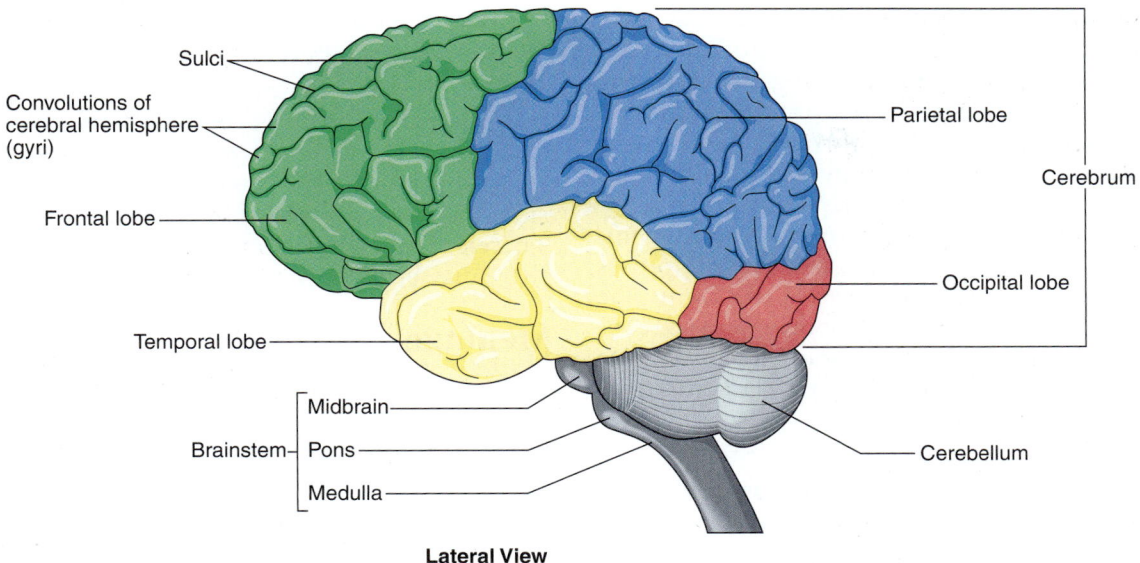

Lateral View

FIGURE 11-38A   The parts of the brain

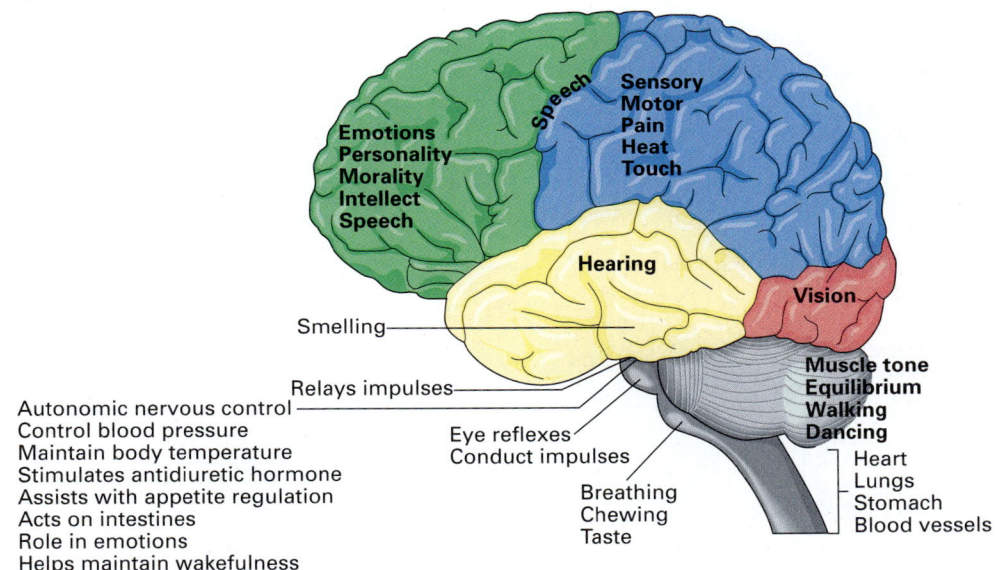

FIGURE 11-38B   Areas of brain function

lobe that receives impulses from receptors in the hands, feet, and tongue, among others, and sends impulses that cause movement in all these parts in response. This area also receives nerve impulses from sensory receptors for pain, touch, heat, and cold. A small **temporal** lobe lies on the side of the cerebrum. The **auditory** nerve association area is here, which provides us with the sense of hearing. The **olfactory** area, which provides our sense of smell, is within a small projection under the temporal lobe. It is connected by nerve fibers to receptors in the nasal cavity.

Beneath the cerebrum lies the part of the brain known as the **cerebellum**. This section is responsible for

smooth muscle movement, muscle tone, and coordination of sensory impulses with muscular activity, particularly for equilibrium, walking, and dancing. If the cerebellum is damaged, many activities requiring coordination of muscles cannot be performed.

The **medulla oblongata** is the part of the brain that adjoins the spinal cord. The medulla influences, through the autonomic nervous system, the function of the heart and lungs, stomach secretions, and the size of the openings in blood vessels.

Just above the medulla is the **pons**. This part of the brain also helps to regulate breathing. It is the reflex center for chewing, tasting, and secreting saliva. A small part called the **midbrain** is superior to the pons. This area is the control center for some of the reflex movements of the eyes, such as blinking and changing the size of the pupil. It also conducts impulses between the brain parts above and below it.

In an area between the cerebrum and the midbrain are two major structures, the **thalamus** and the **hypo-thalamus**. The thalamus acts as a relay station for impulses going to and from the brain and those impulses from the cerebellum and other parts of the brain. The hypothalamus lies below the thalamus and is connected to the pituitary gland, midbrain, and thalamus by a bundle of nerve fibers. The hypothalamus performs many vital functions:

1. Controlling the autonomic nervous system.
2. Controlling blood pressure by regulating the heartbeat and blood vessel constriction and dilation.
3. Maintaining body temperature.
4. Stimulating the production of an antidiuretic hormone to conserve water in the body and to cause thirst to maintain normal water balance.
5. Assisting in the regulation of appetite.
6. Increasing secretions and motility in the intestinal tract.

7. Playing a role in emotions such as fear and pleasure.
8. Helping maintain wakefulness when it is necessary.

The midbrain, the pons, and the medulla make up the brainstem. Doctors learned long ago that nerve fibers from the right side of the body cross over in the brainstem to the left side of the brain. The body's left side is likewise controlled by the right side of the brain. Therefore, when a person is paralyzed on the right side, there may be damage to the left side of the brain.

Meninges

Because of their common origin, the brain and the spinal cord are covered with the same meninges (membranes) (Figure 11-39). Three membrane layers make up the meninges. The innermost layer is called the **pia mater**, a delicate, tight-fitting covering containing blood vessels to nourish the nerve tissue. The middle layer, the **arachnoid**, is a delicate, lacelike membrane. The outer layer, called **dura mater**, is a tough, fibrous tissue that protects the CNS from being damaged from contact with the bony surfaces of the skull and spine. The space between the dura mater and the arachnoid is called the **subdural** space. The **subarachnoid** space is between the arachnoid and the pia mater.

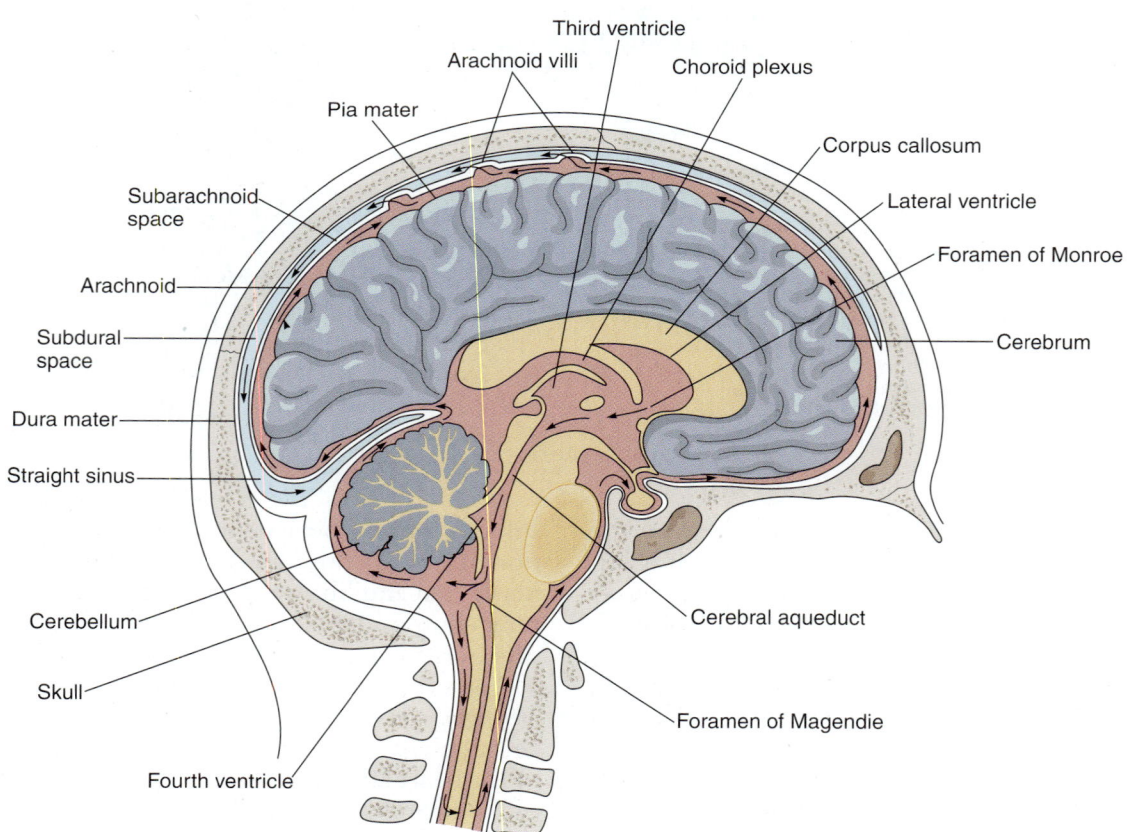

FIGURE 11-39 A diagrammatic representation of the meninges and the circulation of the cerebral spinal fluid from its formation in the choroid plexus until its return to the blood in the cranial sinus.

Cavities of the Brain and Spinal Cord

Within the brain are several hollow areas called **ventricles**. They extend into the lobes of the cerebrum and into contact with the other sections of the brain by means of small passageways. The central canal of the spinal cord is directly associated with the most inferior ventricle. There are also connections from the ventricles into the subarachnoid space of the meninges.

Cerebrospinal Fluid

The hollow cavities within the brain and spinal cord are filled with a liquid called **cerebrospinal fluid** (CSF). This fluid acts as a watery cushion or shock absorber to provide additional protection for the delicate tissues of the CNS. The fluid transports nutrients, primarily proteins, and carbohydrates to the brain and spinal cord. CSF is formed continuously within the ventricles of the brain at the rate of 450 mL (15 oz) per day. Only 150 mL are present at any one time in a normal adult. The fluid circulates within the cavities of the brain and spinal cord and the subarachnoid space, being reabsorbed into the blood vessels in special structures called *arachnoidal villi*.

DIAGNOSTIC TESTS

Diagnosis of neurologic disorders and diseases may require the use of specific tests. Some of the more common tests and a few possible findings are as follows:

- **Arteriography** (cerebral **angiography**)—A catheter (small tube) is inserted into an artery and threaded up to the carotid artery in the neck. A dye is injected through the catheter to show the cerebral blood vessels when x-rays are taken. This test can detect an aneurysm, hemorrhage, evidence of a cerebrovascular accident, and arteriosclerosis.

- **Coma scale**—The Glasgow Coma Scale (GCS) is an assessment tool used to describe the level of consciousness (Figure 11-40). Terms often used to indicate this state are semicomatose, stupor, lethargic, comatose, and others. The tool was developed in 1974 at the University of Glasgow to standardize what observers were reporting as evidence of the state of "coma" with head injury patients. The method is now acceptable in both European and American neurologic centers as a quick, accurate, and simple tool for evaluating neurologic status. The scale assesses three things: eye movement, verbal response, and motor response. The scale is based upon the need for more stimulation to induce a response in the patient. Paramedics may be trained to perform the grading at the accident scene or en route to alert the emergency room staff to the severity of the injury of the incoming patient. (This probably would not be encountered in the physician's office, but knowledge of the scale will be helpful in personal understanding and patient teaching.)

- **Computerized axial tomography (CAT or CT scan)**—A series of x-rays of layers of the brain to construct a three-dimensional picture. Useful for identifying tumors, bleeding, a blood clot, decrease in brain size, and brain edema. The machine is doughnut-shaped and was developed in the early 1970s. Today, CT scans can be equipped with spiral imaging to make images in seconds. The patient will have to remove earrings, any hair ornament, removable dental work, hearing aids, glasses, and any other item that might interfere with the test. After being positioned on the CT scan table, a special contrast material may be injected into the vein so that certain structures will appear on the CT scan images. The patient's head will then be positioned within the CT scan ring and immobilized with a band. The table moves slightly be-

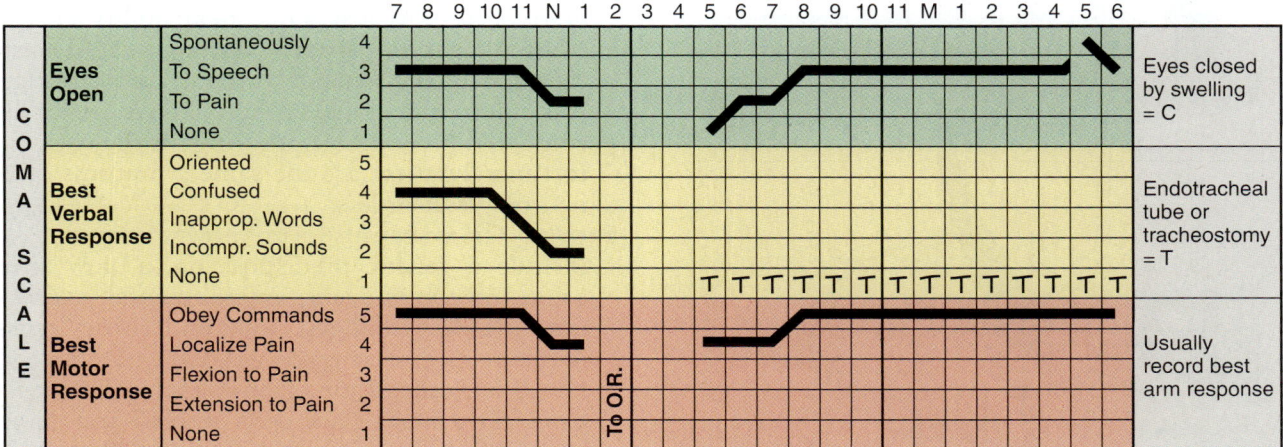

FIGURE 11-40　The Glasgow Coma Scale (GCS) includes three parts: assessment of eye opening, verbal response, and motor response. Each can be assessed hourly, given a numerical value, and plotted graphically.

tween each scan. It takes about 15 minutes to complete a head CT scan. (See Chapter 16, Unit 4.)

- **Electroencephalography (EEG)**—A brain wave test that measures the brain's electrical signals, both normal and abnormal. It can pick up abnormalities caused by epilepsy, a tumor, a stroke, a head injury, or infection. It can also document sleep disorders. It cannot detect mental retardation unless it is associated with seizures or brain atrophy. An EEG in retardation as well as in psychologic disorders is normal unless they are caused by a disease such as lupus. New technology has developed an ambulatory EEG monitor that helps diagnose neurological conditions, including fainting "spells" and seizures, by permitting continuous monitoring.
- **Electromyography** (EMG) and nerve conduction studies (NCS)—Electromyography (EMG) demonstrates the electrical activity of the peripheral muscles at rest and when activated by electrical stimulation of a small needle inserted into the muscle. NCS are done in conjunction with an EMG to measure the speed of nerve conduction. NCS are used to diagnose disorders like diabetic neuropathy and carpal tunnel syndrome.
- **Lumbar puncture**—A spinal needle is inserted into the subarachnoid space between the vertebrae of the lower back, and CSF is removed for examination (Figure 11-41A and B). The procedure is indicated when infection is suspected, when there is hemorrhage from injury, or when the fluid pressure must be measured. When measurement is desired, a calibrated glass tube is attached to the needle, and the level of the fluid is observed and recorded.
- **Magnetic resonance imaging (MRI)**—MRI was pioneered in 1977. The machine resembles a large white tube and uses radio waves and powerful magnets to make pictures. When images of the brain and spine are needed, MRI is the method of choice. Its main advantage is that it can image from numerous angles. (See Chapter 16, Unit 4.)
- **Myelography**—A lumbar puncture is performed to remove CSF and instill a dye to outline the structures on the x-ray. This will show irregularities or compression of the spinal cord.
- **Positron emission tomography (PET scan)**—A newer form of imaging that allows visualizing the physiologic performance of the body. An "agent" is labeled or "mixed with" a radioactive substance. Agents can be many things, such as glucose or any number of hormones. After the material is injected into the blood, images are recorded to measure where the material ends up in the body. The images are further enhanced by the use of color, which can be selected by the operator. The brighter the shade of the color, the greater the amount of uptake. The PET scan has been useful with conditions such as epilepsy and Alzheimer's disease.
- **Skull x-ray**—To identify fractures and dense areas that indicate a tumor or increased pressure within the skull.

DISEASES AND DISORDERS

Alzheimer's Disease (Alts'-hi-merz)

Description—This is a progressive, degenerative disease that attacks the brain and results in impaired memory, thinking, and behavior. It affects an estimated 4 million American adults. It is the most common form of dementia (loss of mental function). Alzheimer's is the 8th leading cause of death in United States, with 58,866 deaths recorded in 2002 by the Centers for Disease Control and Prevention.

Signs and symptoms—Evidence of the disease includes a gradual memory loss, a decline in ability to perform routine tasks, impairment of judgment, disorientation, personality change, difficulty in learning, and loss of language skills. The individuals eventually become totally incapable of caring for themselves. Unfortunately, these are the same symptoms of other neurologic disorders.

Etiology—The exact cause is unknown. Suspected causes include a genetic predisposition, a slow virus or other infectious agent, environmental toxins, and immunologic changes. The underlying cause of Alzheimer's disease is the gradual extinction of certain brain cells. Brains from people who have died from Alzheimer's have been studied and show abnormalities called amyloid plaques and neurofibrillary tangles. About 20% of all cases are inherited, and these people tend to develop symptoms earlier in life

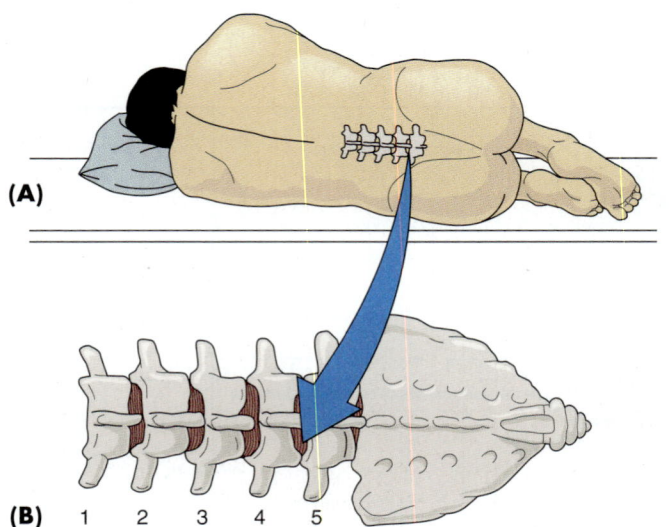

(A)

(B) 1 2 3 4 5

FIGURE 11-41 (A) Positioning of patient for limbar puncture; (B) site of lumbar puncture

than others. Scientists have also recently discovered several mutated genes that can cause the inherited form.

Treatment—There is no cure for Alzheimer's disease. Scientists are working on preventing the death of nerve cells. Unlike other types of cells, nerve cells cannot reproduce themselves—they were meant to last a lifetime. It is normal for some brain cells to be gradually lost, but when a large population of a certain type die over time, it causes problems. Researchers are looking at neuroprotectors to keep cells alive even when there is a stroke or spinal cord injury. Cells manufacture several neuroprotectors on their own. It is their hope to develop neuroprotective drugs that could guard brain cells against damage and death or perhaps even help them regenerate. In the meantime, appropriate medication continues to be used to lessen agitation, anxiety, and unpredictable behavior; improve sleeping; and treat depression. Physical exercise, social activity, good nutrition, and health maintenance are important. A calm and well-structured environment may help maintain the patient's sense of well-being. It is especially important to support and assist the family in dealing with this devastating disease. The course usually runs from 2 to 10 years, but it can take as long as 20 years. The roll of the caretakers is difficult and exhausting.

Currently, positive diagnosis of Alzheimer's is not possible until after death, when the brain can be examined for the telltale signs of amyloid plaque; therefore, there is no way to rule out other degenerative diseases. Recently, a cell abnormality in Alzheimer's patients has been found and may lead to early diagnosis and treatment. The cells were grown and tested in the laboratory and showed collapsed potassium channels in their membranes, a finding that occurred only in the Alzheimer's patients. Preliminary results are fairly reliable, and if after extensive clinical tests it appears to be diagnostic, it could save millions of dollars annually in diagnostic evaluations. Within the next 20 years, as the population ages, the incidence of the disease is expected to rise from the current level of about 4 million to approximately 12 million.

Although there is not yet a proven way to reverse or stop the disease, some promising treatments are being tested. A vaccine (AN-1792) is undergoing clinical tests in humans. The drug donepezil (Aricept), the herb ginkgo, and vitamin E have shown a slight slowing in the progress of the disease. In view of this, a recent panel's findings seem very important. After reviewing the current research on Alzheimer's, they came up with three "keys to cognitive vitality": (1) build reserve brain capacity, (2) acquire more knowledge, and (3) protect your brain from various forms of damage. It is possible to reduce the risk of Alzheimer's by following the eight steps to keep the brain function sharp:

1. Establish a brain reserve; think of it as a brain bank.
2. Exercise the body; it improves blood supply to the brain.
3. Eat well; it will protect against four potential causes: inflammation, oxidative stress, elevated homocysteine levels, and small strokes.
4. Consider a daily aspirin; some studies have identified it as a link to reduced risk.
5. Get enough folic acid through fortified foods or supplements because it keeps down serum levels of homocysteine. Alzheimer's patients have a higher than normal level.
6. Maintain a positive attitude, because it may help hold off cognitive decline.
7. Avoid tobacco and excess alcohol. Smokers are more than twice as likely to develop Alzheimer's. Alcohol appears to be protective if only consuming one to two drinks per day.
8. Treat chronic conditions that can affect cognitive function such as hypertension, heart disease, high cholesterol, diabetes, or depression.

The Alzheimer's Association publishes a list of 10 warning signs of the disease of which you should be aware. They are as follows:

1. Recent memory loss that affects job skills
2. Difficulty performing familiar tasks
3. Problems with language
4. Disorientation of time and place
5. Poor or decreased judgement
6. Problems with abstract thinking
7. Misplacing things (putting things in an inappropriate place, such as an iron in the refrigerator)
8. Changes in mood or behavior
9. Changes in personality
10. Loss of initiative

With the identification of genes that are believed to be involved with Alzheimer's, genetic engineering and manipulation may effectively correct or replace the defective gene to stop the progression and restore former function.

Amyotrophic Lateral Sclerosis (ALS) (A-mi-o-trof'ik) (Skle-ro'-sis) (Lou Gehrig's Disease)

Description—ALS is a progressive, fatal neurologic disease that causes degeneration of motor neurons of the brain and spinal cord. It strikes between ages 40 and 70 and causes muscle weakness, which leads to paralysis and death usually within 2 to 5 years of diagnosis. It affects 5,600 new people each year, with approximately 25,000 Americans having the disease at any given time. ALS is 20% more common in men than women, but with increasing age, it is more equally represented. About 10% of ALS cases are familial and can be passed on to children. The remaining 90% are known as sporadic ALS.

Signs and symptoms—The onset if insidious (slow and unnoticed) muscle weakness or stiffness are the early symptoms. As the weakness progresses, the muscles atrophy and paralysis begins as well as problems with speech, chewing, and swallowing. If the brainstem is involved, respirations will be affected, and occasional choking and excessive drooling will result. Mental deterioration does not usually occur; therefore, the patient is acutely aware of the progressive physical deterioration, so depression caused by the consequences of the disease may develop.

Etiology—The cause of sporadic ALS is unknown. There is much speculation about a combination of genetic and environmental factors that perhaps cause a mutation that leads to the disease. On the other hand, some cases of familial ALS (FALS) have been shown to be linked to a defective gene on chromosome 21 that produces excessive copper-containing enzymes that appear to lead to the death of nerve cells in the brain and spinal cord. Studies have indicated that over 60 mutations can interfere with the enzyme's ability to protect against free radical damage. FALS seems to run in families and can be passed on to children; however, there is no definite hereditary pattern. Scientists hope to soon identify what causes the mutant proteins to produce chemicals (oxidants) that interfere with the cell's ability to protect itself.

Treatment—No effective treatment is available, only methods to control symptoms and provide emotional and physical support. Rehabilitation techniques, assistive devices, and respiratory support can enhance the quality of life. Late in 1995 a drug called Rilutek was approved. It has shown scientifically that it can prolong the life of persons with ALS by at least a few months. The drug, the first to alter the course of the disease, slows the progress of ALS, allowing the patient more time in the higher functioning state of the disease.

Bell's Palsy (Pawl'-ze)

Description—This disease affects the seventh cranial nerve of the face. It occurs suddenly and will usually spontaneously subside within 1 to 9 weeks.

Signs and symptoms—The affected nerve results in weakness or paralysis on one side of the face, which causes the mouth to droop on the affected side, resulting in the drooling of saliva. There is a distorted sense of taste and an inability to close the affected eye. Occasionally, pain in the area of the jaw's angle may be present.

Etiology—The cause is unknown for certain, but most scientists believe it results from a viral infection that inflames the facial nerve.

Treatment—Early treatment with steroids and an antiviral medication, such as valacyclovir (Valtrex), may shorten the course. Prednisone is usually prescribed in a high dose and then quickly reduced over 7 to 10 days. Moist heat applied to the face and jaw helps relieve any pain, but care must be taken to avoid burning the skin. It may be advisable to protect the eye with an eye patch while outdoors, or if exposed to dust or pollutants, and while sleeping.

Cerebral Palsy (Se-re'-bral)

Description—This disorder is a nonprogressive brain injury that occurs during fetal development, perinatally, or in early infancy. Its incidence is at the rate of 2.5 per 1,000 live births, or about 8,000 per year. There are four forms of the disorder: spastic (50% to 75% of the cases), athetoid (15% to 20%), atonic (10%), and mixed.

Signs and symptoms—Characteristics of the spastic form are hyperactive tendon reflexes, rapid alteration between muscular contraction and relaxation, contracture tendency (permanent muscle shortening), and underdevelopment of the affected extremities. Approximately 40% of the children affected are also mentally retarded, 25% have seizures, and 80% have speech impairment.

Etiology—Cerebral palsy is probably caused by conditions that resulted in a lack of oxygen to the brain, hemorrhage, or brain damage. Prenatal conditions that may be associated with cerebral palsy include rubella (German measles), toxemia, maternal diabetes, and malnutrition. Cerebral palsy may be caused by hypoxia during fetal development, infections, or trauma. There is a higher incidence in low birth weight and premature infants. Maternal smoking and alcohol are risk factors.

Treatment—There is no cure for cerebral palsy, only supportive treatment including physical, occupational, and speech therapy; psychologic assistance; braces or splints; perhaps orthopedic surgery for severe contractures; muscle relaxers; and, when indicated, barbiturates and anticonvulsants to control seizures.

Encephalitis (En-sefa-li'tis)

Description—This is a severe brain inflammation that causes edema and nerve cell destruction. The onset is sudden and acute.

Signs and symptoms—Symptoms include fever, headache, and vomiting with progression to stiff neck and back, drowsiness, and eventually restlessness, convulsions, and coma.

Etiology—It is usually caused by a virus-bearing mosquito or tick. It can also be contracted from viruses that cause chickenpox, herpes, or mumps or following measles, rubella, or mononucleosis.

Treatment—The disease is treatable with supportive drug therapy to control restlessness and convulsions, reduce edema, and relieve headache. Antiviral agents are ineffective except against herpes virus encephalitis.

Epilepsy (Ep'-i-lep-se)

Description—This seizure disorder affects 1% to 2% of the population. It is associated with abnormal electrical impulses from the neurons of the brain.

Signs and symptoms—The disorder is characterized by either petit or grand mal seizures. Petit mal seizures are of short duration and mild. Grand mal seizures may last up to 5 minutes with convulsions, loss of control of bodily functions, and unconsciousness.

Diagnosis is made based on evidence of seizure characteristics, a positive EEG, and various x-ray procedures.

Etiology—It is believed to be caused by either abnormal brain chemistry or several other possibilities, including prematurity, anoxia (lack of oxygen), meningitis, encephalitis, ingestion of toxins (mercury, lead, carbon monoxide), brain tumor, PKU, head injury, and stroke.

Treatment—Treatment consists of drug therapy to control the seizures and psychological support.

Essential Tremor

Description—This is the most common movement disorder: an involuntary shaking of the hands and head, which is made worse by action or movement. It affects between 3 and 4 million people in the United States, usually beginning in the 30s or 40s with mild symptoms and becoming troublesome by the 50s. This common and benign condition is often confused with Parkinson's disease even though symptoms differ.

Signs and symptoms—Initially, mild shaking is noticed when trying to hold silverware to eat, thread a needle, drink from a glass, or perform writing tasks. The hands shake when trying to make movements, and the head may move in a yes-yes or no-no motion. The voice may also become shaky. Symptoms may worsen, but fortunately they can be controlled with medication. With Parkinson's, the hands shake at rest, and head motions are very infrequent. Also,

writing with essential tremor results in large and scrawled letters, whereas Parkinson's causes progressively smaller and shakier handwriting within a piece of correspondence.

Etiology—The cause is unknown, but it is generally accepted to be a disorder of the nervous system. It is usually inherited, and each child of a person with essential tremor has a 50% chance of developing the disorder.

Treatment—The disorder can be treated with the beta-blocker propanolol (Inderal) or an antiseizure medication such as primidone (Mysoline). These can be taken daily or may be used only on occassions such as dining out. The severity of tremors is reduced about 60% by the drugs. Other antiseizure drugs and tranquilizers can also be tried. If the tremors become severe, a device can be implanted in the brain that delivers a mild electrical stimulation to block the signals causing the tremor. An unusual treatment may be the therapeutic use of alcoholic beverages. Essential tremor is usually relieved by alcohol and in fact alcohol can be used as a low-tech way to rule out other causes of tremor. Some doctors hesitate to recommend alcohol as a treatment because of the potential for abuse, but with no history of alcoholism, liver, or kidney disease, one to two drinks a day can relieve the tremor.

Headache

Headaches are commonly classified as vascular, muscle contraction (tension), or traction-inflammatory. Both muscle contraction and traction-inflammatory types cause dull, persistent aching and a feeling of a tight band around the head, with tender spots on the head or neck. Most chronic headaches result from tension that may be caused by emotional stress, fatigue, or environmental conditions. Other causes include inflammation of the sinuses, diseased teeth, and muscle spasms of the neck and shoulder.

Vasodilators, such as nitrates, alcohol, and histamine, expand arteries, causing pressure against the brain's nerve endings, and are often the causative factors. Many people are affected by anything aged or fermented, such as cured or processed meats and wine, especially red wine. Other foods or additives cause headaches by the vasoconstricting action of amines in such things as MSG, chocolate, and aspartame. A condition known as hypoglycemia (low blood sugar) can result in vasodilation and headaches but can be easily avoided by eating three meals a day, preferably five smaller ones.

Headache—Migraine (Mi'-gran)

Description—This is a severe throbbing pain that occurs more frequently in people with compulsive personalities and within families. About 16 to 18 million Americans suffer from **migraines**; approximately 75% are women.

Signs and symptoms—It is frequently characterized by prodromal (beginning) symptoms, which may include fatigue, visual disturbances (such as zig-zag lines and bright lights), sensory symptoms (such as tingling of the face and lips), and sometimes motor symptoms like staggering. Usually the extreme pain is accompanied by sensitivity to light, nausea, and vomiting. It is usually on one side of the head, can occur suddenly, and will last from a few hours to a few days.

Etiology—The headache is caused by the initial constriction and then dilation of the blood vessels in the brain. There are "triggers" that seem to initiate migraines, which must be avoided if possible. They include chocolate, red wine, bright light, and sleeping late.

Treatment—Migraine incidence and severity can be decreased by diet and exercise. Medication can also reduce frequency and intensity. Ergotomine, especially with caffeine, seems to be fairly effective if taken early; it is available in suppository form if vomiting prevents oral administration. There is no cure for migraine headaches, only control. Drugs known as beta blockers and tricyclic antidepressants appear to be effective in prevention.

The drug sumatriptan (Imitrex) is considered to be nearly "diagnostic" in that if the headache is a migraine, the medication is effective. It is non-narcotic and will stop a full-blown migraine. Previously, the drug required injecting, but now it is available in an oral and nasal spray form. The sumatriptan in pill form will stop the migraine within 2 hours for 50% to 70% of the sufferers and by injection within 1 hour, with effectiveness rate up to 80%. A second dose, by either means, is usually necessary within 24 hours to keep the migraine from returning. Another drug called dihydroergotamine mesylate (DHE), usually given only in emergency rooms, is now available in a nasal spray form. The spray DHE is effective in 60% to 70% of people within 3 hours. People usually repeat the spray every 20 to 60 minutes, up to six or eight times, in order to get full relief. There are specific limitations and significant side effects that must be considered.

When an attack occurs it seems best to lie quietly in bed in a darkened room until the symptoms subside. Limited relief may be obtained from regular analgesics, and some people feel an ice bag to the head and a wet cloth over the eyes and forehead are beneficial. Usually, it is just a matter of waiting out the episode.

When headaches are frequent, unusual (such as causing awakening in the middle of the night), persistent, or become increasingly more intense, medical attention should be sought. It is important to rule out the presence of pathology such as an aneurysm, abscess, intercranial bleeding, or tumor.

Herpes Zoster (Her'-pez Zos'-ter) (Shingles)

Description—This is an acute usually unilateral inflammation of the dorsal root ganglion (see Unit 4).

Signs and symptoms—It is characterized by fluid-filled vesicle lesions on the skin and severe pain from the affected nerve. The onset is characterized by fever and discomfort followed by severe deep pain, itching, and abnormal skin sensations. The vesicles erupt in about 2 weeks, spreading around the **thorax** or vertically on the extremities. The episode may last from 1 to 4 weeks.

Etiology—Shingles is caused by the same herpes virus that causes chickenpox. The virus has reactivated after lying dormant in the ganglion since a previous episode of chickenpox. Why this occurs is not clear; however, it may follow trauma, malignancy, and local radiation and is commom in individuals with diabetes. Occasionally, there is no known factor.

Treatment—Treatment consists of medication, sometimes even narcotics, to relieve the pain and itching, plus an antiviral to reduce the length of viral shedding.

Hydrocephalus (Hi-dro-sef'-a-lus)

Description—This excessive accumulation of CSF within the ventricles of the brain occurs most frequently in newborns. The increased fluid compresses the brain tissue against the skull, resulting in brain damage.

Signs and symptoms—Hydrocephalus is characterized by an abnormally enlarged head; distended scalp veins; fragile, shiny scalp skin; a high-pitched, shrill cry; irritability; and vomiting.

Etiology—Hydrocephalus results from either the overproduction of CSF or the lack of its absorption. Either results in excessive fluid and the enlargement of the brain. Because the newborn skull is not completely hardened, it expands to accommodate the extra fluid, resulting in the characteristic appearance.

Treatment—Surgery is the only treatment for hydrocephalus. A shunt (passageway) is inserted into a ventricle in the brain to drain off excess fluid into either the peritoneal cavity of the abdomen or the atrium (upper chamber) of the heart for absorption by the body (Figure 11-42A). The ventriculoperitoneal (VP) shunt is the most common (Figure 11-42B).

Meningitis (Men-in-ji′-tis)

Description—This is an inflammation of the meninges of the brain and spinal cord. It may be viral or bacterial. Mortality is 70% to 100% if bacterial meningitis is left untreated.

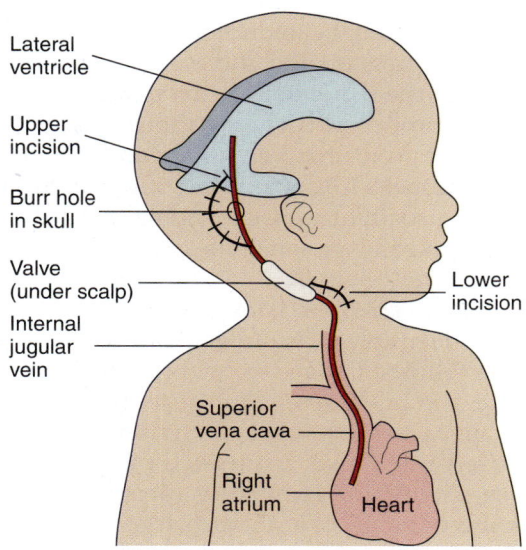

FIGURE 11-42A   The ventriculoatrial shunt drains spinal fluid into the circulation in the heart.

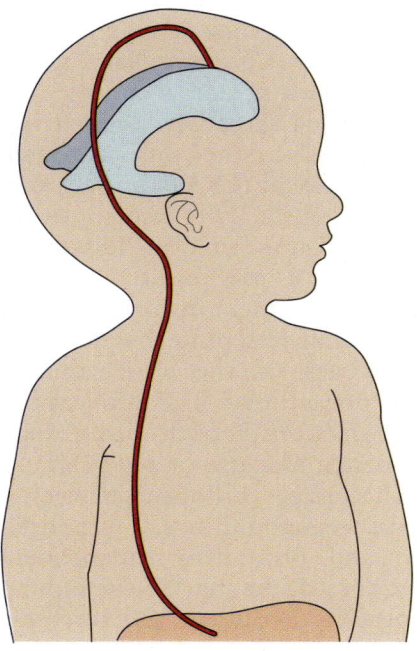

FIGURE 11-42B   The ventriculoperitoneal (VP) shunt drains spinal fluid into the peritoneum.

Signs and symptoms—Meningitis is characterized by a high fever, chills, headache, vomiting, and specifically by positive Brudzinski's and Kernig's signs (Figure 11-43). Brudzinski's sign is demonstrated by the flexing of the hips and knees when the head and neck of a dorsal recumbent person are raised and pulled forward. Kernig's sign is demonstrated by pain and resistance when the knee is straightened after flexing at the thigh and knee.

Diagnosis of meningitis is confirmed by a lumbar puncture that shows elevated pressure, cloudiness from the excess white cells, and identification of the causative organism after culturing.

Etiology—Meningitis is usually caused by a bacterial infection from the ears, sinuses, or lungs (pneumonia) or an abscess of the brain. Aseptic meningitis may result from a virus or other microorganism. At times, the cause is unknown.

Treatment—Treatment consists of antibiotics, medication to reduce cerebral edema, pain relievers for headache, and an anticonvulsant. Isolation may be indicated in certain instances.

Multiple Sclerosis (MS) (Skle-ro′sis)

Description—This is a demyelinating disease of the nervous system that attacks young men and women in the prime of life. It affects the central nervous system

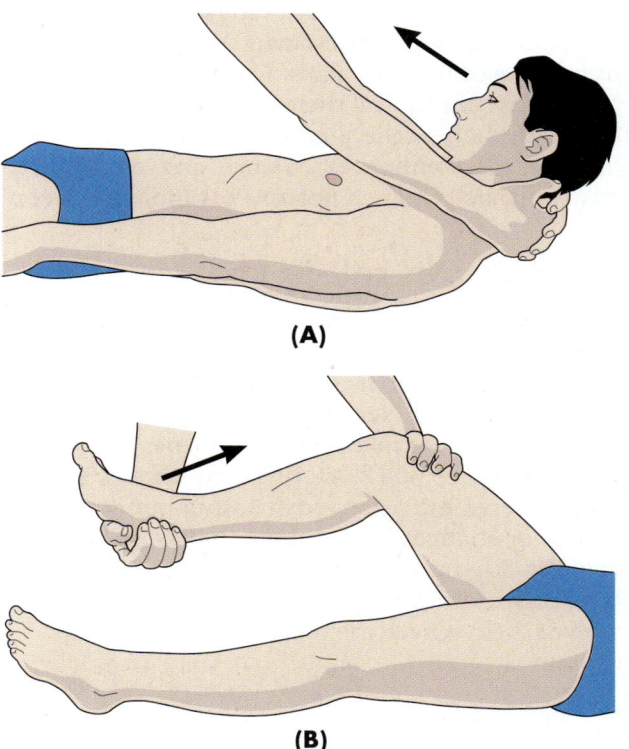

FIGURE 11-43   Two telltale signs of meningitis: (A) Brudzinski's sign; (B) Kernig's sign

and is usually first diagnosed between the ages of 20 and 40. It is estimated that 500,000 Americans have MS or a related disorder. It causes a heavy economic burden on affected families because a great many people with MS are unable to work.

Signs and symptoms—The symptoms depend upon the site of nerve damage but may include paralysis, numbness, double vision, foot dragging, loss of balance, extreme weakness, hand tremors, speech and hearing difficulties, bladder and bowel problems, and "pins and needles" sensations. Multiple sclerosis patients may go into remission after just one episode, but most patients have a history of remissions and exacerbations with eventual progressive worsening.

Etiology—The disease attacks the myelin sheaths of the nerves, destroying patches that are replaced by scar tissue that distorts or interrupts the passage of nerve impulses. Much of the current research is based upon the idea that the disease is probably the result of a reactivated, dormant, slow-acting virus; an autoimmune response; or both. There is evidence that environmental factors play a role, but genetic factors may also determine a predisposition to MS. Viruses currently being considered are those from measles, mumps, chickenpox, and parainfluenza.

Treatment—Treatment consists of adrenocorticotropic hormone (ACTH) and steroids to relieve symptoms and hasten remission. Drugs for the emotional swings, urinary problems, and muscular spasticity are used as required. Bed rest to prevent fatigue is important during acute phases. The new drug Avonex, an interferon, is being used to treat relapsing forms of the disease.

The use of physical therapy is helpful. It optimizes strength, helps relieve some of the stiffness in the muscles and enhances balance and endurance. It also appears to have a positive psychologic effect.

Neuralgia (Nu-ral'-je-ah)

Description—This is a term used to describe general nerve pain. It is further classified in relation to the area of the body that is affected.

Signs and symptoms—Neuralgia causes severe pain along the course of the involved nerve or nerves.

Etiology—This results from pressure on nerve trunks, faulty nerve nutrition, toxins, inflammation of the nerve, or changes in the root ganglia.

Treatment—Medications, the use of heat, physical therapy, rest, or stretching, depending upon the nerve involved, help relieve the pain.

Paralysis

Paralysis is a term used to describe the temporary or permanent loss of voluntary function in a portion of the body. Any voluntary movement depends on the integrity

of the motor neurons—the upper neurons in the brain, the lower neurons in the spinal cord, and those axons passing to the muscle. Paralyses are divided into two general groups: spastic, if caused by upper motor neurons, and flaccid, if caused by lower motor neurons. There are many forms of paralysis, but for the purpose of this unit, the term is being used to identify the condition following an injury or destruction of nerve tissue in the brain or spinal cord. Three general classifications will be discussed: hemiplegia, paraplegia, and quadriplegia. *Caution:* It is extremely important to prevent damage to the brain and spinal cord. The possibility of a stroke, which damages the brain, can be reduced with proper exercise, healthy blood pressure and cholesterol, refraining from smoking, and the reduction in stress. Injury can be prevented with proper instruction, applying safety principles, the use of protective gear, not driving after drinking, and using seat belts. Unfortunately, once damage has occurred, it is usually irreversible. Spinal cord damage is devastating and changes one's life *forever*.

Hemiplegia (Hem-e-ple'je-a)

Description—Hemiplegia is unilateral (one-sided) paralysis that follows damage to the brain. Because nerves cross in the brainstem, damage to the right side of the brain causes left-sided paralysis, whereas damage to the left side causes right-sided paralysis.

Signs and symptoms—Hemiplegia produces unilateral weakness or paralysis of the arm, leg, face, and tongue. It may be sudden, if caused by a stroke or injury, or gradual, if caused by a tumor or disease. The paralysis begins as flaccid but often progresses to spastic. Hemiplegics often have difficulty understanding oral or written language, may develop muscle shortening and foot drop, have a decreased level of consciousness, and may experience problems eating.

Etiology—Hemiplegia is caused by any injury to the brain or one side of the spinal cord, such as cerebrovascular accident (CVA or stroke), a tumor, CNS infection, a degenerative disease, or trauma (see CVA, Unit 8). If the damage is less severe, weakness instead of paralysis may result.

Treatment—Early treatment involves preventing further involvement and lessening the effects of the damage, which varies with the cause. Later treatment focuses on prevention of complications such as muscle contractions, foot drop, and spastic muscular movements. The use of physical, occupational, and speech therapy; orthopedic devices; and modifications in the surroundings are important to rehabilitation and promoting independence (Figure 11-44). At age 44, the man in the Figure 11-44 suffered a near-fatal rupture of a cerebral aneurysm, which severely damaged the left side of his brain. Initially he was not expected to survive, but with time he regained some physical functions. He was

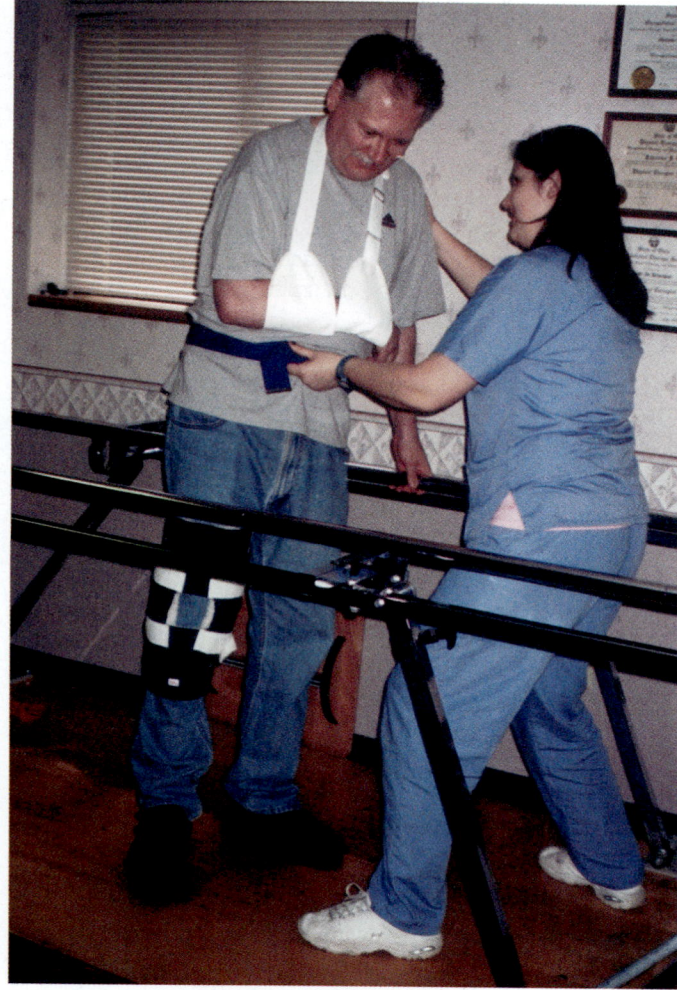

FIGURE 11-44   Physical therapy can be helpful for the hemiplegic patient following a stroke on the left side of his brain that affected the right side of his body. *(Courtesy Mayfair Village Nursing and Rehab Center, Dublin, OH)*

Signs and symptoms—The onset of total or partial paralysis is immediate in most patients, with the loss of motion, sensation, and reflexes below the level of damage. With complete spinal cord injury, there is lack of sensation or voluntary muscle control that persists for 24 hours; any return of functional muscle activity below the injury is unlikely. There is usually loss of bladder, bowel, and sexual function. With incomplete damage, the patient can still sense the perianal area, flex the toes, and control the bladder and bowels.

Etiology—Paraplegia usually results from trauma that occurs with automobile, motorcycle, and sporting accidents; gunshot wounds; and falls. Conditions such as spina bifida and cerebral palsy may also cause paralysis.

Treatment—It is important that treatment starts at the time of the accident. The patient must be strapped on a board before any movement occurs to prevent additional spinal cord injury. The spine must be realigned and any fractures reduced. Compression of the cord and nerves must be relieved. Surgery may be required to repair fracture dislocations and remove bone fragments. A urinary catheter is installed to drain urine. Extensive care to maintain the skin, monitor fluids, and promote good nutrition and medications to prevent infection and control muscle spasms are required. Rehabilitation to promote as much activity as is possible begins early. Psychological support is very important. The final extent of paralysis cannot be accurately evaluated until 2 years following the injury.

Quadriplegia (Quah-drih-plee'-jee-ah)

Description—The devastating permanent paralysis affecting all body systems, the arms, the legs, and all of the body below the level of the injury to the spinal cord. The injury is usually the result of a trauma. It affects about 150,000 Americans, most being men between the ages of 20 and 40.

Signs and symptoms—Quadriplegia is evidenced by the flaccid or spastic appearance of the arms and legs and the loss of sensation and movement below the level of the injury. If the cord is damaged above the fifth cervical vertebrae of the neck, body systems also will be dramatically affected. This type of injury would produce symptoms such as:

Low blood pressure from the blocking of the sympathetic nervous system

Low body temperature caused by dilated surface blood vessels, which allows heat to escape

Slow heart rate caused by absence of sympathetic system inhibiting action

Respiratory system involvement, which may require mechanical support

Etiology—Paralysis results from spinal cord injury in the cervical vertebrae. It is usually the result of automo-

unable to stand. With therapy he managed to go from a wheelchair to a walker and then to a cane. Now 6 years later, he can walk alone and wears only a small brace on his right ankle. He has lost most of the use of his right hand.

Paraplegia (Par-a-ple'-je-a)

Description—This is the loss of motor or sensory function in the lower extremities, usually from trauma, with or without involvement of the abdominal and back muscles. The paralysis may be permanent or temporary, spastic or flaccid. Almost half of the 10,000 to 12,000 spinal cord injuries each year result in paraplegia. It occurs twice as often in males as in females, with the highest incidence between the ages of 16 and 35.

bile, motorcycle, or sporting activities accidents; gunshot wounds; or falls. Diving and gymnastics are common causes. The dangers of horseback riding became apparent in 1995 with the extensive injury to actor Christopher Reeve, which in a few seconds changed his life forever.

Treatment—Again, treatment begins at the scene of the accident with immobilization of the neck and spine. Following hospitalization, tongs or a halo traction are attached to the skull to pull the neck into alignment and stabilize the spine. Treatment is aimed at reducing the edema (swelling) of the spinal cord, thereby relieving pressure on the spinal nerves. An artificial airway will be required if injury is above the 5th vertebra, and ventilation assistance will be necessary. After about 10 days, surgery is done to fuse vertebrae and remove any fragments. Unfortunately, many functional problems will occur. Some of the more common are:

- Maintaining open airway and adequate respiration
- Providing adequate fluids and nutrition
- Excessively slow heart rate and resulting low blood pressure
- Low body temperature, perhaps to less than 90° F, which will require warming with blankets
- Extremely high blood pressure, which may lead to heart failure and intracranial bleeding when injury is above the 4th vertebra

The greatest challenge comes from the enormous change in the individual's life. If there is an artificial airway, the patient may not be able to even speak. Paralysis requires extensive emotional, physical, and social support, not only for the affected individual but also for the entire family and circle of friends.

Extensive research continues to find ways of restoring function to damaged nerves. A great deal of discussion regarding the possibilities of stem cell applications is giving these individuals some glimmer of hope.

Parkinson's Disease

Description—This is a common progressive crippling disease affecting about one in every 100 people over age 60, which translates to about 60,000 new cases annually in the United States. It affects men more often than women. It progresses for about 10 years until pneumonia or another infection results in death.

Signs and symptoms—The main symptoms are the muscle rigidity and tremor of the hand, described as "pill-rolling." The disease produces a high-pitched, monotone voice and a masklike expression. As it progresses, the condition is characterized by severe muscle rigidity, a peculiar gait, drooling, and a progressive tremor. The body becomes bent forward, with head bowed. The steps become faster and faster with increasing forward body inclination, which often results in falling.

Etiology—The cause of Parkinson's disease is unknown; however, it has been established that a deficiency in dopamine prevents affected brain cells from functioning properly. Some researchers have noted some forms may be caused by a viral infection experienced many years earlier.

Treatment—There is no known cure for the disease, although a drug called levodopa relieves most of the symptoms until the necessarily increased dosage begins to cause serious side effects. In selected patients, surgical procedures can either freeze, electrically coagulate, or radioactively destroy a small area of the brain to prevent the involuntary motions.

Surgical options are appropriate only for those in good health, who are relatively young (under age 70), no longer able to tolerate medication, and have specific symptoms. A thalamotomy, which destroys a specific group of cells in the thalamus, is appropriate for 5% to 10% of patients with severe tremor of the hand and arm. It results in immediate improvement in 80% to 90% of the patients. A pallidotomy destroys a specific group of cells within the globus pallidus (movement center of the brain). It is used for patients with slow movement, tremor, imbalance, and drug side effects. The results are about the same as with thalamotomy. *Note:* The surgery will not cure the disease; it only relieves the symptoms and decreases need for medication. The disease will progress.

Again a well-known person is giving urgency to research into treatment and a cure for this debilitating disease. Popular actor Michael J. Fox was diagnosed with Parkinson's disease in 1991, many years before he reached the "average age" of incidence. The involvement of well-known people like Christopher Reeve and Michael J. Fox in forming foundations for research and education into these tragic conditions is having a very positive impact on the urgency for answers and treatments.

Reye's Syndrome

Description—This acute childhood illness is characterized by fatty infiltration of the liver and increased intracranial pressure (ICP). Further damage from fat infiltration occurs in the kidneys and possibly the muscle of the heart. The **syndrome** (group of symptoms) affects children from infancy to adolescence, occurring equally in males and females, but affects whites more than blacks. It is rare, affecting about one in a million.

The syndrome prognosis depends on the degree of CNS depression from ICP. At one time, mortality was 90%; now with early treatment and ICP monitoring, the rate has been reduced to 20%. Death usually results from cerebral swelling, respiratory arrest, or coma.

Signs and symptoms—The symptoms occur in stages of severity, beginning with vomiting, lethargy, and liver dysfunction and then progressing to hyperventilation, delirium, hyperactive reflexes, and coma. The condition worsens as symptoms of rigidity; deepening coma; large, fixed pupils; seizures; and eventual respiratory arrest occur.

Etiology—Reye's syndrome almost always follows within 1 to 3 days of an acute viral infection, such as upper respiratory infection, type B influenza, or chickenpox. A correlation exists between the use of aspirin in children and the incidence of influenza and chickenpox. Even though it may not be causative, aspirin is therefore not recommended for any pediatric patient with viral illness.

Treatment—Proper treatment is essential. With increased ICP, the prime concern is to reduce the pressure and brain edema to prevent damage. Aggressive action involves medications to reduce body fluid, prevent seizures, and maintain appropriate levels of vitamin K and glucose. If the condition worsens, the ICP is monitored, and mechanical ventilation may be necessary. As a final effort, coma may be induced with barbiturates, dialysis may be used to extract fluids and built-up elements, and a section of skull may be removed to relieve brain compression.

Sciatica (Si-at'i-ka)

Description—**Sciatica** is the inflammation of the sciatic nerve of the leg. It is usually unilateral and is more common in males and in middle age.

Signs and symptoms—A sharp, shooting pain that may begin gradually or abruptly and runs down the back of the thigh and into the lower leg. It may seem to originate deep within the buttocks. It is often intensified with movement. The pain may become worse at night or when the atmosphere changes with the approach of a storm. It may be difficult to achieve comfort while sitting or standing.

Etiology—The nerve roots that comprise the sciatic nerve may have been injured or irritated by impingement by spinal arthritis or a herniated disk. Gradually occurring pain can result from unequal leg length, causing improper vertebral alignment. The nerve may become damaged by accidental stretching during strenuous activities or pelvic tumors or scarring.

Treatment—Activities causing discomfort will need to be curtailed temporarily. Treatment consists of bed rest, if needed, although activities as tolerated are recommended; heat; medication for pain; and sometimes the use of traction. Some people find that the application of cold instead of heat is beneficial. An adjustment to a shoe may be helpful in leveling the legs. Often, the use of specific stretching exercises, begun gently, will gradually solve the problem. The discomfort may persist for an extended period of time. It may become chronic and cause atrophy (wasting away) of the affected muscles, although that is unusual. Surgery may be indicated in severe cases that do not respond to conservative measures.

Spinal Cord Defects

Description—Spinal cord defects result from failure of tissues to properly close during the first 3 months of pregnancy. They occur most frequently in the lumbosacral area.

The incidence is approximately 5% of live births or about 100,000 infants per year and is highest among persons of Welsh or Irish descent.

Signs and symptoms—**Spina bifida occulta** (spi'-na bif'-i-da oc-cult'-ah) is the most common type of the defects. It is characterized by the incomplete closure of one or more vertebra but without protrusion of the spinal cord or meninges (Figure 11-45). There is usually a depression, a tuft of hair, a port wine nevus, or a combination of these signs over the defect. In spina bifida with meningocele (men-in'-go-sel), a protruding sac contains meninges and CFS. With myelomeningocele (mie-lo-men-in'-go-sel), the meninges, CFS, and a portion of the spinal cord or distal nerve roots are within the sac. The defects usually occur in the lumbosacral area but are occasionally found in the thoracic and cervical areas. Neurologic symptoms range from minimal weakness of the feet and some bladder and bowel problems to permanent neurologic dysfunction, such as paralysis, inability to control the bladder and bowels, hydrocephalus, clubfoot, and sometimes mental retardation.

Etiology—A congenital defect caused by the failure of the neural tube of the embryo, which becomes the brain and spinal cord, to close properly. Normally, by about the 23rd day, it is completely closed, except for the openings at each end. A recent finding revealed that lack of folic acid is a contributing factor. All pregnant women should take a supplement containing the element as soon as pregnancy is known. Ideally, it should be started prior to conception. Viruses, radiation, the environment, and genetic factors may also be responsible.

Treatment—Treatment and prognosis depend on the extent of the defect. Spina bifida occulta usually requires no treatment. If CSF and meninges are involved, surgical closure is required to prevent further injury. Unfortunately, the neurologic condi-

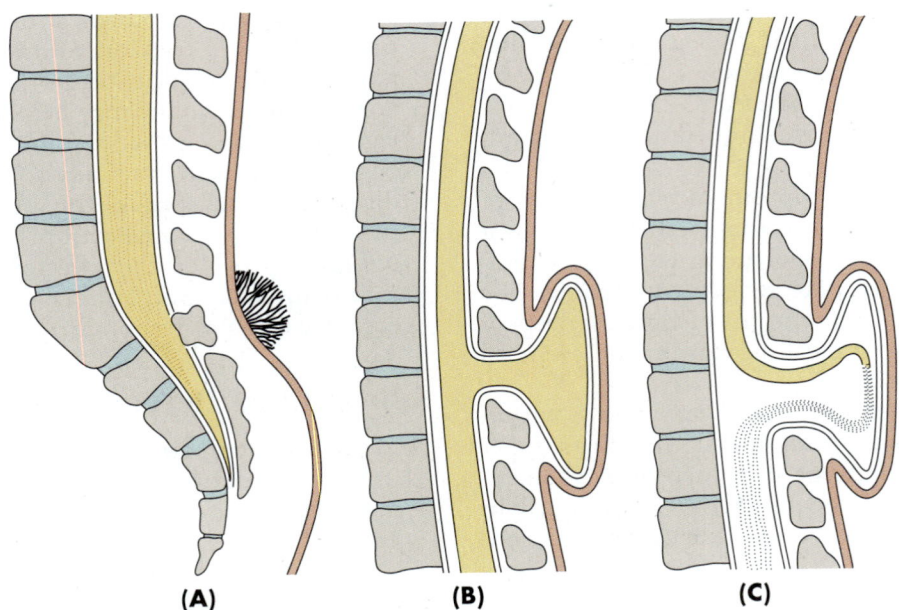

FIGURE 11-45 Spinal cord defects: (A) spina bifida occulta, (B) meningocele, (C) myelomeningocele

tions cannot be reversed. If hydrocephalus is also present, a shunt will be implanted to relieve the fluid pressure. Supportive measures to promote independence may involve leg braces, crutches, walkers, and wheelchairs. *Note:* With paralysis and spinal cord defects, there are bladder and bowel concerns.

Subarachnoid Hemorrhage (Sub-a-rak'-noyd)

Description—This is a collection of blood in the subarachnoid space, usually caused by the spontaneous rupture of a weakened blood vessel.

Signs and symptoms—The patient may complain of a sudden, severe headache and experience nausea and projectile vomiting. This may be accompanied by motor disturbances, seizures, and deviations in sensory perception, particularly in vision.

Etiology—Precipitating factors include hypertension, oral contraceptives, malformations of cranial blood vessels, and family history.

Treatment—Treatment varies with the causative factor. With hypertension, efforts would be made to lower the blood pressure. If contraceptives are suspected, they would be discontinued.

Subdural Hematoma (Sub-dur'-al He-ma-to'-ma)

Description—This is a collection of blood within the subdural space. It is usually a slow process in which the gradually accumulating blood causes progressive symptoms.

Signs and symptoms—There are disturbances in motor activities and a progressive facial weakness on the side opposite the hematoma. With progression, there may be seizures and a decreased level of consciousness. Because the blood accumulates slowly, symptoms may not occur until days after the injury.

Etiology—Hematoma results from blood leaking into the subdural space as the consequence of a head injury.

Treatment—Surgical intervention is indicated to remove the pressure on the brain tissues caused by the hematoma when symptoms and intracranial pressure reach a significant level.

Tourette Syndrome (Tur'-et)(Sin'drom)

Description—Tourette syndrome (TS) is a neurologic disorder characterized by "tics"—the involuntary, rapid, sudden movements that occur repeatedly in the same way. The onset is before the age of 21. The incidence in the United States has not been determined; however, the National Institutes of Health estimate there are 100,000 people with the affliction, and the incidence may be as high as one in every 200 if chronic and transient childhood tics were included. Most tics are benign.

Signs and symptoms—The most common first symptom is a facial tic, such as rapidly blinking eyes or twitches of the mouth. Another tic involves the voice, which may result in barking noises and tongue clicking. Some people vocalize socially unacceptable words and echo things just heard. People with TS do have some control, repressing the symptoms until a more socially accepted time; however, this causes a more severe outburst when expressed. Tics of the limbs may also be an initial sign. Motor tics may cause jumping, touching other people or things, twirling about, and self-injurious actions such as hitting or biting oneself. There is no diagnostic test to confirm TS; only history and observation can be used to diagnose.

Etiology—The cause of TS has not been definitely identified. There is evidence that it is caused by the abnormal metabolism of at least one brain chemical called dopamine. Others are suspected. Genetic studies show that TS is from an inherited dominant gene that can produce different symptoms in different family members.

Treatment—Most persons are not significantly affected to require treatment. There are medications to control the outbursts when necessary. The dosage must be determined individually. Psychotherapy can assist persons and their family to cope with the strange condition. Relaxation techniques and biofeedback help reduce stress that causes tics to increase. Affected people may be ridiculed and rejected. Children can be excluded from school activities and experience difficulty in interpersonal relationships.

Transient Ischemic Attack (Trans'-e-ent Is-ke-mick)

Description—A transient ischemic attack (TIA) is a recurring strokelike event that lasts from a few seconds to hours, then disappears after 12 to 24 hours. It is considered to be a warning sign of impending stroke. The age of onset varies but rises dramatically after age 50. It is highest among blacks and men. TIAs have occurred in 50% to 80% of patients who experience a stroke from a blood vessel blockage.

Signs and symptoms—It is characterized by symptoms such as double vision, slurred speech, dizziness, staggering gait, and falling. TIA is a warning sign of impending thrombotic CVA (stroke from a blood clot).

Etiology—A microembolus (tiny circulating mass) is released from a thrombus (blood clot) and probably interrupts blood flow in the tiny arteries of the brain. This causes symptoms similar to those of a stroke to develop; however, they are transient (passing quickly) in nature.

Treatment—Treatment includes the use of aspirin and an anticoagulant to reduce blood clot formation and to minimize the risk of thrombosis and the resulting CVA.

Trigeminal Neuralgia (Tri-gem'-in-al Nu-ral'-je-a) (Tic Douloureux) (tick dol-o-roo')

Description—This is a disorder of the fifth cranial nerve, usually on one side of the face.

Signs and symptoms—It produces episodes of excruciating facial pain on stimulation of a trigger zone. It frequently follows exposure to heat or cold, a draft from air, smiling, or drinking hot or cold liquids. The episodes may last from 1 to 15 minutes, recurring from several times daily to a few times a year. Persons with the disorder live in fear of the next attack. It occurs mostly in people over the age of 40, in women more than men, and more frequently on the right side of the face.

Etiology—The exact cause is still under investigation. However, such things as compression on nerves by tumors, an aneurysm, and an afferent reflex condition can cause it. Occasionally it is associated with multiple sclerosis or herpes zoster. The pain is probably the result of an interaction or short-circuiting of touch and pain fibers.

Treatment—Treatment consists of oral medication or the injection of alcohol or phenol into the nerve branch. With frequent, severe attacks, a surgical procedure is indicated that severs the nerve, thereby relieving the pain but also resulting in loss of sensation to the innervated area. Care must be taken afterward to protect the affected eye, avoid burns from hot food, guard against dental decay, and avoid biting the inner cheek and lip.

Tumor

Description—Tumors can occur anywhere in the body. However, those in the brain that are malignant are especially difficult to treat. There are several types with differing age and sex preferences, but almost all limit life from 6 months to 6 years following diagnosis. They are slightly more common in men than women, with an incidence of 4.5 per 100,000 people. They are most prevalent between the ages of 40 and 60 in adults and between 2 and 12 in children. They are one of the most common causes of death from cancer in children.

Signs and symptoms—Tumors cause changes in the CNS because of the destruction of tissue; the compression of the brain, cranial nerves, and blood vessels; cerebral swelling; and increased intracranial pressure. Specific symptoms vary with the type of tumor, its location, and the extent of involvement. Common symptoms are nausea, vomiting, headache, seizures, facial nerve palsies, dizziness, visual and hearing changes, weakness, and many others. The symptoms are usually insidious (slow) and often misdiagnosed.

Etiology—The cause of brain tumors is unknown.

Treatment—A resectable tumor is removed; a nonresectable tumor is debulked if possible. The type of therapy depends upon the cellular structure, its sensitivity to radiation, and its location. Surgery, radiation, chemotherapy, and relief of ICP by diuretics or shunting are the usual treatments.

A CHIEVE UNIT OBJECTIVES

■ Complete the Workbook activities to meet the learning objectives.

■ Apply your knowledge at the end of this chapter in completing the Critical Thinking Challenge and Activities, as well as the StudyWARE on your Student CD-ROM.

UNIT 3
THE SENSES

OBJECTIVES

Upon completion of this unit, you will be able to achieve the following:

L EARNING Objectives

1. Spell and define, using the glossary at the back of the text, all the Words to Know in this unit.

2. Name the senses of the human body, identifying the corresponding organ(s) responsible for perception.

3. Identify on an anatomical illustration the structures of the eye, ear, nose, tongue, and skin.

4. Trace the path of a visual image from the cornea to the visual center of the brain.

5. Explain the effects of the lens and cornea upon the focusing of images.

6. Trace the path of sound from the entrance of the ear to the auditory center of the brain.

7. Explain the balance function of the inner ear.

8. Describe the anatomy of the olfactory organ, and explain how an odor is perceived.

9. Name the types of contact receptors found in the skin.

10. Describe 17 diseases or disorders of the eye, eight of the ear, three of the nose, and three of the mouth and tongue.

WORDS TO KNOW

accommodation	hyperopia	presbyopia
amblyopia	incus	pupil
aqueous humor	insidious	receptor
astigmatism	iris	retina
auditory	lacrimal	retinopathy
cataract	lens	sclera
cerumen	malleus	semicircular
choroid	Ménière's	canals
cochlea	disease	sensorineural
conjunctiva	myopia	stapes
cornea	optic disc	strabismus
enucleation	organ of Corti	tinnitus
epistaxis	otitis	tympanic
eustachian tube	otosclerosis	membrane
fovea centralis	polyps	vitreous humor
glaucoma	presbycusis	

CERTIFICATION CONNECTION

CMA
Diagnostic procedures
Common diseases and
    pathology
Anatomy and physiology

CMAS
Anatomy and physiology

RMA
Anatomy and physiology

The human being is able to communicate with the surrounding environment because of a miraculous network of nerves coordinated with the organs of the five special senses, which allow us to see, hear, taste, smell, and touch. Knowledge of the environment requires the cooperation of three factors: the sense organs to perceive, intact cranial nerves to transmit, and a functioning area of the brain to interpret the received stimuli.

A stimulus is anything the body is able to detect by means of its **receptors**. Receptors are the peripheral nerve endings of sensory nerves that respond to stimuli. They are not all alike and do not respond to the same kinds of stimuli. Some respond to environmental chemical energy from ions or molecules that are dissolved in body fluids. These are chemoreceptors and are associated with the sense of taste and smell. Changes in position or pressure or the effects of acceleration create mechanical energy, which is detected by mechanoreceptors. These are associated with touch, hearing, and equilibrium. The detection of energy from light is possible as a result of the photoreceptors in the eyes. Thermoreceptors detect radiant energy from heat and are in the skin or connective tissue.

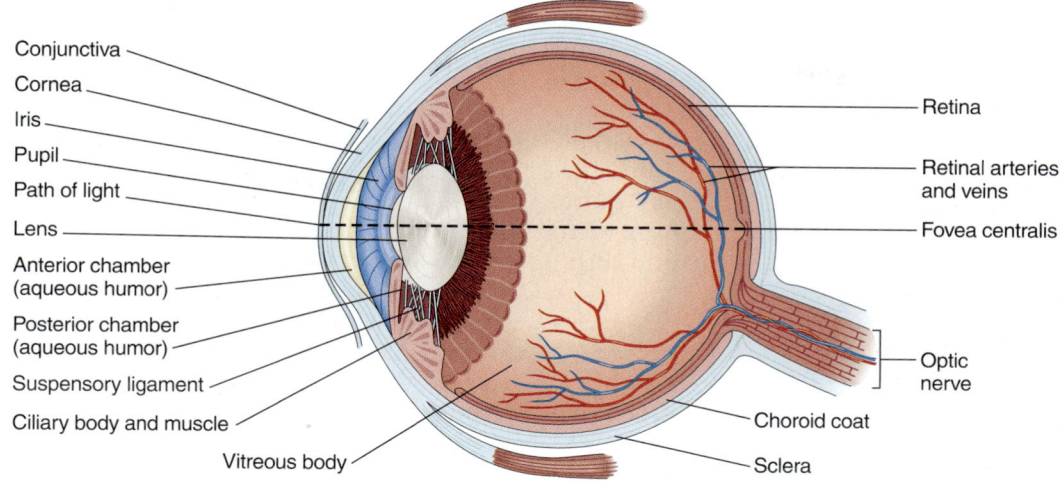

FIGURE 11-46   Cross-section of the eye

The stimulus, regardless of its form, is converted into energy. If the stimulus is sufficient enough to cause an action potential in the neuron, the message will travel along the sensory nerve to the brain. The reason messages are interpreted differently (such as being hot, a color, or an odor) is that certain nerves always end up in the same specific part of the brain. In other words, the sensation of heat or pain and the "seeing" of a color actually occurs in the brain, not at the point of stimulus. The ability to distinguish between hot, cold, red, or blue, for example, is the outcome of messages being received in an appropriate section of the brain, undergoing routing, being compared with stored past experiences, and producing the interpretation of the stimulus.

The primary organs of the senses are familiar: the eye and the sense of sight; the ear and the sense of hearing; the tongue and the sense of taste; the nose and the sense of smell; and the skin and the sense of touch. However, these organs cannot perform their functions without the cooperation of the corresponding nerves and the section of the brain.

THE EYE AND THE SENSE OF SIGHT

The structure of the eyeball is frequently compared with that of a camera. The outside of the camera is made of a strong plastic or metal to protect its interior structures. Well-protected, the eye is located within the bony orbital cavity of the skull. For additional protection, the outside of the eye is covered with tough, white fibrous tissue called the **sclera** (Figure 11-46). The sclera helps maintain the shape of the eyeball. Six extraocular or extrinsic (outside) muscles are attached to the sclera and anchored in the skull; these contract or relax as pairs to move the eyeball within its cavity. This permits the eyes

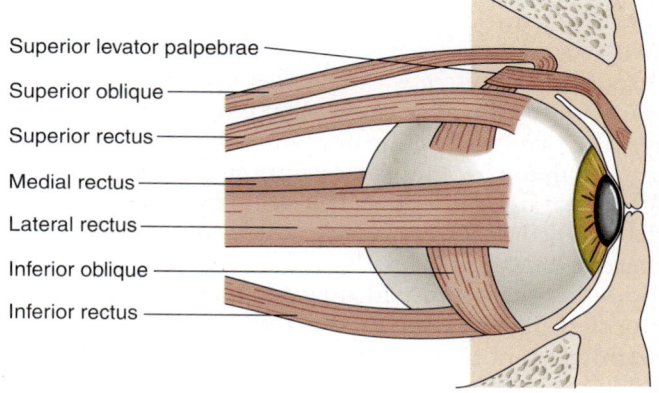

FIGURE 11-47   Extraocular (extrinsic) muscles of the eye

to roll up and down, in and out, and in combinations of these directions, thereby permitting a large field of vision without moving the head (Figure 11-47). A 7th muscle, the superior levator palpebrae, does not move the eyeball but is attached to and moves the eyelid. Under the sclera is another covering called the **choroid**, which contains the blood vessels that serve the tissues of the eye. This layer has a nonreflective pigment that makes it dark and opaque and prevents light from reflecting within the eye.

Focusing the Image

Both the eye and the camera have a lens to focus an image onto a surface for "recording." In the camera this surface is the film or the sensors in a digital camera. In the eye it is the **retina**. In the camera, the distance between the film and the camera lens is adjusted to bring the picture into focus before it is recorded on the film. In the eye, the shape of the elastic **lens** is automatically altered by ciliary muscles of the ciliary body to focus objects onto the retina. When the ciliary body contracts, the lens becomes rounder in a process known as **accommodation** to permit near vision. With relaxation, the lens thins out to accommodate focusing on distant objects. The shape of the lens is convex on both the anterior and posterior surfaces. The shape is quite rounded in childhood but becomes more convex with age until it is nearly flat in the elderly, causing difficulty accommodating for near vision.

Controlling Light

The aperture of the camera is similar to the **iris** of the eye; the size of their openings is adjusted to allow varying amounts of light to enter. The iris is the colored circular muscle that surrounds the central opening called the **pupil**. The amount of melanin (color) and its location in the iris determines the color of the eye. When melanin is present only in the posterior area, the iris appears blue; if melanin is scattered throughout, eye color ranges from green to brown to black, depending on the amount of pigment. In the eye, the two intrinsic (inside) muscle structures of the iris regulate the amount of light that enters the eye. When the light is bright, the circular muscle fibers of the iris contract, reducing the size of the pupil, thereby permitting less light to enter. If it is dark or dimly lit, the pupil will dilate (enlarge) as the radial muscle fibers of the iris contract to pull it outward, permitting more light to enter.

The Cornea

The **cornea** is a transparent extension of the sclera that lies in front of the pupil. This covering has no blood vessels to interfere with vision, so the tissue is nourished by lymph fluid circulating through the cellular spaces. It has both pain and touch receptors, which cause it to be extremely sensitive to any foreign body that touches its surface. If an injury to the cornea results in scarring, vision will be impaired.

The curvature of the cornea "corrects" some of the unclear image that the edge of the lens projects. If the cornea develops an abnormal shape, vision becomes blurred, and the result may be a disorder known as **astigmatism**.

Surface Membranes

A mucous membrane called the **conjunctiva** lines the inner surfaces of the eyelids and covers the anterior sclera surface of the eye. At the margin of the cornea, the conjunctiva merges with the transparent epithelium covering that protects the cornea. The conjunctiva

and cornea are lubricated by tiny glands that secrete an oily substance. Further protection for the eye is provided by **lacrimal** glands, which secrete tears to moisten and cleanse the surface of the membrane.

Cavities and Humors

The eyeball is divided into two main areas separated by the lens and its supporting ciliary body structures. The more anterior area is subdivided into the anterior chamber, which is between the cornea and the iris, and the posterior chamber, which lies between the iris and the lens. A salty, clear fluid known as the **aqueous humor** fills and circulates between the chambers. It maintains the curvature of the cornea and assists in the refraction process. It is made by the ciliary processes and circulates from the posterior chamber past the iris to the anterior chamber. It then drains through the tiny holes of the trabecular meshwork into the venous system. The space where the drainage holes are located is between the cornea and the iris inside the anterior chamber and is known as the drainage angle (see Figure 11-53).

The eyeball behind the lens, sometimes called a vitreous chamber or vitreous body, is filled with a thick, jellylike substance called the **vitreous humor**. This material not only aids in refraction but also maintains the shape of the eyeball. Injury with the loss of an appreciable amount of the vitreous may cause damage to the eyeball, which could necessitate surgical removal of the eye by a procedure called **enucleation**.

The Retina

The inside layer of the eyeball is the retina, a multilayered nervous tissue. Specialized nerve cells called rods and cones transmit the stimuli focused on the retinal surface through the optic nerve to the visual center in the brain where the image is "seen." The cones, about 7 million in number, are sensitive to colors and function only in well-lighted environments. Most of them are located in a depression on the posterior surface of the retina called the **fovea centralis**, the area of sharpest vision. There are about 100 million rods in the more peripheral areas of the retina. The rods are very sensitive to light and permit us to see, without color, in dimly lit or nearly dark surroundings.

Optic Disc   Two other types of nerve cells in the retina relay impulses from the rods and cones. The axons of one type form the fibers of the optic nerve. Where the optic nerves exit the retina, there are neither rods nor cones, so this area is referred to as the **optic disc** or blind spot.

The Path of Light

The process of sight begins with the passage of light rays through the cornea; on through the aqueous humor, the pupil, and the lens into the vitreous humor; and finally focusing at the back of the eyeball on the retina. Here the image is picked up by the rods and cones, transformed into nerve impulses, and transmitted over the optic nerve to the thalamus. Here some of the fibers cross over to the nerve tract of the other eye. From the thalamus, other neurons relay the impulses to the visual center in the occipital lobe of the cerebrum, where the impulses are "developed" into pictures and "seen."

Refraction Error

Each part of the eyeball refracts (deflects) the light to cause the image to focus on the retina (Figure 11-48A). However, this does not always occur correctly. When the image is improperly refracted and focuses in front of the retina (B), the person is said to be nearsighted, or to have **myopia**. When the image focuses behind the retina (C), the person is said to be farsighted, or to have **hyperopia**. These conditions may result from abnormal curvature of the lens or cornea or from an abnormally shaped eyeball. Note that images are inverted when

they pass through the lens because of the curvature deflecting the image. Eyeglasses provide a means of refracting light to correct abnormal deflection of the image. They perform artificially what the eyes' structures fail to do.

DISEASES AND DISORDERS OF THE EYE

Age-Related Macular Degeneration (ARMD) (Mak'-u-lar De-jen-er-a'-shun)

Description—A disease that affects the macula, the small central point of light-sensing retina in the back of the eye, and alters the center of the visual field. Ten million Americans have some loss of vision from age-related macular degeneration (ARMD). It causes 90% of new legal blindness in the United States.

Signs and symptoms—This is a gradual loss of central vision; however, side or surrounding vision is often maintained. There is a blurred, distorted, dark, or empty area in the center of things viewed. If both eyes are involved, it makes things like threading a needle and reading virtually impossible. The condition can be easily diagnosed by having the patient look at a square grid that resembles graph paper but has a small dot in the center. The appearance of crooked lines or other visual symptoms around the dot is diagnostic.

Etiology—It results from damage to the blood vessels supplying the retina. It takes many years to develop, eventually causing the thinning of the macula. Although the specific cause is not known, it seems that aging is the most significant risk factor. Other identified risk factors are heredity, blue eyes, high blood pressure, cardiovascular disease, and smoking. A recent study of the diets of 2,000 people from 45 to 84 years old showed a relationship between dietary fat and ARMD. Signs of the disease were 80% more common with those people who had consumed the most saturated fat within the past 10 years. Researchers believe that the saturated fat clogs the arteries and reduces the amount of blood that reaches the retina. This form of degeneration is also known as "dry," "atropic," or "involuntional" macular degeneration and represents about 90% of the macular-related disease.

Another form known as "wet" macular degeneration accounts for the remaining 10% of cases. Although wet ARMD is less common, it is more serious. Abnormal blood vessels grow in a layer beneath the retina. They leak blood and fluid, creating distorted vision or a large blind spot of scar tissue in the center of the visual field.

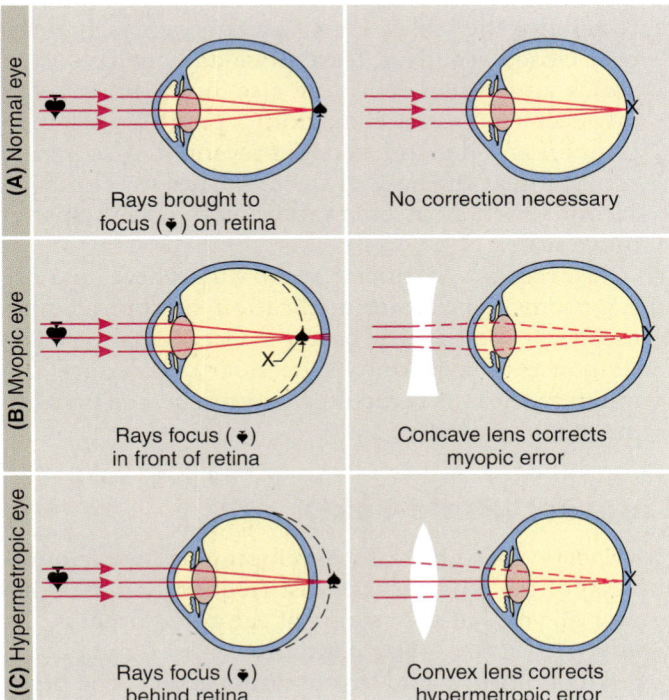

(A) Normal eye	Rays brought to focus (♠) on retina	No correction necessary
(B) Myopic eye	Rays focus (♠) in front of retina	Concave lens corrects myopic error
(C) Hypermetropic eye	Rays focus (♠) behind retina	Convex lens corrects hypermetropic error

FIGURE 11-48 The refraction of an image in (A) normal vision, (B) nearsightedness, (C) farsightedness and the type of lens required to correct the vision

Treatment—There is no cure for the dry form of macular degeneration; however, assistance with ways to cope with the visual impairment is available. There are various optical devices including magnifying lenses, closed circuit TV, large-print reading materials, and special lighting to assist with vision.

Although not a cure, recent studies have shown that using dietary supplements of vitamins C, E, beta carotene, and zinc lowers the risk of the disease progressing. The wet form can also be helped with low-vision optical devices. In addition, if the blood vessels are not growing directly under the macula, laser surgery can be performed and is the only proven effective treatment. The surgery does not improve vision but it prevents further loss. The laser beam is focused to seal the leaking blood vessels. The surgery does make a permanent dark "spot" at the laser area, but it will retard damage and preserve more sight overall.

Scientists are perfecting an artificial retina that will permit limited vision of light and large objects. The technology involves the use of a bionic silicon chip and is being used in patients with retinitis pigmentosa, a genetically induced form of blindness. It is anticipated that it may also be applicable to macular degeneration. Researchers believe that a dietary regimen that protects against heart disease may also preserve vision in later life.

Amblyopia (Am-ble-o'-pe-a) (Lazy Eye)

Description—**Amblyopia** is a condition known as lazy eye because it causes the turning eye to become "lazy." It is most prevalent in children under the age of 5.

Signs and symptoms—Observation reveals one eye turns inward, causing blurred vision. The brain suppresses the visual impulses from the inward-turning eye.

Etiology—Amblyopia is caused by any condition that affects normal use of the eyes and their development. The three major causes are strabismus because of misaligned eyes, unequal focus caused by refractive errors, and cloudiness in the normally clear eye tissues. Strabismus is the most common cause because the crossed eye "turns off" to avoid double vision and becomes amblyopic. (See Strabismus on page 368 in this unit.)

Treatment—The condition is treated by covering the "good eye," thereby stimulating the development of the "lazy eye." For a good prognosis, therapy should begin before the age of 8; otherwise, eventual blindness of the affected eye may result. Sometimes surgery is required to correct the eye.

Arcus Senilis (Are'-cuss Se-nill'-us)

Description—The condition accompanies normal aging and is included in this discussion because it is so prevalent. It results in a thin grayish-white arc or circle not quite at the edge of the cornea. If it is present in young people, it may suggest hypercholesterolemia (high level of cholesterol in the blood).

Blepharitis (Blef-ar-i'-tis) (Lid Margin Disease)

Description—This is a persistent inflammation of the edges of the eyelids involving the hair follicles and glands. The condition is usually associated with seborrhea of the scalp (dandruff), oily skin, or dry eyes.

Signs and symptoms—The person experiences itching and burning sensations, which causes continuous blinking and rubbing of the eyes, resulting in red-rimmed eyelid margins. The person develops greasy scales and sticky, crusted eyelids. Ulcerated lid margins, loss of lashes, and the presence of nits (eggs of lice) with pediculosis are possible.

Etiology—There are bacteria and excess secretions from the hair follicles of the eyelids. It may also develop from pediculosis of the brows and lashes.

Treatment—Treatment depends on the cause. It consists of frequent shampoos of the hair and daily cleansing of the eyelids with a mild baby shampoo to remove the scales. Placing warm wet washcloths over closed eyelids at least twice daily helps soften scales and other debris. It also helps liquefy the oily secretions so a chalazion, a painful, inflamed lump in an oil gland, can be prevented. Also gently scrubbing at the base of the eyelashes for about 15 seconds with a cotton swab or washcloth helps remove scales.

If necessary, artificial tears will relieve dry eye symptoms. Antibiotic medication or topical ointment will decrease the bacteria. Occasionally, short-term use of a steroid is necessary to reduce the inflammation. If pediculosis is present, the parasite must be removed.

Cataract (Kat'a-rakt)

Description—This gradually developing opacity (cloudiness) of the lens occurs most frequently in persons over 70 years of age as part of the aging process.

Signs and symptoms—The condition causes a painless, gradual blurring and loss of visual acuity. The pupil turns from black to a milky white as the lens becomes cloudy (Figure 11-49). People with cataracts frequently complain of seeing halos around lights or being blinded at night by oncoming automobile headlights. This is because as the lens becomes

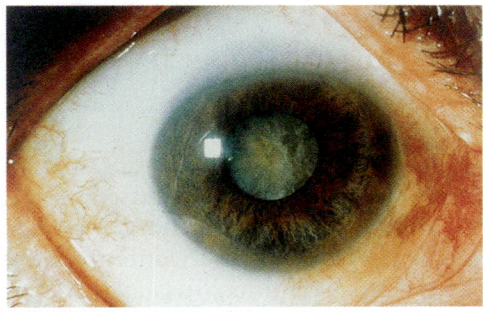

FIGURE 11-49   Cataract *(Courtesy of National Eye Institute, NIH)*

Etiology—The probable cause of **cataracts** is a change in the composition of the proteins of the lens. Aging is the underlying cause. Other things such as trauma, medications such as steroids, systemic diseases such as diabetes, and prolonged exposure to ultraviolet light can cause cataracts. Babies are occasionally born with a cataract.

Treatment—Vision cannot be improved with glasses or contact lenses. Reducing the amount of exposure to ultraviolet light by wearing sunglasses may lessen the risk, but once a cataract is developed, there is no cure. The treatment of choice is surgery. The surgeon makes a very tiny incision (Figure 11-51), to remove the lens and allow insertion of the intraocular lens (IOL). A special instrument uses sound waves to break up the lens and remove the pieces. The capsule that held the natural lens is left in place, and a tiny new IOL (Figure 11-52A) is inserted through the incision and held in position in the capsule by flexible

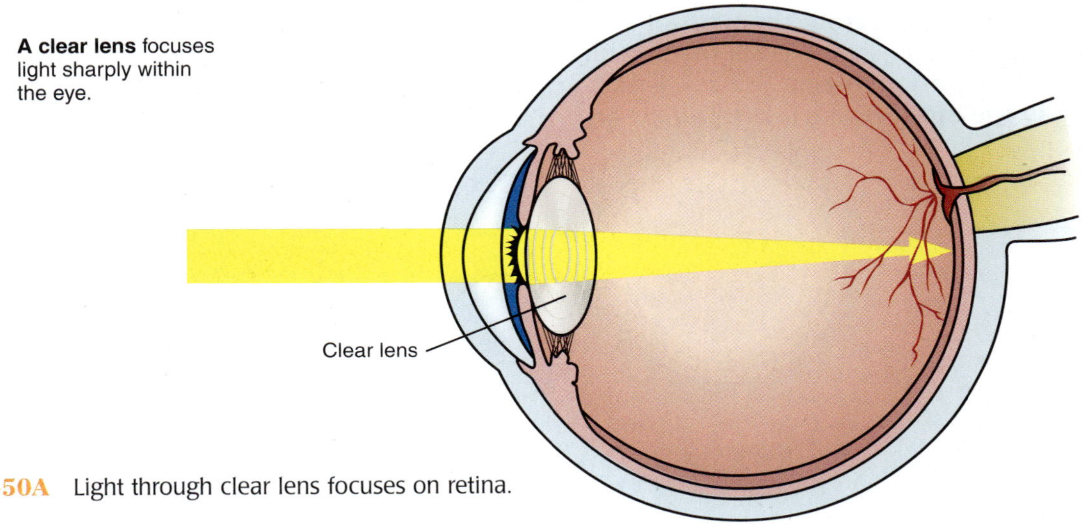

cloudy, it no longer sharply focuses light on the retina (Figure 11-50A), but instead the cataract either blocks or scatters the light coming into the eye around the retina (Figure 11-50B), causing blurring of the vision.

A **clear lens** focuses light sharply within the eye.

Clear lens

FIGURE 11-50A   Light through clear lens focuses on retina.

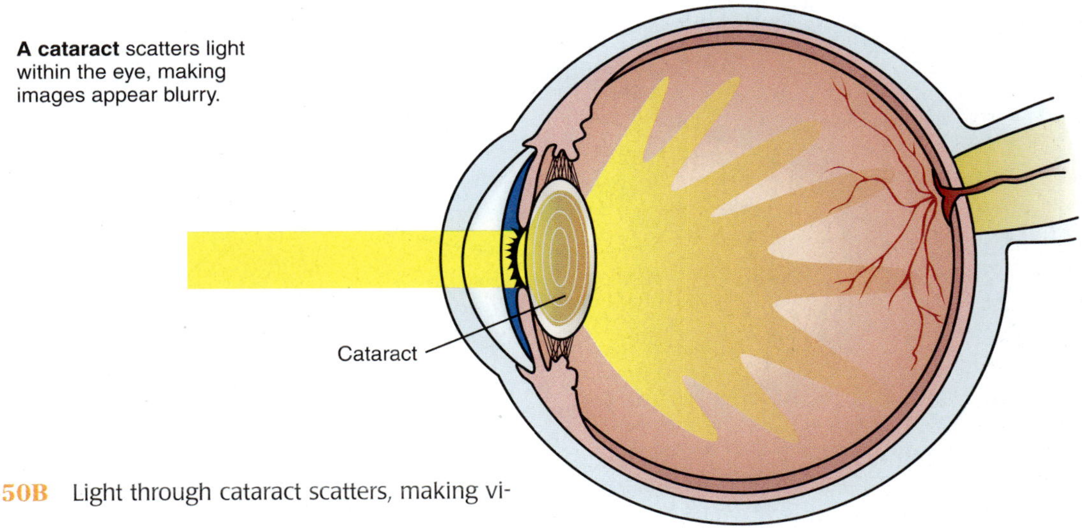

A **cataract** scatters light within the eye, making images appear blurry.

Cataract

FIGURE 11-50B   Light through cataract scatters, making vision blurry.

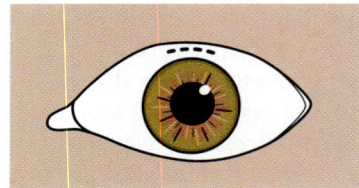

FIGURE 11-51 Incision size to remove a cataract

tabs (Figure 11-52B). (*Note:* Some newer IOLs do not have tabs but maintain their position without them). The incision may be self-sealing, or a stitch or two may be used if the patient is very active. The new IOL has the necessary individualized correction to allow the patient to see well almost immediately and normally lasts a lifetime. Cataract surgery is now being done on an outpatient basis, with the patient detained only an hour or two.

Sometimes after surgery, the posterior capsule, which is now supporting the IOL, may become clouded, once again obstructing the path of light into the eye. This problem can be easily solved without invasive surgery, using a laser beam to make a tiny opening in the capsule, which lets in light and restores vision.

Conjunctivitis (Kon-junk-ti-vi'tis) (Pinkeye)

Description—This condition is caused by inflammation of the conjunctiva. It usually begins in one eye, spreading rapidly to the other from contamination by a wash cloth or by the hands. Because it is highly contagious, other family members should not share towels, wash cloths, or pillows with the infected person.

Signs and symptoms—Conjunctivitis causes redness and a "bloodshot" appearance. Pain, swelling, and occasionally a discharge from the eyes may be present.

Etiology—It is usually caused by an infectious organism, such as bacteria (streptococcus or staphylococcus) or a virus (herpes simplex). Allergic reactions and environmental irritants can also cause the condition.

Treatment—Bacterial conjunctivitis responds to antibiotics and sulfa drug therapy; the herpes viral type does not.

Corneal Abrasion (Kor'ne-al A-bra'-zhun)

Description—A scratch or trauma to the cornea, usually from a foreign body in the eye. Even if the eye waters profusely to cleanse the surface, the scratch (abra-

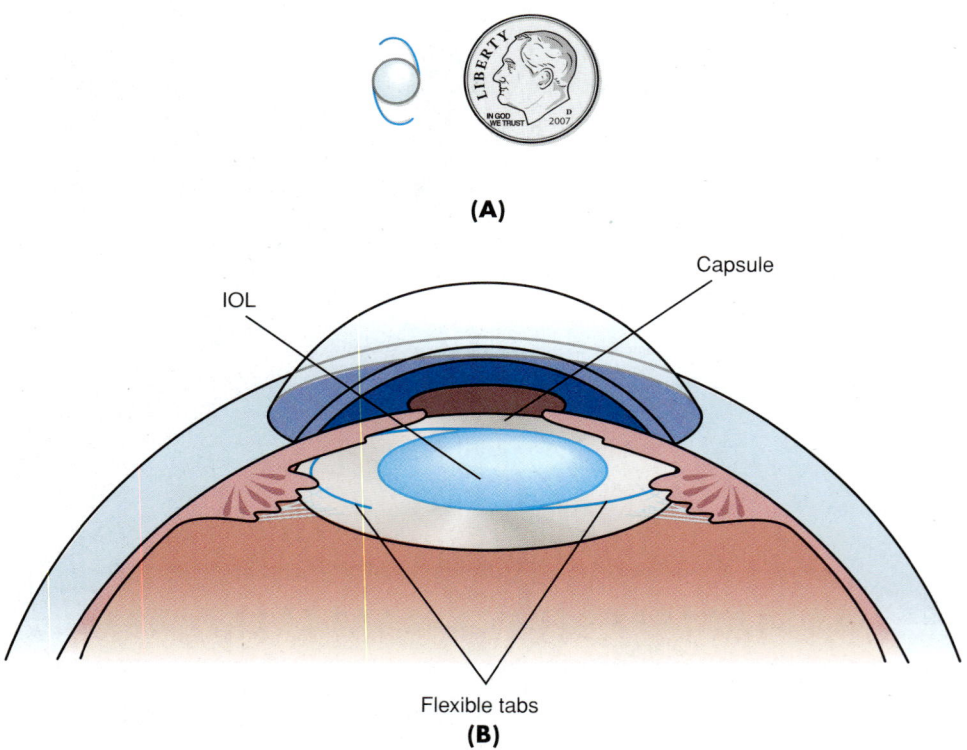

(A)

FIGURE 11-52 The intraocular lens (IOL) size (A) and location (B).

sion) remains. Vision may be affected if the location and extent of injury are significant.

Signs and symptoms—The presence of redness, tearing, and irritation that causes excessive blinking.

Etiology—It is most often caused by dirt or small pieces of wood, metal, or paper that become embedded under the eyelid or an injury from a fingernail. Abrasions may also occur from falling asleep while wearing contact lenses.

Treatment—Foreign bodies embedded in the cornea require removal following application of a topical anesthetic. Treatment consists of antibiotic eyedrops or ointment. Corneal epithelium heals rapidly within 24 to 48 hours.

Corneal Ulcers (Kor'ne-al Ul'-ser)

Description—An acute disease causing a break in the cornea of the eye.

Signs and symptoms—The first signs are pain, aggravated by blinking, and excessive tearing. Blurred vision results from the ulcerations, the corneal surface appears irregular, and exudate (pus) may be present. Instillation of an ophthalmic dye will permit confirmation of the diagnosis.

Etiology—Corneal ulcers result from bacterial, viral, or fungal infections.

Treatment—A culture of the drainage to determine the causative organism will indicate appropriate medication. Broad-spectrum antibiotics are used initially to prevent corneal scarring and the resulting impairment of vision. Certain bacterially caused ulcers progress so rapidly that, without proper treatment, the cornea will perforate (be pierced with holes), and vision in the eye will be lost within 48 hours.

Diabetic Retinopathy (Di-a-bet'ik Retin-op'a-the)

Description—This form of vascular **retinopathy** results from juvenile or adult diabetes. Approximately 75% of patients with juvenile diabetes develop diabetic retinopathy within 20 years after the onset of diabetes. Incidence in adults with diabetes increases with the length of time a person is diabetic. About 80% of patients with diabetes of 20 to 30 years' duration develop retinopathy. It is the leading cause of acquired blindness in adults.

Signs and symptoms—Symptoms result from an edematous retina, which causes light to scatter. Tiny capillary walls thicken and show evidence of dilation, twisting, and hemorrhage. This causes glare, blurred vision, and reduced visual acuity. If diagnosed and treated early, prognosis is good for simple forms; in

extensive forms, prognosis is poor, with 50% becoming blind within 5 years.

Etiology—The condition is a result of an interference with the blood supply to the eyes.

Treatment—Treatment consists of sealing holes that have developed in the retina and coagulating the leaking vessels with a laser beam. If new abnormal vessels have grown onto the retina and into the vitreous body, it is possible for the retina to detach from the choroid layer, resulting in vitreous hemorrhage and blindness. With this advanced condition, open surgery will be required.

Glaucoma (Glaw-ko'-ma)

Description—This condition of excessive intraocular pressure results in atrophy (wasting away) of the optic nerve. **Glaucoma** causes severe visual impairment and eventually blindness. It occurs in 2% of adults over age 40 and accounts for 15% of all blindness in the United States. It is the most easily prevented cause of blindness.

There are two main forms of glaucoma: open-angle (most common) and closed-angle. Each form has its own parameters. Glaucoma causes severe visual defects because the increased intraocular pressure within the eyeball causes pressure against the blood vessels of the retina, reducing the blood supply and destroying retinal nerve fibers. Glaucoma is diagnosed with evidence of increased intraocular pressure as measured by a tonometer. The pupil of the eye is then dilated in order to examine the optic disc. Millions of nerve fibers go from the retina to the optic nerve. They meet at the optic disk, the "blind spot" at the back of the retina. As the nerve fibers are destroyed, the disc begins to change and appears to hollow out. This is referred to as "cupping." As more fibers die, the cup becomes deeper, and more vision is lost (Figure 11-53).

The fluid that exerts pressure within the eye can result from either an overproduction of the aqueous humor produced by the epithelium of the ciliary body or the obstruction of its outflow circulating mechanisms to the canal of Schlemm for absorption into venous circulation (Figure 11-54).

Glaucoma—Open-angle

Signs and symptoms—The symptoms are **insidious** (gradual), bilateral, and often not recognized until late in the disease. They include mild aching, a loss of peripheral (side) vision, seeing halos around lights, and difficulty seeing at night or in darkened places.

Etiology—With this type of glaucoma, the drainage angle is wide but the circulating aqueous humor cannot drain because of a blockage of the trabecular

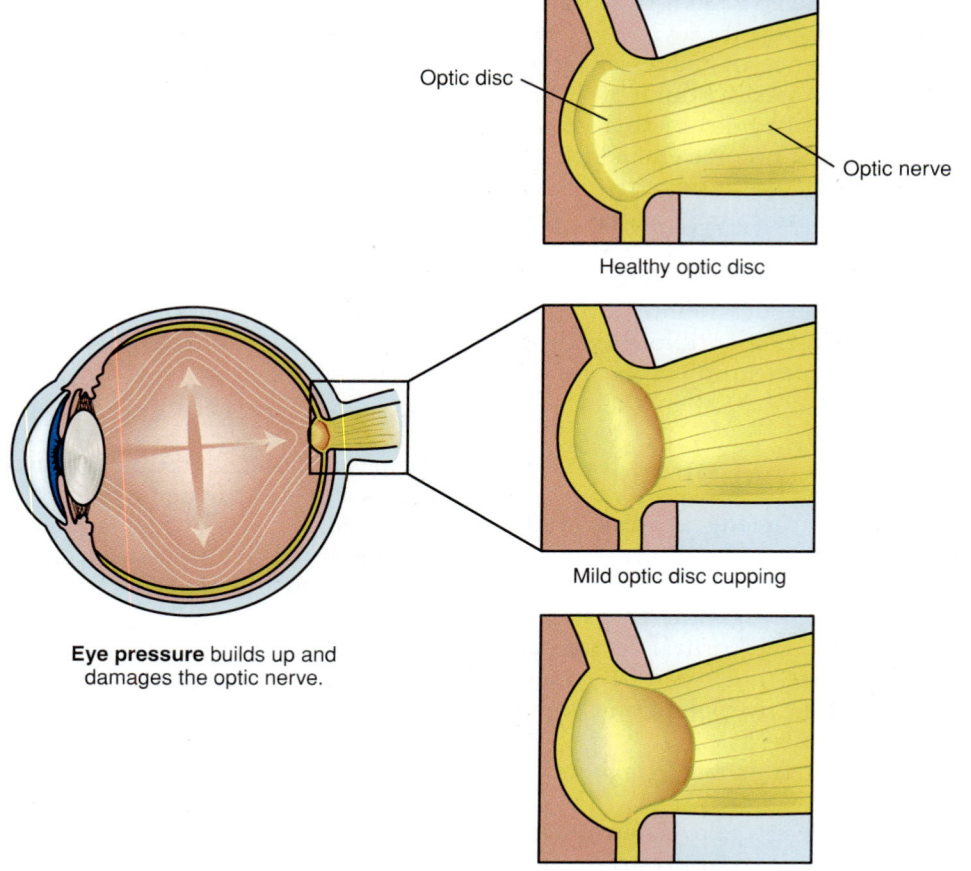

Eye pressure builds up and damages the optic nerve.

FIGURE 11-53 How glaucoma affects the optic disc

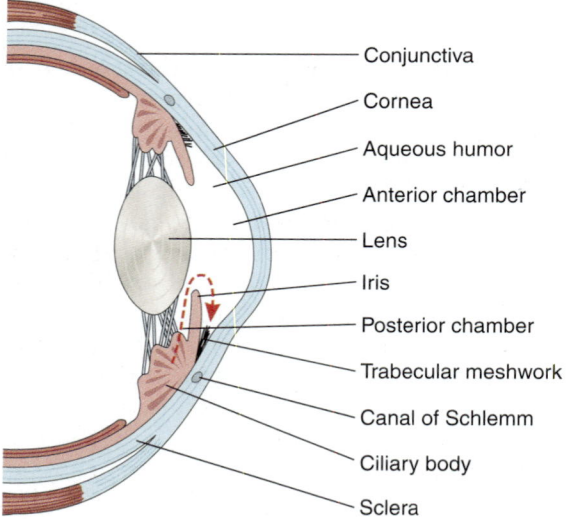

FIGURE 11-54 Normal flow of aqueous humor

meshwork, the canal of Schlemm, or the aqueous veins. Pressure rises slowly.

Treatment—Treatment is aimed at reducing the production of aqueous humor by the use of medications and eyedrops to encourage the circulation. With in-adequate response, a laser procedure to create openings for the aqueous outflow is indicated. The tra-beculoplasty procedure focuses the laser beam at areas around the drainage holes. The laser stimulates the area to enlarge the holes and therefore increase drainage.

Glaucoma—Closed-angle

Signs and symptoms—There is pain and redness of the affected eye with a feeling of pressure. The pupil is moderately dilated and nonreactive to light. There is blurred and decreased visual acuity and sensitivity to light. Unless the pressure is relieved quickly, blindness may occur within 24 hours.

Etiology—This type results from obstruction of the drainage holes resulting from anatomically narrow angles, shallow chambers, and a thickened iris that closes the passages. There is a rapid onset of symptoms, and it is considered an emergency.

Treatment—Usual treatment consists of aggressive drug therapy and a peripheral iridotomy (laser removal of a piece of the iris) to permit outflow of the aqueous humor.

Laser surgery is a quick, less expensive, and relatively painless solution to both open- and closed-angle glaucoma. In open-angle, if medication is ineffective, a laser beam is directed to open the trabecular meshwork. In closed-angle, the laser makes a tiny opening in the iris to allow the fluid to drain. A second treatment may be necessary in closed-angle glaucoma. Laser eye surgery is more effective in the early stages of the disease. Both eyes may be treated to prevent an attack in the other eye.

Hordeolum (Hor-de'o-lum) (Stye)

Description—This localized infection of a gland of the eyelid produces an abscess around an eyelash.
Signs and symptoms—The eye is red, painful, and swollen.
Etiology—The causative organism is staphylococcus.
Treatment—Treatment consists of applying warm, wet compresses to relieve pain and promote drainage and the use of eye drops or ointment to treat the infection.

Iritis (I-rit'-is)

Description—An inflammation of the iris.
Signs and symptoms—Iritis produces moderate to severe eye pain, photophobia, and a small nonreactive pupil caused by the spasm of the iris.
Etiology—It is often caused by an improperly healed corneal abrasion, especially if damage is from a sharp object.
Treatment—Prompt treatment is required to prevent complications. The pupil is dilated with mydriatics to allow the eye to rest to prevent the formation of posterior synechiae (adhesions of the iris to the lens). Corticosteroid drops are used to reduce the inflammation.

Myopia (Miop'-e-a)

Description—This condition is a defect in vision that is also known as nearsightedness. Objects can be seen distinctly only when close to the eyes. The rate of incidence is believed to be around 11 million Americans.
Signs and symptoms—There is a blurring of vision when looking at objects beyond immediate surroundings.
Etiology—The primary cause is a misshapen eyeball. When the cornea is too convex, objects are refracted in front of the retina.
Treatment—Myopia is normally treated with the application of glasses or contact lenses to alter the refraction of images and to bring them to focus on the retina. A procedure called radial keratotomy (RK) provides an alternative method of correction. It is a surgical procedure that requires extreme precision. Small cuts are made in the cornea to flatten it so that the focal point is corrected. It can be done only after

the individual has passed young adulthood because myopia may worsen into the early 20s. The newest form of RK is a computerized procedure using an excimer (or cold laser).

This variation of keratotomy procedure is called photorefractive keratectomy (PRK). It removes a thin layer of tissue from the surface of the cornea to flatten and reshape it to the desired correction. The actual laser treatment takes only 15 to 40 seconds. One eye at a time is usually done in order to evaluate the results before treating the second eye. PRK is appropriate for people who have stable vision with low to moderate myopia and no other eye problems.

The newest method, which provides an alternative to surgery, reshapes the corneas with cornea-flattening *reverse-geometry* contact lenses. The lenses are worn at night for about 60 days and reportedly produce dramatic improvement with results equal to radial keratotomy.

Presbyopia (Prez-be-op'e-a)

Description—This condition is characterized by inability of the lens to accommodate for near vision. **Presbyopia** occurs as part of the normal aging process.
Signs and symptoms—The first symptom is usually the inability to read smaller print without straining and the use of a bright light. With advancement, all normal size print is out of focus at the normal reading distance.
Etiology—Presbyopia is caused by the loss of elasticity of the lens. It is no longer able to adjust to focus images on the retina properly.
Treatment—The condition can be corrected by the fitting of contact lenses or eyeglasses.

Ptosis (To'-sis)

Description—Ptosis is the drooping of the upper eyelid.
Signs and symptoms—This condition is evident upon observation. Eyes appear to be only partially open. The individual has a "sleepy" appearance.
Etiology—Ptosis may be a congenital condition or the result of aging, the presence of an excess fatty fold, or a neurologic factor.
Treatment—Treatment may be required if vision is restricted or the appearance is cosmetically undesirable. A surgical procedure on the eyelid muscles will correct the disorder, or a device can be attached to the eyeglass frame to elevate the eyelid.

Retinal Detachment (Ret'-i-nal)

Description—This disorder is characterized by the separation of the retina from the choroid layer of the eyeball.

Signs and symptoms—Diagnosis can be made from the patient's complaints of seeing floating spots, flashes of light, and a gradual vision loss. Confirmation is possible after pupil dilation and ophthalmoscopy reveal a gray and opaque retina with indefinite margins in the affected areas. Folds, tears, and a ballooning inward of the retina may be seen.

Etiology—The separation may occur with aging, which causes the normal vitreous support to shrink away. This results in a small hole or tear that permits the humor to seep between the layers and cause separation. Other causative factors include severe high blood pressure, diabetes, trauma, and other systemic diseases.

Treatment—Treatment consists of limiting eye movements with a patch, bed rest, sedation, and appropriate positioning of the head. Spontaneous reattachment is rare. A coagulation laser beam can repair simple tears in the retina by "spot welding" the area with several rows of "welds," but once separation has occurred, other treatment will be necessary. Both heat and cold therapies are used to create a sterile inflammatory reaction that causes the retina to readhere. A tight band is placed around the eyeball, inside the sclera layer, which makes the choroid "indent" against the retina to maintain its closeness. Various surgical procedures to reattach the retina to the choroid can be performed.

Strabismus (Stra-biz'-mus)

Description—This is a condition in which one eye deviates with the gaze being abnormally inward or outward, higher or lower than the other eye (Figure 11-55). An abnormally inward gaze (convergent or "crosseye") is also called esotropia, and an abnormally outward gaze (divergent or "walleye") is also known as exotropia.

Signs and symptoms—This condition is obvious upon examination. The deviation and absence of coordinated eye movement cause complaints of double vision and the inability to see objects clearly. **Strabismus** is frequently associated with Down syndrome, cerebral palsy, and mental retardation.

Etiology—The disorder results from eye muscle imbalance or attempts to compensate for farsightedness.

Treatment—Conservative initial treatment consists of a patch on the normal eye, corrective glasses, and specific eye exercises. Surgery to adjust the muscles that control eye placement and movement may be indicated. If strabismus develops before age 5, the deviated eye may be suppressed, resulting in amblyopia that could cause loss of vision if not treated.

Eye Protection

The Prevent Blindness America Association promotes many programs stressing the importance of protecting eyes from injury. Many occupations require the use of goggles or safety glasses. The association recommends the use of impact-resistant glass or plastic in all eyeglasses and sunglasses. A 1972 federal ruling requires that the lens be able to withstand the impact from a $5/8$-inch-diameter steel ball dropped from a height of 50 inches. Individuals with sight in only one eye should use industrial-quality safety lenses and frames. When engaging in do-it-yourself work, sports, or hobbies that involve visual hazards, protective eye wear should be worn. It should be noted that contact lenses do not provide protection for the eyes, and the use of protective eye wear is necessary.

If injury should occur, initial treatment is important in order to prevent further damage. If something is splashed or blown into the eye, it should be rinsed thoroughly, with the eye held open. If caustic, rinse for several minutes. A physician should examine the eye as soon as possible. Foreign bodies that are not embedded may be removed with a fold of a wet tissue or a moistened cotton swab. Objects that are embedded into the surface require medical attention. See Foreign Bodies, Chapter 19.

THE EAR AND THE SENSE OF HEARING

The ear is capable of receiving vibrations in the air and translating them into the sounds we recognize: the more vibrations per second, the higher the frequency, or pitch, of the sound; the stronger the vibration, the louder the sound.

The Outer Ear

Vibrations are picked up by the pinna (auricle) of the outer ear and directed down the external **auditory** canal to the **tympanic membrane** (eardrum) (Figure 11-56).

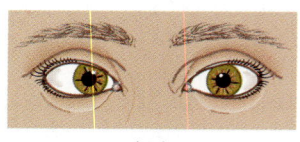

(A)

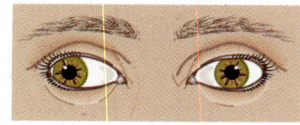

(B)

FIGURE 11-55 Strabismus: (A) convergent or esotropia; (B) divergent or exotropia

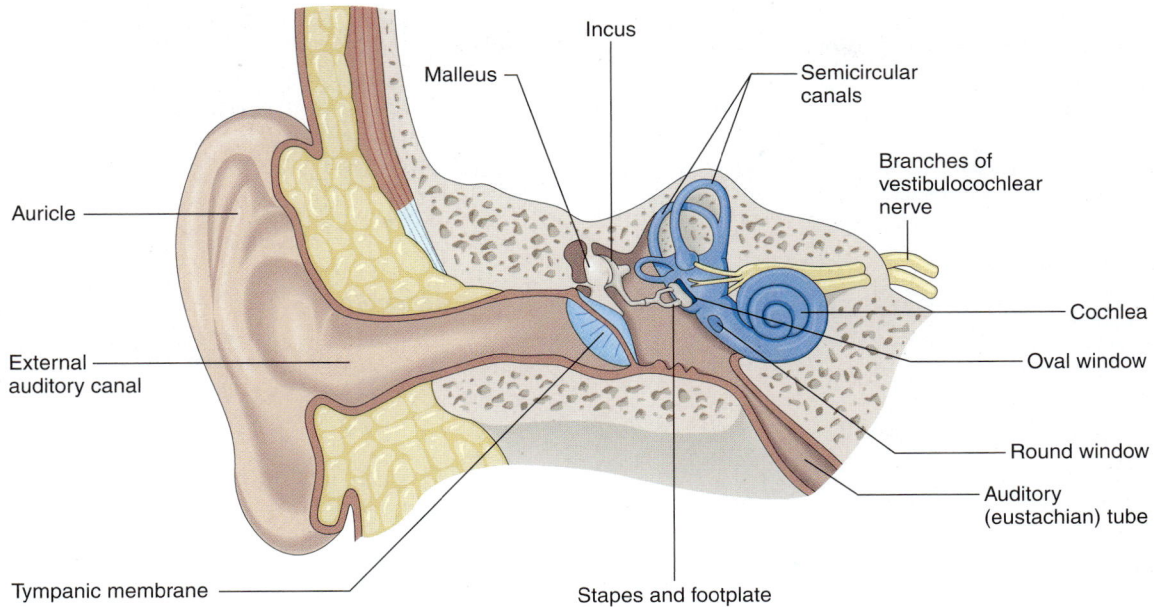

FIGURE 11-56   The ear

The Middle Ear

The sound waves vibrate the membrane and the **malleus** (hammer) attached to its inner surface. The malleus in turn "strikes" the **incus** (anvil), which moves the **stapes** (stirrup). These three small bones and the space around them are called the middle ear. The middle ear communicates the vibrations to the inner ear by the stapes pushing against the fluid in the vestibule of the inner ear through the oval window.

The middle ear is connected by means of the **eustachian tube** to the throat. The tube is responsible for equalizing air pressure in the middle ear with the outside atmospheric pressure. Unfortunately, infections from the throat often pass through the tube into the middle ear. Rapid changes in altitude, harsh blowing of the nose, or a forceful sneeze may cause temporary air pressure imbalances or inequality.

The Inner Ear

The vibrations from the middle ear continue through the coiled **cochlea**, which contains the **organ of Corti**, a collection of specialized nerve cells (Figure 11-57). These cells transmit the impulses to the auditory nerve, which passes them on to the auditory center of the temporal lobe of the cerebrum for interpretation.

The inner ear also contains three **semicircular canals**. These structures are responsible for maintaining equilibrium (balance). Inside the canals, hairlike nerve cell receptors are embedded in a gelatin-like material. When the head moves, the material pushes against the receptors, which transmit to the brain the change in position.

Another nerve receptor network in the semicircular canals is similarly constructed inside two small sacs. The gelatin surface here is covered with a layer of tiny limestone grains. When the head moves, the grains shift, causing the hair cells to send out impulses.

The inner ear, therefore, carries out two important functions for the body: It transmits vibrations to the auditory nerve so that we can hear, and its semicircular canals allow us to maintain our balance.

DIAGNOSTIC TESTS

Routine diagnostic examinations for the ear, such as audiometry, Weber, and Rinne, are discussed in Chapter 14.

Electronystagmograph

The electronystagmograph (ENG) is a special examination that evaluates balance function. Because eyes and ears work together through the nervous system, measurement of eye movements are used to evaluate the balance system. The test is performed in a darkened room with electrodes placed near the eyes. Wires from the electrodes attach to a recording machine. Warm and cool water or air are gently introduced into each ear canal. Patients are asked to identify locations of visible objects when shown. Coordination is evidence of balance function and will be affected by the involved ear.

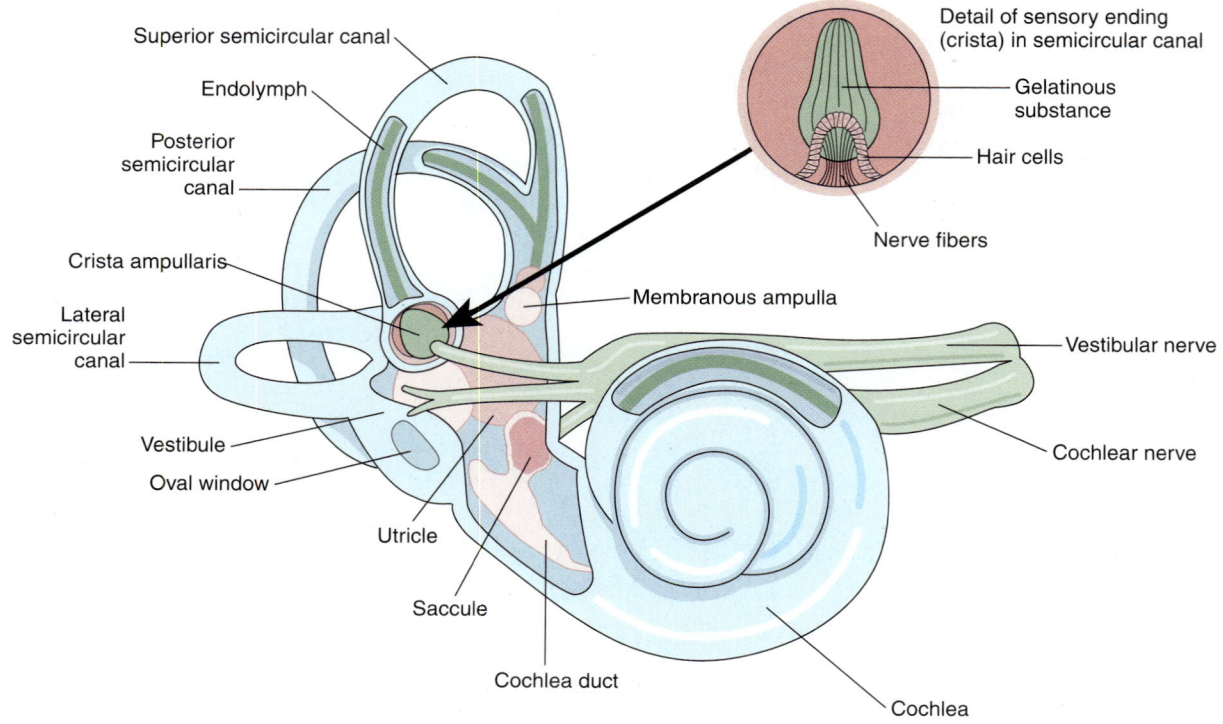

FIGURE 11-57 The inner ear

MRI

MRI of the brain with special emphasis on the inner ear can be used to identify pathology.

DISEASES AND DISORDERS OF THE EAR

Auditory Canal Obstruction

Description—This refers to anything in the ear canal that in some manner occludes the opening.

Signs and symptoms—Symptoms vary with the obstruction. Insects may produce sounds or movement, or objects can cause discomfort, a degree of hearing loss, or annoyance.

Etiology—The auditory canal can be obstructed by impacted **cerumen** (ear wax) or a foreign body such as a bean, pea, pebble, bead, or insect. Children often put objects into their ears.

Treatment—Treatment consists of a removal technique appropriate to the obstruction. Cerumen can be removed by gentle scraping with a cerumen spoon and irrigation by syringe or an aerated water jet (see Chapter 14). Irrigation should be stopped immediately if it causes pain. Removal of insects can be accomplished after killing with an instillation of 70% alcohol. Similar objects can also be removed after irrigation with alcohol if they cannot be reached with forceps. Water

must be avoided if it may cause swelling of the object, such as a bean or pea. Any object that cannot be removed easily should be referred to an otorhinolaryngologist for consultation.

Hearing Loss

Description—This is a condition of reduced ability to perceive sound at normal levels.

Signs and symptoms—The loss can be gradual or sudden. The person has difficulty perceiving sounds in their environment. Hearing loss is classified as conductive if it is caused by the inability to carry sound waves through the ear structures. It is known as **sensorineural** if it is the result of nerve transmission failure within the inner ear or the auditory nerve. Some hearing loss can be caused by a combination of factors. The gradual loss of hearing that occurs normally as part of the aging process is known as **presbycusis**.

Etiology—Conductive loss may be caused by an obstruction from a buildup of cerumen (wax), a foreign body, swelling within the auditory canal, middle ear infection, or otosclerosis.

Sudden loss of hearing without prior impairment is considered a medical emergency, because prompt treatment may restore hearing. Common causes are acute infection, head trauma, brain tumor, toxic drugs, or metabolic and vascular disorders.

Hearing loss can also be noise-induced and can be temporary or, over time, permanent. It follows prolonged exposure to noise in excess of 85 to 90 db (see Chapter 14). It is common among people who work in constant industrial noise, military personnel, and rock musicians. This loss is preventable with the enforcement of the use of protective devices, such as ear plugs, as mandated by law in occupational exposure.

Bone and air conduction hearing loss is assessed by the Rinne and Weber tests. An audiometer can be used to give a pure tone audiometry examination to measure the threshold and degree of loudness at which sound can be perceived (see Chapter 14).

Treatment—The form of treatment depends upon the causative factor. Removal of obstructions will correct the related conductive loss. With sudden loss, treatment may involve medication, surgery, or antidotes to toxins. Loss caused by aging can usually be improved with the use of modern hearing aids; providing sound amplification is all that is required. A new cochlear implant can improve severe hearing loss that is not benefitted by a hearing aid. The implant involves a mini-microphone behind the ear, a calculator-sized processor that can be worn on a belt, a receiver surgically implanted in the ear, and electrical contacts that run through the cochlea. To be approved for the implant, patients must have an intact auditory nerve and a hearing loss in which less than 30% of speech is understood, even with a hearing aid. Most will gain at least modest communication ability; some are even able to use a phone. Implant failure rate is about 2% and unfortunately causes patients to lose any natural hearing they may have had prior to the surgery.

Ménière's Disease (Mane-arz')

Description—This disease is a disorder of the inner ear, usually affecting only one ear; however, 15% of patients may have both ears affected. It typically begins between the ages of 20 and 50, affecting men and women equally.

Signs and symptoms—The condition known as **Ménière's disease** is characterized by severe vertigo (dizziness) and **tinnitus** (ringing in the ears). Violent attacks may last from 10 minutes to hours and cause severe nausea, vomiting, and perspiration. Occasionally the vertigo causes loss of balance and results in the person falling. There is intermittent hearing loss early in the disease, but over time a fixed loss may develop, probably as a result of the degeneration of hair cells in the cochlea.

Etiology—The cause is unknown, but it probably results from an abnormality in the fluids of the inner ear.

Treatment—Treatment consists of drugs to reduce fluid, antihistamines, and mild sedation. Anti-vertigo and anti-nausea medications may be used. Patients are advised to avoid caffeine, smoking, and alcohol. Excessive fatigue and stress may aggravate the disease. Patients who experience vertigo without warning are advised not to drive or engage in any type of potentially hazardous activity because of the possibility of an accident. If attacks are not controlled conservatively and become disabling, a surgical procedure may be indicated. Options range from a shunt to remove excess fluid to the cutting of the balance nerve (which will usually control the vertigo while still maintaining hearing) to a labyrinthectomy (which destroys both the balance mechanism and hearing on the affected side, but will control the attacks). Medical labyrinthectomy with vestibule-toxic drugs is appropriate in some cases. There is only a cure for vertigo, not for Ménière's disease.

Motion Sickness

Description—A condition that occurs when engaging in activities involving movement, such as riding in automobiles, boats, planes, or amusement rides.

Signs and symptoms—This is characterized by loss of equilibrium, perspiration, headache, nausea, and vomiting brought on by irregular motion.

Etiology—The disorder probably results from excessive stimulation of the inner ear receptors or confusion in the brain between the visual stimulus and movement perception.

Treatment—Treatment consists of avoiding the causative motions, lying down, and closing the eyes. When avoidance is not possible, the head should be kept still and vision focused on distant and stationary objects. Medications to prevent nausea and vomiting, such as valium, scopolamine, and antihistamines, are usually beneficial if taken prior to the trip. Symptoms can also be controlled by applying medication in a patch form to the skin behind the ear.

Otitis: Externa (O-ti'-tis)

Description—An infection of the external auditory canal.

Signs and symptoms—**Otitis** causes pain and hearing loss.

Etiology—Otitis externa can result from contaminated swimming water (swimmer's ears); cleaning the canal with bobby pins or introducing an organism on a cotton swab; regular use of earphones or plugs, which can trap moisture, creating optimal growing conditions; and scratching the ear canal with a fingernail.

Treatment—It is best treated with pain medication and antibiotic ear drops, following thorough cleaning.

Otitis: Media

Description—An infection of the middle ear often associated with respiratory infections.

Signs and symptoms—Otitis media is characterized by a severe, deep, and throbbing pain; fever and hearing loss. The tympanic membrane may be reddened and bulge into the external canal. Excessive pressure may cause it to rupture, resulting in drainage into the canal. Recurring episodes may scar and thicken the membrane, causing a conductive hearing loss. Holes and tears from a rupture will also cause a loss of hearing.

Etiology—Otitis media usually occurs from an organism that has caused a sore throat or cold. However, it can also be caused by obstruction of the eustachian tube that results in a negative pressure within the ear that "pulls" serous fluid from the blood vessels into the middle ear.

Treatment requires antibiotics, such as penicillin or erythromycin (with a sulfa drug if allergic to penicillin), in addition to pain medication. A myringotomy (incision of the tympanic membrane) may be indicated if bulging and severe pain are present.

Note: Young children and infants are prone to ear infections. Anatomically, their eustachian tubes lie horizontally, which makes it more difficult for them to open and ventilate the middle ear. Infants who are allowed to take a bottle while lying down may get fluid and bacteria into their eustachian tubes from reflux or from obstruction, causing negative pressure to extract fluid.

Treatment—With chronic fluid collection caused by obstruction, it may be necessary to insert a tiny polyethylene tube through the tympanic membrane to temporarily equalize the pressure. This procedure is known as a tympanoostomy. Tubes usually fall out after about 6 to 12 months. *Caution:* Untreated middle ear infection can lead to severe complications, such as mastoiditis, brain abscesses, or meningitis. With today's antibiotics, these complications are rare. Sudden hearing loss, headache, dizziness, chills, and fever are possible warning signs.

Otosclerosis (O-to-skle-ro'sis)

Description—The most common cause of conductive deafness is **otosclerosis**. It is characterized by the formation of spongy bone that immobilizes the stapes in the oval window of the vestibule, disrupting the conduction of vibrations from the tympanic membrane to the cochlea.

Signs and symptoms—Otosclerosis is a condition characterized by the slow and progressive loss of hearing and may be accompanied by tinnitus.

Etiology—It appears to result from a genetic factor and often occurs among family members. Incidence in Caucasians is at least 10%, affecting twice as many females as males, usually between 15 and 30 years of age.

Treatment—Treatment for otosclerosis consists of surgically removing the stapes (stapedectomy) and inserting an artificial substitute, which results in partial to complete return of hearing. An appropriate hearing aid is helpful if a stapedectomy is not possible.

Presbycusis (Prez-bi-ku'-sis) (Senile Deafness)

Description—This hearing loss is an effect of aging. It is sensorineural in nature.

Signs and symptoms—The deafness normally manifests itself through the loss of high-frequency sounds. It is usually accompanied by an annoying tinnitus. The patient has difficulty understanding the spoken word and may become depressed because of inability to communicate.

Etiology—The loss is caused by the deterioration of the auditory system and a loss of the hair cells in the organ of Corti.

Treatment—Presbycusis is irreversible but can be helped with an effective and properly fitting hearing aid.

THE NOSE AND THE SENSE OF SMELL

The sense of smell is due to the olfactory organ in the top of the nasal cavity (Figure 11-58). The nerve fibers in the organ are chemoreceptors that respond to stimuli from ions or molecules dissolved in the moisture from the mucous membranes. The organ is connected by nerve fibers, which run through tiny holes in the skull bone above the nasal cavity, to the olfactory center in the brain. The nerve fibers connect with receptor cells in the mucous membrane of the nose. These odor detectors can "smell" something only after it is dissolved in the mucus secretions.

DISEASES AND DISORDERS OF THE NOSE

Epistaxis (Epi-stak'-sis) (Nosebleed)

Description—Bleeding from the nose.

Signs and symptoms—The presence of blood coming from the nose is evidence of epistaxis. However, blood originating from the nose may be expectorated from

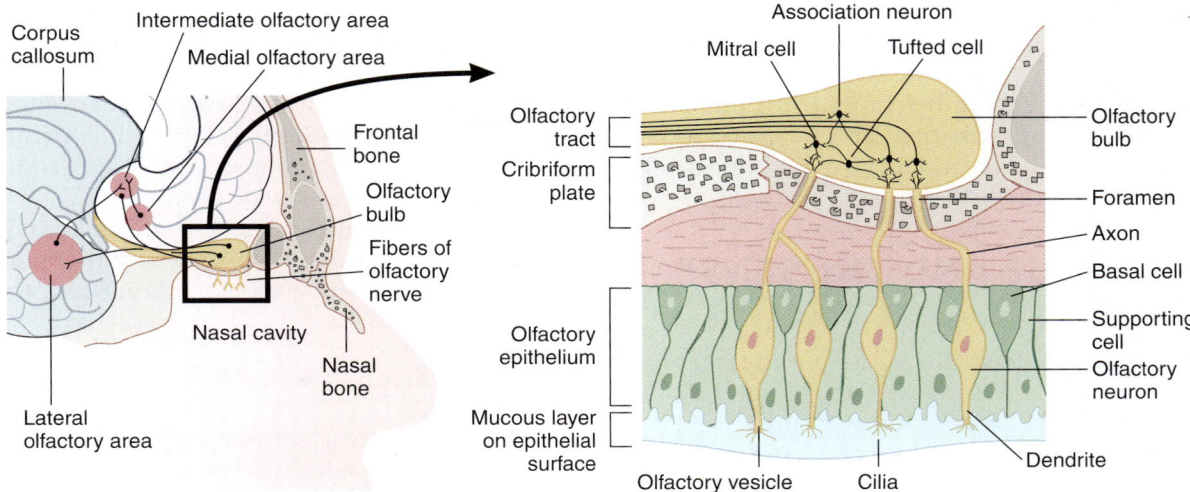

FIGURE 11-58   The sense of smell

the mouth or swallowed into the throat. Symptoms other than visible blood may be lightheadedness, a drop in blood pressure, rapid pulse, dyspnea, pallor, and other indications of shock.

Etiology—This usually occurs after injury, either external or internal, such as a blow to the nose, nosepicking, or foreign body insertion. Less frequent causes of **epistaxis** are chronic conditions, such as nasal or sinus infection that results in capillary congestion and bleeding, or the inhalation of irritating substances. Predisposing systemic factors include high blood pressure; anticoagulation drugs; chronic aspirin use; and blood diseases, such as anemia, hemophilia, and leukemia.

Treatment—Treatment varies depending on the cause, location, and severity. Even moderate bleeding is considered severe if it persists longer than 10 minutes after pressure is applied. Initial first aid treatment may consist of elevating the head, compression of nostrils against the septum continuously for 5 to 10 minutes, application of ice or cold compresses to nose, preventing the swallowing of blood (to determine the amount lost), avoiding talking or blowing the nose, and observing for amount of blood loss and signs of shock.

Advanced treatment depends on location. For anterior bleeding, apply an epinephrine-saturated cotton ball or gauze to the bleeding site and use external pressure, followed by cauterization by electric cautery or silver nitrate. For posterior bleeding, the insertion of a nasal balloon for 48 to 72 hours may be required. Small catheters with balloons are passed through the bleeding side of the nose into the nasopharynx. The ballons are inflated, creating pressure against the leaking blood vessels. If necessary, anterior bleeding can be treated by packing for 24 to 48 hours. Other treatment may include supplemental vitamin K, blood

transfusions, and surgical ligation (tying) of the bleeding artery. Embolization of blood vessels (clotting) by x-ray guided catheters is also effective.

Nasal Polyps (Pol'ips)

Description—These usually benign growths, most often multiple, and in both sides of the nose, may occur in large enough numbers and size to obstruct the airway.

Signs and symptoms—Patients usually complains of obstruction and "something" in the nose. They experience difficulty breathing. Diagnosis is made by visual observation through a nasal speculum or by x-rays of the nasal passages and the sinuses.

Etiology—They are thought to be caused by prolonged mucous membrane edema associated with allergies, chronic sinusitis, rhinitis, and recurrent nasal infections.

Treatment—If infected, treatment with steroids and antibiotics will temporarily reduce the size of the **polyps**. However, surgical removal is the treatment of choice and is usually necessary.

Rhinitis (Allergic) (Ri-ni'-tis)

Description—Allergic rhinitis is a reaction to airborne allergens.

Signs and symptoms—It causes sneezing, profuse watery discharge, itching of the eyes and nose, conjunctivitis, and tearing. Many symptoms are the result of the body's attempt to dilute or remove irritants coming into contact with its mucous membranes.

Etiology—Any antigen occurring in the environment can be an irritant and cause allergic rhinitis. Some of the most common are dust, ragweed, pollens, and cat dander.

Treatment—Treatment consists of eliminating environmental antigens when possible and the use of antihistamines and topical corticosteroids. Long-term management includes injections of the offending allergens to cause desensitization, the use of air conditioning, and, if severe and persistent, relocation to a safe environment.

THE TONGUE AND THE SENSE OF TASTE

The ability to taste flavors is located in the receptors of the taste buds on the tongue. They are located at the tip, sides, and back. Like the sense of smell, taste is possible because of the chemoreceptors that receive stimuli from ions or molecules and initiate the impulses. As with smell, taste is not possible unless the substance is moistened. This moisture is supplied by the salivary glands in sufficient quantities to affect taste.

DISEASES AND DISORDERS OF THE MOUTH AND TONGUE

Candidiasis (Kan-di-dia'-sis) (Thrush)

Description—This disease is a fungal infection of the mucous membranes of the mouth and throat. The organism can cause infection in other locations, such as nails, skin (diaper rash), vagina, and the gastrointestinal tract.

Signs and symptoms—Evidence of the disease is cream-colored or white patches of exudate on the tongue, mouth, or throat that cannot be scraped off (Figure 11-59). The infected areas may swell, causing respiratory distress in infants. Occasionally they are painful, but they usually cause a burning sensation in the throat and mouth of adults.

Etiology—It is caused by a fungal organism of the *Candida* species. These organisms are normally present

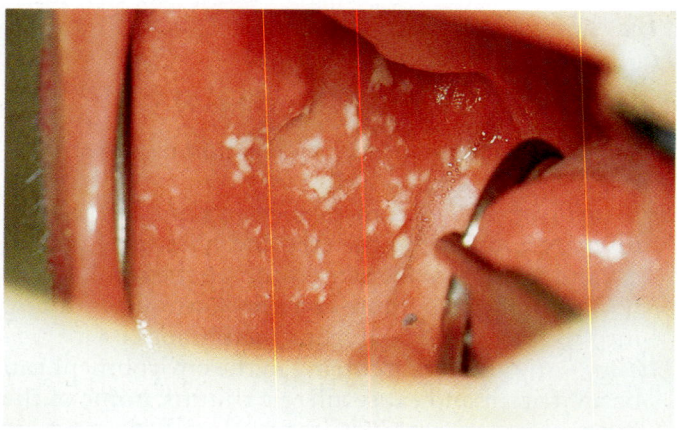

FIGURE 11-59 Candidiasis (thrush) *(Courtesy of Dr. Joseph Konzelman, School of Dentistry, Medical College of Georgia)*

in the body but cause infection when their sudden growth is permitted by some change, such as an illness, a suppressed immune system, drug abuse, or from the use of broad-spectrum antibiotics that alters the body's normal flora, which permits candida to increase. Infants may acquire thrush during birth or from unclean bottle nipples.

Treatment—Initial treatment is aimed at improving the underlying cause, then swabbing the mouth with an oral nystatin suspension or oral antifungal medication.

> **PEDIATRIC PERSPECTIVE**
>
> If the mother is breast-feeding, she must also treat her nipples with an antifungal medication.

Glossitis (Gloss-i'-tis)

Description—Inflammation of the tongue.

Signs and symptoms—The condition results in a red, swollen tongue, pain on chewing, difficult speech, and occasionally an obstructed airway.

Etiology—It is caused by an organism, irritation, injury, or nutritional deficiencies. Agents such as tobacco, alcohol, spicy foods, and jagged teeth may cause glossitis.

Treatment—Treatment includes topical anesthetic mouthwash, systemic pain medication, good oral hygiene, and the avoidance of alcohol and hot, cold, or spicy foods.

Oral Cancer

Description—In recent years, a significant increase in the incidence of oral cancer has been noted. There seems to be evidence that some people have switched from cigarettes to smokeless forms of tobacco in an effort to avoid the development of lung cancer. Oral cancer is linked to alcohol and tobacco ingestion.

Signs and symptoms—Any lesion or growth within the mouth is not normal and should be examined by a physician or dentist. They can be of varying shapes and types and may present no evidence of pain or discomfort.

Etiology—No one knows for certain the exact cause for cancer, but there are strong correlations between substances and the development of malignant lesions. Normal cells are affected by something in their environment that causes their normal growth-limiting control to fail and excessive cell production to begin. The use of products such as chewing tobacco and snuff causes extensive disease of the gums, tongue, and other oral structures and often results in the development of cancer within the oral cavity.

Treatment—The use of surgical excision as a treatment depends upon the form of cancer developed. Quite disfiguring results arise from removal of part of the mouth, and often speech is affected when the tongue is involved. Chemotherapy and radiation are appropriate.

THE SKIN AND THE SENSE OF TOUCH

The sense of touch requires direct contact with the body through contact receptors (Figure 11-60). The sense of touch involves mechanical energy, such as pressure or traction, which activates mechanoreceptors. Radiant energy, such as heat or cold, activates thermoreceptors. The design of the receptor varies with its location on the body. Touch receptors are most concentrated in the fingertips. Pain receptors are simply bare nerve endings in the skin and other organs. Separate skin receptors perceive heat and cold. Each of the contact receptors in the skin has its own perceptive function, enabling us to feel the many different sensations of pain, touch, pressure, heat, cold, traction, and tickle. This sense aids us in protecting ourselves, identifying injury, feeling pleasure, and maintaining contact with our environment. The skin is the subject of the next unit.

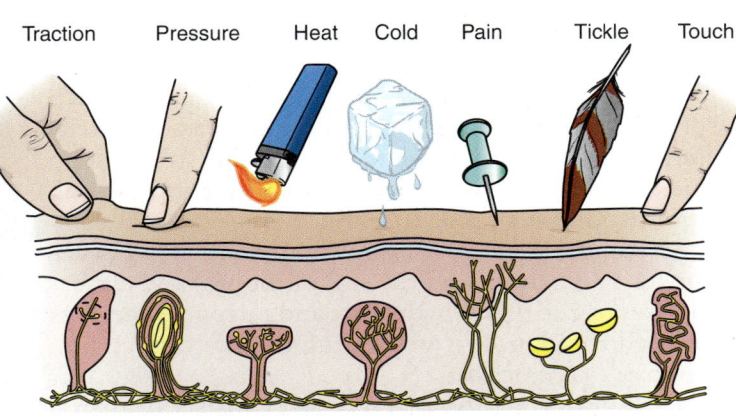

Traction   Pressure   Heat   Cold   Pain   Tickle   Touch

FIGURE 11-60   The sense of touch

ACHIEVE UNIT OBJECTIVES

- ☐ Complete the Workbook activities to meet the learning objectives.
- ☐ Apply your knowledge at the end of this chapter in completing the Critical Thinking Challenge and Activities, as well as the StudyWARE on your Student CD-ROM.

UNIT 4
THE INTEGUMENTARY SYSTEM

OBJECTIVES

Upon completion of this unit, you will be able to achieve the following:

LEARNING Objectives

1. Spell and define, using the glossary at the back of the text, all the Words to Know in this unit.
2. List the five functions of the skin.
3. Explain how the skin regulates body temperature.
4. Describe how the body cools its surface.
5. Name the three layers of skin tissue and the characteristic structures of each layer.
6. Describe the process that causes wrinkles.
7. Explain what causes a suntan to develop.
8. Describe the distinguishing features of basal cell and squamous cell carcinoma lesions.
9. Identify the ABCDE rules and other warning signs of melanoma and the factors that contribute to its development.
10. Explain what causes blushing, birthmarks, moles, and albinism.
11. Identify 20 diseases or disorders of the skin.

WORDS TO KNOW

acne	herpes simplex	pustule
albino	herpes zoster	receptors
alopecia	integumentary	sebaceous
carbuncle	keloid	sebum
constrict	lesion	slough
dermatitis	Lyme disease	subcutaneous
dermis	macule	transdermal
dilate	melanin	urticaria
eczema	melanocytes	verrucae
epidermis	papule	vesicle
erythema	pediculosis	viral shedding
follicle	perception	wheals
folliculitis	pigment	whorl
furuncle	psoriasis	

CERTIFICATION CONNECTION

CMA
Diagnostic procedures
Common diseases and
    pathology
Anatomy and physiology

CMAS
Anatomy and physiology

RMA
Anatomy and physiology

The word **integumentary** refers to an external covering or skin. You may never have thought of the skin as a "body system," but according to the definition of a system in Unit 1, the skin with all its structures qualifies: it is many tissues (nerve, connective, muscle, epithelial), forming organs (sweat and oil glands), to perform a function. The skin is not usually listed as one of the body's systems, however. Most anatomists classify the skin as an organ. When listed in this category, it becomes the largest organ of the body. An average adult has about 3,000 square inches of skin surface. The skin makes up about 15% of the total body weight, which would be approximately 20 pounds of a 145-pound person. The skin varies in thickness from very thin on the eyelids to quite thick on the soles of the feet.

The skin is so important to survival that the loss of even a small percentage of its vital function is a cause for concern. If about one third of the skin of a healthy young adult is lost, death may result. Skin covers all the body's surface, preventing the tissue fluids from escaping and foreign materials in the environment from entering. At the openings to the body, such as the nose, mouth, or anus, it joins with the mucous membranes that line the openings into the respiratory and digestive systems to make a continuous internal and external covering.

FUNCTIONS

The skin performs five important functions for the body: protection, perception, temperature control, absorption, and excretion. The skin protects against the invasion of bacteria by serving as a barrier. It is effective, however, only as long as it remains intact. A cut or scrape of the surface allows bacteria to enter. It also protects the delicate underlying tissues from injury by the damaging rays of the sun. Equally important, it protects the body's tissues from loss of fluid. This is of great concern when large areas of skin are lost as a result of burns, for example, which allows fluids to escape and bacteria to enter.

The skin serves as an organ of **perception** in cooperation with the nervous system and the sense of touch. A square inch of skin contains about 72 feet of nerves and hundreds of **receptors** registering pain, heat, cold, and pressure.

In that same square inch are about 15 feet of blood vessels, which provide nutrients and oxygen and also regulate the body's temperature. This function is of such importance to the body that the skin receives approximately one third of the blood circulating throughout the body. When the body's temperature control center in the brain senses the body is becoming too warm, the nervous system sends messages to the surface vessels to **dilate**, which allows heat from the blood to escape through the skin's surface and therefore cool the body. If heat must be retained, the vessels are ordered to **constrict** to reduce the loss of heat so that body temperature can be maintained at an adequate level. This important function is discussed in greater detail in Chapter 13, Unit 3.

The skin also contains sweat glands, which are likewise controlled by the heat regulator in the brain. When the air temperature rises, the body produces sweat, which evaporates from its surface to provide a cooling effect and thereby reduce the amount of heat within the underlying blood vessels.

The skin is capable of absorbing some materials from its surface through the hair **follicles** and the glands. This function can be of use to the physician in treating certain conditions. Perhaps the two most common applications are anti-motion sickness medication in a patch form, which is placed on the skin's surface behind the ear, and in a medicated paste form, which is placed on the chest to treat certain heart conditions. A trend seems to be developing toward a greater amount of medications being administered through the skin. Primarily the advantages are "timed release," which spreads medication evenly over a long period, thereby eliminating repeated dosage and the digestive system side effects from certain oral drugs. This form of drug administration is called **transdermal**.

Several substances known as lipid-soluble (e.g., vitamins A, D, E, and K and the sex hormones) and almost all gases (e.g., oxygen, hydrogen, and nitrogen) can pass through the skin. It is interesting to note that carbon monoxide cannot pass.

The skin's function of excretion consists primarily of eliminating water and salt plus a minute amount of other waste products. Excessive fluid loss as a result of strenuous activity or a highly elevated temperature can be a matter of concern. Fluid must be replaced to maintain a proper fluid balance. The skin also combines the ultraviolet rays from sunlight with compounds normally present in the skin to produce vitamin D.

A great number of microscopic skin structures are located within an area of only 1 square centimeter. This is illustrated in Figure 11-61 as a small circle on the back of the hand. It seems inconceivable that this large group of anatomical structures could be located in such a small area. These microscopic wonders perform an invaluable service for the body.

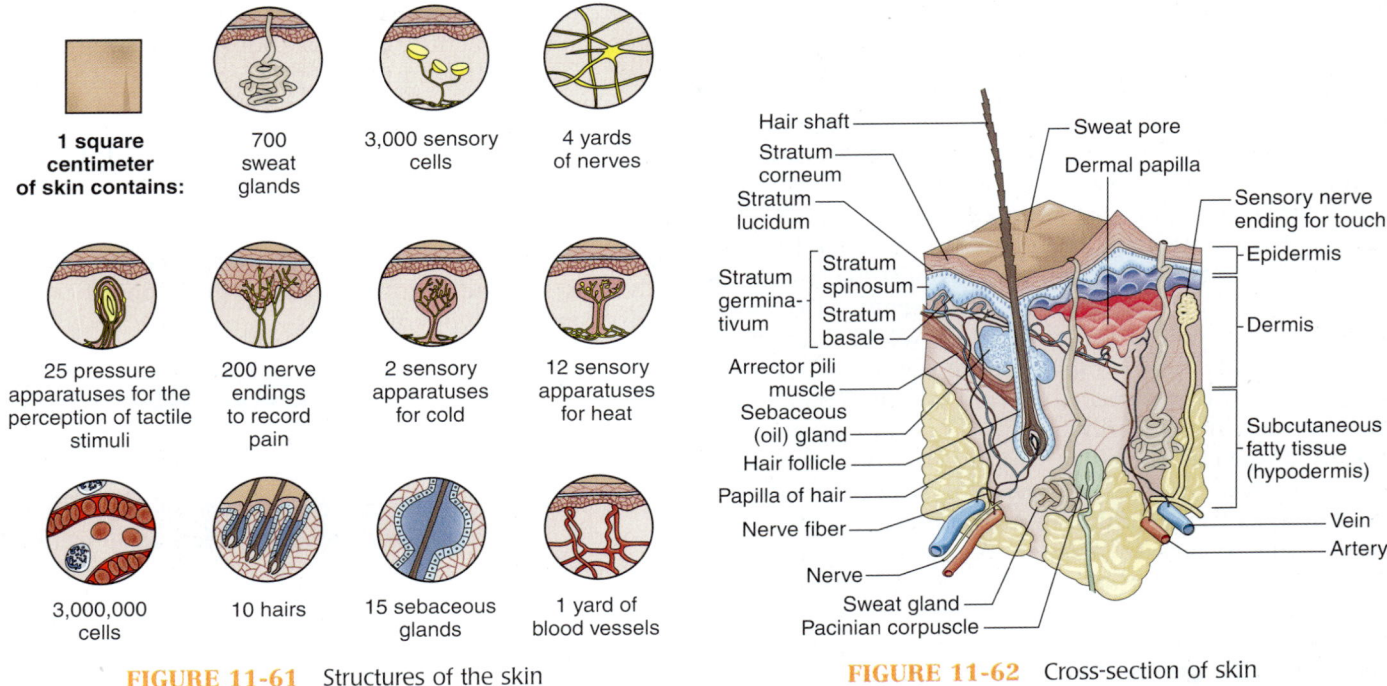

1 square centimeter of skin contains:

700 sweat glands

3,000 sensory cells

4 yards of nerves

25 pressure apparatuses for the perception of tactile stimuli

200 nerve endings to record pain

2 sensory apparatuses for cold

12 sensory apparatuses for heat

3,000,000 cells

10 hairs

15 sebaceous glands

1 yard of blood vessels

FIGURE 11-61   Structures of the skin

FIGURE 11-62   Cross-section of skin

Figure 11-62 labels: Hair shaft; Stratum corneum; Stratum lucidum; Stratum germinativum [Stratum spinosum, Stratum basale]; Arrector pili muscle; Sebaceous (oil) gland; Hair follicle; Papilla of hair; Nerve fiber; Nerve; Sweat gland; Pacinian corpuscle; Sweat pore; Dermal papilla; Sensory nerve ending for touch; Epidermis; Dermis; Subcutaneous fatty tissue (hypodermis); Vein; Artery

STRUCTURE OF THE SKIN

The skin is composed of three layers: the **epidermis** on the top, the **dermis** in the middle, and the **subcutaneous** layer on the bottom (Figure 11-62). The subcutaneous layer is filled with fat globules, blood vessels, and nerves. The dermis contains blood vessels, nerves, hair follicles, and sweat and oil glands. This layer is usually referred to as the "true skin." The top of the dermis is covered with cone-shaped papillae, which create an uneven surface. The epidermis is full of ridges that fit snugly over the papillae on top of the dermis. These ridges form the **whorls** and patterns on the fingertips that we call fingerprints. Because no two people have exactly the same pattern of ridges, they will not have the same fingerprints, making this characteristic a suitable means of identification. Similar patterns of ridges appear on the soles of the feet and are used for identification of newborns. New cells are formed deep in the epidermis. Here rapid cell division pushes cells toward the surface of the skin to replace those that wear away, die, and flake off. The process from division to flaking off takes about 28 to 60 days. Because of the skin's ability to reproduce cells rapidly, it can repair itself quickly following cuts and abrasions.

The skin is strong, soft, flexible, and elastic in young people because of the presence of keratin in the epidermis and collagen fibers in the dermis. With age, elastic fibers in the dermis increase in size, and collagen in the dermis degenerates. The support for the epidermis is decreased, and as a result, wrinkles occur. This is especially noticeable in areas where there is more facial movement, such as around the eyes and mouth.

The skin has four appendages. These are the sweat glands, oil glands, hair, and nails. The dermis contains the sweat and **sebaceous** (oil) glands. Sweat glands are tiny coiled tubes deep in the dermis and corkscrew tubules leading to the surface. Oil glands are located in or near hair follicles over the entire skin surface, except for the palms of the hands and the soles of the feet.

A sebaceous gland produces an oily substance that helps prevent the hair and skin from becoming dry and brittle. Unfortunately, oil glands often become plugged by cell overgrowth. The gland continues to produce oil, which fills the duct and results in development of a blackhead or pimple. This results in a condition known as **acne**.

Every hair has a root, which is inside a follicle (shaft) that extends deep into the dermal layer. With long hair, the root extends into the subcutaneous layer. Attached to each follicle is a small involuntary muscle. With certain emotions or sensations of coldness, the muscle contracts, causing the hair to stand erect and producing what we call "goose flesh." An inner layer of cells in the shaft of hair contains a **pigment** that gives the hair its color. Hair that is white has cells that contain little pigment.

The hair and nails are composed of hard keratin (soft keratin is found in the epidermis). The keratins are similar, but the hard keratin is more permanent and does not **slough** (drop) off, which means they must be cut occasionally.

Skin Color

A brown-black pigment called **melanin** is produced by cells called *melanocytes,* which are present in the epidermis. They protect the underlying tissues from damage by the sun. The amount of melanin affects the color of the skin, as does another pigment, carotene, which is yellow. In light-skinned people, melanin is found at the bottom of the epidermis. In people with darker skin, it is found throughout the epidermis. The presence of blood vessels in the dermis also contributes to the coloration of the skin. When the skin is exposed to the sun, it may become reddened because of dilation of the superficial blood vessels. The condition is known medically as **erythema**, but it is commonly known as sunburn. If it is not severe, the skin will acquire a brown coloration or suntan, which is produced by the melanin pigment increasing and moving to the surface to protect the underlying tissues. New melanin will replace the old in the lower cell layer. Freckles are actually small areas of melanin pigment.

Skin coloration is affected by many factors. When we blush, the rich supply of blood vessels causes reddening of the skin caused by dilation. Birthmarks may be caused by coloration from a concentration of blood vessels or from patches of skin pigment. Moles are also pigmented patches. A person whose skin has little or no pigment to give it color is said to be an **albino**. An albino's hair also lacks pigment and will be pale yellow or white. Because pigment is also lacking in the coloration of the eyes, the sun and artificial light cannot be filtered out. Therefore, the eyes of a person with albinism are a red color as the result of translucent irises and are very sensitive to light. People with this disorder must wear sunglasses or tinted lenses for comfort and to prevent eye damage. They also need to protect their skin, as their lack of pigment places them at high risk for skin cancer.

THE SKIN AS A DIAGNOSTIC TESTING SITE

The skin is often used to test and diagnose disorders and diseases of the body, specifically in the area of allergies. Because of its natural capacity to defend the body from foreign substances, it makes an excellent medium for testing the reaction to minute amounts of allergens. Following injection of common substances, usually on the patient's back or the inner surface of the forearm, the skin will form various-sized areas around the injection sites, reacting to those materials that initiate an allergic response. Besides injecting allergens, the skin can also be used for patch tests. Tiny amounts of allergens are placed on stainless steel discs and applied to the back. Forty-eight hours later the skin under the discs is assessed for reaction. Based upon these findings, physicians can then identify causative substances and recommend measures to reduce the problems associated with the allergic disorder. (See Chapter 16).

Skin Appearance

Conditions of the skin cause changes in its appearance. These changes are known as **lesions** and manifest themselves as specific eruptions. Table 11-3 identifies the most common types of lesions.

DISEASES AND DISORDERS

Acne Vulgaris (Ak'ne Vul-gar'is)

Description—This inflammatory disease of the follicles of the sebaceous glands mainly affects adolescents.

Signs and symptoms—The acne may appear as a closed comedo or whitehead if it does not protrude from the follicle and is covered by the epidermis. If it protrudes and has black coloration caused by the melanin or pigment from the follicle, it is known as a blackhead or open comedo. Eventually, the enlarged plug leaks or ruptures, spreading into the dermis and resulting in inflammation and the development of pustules and **papules**.

Etiology—The cause is multifactorial (many factors). Research has determined that dietary habits appear to be less of a factor than originally thought. Present findings seem to suggest that hormonal dysfunction and an oversupply of **sebum**, oil from the sebaceous glands, are the probable underlying causes. It collects at the openings to the glands, hardens, and closes off the natural flow of oily secretion, causing blackheads or cysts to develop. Sometimes the area will become filled with leukocytes that cause pus to accumulate and pimples develop. Trapped bacteria within the follicle are also a contributing factor.

Treatment—Usual treatment for severe acne includes a topical antibacterial product either alone or in combination with a topical retinoid product. Antibiotics applied to the skin are helpful. Systemic antibiotics decrease bacterial growth within follicles. Accutane is reserved for use in those patients with severe scarring acne. Oral contraceptives are used in women.

Alopecia (Al-o-pe'she-a)

Description—This is loss of hair, usually occurring on the scalp. There are two types of **alopecia**: a scarring type, which causes irreversible hair loss, and a nonscarring type, which usually is reversible.

TABLE 11-3   Types of Skin Lesions, Their Characteristics, Size, and Examples

Type of Skin Lesion	Characteristics	Size	Example
Bulla (blister)	Fluid-filled area	Greater than 5 mm across	• A large blister
Crust	A collection of dried serum and debris	Varies in size	• Impetigo or eczema
Excoriation	Area missing the epidermal layer	Varies in size	• Scrape or burn
Fissure	Linear crack from epidermis to dermis	Varies in size	• Athlete's feet, hand dermatitis
Macule	A round, flat area usually distinguished from itssurrounding skin by its change in color	Smaller than 1 cm	• Freckle • Petechia (small hemorrhage spot)
Nodule	Elevated solid area, deeper and firmer than a papule	Greater than 5 mm across	• Wart • Epidermal inclusion cyst
Papule	Elevated solid area	5 mm or less across	• Elevated nevus (mole)
Pustule	Discrete, pus-filled raised area	Varying size	• Acne
Ulcer	A deep loss of skin surface that may extend into the dermis that can bleed periodically and scar	Varies in sizes	• Venous stasis ulcer
Tumor	Solid mass of cells that may extend deep through cutaneous tissue	Larger than 1–2 cm	• Benign (harmless) epidermal tumor • Basal cell carcinoma (rarely metastasizing) • Lipoma
Vesicle	Fluid-filled raised area	5 mm or less across	• Chickenpox • Herpes simplex
Wheal	Itchy, temporarily elevated area with an irregular shape formed as a result of localized skin edema	Varies in size	• Hives • Insect bites

Scarring Alopecia

Signs and symptoms—The main symptom is the continual loss of hair, resulting in gradual thinning and the eventual absence of hair.

Etiology—This is usually an irreversible loss of hair resulting from the destruction of the hair follicles. It is caused by physical or chemical trauma or the chronic tension on the hair shaft from braiding or tight rolling of the hair. Certain diseases like lupus erythematosus, bacterial or viral infections, and skin tumors may also cause this type.

Treatment—This depends upon the cause. A change in the way the hair is cared for and the control of infection could prevent further loss but may not restore lost follicles.

Nonscarring Alopecia (Several Forms)
Male-pattern baldness

Signs and symptoms—The most common form of nonscarring alopecia is the evidence of hair loss with male-pattern baldness. It often begins around age 30 with a receding front hairline and loss of hair on the top and back. In some men, the areas eventually meet, leaving hair only on the sides (Figures 11-63A and B).

Etiology—It seems to be primarily caused by aging and the level of androgen (male hormone). There is a tendency for genetic influence, and it will often be displayed among male family members. Women may also exhibit the male pattern but at a lesser degree.

Treatment—There is no known "cure"; however, the use of Rhogaine and Propecia seems to prevent further loss and encourage regrowth in some men. Surgical grafting of hair follicles from other parts of the scalp have proved successful.

Physiologic

Signs and symptoms—A normal temporary hair loss that may occur immediately following or up to 4 months after giving birth.

Etiology—Prolongation of the growing phase.

Treatment—None required.

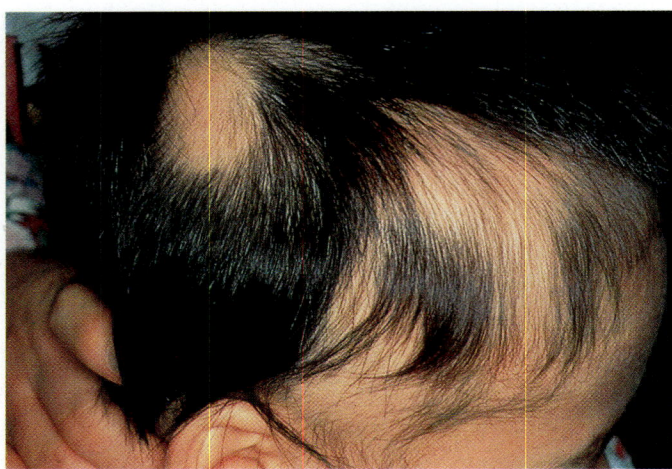

FIGURE 11-63A Alopecia *(Courtesy of Robert A. Silverman, MD, Clinical Associate Professor, Department of Pediatrics, Georgetown University)*

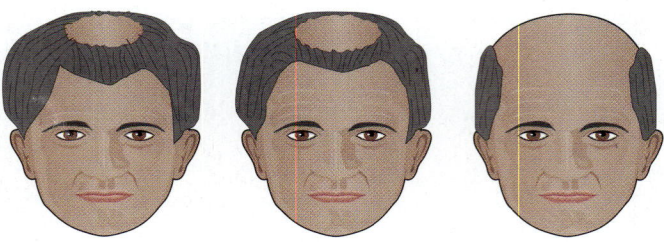

FIGURE 11-63B Male-pattern baldness

Areata (idiopathic)

Signs and symptoms—This type is self-limiting and reversible, occurring among both sexes from young to middle-age adults. It usually affects small patches but can involve the entire scalp and body.

Etiology—Unknown, but some feel it may be linked to stress.

Treatment—None. Regrowth is normally spontaneous. Solutions and local injections of Kenalog as well as topical steroid creams may also be used.

Trichotillomania

Signs and symptoms—This hair loss is characterized by patchy, incomplete areas of hair loss with many broken hairs, primarily on the scalp, but can also involve other areas, such as the eyebrows. It is more common in children.

Etiology—This loss is the result of it being pulled out because of compulsive behavior.

Treatment—Some form of psychotherapy may be necessary. Dressings over the areas aid in behavior change to encourage normal growth.

Chemotherapy related

Signs and symptoms—There is a sudden loss of most of the hair.

Etiology—Certain chemical agents destroy the cells of the hair, which result in the massive loss of hair over a 2- or 3-day period soon after the initiation of the drug. Normally, some fine hair will remain but is very sparse.

Treatment—Fortunately, about 3 months after treatments end, hair will begin regrowth, sometimes a different color or texture.

Cancer

Description—The skin may be the site of different forms of cancerous lesions, such as basal cell carcinomas, squamous cell carcinomas, and malignant melanomas. Nevi (moles) are considered to be potentially malignant and require careful observation.

Signs and symptoms—Bleeding; itching; or a change in color, size, shape, or texture of a mole suggests a possible conversion to a malignant state. A new, nonhealing lesion that bleeds easily should also raise suspicion.

Basal Cell Carcinoma
This is a slow-growing, locally destructive skin tumor. They occur where there are abundant sebaceous follicles, especially on the face. It is more prevalent in persons over the age of 40, especially those who are blond, blue-eyed, and fair skinned (Figure 11-64A). It is the most common malignant tumor affecting Caucasians. There are basically three types of basal cell carcinoma lesions, each with its own distinctive characteristics and usual location. They are diagnosed by appearance and surgical biopsy.

1. *Nodulo-ulcerative* lesions occur most often on the face and are small, smooth, pinkish, and translucent papules. As they enlarge, the centers become depressed and the borders elevated and firm.

2. *Superficial* basal cell carcinomas are often multiple and commonly occur on the chest and back. They are oval or irregularly shaped with sharply defined, threadlike borders that are slightly elevated.

3. *Sclerosing* basal cell lesions occur on the head and neck. They appear yellow to white, are waxy, and do not have distinct borders.

Etiology—Basal cell carcinoma is caused primarily by prolonged exposure to the sun.

Treatment—Treatment depends upon the extent of the lesion. It can include surgical excision, irradiation, chemosurgery, or curretage and electrodesiccation.

Squamous Cell Carcinoma (Skwa'-mus)

Description—This is an invasive tumor with metastatic potential. Its incidence is highest in fair-skinned Caucasian males over the age of 60. Living in sunny

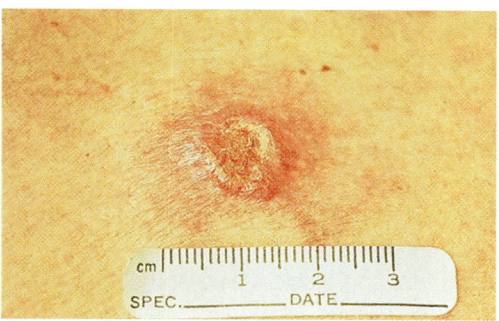

FIGURE 11-64A   Basal cell carcinoma *(Courtesy of Robert A. Silverman, MD, Clinical Associate Professor, Department of Pediatrics, Georgetown University)*

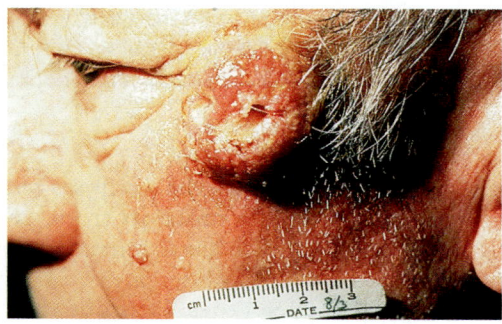

FIGURE 11-64B   Squamous cell carcinoma *(Courtesy of Robert A. Silverman, MD, Clinical Associate Professor, Department of Pediatrics, Georgetown University)*

climates, working in outdoor employment, and smoking greatly increase the risk of development.

Signs and symptoms—This form of carcinoma is commonly found on the face, the ears, the back of the hands, and other sun-damaged areas. The lesions have a tendency to metastasize, with those located on unexposed skin having the greater incidence. Lesions of the lower lip and ears are exceptionally metastatic (Figure 11-64B).

Etiology—This type is predisposed by sunlight, the presence of premalignant lesions, x-ray therapy, environmental carcinogens, and chronic skin irritation.

Treatment—The treatment varies with the size, location, and invasiveness of the lesion. Options include wide surgical excision, scraping and electrodesiccation, radiation, and chemosurgery.

Malignant Melanoma (Ma-lig'-nant Mela-no'ma)

Description—A neoplasm that develops from the pigment-producing **melanocytes**. The peak of incidence occurs between 50 and 70 years of age. The incidence is more common in women. There are four clinical types: superficial spreading melanoma, nodular melanoma, lentigo maligna melanoma, and acral lentiginous

melanoma. Superficial lesions may be curable with wide local excision. Deeper lesions may metastasize through the lymphatic and circulatory systems. Prognosis depends on the depth of the lesion, as measured in millimeters by the pathologist.

The American Cancer Society releases facts about the incidence of malignant melanoma. In 1993, 32,000 people were diagnosed; about 6,500 died. This translated into a lifetime risk of 1 in every 105 United States residents (compared with only 1 in every 1,500 in 1935). According to a Harvard Medical College article in September 2001, they were predicting about 51,400 new cases with approximately 7,800 deaths for that year. The lifetime risk of developing melanoma is now about 1 in every 75 people. The American Academy of Dermatology views this prevalence as an undeclared epidemic. The American Cancer Society, in its most recent release, estimated that there would be 62,190 new cases and 7,910 deaths in 2006.

Signs and symptoms—The information and photos in Figure 11-65 and Table 11-4 shows the ABCDE rules and appearance signs of melanoma.

Etiology—The major cause of malignant melanoma is exposure to the sun. The sun produces ultraviolet rays, mainly UVA and UVB. UVBs cause sunburn, premature aging of the skin, and skin cancers. Most sunscreens provide a degree of protection against this ray. However, recent evidence suggests that the

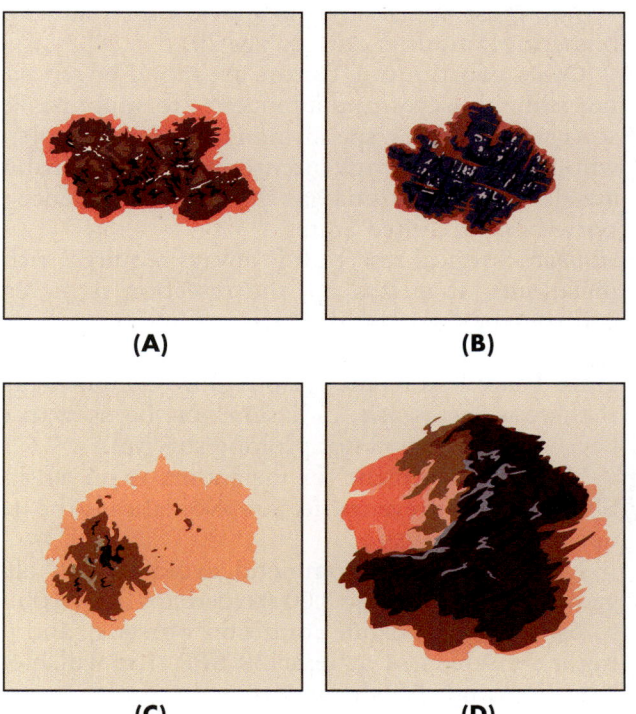

(A)   **(B)**

(C)   **(D)**

FIGURE 11-65   The signs of melanoma: (A) asymmetry, (B) border irregularity, (C) color, (D) diameter. Also see Table 11-4.

TABLE 11-4	Ordinary Moles versus Melanoma	
	Ordinary Mole	**Melanoma**
Shape	Symmetrical, round or oval	**Asymmetrical**—one side does not match the other (Figure 11-65A)
Border	Sharply defined **borders**	Edges are ragged, notched, or blurred (Figure 11-65B)
Color	Evenly **colored** brown, tan, or black	Shades of brown, tan, and black. May also have shades of red, white, or blue (Figure 11-65C)
Diameter	Generally less than 6 mm in diameter	Greater than 6 mm in **diameter** (Figure 11-65D)
Development	Once developed, remains the same size, shape, and color. Moles may fade with age.	**Evolving.** The surface of a mole may change to be scaly, oozing, or bleeding. A bump may appear. Pigmentation may spread past the mole border into the surrounding skin, and redness or swelling may occur. The mole may itch, swell, and feel tender. The person may even experience pain.

Adapted from The American Academy of Dermatology

UVA rays may also be damaging the skin, perhaps aiding the cancer-forming ability of UVB.

The Cancer Society cited the primary reasons for the melanoma increase to be weekend-packed leisure time, which results in intense bursts of exposure to UVB; the loss of the ozone layer protection; UVA rays not being blocked by sunscreens; and the tendency of people to purposely lie flat in the sun for hours at a time, which allows deeper penetration of the rays. People most at risk are those who have had severe blistering sunburns prior to age 20.

Other contributing factors are blond or red hair, fair skin, blue eyes, and a tendency to sunburn. Persons who work or spend many hours outdoors or who live in places with intense year-round sunshine are also at risk. Arizona has the highest incidence reported in the United States.

Treatment—Surgical resection is always required with a melanoma. If it is deep, the resection is at least 2 inches beyond the primary lesion's borders and into the deep tissues. Closure often requires a skin graft. Large lesions may also require chemotherapy. If there is metastasis, radiation may be used to relieve pain, but it will not prolong survival.

The best treatment for melanoma is prevention. Skin cancer is preventable. Sun avoidance is the best defense.

Dermatologists recommend avoiding sun altogether from 10:00 AM to 3:00 PM (perhaps from 8:00 AM to 6:00 PM if the ozone condition worsens), and using a sunscreen of at least 30 SPF that will block both UVA and UVB during exposure. Sunlamps, tanning pills, and tanning salons should be avoided.

The practice of monthly self-examination should be established to observe for any developing lesion so that it can be caught in the early stages. While standing in a brightly lit room in front of a full-length mirror and using a hand mirror, completely examine the body. Check under arms, on backs of legs, on feet, and between toes. Examine the back of the neck, and part the hair to check the scalp. If any growth, mole, sore, or discoloration appears suddenly or begins to change, it needs to be seen by a physician.

Cellulitis (Sel-u-li'-tis)

Description—The acute diffuse or spreading inflammation of the skin and subcutaneous tissue.

Signs and symptoms—It is characterized by localized swelling, pain, heat, and redness (Figure 11-66).

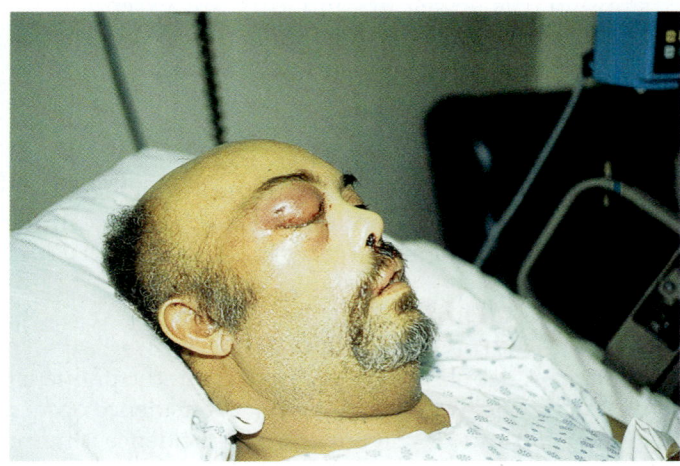

FIGURE 11-66 Cellulitis *(Courtesy of Dr. Mark Dougherty, Lexington, KY)*

Etiology—The cause of cellulitis is usually the *Strepto-coccus* or *Staphylococcus aureus* bacteria. It is potentially dangerous and may be deadly. There are antibiotic-resistant strains that require prompt treatment.

Treatment—It is usually treated successfully with oral antibiotics if diagnosed early. Severe cases require hospitalization and IV antibiotics.

Dermatitis (Der-ma-ti′-tis)

Description—The term means inflammation of the skin and can refer to any form of skin condition such as seborrhea, eczema, contact **dermatitis** (from irritants), exfoliative dermatitis (large pieces of peeling skin), or stasis (from lack of blood supply).

Signs and symptoms—Common symptoms are dry skin, redness, itching, edema, formation of lesions, and scaling.

Etiology—Dermatitis is often caused by allergens, such as wool; detergent; cosmetics; pollen; or foods, such as eggs, milk, seafood, or wheat products. Irritants to the skin; lack of moisture in the environment; harsh soaps; and long, hot showers also contribute to dermatitis.

Treatment—It is treated by avoiding known allergens and irritants; using emollients, hydrocortisone creams and ointments, systemic steroids, and antihistamines; and taking other dermatitis-specific measures.

Eczema (Ek′-ze-ma)

Description—This noncontagious skin disease can be acute or chronic.

Signs and symptoms—This condition is characterized by dry, red, itchy, and scaly skin. There may be the presence of a watery discharge if it becomes chronic (Figure 11-67).

Etiology—Several things may initiate **eczema**, such as diet, cosmetics, clothing, medications, soaps, occupational or environmental substances, and emotional stress.

Treatment—Treatment consists primarily of removal of the causative agent where possible and the local application of ointments to alleviate the symptoms. Topical steroids are indicated to reduce inflammation, and antibiotics are used if secondary infection is present. The noncortisone cream *tacrolimus* (Protopic) is the most effective remedy yet developed, usually providing results within several weeks. *Note:* The FDA has issued a warning about Protopic, so watch for additional information. This and other eczema medications are available by prescription only.

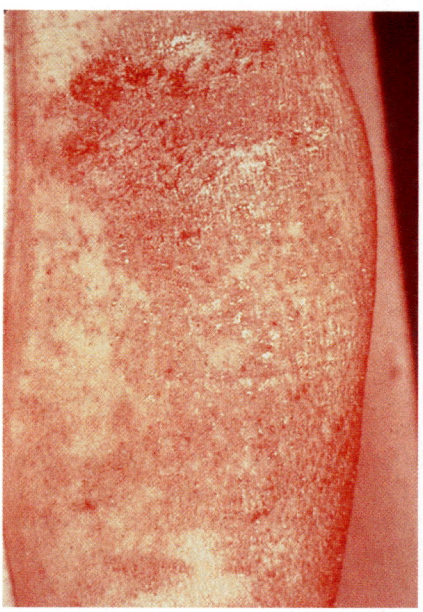

FIGURE 11-67   Eczema *(Courtesy of the Centers for Disease Control and Prevention, Atlanta, GA)*

Folliculitis (Fo-liku-li′tis)

Description—**Folliculitis** is an infection of the hair follicle with the formation of a pustule. It can be of a superficial form, involving only the surface area around a single follicle, or deep, involving the total hair follicle.

Signs and symptoms—The presence of redness and pustules around a single follicle on the scalp, arms, and legs, and on the face of bearded men (Figure 11-68).

Etiology—The most common cause is *Staphylococcus aureus*.

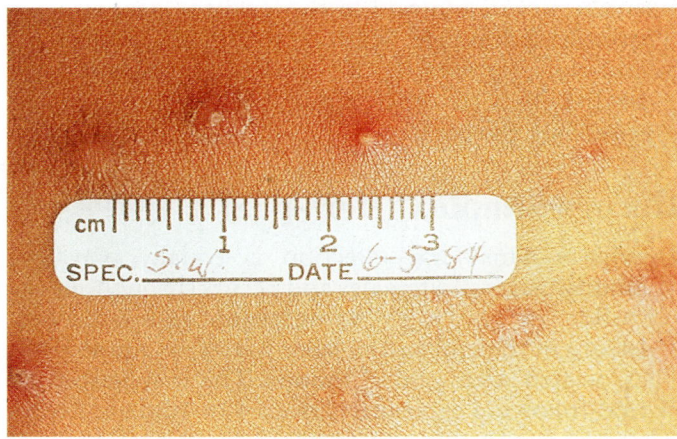

FIGURE 11-68   Folliculitis *(Courtesy of Robert A. Silverman, MD, Clinical Associate Professor, Department of Pediatrics, Georgetown University)*

Treatment—Treatment consists of thorough cleansing of the area, the application of moist heat to promote drainage from the lesion, and the use of topical antibiotics. Systemic antibiotics are usually indicated.

Furuncles (Fu′rung-kl)

Description—Folliculitis may lead to the development of **furuncles** (boils).

Signs and symptoms—They are hard, painful nodules that enlarge over several days' time until they rupture, releasing pus and dead cells through one draining point. The area remains red and swollen for a short time, but the pain lessens.

Etiology—Furuncles may be caused by irritation, pressure, friction, or infection with *Staphylococcus aureus*.

Treatment—Treatment consists of the measures used for folliculitis with moist heat to relieve pain and encourage "ripening" of the lesion. Often, incision and drainage are required to allow complete expulsion of the material. Patients must be cautioned not to squeeze a boil because it may rupture into the surrounding tissues. Systemic antibiotics are necessary if there is surrounding erythema or a fever. A patient with recurring furuncles should see a physician to rule out any underlying cause, such as diabetes.

Carbuncles (Kar′-bung-k′i)

Description—A **carbuncle** begins as a nodule, then enlarges to involve several adjacent hair follicles.

Signs and symptoms—It is characterized by deep follicular abscesses of several follicles with multiple draining points. It is extremely painful and usually associated with fever and general malaise.

Etiology—Usually caused by a persistent staphylococcal infection and often follows a furuncle.

Treatment—Carbuncles require treatment with systemic antibiotics in addition to the localized heat applications and drainage. Washcloths, towels, bed sheets, and clothing used by the infected person must not be shared with other family members to prevent spreading the bacteria.

Herpes Simplex (Her′-pez)

Description—This viral infection is equally prevalent among males and females and occurs throughout the world. **Herpes simplex** I is most often associated with lesions in the oral and nasal area. Herpes simplex II is associated with genital lesions. The incubation period following exposure is from 4 to 10 days. A prodrome (symptom of approaching disease) of pain, tingling, and itching signals the oncoming **vesicle**.

Signs and symptoms—The presence of small, grouped, painful, clear vesicles on an erythematous base (Figure 11-69).

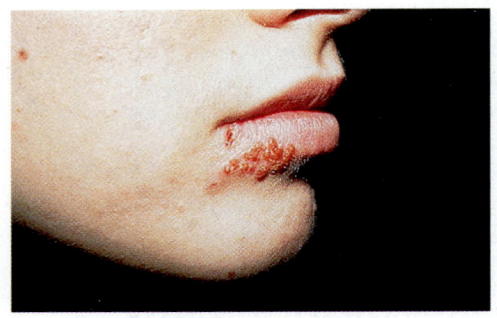

FIGURE 11-69 Herpes simplex 1 virus *(Courtesy of Robert A. Silverman, MD, Clinical Associate Professor, Department of Pediatrics, Georgetown University)*

Etiology—It is caused by the herpes virus.

Treatment—The most effective treatment is an oral antiviral medication. It has shown some decrease in pain and new lesion formation and a shortened period of viral shedding and healing time. Some relief from minor outbreaks may occur with the application of various over-the-counter topical preparations.

(*Note:* The term **viral shedding** refers to that period of time when a virus is the most active and most contagious.)

Herpes Zoster (Her′-pez Zos′-ter)

Description—**Herpes zoster** is an acute infectious process also known as shingles (Figure 11-70).

Signs and symptoms—It causes severe neuralgic pain along the area of the involved nerves. It is characterized by fever, malaise, and the eruption of vesicles in

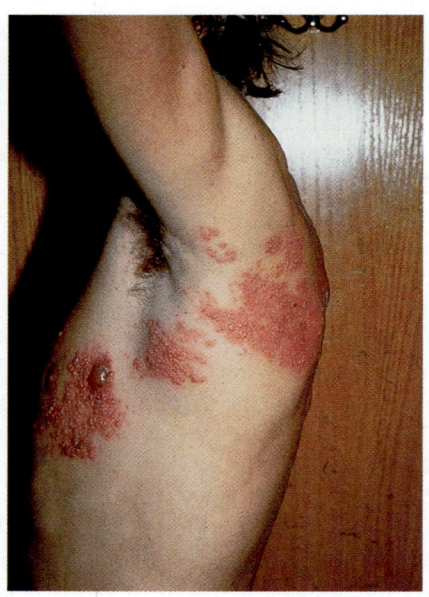

FIGURE 11-70 Lesions of herpes zoster (shingles); note how vesicles follow a nerve pathway. *(Courtesy of Robert A. Silverman, MD, Clinical Associate Professor, Department of Pediatrics, Georgetown University)*

the painful area, which spread unilaterally around the back, chest, or back of neck or vertically on the extremities. (See Unit 2.)

Etiology—It is caused by the varicella zoster virus, which also causes chickenpox.

Treatment—Usually the patient requires an analgesic and antipyretic to reduce fever and relieve pain. Antiviral drugs decrease acute pain, new lesion formation, viral shedding, healing time, and rates of dissemination (spreading), and incidence of postherpetic pain.

Hirsutism (Hur'-sut-izm)

Description—This disorder usually appears in women and children. Excessive body hair develops in an adult male pattern of growth.

Signs and symptoms—The most common symptom is growth of facial hair, but other masculinization signs, such as deepening voice, increased muscle mass, menstrual irregularity, and breast size reduction, may be exhibited.

Etiology—There may be a family history of the disorder, or it could be related to an endocrine problem resulting from either pituitary dysfunction, ovarian lesions, or adrenal gland enlargement.

Treatment—Treatment consists of hair removal by shaving, depilatory creams, or waxing as well as bleaching to minimize the appearance of hair. Electrolysis will permanently destroy the hair follicles but is slow and expensive. Laser hair removal may be effective. A new topical cream is available to treat increased hair growth on the face. If hormonal causes are evident, treatment may involve counteracting or controlling endocrine secretions in specific situations.

> **P**EDIATRIC PERSPECTIVE
>
> Referral to an endocrinologist is necessary to reduce or prevent masculinization and encourage appropriate sexual development.

Impetigo (Im-pe-ti'go)

Description—This is a contagious, superficial skin infection that is usually seen in young children.

Signs and symptoms—If the cause is streptococcal, the small red **macule** (flat area with definite edges) turns into a vesicle (raised lesion containing serous fluid) and then to a **pustule** (lesion with purulent material) within a relatively short time. (The terms macule, vesicle, and pustule refer to any skin lesion that demonstrates these descriptive characteristics, not to impetigo alone.) When the lesions break, a characteristic yellow crust develops from the exudate (drainage) (Figure 11-71). Other sites develop from contact with the lesions

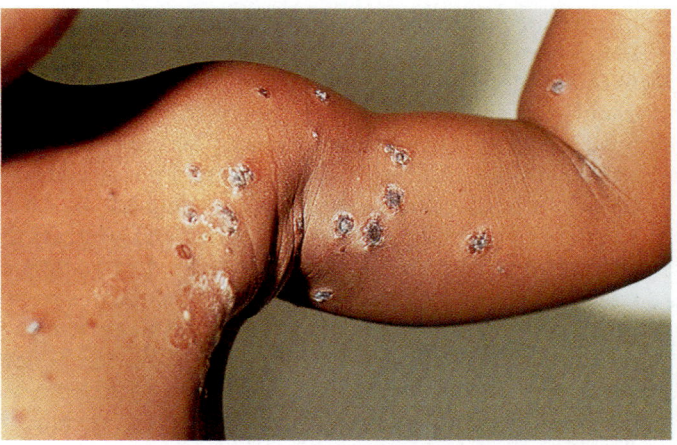

FIGURE 11-71   Impetigo *(Courtesy of Robert A. Silverman, MD, Clinical Associate Professor, Department of Pediatrics, Georgetown University)*

or the drainage. The staph lesion is characterized by a thin-walled vesicle that forms a thin, clear crust from the exudate. Both forms characteristically have a clear central area and definite outer rims. The lesions appear primarily on the face, neck, and other exposed areas of the body. Contamination of others is prevented by avoiding contact through washcloths, towels, and bed linens. Scratching of the lesions must be prohibited.

Etiology—It is caused by streptococcus or *Staphylococcus aureus* bacteria.

Treatment—Good hygiene is essential. The exudate can be removed by washing with soap and water two to three times a day. An oral systemic plus a topical antibiotic is indicated.

Keloid

A scar that developed excess dense tissue as it progressed through the healing process is known as **keloid**. (See Chapter 11, Unit 1.)

Lyme Disease (Lime)

Description—A tick-borne disease named after Old Lyme, Connecticut, where it was first reported in 1975. It has since been reported in 45 states, but over 90% of the cases occur within distinct areas: the East Coast from Massachusetts to Maryland, the upper midwest, the South and Southeast, and northern California and Oregon. Incidence is increasing dramatically. In 1986, only 700 cases were reported. In 1988, there were 5,000 reported. In 1994, New York alone reported 3,098 new cases. The most recent incidence reports issued for 2004 indicate 19,804 cases. The disease is spreading primarily because people are moving into suburban and rural areas, and the explosive deer population is moving into habitated areas. Both humans and pets can become infected. *Note:* If you live or work in one of the high-incidence areas, find out more about Lyme disease.

Signs and symptoms—The early stage of **Lyme disease** is usually marked by flu-like symptoms: fatigue, chills, fever, headache, muscle and joint pain, and swollen lymph nodes. In 60% of the cases, there is a characteristic circular, red skin lesion caused by the spirochete (corkscrew-shaped bacterium) migrating through the skin in all directions. This can appear from 3 days to 1 month after a bite. It enlarges to as much as several inches across and develops a clear center, giving it the appearance of a bull's eye; hence the name, "bull's eye rash." Diagnosis is difficult in the remaining 40% who do not develop the rash and therefore may not get diagnosed and treated early. Their first symptoms are usually arthritis, fatigue, and memory loss. Later, nervous system symptoms develop. These may include numbness and pain, Bell's palsy, poor motor coordination, insomnia, irritability, heart arrythmia, headaches, and depression.

Etiology—Lyme disease is caused primarily by the bite of a spirochete-infested deer tick. It is an unusual three-host tick with a 2-year life cycle. It begins when adult ticks feed and mate on deer and then drop off to lay eggs. The eggs hatch and the young ticks, called nymphs, attach and feed on small rodents that carry the spirochete and infect the tick. The mice carry the nymphs through the woods and fields and into human habitats: the grass, shrubs, wood piles, garages, and homes. From contact they attach and feed on dogs, squirrels, and humans. Bites seem to occur most often between May and September. The tick, in its unfed state, is about the size of a pinhead. It looks like a pear-shaped crab and has eight legs. Ticks insert their barbed mouth parts into the skin, deposit spirochetes, suck blood until satisfied (usually 2 to 4 days), and then drop off. The longer a tick feeds, the larger it becomes and the greater the chance for infection. If the tick is removed before the first 24 hours, infection is unlikely. (Not all ticks carry the spirochete; approximately 30% to 60% of northeastern ticks test positive.)

Treatment—The best treatment is prevention. Avoid tick-infected areas especially from May through September. Dress in light-colored clothing to make ticks more visible—they are not easily seen. Long sleeves and long pants tucked into light-colored socks or boots are highly recommended. Spray clothing with a tick repellent, and allow to dry before wearing. Applying a repellent containing up to 30% DEET directly to the skin (according to directions) is advisable for adults but unsafe for children because of its chemical composition. Check your entire body at the end of the day, paying particular attention to ankles, knees (especially backs), groin, armpits, under breasts, scalp, ears, and the back. Check all pets *before* bringing them into the house. *Do not* let pets sleep in or on the bed.

Before washing, put outdoor clothing in the clothes dryer on the highest temperature for 30 minutes to kill hiding ticks. They can survive laundering.

If a deer tick is found, remove it and show it to a doctor, or send it to health authorities for positive identification. (See "How to Remove a Tick.") Its size is important because it is evidence of the length of time attached. Ticks that are to be tested should be put in a clean glass container and placed in the refrigerator until they are sent to health authorities. Results take about 2 weeks. Ticks, dead or alive, can be tested using a polymerase chain reaction test that detects the DNA of the spirochete, which will identify the type of tick, confirm the spirochete's presence, and therefore determine treatment. If identification can be made without testing, dispose of the tick by dropping it in 70% alcohol or diluted bleach. Do not "treat" ticks that are going to be tested.

If symptoms or a positive test result indicate Lyme disease, a course of antibiotics are prescribed for 3 weeks, with 1 week off, and then another 3-week course of antibiotics, which effectively treats the infection. If diagnosis is not made until later-stage disease, then other systemic conditions require treatment in addition to antibiotics. Recent discovery of a specific antibody in patients with the disease may lead to immediate diagnosis and earlier treatment. Current blood tests are not conclusive. Dogs, cats, cattle, and horses can also become infected and treated with antibiotics if detected early. Prevention in dogs is possible with a good tick collar and a vaccine. Two human vaccines have been tested that may provide protection for uninfected people when available.

Pediculosis (Pe-dik-u-lo'-sis)

Description—There are three types of **pediculosis** resulting from three varieties of parasitic lice: capitis from head lice, corporis from body lice, and pubis from

---

P **PATIENT EDUCATION**

HOW TO REMOVE A TICK

Removal is done with forceps or tweezers at the mouth parts. Pull gently until it releases its hold. The entire head should be removed. If tweezers are not available, cover with a tissue. Never use bare fingers. A ruptured tick can release infectious material onto a cut in the skin and transfer its disease. If a part remains, see a physician immediately. After removal, wash the area and your hands thoroughly and treat the area with 70% alcohol. Companies such as IMUGEN can provide testing services once a tick is removed. For more information, go to www.imugen.com or call 1-800-246-8436.

pubic lice. The lice feed on human blood and lay eggs known as nits on body hairs or fibers of clothing. The nits hatch and will die in 24 hours unless they feed on a host. Nits mature in 2 to 3 weeks.

Pediculosis Capitis

Description—It is the most common form and is found primarily among children, especially girls. It spreads through shared combs, brushes, clothing, and hats.

Signs and symptoms—It is identifiable as an oval, grayish, dandruff-like fleck that cannot be shaken off. Its symptoms are itching and scalp abrasions, with matted, foul-smelling hair in severe cases.

Etiology—Pediculosis is caused by parasitic forms of lice that are found in overcrowded conditions and with poor personal hygiene.

Treatment—Treatment consists of gamma benzene hexachloride (GBH) cream rubbed into the scalp at night, then rinsed out with GBH shampoo the next morning. Treatment is repeated the second night. A fine-toothed comb dipped in vinegar helps remove nits from the hair.

PEDIATRIC PERSPECTIVE

Parents have the option of purchasing over-the-counter medication if they choose; it is similar to prescription medication and provides effective treatment.

Pediculosis Corporis

Description—Pediculosis corporis lives in clothing seams, except when feeding on the host.

Signs and symptoms—Initially, small red papules appear, which itch. The resulting scratching causes rashes and wheals to develop.

Etiology—Prolonged wearing of the same clothes, overcrowding, and poor hygiene. It is spread through shared clothing and linens.

Treatment—Pediculosis corporis can be removed by bathing unless infestation is severe. Clothing and bed sheets must be washed, ironed, or dry cleaned. A prescription medication may be ordered if necessary.

Pediculosis Pubis

Description—Pediculosis pubis, commonly called crabs, is found attached primarily to pubic hair.

Signs and symptoms—The lice cause itching, which results in skin irritation from scratching.

Etiology—It is transmitted through sexual intercourse or contact with infected clothes, bedding, or towels.

Treatment—Pediculosis pubis is treated with a prescription medication and left on for 24 hours or with shampooing the affected area. Treatment must be

repeated in 1 week. The sexual partner must also be treated or reinfestation will occur. This type of infestation is also treated with a prescription drug.

Poison Ivy

Description—This is a dermatitis caused by contact with the poison ivy plant.

Signs and symptoms—Initially, poison ivy causes moderate itching and burning that is soon followed by small blisters. As blisters increase, some break and skin is covered with a coating of serum. Marked discomfort and intense itching may be present (Figure 11-72).

Etiology—It is caused by the sap of the three-leafed poison ivy plant, fresh or dry.

Treatment—The best treatment is prevention. Learn to recognize and avoid contact with the plant. Especially susceptible people can be given injections to prevent its development. Different preparations are available to control the itching and to "dry up" the lesions. Treatment depends upon the extent of involvement. Oral steroids or topical steroid cream is usually sufficient.

Psoriasis (So-ri'-a-sis)

Description—This is a chronic inflammatory condition that is recurrent, with alternating periods of remission or increased severity. The episodes are affected by the environment (cold weather causes flare-ups), endocrine changes, pregnancy, and emotional stress.

Signs and symptoms—**Psoriasis** is a chronic disease characterized by red papules that are covered with silvery scales (Figure 11-73). The lesions are dry, cracked, and encrusted, sometimes covering large areas of the body. The scales either flake off or build up, covering the lesion.

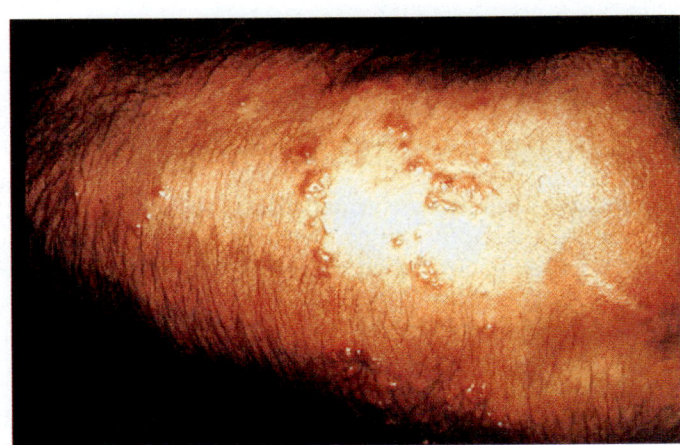

FIGURE 11-72 The fluid-filled vesicles of poison ivy *(Courtesy of the Centers for Disease Control and Prevention, Atlanta, GA)*

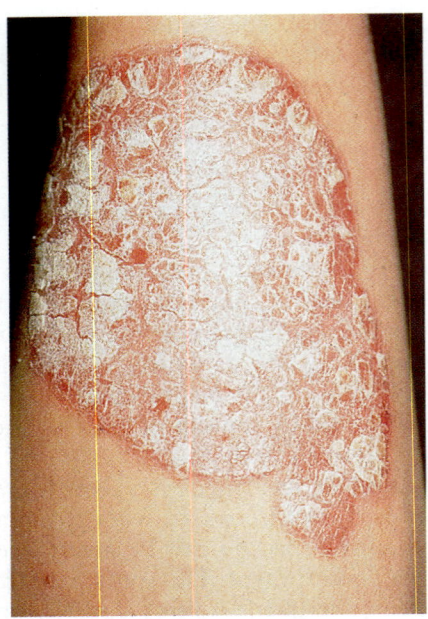

FIGURE 11-73   Psoriasis *(Courtesy of Robert A. Silverman, MD, Clinical Associate Professor, Department of Pediatrics, Georgetown University)*

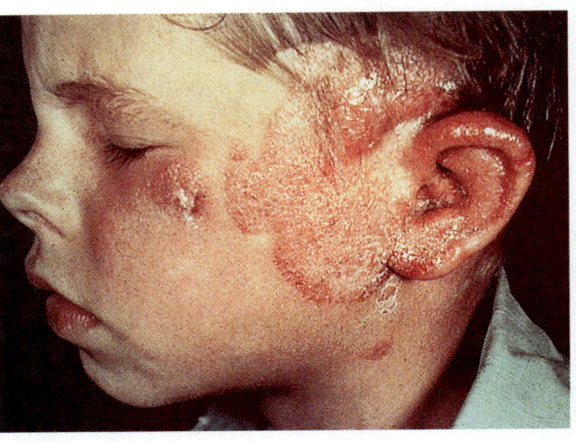

FIGURE 11-74   Ringworm (tinea corporis) of the face and scalp *(Courtesy of Robert A. Silverman, MD, Clinical Associate Professor, Department of Pediatrics, Georgetown University)*

Etiology—The appearance is caused by the overgrowth of skin cells. Normally, a cell takes 14 days to move from the basal layer to the surface, where after another 14 days of wear it is sloughed off. The life cycle of a psoriatic skin cell is only 4 days, during which it produces a surface of immature cells causing a thick and flaky appearance.

Treatment—Psoriasis cannot be cured, but it may be controlled. Initial therapy is with topical hydrocortisone preparations. Then, topical retinoids, vitamin A or D creams, topical tar, and salicylic acid preparations are also used. Ultraviolet light in a controlled, prescribed setting slows the cell turnover. Oral medications in the form of antimetabolites, retinoids, and immunosuppressives are used in extensive severe cases. The new eximer laser is effective in treating localized psoriasis.

Ringworm

Description—This fungus may affect the scalp (tinea capitis), the body (tinea corporis), or other areas, such as the groin, beard, or feet (tinea pedia, or athlete's foot).

Signs and symptoms—On the body, it is characterized by flat lesions, which are dry and scaly or moist and crusty. When they enlarge, clear central areas develop, leaving an outer ring from which it gets its name. On the scalp, small papules occur causing scaly patches of baldness (Figure 11-74).

Etiology—Fungi dermatophytes.

Treatment—Treatment consists of systemic medication or the topical applications of antifungals. Because the disease is contagious, care must be taken to prevent its spread by refraining from sharing bed linens, combs, and towels.

Rosacea (Ro-za'-se-a)

Description—It is a chronic skin eruption that makes the face, especially the nose and cheeks, look flushed. It occurs most often in Caucasian women between 30 and 50 years old. It also occurs in men but is usually more severe and associated with rhinophyma (dilated follicles with an enlarged red nose).

Signs and symptoms—There is the characteristic coloration of the face that may also exhibit papules and pustules like acne but without the comedones.

Etiology—The condition results from the dilation of small blood vessels that causes the flushed, red appearance. The exact cause is unknown. Stress, infection, vitamin deficiency, and endocrine problems do aggravate the condition. Certain foods, such as spicy things and hot beverages, also cause problems. It is also affected by alcohol, physical activity, sunlight, and extreme temperatures.

Treatment—Topical use of cortisone ointment to reduce erythema may be helpful. Oral doses of tetracycline given in decreasing amounts as symptoms subside and electrolysis may destroy the large or dilated blood vessels.

Figure 11-75 shows a female who has had rosacea for 20 years. Her skin will react to temperature changes and becomes flushed with drinking hot liquids or alcohol. She also tends to develop pustules, and her skin becomes very sensitive. She uses an ointment called MetroGel to alleviate symptoms.

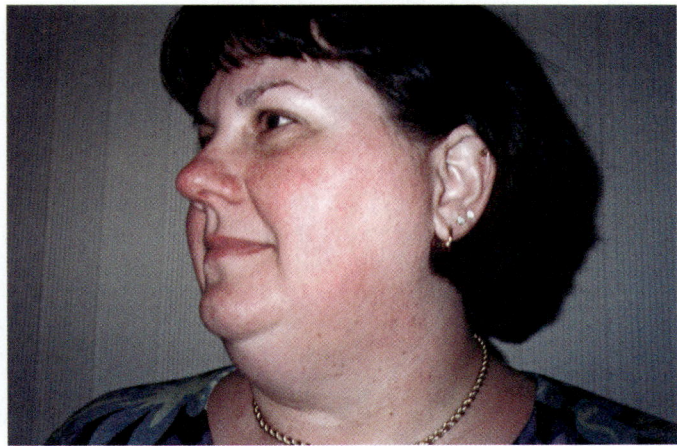

FIGURE 11-75   Female with rosacea

Scabies (Ska′-bez)

Description—This skin infestation is caused by the itch mite.

Signs and symptoms—The condition causes an itching that becomes intense at night. The lesions are characteristically threadlike red nodules, approximately ⅜-inch long. They occur between fingers, at the inner wrist area, on the elbows, in axillary folds (armpit), around the waist, on genitalia (external sex organs) of males, and on the nipples of females. The infestation is spread by skin contact or sexual activity.

Etiology—It is caused by the itch mite, which burrows into the skin to lay eggs. The larvae emerge to mate and then reburrow under the skin. It can be associated with overcrowding and poor personal hygiene.

Treatment—Treatment consists of an application of pediculicide such as the prescription drug Elimite, which must remain on the skin from 6 to 8 hours or overnight. The treatment is then followed with a bath. An antipruritic (against itching) or steroid may be applied topically to help reduce the itching.

Urticaria (Ur-ti-ka′re-a) (Hives)

Description—This is a self-limiting reaction to allergens. **Urticaria** often occurs during especially stressful or emotional times or during a viral infection.

Signs and symptoms—The reaction produces distinct, raised **wheals** surrounded by a reddened area. They may be few in number or cover the entire body. They may or may not cause itching, burning, and tingling (Figure 11-76).

Etiology—Urticaria are caused by allergy to drugs, food, insect stings, and occasionally inhaled allergens from animal hair, cosmetics, and flour. Nonallergic urticaria can be caused by the body's release of histamine for unknown reasons.

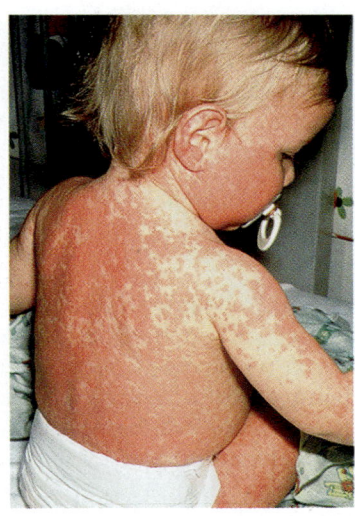

FIGURE 11-76   Urticaria *(Courtesy of Robert A. Silverman, MD, Clinical Associate Professor, Department of Pediatrics, Georgetown University)*

Treatment—Urticaria is treated by eliminating or limiting the causative allergen or, when that is not possible, by gradual desensitization through interdermal injection of the allergen. An antihistamine is used to reduce itching and swelling. A tranquilizer may be required when the causative factor is emotional stress.

Verrucae (Ver-roo-ka) (Warts)

Description—This is a benign (noncancerous) viral infection of the skin.

Signs and symptoms—Common **verrucae** are characterized by a rough, elevated, rounded surface, usually on the extremities, especially the hands and fingers. They can also occur on the elbows, knees, and face and scalp.

Etiology—Warts are caused by a family of viruses known as human papillomavirus, which is spread by direct contact. It invades skin cells where the surface is broken and "encourages" the creation of more infected cells. In most cases, the body's immune system eventually eliminates the wart. It is estimated that a wart will die off within about 5 years. Plantar warts occur primarily at pressure points on the soles of the feet. Condyloma accuminatum (venereal warts) are moist, soft, pink to red warts occurring singly or most often in large clusters on the penis, vulva, or anus. They grow rapidly in groups, often accumulating into large clusters. Genital warts spread by sexual contact and are highly contagious. They are associated with an increased risk of cervical cancer in women.

Treatment—Treatment of warts varies with the type, size, and location. Common types often disappear spontaneously. When removal is necessary, they can be destroyed by methods using electricity, acid, liquid nitrogen, or solid carbon dioxide. Genital warts must be treated promptly. Partners must also be evaluated by a physician for evidence of the virus and treated if present or the infection will be reacquired upon renewed contact.

Wrinkles

As people age, the skin begins to develop wrinkles, particularly on the face and back of the hands. This is primarily caused by years of exposure to the environment and the diminishing layer of collagen beneath the skin. Many forms of treatment can be performed to remove or reduce their presence and at least temporarily improve the patient's appearance. Because there is such an interest in the procedures, a brief discussion of the most common forms of correction follows.

Dermabrasion   This is the controlled scraping of the top layers of the skin to remove scars from acne or accidents and to smooth out fine facial wrinkles, such as those around the mouth. Local anesthesia and a sedative are used during the procedure. It involves the use of a high-speed, hand-held rotary instrument with a rough wire brush or diamond impregnated burr. Afterward, the skin is treated with ointment, a wet dressing, a dry treatment, or some combination. There is redness, swelling, and some pain, tingling, burning, or itching, which is controlled by medication. The side effects subside within a few days. It is rarely performed since newer techniques have been developed.

Microdermabrasion   This is a noninvasive, non-surgical procedure. A controlled spray of fine aluminum oxide crystals is applied to remove the outer layer of the skin. This gives the skin a fresher appearance. There are varying depths of treatment available. It may improve the appearance of fine wrinkles, superficial age spots, and sun-damaged skin.

Chemical Peel   This is known as chemosurgery and can be done at three levels: light, medium, and deep. Medium and deep peels require the use of medication during the treatment to relieve tension and discomfort. They involve the application of varying concentrations of an acid that strips away old, damaged skin cells, causing the body to replace them with healthy new ones. With deeper peels, collagen is stimulated, which "pumps-up" the new skin.

Light peel   This type affects only the top layer and can be done in about an hour. It produces only mild redness and will make the skin appear softer, reduce the size of pores, produce a more even coloring, and may reduce some fine lines. It may need to be repeated to achieve desired results.

Medium peel   This type affects surface and some underlying cells. It also stimulates collagen and elastin, the fibers that act as the skin's support structure. This results in much smoother skin and the reduction of wrinkles. Some precancerous lesions may be removed. It takes from 7 to 10 days for the swelling, redness, and peeling to subside after the application.

Deep peel   This type requires a strong acid and destroys all the top layers of skin and sometimes a part of the dermal layer. This results in removing all the signs of skin aging except deep forehead furrows and the nose-to-mouth grooves from sagging. Pigmentation problems and precancerous lesions can be removed. The procedure requires expert application and produces considerable pain for 12 hours, which requires medication, followed by discomfort for a few days. There is considerable swelling, redness, and peeling for a few weeks. It also results in the loss of pigment, which causes a waxy, lighter face that may not match the body.

Laser Resurfacing   This is the newest form of repair and involves the use of a controlled, pulsed laser beam to vaporize the skin's surface. The depth of the beam can be set to go light on the thin skin around the eyes and deeper into thicker skin around the mouth. Surface blemishes, sun-damaged skin, and the wrinkled surface are removed. It also stimulates the development of new cells and collagen for new, smoother, younger-looking skin and produces a tightening effect on the skin as it removes or reduces the wrinkles. Small areas to be treated can be injected with local anesthetic; full face treatment may require general anesthesia. Immediate visual change can be observed as the beam penetrates the skin, leaving behind a puff of mist and a fine ash, which is "vacuumed" away as the skin tightens and the wrinkle disappears. The odor of burnt flesh is apparent. The procedure's immediate results are like a bad sunburn, with some swelling of the area. The burned skin is tender, very red, and oozes fluid initially. Crusts form, which can be gently removed. The area is covered with antibiotic ointment to relieve any surface drying and to prevent infection. Medication is prescribed for pain relief. The swelling and excessive redness subsides within a few days. It may take a few weeks for all the coloration to fade. The results are usually considered well worth the discomfort and temporary inconvenience.

Plastic Surgery   This term is derived from a Greek word meaning to mold or give form. Plastic surgery is also known as cosmetic surgery and involves the reshaping of the facial features to improve appearance. The procedure demands a skillful surgeon to achieve the desired results. The procedures can remove "bags" under the eyes, lift drooping upper lids, and tighten up skin around the eyes. The repair of both upper and lower lids is known as quadrilateral blepharoplasty. The procedures to raise sagging jaws and forehead and pull back the sides of the face is commonly referred to as "a face lift." These procedures can be performed under general or local anesthesia in connection with sedation. Pain, marked swelling, and bruising will require medication for a few days. The recovery time varies, but most swelling and significant bruising are sufficiently gone after 2 to 3 weeks to allow the patient to go out in public.

A new face lift technique known as "thread lift" is being marketed as less invasive and less expensive. It involves using a special suture with "barbs" to stitch through subcutaneous tissue and make loops at various points to pull surface tissue upward toward the temple. It reportedly costs about $300 per suture and will require at least three to four sutures to accomplish. The recovery time may be less, but it means the skin tissue must "reposition" itself after being "gathered up," which may ultimately take longer than the traditional face lift. Again, nothing is lifted beneath the surface, so results and length of effect are anticipated to be about 5 years. This technique may allow other surgeons and dermatologists to enter the field of plastic surgery without the extensive surgical training and experience.

ACHIEVE UNIT OBJECTIVES

- ■ Complete the Workbook activities to meet the learning objectives.
- ■ Apply your knowledge at the end of this chapter in completing the Critical Thinking Challenge and Activities, as well as the StudyWARE on your Student CD-ROM.

UNIT 5
THE SKELETAL SYSTEM

OBJECTIVES

Upon completion of this unit, you will be able to achieve the following:

LEARNING Objectives

1. Spell and define, using the glossary at the back of the text, all the Words to Know in this unit.
2. Name the two divisions of the skeletal system and the bone groups in each division.
3. Describe the structure of the long bones.
4. Explain how long bones grow.

5. Identify the elements that make up bone tissue.
6. Identify the major bones of the body.
7. List the six functions of the skeletal system.
8. Name the divisions of the spinal column and the number of vertebrae in each division.
9. Describe fontanels and explain why they are essential.
10. Describe the structure of the rib cage and its primary function.
11. Identify three kinds of synovial joints, and give examples of each.
12. List the parts of a synovial joint, and identify the purpose of each part.
13. Name the seven types of fractures and the characteristics of each.
14. Outline the treatment of a fracture.
15. Describe the healing process of a fracture.
16. Define the term fatty embolus, explaining its origin and what might occur.
17. List situations predisposing to amputation.
18. Define the phantom limb sensation.
19. Describe four diagnostic examinations.
20. Explain why the symptoms of carpal tunnel syndrome occur.
21. Name the three types of spinal curvatures, describing their physical characteristics.
22. Identify 20 diseases and disorders of the skeletal system.

WORDS TO KNOW

alignment	cervical	fibula
amputate	clavicle	fracture
appendicular	coccyx	greenstick
arthritis	comminuted	humerus
articulation	compound	ilium
axial	cranium	impacted
bunion	depressed	intervertebral
bursa	diarthrosis	ischium
callus	dislocation	kyphosis
cancellous	embolus	laminectomy
carpal	epiphysis	ligament
cartilage	femur	lordosis

marrow	radius	sternum
metacarpal	reduce	symphysis pubis
metatarsal	sacrum	synovial
osteoporosis	scapula	tarsal
patella	scoliosis	tibia
periosteum	simple	traction
phalanges	skeletal	ulna
phalanx	spinal fusion	vertebrae
phantom limb	spiral	xiphoid
prosthesis	sprain	

 CERTIFICATION CONNECTION

CMA
Diagnostic procedures
Common diseases and
    pathology
Anatomy and physiology

CMAS
Anatomy and physiology

RMA
Anatomy and physiology

The **skeletal** system consists of organs called bones. It may be difficult to think of bones as living, functioning organs that use food and oxygen and perform functions just as other organs do.

The skeleton is divided into two sections. The spinal column, skull, and rib cage make up the **axial** skeleton. The bones of the arms, hands, legs, feet, shoulders, and pelvis make up the **appendicular** skeleton (Figure 11-77).

The primary purpose of the skeletal system is to support the body. This support must be strong yet not heavy. Bone is said to be as strong as cast iron, yet it is much lighter and more flexible. The skeleton must be flexible enough to endure pressure, stress, and shock without shattering.

BONE STRUCTURE

Over 20% of the weight of bone is water. Two thirds of the remainder are minerals and one third, organic matter. The main minerals are calcium, phosphorus, and magnesium. The organic matter is primarily collagen, a

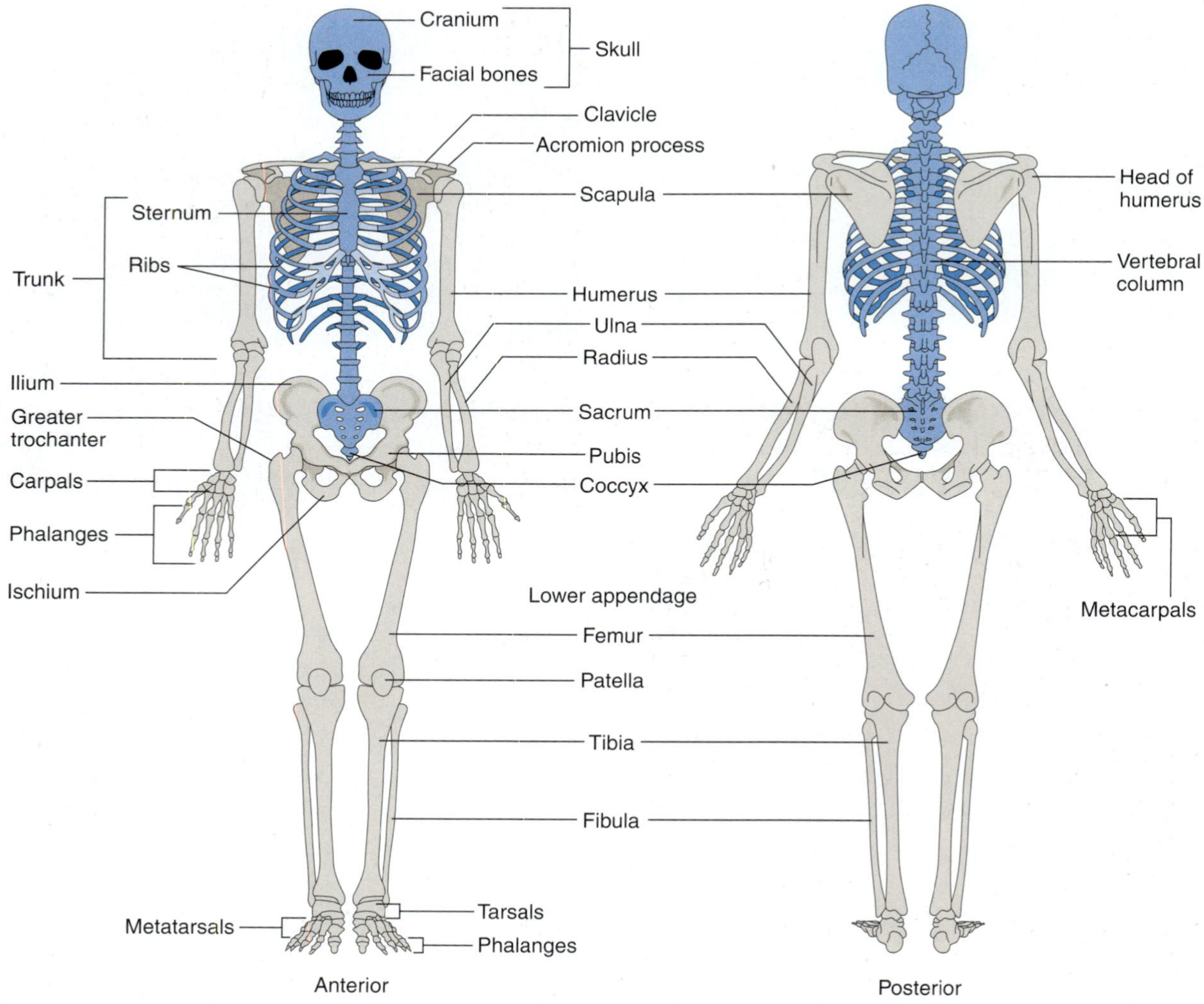

FIGURE 11-77   Bones of the skeleton (axial in blue, appendicular in gray)

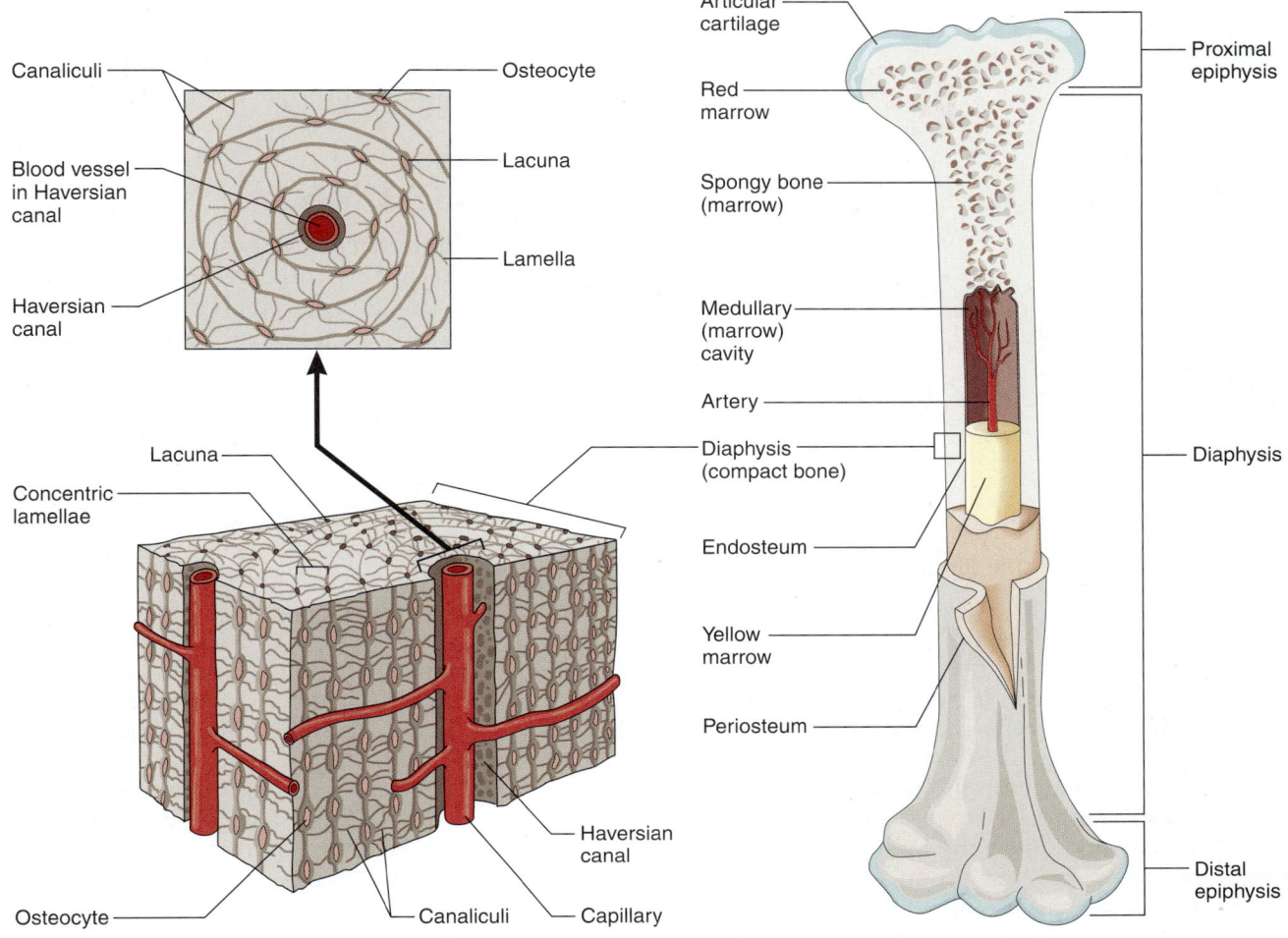

FIGURE 11-78 Structure of a long bone

type of protein fiber that forms the matrix (intercellular substance) of the bone.

The ends of long bones have articulating (connecting) surfaces that fit together with other bones to form joints (Figure 11-78). These ends are separated by cartilage to facilitate movement. The ends and parts of the shaft are filled with a meshlike network of spongy **cancellous** bone. The openings in the spongy bone are filled with red **marrow**. The inside of the shaft of the bone is filled with a fat or yellow marrow. Dense bone called cortical bone makes up the outside of long bones.

A tough membrane called **periosteum** covers the surface of the bone. Blood vessels and nerves pass through the periosteum and into the bone through a network of openings called Haversian canals. Some larger vessels pass directly into both the yellow and red marrow.

NUMBER OF BONES

At birth, a baby has 270 bones. As the child grows, some of the bones fuse together so that in adulthood there are only 206. For example, at the lower end of the spinal column, five **vertebrae** have fused to form the **sacrum**, whereas the last four have fused into the **coccyx** (tailbone) (Figure 11-79). The smallest bones in the body are the malleus, incus, and stapes of the middle ear.

FUNCTIONS OF THE SKELETON

The skeleton serves at least six functions for the body. One, as previously indicated, is to support the body. The bones provide a framework for the distribution of the body's fat, muscles, and skin.

Two, the bones also serve to protect the body's vital organs. The brain and spinal cord are both located within bony cavities. The cranium also provides protection for the inner ear and parts of the eye. The heart and lungs are positioned within the rib cage. The internal reproductive organs and the urinary bladder lie within the bony pelvis.

Third, the bones are the points of attachment for skeletal muscles. When the muscles contract, they allow the joints of the skeleton to rotate, bend, or straighten, thereby providing for movement and flexi-

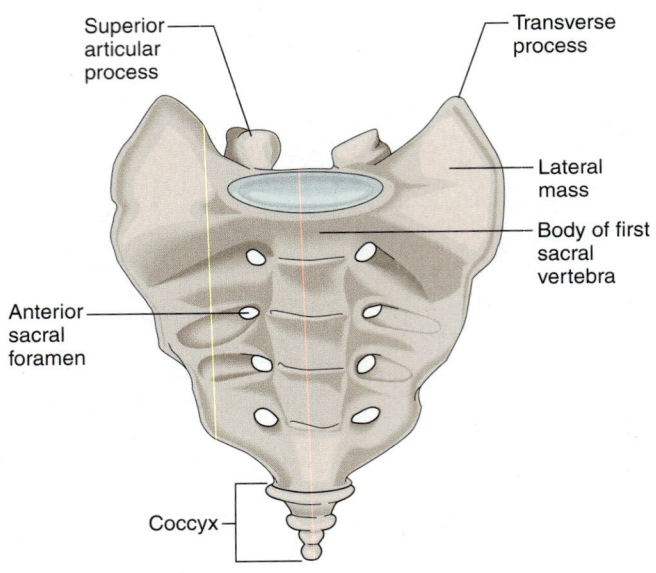

FIGURE 11-79 The sacrum and coccyx

bility. Fourth, the bones, along with the muscles, give shape to the body.

A fifth and vital function of bone is the formation of the red and white blood cells and the platelets. The red marrow in the spongy areas of the long bones, the ribs, and the vertebrae produces millions of red blood cells a minute. This rate is necessary to replace the cells, which live only a few weeks. When the body needs more red cells than the red marrow can produce, some of the yellow marrow is converted to red.

Finally, bones store most of the body's supply of calcium. Calcium is needed by the heart to beat, by the muscles to contract, and by the blood to clot.

When the calcium in the body is inadequate for all its needs, the blood takes calcium from its storage in the bone. The bone minerals are constantly being borrowed and replaced through the blood flow within the body.

SPINAL COLUMN

The spinal column is a stack of vertebrae that supports the head and keeps the trunk erect. As noted earlier, it provides protection for the spinal cord, which descends from the brain through its canal. The bones of the column are separated by **intervertebral** cartilage disks between their rounded front portions, the vertebral bodies (Figure 11-80). The disks permit the column to bend or twist and also absorb much of the shock received from walking, running, or jumping. The vertebrae in the column are named for the area of the body in which they are located: **cervical** (neck), thoracic (chest), lumbar (back), sacral (posterior pelvic girdle), and coccygeal (tailbone) (Figure 11-81).

The spinal nerves enter and leave the spinal cord through foraminae (openings) between the vertebrae. The disks maintain adequate spacing between vertebrae to prevent damage to the spinal nerves from bone-to-bone contact.

Typical vertebrae, as shown in Figure 11-80, have descriptive parts, mainly the large solid part called the *body,* the winglike side projections called the *transverse processes,* a posterior projection called a *spinous process* (the part you can feel if you arch your back), and the *foramen* through which the spinal cord passes. Other processes called *articular* are where parts of two vertebrae touch.

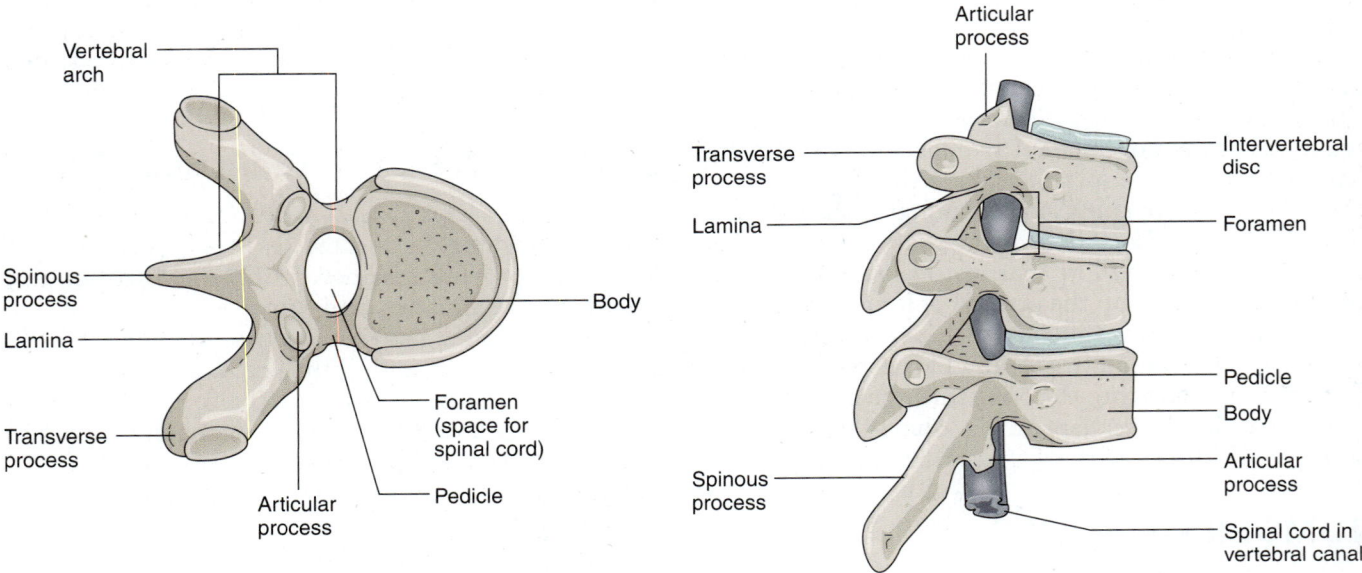

A typical vertebra

FIGURE 11-80 Vertebrae structure

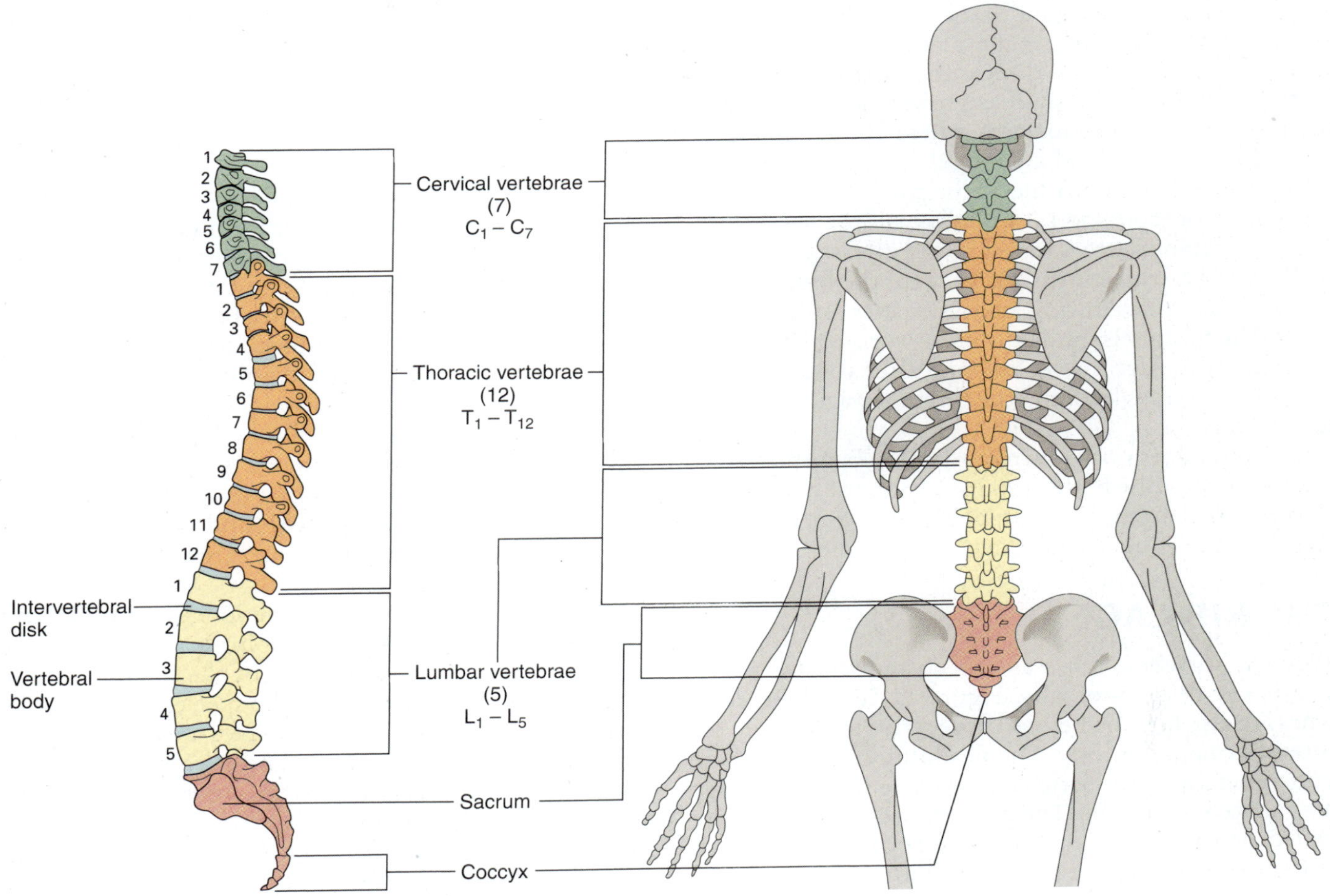

1
2
3
4
5
6
7
1
2
3
4
5
6
7
8
9
10
11
12
1
2
3
4
5
Intervertebral disk
Vertebral body
Cervical vertebrae (7) C1 – C7
Thoracic vertebrae (12) T1 – T12
Lumbar vertebrae (5) L1 – L5
Sacrum
Coccyx

FIGURE 11-81 The spinal column

THE SKULL

The skull is the bony structure of the head. It consists of a cranial and a facial portion. The **cranium** is actually a fusion of eight cranial bones, with the vital function of protecting the brain from injury (Figure 11-82). The main bones of the cranium are the frontal (the forehead and upper eye sockets), two parietal, two temporal, and the occipital (back of the skull). The facial bones are the mandible (lower jaw), the maxillae (upper jaw), the zygomatic (cheek bones), and the several small bones around the eyes, nose, and palate.

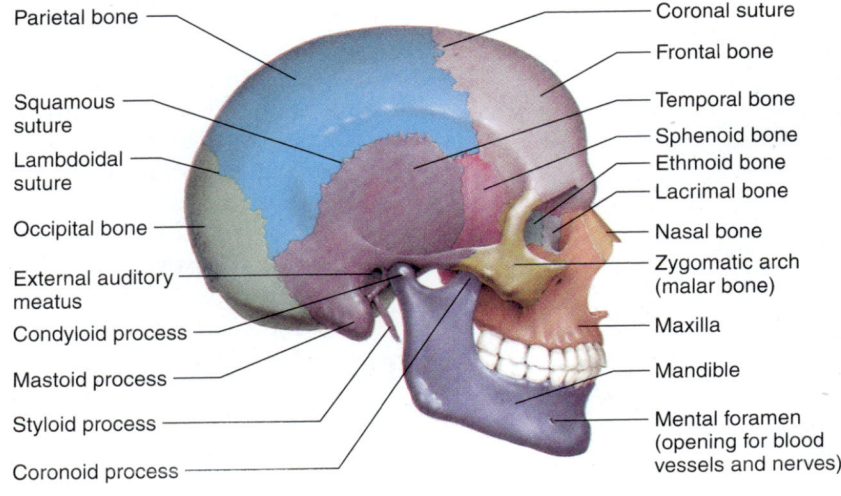

Parietal bone
Squamous suture
Lambdoidal suture
Occipital bone
External auditory meatus
Condyloid process
Mastoid process
Styloid process
Coronoid process
Coronal suture
Frontal bone
Temporal bone
Sphenoid bone
Ethmoid bone
Lacrimal bone
Nasal bone
Zygomatic arch (malar bone)
Maxilla
Mandible
Mental foramen (opening for blood vessels and nerves)

FIGURE 11-82 The skull

The cranium is not solid bone at birth. Spaces between the bones are soft, incomplete bone to allow for the molding of the skull during the birth process and for enlargement of the skull as growth occurs. A large, diamond-shaped anterior area where the frontal and parietal bones meet and a triangular space posteriorly where the occipital bone meets the parietals are known as *fontanels,* or "soft spots," and can easily be felt. Other smaller fontanels are located along the sides of the skull. Without these areas for growth, the brain could not increase in size during late pregnancy and early infancy. The fontanels gradually close, turning the membrane and cartilage into solid bone after about 2 years. The irregular lines marking the former growth areas are called *sutures.*

The skull does not grow remarkably when compared with the rest of the body. It makes up about one fourth of the total length of the infant's body but only one eighth of the adult's total length.

THE RIB CAGE

Thoracic vertebrae serve as the posterior attachment points for 12 pairs of ribs (Figure 11-83). The top 10 pairs are also attached by cartilage strips to the **sternum** (breast bone) anteriorly. The flexibility of the cartilage attachment allows the rib cage to move when the lungs are inflated to breathe. The bottom two pairs of ribs are called floating ribs because they are attached only to the spinal column and not the sternum.

The rib cage is sometimes described in terms of true and false ribs. When this division is made, the first seven pairs of ribs are considered "true" ribs because of their posterior and direct anterior attachment. The last five pairs are "false" ribs because they attach anteriorly to the cartilage of the rib above or have no anterior attachment.

Three other bony features of the thoracic area should be mentioned. They are the **clavicle** (collar bone), located anteriorly, and the **scapula** (shoulder blade), located posteriorly. The inferior portion of the sternum is a small bony process called the **xiphoid** process.

LONG BONES

The long bones of the body are found in the extremities. To a great extent, the long bones of the lower extremities determine height. Long bones are generally shaped like hollow cylinders to be strong with the least amount of weight. A typical long bone has three distinct regions: diaphysis, epiphysis, and metaphysis. The middle shaft (diaphysis) is connected to the ends (**epiphysis**) by a transitional segment (metaphysis). Early in life the epiphysis is mainly **cartilage**. Later the cartilage becomes a strip or "growth plate" that permits new tissue growth and bone length. At maturity, growth stops and the cartilage is replaced by bone.

The **femur** (thigh bone) is the longest bone in any species, extending from the hip joint to the knee. (Refer to Figure 11-77.) The thickness of the femur wall depends on the size and needs of the species. For example, large animals, such as the bear, have a thick, heavy femur to support their weight and accommodate slow movements, whereas the deer has a very thin and light femur to permit speed. The **tibia** (shin bone) and **fibula** complete the long bones of the leg. The small bone at the knee is known as the **patella**.

The long bones of the upper extremities are the **humerus** of the arm and the **radius** and **ulna** of the forearm. The radius extends from the thumb side of the wrist to the elbow, whereas the ulna extends from the little finger side to the elbow joint.

BONES OF THE HANDS AND FEET

The bones of the hands and feet are similar in structure (Figure 11-84). The wrist has eight bones, known as **carpals**, whereas the ankle has seven, called **tarsals**. In the palm area of the hand, there are five **metacarpals** that correspond to the five **metatarsals** of the instep of the foot. The **phalanges** (fingers and toes) are further subdivided into individual sections called a **phalanx**. There are three phalanx sections in each finger and toe, except in the thumb and great toe, which have only two. The section of a phalanx is identified as distal, middle, or proximal by its relationship to the metacarpals or metatarsals.

THE PELVIC GIRDLE

The pelvic girdle provides the structure for the hip area. Two large bones called *os coxae* (hip bones) are joined posteriorly with the sacrum. The top blade-shaped portion is called the **ilium** (Figure 11-85). The anterior

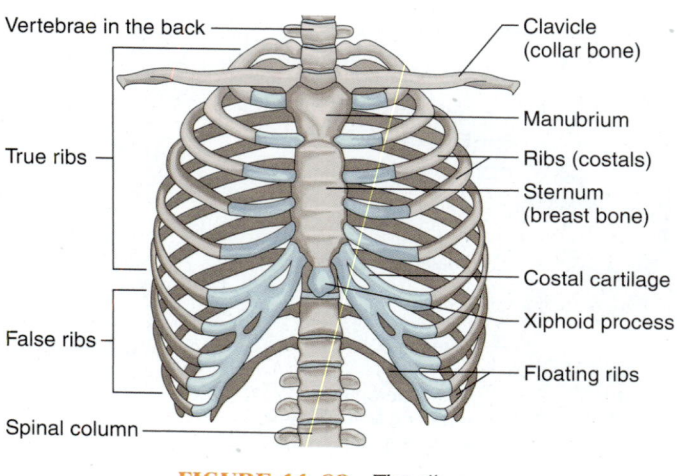

Vertebrae in the back — Clavicle (collar bone)

Manubrium

Ribs (costals)

Sternum (breast bone)

Costal cartilage

Xiphoid process

Floating ribs

True ribs

False ribs

Spinal column

FIGURE 11-83   The rib cage

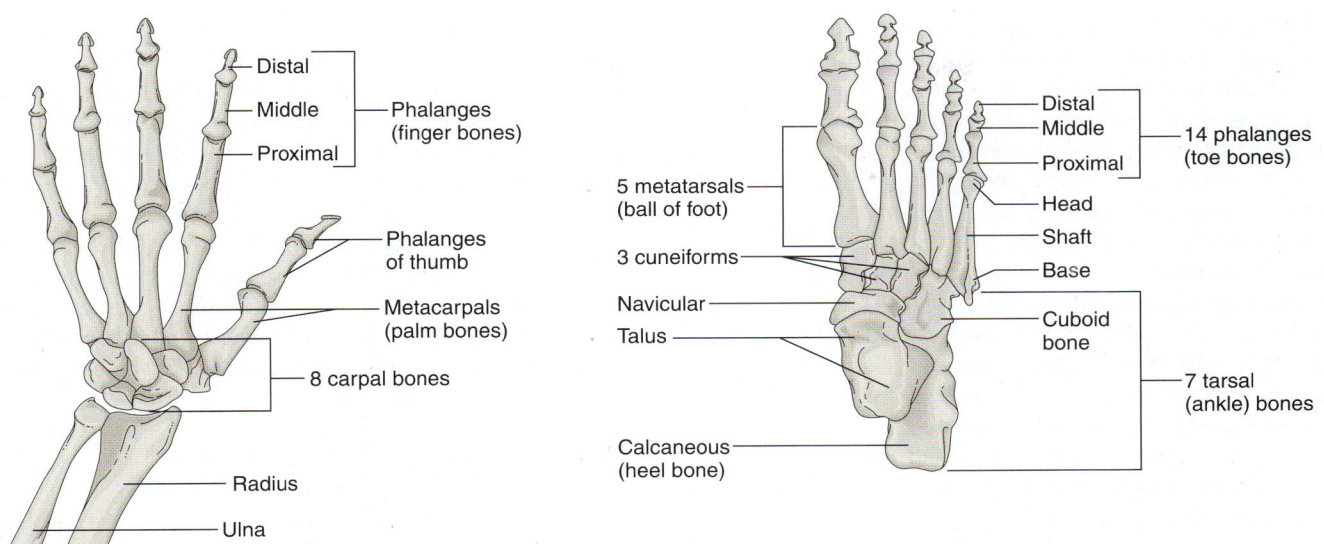

FIGURE 11-84   Bones of the hand and foot

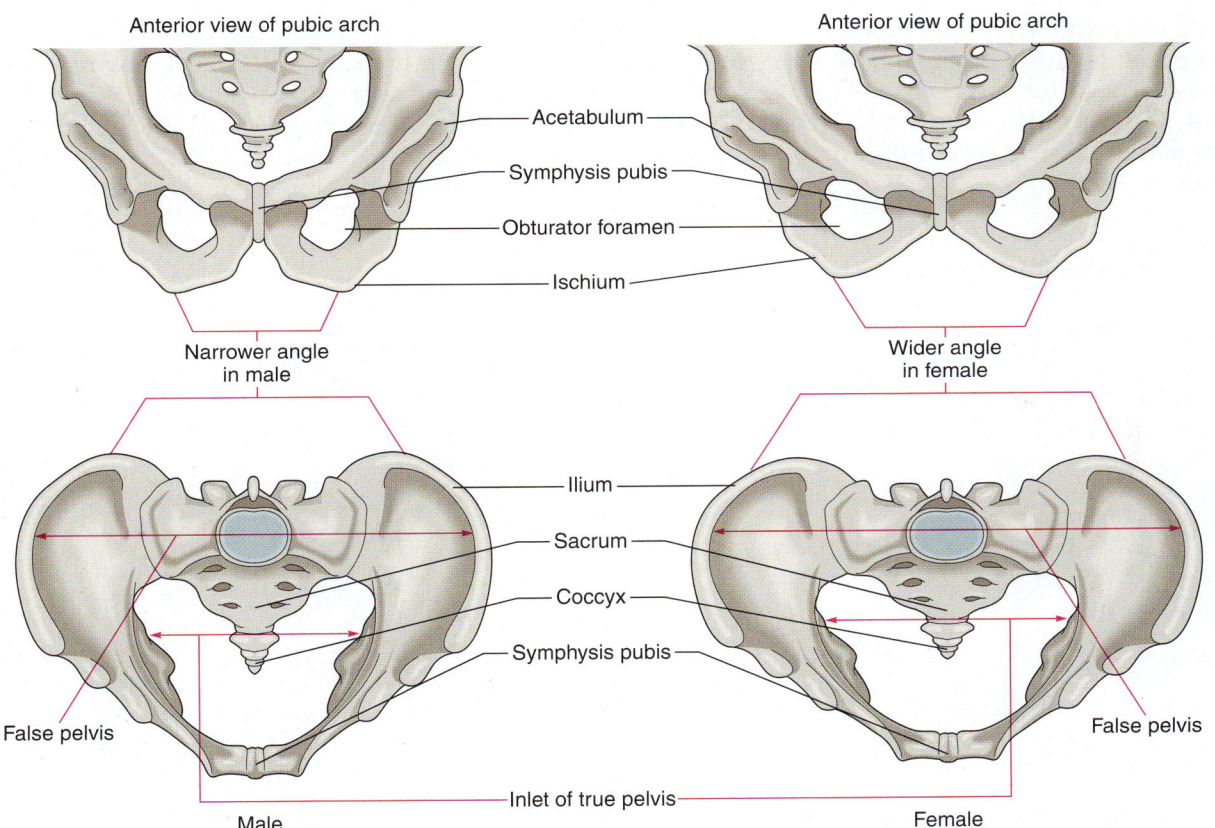

FIGURE 11-85   The pelvic girdle

lower portion is called the pubis, and the point of attachment (right and left pubis) is called the **symphysis pubis**. The posterior lower portion of the bone is called the **ischium**. The hip bone provides the recessed area where the head of the femur fits. The anatomical name for the socket is *acetabulum*.

JOINTS

The place where two or more bony parts join together is known as an **articulation** or joint. Strong, flexible bands of connective tissue called **ligaments** hold long bones together at joints. Ligaments can stretch and often become torn as a result of injury.

There are three main types of joints, classified primarily by their degree of movement. A movable joint, such as the knee or elbow, is called a **diarthrosis** or **synovial** joint. A partially movable joint, like where the ribs attach to the spine or between the vertebrae, is known as *amphiarthrosis* or *cartilaginous*. An immovable joint, such as a cranial suture, is called *synarthrosis* or *fibrous*.

Most of the body's joints are diarthrotic. They may have three distinct parts: articular cartilage, a **bursa** (saclike capsule), and a synovial cavity. The articulating joint surfaces of bones are covered with the articular cartilage, which provides a slippery, smooth surface and enables the joint to absorb shock. An articular capsule of tough, fibrous tissue encloses the articulating surfaces and is lined with a synovial membrane, which secretes synovial fluid into the cavity, lubricating the joint and reducing friction.

The joint is surrounded by ligaments, tendons, and muscles that hold the joint together but still allow for movement. Some synovial joints have cushionlike sacs called bursa, which form from the synovial membrane and are filled with synovial fluid. These are generally located between tendons and bones. In addition, synovial membranes may also form sheaths that wrap around the tendons. Bursae and tendon sheaths cushion and lubricate tendons and help reduce friction between the tendons and the bone.

The synovial joints of the body have been copied by man to develop many useful devices (Figure 11-86). The ball and socket joint found in the hip or shoulder can be seen in the movement of a desk pen set. The action of the fingers, knees, and elbows is like that of a hinge. An unusual pivot joint appears at the wrists and elbows. When the palm of the hand is up, the radius and ulna are side by side. As the palm is turned down, the radius crosses over the ulna in a pivoting action. This type of motion is independent of the elbow's hinge action. Joints found in the wrists and ankle are formed by bones with curved surfaces, which allow for various angular movements.

FRACTURES

The bones of children contain a high percentage of cartilage and are much more flexible than those of an adult. Frequently, the bone will crack under pressure but will not break all the way through. This type of break is known as a **greenstick fracture**.

A complete bone break in which there is no involvement with the skin surface is known as a **simple** or "closed" fracture (Figure 11-87). When broken bone protrudes through the skin's surface, it is known as an open fracture, formerly called a **compound** fracture. This causes additional concerns because of the

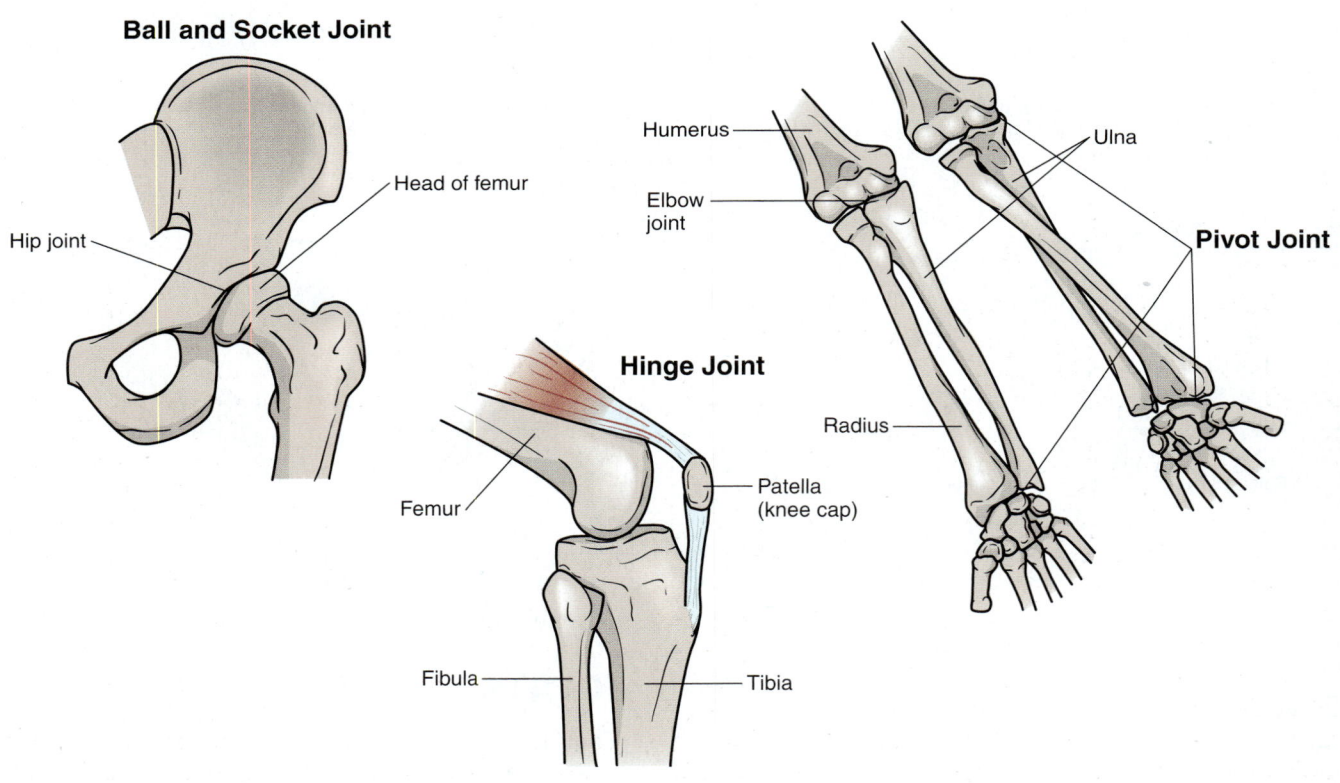

Ball and Socket Joint

Hip joint

Head of femur

Hinge Joint

Femur

Patella
(knee cap)

Fibula

Tibia

Humerus

Elbow
joint

Ulna

Pivot Joint

Radius

FIGURE 11-86 Types of joints

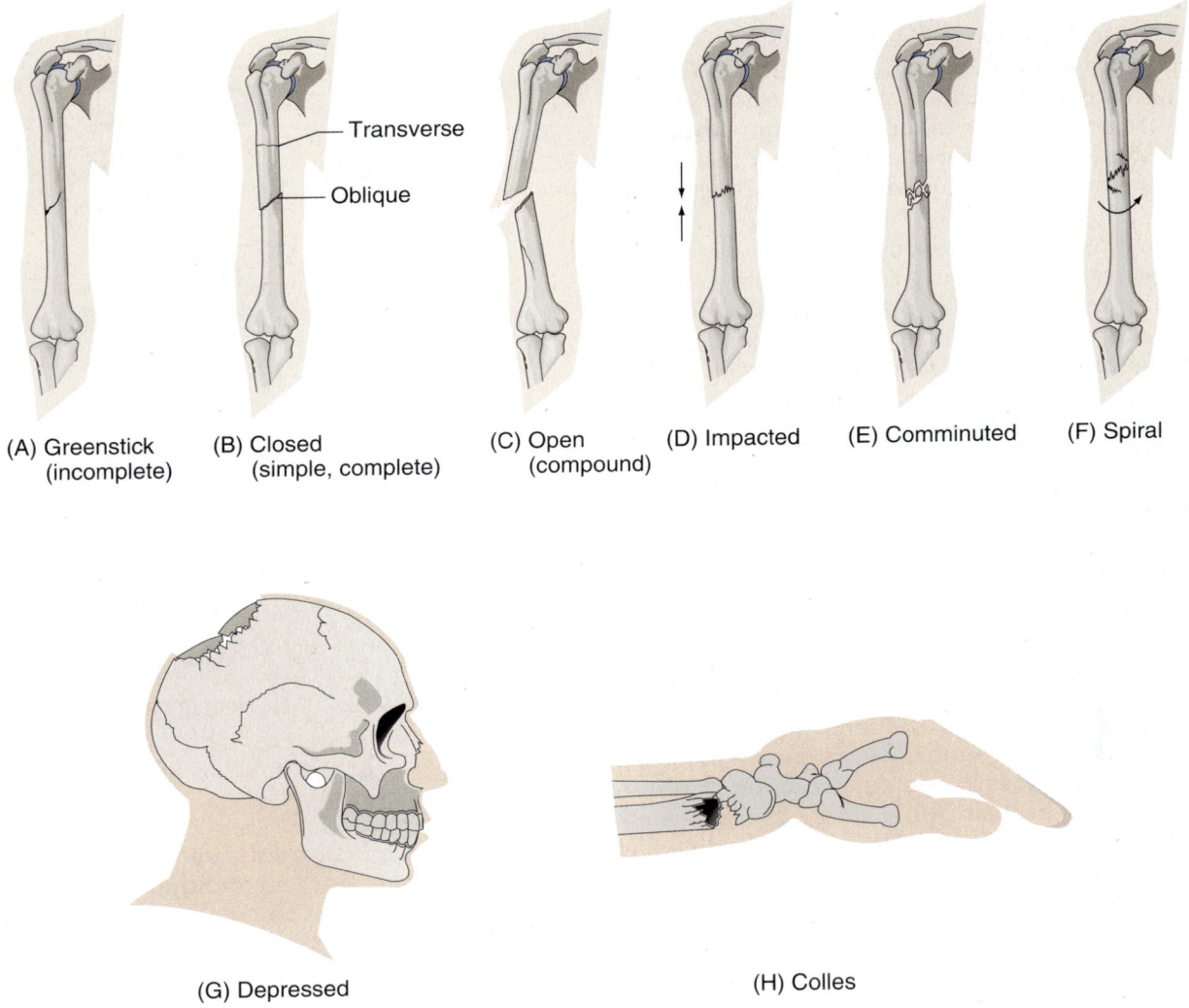

(A) Greenstick
(incomplete)

(B) Closed
(simple, complete)

Transverse

Oblique

(C) Open
(compound)

(D) Impacted

(E) Comminuted

(F) Spiral

(G) Depressed

(H) Colles

FIGURE 11-87   Types of fractures

possibility of infection to the area. A more involved type of fracture is called **impacted**, which indicates that the broken ends are jammed into each other. A **comminuted** fracture is one with more than one fracture line and several bone fragments. A **depressed** fracture may occur with severe head injuries in which a broken piece of skull is driven inward. A **spiral** fracture may occur with a severe twisting action, such as in a skiing accident, causing the break to wind around the bone.

A common injury among children is the Colles fracture. This involves the breaking and dislocating of the distal end of the radius, causing a characteristic bulge at the wrist. Often, the ulna is also fractured, resulting in a greater wrist deformity and a limply hanging hand. It is a common fracture of children from injuries while skating, riding bikes, and

climbing. It is generally the result of falling on an outstretched hand.

In treating fractures, immobilization of the affected part and prevention of shock are the main concerns. The extremity is splinted extending above and below the area of fracture. Elevation of the part and application of a cold pack or ice help prevent swelling. When there is also extensive damage to the surrounding tissues, especially to the exterior, control of bleeding may be indicated. This may require direct pressure over the wound.

When long bones are broken, they are usually pulled by the muscles attached to their surfaces into abnormal positions, often causing overlapping of their broken parts. Before the bone can be set, **traction** (pulling)—either manually or by a system of ropes and pulleys—must be used to stretch the muscles and pull the bone pieces back into **alignment**. This procedure is known as **reducing** the fracture. Once the ends fit together properly, a splint or cast can be used to maintain the position until the bone has healed. Occasionally, an external fixator is used to maintain alignment of the fracture. An external fixator is a device that includes a frame through which pins or wires are attached to the bones.

With involved fractures, such as compound or comminuted, an additional surgical procedure is often necessary either to repair the skin and surrounding tissues or to place all the small bone fragments in position. This procedure is called an *open reduction* because it involves an opening into the fractured bone through the skin and overlying tissues to achieve alignment of the bone. Typically, open reduction includes the placement of pins, wires, plates, or screws to hold the fracture in the proper position. When the hardware is used internally, it is covered by the normal soft tissues of the body and is known as an internal fixation.

Bone Healing Process

When a fracture occurs, a collection of blood (hematoma) forms around the fracture site. The hematoma begins an inflammatory reaction that initiates the healing process. A fibrous bridge is formed between the fracture fragments. Some of the cells in this fibrous mesh differentiate into cartilage cells and begin to accumulate calcium, forming a **callus** (Figure 11-88). As time passes, the callus turns first to cartilage and then to bone. Certain bone cells build the new bone tissue, whereas others remove the cartilage and then slowly smooth the repaired section back to its approximate original size.

A complication that may occur after the fracture of a long bone is a fat **embolus**. An embolus is a mass of foreign material circulating within the blood vessels. This potentially fatal complication may follow the release of fat droplets from the marrow of the long bones. The trauma of the event can also cause the body to release catecholamines (organic compounds and hormones), which in turn activate fatty acids. The fatty acids can develop into a fatty embolus and circulate in the blood, interfering with circulation in the lungs or even the brain. This interference may cause hypoxia (lack of oxygen), a change in the mental status, and even death.

Usual symptoms and signs include apprehension, sweating, fever, rapid heart rate, pallor, difficulty breathing, bluish discoloration of the skin, convulsions, and coma. If the complication occurs, it is usually within 24 to 48 hours, but it may occur as late as 3 days after the fracture.

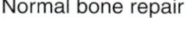

Normal bone repair

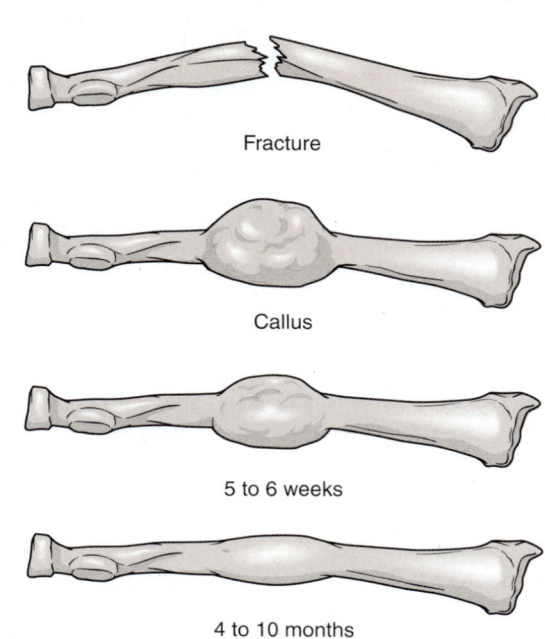

Fracture

Callus

5 to 6 weeks

4 to 10 months

FIGURE 11-88 Normal bone repair

AMPUTATION

Severe trauma, a malignant tumor, lack of circulation, or complications of other conditions, such as diabetes, may result in the need to **amputate** an extremity. The change in the patient's body image and function causes emotional and physical difficulties in coping with daily activities. Following amputation, a condition often occurs known as **phantom limb**, the sensation that the missing extremity is still present. It is often described as an itching or tingling sensation. This may last for quite some time but will usually subside eventually. It is considered normal to experience the sensation.

When the amputated stump has healed sufficiently, a **prosthesis** (artificial part) may be fitted. Lower limbs are either attached directly to the remaining extremity, fastened by means of straps or belt to the waist, or hung from the shoulder. The method depends to a great extent on the amount of the remaining extremity. Upper limbs may be replaced by a "hook" device that can be opened and closed to grasp objects. A prosthesis that closely resembles a real arm and hand cosmetically is often desired, even though it lacks the flexibility of the "hook."

DIAGNOSTIC EXAMINATIONS

● Arthroscopy—This endoscopic procedure permits direct visual inspection of a joint, most often the knee (Figure 11-89). In an arthroscopic examination, a surgeon makes a small incision in the patient's skin and then inserts pencil-sized instruments that contain small lenses and lighting systems to magnify and illuminate the structures inside the joint. Light is transmitted through fiber optics to the end of the arthroscope that is inserted into the joint. By attaching the arthroscope to a miniature television camera, the surgeon is able to see the inside of the joint through this very small incision. It is frequently used to evaluate injuries suffered by athletes. Arthroscopy is useful in detecting **arthritis**, torn meniscus, cysts, or loose pieces of tissue. The display of the image on the television screen allows the surgeon to look throughout the knee to determine the amount or type of injury. Many surgical procedures can be performed through the scope, thereby eliminating open surgery.

- Bone scan—This is a precise nuclear medicine procedure using small amounts of a radioactive substance that are injected into a vein to help diagnose the presence of disease based on structural appearance. A scintillation or gamma camera positioned over the area obtains images by detecting the substance in the bones and recording it on a computer or film. Usually the procedures is done in two parts. The injection is given first, and the medium is carried in the blood to the skeleton and distributed throughout the bones. After the injection, the patient may leave the area for about 2 hours while the bones thoroughly absorb the medium. After the time has passed, the patient returns and is placed on the imaging table, and the camera is positioned over the patient. It slowly moves up or down a framework over the body, taking the images for at least 30 minutes. It is important that the patient remains still throughout the scanning process.

- Computed tomography (CT) scan—This is a special x-ray in that the x-ray tube moves around the patient. A computer takes the information and reconstructs a cross-sectional (axial) "slice" of the patient. Multiple slices are taken that allow the physician to determine the anatomy in three dimensions.

- Magnetic resonance imaging (MRI)—This process uses strong magnets that cause all of the protons in the field to "line up." Radio waves are then passed through the patient, causing the protons to resonate. A computer takes this information and constructs images in any plane. This technology has three advantages over CT scans: (1) There is no ionizing radiation (x-ray) used, (2) soft tissues are seen in more detail, and (3) images can be constructed in any plane (not just axial). The major disadvantage is that the technique is expensive. There are also some factors that prevent many patients from being candidates for the procedure, such as obesity or claustrophobia.

- X-ray—This is a frequently used test that evaluates the condition of bones in cases such as dislocations, sprains, and fractures. X-ray can also be used to determine bone structure changes like those occurring in some metabolic conditions such as acromegaly (gigantism) and **osteoporosis** or with Paget's disease.

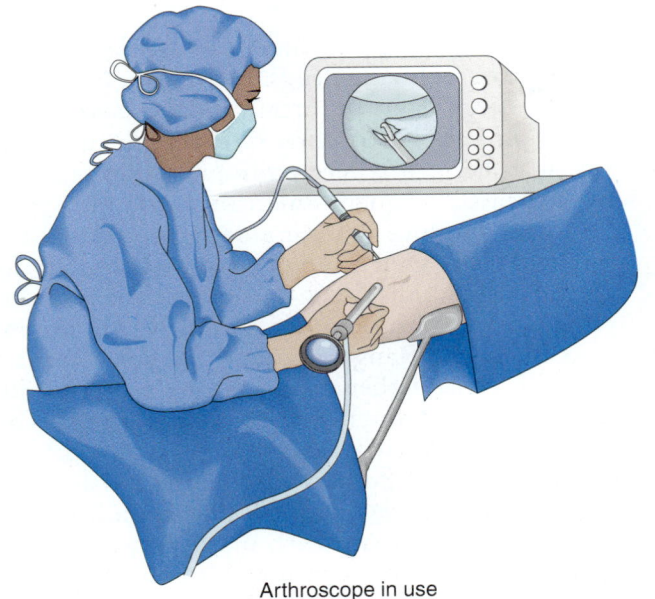

Arthroscope in use

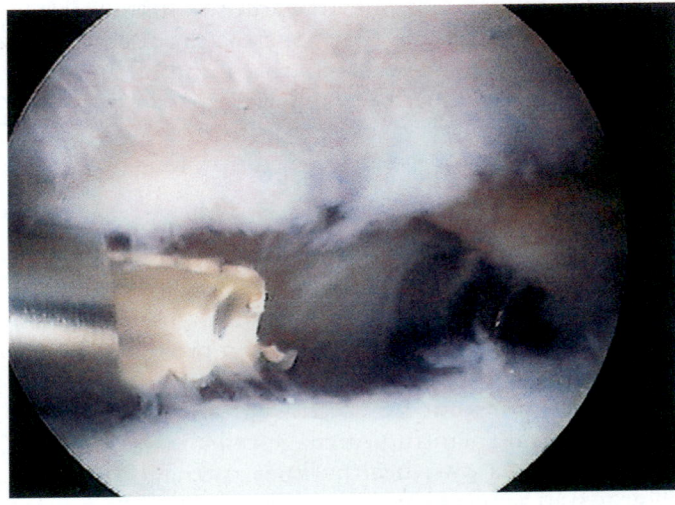

FIGURE 11-89   View of the inside of a knee through arthroscope

DISEASES AND DISORDERS

Arthritis (Ar-thri'-tis)

The word arthritis means joint inflammation. There are more than 100 different forms of arthritis. Currently it affects about 40 million Americans, the larger percentage being women. The most common forms are osteoarthritis, rheumatoid arthritis, gout, fibromyalgia, and lupus. It is important to identify the type a patient has, because different types require different approaches to treatment.

Osteoarthritis (Os-te-o-ar-thri'tis)

Description—This common form of arthritis results in progressive deterioration of joint cartilage, most often at the hips and knees. It affects many people as they grow older. Symptoms result from the breakdown of cartilage between bones and of the bones themselves. It is also known as degenerative joint disease. There is no cure.

Signs and symptoms—It is accompanied by joint pain, stiffness, aching (particularly with weather changes), "grating" during joint motion, and fluid around the joint.

Etiology—Osteoarthritis was believed to be caused by joint wear-and-tear from years of use. However, recent research suggests that a mild, slow-moving inflammation or a metabolic disorder is the root of the problem.

Treatment—Osteoarthritis is best treated with aspirin and other nonsteroidal anti-inflammatory drugs (NSAIDs), intraarticular joint injections of steroids, and reducing pressure on joints through the use of a cane, crutches, or a cervical collar. One popular drug used to treat arthritis is Celebrex. It is from a class of drugs called COX-2 inhibitors, which means they block an enzyme that causes inflammation but not the enzyme that controls production of a prostaglandin that protects the lining of the stomach. They are effective in relieving discomfort without the significant risks of the gastric side effects of Tylenol or the NSAIDs (e.g., ibuprofen, naproxen, and Feldene).

If the COX-2 drugs do not work, new injectable drugs containing hyaluronic acid can be used. The acid is a gooey fluid found in joint cavities that normally lubricates and absorbs shock. A series of several injections is necessary but can provide relief for up to a year. Initially, the injections were approved for the knee joint only. Other promising therapies involve transplanting cartilage cells harvested from the patient's own healthy knee cartilage. They are grown in a culture and then injected into the injured area to make new tissue. A third therapy uses stem cells harvested from the patient and grown and implanted in defects where cartilage is worn. A fourth removes a cylindrical plug of cartilage and bone from a healthy area within the knee and fits it into a drilled hole in the damaged cartilage. All these rely on the body's ability to repair itself if given the necessary materials. Occasionally, disability and uncontrollable pain will require surgical intervention. This can range from scraping deteriorated bone fragments from the joint to replacing joint bone parts with prosthetic appliances (artificial joints). (See Figure 11-93.)

Rheumatoid Arthritis (Roo'ma-toyd)

Description—A chronic systemic inflammatory disease attacking joints and surrounding tissues, this is an intermittent disease with periods of remission. It is three times more common in females than males, most often striking between the ages of 35 and 45.

Signs and symptoms—The disease attacks the joint synovial membrane, causing edema and congestion. Tissue layers become granulated and thicken, eventually involving the cartilage and destroying the joint capsule and bone. Scar tissue formation, bone atrophy, and malalignment cause visible deformities, pain, and often immobility. Figure 11-90A shows hands with rheumatoid arthritis, and Figure 11-90B shows the appearance of the thumb that is characteristic with rheumatoid arthritis.

Etiology—Rheumatoid arthritis is caused by a fault in the immune system that causes it to attack the joint membranes. The attack not only triggers inflammation but also stimulates the abnormal growth of cartilage and bone. It can affect persons of all ages.

Treatment—Treatments include anti-inflammatory and disease-modifying drugs, exercise, heat or cold, saving energy, joint protection, and sometimes surgery. Injections of cortisone directly into the joint may help to relieve pain and swelling; however, repeated frequent injections into the same joint can produce undesirable side effects. Researchers using genetic engineering techniques developed a drug called cA2 that blocks the immune system action. Maintaining a normal weight lessens stress on joints. Range of motion and low-impact aerobic exercise is beneficial and helps maintains flexibility. Warm water exercise is especially easy on joints. The woman whose hands are pictured in Figure 11-90 was diagnosed with rheumatoid arthritis 16 years ago at 34 years of age. She initially experienced debilitating pain with marked swelling and heat in her joints and considerable deformity. Current treatments have greatly improved her condition. One day a week she takes six tablets of

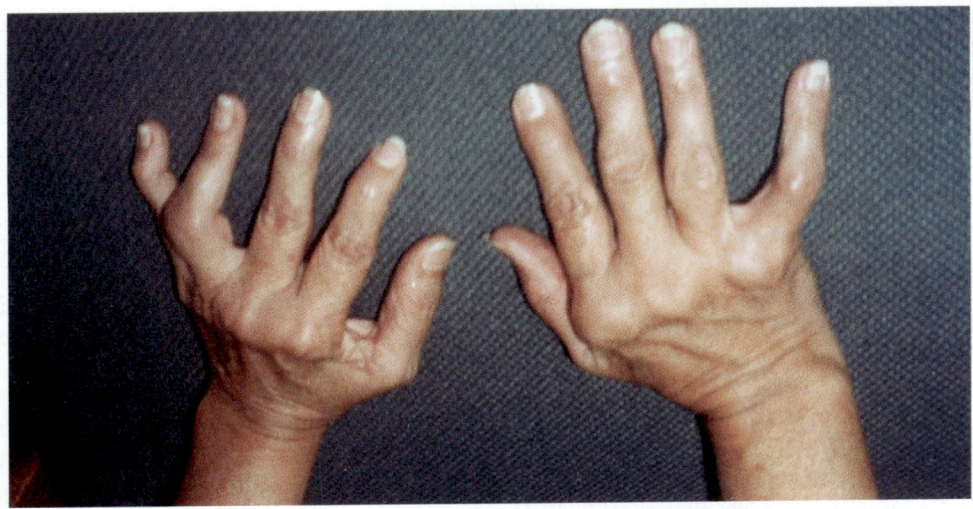

FIGURE 11-90A Rheumatoid arthritis of the hands

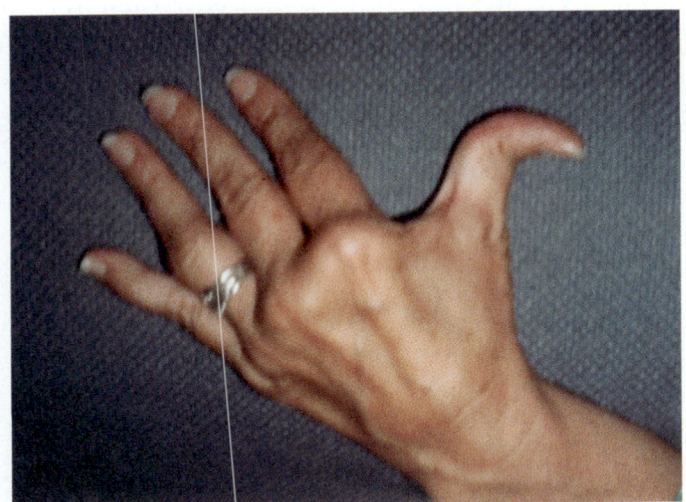

FIGURE 11-90B Characteristic thumb position of rheumatoid arthritis

methotrexate, and she also gets injections of Enbrel twice a week, plus daily prednisone. These medications require frequent lab work due to the possibility of liver damage. Her treatments cost her approximately $14,000 a year.

Gout (Gouty Arthritis)

Description—This metabolic disease results in severe joint pain, especially at night. It most often affects the great toe but can involve other joints. The pain results from deposits of urates (uric acid salts), which are overproduced or retained by the body. Often gout is associated with another disease, such as leukemia, because of cell destruction by chemotherapy. Gout may also follow drug therapy that interferes with urate excretion.

Signs and symptoms—Gout can be a progressive disease, initially causing severe pain and a hot, tender, inflamed joint. This attack will be followed by a symptom-free period of approximately 6 months to 2 years, when a second episode will occur. Additional attacks usually involve other joints of the feet and legs. Eventually the condition becomes chronic (ongoing), involving many joints that are persistently painful and become degenerated, deformed, and disabling.

Etiology—The exact cause of gout is unknown, but it seems linked to a genetic defect in purine metabolism that causes overproduction of uric acid, retention of uric acid, or both. This interferes with urate excretion, leading to urate deposits that cause local tissue destruction.

Treatment—Gout is best treated with medication to suppress uric acid formation and promote excretion of the urates. Dietary restrictions must be followed, such as avoiding alcohol, primarily beer and wine, and purine-rich foods, such as liver, sardines, kidneys, and lentils.

Bursitis (Bur-si′tis)

Description—This is a painful inflammation of the bursa. A bursa is a sac located around a joint containing lubricating fluids that allow muscles and tendons to move freely over bony surfaces. Bursitis occurs most frequently at the hip, shoulder, or knee.

Signs and symptoms—The most common sign is pain upon movement and limited motion of the affected joint. The pain can be gradual or sudden. Symptoms vary according to the joint involved.

Etiology—It usually occurs in middle age and is the result of recurring trauma that stresses or pressures a joint. It can also be the result of an inflammatory joint disease. A chronic form develops from repeated attacks of acute bursitis or repeated trauma and infection.

Treatment—Treatment consists of joint rest, often immobilization, a pain medication, and joint injection with a steroid combined with an anesthetic. It may be necessary to remove joint fluid by aspiration (withdrawal through a needle) and the institution of a program of physical therapy to preserve joint motion.

Carpal Tunnel Syndrome

Description—This condition results from the compression of the median nerve at the wrist. The carpal tunnel is a passageway for nerves, blood vessels, and flexor tendons to the fingers and thumb. It is formed by the carpal bones and the transverse ligament. The tendon sheaths become inflamed, causing swelling, which presses the median nerve against the transverse ligament.

Signs and symptoms—There is pain, tingling, numbness, and weakness of the hand. It involves only the thumb and index and middle finger. The patient will be unable to make a fist.

Etiology—Persons most likely to develop the syndrome are individuals who use vibrating hand tools, such as dental hygienists, and striking tools, such as a cleaver by a meat cutter. Systemic conditions that cause the carpal tunnel to swell are diabetes mellitus, pregnancy, menopause, hypothyroidism, and benign tumors.

Diagnosis can be made based on an examination that reveals decreased sensitivity of the first two fingers and the thumb on pricking with a pin and an electromyogram showing delayed motor nerve conduction. Patients may also have an *atrophy* (shrinking) of the muscle on the palm side of the thumb because of decreased innervation.

Treatment—If the syndrome is of short duration, treatment will consist of immobilizing the hand and forearm in a splint, local injections of corticosteroids, and systemic anti-inflammatory medication. It may be necessary to seek new employment if a work-related connection is determined. If conservative treatment does not correct the problem, a surgical procedure may be indicated to section the transverse ligament and "free-up" the nerve.

Congenital Hip Dysplasia (Kon-jen'-i-tal Dis-pla'-je-a)

Description—This abnormality of the hip joint is present at birth. It is the most common hip disorder of children, affecting one or both joints. It is present in three forms: unstable, with the hip in place but easily dislocated by manipulation; incomplete dislocation, with the head of the femur on the edge of the acetabulum; and complete dislocation, with the head totally outside the hip socket.

Signs and symptoms—Signs of hip dysplasia include the appearance of one leg being shorter than the other or one hip being more prominent. The child has a characteristic "duck waddle" if both hips are involved, or, if one hip only, a limp.

Etiology—The exact cause of dysplasia has not been proven. It is believed that hormones that relax maternal ligaments at the time of labor may also cause the infant ligaments to relax around the hip joint capsule. There is also an association of dislocation and a breech delivery.

Treatment—Early treatment is essential to normal development. In infants, a splint device is used for 3 to 4 months to maintain proper positioning. Older babies may be placed in traction, or the hips may be reduced and a cast applied for a period of 4 to 6 months.

Dislocation

Description—Displacement of bones at a joint so that the regularly articulating surfaces are no longer in contact is a **dislocation**. This occurs most frequently at joints of the finger, shoulder, knee, and hip.

Signs and symptoms—It is extremely painful and is often accompanied with joint surface fractures. Dislocation produces deformity around the joint, changes the length of the involved extremity, interferes with motion, and causes joint tenderness.

Etiology—Dislocation can be congenital, or it may follow trauma or disease of the surrounding joint.

Treatment—Prompt reduction (relocation) is essential to limit damage to surrounding tissues. Following reduction, a splint, cast, or traction (depending on the joint involved) to immobilize the area is indicated. Two to eight weeks will be needed to allow surrounding ligaments to heal completely.

Epicondylitis (Ep-i-kon-dil-i'-tis) (Tennis Elbow)

Description—This is an inflammation of the forearm extensor tendon at its attachment to the humerus or less commonly, the flexor tendon at its attachment to the humerus.

Signs and symptoms—Pain occurs at the elbow and becomes intense. There is tenderness over the area where the radius articulates with the humerus.

Etiology—The condition probably begins as a tear and is common among people who grasp things forcefully or twist the forearm. Untreated epicondylitis can become disabling.

Treatment—The condition is best treated with an injection of a steroid and a local anesthetic, aspirin, an immobilizing splint, heat, or cold and physical therapy. Epicondylitis usually resolves with or without treatment.

Hallux Valgus (Hal'-uks Val'-gus)

Description—Common in women, this is a lateral deviation of the great toe with enlargement of the first metatarsal head and a **bunion** formation. A bunion may be associated with a painful bursa.

Signs and symptoms—The bursa becomes inflamed, filled with fluid, and tender. The overlying skin is red.

Etiology—It may be congenital but is usually acquired from degenerative arthritis or the prolonged pressure on the foot from narrow, high-heeled shoes. Hallux valgus will cause bone deformity, and the change will alter the person's weight-bearing pattern.

Treatment—Early treatment with proper shoes, the use of padding and straightening devices, and exercises may correct the situation. A severe deformity and disabling pain will require surgical removal of the bunion.

Herniated Disk (Her-ne-a'-ted) (Ruptured Disk)

Description—In this situation, the soft gel-like material within an intervertebral disk has been forced through its outer surface. The extruded material may cause pressure on a spinal nerve exiting the spinal cord or may impinge on the spinal cord itself.

Signs and symptoms—The classic symptom is severe lower back pain, frequently radiating deep into the buttocks and down the back of the leg. It is usually unilateral (one sided). Sensory loss results from nerve compression, and the patient experiences numbness, muscle spasm, motor difficulty, and eventually weakness and atrophy of the leg muscles.

Etiology—A herniated disk may result from severe trauma or strain, but it is frequently related to de-

generation of the intervertebral joints. It occurs most often in the lumbar or lumbosacral regions. Herniated disk usually occurs in adults, mainly men, under age 45. In elderly people with disk degeneration, herniation can occur from a minor trauma.

Treatment—Conservative treatment consists of avoidance of painful activities, light exercises, frequent resting, analgesics as appropriate for pain, and anti-inflammatory medications, both steroidal and non-steroidal. A **laminectomy** is indicated if there is neurologic involvement that does not improve with conservative therapy. This procedure involves removing a portion of the lamina (flattened portion of the vertebral arch) to remove the protruding disk material.

If symptoms persist, a surgical procedure, **spinal fusion**, is performed to stabilize the adjoining vertebrae. A spinal fusion is typically accomplished by placing a screw and rod assembly into the spine to achieve a stable internal fixation. A piece of bone for a graft can be harvested from the pelvis or obtained from the bone bank. It is placed within a prepared space in the vertebra in conjunction with the hardware to achieve a solid fusion. When the bone heals, the joined vertebrae can no longer move independently to impinge on the nerve or spinal cord.

Kyphosis (Ki-fo'-sis) (Roundback, Humpback)

Description—This is a bowing of the back, usually at the thoracic level, resulting from improper vertebral alignment (Figure 11–91A). There are two types of **kyphosis**: adolescent and adult.

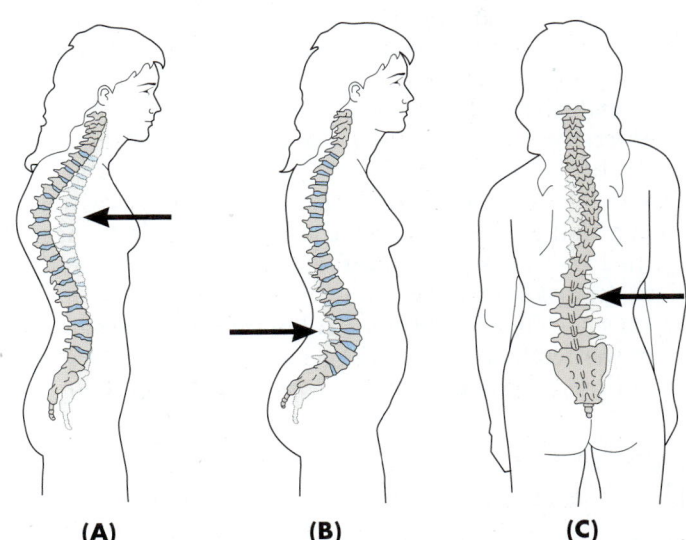

(A)   **(B)**   **(C)**

FIGURE 11-91   Abnormal curvatures of the spine; (A) kyphosis; (B) lordosis; (C) scoliosis

Signs and symptoms—With adolescent kyphosis, the condition is essentially without symptoms except for the visible curving of the back. Some adolescents may have mild pain, fatigue, localized tenderness, stiffness in the involved area, and tightening of the hamstring muscles of the posterior thighs because of compensating posture. In adult kyphosis, there is the characteristic rounded back, possible pain, weakness of the back, and fatigue.

Etiology—In children and adolescents, kyphosis may be caused by growth retardation or the result of rapid growth periods with improper epiphysis development. Poor posture and excessive sports activity can also result in curvature. In the adult form, it is caused by aging and the degeneration of intervertebral disks or the actual collapse of vertebrae resulting from osteoporosis.

Treatment—Kyphosis as a result of poor posture during childhood can be treated by therapeutic exercise, a firm mattress, and a Milwaukee brace to straighten the spine until spinal growth is complete. If neurologic damage or disabling pain occurs in adolescents and adults (which happens rarely), a surgical procedure may be indicated, which involves posterior spinal fusion, bone grafting, and casting to straighten the severe curvature. With full skeletal maturity and debilitating curvature, a posterior spinal fusion can be accomplished with the use of a stainless steel Harrington rod mechanism to align the vertebrae.

Lordosis (Lor-do'-sis)

Description—This abnormal anterior convex curvature of the lumbar spine is commonly referred to as swayback (see Figure 11-91B). The body's spine normally curves in at this point; however, if it is exaggerated, it is considered to be **lordosis**.

Signs and symptoms—The obvious visual symptom is the excessive inward curvature of the lumbar portion of the back.

Etiology—It is usually caused by poor posture. The wearing of high heels causes the inward positioning of the lower back to counteract the position of the feet to maintain balance.

Treatment—This condition can be improved, or at least prevented from progressing, by appropriate exercises, improving posture, and wearing proper footwear.

Lumbar Myositis (Lum-bar Mi-o-si'tis)

Description—An inflammation of the lumbar region muscles of the back.

Signs and symptoms—Low back pain.

Etiology—It is common and is primarily caused by a straining of the back muscles.

Treatment—The condition is best treated with rest, mild analgesics, and muscle relaxers. When improved, a program of stretching exercises is prescribed to condition and strengthen the muscles.

Osteoporosis (Os-te-o-por-o'-sis)

Description—A metabolic bone disorder, characterized by acceleration of the rate of bone resorption while the rate of bone formation slows down, which results in a loss of bone mass. The loss of calcium and phosphate from the bone allows it to become porous, brittle, and prone to fracture. There are two forms of osteoporsis: primary and secondary. Primary is also known as senile or postmenopausal osteoporosis because it affects primarily elderly, postmenopausal women. Of the 25 million older Americans with osteoporosis, only 5 million are men. Secondary osteoporosis can occur following prolonged steroid therapy, bone immobilization or lack of use (with paralysis), malnutrition, excessive alcohol intake, scurvy, and hyperthyroidism. It is usually discovered following injury from bending to lift something.

Signs and symptoms—The individual feels instant pain in the mid thoracic to lumber spine. The pain is from the collapse of a vertebra. Other common signs of osteoporosis are slowly developing kyphosis with loss of height, fractures of the forearm or hip from minor falls, and additional spontaneous vertebral fractures. Figure 11-92A illustrates the progression of spinal curvature caused by osteoporosis and the resulting loss of height. (Note height measurements.)

Etiology—The cause of primary osteoporosis may be the combination of aging, prolonged inadequate dietary intake of calcium, faulty metabolism because of estrogen deficiency, or a sedentary lifestyle. Females with small, thin frames are more likely to develop it. Males with low levels of testosterone are also more prone. The use of tobacco and a family history of osteoporosis also increases the risk.

Treatment—The condition is treatable to prevent additional fracturing by increasing exercise, giving an estrogen supplement, and taking calcium and vitamin D to support normal bone metabolism.

Today there are four new approved treatments. A drug called Miacalcin, which decreases bone loss, has been in use in injectable form but is now available as a nasal spray. Fosamax, Slow Sodium, and Citracel are also able to increase bone mass.

The most significant development is the ability to determine the disease before fractures occur. There are seven different techniques for measuring bone density in various body locations. The most used form of densitometry is called dual energy x-ray absorptiometry (DEXA). It can measure bone density

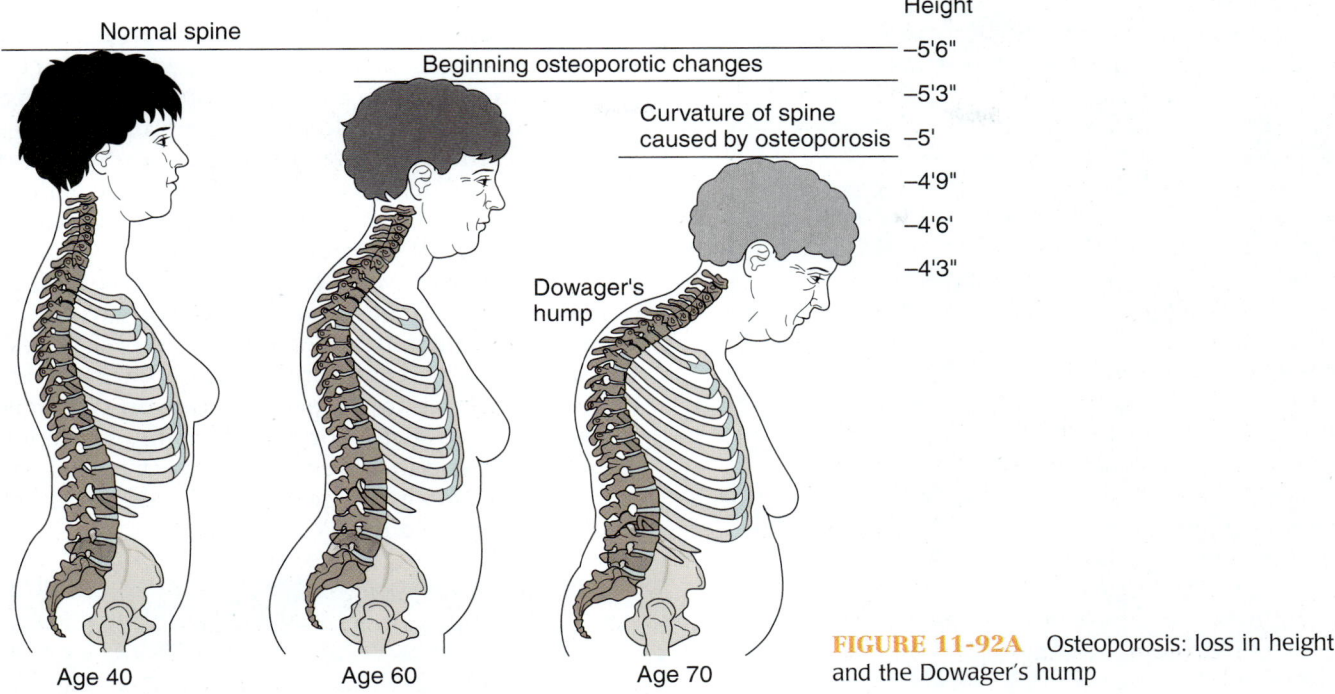

Height
- −5'6"
- −5'3"
- −5'
- −4'9"
- −4'6'
- −4'3"

Normal spine

Beginning osteoporotic changes

Curvature of spine caused by osteoporosis

Dowager's hump

Age 40　　　　Age 60　　　　Age 70

FIGURE 11-92A　Osteoporosis: loss in height and the Dowager's hump

and also estimate fracture risk. The procedure is relatively fast, uses a low level of radiation, and is fairly inexpensive. Another even simpler method screens for the rate of bone loss with a urine test called Osteomark, or the NTX test. The purpose of all procedures is early detection so that preventive therapies can be prescribed. Figure 11–92B shows an x-ray of the thoracic spine with osteoporosis changes and compressed vertebra.

Recently, scientists in Philadelphia, using new biotechnology equipment, believe they have discovered the cause of postmenopausal osteoporosis. They have linked the condition to a defect on chromosome 7, leading them to think that it may be possible to develop a test that will predict who will develop osteoporosis so that preventive measures may be taken long before the symptoms would become evident.

The National Osteoporosis Foundation is trying to educate people about the condition, because osteoporosis is a "silent" disease, meaning there are no warning symptoms. Often, by the time it is diagnosed, there has been significant loss of bone strength leading to irreversible damage and probable disability. A risk analysis assessment (see the following box) provides a means of determining the probability of developing osteoporosis.

Scoliosis (Sko-le-o'-sis)

Description—A lateral curvature of the spine, usually in the thoracic region, associated with rotation of the spinal column. It may also be lumbar or involve both (see Fig-

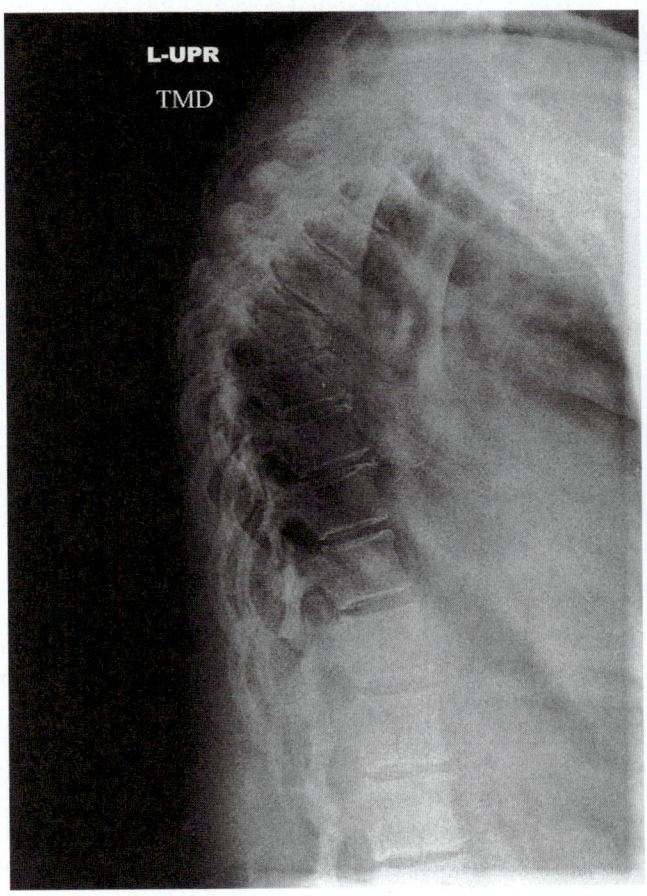

L-UPR

TMD

FIGURE 11-92B　X-ray of the thoracic spine showing osteoporotic changes and compression of vertebra. *(Courtesy of John S. Wolfe, MD, orthopedic surgeon)*

ure 11–91C). The thorax usually curves to the right while the lumbar curves left. Because the body has to maintain balance, the cervical spine will also curve left, which gives the spine an "S" curve appearance.

There are different types of **scoliosis**. An infantile type of transmitted scoliosis occurs primarily in boys from birth to age 3 and causes left thorax and right lumbar curves. Another type, known as juvenile scoliosis, affects both sexes between the ages of 4 and 10. The third type, called adolescent, primarily affects girls between 10 and maturity of the skeleton and results in varying types of curvatures.

Signs and symptoms—Adolescent scoliosis can be easily diagnosed. Classic symptoms are uneven hemlines or unequal pants legs, one hip appearing to be higher than the other, and one shoulder appearing higher and perhaps the scapula more pronounced.

Etiology—Different types have different causes. Some are from congenital defects of the vertebra, muscular dystrophy, paralysis, or a transmitted trait that develops during the growth process. Others are the result of poor posture or uneven leg lengths. Most scoliosis is of idiopathic (without apparent cause) origin.

Treatment—Treatment includes observation, exercises, and a brace. With curvature beyond 60 degrees, an immobilizing cast or preoperative traction system is followed by surgical correction using posterior spinal fusion and insertion of a Harrington rod for stabilization. Note the parent teaching aid box titled "How to Detect Scoliosis."

Sprain

Description—The complete or incomplete tear in the supporting ligaments of a joint.

Signs and symptoms—**Sprains** are characterized by pain, swelling, and a black-and-blue discoloration. The ankle is the most common site.

Etiology—Sprains follow a severe twisting action of a joint.

Treatment—Care of sprains should follow the easy to remember R.I.C.E. method—Rest, Ice, Compression, and Elevation. Treatment consists of (1) controlling pain and swelling by elevating the joint and applying ice intermittently for the first 12 to 24 hours, (2) immobilization using an elastic wrap or, if very severe, a soft cast, and (3) the use of crutches to eliminate stress on the joint. If healing does not occur normally in 3 to 4 weeks, the torn ligaments may require surgical repair, especially if sprains recur.

Subluxation (Sub-luks-a'-shun)

Description—The partial or incomplete dislocation of the articulating surfaces at the joints.

Signs and symptoms—There is joint deformity, impaired motion, pain, and change in length if an extremity is involved. Common sites are shoulders, elbows, wrists, knees, fingers and toes, hips, and ankles. Diagnostic x-ray is usually indicated to rule out or confirm accompanying joint fracture.

Etiology—Subluxation is caused by an injury or a disease process of a joint. Often with an injury there is also involvement of the surrounding nerves, blood vessels, ligaments, and soft tissues that results in pain, swelling, and joint deformity.

Treatment—Treatment consists of reduction as soon as possible to minimize swelling and muscle spasms, which make reduction difficult. The use of medication to control muscle spasm and pain and possibly a splint or cast to provide joint immobilization and support while ligaments heal depend on the joint involved.

Temporomandibular Disorders (TMD) (Tem-po-ro-man-dib'-u-lar)

Description—This is a condition of the jaw that is described as a feeling that the jaw has come unhinged. For unknown reasons, 90% of sufferers are women.

Signs and symptoms—The symptoms include a grinding or clicking sound and pain and discomfort when opening the mouth. Jaw muscles become sore, chewing is difficult, and pain spreads to the facial and neck muscles. Symptoms persist continuously. Headaches, toothaches, and earaches may also be part of the disorder.

Etiology—The cause is not certain. Some feel it is emotional stress, others that the joint is very complicated and is a manner of many factors adversely affecting the joint. Teeth grinding and clenching cause muscle spasm and can be caused by it. A malocclusion of the teeth can throw the jaw out of line. Bad posture that thrusts the chin forward can strain the neck and jaw muscles. Certain orthopedic problems, such as arthritis and bone degeneration, can contribute. Other causes may be excessive chewing of gum or chewy foods or a blow to the jaw. A common cause is prolonged gripping of a phone between the shoulder and cheek or carrying a heavy shoulder bag that strains neck and shoulder muscles.

Treatment—First is self-treatment, such as a soft diet and an analgesic for the pain, and eliminating activities known as causes. Hot or cold compresses, gentle exercises, controlling yawns (with the hands), and resting of the jaw may help. If malocclusion is present, a simple grinding of teeth surfaces by a dentist may correct the problem. Bite splints or plates fitted over the teeth can also stabilize the bite and eliminate night grinding. Taking muscle relaxers and eliminating the source of stress may be necessary.

REPLACING BONE AND JOINTS

When bone is destroyed by injury, cancer, or an infectious process, doctors may use bone taken from other places in the body. However, there is a limit to the amount that can be "borrowed." When desperate, bone can be salvaged from cadavers, but the problems of inflammation and infection are a concern. Surgeons have discovered that coral from the ocean is uniquely compatible with bone and makes an excellent framework upon which bone cells can construct new bone. Certain species of coral have an almost identical physical makeup as bone. It unites, almost without seams, with the human skeleton. In addition, it does not activate the body's inflammation or immune responses. Once the surgery has healed, the strength of the resulting bone composite is excellent. The coral is available in blocks of different sizes, which doctors carve into the shapes they need for surgery.

Replacing worn or damaged joints is a commonly performed procedure. The knees and hips are the joints most often affected by the wear and tear of movement and supporting the body. Articulating surfaces at joints normally have protective coverings of cartilage that allow the surfaces to move against each other easily. When this cartilage wears thin, is damaged, or breaks up, it causes pain within the joint from the fragments and the bones rubbing together. Figure 11-93A shows a knee with the

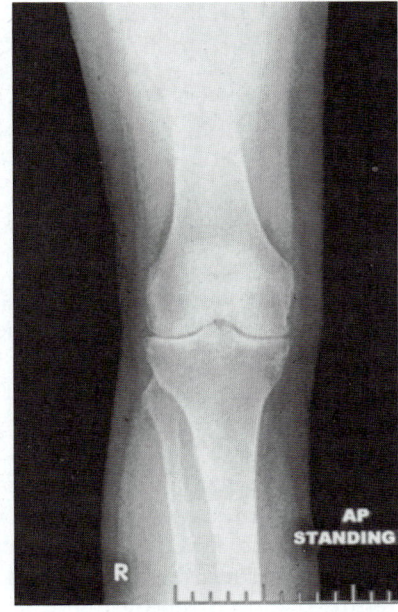

FIGURE 11-93A   Preoperative knee with cartilage destroyed by rheumatoid arthritis

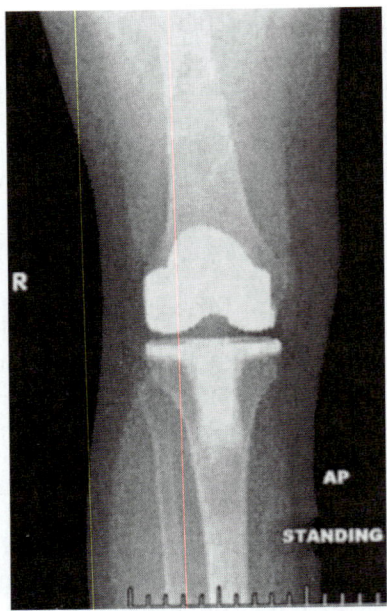

FIGURE 11-93B Postoperative knee with replacement artificial joint

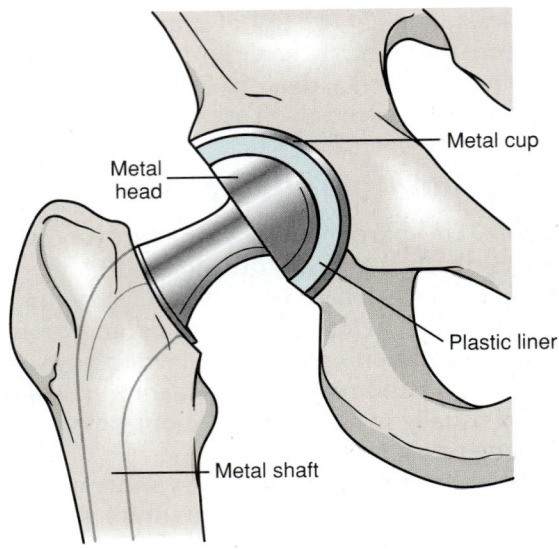

FIGURE 11-93D Postoperative artificial hip joint

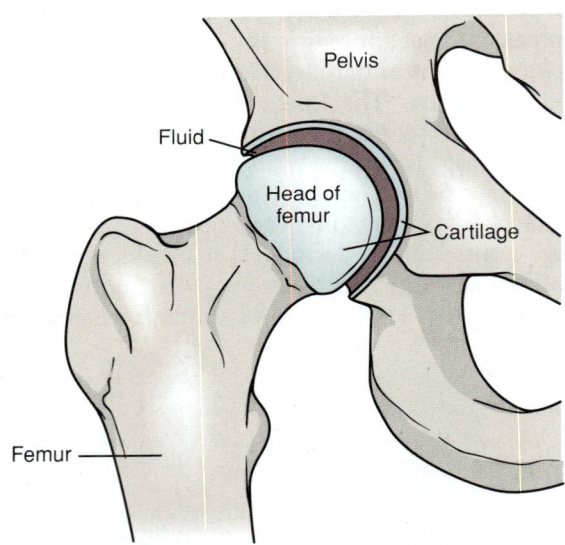

FIGURE 11-93C Preoperative hip joint

loss of cartilage from rheumatoid arthritis. Note the bones at the joint have no space between them and are therefore painful upon movement. In Figure 11-93B, the damaged knee is replaced with an artificial joint. The ends of the natural bone are modified to attach and insert the new metal surfaces.

In Figure 11-93C, the head of the femur is damaged. Usually the head will not stay within the socket of the pelvis due to years of movement and the weakening of the supporting joint structures. In Figure 11-93D, the head of the femur has been removed and a metal shaft inserted into the femur. The corresponding socket has been implanted into the pelvic bone. This new joint will

last for 10 to 15 years but will eventually wear out and require replacement.

Research continues to identify new materials and techniques to prolong the life of artificial joints. Replacement is usually delayed as long as possible, particularly in younger people. Joints can be redone, but the risk of complications increases with repeat operations.

ACHIEVE UNIT OBJECTIVES

- ☐ **Complete the Workbook activities to meet the learning objectives.**
- ☐ **Apply your knowledge at the end of this chapter in completing the Critical Thinking Challenge and Activities, as well as the StudyWARE on your Student CD-ROM.**

UNIT 6
THE MUSCULAR SYSTEM

OBJECTIVES

Upon completion of this unit, you will be able to achieve the following:

LEARNING Objectives

1. **Spell and define, using the glossary at the back of the text, all the Words to Know in this unit.**

2. **Explain how muscular activity increases body heat.**

3. **List six functions of skeletal muscles.**

4. **Name and describe the three types of muscular tissue and the purpose of each.**

5. **Describe the purpose of a muscle team, and give an example.**

6. **Explain what muscle tone means.**

7. **Describe the structure and function of a tendon, and identify the body's strongest tendon.**

8. **Explain the terms *origin* and *insertion*.**

9. **Describe a muscle sheath and a bursa and the purpose of each.**

10. **Identify the muscles of respiration, and describe how their function results in breathing.**

11. **Name the major skeletal muscles of the body.**

12. **Describe the smooth muscle action of peristalsis.**

13. **Explain the structure and function of a sphincter.**

14. **Describe four disorders or diseases of the muscular system.**

WORDS TO KNOW

abduction	gluteus maximus	sartorius
Achilles' tendon	hamstring	sheath
adduction	hiccough	spasm
anchor	insertion	sphincter
aponeurosis	intercostal	sternocleido-
atrophy	latissimus dorsi	mastoid
biceps	muscle team	strain
contracture	muscle tone	tendon
cramp	musculoskeletal	tendonitis
deltoid	origin	tibialis
dystrophy	pectoralis	anterior
extensor	major	torticollis
fascia	peristalsis	trapezius
flexor	quadriceps	triceps
gastrocnemius	femoris	

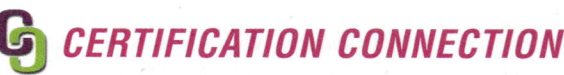

CERTIFICATION CONNECTION

CMA	**CMAS**
Diagnostic procedures	Anatomy and physiology
Common diseases and	
pathology	**RMA**
Anatomy and physiology	Anatomy and physiology

There are approximately 600 muscles in the human body. Muscles are composed of muscular tissue, which is constructed of bundles of muscle fibers about the size of a human hair. The larger the muscle, the greater the number of fibers. Muscles perform their duties by alternately contracting and relaxing. All muscle activity is influenced by the nervous system. Motor neuron axons innervate several muscle cells within a muscle. Signals from the brain go through the axons and cause all the cells under their control to contract at the same time. That group of cells and its motor neuron are called a *motor unit*. When only one stimulus acts on the unit causing a contraction, it is called a *twitch*. This quick, simple contraction naturally occurs occasionally as a spontaneous event in a muscle. Scientists can study these units by using an electrical stimulus, which will also activate the motor unit. A muscle contraction is a quick progression of events following a stimulus—a very brief interval before the contraction begins, then it intensifies to a peak, and decreases to relaxation. If a second stimulus is received before the first is completed, the contraction will strengthen. When repeated stimulation occurs without a relaxation time, the muscle is maintained in a state of contraction called *tetanus* (not to be confused with the disease of the same name). This occurs when we experience muscle **cramps** and **spasms**.

At all times, motor units are alternately either contracted or relaxed; there is no other state in which they exist. The units that make up the muscles are contracted in sufficient number to meet whatever need is necessary. During sleep, for instance, only a few would be contracted at a given time, yet during strenuous activity, a great number would be called on to contract, a process known as *muscle recruitment*.

Some muscles work in partnership with the bones and can be controlled voluntarily by the motor nerves of the peripheral nervous system to achieve movement. Other muscles function continuously without the slightest conscious concern. The autonomic nervous system directs their activities to provide the body with essential services. It is the action of these muscles that causes us to breathe and our blood to circulate.

MUSCLE FUEL

All body tissues must have food and oxygen to survive. The muscles receive an ample supply of both because of their importance to the body's safety and well-being.

The body stores carbohydrates in its muscles in the form of a starch called *glycogen*. When muscles function, they use the stored glycogen, changing it to glucose, as their source of energy. Heat is released as this fuel is used, thereby warming the body. Strenuous exercise burns a great deal of stored glycogen and therefore often results in overheating the body.

FUNCTIONS OF MUSCLE

In addition to providing heat and the ability to move, muscles support the structures of the body and hold the body upright. The muscles along the back, shoulders, and neck hold the trunk and head erect while permitting great flexibility in movement.

The structure of the skeletal muscles protects the blood vessels and nerves that lie throughout the body. The contraction of lower leg muscles aids in the return flow of blood to the heart by squeezing the veins of the legs. Muscles also provide protective padding to shield delicate internal organs and structures from injury.

Visually, the muscles add greatly to our appearance by giving shape to the body. Body-building enthusiasts spend years developing the degree of muscle enlargement and definition they feel is desirable. Muscle fiber, and therefore the muscle, hypertrophies (grows larger) with exercise; the number of fibers does not increase, however.

MUSCLE GROWTH

Muscle tissue changes slightly with age. During infancy, muscles have little connective tissue, often being attached to the bone directly. With maturity, the connective tissue increases, as do the elastic fibers. Muscles grow in relation to the structures to which they are attached. Muscles of the eye, for example, grow very little, whereas the large muscles of the lower extremities grow considerably.

TYPES OF MUSCLE TISSUE

There are three types of muscle tissue (Figures 11-94A through C). First, there is the *skeletal* type. Skeletal muscles are attached to bones and therefore permit movement. Because we have some control over movements, this type of muscle tissue is also called voluntary. Skeletal muscle cells are long and strong, some reaching lengths up to 12 inches. These cells are held together by connective tissue to form a muscle bundle. The bundles in turn are enclosed in a tougher connective tissue **sheath** to form the muscle organs such as the **biceps** of the arm. The larger the muscle organ, the greater the number of fibers.

The second type of muscle tissue is *smooth*. Smooth muscle tissue is made of small, delicate muscle cells

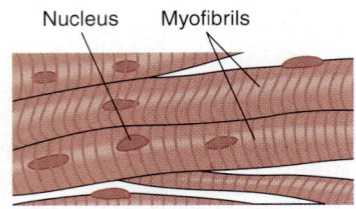

FIGURE 11-94A Skeletal muscles are attached to the skeleton (bones, tendons, and other muscles).

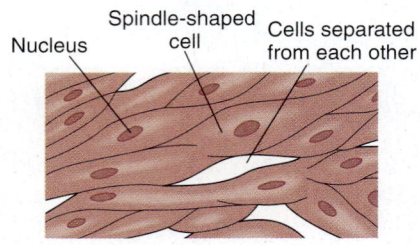

FIGURE 11-94B Smooth muscles make up the walls of the digestive, genitourinary, and respiratory tracts; blood vessels; and lymphatic vessels.

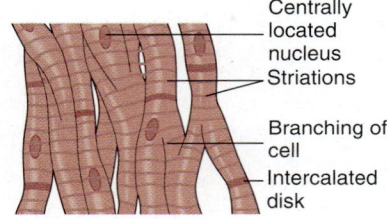

FIGURE 11-94C Cardiac muscles make up the walls of the heart.

and is found throughout the internal organs of the body, except for the heart. Smooth muscle activity occurs continuously in such actions as breathing, moving food through the intestinal tract, changing the size of the pupil of the eye, and dilating or constricting blood vessels. These muscles function without conscious direct control, so they are also called involuntary.

The third type is *cardiac* muscle tissue. As the name implies, this type is found in the heart. These cells are joined in a continuous network without sheath separation. The membranes of adjacent cells are fused at places called *intercalated disks*. A communication system at the fused areas will not permit independent cell contraction. When one cell receives a signal to contract, all neighboring cells are stimulated and they contract together to produce the action of a heartbeat. This type of muscle tissue is also involuntary, which is fortunate. It would be a full-time job to consciously contract the heart muscle 70 times a minute, 100,800 times a day.

SKELETAL MUSCLE ACTION

When muscles contract, they become shorter and thicker. A good example is the skeletal muscle of the upper arm, the biceps. When the biceps contract to bend the elbow, the shorter and thicker muscle causes a bulge in the upper arm (Figure 11-95).

The skeletal muscle that bends a joint is called a **flexor**, whereas the action of straightening the joint is done by the **extensor** muscle. The extensor muscle that straightens the elbow is the **triceps**. The flexor and its partner, the extensor muscle, form what is known as a **muscle team** to bend and straighten joints (Figure 11-96). Muscles also contract to move extremities away from the body's center line, which is known as **abduction**, or toward the center line, which is known as **adduction** (Figure 11-97).

MUSCLE TONE

Most skeletal muscles are partially contracted at all times to maintain the body's erect position. It is believed that some fibers contract while others rest and that they then exchange roles. This constant state of contraction is known as **muscle tone**. Physicians frequently refer to muscle tone when examining patients. Evaluation of muscle tone aids in determining the sta-

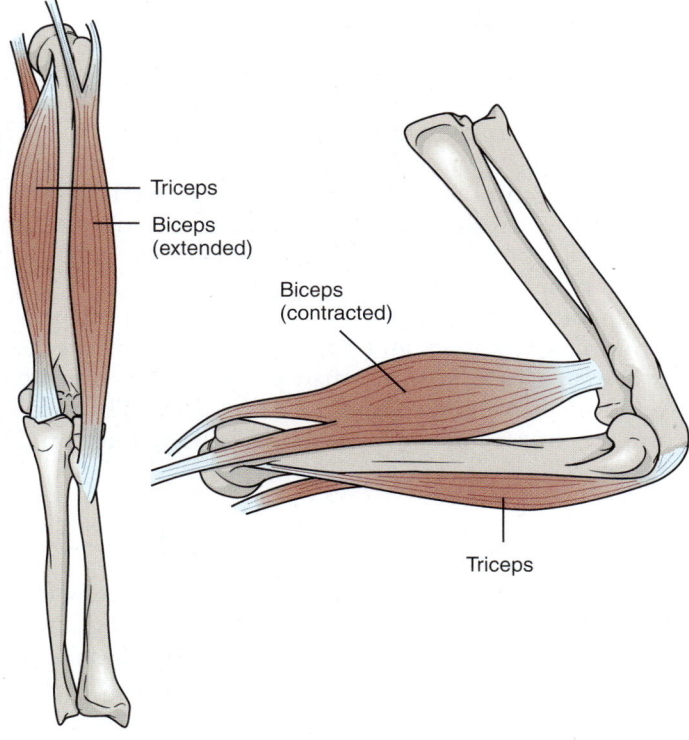

FIGURE 11-95   Action of the biceps/triceps muscle team

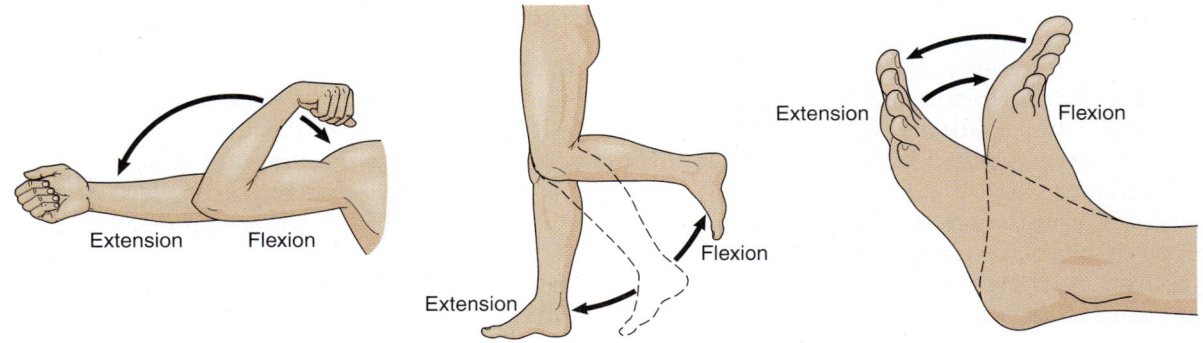

FIGURE 11-96   Flexor/extensor muscle team action

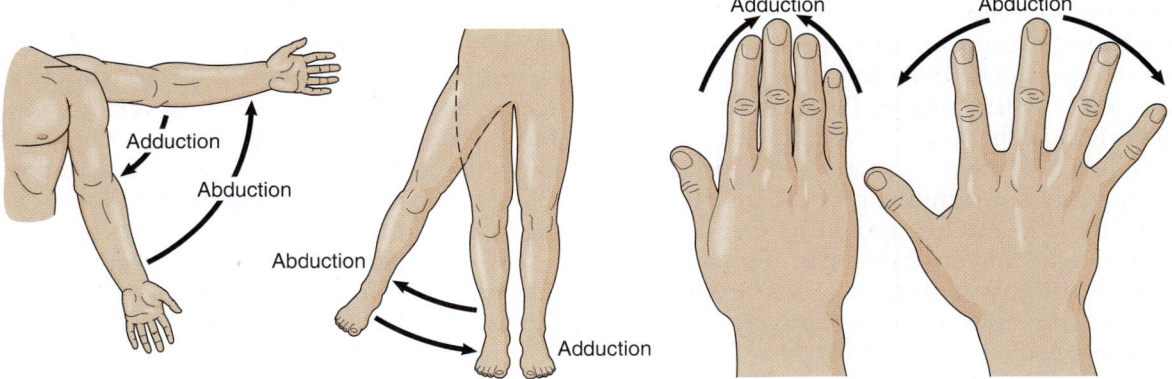

FIGURE 11-97   Abduction/adduction muscle team action

tus of the CNS and the motor function of the peripheral nerves.

Loss of muscle tone can occur when muscles are not used, as with severe illness, elderly people, paralysis, or temporarily when an extremity has been immobilized in a cast. With prolonged lack of use, muscles will **atrophy**, which is a progressive wasting away of the muscle tissue. Another muscular condition that develops from lack of use is called **contracture**. Here flexor muscles become shorter and permanently bend the joints. This is a common condition with paralyzed or unconscious patients. The most common sites are the fingers, elbows, knees, and hip joints.

MUSCLE ATTACHMENT

Skeletal muscles are attached to bone in various ways. In some instances the connective tissue within the muscle is attached directly to the bone periosteum. Some muscular connective tissue sheaths extend to form a strong fibrous structure known as a **tendon**, which is attached to rough surfaces on a bone. Tendons are extremely strong and do not stretch. A 1-inch thick tendon reportedly will support 9 tons of weight. Because of this characteristic, a bone will sometimes fracture before the tendon attached to it will separate. The thickest and strongest tendon in the human body is the **Achilles tendon**, which attaches the **gastrocnemius** muscle in the calf of the leg to the heel bone.

A similar type of connective tissue is called a ligament, but it does not perform the same function. A ligament is a flexible, fibrous tissue that supports organs and connects bone to bone at joints. Ligaments, unlike tendons, do stretch.

Another form of muscular attachment is by **fascia**, a sheetlike, tough membrane that forms sheaths to cover and protect the muscle tissue. The term **aponeurosis** designates either a fascia or a flat tendon type of muscle attachment.

Origin or Insertion

When skeletal muscles join bones that meet at joints, one of the bones becomes the **anchor** on which the muscle has its **origin**. The bone to be moved becomes the **insertion** end for the muscle. For example, the biceps has its origin at the shoulder and its insertion on the radius. When the biceps contracts, being firmly anchored at the shoulder, it pulls upon the insertion location on the forearm, and the arm flexes (bends).

The terms origin and insertion can also apply to muscle attachments other than at joints. Essentially, the end nearest the center of the body is described as the origin, whereas the distal end is referred to as the insertion. Usually the origin is relatively immobile, whereas the insertion is into a movable structure.

SHEATHS AND BURSAE

To protect the moving parts of the muscles, muscle groups are separated from each other by membranes called *sheaths* to reduce the friction from movement. Within muscle groups, individual muscles are also separated by membranes. The tendons that extend from the muscle group are also enclosed in lubricated sheaths to protect them from damage by rubbing against other tendons, bone, or cartilage.

A sheath that is shaped like a sac and has a slippery fluid lining is known as a bursa. A bursa functions as a watery cushion to minimize pressure and friction over bony prominences and under tendons. The most common bursae are located at the elbow, knee, and shoulder.

MAJOR SKELETAL MUSCLES

The muscle most important in breathing divides the chest cavity from the abdominal cavity. This muscle is called the *diaphragm* (Figure 11-98). It is a dome-shaped muscle with tendons that attach it in the back to the spinal column, in the front to the tip of the sternum, and along the sides to the cartilage edge of the ribs. When the muscle contracts, it becomes shorter and therefore flatter, creating a vacuum that causes the lungs to draw in air. When the muscle relaxes, it returns to its dome shape and forces air out of the lungs. The diaphragm also plays a role in coughing, sneezing, or laughing. Spasmodic contractions of the diaphragm, followed by spasmodic closure of the space between the vocal cords, cause the common **hiccough**.

The orbicularis oculi and orbicularis oris are circular muscles around the eye and mouth (Figure 11-99). Their contraction enables us to squint or wink and to whistle or pucker the mouth. The **sternocleidomastoid** and the **trapezius** are the major muscles of the neck and upper back that hold the head erect and assist with its movement (Figure 11-100). The trapezius not only supports the head but extends down the back and shoulders, giving us the ability to raise and throw back the shoulders.

The **pectoralis major** is the main upper chest muscle. It extends from the sternum to the head of the humerus, enabling us to flex the arm across the chest. The **intercostal** muscles lie beneath the pectoralis major, between the ribs. These serve as accessory muscles to the diaphragm by enlarging the thoracic cavity during inspiration.

The abdomen is covered by three main muscle layers that run in different directions to make a strong wall to protect the abdominal organs. The external oblique is first, the internal oblique is beneath, and the transversus abdominis is the innermost layer. A long, narrow muscle, the rectus abdominis, extends from the pubis

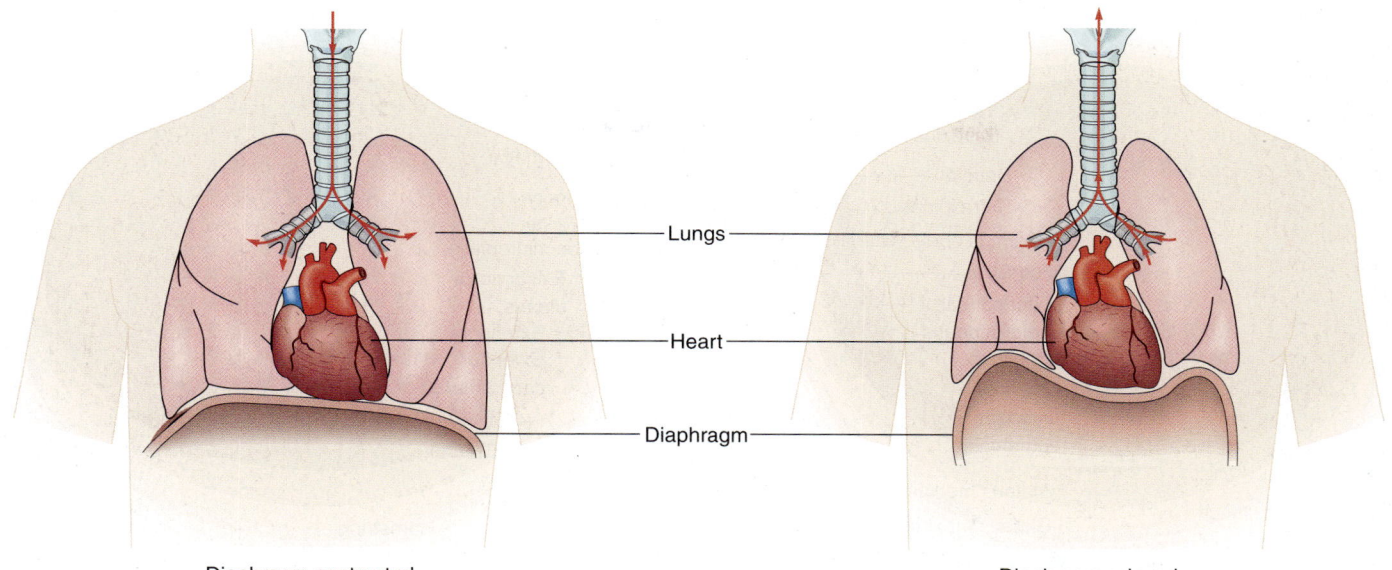

Diaphragm contracted

Diaphragm relaxed

FIGURE 11-98   The action of the diaphragm muscle

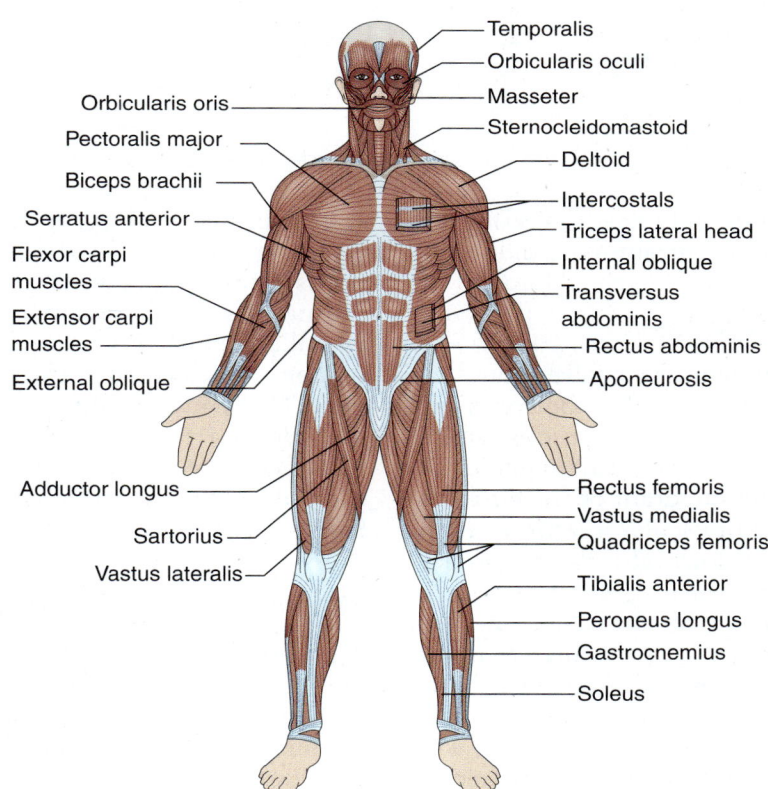

FIGURE 11-99   Principal muscles (anterior view)

to the bottom of the rib cage in the center of the abdomen. It overlies and is surrounded by connective tissue layers from the other three muscles.

The back is covered by a large muscle called the **latissimus dorsi**. Its main function is to extend and adduct the arm, as when swimming. Thick vertical groups of four different muscles overlap and extend from the occipital bone and upper cervical vertebrae to the sacrum and lower vertebrae to support and move the spinal column.

The shoulders are protected by a triangle of muscle called the **deltoid**, which abducts the arm. The deltoid,

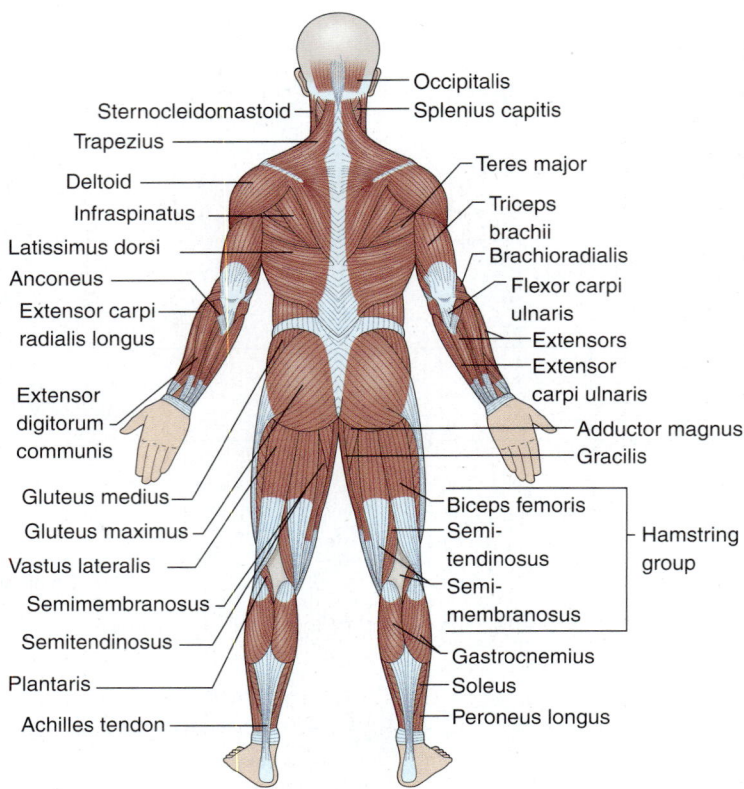

Occipitalis
Splenius capitis
Sternocleidomastoid
Trapezius
Teres major
Deltoid
Triceps
Infraspinatus
brachii
Latissimus dorsi
Brachioradialis
Anconeus
Flexor carpi
Extensor carpi
ulnaris
radialis longus
Extensors
Extensor
carpi ulnaris
Extensor
digitorum
Adductor magnus
communis
Gracilis
Gluteus medius
Biceps femoris
Gluteus maximus
Semi-
tendinosus
Hamstring
Vastus lateralis
group
Semi-
Semimembranosus
membranosus
Semitendinosus
Gastrocnemius
Plantaris
Soleus
Peroneus longus
Achilles tendon

FIGURE 11-100   Principal muscles (posterior view)

if of adequate size, may be used for small injections of medication that must be given intramuscularly.

Lower Extremity Muscles

The muscles of the lower extremities involve about half of the body's total muscle mass. The buttocks are formed by the large **gluteus maximus** muscles, which support much of the body's weight and enable us to stand erect. The upper outer quadrant of the buttocks is the site of choice for intramuscular injections, especially for large amounts of a slowly absorbing material.

The front of the thigh has the longest muscle of the body, the **sartorius**. It anchors on the iliac spine and crosses diagonally down the front of the thigh to insert on the medial surface of the tibia. The sartorius flexes the hip and knee joints to turn the thigh outward, making it possible to sit cross-legged on the floor. The **quadriceps femoris**, with four separate parts (rectus femoris, vastus lateralis, vastus medialis, and vastus intermedius), makes up the bulk of the anterior thigh musculature. It is a powerful extensor of the knee and is used when we rise from a sitting position, kick a ball, or swim.

The **tibialis anterior** is in the front of the leg. When it is flexed, it is possible to walk on your heels with the rest of the foot off the ground. It also serves to invert the foot, turning it toward the other foot.

The posterior thigh is the site of the **hamstring** group, which includes the biceps femoris, semitendinosus, semimembranosus, and a portion of the adductor magnus. Their primary function is to flex the knee by pulling on the insertion at the fibula and tibia. The tendons are easily identified by palpation behind the knee. The gastrocnemius is the main muscle in the calf of the leg. Its tendon, the Achilles, has been mentioned. Contraction of the gastrocnemius permits you to stand to tiptoe because it acts as the flexor of the plantar surface (sole) of the foot.

Muscles of Expression

A number of muscles in the face enable us to show our feelings. The frontalis (forehead) can be raised to express surprise or lowered to show a stern gaze. Raising one side of the obicularis oris about the upper lip will result in a sneer. The obicularis oris also allows us to whistle, kiss, smile, grin, grimace with pain, or pout.

The obicularis oculi around the eyes help complete the frown and enable us to squint or wink. The large muscle of the lower jaw, the masseter, in cooperation with other smaller muscles, opens and closes the mouth to express emotions of surprise and disbelief but also is powerful and is responsible for our ability to chew and grind the food we eat.

MUSCLE STRAIN AND CRAMPS

Occasionally, too much stress is applied to skeletal muscles while exercising or participating in athletic activities. This may result in a **strain**, but the muscles will recover with a period of rest. Athletes frequently "pull" their hamstring group during strenuous competition. Another frequent occurrence is a muscle cramp or spasm, caused by a muscle that has contracted but cannot relax. It can usually be relieved by stretching the muscle or causing it to bear weight.

Muscle Fatigue

Prolonged strenuous exercise can result in muscle fatigue. Muscles require large amounts of oxygen to sustain the conversion of glycogen stored in the muscle into energy (adenosine triphosphate or ATP), a function of the many mitochondria within muscle cells. Vigorous exercise is believed to cause an oxygen deficit within the muscle because the body cannot take in and circulate oxygen fast enough to keep up with the demand. When this occurs, lactic acid begins to accumulate, the glycogen is depleted, and the muscle's supply of ATP runs low. The muscle loses its ability to contract effectively and finally becomes incapable of reacting at all to the stimulus to contract. This occurs primarily in marathon runners who sometimes even collapse from muscle fatigue. Most of us simply stop our activities long before this happens.

Oxygen debt is "paid back" by the rapid and deep breathing that follows exercise. When the accumulated lactic acid is removed and the amount of oxygen is restored to once again produce ATP, the muscle can again respond to a stimulus and contract.

SMOOTH MUSCLE ACTION

Smooth, involuntary muscles can be found throughout the internal organs and structures of the body. They are controlled automatically by signals from the autonomic nervous system.

In the esophagus (the structure that connects the mouth with the stomach), the muscle tissue changes from voluntary muscles at the top that assist in swallowing, to smooth, involuntary muscles that move the food to the stomach. A two-layer muscle structure in the lower esophagus continues into the stomach and intestines. One layer of smooth muscle is circular and contracts to narrow the tube. Another layer is longitudinal and contracts to shorten the tube. The alternating action of both layers, contracting and relaxing, works the food through the body in a wavelike action called **peristalsis** (Figure 11-101). The stomach has a third layer in the muscle wall because of its need to break up and churn the food that is swallowed, which

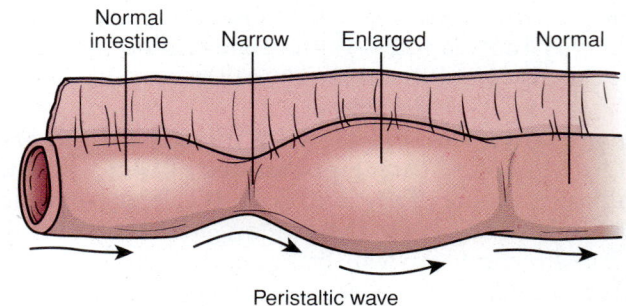

FIGURE 11-101　Peristaltic action

must be in a near-liquid state before it can be passed on to the small intestine.

Sphincters

Throughout the digestive system and inside the blood vessels of the body are smooth, donut-shaped muscle structures called **sphincters**. These pinch shut intermittently to control the flow of food, liquid, or blood. Sphincters in the digestive system are capable of remaining contracted for hours if necessary. Both ends of the stomach have sphincter muscles to hold the contents securely inside while muscular action and chemical processes digest food. When the food is in the proper state, the lower sphincter opens slightly to allow small amounts of the liquid to escape into the small intestine.

An example of smooth muscle sphincter action that can be easily observed is the pupil of the eye. When available light is decreased, the radial muscles of the iris contract to enlarge the pupil, permitting more light to enter, thereby increasing the ability to see. When light is focused on the eye, the circular sphincter muscles of the iris that surround the pupil contract, making the pupil smaller, thereby limiting the amount of light striking the retina. The physician will usually check light reflex action of the eyes in assessing the condition of the brain and autonomic nervous system.

DISEASES AND DISORDERS

Bursitis/Tendonitis (Bur-si'-tis/Ten-dun-i'-tis)

Description—**Tendonitis** is a painful inflammation of the tendon and tendon-muscle attachments to bone, usually at the shoulder, hip, heel, or hamstrings. Bursitis is an inflammation of the bursa that covers and lubricates the muscles and tendons and occurs most often at the shoulder, elbow, or knee. (See Unit 5.)

Signs and symptoms—Pain at joints or at the muscle attachment that results in limited motion.

Etiology—Tendonitis normally follows a sports-related activity that damages the muscle-tendon structure. It can also result from misaligned posture and other **musculoskeletal** disorders.

Treatment—With injury, apply ice initially for the first 12 to 24 hours. Later, applications of heat will usually aid in relief of the joint pain. If calcium deposits have formed within the tendon, it becomes weak, and the condition will be aggravated by heat. The calcium deposits are visible on x-ray to confirm the diagnosis. Application of ice packs will help relieve discomfort from calcified tendonitis.

Both conditions may be treated by resting the joint, oral doses of pain medication, and intraarticular injections of a mixture of corticosteroid and a local anesthetic. If fluid has accumulated within the area, it may require aspiration prior to the injection treatment. When pain has subsided, a physical therapy regimen may be indicated to maintain joint function and prevent muscular atrophy.

Epicondylitis (Epi-kondi-li′tis) (Tennis Elbow)

Description—This is inflammation of a forearm tendon at the attachment on the humerus at the elbow. (See Unit 5.)

Signs and symptoms—The initial elbow pain gradually worsens and often involves the forearm and the back of the hand when an object is grasped or the elbow is twisted. There is tenderness over the head of the radius and the projection of the humerus at the elbow joint.

Etiology—Epicondylitis probably begins as a partial tear of the tendon from its attachment.

Treatment—Injection of the area, as with tendonitis, is effective. Immobilization, heat therapy, and manipulation of the tendon attachment are used before resorting to surgical excision of the tendon for recurring and continual inflammation.

Fibromyalgia Syndrome (Fibro-mial′-ja)

Description—Fibromyalgia is a chronic musculoskeletal condition characterized by widespread pain. It was once called fibrositis. It affects people of all ages. It is estimated that at least 3.7 million people have the syndrome. Fibromyalgia occurs frequently in people with autoimmune and arthritis disorders.

Signs and symptoms—The prime symptom is widespread pain and the presence of tender points or trigger points at specific sites on the body (Figure 11-102). Diagnosis is considered positive when 11 of the 18 points are painful. Besides pain and muscle stiffness, patients may experience fatigue, an inability

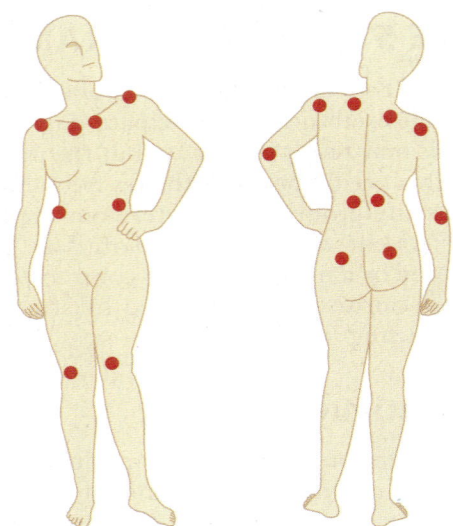

FIGURE 11-102   The tender point sites of fibromyalgia

to concentrate, sleep disturbances, dry eyes and mouth, frequent urination, irritable bowel syndrome, headaches, numbness or tingling in the arms or legs, bursitis, tendonitis, and depression. All are symptoms of an alteration in the body's sympathetic nervous system.

Etiology—The cause is unknown. There seems to be some familial tendency, but a genetic connection has not been proven. It appears to be affected by many things, such as the weather, stress, and a poor state of physical fitness. Symptoms come and go, but the syndrome persists.

Treatment—There is no cure, only methods to make it possible to cope with the symptoms. The use of biofeedback, massage, warm showers or baths, gentle aerobic exercise, and adjustments to reduce stress are helpful. Other treatments include injection of the tender points, spraying the skin with ethyl chloride and then stretching the muscles, physical therapy, ultrasound, heat and cold applications, a jacuzzi, and medication to relax muscles and relieve pain. Currently used drugs include low doses of tricyclic medications, such as Elavil and Flexeril. Other similar drugs are used that increase the level of serotonin, a neurotransmitter. When the serotonin level is low, there is an increase in depression, sensitivity to pain, and difficulty with sleeping. The best course of treatment is becoming physically fit, achieving a good body weight, and acquiring restful sleep.

Muscular Dystrophy

Description—This group of congenital disorders results in progressive wasting away of skeletal muscles. There are several types of muscular **dystrophy**.

Duchenne's Dystrophy This disorder represents about 50% of all the cases. In this genetic disease, the gene is carried by the female but affects only males; it can affect multiple members of the family. The onset is in early childhood, with death occurring after 10 to 15 years. It is usually first recognized when the child is about 1 year of age.

Signs and symptoms—Initially, the leg and pelvic muscles are affected, making all activities involving the lower extremities difficult. Children are usually confined to a wheelchair by ages 9 to 12. The disease progresses from skeletal to smooth muscles, affecting the heart and diaphragm and eventually resulting in cardiac or respiratory failure.

Etiology—Duchenne's is an X-linked chromosome disorder affecting only males.

Treatment—None available. However, orthopedic appliances, exercise, physical therapy, and surgery to correct muscle contractures can help preserve mobility.

Erb's or Juvenile Muscular Dystrophy

This type progresses slowly and occurs later in childhood or adolescence. It affects both sexes. It does not reduce life expectancy.

Signs and symptoms—Erb's main symptoms are weakness of the upper arm and pelvic muscles. Other symptoms include winging of the scapulae, lordosis with protruding abdomen, waddling gait, poor balance, and the inability to raise the arms.

Etiology and Treatment—Same as Duchenne's.

Mixed Dystrophy

Mixed dystrophy does not appear to be inherited and affects both sexes. It generally begins between ages 30 and 50. Progressive deterioration is rapid and is usually fatal within 5 years after onset.

Signs and symptoms—This type affects all voluntary muscles. A positive diagnosis can be made from a typical medical history and evaluation of voluntary muscle movements. Confirmation is possible by a biopsy of the muscle tissue, which shows characteristic deposits of fat and connective tissue.

Torticollis (Torti-kol'is) (Wryneck)

Description—This neck deformity bends the head to the affected side and rotates the chin toward the opposite side. It can be congenital or acquired.

Signs and symptoms—The obvious positioning of the head.

Etiology—Torticollis is caused by shortening or spasm of the sternocleidomastoid neck muscle. The congenital form usually follows a difficult (breech) birth and occurs mostly in firstborn females. It is thought to develop from malposition before birth, prenatal injury, or the rupture of muscle fibers with resulting scar tissue development. Acquired **torticollis** results from muscle damage by disease, a cervical spine injury, or muscle spasms.

PEDIATRIC PERSPECTIVE

Infants younger than 6 months of age with poor neck control can rupture the sternocleidomastoid muscle. The muscle heals over time. Pain relievers, such as Tylenol, can be used.

Treatment—Treatment of the congenital type consists of stretching the shortened muscle through passive exercises and positional arrangement of the head during sleeping. Surgical correction of the muscle can be accomplished if conservative methods are not effective. Acquired torticollis is treated by correcting the underlying cause whenever possible. Application of heat, cervical traction, a neck brace, exercise, psychotherapy, and massage are indicated.

ACHIEVE UNIT OBJECTIVES

- ☐ **Complete the Workbook activities to meet the learning objectives.**
- ☐ **Apply your knowledge at the end of this chapter in completing the Critical Thinking Challenge and Activities, as well as the StudyWARE on your Student CD-ROM.**

UNIT 7
THE RESPIRATORY SYSTEM

OBJECTIVES

Upon completion of this unit, you will be able to achieve the following;

LEARNING *Objectives*

1. **Spell and define, using the glossary at the back of the text, all the Words to Know in this unit.**
2. **Describe the source and importance of oxygen.**
3. **Trace the path of oxygen to an internal cell.**

4. **Describe the structure and function of the nose, pharynx, epiglottis, larynx, trachea, bronchus, bronchiole, and alveolus.**

5. **Explain how voice sounds are produced.**

6. **Differentiate between external and internal respiration.**

7. **Describe the structure and function of the pleural coverings of the lungs and chest cavity.**

8. **Describe the relationship of the diaphragm and brain to breathing.**

9. **Describe five normal occurrences that alter breathing patterns and explain why they occur.**

10. **Identify diagnostic examinations for respiratory assessment.**

11. **Explain the role of surfactant in the lungs.**

12. **Differentiate between perfusion and ventilation scans.**

13. **Describe the diseases or disorders of the respiratory tract.**

WORDS TO KNOW

allergic rhinitis	empyema	orthopnea
alveoli	epiglottis	oxygen
angiography	epistaxis	perfusion
apnea	expectorated	pharynx
arteriography	expiration	pleura
asthma	fibrosis	pleurisy
atelectasis	hemothorax	pneumonia
bleb	hiccoughs	pneumo-
bronchi	hiccup	noconiosis
bronchiole	histoplasmosis	pneumothorax
bronchitis	hypoxia	pulmonary
carbon dioxide	influenza	pulmonary
chronic	inspiration	edema
obstructive	intubation	pulmonary
pulmonary	laryngectomy	emboli
disease	laryngitis	respiratory
cilia	larynx	rhinitis
cyanosis	legionnaires'	septum
diaphoresis	disease	sinusitis
dyspnea	liter	spirometer
emphysema	lung	spontaneous

sputum	surfactant	upper respiratory
sudden infant	trachea	infection
death	tracheotomy	ventilation
syndrome	tuberculosis	vital capacity

CERTIFICATION CONNECTION

CMA
Diagnostic procedures
Common diseases and
pathology
Anatomy and physiology

CMAS
Anatomy and physiology

RMA
Anatomy and physiology

In the environment, **oxygen** (O_2) is provided continuously by plants on land and in the sea. Plants use sun, water, and **carbon dioxide** (CO_2) to make oxygen, which they release into the air. Humans breathe O_2 and exhale CO_2 and water. This cycle provides the means for supporting life.

Oxygen in the air is essential to the survival of living cells. An adult human being carries 2 quarts of O_2 in the blood, lungs, and tissues. This supply is adequate to sustain life for about 4 minutes. The respiratory system is responsible for taking in air, removing the oxygen, and sending it through the blood to the cells of the body. The oxygen concentration of inhaled air is about 21%.

The respiratory system must also take from the blood the waste product CO_2 and exhaust it from the lungs. Exhaled air still contains about 16% oxygen. When the level of CO_2 in the blood rises to a certain point, the respiratory center in the brain is triggered and a breath is taken. This function is so vital to life that its interruption for just a few minutes will result in death.

THE PATHWAY OF OXYGEN

The Nose

Air enters the body through the nose (Figure 11-103). Here the air is filtered, warmed, and moistened by the structures within the nasal cavity. The nose is divided by a wall of cartilage called the **septum**. Near the middle of the nasal cavity, on each side, are a series of three scroll-like bones called conchae or turbinates. The conchae are covered with mucus-producing epithelium, which adds moisture to the air, and are supplied with abundant blood vessels, which warm the air. Just inside the nostrils are hairs called **cilia**, which trap particles in the air so that they do not enter the lungs.

The mucus from the lining also helps trap dust and bacteria. When irritating substances come in contact with the lining, extra mucus is produced to dilute the irritant. This is why sneezing occurs and the nose "runs." Both actions are methods of removing irritants.

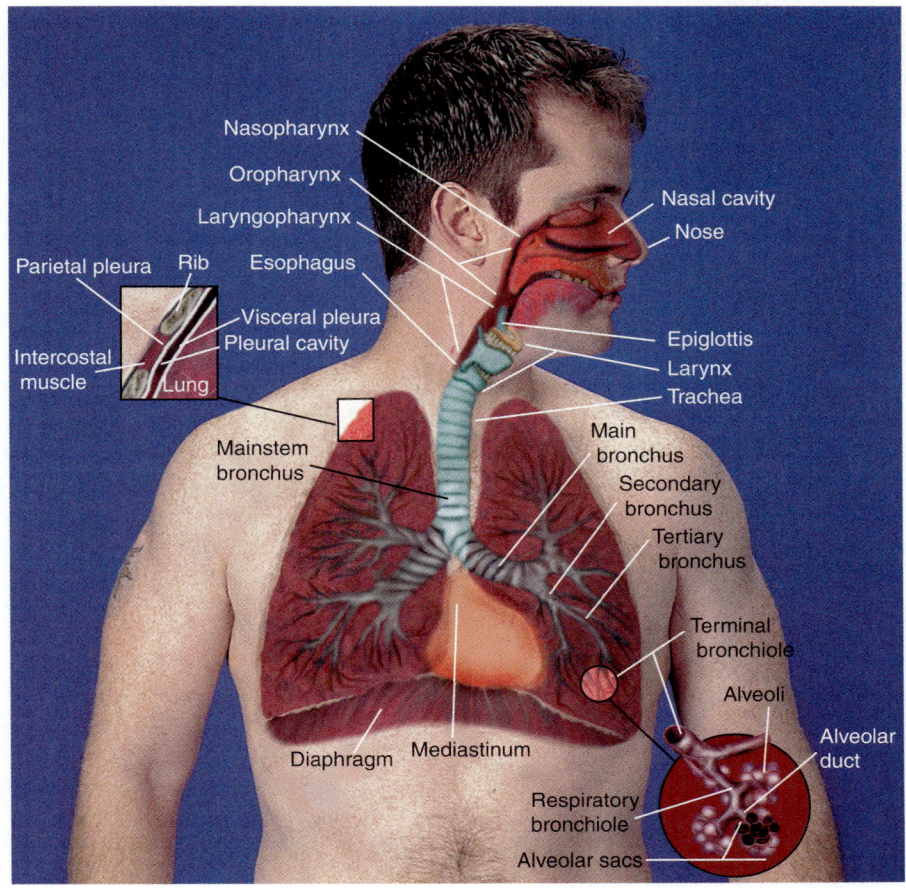

FIGURE 11-103 The respiratory system

Ciliated mucosa in the posterior portion of the nose and in the pharynx (throat) help propel inhaled particles into the back of the pharynx to be swallowed. Particles inhaled into the trachea and bronchi must first be propelled upward past the epiglottis, in an action called *mucus streaming*. The particles can then be directed toward the esophagus and swallowed. The constant beating action of the cilia and the flow of the mucus secretions cleanse the air passages. This beneficial function is temporarily halted by the effect of smoking, which paralyzes the cilia and mucus streaming action, thereby allowing foreign particles to enter the lungs. The paralysis lasts for several minutes.

The sinuses of the head are lined with the continuation of the nasal membranes (Figure 11-104). This explains why **sinusitis** occurs frequently with nasal infections.

The Pharynx, Larynx, and Epiglottis

After the air is filtered, warmed, and moistened in the nose, it enters the **pharynx**. The pharynx serves as a passageway for both air and food. Except for an occasional mistake, it is not possible to swallow food and breathe at the same time. When this does occur, the result is choking, which can be very serious.

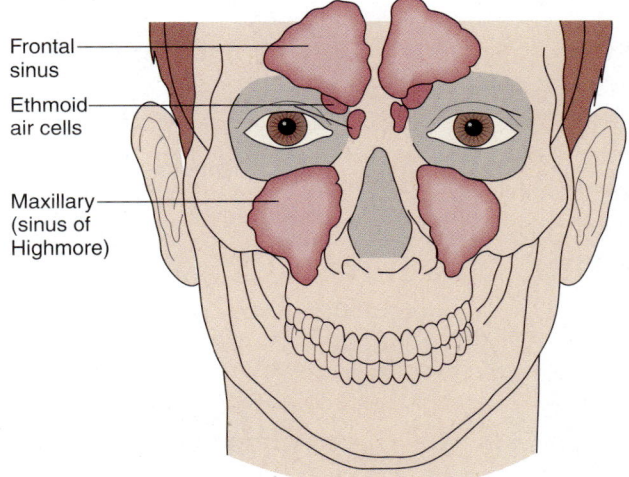

FIGURE 11-104 Paranasal sinuses (frontal view)

Normally, when food is swallowed, a cartilage "lid" called the **epiglottis** is pushed by the base of the tongue to cover the opening into the **larynx**. At the same time, the larynx moves up to help close the opening. With the opening to the larynx covered by the epiglottis, food is directed down the esophagus into the stomach.

When air passes under the open epiglottis, it enters the larynx, commonly called the voice box. The larynx is a tube with a series of nine separate cartilages to maintain its opening (Figure 11-105A). The thyroid cartilage is the largest and is located anteriorly. Its prominent projection is known as the Adam's apple, and its action can be observed when a person swallows. The larynx is lined with mucous membrane, which also forms two folds called the vocal cords. The cords are attached to the front of the larynx wall by cartilage. Muscles attach to the cartilage, and when they contract or relax, the vocal cords move either toward or away from the center of the larynx (Figure 11-105B).

During breathing, the vocal cords are near to the wall of the larynx so that air can pass freely in and out. During speaking, the vocal cords move across the larynx and are held tense by the contracting muscles. The degree of tension and the length of the cords, determine the pitch of the voice. The tighter and longer the cords the higher the pitch. The pressure on the air being expelled from the lungs determines the volume or loudness of the voice as it vibrates the vocal cords. Note that speech is most easily accomplished during the exhaling of air. Inhaling does not create sufficient air pressure, nor can it be sustained long enough to produce speech.

Part of the mucous membrane lining of the larynx is loosely attached and of a different type of epithelium. With a severe infection, it may become swollen, actually preventing respirations. In this emergency situation, an airway may be achieved by **intubation** (passing a tube through the mouth and larynx and into the trachae) or by making an external opening into the **trachea**, called a **tracheotomy**, and inserting a tube to permit air to enter.

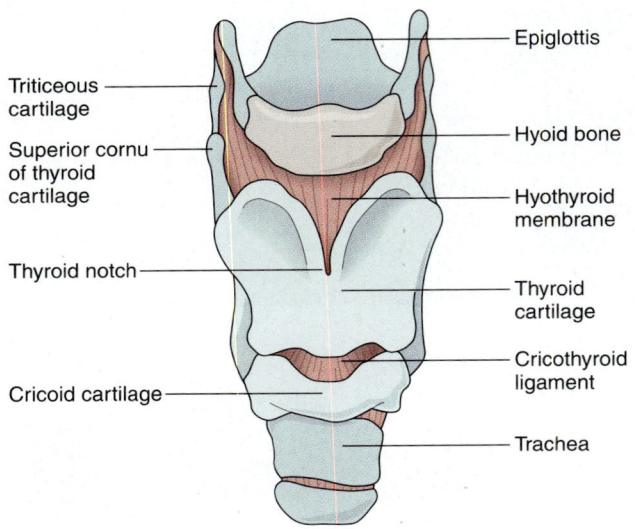

FIGURE 11-105A Larynx (anterior view)

Triticeous cartilage
Superior cornu of thyroid cartilage
Thyroid notch
Cricoid cartilage
Epiglottis
Hyoid bone
Hyothyroid membrane
Thyroid cartilage
Cricothyroid ligament
Trachea

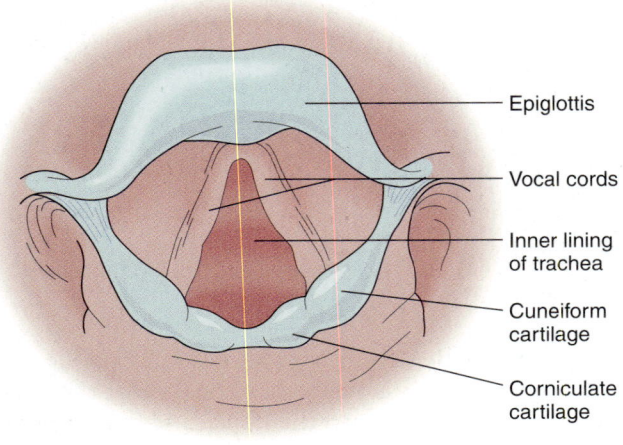

FIGURE 11-105B The vocal cords in the larynx

Epiglottis
Vocal cords
Inner lining of trachea
Cuneiform cartilage
Corniculate cartilage

The Trachea, Bronchi, and Bronchioles

The next passageway for air is the trachea (Figure 11-106). It is commonly called the windpipe and extends from the neck into the chest, directly in front of the esophagus. The trachea is held open by a series of C-shaped cartilage rings. The wall between the rings is elastic, enabling the trachea to adjust to different body positions.

About the middle of the sternum, the trachea divides into two sections called the right and left **bronchi**. The structure of the two main bronchi is similar to that of the trachea, with incomplete cartilage rings to maintain the air passageway. Each bronchus divides and subdivides into many increasingly smaller bronchi, each with the cartilage-ringed structure, until they are barely visible without a microscope. These tiny air passageways have walls of muscle cells and are called **bronchioles**.

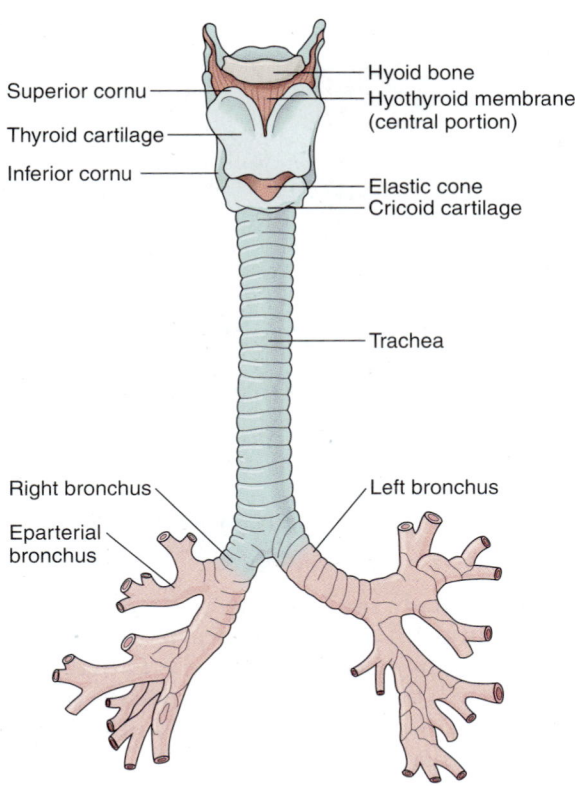

FIGURE 11-106   The larynx, trachea, and bronchi

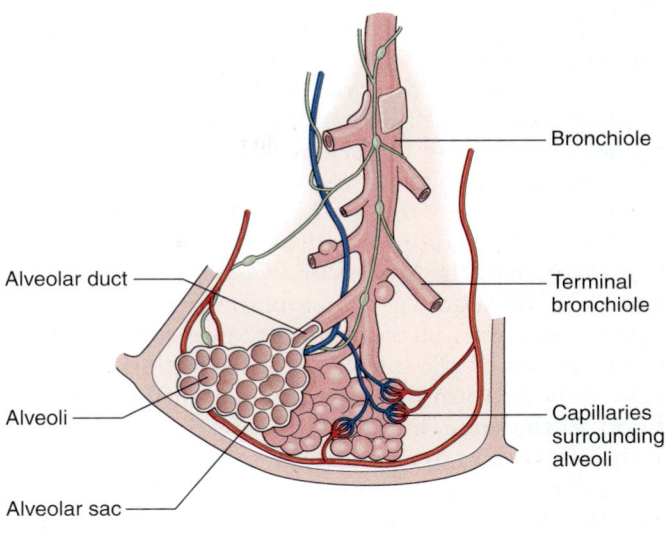

FIGURE 11-107   Alveoli

The Alveoli

Each bronchiole ends in a grapelike cluster of microscopic air sacs called **alveoli**. It is estimated that the body contains about 500 million alveoli, approximately three times the amount necessary to sustain life. The membrane walls of the alveoli are only one cell thick and are surrounded by a network of microscopic blood vessels called capillaries (Figure 11-107).

RESPIRATION

The structure of the **respiratory** apparatus has been compared with an upside-down tree, with the trunk, branches, twigs, and leaves corresponding to the trachea, bronchi, bronchioles, and alveoli.

On **inspiration**, air enters the body, eventually arriving in an alveolus. Here O_2 passes through the wall of the alveolus into the surrounding capillary as CO_2 leaves the capillary and enters the alveolus. When **expiration** occurs, CO_2 exits from the bronchial tree and is exhaled from the body. The process of getting O_2 from the nose to the alveolus and into the capillary and the return of CO_2 to the nose is known as *external respiration* (Figure 11-108A).

At the same time, oxygen from the alveolus is circulating through the body to every cell. First, the oxygen

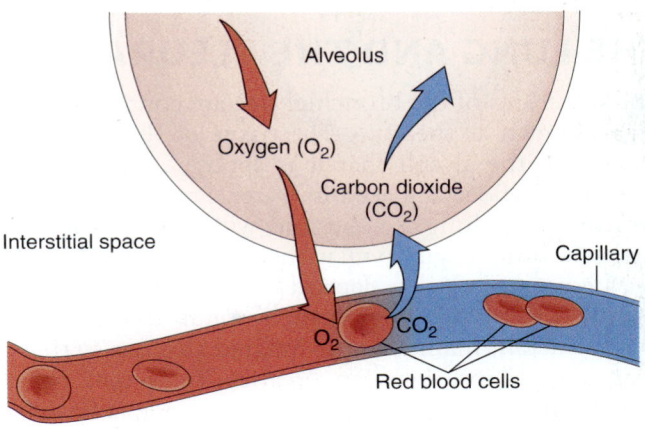

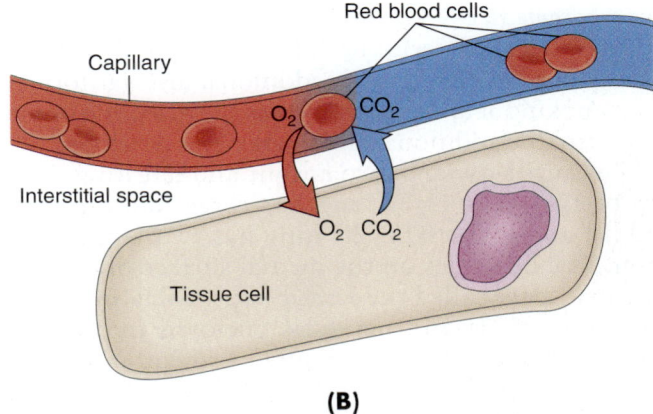

FIGURE 11-108   Simplified external and internal respiration: (A) external respiration in the lungs and (B) internal respiration at the cell

enters the capillary surrounding the alveolus, then it circulates through a venule, a vein, back to the heart, out an artery, to an arteriole, and into a capillary next to a tissue cell. Here the O_2 in the blood is given to the cell while CO_2 from the cell is picked up by the capillary. The exchange of O_2 and CO_2 at the cell is known as *internal respiration* (Figure 11-108B).

Oxygen and carbon dioxide in the alveolus and the cell exchange by the process of *diffusion*. Remember that materials move across a membrane from an area of higher concentration to an area of lower concentration. In the alveoli of the lung, O_2 concentration is greater than in the surrounding capillary, so it diffuses into the blood. At the same time, CO_2 is in higher concentration in the blood than in the alveolus, so it leaves the blood, enters the alveolus, and is exhaled during the next respiration. At the tissue cell, the O_2 content in the capillary is greater than that within the cell, so the O_2 leaves the blood and enters the cell. On the other hand, the CO_2 level within the cell is greater than in the capillary, so CO_2 diffuses out of the cell into the blood. This process of external and internal respiration is continuous throughout the life span of a person.

THE LUNG AND THE PLEURA

The structures of the bronchial tree are contained in an organ known as the **lung**. The tissue of the lung is so filled with the alveoli that it is spongy and extremely light. It will float if placed in water. Prior to birth and breathing, the lung is solid and will sink in water. At birth, the lungs begin to fill with air, inflating the alveoli. The degree of inflation depends on the presence of **surfactant**, a fatty molecule on the respiratory membrane. The surfactant maintains the inflated alveolus so that it does not collapse between breaths. Surfactant is not present in sufficient amounts to cause adequate inflation in premature infants and sometimes also in those born with other conditions. This results in *respiratory distress syndrome* (RDS) or hyaline membrane disease (described in detail later). The lungs continue to mature throughout childhood, with additional alveolar formation. Smoking at an early age retards the maturing of the lungs, and the additional alveoli are never developed.

The lung is divided into a right and left lung (Figure 11-109). The right lung has three lobes: upper, middle, and lower. The left lung has two: upper and lower. The heart lies on the medial surface of the left lung in a space called the *cardiac notch*. Each lung with its blood vessels and nerves is enclosed in a membrane called the visceral **pleura**. A membrane also lines the thoracic cavity and is called the parietal pleura. The airtight space between the pleural membranes is known as the pleural space or cavity. It contains a lubricating fluid to prevent friction as the membranes rub together during respiration. The

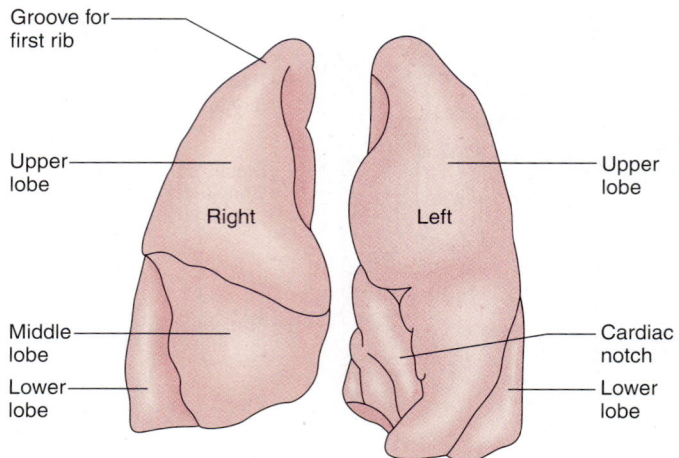

FIGURE 11-109 Anterior lung surface

"space" is virtually nonexistent in healthy lungs because the lungs fill the thoracic cavity within the rib cage, pressing the visceral against the parietal pleura. However, as will be discussed later, certain conditions and diseases cause an abnormal presence of fluid or air within the pleural space.

THE MUSCLES OF BREATHING

The action of the diaphragm and the muscles of the rib cage were discussed in Unit 6. The diaphragm is the principal breathing muscle, and when it contracts, it produces a vacuum within the thoracic cavity, causing air to be drawn in. When this begins, there is a negative pressure within the lungs; the pressure inside is less than the atmospheric pressure outside. When the inside pressure exceeds outside atmospheric pressure, it becomes positive and causes expiration to again equalize inside and outside pressure. When the diaphragm returns to its relaxed state, air is forced out of the lungs (Figure 11-110).

Breathing action is controlled by the respiratory center in the brain. An increase of CO_2 or a lack of O_2 in the blood will trigger the center. Because we can somewhat voluntarily control breathing, it is possible to force rapid respirations, temporarily interrupting breathing and possibly losing consciousness. Children will occasionally hold their breath to frighten their parents and receive concessions. Usually, there is no need to be overly concerned, because sooner or later a breath has to be taken. If consciousness is lost, the automatic system resumes control, and breathing returns to normal.

Other situations can alter a breathing pattern for perfectly normal reasons, such as:

● Coughing—When a deep breath is taken followed by a forceful exhalation from the mouth to clear something from the lower respiratory structures.

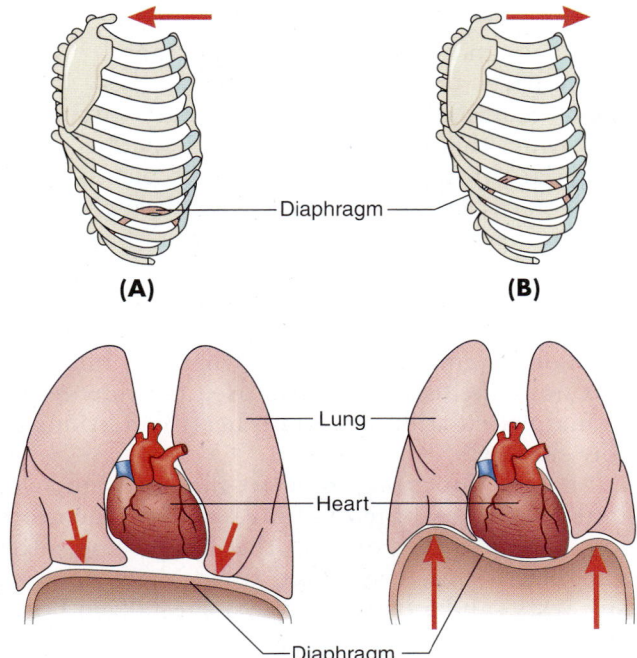

FIGURE 11-110 Position of diaphragm and ribs during (A) inspiration and (B) expiration

- **Hiccoughs** (also spelled **hiccups**)—Caused by a spasm of the diaphragm and a spasmodic closure of the glottis (space between the vocal cords). It is believed to be the result of an irritation to the diaphragm or the phrenic nerve, which innervates the diaphragm.
- Sneezing—Occurs like a cough except air is forced through the nose to clear the upper respiratory structures. Usually results from mucous membrane contact with an irritant.
- Yawning—A deep prolonged breath that fills the lungs.
- Crying (or laughing)—Alters the breathing pattern in response to emotions.

DIAGNOSTIC EXAMINATIONS

- Arterial blood gases—Blood taken directly from an artery to evaluate the exchange of O_2 and CO_2 in the lungs. The test measures the partial pressures of both gases and determines the pH of the blood. The PaO_2 (partial pressure of oxygen) indicates how much oxygen the lungs are delivering to the blood. The $PaCO_2$ (partial pressure of carbon dioxide) indicates how efficiently the lungs eliminate carbon dioxide. The pH determines the acid–base level, which indicates the hydrogen (H^+) ion content. If acidic, there is excess hydrogen ion; alkalinity indicates a deficit. Results aid in the medical management of many disorders and conditions, such as CNS depression from drugs or injury, pneumonia,

chronic obstructive pulmonary disease (COPD), respiratory distress, certain kidney diseases, and many others.
- Bronchoscopy—The insertion of an instrument called the bronchoscope into the trachea and bronchial tree to view the airways, obtain a secretion or tissue sample, or remove a foreign body.
- Chest CT scan—A very sensitive computer-generated image that gives much more detail of the lungs and other structures in the chest than a chest x-ray. The scan is done with an electron beam tomography scanner (Figure 11-111A). The examination is four times more sensitive in detecting lung cancer than conventional x-rays. It can be used as a screening examination to identify disease long before symptoms occur. Unfortunately, about 85% of lung cancer is discovered after it has begun to spread. The high-speed scan takes only a few seconds and does not require removal of clothing. Figure 11-111B is a photo of a lung scan showing a nodule in the left upper lobe.
- CT scan of pulmonary arteries—A scan used to rule out pulmonary embolus. High-resolution CT scan (HRCT) is used to evaluate lung tissue in greater detail than a standard CT scan. This is useful in evaluating pulmonary fibrosis.
- CT-guided needle biopsy—Done by a trained radiologist. Using the CT scan as a guide, the radiologist inserts a needle into the chest cavity to biopsy a lung mass.

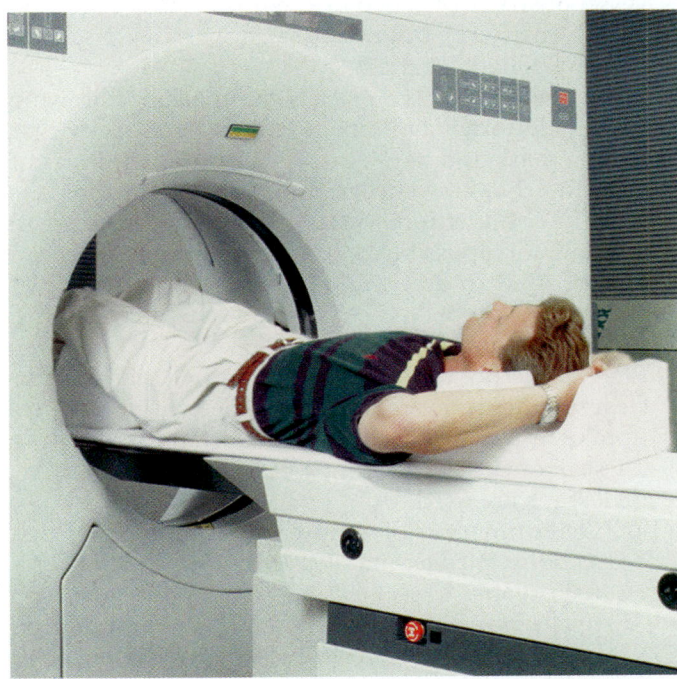

FIGURE 11-111A High-speed CT scanner *(Courtesy of CAT SCAN 2000)*

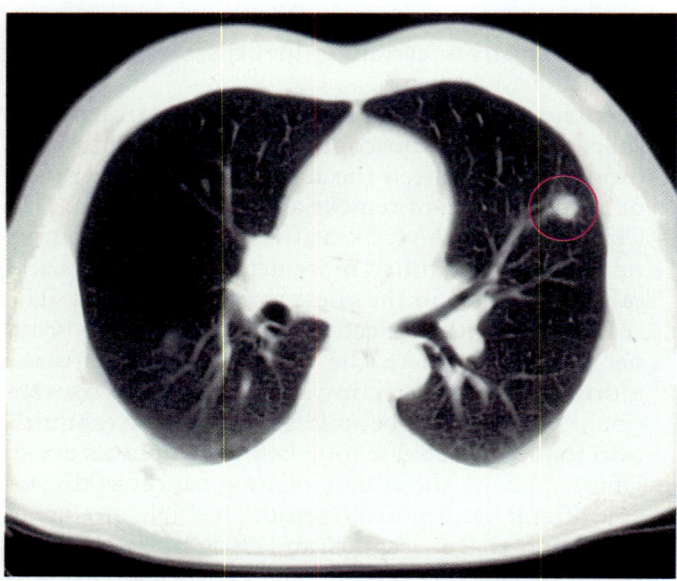

FIGURE 11-111B Lung scan showing a nodule in the left upper lobe. *(Courtesy of CAT SCAN 2000)*

- Chest x-ray—A radiologic examination to determine the general health of lung and surrounding tissues or to identify a disease process, such as pneumonia.
- Lung **perfusion** scan—An examination of the lung following intravenous (IV) injection of a radioactive contrast medium to provide a visual image of pulmonary blood flow. It is useful in diagnosing blood vessel obstruction, such as **pulmonary emboli** (blood clot in an artery), but not as sensitive as a CT scan of the pulmonary arteries.
- Lung **ventilation** scan—An examination following the inhalation of a mixture of air and radioactive gas from a mask and bag. The test indicates the areas of the lung that are ventilated during respiration. It is used in conjunction with a lung perfusion scan to evaluate for a possible pulmonary embolus. This can also be used to determine the amount each lobe of the lung is perfusing, for example, before performing a lobectomy.
- PET (positron emission tomography) scan—A nuclear medicine examination to determine cellular uptake in parts of the body. It is often fused with a CT scan of the chest. From a pulmonary perspective, PET scans are used for:
  1. Determination of lung cancer metastasis, such as bone, mediastinal lymph nodes, and abdominal organs
  2. Evaluation of a solitary pulmonary nodule that is greater than 1 cm in patients that are a high risk for biopsy
  3. Early detection of recurrent cancer. Areas of the body that are positive for uptake of the injected

material are consistent with a potential malignancy and warrant further evaluation.
- Pulmonary **angiography/arteriography**—A radiologic examination of the pulmonary circulation following the injection of a radiopaque iodine material through a catheter that is placed in the pulmonary artery or one of its branches. The catheter is inserted into a vein at the inner surface of the elbow or in the groin and passed through the veins and through the first half of the heart into the pulmonary artery. The test aids in diagnosing pulmonary emboli, especially when the lung scan was not conclusive. It is also used to evaluate pulmonary circulation in certain heart conditions before surgery.
- **Pulmonary** function tests—To measure lung volume in a normal breath, lung capacity when forcing air into and out of the lungs, and other variables within a specified time. Many noninvasive tests can be performed in a specialized hospital pulmonary laboratory; however, the most common test and one that is appropriate to the physician's office uses a **spirometer** to measure ventilation function. Spirometry is used to evaluate a patient's **vital capacity**, or the amount of air available in the lungs for respiration. It is also used to evaluate how quickly a patient can get air out of the chest and thus is useful to test for airflow obstruction. Spirometry is most often used to assist with the diagnosis of asthma or COPD. (See Chapter 14 for additional information.)
- Pulse oximeter—The pulse oximeter is a small electronic device that fits over the end of the index finger and is connected by a wire to a machine. The device determines the amount of oxygen in the blood and displays it digitally in the window of the machine. Frequently, postoperative patients and patients with cardiac and respiratory conditions are monitored for oxygen content. If the pulse oximeter indicates the oxygen level is too low, oxygen will be administered at a proper amount to supplement that being circulated by the body.
- **Sputum** analysis—A laboratory examination of material coughed up from the bronchial tree or trachea. If properly prepared, it can aid in the diagnosis of infectious organisms or cancer cells.
- Thoracentesis—Withdrawing of fluid from the pleural space by needle aspiration following local anesthetic (Figure 11-112). Fluid may be present as a result of excessive production or inadequate reabsorption of the pleural fluid that may be associated with cancer, tuberculosis, heart failure, trauma, or a blood or lymphatic disorder. A specimen is often withdrawn for analysis to determine the presence of organisms, malignant cells, blood, or lymph fluid properties.

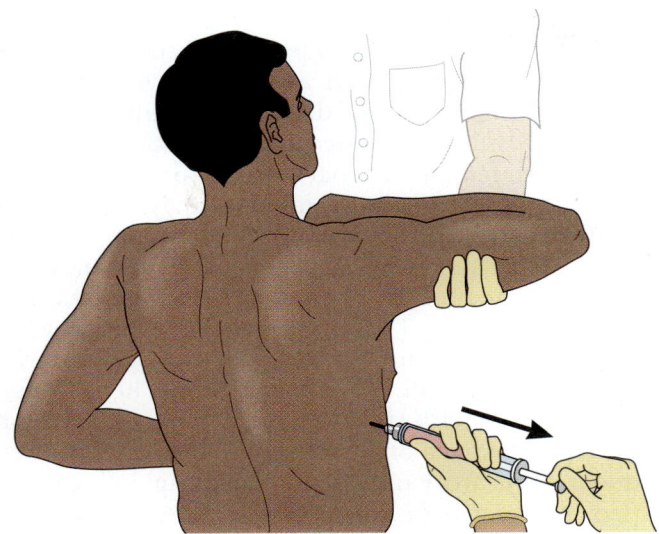

FIGURE 11-112   Thorocentesis. Fluid is being removed from the pleural cavity.

DISEASES AND DISORDERS

Allergic Rhinitis (Ri-ni'-tis)

Description—A reaction of the eyes, nose, and sinuses to airborne allergens.

Signs and symptoms—Sneezing, profuse watery nasal discharge, itching of the eyes and nose, red and swollen eyelids, and nasal congestion.

Etiology—**Allergic rhinitis** may be seasonal, as with hay fever, or perennial, caused by dust, mold, cigarette smoke, and animal mites.

Treatment—Treatment consists primarily of administering antihistamines, topical nasal steroids, and decongestants and avoiding the allergens. The use of air-conditioning filters allergens, keeps down dust, and removes excess moisture from the air. The use of steroid nasal sprays to reduce inflammation may also be helpful. Desensitizing injections of the allergens before or during the season may be indicated for long-term management. In severe or persistent cases, it may be necessary to relocate to a relatively pollen-free environment.

Asthma (Az'-ma)

Description—**Asthma** is a chronic disorder characterized by swelling, inflammation, and constriction of the bronchi and bronchioles.

Signs and symptoms—Wheezing, coughing, and shortness of breath are the most common symptoms. With a severe attack, there can be significant bronchospasm (narrowing of the bronchioles) and mucous production, markedly limiting airflow. This can result in respiratory distress, causing anxiety and a feeling of suffocation. Following an acute episode, accumulated mucus is coughed up and **expectorated**.

Etiology—Asthma is commonly caused by an allergic reaction to allergens, such as pollen, dust, animal hair, certain foods, and a number of other substances. However, it can also result from nonspecific irritants to the airway, such as cigarette smoke and other unknown causes. It can develop at any age.

Treatment—Determination of the offending allergens can sometimes be accomplished with a series of skin tests. Minute amounts of the most common causative agents are introduced just below the skin by a needle prick or applied as patches to the skin surface. The presence of a reddened area around a site after a specified time is evidence of sensitivity. (See Chapter 16, Unit 1.)

The treatment of choice for allergic asthma is prevention by eliminating allergens. Drugs to prevent or control attacks, such as inhaled steroids, long-acting bronchiodilators, and leuketriene modifiers block asthma response to allergen and exercise triggers. Other drugs are used to provide quick relief of an episode. The bronchodilating drugs albuterol and ipratropium open airways almost instantly and are considered rescue medications. The goals of asthma treatment are to prevent or reduce symptoms, maintain normal activity levels, and prevent flare-ups of asthma. During severe attacks, O_2 may be administered at approximately 2 **liters** per minute to ease breathing and increase O_2 within the arteries. In addition, an albuterol nebulizer treatment and an oral, IM, or IV steroid burst may be required.

Atelectasis (Ate-lek'ta-sis)

Description—This is the lack of air in the lungs caused by the collapse of the microscopic structures of the lung; **atelectasis** may occur following abdominal or thoracic surgery or with pressure from pleural effusion (fluid, air, pus, blood, or lymph) in the pleural cavity.

Signs and symptoms—Symptoms vary with the cause of collapse and the degree of hypoxia. There is generally some **dyspnea**. With extensive collapse there is severe dyspnea, anxiety, **cyanosis, diaphoresis** (profuse perspiration), tachycardia (rapid pulse), and retraction of intercostal muscles.

Etiology—It can be chronic, caused by mucous plugs in the bronchial tree in patients with cystic **fibrosis** and in heavy smokers with obstructive pulmonary disease. Bronchial occlusion can also result from cancer or inflamed tissues. Acute (sudden) atelectasis may occur with any condition that causes pain on deep breathing, such as rib fractures, traumatic injury, surgical procedures, or pleurisy.

Treatment—Treatment includes chest percussion, postural drainage, frequent coughing, and deep breathing exercises or intermittent positive pressure breathing (IPPB).

Bronchitis (Brong-ki'tis)

Description—**Bronchitis** can be an acute or chronic disease with inflammation of the bronchial walls with distortion and narrowing of the airways. Chronic bronchitis is a condition in which excessive mucus is secreted in the bronchi during several months a year for several years in a row. The typical patient is middle-aged or older, often with a long history of cigarette smoking. Acute bronchitis is associated with an infection. It occurs abruptly and lasts several days or weeks.

Signs and symptoms—The presence of a cough that produces yellowish-gray or green mucus is one of the main symptoms of acute bronchitis. Other symptoms may include those common with upper respiratory disease such as sore throat, slight fever, soreness or feeling of constriction in the chest, and general malaise. Chronic bronchitis sufferers also produce thick mucus with a constant "smoker's cough," have recurring respiratory infections, and may have weakness and weight loss. Wheezing and prolonged expiration time may be observed.

Etiology—Acute bronchitis is caused by a viral or bacterial respiratory infection. You can also develop bronchitis from exposure to your own or someone else's cigarette smoke and even pollutants such as household cleaners and smog. Bronchitis can also occur when acids from the stomach consistently back up into the esophagus, a condition known as gastroesophageal reflux disease (GERD, see Unit 10), which causes a reflex mechanism. Chronic bronchitis is caused by damaged cilia, enlarged mucous glands, and chronic inflammation. The severity of chronic bronchitis is related to the amount and duration of smoking.

Treatment—Acute bronchitis is managed with expectorants to help remove excessive mucus and by avoiding smoking. Antibiotics are sometimes needed if bacterial infection is suspected. Chronic bronchitis requires bronchodilators, respiratory therapy to loosen mucous secretions, smoking cessation, and corticosteroids in some cases. Adequate fluid intake is important.

Chronic Obstructive Pulmonary Disease (COPD)

Description—This is a condition characterized by chronic obstruction of the airways. COPD is an umbrella term that includes conditions such as emphysema, chronic bronchitis, and asthma. It is a progressive disease. Symptoms occur gradually and become worse with age. COPD is the most common chronic lung disease, affecting an estimated 17 million Americans. It affects males more often than females, probably because until recently men were more likely to smoke heavily. COPD is a leading cause of death in both men and women; however, there has been a significant increase recently in the number of women with the disease.

Signs and symptoms—The first signs are a decline in the ability to exercise or do strenuous work. A productive cough will begin to develop. These symptoms worsen with time, and eventually the patient develops dyspnea on minimal exertion and has frequent respiratory infections, wheezing, hypoxemia (lack of oxygen in the blood), and grossly abnormal pulmonary function studies. Difficulty with breathing makes eating difficult, so weight loss and lack of appetite is common. With advanced disease, the patient must work so hard to breathe that they may consume up to 20% of their resting energy. Thoracic deformities develop (usually a barrel chest from muscular changes caused by struggling to breathe). Eventually there is overwhelming disability, severe respiratory failure, and death.

Etiology—The primary cause of COPD (80% to 90%) is long-term cigarette smoking, which impairs the ciliary action, causes inflammation in airways, destroys alveolar walls, and results in the formation of scar tissue around the bronchioles. COPD is the result of emphysema, chronic bronchitis, asthma, or any combination of these disorders. It can also develop from chronic respiratory infections and allergies.

Treatment—Treatment consists of methods to halt the progression of the disease and control symptoms. Prime emphasis is placed on stopping smoking and avoiding other respiratory irritants. The main focus of treatment involves the use of bronchodilators, prompt treatment of respiratory infections, effective breathing and coughing instructions, proper diet, the use of O_2 as indicated, and exercise rehabilitation programs. Lung volume reduction surgery and lung transplant are options for a select group of patients. The woman in Figure 11-113 began having significant respiratory problems about 5 years ago, experiencing severe acute episodes of asthma. Her condition became chronic and is now considered COPD. She requires the use of oxygen continuously. While at home she uses a machine that concentrates oxygen from the room, but when she leaves, she must use a portable tank to provide her with supplemental oxygen.

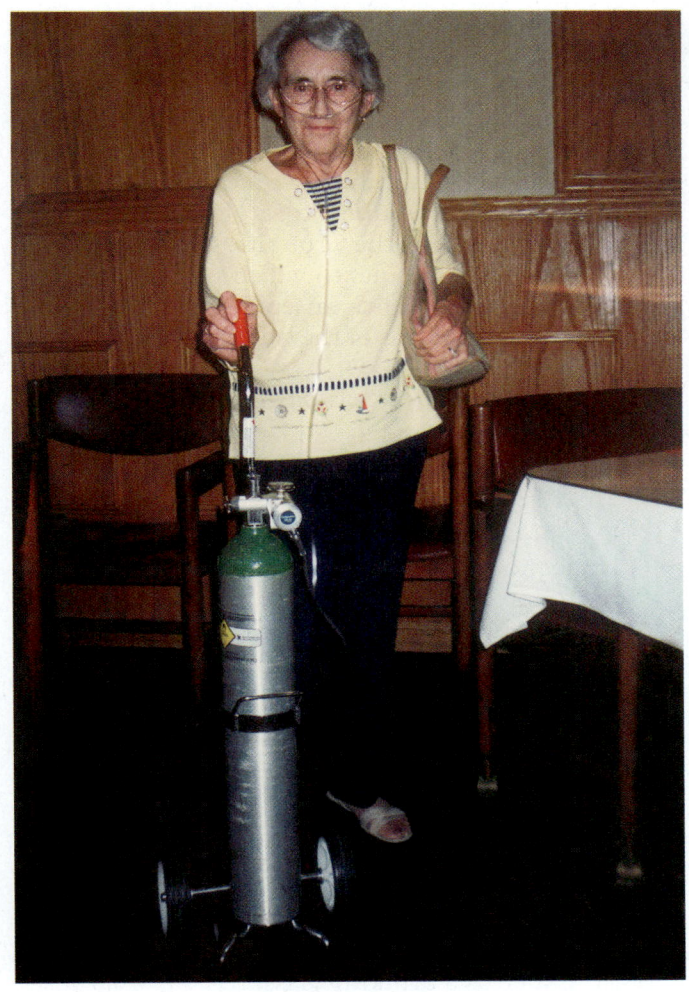

FIGURE 11-113   Individuals with COPD often need a portable oxygen tank to assist with breathing, allowing them to leave home.

Emphysema (Em-fi-se-ma)

Description—This is the irreversible enlargement of the air spaces in the lungs caused by the destruction of the alveolar walls. **Emphysema** results in the inability to exchange O_2 and CO_2 in the affected areas and to exhale stale air from the lungs. The lungs may actually be enlarged, but at the same time they are not efficient because of the decreased surface area for exchanging oxygen and carbon dioxide. Figure 11-114 is a photo of a CT scan showing the **blebs** (bubbles) of destroyed alveoli around the outer lung areas of a patient with emphysema. These are visible as large white-edged black areas.

Signs and symptoms—Emphysema is characterized by a chronic cough, weight loss, fatigue, barrel chest, the use of accessory muscles to breathe, pursed lips, cyanosis, and eventually respiratory failure, heart enlargement and failure, and death.

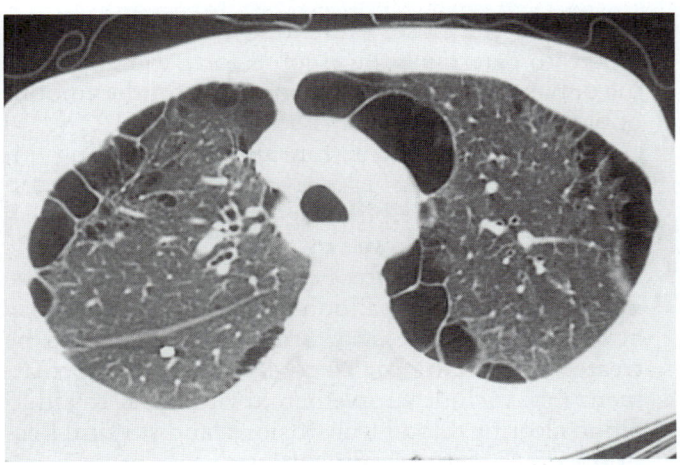

FIGURE 11-114   CT scan showing the large blebs (bubbles) of emphysema. They are identifiable as the large dark areas with white borders on the outer edges of the lungs. *(Courtesy of Philip T. Diaz, MD, pulmonologist)*

Etiology—The prime cause is cigarette smoking. Emphysema can also develop from chronic infection or irritation from environmental factors.

Treatment—The treatment is the same as for COPD: smoking cessation, the use of bronchodilators, prompt treatment of respiratory infections, effective breathing and coughing instructions, proper diet, and the use of O_2 as indicated.

Epistaxis (Epi-stak'-sis) (Nosebleed)

Description— Epistaxis is the loss of blood through the nose. (See Unit 3.)

Signs and symptoms—The visible presence of blood coming from the nose or the patient experiencing bleeding posteriorly into the throat.

Etiology—Nosebleeds usually follow injury, either external or internal, such as a blow to the nose, nosepicking, or foreign body insertion. Less frequent causes of **epistaxis** are chronic conditions, such as nasal or sinus infection that results in capillary congestion and bleeding, or the inhalation of irritating substances. Predisposing systemic factors include high blood pressure; anticoagulation drugs; chronic aspirin use; and blood diseases, such as anemia, hemophilia, and leukemia.

Treatment—Treatment varies depending on the cause, location, and severity. Even moderate bleeding is of concern if it persists longer than 20 minutes after pressure is applied. Symptoms of severe blood loss may include lightheadedness, a drop in blood pressure, rapid pulse, dyspnea, pallor, and other indications of shock. Initial first aid treatment may consist of elevating the head, compressing the nostrils against the septum continuously for 5 to 10 minutes, applying ice or cold compresses to the nose, preventing the swallowing of blood (to determine the amount lost), avoiding talking or blowing the nose, and observing for the amount of blood loss and signs of shock.

Advanced treatment for anterior bleeding includes applying an epinephrine-saturated cotton ball or gauze to the bleeding site and the use of external pressure, followed by cauterization by electric cautery or silver nitrate. For posterior bleeding, the insertion of a nasal balloon for 48 to 72 hours may be required. If necessary, anterior bleeding can be treated by packing for 24 to 48 hours. Other treatment may include supplemental vitamin K to aid in blood clotting, blood transfusions, and surgical ligation (tying) of the bleeding artery.

Histoplasmosis (His-to-plaz-mo'-sis)

Description—This is a fungal infection that occurs worldwide. In the United States, histoplasmosis occurs in three forms: primary acute, progressive disseminated, and chronic pulmonary.

Signs and symptoms—Symptoms vary with the form contracted. The primary acute form resembles a severe cold. The progressive form involves the liver, spleen, and lymph glands, and it may cause inflammation of the heart muscle, the pericardium (covering membrane), and the meninges of the brain and spinal cord. The chronic form resembles tuberculosis, causing a productive cough, dyspnea, weakness, hemoptysis (spitting up blood), fever, and cyanosis.

Etiology—**Histoplasmosis** is caused by an organism found in droppings from birds or bats, or in soil near their roosts, as in barns, caves, chicken coops, around buildings, and under bridges. It may also come from cat feces because of ingested birds.

Treatment—The acute form generally does not require treatment. With the progressive disseminated or chronic pulmonary forms, a high dose or long-term treatment with an antifungal such as amphotericin B or itroconozole is indicated. Surgery to remove pulmonary nodules and a shunt to relieve intracranial pressure may be necessary. Oxygen can be given to reduce respiratory distress. Additional treatments are indicated if other severe conditions develop.

Hyaline Membrane Disease (HMD) (Hi'-a-lin)

(See Respiratory Distress Syndrome.)

Influenza (In-flu-en'-za) (Flu)

Description—This acute, highly contagious respiratory infection usually occurs in colder months and in infrequent epidemics (widespread incidence, not of local origin). It is more prevalent in school children aged 6 to 14 and adults over age 40. **Influenza** can be fatal to the elderly or people with chronic heart, lung, or kidney disease. Influenza viruses have the ability to alter their influence on the population. As people develop immunity to a virus after coming into contact with it, the virus alters its composition and a new strain results to which people have little or no resistance. Hence an epidemic or pandemic (present in many areas of the world at the same time) can develop.

Influenza viruses are classified into three types:

- Type A—The most lethal, occurring every 2 to 3 years, with a major new strain developing every 10 to 15 years
- Type B—Occurring every 4 to 6 years, resulting in epidemics (types A and B combined are responsible for 50% of viral pneumonia cases.)
- Type C—Endemic (of local origin) and causing infrequent cases

Signs and symptoms—Symptoms of flu are the sudden onset of chills and a fever of 101° to 104°F (38° to 40°C), headaches, muscle aches, a nonproductive cough, and **rhinitis**. Pneumonia is the most common complication, developing 3 to 5 days after infection begins.

Etiology—The disease is directly transmitted by droplets inhaled from an infected person's sneezing or coughing or by indirect contact with contaminated objects, such as a drinking glass.

Treatment—Treatment consists of bed rest, adequate fluid intake, and aspirin or similar medication to relieve the pain and fever. Antibiotics have no effect on the virus and should not be used unless there is secondary bacterial infection. Flu immunizations, which provide protection for 3 to 6 months, are recommended for the high-risk population. However, the vaccine is only 75% effective. At the time of this writing, avian influenza (bird flu) is of concern to public health officials and the World Health Organization. Avian influenza is an infection caused by a flu virus that occurs naturally in birds. Wild birds carry the viruses in their intestines but normally are not affected by it. Infected birds shed the viruses in feces, nasal drainage, and saliva. Other birds become infected by coming into contact with the secretions; infected fowl; or contaminated surfaces, feed, or water. It is very contagious among birds and can infect *domestic* birds, chickens, ducks, and turkeys, causing a mortality rate of 90% to 100%, often within 48 hours.

One type of bird flu is caused by the avian influenza A (H5N1) virus, which can cause infection in birds and humans. There are many different subtypes of type A viruses; to date 16 HA types and 9 NA subtypes have been identified, and all can be found in birds. Infection from these viruses can occur in humans, but the risk is low. There have been confirmed cases of humans being affected by subtypes of the virus since 1997. Most cases resulted from direct contact with infected poultry or surfaces contaminated by birds. Avian flu spread from one person to another is very rare, and transmission has not occurred beyond one person.

All influenza viruses are capable of change, and the H5N1 virus is believed to have genetic parts that came originally from birds. Influenza A viruses are constantly changing and may over time adapt to infect and spread among humans. If this should happen, a pandemic may occur. Symptoms of avian flu in humans are like typical human flu: fever, cough, sore throat, and muscle aches. In addition, eye infections, pneumonia, severe respiratory diseases, and other life-threatening complications may occur depending upon which virus causes the infection. Because these viruses are not common among humans, there has been no build up of immunity in the population.

Worldwide attention has focused on this new disease. To date all cases have occurred in Asia, Africa, the Pacific, Europe, and the near East. Since first reported in 2003 there have been 228 confirmed cases with 130 deaths. The World Health Organization has responded immediately to any new case, and the spread has been contained. There is a ban on all poultry and eggs from any country having any disease. Research studies began in April 2005, and clinical trials are under way to develop a vaccine to protect humans. There are current antiviral medications that are thought to be effective against the virus, but studies have not been completed. For up-to-date information, go to www.cdc.gov/flu/avian/gen-info/facts.htm.

Laryngectomy (Larin-jek′to-me)

This is not a disease or disorder but a surgical solution to a life-threatening situation. It is the surgical removal of the larynx and is usually performed to treat throat cancer caused by smoking. The earliest symptom of internal disease of the larynx is persistent hoarseness. With involvement externally, it is a lump in the throat or pain, or burning when drinking hot liquids or citrus juices.

Diagnosis can often be made by viewing the larynx with a laryngoscope. This examination is often followed with radiological studies to confirm the diagnosis. With positive diagnosis, the larynx may be partially or totally removed. With total removal, a permanent opening called a stoma is made in the neck through which air can be taken in and exhaled (Figure 11-115). Coughing results in material being expelled through the stoma.

A great deal of patient support is necessary to assist in developing alternative methods of communication prior to surgery. The patient may need psychiatric assistance to cope with the loss of speech, sense of smell, ability to blow the nose, and related problems. Much support can be obtained from organizations established to aid in rehabilitation of **laryngectomy** patients. Local chapters of the "Lost Chord Club," made up of persons who have lost their larynx, volunteer their services to speak with new patients and help them learn techniques of producing speech. The American Cancer Society and the International Association of Laryngectomies also provide assistance with speech methods that use esophageal air that is swallowed and released slowly, the artificial larynx, and other mechanical devices.

The individual in Figure 11-115A has a Blum finger voice prosthesis inserted into the stoma (Figure 11-115B shows an inserter). By placing his finger over the opening in the prosthesis, he is able to produce a good quality of speech. A "patch" of thin foam is worn over the opening to prevent inhaling foreign materials. The foam is porous and permits easy exchange of air.

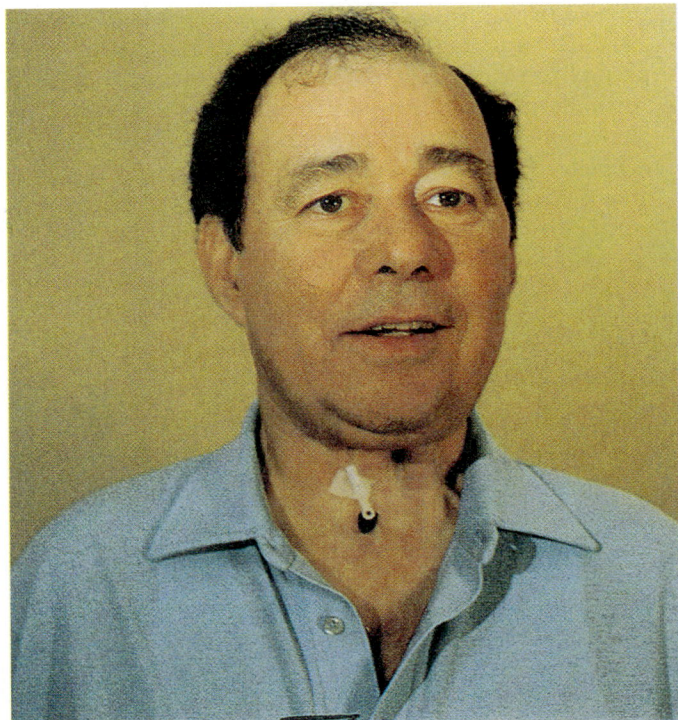

FIGURE 11-115A Laryngeal stoma following laryngectomy with an inserted Blum finger prosthesis

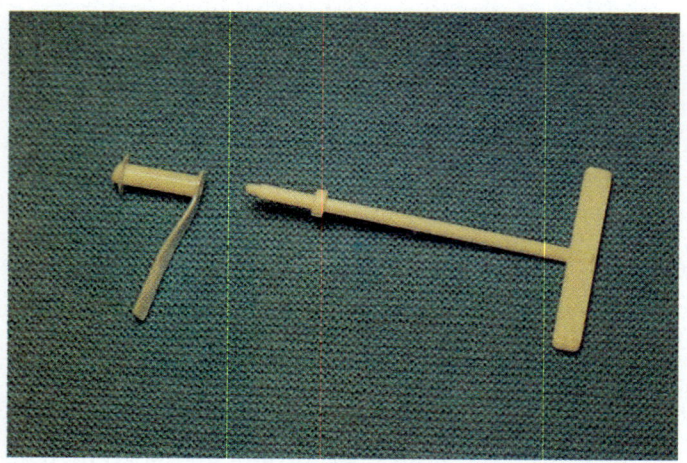

FIGURE 11-115B An inserter

Laryngitis (Lar-in-ji'-tis)

Description—This inflammation of the vocal cords occurs in both acute and chronic forms.

Signs and symptoms—Acute **laryngitis** usually begins as hoarseness, with either minimal or complete loss of voice. There may be some pain when talking or swallowing, a dry cough, fever, and malaise. With chronic laryngitis, the only symptom is persistent hoarseness.

Etiology—Acute laryngitis usually results from an infectious process, excessive use of the voice, inhalation of smoke or fumes, or accidental aspiration of chemicals. Chronic laryngitis develops from other preexistent chronic conditions (such as sinusitis, bronchitis, and allergies) or from smoking, abuse of alcohol, or continual exposure to irritants.

Treatment—Laryngitis is treated by resting the voice, using medication for underlying infection, if present, and eliminating coexistent causes (in the case of chronic laryngitis).

Legionnaires' Disease (Le'-jun-airs)

Description—This is an acute bronchopneumonia that derived its name from a highly publicized incident in which 182 people developed the disease at an American Legion Convention in Philadelphia in 1976. **Legionnaires' disease** usually occurs in late summer or early fall.

Signs and symptoms—Symptoms are nonspecific and include diarrhea, lack of appetite, headache, chills, weakness, and an unremitting fever that develops within 12 to 48 hours. Temperature may reach 105°F (40.5°C). A cough then develops, which becomes productive, with grayish sputum. Other symptoms are nausea, vomiting, confusion, dyspnea, and chest pain. Severe symptoms are evidence of complications and include low blood pressure, irreg-

ular heartbeat, respiratory failure, kidney failure, and shock (which is usually fatal). Smokers are three to four times more likely to develop legionnaires' disease than nonsmokers.

Etiology—It is caused by the bacteria *Legionella pneumophilia* and is transmitted through water that is contaminated with the bacteria. In past epidemics, it was spread through air-conditioning systems and cooling towers. It does not spread person to person.

Treatment—Treatment consists of antibiotics, medication to reduce the fever, maintaining fluid balance, and measures to support adequate respiration, such as oxygen and mechanical ventilation.

Lung Cancer

Description—This is the leading cause of cancer deaths among men and women, despite the fact that it is largely preventable. It is the progressive cellular degeneration of lung tissue. It usually develops within the wall or lining of the bronchial tree. There are different types of lung cancer: squamous cell, small-cell, adenocarcinoma, and large-cell. Approximately 172,570 new cases of lung cancer were estimated in 2005. This represents 13% of all cancer diagnoses. There is a significant decrease in the number of cases per 100,000 people for the first time in many years. However, lung cancer is still the leading cause of cancer-related deaths, with an estimated 163,510 deaths, or 29% of all cancer deaths, in 2005.

Signs and symptoms—There are often minimal symptoms that are usually not associated with cancer, such as cough, fatigue, and shortness of breath. This frequently results in diagnosis at the late stages when the disease is far advanced, offering little hope for survival. The symptoms of squamous and small cell carcinomas are smoker's cough, sneezing, dyspnea, hemoptysis, and chest pain. Symptoms of adenocarcinoma and large cell types include fever, weakness, weight loss, and anorexia. Unfortunately, there is no proven screening test for lung cancer.

Etiology—It is attributed to inhalation of carcinogens in tobacco and the environment. The inhalation of carcinogens causes damage to the cells of the lungs, which then causes uncontrolled abnormal growth when these cells become cancerous. There is a correlation between the risk of cancer and the number of cigarettes smoked daily, the depth of inhalation, the age at which smoking began, and the nicotine content of the tobacco. An individual over 40 who began smoking as a teenager and has averaged a pack a day for at least 20 years is most susceptible. Lung cancer can take 20 to 30 years to develop. Less than 10% of lung cancers occur among nonsmokers.

Other inhalants that increase *susceptibility* to cancer are industrial air pollutants, such as asbestos, arsenic, iron oxides, chromium, radioactive dust, vinyl chloride, and coal dust. There also is an indication that there is a familial tendency link to lung cancer. The combination of industrial pollutants and cigarettes is very risky. For example, asbestos workers who also smoke increase their risk of developing lung cancer by 60 times.

Involuntary smoking, which the nonsmoker receives "second hand" from a spouse or others, is less concentrated but still contains the same harmful substances. For example, wives exposed to husbands who smoke 20 or more cigarettes a day at home have double the risk of lung cancer when compared with wives of nonsmokers. Cancer caused by second-hand smoke kills 3,400 nonsmokers per year. Children of smoking parents are also affected. They are more prone to respiratory and middle ear infections, asthma, and sudden infant death syndrome (SIDS).

The prognosis for lung cancer patients is very poor because by the time a diagnosis is made, two thirds of the patients have passed the stage where it might be curable. Only 13% of all lung cancer patients (all races and all stages) live 5 or more years after diagnosis. This is primarily the result of delayed diagnosis because of lack of symptoms. The disease metastasizes to many other sites within the thoracic cavity and throughout the entire body.

Treatment—Treatment consists primarily of surgical excision when appropriate, radiation, and chemotherapy. Often the disease is advanced before treatment begins, and little more than alleviation of symptoms is possible. The best treatment is obviously prevention. Quitting smoking or never starting is the best defense against lung cancer.

Pleurisy (Ploo′ris-e)

Description—This is an inflammation of the visceral and parietal pleura in the thoracic cavity. **Pleurisy** develops as a complication of viral infections, pneumonia, tuberculosis, chest injury, and other factors.

Signs and symptoms—Sharp, stabbing pain is experienced on respiration because of irritation of the pleural nerve endings as the lungs move, rubbing against the inner chest wall. As a result, lung movement on the affected side may be limited, and dyspnea occurs.

Etiology—Pleurisy pain is caused by the inflammation or irritation of sensory nerve endings in the parietal pleura. It begins suddenly as a complication of pneumonia, a viral infection, or other causes.

Treatment—In the case of a viral infection, treatment is generally symptomatic, with bed rest and medications to reduce the inflammation and relieve the pain. If fluid collects within the pleural space (see Pleural Effusion), a thoracentesis is indicated to prohibit lung compression by the fluid or to determine,

by laboratory examination, a causative agent (see Figure 11-112).

Paroxysmal Nocturnal Dyspnea (PND) (Parok-sizmal Nok-turn-al)

Description—This is a symptom associated with chronic lung disease or left ventricular failure (heart disease).

Signs and symptoms—It occurs at night. Individuals awaken from sleep with a feeling of suffocation. They often run to open a window and gasp for air. Just sitting upright will help some people because of the effect of gravity on fluid in the lungs.

Etiology—This is associated with chronic lung disease and left ventricular heart failure probably caused by the accumulation of fluid in the lungs.

Treatment—The episode will often resolve within a few minutes; however, the symptom of PND indicates a serious underlying condition that requires treatment.

Pleural Effusion (Plooral E-fu′-zhun)

Description—This is the presence of excess fluid in the pleural space (Figure 11-116).

Signs and symptoms—When the effusion becomes symptomatic, it compresses lung tissue and reduces the lungs' ability to exchange O_2 for CO_2, and **hypoxia** (lack of O_2) results. If the fluid is a result of an infec-

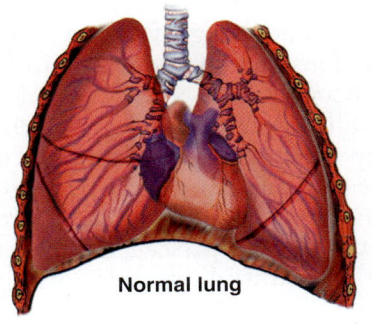

Normal lung

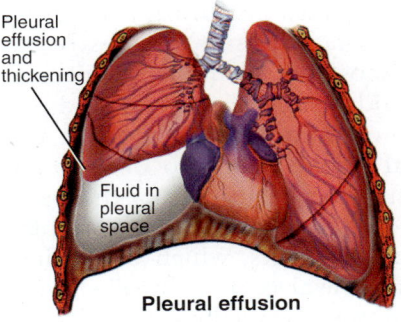

Pleural effusion and thickening

Fluid in pleural space

Pleural effusion

FIGURE 11-116 Comparison of a normal lung with pleural effusion.

tious process, exudate (pus) and dead tissue may be present, and the effusion is known as **empyema**.

Etiology—Pleural effusion results from the overproduction or the inadequate reabsorption of the pleural fluid. Some effusions result from chronic diseases, such as congestive heart failure, liver disease, tuberculosis, malignancy, lupus, and rheumatoid arthritis.

Treatment—Oxygen is administered to increase concentration to the remainder of the lung. Drainage of the material by thoracentesis and insertion of chest tubes may be necessary. Antibiotics may be required if the effusion is infectious in origin. Effusion that contains blood is called a **hemothorax** and will require drainage to prevent fibrothorax (scar tissue) formation.

Pneumonoconiosis (Nu mo-kone-o'sis)

Description—These are lung diseases developed after years of contact with environmental or occupational causative agents. Basically, there are three types of **pneumonoconiosis**: silicosis, asbestosis, and black lung disease.

Signs and symptoms—Some symptoms, common to all forms of pneumonoconioses, are rapid respirations, dry cough, dyspnea upon exertion that becomes worse, pulmonary hypertension, right ventricular involvement, and recurrent respiratory infections.

Silicosis
This occurs from exposure to silica sand dust in occupations such as sand blaster and foundry worker; in manufacturing of ceramic and sandstone products and construction materials; and in mining of gold, lead, zinc, and iron. Nodules develop where specific disease-fighting cells have ingested the silica particles but then are unable to dispose of the ingested material. The cells die, causing the release of an enzyme that attracts more cells to assist in destroying the invading material. A fibrous (scar) tissue results, and the process continues until large areas of the lung tissue are destroyed.

Asbestosis
This condition can develop 15 to 20 years after regular exposure to asbestos has ended. Asbestosis is most prevalent in the construction, fireproofing, and textile industries and in brake and automotive occupations dealing with clutch linings. The general public may also develop the condition from exposure to fibrous dust or the waste piles of asbestos factories. Asbestosis is the result of inhaling minute asbestos fibers, which enter the bronchioles and penetrate the alveolar walls. The fibers become encased, and fibrosis of the lung tissue develops, obliterating the air passages. Fibers also cause fibrotic changes in the parietal pleura.

Coal Worker's or Black Lung Disease
This is a progressive nodular type found in two forms: simple, which produces small lung lesions, or complicated, which produces masses of fibrous tissue. The development usually occurs after 15 years or more of exposure and depends to some extent on the amount of dust, the type of coal mined, the silica content, and the location of the mine.

Initially, the body's fighting cells ingest the dust and become filled, forming macules in the terminal bronchioles, which are surrounded by dilated alveoli. The supporting tissue atrophies (wastes away), resulting in permanent dilation of the small airways. When the disease changes from a simple to a complicated form, one or both lungs can become involved. The fibrous tissue masses enlarge, causing destruction of the alveoli and airways.

Treatment—Treatment of all types is essentially the same: avoid respiratory infections, use bronchodilators to aid in respiration, supplement oxygen when indicated, and other use respiratory therapy to improve removal of bronchial secretions.

Pneumonia (Nu-mo'ne-a)

Description—This is an acute infection of the principal tissues of the lungs, which may impair the exchange of O_2 and CO_2. Chances for recovery from **pneumonia** are good for persons with normal lungs, but pneumonia is a very common cause of death in debilitated (weakened) patients.

Pneumonia is classified in several ways: by microbiological origin (bacterial, viral, or fungal), by location (bronchial or lobar), or by type (primary or secondary).

Signs and symptoms—Symptoms include coughing, sputum production, pleural chest pain, chills, and fever.

Etiology—Pneumonia can be caused by inhaled pathogens, an inhaled chemical, or an infection spread from another area of the body. It often occurs with a chronic weakening illness (such as cancer or AIDS) or following surgery. It is also associated with malnutrition, smoking, COPD, advanced age, and with a decreased level of consciousness.

Treatment—Treatment consists of bed rest, antibiotics for bacterial pneumonia, adequate fluid intake, respiratory support measures (such as oxygen or mechanical breathing therapy), and medication for pain.

Pneumothorax (Nu-mo-tho'raks)

Description—In this condition, air or gas has accumulated between the parietal and visceral pleurae, causing some degree of collapse of the lung tissue. Figure 11-117 shows an accumulation of air at the

ACHIEVE UNIT OBJECTIVES

- ☐ Complete the Workbook activities to meet the learning objectives.
- ☐ Apply your knowledge at the end of this chapter in completing the Critical Thinking Challenge and Activities, as well as the StudyWARE on your Student CD-ROM.

UNIT 8
THE CIRCULATORY SYSTEM

OBJECTIVES

Upon completion of this unit, you will be able to achieve the following:

LEARNING Objectives

1. Spell and define, using the glossary at the back of the text, all the Words to Know in this unit.
2. Name the four main parts of the circulatory system.
3. Describe the anatomy of the heart, identifying the internal and external structures.
4. Differentiate between pulmonary, systemic, and portal circulation.
5. Describe the heart sounds, including the actions producing the sounds and where they can be auscultated.
6. Locate the pacemaker, explain its action, and tell how the heart rate is influenced by the body.
7. Explain how the cardiac conditions of heart block and fibrillation relate to the pacemaker.
8. Explain the purpose of an artificial pacemaker and how it functions.
9. Name the five types of blood vessels and their purpose and structure.
10. Describe the function of a capillary bed.
11. Trace the pathway of blood through the pulmonary and systemic circulation.
12. Explain the function and structure of the lymphatic system.
13. Name the components of whole blood and the role of each.
14. Describe the clotting process.
15. Name the blood types, and explain their importance to recipients of transfusions.
16. Explain the importance of the Rh factor in pregnancy and transfusions.
17. Identify nine cardiovascular tests and the reasons for giving them.
18. Describe 26 diseases or disorders of the circulatory system.

WORDS TO KNOW

accelerator	coronary	myocardial
acute phase	cross-match	infarction
adenitis	diastole	(MI)
ambulatory	electrocardio-	myocardium
anemia	graph (ECG)	nodes
aneurysm	embolism	pacemaker
angina	endocardium	papillary
angioplasty	erythrocyte	muscles
anticoagulant	exudate	pericardium
aorta	fibrillation	phlebitis
arrhythmias	heart block	plasma
arterioles	hemoglobin	platelet
arteriosclerosis	hemorrhage	portal
artery	Holter monitor	Rh factor
atherosclerosis	hypertension	SA node
atrium	hypotension	semilunar
AV node	infarction	septum
bicuspid	ischemia	sickle cell
bradycardia	leukemia	anemia
capillary	leukocyte	spleen
cardiac	lubb dupp	stasis ulcer
cardiovascular	lymph	systole
cerebrovascular	lymphatic	tachycardia
accident	system	thrombophlebitis
cholesterol	lymphocyte	thrombosis
chronic leukemia	metastasize	transfusion
compatible	mitral	transient
congestive heart	MUGA scan	ischemic
failure	murmur	attack

tricuspid   valve   vena cava
triglycerides   varicose   ventricle
vagus   vein   venule

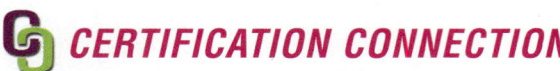

CERTIFICATION CONNECTION

CMA

Diagnostic procedures

Common diseases and
  pathology

Anatomy and physiology

CMAS

Anatomy and physiology

RMA

Anatomy and physiology

The circulatory system transports oxygen and nutrients to the body's cells, and it transports carbon dioxide and other waste products from the cells to be eliminated from the body. The blood, which flows through a closed circuit of vessels, is the transportation vehicle. A very efficient muscle, the heart, is the force behind the system. A few minutes' interruption of the circulatory system can result in death.

The circulatory system is composed of four main parts: (1) a pump, the heart; (2) the plumbing, the blood vessels; (3) the circulating fluid, the blood; and (4) an auxiliary fluid system, the **lymphatic system**. Each day the heart pumps the equivalent of 4,000 gallons of blood, at 40 miles per hour, through an estimated 70,000 miles of blood vessels. To achieve this, the heart must forcefully contract, squeezing out blood, at an average rate of 72 times per minute or about 100,000 times each day. In a year's time, the heart will contract 40 million times, resting only a fraction of a second between beats. To appreciate this phenomenal organ, alternately open and close your fist a little more often than once a second for just 1 minute by the clock. You will notice that not only your hand but also your forearm muscles begin to tire. Scientists have estimated that the work of the heart is about equal to the energy needed to lift a 10-pound weight 3 feet off the floor twice a minute for a lifetime. The condition of the blood vessels and the composition of the blood are major factors in the amount of force the heart must exert to circulate the blood.

THE HEART

The heart is about the size of a clenched fist and is located behind the sternum, between the lungs, with two thirds of it on the left side of the chest. It is constructed of several layers of muscles arranged in both circular and spiral fashion. When the muscles contract, blood is squeezed out of the heart chambers. During the relaxation phase, the heart fills with blood entering from the great **veins**. There is a considerable difference in the size of the heart during the phases, as shown in Figure 11-118.

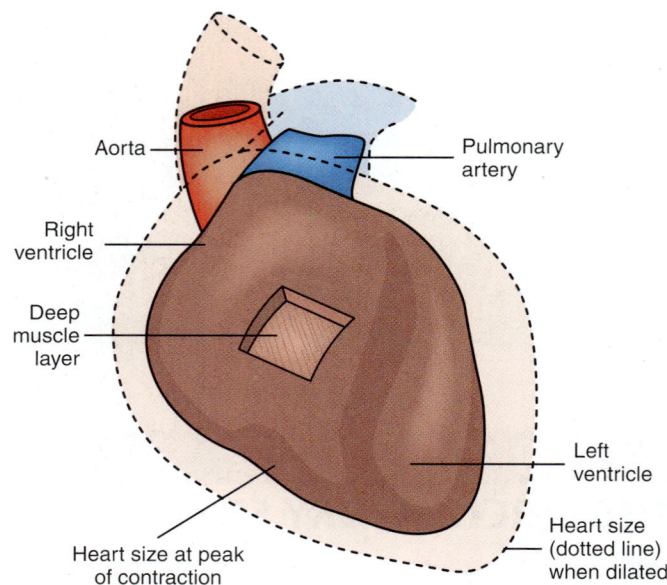

FIGURE 11-118   Heart size during contraction and filling actions

The contraction phase is known as **systole**, and the relaxation phase is called **diastole**. Systole is the period when the heart exerts the greatest pressure on the blood. This corresponds to the beat phase of the heart and can be heard over the heart with a stethoscope or felt as the pulse in an **artery**. The systolic pressure can be determined by measurement with blood pressure equipment and is represented by the larger or top number of the blood pressure reading. Diastole is the period of least pressure and is the time when the heart rests. This phase cannot be felt as a beat, but the diastolic pressure can be heard and determined by measurement. It is represented by the smaller or bottom number of the blood pressure reading.

External Heart Structures

The outer wall of the heart is surrounded by a sac called the **pericardium**. Like the pleura of the lungs, the pericardium has one layer called the parietal, which lines the sac, and another layer called the visceral, which covers the heart itself. The pericardial fluid between the layers prevents friction when the heart beats. The heart structure does not receive its blood supply from the blood pumped through its interior but from a number of small blood vessels that cover the surface of the heart (Figure 11-119). These blood vessels, called the **coronary** arteries and veins, carry oxygen, nutrients, and waste products to and from the heart muscle. The right and left coronary arteries enter the top of the heart from the **aorta**. Blood from the coronary veins returns to the right atrium by a small opening called the coronary sinus.

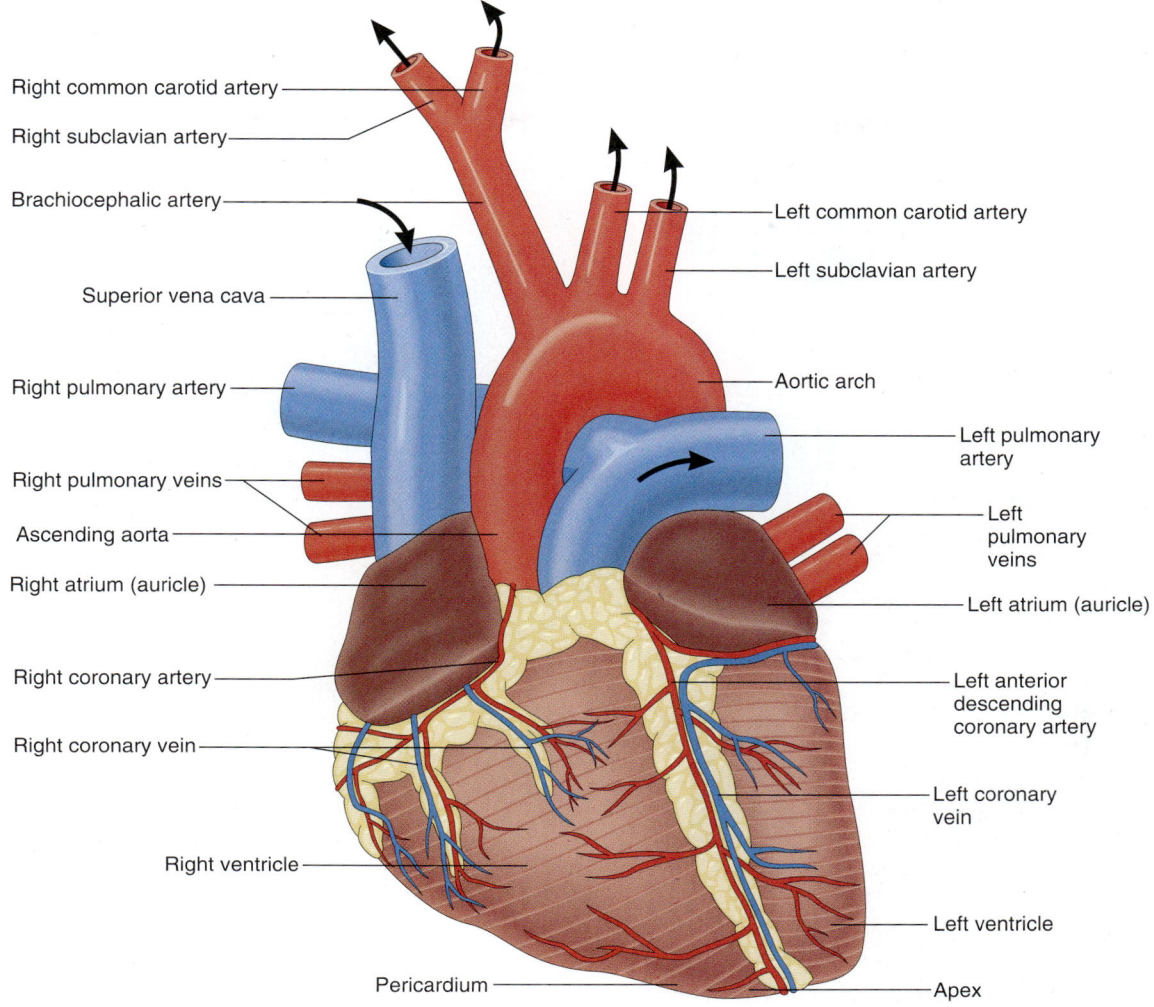

Right common carotid artery

Right subclavian artery

Brachiocephalic artery

Superior vena cava

Right pulmonary artery

Right pulmonary veins

Ascending aorta

Right atrium (auricle)

Right coronary artery

Right coronary vein

Right ventricle

Pericardium

Left common carotid artery

Left subclavian artery

Aortic arch

Left pulmonary artery

Left pulmonary veins

Left atrium (auricle)

Left anterior descending coronary artery

Left coronary vein

Left ventricle

Apex

FIGURE 11-119　External heart structures

The muscle wall of the heart is called the **myocardium**. The wall of the left lower chamber is thicker because it must pump blood through the entire general or systemic circulation, as discussed later.

Internal Heart Structures

A tissue known as **endocardium** lines the interior surface of the heart (Figure 11-120). The lining also covers the heart valves and the interior surface of the blood vessels to allow for the smooth flow of blood. Internally, the heart is a double pump, divided into a right and left side by a muscular wall called a **septum**. The septum prevents the blood on the right side from mixing with that on the left. The sides are further divided into upper and lower chambers. The right upper chamber is called the right **atrium**, and the lower is the right **ventricle**. The left side is similarly divided into a left atrium and left ventricle.

The chambers are separated by one-way **valves** that keep the blood flowing in the right direction. The **tricuspid** valve is between the right atrium and ventricle, and the **bicuspid** or **mitral** valve is between the left atrium and ventricle. **Papillary muscles** are attached by cords to the undersurfaces of the valve cusps or leaflets. When the atria contract, the papillary muscles also contract to pull open the valves, allowing the blood from the atria to enter the empty ventricles. Then the muscles relax, which allows the valves to close as the atria refill. The closed valves prevent the blood from reentering the atria when the ventricles contract.

When the ventricles contract, blood is forced out to the great arteries of the body. The right ventricle sends the blood through a **semilunar** valve into the pulmonary artery on its way through the pulmonary circulation in the lungs for a supply of oxygen. The left ventricle forces the blood past a semilunar valve into the aorta to be distributed throughout the general or systemic circulation of the body.

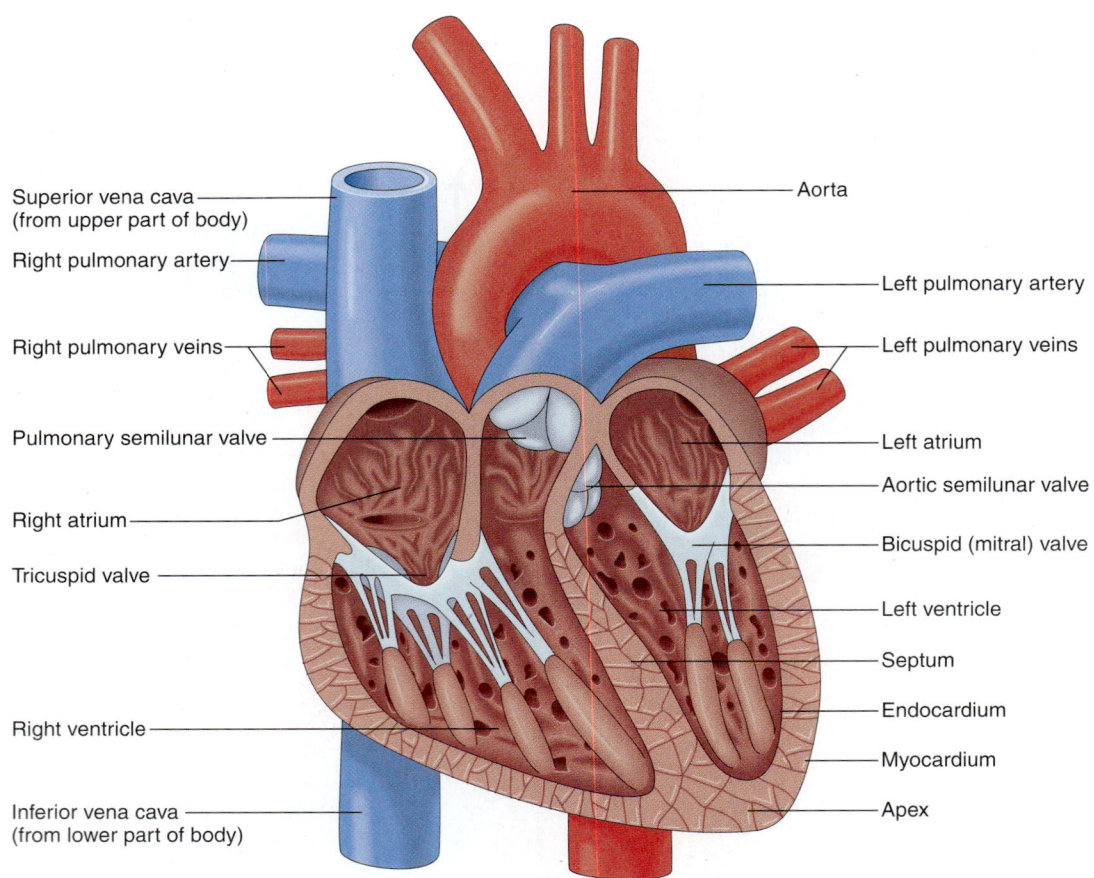

Superior vena cava
(from upper part of body)

Right pulmonary artery

Right pulmonary veins

Pulmonary semilunar valve

Right atrium

Tricuspid valve

Right ventricle

Inferior vena cava
(from lower part of body)

Aorta

Left pulmonary artery

Left pulmonary veins

Left atrium

Aortic semilunar valve

Bicuspid (mitral) valve

Left ventricle

Septum

Endocardium

Myocardium

Apex

FIGURE 11-120 Internal heart structures

A specific sequence of events occurs within the body as the blood is circulated. Blood flow occurs in two distinct patterns: *pulmonary circulation* between the heart and the lungs and *systemic circulation* between the heart and the rest of the body. Figure 11-121 and the following material describe the flow of blood through the pulmonary system.

Pulmonary Circulation

1. Deoxygenated (without O_2) blood carried in the superior vena cava from the arms, neck, and head and carried in the inferior vena cava from the lower extremities and internal organs (except the heart itself) enters the right atrium. Circulation from the heart also empties into the atrium by way of the coronary sinus.

2. The right atrium contracts, squeezing blood through the tricuspid valve, which is opened by the papillary muscles, into the right ventricle. Then the valve closes.

3. The right ventricle contracts, sending blood out through the semilunar valve into the pulmonary

artery. (Remember, this artery carries deoxygenated blood but is still an artery because it is leaving the heart.)

4. The pulmonary artery divides into a right and left branch, one going to each lung. The division continues into smaller arteries, arterioles, and then to the capillaries in the alveolar sacs. Here the deoxygenated blood gives up its CO_2 and picks up O_2.

5. With a fresh supply of O_2, the capillaries join the venules, then become veins and reenter the heart as four pulmonary veins, two from each lung, emptying into the left atrium. (This is the only time veins carry oxygenated blood, but they are still veins because they are returning to the heart.)

6. The left atrium contracts, forcing blood through the mitral or bicuspid valve into the left ventricle, and the valve immediately closes.

7. The left ventricle contracts forcefully, sending blood racing out of the heart past the semilunar valve into the aorta.

The action of the chambers of the heart just described occurs simultaneously in both sides of the heart. In other words, both atria contract at the same time, as

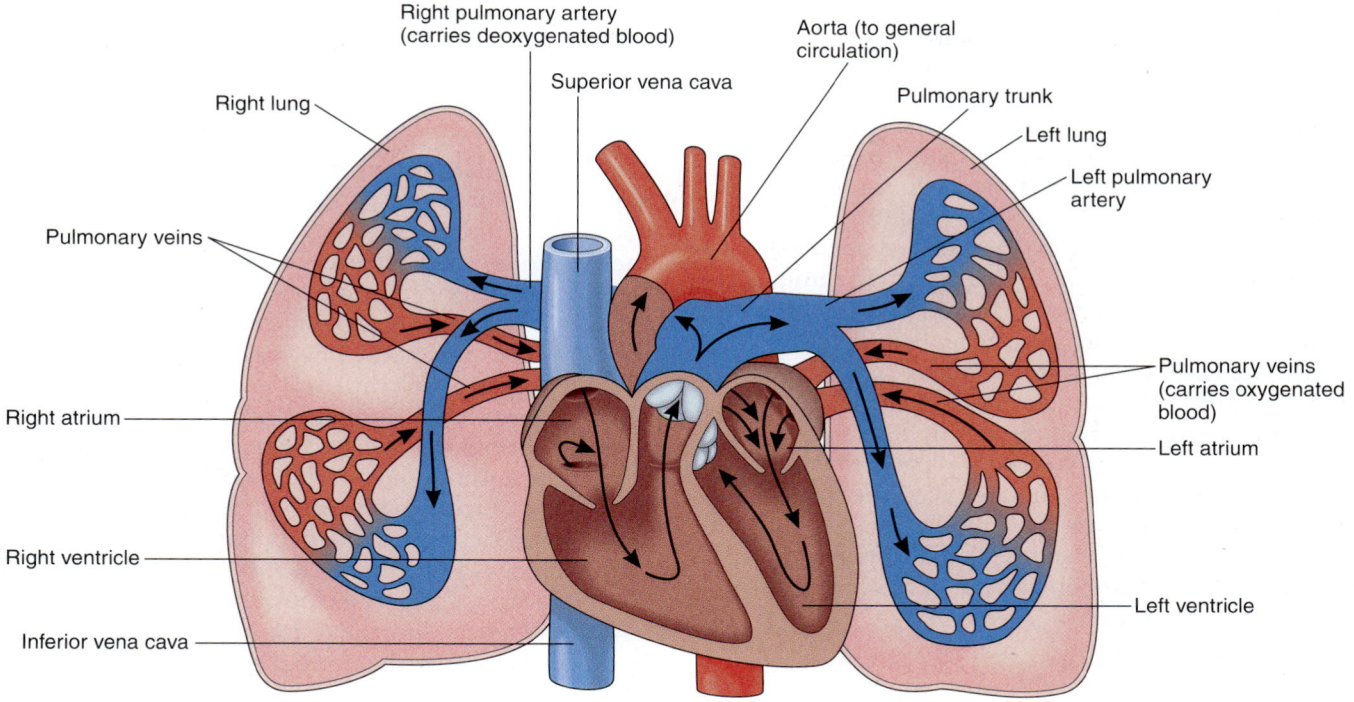

FIGURE 11-121 Pulmonary circulation

do the ventricles. The chambers must work in unison, or blood being pushed forward would have no place to go (this situation does occur in certain cardiovascular disorders and will be discussed later). The total action just described occurs each time the heart beats.

Heart Sounds

The physician listens at specific locations on the chest wall to hear specific functions of the heart. Figure 11-122 illustrates the anatomical location of the valves and the corresponding auscultatory areas. When a stethoscope is used to listen to the heartbeat, two distinct sounds can be heard. They are referred to as the **lubb dupp** sounds. The lubb sound, which is heard first, is caused by the valves slamming shut between the atria and the ventricles. The physician refers to this sound as the S_1. It is heard loudest at the apex of the heart.

The dupp, heard second, is shorter and higher pitched. It is caused by the semilunar valves closing in the aorta and the pulmonary arteries. This sound is known as the S_2. It is loudest at the second intercostal space on each side of the sternum. With a little practice, the valves' condition and level of function can be evaluated from their sounds.

Certain conditions cause changes in the action of the heart valves. Normally, the right heart valves close a fraction of a second before the left because of the lower pressure in the right side of the heart. When the ventri-

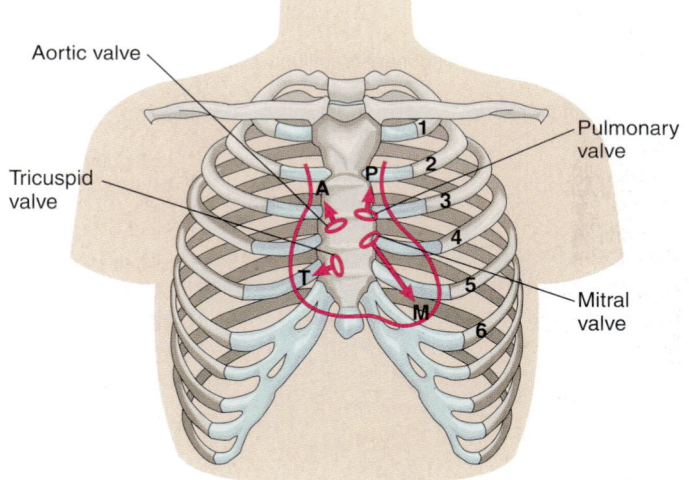

FIGURE 11-122 Anatomical location of the heart valves and the corresponding auscultatory location. Valves are shown as oval structures and the auscultatory locations by the letters A, T, M, and P. The rib levels are numbered.

cles are distended, an audible vibration may occur, which is referred to as an S_3 or a ventricular gallop. Occasionally, just before S_1 at the end of diastole, the atria may contract, forcing blood into an already filled ventricle. This causes a rise in the ventricular pressure and vibrations known as atrial gallop or S_4.

The Pacemaker

The normal heart beats rhythmically as long as the cells receive the correct balance of sodium, calcium, and potassium and an adequate supply of oxygen and nutrients. Another essential element is the "spark" from the group of nerve cells in the right atrium called the sinoatrial or **SA node**, also called the **pacemaker** (Figure 11-123). The node generates the electrical impulse that starts each wave of muscle contraction in the heart. The impulse in the right atrium spreads over the muscles of both atria, causing them to contract simultaneously, sending blood into the ventricles. The impulse apparently triggers the atrioventricular or **AV node**, located between the atria and the ventricles, even though there is no direct connection between the nodes. The AV node has nerve fibers that extend through the septum and are called the *bundle of His*. The bundle divides into a right and left branch, infiltrating the muscles of each ventricle with a system of Purkinje fibers, which cause contraction of the ventricles.

Rhythm Disorders

The self-generating impulse of the heart is one of the body's miracles. Even if the heart were removed from the body, it would continue to beat as long as it was supplied with the necessary nutrients. In a **cardiac** condition known as **heart block**, there is an interruption in

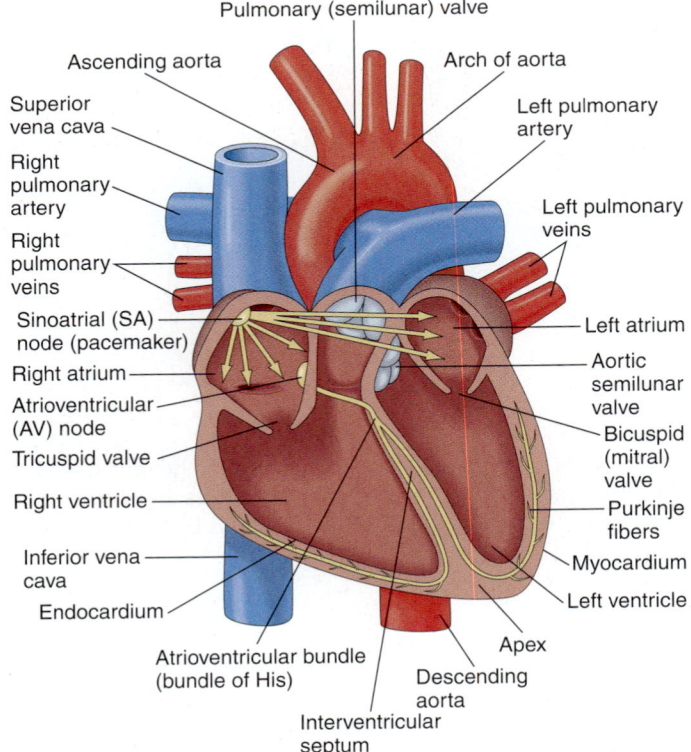

FIGURE 11-123   SA and AV nodes and the conduction pathway of the heart's electrical impulse

Pulmonary (semilunar) valve
Ascending aorta
Arch of aorta
Superior vena cava
Left pulmonary artery
Right pulmonary artery
Left pulmonary veins
Right pulmonary veins
Sinoatrial (SA) node (pacemaker)
Left atrium
Right atrium
Aortic semilunar valve
Atrioventricular (AV) node
Bicuspid (mitral) valve
Tricuspid valve
Right ventricle
Purkinje fibers
Inferior vena cava
Myocardium
Endocardium
Left ventricle
Atrioventricular bundle (bundle of His)
Apex
Descending aorta
Interventricular septum

the message from the SA node to the AV node. The interruption can occur in varying degrees. The abnormal rhythm patterns can be viewed on an **electrocardiograph** (**ECG,** heart action recording). *First degree block* is characterized by a momentary delay at the AV node before the impulse is transmitted to the ventricles. *Second degree block* can be of two forms. One occurs in cycles of delayed impulses until the SA node fails to conduct to the AV node, then returns to near normal. A second form is characterized by a pattern of only every second, third, or fourth impulse being conducted to the ventricles. This causes a marked decrease in heart output and usually progresses to the third degree. *Third degree heart block* is known as "complete heart block." There is no impulse carried over from the pacemaker. Because the heart is essential to life, there is a built-in safety factor. The atria continue to beat at 72 times per minute while the ventricles contract independently at about half the atrial rate; this is adequate to sustain life but results in a severe decrease in cardiac output.

Other rhythm disorders are known as **arrhythmias** (any deviation from the normal electrical rhythm of the heart). Premature contractions cause arrhythmia and occur when an area of the heart (not the SA node) "sparks" and stimulates a contraction of the rest of the myocardium. This area is known as an ectopic (abnormal place) pacemaker. There are three types of premature contractions, each identified by the area of its location: atrial, ventricular, or AV junctional.

Atrial are known as *premature atrial contractions* (PACs) and cause the atria to contract ahead of the anticipated time. *Premature junctional contractions* (PJCs) have the ectopic pacemaker focused at the junction of the AV node and the bundle of His. Usually PACs and PJCs are of no clinical significance and are caused by nicotine, caffeine, fatigue, or tension.

Premature ventricular contractions (PVCs) are a different matter. They originate in the ventricle and cause contraction ahead of the next anticipated beat. They can be benign or deadly. If frequent (five to six per minute) or in pairs, they may require immediate intervention to decrease the irritability of the cardiac muscle to maintain cardiac output. If the PVCs occur every other beat, it is a *bigeminal rhythm;* if they occur every third beat, it is a *trigeminal rhythm.* PVCs can be caused by electrolyte and acid-base imbalance, drug therapy, myocardial infarction (see diseases), or oxygen deficit.

Artificial Pacemaker

When the natural pacemaker of the heart fails to maintain a normal heart rate and cardiac drug therapy designed to cause effective, regular beats fails to correct the situation, an artificial pacemaker may be indicated. The device consists of a small battery-powered pulse generator with electrode catheters (Figure 11-124). The

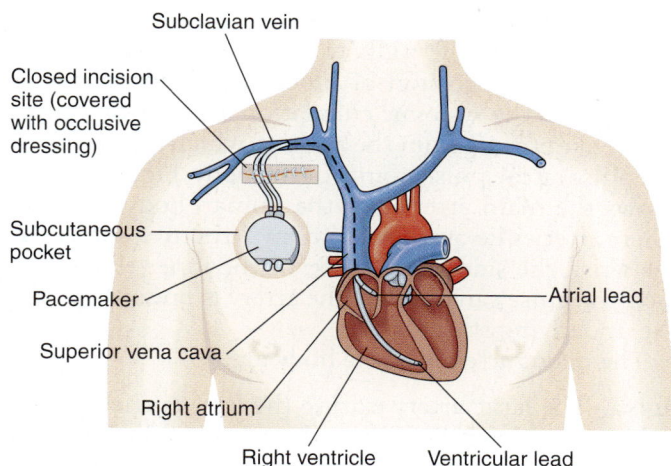

FIGURE 11-124   Artificial pacemaker with atrial and ventricular leads

electrodes are inserted into a vein and threaded through the vena cava, one to the right atrium, the other into the right ventricle at the apex. The procedure is accomplished while observing the path of the electrodes by fluoroscopy. The action of the heart throughout the procedure, and for at least the first 24 hours following, is monitored carefully by frequent ECG tracings. The stimulation threshold of the pacemaker to maintain myocardial contractions is determined by noting the number of milliamperes (MA) that produce the desired QRS complex (ECG tracing of contraction). This MA and the desired rate can be set in the pacemaker with a hand-held radio transmitter.

It should be noted that when the heart is totally dependent on artificial pacing, the heart rate may always be that which is artificially set. Newer artificial pacemakers can increase the rate to meet the needs of increased activity by sensing body motion.

A pacemaker is permanently inserted surgically into a muscular pocket on the chest wall. Permanent units are self-contained and will operate for about 3 to 12 years. Pacemakers can also be of either the fixed or the demand type. Fixed units fire continuously at a predetermined rate. Demand types sense the person's own rate and fire only when required. An external unit can be programmed to change the mode of firing of some implanted types. Battery failure requires replacement of the entire generating unit.

Pacemakers are of benefit to patients with a slow, irregular heart rhythm, complete heart block, or a slow ventricular rate resulting from congenital or disease conditions.

In another malfunction of the impulse mechanism known as ventricular **fibrillation**, the rhythm breaks down and the muscle fibers contract at random without coordination. This results in very ineffective heart action and is a life-threatening condition. An electrical device called a *defibrillator* is used to discharge a strong electrical current into the patient's heart through electrode paddles held against the bare chest wall. The shock should interfere with the uncoordinated action and allow the SA node to resume its control.

A type of artificial pacemaker, known as an implantable cardioverter defibrillator, can also affect the rhythm of the heart. The defibrillator is used to reestablish effective heart action with patients who have episodes of potentially fatal ventricular fibrillation. This device consists of a small power pack about the size of a pager. It is implanted in the chest wall near the clavicle and attaches to electrode tubes that are threaded through veins to permanent positions in the heart, much like an artificial pacemaker. It includes a microcomputer that monitors the heart's rhythm and responds with a low-energy "shock" for a minor problem or gives a high energy jolt, similar to one given with external defibrillator paddles, to automatically correct fibrillation. Use of the implanted defibrillator is becoming more common, especially with patients who have an increased risk of heart rhythm problems following a heart attack. In 2001, over 60,000 Americans were implanted with the sophisticated electronic device.

Controlling the Rate

Two nerves, the **vagus** and the **accelerator**, have fibers in the muscle of the heart and have some control over the natural rate of the heartbeat (Figure 11-125). The vagus nerve, also called the decelerator, slows down the heart rate, whereas the accelerator nerve increases the rate. The nerves, however, are stimulated by many things. Heart rate can increase as the result of fear, anger, or

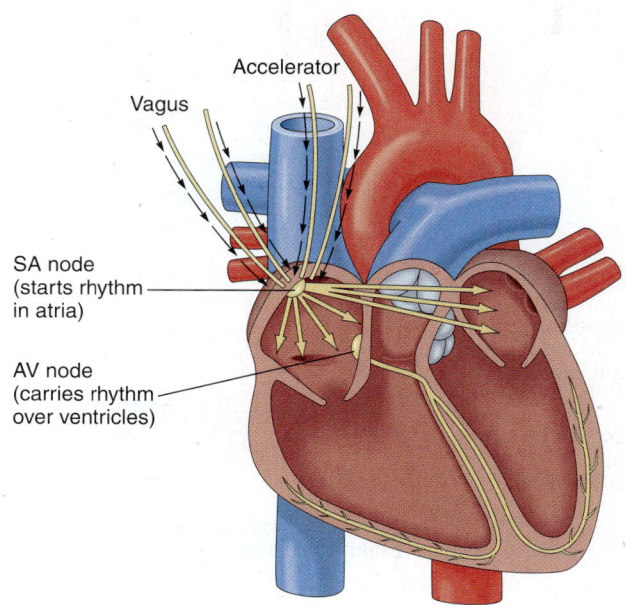

FIGURE 11-125   Nerves influencing the heart rate

excitement and can decrease with severe depression. The amount of oxygen, carbon dioxide, and electrolytes (sodium, potassium, magnesium, phosphates, and chlorides) present in the blood affect the rate of the heart. A heart rate that is consistently rapid (over 100 beats per minute) is known as **tachycardia**. When the rate is consistently slow (less than 60 beats per minute), it is referred to as **bradycardia**.

THE BLOOD VESSELS

Blood vessels are divided into three main types: arteries, veins, and **capillaries** (Figure 11-126).

Arteries

An artery always carries blood *away* from the heart and usually carries fresh, oxygenated blood. The one exception is the pulmonary artery, which leaves the right ventricle of the heart on its way *to* the lungs to pick up oxygen. Arteries are constructed with layers of elastic fibers that allow the walls to expand and recoil in response to the injection of blood when the ventricles contract. In the systemic circulation, this action causes a wavelike effect within the arteries, which can be felt as the pulse at the pulse points of the body. Figure 11-127 shows the main arteries of the human body. In areas where arteries lie over firm or bony structure, such as at the wrist, the side of the neck, or the inner elbow surface, the pulse can be felt if the artery is pressed against the underlying structure.

The major arteries of the body are:

Aorta—The large artery exiting the left ventricle of the heart and extending down the center of the body. All other arteries branch off the aorta.

Carotid—Extends up the side of the neck into the head

Pulmonary—Extends from the right ventricle to the lungs

Brachial—Extends down the arm

Radial—Extends on the thumb side of the forearm

Ulnar—Extends on the little finger side of the forearm

Common iliac—Branches off the abdominal aorta and extends down through the pelvis

Femoral—Extends to the thigh

Tunica interna, or intima
endothelium, areolar, and elastic tissue

Tunica media
smooth muscle

Tunica externa, or adventitia
connective tissue

Elastic fibers

Endothelium

Capillary

Valve

Lumen

Artery

Vein

Endothelium

Internal elastic membrane

External elastic membrane

Tunica media (muscle tissue)

Lumen

Tunica adventitia or externa (connective tissue)

Artery Vein Capillary

Types of blood vessels and their general structure

FIGURE 11-126 Comparative structure of blood vessels

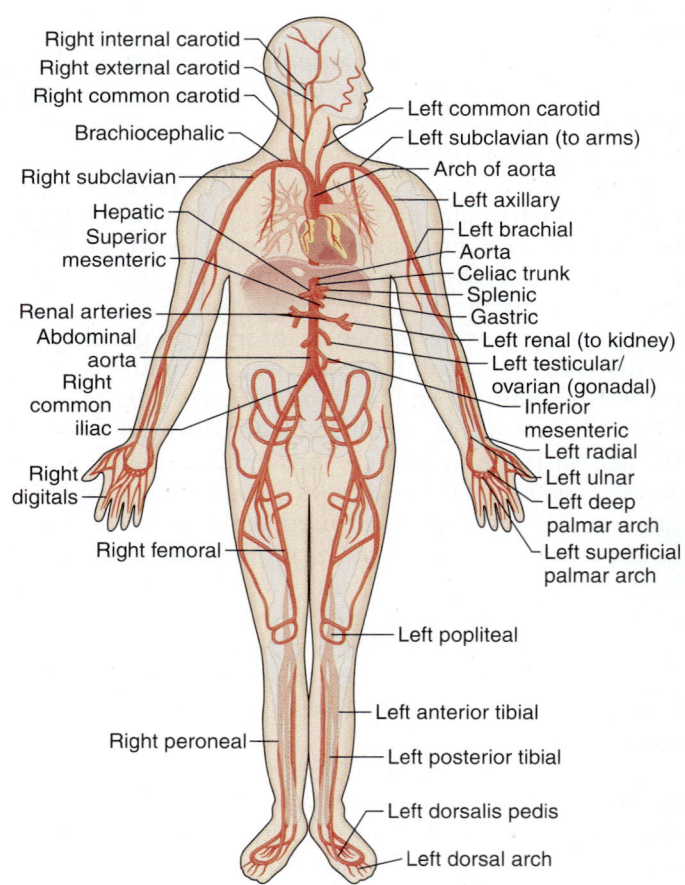

Right internal carotid
Right external carotid
Right common carotid
Brachiocephalic
Right subclavian
Hepatic
Superior mesenteric
Renal arteries
Abdominal aorta
Right common iliac
Right digitals
Right femoral
Right peroneal

Left common carotid
Left subclavian (to arms)
Arch of aorta
Left axillary
Left brachial
Aorta
Celiac trunk
Splenic
Gastric
Left renal (to kidney)
Left testicular/ovarian (gonadal)
Inferior mesenteric
Left radial
Left ulnar
Left deep palmar arch
Left superficial palmar arch
Left popliteal
Left anterior tibial
Left posterior tibial
Left dorsalis pedis
Left dorsal arch

FIGURE 11-127 Major arteries of the body

Tibial—Extends from the femoral through the lower leg

Dorsalis pedis—Extends along the top of the foot

As the arteries divide and branch off into smaller and smaller vessels, they become known as **arterioles**. Eventually, the arterioles join the microscopic blood vessels known as capillaries. When the blood enters the vast network of capillaries, called a capillary bed, it is so dispersed that the rate of flow is reduced to a slow trickle, permitting time for O_2 and nutrients to enter the tissue cells in exchange for CO_2 and waste products (Figure 11-128).

Capillary walls are thin, one-cell structures that allow the passage of molecules into the fluid-filled tissue spaces surrounding the cells. The molecules pass through the fluid to enter either the cell or the capillary. Tiny openings in the capillary walls permit white blood cells to leave the blood and enter the fluid of the tissue spaces to destroy bacteria. **Plasma** also seeps through the capillary walls, adding to the amount of tissue fluid. Excess fluid, certain waste products, and other substances are removed by an adjoining capillary of the lymphatic system, an action that will be discussed later in this unit.

The vast number of capillaries within the body would be more than capable of holding all the body's supply of blood. Therefore, an automatic system is in effect that permits a group of cells being served by one section of a capillary bed to receive blood for only a short period of time. Then another section is served, and the first section must wait for another turn. This control is maintained by a series of capillary sphincters that open and close the entrances to the capillary beds.

Body cells, in order of importance, have a predetermined priority for receiving the available blood supply. At any given time, only two of the three major body functions can be served. The brain and other central nervous system structures always have first priority. Next come the skeletal muscles that enable us to move

and therefore provide a degree of protection to the body with the flight/fight options. Last is the supply to the internal organs of the digestive system. This means that if you have eaten recently and you decide to run, swim, or exercise strenuously, your stomach may complain with cramps because the muscles are not getting enough blood supply to digest its contents.

When the blood leaves the capillary bed, it carries CO_2 and waste products from the cells to be circulated to the proper organ for disposal. Capillaries join with **venules**, which are tiny branches of the veins. As they return blood toward the heart, venules join together, forming veins that eventually enter the heart from the lower body by the inferior **vena cava** and from the upper body by the superior vena cava.

Veins

Veins are similar to arteries in construction, except the walls are thinner and they lack the elastic fiber lining that lets arteries alter the size of their openings. The pressure that is present in arteries is absent in veins, and therefore they can collapse when they are not filled. The major veins of the body are shown in Figure 11-129.

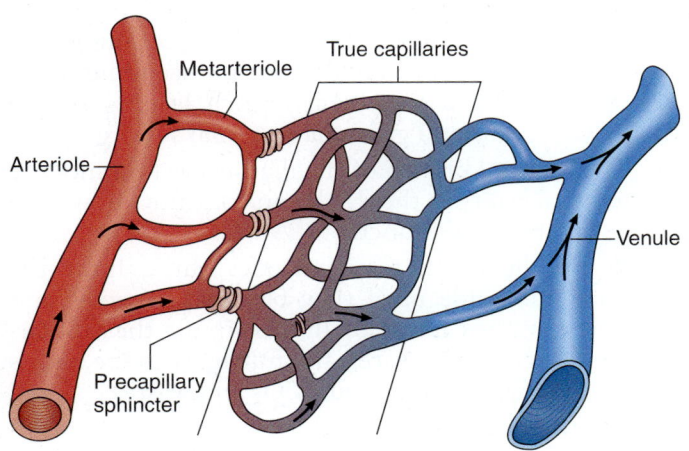

FIGURE 11-128   Capillary bed connecting an arteriole with a venule

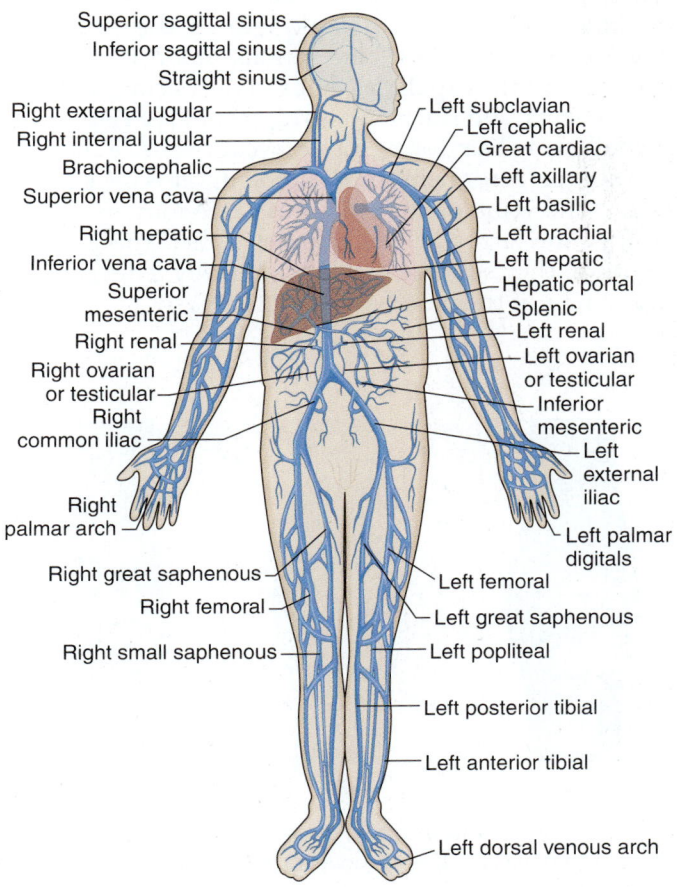

FIGURE 11-129   Major veins of the body

The major veins of the body are:

Tibial—From the feet to the thigh
Saphenous—In the thigh from the knee into the pelvis
Femoral—In the thigh from the knee into the pelvis
Common iliac—From the saphenous and femoral to the inferior vena cava
Inferior vena cava—All lower body veins to the right atrium of the heart
Jugular—From the head and neck
Brachial—From the arm to the brachiocephalic
Cephalic—From the arm to the brachiocephalic
Superior vena cava—All upper body veins to the right atrium of the heart
Pulmonary veins—From the lungs to the left atrium

Veins carry deoxygenated blood back to the heart to be sent to the lungs for exhaling of CO_2 and to pick up a new supply of O_2. Every time the heart beats, blood is forced through the arteries and arterioles to the capillaries, where the pressure from the heart is dissipated in the vast capillary network. With each successive beat, additional blood is forced through the capillaries into the venules and veins, which move it back toward the heart. Special valve structures are located throughout the veins to maintain the flow of blood in the proper direction (Figure 11-130). Veins in the lower extremities especially contain many valves because they are returning blood "uphill" so to speak. During the relaxation phase of the heartbeat, the venous blood could flow back toward the capillaries, but the valves close as relaxation begins, and the blood is trapped in the veins until the following beat forces it to move forward.

Another factor helps move blood in veins back to the heart. The veins of the extremities are located in and around the large skeletal muscles. When the muscles contract, they squeeze the veins, thereby aiding in the movement of the blood (Figure 11-131).

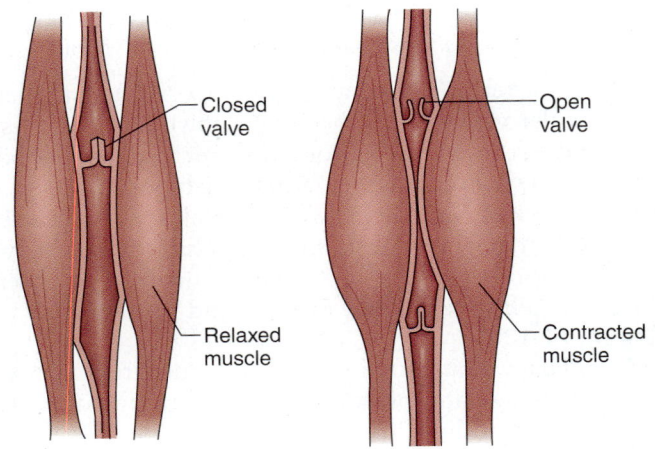

FIGURE 11-131   How muscles help move blood through internal veins

Blood flows to every cell in the body through the systemic circulation. Refer to Figures 11-127 and 11-129 as you read the following description of the flow through the major arteries and veins.

Systemic Circulation

1. As the blood leaves the left ventricle, it enters the huge aorta. Immediately, the right and left coronary arteries to the heart exit from the aorta at its arch. Other great arteries, the common carotid, the subclavian, and the innominate (which becomes the brachial and radial arteries of the arm), also exit from the arch, divide into right and left branches, and supply blood to the head, neck, and upper extremities.

2. As the aorta descends through the body, the thoracic and abdominal portions give origin to the large arteries supplying the organs of the thorax and abdomen.

3. When the aorta reaches the level of the fourth lumbar vertebra, it divides into two large common iliac arteries with the external branch descending down the legs and the internal branch leading to the pelvic organs and genitalia (external sex organs).

4. The external branch of the iliac artery becomes the femoral artery in the thigh and continues down the leg as the tibial branch.

5. Eventually all systemic arteries throughout the body subdivide until they become arterioles and then join the capillaries. In this circuit, the capillaries deliver the O_2, water, and nutrients to the body's cells and pick up the cells' CO_2 and wastes.

6. Upon leaving the capillaries, the blood is considered deoxygenated. The capillaries join venules, which eventually become veins.

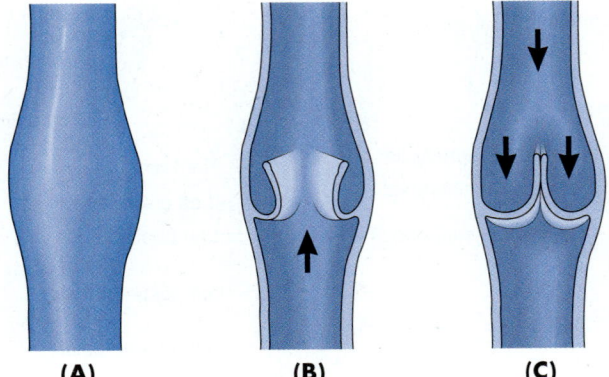

FIGURE 11-130   Vein valves: (A) external view showing dilation at site of valve; (B) veins opened and valves opened; and (C) valves closed to prevent backflow of blood.

7. The major lower extremity veins are the anterior and posterior tibial, the small and great saphenous, the popliteal, and the femoral. These join with pelvic veins and enter the inferior vena cava.

8. The major veins of the upper extremities are the basilic, median, and cephalic. These join with the subclavian, internal and external jugular, the innominate, and the sinuses from the head to enter the superior vena cava.

9. The superior vena cava and inferior vena cava empty into the right atrium of the heart, and systemic circulation is completed.

Portal Circulation

The preceding was a simplified description of the body's general circulation. However, there is another "circuit" that leaves and reenters the system just described. It is called the **portal** circulation (Figure 11-132). The details of its function are beyond the scope of this text, but it can be described in general terms.

As the aorta descends through the abdomen, arteries branch off to the internal organs: the stomach, liver, spleen, pancreas, kidneys, etc. Each organ receives substances on which it reacts. These substances may be sugar, salt, hormones, a toxic chemical, nutrients, or waste products from the cells of other organs. Everything you eat, drink, inhale, or inject into your body eventually enters the circulatory system.

The blood leaving certain organs (ones without a pair) empties into the special portal circulation and eventually the portal vein. This vein goes to the liver to permit the blood from the large and small intestines, stomach, pancreas, and spleen to come into contact with the liver's specialized cells. Many life-preserving functions are performed by these liver cells. For example, here nutrients that enter the blood from the digestive system are altered, stored, or released into the main circulatory system as needed. After passing through the liver, the blood is carried by the venous system to the inferior vena cava and is recirculated.

THE LYMPHATIC SYSTEM

The lymphatic system consists of **lymph** (a straw-colored fluid similar to blood plasma), lymph **nodes**, lymph vessels, and the **spleen**. In addition, the lymphatic tissue, which produces **lymphocytes** (a type of blood cell), is often considered to be part of the system. This includes the tonsils, the thymus gland, and the intestinal lymphoid tissue.

Lymph

Lymph is composed of blood plasma that filters out of the capillaries, lymphocytes, hormones, and many other substances that are the products of cellular activity, such as water, digested nutrients, salts, oxygen, carbon dioxide, and urea (Figure 11-133). It is a continuous-forming process. Lymph fills the spaces between the cells and is also referred to as intercellular or *interstitial fluid*. Lymph acts as the "bridge" between cells and capillaries. Lymph is moved through the lymph vessels primarily by contraction of the skeletal muscles. There is no pump like the heart to move lymph. Lymph vessels are constructed like veins, however, with valves to prevent the backflow of fluid.

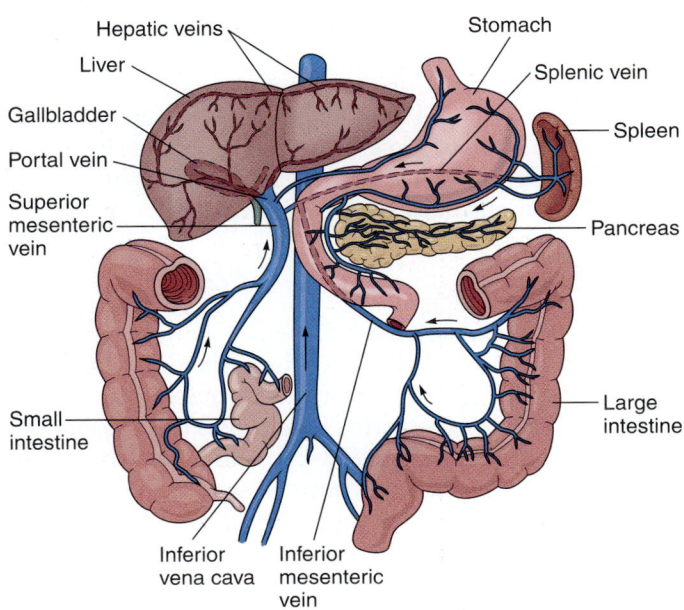

FIGURE 11-132   Portal circulation

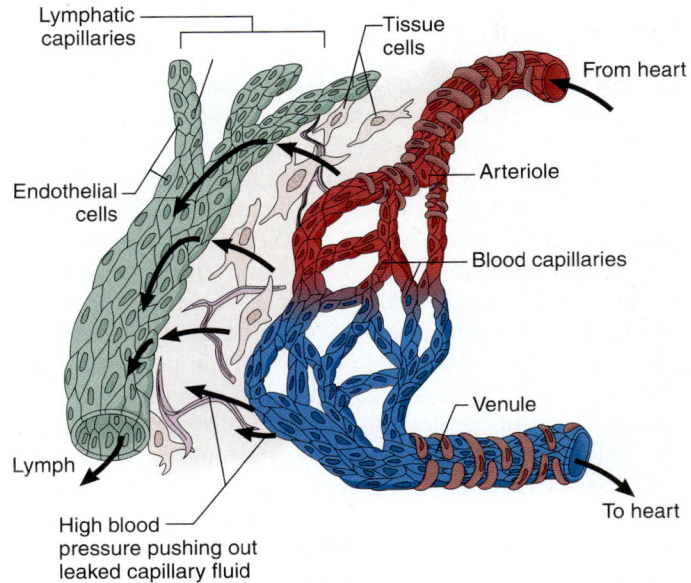

FIGURE 11-133   Leaked blood capillary fluid enters the lymphatic capillaries and becomes lymph.

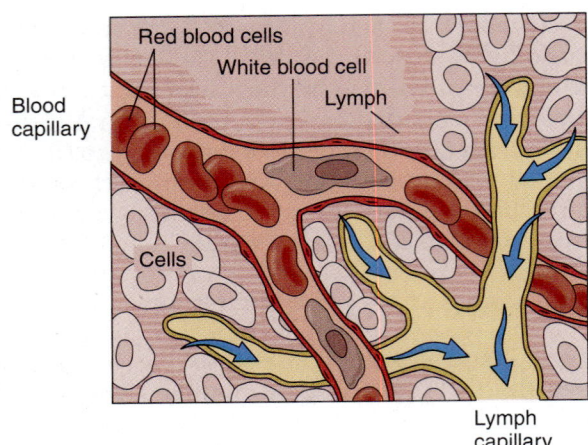

FIGURE 11-134   Lymph capillary

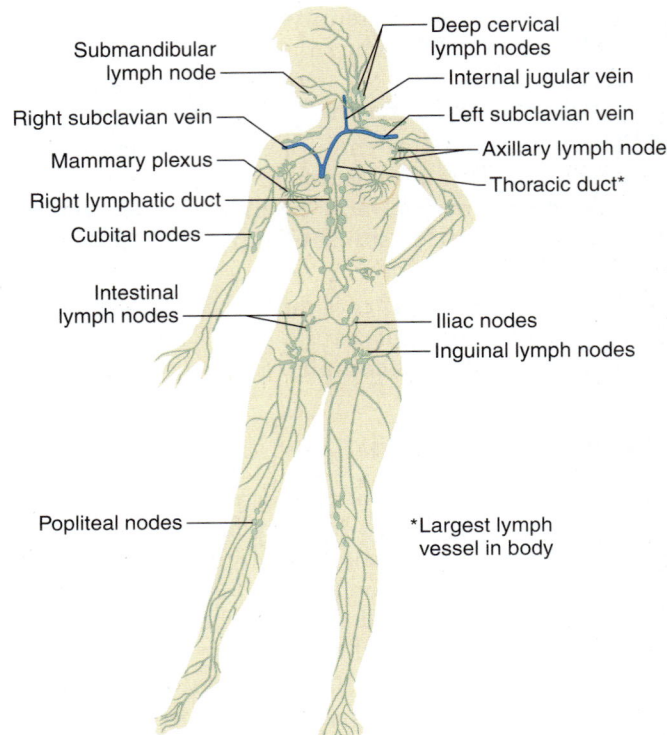

FIGURE 11-135   The lymphatic system

Lymph Vessels

Vessels carrying lymph are located throughout the body, somewhat like veins. Lymphatic capillaries absorb fluid and other substances from the tissues and return them to the circulatory system (Figure 11-134). However, it is a one-way system only, from the cells toward the heart. There are no separate vessels bringing lymph to the cells.

The vast network of lymph capillaries joins to form small lymph vessels that in turn form larger vessels called *lymphatics*. Lymphatics eventually form two main ducts. The right lymphatic duct receives lymph from the right side of the head, the right arm, and the upper right trunk. The thoracic duct receives lymph from the rest of the body (Figure 11-135).

Lymph Nodes

Lymph nodes are small, round or oval structures located usually in clusters along the lymph vessels at various places in the body. Lymph enters the nodes from four afferent lymph vessels, filters through a mesh of sinuses, and leaves by way of a single efferent vessel. Lymphocytes, a type of white blood cell, are derived from stem cells in the bone marrow. They enter the bloodstream and go to the lymph tissue to "live." Their action is essential to the immune system of the body. When needed, they divide by mitosis, greatly increasing in number. Phagocytes, another type of white blood cell, can also be found in lymph nodes. The structure of the nodes and the cell's function purify the lymph by removing harmful substances, such as bacteria or malignant cells. The nodes increase and decrease in size in relation to the amount of material being filtered. In acute infections, they become swollen and tender because of the collection of cells gathered to destroy the invading substances. This condition is known as **adenitis**. With extensive in-

volvement, the node may break down, and an abscess will form.

Physicians palpate for nodes when patients have infectious conditions or when a malignancy is known or suspected. With malignancy, the cancer cells are abnormal and so are identified by the cells in the lymph node to be removed from the circulating fluid. As more cells accumulate, the node becomes enlarged and is therefore palpable. Early detection of lymph node involvement is critical to the prognosis of patients with cancer, for it is through the lymphatic system that a malignancy often **metastasizes** (spreads) to other sites. The extent of lymph node involvement is an important indicator of the ultimate prognosis of the patient.

The Spleen

The spleen is an organ composed of lymphatic tissue that lies just beneath the left side of the diaphragm, in back of the upper portion of the stomach. The spleen produces lymphocytes, stores red blood cells, keeps the appropriate balance between cells and plasma in the blood, and removes and destroys worn-out red cells. The organ functions like a large lymph node. It is soft and elastic and varies in size according to the flow of blood through the organ. During an acute infection, it will become enlarged and tender. Patients with leukemia may have an enlarged, firm spleen that is palpable on examination. The spleen is filled with excess immature cells to be destroyed.

THE BLOOD

Blood is the life-giving fluid of the body. It flows through the blood vessels, transporting substances essential to the maintenance of life. The average adult has 8 to 10 pints of blood. A loss of 2 pints, or about 20%, is cause for concern. The blood carries oxygen from the lungs to the body's cells, nutrients from the digestive system to the cells, and cellular wastes from the cells to the appropriate organ for excretion. It picks up hormones excreted from endocrine glands and distributes them throughout the body to the appropriate receiving organ. Blood also delivers the minerals necessary for muscular contraction, heartbeat, stimulation of the respiratory system, and the homeostasis of cells. This vital substance is composed of only two main parts—the plasma and the cells—but each part has many essential components (Figure 11-136).

Plasma

Plasma is a straw-colored liquid that makes up a little over half the volume of blood. It is about 90% water, the remainder consisting of minerals, such as calcium, sodium, potassium, phosphorus, and bicarbonates.

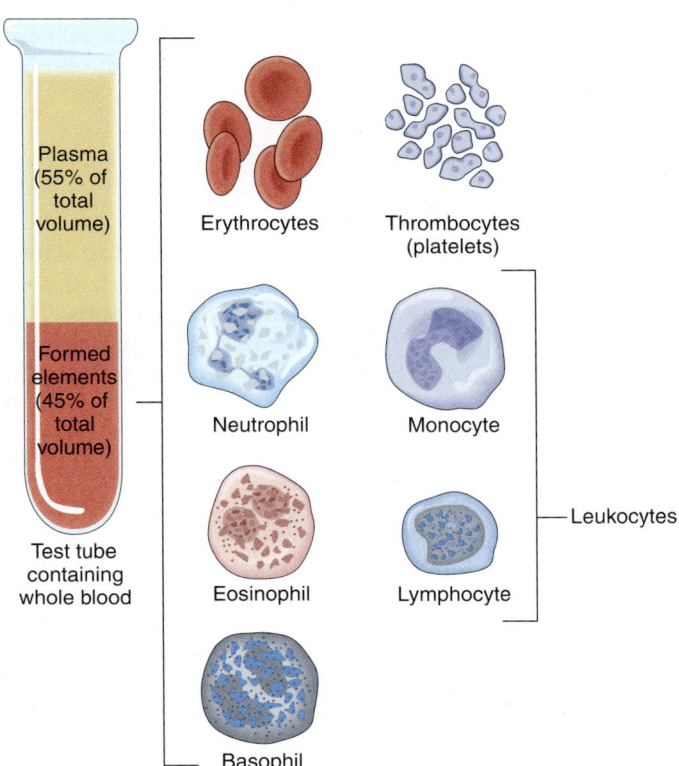

Plasma (55% of total volume)

Erythrocytes

Thrombocytes (platelets)

Formed elements (45% of total volume)

Neutrophil

Monocyte

Eosinophil

Lymphocyte

— Leukocytes

Test tube containing whole blood

Basophil

FIGURE 11-136   Major components of the blood

The minerals are commonly referred to as *electrolytes.* These elements are processed by the body from the foods that are eaten and play a major role in maintaining the acid-base balance of the blood.

Plasma contains other vital substances, such as vitamins, hormones, enzymes, and nutrients absorbed from the digestive system (i.e., glucose, fatty acids, and amino acids). Oxygen, carbon dioxide, and other waste products from the cells are also carried in the plasma.

In addition, three important proteins are found in plasma: fibrinogen, which is necessary to clot blood; serum albumin, which aids in maintaining blood pressure by regulating the exchange of water between the cells and the blood; and serum globulin, which assists in the formation of antibodies. A substance called prothrombin is a type of globulin formed by the liver with the aid of vitamin K. It plays an important role in the clotting of the blood.

Cells

The cellular portion of the blood can be divided into three types of cells: red, white, and platelets.

Red Blood Cells   **Erythrocytes** (red blood cells) are biconcave disks with very thin centers to enable them to fold over if necessary to pass through a narrow opening. Red cells number about 25 trillion in the body or about 5 million to a cubic millimeter of blood. It is the red cells that give blood its color. A red blood cell lives about 4 months. They are produced in the bone marrow at a rate of about 1 million a second, the same rate at which they wear out.

Erythrocytes obtain their color from **hemoglobin**, which is a combination of a protein and an iron pigment. It is hemoglobin that attracts and carries the oxygen and carbon dioxide in the blood. When hemoglobin is carrying a lot of oxygen it is bright red in color. As the oxygen is given up to the cells and exchanged for carbon dioxide, the color changes to the dark reddish blue that is visible in surface veins.

White Blood Cells   White blood cells are called **leukocytes**. Leukocytes are present in the blood at approximately 5,000 to 9,000 per cubic millimeter, or about 1 white cell for every 600 to 700 red blood cells. White cells are about twice the size of red blood cells. Leukocytes play a vital role in defending the body against invasion, moving through capillary walls into the tissue fluid to chase down bacteria.

Leukocytes are divided into two major groups, granulocytes and agranulocytes, depending upon the presence of granules and certain staining characteristics.

Granulocytes are produced in red bone marrow and live for only a few days. There are three types. *Neutrophils* phagocytize (destroy) bacteria by surrounding, swallowing, and digesting them. *Eosinophils* are thought to consume the toxic substances in tissues because they are found in increasing numbers when the body has had a foreign protein injected, has an allergic reaction, or has been infected by a parasite. The third type, the *basophils,* are also thought to participate in phagocytosis because their numbers increase with chronic inflammation or during healing from an infection.

Agranulocytes are of two types: *lymphocytes,* which are produced by bone marrow and lymphoid tissues (such as the nodes and spleen), and *monocytes,* which are formed in the bone marrow. Lymphocytes primarily specialize in providing immunity for the body by attaching themselves to foreign bodies and destroying them and by developing antibodies. The monocyte assists with phagocytosis. Some enlarge greatly when they enter tissue and become fixed.

When an inflammation occurs, white cells can divide and proliferate into capsule-like structures around foreign objects that cannot be digested, such as silica dust and carbon particles, or causative organisms of infections, such as tuberculosis. This action effectively walls off involved tissue in an attempt to contain the foreign material or prevent the spread of disease. The evidence of a phagocytic reaction to invading bacteria or a foreign object is the presence of **exudate** (pus). Exudate is composed of lymph, bacteria, and dead white blood cells.

Platelets   The third kind of cell is the **platelet**. These cells are the smallest of the three and are present in the blood at a rate of 200,000 to 400,000 per cubic millimeter. They are also formed in the bone marrow from cell fragments.

Platelets function in the life-saving process of clotting blood. When a blood vessel is cut or damaged, it is believed that the rough surface may catch or attract platelets to the area. This reaction occurs only when there is an incidence of bleeding; otherwise, the clotting process would stop circulation within the blood vessels. When there is a cut, platelets pile up at the site to form a small mass. Once attached firmly to the damaged area, they release the chemical serotonin, which causes the blood vessel to spasm, resulting in a narrowing of the vessel and a decrease in blood loss until the clot can be formed (Figure 11-137). At the same time, platelets and injured tissues release thromboplastin, which triggers the clotting process to begin. The thromboplastin cooperates with calcium ions and other blood clotting factors in the blood to convert prothrombin (present in plasma) into thrombin. The thrombin acts on another protein in the plasma called fibrinogen. This reaction results in the formation of fibrin, tiny threads that form a network of fine mesh fibers over the cut. This net begins to catch the red blood cells, other platelets, and plasma, forming the

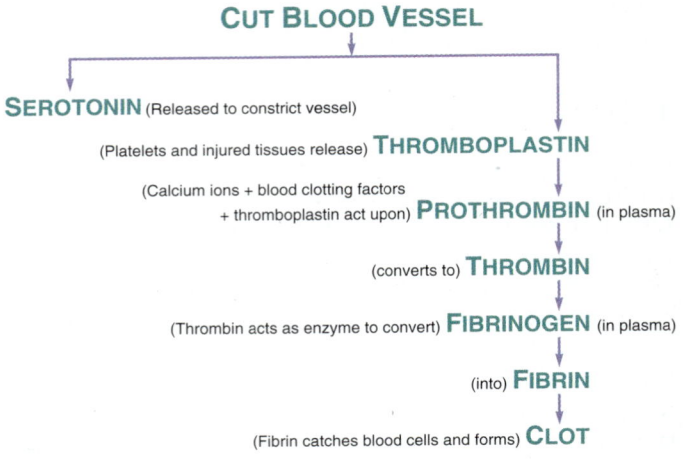

FIGURE 11-137   Process of blood clot formation

clot. It should be remembered that unless the cut blood vessel is small, a clot may not be able to form. The force of the flow of blood will wash away the body's efforts to form fibrin nets and therefore will be unable to collect the ingredients of the clot. Clotting can be assisted by applying pressure over the area to stop the blood flow until a clot can form. When major vessels are cut, it may be necessary to surgically close the opening with sutures to control the bleeding. Fortunately, internal bleeding vessels can also undergo the clotting process. Complications can occur from the clotted mass, especially if the clot or its fragments break loose and enter the circulation before the body's natural "housekeeping" function can gradually remove it from the blood vessel.

Bleeding Time

The length of time required for blood to clot from an induced puncture wound is useful information when preparing a patient for a surgical procedure or evaluating the effects of certain disorders or medications. The normal range of bleeding time for the template puncture method is from 2 to 8 minutes. The length of time varies with the method used.

Blood Types

There are four types of blood: A, B, AB, and O. The type of blood a person has depends on the presence of a protein factor called agglutinogen or antigen on the surface of the red blood cell. Type A blood has an A agglutinogen, type B has a B agglutinogen, type AB has both agglutinogens, and type O has neither (Figure 11-138).

Similarly, a protein known as agglutinin or antibody is present in blood plasma. Type A blood has a *b* agglutinin, type B blood has an *a* agglutinin, type AB has no agglutinins, and type O has both *a* and *b*.

Blood Type	Percent of Population	Antigen/Agglutinogen on Red Blood Cells	Antibody/Agglutinin in Plasma	Can Receive	Can Donate To
A	41%	A	Anti-B	A or O only	A or AB only
B	12%	B	Anti-A	B or O only	B or AB only
AB	3%	A and B	None	A, B, AB, O Universal recipient	AB only
O	44%	None	Anti-A and B	O only	A, B, AB, O Universal donor

FIGURE 11-138   Blood types

The term *agglutinate* refers to the process of clumping or sticking together. Blood clumps and forms clots in the blood vessels if agglutinins and agglutinogens of the same type are mixed together. This reaction can be fatal. Therefore, it is extremely important to determine the blood types of both the recipient and the donor when blood **transfusions** are required. A laboratory test known as type and **cross-match** is necessary to make this determination prior to the administration of either whole blood or packed cell transfusions. Not only is the blood typed, but it is also mixed and observed to ensure that agglutination does not occur. Cross-matching will also detect the presence of subtypes and an agglutinogen known as H.

Figure 11-139 shows how the different types of blood would be distributed through 100 people as identified by the American Red Cross. The need for blood from donors is a constant concern for patients

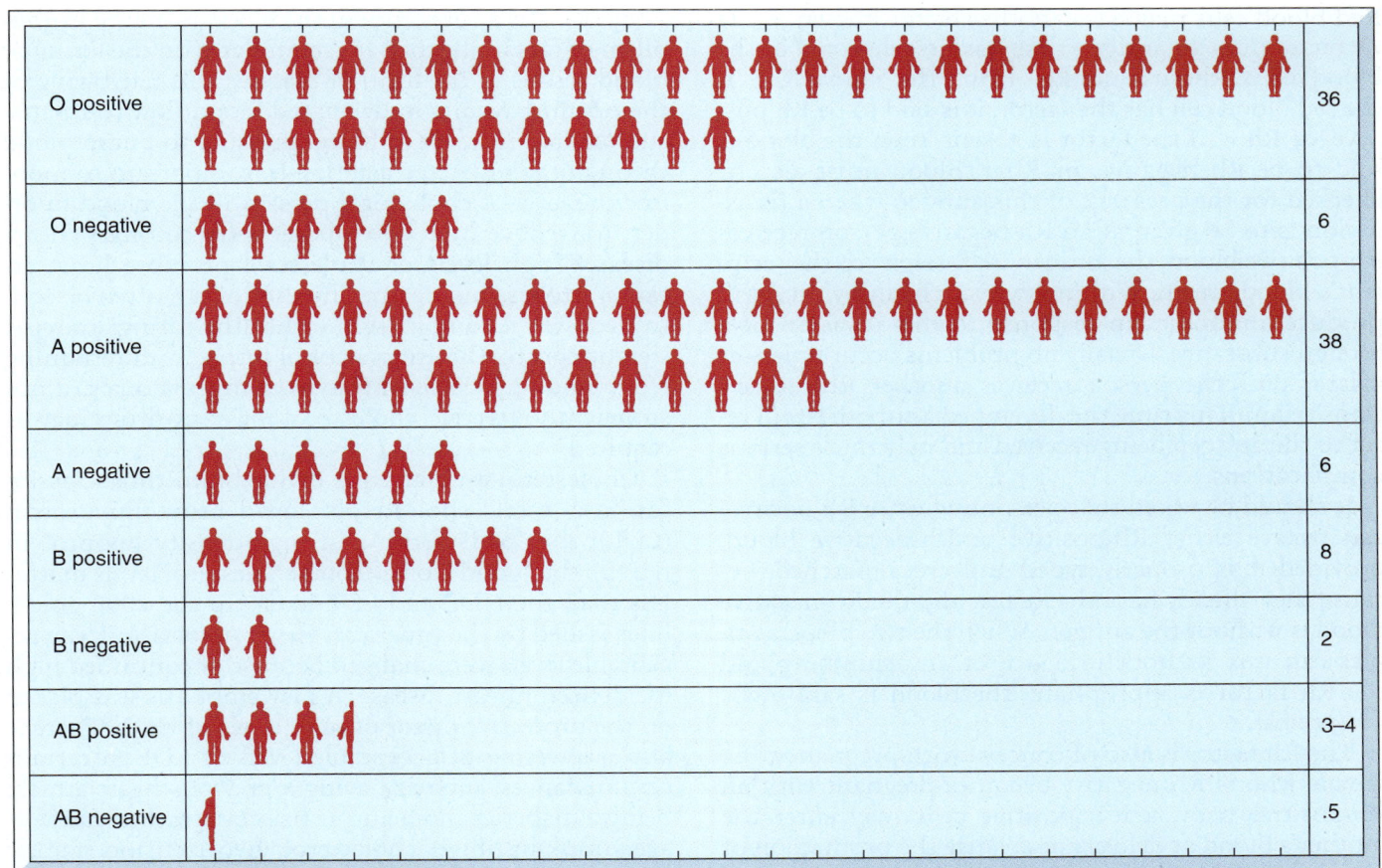

O positive	36
O negative	6
A positive	38
A negative	6
B positive	8
B negative	2
AB positive	3–4
AB negative	.5

FIGURE 11-139   The occurrence of blood types within 100 people as identified by the American Red Cross

and their physicians. Information from the central area of a midwestern state indicates that 550 donors are needed each day. That translates to 16,775 per month or over 200,000 a year. A recent survey showed that 33% of Americans feel there is a great risk of getting AIDS or hepatitis from a transfusion. Currently, with the methods used to screen donors and the tests performed on the blood, it is highly unlikely. The risk of blood-borne AIDS is now only one in 420,000 units of blood; hepatitis is far smaller. A new form of hepatitis called hepatitis "G" has now been identified, so testing for it will be developed. To this point, six types have been found, and more are suspected. Scientists have been trying to develop an artificial blood as a substitute. One firm is now ready to test its product. Another research project has led to the creation of three pigs that carry genes that produce human hemoglobin that can be extracted, chemically modified, and then pasteurized for human use. It has a longer storage life, does not require refrigeration, avoids the risks of human viral diseases, and works in all blood types. At this point, it is in the testing stage.

Rh Factor

Red blood cells may have another factor known as the **Rh factor**. It is an antigen that was first detected in the blood of a Rhesus monkey (thus the name Rh). If the red blood cell has the factor, it is said to be Rh positive, or Rh+. If the factor is absent, then the blood is said to be Rh negative, or Rh−. Blood must also be checked for the presence of this antigen when a transfusion is to be given. If an Rh negative person receives Rh-positive blood, the antigen is "foreign" to the recipient's bloodstream. Within 2 weeks, the individual will produce antibodies in response to this invasion of a foreign substance. Usually no problems occur unless at a later date the person receives another Rh-positive transfusion. This time the developed antibodies will react to the antigen being received and may cause serious complications.

It should be noted that persons who are Rh positive can receive either Rh-positive or Rh-negative blood, provided it is properly typed and cross-matched, because they already have the factor, and the Rh-negative blood is without the antigen. When the two blood samples can mix without evidence of any clumping and the Rh factor is appropriate, the blood is said to be **compatible**.

The Rh factor is also of concern with pregnancy. If a female who is Rh negative becomes pregnant with an Rh-positive baby, a few positive cells may enter the mother's blood at delivery and cause the production of antibodies. The firstborn will not be affected, but if later pregnancies are Rh positive, they may be affected by the antibodies that have been developed. These anti-

bodies slowly filter into the fetal circulation and destroy the Rh-positive red blood cells, making the newborn profoundly anemic and jaundiced. The situation must be treated vigorously with steps taken to alter the infant's blood.

This potentially fatal situation can be avoided by determining the Rh factor of the mother. If she is negative, then the father's factor must be determined before the first child is born. At the time of delivery, if the baby is positive, the Rh-negative mother is given an injection of an Rh(D) immune human globulin, which prohibits the production of antibodies against the baby's Rh-positive blood. Only when the mother is negative and the fetus positive is there cause for concern. If the father is also negative, there is no need to treat for the antibodies unless the mother could have, at some previous time, received an Rh-positive blood transfusion.

The next unit on the immune system takes a deeper look into the function of leukocytes and how they maintain immunity and discusses more about the antigen and antibody process.

Cholesterol

Cholesterol is a substance in the blood from the metabolism of fats in the diet. It accumulates on the lining of blood vessels in the form of plaque. This narrowing of the opening results in decreased blood flow to the tissues and an increase in blood pressure to pump blood through the restricted arteries. It is important to monitor the level of cholesterol present in the blood in order to reduce the development of coronary heart disease. High levels of cholesterol promote heart attacks, strokes, and death. Cholesterol can often be controlled with a combination of healthy eating, exercise, weight control, limiting alcohol intake, and refraining from smoking. When lifestyle changes alone are not sufficiently effective, cholesterol-lowering drugs may be required.

Cholesterol evaluation is divided into three classifications: total cholesterol; low-density lipoprotein (LDL), the "bad" form; and high-density lipoprotein (HDL), the "good" form. Total cholesterol levels matter less than the HDL and LDL levels. In the 2006 guidelines issued by the American Heart Association, the acceptable levels were changed because of continued high incidence of heart disease. A new emphasis was placed on the protective factor of high levels of HDL. There is also a lowering of acceptable levels of LDL in certain circumstances, such as having a previous heart attack; being a diabetic; and being at risk for attack because of age, smoking, high cholesterol, hypertension, family history, and obesity. Diabetes is now considered such a potent risk factor that it automatically places an individual in the lower level category.

The new general guidelines for cholesterol levels are as follows:

TOTAL CHOLESTEROL	
Desirable	Less than 200 mg/dL
Borderline-high	200–239 mg/dL
High	240 mg/dL and above
LDL CHOLESTEROL	
Optimal	Less than 100 mg/dL
Desirable	100–129 mg/dL
Borderline-high	130–159 mg/dL
High	160–184 mg/dL
Very high	190 mg/dL and above
HDL CHOLESTEROL	
Low (risk factor)	Less than 35 mg/dL
High (protective)	60 mg/dL

Interpretation of the results can take several factors into consideration. For example, if the total cholesterol level is high and the HDL level is also high, then it will compensate for a higher LDL level and the overall level may be acceptable. However, a low HDL, regardless of the other levels, is considered a major concern. High LDL cholesterol levels respond well to a group of drugs called statins. The most common are Lipitor, Zocor, Mevacor, Pravachol, and Lescor. They have proven to reduce the risk of coronary artery disease. Many people take drugs as a preventive measure when family history of heart disease is present.

Drug therapy may be considered at certain levels of cholesterol, for example:

● People without coronary heart disease but with two risks factors or less and an LDL level of 190 or higher
● People without coronary heart disease and two or more risk factors with a level of 160 mg/dL or higher
● People with heart disease may begin with a level of 130 mg/dL

Triglycerides

Triglycerides are common types of fats that are good for you in normal amounts. They are present in food and are also manufactured by the body. Abnormally high levels are associated with some common diseases and disorders such as cirrhosis of the liver, underactive thyroid, and inflammation of the pancreas. High levels are also known to be associated with high LDL cholesterol, low HDL cholesterol, and obesity, risk factors for heart disease. It is believed triglycerides contribute to the thickening of arterial walls, which is a predictor of atherosclerosis.

High triglyceride levels are a warning sign of heart disease risk. It is important to lose weight, exercise, stop smoking, limit alcohol intake, control diabetes, and follow a diet low in saturated fat and with a limited intake of carbohydrates. The U.S. National Heart, Lung, and Blood Institute released the following classifications for triglyceride levels in September 2005.

TRIGLYCERIDE LEVEL	CLASSIFICATION
Less than 150 mg/dL	Normal
150–199 mg/dL	Borderline high
200–499 mg/dL	High
500 mg/dL and higher	Very high

CARDIOVASCULAR TESTS

Many sophisticated tests can be performed on the circulatory system, but most of them are best studied at a more advanced level. A few of the more frequently encountered **cardiovascular** diagnostic procedures will be discussed briefly here. Common studies done on blood are discussed in Chapter 15.

● Arteriography (angiography)—A radiologic examination of an artery or arteries after the injection of a contrast medium. The test is used to indicate the status of blood flow, collateral circulation, malformed vessels, an aneurysm, or the presence of **hemorrhage**. Figure 11-140 is an example of an artery following injection. It is often done in connection with cardiac catheterization. A heart catheterization is very helpful in diagnosis. It can reveal faulty motion of the

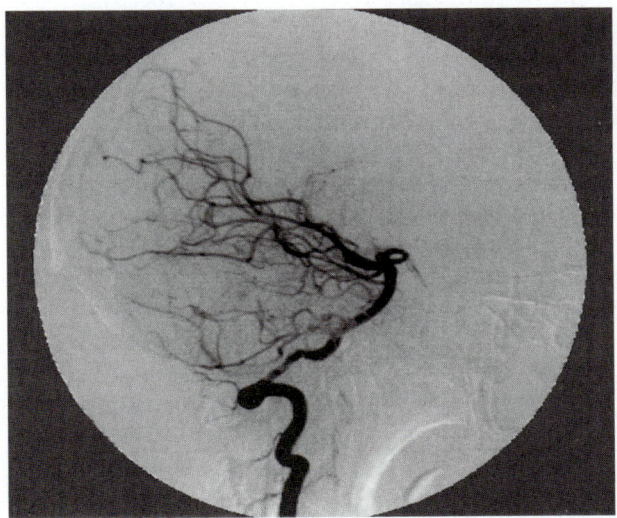

FIGURE 11-140   Example of an angiogram (angiograph) of the brain

heart wall, leakage of blood back through diseased valves, or a hole between the right and left sides. In the coronary arteries, angiography can help locate blockages, which can then be treated with an angioplasty procedure or identified for bypass surgery. About 1 million angioplasties are performed in the United States each year.

- Cardiac catherization—A catheter to the right side of the heart is inserted into a vein at the antecubital space of the right or left arm. A catheter to the left side of the heart is inserted into the brachial artery at the left or right antecubital space. The femoral artery or vein may also be used. The catheter is passed through the blood vessels until it reaches the heart. When it is determined by fluoroscopy that the catheter is properly positioned, a contrast medium is injected to permit visualization. The heart's chambers and valves and the coronary arteries or the pulmonary artery may be viewed, depending on the site being catheterized. The procedure can also be used to measure blood pressure within the pulmonary artery and some portions of the heart. It is used in connection with coronary angiography. Figure 11-141 illustrates the usual points of insertion of the cardiac catheter. Notice the different shapes of the catheter tips that help to guide the catheter into the desired position.
- Dobutamine stress test—This is a variation of the cardiac stress test that also combines the information from an echocardiogram. A resting state echocardiogram is performed first to evaluate the myocardium, the valves, the blood flow, and the action of the heart. Then, dobutamine is given intravenously in ever-increasing amounts to "stress" the

heart chemically without the need for exercise. During the test, additional echocardiogram findings are taken and the blood pressure is monitored. At peak stress, additional echocardiogram pictures are taken. A continuous ECG records the activity of the heart throughout the examination. Upon completion, the effects of dobutamine gradually subside, and the patient's heart rate returns to normal. This combination of diagnostic tools gives the cardiologist a fairly complete picture of structural and functional aspects of the heart. Other drugs, such as Persantine or Adenostine, are used with a radioactive tracer (such as Cardiolite) and a special camera to produce similar studies of the heart.

- Doppler ultrasonography—Sound waves are transmitted through the skin and are reflected by the cells in the blood moving through the blood vessels (Figure 11-142). This diagnostic tool can evaluate the major blood vessels of the body to determine deep vein **thrombosis** (DVT), peripheral arterial **aneurysms**, and occluded carotid arteries.
- Echocardiogram—This is a noninvasive test that uses ultrasound (high-frequency sound waves) to make images of the internal structures of the heart. A special gel is applied to the chest wall, and a hand-held device called a transducer is maneuvered over the heart area. Sounds waves are transmitted through the skin and strike the structures of the heart, sending echoes back to the transducer. The machine converts the information into images that are displayed on the screen and produce an image or picture of the structures of the heart and its chambers. The test evaluates cardiac function and structure and can reveal valve ir-

Possible points of insertion

Femoral artery

Femoral vein

Upper thigh insertion

Arm insertion

Brachial artery

Antecubital vein

(A)

Commonly used catheters

Right heart catheter

Left coronary artery catheter

Catheter used for injections

Right coronary artery catheter

(B)

FIGURE 11-141   (A) Points of insertion for a cardiac catheter; (B) commonly used catheters

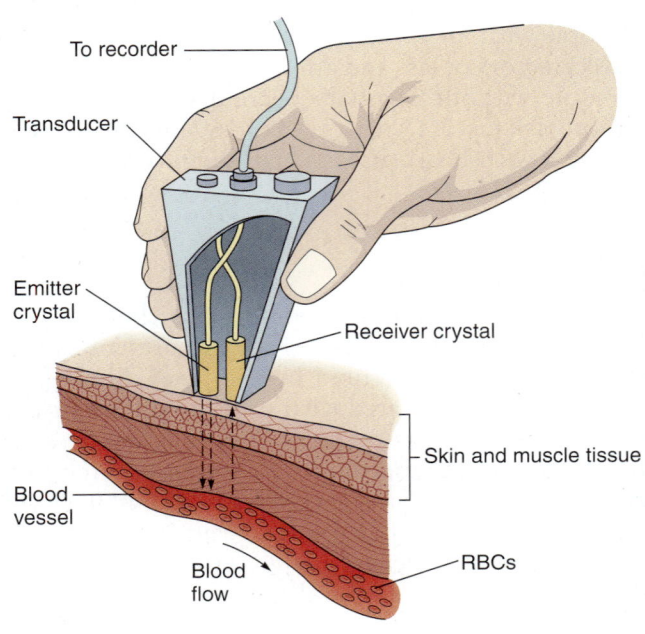

How the Doppler probe works

To recorder

Transducer

Emitter crystal

Receiver crystal

Skin and muscle tissue

Blood vessel

Blood flow

RBCs

FIGURE 11-142   Doppler ultrasound

regularities, defects in the interior walls, and the presence of fluid between the layers of the pericardium.

- Electrocardiograph (ECG)—This test is also called EKG. It is perhaps the most common tool used to evaluate heart performance. The ECG is a graphic recording of the electrical activity of the heart. It identifies rhythm, abnormalities in conduction, and electrolyte imbalance. The graph is useful in documenting diagnosis and provides a method of measuring progression of cardiac disease conditions. The ECG also helps evaluate the effectiveness of an artificial pacemaker and cardiac medications.

The test may be taken while the patient is lying in a comfortable position or in an exercise mode, such as bicycling or walking a treadmill. The exercise mode measures the effects of controlled physical stress and is referred to as a *stress ECG*. Frequently, abnormalities of cardiac action are more evident upon exertion.

Another type of ECG is called the **Holter monitor** or **ambulatory** (walking) ECG. The ECG electrodes are attached to the patient's chest wall and a portable cassette recorder (monitor) is placed in a belt about the waist. For a 24-hour period, the patient's heart action is recorded, and a diary is kept of daily activities and any associated symptoms. At the end of the test, the recording is analyzed by computer, and a report is printed. This type of test is most beneficial for symptoms that occur irregularly or to evaluate the status of recovering cardiac patients. Another version permits the patient to activate the recording device only when experiencing symptoms. This patient-activated monitor can be worn for several days. (See Chapter 16.)

- Heart scan—This noninvasive test using a high-speed scanner takes accurate pictures of the heart in less than a second. The technology is known as ultra-fast CT scan and is done by an electron beam tomography scanner. (This same technology can also scan the chest, abdomen, and pelvis). The scanner sweeps electron beams across the patient so quickly that it actually freezes the beating motion of the heart. The scan is helpful in screening for calcified plaque in coronary arteries. Figure 11-143 illustrates the presence of cal-

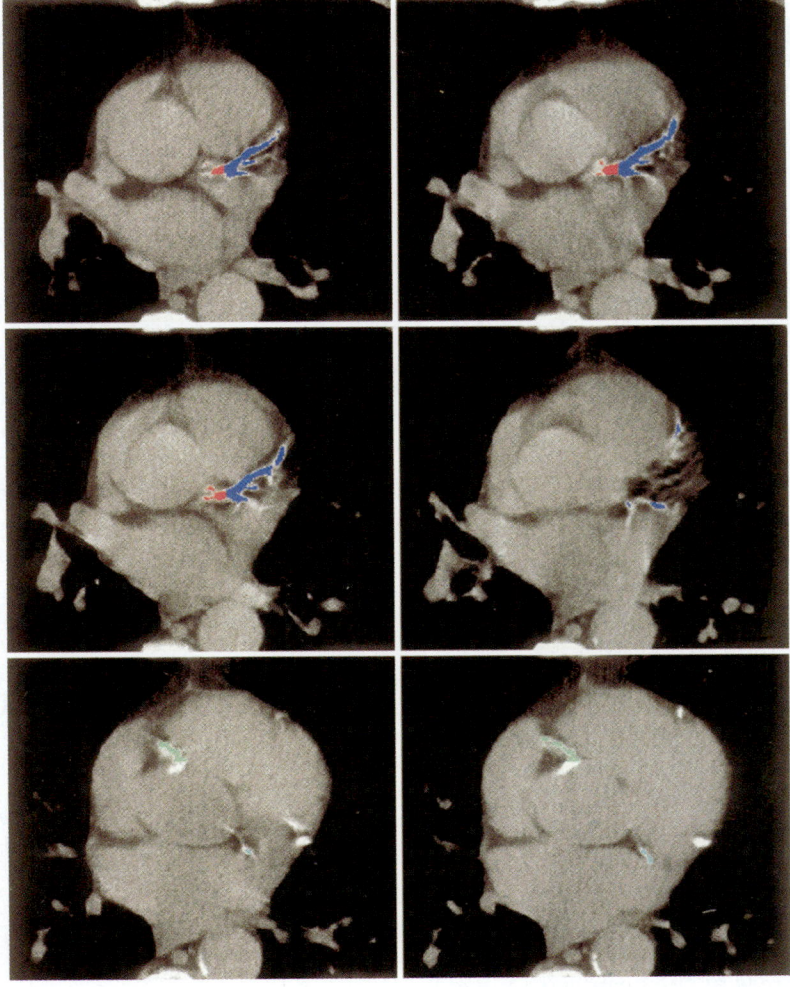

FIGURE 11-143 Heart images showing different amounts of calcified plaque in arteries *(Courtesy of CAT SCAN 2000)*

cified plaque. The amount of calcification is measured and given a score that is an indicator of the degree of coronary artery occlusion. The scan is a screening tool and provides a baseline assessment of coronary artery condition. It can identify coronary disease before symptoms of artery blockage occur, thereby permitting lifestyle changes and treatment to prevent a heart attack. Typically, blockage must be about 50% or more before it can be detected by a stress test.

- **MUGA scan**—MUGA is an acronym for MUltiple Gated Acquisition; it is a test to evaluate the condition of the myocardium of the heart. The test can be done in a resting or exercise mode. Isotopes are injected intravenously and are taken up by the myocardium. The scintillation camera records the motion of the heart. The test permits measurement of ventricular contractions to evaluate the strength of the heart wall. Patients who receive a chemotherapeutic drug that has cardiac toxicity side effects are monitored periodically by MUGA scans because of the drug's tendency to damage the myocardium.

- Myocardial perfusion imaging—This is a test to measure the passage of blood through the coronary arteries to the myocardium. The first part of the test involves "stressing" the heart by dilating the arteries with a special IV medication. This is done over a 6-minute period. (Normal arteries will dilate more than partially or completely blocked arteries.) The heart is monitored during the test by ECG. After dilation, a radioactive imaging material is injected into the IV. The material concentrates in those parts of the myocardium that have the best blood flow. For about 45 minutes, the camera records images that identify any part of the heart that is not getting enough blood. Later, after the dilating drug has worn off, a series of images will be taken to show perfusion of the heart "at rest." The two series are compared to identify the differences in blood flow. A healthy heart will show little difference.

- Stress thallium ECG—This test evaluates myocardial blood flow and the condition of the cells. The ECG electrodes are attached to the patient before performing the stress test on either a treadmill or a bicycle. The blood pressure and pulse rate are carefully monitored. When the patient reaches peak stress, the thallium is injected intravenously into the antecubital vein and the exercise continued for an additional minute to ensure circulation of the isotope to the heart. The ECG electrodes are removed, and within 3 to 5 minutes the patient is positioned under the scintillation camera. The scanner records the amount of thallium uptake by the heart over the next several minutes. Areas of the heart with normal blood supply and healthy cells rapidly take up the isotope. Areas of poor blood flow or damaged cells

do not take up the material and appear as dark spots on the scan; these are known as cold spots.

The test is indicated for assessing myocardial condition, demonstrating the location and extent of a **myocardial infarction (MI)**, diagnosing coronary artery disease, and determining the effectiveness of artery grafts and angioplasty procedures. Persantine thallium is also a type of stress test. It is used for patients with arthritis or any other condition that prevents a patient from exercising. It determines the presence of coronary artery disease.

- Transesophogeal echocardiography (TEE)—In this procedure a transducer device is inserted into the esophagus behind the heart to more thoroughly view portions of the heart. In about 10% of patients, external echocardiography cannot provide a clear enough picture. Chest deformities, chronic lung disease, and obesity are the main reasons for poor-quality imaging. TEE is particularly helpful when valve abnormalities, blood clots, tumors, growths, and aortic dissection (tears in the artery) are suspected. It may also be beneficial in detecting valve hardening, stenosis, and fungus or bacterial infections.

- Venogram—This radiographic examination uses a contrast medium to determine the condition of the deep veins of the legs. It is especially useful in determining the presence of deep vein thrombosis (DVT), which may occlude the vein systems and lead to pulmonary embolism, a potentially lethal situation. DVT may result from vein injury, prolonged bed rest, surgery, childbirth, irregularity in the coagulation process, or the use of oral contraceptives.

- Ultrasound, cardiac—(See Echocardiograph.)

- Ultrasound, carotid artery—This noninvasive test measures the thickness of the carotid arteries of the neck using sound waves to create images. It was discovered that the risk of heart attack and stroke increased in direct proportion to the thickness of the artery walls. The thicker the walls, the greater the buildup of atherosclerotic plaque. The people with the thickest walls had more than double the risk of stroke and heart attack as those with thin-walled arteries.

DISEASES AND DISORDERS

Anemia (A-ne′me-a)

Description—This term indicates that certain elements are lacking in the blood. There are various types of **anemias**.

Iron Deficiency Anemia   This is the most common form of anemia.

Description—This form is characterized by an inadequate supply of iron to form normal red blood cells.

When the body's supply of iron decreases, so does the number of red blood cells and, as a result, the hemoglobin. This reduces the body's ability to carry oxygen to the cells.

Signs and symptoms—Symptoms include fatigue, listlessness, pallor, inability to concentrate, and difficulty in breathing on exertion.

Etiology—Iron deficiency anemia develops from an inadequate dietary intake of iron or inability of the body to absorb iron as the result of diarrhea, partial or total removal of the stomach, or certain diseases. It can also be caused by intestinal bleeding, heavy menstruation, colon cancer, or bleeding ulcers. It is most common among premature infants, children, adolescents (especially girls), and women before menopause.

Treatment—Iron deficiency is treated by first identifying the underlying cause. Once determined, iron replacement can begin. Oral preparations of iron or iron combined with ascorbic acid are given. Intramuscular injections are possible but not desirable because of the discomfort produced. Intravenous infusion is relatively painless and requires fewer injections.

Aplastic Anemia

Description and causes—Aplastic anemia results from injury or destruction of the blood cell formation by the bone marrow.

Signs and symptoms—This disease generally produces symptoms of weakness and fatigue.

Treatment—Treatment for aplastic anemia must first rule out any identifiable cause and follow with transfusions of pack cells. Recovery may take months. Bone marrow transplant is the treatment of choice in severe aplastic anemia and with those needing constant RBC transfusions. The use of corticosteroids and bone marrow stimulants is appropriate in some cases.

Blood Loss Anemia

Description and causes—This term describes conditions of low red blood cell count occurring over extended periods of time. However, low red blood cell count can also occur following an acute blood loss and is referred to by some as acute blood loss anemia.

Signs and symptoms—In this instance, there is a sudden loss of red blood cells and therefore hemoglobin and iron. The rapid loss of blood volume can be fatal.

Etiology—Acute blood loss can result from severe trauma, the inability to coagulate the blood, ruptured gastric or intestinal ulcers, postoperative bleeding, postpartum (after birth) hemorrhage, or a ruptured aneurysm. A loss of 20% to 30% of blood volume causes circulatory insufficiency with symptoms of shock, restlessness, low blood pressure, rapid pulse, perspiration, and cool, clammy skin. With a loss greater than 30%, the circulatory system

may fail and be followed by shock and then coma. Blood loss beyond 40% is life threatening, and the patient will die unless blood volume is immediately replaced.

Treatment—The treatment goal in acute blood loss anemia is to control the hemorrhage and restore blood volume. Prevention of shock is very important. Immediate infusion of IV fluids, electrolyte solutions, and plasma can increase the circulating volume while packed cells or whole blood are being typed and cross-matched for infusion.

Aneurysm (An'u-rism)

Description—This is the ballooning out of the wall of an artery. Often an aneurysm is associated with **atherosclerosis** or **arteriosclerosis** and hypertension.

Etiology—A slight break or weakness in the muscular layer of an artery allows the pressure of the blood to push the walls of the blood vessel out (Figure 11-144). The larger the bulge, the thinner the arterial wall becomes. Eventually, the wall gives way and a hemorrhage occurs. The extent of the bleeding and its effects on the body depend to a great extent on the location of the aneurysm and the size of the involved blood vessel.

Aneurysms are found primarily in cerebral arteries, the thoracic or abdominal section of the aorta, and the femoral and popliteal arteries of the leg. Some aneurysms are without symptoms and are discovered by accident or an x-ray.

Cerebral Aneurysm   This type occurs within the brain.

Description—Depending on its location, it may rupture and cause bleeding within the subarachnoid space, or an artery within the brain tissue itself may rupture. If the hemorrhage is not too massive, the blood clots. Later, the body will slowly reabsorb the blood

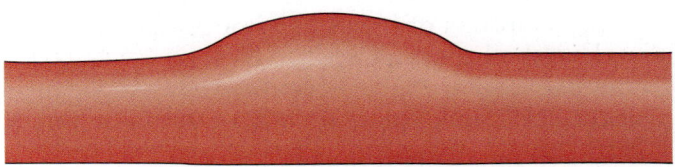

Saccular—unilateral pouchlike bulge

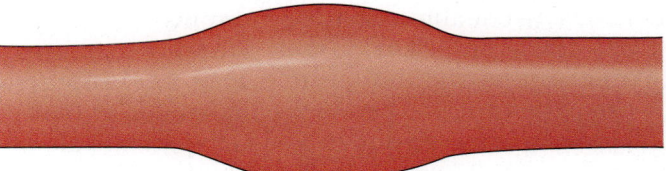

Fusiform—a spindle-shaped bulge of the entire artery wall

FIGURE 11-144   Types of aneurysms

clots, and function will return. Hemorrhage may be fatal, however, because of increased intracranial pressure from the blood, which compresses and damages brain tissue. Remember, the skull does not stretch; therefore, when bleeding occurs, the delicate tissues of the brain are displaced and damaged. Cerebral aneurysms are graded from I to V depending on the amount of bleeding. Rebleeding after 7 to 10 days is not uncommon. When the initial blood has clotted, the body resumes its normal function of removing clotted material, which may lead to a renewed and often fatal recurrence.

Signs and symptoms—Usually the onset is without warning, but headache, nuchal (back of neck) rigidity, stiffness in the back and legs, and intermittent nausea may be present for several days preceding the rupture. Upon rupture, there is a sudden severe headache, nausea, vomiting, and maybe some altered level of consciousness, including coma. Following bleeding, there may be back and leg pain, restlessness, fever, irritability, and occasionally seizures and blurred vision. If there is bleeding into the tissues, there may be paralysis, sensory deficits, difficulty speaking, and visual defects.

Treatment—Treatment is directed toward reducing the risk of rebleeding by repairing the aneurysm surgically. When the patient's condition will not withstand the surgery, a conservative treatment is indicated. This involves bed rest for 4 to 6 weeks; avoidance of coffee, other stimulants, and aspirin; analgesics as needed; a hypotensive drug if there is hypertension; corticosteroids to reduce edema; a drug to delay blood clot destruction; and sedatives to reduce stress.

Thoracic Aortic Aneurysms

Description—These occur as a result of great pressure in the artery. Rupture of the aorta is usually fatal. If the thoracic aneurysm begins by "splitting" of the wall, the person may experience a tearing or ripping sensation accompanied by chest pain, pallor, rapid pulse, shortness of breath, loss of pulses below the neck, and other symptoms.

Treatment—Surgery can remove the damaged segment of the aorta and replace it with a Dacron or Teflon graft.

Abdominal Aortic Aneurysms

Description—Usually without symptoms, this type is detectable on palpation as a pulsating mass in an area around the umbilicus (navel). If it ruptures, the patient may experience pain similar to that of kidney spasms. About 20% of such patients die immediately; however, if the bleeding is in the retroperitoneal space (behind the peritoneal lining of the abdomen), the limited space puts pressure

on the tear as it fills with blood, closing off the opening.

Treatment—An abdominal aneurysm is repaired like an aneurysm of the thoracic aorta. In addition, an external Dacron prosthesis (artificial part) may be applied around the aneurysm and sutured into place to support the weakened wall.

Aneurysms in the lower extremities may interfere with circulation and result in severe **ischemia** (lack of blood) and gangrene (tissue death), which may require amputation of the extremity.

Angina (An'ji-na)

Description—This heart condition causes severe chest pain that radiates down the inner surface of the left arm, usually associated with emotional stress or physical exertion. The episode may last from a few seconds to several minutes.

Signs and symptoms—Symptoms, in addition to the pain, include irregular heart rate, lowered blood pressure, anxiety, and perspiration.

Etiology—The pain is believed to be caused by a spasm or blockage of one or more coronary arteries, which results in ischemia to a portion of the heart muscle.

Treatment—The treatment consists of nitroglycerin, in a tablet form, placed under the tongue. The nitroglycerin dilates the constricted artery or arteries to permit the flow of blood to the heart tissue. When **angina** pain persists after 10 minutes and the use of three sublingual tablets, the patient should go directly to the nearest hospital emergency room.

The patient must be instructed to have nitroglycerin available at all times. Tablets must be kept in a dark, tightly closed bottle, without cotton, and be protected from heat and sunlight. Tablets over 3 months old should be discarded. Nitroglycerin is also available as an oral spray or in the form of a paste that is applied to the skin to permit prolonged release of the drug in measurable doses. Other medications, such as calcium channel blockers and beta blockers, are also used to prevent angina.

A new little-known procedure is being used in specific centers in the United States. It is thought useful in about 5% to 15% of angina sufferers who are *not* candidates for established alternatives. It is called Enhanced External Counterpulsation. It involves the use of "cuffs" positioned around the legs, thighs, and hips. The apparatus is operated by a computer that synchronizes pulsations to the heartbeat and a compressor that inflates the cuffs, forcing blood to the arteries when the heart muscle is relaxed. This increases blood flow to the heart and decreases the workload. It requires daily 1-hour treatments for 35 days. At present, the treatment is limited to patients with stable angina who are not candidates for other treatments. The patients treated have shown a decrease in the frequency and intensity of pain and an increase in exercise tolerance. Some have been able to resume work and even exercise. The treatment is noninvasive but does require a considerable investment in time. At present, insurance will not cover the costs because it is considered experimental.

Arrest (Cardiac)

Description—This is complete, sudden cessation of heart action. The condition is rapidly fatal, producing irreversible brain damage after 5 minutes.

Signs and symptoms—The major symptom is the sudden ending of heart function, hence the absence of heartbeat and pulse.

Etiology—It is believed to result from a failure in the body's ability to transport calcium, which interferes with its electrical and mechanical functions. It is associated with a severe lack of blood to the myocardium. Cardiac arrest can also be caused by heart failure, electrical shock, fibrillation, drowning, anesthetics, respiratory failure, and severe electrolyte imbalances.

Treatment—Arrest is treated initially by external cardiac massage (cardiopulmonary resuscitation [CPR] technique), then supplemented by defibrillation, IV drug therapy, and ventilation procedures. Death is certain if function cannot be restored quickly.

Arrhythmia (A-rith-me-a)

Description—This term is used to identify any abnormal changes in the heart rhythm. Arrhythmias vary in severity from mild to life threatening, as with fibrillation. They are classified according to the origin of the irregularity (e.g., PVC or atrial flutter). The more the heart action is affected, the greater the consequences on the cardiac output and the blood pressure, which in turn determines the clinical significance.

Signs and symptoms—The presence of an irregular heart action pattern.

Etiology—Arrhythmias may be congenital or may result from myocardial anoxia, infarction, hypertrophy of muscle fiber from hypertension, or degeneration of conductive tissue required to maintain normal rhythm.

Treatment—Treatment varies in relation to the cause and severity of the irregularity from no treatment to medication, eliminating known causes, CPR, and the insertion of a pacemaker.

Arrhythmia that produces extra beats, delayed beats, or missed beats often results from caffeine, amphetamine, or a medication reaction and can usually be treated by removing the causative factor.

Arteriosclerosis (Ar-tere-olo-skle-ro'sis)

Description—In this "hardening" of the arteries and arterioles, the muscular and elastic tissue is gradually replaced by fibrous tissue and calcification. Because the vessels are no longer capable of expanding and recoiling with each heartbeat, the heart must exert more pressure on the blood to pump it through the more rigid vessels. Arteriosclerosis results in high blood pressure and may lead to an aneurysm and cerebral hemorrhage.

Signs and symptoms—The major sign is hypertension.

Etiology—The artery and arteriole walls become fibrous and contain calcium deposits.

Treatment—The prime focus of treatment is aimed at preventing the rupture of an aneurysm or a CVA (stroke) by reducing blood pressure.

Atherosclerosis (Ather-oskle-ro'sis)

Description—This condition is characterized by the deposit of fatty material along the linings of the arteries (Figure 11-145). As the material builds up, the opening of the artery may become partially or totally closed, thereby reducing or eliminating the flow of

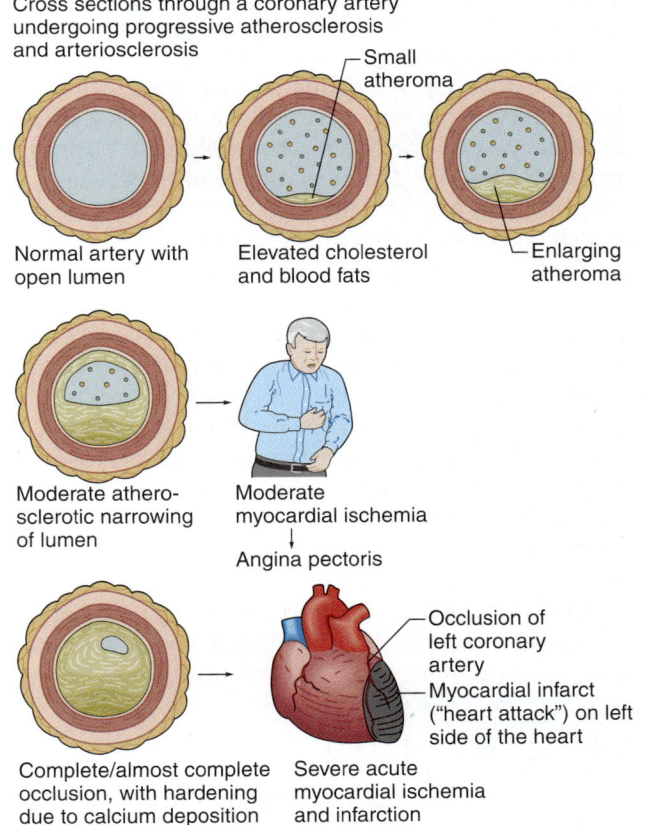

Cross sections through a coronary artery undergoing progressive atherosclerosis and arteriosclerosis

Small atheroma

Normal artery with open lumen

Elevated cholesterol and blood fats

Enlarging atheroma

Moderate atherosclerotic narrowing of lumen

Moderate myocardial ischemia
↓
Angina pectoris

Complete/almost complete occlusion, with hardening due to calcium deposition

Severe acute myocardial ischemia and infarction

Occlusion of left coronary artery

Myocardial infarct ("heart attack") on left side of the heart

FIGURE 11-145   The natural history of coronary heart disease

blood to the area. Atherosclerosis can also result in elevated blood pressure, but the greatest danger is a blocked coronary artery and heart attack. There is also danger from the atherosclerotic plaque deposits that can break loose and circulate through the bloodstream as emboli.

Signs and symptoms—The major symptom is determined by the territory affected by the blocked blood vessel. Examination of the interior of arteries would show plaque of lipids and fat deposits. Decreased circulation symptoms are particularly observable in the carotid, coronary, and lower extremity arteries.

Etiology—Atherosclerosis is linked to many risk factors: family history, hypertension, obesity, smoking, diabetes, stress, sedentary lifestyle, and high serum cholesterol and triglyceride levels.

Treatment—If there is coronary involvement, the goal of treatment is to prevent occlusion of the arteries and prevent myocardial infarction. Dietary restrictions to reduce intake of salt, fats, and cholesterol; abstaining from smoking; and reducing stress are indicated. Angioplasty is used to open the blocked arterial segment. With complete obstruction, bypass surgery may be indicated.

Athletic Heart Syndrome

Description—This is a series of cardiac changes resulting from strenuous exercise. Primarily, the heart enlarges (cardiomegaly), particularly the ventricles, because of its adaptive ability to meet the body's need for increased output. Because the heart is a muscle, it reacts just as the biceps do to physical endurance training. This syndrome is increasing because of the emphasis on physical fitness.

Signs and symptoms—The athletic heart usually produces no symptoms except perhaps pounding or irregularity after strenuous activity. Bradycardia of 40 beats per minute is common and may be considered "normal" because of the heart's increased efficiency upon contraction.

Etiology—The syndrome is probably a physiologic response to maintaining optimal cardiac performance during physical endurance training. The stress placed on the heart causes the left ventricle to enlarge and thicken in order to meet the demand for more oxygen and hence more blood flow.

Treatment—Nothing is required unless there is underlying cardiac disease, which will necessitate discontinuing training.

Carditis (Kar-di'tis)

Description—Literally, it is inflammation of the heart. The term is usually used with one of three prefixes that define the portion of the heart that is involved. The in-flammation results from an infectious process caused by a viral, fungal, or bacterial invasion. Other causes vary with the form of inflammation, as follows.

Pericarditis (Per-i-kar-di'tis)

Description—An inflammation of the pericardium, the fibroserous tissue sac that covers the heart.

Signs and symptoms—It may result in a purulent or bloody exudate forming within the sac, or the tissue may become thickened and fibrous, constricting the filling action of the heart. Pericarditis can follow injury to the heart, an infarction, or cardiac surgery.

Acute pericarditis typically causes sharp, sudden pain that begins at the sternum and radiates across the back to the shoulders and arms. It is similar to pleurisy, becoming more intense on inspiration but decreasing when sitting upright and leaning forward. A very serious condition known as tamponade will occur if the collection of fluid within the pericardium is rapid. Pressure within the sac prevents ventricular filling during diastole, thereby severely decreasing cardiac output and resulting in pallor, hypotension, and eventually cardiovascular collapse and death.

Etiology—Acute pericarditis is caused by bacterial, fungal, or viral infections. It can be caused by noninfectuous etiologies as well.

Treatment—With tamponade, emergency treatment to remove the fluid by needle aspiration or surgical incision will result in a dramatic improvement.

Pericarditis that causes a gradual fluid accumulation allows time for the pericardium to stretch, often to hold 1 to 2 liters of fluid. Chronic pericarditis that results in constriction or recurrent collection of fluid may necessitate partial removal of the pericardium to allow escape of the fluid or, if constriction, a total pericardectomy (removal of the pericardium).

Myocarditis (Mio-kar-di'tis)

Description—An inflammation of the myocardium (heart muscle). It can occur in both acute and chronic forms.

Signs and symptoms—Symptoms produced are generally nonspecific, such as fatigue, palpitations, fever, and dyspnea. It is usually an uncomplicated disease and is self-limiting in nature. Normally, it is associated with a recent upper respiratory infection (URI) and fever.

Myocarditis may produce mild chest soreness and a feeling of pressure, but not the anginal type of pain. Occasionally, myocarditis may initiate a degenerative process of the tiny fibrils (small fibers) in the muscular tissue. This may result in heart failure, enlargement, and arrhythmia.

Etiology—Myocarditis is caused by a viral or bacterial infection, an immune reaction (rheumatic fever), radiation therapy to the chest, and effects of chemicals, such as in chronic alcoholism.

Treatment—Myocarditis is treated with bed rest and appropriate measures for complications that may develop.

Endocarditis (En-do-kar-di'tis)

Description—This is infection of the endocardial lining, heart valves, tissue adjoining artificial valves, or the blood vessel linings. In the infectious process, fibrin and platelets collect where the invading circulating organisms have produced wartlike vegetations on the valves and often the surrounding structures. The vegetative growths may cause serious complications if they embolize to the spleen, kidneys, lungs, or brain.

Etiology—The infecting organism in acute endocarditis is usually a streptococcus, staphylococcus, or pneumococcus. The gonococcus is also capable of causing endocarditis. Intravenous drug abuse may lead to infections from staph or fungi normally present on the skin surface. A subacute form may affect persons with valve or other cardiac lesions that may be acquired or congenital.

Treatment—If endocarditis is left untreated, it usually results in death. Recovery is improved to 70% with proper treatment. When severe valve damage occurs, resulting complications may include insufficient cardiac action and congestive failure caused by improper valve function. Damaged valves can be surgically removed with open heart surgery and replaced with artificial valves. If the infection involves an artificial valve, surgery to replace the prosthesis will be required. Often valves from pigs or cows are used to replace damaged human heart valves and function very effectively.

Cerebrovascular Accident (CVA) (Sere-bro-vas'ku-lar)

Description—A condition commonly known as a stroke, CVA is the sudden impairment of the flow of blood to the brain, thereby diminishing or interrupting the supply of oxygen and causing serious damage or destruction of brain tissue. Because of the urgency for intervention and treatment, strokes are now being referred to as "brain attacks." The phrase "time is brain" also emphasizes the importance of immediate treatment. Strokes are the third leading cause of death and the leading cause of serious long-term disability in the United States. The risk of stroke doubles each succeeding decade of life, beginning at age 55. More men than women have strokes, but women are more likely to die. African Americans and Latinos have a higher rate than whites. Strokes are often referred to as the silent killer because usually no symptoms are noticed in advance.

CVAs are classified according to their cause and effect. **Transient ischemic attacks** (TIAs) are small, temporary interruptions of blood flow. These are referred to as "warning strokes" because they may happen before a major stroke. The symptoms usually last only a few minutes. The most common major stroke is an ischemic stroke, meaning a blood vessel is blocked by a clot and stops all flow of blood to a portion of the brain. A rarer but more dangerous type of stroke is called hemorrhagic, meaning a blood vessel has ruptured, and the escaping blood is damaging brain tissue either by pressure against it or from lack of circulation through the tissue.

Signs and symptoms—Symptoms vary with the area of the brain that is involved. CVAs involving posterior cerebral arteries affect the vision and often result in coma. Anterior artery involvement results in confusion, weakness, loss of coordination, personality changes, and numbness, especially in the legs. If the CVA occurs in the right hemisphere of the brain, symptoms are produced on the left side of the body, and if in the left hemisphere, on the right side. A CVA may leave the patient with many varied symptoms that may include slurred speech, amnesia, dizziness, paralysis (one extremity, one side, or total), inability to speak, coma, double vision, incontinence (inability to control bladder and bowels), and rigidity. In addition, hemorrhagic stroke usually causes severe headache, difficulty breathing, nausea, and vomiting.

Etiology—A **cerebrovascular accident** is the result of high blood pressure, which ruptures an artery; atherosclerosis, which occludes an artery; or thrombosis (a blood clot), which interrupts the flow of blood. When a large enough area is involved, death will result.

All medical personnel should be familiar with the warning signs of stroke as listed in Table 11-6.

Treatment—Remember, with stroke every minute counts. Patients should go to the emergency room immedi-

---

TABLE 11-6   The Warning Signs of Stroke

- The development of difficulty in speaking or in understanding simple statements.
- Sudden blurred or decreased vision.
- Loss of balance or coordination when combined with another warning sign.
- Numbness, weakness, or paralysis of face, arm, or leg—especially on one side of the body.
- Loss of consciousness or severe drowsiness.
- A sudden, severe headache.

These signs could represent a stroke; call 911 or other emergency assistance immediately.

ately either by EMS services, or, if it is quicker, by private car. The patient must NOT drive himself. Upon arrival, a CT scan or MRI will be ordered to identify the type of stroke, the location, and the extent of the damage. With ischemic stroke, a clot buster called tissue plasminogen activator (tPA) is administered intravenously (IV) or directly into the brain by catheter for about 1 hour. It can dissolve about 60% to 80% of the clots and effectively prevent brain damage but ONLY if given within 3 hours of the onset of symptoms. A new clot-busting chemical called prouro-kinase is being tested and has shown to minimize brain damage up to 6 hours after a stroke. Also, a nontoxic form of snake venom was accidentally discovered that is effective up to 6 hours as well. There is always danger from any clot-buster because the blood rushes back in after the blockage is cleared, and the weakened arteries can result in life-threatening bleeding in about 6.5% of patients. An experimental device is being researched as an alternative treatment. It is a tiny pump called an AngioJet that vacuums up a clot almost instantly and without chemicals. It is hoped this proves to be a safer, more effective treatment.

A hemorrhagic stroke is treated differently. Administering tPA could cause life-threatening brain hemorrhage. These patients are treated with methods to control heart rhythm, stabilize blood pressure, and monitor brain function. Unfortunately, little can be done to quickly solve the effects of the hemorrhage.

Research has found that administering neuroprotective materials within 24 hours helps protect the damaged cells. Enzyme-blocking chemicals may be effective for more than a week to prevent damaged cells from dying. After approximately 1 year, little additional progress toward recovery is anticipated.

Scientists have developed many exciting devices to help maximize the patient's ability to function. A "Handmaster" uses voice activation to duplicate brain impulses to move extremities. A minute computer chip has been implanted in the brain to allow brain signals to form a readout on a computer screen so that a person who is paralyzed and mute can communicate. Also, encouraging results are being achieved from infusion of millions of fresh lab-grown neurons into the damaged brain. It was discovered that when cancerous cells in a lab were treated with retinoic acid, they transformed into healthy neurons. Initially, lab rats were induced to have strokes, and following neuron injection, they regained function. A few humans have received these neuron transplants and are showing improvements for the first time since their devastating strokes.

Perhaps the best treatment is prevention. The strongest predictors of stroke are hypertension, irregular heartbeat, diabetes, a sedentary lifestyle, and use of tobacco. Some protective measures may be beneficial. The use of vitamins B_6 and B_{12} and folic acid seems to help because they lower homocysteine levels. It appears that drinking up to two alcoholic drinks per day offers protection against ischemic stroke by increasing HDL cholesterol and tPA levels to keep clots from forming. Higher intake increases risk for hemorrhagic stroke.

Congestive Heart Failure (CHF)

Description—This group of cardiac dysfunctions results in poor performance of the heart with related congestion of the circulatory system. Usually the myocardium of the left ventricle is affected, often as a result of prolonged high blood pressure. **Congestive heart failure** can also be a complication of coronary artery disease or a result of a mechanical disorder involving the heart's valvular functions. It may also be caused by myocarditis and left ventricular dysfunction.

Left-Sided Heart Failure

Description—Cardiac output is decreased; however, the left atrium continues to force blood into the ventricle, resulting in increased pressure and volume within the ventricle. As this backup continues, the left atrium becomes congested, backing up blood into the pulmonary veins and then the pulmonary capillary beds. The fluid in the capillaries fills the alveolar spaces, resulting in pulmonary edema. There is a lack of oxygen exchange and a decrease in the emptying capability of the right ventricle.

Signs and symptoms—Symptoms of left-sided failure are shortness of breath, inability to breathe while lying down, periods of gasping for air, weak and rapid pulse, cool and clammy skin, and an ashen gray or cyanotic skin coloring. Often a cough produces pink, frothy sputum.

Etiology—Congestive heart failure is caused by the increased pressure of blood within the heart, primarily from the poor emptying of the ventricles, which causes fluid from the blood to collect in the tissues. With left-sided heart failure, blood backs up into the lungs, releasing fluid into the alveoli.

Right-Sided Heart Failure

Description—Returning blood flow becomes congested in the systemic circulation, eventually causing fluid to enter the interstitial spaces.

Signs and symptoms—Initially, the fluid can be viewed as edema in the lower extremities, but as the failure continues, edema is present in the upper extremities and in various organs throughout the system. Right-sided failure symptoms include swelling of the extremities, enlarged liver and spleen, and ascites (fluid in the abdominal cavity) caused by filtration from portal circulation venous pressure.

Etiology—When the right ventricle fails to move blood forward into the lungs, the blood backs up into the atrium, which therefore cannot accept incoming blood, so congestion occurs in the lower extremities and abdomen.

Treatment—Heart failure is extremely serious. Treatment involves the use of drugs to quickly increase cardiac output and remove congested fluids. Arterial vasodilators increase the efficiency of heart action. Bed rest is enforced and antiembolism stockings are used to prevent thromboembolism resulting from venous stasis. Continued treatment involves the use of cardiac drugs, frequent periods of rest, the use of elastic support stockings, skin care of the lower extremities, and dietary adjustments to reduce sodium intake and ensure proper nutrition.

Treating the underlying cause of congestive heart failure is the best first step. This may involve diseased heart valves, blocked coronary arteries, or toxins that directly damage heart muscle. Often there is no way to correct the cause, so doctors use an angiotensin-converting enzyme inhibitor (ACE inhibitor), such as Prinivil, Vasotec, or Zestril, to take some workload off the heart. These vasodialators work to relax stiffened blood vessels to make it easier for the weakened heart to push blood through the circulatory system. Diuretics or thiazide diuretics, such as HydroDIURIL, work to decrease edema in the lungs and legs. A weak diuretic, spironolactone, is given to some CHF patients because it helps the body hold on to potassium, whereas Lasix (a powerful diuretic) makes the patient lose potassium, which then causes other problems. Doctors are now using beta blockers, such as Coreg and Toprol XL, that significantly reduce the risk of hospitalization and death in patients with mild to severe heart failure. This type of medication is the standard of care for most patients with heart failure, as well as the ACE inhibitors and angiotensin receptor blocking agents. In some patients, digitalis is used, which helps improve the contractibility of the heart muscle.

Coronary Artery Disease

Description—This is a disease of the arteries that surround the heart, carrying oxygen and nutrients to the myocardium.

Signs and symptoms—The lack of oxygen causes the typical symptoms of angina: tightness of the chest and crushing substernal chest pains radiating to the left arm, neck, and shoulder blades. Other symptoms may be nausea, vomiting, fainting, and perspiring. When angina pain persists, it suggests an infarction.

Coronary artery disease may be diagnosed by the ECG during an attack or during a treadmill or exercise bicycle test. A heart catheterization, also called a coronary angiogram, allows visualization by x-ray examination of the coronary arteries following injection of a contrast medium into the blood vessels.

Etiology—Characteristically it is caused by atherosclerosis that narrows the blood vessel opening, thereby reducing the volume of blood flow to that portion of the heart muscle served by the arterial branch and resulting in angina symptoms.

Treatment—Narrowed, clogged arteries can be treated by three methods. First is the use of nitrates to dilate the vessel. Nitroglycerin in tablet form is placed under the tongue, can be applied in a paste form to the skin surface, or is given in oral form. Beta blockers and calcium blockers can also be used. When medication does not relieve symptoms and arterial openings are considerably narrowed, other treatments are required. Second, an **angioplasty** can be performed during catheterization of the heart. A balloonlike device is inflated to compress the fatty deposits against the arterial walls, thereby opening the constricted vessel. This is called a balloon angioplasty (Figure 11-146A). About 54% of the vessels clog again within 3 years and require a second angioplasty or bypass surgery. Another similar procedure is known as directional coronary atherectomy. It is performed like the conventional balloon procedure except that one side of the tip has a metal cylinder with a cutting blade that is attached to an external motor that rotates the cutter, grinding up the deposits and sucking them out of the catheter (Figure 11-146B). This method is believed to better control the reformation of deposits. A third type of artery procedure is called a coronary stent (Figure 11-146C). A balloon catheter with a stent (stainless steel mesh tube) is inserted into the artery. The balloon is inflated, compressing the deposits toward the sides of the artery and opening up the stent, which expands and stretches the arterial wall. The balloon is deflated and the catheter removed, leaving the stent to keep the vessel open. So far it has produced the best results.

In total, about 700,000 angioplasties are performed each year, often on two or three vessels at a time. Stents are used the majority of the time. Research has shown that 6 months after an angioplasty with a stent in place is performed, patients suffered less pain and less clogging and were less likely to need bypass surgery or additional angioplasty. However, there are some other results. The stent does not seem to decrease the risk of subsequent heart attacks or stroke, primarily because the stents can become blocked with clots, scar tissue, or new fatty deposits. In an effort to improve the results with stents, intra-

(A) Conventional balloon angioplasty

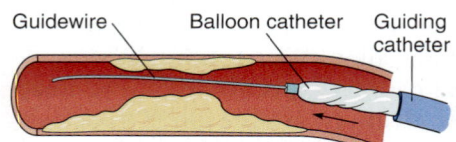

Guidewire   Balloon catheter   Guiding catheter

1. In conventional balloon angioplasty, a guiding catheter is positioned in the opening of the coronary artery. The physician then pushes a thin, flexible guidewire down the vessel and through the narrowing. The balloon catheter is then advanced over this guidewire.

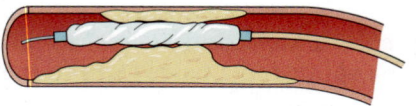

2. The balloon catheter is positioned next to the atherosclerotic plaque.

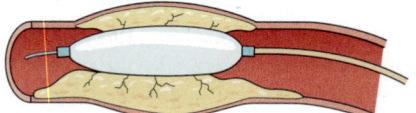

3. The balloon is inflated, stretching and cracking the plaque.

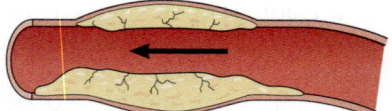

4. When the balloon is withdrawn, blood flow is re-established through the widened vessel.

(B) Coronary atherectomy

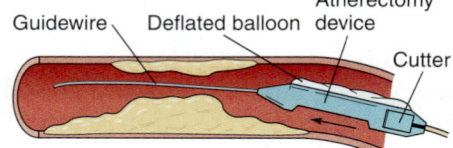

Guidewire   Deflated balloon   Atherectomy device   Cutter

1. In coronary atherectomy procedures, a special cutting device with a deflated balloon on one side and an opening on the other is pushed over a wire down the coronary artery.

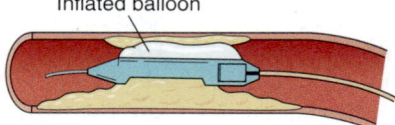

Inflated balloon

2. When the device is within a coronary artery narrowing, the balloon is inflated, so that part of the atherosclerotic plaque is "squeezed" into the opening of the device.

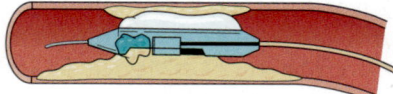

3. When the physician starts rotating the cutting blade, pieces of plaque are shaved off into the device.

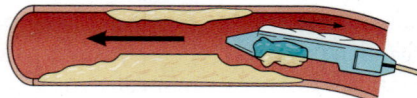

4. The catheter is withdrawn, leaving a larger opening for blood flow.

(C) Coronary stent

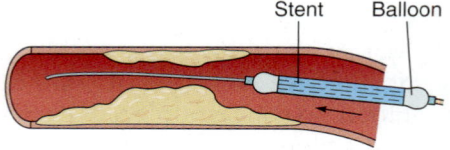

Stent   Balloon

1. To place a coronary stent within a vessel narrowing, physicians use a special catheter with a deflated balloon and the stent at the tip.

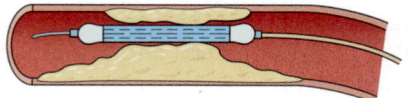

2. The catheter is positioned so that the stent is within the narrowed region of the coronary artery.

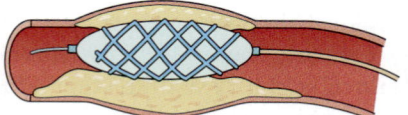

3. The balloon is then inflated, causing the stent to expand and stretch the coronary artery.

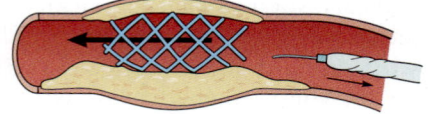

4. The balloon catheter is then withdrawn, leaving the stent behind to keep the vessel open.

FIGURE 11-146 Opening clogged arteries: (A) balloon angioplasty, (B) coronary atherectomy, and (C) coronary stent

coronary radiation has been used when patients have developed restenosis. The radiation technique called brachytherapy reduces the risk of new obstructions. Some researches feel that perhaps radiation alone might be the most effective because blood clots do not seem to appear later. Stents are also being coated to improve their effectiveness. Heparin (an anticlotting agent), rapamycin, or paclitaxel (both drug-eliciting stents) have been used. The drug-eliciting stents have remained open for 8 months in all 30 patients studied, and none have had an additional heart attack, needed a repeat procedure, or died.

Another way to correct clogged arteries is coronary bypass surgery. This entails bypassing clogged arteries by redirecting blood through vein grafts surgically transplanted from the legs to the heart's surface. The replacement vessels, however, are subject to the same disease as the original vessels. Currently, 10% to 15% of bypass surgeries are repeat procedures. A new procedure uses the internal thoracic artery for the graft because it tends to remain free of atherosclerosis longer. Heart surgeons can now operate without opening the chest cavity. The method is called the daVinci Computer-Enhanced Surgical System. Basically, the surgeon sits at a computer keyboard with a monitor and joystick. The doctor controls robotic arms holding specially designed surgical instruments and tiny cameras. The robot performs the surgery through tiny incisions in the chest. The bypass graft is taken from the inside wall of the chest, thereby eliminating harvesting it from the leg. This new minimally invasive procedure greatly reduces pain, postoperative scarring, and recovery time, which can be significant with the open-chest method.

Coronary artery disease is best treated by prevention. That includes weight control; a diet low in salt, fats, and cholesterol; regular active exercise; reduction of stress; and refraining from smoking.

Embolism (Em′bo-lizm)

Description—An embolus is defined as foreign matter that enters and circulates in the bloodstream. Emboli (more than one) can be composed of blood, exudate, fat, or air.

Signs and symptoms—The symptoms vary according to the location of the **embolism**. Obstruction of a cerebral artery has already been described in CVA symptoms. Smaller emboli produce symptoms in relation to the location and size of the mass. The first symptom of pulmonary emboli is usually dyspnea and probably chest pain. Other symptoms include tachycardia, productive cough (often blood-tinged), low-grade fever, and pleural effusion. Signs may include leg edema; massive hemoptysis (coughing up blood); cyanosis; pleural friction; and signs of circulatory collapse, fainting, and coma. A fatty embolus is potentially fatal if it is in the brain or lung. It typically occurs within 24 to 72 hours following an extremity fracture or trauma. Signs are apprehension, sweating, fever, tachycardia, pallor, dyspnea, pulmonary effusion, cyanosis, convulsions, and coma. A distinctive sign is a petechial rash (small purplish hemorrhagic spots) on the chest and shoulders.

Etiology—A thrombus that forms within a blood vessel becomes an embolus when it breaks loose and begins to circulate. An embolus can also result from air introduced into a blood vessel. An infection may produce a circulating clump of exudate, as discussed under endocarditis. Skeletal fractures cause the formation of fat emboli. One theory holds that minute fat globules from the bone marrow enter the damaged blood vessels at the fracture site. The greatest danger of fat emboli is that they may circulate to the capillary beds in the lungs and block the alveolar exchange, resulting in an insufficient supply of oxygen.

An embolus of any type is potentially lethal if the circulating mass is of adequate size to obstruct the blood supply to a significant portion of an organ. The resulting **infarction** (interference with circulation) is especially rapid when it occurs within a major pulmonary artery or in one of the coronary arteries, and it can be fatal. Infarction of a kidney, the spleen, or the brain will produce symptoms related to the degree of tissue damage. If a nonvital organ is extensively destroyed, surgical removal may be indicated.

Treatment—Depending upon the location of the embolus, treatment can include administering oxygen, use of heparin, reduction of pulmonary edema, intubation to restore and support breathing, medications to cause the mass to disintegrate, antibiotic with an exudate, and other supportive measures.

Heart Failure

Description—A condition, particularly prevalent among the older population, in which the heart pumps too weakly to supply the body with blood. With severe failure, life expectancy is shortened. A transplant will correct the problem, but most patients with heart failure are too old or have additional medical conditions. Without the transplant, fewer than half survive for 2 years.

Symptoms—The prime symptoms are weakness, shortness of breath, and others resulting from poor circulation, such as edema.

Etiology—One cause of heart failure is dilated cardiomyopathy, a condition characterized by weakened walls of the left ventricle that allow it to expand outward. Eventually, the expanded walls pull the edges of the mitral valve apart, widening the opening. This results in the valve leaflets being unable to cover the opening, and blood flows backward (regurgitates) into the left atrium when the ventricles contract. This only complicates an already compromised circulation. A variety of conditions can contribute to the development of cardiomyopathy, such as viruses, heart attacks, and high blood pressure.

Treatment—Treatment of regurgitation and the loss of pumping strength involves specific medication, such as Aldactone, Coreg, or digoxin, and an ACE inhibitor, such as Vasotec, Prinivil, or Zestril. Diuretics are given to keep excess fluid from collecting in the lungs and extremities.

If drug therapy proves inadequate, then valve replacement or repair may be indicated. Artificial or animal heart valve replacements have been used for quite some time. Replacement procedures involve a temporary but substantial loss of pumping function because left ventricular tissue around the valve is lost when the valve is removed. This procedure is considered too risky for people with severe failure because their function is already critical. A new procedure called annuloplasty repairs the leaky valve by narrowing the expanded valve opening, which greatly reduces or eliminates regurgitation. The surgeon simply sews a plastic ring around the edge of the mitral valve opening, "cinching" it tighter so that the leaflets overlap. In one study of the procedure, only 1 patient out of 91 died as a result of the surgery. After 1 year, 80% were still alive, and 70% survived 2 years. Additional study is continuing, and the results are encouraging.

Heart Replacement

Perhaps the ultimate treatment for severe heart problems is heart transplant. This procedure involves an enormous amount of physical, financial, legal, emotional, and ethical preparation. Usually, the patient is not a good operative risk because of the extent of disease. There is always an emotional rollercoaster of events while waiting to obtain a donor heart match. Many patients do not survive the wait. Even with the best odds possible, transplantation is not always successful. Some patients have transplant rejections and have been fortunate enough to receive and survive a second successfully. The ability to mentally and emotionally accept the placement of another person's heart into your body can be very difficult. The realization that someone had to die for you to get a chance to survive can be a life-changing experience. Fortunately, trained professionals provide support and counseling to assist in this procedure.

An alternative has been developed that many hoped would provide a solution to the transplant dilemma. In July 2001, a patient with only days to live received the first totally implantable, permanent, artificial heart. The AbioCor is an experimental yo-yo–shaped mechanical heart, a plastic and titanium pump weighing less than 2 pounds. It is powered through the skin by an external battery pack. Earlier, in the mid-1980s, Robert Jarvik developed the Jarvik 7 heart that kept a man alive for more than 600 days. But it was a bulky external machine to which the patient was constantly connected. Jarvik described the AbioCor device as a false hope, a sincere but misdirected effort. The heart is so large it would only fit in people weighing about 200 pounds. He believes many years of experience have proved cutting out the heart is unnecessary.

The new heart was initially tested in five patients across the country. Little information has been given about their progress. The first patient appeared on television in late August 2001 with the main people involved in the experiment. He was very thin but was able to walk into the room and speak briefly. He obviously had a long way to go for recovery. The developing company has stated that every single patient involved in the experiment would die on AbioCor. The initial goal was only 60 days of survival. Only those patients who were ineligible for transplant and who had "end stage" heart disease with less than a month to live were permitted to participate. Patients were just looking for the chance to interact with their families for a little while longer.

The first patient, who had received the artificial heart in July, died November 30, 2001, from complications following a stroke and internal bleeding. He had survived for 5 full months, far exceeding the initial goal of 60 days. Altogether 14 patients were involved in the trials. Only one patient was able to return home and live a somewhat normal life. He survived the longest at 17 months. The last patient implanted was a 73-year-old man. He received the device in November 2004 and lived 166 days, dying from irreversible multiorgan failure. In June 2005, the FDA denied the developer's application to continue the procedure because all 14 patients had suffered in their final days and the FDA felt the device was not ready for wider use. Of the 14, two had died in surgery, another 7 suffered fatal strokes, one was comatose for 53 days after surgery, and the others suffered nonfatal strokes but had irreversible neurologic consequences. All patients were extremely ill and very poor operative risks, so the eventual outcome was anticipated.

Hypertension (Hiper-ten'-shun)

Description—In this condition, blood pressure is consistently elevated above 140/90. In the diabetic population, blood pressure greater than 130/85 is considered hypertensive. These both represent systolic and diastolic hypertension and both need treatment.

Signs and symptoms—The presence of elevated blood pressure readings is the only observable sign of hypertension. Some people may sense that their blood pressure is high and experience headache or "feel" pressure.

Etiology—*Hypertension* may be classified as *essential* (unknown cause) or *secondary* (resulting from another disease or disorder). Essential hypertension is correlated with family history, race, obesity, stress, a diet high in saturated fats and salt, oral contraceptives, and aging.

Secondary hypertension may be the result of kidney disease; thyroid, pituitary, or parathyroid dysfunction; or neurologic disorders that interfere with blood pressure regulation. Treatment of the primary cause will reduce the blood pressure.

Hypertension may also be classified as *benign* or *malignant*. In the benign form, the pressure rises moderately over a fairly long period. Malignant hypertension is characterized by an accelerated, rapid, and severe increase, which may not respond to treatment.

Hypertension is the foremost contributing factor to CVAs, kidney damage, and various cardiac conditions.

Treatment—Treatment of hypertension is directed at reducing the elevated pressure and maintaining an acceptable level of blood pressure. It is of great importance to prevent complications of the disease. Treatment focuses around diet, the control of sodium (currently being questioned), the use of diuretics to encourage elimination of retained body fluids, and antihypertensive drugs to reduce vasoconstriction or increase kidney filtration. It is of the utmost importance that the patient maintain the treatment regimen because hypertension is not curable, only treatable. Patients must be encouraged to continue with their medication even if they have no symptoms of hypertension. Compliance with dietary and drug therapy is the only means of preventing life-threatening complications.

Hypertrophic Cardiomyopathy (Hiper-tro′fik Karde-o-mi-op′a-the)

Description—This is a disease in which the walls of the ventricles of the heart are markedly thickened, sometimes to three times their normal width. The "muscle-bound" heart is stiff and cannot fill with blood and pump efficiently. It affects an estimated one in every 2,000 people in the United States. It is recognized as an important cause of heart failure and sudden death. Some prominent victims have been young athletes who collapse and die during sports events. The enlargement is for no apparent reason and is not caused by increased workload as with hypertension or aortic narrowing. (Those problems result in left ventricular hypertrophy.) This disease is not to be confused with athletic heart syndrome.

Signs and symptoms—Some signs include lightheadedness, fainting, shortness of breath, heart palpitations, and occasionally chest discomfort like angina. Many patients have a heart murmur. There may also be arrhythmia of the atria and sometimes of the ventricles as well. Rapid ventricular arrhythmia or fibrillation causes fainting and sudden death in about 2% of patients annually.

Etiology—In some cases the disease is caused by a defective gene located on the 14th chromosome. This form results in a 50% chance their children may develop the condition. Other causes are unknown. Diagnosis is confirmed by echocardiogram.

Treatment—Most patients are placed on medication to slow the heart to encourage a relaxation phase using beta and calcium channel blockers. Some patients also require medication to control arrhythmia. Defibrillation treatment may be indicated. Often, strenuous activity is to be avoided. A new experimental therapy involves the use of a permanent pacemaker to change the heart contraction and improve blood flow to prevent sudden death.

Hypotension (Hipo-ten′-shun)

Description—Defined as blood pressure below the normal range, **hypotension** may become life-threatening when the circulation of blood becomes impaired and the exchange of gases is inadequate.

Etiology—Hypotension can result from an acute blood loss, heart failure, shock, kidney failure, thyroid disease, and other infectious conditions.

Treatment—The treatment of hypotension is determined by the underlying cause. Options include transfusion and intravenous fluid replacement, car-diac stimulants, thyroid medication, and other appropriate drugs.

Leukemia (Loo-ke′me-a)

Description—This is a malignant disease of the bone marrow (myelogenous) or lymphatic tissue (lympho-cytic). **Leukemia** can be present in either an acute or chronic form. Leukemia will strike 94,200 Americans this year and will cause the death of 51,650.

Signs and symptoms—In the **acute phase**, a great number of immature white blood cells are produced in the bone marrow or lymph tissue. The excessive amount of white blood cells causes pressure and discomfort within the bones, swelling and pain in the lymph nodes, and greatly elevated white blood cell count in the blood. The earliest symptoms of the disease are fever, pallor, fatigue, swelling of lymphoid tissue (spleen, liver), and a tendency toward large bruises.

Even in the presence of great numbers of leukocytes and lymphocytes, the body has little defense against infection because of the immaturity of the cells. The major complication of leukemia is infection. The disease process may progress to produce bleeding within the brain and other vital organs. In acute leukemia, the onset is rapid, and death occurs within a few months unless treated aggressively with chemotherapy. Acute lymphocytic leukemia is the form common in children. Typically it is approximately 30% into its course before it is diagnosed. Acute myelogenous leukemia is more common in adults. Both acute forms are ultimately fatal, but long-term remissions in the childhood form and approximately 70% cures are now being reported.

Chronic leukemia differs from acute only in that its onset is more insidious (slow), and its course is more prolonged. The median survival rate is 3 to 4 years.

Signs and symptoms—Often the first symptoms are a general malaise (vague discomfort, feeling "bad") and weight loss. Anemia, fatigue, and greatly enlarged spleen and lymph nodes are typical symptoms. Chronic myelogenous leukemia is almost always associated with a chromosome irregularity known as the Philadelphia chromosome. Chronic myelogenous leukemia is characterized by two distinct phases: the chronic phase, which is insidious, lasting an average of 3 to 4 years, and the eventual acute phase, an immature cell crisis, lasting only a few weeks or months before death occurs.

Diagnosis can be confirmed initially by blood studies in addition to typical clinical findings. Differentiation of type and positive identification of acute or chronic forms is possible through cellular and chromosomal analysis of bone marrow aspirates. The bone marrow sample can be withdrawn through a large-gauge needle introduced into the sternum or preferably the posterior superior iliac spine.

Treatment—Treatment varies with the type and form of leukemia. Systemic chemotherapy is used to destroy abnormal white blood cells and induce a remission so that more normal function of the bone marrow will occur. The side effects of the drugs are loss of hair, nausea, vomiting, gouty arthritis, and a number of other complications. Some success has been achieved with bone marrow transplants among siblings, particularly twins. This procedure is especially indicated in treatment of children and younger adults. Before the marrow is given, the patient is medicated with large doses of drugs to completely suppress the body's ability to react to foreign material. Total bone radiation treatments are used to induce marrow aplasia (lack of function) and aid in lowering the body's resistance to the transplant. Approximately 1 liter (1,000 mL) of bone marrow is removed from the pelvic bones of the donor. The marrow is processed and then given to the recipient intravenously. To prevent contact with any microorganisms, the patient is placed in a reverse isolation unit. The patient is in an extremely vulnerable state, and a prolonged hospital stay is inevitable. Barring complications, which are numerous, chances for recovery are good.

Murmur

Description—The abnormal sound of blood flowing through a heart valve can be heard with a stethoscope and is known as a **murmur**. The murmur is named for the valve which is "leaking" or stenotic.

Signs and symptoms—The mitral valve is the one most frequently affected, and the gurgling or swishing sound is called a mitral murmur. Murmurs are further identified as systolic or diastolic. This classification specifies whether the sound is heard during the contraction or relaxation phase of the heartbeat.

Etiology—Valve damage that results in murmurs can be caused by rheumatic fever, an inflammatory disease that follows a streptococcal infection. The valves may become inflamed and in time thicken and develop scar tissue. Hence the valves lose their flexibility and no longer close completely.

Endocarditis is another condition that may lead to valve damage. As previously discussed, bacteria circulating through the heart collect on the valvular surfaces, causing the growth of vegetation and resulting in ulceration and death of some tissue. In its damaged state, the valve is no longer capable of normal function. Preexisting valve damage from rheumatic fever, especially of the mitral valve, is quite common in endocarditis.

Treatment—Artificial or pig valve replacement may be indicated to alleviate the problem if severe enough to interfere with circulation.

Myocardial Infarction (MI) (Mi-o-kar′de-al Infar′k-shun)

Description—MI is a complication of coronary artery disease that results from occlusion (partial or complete) of the artery, causing myocardial tissue destruction. MIs are one of the leading causes of death in the United States. Mortality is high when treatment is delayed; approximately 50% of patients will die within an hour after symptoms develop.

Signs and symptoms—It is characterized by severe, crushing pain, which radiates through the chest to the neck and jaw and down the left arm. It is not relieved by rest, as with angina, and is accompanied by nausea, perspiration, a change in blood pressure, hypotension or hypertension, and dyspnea.

Etiology—Predisposing factors include sedentary lifestyle, stressful occupation, obesity, cigarette smoking, hypertension, aging, positive family history, and elevated levels of cholesterol and triglycerides in the blood. An attack can often be precipitated by a heavy meal, physical exertion, or exposure to cold weather.

Treatment—Treatment of MI is directed at relieving the pain with strong analgesic drugs, such as demerol or morphine, and administering extra oxygen to maintain an adequate supply to the tissues. It is important to prevent complications. Heart rhythm must be stabilized to prevent arrhythmia, which can lead to congestive heart failure. Complete bed rest must be enforced to decrease cardiac workload and a possible additional infarction. **Anticoagulant** drugs are given to reduce the tendency to develop thromboembolism. The newest treatment includes the immediate use of a clot-busting drug to open the narrowed or blocked coronary artery in order to restore circulation to the myocardium. In about 20% of cases this fails to work, and if there are associated bleeding ulcers or a stroke, it is prohibited. An angioplasty is now being performed on these selective patients and is being evaluated for use with other MI patients. Immediate accessibility to qualified surgeons and angioplasty within 1 hour is a problem in many areas. In contrast, clot-busting drugs can be administered immediately almost anywhere, possibly even by specially trained emergency vehicle personnel in the future.

Severe complications may occur in the damaged ventricular area in addition to the systemic threat of embolism and heart failure. Unusual and potentially lethal conditions may develop. The ventricular septum may rupture, causing a circulatory defect in which blood flows between the ventricles. The ventricular wall may weaken because of necrosis following infarction. The wall may develop an aneurysm, leading to a ventricular rupture.

The patient who survives an MI will be faced with a lengthy recovery period. Lifestyles may need to be

P PATIENT EDUCATION

HOW TO RECOGNIZE A HEART ATTACK

Any of the following symptoms lasting more than 2 minutes may signal the start of a heart attack.

- **A sensation of uncomfortable pressure, fullness, squeezing, aching, or pain, usually located in the center of the chest.**
- **Pain, aching, or heaviness in the shoulders, neck, jaw, arms, or upper back or spreading to those areas from the chest.**
- **Pain accompanied by lightheadedness, fainting, sweating, nausea, vomiting, or shortness of breath.**

Taking a 325-mg aspirin tablet while waiting for help will help prevent clots from getting any larger. Clot-dissolving drugs, given intravenously within an hour of the first signs of a heart attack, could prevent about 90% of deaths. Unfortunately, half of all people wait more than 2 hours before getting to a hospital, often because they do not realize they are having a heart attack.

altered and dietary and smoking habits changed. An exercise rehabilitation program must be initiated and adhered to for optimum recovery and maintenance of a healthy state.

The following information was reported in "Consumer Reports on Health" in October 1994.

Phlebitis (Fle-bi′tis)

Description—This localized inflammation of a vein causes an alteration in the epithelial lining, which predisposes to the formation of a thrombus. Phlebitis can occur in deep or superficial veins (see Thrombophlebitis for more information).

Sickle Cell Anemia

Description—This is a congenital anemia occurring primarily among blacks, about 1 in 10 of whom carry the abnormal gene. When two carriers have children, there is a 25% chance that each child will have the disease. When two persons with sickle cell anemia have children, all children will have the disease. If only one has the disease and the other is normal, all children will be carriers of the trait.

Signs and symptoms—Sickle cell anemia is characterized by red blood cells with a hemoglobin defect in their molecular structure that causes the cells to become sickle-shaped. Cells of this shape cannot pass easily through blood vessels and they tend to interfere with circulation.

Symptoms are tachycardia, cardiomegaly, cardiac murmurs, chronic fatigue, unexplained dyspnea, chest pain, enlarged liver, jaundice, pallor, swollen joints, aching bones, and leg ulcers. These symptoms begin after about 6 months of age, when the protective excess amounts of hemoglobin present at birth are exhausted.

The most common feature of the disease is a painful crisis, which usually appears first at about age 5. Sickled red blood cells become tangled, causing blood vessel obstruction and a lack of oxygen to the tissues, with possible destruction of the involved area. This tissue infarction causes severe pain to the affected area. Usual sites are the lungs, liver, bones, and spleen. The spleen, particularly, is affected so frequently that the resulting damage and scarring cause it to shrink and become useless. A crisis usually lasts from 4 days to several weeks and recurs cyclically.

Diagnosis can be made from a positive family history and the typical clinical features. It is confirmed by a blood smear that shows the sickled cell structure. At present, research has failed to discover a means to prevent the sickling alteration.

The disease produces long-term complications, such as delayed puberty and a tendency toward delayed growth. If the patient survives to adulthood, the body is described as spiderlike, with a narrow trunk and long extremities, curved spine, elongated skull, and barrel-shaped chest. Premature death may result from repeated infarctions within vital organs or from an infectious process.

Etiology—It is an inherited condition caused by a faulty gene.

Treatment—Treatment focuses on alleviating the symptoms of the disease and on transfusions with packed red blood cells when an aplastic crisis occurs (depression of the bone marrow activity and destruction of RBCs). The most successful treatment may be prevention through genetic counseling of persons known to be carriers. Information is provided to allow individuals to arrive at informed decisions regarding the conception and birth of children.

There is no known cure for sickle cell anemia. However, recently, a cancer drug has been shown to help prevent the attacks. Hydroxyurea (Hydrea) can cut the rate of painful episodes and complication in half, but the drug poses risks, so only adults with the most severe form are advised to take it.

Stasis Ulcer (Sta′sis Ul′ser)

Description—This is a secondary condition resulting from chronic venous insufficiency. The most common site of stasis ulcers is the ankle at the internal malleous area.

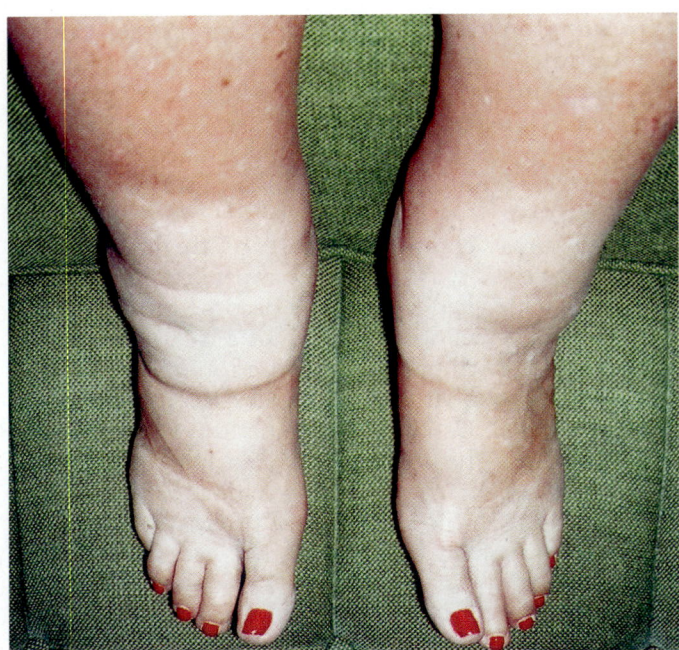

FIGURE 11-147A   Marked edema of the lower legs, ankles, and part of the feet due to venous insufficiency. Also note skin coloration.

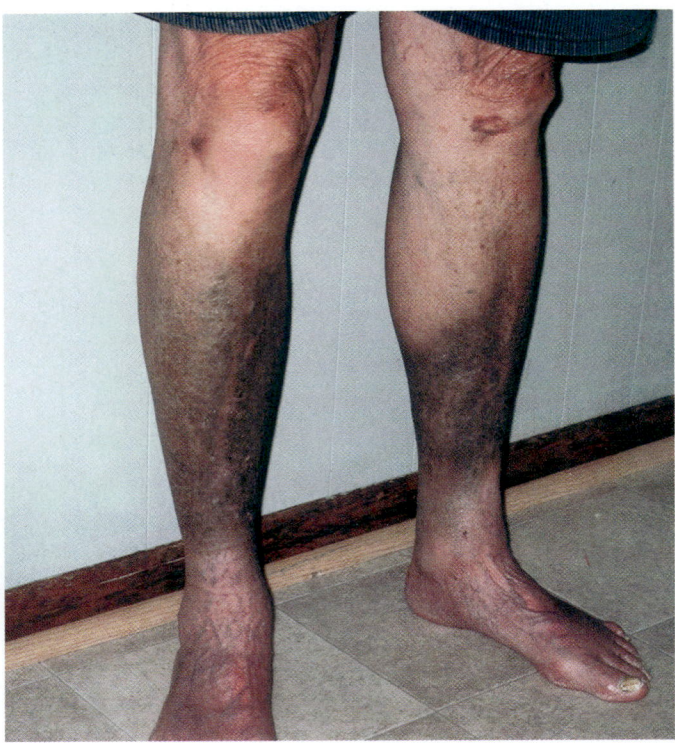

FIGURE 11-147B   Marked discoloration of lower legs from chronic arterial insufficiency

Signs and symptoms—Varicosities and edema are common. Early signs are dusky red deposits in the skin with itching and dimpling of the tissue. Later, there is redness and scaling of large areas of the legs. Then, cracks develop with crusts and ulcers. Figure 11-147A shows edema of the lower legs, ankles, and feet as a result of inadequate *return* of blood by the veins, causing fluid to escape into the tissues. There are also red spots developing on the skin. This woman has venous insufficiency, which may lead to a stasis ulcer if not treated. Currently she wears 40-mm compression hose to the knees, which assist the veins to return fluids and control most of the edema. By contrast, in Figure 11-147B, the dark skin is caused by inadequate blood supply *to* the legs due to chronic arterial insufficiency. This man injured his legs, causing an interruption of the flow of blood. His skin is even hard to the touch.

Etiology—Stasis ulcers develop following deep vein thrombophlebitis that destroys the valve structures. Communicating veins in the affected area fail to compensate for the damaged vein. The venous pressure increases, causing fluid to enter the interstitial tissues and produce edema. The tissue swelling leads to fibrosis and skin discoloration from blood entering the subcutaneous tissues. The poor condition of the skin and the inadequate circulation from the area lead to a breakdown of the surrounding tissues (Figure 11-148). They can also be caused by lower extremity trauma or a skin irritation.

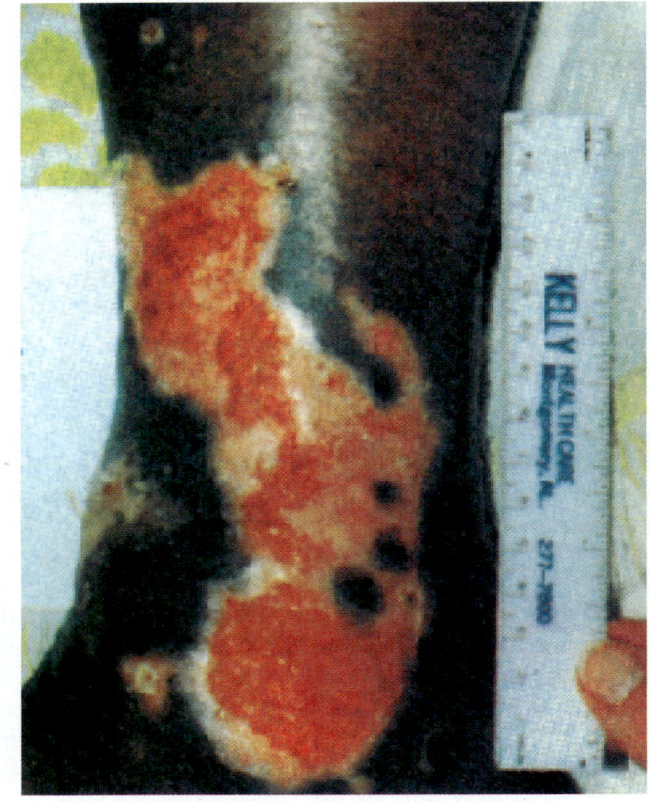

FIGURE 11-148   Venous stasis ulcer *(Courtesy of Carrington Laboratories, Inc., Irving, TX)*

Treatment—Treatment of small ulcers involves elevation of the affected extremity, warm soaks, bed rest, and the use of drugs to counteract infection. When the swelling subsides, pressure is applied by a sponge rubber dressing or an Unna's boot (zinc gelatin boot). Large stasis ulcers not responding to treatment may require removal of the ulcer site followed by a skin graft.

Thrombophlebitis (Thrombo-fle-bi'tis)

Description—This is an acute condition in which the lining of the vein wall becomes inflamed and a thrombus forms. **Thrombophlebitis** can develop within small superficial veins and is usually self-limiting. Deep vein thrombosis (DVT) can affect small or large veins. When there is an alteration of the vein lining, platelets begin to collect at the area. The platelet fibrin catches red blood cells, white blood cells, and additional platelets, forming a blood clot. The thrombus enlarges rapidly, particularly if the blood flow is slow, causing an inflammation that becomes fibrotic. The enlarging clot may completely fill the vein opening, occluding the vessel, or it may break loose, becoming an embolus.

Signs and symptoms—Symptoms of deep thrombophlebitis include severe pain, fever, chills, and possibly edema, with discoloration of the affected extremity. When superficial veins are involved, visible and palpable signs may include heat, swelling, tenderness, redness and discoloration, and induration (hardening) along the affected portion of the vein.

Etiology—DVT usually results from lining damage, but it can also follow accelerated blood clotting and a slow, reduced flow of blood. Conditions that precipitate thrombophlebitis are prolonged bed rest, trauma, childbirth, surgery, and the use of oral contraceptives.

Treatment—Treatment is directed toward preventing complications, controlling the development of thrombi, and relieving the discomfort. The patient is maintained on bed rest, with the affected extremity elevated to aid circulation. Warm, moist soaks are applied to the affected area. Medication is given to relieve pain, and anticoagulants are frequently used to reduce the blood's clotting ability. Antiembolism stockings (tight-fitting, elastic, knee- or thigh-length hose) are indicated to assist the return of blood from the legs to the heart. Individuals who are prone to develop thrombophlebitis should avoid prolonged periods of sitting or standing, especially with little movement, to help eliminate pooling of blood in the lower extremities. When sitting, the legs should be resting on a support that does not cause pressure to interfere with return circulation.

Varicosities (Vari-kos'i-tes)

Description—Veins that become dilated, twisted, and inefficient are known as **varicose** veins. The condition usually results from weakness of the valves in the saphenous vein and its branches, which permits blood to leak backward as a result of incomplete closure. As the blood accumulates, the veins become dilated, the valve is no longer capable of reaching across the opening of the vein, and the situation becomes worse.

Signs and symptoms—Symptoms include a feeling of heaviness, night leg cramps, aching, and a feeling of fatigue. With deep vein involvement, edema may accumulate in the feet and ankles, often associated with the discoloration that precedes stasis ulcers. Superficial varicosed veins can often be seen or palpated behind the knees or on the medial surface of the calf. Varicosed veins are not to be confused with the tiny purplish red surface veins seen on the skin of most adults. These are commonly referred to as spider veins and are evidence of increased venous pressure. They are often associated with varicosities.

Etiology—This stasis (stagnation) of blood is often the result of occupations requiring long periods of standing or of other factors interfering with circulation, such as pressure against the veins during pregnancy.

Treatment—Treatment for mild to moderate varicosities includes an exercise program to improve circulation; use of antiembolism stockings; attention to sitting position; and the elimination of tight-fitting or constricting clothing, such as girdles, garters, elastic bands of clothing, and knee-high or thigh-high hose. More severe varicosities may require injection of a sclerosing agent into small venous areas to scar and harden the vein. Larger involvement will necessitate surgical ligation (tying off) of the involved vein from its branches and stripping the vein from the leg.

ACHIEVE UNIT OBJECTIVES

- Complete the Workbook activities to meet the learning objectives.

- Apply your knowledge at the end of this chapter in completing the Critical Thinking Challenge and Activities, as well as the StudyWARE on your Student CD-ROM.

UNIT 9
THE IMMUNE SYSTEM

OBJECTIVES

Upon completion of this unit, you will be able to achieve the following:

LEARNING Objectives

1. Spell and define, using the glossary at the back of the text, all the Words to Know in this unit.
2. List the body's three main lines of defense against antigens.
3. Define the function of the immune system.
4. Identify the three basic services of the immune system.
5. Describe the origin of blood cells.
6. List the organs of the immune system, and identify their locations.
7. Describe the purpose of MHC.
8. Explain the role of the B cell.
9. Identify the four types of T cells.
10. Tell how NK cell action differs from phagocytic action.
11. Explain what causes an inflammatory response.
12. Tell how immunizations and vaccines work.
13. Explain how the acquired immunodeficiency syndrome (AIDS) virus destroys the immune system.
14. Identify five ways to acquire the AIDS virus.
15. List four high-risk behaviors to avoid.
16. Name the three most common opportunistic diseases.
17. Define cancer.
18. Name the classifications of cancer.
19. Identify six characteristics of a cancerous cell.
20. Identify the basic cause of cancer.
21. Describe grading and staging of cancer.
22. List four types or categories of carcinogens.
23. Identify the three categories of diagnostic testing.
24. List the four major cancer treatment methods.
25. List five symptoms of chronic fatigue syndrome.
26. Explain how lupus affects the immune system and the major body organs it may affect.
27. Identify the symptoms of rheumatoid arthritis.

WORDS TO KNOW

abstinence
acquired immunodeficiency syndrome (AIDS)
allergens
allergies
anaphylaxis
antibody
antibody-mediated
antigen
autoimmune
basophils
benign
biopsy
brachytherapy
cancerous
carcinoembryonic antigen (CEA)
carcinogens
carcinoma
cell-mediated
chemotherapy
clonal
complement

corticosteroids
cytokine
cytotoxic
debilitating
desensitization
discoid
eosinophils
extracellular
histamine
humoral
immune
immunoglobulin
immuno-suppressed
interferon
interleukin
intracellular
lupus erythematosus
lymphedema
lymphocyte
lymphokine
macrophage
malignant
metastasis
monoclonal

monocyte
monogamous
monokine
mutation
neoplasm
neutrophils
oncogenes
opportunistic
permeable
phagocyte
prostaglandin
psychoneuroim-munology
radiation
Raynaud's phenomenon
remission
retrovirus
sarcoma
staging
suppressor
surveillance
thymus
transmission
vaccine
virus

 ### CERTIFICATION CONNECTION

CMA
Diagnostic procedures
Common diseases and pathology
Anatomy and physiology

CMAS
Anatomy and physiology

RMA
Anatomy and physiology

The **immune** system is not usually given the distinction of being identified as a body system. The function of immunity is primarily provided by specific cells and organs of the circulatory system, so it is usually included in that system's discussion. The role of immunity is essential to the health and well-being of humans. When the system misfires or is crippled, a whole host of diseases can develop, such as AIDS, allergy, arthritis, and cancer. Because its function is of such importance, it is being given significance equal to a body system in this text.

We live in an environment full of **antigens**, things that the immune system recognizes as nonself and responds to by destroying or rendering them ineffective. All antigens carry markers that identify them as foreign to the immune system. Foreign materials, bacteria, **viruses**, fungi, and parasites are antigens. Foreign material can be a cell, tissue, a protein, the food we eat, and even particles in the air. Blood from a transfusion or cells and tissue from a transplant are prime examples of foreign material. In abnormal situations, the immune system can mistake self for nonself and attack. This results in the development of an **autoimmune** disease, such as rheumatoid arthritis, diabetes, and lupus. Sometimes, the system responds inappropriately to harmless substances, such as ragweed pollen or cat hair. This kind of antigen is called an **allergen**, and the result is known as an allergy. When one's own cells become **malignant**, their structure changes, making them "different," and a response occurs. Many antigens can cause serious reactions, infections, diseases, and even death.

The body has three main lines of defense against antigens: barriers, the inflammation process, and **antibodies**. The first line of defense are the three types of barriers that prevent entry of antigens. (1) Anatomic barriers are the skin, which covers the body, and the mucous membranes, which line the respiratory, gastrointestinal, and genitourinary tracts. (2) Biochemical barriers are located within the anatomic barriers. Sebaceous glands in the skin secrete antibacterial and antifungal fatty acids and lactic acid. Tears, perspiration, and saliva contain enzymes that attack the cellular walls of gram-positive bacteria. Secretions from certain glands make the skin acidic, which is hostile to bacteria. (3) Mechanical barriers work to eliminate substances. Skin sloughs off, and irritated membranes cause coughing. The acts of urinating and vomiting expel materials.

The second and third lines of defense involve cooperation of various components of the immune response that require additional specific explanation before the defense can be understood. For now, inflammation, the second line, occurs when the barriers have been penetrated. This response begins within seconds of an injury or invasion and results in the familiar warm, red, and swollen area that we recognize as an infection. The third line, antibody defense, is a dual-response system involving the actions of specific cells and other immune system components to attack the antigen. This is our immunity and is our last line of defense.

The function of the immune system is to create effective immune responses to continually defend the body against antigens. To do this, the immune system must be able to provide three basic services: (1) identify self and destroy nonself substances, (2) maintain homeostasis, and (3) conduct continual **surveillance**. To understand how these services work, it is necessary to learn about the way each part of the system contributes to the services. The system includes a variety of cells, the organs, the **complement** system, antibodies, cytokines, and the process of surveillance.

ORIGIN OF CELLS

In the last unit, it was stated that cells within the blood are of three types—red, white, and platelets. The leukocytes (white blood cells) were identified as playing a vital role in defending the body. It is these cells in cooperation with protein molecules that are responsible for immunity.

All blood cells originate in the bone marrow and initially develop from stem cells. They progress through different stages of maturation and differentiation until they become mature, functioning cells. Refer to Figure 11-149 as the origin and maturity of cells is explained. Erythrocytes (RBCs) develop from erythroid stem cells and mature in the bone marrow. White blood cells (WBCs), which become the granulated **eosinophils**, **neutrophils**, and **basophils**, develop from myeloid stem cells. One type of agranulocyte, the **lymphocyte**, develops from a lymphocyte stem cell into two major classes: B cells that mature in the bone marrow and T cells that mature in the **thymus**. A granulated cell means that it has granules within its cytoplasm. If no granules are present, the cell is agranulated. Mononuclear phagocyte stem cells become the **monocytes**.

Monocytes are immature cells that have little ability to fight infection. However, once they enter the tissue, they sometimes swell to as large as 80 micrometers, large enough to be seen by the naked eye. At this stage, they are called **macrophages** and are very effective at fighting infection. The most important function of macrophages is phagocytosis, the ability to engulf and destroy antigens. They can phagocytize as many as 100 bacteria and large organisms or cells, such as whole red blood cells and some parasites. Neutrophils are also phagocytic, but in addition, they carry granules of potent chemicals to destroy microorganisms. They can only engulf small particles, such as bacteria.

Neutrophils make up about 40% to 60% of all white blood cells. They are also known as segmentals (segs) and polymorphonuclear neutrophils (PMNs). They attack

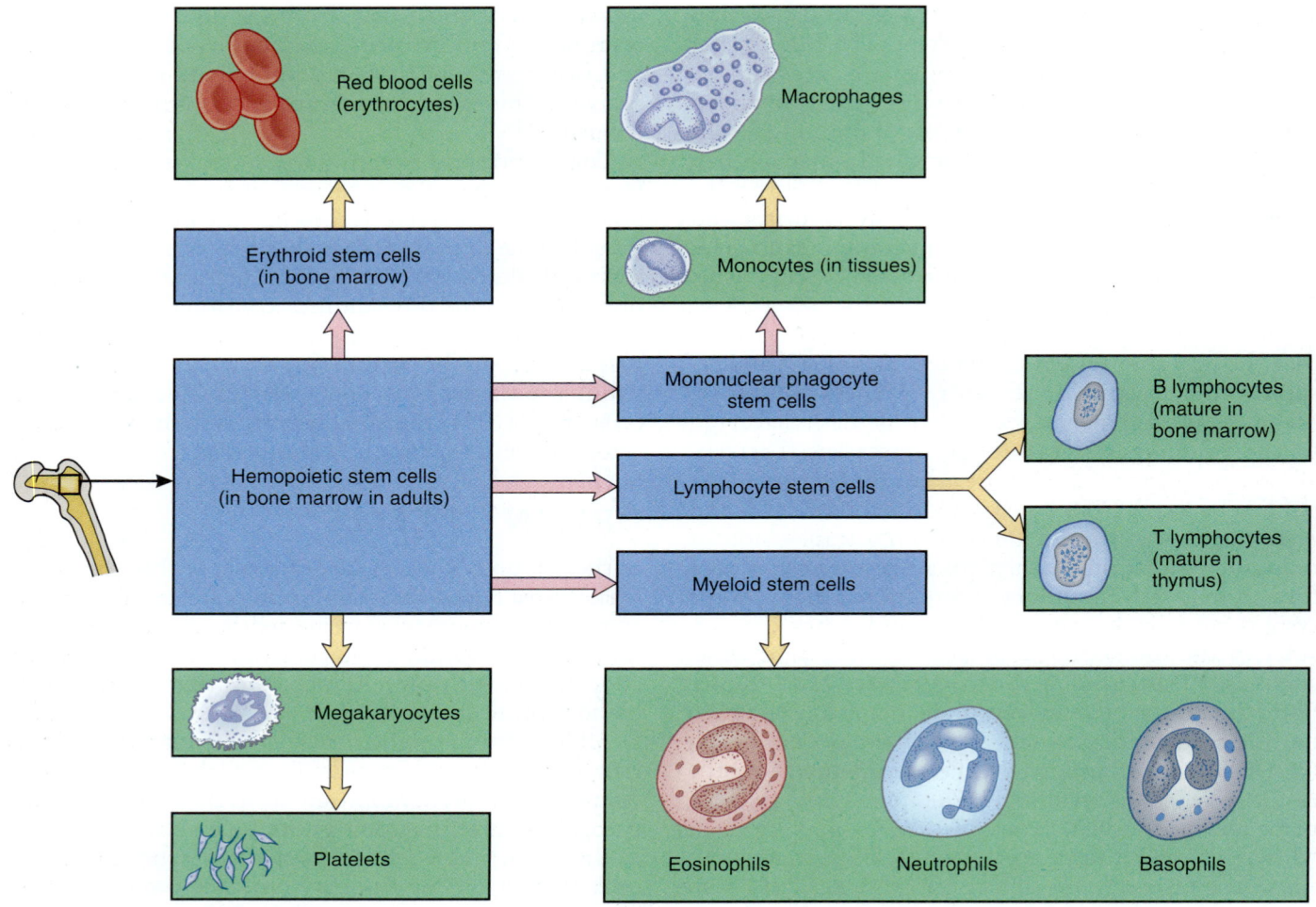

FIGURE 11-149 Origin of cells

and destroy invading bacteria, viruses, and other antigens. Eosinophils make up about 2% to 3% of white blood cells. They are weak **phagocytes** when fighting common infections but are produced in large amounts in response to certain parasitic infections. A high number of eosinophils will be found when there is inflammation or an allergic reaction. Basophils release heparin and histamine, which are essential components of the inflammatory process. Eosinophils and basophils are also granulated cells. They release their chemicals onto harmful cells or microbes in their environment.

ORGANS OF THE IMMUNE SYSTEM

The organs of the immune system are located throughout the body and are generally known as lymphoidal organs because they are where lymphocytes develop, grow, and perform their functions. These organs include the bone marrow, the thymus, lymph nodes, spleen, tonsils, adenoids, appendix, and clumps of lymphoid tissue in the small intestine called Peyer's patches (Figure 11-150). The lymph tissue organs house large numbers of lymphocytes and are located strategically throughout the

body. The lymph tissue in the Peyer's patches is exposed to antigens invading the intestinal tract. The lymph tissue of the tonsils and adenoids intercept antigens invading the upper respiratory tract. The tissues in the spleen and bone marrow are involved in fighting antigens that reach the blood vessels. When the B and T lymphocytes leave the bone marrow and the thymus, they travel throughout the body in the blood. They exit the capillaries and enter the **extracellular** fluid surrounding the cells to patrol the environment. As the lymph flows around the cells and through the body, it carries the lymphocytes, macrophages, and the antigens into the lymph capillaries and vessels. All along the lymphatic vessels are clusters of lymph nodes. A node functions somewhat like a filter. Immune cells and antigens enter the nodes through incoming afferent lymph vessels. Each node contains specialized compartments that store large numbers of B and T cells and others. The antigens are trapped and presented to the T cells for destruction (Figure 11-151). After the response is completed, the lymphocytes leave the lymph nodes in the outgoing efferent lymph vessels that eventually return them to the blood, where they begin the patrolling cycle once again.

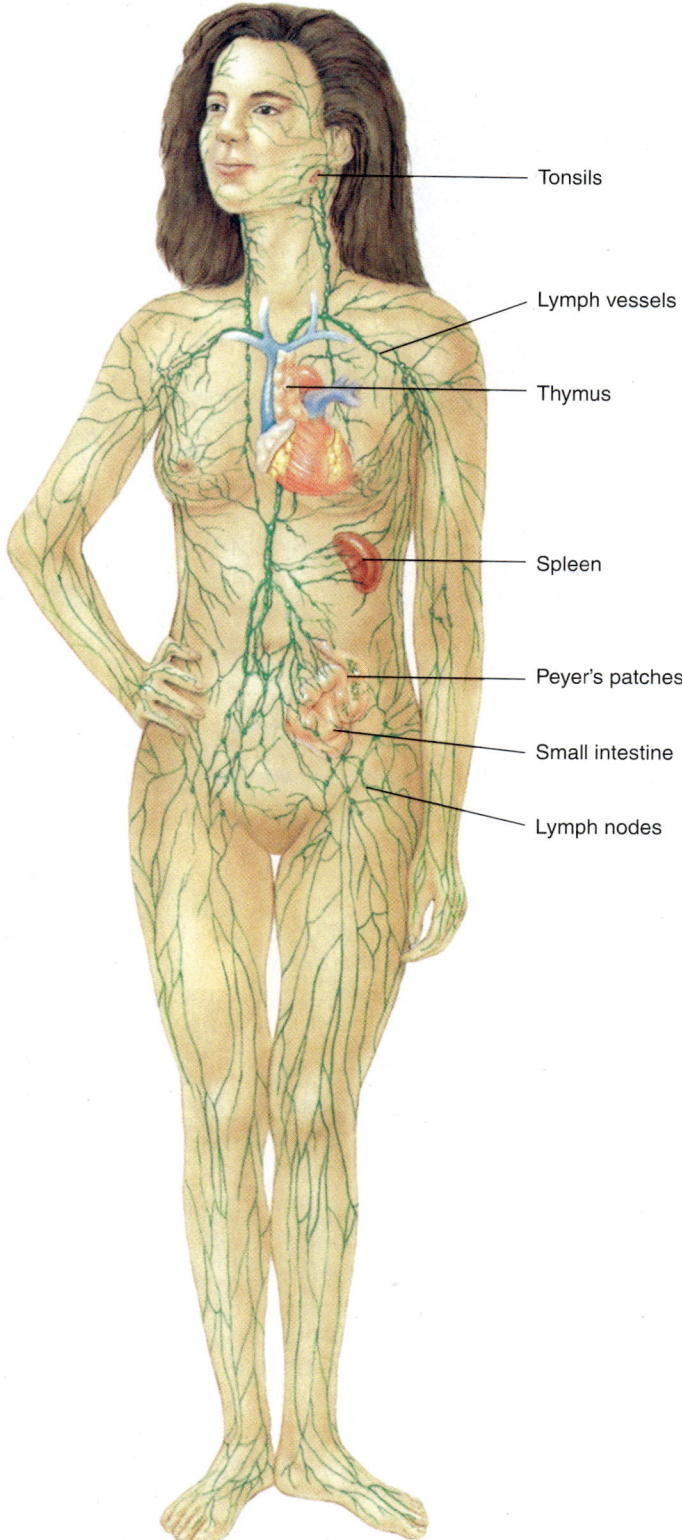

- Tonsils
- Lymph vessels
- Thymus
- Spleen
- Peyer's patches
- Small intestine
- Lymph nodes

FIGURE 11-150   Organs of the immune system

Now that you know how lymph nodes function, it is easy to understand why they become swollen and tender during periods of infection. It is because of the increased amount of cellular activity within the nodes. In the same manner, when malignant cells break away from the primary tumor and begin to circulate in the lymph fluid, they become trapped in the nearest nodes. When the nodes cannot contain all the malignant cells, the cells are able to circulate to another body site and begin to produce another area of malignancy. This is known as metastasis. The amount of lymph node involvement is one of the criteria for determining the extent of the cancer. This assessment is called **staging** and is determined by the size of the tumor, the number of involved lymph nodes, and the metastatic progress. As an example, when a mastectomy is performed for breast cancer, the surgeon also removes the lymph nodes that drain from that area of the breast. The nodes are tested for cancer cells, and the results become one factor in determining the staging of the cancer and the plan of treatment.

CELL MARKERS

Basic to the immune system is the ability of immune cells to determine initially the self or nonself status of encountered cells and molecules. All body cells carry molecules that are encoded by a group of genes known as the *major histocompatibility complex* (MHC). This is like a biochemical "fingerprint" that serves as the "ID" for cells so that they are marked as "self." This allows immune cells to recognize and communicate with each other. The body's immune defenses do not normally attack cells carrying this "self" marker. In addition, the millions of lymphocytes have approximately 100 million different surface receptor molecules that can "read" the surface patterns of virtually all nonself molecules that might invade the body. When they meet molecules carrying foreign markers, they move quickly to destroy them. Any nonself substance capable of triggering an immune response is considered to be an antigen. An antigen announces its foreignness by carrying different kinds of characteristic shapes called *epitopes,* which stick out from its surface. The immune system is capable of recognizing millions of these nonself molecules, or it can produce matching molecules that can counteract and destroy the antigen.

The MHC markers enable the immune system to achieve its function of recognizing self from nonself. The second function, homeostasis, involves the maintenance of the steady state of the system. This is accomplished by destroying damaged or dead cells. An example is the function of the spleen when it destroys damaged and dead red blood cells. The third function, surveillance, involves the recognition and destruction of abnormal cells. It is estimated that 100 to 1,000 mutated cells are formed every day. If not held in check by the immune system, cancer might develop. This is demonstrated by statistics showing that individuals who are immunocompromised have an increased risk of cancer.

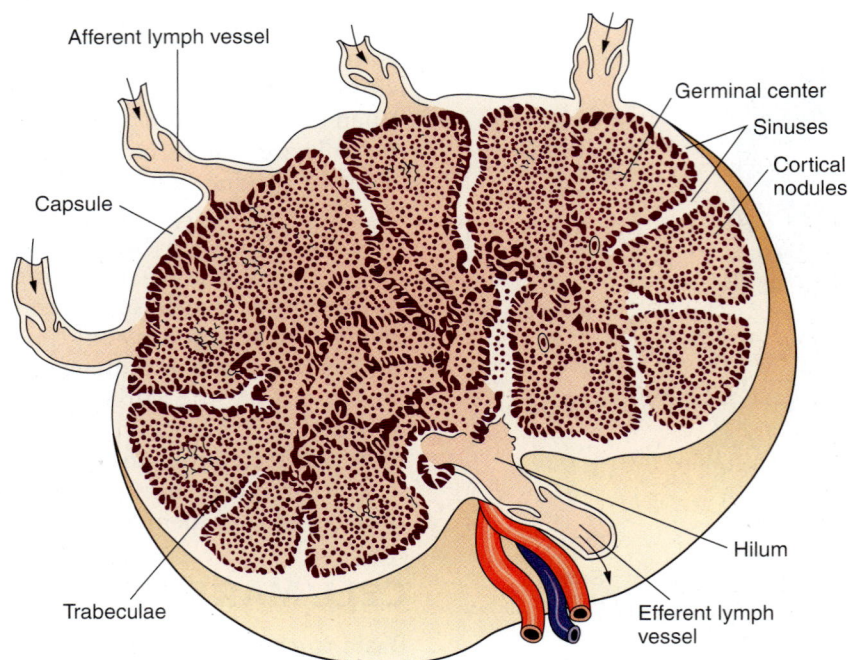

FIGURE 11-151   Lymph node

LYMPHOCYTES

Lymphocytes are the small white blood cells charged with immunity functions. Both T cells and B cells are able to recognize specific antigen targets.

T Lymphocytes

T lymphocytes make up about 80% of all circulating lymphocytes. They are capable of acting directly on their targets by a process called **cell-mediated** *immunity*. They are present in four identifiable types: helper T cells, suppressor T cells, memory T cells, and killer T cells.

- *Helper* T cells produce proteins called **lymphokines** that help other lymphocytes and phagocytes perform their functions. They also help B lymphocytes make antibodies. Helper T cells are identifiable by the CD4+ cell marker. The HIV virus affects the function of the helper T cells, and the severity of the disease is measured by the CD4+ blood counts.
- *Suppressor T* cells stop or turn off the actions of the T cells when the "battle" is under control.
- *Killer T* cells can directly kill infected or malignant cells and those cells carrying a target antigen. They are also known as **cytotoxic** T cells and carry the CD8+ cell marker. One type of killer T cell can attach tightly to its target and secrete perforin and other chemicals, which make holes in the target cell's membrane, destroying it before it can reproduce. Unfortunately, killer T cells will also attack the nonself marker cells of transplant tissues and organs, causing rejection.

- *Memory T* cells have a memory from a previous experience with specific antigens and so are prepared to act immediately upon recontact.

B Lymphocytes

B lymphocytes represent about 20% of the total lymphocytes. They act upon their targets by producing antibodies in a process called humoral immunity. When B cells are maturing, they go through two stages of development. The first begins with the cell inserting numerous molecules of one specific kind of antibody into its cytoplasmic membrane. Each type of B lymphocyte is capable of making only one type of antibody, and only one specific antigen can activate it. There are about 100,000 antibodies on the cell membranes of B lymphocytes. These each have a "combining site" with specific characteristics that will match the same characteristic site on the surface of a specific antigen.

When B cells with their antibody molecules come into contact with antigens, they undergo a second change. When the combining site of a B cell's surface "fits" one of the variety of antigen's surface shapes, they join and are changed into an antigen-antibody complex, and the antibody begins to perform its duties. It causes the antigen to stick to other antigens, forming clumps so the large macrophages can destroy large numbers of them at one time.

It also causes the B cell to begin to divide, rapidly producing many clone cells with the same antibody. Later the cells divide into memory or plasma cells (Figure 11-152). The memory cells go to the lymph nodes

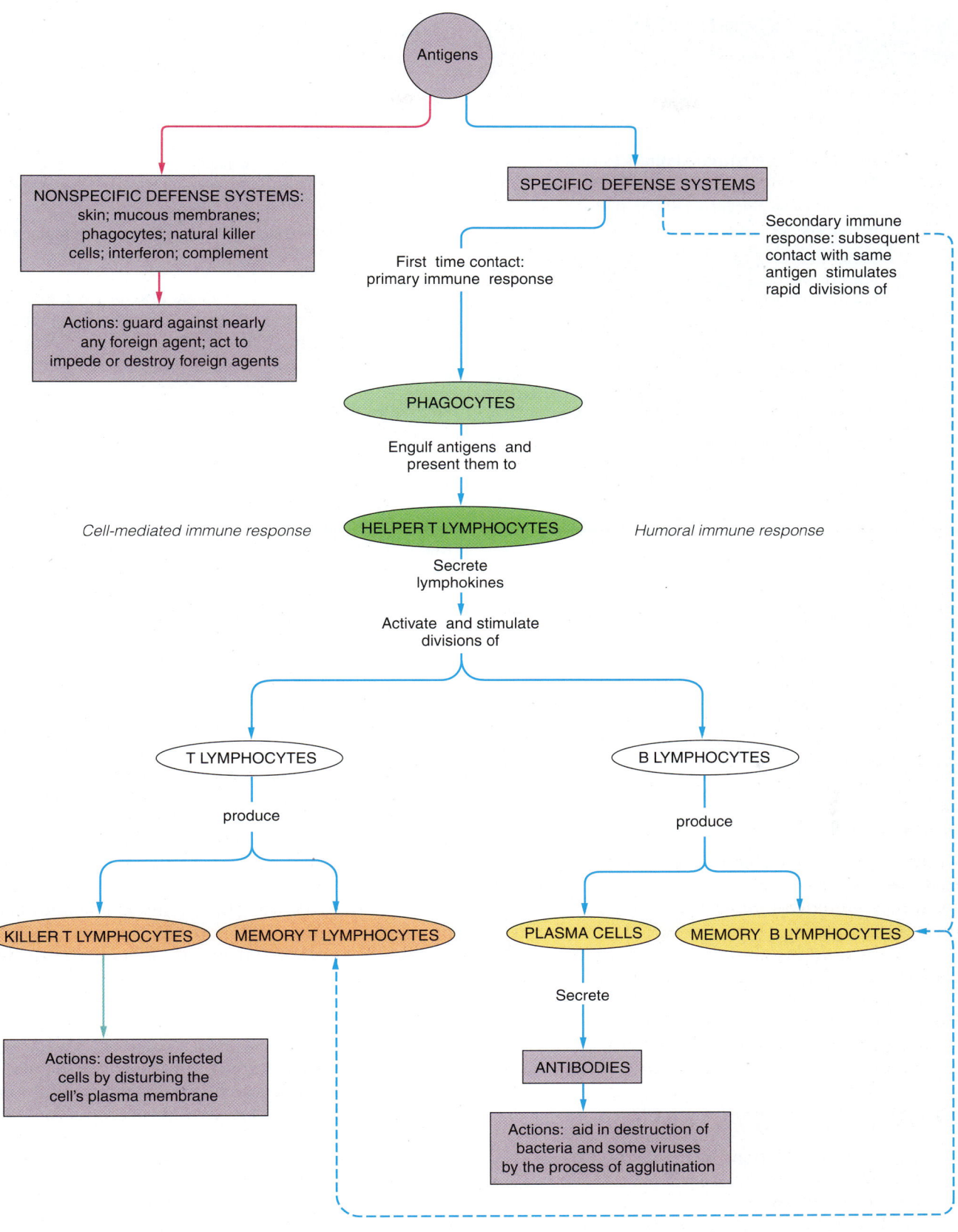

FIGURE 11-152   The body's defense mechanisms

TABLE 11-7	Antibody Class and Function
Class	**Function**
IgA	Concentrated in body fluids, such as tears, saliva, and respiratory and gastrointestinal secretions, to guard the entrances of the body
IgD	Located on B cell membranes. Believed to regulate B cell activity
IgE	Very effective against parasites but also involved in allergic responses, such as hayfever, asthma, and urticaria
IgG	The most plentiful antibody. It coats microorganisms in the tissues to speed up the uptake by other immune system cells. It carries out both antibacterial and antiviral activity. It can cross the placenta barrier.
IgM	Found in the bloodstream and very effective in killing bacteria. It is responsible for initial formation of antibodies once exposed to an antigen.

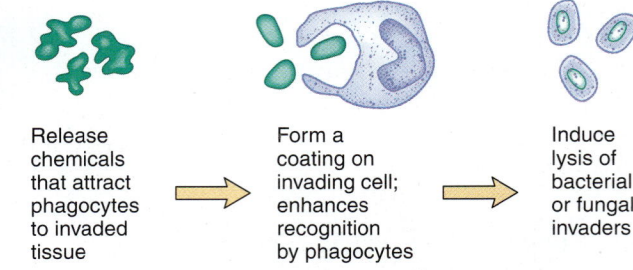

Release chemicals that attract phagocytes to invaded tissue ⟹ Form a coating on invading cell; enhances recognition by phagocytes ⟹ Induce lysis of bacterial or fungal invaders

FIGURE 11-153 Function of proteins in the complement system

to stand by for the next same-antigen invasion while the plasma cells continue to secrete millions of identical antibody molecules.

The immune system stockpiles a huge arsenal of cells, some for general defense, others for specific invaders. To be able to match millions of antigens, the system stores a few of each kind but can produce millions of the type to match the antigen within a very short period.

Antibodies

The antibodies from the B cells are protein substances belonging to a family of large molecules known as **immunoglobulins**. Five classes of human immunoglobulins have been identified and are classified by "Ig" for immunoglobin and a capital letter. The classes are: IgA, IgD, IgE, IgG, and IgM. Their presence in the body can be measured by a blood test called *serum protein electropheresis*. The role of antibodies is summarized in Table 11-7, which lists the antibody classes and key points of their function.

COMPLEMENT SYSTEM

Antibodies may change their shape slightly when they bind with antigens. This change will expose two regions called complement-binding sites. Complement is a group of about 20 *inactive* enzyme proteins normally present in the blood and involved in humoral immunity. When one complement protein meets an antibody-

antigen complex, it will *activate* and begin a chain reaction of attracting the others to "complement" the activity of the antibodies in destroying bacteria. Complement proteins circulate in the blood in an inactive form. When the first of the complement substances is triggered—usually by an antibody interlocked with an antigen—it sets in motion a ripple effect. As each component is activated in turn, it acts upon the next in a precise sequence of carefully regulated steps known as the "complement cascade." This results in the creation of lethal chemicals to attract the phagocytes to the scene, coat the target cell to make it more recognizable, or destroy the antigen by puncturing its membrane. In this way, antibodies and the complement system work together to destroy antigens by the **antibody-mediated** response also known as **humoral** immunity (Figure 11-153).

Inflammation

The events set off by antibody-mediated response and the other chemicals help to develop an inflammatory response. When complement proteins begin to act, basophils and mast cells are also activated. Both cells release the substance called **histamine**, which dilates blood vessels, slowing down the rate of flow. The vessel walls become more **permeable,** which allows fluid to seep into the surrounding tissues. The result is localized warmth, redness, and swelling. The complement proteins and other factors in the fluid can easily leave the blood vessels and attract the phagocytes in the tissues to fight the intruders.

CYTOKINES

Cytokines are nonantibody proteins that regulate the immune response. These substances are diverse and potent chemical messengers. Cytokines produced by T cells are called *lymphokines*. Those produced by macrophages/monocytes are called **monokines**. Another group of cytokines are produced by both lymphocytes and macrophages/monocytes. Lymphokines bind to specific receptors on target cells and set off other actions, such as getting other cells and substances involved, encouraging cell growth, and stimulating macrophages. Two other cytokines are lymphotoxin from lymphocytes and tumor necrosis factor from macrophages. Both of these cytokines kill tumor cells. Many cytokines have been renamed as **interleukins** (IL), which means "messengers between leukocytes." IL-1 from macrophages helps to activate B and T cells. IL-2 is produced by antigen-activated T cells and promotes rapid growth of mature B and T cells and the development of different types of T cells. There are six types of interleukins identified at present.

Some of the first cytokines discovered were **interferons**. They are produced by T cells, macrophages, and some cells outside the immune system. Interferons are a family of proteins that can fight viruses. Interferon from immune cells activates macrophages. The cytokine called tumor necrosis factor, which also comes from macrophages, kills tumor cells and inhibits parasites and viruses. Scientists have genetically engineered genes with cytokines to attack cancer cells. The tumor necrosis factor is measured to determine the effects of chemotherapy on certain cancers.

A summary of the 14 groups of cytokines is included in the Components of the Immune System, a color-treated section of the text following the discussion on immune response.

Natural Killer (NK) Cells

Natural Killer (NK) cells are non-T and non-B lymphocytes. NK cells are numerous in the bloodstream and the reticuloendothelial system. (The tissue macrophages and phagocytes in the blood and lymph.) NK cells kill cancer cells and cells infected with viruses without using antibodies or having prior exposure to the antigen. Like the killer T cell, they contain granules filled with potent chemicals. They bind to their targets and deliver a lethal burst of their chemicals to produce holes in the target cell's membrane, leading to its destruction. NK cells get the name "natural" because they do not need to recognize a specific antigen like other T cells in order to kill the invading antigen. The killing function of NK cells can be boosted by the administration of alpha interferon (a cytokine, nonantibody protein that is produced by T cells). Treatment with alpha interferon is used for many types of cancer, including chronic myelogenous leukemia and renal cell cancer, to increase the ability of NK cells to kill the cancer cells.

IMMUNE RESPONSES

The organs of the immune system, immune cells, cell markers, complement system, and related activities have been discussed. It is time to put it all together in an immune response as it would occur in the body.

The immune response system has two branches, one resulting from B cell activity, the humoral or antibody-mediated immune response, and one resulting from T cell activity, the cell-mediated immune response (review Figure 11-152). The response can also be primary when it is the first encounter with the antigen or a secondary response with subsequent encounters.

Primary Humoral (Antibody-Mediated) Response

In primary humoral response, an antigen enters the body and goes undetected past "virgin" desensitized B cells until it meets one with matching antibody sites. The B cell connects (becomes sensitized) and processes the antigen to attract helper T cells. When the sensitized B cell and the helper T combine, interleukins are released, which cause the cell to begin mitosis. At the same time, other similar antigens have been engulfed by the macrophages. Helper T cells bind with the macrophages, and interleukins are secreted. The secretion of interleukin stimulates the helper T cells to mature and secrete lymphokines to cause a rapid growth and division of the B cells. Some of the differentiated B cells become plasma cells and release identical antibodies in order to bind with more antigens for recognition and destruction. Some B cells convert to memory B cells. They do not produce antibodies at the time of the initial exposure, but they "remember" the encounter until the next exposure to the same antigen.

The immunoglobulins get other cells and substances involved. IgM and IgG activate macrophages and the complement system. IgE stimulates mast cells to release histamine. IgA causes secretions in the first line of defense in the saliva, tears, lungs, and intestines to protect the body's entrances. IgD works in the cell's membranes to regulate activity. A full primary immune response requires 5 to 6 days to develop.

Humoral antibody-mediated responses act against bacteria and extracellular viruses, fungi, and parasites. They *cannot* react to an invader already within a cell's cytoplasm, only those in circulation or attached to a cell's surface.

Secondary Response

In a secondary response, the reaction is much faster, taking only 2 to 3 days. This is possible because leftover **clonal** lymphocytes with memory are able to attack the antigen. Once one of the cells meets the same antigen, mitosis is immediate, and large numbers of appropriately matched cells and antibodies are produced to destroy the antigen.

Primary Cell-Mediated Response

Primary response of T cells in cell-mediated response is both quick and direct. Some T cells are vital to the operation of other cells. The helper T cells assist B cells to produce antibodies. Helper T cells identify antigens trapped by macrophages. The processed antigen binds with helper T cells and with B lymphocytes. The helper T cells secrete interleukin, and the B cell carries out humoral immunity. In cell-mediated immunity, the helper T cells' interleukin secretions activate the killer T cells to attack. Macrophages are recruited, and inflammation is triggered. The NK cells are also stimulated into action to directly destroy **cancerous** and virus-infected cells before they can divide and begin growing.

Some T cells will also develop memory and are held in reserve for subsequent invasions. Cell-mediated immune responses attack **intracellular** viruses, fungi and protozoans, cancer cells, and transplant tissue cells.

Killer cells that cause rejection of organ transplants do so because the MHC markers of the donor cells are not identical self-markers unless they are from an identical twin. Individuals who are to receive organs are given drugs to destroy the killer T cells to prevent rejection; however, that leaves the recipient without the ability to have a full immune response to other invaders and can lead to death from infections such as pneumonia.

Both antibody-mediated and cell-mediated immune responses are controlled reactions. When the "battle" is won, the binding sites are saturated with antibodies, and the **suppressor** T cells stop the attack. Without this feedback, immune reactions would go out of control.

The complexity of the immune system makes it very difficult to understand. The two features on the following pages provide summaries, one of the components and another of the surveillance process, to make the immune system a little clearer. This material is taken from a presentation by Elaine Glass, RN, MS, OCN; Clinical Nurse Specialist in Medical Oncology and Hematology. She explains the functions of the components of the immune system and relates them to the familiar roles of a police and military force (shown in italics). The cell-mediated responses are the duties of the police, whereas the antibody response is the job of the army. There is even one firefighter who is involved. Note that there are also statements in italics and parentheses concerning emotions, exercise, and personal interactions and their effect upon the immune system. This connection is now being recognized as important and as evidence of the impact of diet. Because these effects are often based on multiple and difficult to measure factors and usually cover long periods, studies require long-term commitments from participants and extended time to identify and validate apparent cause and effect relationships in the development of disease.

COMPONENTS OF THE IMMUNE SYSTEM

AGRANULOCYTES

A. Macrophages/Monocytes

The cop on the beat

Monocytes circulate in the blood; macrophages infiltrate the tissues. They engulf antigens and summon other cells to analyze them.

(Stress causes release of cortisol that renders the macrophage unresponsive.

Exercise increases endorphins [natural brain analgesic], which may increase macrophage activity.)

B. Lymphocytes

A collective label for T and B immune cells

1. T CELLS

Involved in the cellular immune system response.
Mature in the thymus gland.

a. Helper T cell

The detective

Identifies the antigens trapped by macrophages or monocytes and stimulates other cells to destroy them. Does not attack or destroy by itself.

b. Activated helper T cell

Helps destroy identified antigens by producing interleukin-2, which stimulates other helper and killer T cells to multiply.

c. Killer T cell

SWAT team member

Destroys cells that have been invaded by antigens. They can trigger a process that punctures a cell membrane and destroys it before the invading virus inside has a chance to grow.

d. Natural killer T cell

Rambo or a vigilante

Attacks cancerous or virus-infected cells without previous exposure to the antigen. NKs are stimulated by interferon. They can recognize artificial antigens created in a lab to which humans have never come into contact.

(In one study, patients with a lot of support from their "significant others" and doctors had higher levels of NK cells.)

e. Suppressor T cell

The police chief

Slows down or stops other immune cell activity after antigens are destroyed.

2. B CELLS

Produces antibodies against antigens; involved in the humoral immune response.

a. Plasma cell

The army sergeant

Descends from B cells to produce antibodies. They make thousands of antibodies per second.

b. Antibodies

The foot soldiers

Proteins that neutralize antigens and destroy other cells where the antigen has invaded.

1) IgG

The most common protein antibody in the blood and tissue spaces, where it coats antigens, speeding their uptake by other immune cells.

2) IgM

A protein antibody that circulates in the bloodstream in star-shaped clusters; very effective in killing bacteria.

3) IgA

A protein antibody in body fluids (tears, saliva, respiratory and digestive tracts) to guard body entrances.

(College students who watched a video of Mother Teresa had higher levels of IgG and IgA than students who watched a video that did not stimulate positive emotions.)

4) IgE

A protein antibody that attaches itself to mast cells and basophils. When it encounters its matching antigen, it stimulates the cell to pour out its contents. It provides protection by coating bacteria and viruses.

5) IgD

A protein antibody that inserts itself into the membrane of the B cell to regulate the activation of the cell.

c. Complement

Flying Aces

A series of 20 proteins that circulate in the blood in an inactive state until they are triggered by contact with antigen-antibody complexes or by contact with the cell membrane of an invading organism.

T cells = Police chief with a history on the force

B cells = Army sergeant with a history in the service

T and B cells that have been activated by an antigen and continue to circulate within the body, ready to attack an antigen if it reinvades. (These cells are the basis of how vaccines work.)

GRANULOCYTES

A group of immune cells filled with granules of toxic chemicals that enable them to digest microorganisms.

A. Neutrophil

Like cop on beat but more heavily armed

A circulating WBC that destroys foreign matter and cell debris by phagocytosis, by digesting cellular membranes, and by releasing chemotactants and pyrogenic substances that cause fever.

B. Basophil

A firefighter

A circulating WBC that is responsible for allergy symptoms by releasing heparin, histamine, bradykinin, and serotonin from its granules, to cause vasodilation and permeability.

C. Eosinophil

A circulating WBC that can digest microorganisms, especially parasites, and assists in allergic reactions by detoxifying some of the inflammation-inducing substances to prevent the spread of the local inflammatory process.

D. Mast cells

Special member of police force that is armed with chemicals.

Special cells found in tissues that contain granules of chemicals that produce redness, warmth, and swelling (allergy symptoms).

CYTOKINES

All nonantibody proteins that regulate the immune response. Cytokines produced by T cells are called *lymphokines*. Cytokines produced by macrophages/monocytes are called *monokines*.

A. Lymphokines

A number of proteins produced by T cells

1. Granulocyte-macrophage colony-stimulating factor (GM-CSF)

GM-CSF stimulates the growth of neutrophils, eosinophils, and macrophages. It increases the ingestion of bacteria and the killing of tumors coated with antibody. It activates mature granulocytes and macrophages.

2. Interferons

A class of lymphokines with important immunoregulatory functions, especially improving the activities of macrophages and NK cells. *Exercise may increase the production of interferon.*

a. Alpha (IFN-α)

Is produced by leukocytes in response to viral infections. It also increases NK activity and the numbers of cytotoxic T cells and starts the tumoricidal activity of macrophages.

b. Beta (IFN-β)

Its activity is similar to IFN-α.

c. Gamma (IFN-γ)

Is produced by T and NK cells. It (1) activates killer T cells; (2) increases the ability of B cells to produce antibodies; (3) keeps macrophages at the site; and (4) assists them in digesting bacteria and cancerous cells they engulf. IFN-γ also regulates other lymphokines, increases NK activity, and starts the production of T cell suppressor factor.

3. IL-2 (Interleukin-2)

Is produced by helper T cells and NK cells, which stimulates other helper, killer, and suppressor T cells to multiply. It starts cytokine production by T cells and monocytes. It improves NK cell activity.

4. IL-3

   Is produced by activated T cells. It is a growth factor for mast cells and most bone marrow progenitor (after stem) xcells.

5. IL-4

   Is called B cell growth factor and causes B cells, mast cells, and resting T cells to multiply. It increases toxicity of killer T cells and macrophages. It is produced by helper T cells.

6. IL-5

   Is produced by activated T cells. It is an important factor in the final differentiation of eosinophils and activated B cells. It increases IgA, IgM, and IgE development and secretion. It begins the appearance of IL-2 receptors on B cells.

7. Soluble immune response suppressor (SIRS)

   SIRS is released by suppressor T cells and may slow down immune cell activity.

B. Monokines

Proteins produced primarily by monocytes

1. Granulocyte colony-stimulating factor (G-CSF)

   G-CSF stimulates the growth and activity of neutrophils. It is produced by monocytes and some other nonblood cells.

2. Macrophage colony-stimulating factor (M-CSF)

   M-CSF stimulates the growth and activity of macrophages. It is also produced by monocytes and other nonblood cells.

   (GM-CSF, G-CSF, IL2, and interferon are now produced synthetically and are being used as anticancer drugs. They have shown promise in the treatment of some types of malignancies.)

C. Other cytokines

(Produced by both lymphocytes and macrophages/monocytes)

1. IL-1

   Is produced by macrophages, T cells, granulocytes, and NK cells. It activates helper T cells and raises the body's temperature. (Fever increases immune cell activity). It stimulates the production of lymphokines and activates macrophages to immobilize cancer cells. It starts the differentiation of stem cells and activated B cells and increases the number of activated B cells. Exercise may increase IL-1 production.

2. IL-6 (B cell differentiation factor)

   Is called BCDF and causes some B cells to stop dividing and to start making immunoglobin and antibodies. Improves the differentiation of killer T cells. Is produced by helper T cells, monocytes, and fibroblasts. It also stimulates the production of platelets.

3. Tumor growth factor-beta (TGF-β)

   TGF-β is produced by T cells, macrophages, and tumor cells. It suppresses T and B cell growth and differentiation and antibody secretion.

4. Tumor necrosis factor-B (TNF-B)

   TNF-B, also known as lymphotoxin, is produced by B cells, T cells, mast cells, and macrophages. It makes some cells more vulnerable to lysis by NK cells.

5. Tumor necrosis factor (TNF)

   TNF is produced by monocytes, activated macrophages, NK cells, and mast cells. It can kill tumors or retard their growth. It causes some tumors to bleed and die. It stimulates the production of lymphokines and activates macrophages.

By now, you must be amazed at the complexity and function of the immune system. The previous outline of the duties of its components causes one to wonder how all that coordinated effort ever gets accomplished. And yet, so much more is not understood.

To give a brief overall picture of what happens when an immune system cell comes into contact with an antigen, consider the following box. In italics within parentheses are descriptions of the cartoon slides Glass uses to summarize her discussion of the surveillance process of the immune system. She again uses the police and military roles in the scenarios. If you can visualize the scene, it may help you to get an understanding of the immune process.

IMMUNE SYSTEM SURVEILLANCE PROCESS

1. A macrophage (or complement protein, NK cell, or memory cell) recognizes an antigen.
   (A cop begins to struggle with an alien.)
2. Helper T cells bind to the macrophage and become activated by the cytokine, IL-1, which also causes fever.
   (The detective sees the cop and alien struggling and calls for help.)
3. Activated helper T cells produce a lymphokine, IL-2, which stimulates other helper and killer T cells to multiply.
   (Help arrives as detectives, SWAT team, and a few army sergeants.)
4. Helper T cells also secrete a lymphokine, IL-4, which causes B cells to multiply.
   (The detective decides more army personnel are needed and calls in the troops. The army comes marching in.)
5. Helper T cells also secrete a lymphokine, IL-6, which causes some B cells to stop dividing and start making antibodies.
   (The sergeant calls the foot soldiers into duty.)
6. Helper T cells also produce the lymphokine interferon, which activates killer T cells, increases the ability of B cells to produce antibodies, and keeps macrophages at the site and assists them in digesting the cells they engulf.
   (The detective calls out words of encouragement to the SWAT team, the sergeants, and the street cops.)

7. Killer T cells destroy the cells where antigens have invaded.
   (The SWAT team member nails an alien inside a phone booth.)

8. Antibodies neutralize the antigen and destroy other cells that have also been infected.
   (A foot soldier punches out an alien.)

9. Complement proteins, triggered by antigen-antibody complexes, or the cell membranes of some invading microorganisms:
   (The flying aces come into the action.)
   - Cause chemotaxis of macrophages and neutrophils to the area. *(An ace calls in the street cop.)*
   - Increase phagocytosis of macrophages and neutrophils. *(The street cops look mean and ugly.)*
   - Activate basophils and mast cells to release immobilizing chemicals and other products that increase inflammation. *(The firefighters and cops with chemicals soak the aliens.)*
   - Change the invader's cell surface, causing them to stick together. *(The aliens get stuck.)*
   - Attack the invader's structure and make it inactive. *(The aces crop-dust the aliens.)*
   - Rupture the invader's cell membrane. *(The ace's gunner blows a hole through the alien.)*

10. Suppressor T cells halt the immune response after the antigen is destroyed.
    (The police chief enters the scene and halts the action once the aliens are destroyed.)

11. Memory T and B cells are left in the blood and lymph system to defend against another attack.
    (The detectives and the army sergeants have the alien's ID in case future attacks occur.)

Note: Scientists have made great progress in understanding the functions of the many components of the immune system, but a great deal still remains a mystery. It is an unbelievably complicated interaction of cells, antibodies, and proteins against antigens and allergens. Recently, it has been recognized that the brain, nervous system, and hormones also have a relationship with the immune response. A new science called **psychoneuroimmunology** involves researching the connection between the brain, behavior, and immunity. Scientists have discovered that the brain produces over 50 neuropeptides that have receptors on WBCs and can affect the cell's activity. For example, people who feel hopeless have sluggish macrophages. Laughter increases NK activity, lymphocyte proliferation, migration of monocytes, and the production of IL-2 and IgA. It would seem we may have the power to influence our own immune system if we can learn how.

IMMUNIZATION

With the knowledge of immune reactions, it is easy to understand how immunizations (shots) and vaccinations provide protection against antigens. The smallpox **vaccine**, for instance, was the deliberate introduction of the smallpox antigen into the body in a state that caused only minor reaction but was sufficient for the body to produce an antigen-antibody complex and eventually memory cells against the disease. Other examples of purposeful antigen introduction are measles, mumps, diphtheria, poliovirus, varicella, hepatitis A and B, pneumonia, pertussis, and tetanus toxoid (given routinely to infants and children).

Vaccines are given in initial and in "booster" doses to provide memory cells and antibodies for longer periods. These methods provide active immunity because the recipients make their own immunity. Another form is known as passive immunity and is given to people already exposed to a disease, such as tetanus. Antibodies from another source are injected into the person to provide a temporary immunity to counter the immediate attack of pathogens. This immunity is short lived. The tetanus antitoxin given after certain injuries or animal bites is an example of this type of vaccine.

DISEASES AND DISORDERS

Acquired Immunodeficiency Syndrome (AIDS) (Imu-no-de-fish'en-se)

*Description—***Acquired immunodeficiency syndrome (AIDS)** is a worldwide epidemic caused by the human immunodeficiency virus (HIV). The term AIDS refers to the most advanced stages of HIV infection. It is estimated that there are 40 million people in the world living with HIV infection. The AIDS epidemic is greatest in sub-Saharan Africa. In Zimbabwe the prevalence is estimated at 20% of the population. The impact is great on the work force and families, especially the large number of orphans. In South Africa in 2004, over one in five teachers between 25 and 34 years of age were HIV positive. The epidemic has slowed somewhat from 1.5 million new HIV infections per year in the 1990s to 1.1 million for the last 3 years.

Globally, HIV prevalence is still increasing over time as the epidemic spreads to different countries. Data are very difficult to obtain in developing countries due to lack of contact with the medical community and ineffective means of collection. Also, intense and even life-threatening stigma and discrimination in some cultures leads to denial and underreporting.

The beginning of AIDS in the United States is well documented. Between October 1980 and May 1981, five young, previously healthy homosexual men were treated for a pneumonia caused by *Pneumocystis carinii*. They were treated at three different hospitals in Los Angeles. Doctors and health care professionals were curious because usually *P. carinii* pneumonia occurred only in immunosuppressed patients, especially those receiving cancer therapy. At the same time, a rare and unusual blood vessel malignancy called Kaposi's sarcoma was being diagnosed with increasing frequency in young homosexuals in California and New York (Figure 11-154). By July 1981, 26 cases of Kaposi's sarcoma had been diagnosed. Seven of these men also had serious infections; four had *P. carinii* pneumonia. These cases were an early indication of an epidemic of a previously unknown disease. Later it was called the acquired immunodeficiency syndrome, or AIDS. As of 2004, a total of 944,305 cases have been reported—934,862 adults and adolescents, with 756,399 being male and 178,463 being female. Of these cases, the total number of reported deaths is 523,598, about 58% of the infected.

The data in Table 11-8 and 11-9 are adapted from CDC HIV/AIDS Surveillance Report: HIV Infection and AIDS in the United States, 2004.

TABLE 11-8	AIDS Cases		
Age	New AIDS Cases in 2004	Number of AIDS Cases, through 2004 (Estimated)	Cumulative Cases, by Ages
<13	48	9,443	9,443
13–14	60	959	10,402
15–19	326	4,936	15,338
20–24	1,788	34,164	49,502
25–29	3,576	114,642	164,144
30–34	5,786	195,404	359,548
35–39	8,031	208,199	567,747
40–44	8,747	161,964	729,711
45–49	6,245	99,644	829,355
50–54	3,932	54,869	884,224
55–59	2,079	29,553	913,777
60–64	996	16,119	929,896
65	901	14,410	944,306

PEDIATRIC PERSPECTIVE

There have been 9,443 AIDS cases reported through 2004 in children younger than 13. During the same time, 5,515 children under age 13 died, also about 58% of the infected.

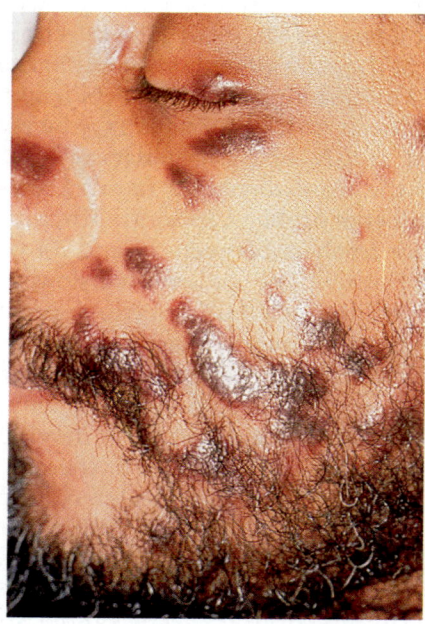

FIGURE 11-154   Typical skin lesions of Kaposi's sarcoma *(Courtesy of Robert A. Silverman, MD, Clinical Associate Professor, Department of Pediatrics, Georgetown University)*

Table 11-8 lists the cumulative AIDS cases by age. Observe that a very large number of patients, 729,711 (approximately 77%), are younger than 45 years old. This translates into a lifelong battle against the disease for a lot of people. It also translates into billions of dollars needed for their care.

The Centers for Disease Control and Prevention estimated at the end of 2003 that 1,185,000 persons in the United States were living with HIV/AIDS, and another 24% to 27% were undiagnosed and unaware of their HIV infection.

Etiology—AIDS is an infectious disease caused by the human immunodeficiency virus (HIV), which renders the body's immune system ineffective. The virus has been found in many body fluids but survives well only in those with numerous WBCs, such as in blood, semen, and vaginal secretions. The virus invades the helper T cells and macrophages, hiding within their membranes. Because both stimulate one another at different times in the immune response, when the helper Ts are "disabled," they do not cause the macrophages to act, which results in the diversion of B cell antibody production and the absence of NK cell formation. HIV is a **retrovirus**: its genetic material is RNA instead of DNA. It wraps itself in components from the host helper T cell membrane. Once inside the host, an enzyme uses the viral RNA as a "pattern" for making DNA and inserts these new instructions into the host's chromosome.

The virus hides in the cells for months or even years. It is difficult to determine its average or maximum incubation period. The onset of AIDS following infection with the HIV virus has been observed from as little as 6 months to as many as 10 years or more. The average onset of symptoms of AIDS appears to be 10 years. At some time, the body makes a secondary response, and the infected cells are activated. They copy their new DNA with the viral RNA, and new virus particles are assembled. They form "buds" on the helper T cell membrane and separate. This process continues until the helper T cells are depleted and the immune system is destroyed, leaving the person vulnerable to opportunistic infections that may eventually cause death.

The HIV virus requires certain conditions to be able to transfer to a new host. Avoiding these situations will decrease the risk of becoming infected. The virus can be transmitted by the following methods:

- Unprotected sex with an infected partner. **Transmission** can occur through the vagina, vulva, rectum, penis, and mouth during sex.
- Sharing drug needles or syringes with a person infected with HIV.
- Women with HIV can transmit the virus to their babies during pregnancy, birth, and breast-feeding. Twenty-five to thirty-three percent of infected mothers will transmit the infection to their babies. (The medication AZT [zidovudine] and delivery by cesarean section can significantly reduce the transmission rate.)
- The risk of getting HIV from blood transfusions is extremely low. All blood in the United States is screened for HIV.
- The risk to health care professionals of obtaining HIV from accidental needle sticks and contact with blood and body fluids are eliminated by following protective Standard Precautions when providing care.

Table 11-9 identifies the method of contact for the estimated number of cases in 2004. At best these are estimates, because there is a considerable lapse of time between exposure and development of AIDS.

There are some people who fear that HIV can be transmitted in other ways, but it has not been proven by research. The most common misconceptions are:

- Casual contact with an infected person through sharing food utensils, towels, toilet, telephones, bedding, or swimming pools.
- Closed-mouth kissing. The CDC does recommend eliminating open-mouth kissing, although the risk is very low.
- Mosquitoes, bedbugs, or other biting insects.
- Tattooing and body piercing could theoretically transmit the virus if the open skin area comes into contact with the organism or if contaminated instruments are used. There have been no instances of HIV transmission in the United States from either activity.

TABLE 11-9 Estimated Number of AIDS Cases by Exposure Category in 2004

Exposure Category	Male	Female	Total
Male-to-male sexual contact	17,691	—	17,691
Injection drug use	5,968	3,184	9,152
Male-to-male sexual contact and injection drug use	1,920	—	1,920
Heterosexual contact	5,149	7,979	13,128
Other (includes hemophilia, blood transfusion, perinatal, and risk not reported)	298	279	577

Early signs and symptoms—Many people who are infected with the virus do not have any symptoms when first infected. Within a month or 2 after exposure, however, they may have a flulike illness that includes headache, fever, fatigue, and enlarged lymph nodes. The symptoms usually subside within a week. During this flulike period, the HIV virus is present in high concentrations in genital fluids, and infected persons are highly contagious.

Later signs and symptoms—Severe symptoms of HIV infection may not appear for 10 or more years in adults and 2 or more years in children. However, during this asymptomatic period, the infected person is still capable of passing on the virus, and the T helper cells are being systematically destroyed. The numbers decline (as measured by the CD4 [T4] counts) and infections and other symptoms begin to occur, such as:

- Enlarged lymph nodes
- Fatigue
- Pelvic inflammatory disease
- Fever, sweats
- Weight loss
- Yeast infections
- Rashes, dry skin
- Short-term memory loss

Late signs and symptoms of AIDS—The signs and symptoms of AIDS are related to the effects of infections and cancer.

The presence of the opportunistic infections, such as *Pneumocystis carinii pneumonia*, are indicated by a fever, cough, and difficulty breathing; by *Kaposi's sarcoma*, a form of cancer appearing as purplish blotches on the skin (see Figure 11-154); by *candidiasis*, a yeast infection that is sometimes present in the mouth, esophagus, and vagina; and by the usual infections. There are over 20 opportunistic infections that people with AIDS may experience, such as other forms of pneumonia, meningitis, encephalitis, esophagitis, persistent diarrhea, and skin inflammation. These are often resistant to treatment. About 60% of AIDS patients have neurologic symptoms, including motor problems, inability to concentrate, memory loss, and progressive mental deterioration. They are believed to be caused by brain infection or cancer.

Diagnosis of HIV Infections

Early HIV infection usually has no signs or symptoms; therefore, it can only be detected by a blood test or by testing saliva. Blood tests detect antigens found on the virus or detect antibodies made against HIV. The antibodies may not be detectable for 1 to 4 months after infection, and it may be as long as 6 months before enough antibodies are present in the blood to test positive.

There are two different tests for HIV antibodies, the *ELISA* (enzyme-linked immunosorbent assay) and the *Western blot.* A general guideline used is if the ELISA test is reactive, it is repeated two more times. If it is positive three times, a Western blot test is performed. The Western blot is used to confirm the diagnosis because a small number of ELISA tests may show a false positive. Another test called the Coulter HIV-p24 Antigen Assay can detect the presence of HIV antigens. In the clinical setting, it is used when patients are highly suspected to be positive but show negative tests on both the ELISA and Western blot tests.

Home testing for HIV is available and is increasing the process of testing, primarily because it protects the patient's identity. Some tests use a blood sample, whereas another, called the Orasure, uses a treated cotton pad to collect an oral sample between the gum and cheek.

Physicians can now predict the risk of HIV progressing to AIDS by monitoring the HIV virus levels in the blood. The test is based on studies that have shown that higher levels of the virus in the blood correlate with an increased risk of the disease progressing to AIDS and AIDS-related infection or death.

Diagnosis of AIDS

The CDC diagnosis for AIDS requires a positive confirmed test for HIV and at least one of the following:

- CD4 count less than 200 per cubic millimeter of blood or a CD4 count of less than 14% of the total number of lymphocytes. The CD4 count measures the number of helper T lymphocytes.
- The presence of an **opportunistic** infection, such as pneumocystis pneumonia.
- An AIDS-related cancer, a severe wasting, or dementia.

Table 11-10 lists the clinical conditions in patients that indicate AIDS.

TABLE 11-10   Clinical Conditions in Patients with AIDS

AIDS Indicator Diseases

Opportunistic Infections

Candidiasis: bronchi, esophageal, trachea, lungs

Coccidioidomycosis

Cryptococcosis, extrapulmonary

Cryptosporidiosis, chronic intestinal greater than 1 month in duration

Cytomegalovirus, other than liver, spleen, or nodes

Cytomegalovirus retinitis with loss of vision

Disseminated histoplasmosis

Herpes simplex: chronic ulcers more than 1 month in duration or bronchitis, pneumonitis, or esophagitis

HIV encephalopathy

Isosporiasis, chronic

Mycobacterium avium complex or *M. kansasii,* disseminated or extrapulmonary

Mycobacterium of other species

Pneumocystis carinii pneumonia

Pneumonia, recurrent in 12-month period

Progressive multifocal leukoencephalopathy

Salmonella septicemia

Toxoplasmosis of the brain

Tuberculosis, extrapulmonary

Tuberculosis, pulmonary

AIDS-Related Cancers

Burkitt's lymphoma

Immunoblastic lymphoma

Lymphoma, primary brain

Invasive cervical cancer

Kaposi's sarcoma

Other

HIV wasting syndrome

AIDS Prevention

AIDS can be prevented by practicing personal measures to protect oneself. The disease is contracted primarily through contact with an infected person's blood, semen, or vaginal secretions. The virus enters through the vagina, penis, rectum, or mouth (in oral sex). The safest lifestyle is sexual **abstinence** or a faithful **monogamous** relationship. If these conditions are not absolutely certain, then precautions must be taken.

1. Avoid high-risk sexual activities. Behaviors that may cause you to acquire the virus are very clear:
   - Having unprotected sex, homosexual or heterosexual, with an HIV-infected person (oral, vaginal, or anal).
   - Using IV drugs and sharing needles.
   - Having many sexual partners; risk increases with number of partners.
   - Having other sexually transmitted diseases, such as gonorrhea, syphilis, or genital herpes.

2. Use a latex condom *properly* to maintain a barrier to the transmission of the virus. It must stay intact and be in place from the beginning to the end of vaginal, anal, or oral sex. The use of a spermicide provides additional protection. The condom must be carefully removed and disposed of properly. Condoms must never be reused.

Treatment—Unfortunately, no vaccine, antitoxin, or drug "cures" AIDS. In 1981, when AIDS was first diagnosed in the United States, there were no effective medications to treat the disease. Over the past 10 years, researchers have developed drugs to fight the virus, the associated infections, and the cancers. A number of medications to treat HIV infection have been approved by the Food and Drug Administration (FDA). The virus can become resistant to any of these drugs; therefore, combinations of medications are used. All medications and combinations used to treat HIV have numerous side effects, including bone marrow suppression, nausea, and nerve damage. The side effects decrease the individual's compliance to taking the medications.

Medications to Treat HIV and AIDS

The following medications are used to treat HIV and AIDS.

- Nucleoside reverse transcriptase (RT) inhibitors—These drugs were the first to be approved to treat HIV infection. They are incorporated into the DNA of HIV and stop the building process. They can slow the spread of HIV and delay the onset of opportunistic infections. Examples are AZT (zidovudine or ZDV), ddC (zalcitabine), ddI (didanosine), and d4T (stavudine).
- Non-nucleoside reverse transcription inhibitors (NNRTIs)—These drugs prevent HIV replication by inhibiting a viral protein. Examples include efavirenz (Sustiva), nevirapine (Viramune), and delavirdine (Rescriptor).
- Protease inhibitors—The inhibitors interrupt virus replication at a later stage in the life cycle. Examples include ritonavir (Norvir), saquinivir (Invirase), and indinavir (Crixivan).
- Entry inhibitors—These newer drugs prevent HIV from entering healthy T cells. The first drug approved in this class is enfuvirtide (Fuzeon).

- Highly active antiretroviral therapy (HAART)—HAART is a treatment regimen that combines reverse transcriptase inhibitors and protease inhibitors. It is considered highly effective and is believed to be responsible for reducing the number of deaths from AIDS by almost half in the United States. Patients who are newly infected with HIV and those with AIDS can take HAART. It has been found to decrease the amount of circulating virus to almost undetectable levels. However, it still cannot eliminate HIV from the body.

Treatment of Opportunistic Infections and Cancer

A variety of at least 22 FDA-approved medications are available to prevent and treat the many opportunistic infections and cancers experienced by patients with AIDS. Table 11-11 lists some of most common.

HIV Vaccines

Research is being conducted in the United States and throughout the world to develop a safe and effective vaccination against HIV infection. The vaccines are designed to induce the development of antibodies to different strains of HIV.

Needless to say, AIDS must be prevented. To obtain a free brochure, materials, and confidential AIDS counseling, call the toll-free National AIDS Hotline (800–342–AIDS). Information is also abundant on the Internet. Search under various sites, such as CDC, AOL Health, and AIDS organizations.

Allergies (Al'er-jees)

Description—Sometimes the immune system can damage instead of protect the body. A secondary response to a normally harmless substance is seen in

TABLE 11-11 Management of Opportunistic Infections in AIDS	
Acyclovir	Herpes infection
Amphotericin B	Candida and aspergillus fungal infections
Fluconazole	Candida infections
Foscarnet	Cytomegalovirus infections of the eye
Gancyclovir	Cytomegalovirus infections of the eye
Interferon alfa-2a	Kaposi's sarcoma
Interferon alfa-2b	Kaposi's sarcoma
Pentamidine	*Pneumocystis carinii* pneumonia
Trimethoprim/ sulfamethoxazole	*Pneumocystis carinii* pneumonia

allergies and may actually damage tissues. About 15% of humans are predisposed to become sensitive. Allergies may affect different areas of the body.

In the nose—as hay fever or allergic rhinitis

In the lungs—as asthma

In the eyes—as conjunctivitis

On the skin—as eczema, contact dermatitis, or hives

In the digestive tract—as cramps, vomiting, and diarrhea

When exposed to the sensitive allergens, the antibody IgE is produced, resulting in allergic symptoms. With each additional exposure to the allergen, IgE antibody is produced and becomes attached to the mast cells or basophils, which in turn release histamine and **prostaglandins** (Figure 11-155).

Signs and symptoms—The histamine causes the mucous membranes to secrete and capillaries to become more permeable. Prostaglandins constrict smooth muscle in some organs, such as the bronchioles of the lungs. The two initiate a local inflammatory response. With hay fever or asthma, for example, there is sneezing, runny nose, congestion, and difficult breathing.

Exaggerated reactions to allergens can be life-threatening. For instance, some people are very sensitive to bee stings and certain drugs. The histamine and prostaglandins cause extensive bronchial constriction, mucus production, and excessive capillary permeability. Breathing is difficult, and extensive loss of blood plasma drastically lowers the blood pressure, leading to circulatory collapse and death. This reaction is known as **anaphylaxis**, and the situation is called *anaphylactic shock*.

Etiology—The most common causative substances are dust, animal hair, certain foods, pollen, insect stings, and drugs. Other factors, such as emotional state, air pressure or temperature change, and infections, can either trigger or complicate allergic reactions.

Diagnostic procedures to confirm allergies consist of blood counts to determine eosinophil numbers (an increase denotes allergy), chest x-ray to determine congestion and perhaps focal atelectasis (mucous plugs with asthma), and pulmonary function test to evaluate lung condition. Often there is a family history of sensitivity. A series of skin tests can identify allergic substances (see Chapter 16).

Treatment—Treatment consists of eliminating contact with allergens and other causative factors as much as possible. **Desensitization** to specific allergens may be helpful. By injecting minute amounts of the allergen intradermally and gradually increasing the amount, the body can be caused to produce IgG antibodies that circulate and bind with the allergen, prohibiting its interaction with IgE. In addition, antihistamines, bronchodilators, antibiotics for secondary infection, and sometimes corticosteroids are helpful.

Cancer

Description—Cancer is a group of diseases characterized by uncontrolled growth of abnormal cells. These cells accumulate and form tumors that may compress, invade, or destroy normal tissue. Cells have the potential to break away from a tumor and travel to other areas of the body. The spread of a tumor to a new site is called **metastasis.** It is the second leading cause of death in adults and the leading cause of death among children ages 1 through 14 in the United States. The American Cancer Society statistics for 2006 estimated that 1,399,790 Americans would be diagnosed with cancer and 564,830 would die during the year. One out of every four deaths in the United States is from cancer. With proper treatment, 65% will survive 5 or more years after their diagnosis. Medical and surgical oncologists, physicians with specialized education in the management and treatment of cancer, are best suited to deal with this complicated disease. Figures 11-156A and B illustrate the leading sites of new cancer and deaths estimated for the year 2006 by the American Cancer Society.

PEDIATRIC PERSPECTIVE

Childhood cancer, though rare, is the chief cause of death by disease in children between birth and age 14. An estimated 9,500 new cases and 1,560 deaths were expected to have occurred in 2006. Early detection of cancer in children is often difficult.

Characteristics of Cancer Cells   The word **neoplasm** is defined as new growth and can refer to both **benign** and malignant tumors. Both types of tumors contain growing tumor cells, connective tissue, and blood vessels. Benign tumors are usually slow growing, do not invade other tissues, and do not spread to other parts of the body. Usually they do not cause

Allergy

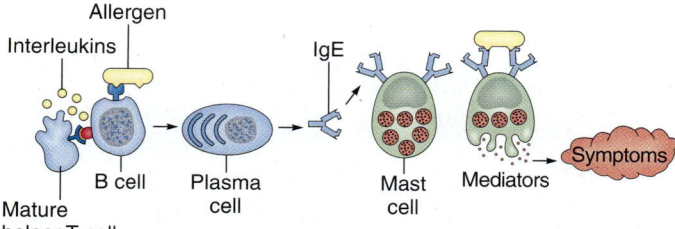

FIGURE 11-155 Response to allergens *(Courtesy of the United States Department of Health and Human Services)*

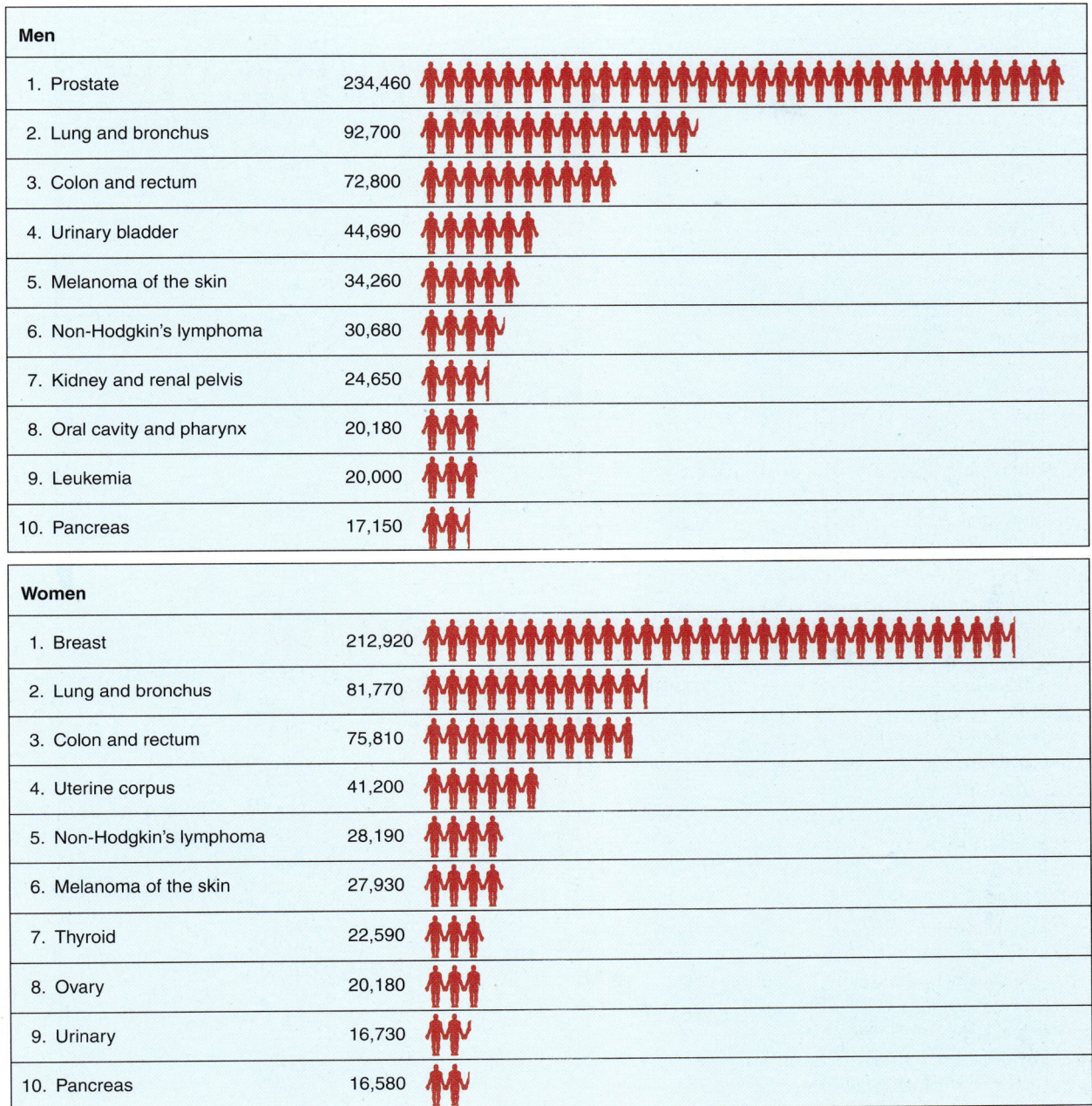

FIGURE 11-156A Ten leading sites of new cancer cases—2006 estimates (*Adapted from the American Cancer Society*)

any problems unless they are growing in a confined space, such as in the brain. Malignant tumors are cancerous and differ from benign in several ways:

- Cancer cells have an altered cell structure that includes an increased nuclear size, irregular chromatin distribution, and prominent nucleoli.
- Cancer cells lack normal growth controlling mechanisms; growth is unorganized and disorderly.

- Cancer cells lack contact inhibition (normal cell growth stops when other cells are contacted). They continue to grow and invade into other tissue.
- Cancer cells do not respond to growth factors that stimulate or inhibit growth of normal cells. They can grow rapidly with reduced growth factors.
- Cancer cells frequently escape immune surveillance.
- Cancer cells are invasive, causing destruction of normal tissue.

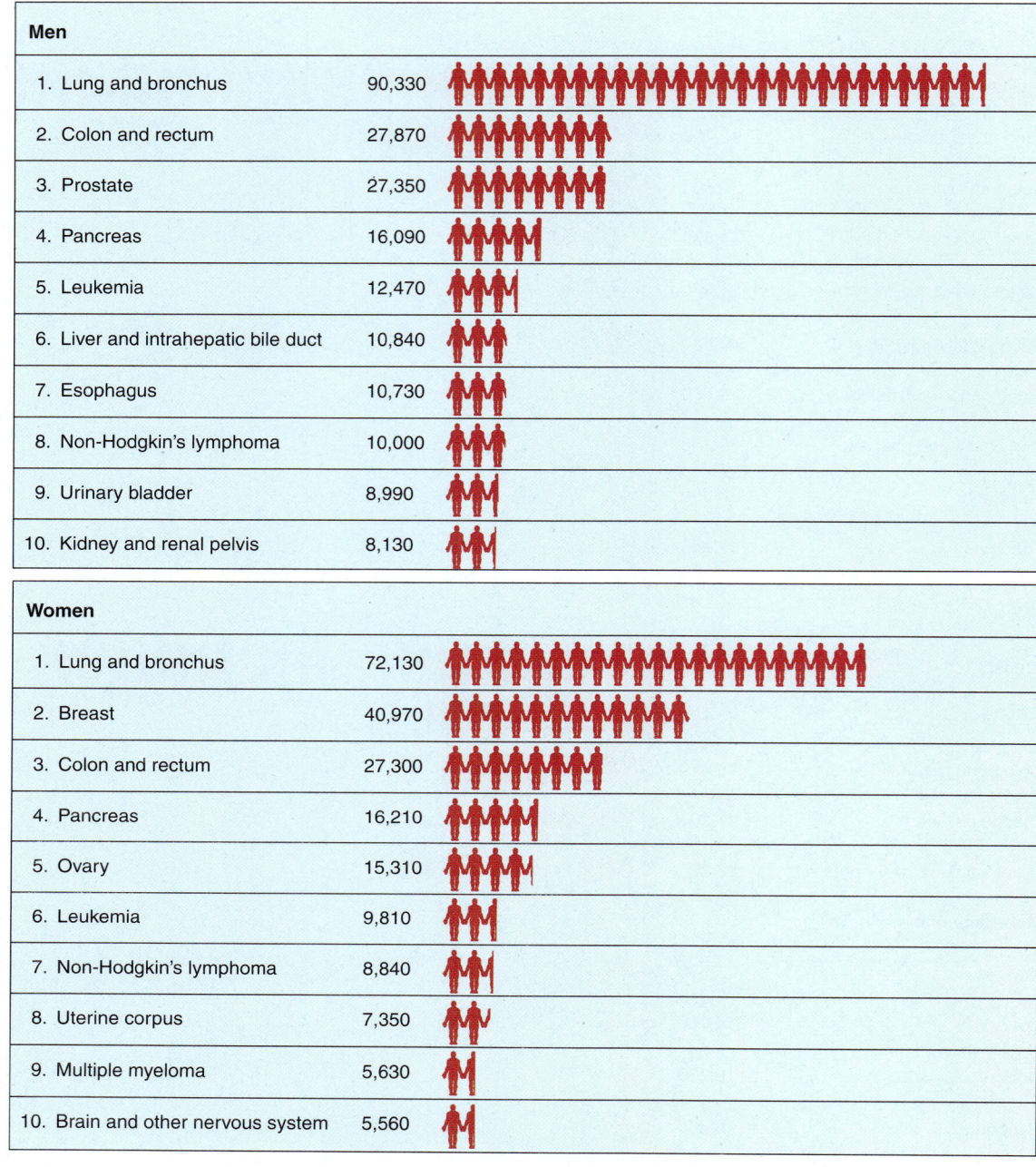

Men		
1. Lung and bronchus	90,330	
2. Colon and rectum	27,870	
3. Prostate	27,350	
4. Pancreas	16,090	
5. Leukemia	12,470	
6. Liver and intrahepatic bile duct	10,840	
7. Esophagus	10,730	
8. Non-Hodgkin's lymphoma	10,000	
9. Urinary bladder	8,990	
10. Kidney and renal pelvis	8,130	

Women		
1. Lung and bronchus	72,130	
2. Breast	40,970	
3. Colon and rectum	27,300	
4. Pancreas	16,210	
5. Ovary	15,310	
6. Leukemia	9,810	
7. Non-Hodgkin's lymphoma	8,840	
8. Uterine corpus	7,350	
9. Multiple myeloma	5,630	
10. Brain and other nervous system	5,560	

FIGURE 11-156B   Ten leading sites of cancer deaths—2006 estimates *(Adapted from the American Cancer Society)*

- Cancer cells can metastasize by traveling through the lymphatic or blood vessels and implanting into other body sites and creating additional tumors.
- Cancer cells have increased metabolic rate.

Classifications of Cancer

Cancer can be classified according to its cellular origin. Cancers arising from epithelial tissues are known as **carcinomas**, whereas those from connective tissues are called **sarcomas**. Cancers of the blood and blood-forming organs are called leukemias, and those from the lymph tissue are lymphomas. Table 11-12 lists benign and malignant tumors according to their cellular origins.

Cancers can also be described according to their degree of differentiation. This refers to how similar the cancer cell appears to the normal cell from which it was derived. A well-differentiated cancer cell looks similar to a normal cell, and a poorly or undifferentiated cancer cell appears very abnormal. Sometimes it is so poorly differentiated that it is difficult to tell from what type of cell it originated, these cancers are termed "carcinomas of unknown primary." Grading refers to

TABLE 11-12   Cellular Origins of Benign and Malignant Diseases

Cell or Tissue of Origin	Benign	Malignant
Tumors of Epithelial Origin		
Squamous cells	Squamous cell papilloma	Squamous cell carcinoma
Basal cells	—	Basal cell carcinoma
Glandular or ductal epithelium	Adenoma	Adenocarcinoma
Transitional cells	Transitional cell papilloma	Transitional cell carcinoma
Melanocytes	Nevus	Malignant melanoma
Germ cells (testes/ovaries)	—	Seminoma (of testes), embryonal carcinoma, yolk sack carcinoma
Tumors of Blood and Blood-Forming Organs/Lymphoid Tissue		
Bone marrow and blood	—	Leukemia
Lymph tissue and organs	—	Hodgkin's disease
Plasma blood cells (B lymphocytes)	—	Multiple myeloma
Lymph tissue and organs	—	Non-Hodgkin's lymphoma
Tumors of Connective Tissue		
Fibrous tissue	Fibromatosis (desmoid tumor)	Fibrosarcoma
Fat	Lipoma	Liposarcoma
Bone	Osteoma	Osteogenic sarcoma
Cartilage	Chondroma	Chondrosarcoma
Smooth muscle	Leiomyoma	Leiomyosarcoma
Striated (skeletal) muscle	Rhabdomyoma	Rhabdomyosarcoma
Endothelial and Related Tissues		
Blood vessels	Hemangioma	Angiosarcoma
Lymph vessels	Lymphangioma	Lymphangiosarcoma
Synovium	—	Synovial sarcoma
Mesothelium	Meningioma	Malignant mesothelioma
Meninges	Meningioma	Malignant meningioma
Neural and Retinal Tissue		
Nerve sheath	Neurilemoma Neurofibroma	Malignant peripheral sheath tumor
Nerve cells	Gangioneuroma	Neuroblastoma
Retinal cells (cones)	—	Retinoblastoma

the degree of differentiation of the cancer cell. The grading system goes from Grade 1, which is a well-differentiated cell, to Grade IV, which is undifferentiated. The grading and staging findings allow for the determination of an anticipated prognosis.

Cancer Staging   Staging is a term used to identify the extent of spread. It is a system that is accepted worldwide for primary site evaluation. It provides a standardized description for planning treatments, eval-

uating outcomes, and estimating prognosis. It is also a criterion for patient eligibility for individual clinical trials. The method is known as the TNM system and uses standardized measurement criteria:

(T)—the size or extent of local spread of the primary tumor
(N)—the presence or absence and extent of regional lymph node metastasis
(M)—the presence or absence of distant metastasis

Numbers are added to the three components to indicate the clinical extent of the disease to show an increase in tumor size, local involvement, regional lymph node spread, or distant metastasis:

Tumor size	T0	T1	T2	T3	T4
Nodal involvement	N0	N1	N2	N3	
Metastasis	M0	M1			

In addition to the letters and numbers, four staging classifications are also used:

c— Clinical based on acquired evidence from exams and studies
p— Pathologic based on information after a surgical procedure
r— Retreatment based on disease-free interval with planned new treatment
a— Autopsy based on pathology after death

In the future, multiple biologic factors, such as hormone receptors, genetic markers, cellular proliferation, and metastasis potential, will probably be used to further classify cancer.

Signs and symptoms—The signs and symptoms vary according to the type of cancer, its location, and the individual affected. The American Cancer Society has developed the warning signals for cancer in adults and children (Tables 11-13 and 11-14). Unfortunately, these are often signs of fairly advanced disease. Many individuals have no symptoms, and the possibility of cancer is detected through routine cancer screening tests. (Chapter 14, Units 3 and 4, discuss recommended screening tests.)
Etiology—Cancer is believed to be caused by cellular **mutation** or abnormal activation of cellular genes that control cell growth and division. These abnormal genes are called **oncogenes**. In cells, proto-oncogenes and tumor suppresser genes are normal genes that

TABLE 11-13   The Seven Warning Signals of Cancer

- Change in bowel and bladder habits
- A sore that does not heal
- Unusual bleeding or discharge
- Thickening or lump in a breast or elsewhere
- Indigestion or difficulty swallowing
- Obvious change in a wart or mole
- Nagging cough or hoarseness

TABLE 11-14   Warning Signals of Childhood Cancer

- Unusual mass or swelling
- Unexplained paleness and loss of energy
- Sudden tendency to bruise
- Persistent, localized pain or limping
- Prolonged, unexplained fever or illness
- Frequent headaches, often with vomiting
- Sudden eye or vision changes
- Excessive, rapid weight loss

regulate the growth and repair of cells. If a proto-oncogene is mutated, it may be left permanently in the "on position," causing continuous cell growth. If the tumor suppresser gene is mutated, it may be left permanently in the "off" position, also allowing continued cell growth.

One of the most common known mutated genes in human cancers is the *p53* tumor suppresser gene. This gene normally stops cell proliferation and promotes DNA repair of damaged cells. Some clinical trials using gene therapy are looking at ways to interact with the *p53* tumor suppresser gene.

Only a small fraction of cells that mutate ever lead to cancer (remember it is estimated that 100 to 1,000 mutated cells are formed every day). Many of the mutated cells cannot survive because they are so defective. Others are destroyed by the immune system, particularly the NK cells. The probability of mutations is increased when a person is exposed to certain chemical, physical, or biologic factors called **carcinogens**. Carcinogens are usually categorized under chemical, viral, physical, and familial headings. Table 11-15 lists the types of known carcinogens and the resulting cancers.

PEDIATRIC PERSPECTIVE

There is evidence that some tumor suppressor gene defects are inherited. Patients with inherited retinoblastoma, a rare pediatric tumor of the eye, are known to have a defective tumor suppressor gene.

Some other reasons for failure of the immune system to destroy mutated cells have been suggested:

- A decrease in antibodies and lymphocytes caused by cytotoxic drugs or steroids
- Stress, which stimulates production of *cortisol*, a lymphocyte destroyer

TABLE 11-15   Types of Known Carcinogens and the Resulting Cancers

Carcinogen	Type of Cancer
Chemical Carcinogens	
Alkylating chemotherapy agents (e.g., nitrogen mustard, cyclophosphamide)	• Leukemia
Arsenic	• Liver • Lung • Skin
Benzene	• Leukemia
Chewing tobacco	• Oral cancer
Cigarette smoking	• Oral cancer • Head and neck cancer • Lung cancer • Bladder cancer • Cervical cancer
Vinyl chloride	• Liver cancer
Viral Carcinogens	
Epstein–Barr virus	• Burkitt's lymphoma in Africa • Nasopharyngeal cancer
Hepatitis B virus	• Hepatocellular liver cancer
Human T cell leukemia/ lymphoma virus (HTLV-1)	• T cell leukemias and lymphomas
Human papilloma virus (HPV-16 or HPV-18)	• Found in at least 70% of cases of cervical cancer
Physical Carcinogens	
Asbestos	• Bronchogenic lung cancer • Mesothelioma
Ionizing radiation	• Leukemia • Lymphoma • Potentially all solid tumors
Ultraviolet radiation	• Melanoma • Skin cancers
Familial Carcinogenesis	
Dysplastic nevus syndrome	• Melanoma
Fanconi's anemia	• Leukemia
Familial polyposis	• Colorectal cancer
Gardner's syndrome	• Colorectal cancer
Neurofibromatosis	• Brain tumors • Endocrine cancers
Xeroderma pigmentosum	• Melanoma • Skin cancer

- Severe infection, which depresses the immune system
- Cancer itself causes suppression of the immune system and predisposes to other cancers.
- Increased infection caused by radiation, toxic drug therapy, and bone marrow depression, which interferes with leukocyte production

Some scientists believe that the mutated cancer cell's surface markers either did not change (still say self), are disguised, or even are released and cause immune fighters to miss destroying the cell.

Diagnostic Tests

Additional tests are indicated when a patient has a positive screening test or has symptoms of cancer. The diagnosis of cancer can only be considered 100% accurate if a sample of cells are removed and examined microscopically. The major goals of the diagnostic evaluation are to determine:

- The tissue type of the cancer (e.g., carcinoma, sarcoma)
- The primary site (e.g., breast)
- The grade of the cancer (the degree of differentiation)
- The extent of the disease in the body (stage)

Diagnostic tests for cancer can be categorized into biopsies, laboratory tests, and tumor imaging.

Biopsies   A **biopsy** is the removal of a sample of tissue from the body for microscopic examination to determine a diagnosis. Treatment decisions for cancers arising from the same organ differ based upon the type of cell involved. For example, adenocarcinoma of the lung is treated very differently than a sarcoma of the lung. Common techniques for biopsies are needle, incisional, excisional, and bone marrow aspiration. During a needle biopsy, a needle is inserted into the tumor and cells are withdrawn. Incisional biopsy involves removing a portion of the tumor for testing. The entire tumor is removed during an excisional biopsy. A bone marrow aspiration is used to test for leukemia and cancers that involve the bone marrow. A bone marrow aspiration requires the patient to lie prone. A local anesthetic is injected over the iliac crest, and a long needle is inserted through the bone and into the marrow where blood cells are made.

Sentinel lymph node biopsy is a newer technique used to remove and sample lymph nodes that may be cancerous. It is most commonly used for breast cancer and melanoma. The sentinel lymph node (SLN) is the first lymph node that drains the area of the cancerous tumor. The patient is injected with a radioactive material. SNLs will have a higher uptake of the material than other lymph nodes, identifying them for removal. A blue dye is also simultaneously injected for visual correlation at the time of surgery. The advantage of SLN biopsy is that fewer nodes are removed, resulting in fewer complications.

Stereotactic breast biopsy is used for breast tumors that are difficult to locate. The biopsy is done while the patient is having a mammogram or ultrasound, allowing the surgeon to see the location of the tumor in order to obtain the biopsy.

Laboratory Tests

Different laboratory tests of the blood, serum, urine, and other body fluids help establish the diagnosis of cancer. In addition to standard tests, tumor markers and genetic testing can be done for different types of cancer.

Tumor markers are proteins, antigens, genes, hormones, or enzymes produced by the tumor and released into the blood. Tumor markers can help establish the diagnosis of cancer and its response to treatment. For example, if a patient has an elevated tumor marker, then the number should decrease with cancer treatment. Tumor markers, however, are not always specific for cancer and can be affected by other factors. **Carcinoembryonic antigen (CEA)** is a tumor marker often elevated in patients with colon cancer; however, it can also be elevated in smokers.

Genetic Testing

Conducting genetic testing is appropriate for some types of cancer and for individuals at high risk for developing inherited cancers. The ethical, social, and legal issues need to be considered. There are two examples of genetic testing: breast cancer genes *BRCA1* and *BRCA2*. Defects in these genes are believed to be responsible for up to 80% of *inherited* breast cancers. (*Note:* Fewer than 5% of all breast cancers have a direct genetic link.) *BRCA1* and 2 are present in everyone; however, when the genes mutate, the risk for breast and ovarian cancer increases. *BRCA1* and *BRCA2* mutations have also been linked to prostate cancer and possibly to colon cancer. Both men and women can inherit and pass on the genes. Women who inherit the *BRCA1* and *BRCA2* mutated gene have a 50% to 80% chance of developing breast cancer.

Tumor Imaging

A variety of different radiology and imaging tests are used to aid in the diagnosis and staging of cancer, including x-rays, CT scans, MRIs, endoscopy, ultrasound, and nuclear medicine. X-rays include mammography used to screen for breast cancer. CT scans are commonly used to aid in the diagnosis of lung, liver, and head and neck cancers. MRIs are used to diagnose and stage cancers such as brain and musculoskeletal cancers (e.g., sarcomas).

Endoscopy is used to visualize the interior of hollow organs. After a hollow tube is inserted into the organ, images may be taken, and tissue samples can be obtained through the scope. Bronchoscopy is used for diagnosis of lung cancers. Sigmoidoscopy and colonoscopy are used for the screening and diagnosis of colorectal cancer. Ultrasound is used to distinguish between a fluid-filled cyst and a solid tumor.

Nuclear medicine imaging involves the injection or ingestion of radioactive substances, followed by imaging of the organ or organs that concentrate the radioactive material. Common nuclear medicine scans include bone, liver, spleen, brain, thyroid, and kidney.

Positron emission tomography (PET) scan is a type of nuclear medicine test that has only recently been used to detect cancer. PET scans are computerized images of the metabolic activity of the body tissues by measuring glucose uptake and can suggest the presence of cancer.

Radiolabeled **monoclonal** *antibodies* include Prosta-Scint scans used for the early detection of prostate cancer. With this technology, antibodies are made for specific tumor types and labeled with a radioactive substance. The radioactive antibody searches for the specific tumor antigen and is detectable by the scan. *Radiolabeled peptides* are most commonly used to detect neuroendocrine tumors.

Ductal Lavage

A new experimental diagnostic examination called ductal lavage is being tried on women at high risk for developing breast cancer. It is a way to detect early changes in the cells of the breast ducts before cancer would be evident on a mammogram or by breast examination. It is showing promise for early detection. In December 2000, Johns Hopkins Medical Center did a study on 500 high-risk women at 19 different breast centers in the United States. These women had a history of breast cancer, a positive *BRCA1/BRCA2* gene mutation, or a first degree or two or more close relatives with breast cancer. Atypical or suspicious cells were detected in 15% of the participants, and cancerous cells were found in 5% of them. All had normal mammograms within the past year.

The procedure is minimally invasive. An anesthetic cream is applied to the nipple area. A nursing pump is attached to the breast to draw a small amount of fluid to the surface in order to locate the milk ducts. A hair-thin catheter is inserted into the duct, and a small amount of anesthetic mixed with sterile saline is injected into the duct. The breast is massaged to mix the saline with the fluid in the duct that contains ductal epithelial cells. The saline and the cells are withdrawn through the catheter and sent to a cytology lab for analysis. The procedure takes about 30 minutes to complete. The test may sound very uncomfortable, but the women who participated reported only mild discomfort.

This type of test seems worthwhile because most breast cancers begin in the cells lining the milk ducts and have been growing for years before they were identifiable by mammogram or examination. Interpreting the results of lavage studies is being evaluated. The presence of cells does not mean that cancer is inevitable. Most atypical cells do not progress to cancer. For the present, it presents the woman with a dilemma because the location within the breast where the cells came from is not known. Women at high risk have the option to watch and wait or to decide on preventive strategies, such as taking tamoxifen, having surgery to remove the ducts, or undergoing a preventive mastectomy.

Treatment—The treatment of cancer is based upon the type, grade, and stage of the cancer. In addition, treatment considerations include the risk or probability that the cancer will metastasize or recur after a "cure." The planning sequence for treatment is as follows:

> The patient presents with a symptom or has a positive screening test
> ↓
> History, physical examinations, laboratory work
> ↓
> Biopsy
> ↓
> Biopsy positive for cancer
> ↓
> The cancer is classified according to cell type and is graded according to the degree of differentiation
> ↓
> The extent of the disease is determined (staging)
> ↓
> Cancer treatment
> ↓
> Cancer re-evaluated
> ↓
> Need for additional therapy evaluated

Goals of Cancer Therapy

The goals of therapy—cure, control, or palliation—are based on the patient's type and stage of cancer. Cure means that there will be no evidence of disease for a specified time. Control indicates that the disease cannot be cured but can be controlled for a period using the identified therapy. Palliation means that the disease cannot be cured or controlled, and palliative treatments will be used to control symptoms only.

Local Versus Systemic Treatment

The major treatment methods for cancer are surgery, **radiation**, **chemotherapy**, and biologic response modifiers. Treatments can have local or systemic effects. A local treatment effects only the area of the therapy and any side effects that occur within that area. An example of local therapy is surgery. Systemic therapy travels throughout the body to treat cancer cells in different locations. Side effects will be systemic as well. An example of systemic therapy is chemotherapy. Most patients receive a combination of local and systemic therapies, especially if they already have or are at increased risk for metastasis.

Table 11-16 lists the types of treatment and their key points.

Surgery is the oldest form of treatment for cancer. About 60% of all patients with cancer will have some type of surgery. It can be used for the purpose of diagnosis, treatment, or palliation of symptoms.

Radiation therapy is the use of high-energy particles or waves, such as x-rays or gamma rays, to destroy or damage the DNA or RNA of cancer cells. It is most effective on dividing cells. Radiation therapy can be delivered by external beam or brachytherapy. External beam therapy is delivered externally through the skin to the area. **Brachytherapy** uses radioactive isotopes that are placed directly on or very near the tumor. Brachytherapy can be delivered interstitially, using seeds "planted" into the tissues, or intracavitary, using a tube or catheter to instill the material. This is commonly used for prostate and breast cancer. General side effects of radiation therapy include fatigue and weakness.

Chemotherapy involves the use of potent medications to treat cancer cells by altering cell division; therefore, it effects both rapidly dividing cancer cells and normal tissues. It can be administered orally, intravenously, subcutaneously, intramuscularly, intra-arterially, topically, intraperitoneally, and into the central nervous system.

The route is dependent upon the type of chemotherapy and the type of cancer. Patients can receive one type of chemotherapy or combinations of chemotherapy. The patient in Figure 11-157 is receiving one of a combination of chemotherapeutic agents. Note there are three small bags of medication along with a larger bag of sterile fluid to help dilute the agents. The tubing combines and flows through an IV pump to regulate the flow. The blue cold compress over the injection site helps to lessen the discomfort from the drugs.

Although drug specific, common side effects of chemotherapy include hair loss, skin changes, mouth sores, and bone marrow depression. Bone marrow depression can lead to anemia, increased risk of infection, and increased risk for bleeding.

Biologic response modifiers (BRM) are defined as any substance that is capable of altering the immune system by either stimulating or suppressing its action. BRMs are also referred to as immunotherapy or biotherapy. The action of BRMs can be divided into three categories:

1. Agents that restore, augment, or modulate the host's immune response
2. Agents that have direct antitumor activity
3. Agents that have other biologic effects, such as affecting tumor growth, differentiation, or the ability of the tumor to metastasize

TABLE 11-16   Types Of Cancer Treatment

Type	Key Points
Surgery	• Most common treatment • Local treatment • Diagnosis and staging • Treatment • Palliation of symptoms
Chemotherapy	• Most routes: systemic treatment • Affects cell division in cancer and normal cells • Most effects, seen in rapidly dividing normal and cancer cells • Side effects: nausea, vomiting, bone marrow depression, hair loss, stomatitis (mouth sores)
Radiation: external beam therapy	• Local treatment • Affects cell division of cancer and normal cells • Side effects: fatigue, skin reactions, other side effects dependent upon site treated
Radiation: brachytherapy	• Local treatment • Radioactive isotope placed near site of cancer • Most common uses: cervical cancer, lung cancer, prostate cancer
Radiation: radiosurgery	• Radiation used to directly target a small area • Most common uses: brain tumors
Biologic response modifiers	• Also called immunotherapy • Examples: alpha interferon, interleukins, monoclonal antibodies, tumor necrosis factor, colony-stimulating factors • Side effects: fatigue, fever, chills, muscle and joint aches, anaphylaxis
Gene therapy	• Investigational • Affects growth-controlling factors of tumors
Complementary therapy	• Complements standard therapies • Examples: massage therapy, biofeedback, music therapy, art therapy
Alternative therapy	• Not approved by the Food and Drug Administration • Examples: shark cartilage, laetrile, megadoses of vitamins, herbs

There are numerous BRMs. Examples include colony-stimulating factors, interferons, interleukins, monoclonal antibodies, and tumor necrosis factor. *Colony-stimulating factors* (CSFs) are cytokines that regulate hematopoiesis, the growth and maturation of blood cells. The CSFs work on different blood cell lines. For example, granulocyte colony-stimulating factor works to promote the maturation of granulocytes, important white blood cells for fighting infection. Erythropoietin targets only red blood cell maturation. Other CSFs regulate stem cell growth and platelet growth. CSF is used to treat granulocytopenia (lack of granulocytes) and allow increased doses of chemotherapy to be given without the risk of long-term granulocytopenia. It is administered subcutaneously or intravenously.

Interferons are naturally occurring cytokines that have antiviral, immunomodulatory, and antiproliferative effects. Interferon interacts with T cells to increase the activity of NK cells to have direct cytoxic affects on cancer cells. Alfa interferon is used to treat a variety of cancers, including renal cell cancer, hairy cell leukemia, melanoma, lymphomas, and Kaposi's sarcoma. It is administered intravenously or subcutaneously. Side effects include flulike symptoms, such as fever, chills, fatigue, rigors, and headache.

Interleukins are important regulatory proteins produced naturally by lymphocytes and monocytes. The most commonly prescribed interleukin is interleukin-2 (IL-2). It is produced by helper T cells. An important function of IL-2 is to stimulate and activate NK cells, which have a cytotoxic affect on cancer cells. IL-2 has been used to treat renal carcinoma, melanoma, and lymphoma. It is administered intravenously or subcutaneously. IL-2 has numerous side effects, including severe flulike symptoms and a change of fluids, which can lead to hypotension, ascites (fluid in the abdomen), and pleural effusion.

Monoclonal antibodies are antibodies directed at specific tumor antigens. They can be used alone to directly

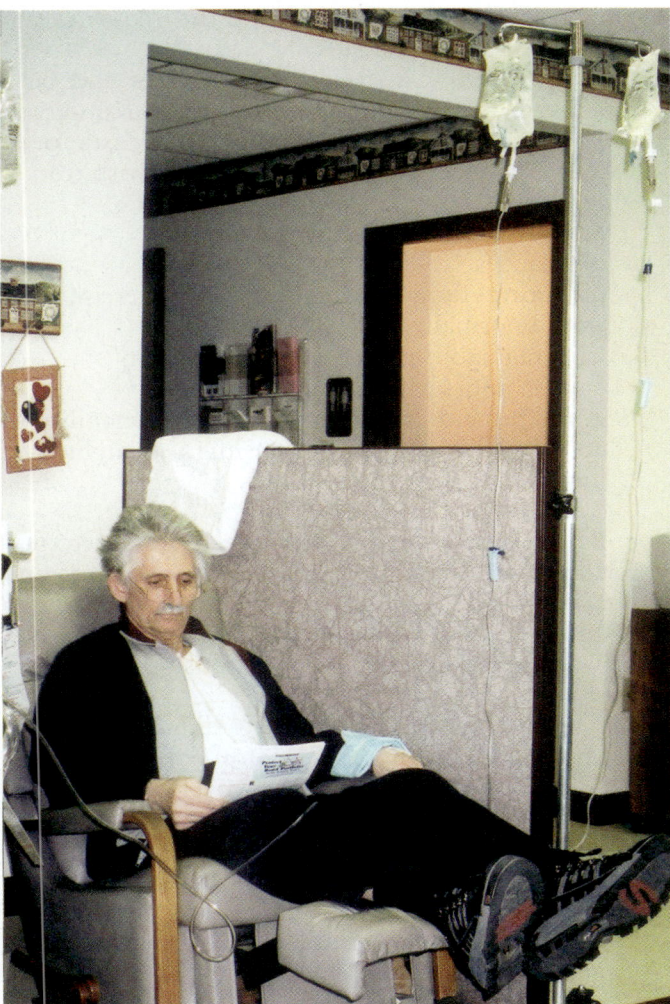

FIGURE 11-157 Patient receiving intravenous chemotherapy. Note cold compress at site to lessen the discomfort from the drugs. *(Courtesy of Carol A. Martin)*

activate the host's immune system or can be attached to a chemotherapeutic agent for direct delivery to the cancer cell. Monoclonal antibodies are currently being used to treat a variety of cancers, including breast, B cell lymphoma, and melanomas.

Alternative Therapies

Alternative therapies are promoted as cancer cures; however, they have not been proven because they have not been scientifically tested or were tested and found to be statistically ineffective. Alternative therapies have not been approved by the Food and Drug Administration as treatments for cancer. Some examples include:

- Shark cartilage
- Laetrile
- Immunoaugmentive therapy
- Megadoses of vitamins

Complementary Therapies

Complementary therapies refer to supportive methods that are used to complement or add to recognized treatments, such as chemotherapy, radiation, and surgery. They are not given to cure cancer but to help control symptoms and improve well-being. Examples of complementary therapies are:

- Art therapy
- Biofeedback
- Imagery
- Massage
- Meditation
- Music therapy
- Pet therapy
- Relaxation
- Yoga

Cancer Vaccine

Researchers have worked diligently for the past 4 decades trying to develop a vaccine for cancer. They were hampered by the lack of knowledge about the immune system. With the mapping of the genes, much has been learned about cellular structure and function. We now know the body's natural defense from the immune system fails to work because cancer cells are mutated from normal cells and the immune system does not recognize them as "foreign."

Researchers have been able to develop vaccines to make these cells visible. Tumor cells are taken from the patient and fused with specialized white cells and injected back into the patient's lymphatic system. The fused cells trigger an immune reaction, and cells are carried back to the lymph nodes. Here, the antigen-specific B and T cells are activated and mass produced. T cells go out to travel the body, identifying and destroying the tumor cells. B cells are activated to make antibodies to attack the antigens.

Another form of vaccine uses viruses to deliver genes to boost the immune system function. Some viruses are even manufactured to infect white blood cells and then trained to kill the tumor cells. The future of vaccines is considered to be another form of cancer treatment to supplement chemotherapy, radiation, and surgery, but with less-invasive procedures and fewer side effects. The effect of vaccines so far depends on the response of a healthy immune system, something few cancer patients have.

It is still a few years away, but it is anticipated that vaccines for melanoma, cervical, and prostate cancer, which are being considered now, will be approved soon. Since cancer exists in many different forms and is associated with unknown numbers of genes, it appears vaccines may have to be developed for specific cancers. One research team identified over 30 genes associated with melanoma and altered their vaccine to attack each type. Since there are over 100 different forms of breast cancer, for instance, individual vaccines might need to be developed for each type.

Researchers believe that if they can identify a gene, they can go in and 6 months later get an antibody and a vaccine; however, the required testing and trials make the process take at least 5 to 6 years before approval. Vaccine therapy is promising. At present efforts are primarily aimed at preventing recurrence. However, efforts are also being made to develop a vaccine to boost the immune system to keep some cancers from forming in the first place. These often develop when patients are immune suppressed for organ transplants, for example. The thought is to have many extra immune cells to fight off the virus cells, already present in most people's bodies, which trigger tumor cell development. Scientists believe we may always have cancer, but the goal is to make it a chronic disease instead.

Infection with the human papillomavirus (HPV), a sexually transmitted disease, has been shown to be responsible for most cervical cancers. A newly approved vaccine targets HPV and will cause a dramatic reduction in the current 3,700 annual death from cervical cancer. As of June 2006, a federal advisory panel recommended that all girls be routinely given the vaccine at 11 or 12 years of age. Three injections are given over a 6-month period and are most effective when administered before the girls become sexually active. The panel also believes girls and women between 13 and 26 would benefit from immunization.

The vaccine appears effective against two strains of the virus that are responsible for about 70% of all cervical cancers and against two others strains that cause almost 90% of the cases of genital warts. It is important to note that PAP tests are still recommended for the early detection of cervical cancer and the precancerous lesions of other HPV strains.

Clinical Research Trials

Clinical trials are research studies that determine the effectiveness and safety of a cancer treatment regimen. Before a treatment can be used for patients, it goes through many years of investigation—first through laboratory trials and then in animal trials. If the treatment is found effective and safe, it is then tested on humans. Patients with specific criteria in their disease are permitted to participate in the trial treatment. After the studies are completed and there is evidence that the new therapy is more effective and safe, it is evaluated by the Food and Drug Administration to be used in mainstream therapy.

Chronic Fatigue Syndrome (CFS)

Description—This **debilitating** disorder was officially recognized and reported in 1984 by two doctors near Lake Tahoe, Nevada. It was officially declared a disease in 1988. The CDC started a surveillance pro-gram costing $1.5 million to track the frequency and impact of the disorder.

Signs and symptoms—The following guidelines have been established to help physicians diagnose the condition.

- Persistent overwhelming fatigue that lasts for at least 6 months and does not go away with rest
- Low-grade fever
- Sore throat or swollen lymph nodes
- Headaches
- Lingering fatigue after levels of exercise that would normally be easily tolerated
- Unexplainable muscle weakness or pain
- Pain in joints without swelling
- Forgetfulness, irritability, confusion, inability to concentrate, depression, sensitivity to light, and impaired vision
- Sleep disturbances

Patients experience varying levels of ability to perform activity, from profound fatigue to being completely bedridden. CFS affects twice as many women as men, particularly between 25 and 45 years old. However, children and senior citizens have also been diagnosed.

The disorder begins suddenly like the common flu, but the CFS symptoms last for 3 or 4 years. Only about 15% to 20% seem to recover fully; 5% are homebound or bedridden.

Etiology—The cause of the disorder is unknown. Current theories suggest that a virus, bacteria, allergen, or environment chemical enters the body but does not set off the normal immune response to fight the invasion. Instead, the system continues to make symptom-producing chemicals. A second theory suggests that some unidentified organism weakens the immune system, allowing normally dormant viruses to become activated. This theory is supported by the presence of high levels of antibodies to Epstein–Barr virus and others.

Physicians still do not know much about the disorder; some deny its existence because it cannot be detected by a blood test. Diagnosis requires a thorough physical examination and laboratory tests to rule out other conditions with similar symptoms.

Treatment—Many treatments have been tried, but only cognitive behavioral therapy and graded exercise have proved effective. Cognitive behavioral therapy involves a series of 1-hour sessions designed to alter beliefs and behaviors that might delay recovery. Treatment for insomnia, pain, and symptoms of depression is also important.

Lupus Erythematosus (Lu'-pus Eri-thema-to-sis)

Description—**Lupus erythematosus** is a chronic disease of unknown cause in which striking changes occur in the immune system. It causes inflammation of various parts of the body. It can involve only a few body organs or cause serious life-threatening problems. Lupus can affect the skin, joints, kidneys, lungs, heart, nervous system, and other body organs and systems.

In lupus, the usually protective antibodies are produced in large quantities but react against the person's own normal tissue; therefore, it is called an autoimmune disease. There are three main types of lupus:

- Discoid lupus erythematosus (DLE)—Cutaneous or **discoid** lupus is confined to the skin and causes a persistent flush of the cheeks or discoid lesions on the face, neck, scalp, and other areas exposed to ultraviolet light. The lesions of the face are referred to as a butterfly rash. The rash is usually scaly and red but not itchy. If not treated, scarring may result, and if on the scalp, bald spots.
- Systemic lupus erythematosus (SLE) inflames the organs of the body. Some persons also have skin and joint involvement; in others, skin, lungs, kidneys, or blood may be affected. The disease is characterized by periods of **remission**, when few if any symptoms are evident, and other periods of active disease and symptoms.
- Drug-induced lupus can be caused by certain medications and is similar to SLE. The most common offenders are hydralazine for hypertension and procainamide for cardiac arrhythmia. The symptoms fade when the drugs are stopped.

The prevalence (everyone affected currently) of SLE in the United States is approximately 40 to 50 cases per 100,000 population according to a publication by an arthritis journal published in 1998. The Lupus Foundation of America believes that total prevalence may be as many as 500,000 people in the United States. Regardless, we do know SLE affects women nine times more often than men, most frequently during the childbearing years. Lupus is more common in African, Asian, and Native Americans. About 16,000 new cases are diagnosed each year.

Signs and symptoms—Symptoms of lupus are:

fever	loss of appetite
weight loss	nausea and vomiting
headache	easy bruising
fatigue	hair loss
swollen glands	edema
depression	

Suggestive signs of lupus include:

a rash over cheeks and bridge of nose	discoid lupus lesions
	ulcers inside mouth
rashes developing after being in the sun	pleurisy
	anemia
arthritis in two or more joints	**Raynaud's phenomenon** (fingers turn white or blue in the cold)
seizures	
bald spots	

Diagnosis is made from symptoms and blood tests for evidence of autoantibodies. Urine is checked for protein, RBCs, and WBCs. A specific antibody test called ANA (antinuclear antibody) looks for antibodies to the nuclei of cells. Over 99% of people with lupus will have a positive test; however, only 33% of people with a positive ANA have SLE.

Etiology—Unknown immune system change.

Treatment—Treatment of SLE consists of assuring patients they can live near-normal lives. Limits on activities are dictated by the disease. Rest when needed, but otherwise engage in normal employment and exercise. Sun exposure should be avoided at peak hours (10:00 AM to 2:00 PM), otherwise, as tolerated. Sunscreens of at least SPF 15 are advisable. No medication has been developed to cure lupus. Joint and muscle pain is controlled with anti-inflammatory and analgesic drugs, such as aspirin, ibuprofen, Naprosyn, and Tylenol. During flareups or if major organs are involved, steroids, such as prednisone, are often used to suppress inflammation. The steroid also interferes with the proliferation and interaction of the cells in the immune system and causes T cells to gather in the lymph nodes, which removes them from concentrating at the inflammation sites. The drugs chloroquine and Plaquenil (antimalarials) are valuable in managing the skin lesions and also help control arthritis symptoms.

Many new treatments are being tested, several dealing with self-antigens, immunoreplacement therapy, and even plasmapheresis (the removal of blood plasma, and hence antibodies). It is believed with further understanding of the immune system, an effective treatment of lupus will be discovered.

Lymphedema (Limf-e-de′ma)

Description—**Lymphedema** is swelling in the tissues of the body caused by an accumulation of lymphatic fluid. Approximately 20% of women who have had breast cancer surgery develop the condition. It may begin as soon as a few months or as late as several years after surgery.

Signs and symptoms—A swelling within the fatty tissue just under the skin of the arm and hand. When it first begins, the arm may seem normal in the morning, but the hand or arm will swell during the day. If it occurs following overuse of the arm in the first year or year and one-half after surgery, it can often be reversed with aggressive treatment. If it occurs 2 or more years after surgery, complete reversal is unlikely, but the condition can be controlled. With chronic marked swelling in the arm, serious complications can arise, such as infection, loss of function, and skin breakdown.

Etiology—Normally lymph fluid circulates easily through the vessels and is filtered in the nodes. However, when the system is altered or damaged it cannot handle the amount of fluid. This is especially true when lymph nodes in the axilla are removed during surgery for breast cancer. Damage can also result from radiation therapy. The more extensive the damage, the greater the risk of developing lymphedema.

One way to reduce the risk from surgery is to perform the sentinel node biopsy procedure. A dye material is injected at the site of the tumor to identify the first node along the lymph vessel that drains the area. This node is biopsied to determine if cancer cells are present. If cancer is not found then, no other lymph nodes are removed.

Treatment—The most comprehensive treatment for lymphedema is complete or complex decongestive physiotherapy (CDP). This involves massage, exercise, hygiene training, and compression bandages or clothing. A trained therapist is required to provide manual lymph drainage. This requires daily massage over a 1- to 4-week period. The massage removes excess fluid by stimulating the lymph vessels to dilate to drain fluid and to open new passageways. After each massage, the affected limb is wound in compression bandages to prevent the build-up of fluid.

Exercise and skin care techniques are also used during the maintenance phase of CDP. Compression bandages may be required for 24 hours a day at the beginning, but once edema has decreased, a compression sleeve that is worn during periods of activity may be adequate. The sleeve is also necessary when exercising or traveling in a plane. CDP may not be appropriate for people under treatment for congestive heart disease. Diuretics are contraindicated because they contribute to protein build-up and may further affect the tissues.

Precautions—Physicians advise patients to take precautions to reduce the risk of lymphedema by observing the following advice:

- Avoid any injury to the arm or puncture to the skin.
- Avoid infection from cuts, burns, or insect bites by applying or taking antibiotics.
- Protect the affected arm by avoiding injections, vaccinations, blood withdrawal, or intravenous procedures. Avoidance of blood pressure readings may be advisable.
- Avoid constricting clothing or jewelry.
- Avoid an activity that might cause heat in the arm or chest, such as tanning, saunas, hot tubs or baths, and vigorous exercise.
- Wear compression bandages or garments when exercising or flying.

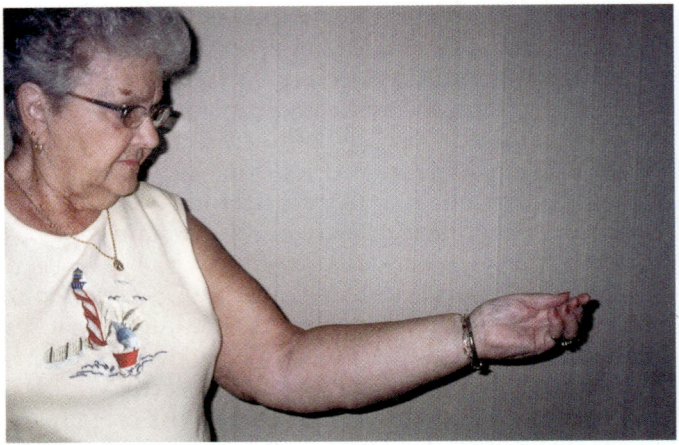

FIGURE 11-158A Woman with lymphedema of the left arm following mastectomy and removal of lymph nodes

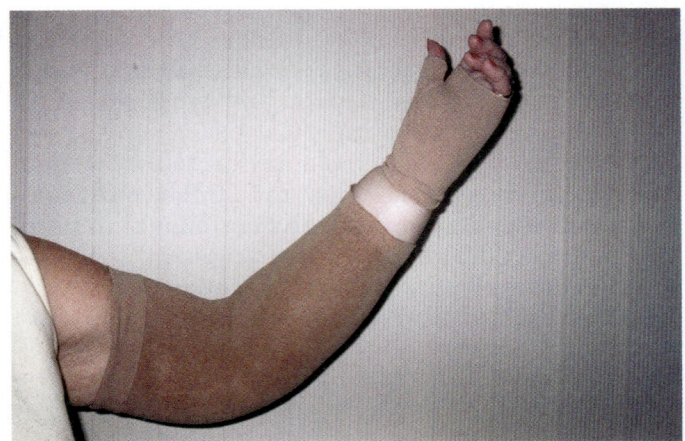

FIGURE 11-158B Compression sleeve and glove

- The woman in Figure 11-158A has lymphedema of her left arm, primarily in the forearm, following a mastectomy with lymph node removal. She stated at times it is much worse, becoming larger, warm, and sometimes developing skin lesions. The compression sleeve and glove (Figure 11-158B) helps to return lymph fluid and reduce swelling.

Rheumatoid Arthritis (Room′a-toyd Ar-thri′tis)

Description—This chronic systemic inflammatory autoimmune disease affects the joints and surrounding muscles, tendons, ligaments, and blood vessels. It affects women three times more often than men. It occurs primarily between the ages of 20 and 60, with a peak onset period between 35 to 45.

Signs and symptoms—The symptoms develop insidiously, then become localized in joints, usually bilaterally. Following inactivity, the affected joints stiffen, swell, and may show beginning signs of deformity. They eventually become tender, painful, hot, and enlarged and have marked deformities and decreased function.

This disease was discussed in the unit on the skeletal system; however, it is believed there is a connection to the immune system. Recent findings suggest a link to genetic defects, which cause the cells to display a specific cell marker. Patients may also have an autoantibody known as *rheumatoid factor*, which locks onto the body's own IgG molecule as if it were an antigen. These antigen-antibody complexes seem to be deposited on the synovial membranes of the joints and are the targets of the inflammatory response.

Etiology—The etiology of rheumatoid arthritis in unknown, but it results in an inflammatory response by the immune system. When the complement system is activated, the macrophages gather at the joint. The inflammatory response dilates the blood vessels, and fluid accumulates in the joint cavity. The cells of the membrane proliferate in response, thickening the joint membrane and causing more swelling. These events continue in cycles and result in the destruction of the joint.

Treatment—Treatment is varied depending on the severity of symptoms. Initially, therapy includes salicylates, **corticosteroids** (prednisone), nonsteroidal anti-inflammatory agents (ibuprofen), gold salts, and antimalarial drugs (chloroquine) and chemotherapy (methotrexate). Patients need periods of rest during the day and 8 to 10 hours of sleep every night. Activities that may be helpful are range of motion exercises, application of heat during chronic episodes, and ice packs with acute phases. Newer therapies include monoclonal antibodies such as etanercept (Enbrel), infliximab (Remicade), and adalimumab (Humira), which are anticytokine therapies that either enhance or inhibit the immune response of the disease.

ACHIEVE UNIT OBJECTIVES

- Complete the Workbook activities to meet the learning objectives.

- Apply your knowledge at the end of this chapter in completing the Critical Thinking Challenge and Activities, as well as the StudyWARE on your Student CD-ROM.

UNIT 10
THE DIGESTIVE SYSTEM

OBJECTIVES

Upon completion of this unit, you will be able to achieve the following:

LEARNING Objectives

1. Spell and define, using the glossary at the back of the text, all the Words to Know in this unit.
2. Name the four phases of the digestive process.
3. Define digestion.
4. Name the raw materials required for a healthy body.
5. Trace the pathway of food through the alimentary tract.
6. Describe the structures of the mouth and the digestive processes that occur there.
7. Explain the process of swallowing.
8. Describe how the esophagus propels food toward the stomach.
9. Describe the structure and function of the stomach.
10. Describe the structure and function of the small intestine.
11. Tell why the duodenum is a vital link in the digestive system.
12. List the functions of the liver, including the portal circulation connection.
13. Describe the role of the gallbladder and its association with the liver.
14. Describe the location and function of the pancreas.
15. Explain how and where nutrients are absorbed.
16. Name the sections of the colon, and describe its function.
17. Describe the function of the rectum.
18. Describe the structure and function of the anal canal.

19. **Describe the diagnostic examinations of the digestive tract.**
20. **Describe the disorders and diseases of the digestive system.**

WORDS TO KNOW

alimentary canal	enzyme	mesentery
anal	esophagus	mouth
anus	fecal	nausea
appendectomy	fissure	pancreas
appendicitis	fistula	pancreatitis
ascending	flatus	paralytic ileus
bile	gallbladder	peptic
bolus	gastric	peristalsis
bowel	gastrointestinal	polyp
cardiac sphincter	(GI)	proctoscope
cecum	gastroscopy	pruritus ani
cholecystectomy	hemorrhoid-	pyloric
cholelithiasis	ectomy	rectum
chyme	hemorrhoids	reflux
cirrhosis	hepatic	saliva
colitis	hepatitis	salivary glands
colon	hernia	sigmoid
colostomy	herniorrhaphy	sigmoidoscopy
common bile	hiatus	stenosis
duct	hydrochloric	stomach
constipation	acid	stool
Crohn's disease	ileocecal	tongue
cystic	ileostomy	transverse
defecate	ileum	ulcer
descending	impaction	varices
diarrhea	incontinent	vermiform
digestion	insulin	appendix
digestive	intestine	villi
diverticulitis	jaundice	villous adenoma
duodenum	jejunum	vomit
emesis	liver	

CERTIFICATION CONNECTION

CMA
Diagnostic procedures
Common diseases and
pathology
Anatomy and physiology

CMAS
Anatomy and physiology

RMA
Anatomy and physiology

The **digestive** system is the group of organs that changes food that has been eaten into a form that can be used by the body's cells. The system is also known as the **gastrointestinal (GI)** tract or system, and the connecting chain of organs is sometimes referred to as the **alimentary canal**. The digestive process can be divided into four phases: *ingestion, digestion, absorption,* and *elimination*. Food that is consumed is acted on by various mechanical and chemical means as it progresses through the body. Each organ, whether main or accessory, plays an important role in physically or chemically altering the composition of the food, selectively absorbing the elements, or eliminating the remains.

The main organs of the system are those through which the food passes. These organs form a continuous tube from the entrance to the exit of the body. They are the mouth, pharynx, esophagus, stomach, small intestine, and large intestine. As important as these organs are, it is the accessory organs that play a major role in the digestive process. In the mouth, there are the teeth, salivary glands, and tongue. The liver, gallbladder, and pancreas have access to the small intestine (Figure 11-159).

Digestion is the activity performed by the organs of the digestive system, and it is defined as the process by which food is broken down, mechanically and chemically, in the GI tract and converted into an absorbable form that can be used by the cells of the body. This process cannot occur within the digestive system alone. As with all body functions, an interrelationship of systems is required to achieve the desired results. Digestion requires cooperation from the nervous system, the muscular system, the circulatory system, and the endocrine system.

The human body can be compared with an engine that needs appropriate fuel to operate. The energy we need to function must come from the foods we eat. The right fuel will not only supply the body with energy, but also provide the materials necessary to build and repair the body so that it can operate efficiently. If the wrong fuel is used too often, the machine will eventually break down.

The human body can manufacture the appropriate fuel if it receives an adequate supply of the right raw materials, mainly carbohydrates, proteins, fats, minerals, vitamins, water, and roughage. All these raw materials are available from the basic food groups and should be eaten daily.

Carbohydrates supply about two thirds of the energy calories needed each day. Fats are also an excellent source of energy; in fact, an ounce of fat yields about three times the calories of an ounce of carbohydrate. Unfortunately, the body does not waste excess energy-producing calories but stores them instead. Therefore, when all the calories eaten are not used for energy, they are stored as excess body tissue we may not desire.

Proteins are obtained primarily from plant and animal sources but are not stored by the body. It is espe-

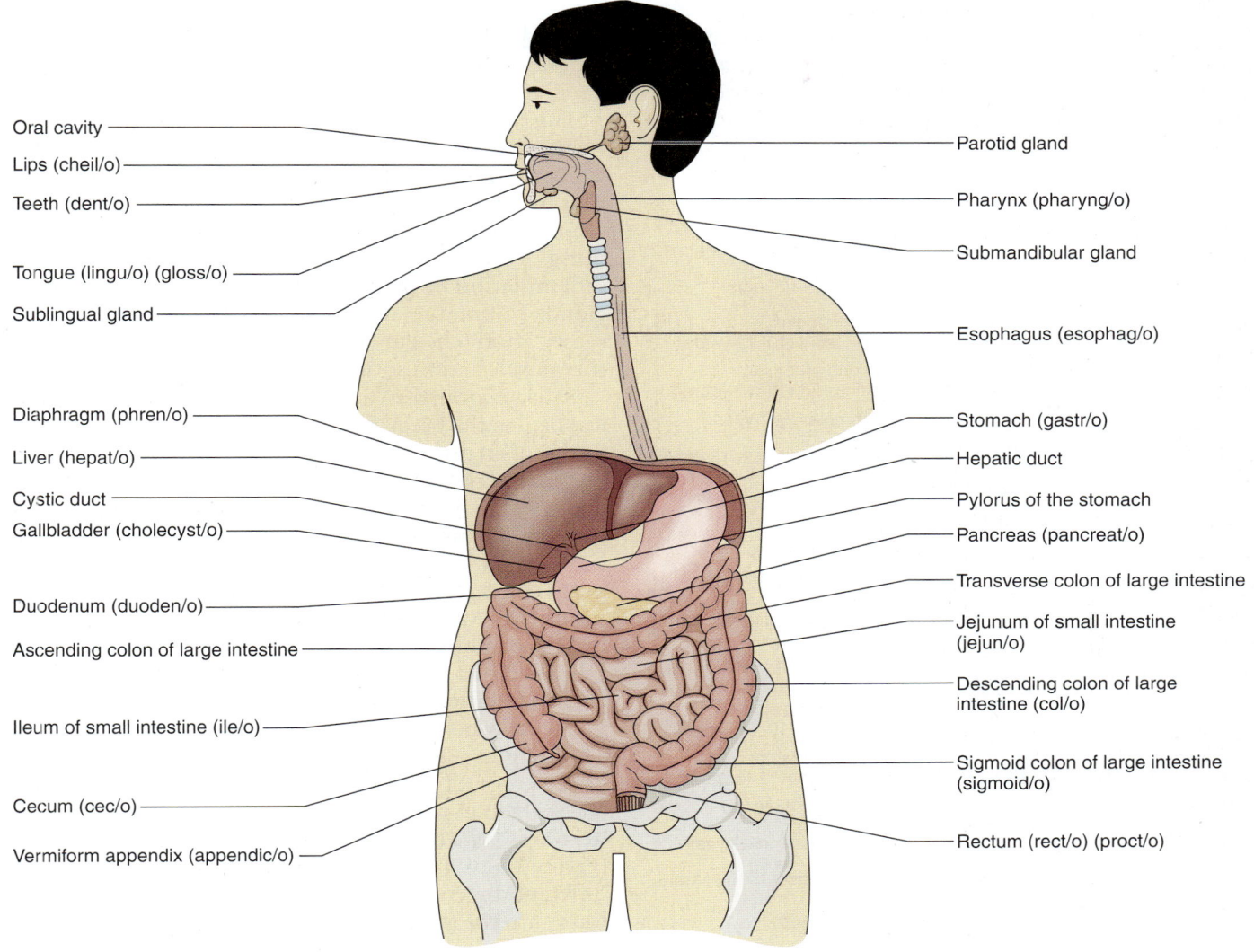

FIGURE 11-159   The digestive system

cially important that they be eaten daily because they are the main ingredients needed to build and repair cells and tissue.

Other raw materials required for a healthy body are vitamins and minerals. Vitamins are regulating chemicals needed for growth and control of body activities. For instance, the chemical that becomes vitamin D must either be absorbed from the intestine or produced in the skin by photosynethsis. The body needs vitamin D to absorb and use calcium. Calcium and another mineral, phosphorus, are needed by the body for the muscles, nerves, blood, teeth, and bones. The formation of red blood cells requires iron and copper. We have already learned that the combination of an iron pigment and a protein forms the hemoglobin of the red blood cells, which enables them to attract O_2 and CO_2 as they move through the body.

All the raw materials the body needs are altered by the digestive system to provide the essential elements necessary for good health. The various stages in this process will become clearer by tracing the pathway of food through the alimentary canal.

THE MOUTH

Food enters the body through the **mouth**. It is held in the oral cavity while the initial digestive process is begun. Teeth break up food into small pieces to make it easier to swallow and also to prepare it for more effective action by digestive enzymes. "Baby" teeth are called *deciduous* and begin to appear at about 6 months. They are gradually exchanged for permanent teeth beginning at about 6 years. Different teeth have specific duties to perform. The incisors bite food with their sharp edges. The canines or cuspids are pointed to puncture and tear. The premolars or bicuspids and the molars are for grinding and crushing (Figure 11-160A and B). The **tongue** aids in the process by moving the food around within the mouth, bringing it into contact with the teeth. The tongue is a muscle and can alter its shape to reach all areas of the mouth. The surface of the tongue contains the taste buds, located within the papillae projections.

The **salivary glands** excrete the fluid known as **saliva**. It is released from three pairs of glands: the parotid, the submandibular, and the sublingual (Figure 11-161). Certain foods cause the glands to excrete profusely, often producing some discomfort, as when eating something sour. The disease called mumps is the inflammation of the parotid glands. A virus causes the glands to enlarge and become painful. With mumps, mastication (chewing) causes great discomfort because the muscle action squeezes the swollen glands.

Saliva contains an **enzyme** called ptyalin. This chemical begins the break down of carbohydrates into sugar. Saliva also provides moisture that enables the taste buds to perceive the sensations of sweet, sour, bitter, and salty. In addition, saliva aids in cleansing the teeth by washing away food particles that might allow bacteria to grow. The presence of saliva in the oral cavity keeps the surfaces moist and flexible, which aids in the production of speech.

The combination of mashed food substances and saliva is called a **bolus**. When it has been mixed well and contains sufficient moisture, it can be easily swallowed. For this to occur, several muscles must work together. The tongue presses upward and backward against the palate (roof of the mouth), while the muscles in the cheeks help in the formation of a chute to direct the bolus toward the back of the mouth and into the pharynx (Figure 11-162). At this point, the bolus could go in three different directions: into the nasal cavity, down and forward into the trachea, or down into the **esophagus**.

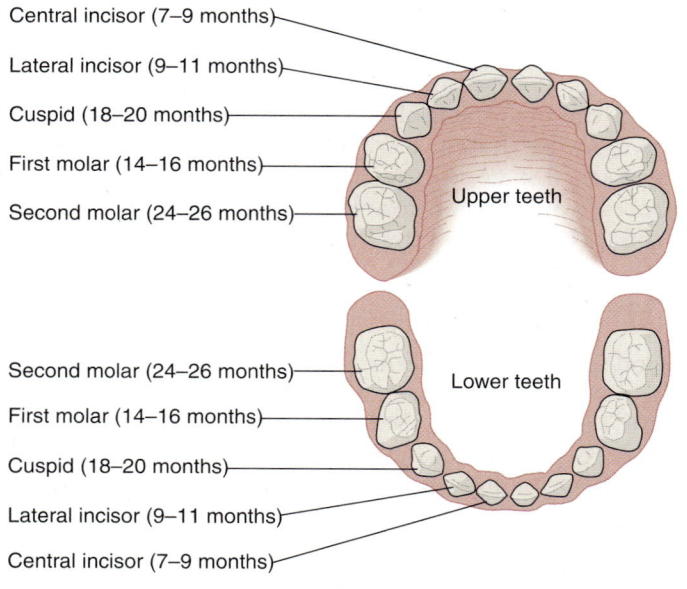

Central incisor (7–8 years)
Lateral incisor (8–9 years)
Cuspid (9–10 years)
First premolar, or bicuspid (10–12 years)
Second premolar, or bicuspid (10–12 years)
First molar (6–7 years)
Second molar (12–13 years)
Third molar (17–25 years)

Upper teeth

Third molar (17–25 years)
Second molar (12–13 years)
First molar (6–7 years)
Second premolar, or bicuspid (10–12 years)
First premolar, or bicuspid (10–12 years)
Cuspid (9–10 years)
Lateral incisor (8–9 years)
Central incisor (7–8 years)

Lower teeth

FIGURE 11-160A Permanent teeth

Central incisor (7–9 months)
Lateral incisor (9–11 months)
Cuspid (18–20 months)
First molar (14–16 months)
Second molar (24–26 months)

Upper teeth

Second molar (24–26 months)
First molar (14–16 months)
Cuspid (18–20 months)
Lateral incisor (9–11 months)
Central incisor (7–9 months)

Lower teeth

FIGURE 11-160B Deciduous teeth

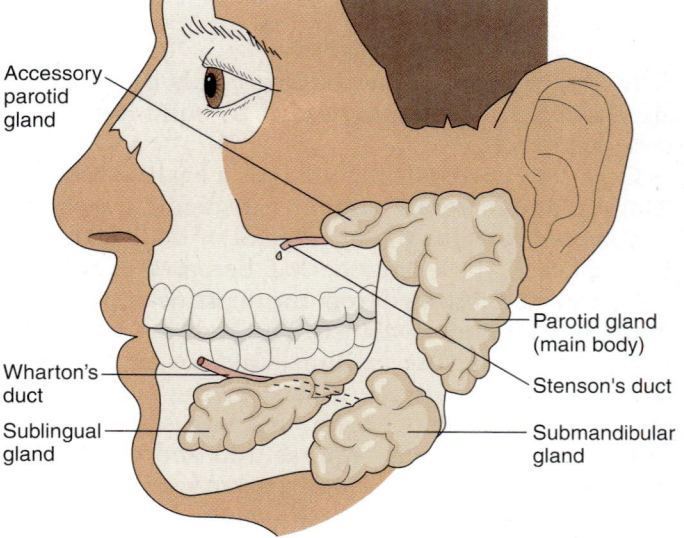

Accessory parotid gland

Wharton's duct

Sublingual gland

Parotid gland (main body)

Stenson's duct

Submandibular gland

FIGURE 11-161 Salivary glands

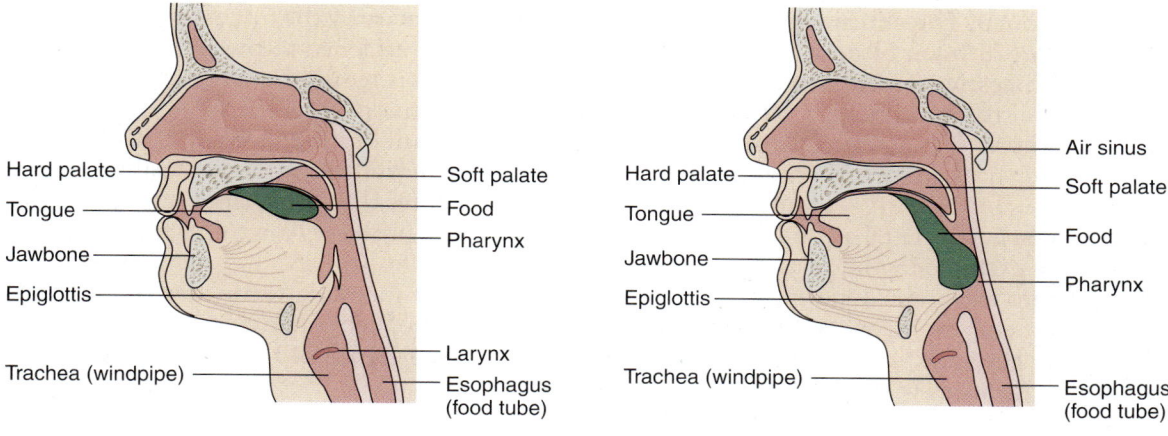

FIGURE 11-162   The process of swallowing

The directing of the bolus is accomplished by a complex combination of "lids" and muscles, which operate automatically. As the bolus is swallowed, it raises the soft palate, closing off the nasal cavity. At the same time, the epiglottis, a cartilage lid attached at the top of the larynx, moves across the opening into the larynx when the tongue pushes the bolus against the palate. At the moment of swallowing, the larynx moves upward against the epiglottis to close the opening. Usually, this reflex action works perfectly, but when the timing is slightly off, food may enter the larynx, triggering the cough reflex (to remove the material). We say, "It went down the wrong pipe."

THE ESOPHAGUS

Once food is swallowed, its movement through the body is maintained by the smooth, involuntary muscle action called **peristalsis**. The esophagus has two layers of involuntary muscles. The inner layer forms circles around the esophagus, whereas the outer layer runs longitudinally along its approximately 10-inch length. When food enters the esophagus, the muscles alternately contract and relax, squeezing the bolus. Together they create the peristaltic "milking action," which moves the bolus to the **stomach**. The whole process only requires about 5 seconds. Because peristaltic action moves material in one direction only and this process does not depend on gravity, it is possible to drink a glass of water while standing on your head.

THE STOMACH

The upper opening to the stomach is controlled by a circular muscle called the **cardiac sphincter**. As the peristaltic wave approaches, the sphincter dilates, allowing the food to enter. Once the food is inside, this one-way "gate" closes to prevent its escape.

The stomach is a 10-inch-long, J-shaped organ constructed of three layers of strong muscle tissue (Figure 11-163). It lies just beneath the diaphragm. The inner lining of the stomach is thick and full of folds called *rugae*. Because muscle tissue is elastic and the folds in the lining can straighten out, the stomach is capable of expanding. It can hold about half a gallon of food and liquid.

Once the material has entered the stomach, the muscular layers begin to contract. A circular layer, a longitudinal layer, and an oblique layer work together in a strong rhythmic motion to break up the food into tiny particles. The stomach continues the digestive process

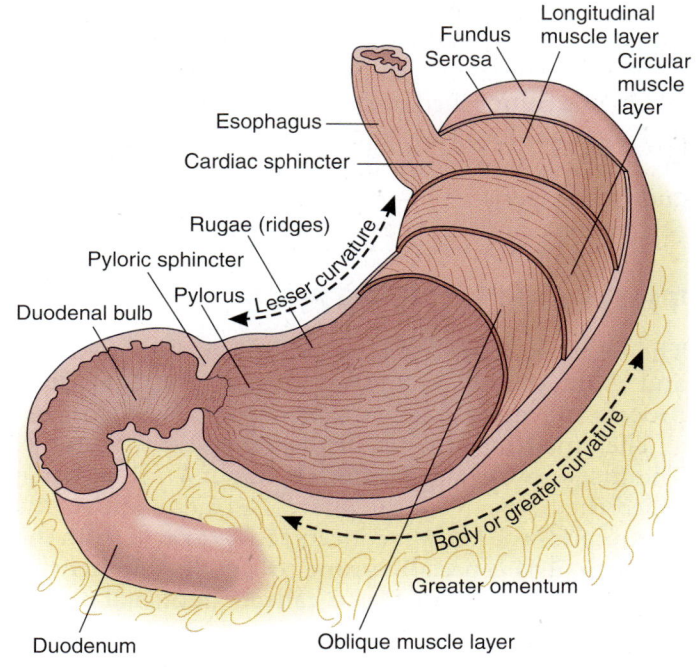

FIGURE 11-163   The stomach

that began in the mouth. The churning action is prolonged and made more difficult by poorly chewed food.

The mechanical digestive process is assisted by a chemical process. The stomach lining is formed of mucous membrane, whose glands secrete mucus. The stomach lining also has about 35 million **gastric** glands, which secrete **hydrochloric acid** and several enzymes. As the stomach contents are being kneaded, acid and enzymes are excreted by the gastric glands and thoroughly mixed into the bolus. One enzyme, rennin, curdles milk. Another enzyme, lipase, splits certain fats, while pepsin digests the milk curds from the rennin. The hydrochloric acid unites with protein to form another chemical, which in turn is split by the pepsin.

Because hydrochloric acid burns holes in most things it touches, you may wonder why it does not destroy the stomach. This is because the mucus layer protects the gastric cells from acid injury. However, when a sufficient amount of excess acid is present for a sufficient length of time, break down of the mucus layer can lead to an **ulcer** (open sore), usually along the posterior wall near the pylorus. An ulcer in the stomach that is caused by acid is known as a gastric (stomach) or **peptic** ulcer.

The partially digested food in the stomach is changed into a semiliquid state called **chyme** in 3 to 5 hours. Liquids, on the other hand, pass through the stomach in a matter of minutes. Of the solid foods, carbohydrates are digested first, proteins second, and fats last. When the consistency of the chyme is right, the **pyloric** sphincter, at the end of the stomach, allows the chyme to spurt through the sphincter into the small **intestine**.

Because of the two sphincters, food is held in the stomach until it is properly prepared to leave. But occasionally, when you suffer from **nausea** and **vomit**, it is obvious the material did not go in the right direction. This action is accomplished by the contraction of the abdominal muscles, forcefully squeezing the stomach as it is pushed downward by the diaphragm. With this pressure and reverse peristaltic waves, the contents of the stomach are forced out and **emesis** (vomiting) occurs.

THE SMALL INTESTINE

The small intestine is a tube about 1 inch in diameter and about 20 feet in length. It completes the digestive process and absorbs the nutrients from the chyme.

The small intestine is divided into three sections. The first is a **C**-shaped segment, about 9 inches long, called the **duodenum** (see Figure 11-163). Because this area receives the highest concentration of acid from the stomach, it is especially prone to the development of ulcers. An ulcer in this area is called a duodenal ulcer.

The next segment, the **jejunum**, is about 8 feet in length. The last segment, about 12 feet long, is called the **ileum**. The jejunum and ileum are suspended in the abdominal cavity by the **mesentery**, a fan-shaped fold of tissue that is attached to the posterior abdominal wall.

The ileum is reduced to about half an inch in diameter by the time it joins the large intestine in the right lower quadrant of the abdomen. The junction is marked by a sphincter called the **ileocecal** valve, which allows the chyme to enter the **cecum** (first segment of the large intestine) but prohibits anything from returning to the ileum.

The small intestine completes the digestive process with the aid of accessory organs and intestinal juice secreted by the glands of the small intestine.

The Liver and Gallbladder

The **liver** is the largest gland in the body. It lies below the diaphragm in the upper right quadrant of the abdomen, extending into the upper left quadrant (Figure 11-164). The liver is a vital organ that performs several functions for the body. It secretes **bile** at a rate of over a pint a day, and the bile is continuously excreted through bile passages to the bile duct. Unconcentrated liver bile is a bitter, yellow-orange liquid that is required to digest fats. Bile is composed primarily of water and contains pigment from red blood cells that have been destroyed (carried to the liver from the spleen in the portal vein). The pigment is changed in the intestines and excreted in **fecal** material, giving it its yellow-brown color. The iron from the destroyed cells is reabsorbed into the body.

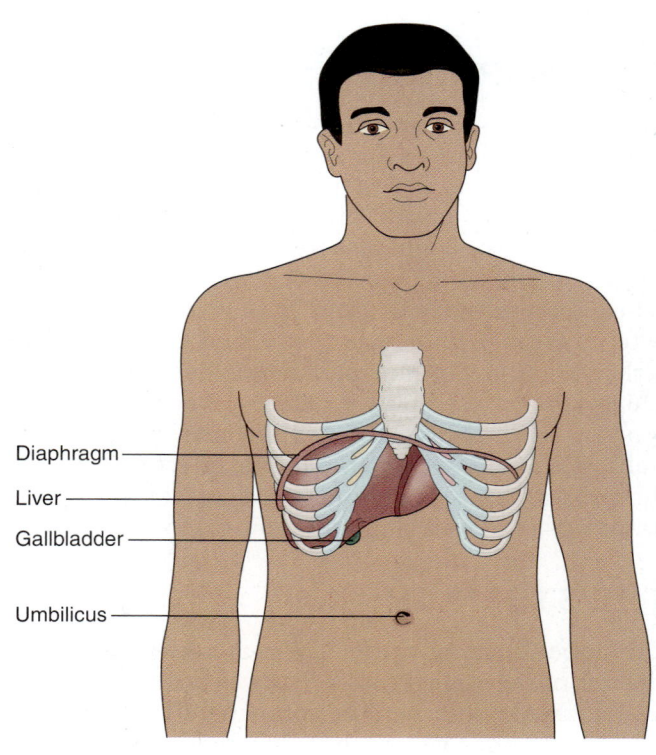

Diaphragm

Liver

Gallbladder

Umbilicus

FIGURE 11-164   The liver and gallbladder

The liver also stores glycogen, a form of glucose (carbohydrate). When the body needs additional blood sugar, it changes the glycogen back to glucose and releases it. In addition, the liver processes proteins from amino acids and either burns fats as fuel or stores them. The liver performs the life-essential service of manufacturing fibrinogen, prothrombin, and other substances required for the process of clotting blood. Antibodies to counteract certain disease organisms are produced in the liver. Also, toxins (poisons) that have been absorbed from the intestine, inhaled, injected, or otherwise taken into the body are circulated in the blood to the liver, where for the most part they are rendered harmless. The liver is also an important storage area for blood and body fluid because of its large size.

The liver receives blood from two separate systems. It receives arterial blood for its own support and preservation from the hepatic artery. It also receives blood from the portal vein that conveys absorbed nutrients and other substances from all the abdominal organs for processing.

The **gallbladder** is a small sac attached to the underside of the liver (Figure 11-165). Its sole purpose is the concentration and storage of bile. When the body needs bile to digest food, the gallbladder releases the concentrated bile to supplement that being currently produced by the liver. Concentrated bile is very bitter and is green-yellow in color. The gallbladder empties its contents via the **cystic** duct. The cystic duct from the gallbladder and the **hepatic** duct from the liver combine to form the **common bile duct**. This common duct empties the bile directly into the duodenum to be added to the chyme during the digestive process. The duodenum is a very vital segment of the digestive system. Not only does it receive chyme from the stomach and bile from the liver and gallbladder, but as we will soon see, it also receives pancreatic juices from the pancreas.

Obstruction of the bile ducts by **cholelithiasis** (gallstones) from the gallbladder is not uncommon. Bile contains certain mineral salts that can become crystallized into "stones" in the gallbladder, perhaps from poor drainage or extended storage. Frequently the stones will be expelled into the cystic duct where they become lodged, causing pain and an inadequate supply of bile and frequently requiring surgical removal. If the stone reaches the common bile duct before becoming lodged, a much more serious situation results. Stones in the commom bile duct are called choledocholithiasis. Now neither the gallbladder nor the liver can empty its bile. The liver maintains its production, but now the bile is absorbed into the bloodstream, producing the yellow discoloration of the sclera, mucosa, and skin known as **jaundice**. The gallbladder itself may become infected or filled with stones and nonfunctional. Periodic "gallbladder attacks" will usually prompt a **cholecystectomy** (surgical removal). The hepatic duct and the common bile duct must remain for the liver to function, however.

A newer surgical procedure to remove the gallbladder and cholelithiasis is called laparoscopic cholecystectomy. It has revolutionized the way gallbladder surgery is performed. The procedure is accomplished with the use of three or more laparoscopes (tiny telescope instruments) inserted into the abdomen. One is placed in the right upper quadrant, one near the umbilicus, and one in the mid-upper abdomen. One scope serves as the source of light and has a camera attachment and a video monitor. Another is an air supply to manipulate tissues, and the third is the one through which the surgery is performed with the aid of the video monitor. The gallbladder and its contents, if any, are excised and removed through the operative scope.

Following surgery, only a few sutures or surgical tape close the small abdominal openings. Previous surgery techniques resulted in a long incision extending down the right side of the abdomen and a considerably uncomfortable postoperative period. The new technique has shortened recovery to 2 weeks or less from the former 6 weeks period.

Occasionally, the endoscopic procedure cannot be completed and an "open" abdominal procedure will be performed. This usually occurs if there is excessive bleeding, the patient is obese or pregnant, the area cannot be visualized, there is excessive scar tissue from previous surgery, or unexpected inflammation is present.

If stones are in the common bile duct, a separate procedure called endoscopic retrograde cholangiopancreatography (ERCP) is done either before or after the laparoscopic cholecystectomy in order to remove them, or an open procedure is substituted.

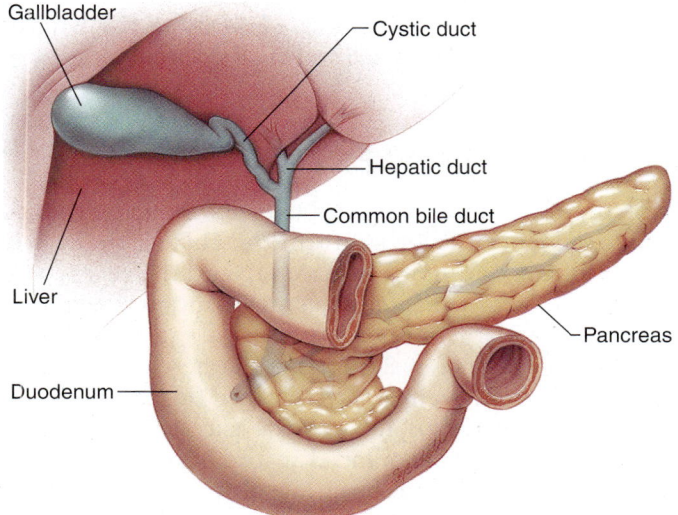

Gallbladder

Cystic duct

Hepatic duct

Common bile duct

Liver

Pancreas

Duodenum

FIGURE 11-165   The gallbladder and cystic, hepatic, and common bile ducts on the underside of the liver

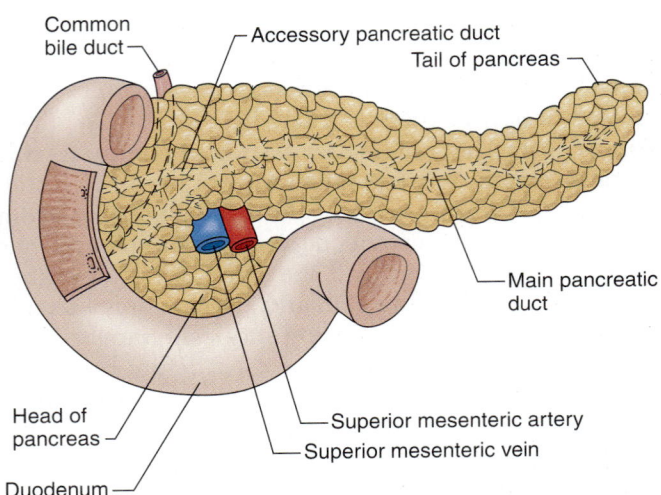

FIGURE 11-166 The duodenum and pancreas. A window has been cut into the anterior wall of the duodenum to show the openings of the common bile duct and the pancreatic ducts into the lumen of the duodenum.

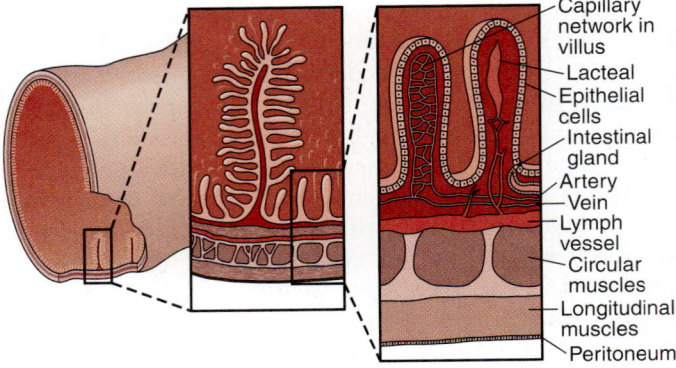

FIGURE 11-167 A magnified view of the inner lining of the small intestine showing the villa with blood and lymphatic capillaries for the absorption of the products of digestion

The Pancreas

The **pancreas** lies behind the stomach, with its head in the curve of the duodenum (Figure 11-166). The pancreas, like the liver, is a gland, but it secretes substances in two different ways. Functioning as an *exocrine gland* (secreting through ducts), the pancreas secretes pancreatic juice via the pancreatic duct directly into the duodenum. The three powerful enzymes in pancreatic juice react chemically on all three types of nutrients to break them down for absorption into the bloodstream. Most of the chemical changes that occur in the intestinal tract are caused by pancreatic juices, which are probably sufficient to digest all foods by themselves. If pancreatic juice is absent, serious digestive problems occur.

Functioning as an *endocrine* (ductless) *gland,* the pancreas also secretes directly into the bloodstream a substance called **insulin**. This function will be covered in Unit 12, The Endocrine System.

It should be clear now why the duodenum is such a critical segment of the digestive tract. Because it receives products from four organs—stomach, liver, gallbladder, and pancreas—it is a vital connective link. When ulceration occurs or a tumor develops in this area, it may interfere drastically with the digestive process. Involvement of the duodenum is a cause for concern.

The Absorption Function

When all the digestive juices and enzymes have been added and the chyme passes into the jejunum, digestion has progressed to the point where absorption of some nutrients and other substances can begin. Absorption is a vital function of the small intestine, oc-

curring primarily in the jejunum and gradually decreasing toward the end of the ileum.

Absorption is accomplished through millions of microscopic structures known as **villi** (Figure 11-167). The villi project from the lining of the major part of the small intestine. These fingerlike structures serve a dual purpose. First, they move continuously, swinging back and forth to keep the chyme thoroughly mixed with the digestive juices. Second, each projection is equipped with blood capillaries and a lacteal (intestinal lymphatic capillary) from the lymphatic system. The external cells of the villi absorb the nutrients, minerals, and water from the chyme. Some fats and all carbohydrates and proteins, in the form of sugar and amino acids, are absorbed into the capillaries of the villi, to be sent by way of the portal vein to the liver. Here, the products are processed and released into the body or stored in reserve. Many fats are absorbed into the lacteals of the lymphatic system to be processed through the lymph nodes and eventually returned to the circulatory system for distribution.

THE LARGE INTESTINE

With digestion completed and the useful nutrients and other substances absorbed from the chyme, the waste products, any undigestible material, and the excess water are sent on to the large intestine through the ileocecal valve. The large intestine is only about 5 feet long, but it is approximately 2 inches in diameter. The **colon**, as it is also called, frames the abdomen (Figure 11-168).

The large intestine absorbs the excess liquid from the chyme through capillaries in the lining. There are no villi in the large intestine. The absorbed water, plus some salts and proteins, are later filtered out of the blood by the kidneys to be eliminated in the urine. The remaining fibrous waste materials are formed into semisolid feces to be eliminated through the **rectum**.

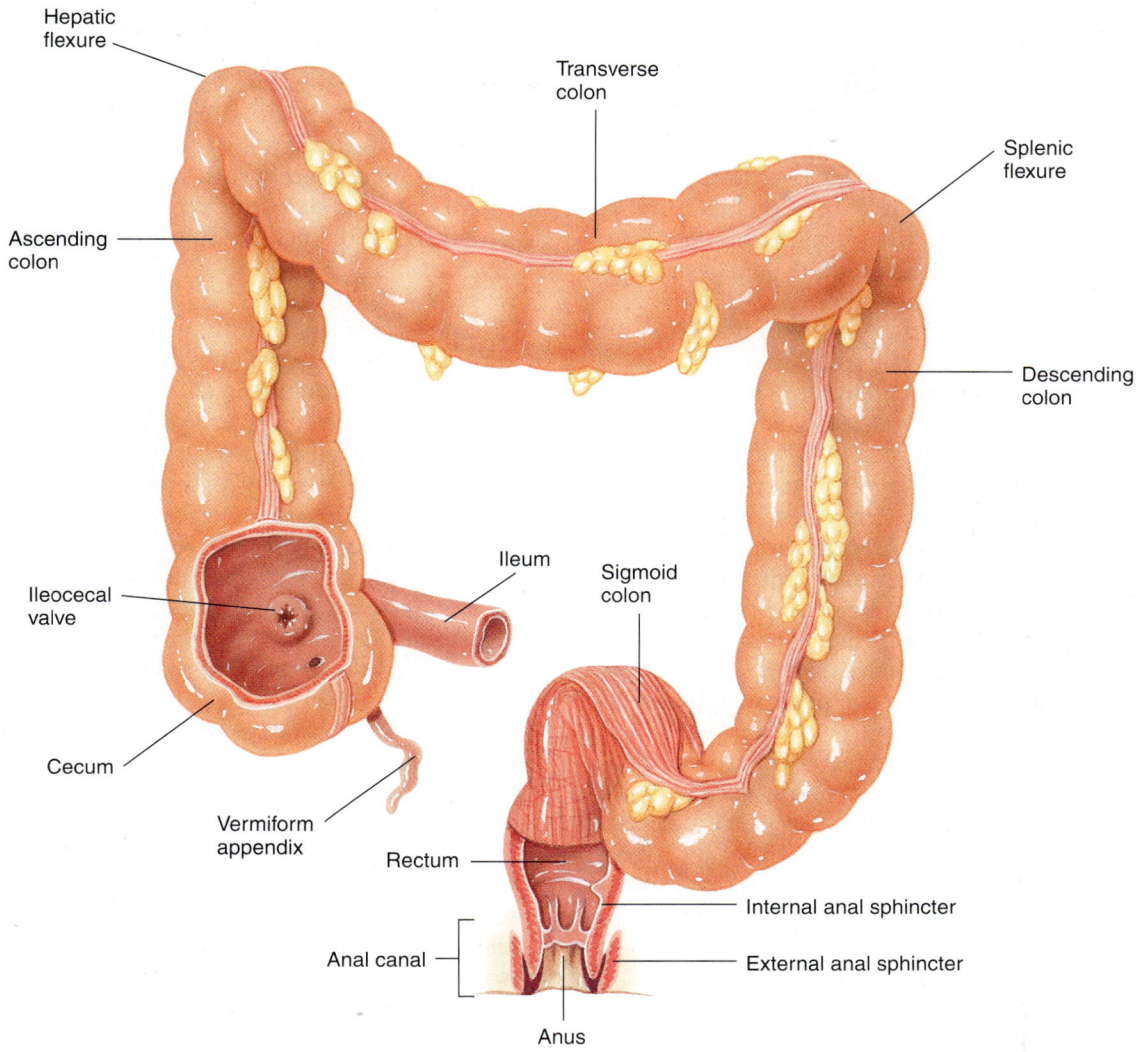

FIGURE 11-168   The large intestine

The Cecum and Appendix

When material leaves the ileum, it enters a small, pouch-like segment of the colon called the cecum. A small projection, the **vermiform appendix**, extends from the cecum. The appendix is a worm-shaped structure about the size of the little finger. It tends to become filled easily but drains rather slowly. Occasionally, a substance causes irritation to the lining, resulting in a painful, inflammatory process known as **appendicitis**. If it persists or progresses, a surgical procedure called an **appendectomy** is indicated.

The Ascending, Transverse, and Descending Colon

The large intestine is divided into **ascending**, **transverse**, and **descending** sections as a means of identification. The ascending section joins the cecum at the level

of the ileocecal valve and continues upward along the right side of the abdomen to the hepatic flexure (bend at the liver). It is generally a little larger in diameter than the descending section. The upper right corner, the hepatic flexure, lies in front of the right kidney and behind the right lobe of the liver. The transverse section begins at the hepatic flexure and extends in a loop across the abdominal cavity to a point below the spleen, the splenic flexure (bend at the spleen). The center section is attached to the mesentery but can move freely. Both the hepatic and splenic flexures are firmly attached to the rear of the abdominal wall, with the splenic attachment being slightly higher.

The descending section begins at the splenic flexure and extends downward along the left side of the abdomen until it reaches the edge of the pelvic cavity. This section is somewhat smaller in diameter. It is firmly anchored to the abdominal posterior wall to maintain its position.

The Sigmoid, Rectum, and Anal Canal

After the large intestine enters the pelvic cavity, it makes two bends suggestive of an **S** and is therefore labeled the **sigmoid** section of the colon. The sigmoid section extends from the left iliac crest over and back to join the rectum. The rectum is 6 to 8 inches long. It serves as a collecting area for the remains of digestion. When enough material is accumulated, sensors are activated, and the urge to **defecate** is felt.

The **anal** canal is a narrow passageway about an inch long, extending from the rectum to the **anus** (opening from the body). Both ends of the anal canal are controlled by sphincter muscles. The internal anal sphincter is an involuntary muscle. When defecation occurs, the nerve endings in the rectum are stimulated to contract, and the internal sphincter is relaxed, allowing the fecal material to enter the anal canal. The external anal sphincter is a voluntary muscle and can be consciously controlled to prevent the rectum from emptying when it is inappropriate. It is unwise to make a habit of delaying defecation unnecessarily, however, as this tends to lessen the urge, which can result in **constipation**.

When a patient's condition interferes with the ability to control the anus, as in a stroke with paralysis, and the rectum empties whenever the nerve impulse is triggered, the patient is said to be **incontinent** of feces. This situation can be extremely embarrassing to a patient who is still capable of being aware of this occurrence. The opposite problem is often the result of prolonged or serious illness causing a loss of muscle tone so that the patient is too weak to expel the contents of the rectum. This results in material becoming more and more solid as fluid content is lost and the mass becoming of such size that it cannot be expelled. This condition is known as a fecal **impaction**. The best solution is manual breakup of the mass followed by an enema to irrigate the rectum and remove the material. A patient may attempt to remove the impaction by taking a laxative. Laxatives work either by increasing the rate of passage through the tract, therefore reducing the water absorption time, or by stimulating the secretion of fluid into the tract. Regardless, the results will not help an impaction but only cause an uncontrollable flow of liquid **stool** around the mass.

The proper function of the digestive system is essential to health. If raw materials cannot be digested and absorbed, the patient will starve. If waste products are not adequately removed, toxins may accumulate and cause illness and even death. This vital function requires a total of about 36 hours from the mouth to the anus. Of course, this time period is influenced by the type of foods eaten and the rate of the peristaltic action.

DIAGNOSTIC EXAMINATIONS

A great many studies can be done on blood to determine the function of the digestive organs. Also, chemical analysis can be performed on secretions withdrawn by catheter from the stomach or small intestine. However, six other types of examinations will be discussed here because they are so frequently used in diagnosis.

- Colonoscopy—An examination to view the entire large intestine using a flexible fiberoptic scope. It is indicated in patients with complaints of diarrhea, constipation, bleeding, or lower abdominal pain. It is usually indicated following negative or inconclusive results from barium enema studies or sigmoidoscopy examination. Preparation for the examination is quite involved. Starting 24 hours prior to the examination, the patient is allowed only clear liquids or things that become liquid when eaten, such as gelatin. If bleeding is suspected, then no liquids that contain red food coloring may be consumed. In addition to the diet, the patient is instructed to take a strong dose of laxative and repeat a liquid laxative until the stool becomes nothing but liquid. Twelve hours before the procedure, nothing can be taken by mouth.

  When the procedure is performed, the patient is sedated and positioned on the left side, and the scope is guided and advanced through the large intestine. The physician may insert air to distend the walls of the intestine to facilitate passage. Manipulation of the abdomen also assists with insertion, and the repositioning of the patient facilitates passage through the splenic and hepatic flexures. It is possible to obtain tissue samples and secretions through the scope to provide cytology studies. Polyps can also be snared, and electrocautery can be performed through the instrument.
- Gastrointestinal series (x-rays)—Radiologic studies of the GI tract are indicated for a wide variety of reasons and concentrated on various portions of the system.

  Barium swallow—If the condition or function of the esophagus is in question, the patient may be asked to drink a radiopaque liquid called barium while the action of the esophagus is observed by fluoroscope. This test is known as a barium swallow. It aids in diagnosing conditions such as hiatus hernia, diverticulosis, and varices. It also detects strictures, tumors, ulcers, and functional disorders. The barium swallow is usually included as part of the more complete GI series.

  Upper GI series—A barium swallow is performed initially to evaluate the esophagus. Sixteen to twenty ounces of additional barium are drunk as the progress of the medium is observed by fluoroscope. X-ray films are taken at specific periods to permit further evaluation. The stomach is compressed to ensure that the barium coats the entire lining. As the barium enters the small intestine, the radiologist manipulates the abdomen to obtain distribution of the barium throughout the bowel loops. The patient is rotated to several positions to record pertinent areas. Spot films may be taken at 30- to 60-minute intervals until peristalsis carries the barium to the ileocecal valve.

An upper GI series is not painful, but the chalky taste and consistency of barium are unpleasant. Preparation for the test may require a 2 to 3 day diet of low-residue foods before the examination. All oral intake must stop at least 8 hours before it is scheduled. The patient must also refrain from smoking. Both a laxative and a cleansing enema may be ordered the evening before the procedure to be certain the tract is empty.

An upper GI series aids in the diagnosis of gastric ulcers, tumors, strictures of the sphincters, inflammation of the lining, motility irregularities, duodenal ulcers, tumors, filling defects, and the like. Following the exam, another laxative may be ordered to aid in removal of the barium from the intestines. Retained barium may cause constipation, obstruction, or fecal impaction.

Lower GI series—To permit viewing of the entire large intestine, the barium mixture is administered as an enema. The medium outlines the interior wall of the colon for detection of mucosal changes, tumors, **polyps**, ulcerated sites, **diverticulitis**, and structural irregularities. The patient must be carefully prepared with a restrictive, low-residue diet for about 2 days, followed by a diet of liquids only the day before examination. A cathartic (strong laxative) is ordered the afternoon preceding the test, and the colon is thoroughly emptied with tap water enemas until no more fecal material is expelled.

A barium enema of 1,000 to 1,500 mL is administered through a tube inserted into the rectum. This tube is often capable of being inflated with a balloonlike section to aid in retention of the medium until the examination is completed. As the medium is instilled, the filling is observed by fluoroscope. The patient is rotated on the x-ray table to assist the flow of the barium. The patient is placed on the left side to fill the descending, on the back to fill the transverse, and on the right side to fill the ascending colon. Periodic x-ray films are taken.

When the procedure is completed, the balloon is deflated and the tube is removed. The patient is instructed to expel as much barium as possible. An additional x-ray may be taken to record the ability of the colon to empty.

- **Gastroscopy**/esophagogastroduodenoscopy (EGD)—Viewing of the esophagus, stomach, and upper duodenum through a flexible scope that is lighted by fiberoptics. This permits observation of the inside of the organs without an exploratory operation. If an unusual area or growth is seen, a biopsy (small piece) can be removed through the scope. The procedure is also used to remove small foreign objects, to obtain cells from the lining, and, with the attachment of a camera, to photograph suspicious areas for later study.

The patient is prepared by spraying the back of the throat with local anesthetic to block the gag reflex and is given a sedative to produce drowsiness. The patient must be awake to swallow the scope. As it is passed into the patient, air is instilled to expand the pathway or flatten out folds. Water may also be instilled to wash off the lens and is removed, along with the air and any other secretions, by suction.

The examination is especially helpful in diagnosing tumors, ulcers, structural abnormalities, damage from ingested chemicals, and esophageal varices. Figure 11-169 shows a fairly large tumor attached to the wall of the stomach. It is clearly visible through the scope and easily accessible for biopsy.

- Nuclear medicine study—Scanning of structures, such as the liver or spleen, is made possible by radioactive materials. A special camera or scanning device may be used to screen the liver for disease processes, infarcts, cysts, tumors, and organ size. The patient is given an intravenous injection of a radioactive material that the body will absorb in the cells of the liver. The scanner is positioned above the patient and passes slowly back and forth in a descending pattern over the area being examined. The resulting pictures outline the organ and indicate ir-

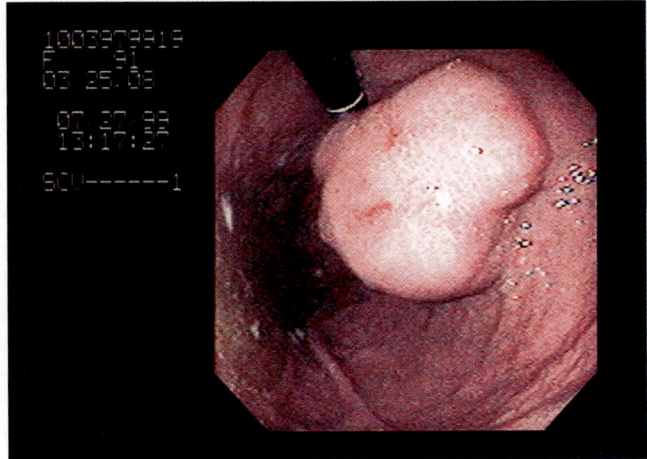

FIGURE 11-169 Tumor in stomach as seen during an esophagogastrosdenoscopy examination *(Courtesy of Thomas C. Ransbottom, MD, Gastroenterologist)*

regularities in its composition. A gamma camera is capable of producing images instantly without the scanning procedure.

Similar studies are accomplished with different types of equipment. Computerized axial tomography studies (CT scans) are multiple x-ray beams passed into tissue to be interpreted and reconstructed by a computer into a three-dimensional picture on a screen. This type of study can be done on the liver, the ducts, and the pancreas.

- Occult blood test—When bleeding from the intestinal tract is not visible because of the small quantity, it can be detected through analysis of the feces. Occult blood studies are frequently used to identify bleeding associated with colorectal malignancy.

Visible blood in the stool has a characteristic coloration that suggests the approximate location of the bleeding. Basically, the nearer the rectum, the brighter red the blood. Dark maroon stool is an indication of bleeding in the ileum or jejunum. Bleeding from the stomach or esophagus will be acted on by gastric juices, which cause it to turn black, resulting in a tarry-looking stool. A simple test involves the use of a Hemoccult slide upon which a thin smear of stool is placed. The Hemoccult Developer is applied to the smear, and results are read within a minute. A trace or change of color to blue is positive for occult blood. Refer to Chapter 15, Unit 4, for additional information.

- Proctoscopy—An examination of the lower rectum and anal canal through a 3-inch-long **proctoscope**. It is preceded by a digital examination to determine anal sphincter condition. The proctoscope permits detection of hemorrhoids, polyps, fissures, fistulas, and abscesses. The patient may need an enema if fecal material is obstructing the view.

- **Sigmoidoscopy**—An examination to view the lower portion of the sigmoid and rectum through a 10- to 12-inch sigmoidoscope. A longer flexible fiber optic scope is capable of manipulation into the descending colon. A digital examination to determine anal sphincter condition precedes insertion of the scope. The patient is examined, preferably on a special jack-knife table, or otherwise in the less comfortable knee-chest position. Sigmoidoscopy aids in the diagnosis of inflammation, infection, or ulcerative conditions. It also permits viewing of tumors, polyps, and other disease processes. Biopsy through the scope permits confirmation of a diagnosis without surgery. The patient must be prepared for the examination with an enema administered a short time before. Soap or other irritants must not be added to the water because they may affect the appearance of the lining. (See Chapter 14, Unit 4.)

- Ultrasound—Ultrasonography uses high-frequency sound waves directed toward the liver, gallbladder, or pancreas. The waves create echos of varying degrees, which are changed into patterns of dots on a screen. The patterns reveal the size, shape, and position of the organ being studied. Ultrasonography is especially useful when liver and gallbladder functions are impaired and the use of contrast media is ineffective.

DISEASES AND DISORDERS

Anorectal Abscess and Fistula (A-no-rek′tal Ab′-ses Fis′tu-la)

Definition—This localized infection is a collection of exudate in the soft tissue adjacent to the anus or rectum.

Signs and symptoms—It is characterized by a throbbing, painful lump, which makes sitting and coughing very uncomfortable.

Etiology—The abscess may be initiated from within the rectum because of a sharp object in the feces, such as a piece of seashell or bone, penetrating the surrounding tissue. Because the feces contain bacteria, an infection develops and an abscess results. The exudate may develop an escape route into the rectum, anal canal, or skin surface, which will periodically relieve the pain and excess pressure. Such a tract is known as a **fistula**.

Treatment—Surgical intervention is indicated to correct the condition by incision and drainage of both the abscess and the tract (Figure 11-170).

Occasionally, an abscess occurs without a fistula. It may appear on the surface of the perineum as a large, firm, red mass, with or without a yellow center. This abscess requires incision to promote drainage and eventual expression of the solid core of material. The application of heat by sitting in a tub of warm water aids in the drainage process and relieves discomfort.

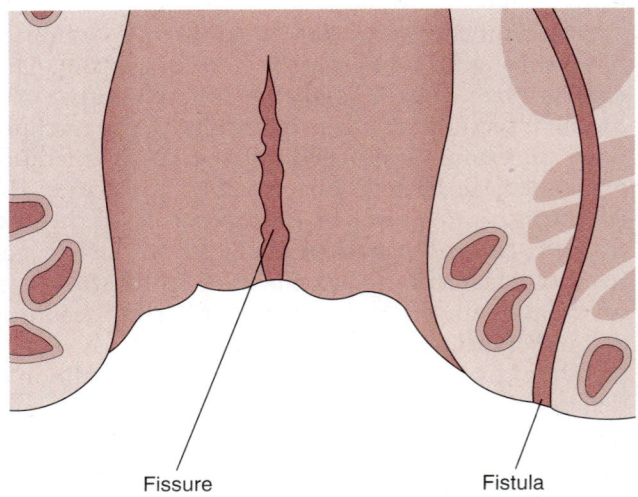

Fissure   Fistula

FIGURE 11-170   Anal fissure and fistula

Appendicitis (A-pendi-si'tis)

Description—An acute inflammation of the appendix probably is caused by an obstruction of the intestinal lumen.

Signs and symptoms—Symptoms of appendicitis begin with generalized abdominal pain that later localizes in the lower right abdomen at a site known as McBurney's point. Increased tenderness, anorexia, nausea, vomiting, and rebound tenderness (produced by slowly compressing the abdomen over the site, then suddenly releasing the pressure) occur. A slight fever may be present. A moderately elevated white blood cell count (12,000 to 15,000) in addition to the physical findings supports the diagnosis. The sudden cessation of symptoms is an indication of infarction or rupture.

Etiology—When obstruction occurs, an inflammatory process begins and leads to infection, thrombosis, destruction of tissue, and eventually perforation of the appendix. On rupture, the infectious material spills into the abdominal cavity and initiates peritonitis, a serious complication. If left untreated, it is fatal.

Treatment—The only effective treatment for appendicitis is surgical removal, an appendectomy. When appendicitis is suspected, abdominal heat, enemas, or laxatives must never be administered because of the risk of causing perforation. Usually pain medication is avoided to prevent masking of the symptoms. Positioning patients on their right side with the knees flexed will usually help to reduce the discomfort.

Cirrhosis (Si-ro'sis)

Description—This chronic disease of the liver causes destruction of the liver cells. The destruction leads to impaired blood and lymph circulation and interferes with the life-preserving functions of the liver.

Signs and symptoms—Early symptoms include a variety of GI tract signs, such as lack of appetite, indigestion, nausea, vomiting, constipation, and **diarrhea**. Later, nosebleeds, bleeding gums, and anemia may develop. The liver becomes enlarged, jaundice is present, and ascites (collection of fluid) occurs within the abdomen. Because the disease interferes with portal circulation, hypertension occurs in the portal system, causing esophageal varices that eventually rupture and bleed.

    Various blood tests support the diagnosis of **cirrhosis**, but positive confirmation can be obtained through a liver biopsy. A liver scan will detect abnormal thickening and a mass.

Etiology—The most frequent cause of cirrhosis is malnutrition associated with alcoholism. Other causative factors are hepatitis or the suppression of bile flow resulting from a disease of the ducts.

Treatment—Treatment consists of taking measures to prevent further damage or complications and dealing with the underlying cause. Dietary changes, supplemental vitamins, rest, and appropriate exercise are indicated. Extra care is required when prescribing drugs because the damaged liver may not be able to process them. Alcohol must be prohibited. It is also important to avoid contact with infections. Mortality is high, with many patients dying within 5 years of diagnosis.

Colitis (Ko-li'tis)

Description—This inflammation of the colon causes tenderness and discomfort. It may be acute, occurring as the result of a bacterial invasion, or chronic, associated with allergy, emotional stress, or other diseases. (See ulcerative **colitis**.)

Colorectal Cancer (Kolo-rek'tal)

Description—This is a malignancy of the colon or rectum. The American Cancer Society estimated 148,610 new cases of colorectal cancer in 2006. It is the third most common cancer in men and women. Incidence rates did decline 1.6% from 1985 to 1997, possibly because of increased screening and polyp removal. (Some polyps tend to become malignant over time.) The Society also estimated 55,170 deaths in 2006, which represented about 10% of all cancer deaths. The 1-year survival rate is 82%, whereas the 5-year rate is 61%. When detected early at the localized stage, the 5-year survival rate increases to 90%; however, only 37% are detected this early. When there is distant metastases, the survival rate drops to only 8%. Figure 11-171A illustrates the percentage of incidence in the common sites and shows that 75% are within viewing distance of the flexible sigmoido-

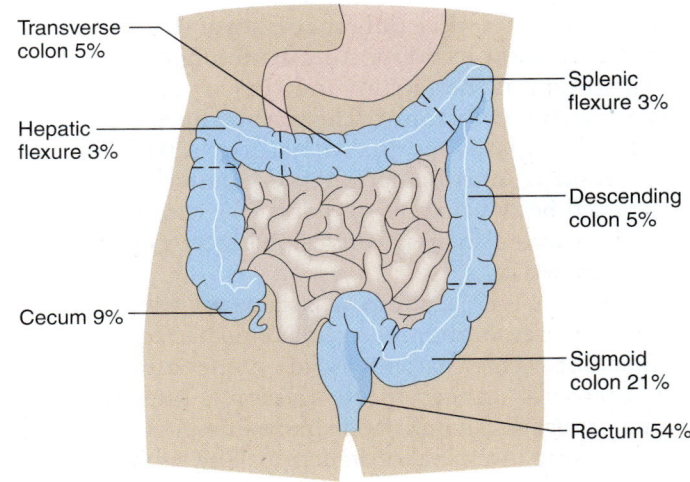

FIGURE 11-171A   Incidence of colorectal cancer by sites

scope. This illustration emphasizes the importance of sigmoidoscopy screening on a regularly scheduled basis as a way of identifying a large percentage of colorectal cancer in its early stage when intervention is most effective.

Signs and symptoms—Symptoms can vary in relation to the area involved. With right side colon involvement there may be black tarry stools, anemia, abdominal aching, pressure, and dull cramps in the beginning. As the disease progresses, weakness, fatigue, dyspnea, vertigo, and eventually diarrhea, anorexia, weight loss, vomiting, and other signs of intestinal obstruction will occur. (Because the wastes are liquid in this section, obstruction is delayed.) With left side involvement, obstruction signs occur earlier because of the formed consistency of the fecal material. There is rectal bleeding, abdominal fullness, cramping, and rectal pressure. Later, there are diarrhea and "ribbon" or pencil-shaped stools. Bright red blood and mucus is in or on the stools. With rectal cancer, the first symptom is a change in bowel habits—often "morning diarrhea" may alternate with obstipation (constipation caused by obstruction). This will be followed by a feeling of incomplete evacuation and later pain and a feeling of rectal fullness.

Etiology—Basically the cause is unknown. However, certain risk factors have been identified.

- A personal or family history of colorectal cancer or polyps
- Inflammatory bowel disease
- Possible relationship to smoking, physical inactivity, high-fat or low-fiber diet, alcohol consumption, and low intake of fruits and vegetables

Recent studies seem to suggest that estrogen replacement therapy and the use of NSAIDs, such as aspirin, may reduce the risk.

Treatment—The most effective treatment is surgery to remove the tumor, adjacent tissues, and any lymph nodes that may be involved. The type of tumor and extent of involvement determine the surgical procedure. It may involve only the removal of a section of the colon and its supporting structures, to total resectioning of the rectum and the construction of a permanent colostomy. Chemotherapy is indicated with metastasis, residual disease, or a recurring inoperable tumor. Radiation and chemotherapy may be used before surgery to reduce the tumor size and activity and also are given following surgery to treat any missed cells.

Figure 11-171B shows a gastostomy tube inserted into a patient's abdomen and connected to a suction machine. This patient is at home after having surgery for cancer (note dressing), but extensive metastasis and lymph node involvement is suspected of causing intestinal obstruction. The tubing can be clamped to allow the patient to take oral medication

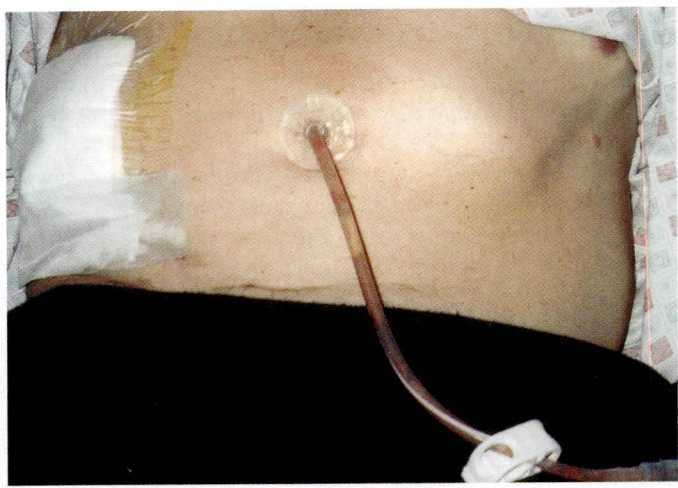

FIGURE 11-171B   Gastrostomy tube to remove stomach contents

and eat or drink fluids. After a period of time, the clamp is opened to remove the remaining fluid.

Colostomy (Ko-los'to-me)

Description—This is an artificial opening of the colon, allowing fecal material to be excreted from the body through the abdominal wall. **Colostomies** are classified according to the portion of the colon involved (for example, transverse colostomy, Figure 11-172). The terms *single* and *double barrel* tell whether only the proximal loop is involved or both the proximal and distal loop. A colostomy can also be temporary or permanent. If a disease process could improve if the colon were not constantly irritated by passing feces, then a temporary colostomy is indicated. By surgically providing for the fecal material to empty through an opening in the colon before reaching the affected area, the area is allowed to rest and heal. After an adequate period, surgery is performed to reattach the ends of the colon.

A colostomy is also indicated when an obstructive growth process, such as a tumor, prohibits the passage of feces. When the growth is close to the end of the rectum, there may not be enough healthy tissue remaining to which a segment of the colon can be attached. There may also be evidence that removal of the affected area, even if possible, would present no advantage. In these cases, a colostomy will be performed for elimination to occur until the disease process results in death.

The colostomy patient has a major emotional adjustment in addition to the physical adjustment to make. The alteration in body image may be difficult to accept. The thought of fecal material being expelled into a pouch attached to the abdomen may be

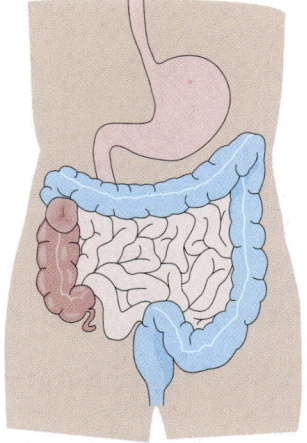

Ascending colostomy

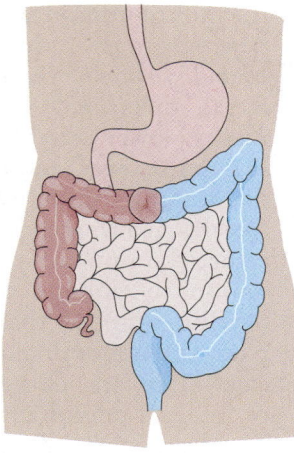

Transverse colostomy

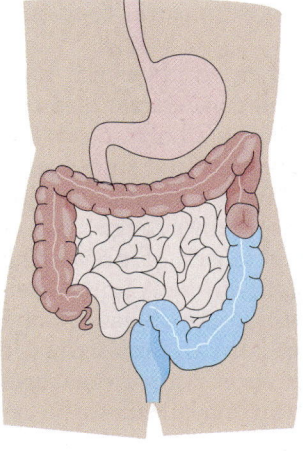

Descending colostomy

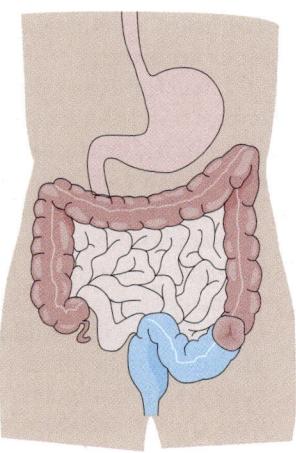

Sigmoid colostomy

Colostomy Sites

FIGURE 11-172 Colostomy sites

very unappealing. Consider also that there is no control over the expulsion of **flatus** (gas) or stool, and it is easy to understand the new patient's rejection. However, with time, diet control, and the use of irrigation, a colostomy can be regulated so that its emptying is at the patient's convenience. Support groups of colostomy patients provide emotional and physical assistance to help new colostomy patients adjust to their changed lifestyle.

Constipation (Konsti-pa′shun)

Description—This is a condition of sluggish bowel action.
Signs and symptoms—It is characterized by dry, hard, infrequent bowel movements.
Etiology—To have normal elimination of body wastes, three things are necessary: a proper diet including bulk, adequate fluid intake, and exercise. When one

or more of these elements is missing, constipation is likely to occur. Other contributing factors are habitual disregard of the impulse to defecate and the chronic use of laxatives or enemas, which dull the impulse stimulation. Constipation is common among the elderly, persons with paralysis, and the chronically ill or bedridden, as a result of lack of activity.
Treatment—Treatment varies with the cause and condition of the patient. If possible, increasing the dietary bulk, fluid intake, and amount of exercise will usually solve the problem. Prompt response to the urge to defecate is necessary. Normally, a person's body will establish a routine schedule given the opportunity. The habitual use of laxatives and enemas must be stopped. The use of bulk-forming products and glycerin suppositories can be substituted until new bowel habits are learned.

PEDIATRIC PERSPECTIVE

Constipation in an infant is commonly the result of early introduction of solid foods, such as cereal, or a switch from breast milk to formula. A history of fussiness, colic, or excessive gas is frequently described in addition to usual symptoms of difficulty and decreased frequency in passing stool. A second common time for constipation to occur is with toilet training because of the pressure the parent or caregiver places on the child to defecate or urinate in the toilet.

Treatment—For infants (less than 1 year of age), adding a fruit juice, such as pear or apple, may resolve the constipation. A glycerin suppository may be needed to soften the stool to reduce the discomfort with defecation. Constipation in infants that does not respond to to soften the stool to reduce the discomfort with defecation. Constipation in infants that does not respond to juice or glycerin suppository needs to be thoroughly evaluated by a physician or gastrointestinal specialist. The parents of a child who is in the process of toilet training should be advised to stop the training until the child is interested in using the toilet or potty chair.

Crohn's Disease (Kron′z)

Description—This is an inflammation of any portion of the GI tract, most common in the terminal ileum. The inflammation involves all layers of the intestinal wall leading to edema, ulceration, narrowing, and the formation of abscesses and fistulas.
Signs and symptoms—Symptoms vary according to the location of the disease. An acute episode often causes appendicitis-type complaints of pain, cramping, and tenderness in the right lower quadrant with flatulence, nausea, fever, and diarrhea. Bloody stools are also possible. Chronic disease is characterized by diarrhea of four to six stools daily, marked weight loss, weakness, and difficulty in coping with everyday stress.

Etiology—The exact cause of **Crohn's disease** is unknown. Some feel it is caused by allergies or immune disorders, obstruction of the lymphatics, or infection.

Diagnosis is made after positive blood tests show increased white blood cells, decreased hemoglobin, and other specific abnormalities. Barium enema studies showing segments of stricture separated by normal bowel, known as *string signs,* supports the diagnosis. Sigmoidoscopy, which reveals patchy areas of inflammation, helps to differentiate Crohn's disease from ulcerative colitis.

Treatment—Treatment is mainly symptomatic and may include dietary supplements, steroids to reduce the inflammation, and the use of antibacterial agents. Most important are changes in lifestyle to obtain more rest and dietary adjustments to eliminate contributing agents. The ingestion of fruits and vegetables must be restricted with intestinal stenosis (narrowing). Surgery may be necessary if certain conditions develop, such as a fistula, bowel perforation, hemorrhage, or obstruction. With extensive disease of the colon, a colectomy with **ileostomy** may be required (see Ileostomy).

Diarrhea (Di-a-re'-a)

Description—This is a condition of repeated passage of unformed wastes.

Signs and symptoms—It is characterized by frequent, liquid stools, which can be very serious in infants and small children because of the excessive loss of body fluid.

Etiology—Diarrhea can be caused by a bacterial, viral, or amebic organism. It can also result from a poor diet, toxic substances, foods such as prunes that stimulate peristalsis, or an irritated colon. Basically, diarrhea occurs because the chyme is moved too rapidly through the colon without sufficient time for the water to be absorbed. When the lining is inflamed, as with colitis, rapid peristalsis occurs as soon as material reaches the affected area. In addition, the lining secretes excess mucus to counteract the irritating material. This response results in a liquid stool with shreds of mucus. Diarrhea can also result from nervousness or anxiety. Again, the peristaltic action is stimulated and the waves move rapidly.

Treatment—Diarrhea is best treated by providing an adequate intake of liquids and taking care of the underlying cause. Medication to slow down peristalsis is helpful, but it will not treat the underlying cause.

Diverticulosis (Diver-tiku-lo'sis)

Description—This is the presence of bulging pouches in the wall of the GI tract where the lining has pushed into the surrounding muscle. The sigmoid colon is the most common site, but diverticuli can occur anywhere from the esophagus to the anus.

Signs and symptoms—Symptoms of diverticulitis (an infected diverticula) include irregular bowel movements, lower left abdominal pain, nausea, flatus, low-grade fever, and an increase in WBCs. Chronic diverticulitis may result in fibrosis and adhesions (tissues growing together) that severely limit or obstruct the lumen. Symptoms progress from constipation to ribbon-like stools, diarrhea, distention (swelling up) of the abdomen, nausea, vomiting, pain, and abdominal rigidity.

Etiology—They are believed to be caused by a high degree of internal pressure and an area of weakness in the intestinal wall. There is a theory that lack of roughage in the diet permits the bowel lumen (opening) to narrow, resulting in higher pressure developing during defecation. The disease is much less common in nations where more natural food and fiber are eaten.

Diverticulitis develops when undigested food mixes with the bacteria normal to the tract and collects in a diverticular sac, forming a hard mass. The mass shuts off the blood supply to the thin-walled sac, followed by inflammation, infection, possibly perforation (a hole), abscess, or hemorrhage.

Treatment—Treatment initially consists of preventing constipation and combating infection. A liquid diet, antibiotics, one medication to soften the stool, and another medication to relieve pain and relax muscle spasms are called for. When conservative measures fail, the affected colon section may need to be removed.

Esophageal Varices (E-sofa-je'al Var'i-sez)

Description—Dilated, tortuous veins in the lower section of the esophagus are called esophageal **varices**.

Signs and symptoms—This results in fluid entering the abdominal cavity, causing ascites. With the veins dilated and therefore thinner and the number of platelets reduced, hemorrhage occurs readily and is often the first sign of the condition. Often massive hemorrhage occurs, producing bloody emesis and stools.

Etiology—They are the result of hypertension within the portal vein. The blood flowing through the portal system in the liver meets with resistance because of cirrhosis, a tumor, thrombosis, or occlusion of the veins. As a result, blood backs up to the spleen, causing it to enlarge, and the blood flows through other veins. The number of platelets decreases, and the other veins dilate.

Treatment—Treatment is limited. To control bleeding, a tube may be inserted into the esophagus to put pressure against the bleeding site. In addition, iced salt water may be instilled into the tube. A drug may be given to control bleeding temporarily. Surgical bypass procedures to correct venous flow may cause from 25% to 50% mortality, and the patient may still die eventually from liver complications instead of hemorrhage. Blood transfusions are also temporary measures. At best, the patient can be kept comfortable until the inevitable massive hemorrhage or coma from liver damage occurs.

Fissure of the Anus (Fish′ur)

Description—An anal **fissure** is a crack or tear in the lining of the anus (see Figure 11-170).

Signs and symptoms—Symptoms of acute fissure are a burning pain and a few drops of blood on the toilet tissue or underwear. The fissure may develop a swelling at the lower end known as a *sentinel pile*. This protrusion may ulcerate, resulting in painful anal sphincter spasms.

A fissure may heal completely or become chronic as a result of partial healing and retearing. Later, scar tissue develops in the area, narrowing the passageway. Because the anus must stretch each time stool is passed, healing is difficult.

Etiology—It is usually the result of passing large, hard stools that stretch the lining beyond its capacity.

Treatment—Treatment consists of digital dilation to prevent stricture, a low-residue diet, stool softeners, adequate liquid intake, hot sitz baths, and a local medication for pain. A chronic condition will require surgical excision of the scar tissue, providing two fresh surfaces that can heal by a gradual regrowth of tissue. Fissures can be prevented by drinking plenty of fluids (eight glasses of water a day), eating a proper diet, and passing stool promptly when indicated.

Gastroenteritis (Gastro-en-ter-i′tis)

Description—This is an inflammation of the stomach and intestines. The term may be applied to such conditions as intestinal flu, traveler's diarrhea, and food poisoning. The inflammation usually subsides within a couple of days and poses no threat to persons in good general health. However, people who are very young, elderly, and generally debilitated are at risk because of the loss of intracellular fluid.

Signs and symptoms—Gastroenteritis is characterized by fever, nausea, abdominal cramping, diarrhea, and vomiting. Other possible symptoms include fever; malaise; and a gurgling, splashing sound over the intestines.

Etiology—There are many possible causes, such as bacteria (associated with food poisoning), amoebas and parasites, viruses (usually with traveler's diarrhea), ingestion of toxic plants, drug reactions (perhaps to antibiotics), and food allergies.

Treatment—It is treated with bed rest, increased fluid intake, and diet. Antibiotics and intravenous fluids to combat dehydration may be indicated for the person at risk. Medication may be needed to control vomiting and diarrhea.

Gastroesophageal Reflux Disease (GERD) (Gastro-e-sofa-jeal Re′fluks)

Description—This is a backflow of gastric and sometimes duodenal contents into the esophagus through the sphincter just above the stomach.

Signs and symptoms—The most common feature is heartburn, which becomes more severe with vigorous exercise, bending, or lying down. There may be esophageal spasms that mimic angina pain, radiating to the neck and arms. **Reflux** may be associated with hiatal hernia. If there is regurgitation of fluids, there may be pulmonary symptoms of aspiration, including nocturnal wheezing, bronchitis, asthma, morning hoarseness, and coughing.

Etiology—It is caused by a faulty lower esophageal sphincter (LES) that is supposed to prevent the backup of gastric contents by creating pressure, which closes the lower end of the esophagus. Normally, the sphincter relaxes after each swallow to allow food into the stomach. Reflux occurs when the pressure is insufficient or the pressure within the stomach exceeds that of the sphincter. Certain other factors may contribute to the condition, such as hiatal hernia, a position that increases intra-abdominal pressure, and any agent that lowers the LES pressure (such as food, alcohol, cigarettes, and certain drugs).

Treatment—Common treatment includes the use of common antacids, such as Alka-Seltzer, Maalox, Mylanta, Rolaids, Tums, and others. These work almost immediately after taken to suppress the symptoms and continue for about 3 to 4 hours. Another group of drugs, such as Pepcid AC, are called H_2-blockers. They suppress the secretion in the first place to prevent the heartburn. Their effects begin after about an hour but last for several. Perhaps the best treatment is prevention:

- Avoid or cut back on foods that trigger heartburn (alcohol, chocolate, fat, peppermint, and spearmint); these tend to relax the sphincter.
- Avoid caffeine; it stimulates gastric acid (caffeine is found in coffee; strong tea; soda pop; and medications, such as Anacin, Excedrin, and No Doz).
- Avoid carbonated drinks; which distend the stomach and increase the pressure.
- Lose weight if overweight.

- If a smoker, quit.
- Use gravity (don't lie down after eating, and raise the head of the bed on 4- to 6-inch blocks at night).

Hemorrhoids (Hem'o-royds)

Description—The anal canal and the lower portion of the rectum contain vertical folds of mucous membrane called anal and rectal columns. The veins in the mucosa of the folds frequently become dilated, resulting in internal or external **hemorrhoids**.

Signs and symptoms—Hemorrhoids may be asymptomatic but characteristically cause painless, intermittent bleeding, which occurs with the passing of stool. There may also be some itching. As they worsen and prolapse, they are still painless as long as they return to the anal canal. With continued progression, constant discomfort may result because of prolapse, which must be corrected by manual reduction. If blood becomes trapped in prolapsed hemorrhoids, it causes thrombosis, which results in sudden rectal pain and a large firm lump that can be felt.

Etiology—Hemorrhoids can result from long periods of sitting or standing, diarrhea, constipation, vomiting, coughing, hepatitis, alcoholism, loss of muscle tone, pregnancy, or anorectal infections. Any condition that increases portal pressure, such as pregnancy or hepatitis, or that leads to a trapping of blood in the veins, as when stool is being expelled, interferes with the return flow of blood. As more blood enters the veins, it causes dilation, and the veins bulge into the anal canal or protrude to the outside, resulting in hemorrhoids. With protrusion comes the possibility of developing a thrombosis. The blood may become trapped externally, forming a painful, hard lump. Once this occurs, it will probably need to be incised to remove the clotted blood.

Treatment—Treatment of mild to moderate hemorrhoids involves regulating bowel habits; limiting sitting time on the toilet; increasing intake of water, raw vegetables, fruits, and fiber; and applying local heat. When swelling and discomfort persist with pain and bleeding on defecation, additional treatment is indicated. A sclerosis agent can be injected into internal hemorrhoids, which causes scar tissue to develop, thus reducing the dilation. More severe involvement requires surgical removal of the dilated vein and the surrounding stretched mucosa in a procedure called a **hemorrhoidectomy**.

Hepatitis (Hepa-ti'tis)

Description—**Hepatitis** is an inflammation and infection of the liver that can result in cell destruction and death. It is caused by a virus that has been identified in several different forms. Hepatitis B, serum hepati-

tis, was the first to be identified over 20 years ago. It is very contagious with a relatively high mortality rate. A vaccine was developed to control its spread. Next hepatitis A, infectious hepatitis, was identified. Type A is also highly contagious but seems to be self-limiting and rather benign. A vaccine also exists for type A hepatitis. After 15 years, a type C (HCV) was identified. It is the most worrisome form. It usually has a silent beginning but develops into a chronic form that causes the liver to scar.

Recently, other strains have been identified. Because they do not meet the criteria for A, B, or C, they have been called D and E. D is like A but not highly prevalent in this country. E is like B. The latest strain, G, appears to be related to C and has been recently added to the family of viruses. There is no F; however, scientists do not believe this is the end of their discoveries.

Etiology—Type A is usually transmitted by the fecal-oral route, meaning organisms from sewage, human, or animal wastes get into the food chain. It is usually transmitted through ingestion of food, water, or milk that has been contaminated, and from seafood taken from contaminated water. Type B is usually transmitted parenterally (other than by mouth). Health care workers are especially prone to it because of contact with human secretions and feces. Universal precautions are indicated when caring for all patients to prevent acquiring or spreading the disease. Like AIDS, hepatitis B can also be acquired through sexual intercourse and contaminated needles, including ear piercing and tattooing. It can be passed from mother to newborn during delivery. But it can be spread by more casual contact through cuts in the skin and in saliva.

In most patients, involved cells will repair themselves, leaving little damage, and in the case of type A hepatitis only, confering a lifelong immunity. When other disorders are present, such as congestive heart failure, diabetes, severe anemia, cancer, and advanced age, complications are more likely and the prognosis is poor.

Type C hepatitis is acquired through blood and body fluids. It seldom causes illness when contracted, but about 75% of those afflicted develop a chronic form that goes undetected for years. Carriers never lose the virus or the ability to transmit it to others. No vaccine has been developed.

Signs and symptoms—Hepatitis produces a variety of symptoms, which appear suddenly with type A; type B symptoms are insidious. Clinical features of stage one include fatigue, malaise, headache, anorexia (lack of appetite), sensitivity to light, sore throat, cough, nausea, vomiting, frequently a fever of 100° to 101°F (37° to 38°C), and possibly liver and lymph node enlargement. These symptoms occur during the preicteric (before jaundice) stage and disappear when jaundice begins. About 6% to 10% of adults and 25% to 50% of children become chronic carriers. These individuals are infectious and can develop potentially fatal complications because of liver degeneration and cancer.

The second, icteric, stage has begun once the urine becomes dark, the stool is clay-colored, the sclera and skin is yellow, and a mild weight loss has occurred. The liver remains enlarged and tender, and the spleen and cervical nodes swell. The jaundice may continue for 1 to 2 weeks. Then, liver enlargement subsides, but the fatigue, flatulence (intestinal gas), abdominal tenderness, and indigestion continue. The third stage, posticteric, usually lasts for 2 to 6 weeks. Full recovery requires 6 months.

Complications may develop, leading to a chronic hepatitis, which occurs in benign or active forms. The active form, known as chronic aggressive hepatitis, has about a 25% fatality rate because of liver failure from cell destruction.

Hepatitis C may be acquired completely without symptoms. Some people, however, do experience nausea, vomiting, fever, and jaundice for a few days, but all symptoms disappear after a couple of days of bed rest. These people are fortunate, because early diagnosis may be made. Diagnosis is made based on history that reveals recent exposure to drugs, chemicals, a jaundiced person, or a blood transfusion and the presence of typical symptoms. Blood tests revealing hepatitis B antigens and the presence of B antibodies confirm type B hepatitis. Antigens are present only in the early phase of the disease, so a false negative result may occur if the blood is drawn too late.

Presence of the antibody (anti-HAV) indicates type A hepatitis. If these antigens and antibodies are absent but the patient still exhibits appropriate symptoms, then type C hepatitis is expected. There is a test to identify antibodies for HCV (type C). People testing positive should be treated before the disease progresses.

HCV can lay dormant for decades before symptoms appear. By then it may have destroyed the liver. It is a silent, deadly virus that infects an estimated four million Americans with 150,000 to 170,000 new cases diagnosed each year. Annually about 10,000 people die, and the number is expected to triple by 2010. One third of all liver transplants in the United States in 1994 were done because of this virus. The new organ will become infected but will not necessarily be seriously damaged. There is no vaccine, and only 10% to 25% become inactive with medical therapy. The carriers never lose the virus or the ability to transmit it to others. Most people discover they are infected when they undergo routine lab tests or when they donate blood. Fortunately, HCV is not highly infectious. Infection is possible from shared manicure tools, toothbrushes, and razors—things that can hold blood. The largest infected group is IV drug users. Sexual activity does not seem to be a very efficient means of transmission, although it increases with the number of partners. Hepatitis G is transmitted through blood but is very rare at this time. Currently, little is known about the strain.

Prevention—Vaccines have been developed to prevent hepatitis A and B and are recommended for the following groups of people:

- IV drug users
- Health workers
- Individuals living with an infected person
- Sexually active homosexuals
- Heterosexuals with multiple partners
- Recipients of certain blood products
- Children born to immigrants from regions where hepatitis B is common, such as Southeast Asia
- Infants born to infected women (Up to 90% of children born to infected mothers become infected and suffer a high death rate.)
- Travelers spending more than 6 months in an area with high incidence

The main problem with the vaccine is it requires three shots over a 6-month period and is relatively expensive in the United States. Many of the targeted groups of people, except for health care workers and infected mothers, are difficult to reach. It is interesting to note several developing countries are immunizing newborns and others at a cost of about $1.

Treatment—There is no cure for hepatitis B; however, there are now many drug treatments such as interferon, lamivudine, and adefovir. Patients are expected to rest and eat small meals with high calorie and protein content. Medication to help relieve nausea and vomiting may be necessary. An effort is made to determine the source of infection or contagion. Hepatitis is one of several contagious diseases that are to be reported to the local public health department.

Health care workers should protect themselves from suspected or confirmed disease by wearing gloves to handle body secretions or draw blood. Hospitalized patients are isolated, with strict techniques used to prevent the spread of the disease.

Treatment of patients with HCV who develop progressive liver scarring usually require powerful drug treatments. Two antiviral agents are the only approved drug therapies of the disease. These are interferon alpha-2b and ribavirin. Interferon is one of the body's lymphokines. It helps boost the immune system and attack viruses. Ribavirin works by blocking the virus's ability to multiply. When they are used together, the drugs can destroy the virus to undetectable levels in about 40% of patients. However, severe side effects of nausea, fatigue, seizures, and even heart or kidney failure make this option suitable only as a life-saving measure. The virus often comes back after treatment is discontinued. A vaccine is in the process of being developed but is not yet available.

Hernia (Hiatus) (Her'ne-a Hi-a'tus)

Description—The protrusion of an internal organ through a natural opening in the body wall is known as a hernia or rupture. One form of hernia involves a defect in the diaphragm that allows a portion of the stomach to move up into the chest cavity through the opening for the esophagus. It is called a **hiatus** or hiatal **hernia**. There are three types of hiatal hernias: sliding, which is most common; rolling or paraesophageal (alongside the esophagus); and mixed, which is a combination of both. This condition is found in up to 50% of the population over 50 years old. If no symptoms occur, no treatment is required.

In all forms of hiatal hernia, some portion of the stomach, the end of the esophagus, or both slip(s) through the diaphragmatic opening (Figure 11-173).

Signs and symptoms—In paraesophageal, a portion of the stomach "rolls" through the opening into the chest but causes few symptoms except a feeling of fullness in the chest and angina-like pain. This type of hernia needs surgical repair. A sliding hernia may cause symptoms, such as heartburn from 1 to 4 hours after eating (which is often aggravated by reclining and occasionally results in regurgitation or vomiting), chest pain (caused by the reflux [return] of gastric

juices), distention and spasms of the stomach, difficulty swallowing (caused by inflammation of the esophagus), or an ulcer. The most serious symptoms are severe pain and shock, which result from incarceration when a large portion of the stomach is trapped above the diaphragm, cutting off circulation to that part of the organ. Because strangulation leads to tissue death, immediate surgery is indicated.

Etiology—It is caused by a portion of the stomach or part of the esophagus protruding up through the diaphragm.

Treatment—Conservative treatment for uncomplicated hiatal hernia involves medication to strengthen the esophageal sphincter muscle; using gravity to decrease the reflux of gastric juices; and a diet of small, frequent, bland meals. Other helpful measures include waiting at least 2 hours after eating to lie down; eating slowly; and avoiding spicy foods, fruit juices, alcohol, and coffee. Smoking is discouraged because it stimulates the production of gastric acid.

Hernia (Inguinal) (Her'ne-a In'gwi-nal)

Description—The wall of the abdominal cavity has normal openings through which blood vessels or other body structures pass. For example, the male's spermatic cords pass through the inguinal rings of the lower abdominal wall to reach the testes, which are external to the body. When a portion of an organ protrudes through an opening, it is known as a hernia.

Signs and symptoms—Diagnosis of a smaller hernia can be made on manual examination of the inguinal ring while the patient is asked to cough. If the examiner feels something touch the examining finger, the patient has a hernia.

Etiology—When the surrounding structure of fibrous tissue, the fascia, becomes weak, it allows a loop of small intestine to protrude through the ring, following the path of the spermatic cord. This type of hernia is called an inguinal hernia, and it often extends into the scrotum when the patient stands.

Treatment—A protruding hernia is visible and can usually be reduced or pushed back into place. Some patients may wear a device called a truss, which exerts pressure directly over the herniated opening, to hold the protruding mass inside the cavity. Occasionally, the mass cannot be reduced and will remain in the hernial sac. It is then possible for additional intestine to enter the sac or the contents to become twisted or trapped, interfering with the circulation of blood to the intestine. This condition is referred to as a *strangulated hernia* and requires a surgical procedure known as **herniorrhaphy** as quickly as possible. The procedure replaces the contents of the sac within the abdominal cavity and closes the opening.

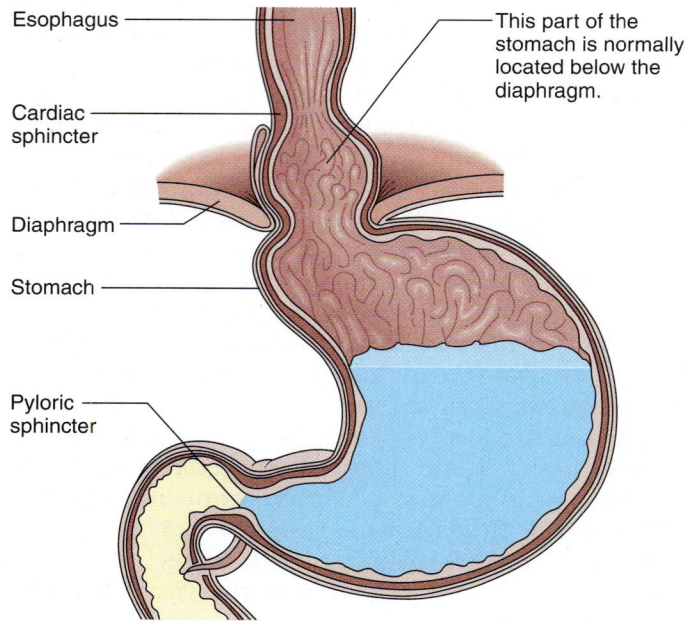

Esophagus

Cardiac sphincter

Diaphragm

Stomach

Pyloric sphincter

This part of the stomach is normally located below the diaphragm.

FIGURE 11-173   Hiatal hernia

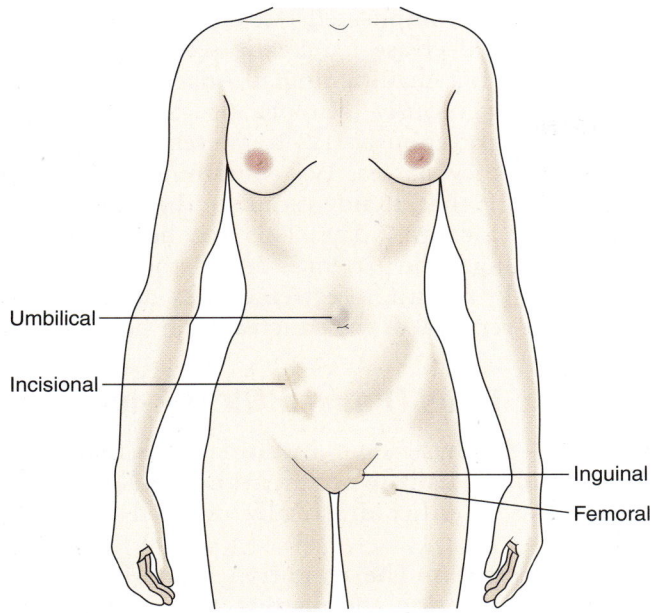

Umbilical

Incisional

Inguinal

Femoral

FIGURE 11-174　Common sites of hernias

Hernias can be the result of weak abdominal muscles caused by a congenital condition or the natural process of aging. Hernias can also develop from increased abdominal pressure caused by heavy lifting, pregnancy, obesity, or straining.

Other types of hernias are femoral, which occurs where the femoral artery exits the abdomen to the legs; umbilical, involving the structure around the umbilicus; and incisional, in an area of previous surgery (Figure 11-174).

Ileostomy (Il′e-os′to-me)

Description—This surgical opening of the ileum allows the chyme of the small intestine to empty through the abdominal wall. This is not a disease but rather a solution to a disease process. An ileostomy is similar to a colostomy except that the chyme is liquid and highly caustic to the skin because of the digestive juices. The patient with an ileostomy has no control over its function and must wear an ostomy appliance (collection bag) attached to a donut-like disk that perfectly surrounds the stoma (mouth or opening). A protective adhesive creates a watertight seal. A belt attached to the disk supports the device. A permanent type of bag may be attached, which must be emptied and cleaned periodically. Disposable plastic bags can also be used. Some disposable types incorporate a deodorizing material; the permanent type requires instillation of a deodorizer.

Etiology—The patient with an ileostomy must accept a great alteration in body image and function. The passing of flatus and the gurgling of liquid stool be-

ing expelled occurs without warning and cannot be controlled. Most patients who have had ileostomy surgery feel better off than before surgery. Many had extensive ulcerative colitis with much pain; bleeding; and excessive, sudden, and frequent diarrhea and were in poor physical condition from the debilitating effects of the disease. The removal of the diseased colon necessitates the ileostomy. Other patients may have been affected by Crohn's disease, which causes inflammation, scarring, and near or complete obstruction of the bowel. These patients experienced pain, nausea, fever, cramping, bleeding, and diarrhea occurring four to six times a day. The freedom from pain and relative increase in control over excretion are often considered to make an ileostomy worthwhile. Many times, these patients have been nearly confined to their homes because of their weakness and the characteristics of the disease. With an ileostomy they can regain fairly good health and live a nearly normal life.

Irritable Bowel Syndrome

Description—This is a common condition marked by chronic or periodic diarrhea and alternating constipation. Irritable **bowel** syndrome is also called spastic colon.

Signs and symptoms—The syndrome is characterized by lower abdominal pain that is relieved by passing flatus or defecation and diarrhea during the day. Stools are often small and contain mucus. There may be abdominal distention and digestion difficulties.

Etiology—It is generally associated with psychologic stress, but it may result from physical factors, such as ingestion of irritants (coffee, raw fruits and vegetables), an abuse of laxatives, food poisoning, a lactose intolerance, diverticular disease, or colon cancer.

Treatment—Treatment is aimed at relieving symptoms and teaching the patient to deal with stress. Elimination of known food irritants, rest, and heat to the abdomen are helpful. The use of sedatives and antispasmodics are recommended for a limited time.

Oral Cancer

Description—The mouth should be examined for oral cancer every time a visit is made to a dentist for routine cleaning and examination. It should also be inspected by the physician as part of a physical examination. People who do not visit a dentist or physician frequently should observe their own mouths for oral cancer.

Signs and symptoms

- Swelling, lump, or growth anywhere in or around the mouth
- White scaly patches inside the mouth

- Any size sore that does not heal
- Numbness or pain anywhere in the mouth area
- Repeated bleeding in the mouth without cause
  Any of these signals should be examined by a physician or dentist.

Etiology—Oral cancer strikes about 30,300 per year, with about 8,000 dying. About 90% of the cancers are squamous cell that develop in the tissue lining or covering of the mouth, lip, tongue, and throat. The single greatest risk factor is the use of tobacco, in the form of cigarettes, cigars, pipe, or chewing tobacco. The use of snuff is clearly linked with cancer of the cheek, tongue, and mouth structures. Abuse of alcohol is also a risk factor. Heavy drinkers who also smoke a pack of cigarettes per day have 24 times the amount of oral cancer risk. Overexposure to the sun is a factor in lip cancer.

Treatment—Oral cancer is usually treated with surgery or radiation or both. With advanced disease, chemotherapy in combination with surgery or radiation is being used. The choice of treatment depends upon the tumor size and location and the patient's willingness to undergo the side effects. Expected survival of 5 years is only 51%.

Oral cancer can result in a disabling and disfiguring condition when areas are excised. If the tongue is involved, speech and the process of eating become difficult.

Pancreatitis (Pankre-a-ti′tis)

Description—This is inflammation of the pancreas, which occurs in both acute and chronic forms. **Pancreatitis** progresses in an unusual manner. The enzymes normally produced and excreted into the pancreatic duct remain and digest the pancreatic tissue. If the cells that produce insulin are destroyed, the condition will be complicated by diabetes.

Signs and symptoms—Mild pancreatitis is characterized by epigastric pain not relieved by vomiting. A severe attack causes extreme pain, persistent vomiting, a rigid abdomen, and rales (noisy, ausculated breath sounds) at the lung bases with pleural fluid on the left side. Tachycardia may occur, as may a fever of from 100° to 102°F (38° to 39°C) with cold, perspiring extremities. Rapidly progressing pancreatitis can cause massive hemorrhage, which results in shock and coma. Mortality is as high as 60% when there is tissue destruction and hemorrhage.

Etiology—The most frequent predisposing factors are alcoholism, trauma to the pancreas, reaction to certain medications, and pancreatic carcinoma. It may also develop as the result of a duodenal ulcer.

Treatment—The complicated treatment consists of methods to decrease pancreatic secretions and relieve pain while maintaining adequate fluids. Shock is treated vigorously by replacing electrolytes and proteins intravenously (IV) to prevent death. After the emergency passes, IVs containing electrolytes and proteins that do not stimulate the pancreas are continued for 5 to 7 days. This may be followed by tubal feeding if the patient is unable to take enough nutrients by mouth. In extreme cases, a pancreatectomy, the removal of the pancreas, may be indicated.

Paralytic Ileus (Para-li′tik Il′e-us)

Description—A physiologic intestinal obstruction, a **paralytic ileus** usually occurs in the small intestine. Peristalsis is either drastically reduced or totally absent.

Signs and symptoms—The condition causes severe abdominal distention and distress, frequently accompanied by vomiting.

Etiology—It is often precipitated by manipulation of the bowel during abdominal surgery or the paralyzing effects of the anesthesia. The ileus usually disappears after 2 to 3 days.

Treatment—If it continues for more than 48 hours, it may be necessary to insert a weighted tube into the small intestine to remove the accumulated fluids and gas. Medication to stimulate colon action may be given.

Peptic Ulcer (Pep′tik Ul′ser)

Description—This is an encircled lesion in the mucous membrane lining of the stomach, lower esophagus, duodenum, or jejunum.

Signs and symptoms—*Duodenal* peptic ulcers cause heartburn, epigastric pain that is relieved by food, a weight gain (caused by extra eating), and a strange feeling of bubbling hot water in the back of the pharynx. Attacks occur whenever the stomach is empty or after drinking alcohol, juice, or coffee. *Gastric* ulcers usually cause heartburn and indigestion, pain in the left epigastrium, and a feeling of fullness. There may be weight loss and repeated episodes of serious GI bleeding. Gastric ulcers tend to cause discomfort after eating because the stomach lining is "stretched," causing pain from the lesion in the membrane lining. Either type of ulcer may develop complications, such as perforation, hemorrhage, and pyloric obstruction.

Etiology—For years, physicians thought ulcers were caused by the overproduction of gastric juices from emotional stimulation. In 1982, an Australian physician drank a concoction with millions of bacteria to prove his theory that ulcers were caused by an organism. A few days later he developed an inflamed stomach lining—the beginnings of an ulcer—and proved that even though the stomach is full of acid, the *Helicobacter pylori* (*H. pylori*) bacteria could survive. The organism itself does not cause the ulcer, but the burrowing of the corkscrew bacteria into the membranes weakens the linings, allowing the stomach acid and the digestive enzymes to create an ulcer. Not everyone who has the organism develops an ulcer, and not every ulcer is the result of the bacteria. However, at least 80% of gastric and 95% of duodenal ulcers are associated with the bacteria, and the remainder are often caused by nonsteroidal anti-inflammatory drugs. Other contributing factors are smoking, drinking alcohol, aspirin taken over long periods, and a hereditary tendency.

Treatment—With the new discovery came a new treatment. If there is bacteria and the existence of an ulcer is confirmed with endoscopy, the infection can be permanently cured with drug therapy involving two antibiotics and a bismuth preparation, such as Pepto-Bismol. Most physicians also add a blocker to relieve symptoms and hasten the healing. A new blood test for *H. pylori* antibodies is probably adequate for people with confirmed ulcer history. Newly diagnosed patients with mild to moderate symptoms may be placed on a couple of months of treatment with newer acid-suppressing drugs and blockers. They will usually heal, and one in three sufferers will not have a recurrence. If the ulcer returns, they are then treated with the antibiotic therapy.

Polyp (Pol'ip)

Description—This is a mass of tissue that results from an overgrowth of upper epithelial cells of the mucosal membrane of the GI tract. There are five varieties, some hereditary, others of common adenoma structure. Most are benign, but **villous adenoma** and hereditary polyps show a tendency to become malignant. Most types develop in adults over 45 years old. Predisposing factors are age, heredity, diet, and infection.

Signs and symptoms—Polyps are difficult to diagnose because they are almost always asymptomatic. They are usually discovered accidentally during a rectosigmoidoscopy or lower GI series x-ray. The most common symptom is rectal bleeding. The structure of the polyps varies from small lesions covering the surface of the rectum or sigmoid to large lesions attached by long, thin stalks. The type of polyp determines its physical characteristics.

Etiology—Overgrowth of epithelial cells.

Treatment—Treatment consists of surgical removal often by electrocautery, especially if benign and pedunculated (on a stalk). If they are villous adenomas, which are invasive and therefore malignant, treatment usually involves abdominoperineal resection (removal of the colon and rectum, including the area around the anus), with a resulting permanent ileostomy. Each type of polyp is dealt with in relation to its current state or its tendency to become malignant.

Pruritus Ani (Proo-ri'tis A'ni)

Description—This is itching of the area surrounding the anus, often associated with irritation and burning.

Signs and symptoms—Classic symptoms are itching after a bowel movement or at night. Scratching can cause reddened, weeping skin or thickened, leathery, darker tissue.

Etiology—The main contributing factors for **pruritus ani** are harsh, vigorous rubbing with soap and a washcloth; poor hygiene; spicy foods; anal skin tags (small pieces of suspended extra skin); excessive perspiration; a systemic disease, such as diabetes; the use of perfumed or colored toilet paper; coffee, alcohol, or food preservatives; a fungus or parasitic infection; an anorectal disease, such as fissure, fistula, or hemorrhoids; and certain skin cancers.

Treatment—Treatment consists of removing the underlying cause, such as a rectal tag, and eliminating irritants to the skin, such as soaps, powders, and colored tissue. The area should be kept clean and dry. Witch hazel applied on wiping pads or cotton balls is soothing. Steroid creams aid in reducing inflammation and controlling itching.

Pyloric Stenosis (Pi-lor'ik Ste-no'sis)

Description—This is a narrowing of the pyloric sphincter, which interferes with the emptying of the stomach. The sphincter is enlarged and often cartilagenous, causing a narrowing of the opening, which results in the dilation of the stomach.

Signs and symptoms—Adults will experience symptoms when there is a delayed action of the stomach to empty its contents, which causes distention. Because of the thickening of the pylorus and the backup of contents, the most common symptom is projectile or forceful vomiting.

Etiology—**Stenosis** can be caused by scar tissue developed during healing of a gastric ulcer.

Treatment—In adult stenosis, the patient may be able to alter the diet and use medication for some time; however, surgical correction will probably be required eventually.

Symptoms of pyloric stenosis usually begin before 4 weeks of age and are considered to be congenital. There is forceful vomiting that may lead to serious dehydration. This condition occurs almost exclusively in infant boys. If vomiting is not too intense, the condition will be observed and may self-correct in time. Otherwise, surgical intervention to open the pyloric sphincter muscle is performed to correct the problem.

Ulcerative Colitis (Ulser-a-tiv Ko-li'tis)

Description—An inflammatory disease, often chronic, that affects the mucosa of the colon. It usually begins in the sigmoid and rectum, extending upward to involve the whole colon. The small intestine is not involved. The disease produces congestion followed by edema, which makes the mucosa fragile. As the lining breaks down, ulcers are formed, which eventually develop into abscesses. The disease can be confined to one area and be known as segmented colitis, or it can spread throughout the colon. Severe colitis may cause a perforation of the colon, which can result in a life-threatening infection called peritonitis and in toxemia (blood poisoning).

Ulcerative colitis primarily affects young adults, mostly female.

Signs and symptoms—The prime symptom of ulcerative colitis is recurrent bloody diarrhea, often containing exudate and mucus. The frequency and intensity will vary with the extent of the disease. Other symptoms include weight loss, weakness, anorexia, nausea, vomiting, irritability, and abdominal pain. The disease leads to other complicating conditions, such as anemia; coagulation defects; liver damage; arthritis; loss of muscle mass; hemorrhoids from frequent stools; and stricture resulting from no solid stool, perforated colon, and toxemia.

Etiology—Predisposing factors are a family history of colitis, a bacterial infection, overproduction of enzymes that damage the mucous membrane, emotional stress, an autoimmune reaction, and allergic reactions to some foods.

Treatment—Treatment consists of controlling inflammation, maintaining nutrition and blood volume, and preventing complications. Patients are usually placed on bed rest, IV fluid replacement, and a clear liquid diet. Drug therapy is used to control the inflammatory process and combat infection. Severe involvement may necessitate antispasmotics and pain medication to relieve the cramping and discomfort. If the patient fails to respond to medical treatment and the symptoms become intolerable, surgical resection (removal) of the colon is indicated, with a colostomy or ileostomy as previously described. Pa-

tients who develop colitis before age 15 and in whom the condition persists for at least 10 years are especially prone to colorectal cancer.

ACHIEVE UNIT OBJECTIVES

- ☐ **Complete the Workbook activities to meet the learning objectives.**
- ☐ **Apply your knowledge at the end of this chapter in completing the Critical Thinking Challenge and Activities, as well as the StudyWARE on your Student CD-ROM.**

UNIT 11
THE URINARY SYSTEM

OBJECTIVES

Upon completion of this unit, you will be able to achieve the following:

LEARNING Objectives

1. **Spell and define, using the glossary at the back of the text, all the Words to Know in this unit.**
2. **Explain the three main functions of the urinary system.**
3. **Identify the organs of the urinary system, and describe their physical characteristics.**
4. **Explain how the urinary system functions with other systems.**
5. **Describe the interior structure of the kidney.**
6. **Name the parts of a nephron, and explain how each part functions.**
7. **Describe the process of dialysis, and name two types.**
8. **Explain the likelihood of success with a kidney transplant.**
9. **List the two main categories of diagnostic examination, and give examples, explaining briefly how each test is performed and for what purpose.**
10. **Describe 10 diseases or disorders of the urinary system.**

WORDS TO KNOW

acute glomerulo-
   nephritis (AGN)
acute renal
   failure
anuria
bladder
Bowman's
   capsule
calculi
calyces
calyx
catheterization
chronic glomeru-
   lonephritis
chronic renal
   failure
cortex
cystitis
dialysis
dribbling
dysuria
elimination

excretion
fistula
frequency
glomerulus
graft
hematuria
hemodialysis
hesitancy
hilum
intravenous
   pyelography
   (IVP)
invasive
   procedure
kidney
lithotripsy
medulla
nephron
nephrotic
   syndrome
nocturia
noninvasive
   procedure

oliguria
peritoneal
polycystic kidney
   disease
polyuria
ptosis
pyelonephritis
renal
residual
retention
secretion
stricture
uremia
ureter
urethra
urgency
urinary
urinary
   meatus
urine
void

CERTIFICATION CONNECTION

CMA
Diagnostic procedures
Common diseases and
   pathology
Anatomy and physiology

CMAS
Anatomy and physiology

RMA
Anatomy and physiology

The **urinary** system removes nitrogenous waste products, certain salts, and excess water from the blood and eliminates them from the body. At the same time, it evaluates the body's acid-base balance and selectively reabsorbs the elements needed to maintain the proper ratio.

The urinary system performs three main functions. The first is **excretion**, the process of removing waste products and other elements from the blood. The second is **secretion**, by which **urine** is produced. The third is **elimination**, the emptying of the urine from its bladder storage.

The major work of the system is performed by two organs called the **kidneys** (Figure 11-175). The well-being of the human body depends heavily on the function of the kidneys. When waste products are not removed from the blood, they build up, producing potentially fatal toxicity. After the kidneys have performed

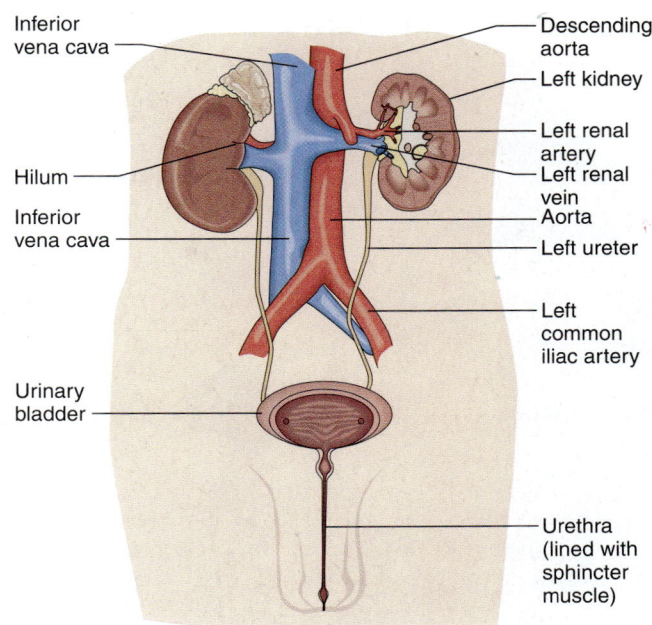

FIGURE 11-175   The urinary system

their functions, the waste material, urine, is carried through the **ureters**, one for each kidney, to temporary storage in the **bladder**. When an adequate amount has been accumulated, the bladder expels the urine through the **urethra**, eliminating it from the body.

As previously stated, no system can function by itself. The urinary system is no exception. Waste products and other substances that are filtered out of the blood must first have been ingested, digested, and absorbed by the digestive system into the circulatory system, to be delivered in the blood to the kidneys. The peristalsis of the muscular system moves the urine through the ureters. The nervous system, in cooperation with a muscular sphincter, controls elimination. The respiratory system and the urinary system cooperate to control the body's acid-base balance and the amount of fluid retained. Pulmonary action influences the amount of O_2-CO_2 exchange and the amount of fluid loss through respiration. Hormones from the endocrine system also influence the amount of urine excreted. The integumentary system works in close relationship to the urinary system to remove or retain body fluid as required. Once again, it is apparent that the body is a complex, interdependent organism.

THE KIDNEYS

The kidneys are shaped like lima or kidney beans. Each kidney is about $4\frac{1}{2}$ inches long, from 2 to 3 inches wide, and about an inch thick, and it weighs about $\frac{1}{4}$ pound. The kidneys are located on each side of the vertebral column, high up on the posterior wall of the abdominal cavity, between the muscles of the back and

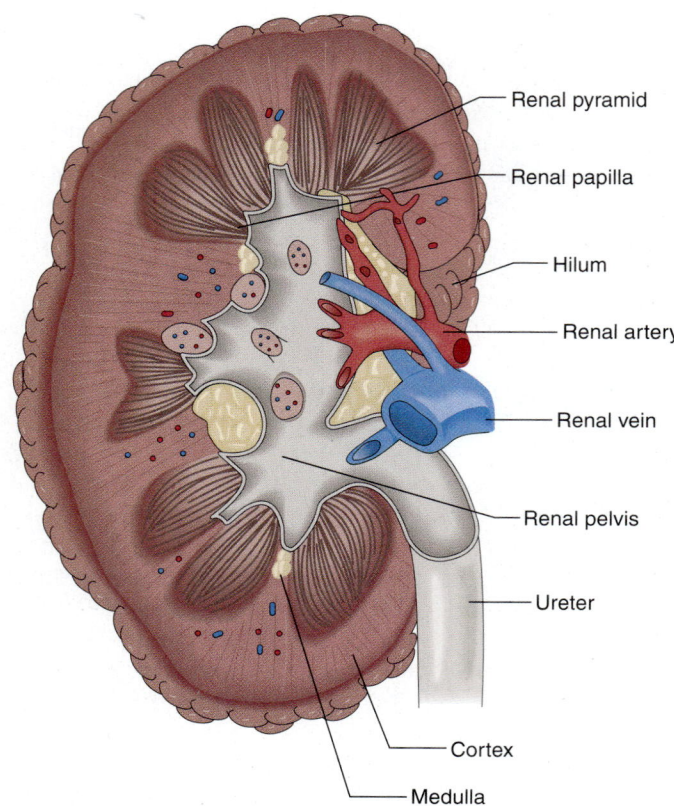

FIGURE 11-176 Internal structure of the kidney

the parietal peritoneum that covers the abdominal organs. Because they are not within the area occupied by the digestive system organs, the kidneys are said to be retroperitoneal (behind the peritoneum). The left kidney is slightly higher than the right, which is displaced by the liver. Normally, a heavy cushion of fat helps keep the kidneys in their proper position. A condition known as **ptosis** (dropping) occurs in very thin persons as a result of an inadequate fatty cushion.

Externally, the kidney is covered with a tough, fibrous capsule. The concave border has a notch called the **hilum** through which the **renal** (kidney) artery enters and the renal vein and renal pelvis of the ureter exits. Internally, the kidney is divided into two sections: an outer layer, the **cortex**, and an inner layer, the **medulla** (Figure 11-176). The medulla is divided into triangular-shaped wedges called renal pyramids with bases toward the cortex and "tops," or renal papillae, emptying into cavities called **calyces** (singular: **calyx**). The pyramids have a striated (striped) appearance; the cortex appears smooth. The cortex extends inward between the pyramids in sections called renal columns.

The Nephrons

The life-preserving service of the kidney is performed by microscopic units called **nephrons**. Each kidney has over 1 million of these units, which altogether contain

roughly 140 miles of filters and tubes. Each minute, the kidneys filter over 1,000 mL of blood, producing about 60 mL of urine per hour. In an average day, a person takes in 2,500 mL of fluid (2½ quarts) and generates another 300 mL (10 ounces) of water, which is formed by the cells in the process of combining oxygen and other materials. About 1,500 mL (1½ quarts) is eliminated as urine each day. Additional fluid is lost through feces and respiration. Some moisture is also lost through the skin, especially when perspiring. Despite the amount of liquid consumed, the kidneys maintain a constant amount of fluid in the body's tissues, excreting the excess as urine. The concentration of the urine is in direct relationship to the amount of liquid consumed.

The process by which the nephrons produce urine is complex. The nephron is a peculiarly shaped structure, resembling a funnel with a long, twisted tail (Figure 11-177). The top of the funnel is a double-walled hollow capsule called the **Bowman's capsule**. Each capsule contains a cluster of about 50 capillaries called the **glomerulus**. The Bowman's capsule and the glomerulus together are known as the renal corpuscle.

Blood enters the glomerulus by way of an afferent arteriole, flows through the glomerular capillaries, and leaves through the efferent arteriole. The efferent arteriole branches into capillaries that surround the renal tubule. The capillaries come back together in tiny veins, which join a branch of the renal vein.

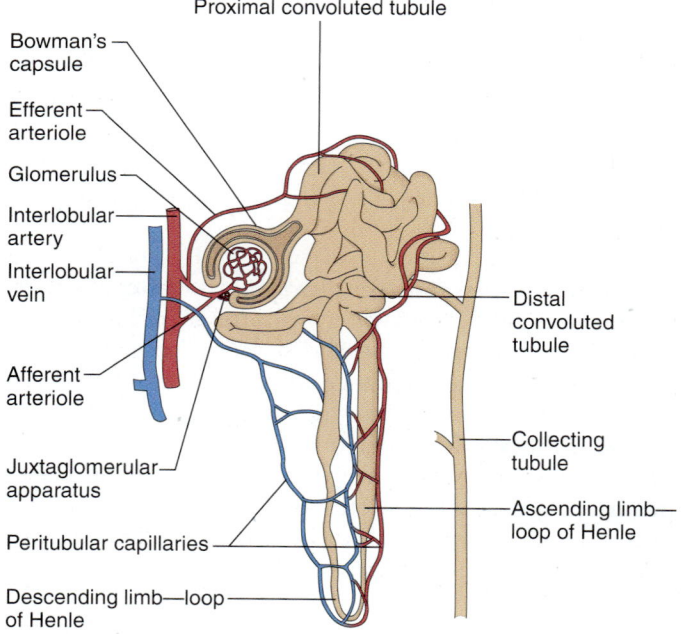

FIGURE 11-177 A nephron unit and related structures. The collecting tubules, which are not microscopic, give the pyramids of the medullary portion of the kidney a striated appearance. As shown, there are some collecting tubules in the cortical portion of the kidney as well.

Beyond the Bowman's capsule is a twisted section of tubule called the *proximal convoluted tubule*. The capsule and this section of tubule descend into the medulla and are called the *loop of Henle*. This loop has a straight descending and ascending limb, but when it returns to the cortex, it changes into another twisted section called the *distal convoluted tubule*. Several distal tubules join into a straight collecting tubule, which empties into the calyx.

Filtration and Reabsorption

Filtration is the first process in the formation of urine. Blood enters the capsule by way of the afferent arteriole, carrying waste products, water, salt, urea, and glucose. The efferent arteriole divides, forming approximately 50 glomerular capillaries. Because so many capillaries are then emptied by a single efferent arteriole, blood pressure increases significantly. This higher pressure forces the fluid to leave the blood by filtration and enter the Bowman's capsule at a rate of about 125 mL a minute. This equals a rate of 60,000 mL (60 liters, or 56.8 quarts) in an 8-hour period.

By a reabsorption process, 99% of the filtrate is returned to the bloodstream. Not only fluid but also useful substances, such as glucose, vitamins, amino acids, electrolyte salts, and bicarbonate ions (base), are reabsorbed. As the filtrate enters the proximal tubule, about 80% of the water is reabsorbed into the surrounding peritubular capillaries along with other substances the body needs to maintain a proper balance. For example, the filtrate contains glucose, which is normally completely reabsorbed. However, when levels exceed normal limits, the selective cells lining the tubules no longer reabsorb glucose but allow it to remain in the tubule to be eliminated in the urine. The term used to describe the limit of sugar reabsorption is the *threshold*. Passing this level is referred to as *spilling over the threshold*. Patients who have diabetes spill sugar frequently and therefore test its presence in their urine to determine the need for additional insulin.

A final reabsorption takes place in the distal tubule. The remaining 10% to 15% of water may be reabsorbed, depending on the body's need. The process is controlled by a hormone that acts upon the nephron.

Secretion

The secretion function of the nephron moves substances directly from the blood in the peritubular capillaries into the urine in the distal and collecting tubules. The substances secreted directly are ammonia, hydrogen ions, potassium ions, and drugs. The elements are selectively secreted to maintain the body's acid-base balance.

Urinary Output

Anything that increases the volume of blood in the capillaries increases the output of urine; conversely, the urine output decreases with a lessening of blood volume. For example, a large fluid intake increases the volume of blood and the output of urine. Hemorrhage or dehydration decreases blood volume and urine output.

Another factor regulating secretion is the amount of solutes in the filtrate. Again considering the diabetic, when there is an increase in the amount of glucose, it spills over into the urine, increasing the urine volume eliminated that day because more liquid is allowed to pass through to dilute the glucose content.

The functional capacity of the healthy kidney is so great that removal of one kidney poses no problem to the body in removing liquid wastes.

THE URETERS

The urine secreted by the nephrons drops out of the collecting tubules into the calyces, then enters the renal pelvis and continues down the ureters into the urinary bladder (Figure 11-178). The ureters begin with a widened upper portion, continuing as a long, slender, muscular tube approximately 10 to 12 inches in length. Peristaltic waves, at a rate of one to five a minute, move the urine down the ureter to enter the lower posterior wall of the bladder. Because of the solutes in urine, some persons tend to form renal **calculi** (stones). As the calculi form in the renal pelvis, they are washed into the ureter by the urine. When a stone is large enough to become lodged in the ureter, severe pain results. Frequently, removal of the stone may be required if it

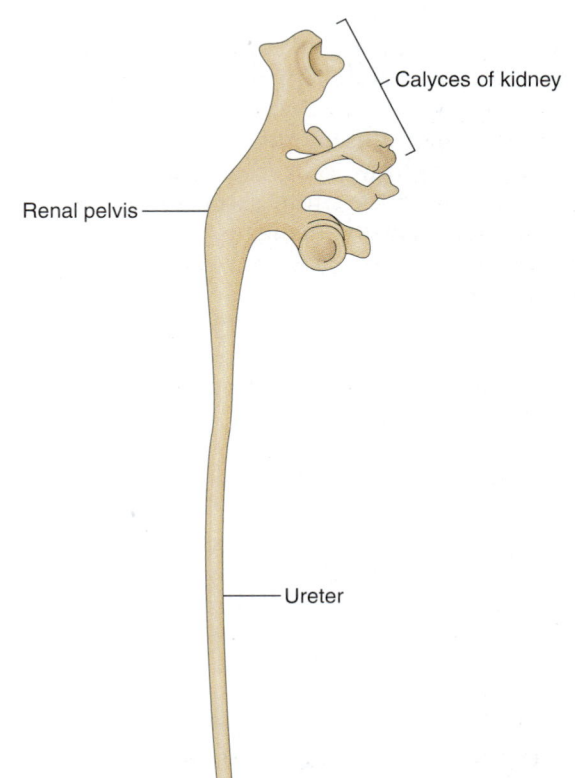

FIGURE 11-178   The ureter, renal pelvis, and calyces

cannot be passed into the bladder. (See Renal Calculi in Diseases and Disorders.)

THE URINARY BLADDER

The bladder is a collapsible bag of muscular tissue lying behind the symphysis pubis. The lining has many folds, giving it the ability to expand. The bladder serves as a reservoir for urine, collecting approximately 250 mL before the urge to **void** (urinate) is felt. The capacity of the bladder is two to three times this amount, and in instances of **retention** (inability to empty bladder) may be in excess of 1,000 mL. In such instances, urine must be removed by inserting a catheter (a tube) through the urethra into the bladder to relieve the distention and discomfort. This procedure is known as **catheterization**.

THE URETHRA

The urethra is a tube leading from the bladder to an exit from the body. In the female, it is a straight tube about 1½ inches in length. It opens externally between the clitoris and the vagina within the folds of the labia minora. The opening is called the **urinary meatus**. Only urine passes through the female urethra. In the male, the urethra is about 8 inches long, extending internally from the bladder down through the prostate gland and out through the penis to the meatus. The male urethra also serves as a passageway for semen.

A circular muscle sphincter within the urethra permits voluntary control of bladder function. This control, however, requires an intact nerve supply and motor area of the brain. Involuntary emptying of the bladder is known as *incontinence.*

Other medical terms commonly used to describe urinary output include **anuria**, an absence of urine; **dysuria**, pain or discomfort associated with voiding; **hematuria**, blood in the urine; **nocturia**, having to urinate at night; **oliguria**, a scanty urinary output; and **polyuria**, excessive urination. Descriptive words used to clarify symptoms are **dribbling**, the involuntary loss of drops of urine; **frequency**, the necessity to void often; **hesitancy**, difficulty in initiating urination; and **urgency**, the sudden need to void.

DIALYSIS

Dialysis is the mechanical process of removing waste products from the blood normally removed by the kidneys. Basically it is a process for purifying blood by passing it through thin membranes and exposing it to a solution that continually circulates around the membranes. The solution is called *dialysate.* Substances in the blood pass through the membrane into the lesser-concentrated dialysate in response to the laws of diffusion. This is called **hemodialysis**.

The term artificial kidney is often used to refer to the kidney dialysis unit. However, the part of the unit that actually substitutes for the kidney is a glass tube approximately 8 inches long and about 1½ inches in diameter. The tube, called the dialyzer, is filled with thousands of minute hollow fibers attached firmly at both ends (Figure 11-179). Blood from the patient flows through the fibers, which are surrounded by circulating dialysate. The dialysate can be individualized for each patient to provide the appropriate levels of sodium, bicarbonate, and other substances. These cross the membrane and enter the blood. At the same time, extra water and waste products leave the blood to enter the dialysate.

The patient is connected to the dialysis unit by means of needles and tubing that take blood from the patient, circulate it through the machine, and return it to the patient. New programmable dialysis management systems, as seen in Figure 11-180, can monitor blood pressure; allow variable control of solution substances; adjust temperature, flow, and filtration rate of the blood; preset the length of treatment time; and perform other functions, all automatically. (On the system pictured in Figure 11-180, the dialyzer is located just left of center; it has black ends with tubing attached to both ends.)

A **fistula** (opening between an artery and vein), or a **graft** (vein inserted between an artery and a vein) is surgically constructed in the patient to provide a site for inserting the large needles required in dialysis (Figure 11-181). The fistulas and grafts are artificial veins that can withstand repeated needle insertions. They lie just under the skin surface and require 2 to 4 weeks for a graft and 8 to 12 weeks for a fistula to completely heal before they can be used.

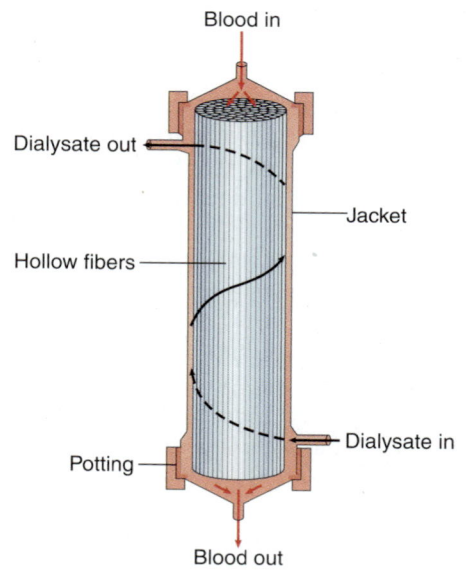

Blood in

Dialysate out

Jacket

Hollow fibers

Dialysate in

Potting

Blood out

FIGURE 11-179 Dialyzer

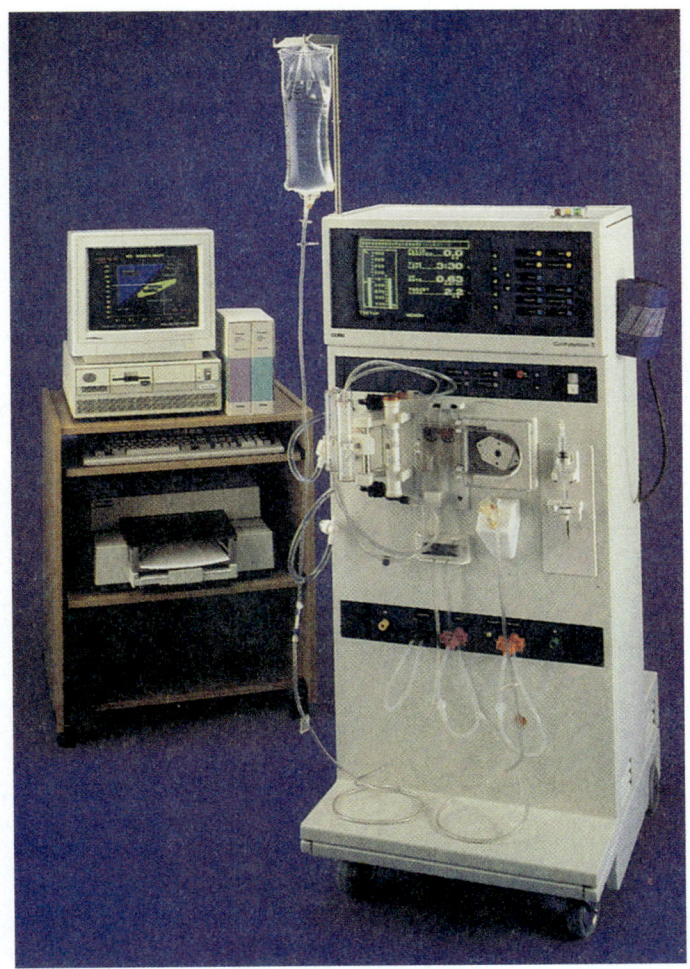

FIGURE 11-180 Hemodialysis unit

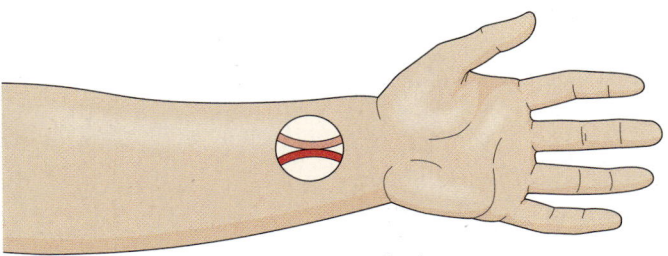

Arteriovenous fistula

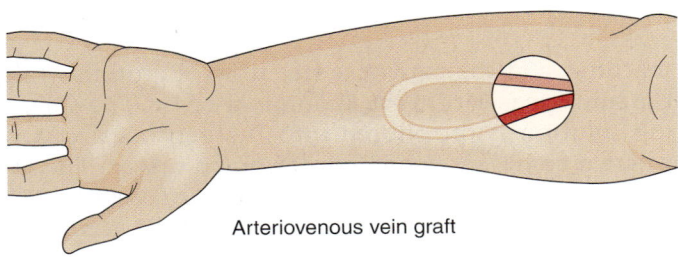

Arteriovenous vein graft

FIGURE 11-181 Hemodialysis sites

The initial site is the nondominant forearm, usually at the radial artery. When this begins to fail, sites are constructed at the brachial artery, then in the dominant arm, and finally grafts at the femoral artery in the groin area. Artificial veins last from 3 to 5 years. Some patients who have had a graft constructed from one of their own veins have had unusually successful sites for as long as 10 years, but this is not the norm. Because dialysis occurs so frequently, the multiple needle insertions not only affect the grafts or fistulas but the overlying skin as well. When too much damage has occurred, the site is no longer usable. The patient must learn to care for the site and protect it from damage. This is truly the lifeline for the patient with renal failure. Nothing, such as tight clothing or elastic cuffs, must constrict the site area. The patient is not allowed to sleep on the involved arm. Women cannot have purse straps across the forearm. Care must be taken when carrying any objects in the arms, such as grocery bags, boxes, firewood, books, and similar articles that could damage the site.

Another access to the bloodstream of patients is through a Permacath, a large double-lumen (two openings) catheter. It can be surgically inserted into either the jugular or subclavian vein to provide temporary access for hemodialysis treatments. Figures 11-182A and B illustrates the catheter insertion sites in (A) the jugular and (B) the subclavian veins. The tubing from the hemodiaysis machine connects with the openings of catheter. The blood exits from the proximal opening on the catheter and goes to the machine for filtering. After being treated through the machine filters, the blood returns through the distal opening of the catheter to the body. The catheter is inserted to provide immediate use of a dialysis access to permit hemodialysis. It is often used while waiting for a fistula or a graft to mature.

Because the rest of the patient's life depends on dialysis, access to a machine becomes critical. Most patients are assigned to dialysis centers for periodic treatment. However, equipment can be obtained for home dialysis if the patient and the family are willing to assume the responsibility. The equipment is similar to that in the centers. The training may take from several weeks to a few months. There are 3 types of home hemodialysis processes. The conventional process is done three times a week for at least 3 to 4 hours each time. A short daily home hemodialysis can be done five to seven times a week with a new type of machine that only needs to operate about 2 hours because the procedure is performed nearly daily. A third process is called nocturnal home hemodialysis. This process is a long, slow treatment during the night while the patient sleeps. This type is usually done nightly or at least every other night. Usually the patient can choose and maybe mix the treatment options, depending upon the machine used and the amount of dialysis needed.

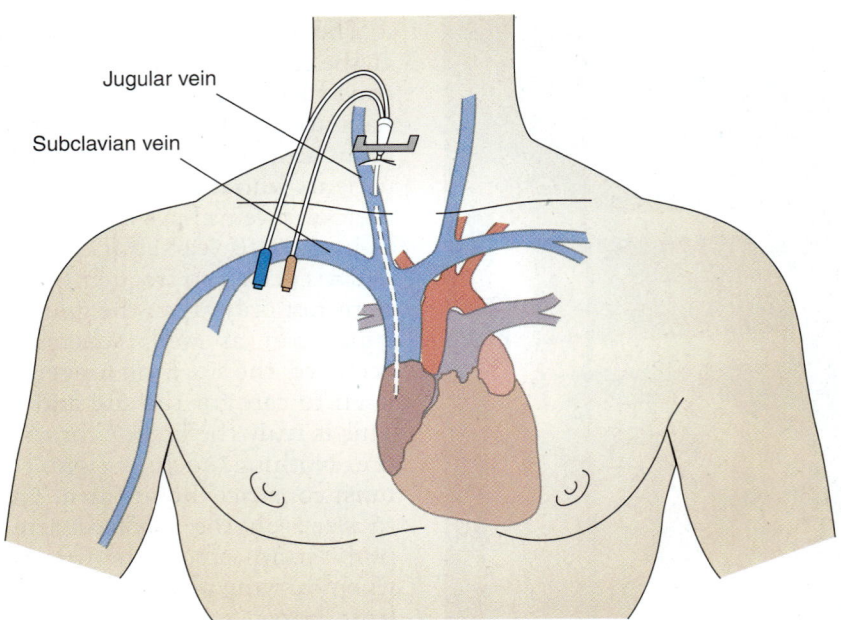

FIGURE 11-182A Catheter insertion sites in the jugular vein.

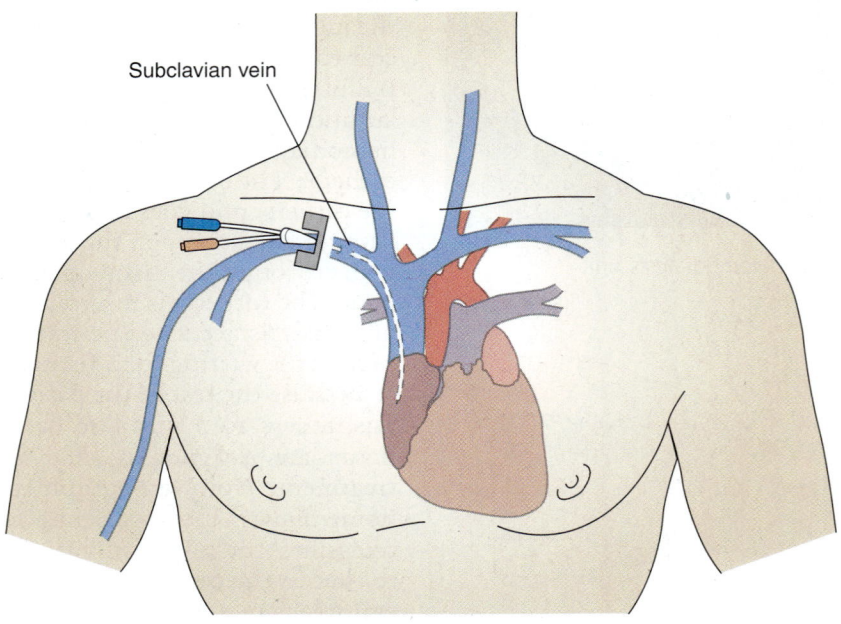

FIGURE 11-182B Catheter insertion sites in the subclavian vein.

An alternative to hemodialysis is **peritoneal** dialysis (Figure 11-183). Instead of an artificial dialyzer to cleanse the blood, the patient's own peritoneal membrane is used (the peritoneum covers the abdominal organs and lines the abdominal cavity).

There are different types of peritoneal dialysis. The most common form is continuous ambulatory peritoneal dialysis (CAPD). This type does not require a machine, and the patient is free to walk around while the solution is within the abdominal cavity. The dialyzing solution is introduced into the peritoneal cavity, where it comes into contact with blood vessels. The solution enters through a catheter permanently implanted into the abdomen. The solution tubing is aseptically attached, and approximately 2 liters of dialyzing solution are infused by the process of gravity by

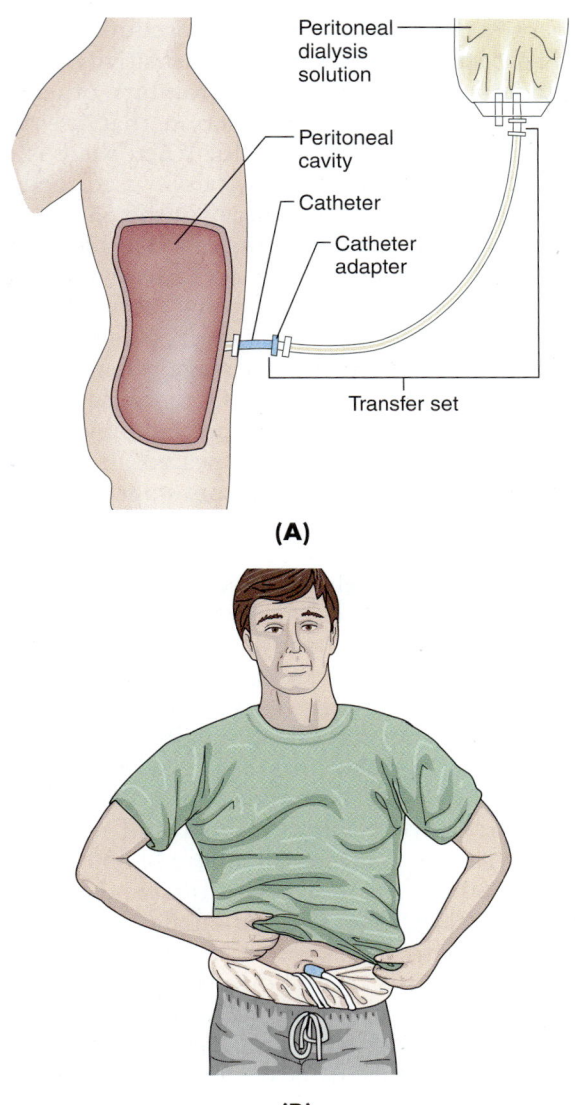

(A)

(B)

FIGURE 11-183   Peritoneal dialysis: (A) infusion of the solution; (B) rolled empty solution container hidden under clothing

suspending the bag at shoulder level. Then the empty bag is rolled up and placed around the waist under the clothing. The solution attracts the waste products and water from the blood, and they are suspended in the solution. After approximately 4 to 6 hours, the bag is unrolled and placed lower than the abdomen, and the waste-bearing dialyzing solution is drained out. Another fresh bag is infused, and the dialysis continues. The exchange process of draining the solution and infusing fresh solution requires from 30 to 45 minutes. This is repeated about every 4 to 6 hours during the day and for an 8-hour period at night.

Another form of peritoneal dialysis is called *continuous cycler-assisted peritoneal dialysis* (CCPD). This is more acceptable to some individuals because the dialysis is accomplished during 6 to 8 hours every night while they sleep. This is especially well suited for children. The patient can completely control peritoneal dialysis, permitting greater freedom of activity.

The CCPD uses an automated cycler to perform three to five exchanges during the night. In the morning, one exchange is instilled, which stays in the abdomen all day.

Yet another type is called nocturnal intermittent peritoneal dialysis (NIPD). This is like CCPD only there are six or more overnight exchanges, and the patient does not have any solution instilled during the daytime. This works for patients whose peritoneum can remove wastes rapidly or who still have adequate remaining kidney function.

The main complication of peritoneal dialysis is peritonitis, an inflammation of the peritonium from accidental contamination of the tubing when connecting and disconnecting solutions. Users of the method must be meticulous in performing the procedure. Peritonitis is painful and can cause scarring of the peritoneum, making it no longer useful for dialysis. Peritonitis can be fatal.

Many considerations must be weighed when dialysis becomes necessary. Routine procedures must be considered: for example, when taking medications, they must be timed after dialysis to prevent removing them from the bloodstream. For additional information about this life-prolonging procedure, contact your local branch of the National Kidney Foundation, inquire at a dialysis center, or consult your physician.

KIDNEY TRANSPLANT

The transplantation of body organs is always at risk of recipient rejection; however, the kidney can usually be successfully transplanted, and the survival of the graft has been markedly improved by the use of the drug cyclosporin. Transplantation is indicated in cases of prolonged chronic debilitating disease and renal failure involving both kidneys; unfortunately, transplantation often is not performed until patients have been on dialysis for a significant time because of a lack of organ donors.

The demand exceeds the supply for healthy organs. In addition, blood and other cellular structures must "match" to ensure the greatest probability for a functioning transplanted organ. There is an anticipated percentage of success within immediate family members. A twin provides the greatest likelihood, with a brother or sister, parent, or child providing decreasing percentages of success in that order. The surgical procedure itself is well established and presents virtually no concern as far as the success of the transplanted kidney. The patient, however, is almost always in a state of relatively poor physical condition because of the effects of the extended illness. This status and the tendency of the body to reject a "substance" that is foreign and not of the same cellular structure sometimes result in the organ not surviving in its new host. The use of drugs to control the body's natural defensive mechanism of rejection increases the rate of success.

Transplant patients need to take medication every day to protect their new kidney. Most patients require three drugs. The primary one will probably be cyclosporine, tacrolimus, or sirolimus. In addition, some form of steroid and either mycophenolate mofetil, azathioprine, or rapamycin will be taken. These patients require frequent medical examination at the transplant location to ensure the health of the new organ.

DIAGNOSTIC EXAMINATIONS

Several procedures and tests are used to determine the physical characteristics of the urinary system and assess its function. Analysis of the blood can determine levels of uric acid and the amount of urea nitrogen present. Urinalysis (analysis of the urine) can determine the presence of blood cells and bacteria; acidity level; specific gravity (weight); and physical characteristics, such as color, clarity, and odor.

● **Noninvasive procedures**—Procedures that attempt to evaluate function deal with urinary output. An *intake-output measurement* involves keeping a record of all fluid, or food that melts to liquid, that is consumed, along with all urine or other fluid loss, be it measured or estimated. For example, emesis would be measured; perspiration estimated as slight, moderate, or profuse; diarrhea indicated as to frequency; and any other loss (such as bleeding, drainage through a stoma, or excessive respiratory activity) evaluated. Hence, intake is compared with output to determine fluid balance within the body.

A *24-hour urine test* collects all urinary output, from a specified hour one day until the same time the next day, in a special container under specific conditions (see Chapter 15). Urine can be collected by various methods, depending to some degree on the purpose for collection. A *routine specimen,* preferably the first of the morning, is simply voided into a clean container. A *clean catch specimen,* usually for culture purpose, pregnancy determination, or microscopic examination, involves specific cleaning of the meatal area and catching the specimen midstream in a sterile container.

An *x-ray* or *plain film* of the abdomen may be taken to determine size, shape, and position of the urinary organs. It may also indicate the presence of calculi. This is usually referred to as a KUB (kidneys, ureter, and bladder) series.

The kidney may also be examined by *ultrasound* to detect abnormalities or to clarify findings from other tests. It is a safe, painless procedure that can be used especially in cases in which sensitivity to the radiological opaque materials prohibits other tests. Examinations for kidney function that use a contrast medium are of little value when there is renal failure. Ultrasound, however, can be used to at least view the structure of the kidney in these instances.

Urine analysis is a new urine test that has been developed that can detect bladder cancer with 95% accuracy. It is capable of finding abnormal DNA material that is evidence of cancer. This makes diagnosis possible at a very early stage, when the 5-year survival rate is 91%. Previously, because no symptoms were present, cancer of the bladder was usually not detected until blood appeared in the urine, which was often too late. At this stage of advanced tumor, the 5-year survival rate drops to only 9%. The current bladder tests detect only 20% to 30% of the patients with early disease because microscopic examination to distinguish malignant from normal cells is very difficult. In addition, early detection requires a cystoscopic examination to obtain the cells from a lesion. This test is invasive, painful, and expensive and is not suitable for bladder cancer screening. However, the new urine test could become a part of a routine physical examination. According to the American Cancer Society, estimates of new urinary bladder cancer cases for 2006 are 44,690 for males and 16,730 for females. The estimated death rate is 8,990 for males and 4,070 for females.

● **Invasive procedures**—Another means of collecting a urine specimen is to withdraw it directly from the bladder through a catheter into a sterile container by strict aseptic (sterile) technique. This procedure, called catheterization, is discussed in Chapter 15 with collection of body fluid specimens.

One of the most common diagnostic procedures is an x-ray series called **intravenous pyelography (IVP)**. The patient is required to fast (no food or water) for approximately 10 hours beforehand. A laxative or cleansing enema removes from the colon any fecal material that might obscure the urinary organs. A contrast medium is injected into a vein, usually at the antecubital space of the arm. After a time, a film is taken to demonstrate the function, location, and position of the kidneys, as determined by the presence of the dye. Subsequent films outline the ureters and bladder as the dye is processed by the system. The film is taken at specific intervals to assess the efficiency of the kidney function. Because the contrast medium is iodine based, it is extremely important to determine if the patient has an allergic response to iodine or seafood before the injection.

Cystourethroscopy is an examination using a lighted instrument inserted into the urethra and bladder to view the interior surface (Figure 11-184). The *amount of* **residual** *urine* left in the bladder after the patient

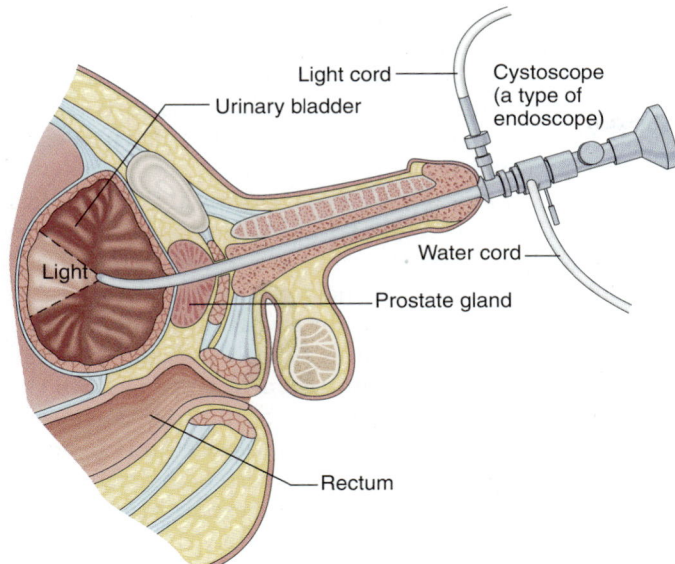

FIGURE 11-184   A cystoscopic examination of the male bladder

has voided (just prior to the examination) may be withdrawn and measured. A local anesthetic (sometimes a general) is given. The scope is lubricated, and as it is inserted, the interior of the urethra is observed. The scope is then advanced into the bladder. A solution is instilled to distend the bladder for observation and to make the ureteral openings visible. At this point, based on findings, other procedures can be performed, such as *catheterization of the kidney(s)* by inserting a catheter up through the ureter(s), *biopsy of a tumor,* or *removal of calculi* in the bladder. It may be possible to crush larger calculi with an instrument and irrigate the pieces out through the scope. When examination of the bladder is completed, the scope is slowly withdrawn as the neck of the bladder and the interior of the urethra are examined.

Other standard procedures performed initially during cystourethroscopy are obtaining a sterile specimen for culture, cytology (for cancer cells), and sensitivity testing.

Other x-ray examinations can be performed in connection with endoscopic examinations. When a catheter is inserted into one of the ureters and passed into the pelvis of the kidney, a radiopaque medium can be instilled. This procedure, known as *retrograde ureteropyelography,* is especially useful for viewing the inside of the kidney when poor kidney function prohibits an IVP procedure. The structure of the ureters can be seen by an additional dye injection as the catheter is withdrawn.

Fluoroscopy and x-ray films aid in determining abnormalities. A delayed film, 15 to 20 minutes following instillation of the dye, can be taken to check for retention indicative of urinary stasis (stagnation). If

an obstruction of the kidney is observed, it can be located by the film to be corrected. When an obstruction prohibits urine drainage, the catheter may be left in position temporarily to ensure adequate drainage. A kidney can be severely, if not permanently, damaged in a relatively short period if pressure from urine builds up because of the inability to drain.

DISEASES AND DISORDERS

Cystitis (Sis-ti′tis)

Description—This inflammation of the bladder usually results from an ascending organism introduced through the meatus.

Signs and symptoms—Symptoms of cystitis are frequent urination, dysuria, spasms of the bladder, nocturia, and often fever and hematuria. Nausea, vomiting, chills, tenderness over the bladder area, and lower-back pain may occur. A frequent complaint is sharp, stabbing pain when voiding, especially at the end of the stream. This discomfort, together with the urge to void small amounts frequently, prompts the patient to seek medical help.

Diagnosis is confirmed by clinical characteristics and the presence of organisms in the urine.

Etiology—The most common cause in women is *E. coli* from the rectum, which may be carried to the meatus by improper cleansing following defecation. Women should be instructed to always cleanse from front to back when washing, wiping, or drying the perineal area. Cystitis can also be caused by organisms from the vagina. Women are far more prone to infection than men, presumably because the urethra is so short. Also, in men, the prostatic fluid acts as an antibacterial shield, thereby providing protection.

Treatment—Cystitis is treated with antibiotics sufficient to sterilize the urine. Usually, medication is given for approximately 5 days. A culture of the urine after 3 days should show no organisms. If bacterial resistance to a certain medication has developed, the drug of choice will need to be changed. The sensitivity studies performed on the urine culture will identify appropriate alterations.

Women who have had cystitis a few times can identify the characteristic symptoms as soon as they begin and start to drink cranberry juice and water. Also, an over-the-counter medication, Phenazopyridine hydrochloride (commonly called pyridium), will relieve the discomfort and pain quickly; however, it will not treat any bacterial infection that may be present.

Urinary tract infections (UTI) are particularly common in patients with neurogenic bladders. The problem stems from the loss of innervation to the bladder, which can cause incontinence, residual retention, spasticity, or flaccidness. Bedfast patients or those confined to wheelchairs are especially susceptible. The use of indwelling catheters to deal with incontinence or the inability to void frequently results in UTI as a result of the direct entrance route for bacteria into the bladder.

Prevention—Women may be able to avoid cystitis by following some simple measures:

- Drink enough water to keep urine a light straw color; this washes out bacteria.
- Drinking 12 ounces of cranberry juice daily may also decrease bacteria.
- Don't use a diaphragm for birth control if you have recurrent UTIs; it boosts the risk for repeat infections.
- Urinate immediately after sex. Often, bacteria in the vagina may be introduced into the bladder, and urination expels the bacteria and decreases the likelihood of infection.

Glomerulonephritis (Glo-meru-lo-ne-fritis)

This inflammation of the glomerulus of the nephron occurs in both acute and chronic forms.

Acute Glomerulonephritis (AGN)

Description—**Acute glomerulonephritis (AGN)** can occur following bacterial infections of the respiratory tract, the urinary tract, or the bloodstream. It affects boys ages 3 to 7 most frequently but can strike either sex at any age. Up to 95% of children and 70% of adults recover fully, with the remainder developing chronic renal failure.

Signs and symptoms—AGN usually begins 1 to 3 weeks after an untreated throat infection. Symptoms include moderate edema, protein in the urine, hematuria, oliguria, and fatigue. Hypertension may develop because of retention of sodium or water from the decreased glomerular filtration rate. Diagnosis is made following a detailed history and clinical assessment. Laboratory findings confirm elevated electrolytes, BUN (blood urea nitrogen), creatinine in the blood, red and white blood cells, and protein in the urine. A throat culture may show a streptococcal organism.

Etiology—AGN results from a collection of antigen-antibodies from streptococcal infections, which become entrapped in the glomeruli membranes. The entrapment causes interference in the glomerular function, damaging the membrane and resulting in the loss of its ability to selectively filter solutes. Red blood cells and protein molecules are allowed to filter out, and the filtration rate drops. Uremic poisoning may result. (See Uremia.)

Treatment—Treatment consists of bed rest, fluid and salt restriction, and correction of the electrolyte imbalance. Diuretics (water pills) may be used to reduce the accumulation of cellular fluid. At this time, the use of antibiotics is controversial. The course of AGN usually resolves in about 2 weeks.

Chronic Glomerulonephritis

Description—This is a slow, progressive disease. It causes scarring and sclerosing of the inflamed glomeruli, gradually leading to renal failure. Unfortunately, sufficient symptoms are not produced to cause early clinical investigation.

Signs and symptoms—The first symptoms are proteinuria (protein in the urine), hematuria, and a specific form of a urine cast. By the time it is diagnosed, **chronic glomerulonephritis** is usually irreversible.

The chronic stage can be asymptomatic for many years, suddenly becoming progressive and producing hypertension, proteinuria, and hematuria. In the later stages, uremic symptoms occur, such as nausea, vomiting, pruritus, dyspnea, fatigue, mild to severe edema, and anemia. Severe hypertension may cause enlargement of the heart, congestive heart failure (CHF), and eventually renal failure.

Etiology—Occasionally, the chronic form follows AGN, but most frequently it is an insidious disease precipitated by other primary renal disorders or systemic syndromes.

Treatment—Treatment consists of measures to treat the symptoms only, such as a diet to restrict sodium, antihypertensive drugs, correction of the electrolyte imbalance, reduction of edema, and prevention of cardiac failure.

Incontinence (In-con'-tin-ence)

Description—This is the uncontrollable loss of urine. It is estimated that at least 20 million people in the United States suffer from incontinence; 85% are women. It interferes with sleep, physical and sexual activity, travel, and daily activities. Many women avoid social activities and are home-bound because of the fear of an accident. Twenty-five percent of women ages 15 to 64 have incontinence. This increases to over 40% for those older than 60. It occurs basically in three forms: stress, overflow, and urge. *Stress incontinence,* the most common, occurs when a person coughs, sneezes, or laughs. Urine may also leak from the stress on muscles when exercising or rising from bed or a chair. *Overflow incontinence* occurs because the bladder never empties completely and its fullness causes leakage. *Urge incontinence* occurs unexpectedly. There is a strong, uncontrollable urge to void requiring immediate emptying of the bladder to prevent wetting.

Males may also be affected by incontinence, but not as frequently as women. The rate among men is 1.5% to 5% but also increases with age. (It may be higher because so many prefer to be silent.) Nearly all older men have "dribbling" of urine when the prostate becomes enlarged and displaces the bladder. (The prostate, shaped somewhat like a donut, lies directly beneath the bladder, with the urethra running through its cen-

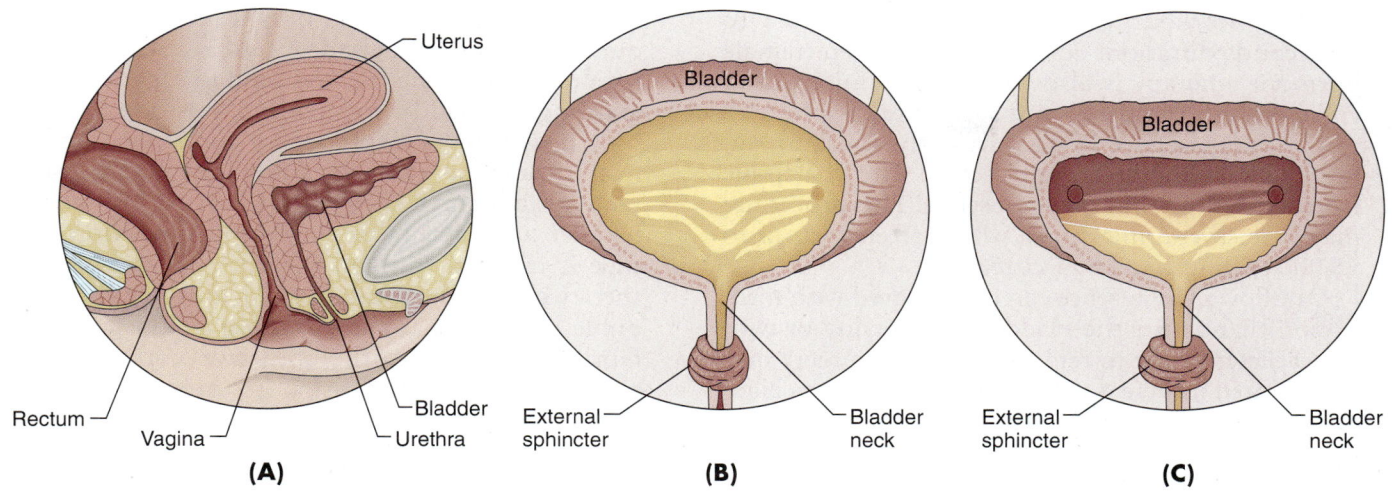

FIGURE 11-185   (A) Structure and function of the urinary bladder. The bladder is located beneath the uterus and in front of the vagina in a female. (B) The sphincter contracts to close the urethra and sends a message to the bladder to relax and the bladder neck to stay closed. (C) To void, the sphincter relaxes and a message goes to the bladder to contract and the bladder neck to open.

ter.) If the prostate is removed, the prostatic portion of the urethra is involved, and control of urine is affected.

Signs and symptoms—The primary symptom is the involuntary loss of urine.

Etiology—Age is not a cause. There are a number of reasons for incontinence; some are specific to one of the forms previously discussed. All involve the physical structure and function of the bladder and urethra. In the female, the bladder lies beneath and is somewhat supported by the uterus and its ligaments (Figure 11-185A). As the bladder fills, a message to void goes to the brain, but if it is not convenient, the external sphincter is contracted and the bladder neck stays closed. This signals the bladder to relax (Figure 11-185B). When it is time to void, the message goes to the external sphincter to relax and it opens; this signals the bladder neck to open and the bladder to contract (Figure 11-185C). With stress incontinence, coughing, sneezing, or laughing increases pressure on the bladder, thereby increasing pressure on the bladder neck, which is not able to stay closed. The external sphincter cannot control urine alone, so it spurts out. With overflow incontinence, the urethra is narrowed, usually by scar tissue or a prolapsed pelvic organ, preventing the bladder from emptying completely. The pressure builds up and overpowers the sphincter, causing leakage. In women, the displacement of the bladder during pregnancy and the pressure during the process of childbirth are definite factors in the development of incontinence. Often, following hysterectomy (removal of the uterus), the bladder will "drop" and protrude into the vagina, causing a cystocele and resulting in improper positioning and the inability to empty completely. With urge incontinence, the urge to urinate is received even though there is little urine, the bladder continues to contract longer than the sphinc-

ter can prevent leakage, and urine is leaked. Menopause is often responsible because the drop in estrogen weakens the urethral sphincter, causing an inability to keep it tightly closed, so a woman feels the urge to void small amounts several times an hour.

Treatment—A variety of things can be done. Many people find it necessary to wear sanitary napkins or specially designed incontinence pads in order to conceal their leakage. Others wear adult-style diapers or waterproof briefs. Some, especially men, wear an external appliance to catch the urine. For stress-related incontinence, exercises of the pelvic floor muscles may be helpful. These muscles act as a sling to keep the bladder and the bladder neck lifted and to control the external sphincter. These exercises are known as "Kegels." They involve contracting and briefly holding the muscles several times a day, which over time can tighten and strengthen the pelvic floor (Figures 11-186A and B). The recom-

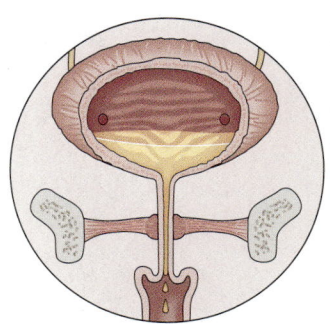

FIGURE 11-186A   Kegel exercises. Beforehand, pelvic muscles are thin, and the sphincter is weak, so the urethra cannot close.

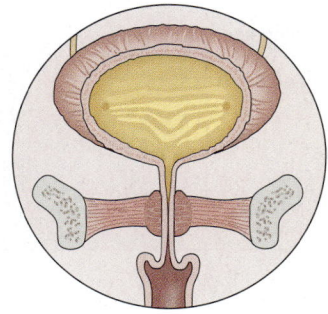

FIGURE 11-186B   After 3 months of exercises, the muscles are thicker and stronger, closing the sphincter.

mended "workout" is 25 to 40 repetitions of 5 to 10 seconds duration. For females, estrogen (female hormone) therapy is also helpful. The injection of collagen into the tissue surrounding the sphincter can be very effective in narrowing the urethra. Figure 11-187 illustrates the injection into the tissue from a needle within the cystoscope. This procedure may take several injections, which often cost up to $5,000 each. It has a 69% cure rate.

Overflow incontinence can be improved with medication that assists the bladder in emptying or with self-catheterization to remove the urine. Surgery may be indicated if there is vaginal prolapse or if the bladder has partially descended through the muscles of the pelvic floor. Urge incontinence is best treated with drugs to relax the bladder contractions and estrogen to improve the sphincter tone. The Kegel exercises are also helpful. Drug therapy costs about $40 to $50 per month and must continue throughout life.

A change in behavior may be sufficient to control incontinence. With stress incontinence, a bathroom trip should be made every 3 hours. Urge incontinence requires bladder training by beginning bathroom trips every hour the first week, then every hour and a half, and eventually every 3 hours. Kegels are used to control the urge. The process is slow and not too successful, helping 54% to 75% but only curing 12% to 16%. Bladder surgery may achieve up to 85%

success but it often lasts only a few years and requires an extended period of time for recovery. The repaired supporting muscles tend to separate again, allowing the bladder to fall out of position.

A newer surgical procedure for stress incontinence known as transobturator tape (TOT) uses a piece of fabric in a slinglike fashion, to support the bladder and urethra in their proper position. The tape is inserted through the anterior vaginal wall, then two small incisions are made through the lower pubic area of the abdomen. Using a laproscope, the fabric is attached to the obturator portion of the pelvis with enough tension to properly support the bladder and urethra. This repair has about a 90% rate of success to correct stress incontinence. The recovery period is from 3 to 6 weeks and has restrictions of lifting no more than 5 pounds and no driving, stairs, or bending over for the first 3 weeks.

In males, exercises following prostate surgery are very important to regain urinary control. The surgical procedure weakens the related muscles and may injure the urethral sphincter. Occasionally, incontinence persists either because of increased bladder pressure or a sphincter problem, or both. If it persists, periurethral collagen injections can be effective. A surgical procedure involving the insertion of an artificial sphincter can also be performed. This device has a valve mechanism that the person can activate to control and expel urine.

There are other health problems that cause incontinence for both sexes. The effects of a stroke and Parkinson's disease, for instance, can damage the nerves, making control impossible. If leakage begins suddenly, it may signify a bladder infection or a medication side effect. High blood pressure drugs called alpha blockers weaken the sphincter. Antihistamines and sleeping pills may also cause problems.

Nephrotic Syndrome (Ne-frot'ik) (Nephrosis)

Description—This noninflammatory disease involving the glomerular membrane allows a large number of protein molecules to leave the blood and enter the urine. As a result, large amounts of water accumulate in the body, causing generalized dependent edema. This often leads to pleural effusion, swollen external sex organs, and ascites (fluid within the abdomen). **Nephrotic syndrome** occurs most often in children, but adults can contract the disease also.

Signs and symptoms—Symptoms range from the dominant clinical feature of edema to hypotension (especially on standing), lethargy, fatigue, lack of appetite, pallor, and depression.

Diagnosis can be confirmed from consistently elevated proteinuria over a 24-hour period, the pres-

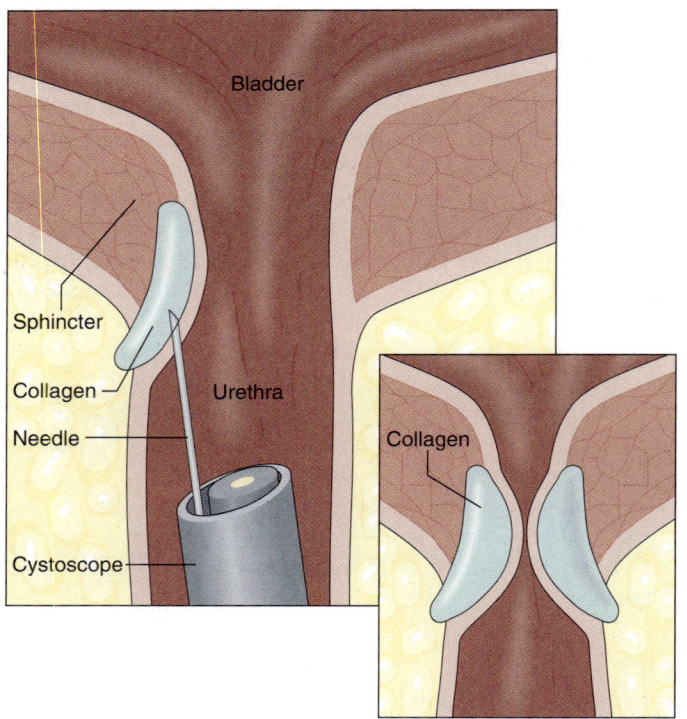

FIGURE 11-187   Injecting collagen near the sphincter narrows the urethra to control leakage.

ence of characteristic fatty casts and oval fat bodies in the urine, and increased serum cholesterol levels with decreased albumin levels.

Etiology—The underlying cause of the disease is usually glomerulonephritis (75% of the cases). The remaining 25% are associated with diabetes; circulatory diseases, such as sickle cell anemia, CHF, and renal vein thrombosis; toxins that affect the nephrons, such as mercury, bismuth, or gold; allergic reactions; and systemic infections, such as tuberculosis.

Treatment—Treatment consists of correcting the underlying cause whenever possible. Supportive treatment involves a high-protein diet, restrictive sodium intake, diuretics for edema, and antibiotics to combat infection. Some favorable results have occurred with the use of corticosteroids, but they are limited to specific uses.

Polycystic Kidney Disease (Pole-sis′tik)

Description—An inherited disorder, **polycystic kidney disease** is characterized by bilateral, grapelike clusters of fluid-filled cysts that replace normal renal tissue (Figure 11-188). The presence of the cysts greatly enlarges the size of the kidney externally and also compresses the nephrons inside, eventually replacing the functioning renal tissue. One form of the disease appears in infants and results in stillbirth or early newborn death. Occasionally, an infant will survive for about 2 years before developing renal failure. The adult form has an insidious onset, usually apparent between ages 30 to 50. The deterioration of the kidney is slower but is nevertheless fatal unless treated by dialysis or transplantation.

Signs and symptoms—Symptoms of the infantile form include a pointed nose, small chin, floppy low-set ears, and folds in the inner eyelids. The kidneys become

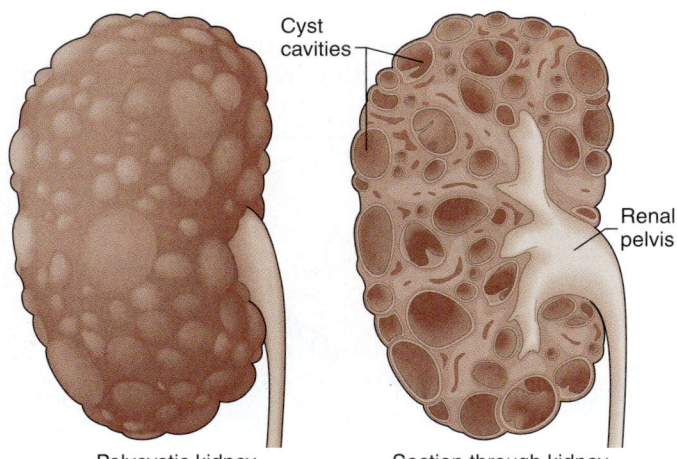

Cyst cavities

Renal pelvis

Polycystic kidney   Section through kidney

FIGURE 11-188   Polycystic disease

huge bilateral masses between the bottom of the ribs and the top of the ileum and are symmetrical, firm, and dense. Usually there is evidence of CHF and respiratory distress. Adult polycystic disease initially presents nonspecific symptoms, such as hypertension, polyuria, and UTI. Eventually additional symptoms appear relating to enlarged kidney masses, such as lumbar pain; widened body; and a swollen, tender abdomen. As the disease advances, the patient develops recurrent hematuria, life-threatening bleeding from cyst rupture, proteinuria, and pain caused by ureteral spasm from the passing of clots or calculi. Ultimately, the insufficiency of the kidney results in failure and uremia.

Etiology—This disease is an inherited disorder.

Treatment—Polycystic disease is not curable, but it can be managed, to a certain degree, by controlling hypertension and urinary infections. Treatment is like that for any chronic, destructive kidney disease.

Pyelonephritis (Pie-lo-ne-fri′tis)

Description—This is one of the most common kidney infections.

Signs and symptoms—Symptoms associated with pyelonephritis include fever, urgency, dysuria, back pain, burning during urination, nocturia, and hematuria. The urine may have an ammoniacal or fishy odor and is usually cloudy in appearance. Other common symptoms include chills, lack of appetite, flank pain, and fatigue. The symptoms generally develop rapidly and may subside within a few days. However, a residual bacterial infection may recur at a later time.

Etiology—Acute pyelonephritis is caused by bacteria that normally inhabit the intestines. The bacteria typically spread from the bladder up the ureters and into the kidney pelvis, causing the development of colonies of bacteria within 24 to 48 hours. **Pyelonephritis** may also result from urinary stasis; the inability to empty the bladder completely; or urinary obstruction caused by strictures, tumors, or enlarged prostate in males.

Diagnosis is confirmed by urinalysis, which shows sediment containing bacteria leukocytes and possibly a few red blood cells. Culture reveals a significant population of bacteria. Specific gravity is below normal because of the temporary inability to concentrate urine.

Treatment—Treatment consists of antibiotics determined by culture and sensitivity tests. A course of treatment is usually 10 to 14 days even though urine becomes sterile after 2 to 3 days.

Reculturing is done 1 week after treatment and periodically for the next year to observe for residual infection. Mechanical problems causing urinary stasis, such as strictures, "dropped" bladder (positioned so that it cannot totally empty), or tumors, should be corrected.

Renal Calculi (Re'-nal Kal'ku-li)

Description—Kidney calculi (stones) are formed from chemicals in the urine, forming crystals that stick together. They may be as small as a grain of sand or as large as a golf ball. Small stones pass out of the kidney with the urine. Some that are larger become caught in a ureter, where they cause severe pain. Still others may pass into the bladder where they continue to enlarge. They will again cause pain if they wash into the urethra and become lodged.

Kidney stones affect primarily young to middle-aged adults, with men being affected four times as often as women. The condition tends to recur.

Signs and symptoms—
- Severe pain, starting suddenly in the kidneys or lower abdomen and moving to the groin area. It may last for minutes or hours, alternating with periods of relief.
- Nausea and vomiting
- Burning and frequent urge to urinate
- Chills, fever, and weakness, probably from infection
- Cloudy or foul-smelling urine
- Blood in the urine
- Blocked urine flow

Diagnosis is made based on symptoms, x-rays (such as KUB or IVP), or ultrasound. Once size and location are determined, then an appropriate course of action can be selected. About 90% can be passed without requiring special treatment or surgery. Often, increasing fluids, being active, and a specific medication to dissolve the stone are sufficient. However, calcium-containing stones, the most common type, cannot be dissolved.

Etiology—The causes of calculi formation are not always clear; however, certain factors seem to contribute to their development:
- Drinking too little fluid
- Chronic UTIs
- Blockage of the urinary tract
- Prolonged limited activity
- Misuse of certain medications
- Certain genetic and metabolic diseases
- Specific foods in certain susceptible people

Treatment—The simplest treatment is chosen first. Many stones, if in the bladder or ureters, can be removed endoscopically either directly or following fracture of the stone with laser or shock waves. Stones in the kidney may be removed by a scope, inserted through the side of the body and directly into the kidney. This allows removal of the stone when it is visualized or fracture of the stone with instruments passed under direct vision.

Another new method of stone removal is called extracorporeal shock-wave **lithotripsy** (ESWL). Shock waves (high-energy pressure waves) similar to sonic booms generated by aircraft are produced outside the body by an electrical spark. The patient, in a disposable swimsuit, is positioned and strapped into a hydraulic chair. Intravenous sedation is given to make the patient comfortable. The chair is positioned within a tank of warm water, so that the stone is in an area where the shock waves can be focused. The waves travel through the water and the body without damaging living tissue because all living tissue is about 80% water. Figure 11-189 illustrates the positioning of the patient for lithotripsy procedure.

It takes about 2,000 shock waves to break up the average stone and requires about 30 minutes to complete the treatment. Most describe the shock feeling as a slapping or tapping sensation. Patients are fitted with headphones to listen to music while the procedure is being done. About an hour after the treatment, most patients are allowed to leave. The small fragments of the fractured stone can easily be passed in the urine. It may take several weeks to completely pass all the fragments.

Most patients experience some abdominal discomfort with or without bruising on the abdomen or back. Frequent, bloody urination is common. Patients are instructed to collect passed stone fragments for analysis and to see their urologists as a follow-up to be certain there is no kidney blockage from the fragments.

Occasionally, people do not qualify for ESWL because of stone location or one of the following:
- Weight in excess of 295 pounds
- Height over 6 feet, 6 inches
- Involved kidney has little or no function
- Uncontrolled urinary infection
- It is the urologist's opinion that another form of treatment is more appropriate

If no other method can be used, the stone will be removed by surgical incision into the kidney. This is considered the final choice to solve the problem because of the risks involved with any major surgical procedure and the length of recovery time required.

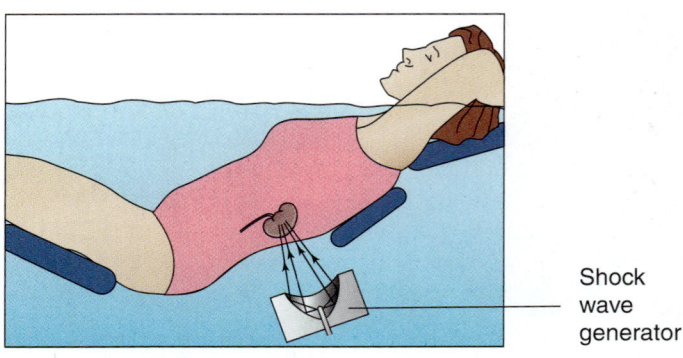

Shock wave generator

FIGURE 11-189 Lithotripsy procedure

Renal Failure

Acute Renal Failure

Description—A critical illness, **acute renal failure** results in the sudden cessation of kidney function. Effective medical treatment usually can overcome the problem. If not, however, it will progress to uremia and death.

Signs and symptoms—Symptoms initially apparent are oliguria and azotemia (nitrogenous products of protein metabolism in the blood). Without filtration, the waste products and excess solutes quickly collect in the blood, resulting in severe electrolyte imbalance, acidosis, and uremia, which interfere with the function of the other body systems. A vast number of other symptoms develop, listed here by body system and in ascending order within the system:

- Gastrointestinal: anorexia, nausea, vomiting, hematemesis (bloody vomitus)
- Nervous: headache, drowsiness, confusion, convulsion, coma
- Integumentary: dryness of the skin, pruritus, pallor, uremic frost (powdery white crystals of urea on the skin)
- Circulatory: hypotension initially, then hypertension, cardiac rhythm irregularities, CHF, edema, anemia, pulmonary edema
- Respiratory: Kussmaul's respirations (fast, deep respirations, over 20 per minute and usually sounding labored, resembling sighs)

Fever and chills, indicators of infection, are an expected complication.

Diagnosis of renal failure is confirmed by blood test findings of greatly elevated quantities of urea, nitrogen, and creatinine and urine samples with casts, protein, and altered specific gravity. Additional verification with diagnostic examinations, such as KUB, IVP, ultrasound, and retrograde pyelography, may be indicated.

Etiology—Renal failure may be caused by an obstruction, inadequate circulation, or damage to the nephrons. Failure caused by bilateral obstruction is usually associated with calculi, blood clots, tumors, strictures, an enlarged prostate, or urethral edema. Inadequate blood flow results from low blood pressure and low volume in the arteries, which eliminates the force required for the kidney to filter water and solutes from the blood. This can result from shock, embolism, hemorrhage, loss of fluid caused by burns, congestive heart failure, and arrhythmias. Nephron damage, which may cause failure, can result from acute glomerulonephritis, sickle cell anemia, bilateral renal vein thrombosis, acute pyelonephritis, renal myeloma (tumor), or toxic substances.

Treatment—Treatment consists of a high-calorie diet that is low in protein, sodium, and potassium. Fluids are controlled. Dialysis may be required.

Chronic Renal Failure

Description—This is an end result of the progressive loss of kidney function.

Signs and symptoms—Symptoms do not develop significantly enough to warrant investigation until almost 75% of glomerular function is gone. The remaining normal nephrons gradually deteriorate, causing symptoms of renal failure and other system involvement. Signs and symptoms initially are related to an imbalance of sodium and potassium and an accumulation of nitrogen from protein metabolism; these may include hypotension, dry mouth, listlessness, fatigue, and nausea. Later the patient will begin experiencing mental dullness and confusion. Symptoms increase as more nephrons fail.

Additional system involvement is similar to that described with acute failure, but a few specific differences do occur with the slower progressive course.

Infertility and amenorrhea (lack of menses) in women, impotence in men, and impaired carbohydrate metabolism also result from improper endocrine action. The skeletal system develops a mineral imbalance that results in bone pain because of parathyroid hormone imbalance. This in turn allows the minerals to be withdrawn from the bones, causing fractures. Calcifications develop in the brain, eyes, joints, myocardium, and blood vessels.

Diagnosis is made in the same manner as for acute renal failure.

PEDIATRIC PERSPECTIVE

Children with chronic failure show stunted growth patterns because of endocrine abnormalities.

Etiology—**Chronic renal failure** can be the result of many preexisting conditions, such as chronic glomerular disease; chronic infections; obstructions; stones; and endocrine diseases, such as diabetes, vascular diseases, hypertension, and chronic overdose of toxic agents.

Treatment—Treatment is almost exclusively dependent on dialysis to correct the chemical imbalance. Other treatment is required for the complications developed in the other body systems. Long-term dialysis requires specific physical and psychologic therapy. Patients must be meticulous in their personal care. The skin must be clean, and lotions should be applied to combat dryness and itching. Good oral hygiene is a must to alleviate bad breath and counteract excessive dryness and bad taste. Diet is extremely critical and requires individual adjustments in relation to dialysis. Daily records of intake and output aid in determining fluid status. If urine is not being excreted, fluid builds up within the body's tissues. Dialysis removes this fluid, causing the patient to express feelings of being "wrung out."

Stricture (Strik'chur)

Description—This is a narrowing of a passageway that interferes with the movement of substances through its interior. For example, the **stricture** of a ureter interferes with the flow of urine to the bladder. A more common stricture occurs in the urethra, particularly in males.

Signs and symptoms—Symptoms of urethral stricture, such as a small urine stream and prolonged urination time, are indicative of a decreased passageway. Stricture of a ureter may not be evident until distention occurs because of the buildup of pressure or until kidney stones develop from urinary stasis. Complete stricture of a ureter will destroy the function of the affected kidney.

Etiology—It may be caused by a congenital abnormality or, in either sex, may be the result of scarring following infection.

Treatment—Urethral strictures can be readily treated by dilation to open up the narrowed passageway. Increasingly larger dilators are inserted into the urethra to stretch the constricted area. The procedure often needs to be repeated periodically to maintain patency (openness), especially with the growing child. If it is not successful, surgery to correct the problem will be necessary.

Uremia (U-re'me-a)

Description—Literally translated, this term means that the products normally found in the urine are instead in the blood.

Signs and symtoms—Blood analysis shows excess protein by-products because urinary disease prevents their excretion in the urine. It is a toxic condition, leading to coma and death if not treated. End-stage uremia may cause "uremic frost," the presence of crystals from the excretion of urine products through the skin.

Etiology—It can be the end result of many acute and chronic kidney diseases. Any condition that renders the kidney unable to regulate the chemical composition of the blood by excretion of waste products causes the wastes to accumulate, slowly building to a toxic level. When renal failure exists, **uremia** is inevitable.

Treatment—Dialysis is the only substitute for kidney function, except for surgical transplantation of another kidney.

ACHIEVE UNIT OBJECTIVES

- ☐ Complete the Workbook activities to meet the learning objectives.
- ☐ Apply your knowledge at the end of this chapter in completing the Critical Thinking Challenge and Activities, as well as the StudyWARE on your Student CD-ROM.

UNIT 12
THE ENDOCRINE SYSTEM

OBJECTIVES

Upon completion of this unit, you will be able to achieve the following:

LEARNING Objectives

1. Spell and define, using the glossary at the back of the text, all the Words to Know in this unit.
2. Differentiate between endocrine and exocrine glands, and give an example of each.
3. Give five examples of body functions affected by hormones.
4. Name and locate the nine glands discussed in the unit.
5. Describe the functions of the pituitary, thyroid, parathyroid, adrenal, pancreas, and thymus glands.
6. Describe the hormones and functions of the gonads.
7. Explain the hormone secretion abnormalities that cause gigantism, dwarfism, acromegaly, goiter, tetany, diabetes, cretinism, Cushing's syndrome, and myxedema.
8. List the symptoms of diabetic coma and insulin shock.
9. Identify the diagnostic examinations used to confirm diabetes, thyroid function, pregnancy, and Cushing's syndrome.
10. Describe briefly the symptoms, characteristics, and usual course of action of endocrine disorders presented in the unit.

WORDS TO KNOW

acromegaly	exophthalmia	luteinizing
adrenal	gigantism	mineralocorticoid
adrenaline	glucohemoglobin	myxedema
adrenocorticotro-	glycosuria	ovary
pic hormone	goiter	parathyroid
(ACTH)	gonad	pineal body
aldosterone	gonadotropic	pituitary
cretinism	hormone	progesterone
Cushing's	hyperglycemia	puberty
syndrome	hyperthyroidism	testes
diabetes mellitus	hypoglycemia	testosterone
dwarfism	hypothyroidism	tetany
endocrine	insulin	thymus
epinephrine	islets of	thyroid
estrogen	Langerhans	thyroidectomy
exocrine		

 CERTIFICATION CONNECTION

CMA
Diagnostic procedures
Common diseases and
   pathology
Anatomy and physiology

CMAS
Anatomy and physiology

RMA
Anatomy and physiology

The **endocrine** system is a group of glands that se-crete substances directly into the bloodstream. En-docrine glands are ductless; in other words, their secretions do not drain into the body by way of a duct but are secreted directly into the capillaries of the cir-culatory system (Figure 11-190A). Glands secreting substances through ducts are **exocrine** glands (Figure 11-190B). The pancreas secretes pancreatic juices by way of a duct into the duodenum, so it is an exocrine gland. However, the pancreas also secretes insulin di-rectly into the blood, which also makes it an en-docrine gland.

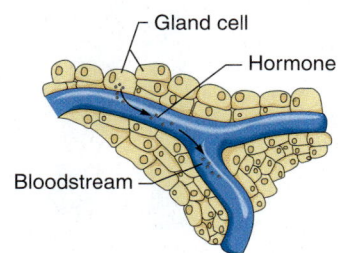

FIGURE 11-190A   Endocrine gland cells secrete hormones into a capillary.

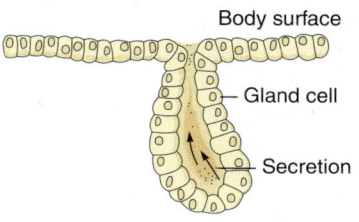

FIGURE 11-190B   Exocrine gland cells secrete substances directly into a duct.

The secretions from endocrine glands are called **hor-mones**. A hormone is a complex chemical that influ-ences actions at distant sites and controls body functions. Hormones are chemical messengers that cause changes. Examples of body functions affected by hormones are growth and development, metabolism, the composition of the blood and bones, sexual matu-rity, and the function of all endocrine glands.

Nine glands or groups of glands will be discussed: the **pituitary**, **thyroid**, **parathyroids**, pancreas (intro-duced in Unit 10), **adrenals**, **ovaries**, **testes**, **thymus**, and the **pineal body** (Figure 11-191). Each gland performs a specific function. The hyperactivity or hypoactivity of the gland causes changes in the body, often altering its appearance, always altering its function, even to the point of death in specific hormonal crises. Hormones either stimulate or inhibit glandular function to main-tain homeostasis.

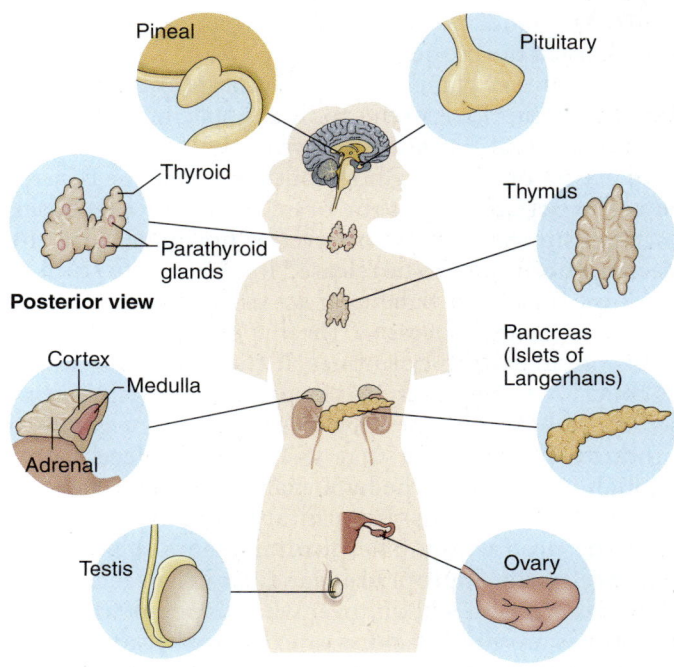

FIGURE 11-191   The glands of the endocrine system

It is important to know that there are hormones secreted from nontraditional endocrine glands. For example, adipose (fat) cells secrete polypeptides that influence appetite and energy metabolism. Leptin is an example of such a hormone that may be used clinically to influence caloric intake and obesity. Also, gastrointestinal hormones are secreted by intestinal cells and have various actions, such as slowing gastric emptying, affecting insulin resistance in diabetes, and inhibiting the secretion of other hormones. Some of these hormones, such as amylin-like products and somatostatin, have recently become available to treat endocrine disorders.

There are many diseases and disorders that develop from either too little or too much hormone influence. Some effects begin in early childhood, others after years of absence or excess of secretions. Fortunately, with appropriate health care, these abnormal conditions are usually discovered early and treated appropriately. In developing nations or when religious beliefs prohibit medical intervention, conditions that develop from too little or too much hormone influence may still be observable.

PITUITARY GLAND

The pituitary gland is considered to be the "master" gland of the body, secreting a large number of hormones that affect other glands, growth, and development.

The gland is attached by a thin stalk to the undersurface of the brain. It is so vital to the body that it is protected within a bony cradle deep within the skull. It sits in a bony depression of the sphenoid bone of the skull, called the *sella turcica,* behind the bony orbits of the eyes at about the level of the bridge of the nose. This tiny gland, not much larger than a pea, secretes nine known hormones.

The pituitary gland consists of a large anterior and a small posterior lobe, each producing specific hormones. A thin sheet of tissue lies between the two lobes. The production of pituitary hormones is under the control of the hypothalamus of the brain by way of a feedback mechanism that senses the level of hormones and the need for hormones to be released in response to stimuli.

This continuous balancing act usually operates well. It is a complex process of the hypothalamus sensing levels of circulating hormones. If the level is too low, a chemical message is sent to the pituitary, which in turn secretes a hormone message to the particular gland to produce the hormone that will raise the level. After enough is produced, the hypothalamus senses the level is sufficient and sends the pituitary another message to stop the production. The pituitary sends a hormone message to the appropriate gland, and the secretion is slowed. Later you will discover what happens when the hormones are either lacking or excessive because something interfered with the balancing act.

Anterior Lobe

The hormones of the anterior lobe of the pituitary are as follows:

1. Growth hormone (GH)—Essential for normal growth of the body's tissues, affects the length of long bones and therefore height. Insufficient production during childhood results in **dwarfism**, whereas overproduction produces **gigantism**. Figure 11-192 is a modern illustration from a 100-year-old photo showing three different sizes of men: a giant, an average-sized man, and a dwarf. The photograph was demonstrating the effects of growth hormone. The average-sized man was probably about 5 feet, 8 inches tall, and perhaps the "giant" was about 7 feet tall. At that time he would have been considered very unusual. Today, many men reach and surpass this height, as evidenced by collegiate and professional basketball players. Not only men but women have grown taller as well. There are many females reaching 6-feet in height, and some are even taller (again, this can be seen among female basketball players). What was once considered excessively tall may not be so today.

   However, overproduction of growth hormone beyond maturity is another thing. Overproduction in adulthood will produce a condition known as **acromegaly**, which is characterized by overgrowth of cartilagenous and connective tissue resulting in

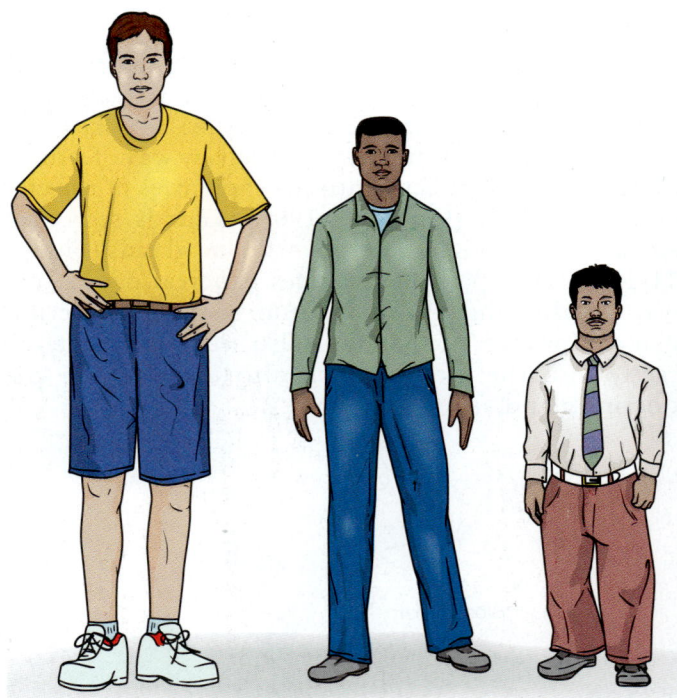

FIGURE 11-192 The effect of growth hormone: a giant, an average-sized person, and a dwarf.

a bulky appearance, protrusion of the eyebrow area, enlargement of the hands and feet, and course features. (See Figure 11-197).

2. Thyrotropin, the thyroid-stimulating hormone (TSH)—Increases the growth and activity of thyroid cells to produce thyroid hormone.

3. **Adrenocorticotropic hormone (ACTH)**—Stimulates the cortex of the adrenal gland.

4. Melanocyte-stimulating hormone (MSH)—Increases skin pigmentation.

5. Prolactin (PR)—Responsible for breast development and the production of milk.

The following **gonadotropic** hormones control the development of the reproductive system in both males and females, including the female menstrual cycle. If production fails before **puberty**, sexual maturity will not occur. If it fails after puberty, secondary sexual characteristics regress.

6. Follicle-stimulating hormone (FSH)—Enlarges the graafian follicle of the ovary to the point of rupture and stimulates the follicle to produce estrogen in the female. FSH stimulates the production of the sperm in the male.

7. **Luteinizing** hormone (LH)—In the female causes the ruptured ovarian follicle to become a corpus luteum that in turn secretes the hormone progesterone. LH in the male stimulates the interstitial cells in the testes to produce testosterone.

Posterior Lobe

The hormones of the posterior lobe of the pituitary are as follows:

1. Oxytocin—Stimulates the contractions of the uterus, especially during childbirth; it also is responsible for the flow of milk from the breast.

2. Vasopressin, or the antidiuretic hormone (ADH)—Acts on the kidney tubule cells to concentrate urine and conserve water within the body. It also stimulates the smooth muscles of blood vessels to constrict.

THYROID GLAND

The thyroid gland has two lobes, one on each side of the larynx, with a connecting central section called the isthmus (Figure 11-193). It is located in front of the upper portion of the trachea in the lower part of the neck. The gland is encased in a capsule of connective tissue.

The thyroid gland produces three hormones: thyroxine (T_4), triiodothyronine (T_3), and thyrocalcitonin. Thyrocalcitonin causes reduction in the level of calcium in the blood. It is synthesized in C cells,

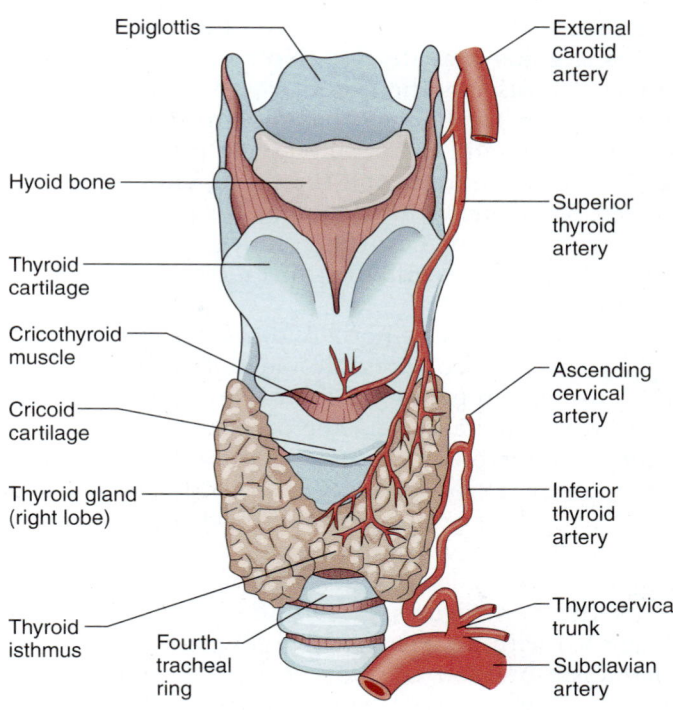

FIGURE 11-193   The thyroid gland

which are nonfollicular cells located in the thyroid gland in humans. Thyrocalcitonin inhibits the bone cells from releasing calcium, making it a useful treatment for conditions associated with increased bone loss, such as osteoporosis. The other two hormones strongly affect metabolism, which influences both the physical and mental activity necessary for normal growth and development. When thyroid activity is below normal, it is called **hypothyroidism**, indicating a decrease in the basal metabolic rate. An overactive thyroid is called **hyperthyroidism** and indicates an increased metabolic rate.

The thyroid gland requires iodine to form the thyroid hormones. Iodine is obtained by eating vegetables grown in soil containing iodine or by eating seafood. Lack of the element causes the thyroid gland to enlarge. When the pituitary receives information from the hypothalamus that the level of thyroid hormones is too low, it secretes TSH to stimulate the thyroid cells and eventually enlarges the entire gland. An enlarged thyroid gland is commonly known as a **goiter**.

The control of hormone release and inhibition by negative feedback is characterized in the relationship between the thyroid and the pituitary gland. When the hypothalamus senses thyroid hormone concentrations are too low, it secretes a releasing factor that travels to the anterior pituitary cells. This thyrotropin-releasing factor stimulates thyrotropin, the TSH secretion, which in turn causes the thyroid gland to synthesize and secrete thyroid hormones. As stated, if this continues, a goiter may develop. Normally, as these hormones increase in the blood, they negatively "feed back" signals to the hypothalamus to reduce the releasing factor, and that results in the pituitary reducing the TSH secretion, and the thyroid hormones are slowed. This finely tuned system is operative in the healthy state to maintain thyroid levels at the appropriate levels for regulating metabolism and other functions.

A person who has hypothyroidism feels cold and fatigued, has low blood pressure and pulse rate, often has a subnormal temperature, and may be overweight due to decreased metabolism. The patient with hyperthyroidism is nervous, restless, and irritable, with heart rate is above normal and elevated blood pressure. The patient may lose weight despite a good appetite. Occasionally the eyes protrude dramatically in a condition called **exophthalmia.**

The man in Figures 11-194 and 11-195 had been diagnosed with an enlarged thyroid gland and hyperthyroidism in 1980 and initially treated with propylthiouracil. In May 2001 he felt pressure in his eye and noticed a change in his vision and the bulging of his eye. He was diagnosed with exopthalmia, but only in one eye, an uncommon condition (see Figure 11-194). By June, he was experiencing increased pressure and having severe pain. The pressure was compressing the optic nerve and would have destroyed his vision. He had his first surgery, an orbital decompression, in June. In this procedure, pieces of the bony orbit are removed to allow for drainage of the fluid and for the eye to recess into the socket. Following this he had a second surgery to adjust the eyelid so his eyes would look similar (see Figure 11-195).

Hyperthyroidism may be treated by removing part or all of the gland or limiting its function by radioactive iodine or antithyroid drugs. The surgical removal of the thyroid is called a **thyroidectomy**. Treatment of hypothyroidism is relatively simple: the thyroid hormone is taken orally as a supplement.

A thyrotoxic crisis or thyroid storm is the extreme clinical development of hyperthyroidism. It produces a greatly accelerated metabolism, severe nervous system malfunction, overheating, and heart failure. The situation is precipitated by stress or a severe infection and can be fatal. Antithyroid drugs propylthiouracil or tapazole are used to treat the condition.

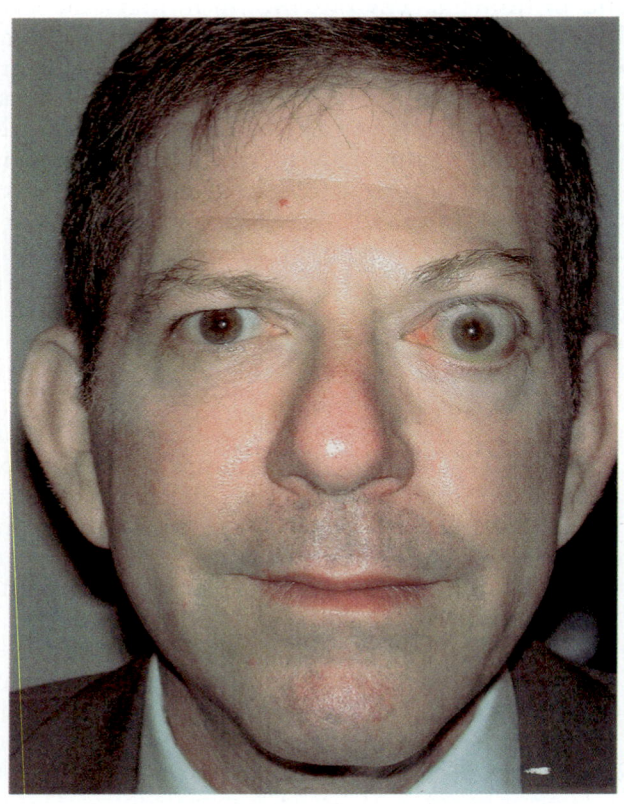

FIGURE 11-194   Male with uncommon unilateral exopthalmus

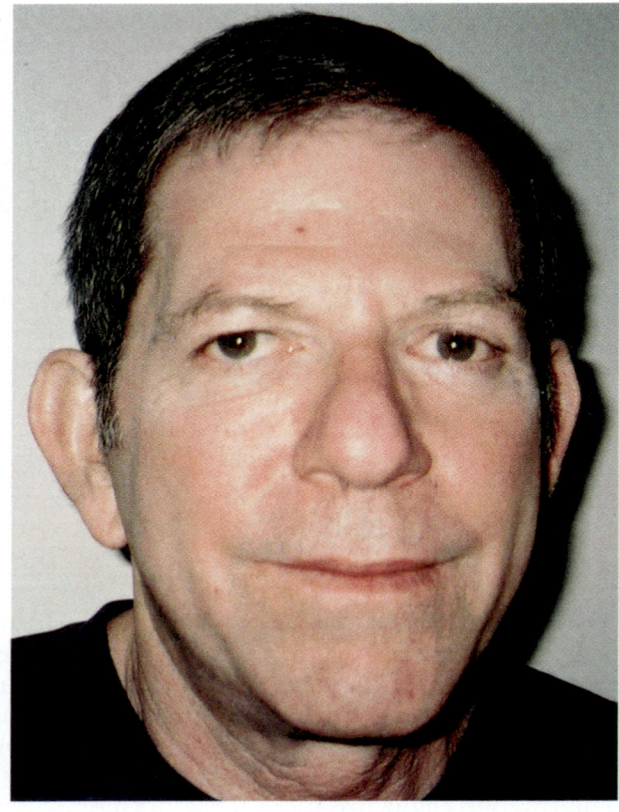

FIGURE 11-195   Male with uncommon unilateral exopthalmus, after surgery

PARATHYROID GLANDS

The parathyroid glands, usually two pairs, are embedded on the posterior surface of the thyroid gland. Their number and size vary greatly, but normally they resemble grains of wheat. The parathyroids are responsible for regulating the calcium content of the blood. The hormone parathromone cooperates with vitamin D to balance the level of calcium in the blood by stimulating the bones to release stored calcium and phosphate into the circulation.

Hyperparathyroidism results in increased levels of calcium in the blood, which causes lethargy and the excretion of large quantities of calcium salts in the urine, leading to the formation of kidney stones. The condition leads progressively to decalcification of the bones and is usually associated with a tumor of one of the glands. Decalcified bones are prone to pathologic fracture.

Hypoparathyroidism is dramatically demonstrated by a condition known as **tetany**, an uncontrollable twitching and spasm of the muscles of the body. This results from hyperirritability of the nervous system in response to the lowered concentration of calcium in the blood. The condition is treated by the addition of calcium. Hypoparathyroidism occurs following damage to or accidental removal of the parathyroids during a thyroidectomy. Inherited hypoparathyroidism is a rare cause of the disorder.

ADRENAL GLANDS (SUPRARENAL)

The adrenal glands sit atop each kidney, hence the additional name *suprarenal*. Each gland is contained in a fibrous capsule and is composed of two parts, each of which acts separately. The outer glandular tissue is called the *cortex,* and the inner tissue is referred to as the *medulla.*

The principal hormone of the medulla is **adrenaline**, also called **epinephrine**. Another hormone, norepinephrine, has a similar action on the body. Together they are considered to be the "flight or fight" hormones because of their effects in emergency situations. The hormones cause an increase in the heart rate, blood pressure, and flow of blood and a decrease in intestinal activity. The adrenal medulla is considered to be nonessential to life.

The cortex of the adrenal gland, however, is essential to life. The cortex produces steroid hormones in three categories: **mineralocorticoids**, glucocorticoids, and sex steroids. The mineralocorticoids, of which **aldosterone** is the principal one, control electrolyte balances through regulating the reabsorption of sodium in the kidney tubules and the excretion of potassium. The glucocorticoids affect the metabolism of protein, fat, and glucose. They stimulate the breakdown of body proteins to amino acids, many of which can be con-

verted to glucose in the liver, thereby increasing blood sugar levels. This process is called gluconeogenesis. They also decrease inflammation by the immune system. ACTH stimulates glucocortocoids to increase in response to stress.

The sex steroids govern certain sexual characteristics, especially those that are male oriented. These steroids are referred to as *androgens.* Excessive secretions cause the virilization and development of masculine secondary sex characteristics in the female and immature male. A mature female's voice will deepen, body hair increases, menstruation will become irregular, and infertility will result.

PANCREAS

The pancreas is a dual-function organ. It has an exocrine function, producing pancreatic juices excreted by way of the pancreatic duct into the duodenum to become part of the digestive juices. It is also an endocrine gland. The hormone *insulin* is secreted by the B cells of the **islets of Langerhans**, often called beta cells (Figure 11-196). There are four cell types located in the pancreas. The alpha cells make up about 25% of the islet cells. Glucagon stimulates new glucose formation by the liver and aids in the breakdown of glycogen to glucose. Thus, its secretion results in a rise in glucose levels. The beta cells are 60% to 80% of the islets and contain the major hormone of the pancreas, **insulin**. Insulin is necessary for the metabolism of carbohydrates. With reduced islet function, the level of blood sugar rises to an abnormal amount, which is referred to as **hyperglycemia**. Conversely, an abnormally low level of blood sugar is known as **hypoglycemia**. When excess glucose is present in the blood, it

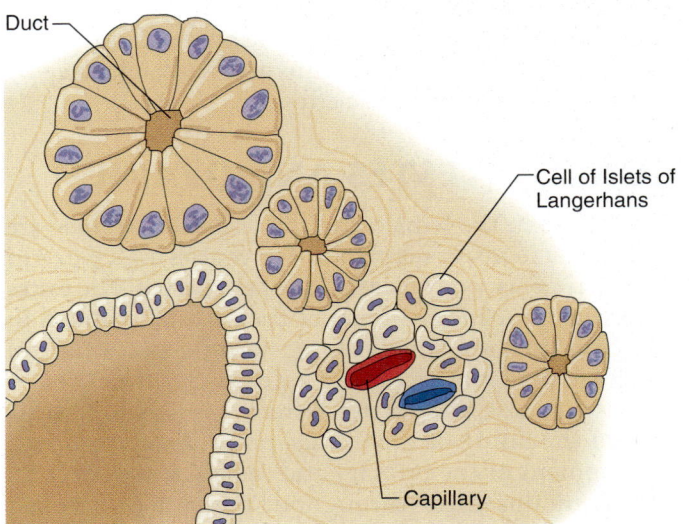

FIGURE 11-196 Pancreatic structure

is excreted in the urine, a finding known as **glycosuria**. Hyperglycemia and glycosuria are the two outstanding characteristics of **diabetes mellitus**.

Type 1 diabetes, also known as juvenile diabetes, is an autoimmune disease that eventually results in severe insulin deficiency. These individuals require insulin replacement to survive. Type 2 diabetics have insulin resistance and are usually overweight. Almost 90% of diabetics are type 2, and their numbers are increasing dramatically due to lifestyles that are associated with inactivity and eating excessive calories. Insulin is also required for the appropriate metabolism of fat and protein.

The other two cell types in islets are delta cells, which contain somatostatin, and pancreatic polypeptide-containing cells, which influence intestinal function.

THYMUS GLAND

The thymus gland is a two-lobed structure located under the sternum. It is composed primarily of lymphoid tissue and is enclosed in a fibrous capsule. The thymus is fairly large during childhood but begins to disappear with the onset of puberty, becoming a small mass of connective tissue and fat in adulthood. It produces active peptides that are involved in T cell maturation, eliminating autoreactive T cells, and selecting T cells that make up the immune system.

PINEAL BODY

The pineal body is a small mass of tissue attached by a slim stalk to the roof of the third ventricle in the brain. The pineal body is believed to produce a substance called melatonin.

This substance plays a role in regulating circadian rhythms. Melatonin levels are highest in the dark and lowest in light. It also has a role in the regulation of the reproductive axis and timing of the onset of puberty. It mainly affects circadian rhythms and regulates sleep by producing a mild hypnotic effect.

GONADS (TESTES AND OVARIES)

The ovaries in the female and the testes in the male are called the **gonads**, or sex glands. The ovaries are located in the pelvic cavity, one on each side of the uterus. The testes are located outside the body of the male, suspended in the scrotum. Both gonads secrete hormones that control the development of secondary sex characteristics.

In the female, the ovaries secrete **estrogen**, which reacts on the lining of the uterus, promotes growth and development of the primary and secondary sex organs, and maintains them throughout adult life. Estrogen also affects the release of other hormones from the pituitary. Another hormone, **progesterone**, is also secreted by the ovaries. It affects the uterine lining and

the development of the secretory portion of the breasts. It aids in maintaining pregnancy.

In the male, the testes produce a hormone known as **testosterone**. This hormone develops the primary male sexual characteristics and the secondary characteristics of a deep voice, muscular development, and body hair distribution. It facilitates maturation of sperm cells.

The gonads are the organs of fertility and reproduction in both sexes. The maturity of the organs and the proper balance of hormonal secretions create the desire for and ability to engage in sexual activity.

See Table 11-17 for a summary of the glands and their functions.

INTERRELATIONSHIP OF THE GLANDS

As stated previously, hormonal secretion is regulated by a feedback mechanism. When the hormone is present or the substance produced by the effect of that hormone on another gland or organ is present, further secretion is affected. For example, the parathyroids increase secretion of parathormone to raise the serum calcium level, taking calcium primarily from the bones. When the serum level rises, a negative feedback message is signaled, and the secretion of parathormone is decreased. A more complicated feedback was described earlier in the control of TSH and the interaction of the hypothalamus, pituitary, and thyroid glands.

In the next unit, the interrelationship of the pituitary and the ovary will be discussed to explain how this complex balance prepares the female for pregnancy.

DIAGNOSTIC EXAMINATIONS

Many diagnostic tests can be performed on blood and urine that either measure the amount of specific hormones present in the body or measure the effectiveness of their function. A few of the more common tests are:

- Blood sugar, frequently measured after fasting (fasting blood sugar, FBS)—To assess the function of the pancreas, including insulin effects
- T_3, TSH, and T_4—To measure the level of the thyroid hormones
- Urine human chorionic gonadotropin (HCG) (pregnancy test)—To measure the presence of a hormone secreted by the placental cells
- Glucose tolerance—To measure the body's ability to process a large dose of glucose. Multiple blood samples are taken at specific intervals following ingestion of the glucose mixture.
- **Glucohemoglobin** (GHB A1c)—A simple blood test that measures how well the glucose level has been controlled over the previous 4 to 6 weeks. The glucose attaches to the hemoglobin of the red blood

TABLE 11-17   ENDOCRINE GLANDS

Gland	Location	Hormone	Principal Effects
Pituitary Anterior lobe	Undersurface of the brain in the sella turcica of the skull	Growth hormone (GH)	Normal growth of body tissues
		Thyroid-stimulating hormone (TSH) (Thyrotropin)	Stimulates growth and activity of thyroid cells to produce and secrete thyroid hormone
		Adrenocorticotropic hormone (ACTH)	Stimulates the cortex of the adrenal gland and the secretion of cortisol
		Melanocyte-stimulating hormone (MSH)	Increases skin pigmentation
		Follicle-stimulating hormone (FSH)	Stimulates the maturity of the graafian follicle to rupture and to produce estrogen in the female. In the male, it stimulates the development of the testes and the production of sperm.
		Luteinizing hormone (LH)	Causes the development of the corpus luteum, which then secretes progesterone in the female. In the male, it stimulates the interstitial cells of the testes to produce testosterone.
		Prolactin (PR)	Develops breast tissue and stimulates secretion of milk from mammary glands
Posterior lobe		Oxytocin	Stimulates contraction of uterus, especially during childbirth; causes ejection of milk from mammary glands
		Vasopressin or antidiuretic hormone (ADH)	Acts on cells of kidney tubules to concentrate urine and conserve fluid in the body; also acts to constrict blood vessels
Thyroid	Lower portion of the anterior neck	Thyroxine (T_4) and triiodothyronine (T_3)	Increase metabolism; influence both physical and mental activity; promote normal growth and development
		Thyrocalcitonin	Causes calcium to be stored in bones; reduces blood level of calcium
Parathyroid	Posterior surface of thyroid gland	Parathormone	Regulates exchange of calcium between the bones and blood and increases blood calcium
Adrenal Medulla	Superior surface of each kidney	Adrenaline (epinephrine)	Increases heart rate, blood pressure, and flow of blood; decreases intestinal activity
Cortex		Aldosterone (mineral corticoid)	Controls electrolyte balances by regulating the reabsorption of sodium and the excretion of potassium
		Glucocorticoids	Affect the metabolism of protein, fat, and glucose, thereby increasing blood sugar; also decrease inflammation
		Sex hormones (androgens)	Govern sex characteristics, especially those that are masculine
Pancreas	Behind the stomach	Insulin	Essential to the metabolism of carbohydrates; reduces the blood sugar level
		Glucagon	Stimulates the liver to release glycogen and convert it to glucose to increase blood sugar levels
Thymus	Under the sternum	Several peptides	React upon lymphoid tissue to produce T lymphocyte cells to regulate immunity
Pineal Body	Third ventricle in the brain	Melatonin	Controls onset of puberty and circadian rhythms
Ovaries	Female pelvis	Estrogen	Promotes growth of primary and secondary sexual characteristics
		Progesterone	Develops excretory portion of mammary glands; aids in maintaining pregnancy
Testes	Male scrotum	Testosterone	Develops primary and secondary sexual characteristics; stimulates maturation of sperm

cells (RBC). A1c is the stable molecule formed when sugar and hemoglobin bind together in the RBC in a process called glycosylation. A1c can be measured. An elevated finding indicates poor glucose control. Measuring A1c reveals a truer picture of blood sugar level control than conventional glucose measurement. If the diabetic patient has not been conforming to diet, except in anticipation of an office visit, the cells will reveal that they have picked up excess sugar.

There are also specific tests measuring hormone levels in the blood to aid in confirming diagnoses, such as:

- ACTH, FSH, growth hormone LH, and TSH—When acromegaly or dwarfism is suspected
- FSH, LH, estrogen, and testosterone—When sex organs fail to develop properly
- ACTH, cortisol—When Cushing's syndrome (chronic excessive glucocorticoids) is suspected
- PTH—When hypoparathyroidism or hyperparathyroidism is suspected

Scanning Tests

The thyroid gland is probably the one most frequently scanned.

- Radioactive iodine uptake test—An oral dose of radioactive iodine is given to the patient. After intervals of 6 and 24 hours, an external detector (scintillation counter) measures the amount of the original dose that is present in the gland. Thyroid function can be determined by the gland's ability to absorb and retain iodine.
- Thyroid scan—The thyroid gland is viewed by a scintiscanner camera following either an oral or IV dose of a radioactive iodine. The scan is indicated by discovery of a palpable nodule or mass, enlarged thyroid gland, or asymmetrical goiter. The camera is capable of photographing the isotopes, which identify the size of the gland, position, and uniformity of absorption. A nodule with poor or no uptake capability shows as a "cold spot," suggesting a possible malignancy. A "hot spot" indicates a hyperfunctioning nodule, possibly a toxic nodular goiter. A total gland picture that shows little uptake is indicative of hypothyroidism; an enlarged gland showing uniformly increased uptake is indicative of hyperthyroidism.
- Ultrasound—Valuable in assessing thyroid size and nodules

DISEASES AND DISORDERS

Acromegaly (Akro-meg'a-le)

Description—This is an uncommon hormonal disorder that occurs when the pituitary gland produces excess growth hormone during adulthood, resulting in

the characteristic changes of overgrowth of connective tissue. The occurrence of acromegaly is about 6 in every 100,000 adults.

Signs and symptoms—The symptoms develop gradually. There is enlargement of the hands, feet, and prominent facial features such as protruding lower jaw and brow, enlarged nose, thickened lips, and teeth that tend to separate. Patients may also complain of headaches and loss of peripheral vision due to an enlarging pituitary tumor.

Etiology—This condition results from the excessive production of growth hormone and is almost always due to a pituitary tumor. An MRI or CT scan can determine the location and size of the tumor.

Treatment—A surgical procedure known as transsphenoidal resection is the treatment of choice. The surgeon goes through the nose and sphenoid sinus to extract the tumor through a scope, unless the tumor is too large. Medications such as Sandostatin and bromocriptine can be used occasionally to decrease the growth hormone secretion. Radiation may also be necessary to destroy any remaining tumor cells.

The man in Figure 11-197 was diagnosed in 1970 when he was in his twenties. His original complaints were a change in his facial appearance, enlarging

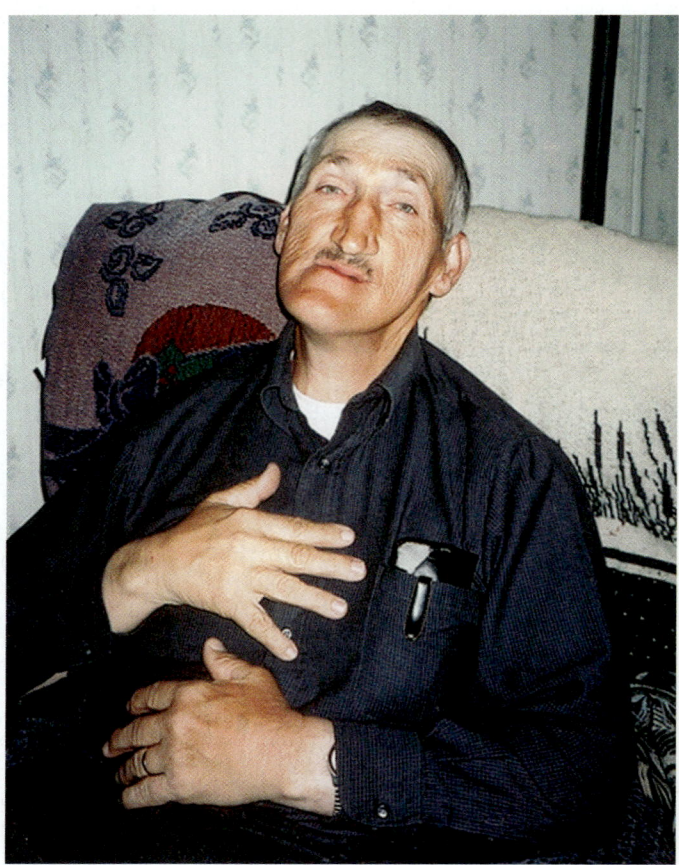

FIGURE 11-197 Male with acromegaly

hands, no energy, headaches, and vision sensitivity to sun or snow. He later developed color blindness. He also noticed his skin became oily and he perspired excessively. A pituitary tumor was discovered and later resected, but a small piece was apparently missed. He had continuing elevated hormone levels and after 3 years received radiation therapy. After surgery and radiation, he noticed a significant change in the size of his hands, reducing by four ring sizes. He has recently developed severe arthritis in his back, hands, and lower extremities, but he attempts to walk 2 to 3 miles a day despite the discomfort and fatigue. He takes prednisone and synthroid medication daily. The main characteristics of acromegaly are evident in the photo.

Addison's Disease

Description—This condition results from a deficiency of adrenal hormones from the cortex of the adrenal gland. This causes significant metabolic changes that can result in serious illness and even death.

Signs and symptoms—Patients gradually develop a pigmented appearance of the skin due to excessive ACTH and melanocyte-stimulating hormone secretion from the pituitary due to low adrenal hormone concentrations in the blood. Weakness, low blood pressure, tiredness, and salt craving are prominent symptoms. The lack of cortisol (a glucocortocoid) and aldosterone (a mineralocorticoid) impairs normal metabolism of proteins and carbohydrates. Electrolyte disturbances, namely a low serum sodium level and high serum potassium, also occur.

Etiology—The most common cause of adrenal insufficiency is autoimmune destruction of the cells producing the hormones. Other causes include infections such as tuberculosis, histoplasmosis, and meningococcemia; hemorrhage into the adrenal glands; and metastasis of malignant tumors.

Treatment—Hormone replacement therapy with hydrocortisone or prednisone and the mineralocorticoid florinef results in a positive outcome. Lifetime treatment is needed, and larger doses are given in stressful situations such as infections or surgery.

Cretinism (Kre'tin-izm)

Description—This is an endocrine disorder of the thyroid gland that has physical and mental ramifications.

Signs and symptoms—**Cretinism** is characterized by lack of mental and physical growth, resulting in mental retardation and a characteristic dwarflike appearance (Figure 11-198).

Etiology—This condition results from a serious lack of the thyroid hormone thyroxine beginning in the early stages of life.

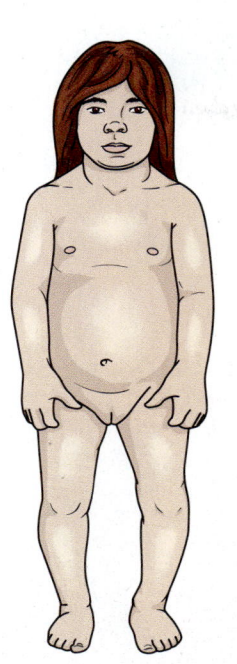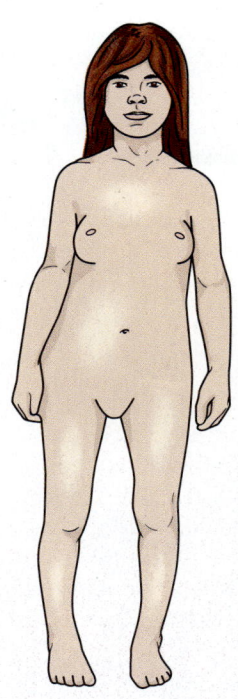

FIGURE 11-198 (Left) Cretinism of a 16-year-old female caused by lack of thyroid hormone; (Right) same female after 2 years of treatment with thyroid extract

Treatment—If thyroid replacement is initiated early enough, normal development may be achieved, but once cretinism has developed, total normal development is not possible. An infant born without thyroid hormones of its own must be treated within a few weeks to prevent irreversible mental retardation.

Cushing's Syndrome (Koosh'ings)

Description—This is an endocrine disorder of the adrenal glands that has physical and physiologic effects.

Signs and symptoms—Symptoms include hypertension, obesity, weakness of the muscles, and a tendency to develop bruises. Typical characteristics result from the rapid deposit of body fat: a deposit of fat between the shoulders, referred to as "buffalo hump," and a rounded face referred to as "moon face." Purple streaks called striae (stretch marks) develop in the skin. The trunk becomes obese, yet the arms and legs are slender.

The excess amount of glucocorticoids, which metabolize protein into glucogen and then into glucose, results in a "steroid diabetes" with hyperglycemia and glucosuria. The urinary system is affected by the hormone imbalance and excretes excessive amounts of potassium, which results in hypokalemia. The lack of potassium results in muscular weakness. Muscle mass slowly wastes away. The decreasing amount of bone structure results in pathologic fractures.

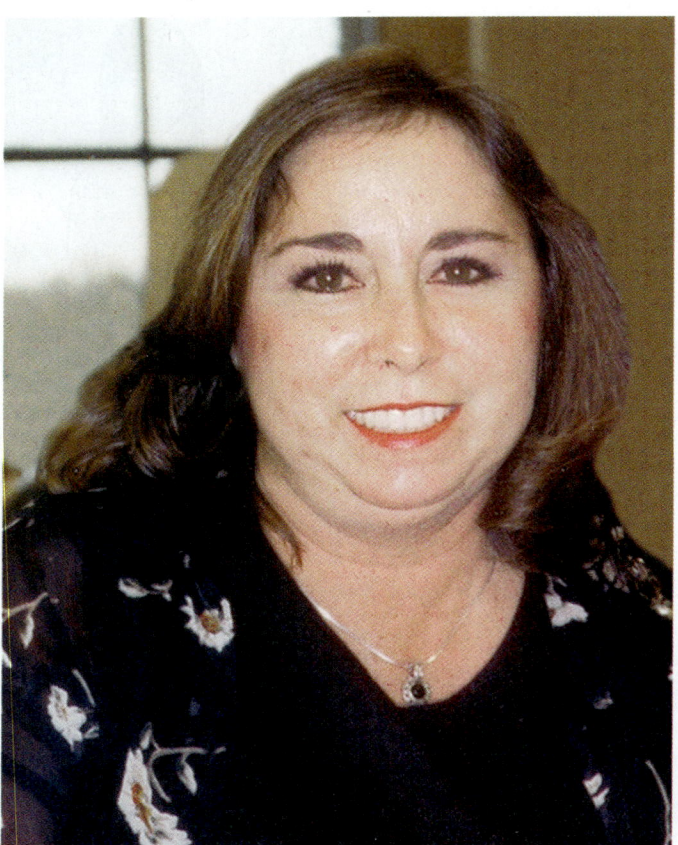

FIGURE 11-199A Female with Cushing's disease

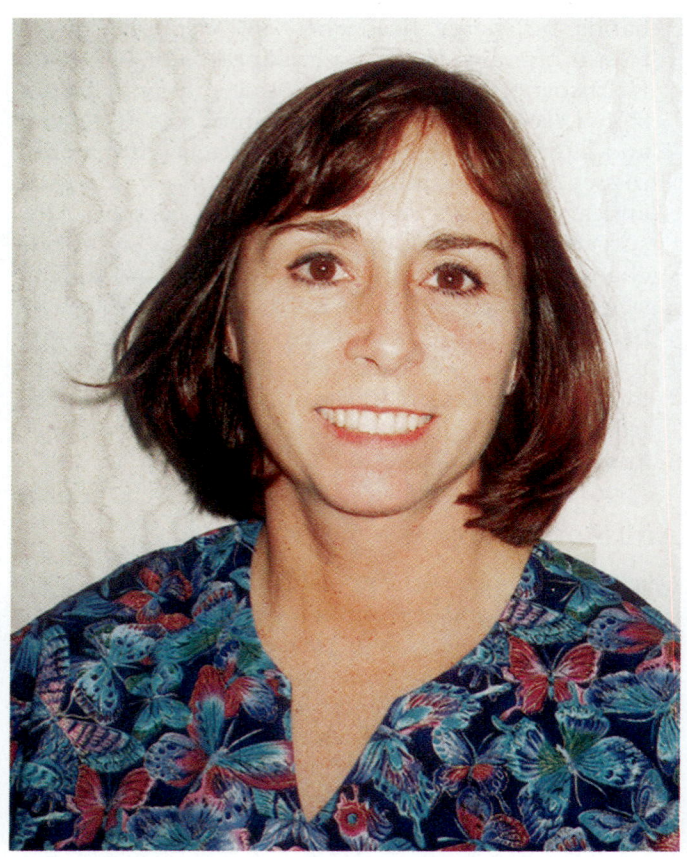

FIGURE 11-199B Female with Cushing's disease, after surgery

Etiology—This disorder is characterized by a group of symptoms that result from the hypersecretion of glucocorticoids from the adrenal cortex caused by excess ACTH production. **Cushing's syndrome** may also be directly related to a tumor of the cortex of the adrenal gland or long-term steroid treatment for a variety of diseases.

Treatment—Treatment is related to the underlying cause. If there is an adrenal tumor, then the adrenal gland must be removed. If both adrenals are removed, replacement steroid therapy must be instituted. If the adrenals are being stimulated because of a pituitary tumor, then the pituitary gland or adenoma must be irradiated or removed. Afterward hormone therapy would be required to replace the pituitary's secretions.

The woman in Figures 11-199A and B was diagnosed with Cushing's disease in 2003. She is a nurse and experienced difficulty convincing physicians that "something was wrong with her." Her 45-pound weight gain and "buffalo hump" were dismissed as too much food and not enough exercise. She also had a blood pressure of 176/100, acne, excessive perspiration, and weakness and was growing facial hair. At her insistence, diagnostic and radiologic tests were performed; they indicated excess ACTH and the presence of a microadenoma of the pituitary. The tumor was removed by transphenoidal resection and proved to be benign. As you can see, 18 months after surgery, her appearance had returned to normal, and her other symptoms had subsided.

Diabetes Mellitus (Dia-be'tez Mell'i-tus)

Description—A chronic disease of insulin deficiency or resistance, diabetes mellitus interferes with the metabolism of carbohydrates, proteins, and fats. Insulin in the blood facilitates the transfer of glucose into the cell to be used for energy or stored as glycogen. It also stimulates the formation of proteins and free fatty acid storage. Without sufficient insulin being secreted by the pancreas, the body's tissues do not have access to essential nutrients for fuel or storage.

Diabetes mellitus affects an estimated 7% of the United States population or over 20 million people. The prevalence of diabetes has increased greatly in the past decade, and more children and teenagers are being diagnosed with both Type 1 (insulin requiring) and Type 2 diabetes. The reasons are multifactorial, but increasing numbers of obese individuals and inactivity are common risk factors. There are many long-term effects of diabetes. Diabetes is the leading cause of new cases of blindness, end-stage kidney disease, and lower limb amputation in the United States. It develops more often in people who are older than 40, and have a family history of diabetes, or are of African-American, Hispanic, or Native-American descent. It more than doubles the risk for stroke and heart disease. The disease also interferes with resistance to organisms, which may result in skin and bladder infections. Diabetic retinopathy results from microvascular changes in the retina of the eye, especially in poorly controlled diabetics. In patients who have had diabetes for 20 or more years, 80% develop retinopathy.

How Insulin Works   Insulin is the hormone made in the pancreas and released into the bloodstream as glucose rises. It helps sugar to enter the body's cells, where it is used as fuel for the cell's activities (Figure 11-200). When the sugar level rises, the pancreas secretes more insulin so that the larger amount of sugar can move out of the blood and into the cells. When the sugar level falls too low, insulin secretion is greatly reduced and the hormone glucagon is released. This causes the liver to release stored glycogen into the blood.

To completely understand the role of insulin, we need to consider a basic fact of life. All living organisms are programmed to withstand cycles of feast and famine and have developed ways of storing energy for lean times. In humans and most animals, it is insulin that allows us to store glucose, protein, and fat in the liver, fat and muscle cells until it is needed. Our bodies are programmed to store glucose and fat that produce excess weight and obesity when excessive calories are consumed, which leads to diabetes and numerous other illnesses. In the United States, obesity is at alarming incidence rates not only for adults but also for children. There is much concern about the future health of our population.

There are two forms of diabetes: a Type 1 DM, or insulin-dependent diabetes mellitus, and a Type 2 DM, noninsulin-dependent diabetes mellitus, often called adult-onset form. Type 1 DM tends to afflict children and young people, and insulin replacement is necessary for survival.

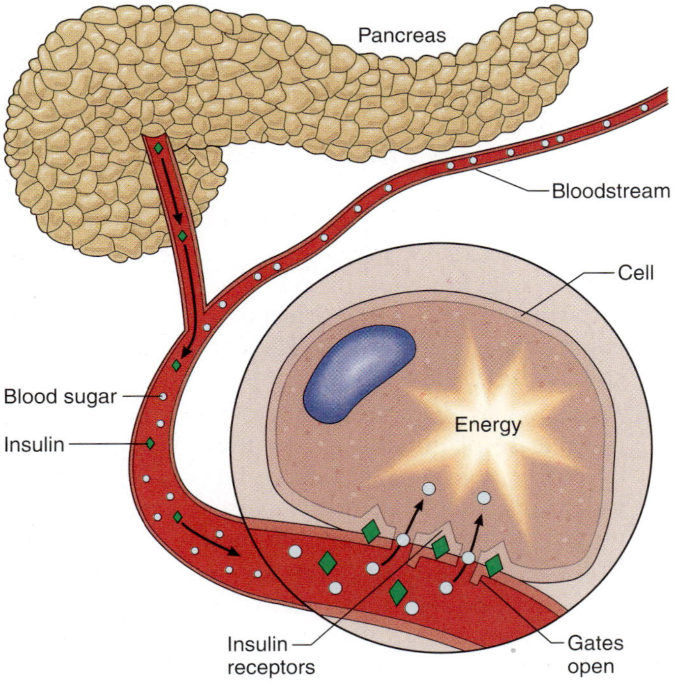

FIGURE 11-200   How insulin works. Insulin is excreted by the pancreas into the blood. It circulates to an insulin receptor on the membrane of a cell. When it binds to the receptor, a signal is sent, and the gates in the cell wall open, allowing blood sugar to enter the cell to be converted to energy.

P PEDIATRIC PERSPECTIVE

Type 1 Diabetes Mellitus (Type 1 DM)

Etiology—Type 1 diabetes can be considered a genetic disease. It is an autoimmune disorder that attacks the cells of the pancreas known as the islets of Langerhans.

Signs and symptoms—The diagnosis of diabetes in childhood is usually straightforward. The parents report an increased thirst, increased urination, and weight loss. The child will appear to be dehydrated and may have a sweet odor to the breath from the ketones (a by-product of fatty acids). A urinalysis will generally reveal a large amount of ketones and is positive for glucose.

Treatment—A child with newly diagnosed Type 1 DM will be admitted to the hospital for stabilization and treatment. Insulin injections or intravenous insulin are required for initial management. During hospitalization, the parents, caregivers, and the child (if of appropriate age) are taught to administer the insulin injections. Commonly, several types of insulin (short-acting, intermediate, and long-acting) will be used to control the elevated blood sugar and complications with childhood diabetes.

Signs and symptoms—Signs and symptoms of diabetes include fatigue and the three *P*s; polyuria, polyphegia, and polydipsea. The elevated glucose level in the blood causes fluid to be withdrawn from the body's tissues. The excess fluid in the blood causes polyuria and dehydration of the cells. The diabetic patient is frequently thirsty and has dry mucous membranes. The lens of the eye becomes affected by the hyperglycemia and edema, which results in visual difficulties. Characteristically, glycosuria is present when the threshold is exceeded to reabsorb glucose (about 180 mg per dL); the excess glucose spills over into urine. This wasting of sugar causes the weight loss and hunger of the Type 1 DM patient.

Etiology—Type 2 DM is the most common form, usually starting from insulin resistance. This is a complex problem arising from the reduced effectiveness of insulin to deliver glucose into the cell. The blood sugar level rises, and to add to the problem, the liver produces more sugar and often releases lipoproteins full of triglycerides that may increase LDL cholesterol and decrease HDL cholesterol. Insulin resistance can also result from genetics, aging, and some medications, but being overweight and lack of exercise are the main nongenetic factors. About 90% of all newly diagnosed diabetics are overweight. Some of the hormones secreted by fat cells, for example resistin, interfere with insulin action. The role of fat cells is being studied specifically because obesity is so often associated with the disease.

In addition to resistance, other factors exist. The pancreas compensates by secreting more insulin. Eventually, the insulin-producing cells can no longer keep up, and glucose builds up in the blood. Over time, this high level of sugar damages blood vessels, nerves, and other body tissues. It also causes a vicious cycle of increasing resistance and further exhausts the pancreas.

Treatment—Treatment begins with a strict diet, planned to meet the nutritional needs of the individual patient and to control the blood sugar level. Diet can have a significant impact on controlling blood sugar and diabetes. Losing as little as 10 pounds will reduce blood sugar levels. A recent study determined that a high-fiber diet lowered blood sugar levels by 10%, a comparable figure to the effect of some medications. Exercise may be the most important intervention. It not only increases glucose metabolism, but it also increases insulin sensitivity, which causes fat and muscle cells to better respond to insulin. Diet and exercise can have a significant effect in preventing diabetes, but as a treatment, they can only go so far. In most people, the problem of insulin production and insulin resistance tend to worsen despite weight loss, diet, and exercise. When diet alone is inadequate, insulin injections or the use of oral hypoglycemic drugs are indicated. Injections may be necessary initially once a day, using a long-acting insulin; when control is more difficult, a short-acting insulin, injected at specific times, may be used. Diabetic patients are taught to evaluate their glucose level by performing a finger stick for blood analysis. The amount of insulin injected is based on the findings. Hypoglycemic drugs are taken orally to aid in the metabolism of sugar. Oral therapy is adequate only for Type 2 DM patients.

The drugs used today address insulin resistance and secretion to reduce blood sugar levels. Physicians are using more drugs and using them more aggressively. Drugs can be categorized according to their actions (see the following).

Increasing Insulin Supplies

1. *Sulfonylureas* stimulate beta cells to release more insulin. This works for a while but then may become ineffective. These drugs can work too well, causing hypoglycemia that can be dangerous for older patients because it causes fainting, falls, and fractures.

2. *Rapid-acting insulin stimulators* are similar to sulfonylureas but faster. They are of short duration and are less apt to cause hypoglycemia. Two drugs in this class are Prandin and Starlix.

3. *Injection of insulin* subcutaneously is the ultimate method of overriding pancreatic dysfunction. Type 1 diabetics who lack insulin are dependent on injections. Patients with Type 2 diabetes often can control their disease with diet, exercise, and medications, but if that fails, insulin is the most potent and effective therapy. They usually require higher doses because of the need to overcome resistance. A form of insulin that can be inhaled is being developed. Initial trials have yielded promising results.

Lowering Blood Sugar by Other Means

1. *Alpha-glucosidase inhibitors* block the action of a digestive enzyme that breaks down carbohydrates into smaller sugars. The effect is to moderate blood sugar surges after a meal. The drug is weaker than some others but very safe.

2. *Biguanides* work to lower sugar levels by blocking the release of glucose by the liver. The only drug currently approved is Glucophage, and it works well in overweight people because it does not cause weight gain or risk of hypoglycemia.

3. Thiazolidinediones (TZD) reduces insulin resistance by modulating activity of nuclear transcription factors. They show promise in improving the lipid profiles and other metabolic factors.

Multi-Drug Approach
More physicians are using a multi-drug approach to management. Previously, they would do one thing at a time: diet and exercise, then drug after drug until ineffective, and then insulin.

However, this method of control was successful in a minority of the patients. By using drug combinations, lower doses of each are effective, and therefore fewer side effects occur. This approach better addresses the new view of diabetes as a syndrome instead of a simple disease of high blood sugar.

A common drug combination is metformin and sulfonylurea. Clinical trial with metformin-T2D combination showed improved effectiveness in control of blood sugar, insulin sensitivity, and islet cell function. When insulin becomes necessary, combining it with oral medications may mean a lower dose of insulin is needed.

Future Treatments

It is hoped that the human genome project will reveal new information on diabetes and its treatment, but researchers realize this will take some time to determine. Some researchers are focusing on preventing the complications associated with diabetes, such as atherosclerosis; others focus on therapies directed at fat cells. Pancreatic and islet transplantations show encouraging promise.

A study also revealed that the simple action of taking an aspirin a day is a very effective health strategy for diabetics and would help those with cardiovascular involvements. Controlling blood pressure and lowering LDL are crucial even if there is no evidence of coronary disease.

Maintaining Health

The glucose level of the blood can be affected by circumstances other than food or insulin. For example, the diabetic requires either less insulin or more food when engaging in a high level of physical activity. Adjustments are also required with illness. A patient who has diarrhea or vomiting may require less insulin. Pregnancy, the use of contraceptives, a fever, and periods of stress all influence the diabetic's need for supplemental insulin or oral hypoglycemic therapy.

Specific symptoms indicate whether the blood sugar is too high or too low. A diabetic must be aware of her physical condition at all times. Should the blood sugar level become significantly low, she may enter into insulin shock; if it goes very high, there is a possibility of a diabetic coma. Both situations require urgent attention. When patients sense impending shock, they will drink orange juice or eat a piece of candy immediately. A patient going into coma needs an urgent blood sugar measurement and injections of insulin. Figure 11-201 illustrates the contrasting symptoms of shock and coma. Become familiar with the signs and be prepared to act.

Diabetic patients must be encouraged to maintain their optimal level of health. They must guard against injury, especially to the lower extremities, because of difficulty healing. They must use extreme caution when cutting toenails and must never try to remove corns or calluses themselves. Diabetics frequently suffer amputations as a result of infection from an injury that would not heal or from the loss of peripheral circulation, which causes tissue ischemia.

Patients should be encouraged to visit an ophthalmologist at least yearly to detect the possibility of retinal changes. Blindness may result from uncontrolled diabetes. The physician must be alert to signs of cardiovascular complications and urinary tract involvement. Cerebral vascular disease, coronary artery disease, and renal failure resulting from vascular deterioration in the kidney are common.

Graves' Disease

Description—This condition is the most common form of hyperthyroidism.

Signs and symptoms—The thyroid gland enlarges and the patient becomes nervous; has an intolerance to heat; loses weight; sweats; and may have diarrhea, tremors, and palpitations. The increased thyroxine may also cause difficulty in concentrating because of the accelerated cerebral functioning. Mood swings and emotional instability may occur. The cardiovascular system is also affected in the form of tachycardia, increased cardiac output, cardiomegaly, and possibly atrial fibrillation (especially in the elderly). The patient may experience dyspnea and an array of musculoskeletal symptoms ranging from weakness and fatigue to localized or generalized paralysis. The dominant feature of exophthalmus may also be present. The woman in Figure 11-202A was diagnosed with Graves' disease in her early 20s. She experienced weak pelvic muscles, dissociation of thoughts, rapid heart rate, and an intolerance to heat. She also had the traditional exopthalmia and an enlarged thyroid gland. (Enlargement is noticeable in the photo). She was treated with propylthiouracil for 1 year, and the thyroid gland was later ablated with radioactive iodine. After about 6 years, she had bilateral orbital decompression to allow fluid to drain from behind the eyes, which permitted them to recess into the bony sockets (Figure 11-202B).

The patient may become seriously ill if the hyperthyroidism escalates into a thyroid storm. The symptoms persist and others develop, such as hypertension, extreme irritability, vomiting, high fever, delirium, and eventually coma.

Etiology—Graves' disease results from an increase in the production of thyroxine that may be caused by a genetic susceptibility to autoimmune factors. The production of autoantibodies arise from a defect in suppressor T lymphocyte function that allows other T cells to make autoantibodies.

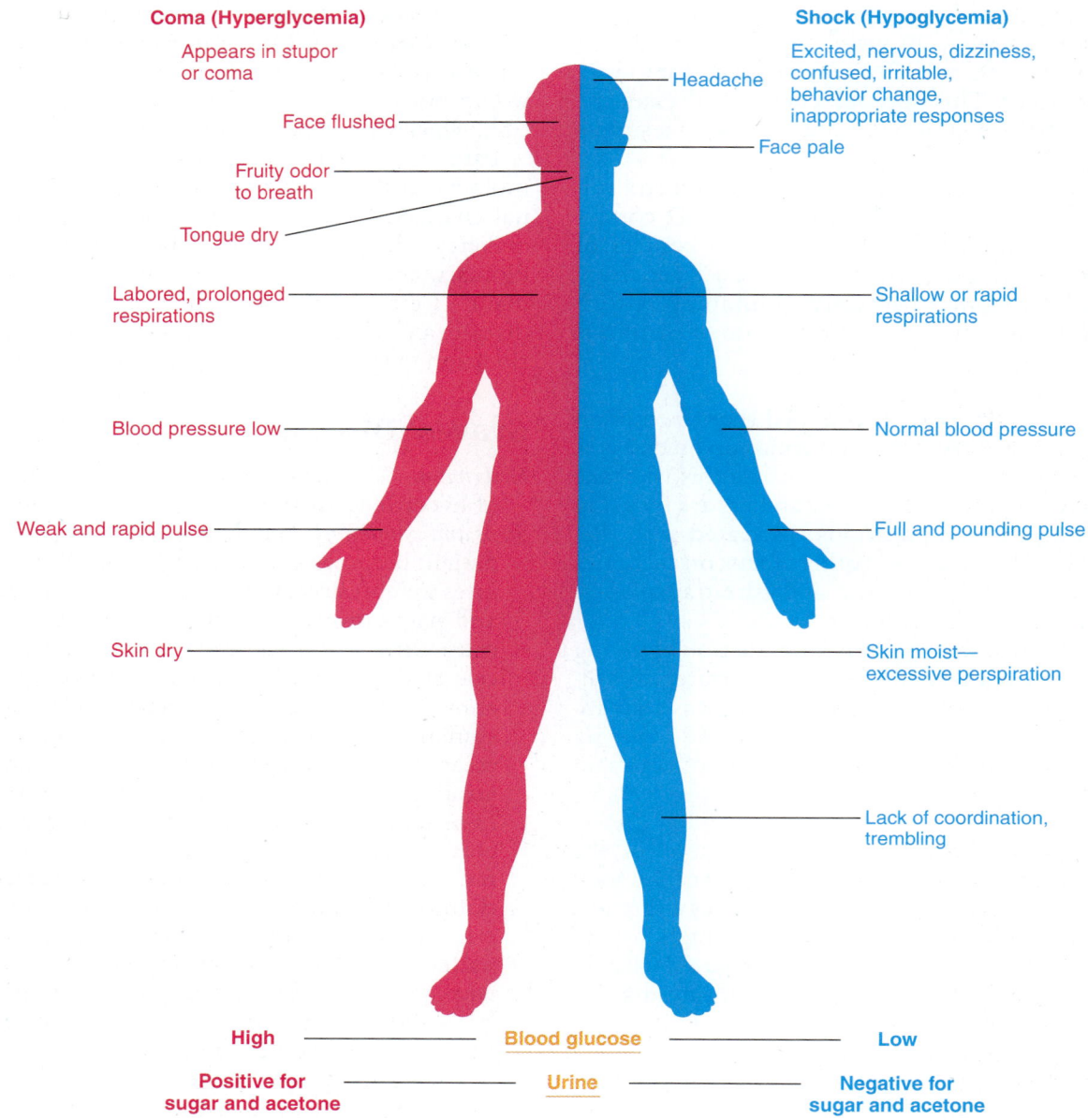

Coma (Hyperglycemia)

Appears in stupor or coma

Face flushed

Fruity odor to breath

Tongue dry

Labored, prolonged respirations

Blood pressure low

Weak and rapid pulse

Skin dry

Shock (Hypoglycemia)

Excited, nervous, dizziness, confused, irritable, behavior change, inappropriate responses

Headache

Face pale

Shallow or rapid respirations

Normal blood pressure

Full and pounding pulse

Skin moist— excessive perspiration

Lack of coordination, trembling

High — Blood glucose — Low

Positive for sugar and acetone — Urine — Negative for sugar and acetone

FIGURE 11-201 Diabetic coma (hyperglycemia) versus insulin shock (hypoglycemia)

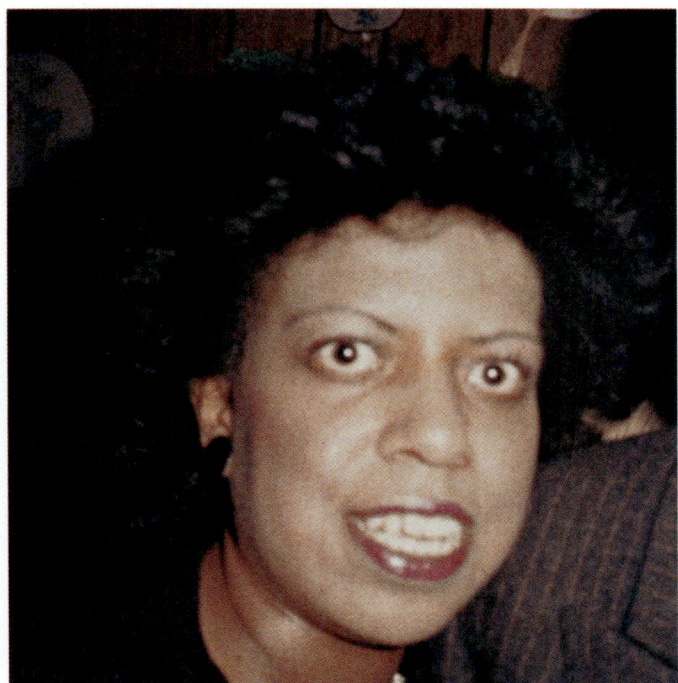

FIGURE 11-202A   Female with Graves' disease

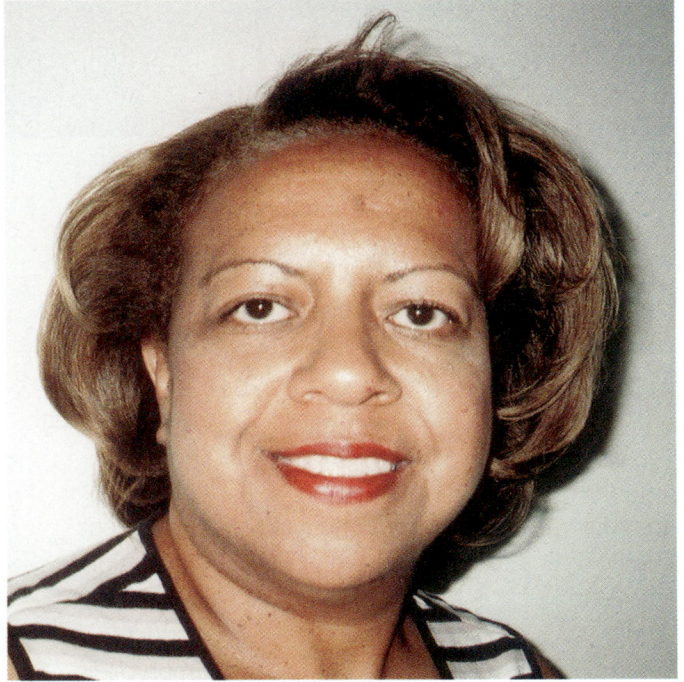

FIGURE 11-202B   Female with Graves' disease, after treatment and surgery

Treatment—A common treatment is the use of antithyroid drugs that block the formation of thyroid hormone. Some patients are candidates for an oral dose of radioactive iodine that concentrates in the thyroid, destroying some cells and reducing the size of the thyroid gland. In addition, a portion or all of the gland can be removed surgically to reduce or eliminate the hormone.

Myxedema (Miks-e-de'ma) (Hypothyroidism)

Description—This is an endocrine disorder of the thyroid gland that is associated with too little thyroid hormone.

Signs and symptoms—Clinically, **myxedema's** characteristics are in relation to the degree of hypothyroidism. If it is mild, the patient will probably complain of forgetfulness, dry skin, and an intolerance for cold. With more severe myxedema, the decreased metabolism causes a marked intolerance for cold and weight gain. Motor function and reflex actions are slowed. The voice becomes low and husky. A characteristic yellowish discoloration of the skin, called *carotenemia*, results from reduction in the conversion of carotene to vitamin A. Levels of cholesterol are increased and may also produce atherosclerosis. Because cardiac function is depressed, the myocardium becomes enlarged and weak. Protein and certain electrolytes accumulate in the tissue spaces, causing edema. Myxedema patients have a characteristic drowsy appearance, with puffiness about the eyes. There is a marked degree of fatigue and weakness. The temperature, pulse, respiration, and blood pressure are all below normal.

Etiology—This condition is caused by a hyposecretion of the thyroid gland. It varies in significance in relation to the amount of secretion. Hashimoto's thyroiditis is a common cause of goiter and hypothyroidism.

Treatment—Treatment consists primarily of thyroid hormone replacement to a level necessary to maintain normal balance.

Hormonal Balance

Diagnosing, treating, and maintaining hormonal balance in patients with endocrine gland malfunctions is a challenging endeavor because of the hormone interactions. For example, what may appear to be a simple overproduction by the thyroid may actually be a pituitary malfunction, a failed hypothalamus, or an inhibitor that did not cause the pituitary to stop secreting a thyroid stimulant. Many possibilities must be considered to explain the symptoms presented by a patient with endocrine dysfunction.

UNIT 13

THE REPRODUCTIVE SYSTEM

OBJECTIVES

Upon completion of this unit, you will be able to achieve the following:

LEARNING Objectives

1. Spell and define, using the glossary at the back of the text, all the Words to Know in this unit.
2. Differentiate between sexual and asexual reproduction.
3. Describe the differentiation of reproductive organs.
4. Explain how sperm are able to fertilize an egg.
5. Describe male prenatal development.
6. Name the male sex organs, and describe their location and function.
7. Explain how pituitary hormones affect the functions of the testes.
8. Identify the male secondary sex characteristics.
9. Trace the pathway of sperm from production to expulsion.
10. Name the components of semen.
11. Describe four diseases and disorders of the male reproductive system.
12. Name the female sex organs, and describe their location and function.
13. Explain the interaction of pituitary hormones with the ovaries and other organs.
14. Identify the female secondary sex characteristics.
15. Describe the maturation and release of an ovum.
16. Compare the internal and external sexual organs of the male and female.
17. Describe the phases of the menstrual cycle and the purpose of menstruation.
18. Explain how fertilization occurs.
19. Describe the events occurring during each trimester of pregnancy as they relate to the woman and the embryo or fetus.
20. Describe the events that occur in the three stages of labor.
21. List the reasons for practicing contraception.
22. Identify the contraceptive methods, stating their relative effectiveness.
23. Describe the diagnostic tests of the female reproductive system.
24. Describe the diseases or disorders of the female reproductive system.
25. Identify the characteristics of the sexually transmitted diseases.

WORDS TO KNOW

ablation	bulbourethral	cryptorchidism
abortion	glands	dilation and
alpha-fetoprotein	cervix	curettage
screening	cesarean	dysmenorrhea
(AFP)	chlamydia	dysplasia
amniocentesis	circumcision	ectopic
amniotic	clitoris	effacement
anteflexed	coitus	ejaculation
anteverted	colposcopy	ejaculatory
areola	conceive	duct
Bartholin's	conception	embryo
glands	contraception	endometrium
benign	contraction	epididymis
hypertrophy	corpus luteum	episiotomy

erectile
erectile
  dysfunction
fallopian tubes
fertilization
fetus
fibroid
foreskin
gamete
genital herpes
genitalia
gonorrhea
graafian follicle
gynecology
hydrocele
hymen
hysterectomy
hysteroscopy
impotence
inguinal canal
inguinal hernia
interventional
  hysterosal-
  pingography
labia majora

labia minora
ligation
mammary
  glands
mammogram
mastectomy
menarche
menopause
menorrhagia
menstruation
moniliasis
mons pubis
myometrium
nonspecific
  urethritis
os
ovulation
ovum
Papanicolaou
  (Pap) smear
penis
perineum
phimosis
placenta
pregnancy

prolapse
prostate
prostatectomy
rectocele
reproductive
retroflexed
retroverted
salpingo-
  oophorectomy
scrotum
semen
sperm
spermatozoan
syphilis
transurethral
trichomoniasis
trimester
uterus
vagina
vaginitis
vas deferens
vasectomy
vulva
womb
zygote

Sexual methods of reproduction are found in multi-celled forms of life, including humans. The methods may vary but certain characteristics are common to all. In each species, there are sexes, namely a male and a female. Each sex has special sex glands, or gonads, which produce sex cells (**gametes**). In humans, the union of the male gamete (a **spermatozoan**) with the female gamete (an **ovum**) forms a new one-celled structure called a **zygote**. The zygote then undergoes mitosis repeatedly to form a new individual.

In Unit 1, the cell was described as having 46 chromosomes, or 23 pairs. Each chromosome has a partner of the same shape and size. One pair of chromosomes are the sex chromosomes. In the female, both chromosomes in the pair are X chromosomes, but in the male, one is an X and one is a Y. When the gonads produce the ovum and spermatozoan cells, the number of chromosomes is reduced to 23 (one half). When the two cells unite as fertilization occurs, the new cell, a zygote, will again have 46 chromosomes. If the spermatozoan carries an X chromosome, the embryo will develop female characteristics. If it carries a Y chromosome, the embryo will develop as a male.

The reproductive organs are the only organs in the human body that differ between the male and female, yet there is still a significant similarity. This likeness results from the fact that male and female organs develop from the same group of embryonic cells. For approximately 2 months, the embryo develops without sexual identity. Then the influence of the X or Y chromosome begins to make a differentiation.

CERTIFICATION CONNECTION

CMA
Diagnostic procedures
Common diseases and
  pathology
Anatomy and physiology

CMAS
Anatomy and physiology

RMA
Anatomy and physiology

The **reproductive** system consists of the organs that are capable of accomplishing reproduction, the creation of a new individual. All living organisms reproduce, some very simply by an asexual method or without the need of sexual contact. An example of asexual reproduction is one of the simplest forms of life, a single cell. In binary fusion, a cell divides into two cells by simple cleavage. In mitosis, a single cell rearranges its chromatin into chromosomes and then divides into two cells (the method by which human cells reproduce). Both methods require that the "parents" become the "children"; therefore both parent and child cannot exist at the same time.

DIFFERENTIATION OF REPRODUCTIVE ORGANS

The gonads of the embryo begin to evolve into the sexual organs of the female at about the 10th or 11th week of pregnancy. The ovaries of the embryo develop high in its abdomen from the same type of tissue as the testes. However, the testes evolve from the medulla of the gonad, whereas the ovaries develop from the cortex. Figure 11-203 illustrates how the undifferentiated external **genitalia** develop into fully differentiated structures. In the male, the tubercle becomes the glans **penis**, the folds become the penile shaft, and the swelling develops into the **scrotum**. In the female, the tubercle becomes the **clitoris**, the folds the **labia minora**, and the swelling the **labia majora**.

Internally, there is also a similarity of structures. The embryonic müllerian ducts degenerate, and the wolffian ducts become the **epididymis**, **vas deferens**, and **ejaculatory duct** in the male. In the female, the wolffian ducts degenerate, and the müllerian ducts develop into the **fallopian tubes**, the **uterus**, and the upper portion of

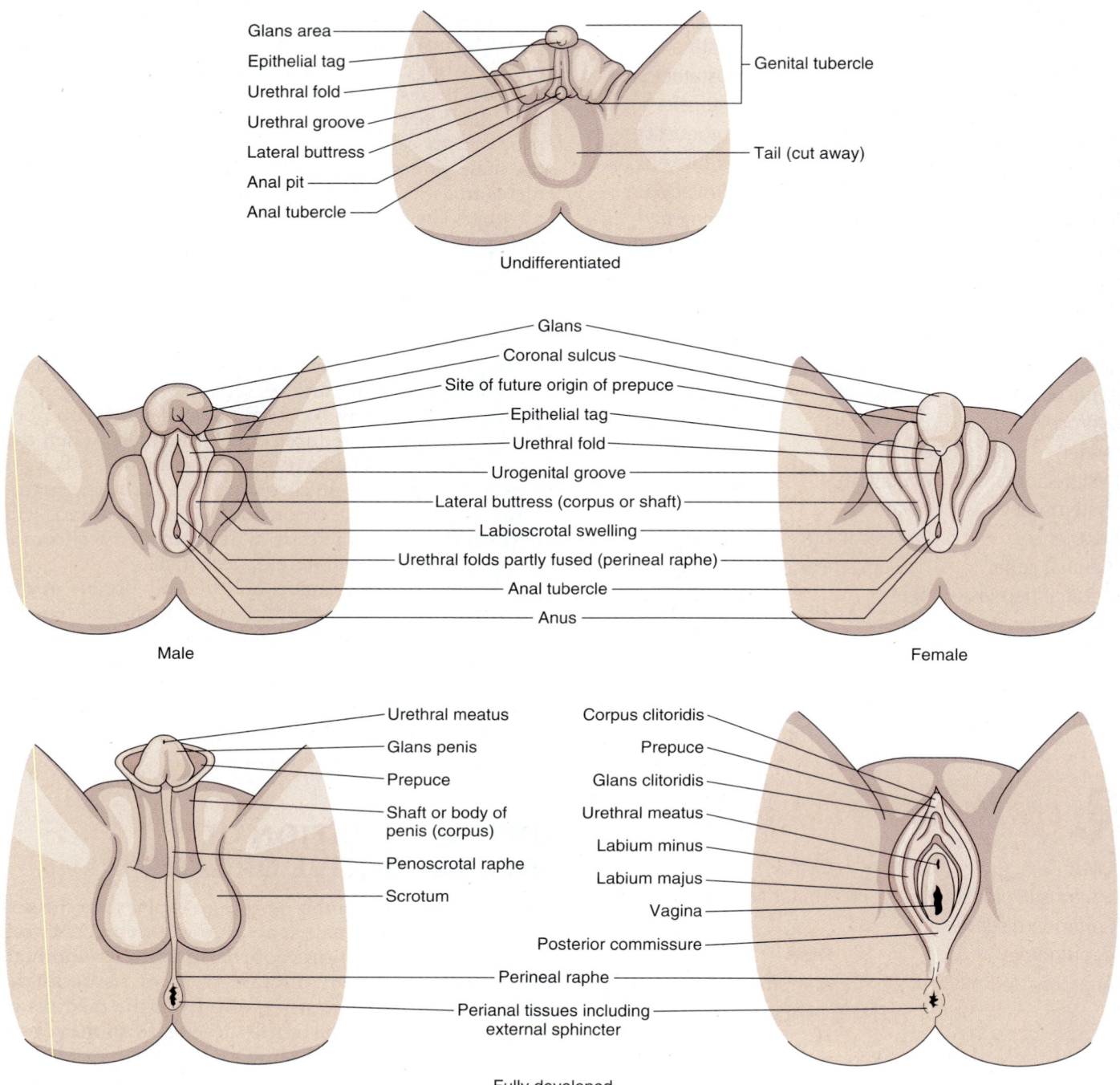

Glans area
Epithelial tag
Urethral fold
Urethral groove
Lateral buttress
Anal pit
Anal tubercle
Genital tubercle
Tail (cut away)
Undifferentiated

Glans
Coronal sulcus
Site of future origin of prepuce
Epithelial tag
Urethral fold
Urogenital groove
Lateral buttress (corpus or shaft)
Labioscrotal swelling
Urethral folds partly fused (perineal raphe)
Anal tubercle
Anus
Male
Female

Urethral meatus
Glans penis
Prepuce
Shaft or body of penis (corpus)
Penoscrotal raphe
Scrotum

Corpus clitoridis
Prepuce
Glans clitoridis
Urethral meatus
Labium minus
Labium majus
Vagina
Posterior commissure
Perineal raphe
Perianal tissues including external sphincter

Fully developed

FIGURE 11-203 Sexual differentiation before birth

the **vagina**. It is believed that the presence of the testes in the male is the differentiating factor in the development. Without the androgens (male hormones) from the testes, a female develops. With the androgens, a male develops. Another substance called the müllerian inhibitor works in partnership with the androgens to produce the sex differentiation.

MALE REPRODUCTIVE ORGANS

When the zygote contains a Y chromosome, a male child will develop. About the 7th or 8th week of pregnancy, the testes begin to develop within the abdominal cavity at about the level of the ileum of the pelvis bone. The sex of the fetus is evident by about the 4th month.

During the 8th and 9th months of pregnancy, the testes move from the abdomen through the **inguinal canal** into the external pouch called the scrotum (Figure 11-204). After the testes pass, the canal closes to prevent the descent of other structures into the scrotum or the return of the testes into the abdomen. When a loop of small intestine descends through the canal because of improper closure or later in life because of relaxed inguinal structures, it is known as an **inguinal hernia** (Figure 11-205).

If the testes fail to descend or if they return to the abdomen, a condition known as undescended testicle (unilateral or bilateral) exists, which must be corrected or sterility will result. An undescended testicle is known medically as **cryptorchidism**. The testes normally produce **sperm**, but sperm cannot be produced or survive in the internal heat of the body. It is this characteristic that necessitates their location outside the body.

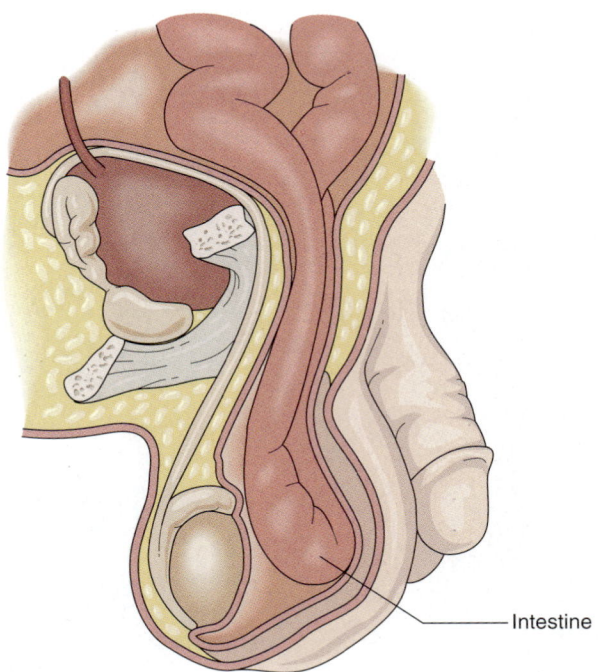

FIGURE 11-205   Inguinal hernia

Intestine

PEDIATRIC PERSPECTIVE

When testes do not descend spontaneously by age 1, surgical correction is generally indicated and is performed before age 6. An orchiopexy secures the testes within the scrotum to prevent sterility and the resulting harmful psychological effects.

The scrotum, which contains the testes, has another function, which is to regulate the temperature of the testes' environment. Sperm are most effectively produced at temperatures 1.5° to 2°C below body temperature. To maintain this difference, the scrotum con-

tains many sweat glands that perspire profusely to dissipate heat. The scrotum also has cremasteric muscles, which can contract to draw the testes closer to the body and increase the temperature or relax to lower them away from the body and reduce it.

Testes

The testes or testicles are the primary sex organs of the male. They are almost of equal size, oval in shape, about $2 \times 1 \times 1\frac{1}{2}$ inches in size, and are suspended in the scrotum, with the left testis usually somewhat lower than the right. A testis has two functions: to produce sperm and to secrete testosterone, the male hormone. These functions begin to occur about age 10 when the hypothalamus releases a hormone that initiates puberty. The hormone stimulates the anterior pituitary gland, which releases the gonad-stimulating hormones to effect change in the testes.

Male gonadotropic hormones secreted by the pituitary are FSH (follicle-stimulating hormone) and ICSH (interstitial cell-stimulating hormones). FSH causes sperm to develop in the male and ova to mature in the female, a very similar function.

Sperm Production   Sperm develop and mature in microscopic tubes in the testes known as *seminiferous tubules* (Figure 11-206). FSH stimulates the production of sperm in the cells that line the tubules. There are about 300 sections of coiled tubules that, if uncoiled, are estimated to extend over a mile. As the sperm develop, they are released into the tubules to start their

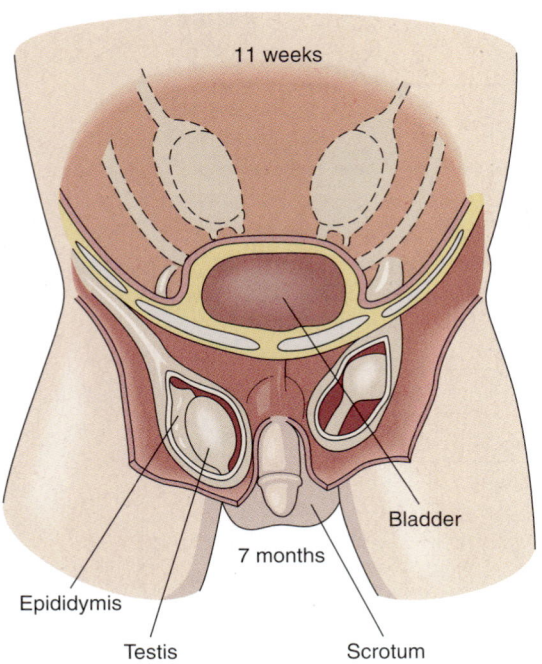

11 weeks

7 months

Bladder

Epididymis

Testis   Scrotum

FIGURE 11-204   The descent of the testes

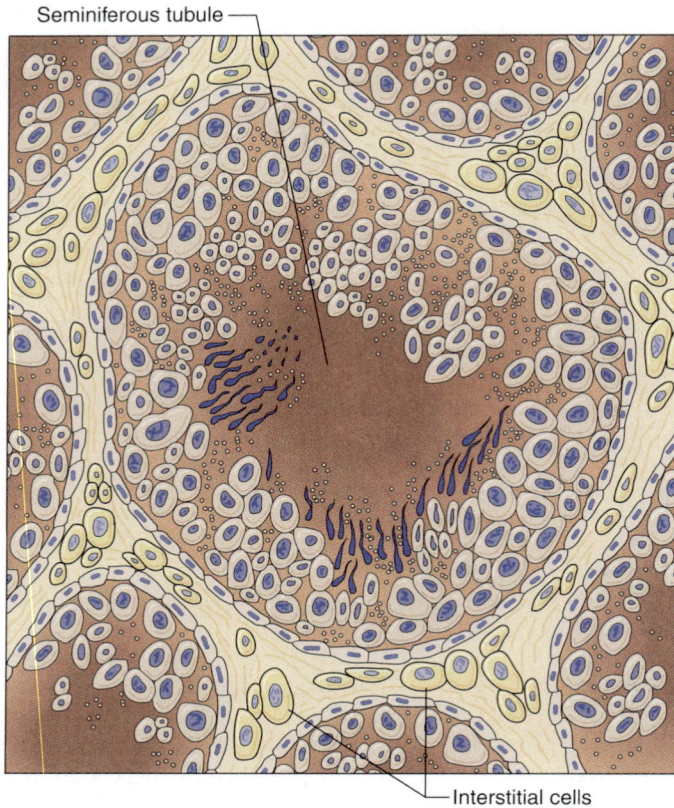

Seminiferous tubule

Interstitial cells

FIGURE 11-206 The production of sperm in the seminiferous tubules and the secretion of testosterone by the interstitial cells

journey from the testes. Sperm formation in an adult male requires about 74 days to maturity. The function normally begins to develop at about age 12, and the first mature sperm are ejaculated at about age 14.

Testosterone As sperm are developing, ICSH is causing the interstitial cells in the network of structures around the tubules to secrete testosterone. Testosterone aids in the maturing of sperm and causes many changes in the male body as it circulates in the bloodstream. These changes are referred to as the development of secondary sex characteristics (Figure 11-207).

In the male, secondary sex characteristics are:

1. Longer and heavier bone structure
2. Larger muscles
3. Deep voice
4. Growth of body hair
5. Development of the genitalia (external sex organs)
6. Increased metabolism
7. Sexual desire

Epididymis, Vas Deferens, and Seminal Vesicles

The epididymis is a coiled structure about 20 feet in length. It is shaped like a half-moon and sits with its head on top of the testes with its tail extending down the side to join the vas deferens (Figure 11-208).

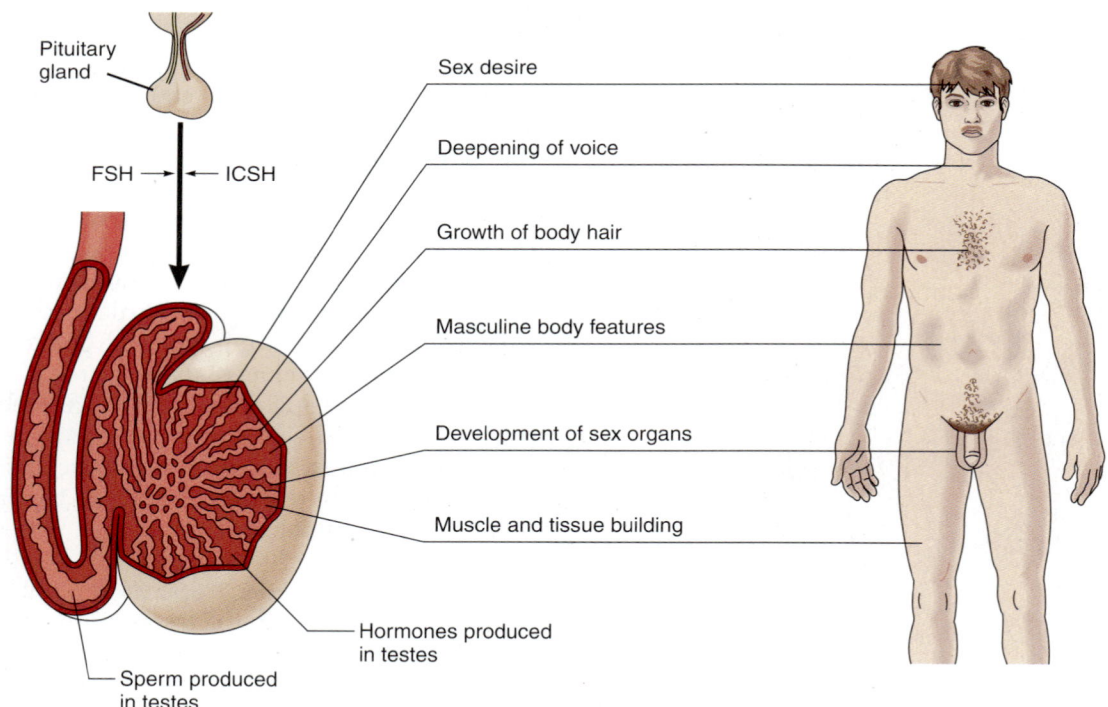

Pituitary gland

FSH → ← ICSH

Sperm produced in testes

Hormones produced in testes

Sex desire

Deepening of voice

Growth of body hair

Masculine body features

Development of sex organs

Muscle and tissue building

FIGURE 11-207 Secondary sex characteristics of the male

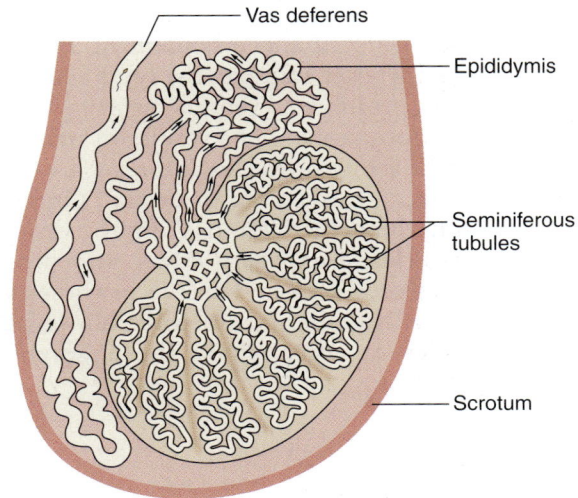

FIGURE 11-208   Seminferous tubules, epididymis, and vas deferens

After sperm are produced in the tubules, they pass into the epididymis, where a small number are stored. The sperm mature in the epididymis for about 18 hours. The fluid secreted by the epididymis adds to the volume of ejaculant.

The vas deferens serves as the passageway for sperm to exit the epididymis. On each side, one vas deferens joins one epididymis extending upward for about 45 cm through an inguinal canal to the base of the urinary bladder. Each vas joins with a duct from a seminal vesicle to form a common ejaculatory duct (Figure 11-209).

The seminal vesicles are a pair of convoluted tubes lying posterior to the bladder. They also empty into the ejaculatory duct. The vesicles secrete a fluid that contains fructose, a simple sugar, which provides nutrition for the sperm. The fluid makes up a major portion of the ejaculant. The ejaculatory duct is a short straight tube that passes through the **prostate** gland to join the urethra.

Prostate Gland, Bulbourethral Glands, and Urethra

The prostate gland is a donut-like pyramidal structure with the urethra extending through its center (see Figure 11-209). The gland is positioned just beneath the bladder. It produces secretions that are drained through tiny tubules into the prostatic section of the urethra. The fluid secreted is alkaline in nature. Its addition to the ejaculant stimulates sperm motility and preserves sperm

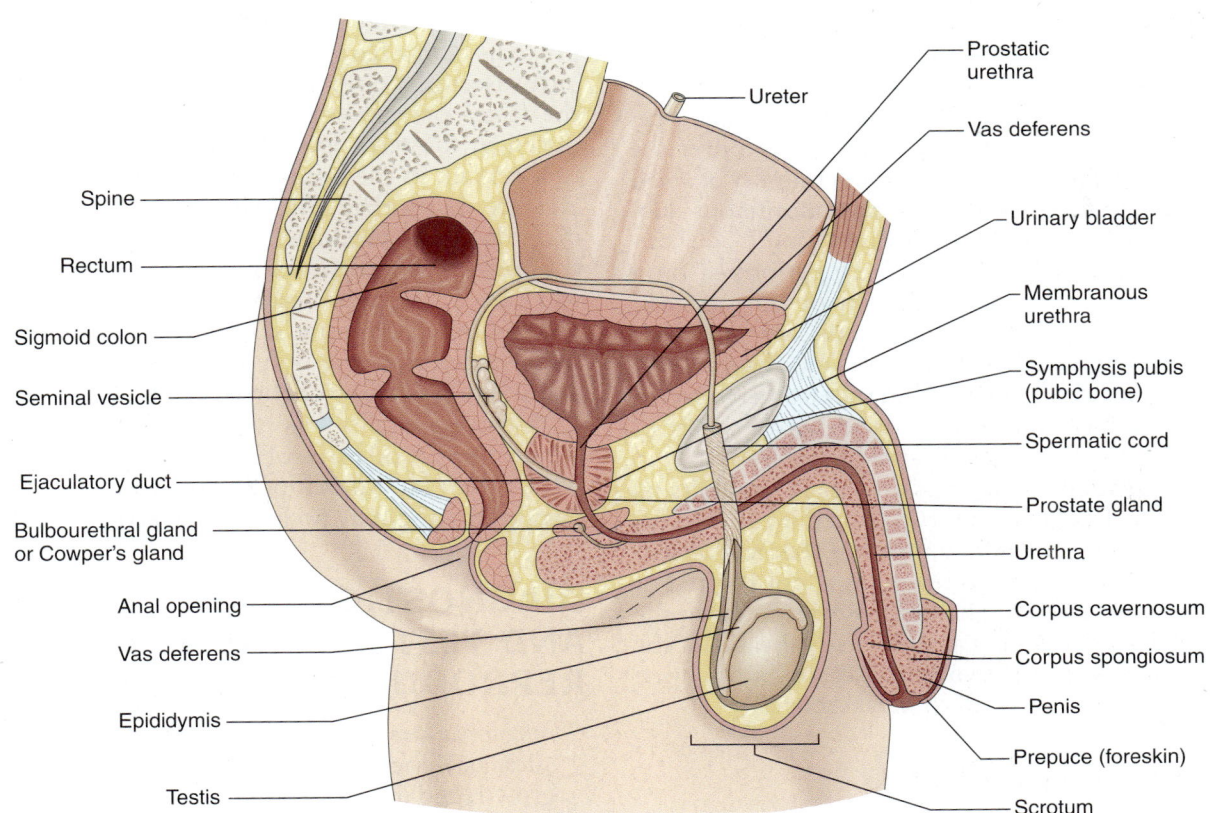

FIGURE 11-209   The organs and ducts of the male reproductive system

life by neutralizing the acidity of the vagina. The prostate is surrounded by muscular tissue that contracts during ejaculation to empty the **semen** (ejaculant fluids and sperm) into the urethra to be propelled from the body.

The **bulbourethral glands** lie beneath the prostate and empty their contents into the urethra. The fluid the glands secrete aids in the movement of sperm and makes the normally acidic male urethra alkaline just prior to **ejaculation**. The secretions may serve as a lubricant for intercourse. Bulbourethral glands are sometimes called Cowper's glands.

Semen

The combined secretions from all the glands and ducts along with the sperm are called the seminal fluid or semen. Approximately 3.5 mL of total fluid are expelled per orgasm (series of rhythmic muscular contractions). Semen is composed of:

- Fluids from the testes and epididymis containing about 350 million sperm (5%)
- Fluid secreted by the seminal vesicles (30%)
- Fluid secreted by the prostate gland (60%)
- Fluid secreted by the bulbourethral glands (5%)

Penis

The penis consists of three columns of **erectile** tissue. Two are the corpora cavernosa and the third, the corpus spongiosum, which contains the urethra. It is surrounded by a layer of subcutaneous tissue and covered with skin. The distal end of the penis enlarges to form the glans penis. A circular fold of skin that extends down over the glans is called the prepuce or **foreskin**. A number of small glands in the foreskin secrete a waxy, odoriferous substance called smegma onto the glans. A **circumcision** (surgical removal of the foreskin) may be performed on a male infant to prevent accumulation of the smegma, thereby avoiding bothersome infections later in life. It also has been observed that circumcised men have a lower incidence of cancer of the penis and that women married to circumcised men have a lower incidence of cancer of the cervix. Circumcision is indicated to correct **phimosis**, a narrowed opening of the foreskin, which prohibits its retraction over the glans. Phimosis contributes to the accumulation of smegma. Many men feel that sexual sensations are heightened when the glans is not covered or restricted by the foreskin. The urethra extends down the length of the penis, opening at the urinary meatus of the glans. The urethra serves two purposes, to empty urine from the urinary bladder and to expel semen.

Erection and Ejaculation

Successful intercourse is dependent on the two cavernosa columns of erectile tissue in the penis. When a male is sexually aroused, nerve impulses cause the erectile tissue to engorge with blood, which makes the erectile tissue increase in size and become firm. Blood entering the dilated arteries squeezes the veins against the penile structures, prohibiting venous return.

After stimulation of the glans results in maximum stimulation of the seminal vesicles, impulses are sent to the ejaculatory center and orgasm occurs. Orgasm is the result of muscular contractions from the vas deferens, seminal vesicles, ejaculatory ducts, and prostate gland. Secretions produced and stored in these structures, along with the sperm, are forcefully expelled through the urethra, after which the engorgement gradually subsides.

Vasectomy

Vasectomy is a simple surgical procedure to prohibit the ejaculation of sperm and effect sterilization of the male. It has become a popular means of birth control. The procedure involves making a small incision in each side of the scrotum. The vas deferens, on each side, is grasped and a loop is withdrawn through the incision. The physician ties the duct in two places and removes a piece of the duct between the ties. The ends are placed back into the scrotum, and the small incision is closed with sutures. The procedure can be performed in the physician's office under local anesthesia or in a hospital outpatient clinic. It is a much simpler means of sterilization than the surgery required to perform a similar procedure on a female.

A vasectomy does not interfere with the function of the testes or with sexual ability. Sperm are still produced in the testes but, because their exit is blocked, they remain in the testes and epididymis until they die and are reabsorbed into the body. Testosterone, the male hormone produced by the testes, gains access to the body by way of the veins in the scrotum. Vasectomy will have no effect on testosterone levels. Most men report as much or more sexual activity after as before their vasectomy. The only negative aspect is that the procedure is likely to be irreversible. Recently, success at restoring fertility has been achieved by surgical reconnection in one out of five attempts. However, the patient may have developed autoantibodies toward his own sperm and may no longer be fertile.

DIAGNOSTIC EXAMS AND TESTS OF THE MALE REPRODUCTIVE SYSTEM

Chromosomal analysis—Tests to determine genetic defects, such as Klinefelter's syndrome, that cause abnormal growth and development of sexual characteristics and chromosome basis for hypogonadism.

Digital rectal examination—A common manual examination involving insertion of a gloved finger into the rectum to palpate the prostate gland for size, density, and nodules or tumors.

Hormonal studies—Measurement of pituitary hormones, such as interstitial-cell stimulating hormone that causes development of testes and sperm production or adrenal cortex androgens that govern sex characteristics and testosterone levels of the testes, to diagnose conditions like hypogonadism, early or delayed sexual development, and infertility.

Prostatic specific antigen (PSA)—A blood test used to measure the amount of antigen present when there is prostate hypertrophy. An elevated amount may be indicative of cancer.

Semen analysis—Analysis of semen and the sperm to determine the volume of semen; the number, maturity, and motility of sperm; the presence of abnormal or immature sperm; and other characteristics. Approximately 40% to 50% of fertility problems are attributed to the male when couples fail to achieve pregnancy.

Testicular biopsy—Examination of testicular tissue to determine unexplained oligospermia, the absence or great decrease in the amount of sperm, when diagnosing infertility.

Testicular self-examination—The American Cancer Society recommends that men perform routine testicular self-examination (TSE) as a means of early identification of testicular cancer. The cancer tends to occur primarily in men from 20 to 40 years old, but it is the most common site of cancer in men 29 to 35 years of age. The Society recommends monthly TSE beginning at 15 years of age (see Chapter 14).

DISEASES AND DISORDERS OF THE MALE REPRODUCTIVE SYSTEM

Epididymitis (Epi-didi-mi'tis)

Description—This is an infection of the epididymis and is an uncommon infection of the male reproductive tract. It may spread to the testicle, causing *orchitis* (inflammation of the testicle).

Signs and symptoms—The primary symptom is intense pain with swelling in the scrotum. Other symptoms include fever, malaise, and a characteristic waddle when walking.

Etiology—The causative organism is usually a coliform bacteria from the intestinal tract and generally follows urinary or prostatic infections. Other causes include trauma, gonorrhea, or syphilis.

Treatment—Treatment may consist of bed rest, elevation of the scrotum on towel rolls, and ice to relieve pain and swelling. A broad-spectrum (inclusive) antibiotic and pain medication are indicated. Therapy must be initiated immediately, especially if there is bilateral involvement, because of the risk of sterility.

Erectile Dysfunction (Impotence)

Description—This is an inability to have or sustain an erection to complete intercourse. Because of the negative connotation of the word "**impotence**," physicians and sex therapists use the term *erectile dysfunction* to identify the occurrence.

Signs and symptoms—Primary **erectile dysfunction** refers to the patient who has never had an erection. Secondary dysfunction refers to the patient who is currently unable to sustain erection but has had intercourse in the past. Transient periods of inability are not considered a dysfunction and probably occur in half the adult male population. The incidence of erectile dysfunction increases with age.

Etiology—Organic factors cause most dysfunction and may result from a chronic illness such as diabetes, renal failure, or cardiopulmonary disease. Spinal cord trauma, the effects of alcohol, or the results of certain drug therapy may also cause organic dysfunction. About 30% may be psychogenic in origin. The usual causes are anxiety, fear of failure, depression, parental rejection, and previous traumatic sexual experiences. Dysfunction may result from stress. Interpersonal factors such as insufficient knowledge of sexual function or lack of communication with a partner may also cause difficulty.

Treatment—Treatment may include sexual therapy to reduce the anxiety and usually involves both partners. The type of therapy chosen depends on the specific cause of the dysfunction. Most often it involves improving communication, reevaluating attitudes toward sex, restricting sexual activity, and encouraging attention to the physical sensations of touching. Many men may benefit from the use of a medication such as Viagra. It can be beneficial for men following prostatectomy where nerves involved in the erection process may be damaged or severed. It is also helpful for men with diabetes or those taking hypertensive medications. It is primarily a trial process to determine whether it will be effective. The medication must be taken 1 hour prior to intercourse for it to be effective. The drug is contraindicated for patients with severe heart problems or those using nitroglycerin products. Additional methods of medicating may be developed, such as a nasal form to be inhaled or a topical ointment and methods with a shortened period to effectiveness. Patients with organic dysfunction may need to develop alternative means of sexual expression. Some patients may benefit from learning to inject one or a combination of drugs into the spongy bodies of the penis. These drugs stimulate a normal erection. Some may use a vacuum device, which pulls blood into the spongy bodies to effect a firm erection. Others may be candidates for the placement of a prosthesis, a device that is implanted into the spongy bodies. There are two basic types of prostheses: a semi-rigid and an inflatable style. The semi-rigid prosthesis will give a constant state of firmness with flexibility at the base so that the penis can be held against the body with underclothing. The inflatable prosthesis can be made erect for intercourse and can be deflated when the man is not engaged in sexual activity.

Hydrocele (Hi′dro-sel)

Description—The presence of an excessive amount of fluid within structures around the testes is called a **hydrocele**.

Signs and symptoms—Enlargement of the scrotum.

Etiology—It may occur following injury or inflammation or may develop as a result of the aging process. It usually is caused by excess production of normal body fluid, lack of reabsorption, or blockage of the circulatory process.

Treatment—Surgical correction is indicated with continued enlargement and discomfort.

Prostatic Hypertrophy (Pros-tat′ik Hi-per′tro-fe)

Description—This enlargement of the prostate gland is common in men over age 50. In **benign** (nonmalignant) **hypertrophy**, the prostate may enlarge sufficiently to constrict the urethra, making it difficult to empty the bladder. Surgery may be indicated to remove the obstructive tissue. A malignant prostate, one of the most common forms of cancer found in men, is a different disease.

Signs and symptoms—Symptoms of hypertrophy vary with the extent of involvement. Usually the initial symptoms are reduced force and size of urinary stream, difficulty in starting a stream, dribbling, a feeling of incomplete voiding, nocturia (having to void at night), and frequent urination. As the hypertrophy increases, symptoms become more pronounced, and eventually hematuria and retention may develop. Diagnosis of hypertrophy can be confirmed by a digital examination to palpate the prostate through the rectal wall (Figure 11-210).

Etiology—It may be caused by a change in hormonal activity.

Treatment—Treatment of benign hypertrophy of the prostate will be conservative until the gland squeezes the urethra and interferes with voiding. Sitz baths, prostatic massage, fluid restriction (for a short time), and several medications can be used, with the addition of antibiotics if an infection develops. Prostatic congestion may benefit from regular sexual intercourse. Conservative therapy is usually only temporary, with a more permanent surgical solution required to effectively relieve urinary retention and other symptoms.

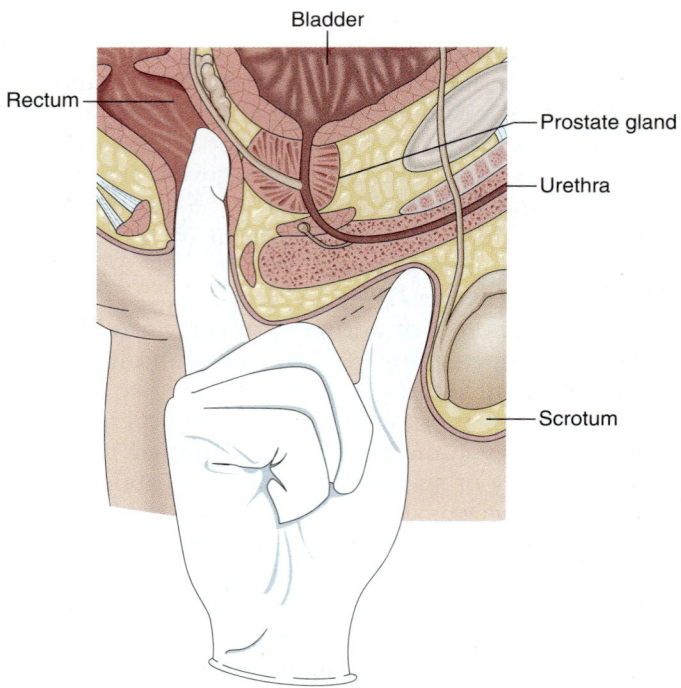

FIGURE 11-210   Digital examination of the prostate gland

A **prostatectomy** (removal of the prostate) can be performed by different methods. An open operation is indicated with a large prostate or with a contained malignancy. An incision is made in the skin above the pubic bone and below the umbilicus. The prostate is exposed as it lies below the bladder and above the penis. The benign tumor of the prostate is removed when no cancer is expected. When cancer is expected, the entire prostate gland and tumor is removed. Another common method is the **transurethral** prostatectomy (TURP). In this procedure, a resectoscope is inserted into the urethra, and the prostate is approached through an incision in the wall of the urethra (Figure 11-211). A wire loop with electric current removes a segment of the gland, thereby interrupting the integrity of the prostate and prohibiting its constricting action.

When there is a malignancy in the prostate, it may cause no symptoms, or the patient may have urinary obstructive symptoms similar to those seen with benign hypertrophy. Cancer may be identified on a rectal examination as a hardened area and may be palpated, or the suspicion of a malignancy may be raised when the patient's prostatic specific antigen (PSA) blood test is abnormal. PSA is a compound that is made only by cells in the prostate, and malignant cells cause this to rise more quickly than is normally seen with an enlarging prostate or with aging.

The incidence of prostate cancer appears to show a family tendency and to be more prevalent in the

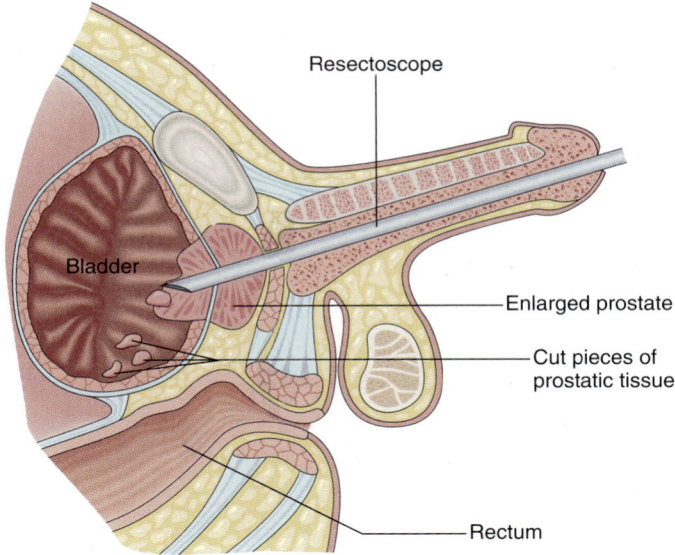

FIGURE 11-211   Insertion of a resectoscope

black race. All men over 50 years should have a rectal examination and a PSA blood test yearly, but those with a family history or who are black should begin annual testing at 40 years.

Treatment of prostatic cancer—Treatment is determined by clinical assessment, expected life span, the stage of the disease, and tolerance for the therapy. Radiation, a prostatectomy, an orchidectomy (removal of testes to stop hormone production), and oral doses of female estrogen are used alone or in combinations, according to the stage of the involvement, to arrest and control the malignancy. Favorable results are obtained from high doses of radiation. Not only does the cancer go into remission, but the associated metastatic skeletal pain, if present, is also relieved.

With the screening for prostate cancer that is now occurring, many younger, sexually active men are being found with prostate cancer, so treatment offers a chance to cure many individuals, and it is anticipated that survival rates will be greatly improved. Unfortunately, the curative treatments available— cryotherapy, radiotherapy, or radical prostatectomy— all have side effects that are disturbing, but they can be overcome. These include incontinence, erectile dysfunction, cystitis, and proctitis (rectal inflammation). If the cancer has spread outside the prostate, making it incurable, it can be controlled by medications or orchidectomy. The cancer can be put into remission for a significant time.

New methods of prevention and treatment are being continuously developed. The National Cancer Institute is sponsoring a study called the Prostate Cancer Prevention Trial (PCPT) to test whether the drug finasteride can prevent prostate cancer. The study involves 18,000 men across the United States over 7 years. To test the drug's effectiveness, only half of the participants are receiving the actual medication; the other half receive a placebo (inactive pill). Not even their attending physicians know which medication their patients are receiving. Hopefully, this will prove beneficial. Prostate cancer currently strikes one out of every seven men age 55 and older and is the second most common cause of cancer deaths.

Two new treatments are being tested. Cryosurgery (freezing) using liquid nitrogen to kill cancer cells is showing promise for some men. It appears to be a good alternative to radiation and is less invasive than traditional surgery. But it still poses risks, including erectile dysfunction and often fails to remove all the cancer cells. It is not considered a good alternative for younger men or good candidates for traditional surgery.

Another treatment uses radioactive seeds, about the size of a grain of rice, implanted in the prostate. The pellets remain permanently in the body, giving off radiation within the prostate for approximately 3 months. It is believed to be more effective than traditional radiation because it delivers about two and a half times the dose without affecting neighboring organs. The seeds are planted through hollow needles that are positioned with the use of a transrectal ultrasound probe.

FEMALE REPRODUCTIVE ORGANS

Because the similarity in function of the male and female reproductive organs is another indication of their common origin, a comparison will be made, when appropriate, as each organ or structure is presented. The order of presentation will be, as with the male, from the formation of the sex cell to its exit from the body.

Ovaries

The embryonic gonadal tissue that is to become the ovaries begins to develop about the 10th or 11th week of pregnancy. The ovaries of the fetus develop high in the abdominal cavity near each kidney but descend to the pelvis as the time for delivery nears. Ovaries are small, almond-shaped glands measuring about $1\frac{1}{2} \times 1 \times \frac{1}{4}$ to $\frac{1}{2}$ inch (Figure 11-212). They are supported by the ligaments, which attach to the uterus and tubes to ensure their position near the fimbriated (fringelike projections) ends of the fallopian tubes. These two organs play a significant role in the life of every female. They have two main roles: to produce the sex cell and the ovum and to secrete hormones. These functions parallel the role of the testes in the male.

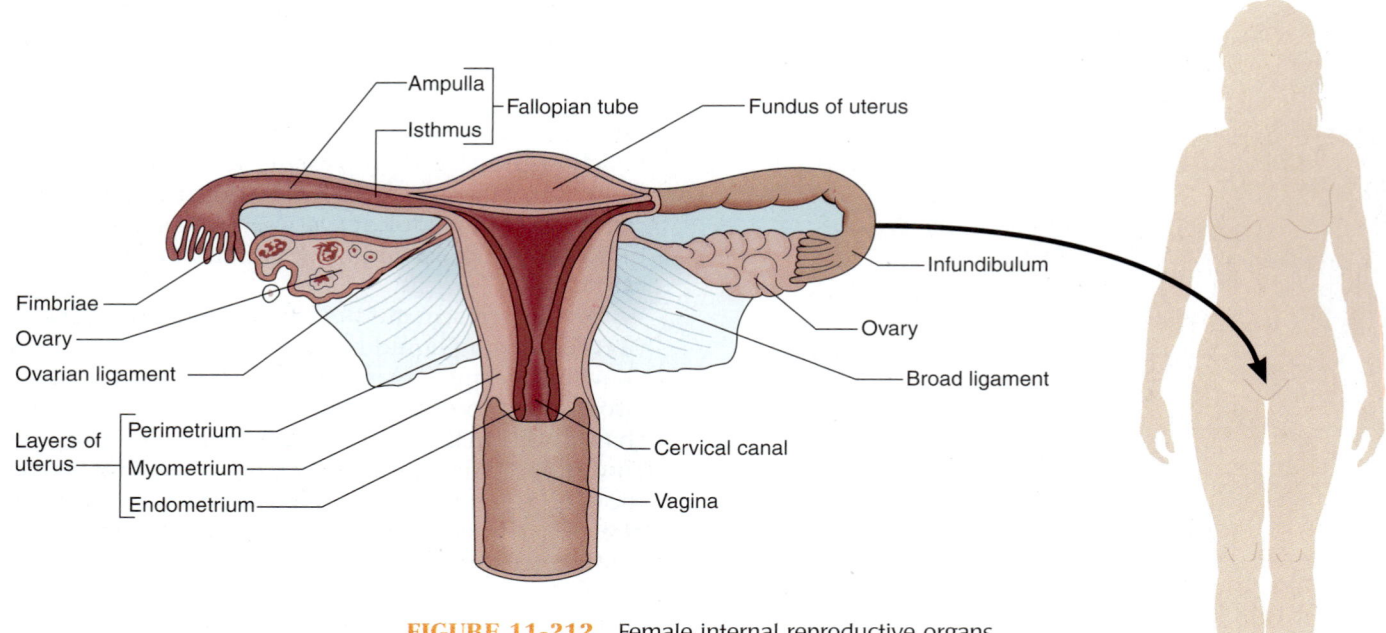

FIGURE 11-212 Female internal reproductive organs

It is estimated that at birth the ovary has between 200,000 and 400,000 primary **graafian follicles** (podlike structures), which contain immature ova. Many follicles never mature and degenerate by puberty. During the reproductive life of a female, about 375 will develop and mature, releasing an ovum. By age 50, most of them have disappeared.

The ovaries are the primary sex organs of the female. When the female is around age 8, the pituitary gland begins to send hormonal messages that puberty is approaching. Within a few years, the messages get stronger, and the pituitary hormone causes the ovaries to begin releasing estrogen into the blood. Estrogen affects the development of the sex organs, such as the fallopian tubes, the uterus or **womb**, and the vagina, causing them to increase in size and maturity.

Estrogen also produces secondary sex characteristics, which alter the shape and appearance of the female body (Figure 11-213). In the female, secondary sex characteristics are:

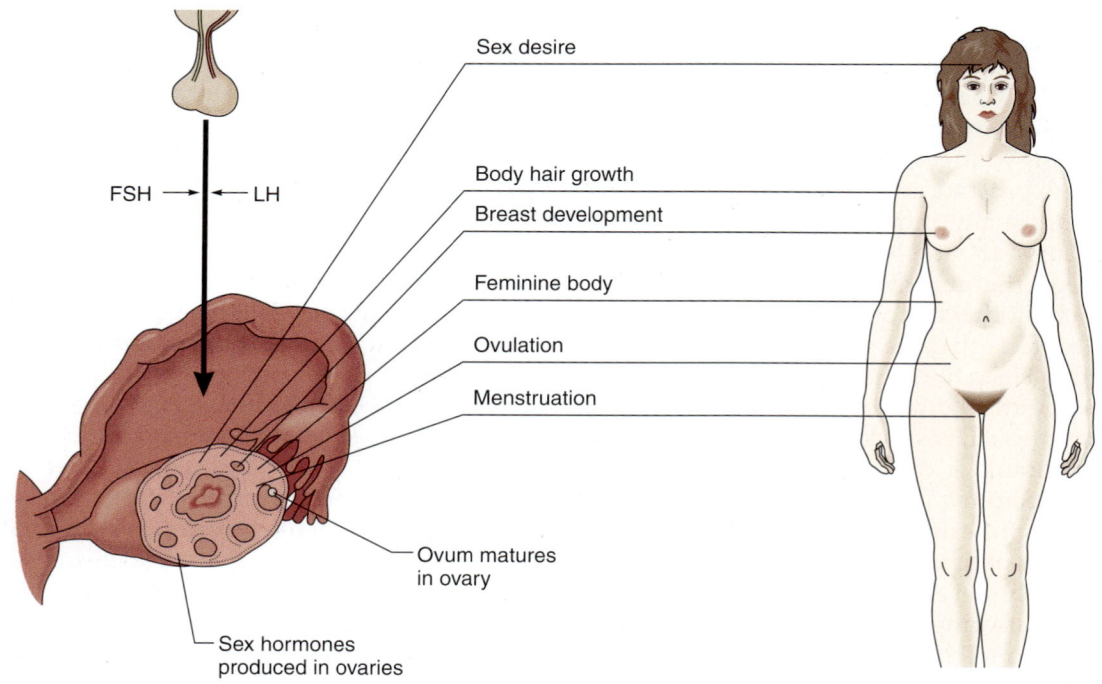

FIGURE 11-213 Secondary sex characteristics of the female

1. Broadening of the pelvis, making the outlet broad and oval (to permit childbirth) (The male pelvic outlet is oblong and narrow.)
2. The epiphysis (growth plate) becomes bone and growth ceases. In the absence of estrogen, females continue to grow, becoming several inches taller than normal.
3. Development of softer and smoother skin
4. Development of pubic hair in a flat upper border pattern
5. Deposits of fat in the breasts and development of the duct system
6. Deposits of fat in the buttocks and thighs
7. Sexual desire

In addition to physical changes, two physiological functions begin to occur, namely **ovulation** and **menstruation**. Ova are produced in the germinal epithelium layer of the ovary (Figure 11-214). There, a "nest" of cells undergo change, with some cells forming a wall around a liquid-filled cavity. Other cells join to thicken one area of the wall. This structure is known as a primary follicle. One of the inner cells will become the ovum. Under the continued influence of FSH and LH from the pituitary, the follicle and ovum mature. Additional fluid collects within the follicle, and it begins to resemble a blister. The follicle moves toward the surface of the ovary and develops a small protrusion called a stigma.

The maturing follicle, called a graafian follicle, produces estrogen, which in turn stimulates the pituitary to release increasing amounts of FSH and LH. When maturity has been achieved and the amount of LH is high, the stigma disintegrates, allowing the follicle to rupture and release the egg into the surrounding area. This action is known as ovulation. At this point, the follicle undergoes change to provide support to the ovum. Under the influence of LH, the follicle fills with a yellow material and begins to function as a temporary endocrine gland, secreting a hormone called progesterone. The follicle is now called a **corpus luteum** (yellowish body).

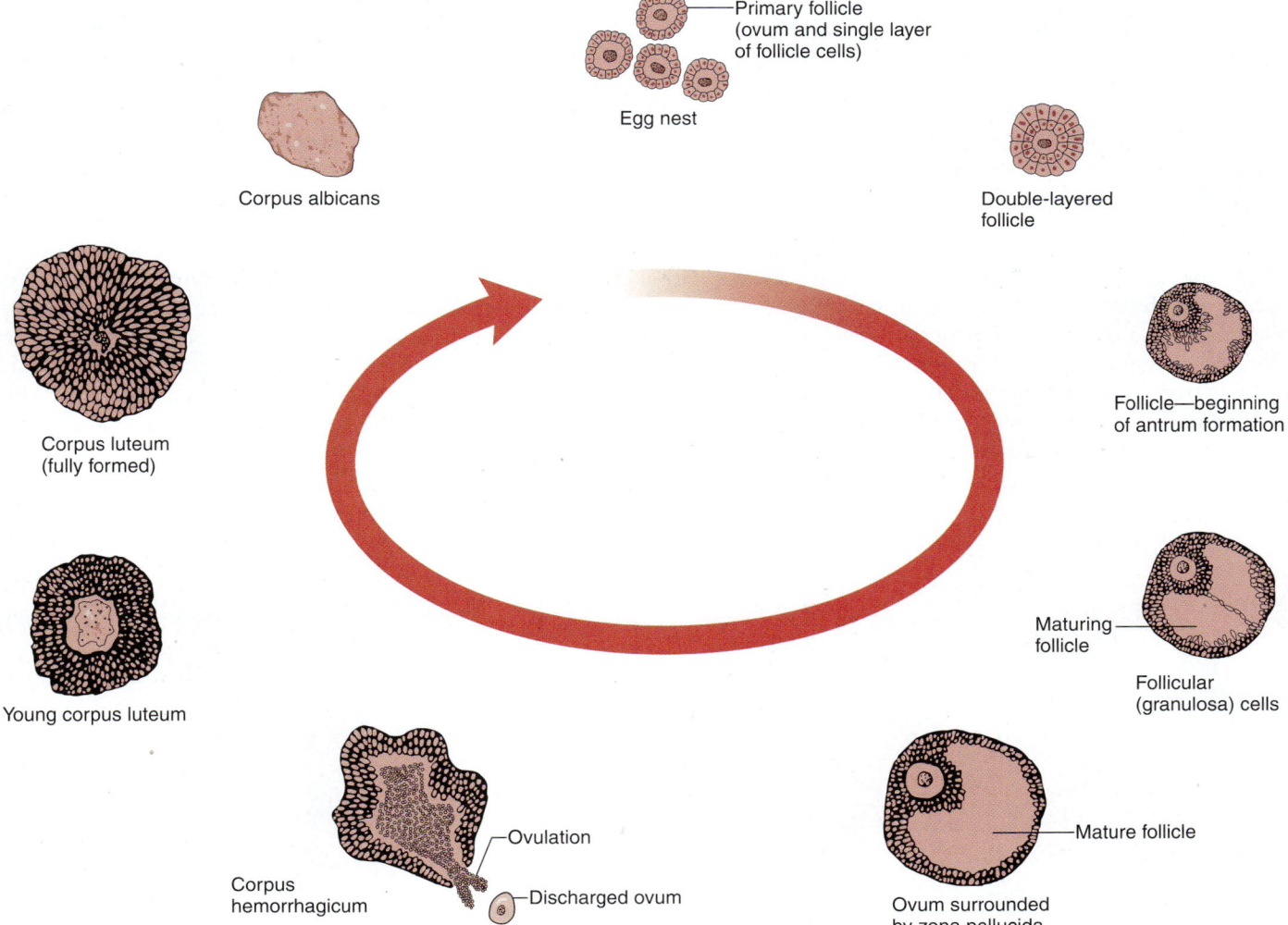

FIGURE 11-214   The lifecycle of an ovarian follicle and the ovum

The high levels of FSH and LH act as a feedback mechanism to prevent the pituitary gland from secreting FSH to mature an additional follicle. The corpus luteum continues to secrete estrogen and progesterone, which prepare the uterus for reception of a fertilized ovum. If fertilization does not occur, the ovum will pass from the body through the vagina, and the corpus luteum, after 10 or 12 days, degenerates and becomes inactive, causing a sharp decline in the hormonal level. This decline stimulates the pituitary to again begin releasing FSH and LH, and the cycle starts again.

Fallopian Tubes

The fallopian tubes extend about 4 inches from the superior lateral surface of the uterus and are attached to the broad ligament (see Figure 11-212). The vas deferens and ejaculatory ducts of the male can be compared with the fallopian tubes of the female. The ducts provide a passageway for sperm, as the fallopian tubes provide a passageway for the ovum to reach the uterus.

The fallopian tubes are constructed of four layers, including a muscle layer and ciliated mucosal layer. The distal ends of the tubes expand into funnel-shaped openings with many fingerlike projections (fimbriae). Upon ovulation, it is believed the fimbriae move the ovum toward the opening of the tube. At the same time, the muscular layer of the tube contracts to produce a vacuum within the tube, and the cilia beat to create a current moving toward the uterus.

The ovary and fallopian tubes lie close together but are not connected. An ovum may be lost within the surrounding abdominal space. Occasionally, sperm will locate and fertilize such an ovum, which will then attach itself to a nearby structure and develop into an abdominal pregnancy. At term, surgical removal of the baby is necessary because no outlet for delivery exists.

Normally, **conception** (**fertilization**) takes place in the outer third of the fallopian tube (Figure 11-215). Upon union, the two cells begin to multiply. The corpus luteum causes secretions to be released from glands within the mucosa of the tubes. The secretions provide nutrition for the new zygote, which must now move into the uterus within 3 to 7 days for implantation and development. However, the opening of the tube narrows in the isthmus section to about 1 mm in diameter near the entrance to the uterus. If the zygote is unusually large or slow, or if there is any constriction of the tube, the zygote may not be able to pass through the opening, and an **ectopic** (abnormal location) tubal pregnancy develops. Because there is no space for growth, pain and discomfort will develop within a few weeks. Surgical removal of the embryo is imperative to prevent rupture of the tube.

Uterus

The uterus is a thick-walled, hollow, muscular organ lying within the pelvis, behind the urinary bladder, and in front of the rectum. It is shaped like an upside-down pear, measuring, before pregnancy, about $3 \times 2 \times 1$ inch (Figure 11-216). The uterus is divided into three parts: the fundus, or rounded upper portion where the fallopian tubes are attached; the body, or middle and main portion; and the **cervix**, or narrowed section that opens into the vagina. The cervix has an internal and an external **os** (opening), with the cervical canal between them. The cavity within the uterus is a small triangular opening.

The uterus has three layers within its walls. The innermost is called the **endometrium**. The structure of the endometrium changes considerably in response to the influence of hormones, as will be discussed under menstruation. The **myometrium** is made up of three layers of muscle fibers running circularly, longitudinally, and diagonally. The outer layer consists of the serous membrane, which covers most of the body and fundus of the uterus.

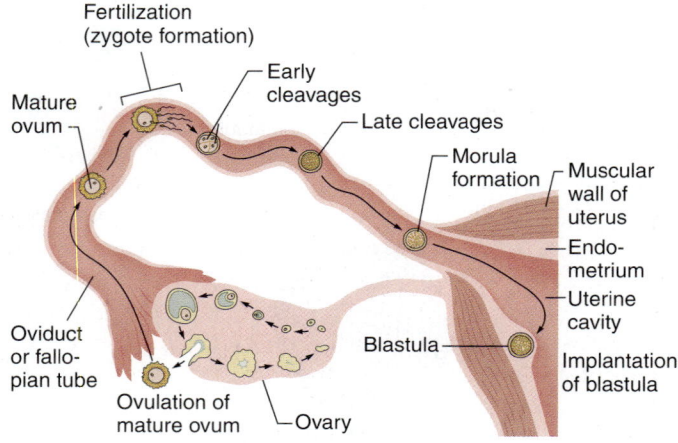

FIGURE 11-215 Pathway of ovum to fertilization and blastula phase implantation in the uterus

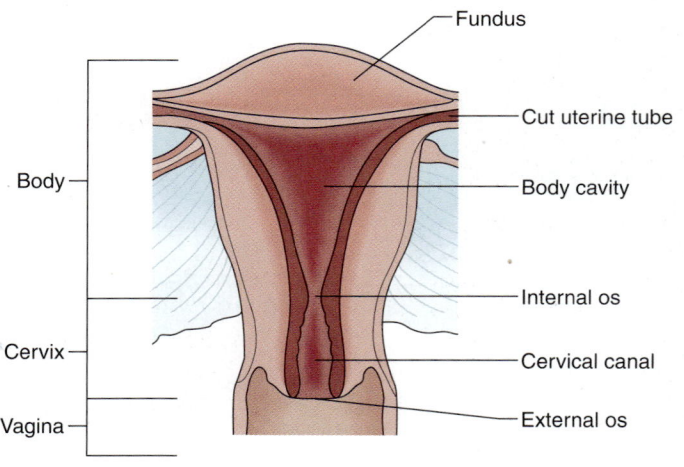

FIGURE 11-216 The uterus

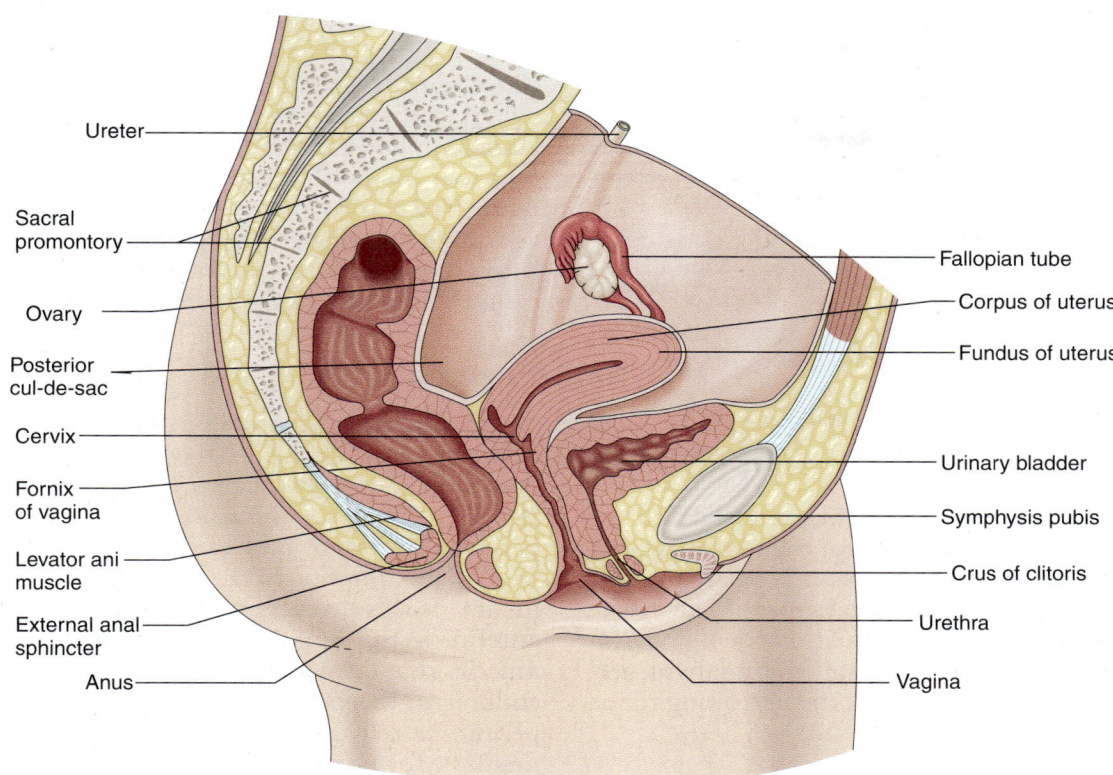

FIGURE 11-217   Female internal reproductive organs with uterus in normal position

The uterus has a great capacity for expansion. During pregnancy, its thick walls stretch and thin out until the fundus touches the diaphragm. Even at this great overextension, the powerful uterine muscles are still able to contract forcefully to produce labor and delivery. In addition, the uterus is flexible in its position, being easily moved in all directions. It is pressed posteriorly when the bladder fills and anteriorly when the rectum is full.

When the uterus is horizontal, at right angles to the vagina, it is in its normal position (Figure 11-217). There are five variances of normal positioning (from anterior to posterior): **anteflexed**, **anteverted**, mid position, **retroverted**, and **retroflexed**. The uterus may also **prolapse**, or drop downward into the vagina. If these positions cause discomfort or interfere with adjoining structures, a device called a pessary can be inserted into the vagina to support the uterus.

Vagina

The vagina is a collapsible muscular tube lined with mucous membrane, which is arranged in folds. The walls of the vagina lie in contact with each other. The posterior wall is 3 to 4 inches long. The anterior wall extends about 2½ or 3 inches to the cervix. The vagina is capable of great expansion. It serves as the passageway for menstruation, an organ of sexual intercourse, and the birth canal for the delivery of an infant.

Behind the vagina and anterior to the rectum is a rectouterine pouch, a space called the cul-de-sac or pouch of Douglas. Infection occasionally develops in this area and necessitates draining. A surgeon can make an incision through the vaginal wall, eliminating the need for abdominal surgery. This is also the area where abdominal ectopic pregnancies usually occur. Though rare, this type of ectopic pregnancy occurs because the fertilized ova goes out the open end of the fallopian tube instead of descending into the uterus. It falls naturally by gravity into the cul-de-sac.

Near the outlet of the vagina is a muscular sphincter that can be detected when inserting tampons or upon examination. The sphincter will maintain a tampon within the vagina and provides a "snugness" for sexual intercourse. The vaginal canal is kept moist by secretions from the uterus and by droplets of mucoid material from the vaginal walls.

Up to this point, all the structures discussed have been internal. Whereas the external genitalia of the male are quite visible, those of the female are practically hidden from sight. Many authorities recommend that women become familiar with their genitalia by making a thorough examination using a mirror and a good light.

The vagina opens onto the surface of the body at the **perineum**, posterior to the urinary meatus and anterior to the anus (Figure 11-218). The external opening is par-

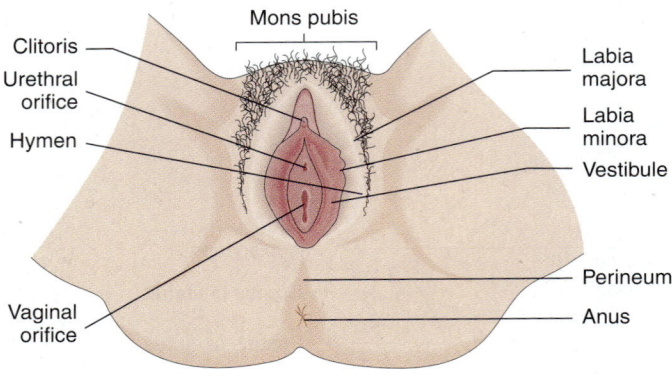

FIGURE 11-218 Female external genitalia

tially covered by folds of mucous membrane called the **hymen**, which border the edges prior to intercourse. Occasionally, the hymen is thicker than normal or covers the entire opening (imperforate hymen). The tissue must be removed prior to menstruation when imperforate. It occasionally requires surgical removal (hymenectomy) to permit intercourse when the narrowing tissue cannot be stretched naturally.

Vulva

The **vulva** is the area of the female external sexual structures. The large pad of fat that is covered with coarse hair on the mature female and overlies the symphysis pubis is known as the **mons pubis**. The labia majora (large lips) are a pair of rounded folds of skin on each side of the vulva and are continuous with the mons pubis. The labia are covered with hair on the exterior surface but with pigmented smooth skin on the inner surface. The labia are composed mainly of fat and numerous glands. The labia majora develop in the female from the same embryonic tissue that becomes the scrotum in the male.

The labia minora (small lips) lie within the labia majora and come together anteriorly in the midline continuous with the prepuce which covers the glans of the clitoris. The labia minora are covered with mucous membrane that is continuous with the lining of the vagina. The female labia minora develop from the same embryonic tissue as the male penile shaft.

The term vestibule is used to denote that portion of the vulva that lies inside the labia minora and posterior to the clitoris. It contains the opening to the urethra and the vagina. The ducts to the vestibular glands (**Bartholin's glands**) open at the base of the labia minora. They secrete a fluid that serves as a lubricant for coitus (intercourse). Posteriorly the labia minora are connected by a thin piece of tissue called the fourchette, which is just posterior to the vaginal opening. The fourchette is destroyed by the birth of the first child.

Clitoris

The clitoris is a rounded mass composed of two small columns of erectile tissue. The clitoris develops in the female similarly to the glans and penis of the male, except that the urethra does not descend through its interior. The clitoris and the glans penis are very sensitive and provide for heightening of sexual excitement. The clitoris becomes enlarged and engorged with blood and is involved in the orgasmic response to sexual arousal.

Perineum

The perineum is identified in two different manners. Some physicians consider the entire pelvic floor as the perineum and apply the term to both male and female. But in **gynecology** (the study of female diseases), the perineum refers to the area posterior to the vaginal introitus and anterior to the anus. In the male, the perineum in this sense is posterior to the scrotum and anterior to the anus. The perineal area is composed of muscles that form a sphincter for the vestibule. During childbirth, the perineum must stretch adequately to permit the delivery of the infant. If it appears the tissue might be torn, the physician will surgically cut the perineum to avoid a ragged tear. This procedure is known as an **episiotomy**. Following delivery, the straight, clean cut is sutured (sewn closed). When the repair heals, the perineum is much smoother, with less scar tissue, than if torn tissue had healed.

Mammary Glands (Breasts)

The mammary glands are secondary sexual structures that develop and function only in the female. The breast consists of lobes separated into sections by connective tissue, somewhat like the structure of a grapefruit half. Each lobe has several lobules composed of connective tissue with grapelike clusters of secreting cells (alveoli) embedded in the tissue. The glandular clusters are drained by minute ducts that unite into a single duct for each lobe for a total of about 15 to 20 in each breast (Figure 11-219). The ducts are arranged like the spokes of a wheel, meeting at the nipple. Here they enlarge slightly to form small reservoirs. The main ducts exit on the surface of the nipple through tiny openings.

Fatty tissue is deposited around the surface of the gland, between the lobes and beneath the skin. A darkened area called the **areola** surrounds the nipple. The color of the areola varies from pink in light blonds and redheads to brown in brunettes. A pink areola will turn brown early in pregnancy and regress somewhat after delivery but will not return to pink. About 3 days after delivery, the glands begin to secrete milk resulting from hormonal stimulation from the pituitary. The hor-

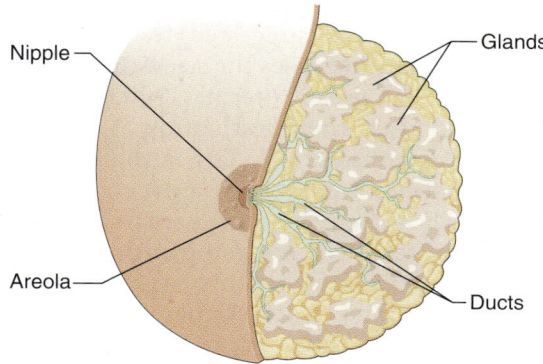

FIGURE 11-219   The structure of the breast

mone prolactin stimulates the production of milk, whereas oxytocin causes it to be ejected in response to the infant's sucking.

Menstruation

When the ovum is not fertilized, and therefore the uterine structures prepared for reception of the embryo are not needed, the lining deteriorates and is discharged from the body in the process called menstruation. Menstruation begins at **menarche** (first cycle) and ends with **menopause** (last cycle). A complete cycle is approximately 28 days in length. If menarche occurs at age 13, the female will experience approximately 455 cycles over the following 35 years. A 28-day cycle is based on a lunar month, not a calendar month; therefore, there are 13 cycles (lunar months) per year.

The menstrual cycle is a result of the interaction of hormones and the endometrium of the uterus. Normally, menstruation is interrupted only by pregnancy or severe illness. The interrelated effects of the hormones and their effects on the sex organs are illustrated in Figure 11-220. The menstrual cycle can be divided into four phases, each characterized by hormonal, ovarian, and uterine changes.

Phase I—The Follicular Phase   Beginning about day 5 in the cycle (counting from the first day of menstruation), the pituitary secretes high levels of FSH to stimulate the ovarian follicles. One follicle ripens an egg and brings about ovulation, at the same time secreting estrogen. About day 10, the pituitary begins to secrete LH in large amounts to react on the follicle. As the estrogen increases, the FSH slows down. The folli-

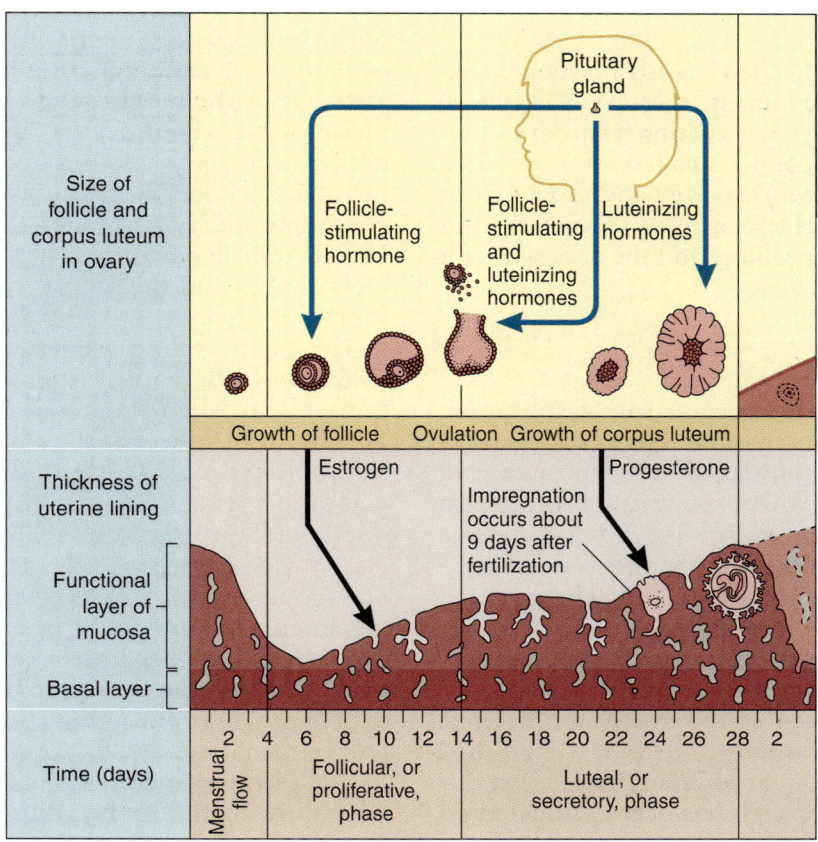

FIGURE 11-220   Menstrual cycle illustrating the levels of pituitary and ovarian hormones, ovarian cycle, and endometrial changes

cle continues to move its maturing egg toward the ovarian surface. At the same time, the endometrium of the uterus has been stimulated by the high level of estrogen and grown a thick lining in preparation for receiving a fertilized egg. This change in the lining is known as *proliferation*.

Phase II—Ovulation
The follicle releases the matured ovum. Estrogen is at a high level; FSH is reduced just prior to ovulation. The high level of estrogen stimulates the release of LH by the pituitary, which causes the follicle to rupture about day 14 in the cycle. The endometrium has continued to grow a thick lining.

Phase III—The Luteal Phase
After the egg is released, the empty follicle undergoes a rapid change caused by the influence of LH. It becomes a glandular mass of cells called the corpus luteum and begins to release progesterone and estrogen. The progesterone reacts on the glands in the endometrium to begin secreting a nourishing substance for the egg. The corpus luteum continues to secrete progesterone for about 12 days until approximately day 26 of the cycle. As the level of progesterone rises, LH is inhibited and the LH level falls. When LH drops, the corpus luteum degenerates, causing the levels of progesterone and estrogen to decline sharply.

Phase IV—Menstruation
With hormonal support gone, the lining buildup in the uterus begins to slough off (shed), causing menstruation from days 1 to 5. The excess endometrium and a small amount of blood pass out through the cervix. Estrogen and progesterone levels are low, but the FSH level is rising to start the next cycle, preparing the uterine lining and the next ovum for the opportunity of pregnancy.

FERTILIZATION

The miracle of reproduction begins with fertilization. In the process of sexual intercourse, sperm at the rate of about 360 million per ejaculation are deposited into the female vagina. From here the microscopic sperm begin an incredible journey toward a single female ovum, which will normally be in the outer one third of one of the fallopian tubes. The ovum must be fertilized within 24 hours after expulsion from the ovary, or fertilization will have to be postponed until the next ovum is ready in approximately 1 month.

The sperm travel at a rate of about 1 to 5 millimeters per minute; their course seems to be in a straight line but in a random direction. Studies on humans are difficult to do, but some research has been conducted. In one study, it was found that sperm deposited in the vagina of a woman just prior to surgery had migrated through the fallopian tubes 30 minutes later. This find-

ing could not be explained based on sperm motility alone. It is hypothesized (suggested) that intercourse or artificial insemination causes the release of a hormonal substance that increases uterine contractions, propelling sperm toward their destination.

The ovum is considerably larger than the sperm, yet it is still only about $1/125$ of an inch in diameter (Figure 11-221). When the sperm reach the egg, they surround its outer surface, attempting to enter. Only the strongest sperm are able to survive the acidity of the vaginal secretions to attack the protective corona radiata that surrounds the ovum. In repeated attacks, the sperm release an enzyme called hyaluronidase, which gradually breaks down the ovum's protection. Eventually, an exposed area of membrane will allow one spermatozoan to penetrate the ovum. The head and middle of the sperm enter the ovum while the tail drops off outside. Immediately, the membrane becomes sealed against additional sperm. The nucleus of the sperm moves to combine with the ovum nucleus, and a zygote is formed. At this time, the traits, which are inherited, and the sex of the new individual are determined and cannot be altered. The father has determined the sex, but the other characteristics are contributed by both parents. At this point, conception has occurred.

Following fertilization, the zygote begins the journey to the well-prepared uterus, arriving about 6 days after ovulation. There it implants itself in the thick wall, and a change in the menstrual cycle begins. At this point, phase III is at about day 20. The endometrium is at its peak. The levels of estrogen and progesterone are high. LH and FSH are low because of the feedback of adequate amounts of hormones; this prevents stimulation of new follicle maturity. The secretions from the fallopian tubes and the uterine glands provide nutrition for the embryo.

The high level of progesterone inhibits the myometrium from contracting; therefore, the embryo cannot be expelled. Progesterone also stimulates development of the ducts of the **mammary glands** (breasts). These effects must be continued to maintain the implantation. If the corpus luteum fails, so does the production of progesterone. Therefore, the developing **placenta** (afterbirth) secretes a hormone, human chorionic gonadotropin (HCG), which maintains the corpus luteum during the early stages of pregnancy. This is the hormone that is detectable on urine pregnancy tests. As the embryo develops, the placenta begins to secrete progesterone and estrogen, and the corpus luteum degenerates and disappears.

The placenta maintains its high level of hormone output throughout pregnancy. When the time for delivery nears, the placenta decreases production of progesterone, which allows the myometrium to begin contracting, and labor begins. With progesterone di-

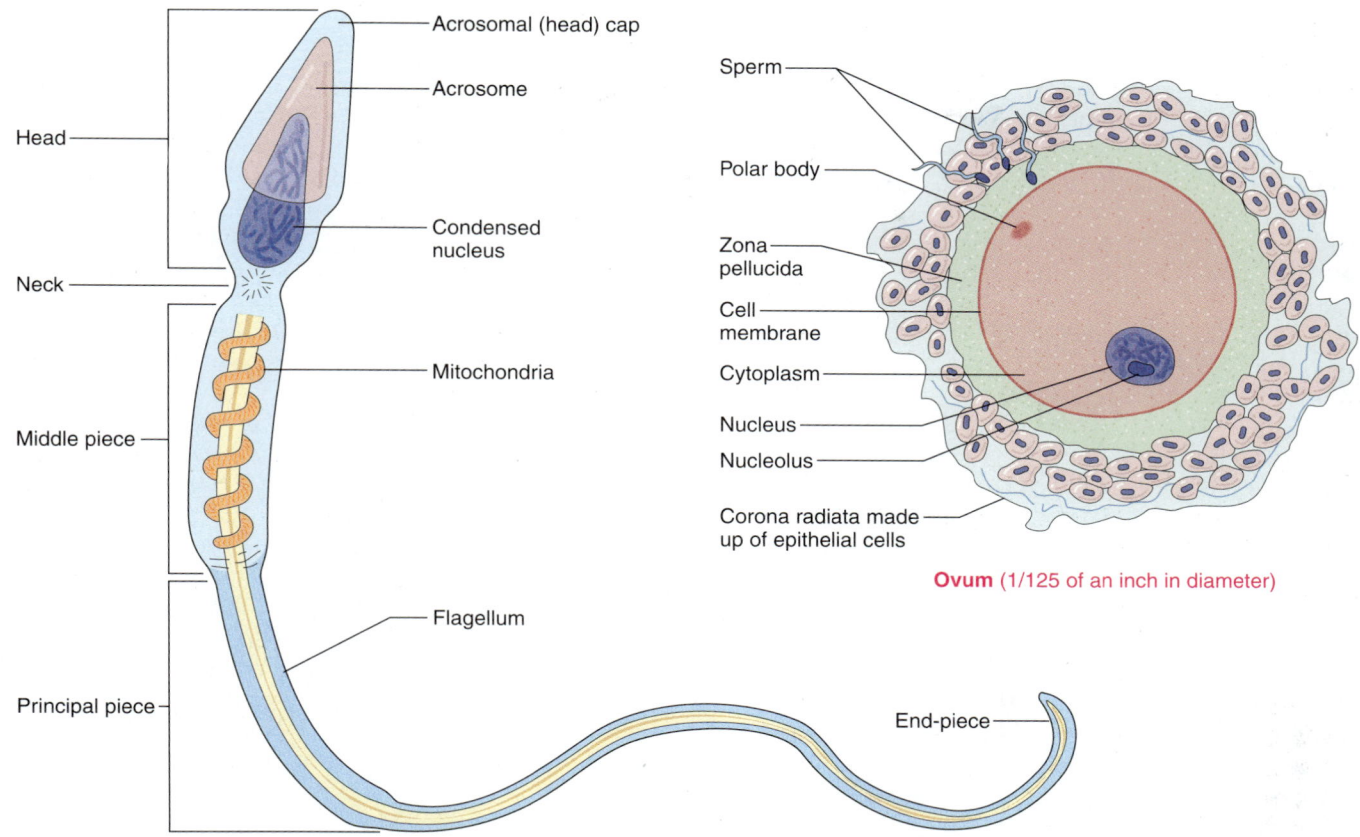

FIGURE 11-221   Sperm and ovum (*Note:* Actual size comparison of sperm entering ovum)

minished, the release of prolactin from the pituitary can occur. Prolactin stimulates the mammary glands to produce, for the first few days, *colostrum,* a thin nutritious liquid, and later, milk. The continued production of milk depends on stimulation from the regular sucking of the infant or the removal of milk by pumping.

PREGNANCY

About 36 hours after fertilization occurs, the zygote begins to grow from its one-cell beginning. It is almost beyond comprehension to realize that everything necessary to the formation of a new life, the bones, muscles, blood vessels, the brain, all the organs, and the skin and hair are all contained in one microscopic cell. In addition, the life-support system of the placenta and umbilical cord and the protective membranes and **amniotic** fluid also develop from this single cell. By about day 6, the small cluster of cells firmly implant within the uterine wall, and it enters the embryonic period (8 weeks) of development when most of the major organ systems are formed at an amazing speed. The group of cells arrange themselves into three layers from which the various organs are formed. One layer, the *ectoderm,* becomes the nervous system, skin, hair, and

parts of the eye. The *endoderm* layer becomes the digestive and respiratory systems. The skeletal, muscular, connective tissue, reproductive, and circulatory systems develop from the *mesoderm* layer.

The **embryo** develops from the head down, which explains why, in Figure 11-222, the head is so large compared with the rest of the body. By the end of the 10th week of **pregnancy**, all systems are completed, even to nails on the fingers. Many of the organs begin limited function by the 7th week. After 8 weeks, the embryo is called a **fetus**. By week 12, the sex can be determined, and the fetus is about 4 inches long and weighs about two thirds of an ounce. This marks the end of the first **trimester** or one third of the total pregnancy period.

It is obvious the fetus has a lot of growing to do, and it does so rapidly. By week 20, movement can be felt and the heartbeat is detectable with a fetascope. By now, the pregnancy is about half way through. A fetus must be carried past the next several weeks to survive. If born in week 23, a little past 5 months, it will weigh less than 2 pounds and has a 1 in 10,000 chance of surviving.

By the 20th week, the fetus opens its eyes, and by week 24, it can hear sounds from inside the uterus. The movements are very vigorous by now, and there

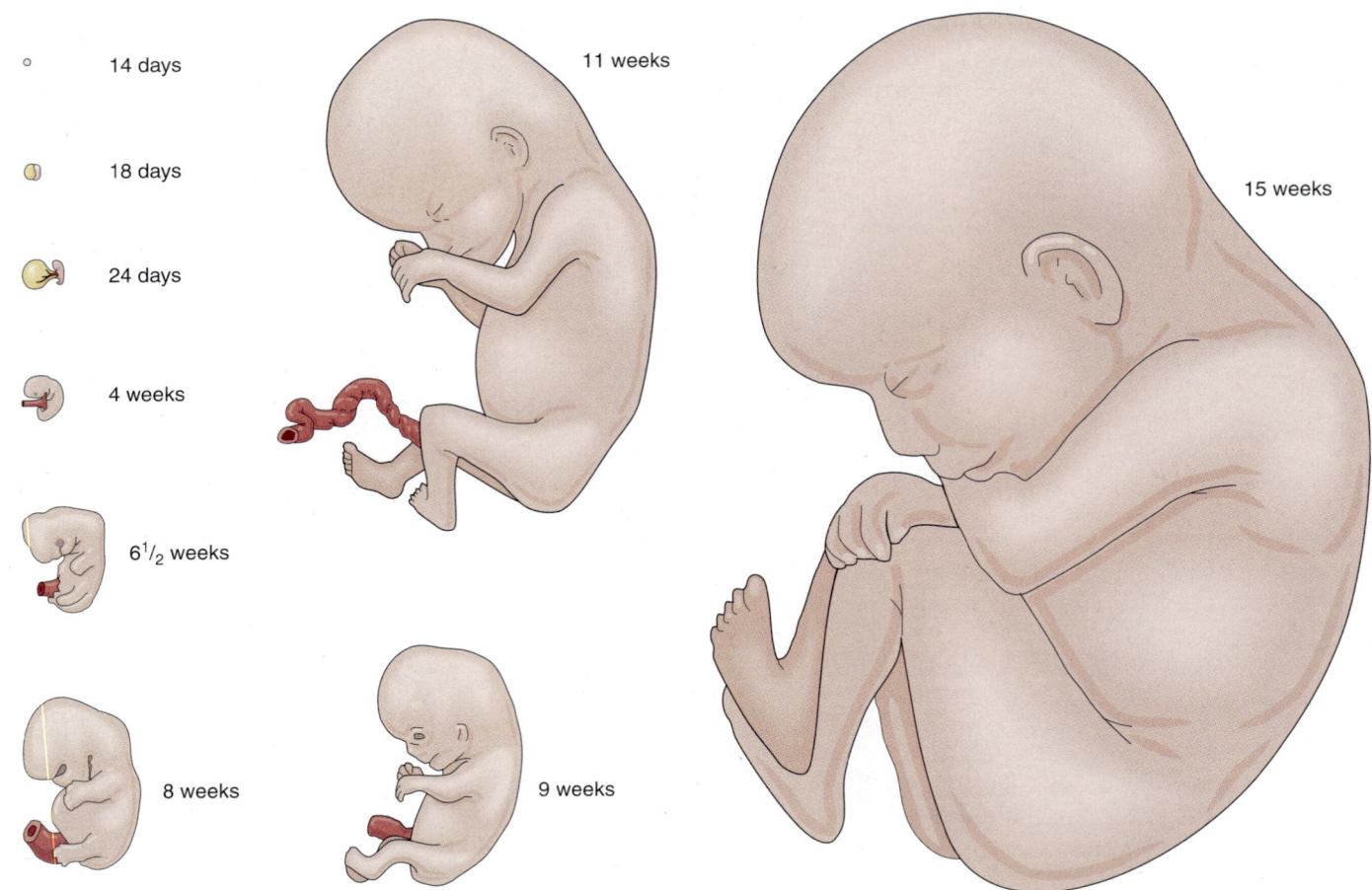

14 days

18 days

24 days

4 weeks

6¹/₂ weeks

8 weeks

9 weeks

11 weeks

15 weeks

FIGURE 11-222 Changes in the body size of the embryo and fetus during development in the uterus (all figures natural size)

are periods of sleep and wakefulness as the second trimester ends.

During the last trimester, the fetus adds greatly to its size. By the end of the 7th month, it has assumed a head-down position and if born would have over a 50% chance of survival. The odds increase to about 95% at 8 months when weight reaches 5 pounds, to 99% at full-term 9 months with average weight being 7½ pounds and a length of 20 inches.

The pregnant woman also undergoes body changes during pregnancy. Initially the first sign is a missed menstrual period. This is a time of joy for couples who have been trying to **conceive** but may be less than welcome to others. Another early sign is breast tenderness caused by the stimulation of hormones. Some women will experience "morning sickness," especially for the first 6 to 8 weeks. Usually there is more frequent urination, fatigue, and the need for additional sleep. By the 8th to 10th week, pregnancy can be detected by manual pelvic examination and the bluish hue of the formerly pale pink cervix. This change is called "Chadwick's sign." Once pregnancy is confirmed, the woman is usu-

ally interested in the expected delivery date. It is calculated using Nagele's rule, which states: Take the first day of the last menstrual period, subtract 3 months, and add 7 days, plus a year. For example, if the first day of the last period was September 1, 2006, the expected day of delivery would be June 8, 2007. Remember, this is only the "expected" date. Babies have a habit of being born when they are "ready." On a percentage basis, 39% are born within 5 days of the projected date and another 55% are within 10 days. The rest obviously are either early or late.

It is important to confirm pregnancy early so that good prenatal care is started. Proper nutrition, such as 1 mg of folic acid daily, is recommended 3 months prior to conception to decrease the risk of neural tube defects of the fetus. If a woman has a history of a previous child with a neural tube defect, she should increase the dose to 4 mg daily prior to conception and continue throughout the pregnancy. Other vitamins and regular exercise are extremely important to promote a healthy baby and an uneventful pregnancy. It is also critical to the health and welfare of the fetus that the mother refrain from the use of tobacco, alcohol, and drugs, all of which cause problems such as low birth weight, drug addiction, and birth defects. The effects of AIDS, hepatitis, or genital herpes from an infected mother is a terrible inheritance. Every pregnant woman should consider it her responsibility to do everything possible to ensure the birth of a healthy baby.

Other symptoms experienced with pregnancy develop as the weeks pass. Usually there are psychological changes, such as the stereotypes of "being radiant," being happy, and having "cravings" (e.g., for dill pickles at unusual times of the day). However, the symptoms of depression and fatigue are also common. In general, the symptoms are influenced by the attitude toward the pregnancy. If there are marriage conflicts or economic problems, or if it is an unwanted pregnancy, it can hardly be a time of joy and anticipation.

As the pregnancy continues, the morning sickness disappears and edema of the hands, face, feet, and legs appears. There may also be constipation caused by pressure on the rectum. Urinary frequency is universal because the bladder is limited in its expansion. As the third trimester progresses, the size of the uterus causes shortness of breath and indigestion because of pressure from displaced organs and the uterus against the lungs and stomach. Hemorrhoids are a common result of constipation and pressure on the blood vessels of the rectum.

Weight gain continues throughout pregnancy. Most physicians prefer to establish a set amount of permissible gain. The total weight of the baby (7½ pounds), placenta (1 pound), enlarged uterus (2 pounds), enlarged breasts (1½ pounds), and additional fat and water (about 6 pounds) add up to about 18 pounds, so 20 pounds is sometimes the recommended amount of gain. Excess weight causes complications such as hypertension, increased stress on the heart, and the problem of weight to be lost after delivery.

THE BIRTH PROCESS

The beginning of the birth process is usually signaled by a show of bloody mucus. This is from the mucous plug that was in the cervix to protect the fetus from organisms in the vagina. There may also be a slow leak or a gush of the amniotic fluid. Irregular **contractions** of the uterus will begin, and stimulation from prostaglandin may initiate labor.

Labor is divided into three stages. The first begins when uterine contractions become regular and proceeds through cervical dilation and **effacement** (thinning out). The cervix must dilate to about 10 centimeters (4 inches) in diameter before the baby can be delivered. Contractions increase in frequency and intensity until they become very strong, uncomfortable, and exhausting. First stage labor varies between as little as 2 to as long as 24 hours; 12 to 15 hours is average for a first pregnancy.

The second stage of labor begins with complete dilation and the entrance of the head (or another part) into the vagina. Continued contractions and bearing down by the woman push the baby through the vagina until it is visible at the entrance; this is known as *crowning* (if it is a head presentation). Strong contractions and pushing force the head through the vaginal opening, then the baby rotates to the side so the shoulders can be delivered. The rest is easily passed, and the second stage is completed.

The baby is suctioned to remove mucus from its mouth and nose, and crying begins to inflate the lungs. The baby's body function changes dramatically. For the first time it must breathe on its own to take in oxygen and begin to circulate its own blood. It changes from a bluish color to a healthy skin tone within a couple of minutes. As soon as the baby's condition is satisfactory, the umbilical cord is clamped, tied, and cut.

To help assess a newborn's condition, a universally accepted evaluation technique called the Apgar scoring system is used. Observation of the newborn is made at 1 and 5 minutes following delivery. The ratings are entered on a chart and the scores totaled. A score of 10 is considered the best possible condition. A score of 7 to 9 is considered adequate, and no treatment is required. A score of 4 to 6 indicates close observation, and some intervention, such as suctioning, is necessary. A score below 4 requires immediate intervention and continued evaluation. Table 11-18 is an example of the Apgar scoring system.

The third stage of labor begins with the detachment of the placenta from the uterine wall, and the *afterbirth* (placenta and its membranes) are expelled. Usually a few more contractions are required to accomplish this stage. After it has emptied, the muscles of the uterus maintain a level of contraction to close off open blood vessels and control bleeding.

In some cases, such as inadequate pelvic outlet, breech presentation (other than head), large baby, ineffective labor, or the development of a serious complication, the baby may need to be removed by **cesarean** section. This involves cutting through the abdomen and into the uterus to remove the baby and the afterbirth. About 18% of all deliveries are cesarean. Pregnancy following a cesarean section may undergo a trial of labor if certain factors are considered. It is commonly called vaginal birth after cesarean (VBAC) and is successful in 60% to 80% of cases. One main concern is the type of *uterine* incision that was made. This may not be the same as that on the surface of the abdomen. If a transverse uterine incision has been made, across the lower, thinner part of the uterus (Figure 11-223), it is the least likely to result in complications in a subsequent vaginal delivery. The low vertical incision is an

TABLE 11-18 APGAR SCORING SYSTEM				Rating	
Sign	0	1	2	1 min	5 min
Heart rate	Not detectable	Below 100	Over 100		
Respiratory effort	Absent	Slow, irregular	Good, crying		
Muscle tone	Flaccid	Some flexion	Active motion of extremities		
Reflex irritability (response to flick on sole)	No response	Grimace, slow motion	Cry		
Color	Blue, pale	Body pink, extremities blue	Completely pink		
			TOTAL		

Scoring system developed by Dr. Virginia Apgar

up and down cut in the lower, thinner area of the uterus, and risks are not well documented. The classic, a high vertical incision in the upper part of the uterus, is not as frequently done now because this type of incision requires that women have repeated cesareans because of the risk of uterine rupture during labor.

INFERTILITY

Infertility refers to the inability to become pregnant after 1 year of sexual intercourse without the use of birth control. It affects one in seven couples in the United States. One cause for infertility may be the delay in childbearing until after age 30. Infertility can be traced to the woman in about one third of the cases, to the man in another third, and to both in the last third. For the woman, the problem is usually a blocked fallopian tube, damaged ovaries, or abnormally developed tubes. Many times, it is the absence or infrequency of ovulation. In the male, it is usually abnormally developed testicles, a low sperm count, or low motility. Sexually transmitted diseases (STDs) account for a large percentage of infertility by silently damaging the fallopian tubes and ovaries. It is very important that young men and women understand the importance of practicing safe sex by using condoms and decreasing the number of sexual partners.

Treatment consists of medications to stimulate egg or sperm production or surgery to repair damaged organs or abnormalities. Other actions such as determining ovulation, intercourse on alternating fertile days (to collect sperm), and the use of boxer shorts for men (this reduces the body heat transferred to the testicles by tight briefs) are indicated. When this is unsuccessful, other methods can be used, such as:

● *Artificial insemination*—The semen is spun down to concentrate the sperm, which are withdrawn and injected into the uterus through a catheter in the cervix. The specimen can be from the women's spouse or another male donor.

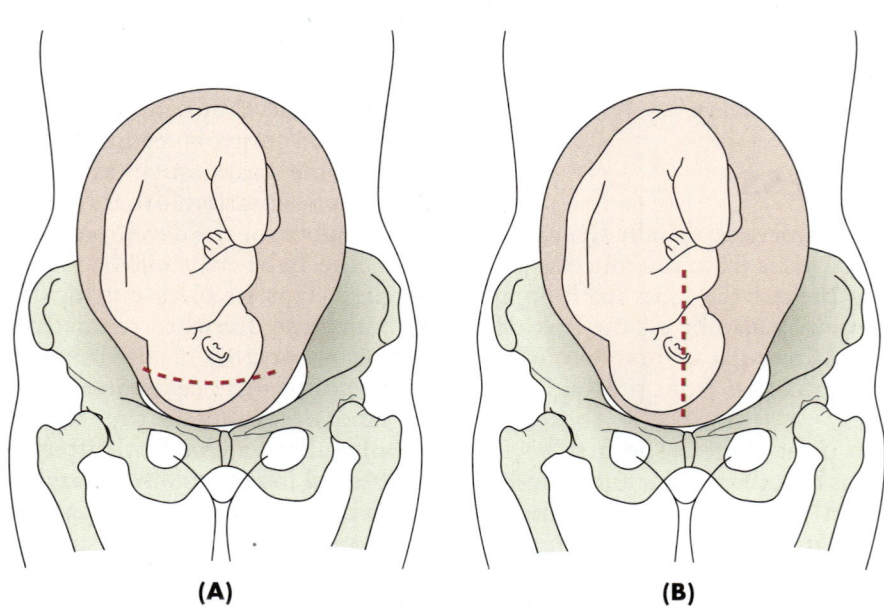

(A) **(B)**

FIGURE 11-223 The types of incision used in cesarean delivery: (A) the transverse incision; (B) the low vertical incision

- *In vitro fertilization*—The eggs are retrieved through a needle inserted into the ovaries, fertilized with sperm in a laboratory, and placed into the uterus.
- *Gamete intrafallopian transfer (GIFT)*—This involves injection of egg(s) mixed with sperm directly into the fallopian tube(s) so that fertilization can occur.
- *Intracytoplasmic sperm injection (ICSI)*—This is a microsurgical procedure involving the direct injection of a single sperm into an egg cell. This procedure is done in instances where only a very few sperm cells are produced or where those sperm cells are incapable of entering an egg on their own. ICSI is also used in those cases where sperm has to be recovered directly from the testes because of blockage of the normal route of sperm cells.
- *Zygote intrafallopian transfer (ZIFT)*—This is a combination of *in vitro* fertilization and gamete intrafallopian transfer. Eggs are fertilized in the test tube, and the resulting embryos are transferred to the fallopian tube by laparoscopy. ZIFT is infrequently used.

Procedures to produce pregnancy are proceeded by medications that increase the maturation of eggs to increase the odds of fertilization. Due to these processes, multiple fertilzations and embryos can occur, resulting in multiple births.

CONTRACEPTION

The authors acknowledge that some religious and ethnic groups oppose birth control, and this text does not ignore that issue; however, this subject matter is presented factually, from a clinical viewpoint, as information required for practice as a medical assistant. As the word implies, **contraception** is literally "against" conception. Several reasons may be given to avoid pregnancy:

- Avoid health risks to the woman. A woman in poor health may not survive a pregnancy.
- Spacing pregnancies. Some women are very fertile and conceive every year or less. The infant death rate is reported to be 50% higher at 1-year intervals than at 2 or more years.
- Avoid having babies with birth defects. Some women have chromosome defects or are genetic disease carriers (or married to carriers) and choose not to risk pregnancy.
- Delay pregnancy early in marriage to allow a time for adjustment to avoid additional stress in the new relationship and establish a strong marriage.
- Limiting family size. It is sometimes a personal decision and other times a reality of limited resources.
- Avoid pregnancy among unmarried couples. Single parenthood is difficult.
- Permit the woman to develop a successful career with planned pregnancies to integrate motherhood.

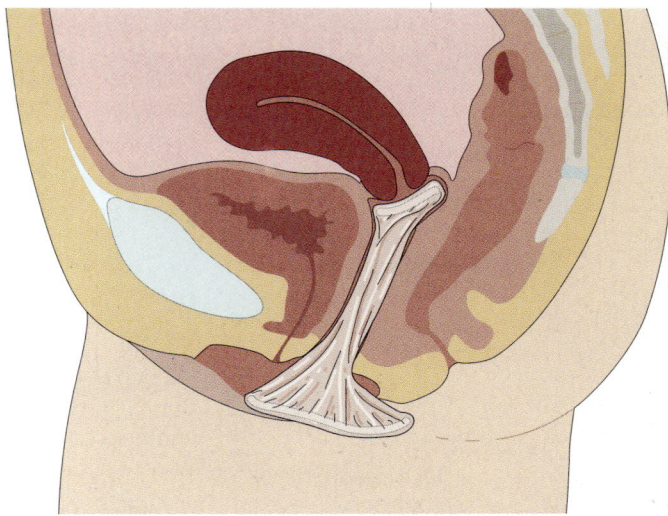

FIGURE 11-224   Female condom placement. The pouch should not be twisted, and the outer ring must be outside the vagina.

- Curbing population growth. The concern over worldwide food supply and supportive environment prompts some to promote contraception. It is expected that the population doubled between 1960 and the year 2000, only 40 years. Each successive doubling time becomes shorter.

Several methods to prevent conception and their relative percentage of effectiveness are listed in Table 11-19. Selection is usually made by the woman in consultation with her doctor. The cost, ease of use, degree of effectiveness, and likelihood of side effects must be taken into consideration when selecting a method. A relatively new product has been introduced into the United States market. It is the female condom. This gives women another method of birth control and protection from sexually transmitted diseases. The device is constructed with a ring at one end similar to a diaphragm, which is fitted internally over the cervix. A latex "tube" extends from the ring to another ring that hangs outside the vagina (Figure 11-224). Intercourse is accomplished within the lubricated latex tube. It is relatively effective, providing that the ring remains outside the vagina and the insertion is within the tube.

Pregnancy Termination

Abortion (A-bore'-shun) (Miscarriage)

Description—This is the spontaneous (unforced) or induced (therapeutic) loss of a pregnancy of less than 20 weeks' gestation.

Signs and symptoms—Symptoms of spontaneous abortion are a pink or brownish discharge for several days followed by uterine cramping and increasing vaginal bleeding. When contractions are sufficient,

TABLE 11-19	Different Methods of Preventing Conception	
% Effective	**Method**	**Description/Comments**
100%	Abstinence	Refraining from sexual intercourse; absolutely most effective.
100%	Sterilization	Tubal **ligation** (cutting of the fallopian tubes) is done in the female. The cut ends can be sewn back in opposite directions or cauterized. The surgical procedure is done through a laparoscope inserted into the abdomen. The procedure is considered permanent. A vasectomy is done in the male, with the ends being sewn in opposite directions. The surgery is performed through a small incision at the base of the scrotum. Vasectomies are usually not reversible; however, in some instances, reconstructive surgery has been successful, especially in cases of shorter duration; sperm production is usually significantly decreased in time. Usually a second marriage and the desire for another child prompt the attempt. The method is relatively expensive initially.
99%	Depo medroxy-progesterone acetate (DMPA) suspension	This is an intramuscular injection that is given quarterly and provides protection for 3 months. The injection is given during the first 5 days of a normal menstrual period and provides contraceptive effects immediately. It is contraindicated if there is a possibility of being pregnant, a history of blood clots in the legs or lungs, known or suspected breast cancer, a liver tumor, or unexplained vaginal bleeding. Some side effects may occur, such as nervousness, dizziness, stomach discomfort, headaches, or fatigue. It may reduce the amount of minerals stored in bones, which could contribute to the development of osteoporosis. The most common side effect is irregular or unpredictable menstrual periods. Some women will stop having periods until 6 to 18 months after stopping the injections. A new warning was issued in 2005 that Depo-Provera should not be used more than 2 consecutive years due to possible bone loss from estrogen suppression.
95%–99%	Birth control pills	Many different kinds are available. They are a combination of hormones that prevent ovulation; no ovum means no pregnancy. Failure occurs when pills are not taken as prescribed. Side effects can be prohibitive for some women. They are available only by prescription and require regular visits to a physician. Cost is a factor to consider.
99%	Contraceptive patch	The contraceptive patch contains hormones similar to those in birth control pills. The patch is just as effective as the pill (99% when used correctly). It is paper thin and as soft as the skin. The patch is changed weekly for 3 weeks, then left off for the 4th week, when a menstrual period will occur. The side effects and warnings are the same as with oral contraceptives. The patch does not protect against sexually transmitted diseases.
99%	Contraceptive ring	The contraceptive ring is a comfortable, flexible ring about 2 inches in diameter that is inserted into the vagina once per month. The ring will release a low level of hormones to prevent conception. The ring is removed after 3 weeks so a menstrual period can occur. A new ring is inserted for the next 3 weeks. The ring is also 99% effective, the same as oral contraceptives, and carries the same risk factors and warnings.
93%–99%	Intrauterine device (IUD)	The intrauterine device is a small piece of plastic or coiled material inserted into the uterus to prevent implantation of a fertilized egg, presumably by providing irritation to the endometrium. Failure can occur if the device is expelled and during the first few months after being inserted. Initial insertion costs and the cost of removal are involved. IUDs are only recommended for women who have had children and who are in monogamous relationships because there is an increased risk of uterine infection with this device. Side effects include increase in menstrual cramping and possible increase in vaginal discharge throughout the month. IUDs are available in two types: one is copper and is effective for up to 10 years. Another contains progesterone and comes in a 5-year form.

(continues)

TABLE 11-19   Different Methods of Preventing Conception (Continued)

% Effective	Method	Description/Comments
90%–99%	Diaphragm	A thin piece of dome-shaped rubber with a firm ring, which is inserted into the vagina to cover the cervix and provide a barrier to sperm. It is most effective when used in combination with a contraceptive cream placed into the dome before inserting. Failure usually results from improper insertion; a defect in the rubber, such as a hole; failure to insert before any penile penetration; or failure to maintain in place at least 6 hours following intercourse. There is an initial cost to examine and fit and purchase. There are side effects. It requires cleaning and inspection after each use.
85%–97%	Condom	A thin sheath of rubber or latex that fits over an erect penis to catch the semen. A properly used condom is very effective. It must be unrolled onto an erect penis *before* any penetration occurs. It is important to leave about $\frac{1}{2}$ inch of free air space at the tip (unless the condom is constructed with a tip) to catch the semen; otherwise, the force of the ejaculant may burst the condom. It must also remain in place throughout intercourse. After ejaculation has occurred, care must be taken to withdraw with the condom in place. It may require grasping with the fingers. This is the only contraceptive that also provides a level of protection against sexually transmitted diseases. It is relatively inexpensive, easy to use, and readily available. Remember, only a latex condom is also effective against the AIDS virus.
75%–97%	Female condom	This is a latex pouch suspended from an inner ring that fits over the cervix. The pouch extends to the outside and has an external ring that holds the opening outside the vagina. The condom provides a barrier for protection against sexually transmitted diseases and contraception. A new condom must be used with each intercourse. Care must be taken to ensure that the penis enters inside the pouch and that the pouch remains in the proper position throughout intercourse.
70%–75%	Spermicides	Contraceptive foams, jellies, sponges, and creams with *sperm-killing* ingredients, inserted by applicator deep into the vagina before intercourse. It must remain for at least 6 to 8 hours afterward. Each application is good for only one act of intercourse. They should not be relied on alone as an effective contraceptive. Combined with a diaphragm or condom, they are effective. They have few side effects (some report allergic reactions), are easily used, and are readily available. They must not be confused with lubricants such as KY jelly or Lubafax, which contain *no* spermicide.
70%–80%	Withdrawal	This method has been practiced since biblical times. It simply requires that the penis be withdrawn and ejaculation occur outside the vagina. It is not very effective because some sperm are deposited in the vagina before ejaculation occurs. In addition, the man may not be able to withdraw in time. It requires a lot of concentration to control. It is also not advised because it may lead to a sexual dysfunction if practiced for a prolonged time.
65%–85%	Rhythm	The practice of abstinence during an 8 day period from days 10 to 17 of the menstrual cycle when conception is theoretically possible. The method works fairly well for women who are extremely regular in their cycles and couples who can practice strong self-control. However, it requires a careful assessment of at least 6 months of cycles to establish ovulation days. If cycles vary in length, the period of abstinence must be increased to cover the longest possible time.
Unknown	Douching	Absolutely not effective. It only takes a couple of minutes for sperm to enter the cervix. Douching in fact, may even assist sperm toward the cervix, thereby increasing the odds of conception.

the cervix dilates and the fetus is expelled. A complete abortion includes expulsion of the fetus, placenta, and membranes, resulting in the end of cramping and minimal bleeding because the uterus contracts to close off the blood vessels. An incomplete abortion results from the retention of some or all of the placenta.

Etiology—A spontaneous **abortion** usually results from one of three factors: (1) *fetal:* defective implantation or development of the embryo (most common cause); (2) *placental:* premature separation or abnormal implantation of the placenta; or (3) *maternal:* endometrial rejection, infection, malnutrition, trauma, drug reaction, endocrine difficulties, or blood group incompatibility. Spontaneous abortions occur in about 30% of all first pregnancies and up to 15% of all pregnancies.

Treatment—If the placenta (or a portion) adheres to the uterine wall, bleeding will persist, necessitating a D & C (**dilation and curettage**) to scrape out the retained placenta and permit the uterus to close off the blood vessels.

A therapeutic abortion is one performed to preserve the mother's mental or physical health in such instances as rape; unplanned pregnancy; or an existing medical condition, such as cardiac or kidney disease.

Diagnostic and Screening Tests in Pregnancy

- **Alpha-fetoprotein screening (AFP)**—This is a blood test taken at about the 15th to 18th week of pregnancy to aid in the detection of birth defects. It can also indicate the presence of multiple births. If the blood level is too high, additional tests will be performed to rule out neural tube defects. These are instances when there is a failure of the brain and skull to develop or there is an opening in the spine, exposing the spinal cord—a condition known as spina bifida. When the blood level is too low, Down syndrome is suspected. The tests are not 100% accurate but serve as a screening device detecting about 85% of open neural tube defects and about 75% of fetuses with Down syndrome in women under 35 years of age. When positive results are obtained, another blood sample, an ultrasound, and an amniocentesis are indicated. Remember that a negative test does NOT guarantee a baby free of birth defects but only that it is unlikely that there is neural tube defect or Down syndrome.
- Amniocentesis—Down syndrome is caused by a chromosomal error (see Unit 1). This occurs in 1 of every 1,000 live births. A test known as an **amniocentesis** can be done on women who apparently are at risk. Amniotic fluid is withdrawn from the amniotic sac in which the fetus is growing (Figure 11-225).

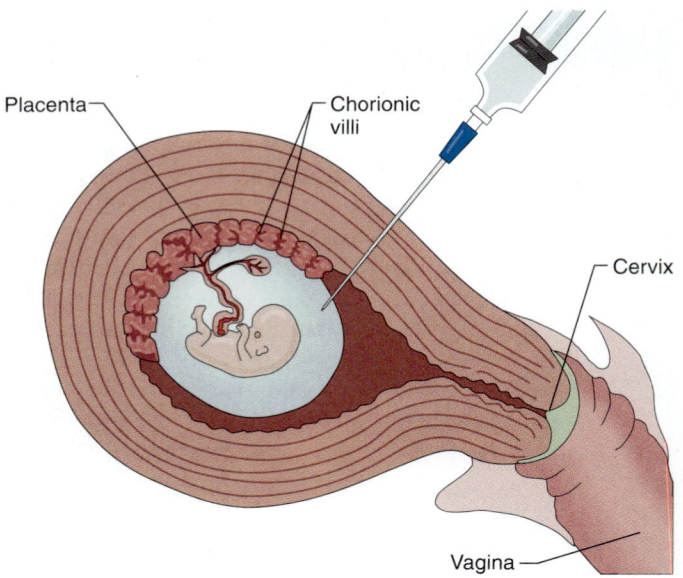

FIGURE 11-225 Amniocentesis

Cells from the skin of the fetus can be grown in a culture and examined for chromosomal abnormalities and neural tube defects. The test is usually done between 13 and 16 weeks, and ultrasound is used to visualize the fetus and amniotic fluid. Amniocentesis is 100% accurate in findings, but it is not without risk. A miscarriage rate of 1 in 200 to 1 in 300 is associated with the procedure. The incidence of Down syndrome correlates to the age of the mother. In her 20s, a woman has only a 1 in 2,500 chance of having a Down syndrome child. That incidence increases dramatically as the woman ages. By age 45, the risk increases to 1 in every 40 births. Figure 11-226 shows the frequency of Down syndrome in relationship to age from 30 to 49 years.
- Chorionic villi sampling (CVS)—A procedure similar to amniocentesis but done by removing cells from the chorionic villi. This procedure is not as common as amniocentesis and is associated with more complications. Like amniocentesis, this is 100% accurate for chromosomal testing.
- Gestational diabetes screening—This test is done between 24 and 28 weeks of pregnancy by drawing a blood sample after drinking a loading dose of glucose. Gestational diabetes only affects pregnant women. It is absent after delivery.
- Group B streptococcus (GBS)—GBS is one of the many bacteria that do not usually cause serious illness. It may be in the digestive, urinary, or reproductive tract, but it is most common in the vagina and rectum. Infected persons who show no symptoms are said to be colonized and usually do not pose any danger to their own health and may not be treated. However, when there is a pregnancy, 1 to 2 out of

DOWN SYNDROME AND MATERNAL AGE	
Maternal Age	Frequency of Down Syndrome
30	1 in 885 births
31	1 in 826 births
32	1 in 725 births
33	1 in 592 births
34	1 in 465 births
35	1 in 365 births
36	1 in 287 births
37	1 in 225 births
38	1 in 176 births
39	1 in 139 births
40	1 in 109 births
41	1 in 85 births
42	1 in 67 births
43	1 in 53 births
44	1 in 41 births
45	1 in 32 births
46	1 in 25 births
47	1 in 20 births
48	1 in 16 births
49	1 in 12 births

FIGURE 11-226   Risk of giving birth to a Down syndrome infant by maternal age

every 100 babies will be infected. Vaginal cultures are used to test during 35 to 37 weeks of pregnancy. This type of bacteria is found in up to 40% of pregnant women. It can be passed on to the fetus during pregnancy, to the baby during delivery, or to the baby after birth. Most babies who get GBS do not have any problems; however, a few will become sick. It can cause major health problems and may even become life threatening. Antibiotics are given during labor to women who test positive for GBS.

- Routine pregnancy screening tests—There are several routine tests that are taken for routine information, such as blood typing, antibody screenings, sexually transmitted disease screening, and urine cultures.

DIAGNOSTIC TESTS OF THE FEMALE REPRODUCTIVE SYSTEM

- **Colposcopy**—An examination and biopsy of the cervix using a colposcope. It is done to rule out cancer when there are abnormal Pap smear results. Often cell structure may be temporarily altered by antibiotics, yeast infections, and other reasons, which might give a false positive Pap smear. The cervix is cleansed with a solution of acetic acid and the scope introduced. The cervix can then be viewed through the colposcope, which magnifies the mucosa and makes cellular structure visible. In most cases, biopsies are taken from the abnormal sites. A Pap smear is a screening test, whereas colposcopy is used to obtain a definitive diagnosis.

- **Hysteroscopy**—A hysteroscope is inserted vaginally into the uterus. It is connected to a monitor that permits viewing of the endometrium. By using instruments through the scope, it is possible to biopsy suspicious areas and remove polyps and fibroid. It is even possible to take photographs or make a videotape for documentation of findings (Figure 11-227). When the hysteroscope is used with a laparoscope, it is possible to increase the visual field and facilitate the performance of surgical procedures. In the Figure 11-227, the use of both scopes permits visualizing both the inside and outside of the uterus at the same time.

- **Interventional hysterosalpingography** (IHSG)—This is a procedure used to evaluate fallopian tubes in cases of infertility. It is an alternative to laparoscopy or laparotomy with tubal resection. It is performed on women with tubal obstruction that has been confirmed with regular HSG. A catheter is placed through the cervix into the uterus while x-ray dye is being injected. The catheter is then pushed into the opening of a blocked tube. Additional dye is injected into the tube. A small, soft wire is pushed into the fallopian tube through the catheter until the tube is reopened and the dye fills the entire fallopian tube. The success rate for opening an obstruction is 75% to 95%. Pregnancy is greater than 50% within 1 year following the procedure. If unsuccessful, a second procedure may result in pregnancy.

The main benefits of the IHSG procedure are that it is relatively inexpensive, and it is a nonsurgical approach to restoring tubal patency.

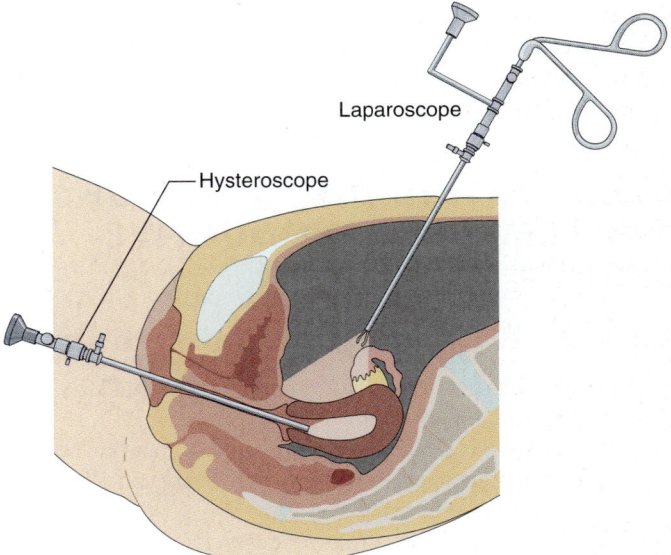

FIGURE 11-227   Laparoscopy performed with hysteroscope

- **Mammogram**—An x-ray of the breast for the detection of malignancy. A mammogram is indicated whenever there are palpable breast masses, breast pain, or nipple discharge. The film can also help differentiate between benign breast disease or breast malignancy. The American College of Radiologists recommends a single baseline mammogram for all women between ages 35 and 40. All women older than 40 should have an annual mammogram. Women at risk require earlier and more frequent examinations. Risk-related factors are fibrocystic disease; history of breast, uterine, ovarian, colorectal, or salivary gland cancer; and a family history of breast malignancy.
- Maturation index—A means of determining hormonal level by examining the percentage of certain types of cells in scrapings taken from the lateral vaginal walls.
- **Papanicolaou (Pap) smear** (test)—A routine examination done on secretions removed from the cervix and upper vagina to determine the presence of cancerous cells.
- Pregnancy test—Conducted on a first-voided morning urine specimen to determine presence of the hormone human chorionic gonadotropin (HCG), which is produced by the developing placenta at the onset of pregnancy.
- Ultrasonography—A test for malignancy. A transducer is used to focus a beam of high-frequency sound waves through the skin into the breast. Sound waves bounce back echos, which are displayed on a computer screen for diagnosis. Ultrasound can detect tumors less than ¼ inch in diameter and can distinguish between cysts and solid tumors. It is anticipated that ultrasonography will eventually replace mammography in breast cancer screening programs.
- Ultrasonography is also used to observe the fetus *in utero*. It can help determine the status of pregnancy, confirm the expected date of delivery, and identify the gender, if desired.

DISEASES AND DISORDERS OF THE FEMALE REPRODUCTIVE SYSTEM

Cervical Erosion (Ser'vi-kal E-ro'shun)

Description—This is an ulceration of the epithelium on a portion of the cervix.

Signs and symptoms—The area bleeds easily when touched during examination and may cause intermenstrual bleeding.

Etiology—It results from chronic cervicitis.

Treatment—Erosion is treated locally by cauterization (burning) to destroy the abnormal tissue growth. Cauterizing agents used can be chemical, such as silver nitrate sticks, or electrical, such as electrocautery. The treatment is administered through a vaginal speculum and produces immediate cramping, which subsides quickly. Vaginal discharge will increase for a few days as the tissue sloughs off.

Cervicitis (Ser-vi-si'tis)

Description—This is inflammation of the cervix.

Signs and symptoms—Often, the only symptoms are a purulent, foul-smelling vaginal discharge and a tenderness of the cervix.

Etiology—It is caused by an invading organism, usually a staphylococcus or streptococcus. Herpes simplex II is a possible cause. A large percentage of patients in whom the cervicitis is associated with pelvic inflammatory disease are infected with the gonorrhea bacteria.

Treatment—Treatment is usually an antibiotic appropriate for the causative organism.

Cystic (Fibrocystic) Breast Disease (Fibro-sis'tik)

Description—This is the presence of multiple lumps within the breast tissue. The lumps may be fibrous tumors that have degenerated or cysts (sacs) containing fluid.

Signs and symptoms—They may occur singularly or in multiple clusters. Fibrous tumors are either round or lobular. They are usually firm, well-defined (with definite borders), freely moveable, and painless. Cysts are also round, soft to firm, elastic, well-defined, moveable, and often tender. Neither type is attached to underlying tissues or to the skin to cause signs of retraction.

Etiology—There is probably no specific "cause" of this disorder. It is not a "disease" as such but rather a condition of normal breast tissue that has just "developed." It tends to occur with aging.

Treatment—Treatment may include needle aspiration of cystic fluid. Often, the cyst will not refill. Women with fibrocystic disease are believed to be at greater risk of developing a malignancy in one of the masses.

Many women naturally have "lumpy" breasts and should not be classified as having a "disease." Young women often have dense breast tissue that feels lumpy all over. This is just a condition of being fibrocystic. Often breasts become fibrocystic as a woman ages. Only professional examination and mammography can accurately diagnose a fibrocystic condition.

Cystocele (Sis'to-sel)

Description—This is the bulging of the anterior wall of the vagina and the bladder into the vaginal canal, sometimes into the introitus.

Signs and symptoms—It can be demonstrated by asking the patient to bear down or strain as the vaginal opening is observed.

Etiology—Cystocele appears in older women because of poor musculature from aging and the effects of childbearing. Other predisposing factors are obesity, lifting of heavy objects, instrument deliveries, and chronic coughing. The displacement of the bladder contributes to improper emptying, which results in cystitis, frequency (because some urine is always in the bladder), urgency, and incontinence, particularly stress incontinence as a result of coughing, sneezing, or laughing.

Treatment—If it causes discomfort or continual urinary problems, it may be necessary to surgically reposition the bladder and repair the vaginal wall.

Dysmenorrhea (Dismen-o-re'a)

Description—This is the lower abdominal and pelvic pain associated with menstruation common among young females and tends to decrease with maturity, particularly after pregnancy. **Dysmenorrhea** in women in their late 20s or early 30s may be a symptom of an organic disease, such as cervical stenosis, pelvic congestion, or endometriosis.

Signs and symptoms—Dysmenorrhea typically begins 12 to 14 hours before the onset of menses and lasts between 24 to 48 hours. It may be associated with headache, nausea, vomiting, fatigue, and diarrhea. Occasionally, pain may be felt in the back and upper legs.

Etiology—It is unrelated to any identifiable cause. However, certain contributing factors are known, such as hormonal imbalances and psychogenic factors. The discomfort probably results from increased secretion of the hormone prostaglandin, which intensifies uterine contractions. Dysmenorrhea is also present with other conditions, such as endometriosis, cervical stenosis, uterine leiomyomas (tumor in the muscle tissue), incorrect uterine positioning, and PID (pelvic inflammatory disease).

Treatment—Treatment consists of analgesics; heat; drugs to decrease uterine contractions; and the use of hormonal therapy, such as oral contraceptives, to suppress ovulation. When discomfort has an organic cause, the underlying condition must be corrected.

Endometriosis (Endo-metre-o'sis)

Description—The presence of endometrial tissue outside the uterus is most commonly found in the pelvic area, affecting the ovaries, ligaments, and peritoneal tissues.

Signs and symptoms—The condition is characterized by dysmenorrhea, with constant pain in the lower abdomen, pelvis, vagina, and back beginning about a week before menses and lasting 2 to 3 days after onset. The degree of pain depends on the location of the endometrial tissue. Other symptoms include excessive, profuse menses when ovarian; hematuria when located in the bladder; rectal bleeding when located in the colon; and nausea, vomiting, and abdominal cramps when located in the small intestine.

Etiology—The cause of endometriosis is unknown, but it is believed to be the result of the following:

- Recent surgery that opened the uterus
- Endometrial fragments expelled through the fallopian tubes at menstruation
- Alteration in the epithelium by inflammation or hormones that changes it to endometrium

Treatment—Treatment consists of conservative methods in younger women, such as analgesics, nonsteroidal anti-inflammatory drugs, and oral contraceptives. Oral contraceptives are the current treatment of choice for long-term therapy because of the action of ovulation suppression. Other injectable medications such as Lupron Depot is used for 6-month therapy. It works by decreasing estrogen and progesterone normally produced by the ovaries. This is mainly used after the diagnosis of endometriosis has been determined, although some physicians are now using Lupron Depot prior to surgery for treatment. After the 6-month therapy, menstrual cycles will return to normal. When ovarian masses exist, they may be surgically removed. In women who no longer desire children, the treatment of choice is **hysterectomy** (removal of the uterus) and bilateral **salpingo-oophorectomy** (removal of both fallopian tubes and ovaries). The condition is not life-threatening, but pain and anemia must be controlled. Because the disease may cause sterility, childbearing should be accomplished as soon as convenient. Endometriosis generally subsides with menopause if surgery is ruled out.

Fibroids (Fi'broyd)

Description—**Fibroids** are known technically as uterine leiomyomas or myomas; they are a common benign, smooth tumor formed of muscle cells, not fibrous tissue as suggested by the name. Usually fibroids do not occur singly and are located most often in the body of the uterus.

Signs and symptoms—The primary symptom associated with leiomyomas is **menorrhagia** (excessive menstruation). Other characteristics are pain, a feeling of heaviness in the abdomen if the mass is large, discomfort from pressure against other organs, possible urinary frequency or constipation, and an irregular enlargement of the uterus. When a leiomyoma is attached to the lining by a stalk and is suspended within the uterine cavity, pain is caused by the uterus contracting in an attempt to expel the mass. The patient is frequently anemic because of excessive bleeding. The diagnosis is usually confirmed by a D & C, showing cells from leiomyoma in the scrapings from the endometrium.

Etiology—The cause of leiomyomas is unknown, but it is believed they are cells that have grown into a tumor, probably stimulated by estrogen and the growth hormone, because following menopause they usually shrink in size and disappear.

Treatment—Treatment depends on several factors, such as the patient's age, general health, and desire for children; the size of the tumors; and the severity of the symptoms. Lupron Depot is used to treat uterine fibroids for 1 to 3 months prior to surgery. The medication shrinks the fibroids, therefore minimizing bleeding with surgery. Small masses can be surgically removed, but a complete hysterectomy is indicated with greater involvement. The ovaries are left intact if possible to maintain hormone levels naturally. Uterine leiomyomas occur in about 20% of all women older than age 35, with leiomyosarcoma (malignancy) developing in only about 0.1% of patients.

Hysterectomy (His-ter-ek'to-me)

Description—This is the surgical removal of the uterus. It is one of the most common procedures performed on female patients. It is not usually done on an elective or request basis but as a solution to a problem, such as endometriosis, leiomyomas, uterine rupture, or malignancy. A hysterectomy can be performed in different ways, depending on the situation. Figure 11-228 illustrates the extent of surgery. Removing the uterus through an abdominal incision is called an abdominal hysterectomy. When the uterus is positioned appropriately, it can be removed through the vagina, called a vaginal hysterectomy.

Endometrial **ablation** is used in cases of excessive bleeding from the buildup of endometrium or benign fibroid. A pen-sized instrument called a resectoscope is inserted into the uterus through the cervix. The procedure removes the lining by electrical cautery, using a loop or rollerball attached to the end of the scope. It requires about 20 minutes to perform, is relatively painless, avoids surgery, takes only a few days' recovery time, and is a fraction of the cost of a hysterectomy. In contrast, a hysterectomy is major surgery, requiring well over an hour to perform, approximately 6 weeks to recover, and a cost between $4,000 and $7,000. The ablation is probably an alternative for 20% to 50% of the annual 600,000 hysterectomies done mainly to stop uncontrollable bleeding. The procedure almost always results in sterilization, which of course would also happen with a hysterectomy. There is a slight chance of per-

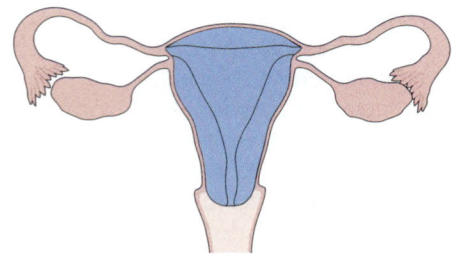

Total hysterectomy

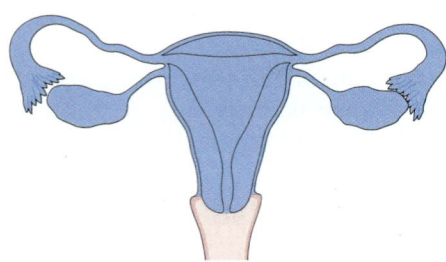

Total hysterectomy with a
salpingo-oophorectomy

FIGURE 11-228 Types of hysterectomies

forating the uterine wall, which may then lead to a hysterectomy.

Ovarian Cyst

Description—This is a sac of fluid or semisolid material on an ovary; it is usually nonmalignant, small, and produces no symptoms. Common cysts include follicular and lutein types that occur in the follicle or the corpus luteum. They can occur any time between puberty and menopause, including during pregnancy.

Signs and symptoms—An ovarian cyst may cause an acute abdomen (a sudden condition, probably requiring surgical treatment) if the ovary is twisted by the cystic mass or the cyst ruptures. Large or multiple cysts may cause pelvic discomfort, lower-back pain, and abnormal uterine bleeding. Symptoms vary according to the type of cyst. Other possible symptoms are acute abdominal pain similar to appendicitis, massive intraperitoneal hemorrhage, and delayed menses followed by prolonged or irregular bleeding.

Etiology—Follicular cysts develop as a result of an overdistended follicle that fails to close off properly. They secrete excessive amounts of estrogen in response to the FSH hormone. Granular lutein cysts are enlargements of the ovaries caused by excessive accumulation of blood during the bleeding phase of the menstrual cycle. Another form of lutein cyst is usually found bilaterally and contains clear, straw-colored liquid.

Treatment—Follicular cysts generally require no treatment because they spontaneously disappear within 60 days. Oral contraceptives or progesterone for 5 days reestablishes the hormonal cycle and induces ovulation. Treatment may also include drugs to induce ovulation or surgery to remove a portion of the ovary if drug therapy fails. Treatment generally consists of observation if the cyst is known to be nonmalignant. Signs of cyst rupture, such as increasing abdominal pain, distention, rigidity, fever, tachypnea, hypotension, and symptoms of intraperitoneal hemorrhage, are carefully watched. Occasionally, a cyst becomes so large that it causes discomfort and surgical removal becomes necessary.

PMS (Premenstrual Syndrome)

Description—This combination of characteristics appears from 7 to 14 days before menstruation and usually subsides with the onset. It is estimated that the syndrome occurs in 30% to 50% of women, particularly between the ages of 25 and 40.

Signs and symptoms—Symptoms include any or a combination of the following:

- Behavioral changes, such as nervousness, irritability, fatigue, and depression
- Neurologic changes, including headache, dizziness, numbness of extremities, and fainting
- Respiratory changes, including increase in colds, exacerbation (aggravation or increase) of allergic rhinitis, and asthma
- Gastrointestinal changes, such as constipation, diarrhea, abdominal bloating, and change in appetite
- General symptoms of backache, palpitations, temporary weight gain, increase in acne, or breast tenderness and enlargement

Etiology—The cause of premenstrual tension is unknown. For some reason, intravascular fluid enters the body tissues and results in secretion of an antidiuretic hormone. This causes fluid retention with characteristic bloating. The tissue edema results in headaches and alterations in mood because of central nervous system changes.

Treatment—Treatment basically is symptomatic. Medication can be used to help relieve emotional symptoms and the physical manifestations.

Polyp (Pol'ip)

Description—This is a growth with a slender stem attachment usually arising from the mucous membranes.

Signs and symptoms—Polyps of the cervix can often be visualized protruding from the external cervical os. They are red, soft, and rather fragile. If only the tip can be seen, it cannot be differentiated from a polyp of the endometrium.

Etiology—Probably result from the unrestrained cell growth of the epithelium.

Treatment—Depending on the location, size, and attachment, removal may be a simple office procedure or an outpatient surgical procedure. Protruding polyps can be chemically cauterized in the office. The procedure causes some immediate discomfort, primarily cramping, but soon subsides.

Rectocele (Rekto-sel)

Description—This is bulging of the posterior vaginal wall, by the rectum, into the vagina.

Signs and symptoms—Inspection of the introitus may disclose a posterior mass, or it may be demonstrable on requesting the patient to bear down. It is most common in postmenopausal women.

Etiology—Contributing factors are believed to be pregnancies, prolonged labor, instrument deliveries, obesity, chronic coughing, and lifting of heavy objects. A **rectocele** of advanced degree may cause difficulty in emptying the rectum.

Treatment—If severe, surgical intervention to repair the vaginal wall and support the rectum can be performed.

Vaginitis (Vaj-in-i'tis)

Description—This is an inflammation of the vaginal mucosa. There are several causes of **vaginitis**, with varying symptoms and treatment.

1. Allergic reaction—This usually happens as a result of douche solutions (especially those that are scented), spermicidal materials, deodorant-treated tampons, or other materials inserted into the vagina. This can be treated easily by discontinuing the causative agent.

2. Bacterial vaginitis—This was formerly called gardnerella or nonspecific vaginitis. It is a complex condition that is not understood well at present. The cause of this infection is thought to be an overgrowth of several different types of organisms. The predominant symptom is an increase in vaginal discharge, often with an unpleasant "fishy" odor. Redness and itching are rare; however, because bacterial vaginitis can occur with other types of infections, other symptoms may be present. Treatment involves oral antibiotics or an antibiotic vaginal cream therapy.

3. Candidiasis—Also called fungus, yeast infection, or **moniliasis**, this is the most common type of vaginal infection that causes irritation symptoms.
   Etiology—It is caused by a fungus like yeast that requires glucose for growth. It can affect any woman but is more frequent among women who are pregnant, diabetic, or obese. These

conditions alter the metabolic balance of the body and the acidity of the vagina, thereby promoting growth of the fungus. The use of antibiotics and birth control pills also increase the risk of the infection.

Signs and symptoms—Many women do not notice a discharge, but if present, it is usually described as odorless with a "cheesy" appearance. The main symptom is intense itching, burning, and redness of the vaginal tissues.

Treatment—With confirmation by exam and lab tests, medication will be prescribed to destroy the fungus. This may include vaginal suppositories or tablets or the insertion of an applicator of cream into the vagina.

4. Vaginal mucosa atrophy—This occurs in menopausal women because of decreased levels of estrogen. This can be treated with estrogen cream inserted into the vagina or by estrogen replacement therapy.

MALIGNANCY OF THE FEMALE REPRODUCTIVE ORGANS

Breast

Description—This is the most common malignancy among females and the number two cause of death. It occurs most often in women older than age 35.

Breast cancer is more common in the upper outer quadrant and in the left breast. It spreads through the lymphatic and circulatory system to the lungs, liver, bone, adrenal glands, kidneys, and brain. Cancer may be classified according to its location and cellular type as adenocarcinoma (from the epithelium) or Paget's disease (cancer of the nipple). In addition, most cancers are classified according to stages to identify the amount of tumor, node, and extent of metastasis.

Signs and symptoms—Specific warning signals that may indicate breast cancer are:
- A lump or mass in the breast tissue
- Change in breast size or shape
- Change in appearance of the skin
- Change in skin temperature (a warm, hot, or pink area)
- Drainage or discharge from a non-nursing woman or discharge produced by manipulation
- Change in the nipple, such as itching, burning, erosion, or retraction

Pain should be investigated but is not usually an early symptom.

Diagnosis is most often made by mammography, ultrasonography, and surgical biopsy. A new technique called Elastography may someday be the diagnostic method of choice, replacing the biopsy. The test uses ultrasound waves and compression to diagnose cancer. The breast lump that is a benign tumor is soft and will compress, whereas a malignant tumor is stiff and holds its shape. In preliminary studies, the technique has been nearly 100% accurate in differentiating between benign and malignant tumors. There are major advantages in that a surgical procedure is eliminated, the test is relatively inexpensive, and it can provide results in a matter of minutes. This greatly reduces the anxiety of waiting several days for a diagnosis while a tissue sample is prepared and a microscopic examination is performed.

The best and most reliable means of detecting breast cancer early is mammography. Numerous studies have shown that early detection saves lives and increases treatment options. The American Cancer Society estimates new cases of breast cancer in women for the year 2006 were 212,920, with an additional 1,720 in men. A total of 41,430 deaths were estimated for 2006.

Etiology—The cause is not known, but estrogen is believed to be in some way responsible. Predisposing factors include a family history of breast cancer, long menstrual cycles, early menarche or late menopause, first pregnancy after age 30, obesity, and drinking alcoholic beverages. There is also a correlation with diet, especially fat intake.

Treatment—The type of surgical treatment selected for breast cancer takes into consideration, first of all, the stage, the woman's age, the medical circumstances, and the patient's preferences. Physicians have become more aware of the woman's fears, attitudes, and feelings about the disfigurement of her body and will, if possible, choose the least radical method of surgery.

A lumpectomy (removal of the tumor only) can be done on a small mass when there is no evidence of lymph node involvement. The next step would be a lumpectomy and removal of axillary lymph nodes but not the breast itself. With additional breast involvement but no node enlargement, a simple **mastectomy** would remove just the breast and no underlying muscles. A modified radical mastectomy removes the breast and axillary nodes. A radical mastectomy removes the breast, axillary lymph node, and muscles from the chest wall. Radical mastectomies are seldom performed because of the lack of statistical data to verify their additional survival benefit. Treatment of ductal carcinoma *in situ* includes local excision, radiation, and tomoxifen.

Recent advances have been achieved in mastectomy surgery. Reconstruction of a breast mound can be provided for most patients. A prosthesis may be implanted after underlying tissues are excised with the skin and breast surface structures being maintained. The approach is determined by the extent of involvement. A mastectomy is disfiguring surgery that alters the patient's body image drastically. Because it can affect a woman's opinion of her sexuality and her relationship with her sexual partner, numerous volunteer support groups and other services are available to assist with the problems of adjustment.

Surgical treatment is usually combined with chemotherapy and/or radiation in an attempt to destroy cells within other structures of the body. Hormone therapy involves the use of androgens, progesterone, or an antiestrogen, depending on the hormone-receptive nature of the tumor.

The 5-year survival rate for localized breast cancer is 97% today. If it has spread regionally, the rate drops to 77%, and with distant metastases, the rate is only 21%. After 5 years, the rate of survival continues to decline, with the best survival being among women with early-stage disease.

Figure 11-229 shows the chest wall of a female who has had a double mastectomy. Twenty-three years ago when she was in her late 40s she was diagnosed with breast cancer and had a modified radical mastectomy. Four years later she had a recurrence in the other breast and had another modified procedure. She is truly a cancer survivor. She has been without disease in any other area since her last mastectomy. She had a very supportive husband and with his help she elected to not have reconstructive surgery. She wears prostheses in her brassiere, and no one is aware she has had surgery. Her only remaining problem comes from lymphedema in one arm due to the removal of many lymph nodes.

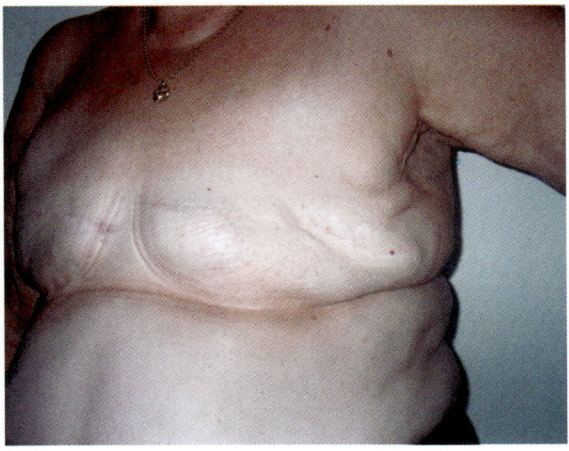

FIGURE 11-229   Female with bilateral modified radical mastectomy (Note the deep scar in the axilla from lymph node removal.)

Inflammatory Breast Cancer

This is an uncommon type of breast cancer, but it is so aggressive that it bears mention. Its symptoms are not what we have been told to observe. The cancer cells block the lymph vessels in the skin of the breast, causing the breast to become red, swollen, and warm. It may also appear bruised or purple, and appear like an orange peel. There may be no lump to be felt and may not be visible with a mammogram. There may be pain and a discharge leaking from the nipple. Diagnosis requires biopsy of the tissue and usually axillary lymph nodes to determine spread.

Inflammatory breast cancer grows and spreads rapidly. Treatment usually involves local treatment to remove the breast and surrounding area followed by radiation. Systemic treatment with chemotherapy and hormonal and even biologic (immune-system stimulation) therapy may also be used prior to surgery to control the disease and swelling within the breast, as well as afterward to destroy cells throughout the body.

Prognosis is guarded; because its progress is rapid and the symptoms are unfamiliar, the disease is often diagnosed late. Researchers are working on effective treatments, and clinical trials are in progress. The National Cancer Institute provides information on their web site or toll-free at 1-800-4-CANCER.

Cervical

Description—This is a cancer of the cervix of the uterus. An estimated 9,710 cases of cervical cancer were expected in 2006 with a death rate of 3,700. The Pap screening has reduced the incidence steadily over the past decades. The Pap test is a simple procedure involving a sampling of cells from the cervix that are easily obtained and examined under a microscope.

Signs and symptoms—It produces no symptoms until the cancer cells penetrate through the membranes and begin to travel through the lymphatic vessels or spread directly to nearby structures. The earliest symptoms are abnormal vaginal bleeding, persistent discharge, and pain and bleeding after intercourse. Cervical cancer can be detected very early by a Pap smear before any clinical evidence is observable. For this reason, the American Cancer Society recommends that all adult women younger than 40 (and sexually active teens) have Pap smears done at least every 3 years, and women older than 40 should be checked annually. The Pap test is not a reliable diagnostic tool for uterine cancer, only cervical. Women at risk require more frequent evaluation.

Etiology—Specific causes are unknown, but certain factors are contributory, such as: early age intercourse, multiple sexual partners, multiple pregnancies, herpes simplex virus II, and other bacterial or viral vene-real diseases.

Treatment—A variety of treatments, surgery, radiation, and chemotherapy, are used depending upon the stage of cancer. More common, especially in younger women, are precancerous cells called **dysplasia**, which are detected by Pap smear or colposcopy. For these preinvasive lesions, cryotherapy is used to freeze the area, or a procedure called LEEP (loop electrical excision procedure) uses electric current to destroy tissue with intense heat. Other methods use laser ablation or localized surgery.

With invasive cancers, surgery, radiation, or both and chemotherapy may be used. The survival rate for patients with preinvasive lesions is nearly 100%. Even invasive cervical cancer survival is at 92% for 5 years when discovered early.

In 2006, research identified the HPV virus as the cause of a large percentage of cervical cancers, and a preventive vaccine was developed. The government issued a policy stating all sexually active females should receive the vaccine. It was recommended that girls even as young as 8 to 10 years old be given the three-injection immunization to establish their protection before sexual activity began.

Ovarian

Description—Ovarian cancer is one of the most common causes of cancer deaths among American women. It accounts for 4% of all cancers among women and ranks second among gynecologic cancers. An estimated 20,180 new cases were expected in 2006 with an estimated 15,310 deaths—more than from any other cancer of the female reproductive system. Prognosis varies with the stage and type of tumor, but only about 25% of patients survive for 5 years. One type, primary epithelial, accounts for about 90% of the cases. Another form strikes children. It is more prevalent in higher socioeconomic women between the ages of 40 and 65 and in single women. Ovarian cancer spreads rapidly by local extension and occasionally through the blood or lymphatics. The most common metastasis is through the diaphragm into the chest cavity. Because of its location, early diagnosis is difficult.

Signs and symptoms—Symptoms are confined to vague abdominal discomfort and mild gastrointestinal disturbances. With progression, urinary frequency, constipation, pelvic discomfort, and distention develop. Symptoms may be confused with appendicitis. Diagnosis requires careful evaluation, complete history, surgical exploration, and lab studies on tissue samples.

Etiology—Risk factors for ovarian cancer increase with age and peak during the 80s. Women who have never had children, who have had breast cancer, or who have a family history of breast or ovarian cancer are at increased risk. Other genetic factors like *BRCA1* and *BRCA2*, a type of hereditary colon cancer, and living in an industrialized country increase the incidence.

Treatment—Treatment generally involves aggressive surgery to remove all reproductive organs, affected lymph nodes, the omentum (the apron of tissue covering the organs), and the appendix. Chemotherapy may be beneficial in early stages, to extend the survival time. Recent therapy is resulting in prolonged remissions in some patients.

Uterine

Description—Uterine cancer is the most common gynecologic malignancy, usually affecting postmenopausal women between ages 50 and 60. Estimates for 2006 were 50,910 cases of uterine body cancer, usually of the endometrium, with an expected death rate of 11,050. The incidence is higher among white women, but the death rate is higher among black women.

Signs and symptoms—The first signs of uterine cancer are uterine enlargement and unusual premenopausal or any postmenopausal bleeding. It may begin as blood-streaked watery discharge but changes gradually to more bloody drainage. The only reliable diagnostic test is biopsy, with a follow-up D & C if the biopsy is negative.

Etiology—The prime risk factor that may lead to the most common form of uterine cancer is a high cumulative exposure to estrogen. This can be from hormone replacement therapy, tamoxifen, early menarche, late menopause, never having children, or a history of failure to ovulate. Other factors include infertility, diabetes, gallbladder disease, hypertension, and obesity. A familial tendency, a history of uterine polyps or hyperplasia of the endometrium, and the normal process of aging are also factors.

Treatment—Surgery is the treatment of choice, removing all reproductive organs. Radiation, either by an implanted internal device or externally administered, is indicated before surgery if the tumor is poorly defined. Chemotherapy and hormonal therapy with progesterone may be used. Both cervical and uterine cancers are rated by stages from 0 to IV, with 0 being suspicious and IV-b indicating metastasis to distant organs. The 1-year survival rate for endometrial cancer is 92%, and the 5-year rate is between 64% and 69%, depending on whether it is discovered early or in a regional stage.

Vaginal

Description—Pertains to the vagina. Vaginal cancer is far less common, occurring primarily in women in their early to mid-50s. It occurs most often in the upper third of the vagina and, like cervical cancer, begins in the epithelial layer, then deepens. It spreads very slowly.

Signs and symptoms—Symptoms include vaginal discharge and bleeding, with an ulcerated, usually firm, lesion of the vagina. Diagnosis is made by the presence of abnormal vaginal cells on a Pap smear. Any visible lesion is biopsied. Involvement of the cervix must be ruled out. Lesions of the vagina are often difficult to visualize because of its physical structure and the presence of the vaginal speculum blades, which obstruct the view.

Etiology—Vaginal cancer appears to be caused by the same factors that contribute to uterine malignancy.

Treatment—Treatment of early stages may be confined to the area alone. Surgery or radiation varies according to the involvement. With extensive disease, surgical exenteration (removal of all pelvic organs) may be required, with construction of a colostomy and an ileal conduit (ureter emptying into the ileum). Radiation is the preferred treatment for vaginal cancer.

Vulva

Description—Pertains to the area of the external genitalia. Cancer of the vulva accounts for 5% of gynecologic malignancies. It occurs usually among older women, most often in their mid-60s, but can occur at any age, even in infancy. Early diagnosis and treatment greatly enhance survival. A 5-year survival rate is possible in 85% of patients without lymph node involvement and 75% when removed nodes are positive.

Signs and symptoms—Symptoms often begin with pruritus, bleeding, and a small surface ulcer that becomes infected and painful. Diagnosis is tentatively made from abnormal cells on a Pap smear and the typical clinical findings. Firm diagnosis requires biopsy of the suspected lesion.

Etiology—Risk factors related to vulvular cancer are chronic pruritus of the vulva with friction, swelling, and dryness and the presence of vulval diseases, including venereal diseases. Also, pigmented moles that are constantly irritated by clothing and perineal pads tend to be predisposing. Other systemic conditions, such as obesity, hypertension, diabetes, and absence of childbirth, present risks.

Treatment—Treatment consists of surgery, which varies with the extent of involvement. Small, confined lesions without lymph node involvement are treated by simple vulvectomy, perhaps on only one side. With node involvement in advanced stages a radical vulvectomy is required. This involves the vulva and superficial and deep inguinal lymph nodes. With adjoining tissue metastasis, it may be necessary to excise the urethra, vagina, and rectum, leaving an open perineal wound requiring 2 to 3 months to fill in and heal. If surgery is prohibited, radiation may be used to make the patient more comfortable.

SEXUALLY TRANSMITTED DISEASES (STDs)

AIDS—Acquired Immune Deficiency Syndrome

Refer to Unit 9 for an in-depth look at this disease.

Chlamydia (Kla-mid'e-a)

Description—This is one of the most frequent sexually transmitted diseases (STDs) in North America, affecting between 3 and 10 million people each year. Approximately 10% of all college students are infected. It is probably present in half of patients with pelvic inflammatory disease (PID).

Signs and symptoms—Symptoms do not easily lead to diagnosis. Men may experience burning on urination and have a mucoid discharge from the penis. They are often misdiagnosed as having gonorrhea. Women experience a vaginal discharge mimicking gonorrhea and have frequent painful urination associated with urinary tract infections. Sometimes chlamydia does not cause any visible signs. If there are visible signs, they will be noticeable within 1 to 3 weeks after having sexual contact with an infected person.

Etiology—This disease is caused by a specialized bacterium that lives as an intracellular parasite. There are two types of bacteria, both of which are pathogenic to humans. One strain causes a type of pneumonia. The other, *Chlamydia trachomatis,* lives in the conjunctiva of the eye and the epithelium of the urethra and cervix.

Treatment—If chlamydia is misdiagnosed, penicillin (for gonorrhea) or a medication for urinary infection may be given, and the chlamydia remains unaffected. Proper treatment requires repeated doses of tetracycline or erythromycin for at least a week to destroy the organism. If left untreated, or mistreated, it usually has no lasting effect on men, but they carry the organism and infect their sexual partners. In women, the bacteria will travel up the reproductive tract, causing inflammation of the fallopian tubes and eventual scarring. The scarring can interfere with pregnancy by causing tubal implantation of the fertilized ova because of the narrowed opening. Complete blockage may also occur, which prevents conception.

The disease, if contracted during pregnancy, will be transmitted to the baby during birth. The infant may develop conjunctivitis or pneumonia. Some evidence suggests that the infection may cause an increase in premature and still births. Two recently developed tests, which are inexpensive and quick to perform, accurately diagnose the disease. Because of its widespread incidence, many physicians routinely treat patients with symptoms and evidence of PID or gonorrhea even without positive chlamydia test results because of the risk of sterility.

Gonorrhea (Gono-re'a)

Description—This is a common venereal disease. The usual sites are the vagina, penis, rectum, mouth, and throat. Because the organism dies almost immediately on exposure to air, it can be spread only by direct sexual contact.

Signs and symptoms—Symptoms vary between the male and female. Men notice burning, itching, or pain on urination; a sore throat with gland involvement; discharge from the anus; or penile drainage that begins as a clear, watery fluid but changes to a thick, milky consistency. Women are usually asymptomatic, but they often develop an inflammation with a greenish-yellow discharge from the cervix. Other common symptoms are similar to those experienced by men, including sore throat, anal discharge, and swollen glands. Women may also develop lower abdominal pain, especially if fallopian tubes and other structures become involved (see PID). Diagnosis can usually be made on visual inspection, but confirmation depends on a microscopic examination of the discharge or a positive culture of the gonococcus organism from the discharge. Treatment is necessary; gonorrhea will not go away by itself.

Etiology—An infection caused by the gonococcus bacteria is known as **gonorrhea**. The organism is fragile and can survive only in a moist, dark, and warm area within the body.

Treatment—Large doses of penicillin or tetracycline are required to destroy the organism. A follow-up examination after treatment is important, because strains of the gonococcus organism have become so resistant to the drugs that one course may not be sufficient. Untreated or undertreated gonorrhea can continue to spread, causing much damage. Men may develop chronic urethritis, long-term urinary tract inflammation, and sterility. Women may develop PID, which damages the reproductive organs and results in sterility.

Women who are infected with gonorrhea when giving birth pose a grave danger to the newborn. The gonococcus organism can infect the delicate tissues of the newborn's eyes and cause permanent blindness. Because of this possibility, all newborns routinely receive silver nitrate solution in their eyes as part of immediate after-birth care.

Gonorrhea can be controlled and prevented with proper education, treatment, and common sense. Knowledge of a partner's sexual frequency and use of protection with others—*before* engaging in sexual activity—can prevent a person from becoming infected in the first place. Since the advent of the contraceptive pill and the IUD, the use of condoms, diaphragms, and foams has diminished. These chemical and mechanical barriers, especially the condom, deterred the spread of the disease. The condom is encouraged as a deterrent to the spread of all sexually transmitted diseases.

Herpes (Her'pez)

Description—Genital herpes is an acute, inflammatory disease of the genitalia. It is one of the most common recurring disorders of the genitalia. Prognosis varies according to the age of the patient, the strength of the immune system, and the infection site. Primary genital herpes is usually self-limiting but may cause painful local or systemic disease. For people with weak immune systems, newborns, and others with widespread disease, genital herpes is often severe, with complications and a high mortality rate. Herpes is passed by direct skin-to-skin contact with your own or someone else's lesions, even 24 hours before they erupt. It is possible to spread your own herpes without being aware of its presence.

Signs and symptoms—Herpes takes from 3 to 7 days to erupt. With **genital herpes**, fluid-filled vesicles appear on the cervix (primary site), labia, vulva, vagina, or perianal skin of the female. The male lesions appear on the glans, foreskin, or penile shaft. Nongenital lesions may cause complications, such as herpetic keratitis of the eye, which may lead to blindness. Vesicles are usually painless at first but may rupture and develop into shallow, painful ulcers with edema, redness, and tender inguinal lymph nodes.

Diagnosis is made by observation and from patient history. Confirmation of herpes simplex II is possible from a culture of the vesicle fluid.

Etiology—The virus causing herpes has two strains: type I and type II. Type I is the typical cold sore on the lip or at the edge of the nose. Type II is the form that appears on the external genitalia, mouth, or anus.

Treatment—Treatment with the usual antiviral medications helps reduce edema and ease discomfort. Antibacterial agents help combat secondary infections. Neither medication will treat the virus, but they will help to speed the healing process of the lesions.

After lesions heal, the virus becomes dormant. It may never recur, but about two thirds of herpes sufferers have additional attacks, some within a few months. Future recurrences decrease in frequency and severity. The best defense is a healthy, well-rested body that can fight the disease organism with its natural defense mechanisms.

Other complications demand attention. Newborns can be infected with herpes during vaginal delivery. Some infants survive, but others develop a brain infection that rapidly leads to death. If a woman has active herpes type II lesions at the time of birth, a cesarean section delivery is indicated. Women with herpes genitalis also have a higher-than-usual rate of spontaneous abortion. One major long-term risk associated with the disease is cervical cancer; therefore, women infected with or exposed to herpes type II should have a Pap smear every 6 months.

Human Papillomavirus (HPV) (Pap-i-lo′mavi′rus) Infection

Description—Human papillomavirus is the common name given to a group of related viruses. HPV is one of the most common STDs. One form, genital warts, has been around for centuries. Today, its increase may result from women having more sexual partners and being less likely to rely on condoms for birth control—hence, there is no physical barrier.

Signs and symptoms—There are different types of HPV. One causes the common warts that appear on the fingers and hands and rarely spread to the genitalia. These are unsightly but do not cause any health problems. Other types of HPV found on the genitalia cause condylomas, or genital warts. These are usually found in clusters growing on the external structures and inside the vagina and on the cervix. However, HPV can be present without the visible warts because the virus can cause changes that cannot be seen by the naked eye. Often the virus is discovered by the Pap test. When the Pap is positive, a visual examination and sometimes a colposcope, a magnifying instrument, may be used to examine the vagina, cervix, and vulva. Suspicious areas are usually biopsied for diagnosis and signs of precancerous changes.

Etiology—HPV is a very small virus that needs to infect cells in order to survive. Once inside a cell, the virus directs the cell to make copies of itself and to infect other healthy cells. The infected cells eventually die and are shed with the virus from the body. When shed, the virus can be passed to another person who then becomes infected. It often takes several months and maybe even years for the person to show signs of infection. The virus can be passed during sex and is therefore considered to be a STD.

Treatment—Some signs of infection may go away, but the following treatments may still be advisable:

- Trichloroacetic acid (TCA) and bichloroacetic acid (BCA) are strong chemicals that can be applied to destroy genital warts.
- Podophyllin is an old treatment that can also be applied with care to warts because it can burn sur-

rounding tissue. It should not be used during pregnancy.

- Interferon is a new drug to treat genital warts. It can be injected into the warts or into muscle. It must also be avoided during pregnancy.
- Cryotherapy destroys the lesions by freezing.
- Laser treatment destroys the warts with a high-intensity beam of light.
- Electrosurgery uses electric current to burn away the lesion or shave it with a loop.
- Excisional biopsy cuts away the tissue.
- TCA, cryotherapy, or a laser are used to treat pregnant patients.

Genital warts are difficult to remove, and repeated treatment may be necessary for several weeks or months. Even after visibly gone, they may return at a later time. The major concern with HPV is the increased risk of other major health problems, such as cancer, especially cervical cancer.

Nongonococcal Urethritis (NGU, NSU) (Non-gono-kokal Ure-thri′tis)

Description—This is a group of infections with similar manifestations that are not linked to a single organism. Sometimes it is also called NSU or **nonspecific urethritis**. In men, it causes urethral inflammation; in women, vaginitis. NGU is transmitted by sexual intercourse. Men can also develop inflammation or allergic reactions from vaginal creams, contraceptive foams, soaps, douching solutions, and deodorants used by their sexual partners.

Signs and symptoms—Symptoms are similar to cystitis: burning on urination, frequency, itching (penile or vaginal), and possibly a thin discharge (penile or vaginal).

Differential diagnosis between NGU and gonorrhea must be made because the symptoms are similar, but the treatment is different. Confirmation is made by absence of the gonococcus from the culture of the discharge.

Etiology—It is usually the result of a bacterial infection. In males, it often results from *Chlamydia trachomatis* infection or from bacteria such as staphylococci, diphtheroids, coliform organism, and *Hemophilus vaginalis*. In females, less is known about nonspecific genitourinary infection. The chlamydia or corynebacterial organisms may also be the cause of infection. The disease often has no obvious cause, but sometimes bacteria or bacteria-like organisms are found in the urethral discharge.

Treatment—Treatment is normally with tetracycline or a similar antibiotic, because NGU does not respond to penicillin therapy. If untreated, it may lead to complications like those associated with gonorrhea. The most serious complication is a scarred urethra, which results in problems with urination. In addition, some strains can cause birth defects in newborns whose mothers have the disease.

Pediculosis Pubis (Pe-diku-lo'sis Pu'bis) (Pubic Lice)

Description—These are little yellowish-gray insects, about the size of a pinhead. They attach themselves to the moist hair roots in the pubic area of humans and feed on the blood of their host, hopping from person to person during sexual contact. It is possible, however, to get lice from contaminated towels, upholstery, clothing, or bedding, because they can survive for about a day without a supporting host.

Signs and symptoms—The prime symptom is an intense itching that cannot be ignored. They are visible on close inspection.

Etiology—Pediculosis is caused by parasitic forms of lice.

Treatment—Treatment is quite simple with a product called Kwell, which is applied to the infected area. All clothing, bedding, and linens must be washed in very hot water and detergent to destroy the nits (eggs) and lice. Nonwashable items can be dry-cleaned or ironed with a hot iron. Lice eggs can survive for a week, so uncleaned items must be avoided.

Pelvic Inflammatory Disease (PID)

Description—This is any acute or chronic infection of the reproductive tract, including the cervix (cervicitis), uterus (endometritis), fallopian tubes (salpingitis), and ovaries (oophoritis). It can also involve the surrounding tissues. Early treatment is important to prevent reproductive damage, infertility, pulmonary emboli, septicemia (blood poisoning), and death.

Signs and symptoms—Symptoms include purulent vaginal discharge, fever, and malaise (especially if gonorrhea-related). There is lower abdominal pain, with severe pain on manipulation of the cervix and adjoining structures.

Etiology—PID is caused by an infection from aerobic or anaerobic organisms. *Gonorrhea coccus* is the most common aerobic organism. It can rapidly destroy the bacterial barrier of the cervical mucus. With the barrier gone, the bacteria present in the vagina can ascend into the uterus and cause infection. Uterine infection can also develop following insertion of an IUD (intrauterine device), which accidentally introduces contaminated cervical mucus into the uterus. Other factors causing PID are abortion, tubal examinations that test patency by inserting air, pelvic surgery, and infection associated with pregnancy. Organisms can enter from the bloodstream, an abscess, an infected tube, or a ruptured appendix.

Treatment—PID can be treated with antibiotics to prevent progressive involvement. Culture of the drainage to identify the organism is important to be certain the appropriate drug is being used. Improper treatment will result in a chronic disease state. If the causative organism is gonorrhea, syphilis may also be present and require treatment. Bed rest, analgesics, and IV therapy may be indicated. Pelvic abscesses may develop, which require drainage. If permitted to rupture, they may cause a life-threatening situation.

Syphilis (Sif'i-lis)

Description—This is a venereal disease that inhabits the warm, moist areas of the genitals and rectum. The organism can be viewed by dark-field microscope examination. Syphilis is spread by direct sexual contact during either the primary, secondary, or early latent stages of infection. Prenatal transmission to the fetus across the placental barrier is possible, resulting in an infant with congenital syphilis. If the mother is in the primary or secondary stage, the infant will probably die before or shortly after birth. If syphilis is diagnosed and treated before the 4th month of pregnancy, the fetus will not develop the disease. Therefore, a blood analysis for syphilis is routinely performed as part of early prenatal care.

Signs and symptoms—Symptoms vary according to the stage of involvement. Primary stage syphilis begins with entrance of the organism through the mucous membrane of the genitals as the result of contact with an infected person. After 3 to 4 weeks, a lesion called a *chancre* appears at the point of entrance. It is an ulcerlike area with a raised, hard edge that looks painful but is not. In the female, it often appears on the cervix and is therefore hidden from sight, going undetected. It may also develop on the vulva and be visible on examination. In the male, the usual site is the glans or corona (ridge) of the penis. It may develop on the penile shaft or scrotum. The bacteria can also enter the mucous membranes of the mouth or rectum during nongenital intercourse, causing chancres to develop on the lip, tongue, tonsils, or around the anus.

The disease progresses through four stages. The primary stage, chancre, even if untreated, disappears within 1 to 5 weeks, giving the infected person a false sense of having healed. Actually, the disease enters an asymptomatic period during which the bacteria circulate through the body in the blood. About 1 to 6 months later a secondary stage begins. This stage is characterized by a generalized painless, nonitching rash. It is particularly distinctive because of its appearance on the soles of the feet and palms of the hands. During this stage, the following may occur: hair loss; a sore throat; headache; loss of appetite; nausea; constipation; persistent fever; and pain in the bones; muscles; or joints. These symptoms could be indicative of any number of illnesses. If the disease is diagnosed accurately and treated, it can be cured without permanent effects. Without treatment, the disease again "goes away" in 2 to 6 weeks, leading to the belief that nothing is wrong, while, on the contrary, a dangerous stage is approaching.

The third stage is the latent stage, which may last for years. There are no symptoms during this stage, but the organism is at work, burrowing into blood vessels, the spinal cord, the brain, and the bones. After the first year, the disease is no longer infectious except to a fetus. About 50% of those who contract syphilis move into the dangerous late or tertiary stage. This stage is further categorized according to the type of involvement: benign late (affecting internal organs); cardiovascular late (affecting the heart and major blood vessels); or neurosyphilis (affecting the brain and spinal cord). Cardiovascular forms can lead to death; neurosyphilis is almost always fatal.

Diagnosis is difficult by history alone, and physical examination at certain periods would be negative. However, a definitive blood test has been developed and is used routinely for suspected infection and as a mass screening test by some states for persons seeking a marriage license. The test is known as a VDRL, named for the Venereal Disease Research Laboratory of the United States Public Health Service. The blood test is fairly accurate, cheap, and easy to perform; however, it does not give accurate results until 4 to 6 weeks after initial infection. About 25% of the tests will be false negatives during the primary stage, but they are completely accurate in the secondary phase.

Etiology—Syphilis is caused by the spirochete *Treponema pallidum*.

Treatment—Penicillin is the treatment of choice for syphilis, which is relatively easily destroyed. Because some of the spirochetes may survive, a large initial dose of long-acting penicillin (1.2 million units) is divided into two injections, one in each buttock. Much greater doses are required for latent, late, or congenital syphilis. A follow-up exam should be done to confirm freedom from organisms.

Trichomoniasis (Triko-mo-ni'a-sis)

Description—This is a protozoal infection of the lower genitourinary tract. It occurs in 15% of sexually active females and 10% of sexually active males.

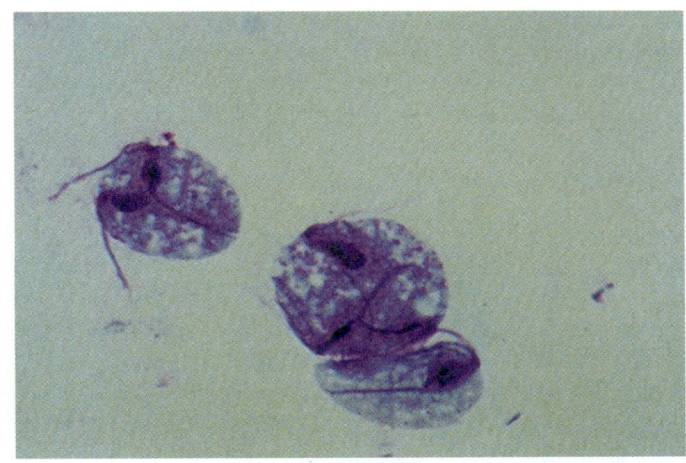

FIGURE 11-230 *Trichomonas vaginalis*

Trichomoniasis can be passed back and forth between sexual partners; therefore, treatment must involve both persons.

Signs and symptoms—The prime and discriminating symptom is abundant, frothy, white or yellow vaginal discharge, which irritates the vulva and has a characteristic foul odor. There are usually no symptoms in the male, except for urethral itching. Diagnosis is made by placing a drop of the secretion on a slide and identifying the organism by microscope. This confirmation rules out ordinary vaginitis from female hygiene products or the presence of rectal *Escherichia coli* in the vagina.

Etiology—It is caused by the single-celled parasitic organism *Trichomonas vaginalis* (Figure 11-230). It is oval in shape, with four hairlike strands protruding from it, which whip back and forth to propel the organism.

Treatment—Treatment of choice is a product called Flagyl, which is taken orally. If left untreated, the female may develop an inflamed cervix and urethra and exhibit abnormal Pap smears. Damaged cells of the cervix may make it more susceptible to cancer. Men develop an infected prostate, testicle, or bladder.

ACHIEVE UNIT OBJECTIVES

■ Complete the Workbook activities to meet the learning objectives.

■ Apply your knowledge at the end of this chapter in completing the Critical Thinking Challenge and Activities, as well as the StudyWARE on your Student CD-ROM.

CRITICAL THINKING CHALLENGE

IMPACTING THE PATIENT, THE PRACTICE, AND YOUR CAREER

Joe is a 68-year-old man of Italian descent. He loves pizza and traditional pasta dishes. He is considerably over-weight and fails to engage in any regular physical activity. He was seen last week with complaints of fatigue, being thirsty, and excessive urination. Today Dr. Stone has reviewed his lab work and informed Joe that he has diabetes. The doctor asked Linda, the medical assistant, to talk with Joe and provide him some patient teaching materials. She is also to set up an appointment with the dietician to instruct Joe on his diet. Joe is not too interested in making any changes in his life. He thinks he is too old and will not live many more years anyhow, so why should he deny himself what he loves just to add a year or so to his life? Linda tried to explain the complications that might develop with diabetes if it is not controlled. She discovered Joe was really concerned that he would have to start taking insulin and he didn't think he could give himself shots. Linda explained to Joe that maybe with adding regular exercise and modifying his diet, he might not need insulin. He finally agreed to talk with the dietician and had Linda schedule an appointment. Linda explained to Joe that his wife needed to be involved in his care since she prepares the majority of his meals. Linda took special care to document what she discussed and to record Joe's remarks. She realized everyone involved in Joe's care would need to keep encouraging him and follow up his progress closely for him to succeed.

QUESTIONS

1. How does the diagnosis of a disease like diabetes affect a patient?
2. How does Joe's attitude affect the practice?
3. What effect does a patient like Joe have on the medical assistant's role?

ACTIVITIES

There has been a great deal of information presented in this special chapter. There may be many topics you would like to explore to learn more about a particular condition or disease. With access to the Internet, resources are readily available and easily obtained. You are encouraged to continue to research and learn about conditions you encounter in your career as you work as a medical assistant.

1. Identify a disease or condition that you, some member of your family, or a friend has that has not been discussed in this text. Prepare a report that describes the disease, its signs and symptoms, any diagnostic tests that apply, the causes, and how it is treated.

2. Look in your phone book business pages listing physicians. Knowing what you do about disease conditions, can you identify specialists who would treat the following conditions: AIDS, asthma, a malignancy, infertility, osteoporosis, severe burns, rheumatoid arthritis, uncontrolled pain, detached retina, GERD, and coronary artery disease? (If you live in a small community you may not be able to match all the specialties.)

3. Work with a classmate to learn the great number of medical terms in this chapter. Identify a particular

unit and take turns playing hangman's noose with the terms. You could also vary the practice by constructing flash cards of the terms with their meanings on the back.

4. Pick out at least two topics in which you are interested that were retrieved from web sites listed in the resources at the end of the chapter. Find three more facts about each topic that you did not know before.

Study WARE™ CHALLENGE

- Study with the flash cards for Chapter 11 to review the key terms in this chapter.
- Complete the image labeling exercises for Chapter 11.
- Solve the hangman activities for Chapter 11.
- Complete the multiple choice quiz in test mode for Chapter 11.

RESOURCES

ALS Association. *All about ALS*. Retrieved March 13, 2006, from www.alsa.org/als/facts.

American Academy of Orthopaedic Surgeons. *Limb lengthening*. Retrieved March 7, 2006, from www.orthoinfo.aaos.org

American Cancer Institute Fact Sheet. *Inflammatory breast cancer.* Retrieved June 30, 2006, from www.cancer.gov

American Heart Association. *What are healthy levels of cholesterol?* Retrieved April 11, 2006, from www.americanheart.org

Annuals of American History. *Approval of stem cell research.* Retrieved July 6, 2005, from www.america.britannica.com

Avian Influenza (Bird Flu). *Key facts about avian influenza (bird flu) and avian influenza A (H5N1) viru*s. Retrieved June 30, 2006, from www.cdc.gov/flu/avian

Bartlett, J. S. (2001, June). Possible solution found for replacing defective C F genes. In *Infectious diseases in children* (p. 67). American Academy of Allergy, Asthma, and Immunology.

Brody, J. E. (2001, May). Better choices in heart bypass surgery. *Bottom Line Health.*

Cable News Network Health (2001, February 12). Landmark gene studies released. Retrieved from www.cnn.com

Cancer facts and figures 2006. Atlanta, GA: Surveillance Research, American Cancer Society, Inc.

The Columbus Dispatch. (2004, October 12). *"Man of steel" Christopher Reeve 1952-2004.* Columbus, OH.

The Columbus Dispatch. (2003, May 15). *Parameters for Blood Pressure Redefined.* Columbus, OH.

Congestive heart failure and beta blockers (2001, August). *Harvard Health Letter, 26*(10).

Diabetes treatment: The tried and true and what's new (2001, April). *Harvard Health Letter, 26*(6), 1–3.

Ductal Lavage (2001, September). *Women's Health Watch,* p. 647.

Eight ways to avoid Alzheimer's disease (2001, August). *Dr. Andrew Weil's Self Healing,* p. 6.

Floria, B. (2001, Spring). Assessing your osteoporosis risk. *Perspective,* p. 7.

Glaucoma Research Foundation. *TGF urges eye exams to detect the disease early.* Retrieved March 8, 2006, from www.glaucoma-foundation.org

Gugliotta, G. (2001, July 1). Doctors implant new heart pump. *The Washington Post.*

Hepatitis C: How to protect yourself against the new blood plague (2001, September). *Bottom Line Health,* pp. 11–12.

HIV Infection and AIDS in the United States, 2004. *CDC HIV/AIDS surveillance report.* Retrieved April 14, 2006, from www.cdc.gov/hiv/topics/surveillance

Krames Health and Safety Education. (2001). Booklets "*Understanding glaucoma* and *Small incision cataract surgery.* San Bruno, CA: StayWell.

Lifesaving asthma secrets. (2001, May). *Bottom Line Health,* pp. 7–9.

Mayo Clinic. *Acromegaly.* Retrieved April 6, 2006, from www.mayoclinic.com/health/acromegaly

Mayo Clinic. *Asthma, bronchitis, emphysema.* Retrieved April 4, 2006, from www.mayoclinic.com/health

Mitral valve repair for severe heart failure (2000, November). *HeartWatch, 4*(10), 1–2.

More iron overload screening recommended (2001, January). *Health and Nutrition Letter 18*(11), 7.

National Institute of Diabetes and Digestive and Kidney Diseases. *Treatment methods for kidney failure; peritoneal dialysis.* Retrieved April 18, 2006, from www.kidney.niddk.nih.gov/kidiseases/pubs/peritoneal

National Institutes of Health. *Misbehaving molecules: 3-dimensional pictures of ALS mutant proteins.* Retrieved March 13, 2006, from www.nih.gov/news

National Kidney Foundation. *Kidney transplant: Home hemodialysis.* Retrieved April 18, 2006, from www.kidney.org

National Library of Medicine. *Genetics home reference: Achondroplasia.* Retrieved March 7, 2006, from www.ghr.nlm.govghr/disease/achondroplasia

New solutions to those too, too embarrassing skin problems (2001, June). *Bottom Line Personal,* p. 11–12.

New treatment for osteoarthritis (2001, January). *Health and Nutrition Letter 18*(11), 4–5.

Robotic arms aid those of physician in heart surgery. (2000, Winter). *The OSU Medical Center Health Connection,* p. 10.

Seven out of 10 stroke patients suffer disability or death: How to beat the odds (2001, August). *Bottom Line Health, 15*(8), pp. 3–4.

Wade, N. (2000, May 9). Another chromosome is decoded. *The New York Times.*

What Is Bell's palsy? (2001, June). *Women's Health Watch,* p. 8.

WEB LINKS

www.aaaai.org (American Academy of Allergy, Asthma, and Immunology)
  Provides information on allergic diseases.

http://cancer.org (American Cancer Society)
  Provides information on cancer.

www.americanheart.org (American Heart Association)
  Provides information on heart diseases, blood pressure, cholesterol, and vascular disease.

http://arthritis.org (Arthritis Foundation)
  Provides information on arthritis.

www.cdc.gov (Centers for Disease Control and Prevention)
  Provides information about all types of diseases and health concerns.

www.mayoclinic.com (Mayo Clinic)
  Affiliated with the Mayo Clinic, this site offers an index of diseases listed A-Z, 11 Condition Centers, and 8 Healthy Living Centers.

www.lymphnet.org (National Lymphedema Network)
  Provides information on lymphedema.

www.nof.org (National Osteoporosis Foundation)
  Provides information on osteoporosis.

www.allthyroid.org (Thyroid Foundation of America, Inc.
  Provides information about thyroid conditions, treatments, and research.

SECTION 4

The Clinical Medical Assistant

Part of the medical assistant's responsibilities in the clinical area is ensuring that transmission of diseases is limited as much as possible. While one may not think that general housekeeping in the office is a job of a medical assistant, it is imperative that the facility be maintained to prevent the spread of disease as well as protect the safety of the patients and their families.

In the reception area, you should do a quick look around to pick up items patients may trip over, as well as items that may be contaminated, such as tissues. This is also important in the clinical area; when you find used tissues, bandages that have been removed by the patient, soiled table paper, trash cans that are full, or biohazardous items in the examination rooms or laboratory areas, it is your responsibility to dispose of them appropriately.

One of the most important things you can do to help reduce the spread of diseases is to wash your hands often and thoroughly. While we tend to concentrate on wearing personal protective equipment to reduce our own exposure to diseases, washing your hands between patients is just as important as donning such equipment.

Recognizing the proper methodology for the care of instruments, from sanitization all the way through sterilization, is essential as well; instruments that are used in the process of examining patients must be disinfected when used on the outside of the body and sterilized if used internally. Just as you would not eat dinner with a fork that still had a food particle on it, you would not expose a patient to an instrument that was not clean. In the case of sterilized instruments, there are indicators to prove sterilization has been achieved; if you encounter a package that does not have the appropriate color change on the indicator, you must repackage the instruments for sterilization for the protection of the patient.

UNIT 1
THE SAFETY AND WELL-BEING OF STAFF AND PATIENTS

OBJECTIVES

Upon completion of this unit, you will be able to achieve the following:

LEARNING Objectives

1. **Spell and define, using the glossary in the back of the text, all the Words to Know in this unit.**

2. **Explain the medical assistant's role and responsibility in maintaining personal safety and well-being of staff and patients.**

3. **List potential hazards and problems in a medical facility and the action that should be taken for each.**

4. **List and name the location of housekeeping items and supplies that should be on hand for use as necessary.**

5. **Describe daily routine care of the medical facility.**

6. **Explain the importance of proper hand washing.**

7. **State the purpose of wearing latex or vinyl gloves.**

8. **Explain how to prevent disease transmission to a patient with a cold.**

9. **List the admirable habits a medical assistant should practice to reduce disease transmission.**

10. **List general guidelines for lab safety.**

11. **Explain the importance of posting informative signs and diagrams for patients and visitors in a medical facility.**

PERFORMANCE Objective

1. **Demonstrate proper hand washing.**

WORDS TO KNOW

asepsis	harbor	pathogens
biohazard	microbes	vigilance
emesis	microorganism	warranted
esthetic		

 ### CERTIFICATION CONNECTION

CMA
Fundamental clinical principles
Prepare and maintain examination and treatment areas
Operational functions
Professionalism
Communications

Principles of infection control

RMA
Asepsis

CMAS
Asepsis in the medical office

In the course of routine daily activities in a medical facility, there should be a scheduled time for inspection of the entire facility. Established guidelines should be followed to maintain a safe and comfortable environment for the safety and well-being of all patients and staff. Establishing and adhering to these standards will help to avoid problem situations regarding potential hazards and possible disease transmission. Foremost in protection for all is cleanliness, which is the best way to prevent the transmission of disease. Because a medical facility is a place where many people, both well and sick, convene, it is a prime target for pathogenic organisms to grow and multiply. Constant and consistent **vigilance** must be upheld to help ensure environmental control and safety. The schedule of duties to perform this important function should be outlined and regulated by the supervisor or office manager on a daily basis.

KEEPING THE ENTIRE MEDICAL FACILITY CLEAN

In the performance of clinical procedures, the medical assistant must be mindful of the necessity of **asepsis**, which is a state of being free from all pathogenic **microorganisms**. Even though there cannot be a completely sterile environment throughout the entire general medical facility, it must be clean and safe for all who enter. Although there is generally a contracted commercial cleaning service (this service is usually referred to as environmental or custodial service) established to do the heavy cleaning and scrubbing of the office walls, windows, furniture, carpets, and so on, it is the staff's job to check dust, debris, and clutter to keep a clean and **esthetic** appearance of the entire facility. Periodic remodeling and redecorating of the facility should be done before furniture and carpets become a safety hazard or an eyesore.

The reception area and the rest of the facility should be a pleasant and comfortable place for those who enter (Figure 12-1). Therefore, all those who are employed in a medical facility have a responsibility to observe, report, and assist in keeping the appearance and safety of the facility ensured. It is your duty to take a good look around to inspect the facility daily before patients arrive.

All surfaces, doorknobs, and plates should be dusted or washed appropriately as necessary and repeated as often as necessary throughout the day, especially in areas where there may be close quarters and where heavily populated. Attention should also be given to water fountains, public restrooms, trash cans, telephones (clean the mouthpiece often), and the areas around them where either periodic re-stocking of supplies or cleanup is indicated. Occasionally, a considerate person may report that more toilet tissue or paper towels are needed in the restroom, but this should be the exception and not the rule. The conscientious medical assistant should already have matters under control in keeping a well cared-for facility. Trash containers are to be lined with disposable trash bags, and this is generally done by the custodial staff. However, there may be times when the container becomes too full, the trash must be disposed of in the appropriate location for trash pick-up, and a new trash bag is placed

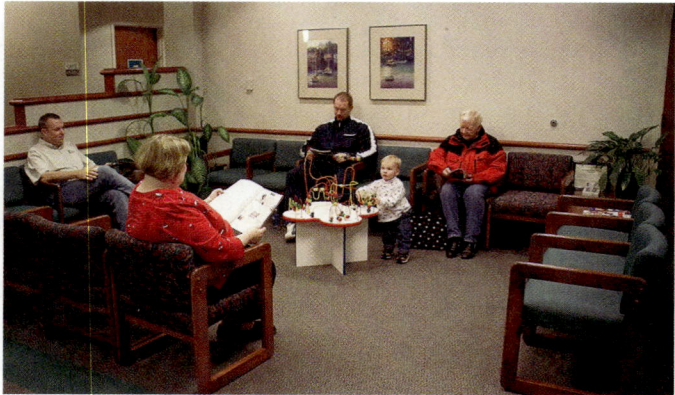

FIGURE 12-1 The reception area should be inviting and comfortable for patients

in the container. The trash containers in the patient restrooms and in the reception area sometimes contain contents that may be unpleasant and should be changed. It is much more attractive in the reception area to have a receptacle with a lid to conceal unsightly trash. In the event that a general cleanup would become necessary (some cleaning services are only contracted on a weekly basis), a standard list of cleaning equipment and supplies should be kept in a convenient place. The following housekeeping list contains standard items that should be kept on the premises:

- Broom and dust pan
- Vacuum cleaner
- Mop and bucket
- Sponges
- Cleaning solutions
- Bleach (including a 10% bleach solution)
- Dust cloths
- Disposable trash bags
- Disposable latex or vinyl gloves
- **Biohazard** puncture-proof containers and bags
- Disposable **emesis** basins
- Glass cleaner
- Disposable paper towels
- Disinfectant spray

Note: A solution of one-fourth cup bleach per gallon of tap water (a 10% dilution of common household bleach) should be made fresh daily and kept readily available for cleanup of accidental spills of blood or body fluids. A disinfectant spray is a good idea to disinfect small areas and to help eliminate odors (a fresh citrus fragrance is very effective against unpleasant odors). In an allergist's practice and for patients' comfort in general, an odorless disinfectant spray should be used.

Proper ventilation and maintaining an ideal temperature of 72° F is necessary. Seating should not be placed directly under, over, or beside blowers or heating or cooling vents. Placing a table or lamp in an area of the room where there may be a draft is a good idea so that patients will not be sitting in an uncomfortable spot. You should also watch for mats near doorways and keep them from buckling so that patients and staff do not trip over them and fall. Absorbent floor mats should be used on rainy days if the floor of the entrance is not carpeted. All furniture, lamps, wires, carpet, and so forth should be periodically inspected and cleaned as necessary. Any repairs or replacements should be made immediately as **warranted**. Keeping all reception room furniture and decor in a neat and clean manner will provide a pleasant and comfortable atmosphere for all patients, helping to make them feel safe, secure, and well cared for as they wait for their appointments.

Cleanliness and Order in the Waiting Areas

Many facilities that provide medical care to children have a play area for the children to occupy while they wait to see the doctor. Even though the babies and children who are very ill will most likely not be playing with anything, it is important to remember to routinely clean and disinfect all items that children play with in the children's area. Remember that the health status of any child cannot be assessed before the physician examines them. This section where toys and games are kept for the entertainment of young patients is a potential source of disease transmission and should be monitored closely. The most efficient way to control this is to have the child bring into the exam room whatever toy he or she played with in the reception area. Then you can clean it before it is placed back out with the other toys and need not worry that other little patients will become infected with whatever the child before them may have had. These toys should be made of a washable plastic or smooth, nonpointed (no sharp edges) metal for children's safety and well-being. Any malfunctioning toys or toys with loose parts should be discarded immediately. Very small toys, such as beads or miniblocks, are not recommended because babies and toddlers tend to put everything into their mouths, and small toys could choke them. The furniture that is used for young patients should also be made of a washable material and be cleaned routinely with a disinfectant solution. Remember to bring in those patients who are feeling very sick or who are in obvious pain or distress as soon as they arrive, because it may be possible to help eliminate further problems and save the patient further stress or embarrassment.

For adult patients, there should be an appropriate assortment of printed materials, such as magazines, newspapers, patient education pamphlets, and booklets. These should be displayed in an orderly fashion for patients to read while they wait. Be sure to straighten up printed material as needed. Periodic checks of these materials should be done, and old or tattered ones should be discarded as necessary. Also, replace light bulbs as necessary so that there is adequate lighting for patients to read easily without eye strain. Patients should be discouraged from eating and drinking in the reception area. Used tissues, paper cups, and other assorted waste items are sometimes left behind, often unintentionally, by patients. As you pick up these trash items, wear disposable gloves or pick them up with a disposable paper towel or tissue so that you do not come in direct contact with the object as you throw it away in the appropriate waste container. Clutter and trash should be removed properly as soon as possible to maintain an attractive environment.

Wearing Gloves

Wearing gloves is necessary when cleaning up blood or bodily fluid in the reception area and in the examination or treatment room. There are three very important reasons why latex or vinyl gloves are worn:

1. To provide protection as a barrier and prevent contamination of the hands when touching any blood or body fluid
2. To reduce the possibility that any **pathogens** present on your hands will be transferred to another
3. To diminish the chance of any pathogens being transmitted from you to patients as you go from one patient to another

Wearing gloves is no substitute for hand washing. Because there is the possibility of gloves having imperfections, such as small holes or tears, or if gloves are ill-fitting, hand washing is a must before and after wearing them. There is also the risk of becoming contaminated during the removal of soiled gloves. Always remember to protect yourself and follow proper procedure (later in this chapter) when it comes to hand washing and gloving.

Avoiding Accidents

In addition to the reception area and examination and treatment rooms, the entire facility should be inspected daily and as you bring patients in to prepare them to see the physician. Even though this may seem like an obvious task, a problem situation could occur at any time; for example, someone could trip and fall over something (a toy, for instance) that was left in the usual walking path of the room. Accidents can and do happen from time to time even in the most cared for facilities. You must be alert to these potential situations and handle them with care and tact. Figure 12-2 provides an example of an accident report form that should be used in case of any accident on the premises. If you are not aware of a problem because of neglect and a patient is injured or becomes ill because of a previously known problem that was never taken care of (such as a natural gas leak or a frayed wire), your facility can be held liable for any injury or illness caused to the patient.

Any and all repairs or replacements should be made or arranged for immediately for safety reasons and to keep the office schedule flowing as smoothly as possible. Because the administrative assistant stays primarily in the business office area and generally sees patients only at the reception window, many of the potential problems are not observed as readily as when the clinical medical assistant opens the door to the reception room to bring patients into the clinical

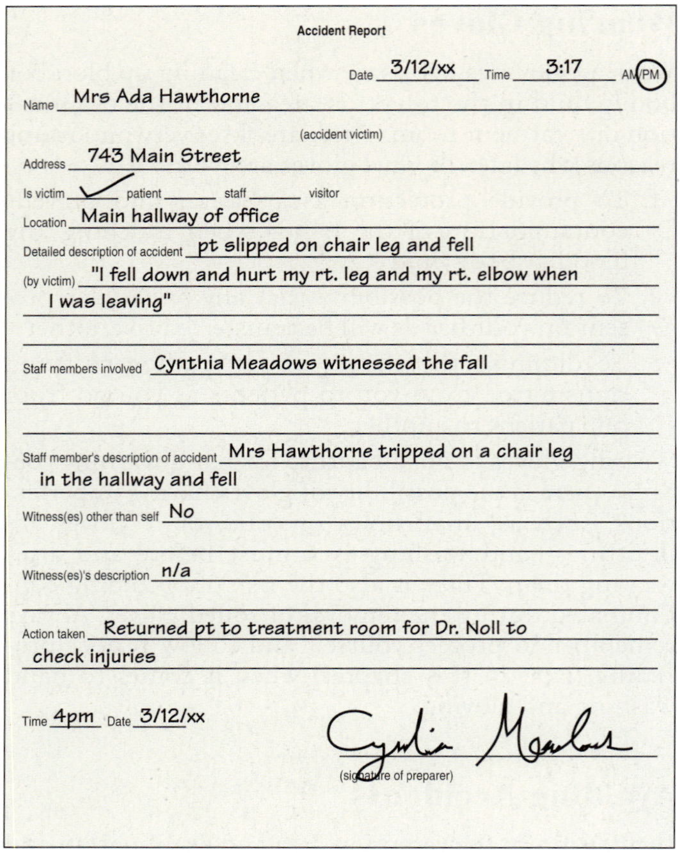

Accident Report

Date 3/12/xx   Time 3:17   AM/PM

Name Mrs Ada Hawthorne

(accident victim)

Address 743 Main Street

Is victim ✓ patient _____ staff _____ visitor

Location Main hallway of office

Detailed description of accident pt slipped on chair leg and fell

(by victim) "I fell down and hurt my rt. leg and my rt. elbow when I was leaving"

Staff members involved Cynthia Meadows witnessed the fall

Staff member's description of accident Mrs Hawthorne tripped on a chair leg in the hallway and fell

Witness(es) other than self No

Witness(es)'s description n/a

Action taken Returned pt to treatment room for Dr. Noll to check injuries

Time 4pm   Date 3/12/xx

(signature of preparer)

FIGURE 12-2   Sample accident report form

For Your Safety and Health

Please:

1. Report any safety hazard or emergency to the receptionist immediately.

2. Use tissues provided to cover your mouth and nose to catch your coughs and sneezes.

3. Dispose of all waste in the plastic-lined waste can.

4. Tell the receptionist if you feel nausea or need to use the restroom.

5. If you are feeling faint, weak, dizzy, nausea, chest pain, shortness of breath, or see another in similar distress, please notify the receptionist immediately.

Thank you.

FIGURE 12-3   A sign that conveys important information such as this one should be displayed in the reception area in clear view for patients and the general public in case of need.

GUIDELINES FOR PREVENTING THE TRANSFER OF DISEASE

How you can be useful in preventing disease transmission and helpful in providing a safe and comfortable environment for staff and patients have been discussed. Yet there are more ways that you can be of help to ensure the health and safety of others. In this unit, you will find important regulations regarding how you can avoid the risks of contracting disease and help in preventing the transfer of disease-causing pathogens to others. Microorganisms that are the cause of disease are called pathogens. They have certain requirements for growth and multiplication. If steps are taken to interrupt and prevent their growth, disease transmission can be reduced. Breaking the infection cycle helps prevent the spread of disease. The requirements of microbial growth are covered in Unit 2 of this chapter.

General guidelines for lab safety follow for your information. These are steps that can be taken to keep yourself and others from coming into contact with contaminated items. Further guidelines are discussed in Unit 2 regarding mandatory Occupational Safety and Health Administration (OSHA) regulations. Once you realize the seriousness of these matters, you will become conscientious about compliance. It is up to each health care provider to be honest and credible about following guidelines. Remember: Some diseases are dangerous and can be fatal. You also have a legal, moral, and ethical responsibility to protect yourself

area. This is a prime time to quickly observe the entire area, make a note of the situation, and then report it to the appropriate person. If you do see a faulty chair or a frayed wire, for example, it is your responsibility to do something about it *before* someone gets hurt. Your initiative and follow-through is necessary to maintain surroundings that are as safe as possible for all concerned.

Additionally, it is a good idea to post a sign in the reception area to alert patients who are waiting about what to do in certain situations. Emergency exits should be clearly posted with easy-to-follow paths for evacuation and security in each of the rooms in the facility where you are employed. There should also be signs clearly posted for public restrooms, water fountains, telephones, and other facilities, such as the lab or pharmacy where patients may need to be sent from your office. Figure 12-3 gives an example of a concise list of advice for patients to follow if there is a problem. This will also give patients clear instructions to follow if they need attention while waiting for their appointment or in case of an emergency.

and others from such preventable problems. Obviously, the best way to do this is to establish a routine and stick to it. It is far better and easier to learn good habits than to break bad ones.

Never put your hands in your mouth (no nail biting), nor any other objects (such as pens or pencils) that could transfer your germs to others who come into contact with these objects. After using tissues, wash your hands to avoid possible spread of pathogens from yourself to others. Promote a good patient education tip by demonstrating to patients how to use tissues when coughing and sneezing to help diminish the transfer of germs. Refer to Figure 12-13 to see how a patient uses tissues to catch the germs of coughing and sneezing and discards the used tissues properly. If you or a coworker has the sniffles or a cold, it is wise to keep from being in contact with patients lest you (or they) contaminate someone. If and when you are sick and feverish, stay home and take care of yourself until you are well, and return to work only after you have been fever-free for at least 24 hours. Being in the health field, your employer should be understanding and appreciate your situation. Working as a cooperative team helps to solve these types of problems that can and do happen from time to time. Also remember that the multi-skilled medical assistant is a well-prepared team member who can fill in when other staff members are absent.

HAND WASHING GUIDELINES

The very first way to prevent the transfer of microorganisms is by washing your hands. This is the responsibility of all health care providers and all people in general to arrest the spread of pathogens. This one task alone could help to eliminate many diseases before they even begin. You must develop the routine of hand washing before you begin your daily work schedule by performing Procedure 12-1 for 2 minutes. Hand washing thereafter should be done for approximately 20 seconds before and after seeing each patient and before and after handling specimens or any soiled or contaminated materials. A 5- to 6-minute hand washing and scrub should be performed before gloving for a surgical procedure. After removing gloves, you should wash your hands for at least 30 seconds. Lotion may be applied to the hands to prevent dry skin. It is important to avoid using lotions that have a petroleum or mineral oil content before putting latex gloves on, because they can break down the latex and could intensify a latex allergic reaction. Those who are allergic to latex should use vinyl gloves. To be safe, it is a good practice to use a water-based lotion without perfume. To protect yourself from the transfer of **microbes**, remember to wash your hands both before and after using the restroom and before and after eating. Proper basic hand washing

helps to remove microorganisms from the skin and from under fingernails. Minimal jewelry should be worn, because it is impossible to eliminate all pathogens from the crevices of jewelry items unless they are sterilized by autoclaving. Autoclaving is not recommended because it is damaging to most jewelry, plus it is highly impractical and time consuming. It is better to wear minimal jewelry or, better yet, none at all.

In places where a sink is not readily available for hand washing between patients, such as in an area designated for allergy injections or blood pressure readings, a practical way to cleanse the hands is by using a commercial foam cleaner preparation. This is a foamed alcohol preparation that is applied and spread over the hands in the same manner as you would use soap and water. It dries in approximately 1 minute. For those who have problems with dry skin, this foam seems to be less drying and irritating than some products used in washing the hands. A supply of hand cream should be readily available. Treating chapped skin with soothing lotions can help prevent a possible infection of the hands.

Carefully adhere to each hand washing step to prevent disease transmission. Even though the hand washing procedure may seem extensive, it takes only a couple of minutes to complete it, and it is done to prevent the spread of disease. Repeated hand washing between your many duties should take 20 seconds and is well worth the time. In Chapter 17, which deals with assisting in surgical procedures, you will learn how to perform a surgical hand washing, which takes considerably longer to complete (approximately 5 to 6 minutes). Learning the correct way to properly wash the hands is outlined in Procedure 12-1. Acquiring this extremely important habit is necessary for your well-being and that of others.

BASIC GUIDELINES FOR LAB SAFETY

1. Proper hand washing before and after every procedure and before and after gloving must become a habit for all health workers for self-protection from disease transmission. (Immediately washing *any* skin surface thoroughly that has been contaminated with any blood or body fluids is vital.)

2. Gloving is always a must when handling *any* blood or body fluid specimens. (If you find that you are allergic to latex gloves, disposable gloves made from materials other than latex are available. Disposable gloves are also available with or without powder.)

3. Cover all scratches, paper cuts, or any breaks in the skin with a bandage after hand washing and before gloving for self-protection against possible contamination.

12-1  Hand Washing

PURPOSE: To reduce pathogens on the hands and wrists, thereby decreasing direct and indirect transmission of infectious microorganisms. Average duration is 2 minutes before beginning to work with patients, 30 seconds following each patient contact.

EQUIPMENT AND SUPPLIES: Sink (preferably with foot-operated controls), soap (preferably liquid soap in a dispenser; bar soap discouraged), disposable paper towels, nail stick or brush, waste receptacle, and water-based antibacterial lotion.

PERFORMANCE OBJECTIVE: The student will stand at a sink with hot and cold faucets and demonstrate each step in the hand washing procedure as specified in the procedure sheet.

Standard Precautions recommend that proper hand washing is performed to avoid the transfer of microorganisms to other patients, yourself, or the environment.

1. Remove all jewelry, including bracelets and rings (wedding rings may be left on but must be scrubbed). **RATIONALE: Jewelry harbors microorganisms.**

2. Stand at the sink and turn faucets on using a paper towel to avoid direct contact with faucets (Figure 12-4A). Adjust water temperature to moderately warm and discard paper towel. Leave water running at desired temperature. **RATIONALE: The sink and faucets are considered contaminated; water temperature must be properly adjusted because once the procedure is begun, the faucets cannot be touched.**

3. Wet hands and press the soap dispenser with the heel of your hand to obtain approximately 1 teaspoon of soap in the palm of one hand. Work soap into a lather, and distribute soap over both palms and backs of hands in circular motions constantly and vigorously for 2 to 3 minutes. Keep hands lower than forearms. **RATIONALE: Circular motion and friction are more effective. Removed soil and water flows into sink, not onto arms (Figures 12-4B and C).**

4. Use the nail brush to dislodge microorganisms around cuticles and under nails (Figure 12-4D).

5. Rinse well, being careful not to touch the inside of the sink or faucets during the procedure (Figure 12-4E).

6. Rinse hands thoroughly. Leave water running, and reach for sufficient paper towels to dry hands completely.

7. Turn off the faucet with a paper towel and discard in the waste container. **RATIONALE: Touching the faucet would contaminate clean hands (Figure 12-4F).**

8. Hand lotion may be applied to prevent skin from becoming dry and chafed.

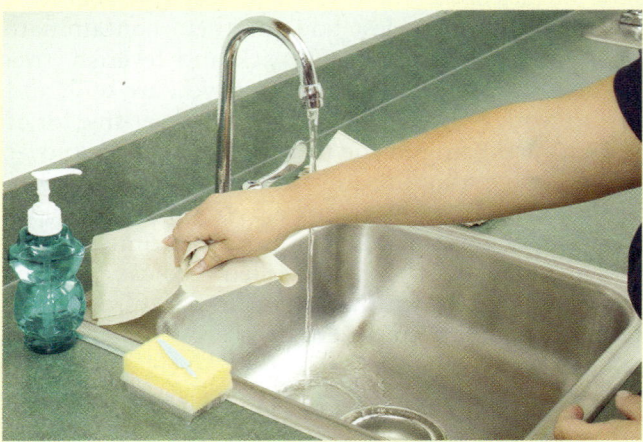

FIGURE 12-4A   A dry paper towel should be used to turn the faucet on (if not lever-operated).

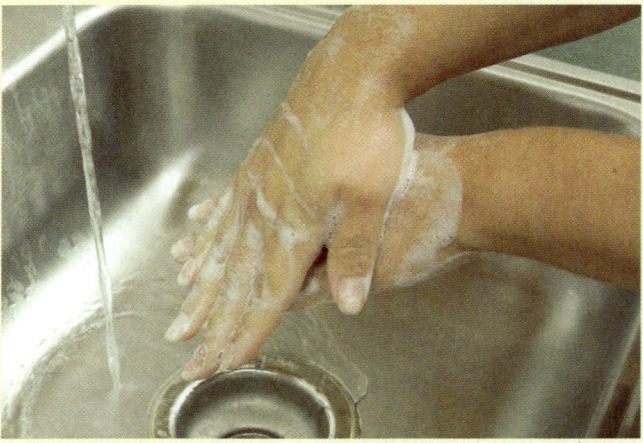

FIGURE 12-4B   Fingertips should be pointed down while washing hands. Use the palm of one hand to clean the back of the other hand.

(continues)

12-1 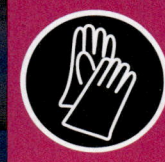 Hand Washing (Continued)

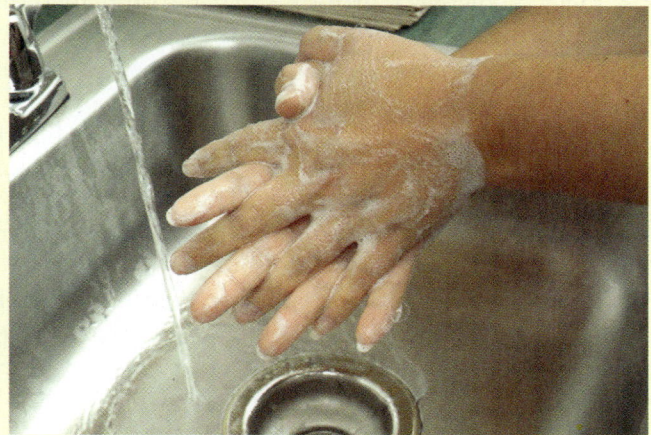

FIGURE 12-4C Interlace the fingers to clean between them.

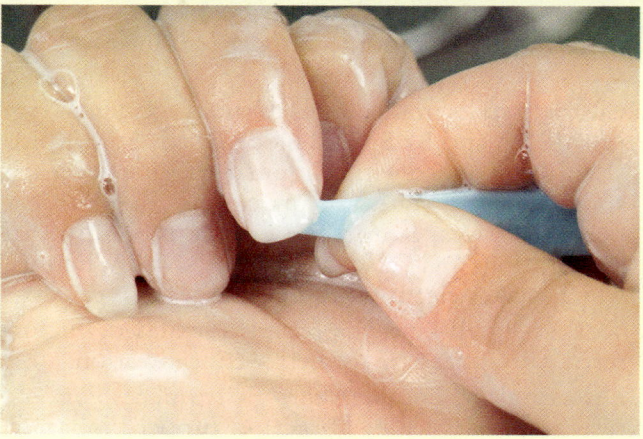

FIGURE 12-4D Clean under the fingernails.

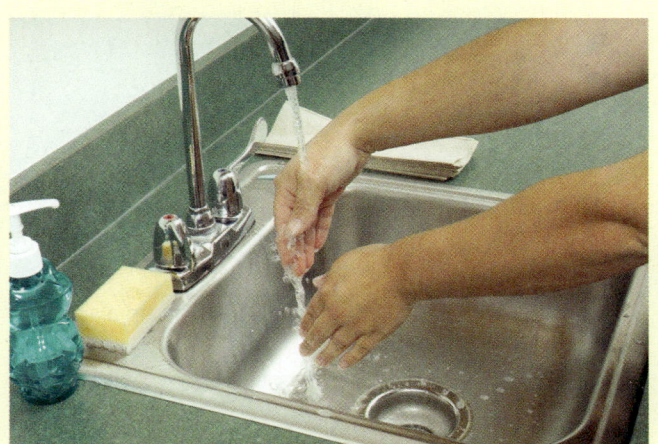

FIGURE 12-4E Rinse the hands thoroughly with the fingertips down.

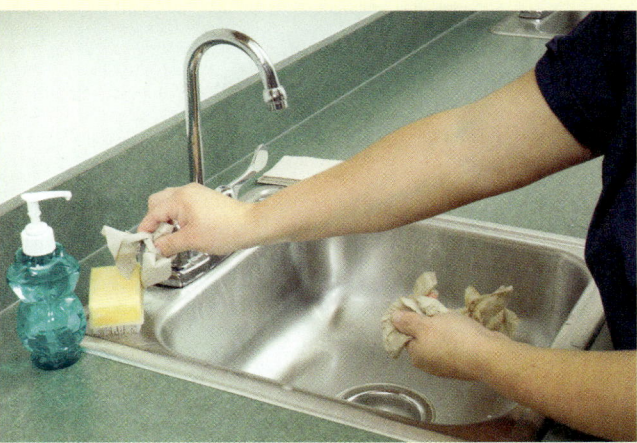

FIGURE 12-4F Use paper towels to dry the hands and turn off the faucet (if not lever-operated).

4. Never eat, drink, chew gum, smoke, place hands or fingers to the mouth, or place any item in your mouth (such as a pen or pencil) while working.

5. Wear protective gloves, a mask, a gown (or apron), and goggles when splashing of any blood or body fluids is possible while you are working (Figure 12-5).

6. Always recap or close bottles, jars, and tubes immediately after desired amounts are obtained to avoid spills, waste, and accidents.

7. Clean up spills immediately to avoid accidents (Figures 12-6A and B). Spilled blood or any body fluids should be flooded with a liquid germicide or bleach solution (a 1:10 ratio) before cleaning up with paper towels (wear latex or vinyl gloves). Commercial preparations may also be used to solidify liquids, which makes cleanup easier.

8. Work in a well-lighted, properly ventilated, uncluttered, and quiet area for better concentration.

9. Discard all disposable sharp instruments, lancets, syringes, and needles (intact) in proper biohazard puncture-proof containers (Figure 12-7). (*Never* break needles off, handle after use, or reuse.) Never put the needle cover between your teeth to remove it when giving an injection. Place reusable metal instruments in a disinfectant solution after rinsing in cold water in preparation for proper cleaning and sterilization.

Package broken glass or any sharp unusable items in a puncture-proof container marked "caution—broken glass" to discard in the proper waste receptacle. (This will protect unsuspecting custodial personnel from injury.)

10. Discard *all* hazardous waste in proper containers (Figure 12-8).

11. Make periodic checks of all electrical appliances and equipment for frayed wires or faulty operation, and tag for repair if needed.

12. Make sure that your hands are dry before using any electrical appliances or equipment.

13. Report all accidents to your supervisor immediately.

14. Clearly post emergency phone numbers near the telephone in the lab (e.g., local fire, police, emergency medical unit, and poison control center, Figure 12-9).

15. Have available (nearby or in the lab) first aid items (e.g., sterile gauze, bandages, tape, and so on) for emergency use.

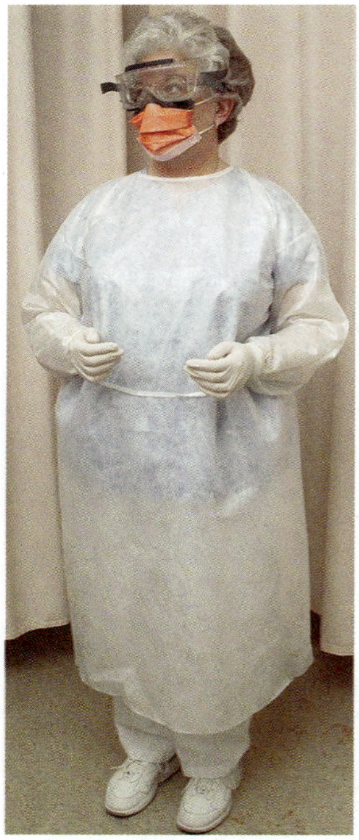

FIGURE 12-5 This medical assistant is wearing personal protective equipment (PPE): goggles, mask, gown, and gloves. PPE prevents possible splashing of blood or other potentially infectious body fluids from coming into contact with the skin or mucous membranes.

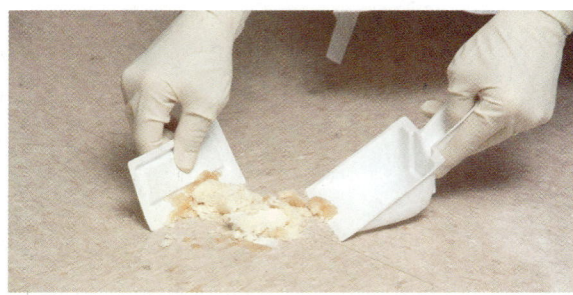

FIGURE 12-6A Wear gloves to clean up a spill.

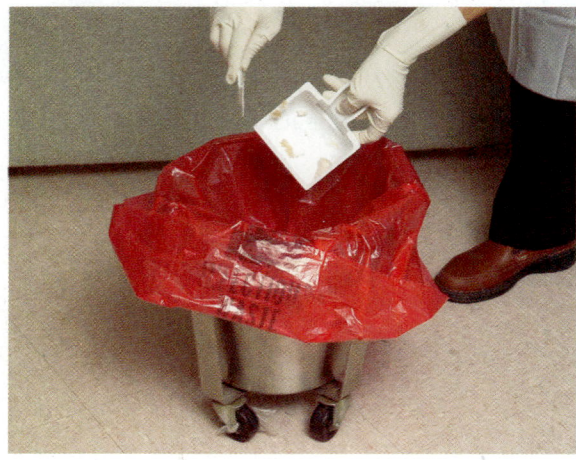

FIGURE 12-6B All materials used to clean up the spill are placed in a biohazard waste bag

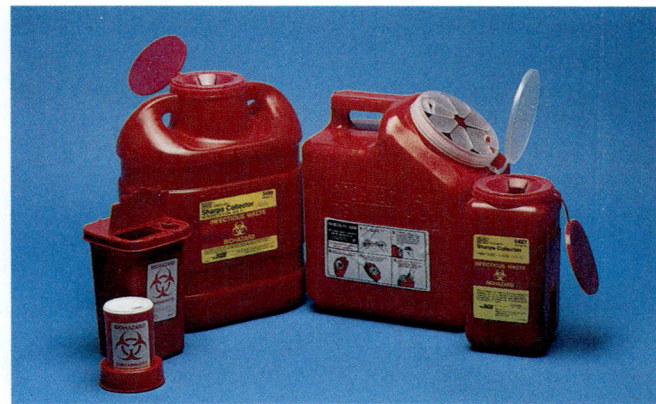

FIGURE 12-7 Various sizes of sharps containers. Note the biohazard material symbols on each to alert you to the potential danger.

16. Post clearly the sign over the functional emergency eye wash station in the lab (Figure 12-10).
17. Do not wear loose-fitting or bulky clothing or jewelry that could contribute to accidents while working with machines or equipment in the lab or any area in the office or clinic.
18. Use gas or air valves and Bunsen burners with caution. Keep flammable chemicals away from them.
19. Use only paper disposable cups for drinking.
20. Designate a "dirty" and a "clean" area in your lab, and enforce this policy.
21. Never lean into the work area when working with flame or chemicals (pour at arm's length) to avoid self-injury or accident.

Another sensible practice is to avoid leaning into sinks or onto equipment or counters that could **harbor**

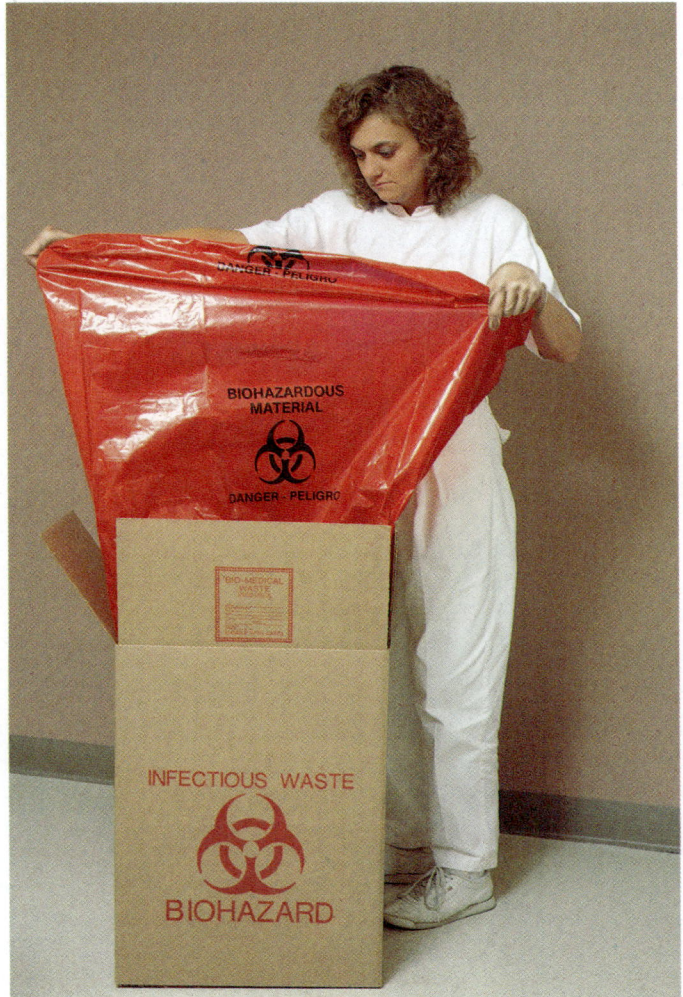

FIGURE 12-8 A sturdy plastic bag marked with the biohazard waste symbol is placed into a durable cardboard box also marked with the waste symbol. An authorized, licensed waste hauler is contracted to dispose of the box and provide documentation of proper disposal of the materials.

EMERGENCY PHONE NUMBERS		
EMS		911
Police		555-1111
Emergency Squad		555-1010
Fire Dept.		555-0000
Rescue Squad		555-5050
Hospital		555-7171
ICU	ext. 210	
CCU	ext. 250	
ER	ext. 265	
Admitting	ext. 200	
Ambulance		555-1818
Poison Control Center		555-6101
Coroner		555-9914
Taxi		555-2222

FIGURE 12-9 Example of recommended phone numbers to post near each phone for emergency assistance.

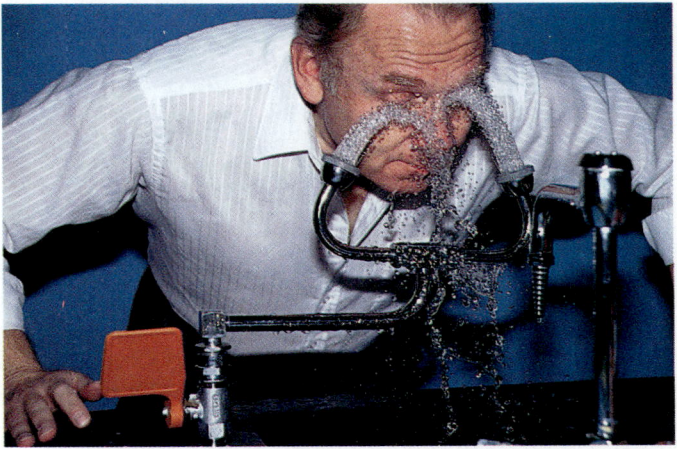

FIGURE 12-10 The emergency eye wash fountain connects to existing plumbing. The two streams of water wash both eyes simultaneously and continuously.

pathogenic microorganisms. Routine housekeeping duties should be performed faithfully, such as scouring and disinfecting sinks and counters. Even if surfaces do not look dirty, you must remember that microorganisms cannot be seen with the naked eye and that preventing the disease is much smarter than taking a chance in getting it.

ACHIEVE UNIT OBJECTIVES

- ■ Complete the Workbook activities to meet the learning objectives.
- ■ Practice the procedures in this unit to meet the performance objectives.
- ■ Apply your knowledge at the end of this chapter in completing the Critical Thinking Challenge and Activities, as well as the StudyWARE on your Student CD-ROM.

UNIT 2
INFECTION CONTROL

OBJECTIVES

Upon completion of this unit, you will be able to achieve the following:

LEARNING Objectives

1. Spell and define, using the glossary in the back of the text, all the Words to Know in this unit.
2. List patient education suggestions to prevent transmitting disease to others.
3. Describe the recommended universal and standard precautions in regard to human tissue, blood, and body fluids.
4. Explain the purpose of the regulatory bodies (OSHA, CLIA) regarding disease transmission in the medical facility.
5. Explain the recommended written statement (and the reason for it) concerning universal precautions that should be posted in the physician's office laboratory.
6. Describe methods of controlling the growth of microorganisms.
7. List the growth requirements of microorganisms.
8. Describe the infection process cycle.
9. Explain what direct and indirect contact is.
10. Describe the body's defense against disease.
11. Explain the difference between sanitization, disinfection, and sterilization.
12. Explain the purpose of sterilization.
13. Explain the purpose of sterilizing all contaminated items before you can safely reuse them (including disposables before discarding).
14. Explain the function of the autoclave.
15. Explain the importance of safety when using the autoclave.
16. Explain the purpose of using sterilization indicators for autoclaving.
17. Explain the preventive measures for health care professionals against the hepatitis B virus.
18. Locate and interpret from the communicable disease chart the means of transmission, incubation time, symptoms, and treatment for a given disease.

PERFORMANCE Objectives

1. Demonstrate the proper procedure for preparing and wrapping instruments to be autoclaved.
2. Demonstrate the proper procedure for sterilization of instruments by use of an autoclave. (*Note:* Many different types of autoclaves are on the market. Pay strict attention to the operating instructions provided by the manufacturer.)

WORDS TO KNOW

aerobe	Clinical	coma
anaerobes	Laboratory	communicable
autoclave	Improvement	confinement
autotrophs	Amendments	debilitated
bacteria	(CLIA)	disinfection

droplet infection	obligate	protozoa
exudative	Occupational	pruritic
fecal	Safety and	pustular
flora	Health	resuscitation
fungi	Administration	sanitization
heterotrophs	(OSHA)	seizures
hygiene	organic	shelf life
incineration	parasite	spores
incubation	personal	sterilization
inorganic	protective	susceptible
invasive	equipment	virulent
malaise	(PPE)	virus
morphology	petechial	vulnerable
nits	pH	

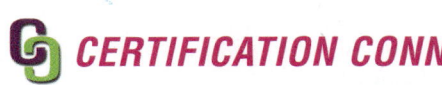

CERTIFICATION CONNECTION

CMA

Principles of infection
   control

CMAS

Asepsis in the medical
   office

RMA

Sterilization

In addition to giving special regard to patients, health care workers have the responsibility of self-protection. It is recommended that standard blood and body fluid precautions be used for all patients, especially when the infection status of the patient is unknown. Appropriate protection against exposure to blood and body fluids should be routine practice for all health care workers. Gloves should be worn when in contact (direct or indirect) with blood or any body fluids, mucous membranes, or nonintact skin; in handling items or surfaces soiled with blood or body fluid; and when performing venipuncture or any other surgical procedure. After each patient contact, gloves should be changed and hands washed. If procedures could possibly generate droplets of blood or other body fluids, the health care worker should wear shields to protect the eyes or face in addition to gloves and gown. This will protect the mucous membranes of the eyes, mouth, and nose.

After gloves are removed, hands should be thoroughly washed. If hands and other skin surfaces have been in contact with blood or other body fluids, they should be washed immediately.

At all times, extreme caution must be used by health care workers in handling needles, scalpels, and other sharp instruments to avoid self-injury. To prevent possible self-injury, it is recommended that needles should never be recapped, broken off, or removed from dis-

posable syringes by hand after use. They should be carefully placed in puncture-proof containers after engaging the safety guard over the needle.

All infectious waste must be disposed of by placing each contaminated item in its appropriate hazardous waste container provided by your employer. Any disposable material that has even a trace of human tissue, blood, or other body fluid on it must be considered as infectious and must be treated with extreme caution. Latex or vinyl gloves must be worn when handling any contaminated item to reduce the possibility of disease transmission, especially the human immunodeficiency virus (HIV) and the hepatitis B virus (HBV). The precautions are recommended for all health care professionals by the Centers for Disease Control (CDC) and the United States Public Health Service.

Note that many of the patients you will serve and possibly some of your coworkers may be highly allergic to latex. A practical way to care for patients with this sensitivity to latex is to make one of the examination rooms free of all latex products. When latex-allergic patients are treated in this way, they may be less likely to have an allergic episode when visiting your office.

DISEASE PREVENTION

Beginning in the mid-1980s, following the frightening reality of the acquired immunodeficiency syndrome (AIDS) epidemic, the ways that health care professionals practice caring for patients has changed dramatically. Regulatory bodies have been established to provide standards for all who are employed with managed care of the public to ensure quality care. Two of the most prominent are the **Occupational Health and Safety Administration (OSHA)**, established long before the epidemic, and the **Clinical Laboratory Improvement Amendments (CLIA)** in 1988. These guidelines have become federal regulations and must be followed not only because of federal mandate, but foremost to protect both health care professionals and the patients whom they serve. These standards, called Standard Precautions (Figure 12-11), have been recommended by the Centers for Disease Control and Prevention since 1987 and pay attention to the welfare of both health care providers and the public regarding health care standards. In each physician's office laboratory (POL) there must be posted a statement in writing that agrees with compliance of the OSHA regulations. Those who do not follow these regulations will be fined. Having this in clear view provides a constant reminder to all who work in the area of health care. Figure 12-12 shows this type of document. This statement must be signed and dated by the employer as well. Knowing that following these regulations can save the lives of so many makes it easier to cooperate. Employees quickly realize the importance of the guidelines and soon respect and

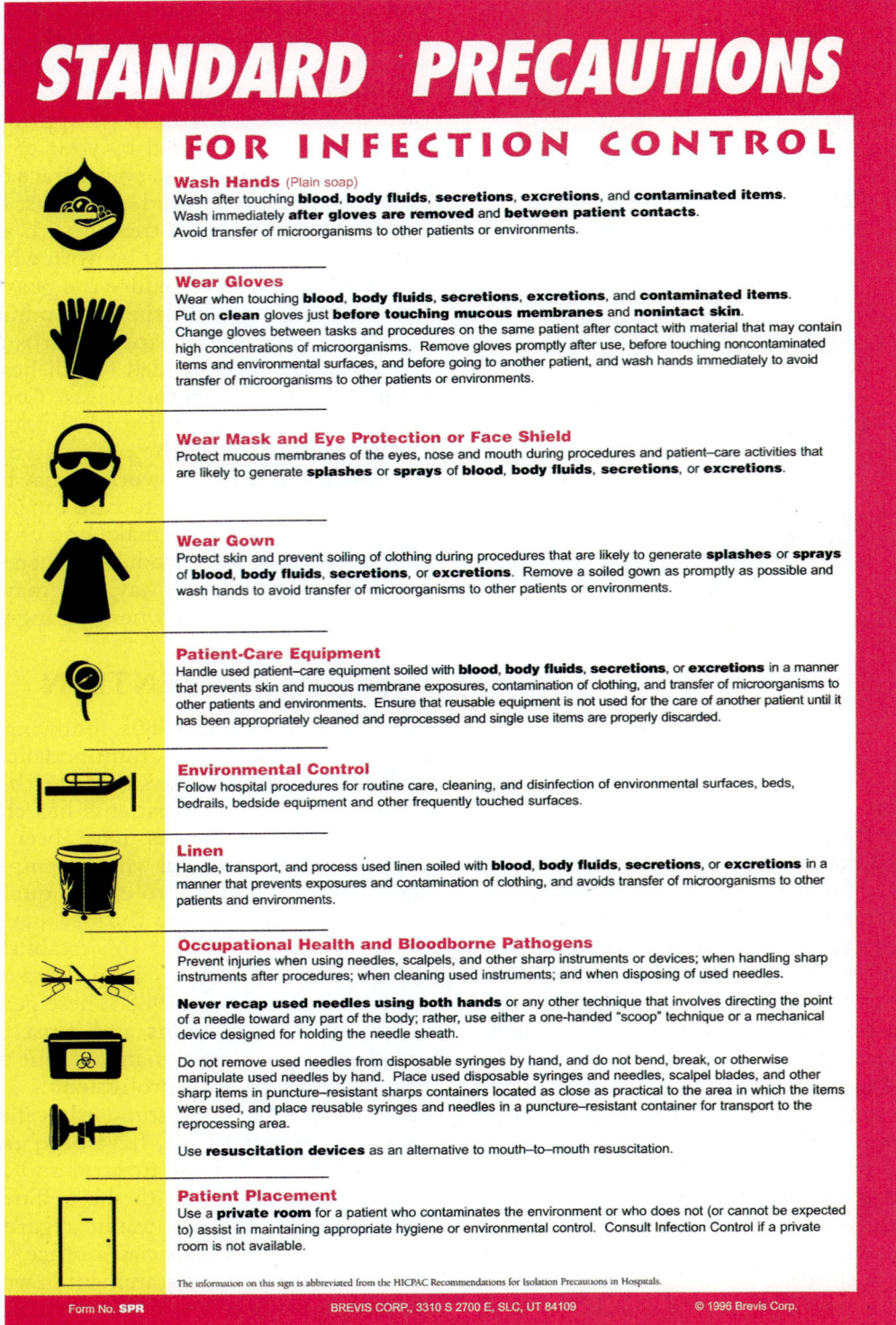

STANDARD · PRECAUTIONS

FOR INFECTION CONTROL

Wash Hands (Plain soap)
Wash after touching **blood**, **body fluids**, **secretions**, **excretions**, and **contaminated items**.
Wash immediately **after gloves are removed** and **between patient contacts**.
Avoid transfer of microorganisms to other patients or environments.

Wear Gloves
Wear when touching **blood**, **body fluids**, **secretions**, **excretions**, and **contaminated items**.
Put on **clean** gloves just **before touching mucous membranes** and **nonintact skin**.
Change gloves between tasks and procedures on the same patient after contact with material that may contain
high concentrations of microorganisms. Remove gloves promptly after use, before touching noncontaminated
items and environmental surfaces, and before going to another patient, and wash hands immediately to avoid
transfer of microorganisms to other patients or environments.

Wear Mask and Eye Protection or Face Shield
Protect mucous membranes of the eyes, nose and mouth during procedures and patient–care activities that
are likely to generate **splashes** or **sprays** of **blood**, **body fluids**, **secretions**, or **excretions**.

Wear Gown
Protect skin and prevent soiling of clothing during procedures that are likely to generate **splashes** or **sprays**
of **blood**, **body fluids**, **secretions**, or **excretions**. Remove a soiled gown as promptly as possible and
wash hands to avoid transfer of microorganisms to other patients or environments.

Patient-Care Equipment
Handle used patient–care equipment soiled with **blood**, **body fluids**, **secretions**, or **excretions** in a manner
that prevents skin and mucous membrane exposures, contamination of clothing, and transfer of microorganisms to
other patients and environments. Ensure that reusable equipment is not used for the care of another patient until it
has been appropriately cleaned and reprocessed and single use items are properly discarded.

Environmental Control
Follow hospital procedures for routine care, cleaning, and disinfection of environmental surfaces, beds,
bedrails, bedside equipment and other frequently touched surfaces.

Linen
Handle, transport, and process used linen soiled with **blood**, **body fluids**, **secretions**, or **excretions** in a
manner that prevents exposures and contamination of clothing, and avoids transfer of microorganisms to other
patients and environments.

Occupational Health and Bloodborne Pathogens
Prevent injuries when using needles, scalpels, and other sharp instruments or devices; when handling sharp
instruments after procedures; when cleaning used instruments; and when disposing of used needles.

Never recap used needles using both hands or any other technique that involves directing the point
of a needle toward any part of the body; rather, use either a one-handed "scoop" technique or a mechanical
device designed for holding the needle sheath.

Do not remove used needles from disposable syringes by hand, and do not bend, break, or otherwise
manipulate used needles by hand. Place used disposable syringes and needles, scalpel blades, and other
sharp items in puncture–resistant sharps containers located as close as practical to the area in which the items
were used, and place reusable syringes and needles in a puncture–resistant container for transport to the
reprocessing area.

Use **resuscitation devices** as an alternative to mouth–to–mouth resuscitation.

Patient Placement
Use a **private room** for a patient who contaminates the environment or who does not (or cannot be expected
to) assist in maintaining appropriate hygiene or environmental control. Consult Infection Control if a private
room is not available.

The information on this sign is abbreviated from the HICPAC Recommendations for Isolation Precautions in Hospitals.

Form No. **SPR**   BREVIS CORP., 3310 S 2700 E, SLC, UT 84109   © 1996 Brevis Corp.

FIGURE 12-11   A poster such as this one should be posted in the physician's office laboratory
to comply with Standard Precautions and to remind employees of safety precautions. *(Courtesy of
Brevis Corp.)*

appreciate their intent. This reminder helps to keep the health care provider alert and reminds them to safeguard against carelessness in the performance of their duties because they may be exposed to blood or other hazardous body fluids or infectious waste in the course of their duties. Each employee must have this statement explained when he is hired and have evidence of this in writing with his signature in a permanent file.

Standard Precautions

All employees in this medical practice must follow standard precautions at all times in performing procedures that may expose them to **bloodborne pathogens** possibly contained in the blood and body fluids from any patient regardless of the patient's health status. All employees must wear protective barriers that are appropriate for the procedure being performed to prevent possible infection. Employees who work with direct patient contact must have HBV vaccine. Any accidental needle sticks, other injuries, or contacts with a potentially infectious body fluid must be reported to the physician at once for treatment and **documentation.**

FIGURE 12-12 This statement regarding Standard Precautions should be posted in clear view.

All items such as mouthpieces, **resuscitation** bags, or any other ventilation supplies necessary for emergency use in mouth-to-mouth resuscitation must be disposable to eliminate any risk of disease transmission—especially in an emergency situation where the health status of the afflicted is unknown. This practice protects both patient and health care provider.

A health care provider who has a skin condition or a laceration that is either seeping or bleeding should refrain from direct patient care until the condition clears up to avoid any possibility of transmitting microorganisms to another. An appropriate bandage that is adequate in covering the affected area should be worn, and the affected provider should follow proper gloving procedures to keep the condition contained. Caution should also be taken in handling all equipment and supplies.

Employees must also be protected from HBV, which is a highly contagious and potentially fatal disease. Preventive immunization involves a series of three injections. Employers must offer this immunization to new employees within their first 14 days of employment, with no cost to the employee; then, documentation of the immunization offer must be filed in the employee's record. If the person has already had the vaccine or refuses to be given the vaccine, documentation must be filed in the employee record. Human nature is imperfect, and the reality is that many serious diseases can be spread by careless acts. Needle-stick injuries are unfortunately common because of human error. Safeguard yourself against this accident by never recapping needles. Always dispose of the entire used needle intact with the syringe to prevent injury. If you ever need to re-cap prior to performing an injection, a needle resheather should be used. Further information can be found regarding this procedure in Chapter 18, Unit 3. Because there are diseases that do carry a fatal risk and there are measures one can take to prevent such a risk, it is obvious that safeguarding from contracting the disease is wise. There are many ways for health care professionals to practice safety in regard to the prevention of disease. Use of barriers, such as gowns and masks, are recommended to avoid possible contamination by splash or spill of blood or blood-containing fluids. Where appropriate, protection should be made with goggles, face shields, or any other protective disposable clothing articles according to the circumstances. These protective barriers are referred to as **personal protective equipment (PPE)** and have been recommended by the Centers for Disease Control and Prevention.

Basic recommended precautions are as follows:

- Routine use of appropriate barriers to prevent contact with mucous membranes, blood, or any other body fluid of a patient (any person)
- Proper routine, thorough hand washing
- Immediate placement of used sharps and needles (intact with syringe) in biohazard puncture-proof containers
- Use of disposables in resuscitation procedures
- Refraining from direct patient care if you have an **exudative** skin condition (or other contagious disease)
- Especially strict adherence to precautions during pregnancy

If all health care workers would follow Standard Precautions to help in the control of contagious diseases, it would set a good example for the public. We all must realize that actions speak louder than words.

Indirect and Direct Contact

The posted guidelines will be a constant reminder to pay special attention to safety. Because diseases can be transmitted in different ways, a brief discussion regarding direct and indirect contact is necessary for you to realize and understand the potential danger that an infected person can have. When a person is sick or infected with a disease, that person is the host of the microorganisms causing the illness. When the person coughs or sneezes, the vapor that is projected from the mouth carries the microbes of the disease with it into the air. This is called **droplet infection** because the vapor contains tiny drops of vapor (moisture) from the person's breath. Depending on the force of the breath, laughing and shouting carry droplets quite far, possibly projecting them up to 20 feet or more. This force is determined by the size and strength of the person and also determines the potential radius of the spread of the microbes. The same is true for sneezing. This is the reason that patient education is so important. When a patient in the reception area is waiting to see the doctor for a routine checkup and another comes in with a terrible coughing and sneezing problem, the entire area is infected with the sick person's germs. It is your responsibility to remove the infected individual immediately to prevent others from being infected with an unwanted disease. Offer the patient instruction on catching the coughs and sneezes in the tissues you provide (Figures 12-13A and B) and show the person where to deposit the waste. Make sure you follow the person's steps with a spray disinfectant to help contain the

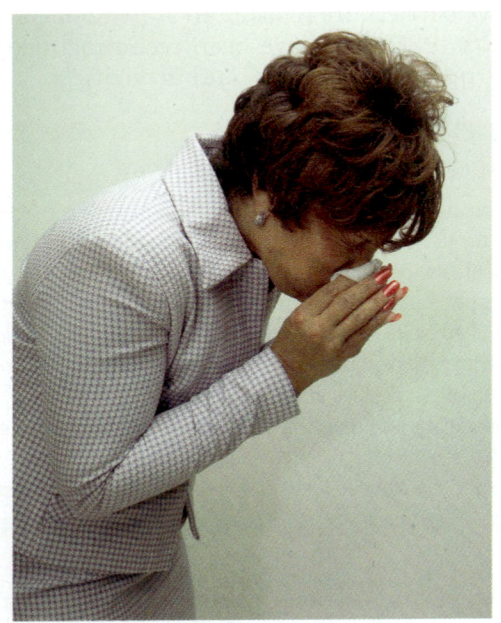

FIGURE 12-13A Teach patients to cough into a tissue.

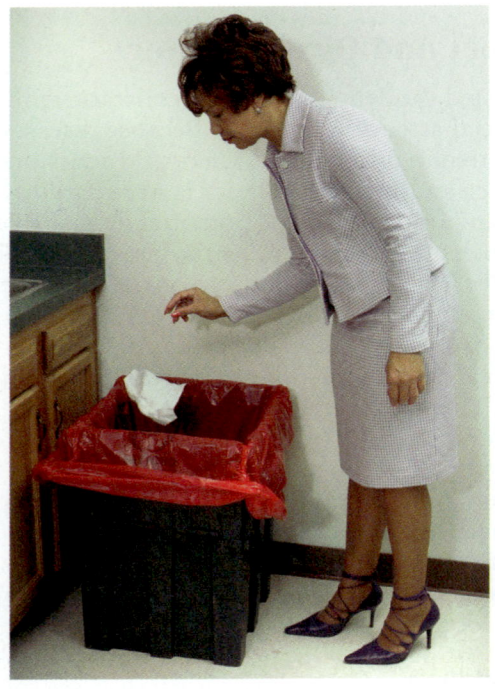

FIGURE 12-13B Remind patients to properly dispose of contaminated tissues.

germs to protect those who will be in that place after the sick patient leaves. If you do not clean up after the person carefully (by gloving to pick up used tissues, for example), there is a risk that you and others may contract the same illness. You and others may catch it by indirect contact. This means that you may contract the disease from having handled soiled tissues, by touching the door knob that the infected patient touched, or that you possibly inhaled the contaminated air following a cough or sneeze of the patient. When you are around a person who is sick, you should not deeply inhale when you breathe, or you may subject yourself to an even greater risk of contracting the disease. In some infectious disease cases, it is wise to wear a face mask that covers the mouth and nose. The physician usually suggests this for protection against disease. These are examples of indirect contact. A direct contact is actual contact with the patient or his body fluids. Direct contact includes eating, drinking, or smoking after another person; touching; kissing; and sexual intimacy.

DISEASE TRANSMISSION

It is suggested that you become familiar with the **communicable** diseases listed in Table 12-1. A description of the disease, the means of transmission, **incubation** time, symptoms, and treatment will inform you about the diseases so that you can be of better service to patients. The incubation time refers to the time between the initial exposure to the disease-causing microbes and the appearance of the first symptoms or signs of the disease. If a person is **susceptible** to a disease, it means that person is receptive, or **vulnerable**, to catching it. Generally, when one is susceptible, the person is weakened because of a pre-existing illness or condition; is overall run down and worn out; or has poor **hygiene** and health habits. All of these points are considered to be factors in one's poor resistance to disease. Study the infection cycle in Figure 12-14. Follow the cycle to see how easily diseases are transferred from one to another unless the cycle is broken. You can be instrumental in the interruption of the cycle by being vigilant in your efforts against the transmission of disease. As you can see, taking care of yourself is extremely important in the scope of disease prevention and protection.

As you learned in Chapter 11, Unit 9, the body's immune system has amazing abilities. Immunity is best when the body is in a state of good physical, emotional, and mental condition. Essentially, this means that defense against disease can be maintained most efficiently by practicing the good health habits of proper exercise, adequate rest, good nutrition, and proper hygiene. Exercise is most helpful in resisting disease because it promotes circulation, encourages nutrition, and reduces stress. Good eating habits that provide a variety of nutrition following the food pyramid guidelines help keep energy levels at a maximum. Getting

TABLE 12-1   Communicable Diseases

Disease	Means of Transmission	Incubation	Symptoms	Treatment
AIDS (acquired immunodeficiency syndrome)*	Direct contact: sexual, anal, or vaginal intercourse, sharing IV drug needles, infected mother to child (childbirth), blood to blood (from cuts, scrapes, punctures of skin). Indirect contact: blood transfusions	Onset of AIDS following infection with human immunodeficiency virus (HIV) from 6 months to 10+ years	Early—loss of appetite, weight loss, fever, night sweats, skin rashes, diarrhea, fatigue, poor resistance to infections, swollen lymph nodes. Later—cough, fever, shortness of breath, dyspnea, purple blotches on the skin	Research and new developments continue in the search for a cure and a vaccine. The current treatment most commonly used is zidovudine (AZT).
Chickenpox* (Varicella zoster virus)	Direct or indirect contact, droplet, or airborne secretion of infected person	2–3 weeks, usually 13–17 days	Crops of **pruritic** vesicular eruptions on the skin, slight fever and headache, **malaise**	Bed rest, topical antipruritics
Common cold (upper respiratory infection—URI)	Direct or indirect contact with infected person	12–72 hours (some viruses 2–7 days), usually 24 hours	Slight sore throat, watery eyes, runny nose, sneezing, chills, malaise, low-grade fever	Rest, decongestant, mild analgesics, increased fluid intake
Conjunctivitis* (pink eye)	Direct or indirect contact with discharge from eyes or upper respiratory tract of infected person	Viral: 24 hours to days; bacterial: 24–72 hours	Redness of eyes, itching, burning of eyes, matted eyelashes	Antibacterial agents, antibiotics, corticosteroids depending on causative agent
Head lice* (pediculosis)	Direct contact with infested person; indirect contact is rare	1 week (**nits**, or eggs, hatch in 1 week, mature in 2 weeks)	Itching of scalp; presence of small, light gray lice and nits (eggs) at the base of hairs	Topical use of 1% lindane shampoo, lotion, or cream (7–10 days); comb nits from hair; launder washable items in hot water with hottest drying cycle, dry-clean or seal in plastic bags nonwashable items (2 weeks); thoroughly vacuum the environment
Haemophilus influenzae type b Hib (H-flu)*	Direct and indirect contact and droplet infection from respiratory tract	3+ days	URI symptoms, fever, aches, sleepiness, no appetite; as disease progresses, child is irritable and fussy	Antibiotics, increased fluid intake, antipyretics, rest, analgesics
Hepatitis A* (acute infective hepatitis)	Direct contact or by **fecal**-contaminated food or water	14–50 days, avg. 25–30 days	Slow onset, fever, malaise, loss of appetite, nausea, vomiting, jaundice, weakness, dark urine, whitish stool	Bed rest, increased fluid intake, proper nourishment (no fats or alcohol)
Hepatitis B* (serum hepatitis)	Contaminated serum in blood transfusion or by use of contaminated needles or instruments	14–50 days	Similar to hepatitis A, but onset is rapid and acute	Same as hepatitis A
Hepatitis C* (formerly non-A, non-B, or NANB)	Direct contact with blood, contaminated needles	14–50 days acute onset	Same as above	Same as above

(continues)

TABLE 12-1   Communicable Diseases (Continued)

Disease	Means of Transmission	Incubation	Symptoms	Treatment
Herpes simplex virus (HSV) (cold sores, fever blisters)	Direct contact with infected person	2–14 days, usually 4–6 days	Painful blisters on lips, which turn **pustular** and then form crusted scabs; oral lesions are small ulcerated areas	Topical applications of drying medications; antibiotics for secondary infections
Impetigo	Direct contact with draining sores	2–10 days	Blisterlike lesions (later become crusted), itching	Cleansing of areas with antibacterial soap and water, topical and/or oral antibiotics
Influenza*	Direct and indirect contact and by airborne secretions	1–3 days	Sudden onset of fever, chills, headache, sore muscles, malaise (commonly runny nose, sore throat, and cough)	Bed rest, increased fluid intake, antipyretics
Meningitis* (aseptic)	Direct contact, fecal-oral route, and respiratory secretions	2–21 days	Sudden or gradual fever, intense headache, nausea, vomiting, stiff neck, irritability, sluggishness	Hospitalization, bed rest, increased fluid intake, antipyretics, analgesics
Meningitis* (bacterial) haemophilus and meningococcal	Direct contact and droplet infection from respiratory tract	1–10 days, usually 3–4 days	Sudden onset of fever, intense headache, nausea, vomiting; sometimes **petechial** rash, irritability, sluggishness (possible **seizures** or **coma**)	Same as aseptic plus antibiotics, by intravenous and/or oral administration
Pinworms (*Enterobius vermicularis*)	Direct transfer of eggs from anus to mouth; indirect contact with eggs in clothing, bedding	3 weeks–3 months	Anal itching, insomnia, irritability	Anthelmintics, initiate scrupulous personal hygiene, shorten fingernails; launder washable items in hottest or boiled water
Pneumonia	Direct and indirect contact	Abrupt onset	High fever, shaking, chills, productive cough	Antibiotics, liquids, rest, antipyretics
Scabies*	Direct contact or indirect contact with infested clothing/bedding	2–6 weeks	Intense itching of small, raised areas of skin that contain fluid or tiny burrows under the skin, resembling a line—may be anywhere on the body	Topical scabicide, oral antihistamines, and salicylates to reduce itching
Strep throat	Direct contact	1–3 days	Fever, red and sore throat, pus spots on back of throat, tender and swollen glands of neck	Antibiotics, analgesics, antipyretics, increase fluid intake
Scarlet fever* (scarlatina) (streptococcal)	Direct or indirect contact	1–7 days	Same as above, plus strawberry tongue, rash of skin and inside mouth, high fever, nausea, and vomiting	Same as above, plus bed rest

*Report these diseases to local health department. Refer also to sexually transmitted diseases in Chapter 11, Unit 13.

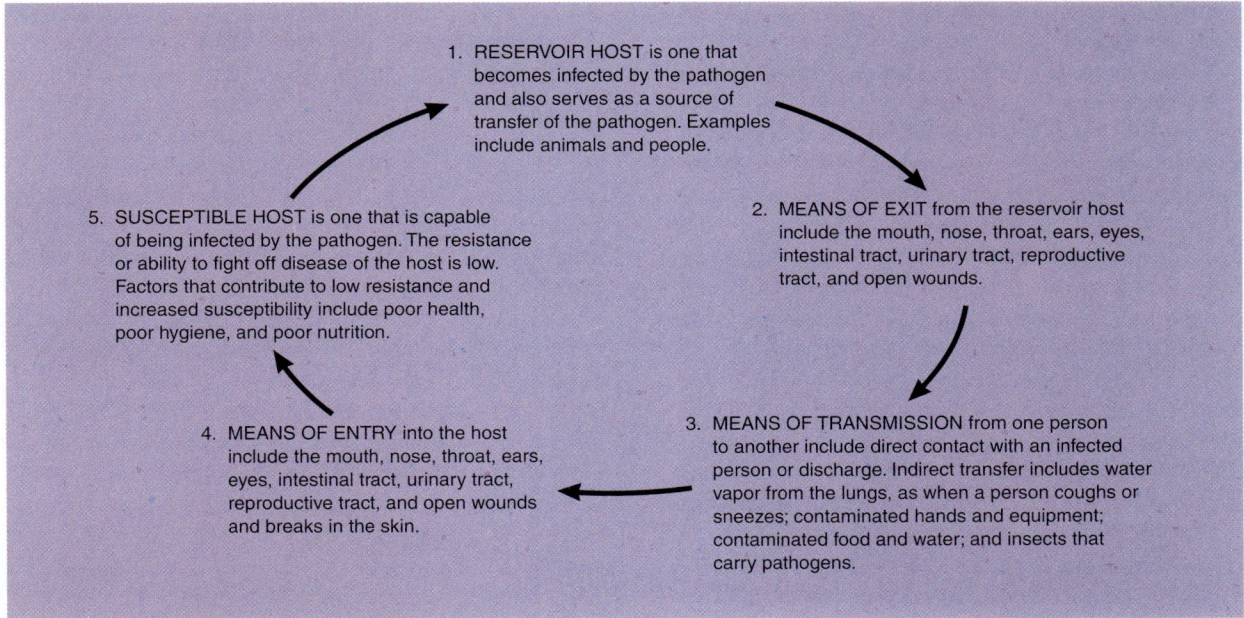

1. RESERVOIR HOST is one that becomes infected by the pathogen and also serves as a source of transfer of the pathogen. Examples include animals and people.

2. MEANS OF EXIT from the reservoir host include the mouth, nose, throat, ears, eyes, intestinal tract, urinary tract, reproductive tract, and open wounds.

3. MEANS OF TRANSMISSION from one person to another include direct contact with an infected person or discharge. Indirect transfer includes water vapor from the lungs, as when a person coughs or sneezes; contaminated hands and equipment; contaminated food and water; and insects that carry pathogens.

4. MEANS OF ENTRY into the host include the mouth, nose, throat, ears, eyes, intestinal tract, urinary tract, reproductive tract, and open wounds and breaks in the skin.

5. SUSCEPTIBLE HOST is one that is capable of being infected by the pathogen. The resistance or ability to fight off disease of the host is low. Factors that contribute to low resistance and increased susceptibility include poor health, poor hygiene, and poor nutrition.

FIGURE 12-14　The infection cycle can be broken if one is aware of the process. It is important to include this in patient education to help prevent disease transmission.

enough rest according to individual needs gives the body time to restore strength and vitality.

The body also has specialized defense mechanisms. The respiratory tract contains hairlike cilia that filter out invading pathogens. Coughing and sneezing are reflexes to rid the body of invaders. Body secretions, such as tears, sweat, urine, and mucus, also wash pathogens from the body. These body secretions have a low **pH**, which discourages bacterial growth. Hydrochloric acid with its low pH discourages the growth of pathogens in the digestive tract.

In the effort to prevent disease transmission, it is helpful to have an idea of what you are trying to prevent. All living organisms have requirements to sustain life and for growth and development. These requirements are oxygen, proper pH and temperature (98.6°F), nutrients, water, and a host to inhabit. Because microorganisms cannot be seen with the naked eye, a brief description follows of the disease-producing microbes, which are **viruses**, **bacteria**, **protozoa**, **fungi**, and **parasites**:

● Bacteria are microorganisms that vary in their **morphology**. These single-celled microorganisms are different from all other organisms because they lack a nucleus and organelles (mitrochondria, chloroplasts, and lysosomes). Bacteria reproduce by cell division approximately every 20 minutes. Figures 12-15A through C show the various forms of bacteria. Many different species of bacteria are pathogenic to humans and animals. For example, *Escherichia coli* causes urinary tract infections (among other illnesses) in humans; *Bordetella per-*

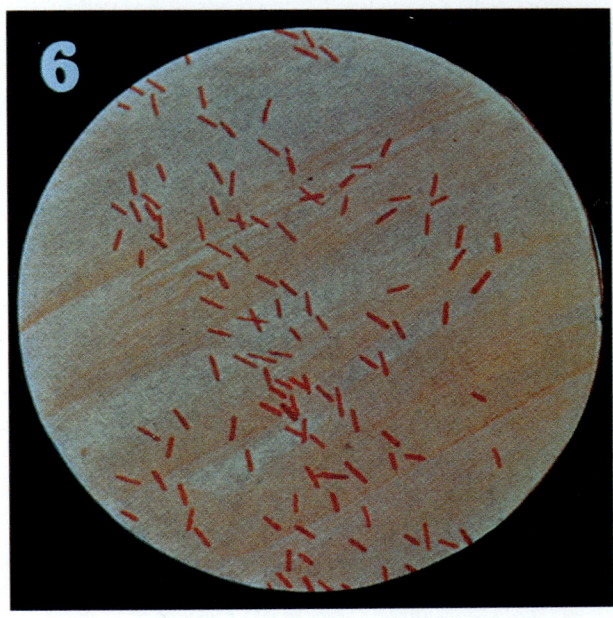

FIGURE 12-15A　Escherichia coli *(Courtesy of the Centers for Disease Control, Atlanta, GA)*

tussis causes whooping cough, which is transmitted by droplet infection; and *Vibrio cholerae* causes cholera in humans who ingest contaminated food and water.

● Viruses, which are the smallest of the microorganisms, may be viewed only by an electron microscope. Figure 12-16 shows a magnified view of a virus. Viruses can only reproduce themselves within a host.

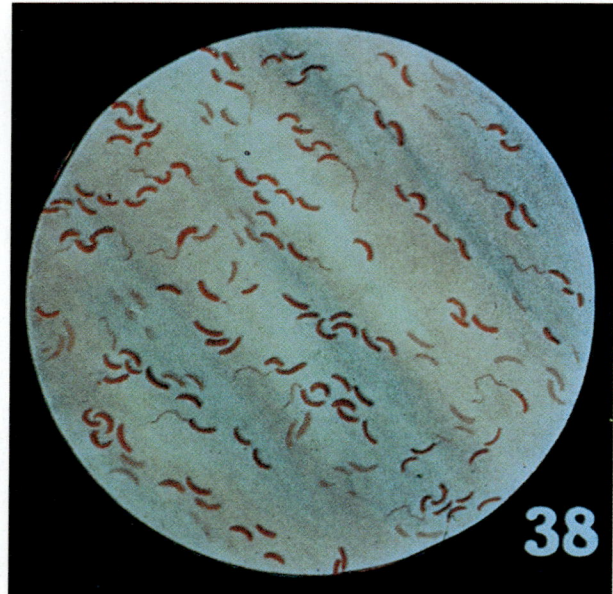

FIGURE 12-15B Hemophilus pertussis *(Courtesy of the Centers for Disease Control, Atlanta, GA)*

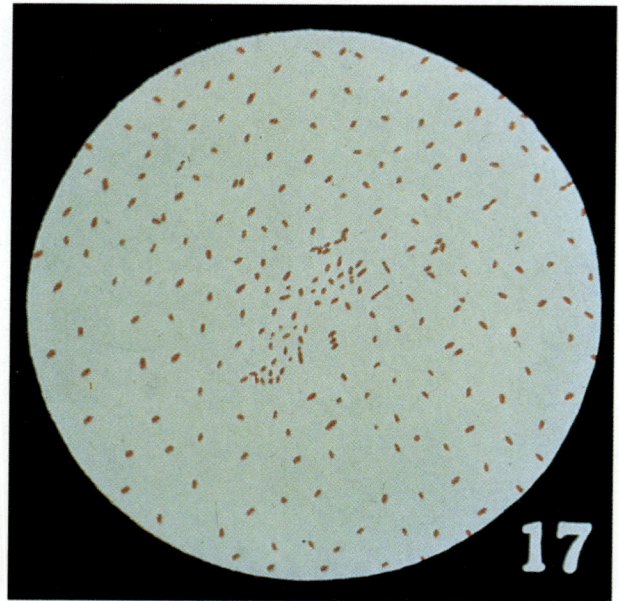

FIGURE 12-15C *Vibrio cholerae (Courtesy of the Centers for Disease Control, Atlanta, GA)*

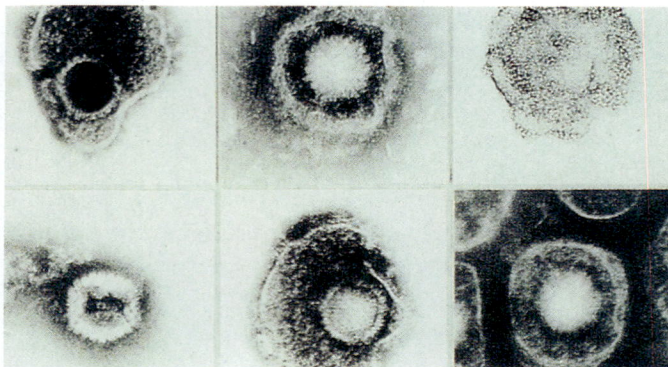

FIGURE 12-16 Electron micrographs of the various types of herpes simplex virus *(Courtesy of the Centers for Disease Control, Atlanta GA)*

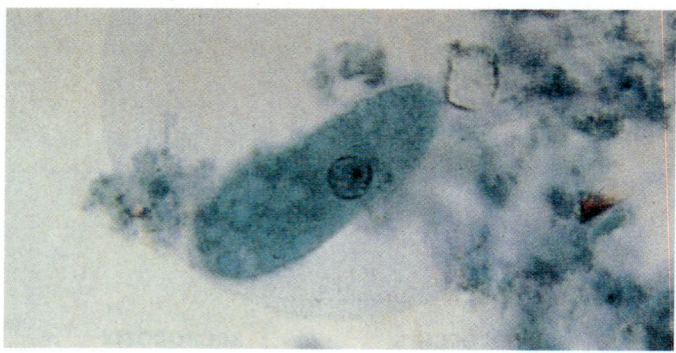

FIGURE 12-17 Intestinal protozoa *Entamoeba coli (Courtesy of the Centers for Disease Control, Atlanta GA)*

Commonly known viruses cause herpes, most childhood diseases, the common cold, and influenza.

- Protozoa are complex, single-celled microorganisms that attach themselves to other organisms (Figure 12-17). Amebic dysentery, malaria, and *Trichomonas vaginalis* are diseases caused by protozoa.
- Fungi are simple parasitic plants (molds) that depend on other life forms for a nutritional source. They reproduce by budding. Multicellular fungi reproduce by spore formation. Approximately 100 different types of fungi are common in humans; however, only 10 of these are pathogenic. Some examples of pathogenic fungus conditions are histoplasmosis, caused by *Histoplasma capsulatum,* and tinea pedis (athlete's foot; Figure 12-18).
- Parasites are organisms that depend on another living organism for nourishment. An **obligate** parasite is one that depends completely on its host for survival. Faculative parasites are able to live independently from their hosts at times. Protozoa, mentioned earlier, are internal parasites because they live within the body of a human or an animal. *External parasites* are those that attach themselves on the outside of the body, such as fleas and ticks on animals. Humans are sometimes troubled with the itch mite (scabies), pinworms *(Enterobius vermicularis)* and hookworms (ancylostomiasis) (Figure 12-19). Other microorganisms are helpful and necessary to normal **flora** in humans and animals because they provide a balance in the body and destroy pathogens. Normal flora is the cohabitation of microorganisms (nonpathogenic and pathogenic in balance) that live in or within an organism to provide a natural

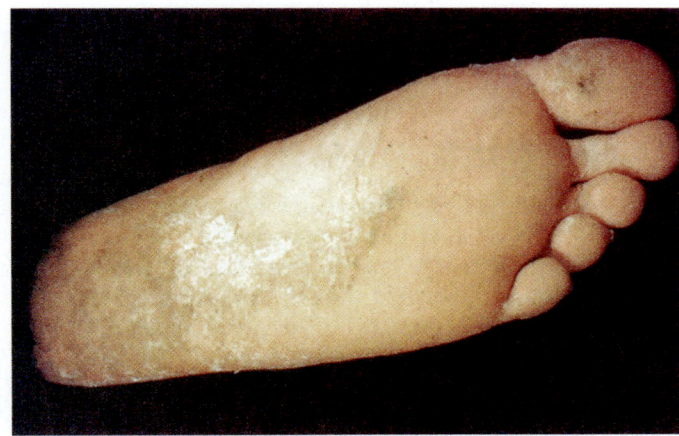

FIGURE 12-18   Athlete's foot (tinea pedis) *(Courtesy of the Centers for Disease Control, Atlanta, GA)*

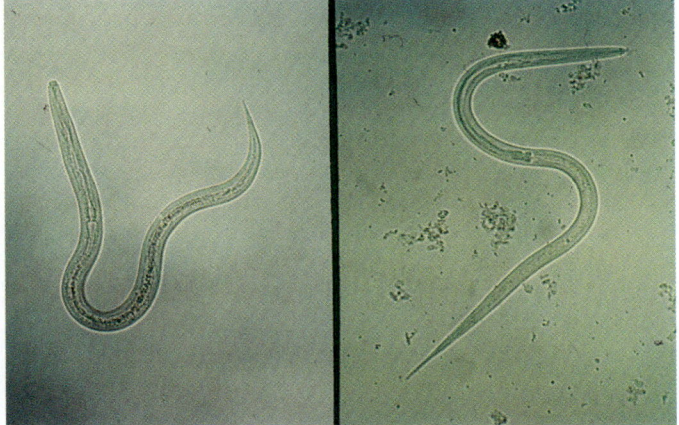

FIGURE 12-19   Strongyloides—filariform larvae of hookworm and strongyloides *(Courtesy of the Centers for Disease Control, Atlanta, GA)*

immunity against certain infections. Infection occurs when this balance is disturbed.

Microorganisms that feed on **organic** matter are called **heterotrophs**; those that feed on **inorganic** matter are called **autotrophs**. Those that need oxygen to grow are called **aerobes**, and those that grow best in the absence of oxygen are called **anaerobes**. Microorganisms grow best at the average body temperature (98.6°F or 37°C). The human body has not only a desirable temperature for microbial growth, but also furnishes darkness and moisture, other growth requirements. In addition, the body has a 6.0 average pH, which is an acidic level high enough to protect the body from microorganism invasion. If the pH level is higher, it indicates that microbial growth is present. As bacteria grow and multiply, the pH level becomes higher in alkalinity. A low pH reading, one less than 6, can be the result of not eating for a long period or ketosis. An environment that is too acidic will not support microbial growth.

Disease begins when a pathogen finds a body (a host) that offers it the conditions necessary for growth. Microorganisms, in the proper growth environment, can be extremely **virulent**, particularly for **debilitated**, aged, or young vulnerable patients. When the microorganism has reached the stage of causing an infection, the patient should take precautions against transmitting it to another. **Confinement** is the best way, but many patients insist on taking their colds and flu to work or play, thereby infecting others. The next step in the cycle, then, is transmission to another person by way of body openings. The microorganisms leave the host through the discharge of body secretions and make either direct or indirect contact with another host. When a patient with a cold coughs or sneezes, the vapor contains the microorganism that is causing the infection. The vapor may be projected through the air as far as 20 feet, and someone else may breathe in that microorganism. The growth requirement is then met by a susceptible host, one whose body resistance may be low because of poor nutritional habits or poor hygiene.

INFECTION CONTROL

Three methods are recommended in addition to the Standard Precautions to diminish the spread of pathogens in the medical facility. They are **sanitization**, **disinfection**, and **sterilization**.

Sanitization is the process of washing and scrubbing to remove materials such as body tissue, blood, or other body fluids. Again, hand washing is the number one step for sanitizing the hands. You should wear latex or vinyl gloves (double-glove as necessary). It is an additional recommendation that utility gloves be worn during the process of sanitization of items and equipment to protect your hands from any possibility of contamination and injury from the articles that you handle. Items should be rinsed in cool water, soaked in a warm detergent solution for generally 20 minutes, washed and scrubbed thoroughly with a brush, rinsed in warm to hot water to remove the detergent, and dried completely. During this process, the gloves also serve to protect your hands from the harshness of repeated contact with soap and water, which may result in chafing and cracking of the skin and possibly lead to infection. Remember to wash your hands before and after gloving. You should use a soothing hand lotion routinely to help prevent dryness caused from excessive hand washing.

Disinfection is a process by which disease-producing microorganisms, or pathogens, are killed. The term *disinfect* pertains to a chemical or physical means of destroying bacteria. It is sometimes referred to as a germicide or bactericide. There are many disinfectant solutions used in medical facilities. Common ones are zephrin chloride and chlorophenyl. Remember that disinfectants are used on objects, not on people. They are chemical solutions that must be changed often (depending on the frequency of use of the container) to ensure the effect intended. Always follow manufacturer's directions for time of exposure and how often to change the solution. Antiseptics are used in preparing the patient's skin for injection or a surgical or invasive procedure. The most commonly used antiseptics are alcohol and Betadine (povidone-iodine).

Sterilization is the process that destroys all forms of living organisms. Disinfectants and antiseptics do not always kill **spores**. Spores are thick-walled, hard capsules formed by some bacteria to remain dormant until conditions for growth are good (Figure 12-20). When the proper growth conditions are present, the bacteria break out of the capsule, grow, and multiply, starting infection. An example of bacteria that produce spores is *Clostridum tetani,* the cause of tetanus, or lock jaw. The only way to be sure that spores are eliminated is to sterilize them. Following the sterilization procedure, generally performed by **autoclaving**, the item remains sterile for 30 days if its packaging is kept dry and intact. This period is referred to as **shelf life**. You should pay attention to the expiration date on all packages to ensure that the contents are sterile. Do not use any sterile package if it is beyond the expiration date (or more than 30 days from the time it was sterilized). If the package is labeled with just the date, it denotes when it was autoclaved. These sterile packages will remain sterile up to 30 days if they are still intact and have not been dampened. Autoclaved packages can also be labeled with "expiration date, 3-10-XX," which is the last date you could use the contents and be assured that they are sterile. If the packaging is torn or punctured, has signs of having been wet (water marks), or is wet, this is an indication that the sterility of the contents has been lost. Microorganisms can enter wrapped or enveloped articles through moisture. Carefully study and practice the procedure of wrapping items for autoclaving within this unit (see Procedure 12-2).

CARE OF INSTRUMENTS

Processing items and instruments for use in procedures that are **invasive** is a vitally important responsibility. When handling any of the instruments or articles that need to be sanitized, disinfected, or prepared for sterilization, you should always wear gloves. This will protect you from becoming contaminated with any possible lingering microorganisms on the item. It will also protect the item from any possible contamination from your hands. Whenever you have a cold or the sniffles, you should wear gloves and a mask to avoid disease transmission. Never sneeze or cough on or over any items you are preparing for any procedure. Always follow Standard Precautions in performing procedures with patient contact.

Because there are microorganisms everywhere, the medical assistant should be ever mindful that pathogens could be present. Practicing proper hand washing and developing good habits is essential in disease control and eliminating the fear of contracting disease.

Many types of sterilization techniques are used in medical practice. The most common method is autoclaving. However, sharp instruments become dull from sterilizing by this method. Rubber or vinyl articles are damaged by intense heat of autoclaving. An alternative method for these items is to place them in a chemical sterilant for at least 20 minutes. Sterilization requires that instruments remain in the sterilizing solution for 10 hours. All instruments must be thoroughly cleaned in a detergent (specifically for this purpose) before placing them into the disinfectant. A way to help prevent injury while cleaning instruments is to wear utility gloves. All instruments, including those with hinges and handles, should be cleaned with a brush and thoroughly dried to prevent diluting the sterilant. The hinges and handles should be kept open to allow all parts to be exposed to the solution. A cover over the sterilant container prevents the evaporation of the solution and keeps the vapor from being inhaled by members of the health care team. This sterilizing solution must completely cover the instruments to be effective. Follow the manufacturer's recommendations regarding sterilant strength and proper disposal. The number of articles placed in this solution will determine how frequently it must be changed. Obviously, the more you use the solution for sterilizing items, the more often it needs to be changed. If this means of sterilizing instruments is only occasional, changing the solution once a week should be sufficient (Figure 12-21).

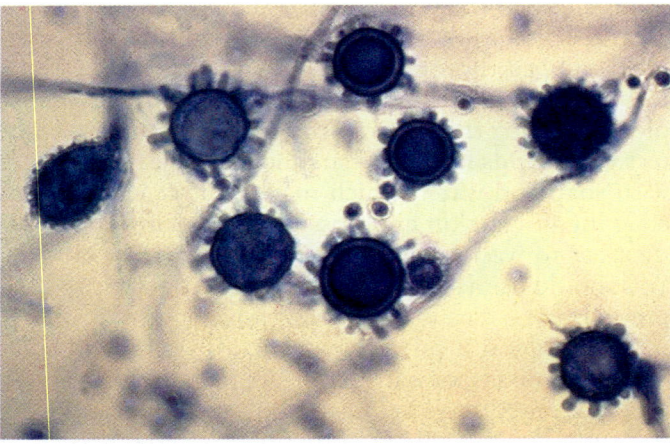

FIGURE 12-20 This picture shows the tough outer wall of spores, which explains their resistance to disinfectants. *(Courtesy of the Centers for Disease Control, Atlanta, GA)*

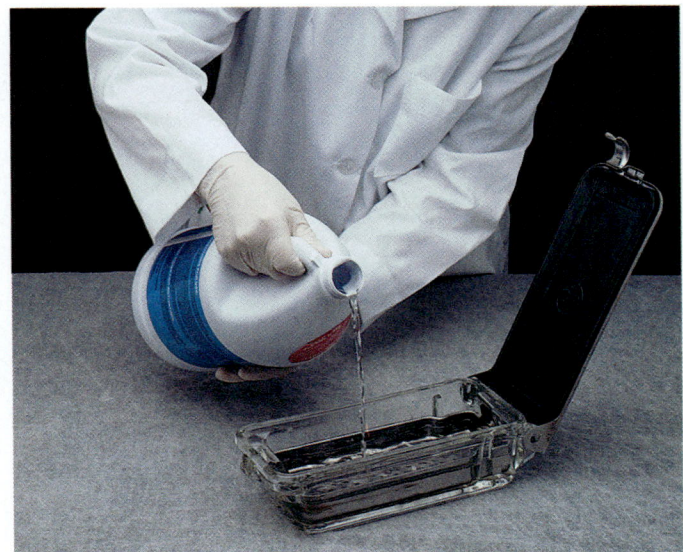

FIGURE 12-21 Chemical sterilizing solutions are used for aseptic control of sharp instruments (dulled by autoclaving) and other articles that can be damaged by the intense heat of autoclaving.

TABLE 12-2 Sterilization Times and Temperatures	
Articles	**Time at 250° to 270°F (121° to 123°C)**
Glassware: empty; inverted	15 minutes
Instruments: metal in covered or open tray; padded or unpadded	
Metal syringe cartridges	
Instruments: metal combined with other materials in covered and/or padded tray	20 minutes
Instruments wrapped in double-thickness muslin	
Dressings: wrapped in paper or muslin—small packs only	30 minutes
Silk, cotton, or nylon: wrapped in paper or muslin	
Treatment trays: wrapped in muslin or paper	

Autoclaving

Many medical practices have an autoclave for sterilization of instruments by steam under pressure, which is a method that guarantees the destruction of spores. The manufacturer's instructions should be followed for the operation and care of the equipment. Instructions are usually printed either on top of the machine or on a tray that pulls out underneath it. It is important that the desired temperature of the sterilizer be maintained for the proper time. Table 12-2 lists the most commonly used articles and the desired times and temperatures for sterilization.

In the process of sterilization, the autoclave exerts approximately 15 pounds of steam pressure per square inch at a temperature between 250° and 270°F. The steam flows through the items and destroys all microorganisms and spores (Figure 12-22).

Articles to be autoclaved must be sanitized and then wrapped in a double thickness of paper or muslin. Envelope packaging is manufactured for some instruments, such as scissors (Figure 12-23). Figure 12-24 shows a medical assistant inserting an instrument into an envelope type of packaging in preparation for autoclaving. A section on the paper envelope permits recording the instrument name, the date, and the initials of the person who sterilized it. Sterilization indicators register proper and complete sterilization (Figure 12-25). Autoclave tape has an indicator stripe that changes color when the proper temperature has been maintained for a long

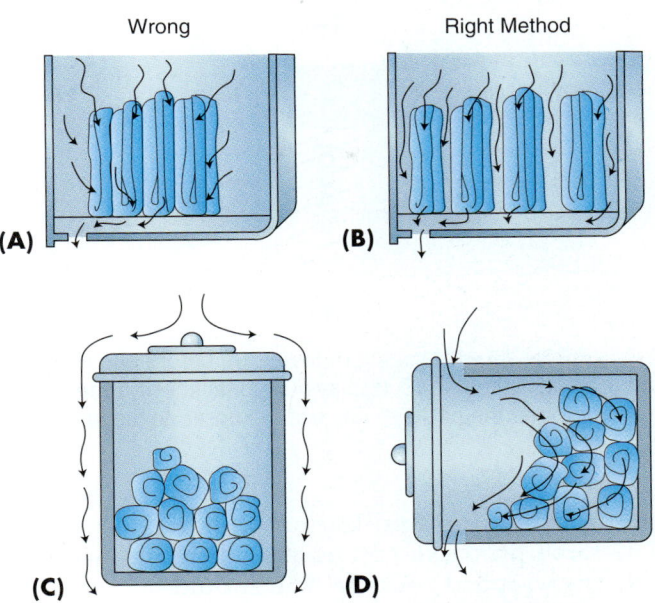

FIGURE 12-22 Packaged instruments should be properly spaced within the autoclave so that the steam can adequately penetrate each pack from all sides. (A) Incorrect method of loading packages in the autoclave; (B) correct method of loading packages in the autoclave. When placing jars in the autoclave, each jar should lie on its side to allow the steam to flow freely through the jar (C) incorrect way; (D) Correct way to place jars in the autoclave. *(Courtesy of STERIS Corporation).*

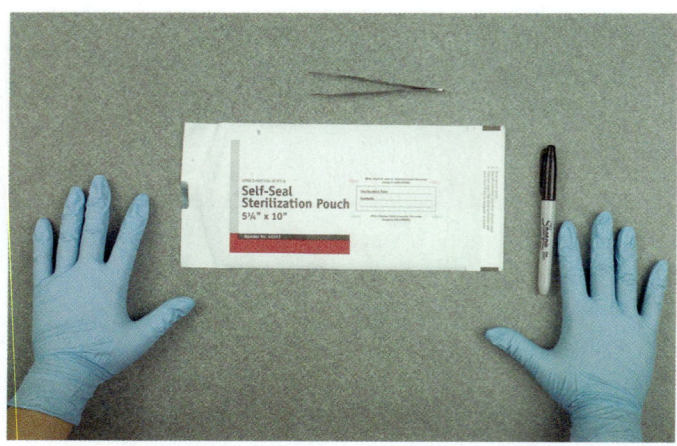

FIGURE 12-23 Envelope-type packaging for autoclaves. Note the color coding to indicate that sterilization has occurred.

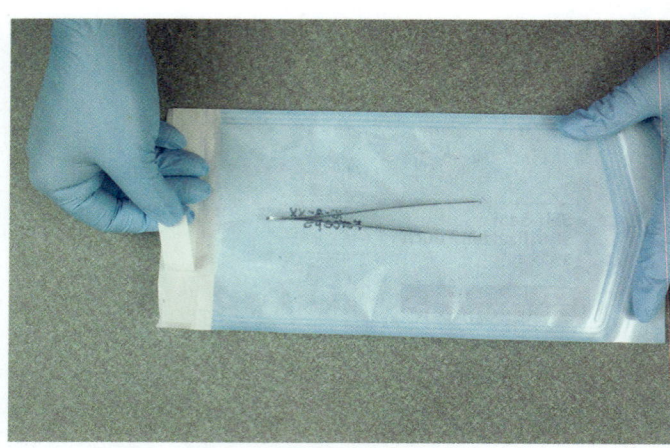

FIGURE 12-24 Placing a single instrument into an envelope autoclave package

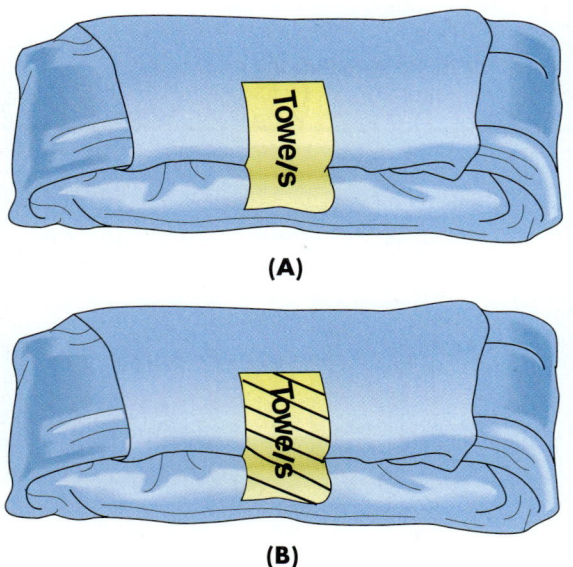

FIGURE 12-25 Packaging of towels (A) before and (B) after autoclaving. Note that (B) displays diagonal lines on the tape, indicating that the package has been exposed to steam.

enough time for sterilization to have taken place. The same principle applies to indicators placed inside the wrapped package. You should be aware that gas sterilizers and steam autoclaves require different indicator tapes. There are also envelopes for both types of sterilizers. The manufacturer can inform you of the proper indicator tape to use when you purchase a sterilizer or can tell you which one(s) to use with your present equipment. You should also clean the sterilizer routinely according to the manufacturer's recommendations.

Study the steps in Procedure 12-2 to learn how to properly wrap items for sterilization by autoclaving. Make sure that you do not put several items together unless they are separated by a gauze square. Items that are up against others during sterilization do not permit the steam to flow properly, and the items do not become sterile. Wrap each package snugly, but not too tight or too loose. If the package is too tight, the steam flow will not be able to get through the package or around each item sufficiently. Packages that are too loose or leave gaps could threaten the sterility of the contents, and they may even come apart. Allow adequate time for the packaging and contents to cool and dry before handling. Special care should be taken to avoid touching the autoclave while sterilization is in progress to avoid an accidental burn. It is a good practice to alert the staff when the sterilizer is operating so that they will also be cautious. When opening the autoclave door after the temperature and pressure are lowered, step to the side to avoid the possibility of a steam burn to the face and upper body. Being careless results in unfortunate injuries. Use caution with any type of sterilizer. You should leave the items in the autoclave with the door partially opened so that the packages can dry. If packs are touched before they are thoroughly dry, they are subject to become contaminated, because microorganisms may enter through the wrap by the moisture.

Some offices or medical centers use the autoclaving service of a hospital. In this case, minimum cleaning is all that is necessary, for all items are properly sanitized before autoclaving.

Study Procedure 12-3 to learn the basic operational steps for use of an autoclave for sterilization.

PROCEDURE PROCEDURE PROCEDURE PROCEDURE PROCEDURE PROCEDURE PROCEDURE

12-2   Wrap Items for Autoclave

PURPOSE: To wrap items to be autoclaved so that they will be protected from contamination after the sterilization process is completed for storage and handling.

EQUIPMENT: Muslin, autoclave paper, disposable paper bags, envelopes, autoclave tape, items to be sterilized or autoclaved, sterilization indicator, pen.

PERFORMANCE OBJECTIVE: Provided with several items to be autoclaved or sterilized, the student will wrap each in autoclave paper or muslin in preparation for the sterilization process. Each item must be wrapped neatly and snugly but not too tightly; the instructor and student will jointly determine if each wrapped item is suitable for autoclaving.

After the paper-wrapping procedure is demonstrated and checked, the paper should be removed from each item and discarded. The above-stated procedure will be repeated using muslin cloth. **(NOTE: When the muslin cloth wrapping procedure is completed, the muslin cloth is retained.)**

1. Wash hands and assemble all necessary items. **NOTE: Work in a clean area where there is sufficient work space.**

2. Check items for flaws and to make sure that they function properly. **NOTE: Items must be sanitized before wrapping for autoclave process. RATIONALE: Instruments must be working properly and materials must be in usable condition.**

3. Wrap item(s) in desired wrap so that there is a double thickness of protection. Make sure that there is no opening and seal with autoclave tape. Wrap item(s) snugly but not too tightly (Figures 12-26A through F). **RATIONALE: Double thickness and complete enclosure prevent pathogenic entry, as illustrated.**

    NOTE: For envelope wrap, place item into envelope, seal, and label. Items suitable for envelope wrap include but are not limited to forceps, hemostats, needle holders, and towel clamps. All hinged instruments must be autoclaved open. RATIONALE: Sterilizing process must reach all parts of the instruments.

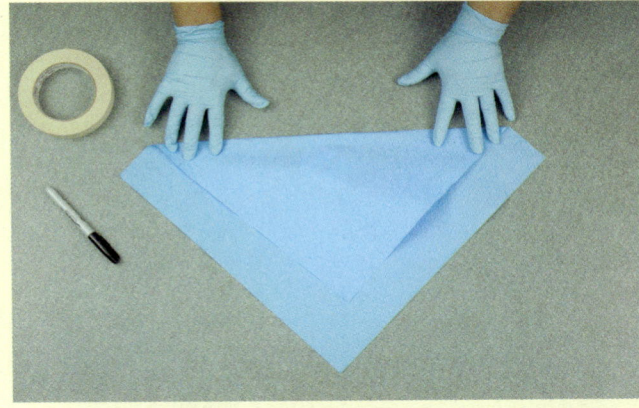

FIGURE 12-26B   Fold the material up from the bottom.

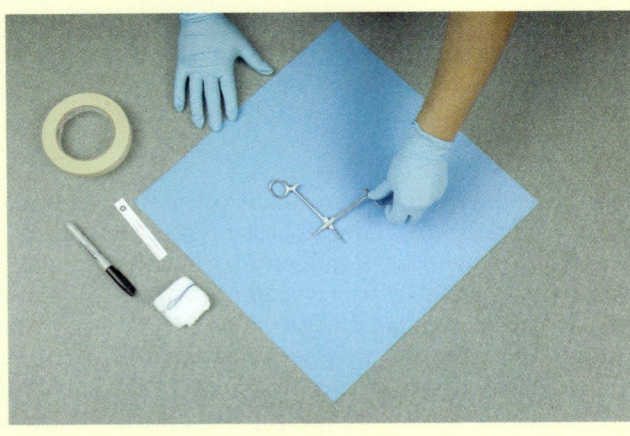

FIGURE 12-26A   To wrap items for autoclaving, start by placing the item(s) in the center of the wrap.

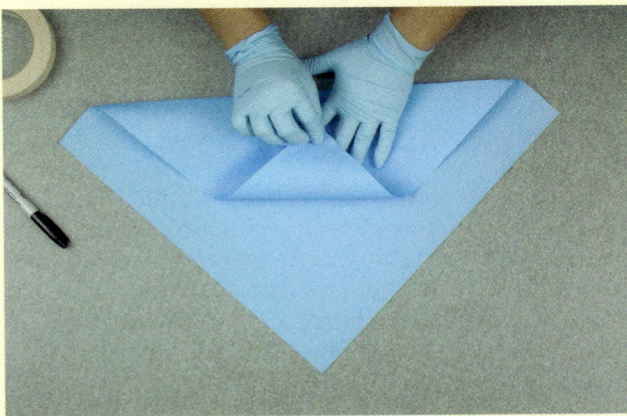

FIGURE 12-26C   Double back a small corner as a tab.

(continues)

PROCEDURE PROCEDURE PROCEDURE PROCEDURE PROCEDURE PROCEDURE PROCEDURE

12-2 · Wrap Items for Autoclave (Continued)

Place spinal needles (small items) in glass test tube with cotton or gauze padding at bottom. Wrap autoclave tape around top to seal, with a pull tab for ease in opening. Label contents on a piece of tape secured to the glass.

4. Make a tab for ease in opening wrapped packages after autoclaving by taping 1 to 2 inches of tape to itself at the edge of the package.

5. Label the contents, and write the date and your initials on the tape. **NOTE: Refer to Table 12-2 for proper time and temperature for items to be autoclaved.**

6. Return all items to the proper storage area when finished.

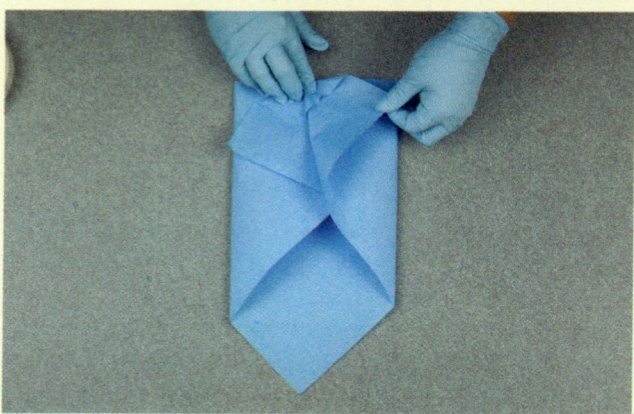

FIGURE 12-26E Then fold the left edge in leaving corners doubled back (as tabs).

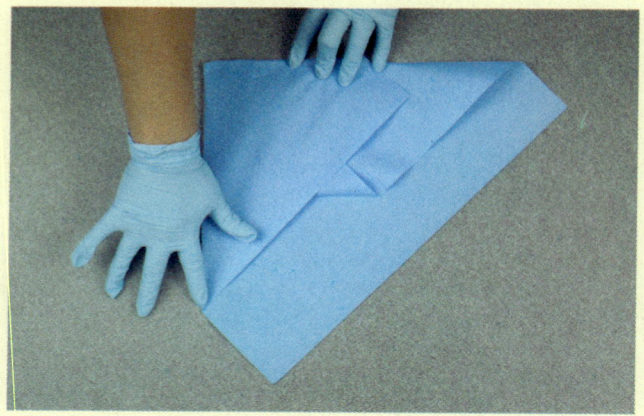

FIGURE 12-26D Fold the right edge in.

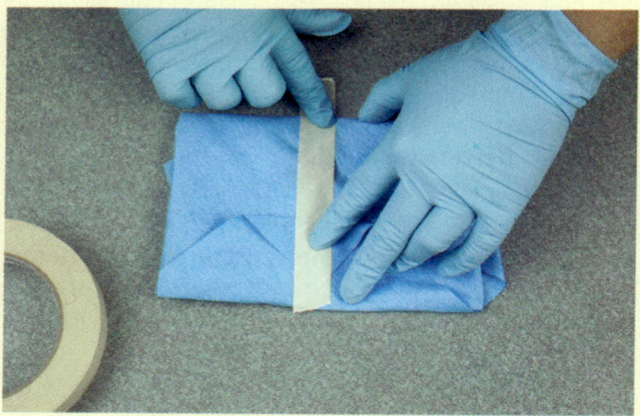

FIGURE 12-26F Fold the pack up from the bottom, and secure with pressure-sensitive autoclave tape.

Incineration

Another type of sterilization is by flame. This is a method for completely destroying disposable items by **incineration**. Items that will be treated in this way must be properly bagged for the procedure so that anyone handling the contaminated articles will not be affected.

Dry Heat Oven

Still another method of sterilization is the *dry heat oven.* Instruments with sharp blades, such as scissors or scalpels, are sometimes sterilized in this way. It is

not the most desirable sterilization method because it is time consuming. The process takes 1 to 2 hours at a temperature of 350°F, depending on the article. It is *not* a way to sterilize items made of rubber. For rubber articles, thorough washing and rinsing is the first step in preparing them for reuse. They must be completely dry before being placed in a disinfectant for chemical sterilization. Spores may still be a threat with this method. Finally, in every medical practice, the policy of the establishment must be followed.

Many companies provide this service for medical facilities with large volumes. They supply containers in

PROCEDURE PROCEDURE PROCEDURE PROCEDURE PROCEDURE PROCEDURE PROCEDURE

12-3  Perform Sterilization through Use of an Autoclave

PURPOSE: To sterilize instruments or supplies that will be used for penetration of a patient's skin or be in contact with otherwise sterile areas of a patient's body.

EQUIPMENT: Items properly sanitized and wrapped or sealed in pouches, disposable gloves, protective mitts, sterile transfer forceps

PERFORMANCE OBJECTIVE: Provided with the listed items, instruments will be loaded into an autoclave and sterilized according to the manufacturer's instructions, allowed to dry, and placed into storage.

1. According to the manufacturer's instructions, preheat the autoclave instrument; some manufacturers require the items to be sterilized and placed in the autoclave prior to preheating.

2. Any quality control procedures required must be performed with the load to be sterilized.

3. Wash your hands and don gloves.

4. Load the wrapped or pouched items in the autoclave wearing disposable gloves, allowing adequate space around the packs to ensure that steam will reach all of the areas.

5. After the correct temperature and pressure have been attained, set the timer for the corresponding amount of time specified by the manufacturer.

6. After the cycle has ended, vent the autoclave door to allow the packs to dry before removing them from the autoclave. The door should only be ajar slightly, $1/4$ to $1/2$ inch.

7. Once the drying cycle is completed, unload the items, making sure not to unload any packs that are damp, since this will result in the item no longer being sterile.

8. Wearing protective mitts, remove the packs from the autoclave. If any individual items have been placed in the autoclave unwrapped, sterile transfer forceps must be used to remove the item and place it in storage to prevent contamination.

9. After placing items into appropriate storage, remove the mitts and wash your hands.

---

various sizes for disposables and schedule periodic pickup of these biohazardous items to take back to the company for sterilization before discarding in general city trash dumps.

Any disposable items, such as needles (never recap), scalpels, suture removal forceps, and scissors, must be placed in the sharps container for company sterilization (Figure 12-27) or wrapped and sterilized before discarding in a general trash receptacle.

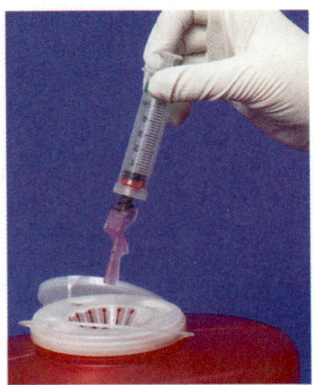

FIGURE 12-27 Discard the entire safety syringe with needle intact into the biohazard sharps container. Secure the lid on the sharps container when three-fourths full.

ACHIEVE UNIT OBJECTIVES

■ **Complete the Workbook activities to meet the learning objectives.**

■ **Practice the procedures in this unit to meet the performance objectives.**

■ **Apply your knowledge at the end of this chapter in completing the Critical Thinking Challenge and Activities, as well as the StudyWARE on your Student CD-ROM.**

CRITICAL THINKING CHALLENGE

IMPACTING THE PATIENT, THE PRACTICE, AND YOUR CAREER

The medical office was very busy with sick patients, and on this particular day, the office was running behind schedule. The medical assistant took a patient presenting with a sore throat and temperature of 102° back to an examination room. The health care provider ordered a strep screen as well as a complete blood count (CBC) to rule out strep throat. The medical assistant, in her haste, did not take the time to don gloves prior to obtaining the throat swab. As the swab was withdrawn from the patient's throat, the patient sneezed on the medical assistant's hand. The medical assistant, instead of washing her hands, only rinsed them and proceeded to the next patient.

QUESTIONS

1. What possible implications may ensue for the subsequent patients the medical assistant encounters during the rest of the day?

2. Are there any implications for the practice as a whole because of this medical assistant's actions?

3. Could this have an impact on the medical assistant's career? Why or why not?

ACTIVITY

1. Go to the Internet and research the CDC guidelines for prevention of transmitting communicable diseases in the medical office.

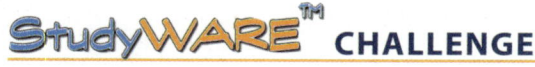 CHALLENGE

- Study with the flash cards for Chapter 12 to review the key terms in this chapter.
- Solve the crossword puzzle for Chapter 12.
- Complete the multiple choice quiz in test mode for Chapter 12.

RESOURCES

Acello, B. (2002). *The OSHA handbook: The guidelines for compliance in health care facilities.* Clifton Park, NY: Thomson Delmar Learning.

Grover-Lakomia, F. (1999). *Microbiology for health careers* (6th ed.). Clifton Park, NY: Thomson Delmar Learning.

Kennamer, M. (2007). *Basic infection control for health care providers* (2nd ed.). Clifton Park, NY: Thomson Delmar Learning.

Neighbors, M., & Jones, R. T. (2006). *Human diseases* (2nd ed.). Clifton Park, NY: Thomson Delmar Learning.

Venes, D. (ed.) (2006). *Taber's cyclopedic medical dictionary* (20th ed.). Philadelphia: F.A. Davis.

WEB LINKS

www.cdc.gov (Centers for Disease Control and Prevention)

Provides information on disease control and prevention.

13 Beginning the Patient's Record

Establishing an accurate database is a very important duty. It is the beginning of the patient's medical record with the physician. Preliminary information is obtained on forms given to patients as they enter the office reception area.

In an effort to combat fraud from identity theft, many physicians, urgent care centers, and hospitals are requiring a photo ID to verify patients are who they say they are. Incidents have occurred in which persons seeking care used stolen health insurance cards and ID to obtain treatment because they had no coverage. A photo ID can also prevent errors when two patients have the same name.

When patients are called into the office, the medical assistant makes the initial personal contact to begin gathering the information that relates to their reason for the office visit. It is important to not appear rushed or as if just performing a routine task. Since this is the patient's first visit, he may be naturally ill at ease and nervous about seeing a new physician, especially if he fears that he may have a serious condition. This in-person screening procedure requires a professional approach and is critical to the patient's perception of the practice.

Following the determination of a clear reason why the patient is there, it is important to obtain an accurate personal and family health history. There are techniques that can assist a patient to remember additional and pertinent information. A complete history is very revealing and a great aid in diagnosing conditions.

After the interviewing process is completed, it is usually customary to obtain basic physical measurements, which become the baseline for future comparisons. The patient will have her height and weight measured as well as a measurement of the vital signs.

With all this data accurately recorded on the patient's chart, or in the electronic health record, it is time for the physician to greet the patient and begin the medical discussion and examination.

It is important to note that medical offices are changing to electronic health records (EHR); therefore, interview data may be obtained and entered directly into the patient's electronic file. Patient-completed forms can be scanned into the file as well. Eventually it is believed patients may sit at a terminal and enter their preliminary information directly into to an EHR instead of on a paper form.

UNIT 1
IN-PERSON SCREENING

OBJECTIVES

Upon completion of this unit, you will be able to achieve the following:

LEARNING Objectives

1. **Spell and define, using the glossary at the back of this text, all the Words to Know in this unit.**
2. **Explain the origin of triage.**
3. **Explain the purpose of screening in today's medical office.**
4. **List the categories for determining the urgency of a patient's condition.**

PERFORMANCE Objective

1. **Perform in-person screening.**

WORDS TO KNOW

carrel	interview	screening
chief complaint (CC)	objective	subjective
	prioritize	triage

CERTIFICATION CONNECTION

CMA
Interviewing techniques
Performing telephone and in-person screening

RMA
Employ active listening skills

CMAS
Basic charting

SCREENING

Screening is the process of obtaining information from patients to determine their medical condition. There is phone screening that occurs in some form every time a patient calls for an appointment, whether for the first or the hundredth time. There is also in-person screening that occurs in the office every time the patient is seen to identify the chief complaint presented as well as secondary conditions. A more intense form of this process was originated during war times and was called triage. It was a concept developed by the military and is particularly applicable to trauma and disaster situations. It referred to the sorting and assessment of soldiers' injuries. The French word *triage* means "to sort." After the medics made a decision regarding the seriousness of the wounds, the soldier was taken as soon as possible for treatment. Those in charge of treatment had a clear description of the nature of the wounds from the initial triage. In addition, triage is a term also used in prioritizing the conditions of the injured following a disaster. The injured were separated into groups according to the seriousness of their needs. Usually they were tagged with a particular color-coded tape or cloth so that the other members of the emergency medical team would know which victims required immediate attention. The rules are that those who have difficulty breathing are always taken first. Chest pain, severe bleeding, head injury, poisoning, open wounds of the chest and abdomen, shock, and some second- and third-degree burns also should be given first priority. The conditions that should be considered next are major (and multiple) fractures, second-degree burns (other than of the neck and face), back injury, and severe eye injuries. Conditions that are not life threatening, such as simple fractures, sprains, and minor injuries, can wait a short time.

Many of the more severe conditions listed would rarely if ever be seen initially in the physician's office in metropolitan areas due to the presence of emergency medical services and hospital emergency rooms. The word "screening" has replaced the term "triage" because it is more appropriate for the process used in the medical office.

PHONE SCREENING

In Chapter 6 the importance of phone screening and scheduling was discussed. It is briefly mentioned here to refresh your memory.

Phone screening is assessing the patient's symptoms over the phone and responding in an appropriate manner. The assistant who speaks to patients over the phone must have knowledge of:

- Medical terminology
- Anatomy and physiology
- Diseases and disorders
- Emergency procedures
- Medications

and must use:

- Communication skills (especially listening)
- Problem-solving methods
- Decision-making skills
- Compassion
- Self-control
- Patience
- Understanding

Taking information regarding a patient's condition by phone requires careful listening and thorough questioning to ascertain the nature and the extent of the problem. In a medical office or clinic, the person who handles the phone and screens the calls is essentially at the heart of the practice. This person is usually the one who controls the schedule. Efficient patient flow and appointment schedules in the medical office are the result of the medical assistant's skill in phone screening. The anticipation of what examinations or procedures may have to be performed, how long it may take, and the seriousness of the patient's condition are all vital.

Communication with the rest of the health care team is essential in meeting the needs of patients who must be worked into the schedule. If the nature of the patient's condition is too serious or complicated to be dealt with in your facility, it should be determined before the patient is advised to come in to be seen by the physician. A true life-threatening emergency should be referred to an emergency medical service (i.e., 911 where applicable) or to an emergency room for treatment.

IN-PERSON SCREENING

Talking to a patient one-on-one and asking questions about his personal condition requires professional communication skills and the assurance of privacy (Figure 13-1). Some offices may have a private area, sometimes called a **carrel**, that is used specifically for **screening**. Other offices conduct the screening and **interview** in the privacy of the examination room. The location is not important, but your ability to obtain and accurately record information received from the patient is. Your goal is to determine why the patient is seeking health care; what she sees as her main problem; any other concerns she may have; and what, if anything, she has done about it.

The purpose of the screening is to help patients focus on their main concern, called the **chief complaint (CC)**, and its related symptoms. After this is established, it may be necessary to continue the screening to obtain and record other health concerns. For example, a work-in patient whose chief complaint is severe muscle spasms of the back may also express concern because of occasional irregular heartbeats and an increasing need to take antacids for indigestion. These complaints need to be recorded and will probably require an additional visit to address due to previous patient scheduling.

The patient's initial visit will require varying amounts of questioning depending upon the reason for the

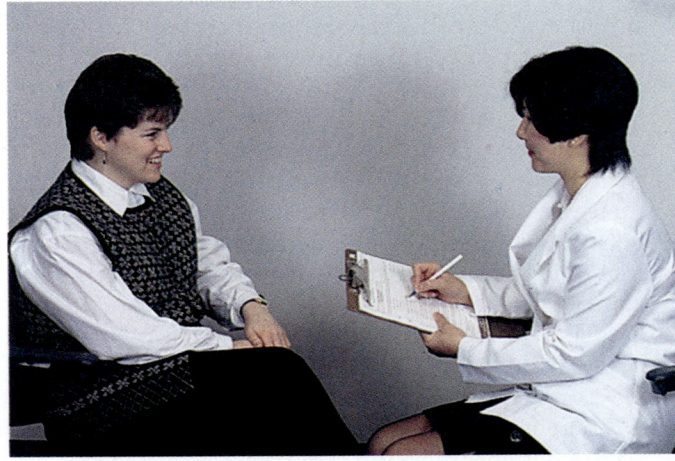

FIGURE 13-1 A medical assistant and patient are in a private area discussing symptoms and assessing the patient's condition. This is called an in-person screening.

visit. Someone requesting a complete physical, but who has no complaints, will not require the in-depth inquiry that someone would who has complaints of intermittent pain, fever, and fatigue for the past 2 weeks. Face-to-face screening is also required when patients return for follow-up visits. The line of questioning then is to determine how they have felt since the last office visit.

Information you receive from patients is based upon symptoms they feel (subjective). **Subjective** symptoms or sensations are those that only the patient can perceive, such as pain, dizziness, itching, or numbness. Information or symptoms that can be observed, in other words, that are perceptible to other people, such as swelling, bruising, vital signs, and physical examination findings, are known as **objective** findings. It is important for you to know the difference. These two distinctions become necessary when you proceed with recording information on the chart. Many physicians use a method called SOAP (subjective, objective, assessment, and plan) for recording data regarding the patient's office visit. The assessment is made by the physician upon examination and the plan refers to what course or courses of action will be taken.

Factors Influencing Screening

Successfully conducting the first interview with a new patient establishes a favorable relationship among the patient, you, and the practice. There are many factors that need to be considered in order to make that experience as beneficial as possible. The following gives you some things to remember when you are talking with the patient.

- *Ensure privacy*—Not only in the setting, but also ensure the patient that the information you are gathering will be protected within the privacy policy of the office.
- *Be aware of your biases*—Our beliefs and behaviors tend to influence how we view others. All patients must be treated with respect without evaluating them as to their race, religion, sexual orientation, ethnic origin, or socioeconomic or educational status. Take care that your value system does not interfere with what you hear or observe.
- *Establish a nonthreatening, relaxed atmosphere—*
  - Greet the patient by name.
  - State your name.
  - Then explain what you would like to do.
  You may say something like this: "Mrs. Green, I am Ginny, Dr. Long's medical assistant. I would like to ask you a few questions about what brought you to the office today. Would you be willing to share this information with me"?

- *Be aware of your own nonverbal messages*—Be attentive and give eye contact so the patient can tell you are interested in who he is and what he has to say. Do not be overly involved with note taking or watching the time.
- *Be sure the patient understands*—Using medical terminology is not appropriate for most patients. Pay attention to their expressions as you talk. Is there a hearing problem or a lack of understanding? Responses to questions will usually indicate any difficulty. Repeating or restating the question will probably be sufficient. If there is a language barrier, it may be necessary to enlist help from a family member or friend. Someone who is hearing or speech impaired will require a person who can sign your questions and speak for her (Figure 13-2).
- *Allow the patient to do most of the talking*—Remember, you are trying to learn about his condition and concerns.
- *Listen attentively to what the patient says*—Be an active listener; ask questions to be sure you understand what was said. You can repeat what you think the patient stated to see if she agrees.
- *Nonverbal communication*—Watch the patient's body language; does it agree with what he is saying? This

HIPAA

Be sure to get the patient's approval to involve another person in the discussion of their private health information. Document the permission; without documentation, it is considered "not permitted."

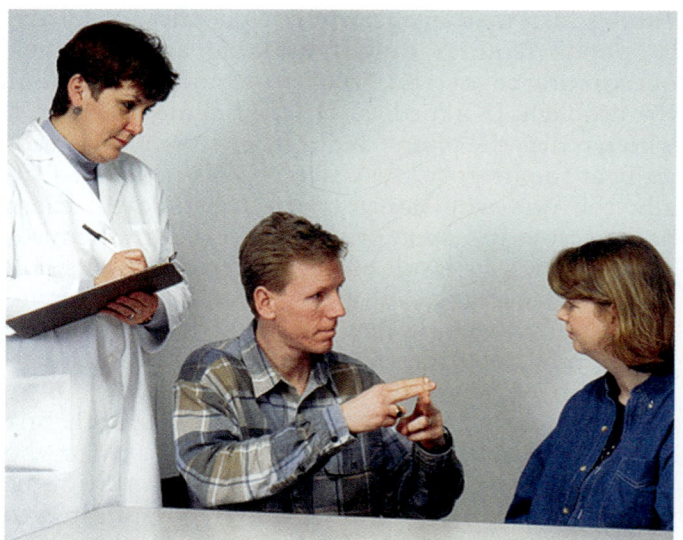

FIGURE 13-2   A person who can sign may be needed to assist with the patient interview.

may take some experience. For example, if the patient does not look at you when answering personal questions, is it because of embarrassment or is he not being truthful? For example, a married person seeking care because of a sexually transmitted disease acquired from an affair may be reluctant to tell anyone other than the physician.

- *Use open-ended questions*—These ask for more than a yes or no answer and provide the opportunity for additional information. Asking, "How would you describe your pain," will get you more information than asking "Do you have pain now"?
- *Focus on the interview*—Do not allow the conversation to go off course.
- *Conclude the screening portion of the interview with a summary*—State to the patient what has been identified and recorded as the chief complaint and any additional concerns in decreasing order of importance. With the patient's agreement, record the CC and other data.

CONDUCTING THE IN-PERSON SCREENING

What is done by the medical assistant during the in-person screening will be determined by the employing physician. Some prefer that the medical assistant do only the chief complaint and they conduct the in-depth interview so they have the advantage of getting the information personally. Other physicians want all preliminary questioning done by the medical assistant so they can review it briefly and begin their examination.

Many offices mail out the preliminary forms so patients can complete them at home and then bring them to their appointment. This gives the patient time to accurately complete the forms and search for specific requested information. Other practices ask new patients to arrive 15 minutes early to complete paperwork before their appointment. In either case, some type of partially or completely filled in form will be the basis for your interview. Before calling the patient in for the in-person screening, you should obtain the form from the receptionist, attach it to a clipboard, and review its contents. (*Note:* It may be worth mentioning that if the form is not completed, the patient may have a language or reading problem. It may be necessary for you to ask the questions and complete the form for such a patient. Use tact when asking if a patient needs assistance with the form. Often the illiterate are very sensitive about their inability to read and write and can be quite clever at disguising their situation. There are also many people in the United States from foreign countries, and learning our language is a major challenge for them.)

After introducing yourself to the new patient, establishing a comfortable environment, and requesting the patient's assistance, it is time to start the interview. Begin by asking what brought the patient to the office today. Look at the health history form to see what the patient listed. Refer to Figure 13-3 for an example of a form. By using questioning techniques, you can arrive at a precise reason for their visit. This chief complaint (CC) will be recorded in the patient's own words, on the chart or entered in the EHR. Have the patient describe this complaint in detail. For example, if the patient says the pain is in his stomach, he may actually be referring to his abdomen. You need to identify the location of the pain, when it began, and whether it is sharp or dull, constant or intermittent. To determine its intensity, ask the patient to describe how severe it is on a scale from 1 to 10, with 10 being most severe.

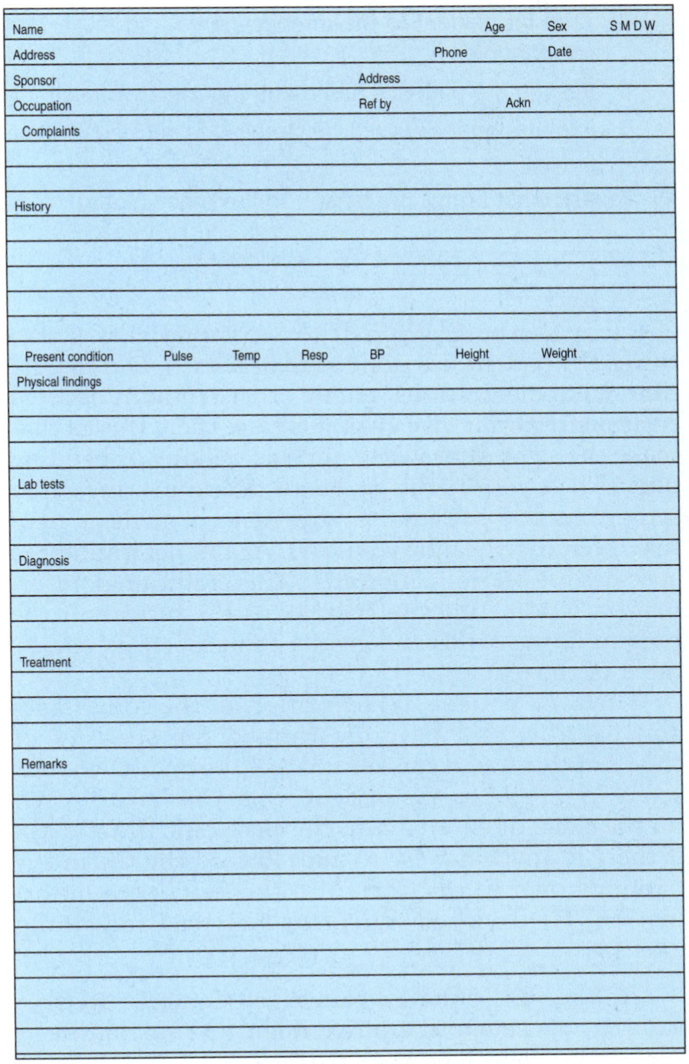
Name Age Sex S M D W
Address Phone Date
Sponsor Address
Occupation Ref by Ackn
Complaints
History
Present condition Pulse Temp Resp BP Height Weight
Physical findings
Lab tests
Diagnosis
Treatment
Remarks

FIGURE 13-3 Example of a basic (general) medical history form

13-1  Perform In-Person Screening

PURPOSE: To identify the patient's reason for seeking medical care

EQUIPMENT: Paper, pen, and patient's chart or computer

PERFORMANCE OBJECTIVE: In a simulated or actual situation, conduct an in-person screening to identify and accurately record the patient's chief complaint (CC) and related symptoms.

1. Select a private location for the interview.
2. Review any completed office forms.
3. Call the patient by name from the reception room.
4. Take the patient to the interview area and make him comfortable.
5. Restate the patient's name and introduce yourself.
6. Explain what you will be doing and request participation.
7. Ask what brings the person to the office today.
8. Use questioning to focus on the CC and its descriptors.
9. Identify the related symptoms and descriptors.
10. Identify and record any secondary concerns.
11. Draft a statement of what you think the patient stated.
12. Obtain the patient's agreement as to the CC, the symptoms, and any other concerns.
13. Record the CC statement and other related information on the chart or electronic record.

CHARTING EXAMPLE

8/6/XX

CC, "I have a pain in my stomach."

RLQ, pain level 6, intermittent, ×3 days, nausea, no vomiting or diarrhea. Some relief from lying down.

G. Jenks, MA

It may also be appropriate to determine what, if anything, the patient has done to treat herself. Did she use heat, cold, medications, or any other self-administered treatment? Did it give any relief? Are there things that make the symptoms worse, such as walking or bending over? Then you might go on to determine any other symptoms the patient has experienced, such as nausea, fever, diarrhea, or vomiting. Again, determine the specifics of those symptoms. This additional information is sometimes referred to as the history of the present illness (HPI) and gives a comprehensive assessment of the CC.

When the patient has identified all the complaints and together you have determined the specifics of the symptoms, you can summarize the results of your screening. Read to the patient what you have written on the chart or entered into the electronic file and ask if there is anything else to add. Record the CC in the patient's own words, then add the descriptive information. The finished statement may read something like this:

8/6/XX CC: "I have a pain in my stomach." RLQ, Pain level 6, intermittent ×3 days, nausea, no vomiting or diarrhea. Some relief by lying down._____G. Jenks, M.A.

Procedure 13-1 provides a generic guide for in-person screening of a patient. With a little experience, you will be able to perform an in-person screening and an interview with confidence.

After obtaining this initial information, you are ready to proceed with reviewing the patient's health history. Completing both these tasks establishes a good basis for not only diagnosing and treating the patient's current condition but also understanding the patient's and the family's past health conditions, which might have some bearing on the present.

ACHIEVE UNIT OBJECTIVES

■ **Complete the Workbook activities to meet the learning objectives.**

■ **Practice the procedures in this unit to meet the performance objectives.**

■ **Apply your knowledge at the end of this chapter in completing the Critical Thinking Challenge and Activities, as well as the StudyWARE on your Student CD-ROM.**

UNIT 2
THE MEDICAL HISTORY

OBJECTIVES

Upon completion of this unit, you will be able to achieve the following:

LEARNING Objectives

1. **Spell and define, using the glossary at the back of this text, all the Words to Know in this unit.**
2. **Identify the 10 categories of information requested on the health history form in Figure 13-4.**
3. **Explain the purpose of obtaining a health history.**
4. **Discuss the genogram and explain why it is useful.**

PERFORMANCE Objectives

1. **Obtain and record a patient history.**

WORDS TO KNOW

adequate	irrelevant	patronize
familial	over-the-counter	remedy
genogram	(OTC)	symptoms

 ### CERTIFICATION CONNECTION

CMA
Interviewing techniques
Patient history interview

RMA
Physical examinations
(medical history)

CMAS
Basic health history
interview

MEDICAL HISTORY

All patients are asked to complete a health history form at their initial visit to a physician's office. As stated before, some are mailed prior to the appointment, usually when referred to a specialist, and others are completed in the office prior to the physician's examination. The forms will vary with the type of practice from short and concise (refer to Figure 13-3) to fairly comprehensive (Figure 13-4). Notice at the end of the comprehensive form there is a statement regarding errors or omissions. The absence of pertinent information could result in a misdiagnosis, a consequence that this form addresses.

As previously mentioned, the medical assistant may need to assist in the completion of the history. There are unfamiliar medical terms and some confusing questions with which the patient may need help. There may be language and literacy barriers that may prevent completion. Assist these patients with respect and without judgment. Some physicians may wish to interview and complete the form themselves as a means to gain insight into the patient's condition. The variables are many.

Reviewing the Information

Even though the patient has completed the form, you must still review all the information for omission and clarity. For instance, if a patient checks "hazardous substances" under occupational concerns, it would be important to identify what those substances are. Another question might arise about who is a "blood relative." You must be thoroughly familiar with the form used by your employer and be prepared to answer any questions. In the sample form in Figure 13-4, notice that not only the patient but also the person reviewing the form must sign and date the document. The validity of this baseline document can become very important later in the patient's course of treatment. The completed forms are filed in the chart or EHR. The patient's medical history is the basis for understanding his present health status. The form is a documentation of current symptoms as well as medical conditions the patient experienced in the past.

Family Health History

Most forms also request information about the health status of the immediate family members. These data, in addition to the physical examination, assist the physician with not only the information necessary to arrive at a diagnosis and treatment for the current complaint but also perhaps to forewarn and possibly prevent future conditions that tend to develop within families. Physician's who treat **familial** disorders and diseases may also use another type of history form called a **genogram**. Figure 13-5 illustrates a family's medical history. Most genograms include at least three generations. This provides visual information to the physician that is helpful in determining the patient's chances of developing a disease that has genetic tendencies.

CONFIDENTIAL HEALTH HISTORY

Name: _____ Date: _____

Birthdate: _____ Age: _____ Date of last physical examination: _____

Occupation: _____

Reason for visit today: _____

MEDICATIONS List all medications you are currently taking	**ALLERGIES** List all allergies

SYMPTOMS Check (✓) symptoms you currently have or have had in the past year.

GENERAL
- ☐ Chills
- ☐ Depression
- ☐ Dizziness
- ☐ Fainting
- ☐ Fever
- ☐ Forgetfulness
- ☐ Headache
- ☐ Loss of sleep
- ☐ Loss of weight
- ☐ Nervousness
- ☐ Numbness
- ☐ Sweats

MUSCLE/JOINT/BONE
Pain, weakness, numbness in:
- ☐ Arms   ☐ Hips
- ☐ Back   ☐ Legs
- ☐ Feet   ☐ Neck
- ☐ Hands ☐ Shoulders

GENITO-URINARY
- ☐ Blood in urine
- ☐ Frequent urination
- ☐ Lack of bladder control
- ☐ Painful urination

GASTROINTESTINAL
- ☐ Appetite poor
- ☐ Bloating
- ☐ Bowel changes
- ☐ Constipation
- ☐ Diarrhea
- ☐ Excessive hunger
- ☐ Excessive thirst
- ☐ Gas
- ☐ Hemorrhoids
- ☐ Indigestion
- ☐ Nausea
- ☐ Rectal bleeding
- ☐ Stomach pain
- ☐ Vomiting
- ☐ Vomiting blood

CARDIOVASCULAR
- ☐ Chest pain
- ☐ High blood pressure
- ☐ Irregular heart beat
- ☐ Low blood pressure
- ☐ Poor circulation
- ☐ Rapid heart beat
- ☐ Swelling of ankles
- ☐ Varicose veins

EYE, EAR, NOSE, THROAT
- ☐ Bleeding gums
- ☐ Blurred vision
- ☐ Crossed eyes
- ☐ Difficulty swallowing
- ☐ Double vision
- ☐ Earache
- ☐ Ear discharge
- ☐ Hay fever
- ☐ Hoarseness
- ☐ Loss of hearing
- ☐ Nosebleeds
- ☐ Persistent cough
- ☐ Ringing in ears
- ☐ Sinus problems
- ☐ Vision - Flashes
- ☐ Vision - Halos

SKIN
- ☐ Bruise easily
- ☐ Hives
- ☐ Itching
- ☐ Change in moles
- ☐ Rash
- ☐ Scars
- ☐ Sores that won't heal

MEN only
- ☐ Breast lump
- ☐ Erection difficulties
- ☐ Lump in testicles
- ☐ Penis discharge
- ☐ Sore on penis
- ☐ Other

WOMEN only
- ☐ Abnormal Pap Smear
- ☐ Bleeding between periods
- ☐ Breast lump
- ☐ Extreme menstrual pain
- ☐ Hot flashes
- ☐ Nipple discharge
- ☐ Painful intercourse
- ☐ Vaginal discharge
- ☐ Other

Date of last menstrual period _____

Date of last Pap Smear _____

Have you had a mammogram? _____

Are you pregnant? _____

Number of children _____

MEDICAL HISTORY Check (✓) the medical conditions you have or have had in the past.

- ☐ AIDS
- ☐ Alcoholism
- ☐ Anemia
- ☐ Anorexia
- ☐ Appendicitis
- ☐ Arthritis
- ☐ Asthma
- ☐ Bleeding Disorders
- ☐ Breast Lump
- ☐ Bronchitis
- ☐ Bulimia
- ☐ Cancer
- ☐ Cataracts

- ☐ Chemical Dependency
- ☐ Chicken Pox
- ☐ Diabetes
- ☐ Emphysema
- ☐ Epilepsy
- ☐ Gall Bladder Disease
- ☐ Glaucoma
- ☐ Goiter
- ☐ Gonorrhea
- ☐ Gout
- ☐ Heart Disease
- ☐ Hepatitis
- ☐ Hernia

- ☐ Herpes
- ☐ High Cholesterol
- ☐ HIV Positive
- ☐ Kidney Disease
- ☐ Liver Disease
- ☐ Measles
- ☐ Migraine Headaches
- ☐ Miscarriage
- ☐ Mononucleosis
- ☐ Multiple Sclerosis
- ☐ Mumps
- ☐ Pacemaker
- ☐ Pneumonia

- ☐ Polio
- ☐ Prostate Problem
- ☐ Psychiatric Care
- ☐ Rheumatic Fever
- ☐ Scarlet Fever
- ☐ Stroke
- ☐ Suicide Attempt
- ☐ Thyroid Problems
- ☐ Tonsillitis
- ☐ Tuberculosis
- ☐ Typhoid Fever
- ☐ Ulcers
- ☐ Vaginal Infections
- ☐ Venereal Disease

CONFIDENTIAL HEALTH HISTORY

FIGURE 13-4 Health history form

(continues)

HOSPITALIZATIONS

Year	Hospital	Reason for Hospitalization and Outcome

Have you ever had a blood transfusion? ☐ Yes ☐ No

If yes, please give approximate dates: _____

OCCUPATIONAL CONCERNS Check (✓) if your work exposes you to the following:	HEALTH HABITS Check (✓) which substances you use and indicate how much you use per day/week.	PREGNANCY HISTORY		
		Year of Birth	Sex of Birth	Complications if any
☐ Stress	☐ Caffeine			
☐ Hazardous Substances	☐ Tobacco			
☐ Heavy Lifting	☐ Drugs			
☐ Other	☐ Alcohol			

SERIOUS ILLNESS/INJURIES	DATE	OUTCOME

FAMILY HISTORY Fill in health information about your family.

Relation	Age	State of Health	Age at Death	Cause of Death	Check (✓) if your blood relatives had any of the following Disease	Relationship to you
Father					☐ Arthritis, Gout	
Mother					☐ Asthma, Hay Fever	
Brothers					☐ Cancer	
					☐ Chemical Dependency	
					☐ Diabetes	
					☐ Heart Disease, Strokes	
Sisters					☐ High Blood Pressure	
					☐ Kidney Disease	
					☐ Tuberculosis	
					☐ Other	

I certify that the above information is correct to the best of my knowledge. I will not hold my doctor or any members of his/her staff responsible for any errors or ommisions that I may have made in the completion of this form.

_____   _____

Signature   Date

_____   _____

Reviewed By   Date

FIGURE 13-4 Health history form (Continued)

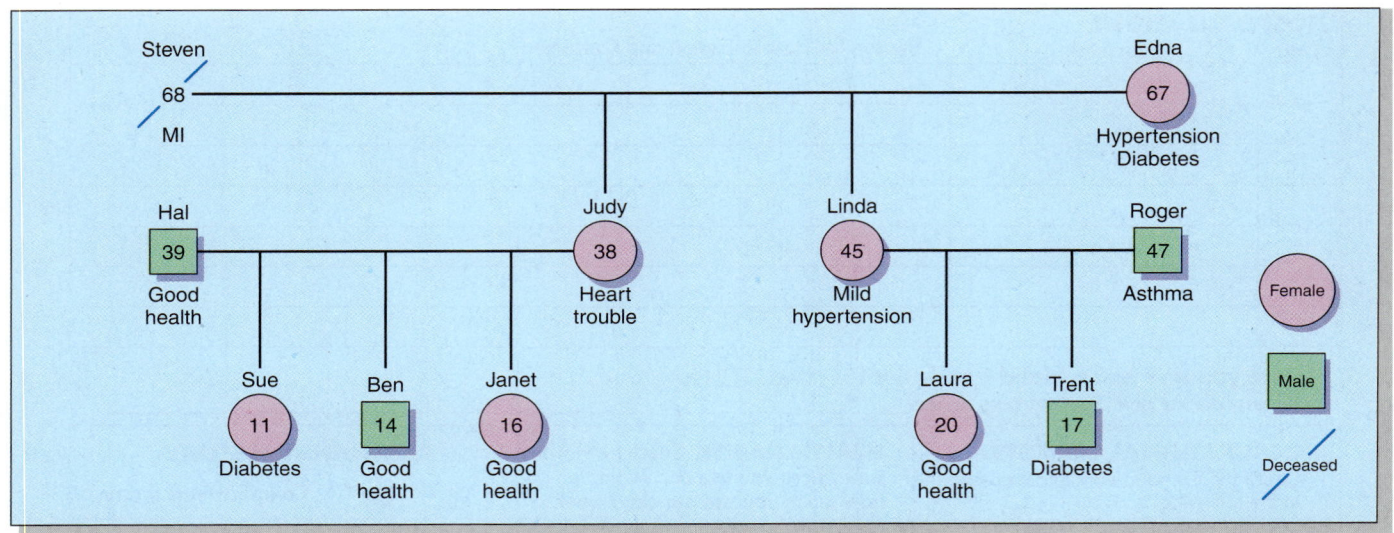

FIGURE 13-5 Example of a genogram tracing a family's medical history

Sections of the Form

Printing companies provide many medical history form designs from which physicians may choose as well as special individual designs to meet specific needs. A four-page history form developed for an oncology practice is included in the Workbook to provide you with an interview experience. Regardless of the form, some information requests are standard. The chief complaint (CC) has already been discussed, as has the present illness (PI) or history of present illness (HPI). These findings need to be recorded on the patient's chart also as previously noted. Other pertinent data concerns what the patient has done for the condition, whether any **over-the-counter (OTC)** medications or home **remedies** were tried and if so, what they were and whether they were effective.

The history form probably also contains a review of the body systems (ROS) in some format. This helps patients to remember previous illnesses or symptoms they may have forgotten. There may also be a past history (PH) or past medical history (PMH) section to identify all illnesses or disorders ever diagnosed. In the example, the sections are divided into **symptoms** during the past year and the history, which refers to present and past *diseases* and *disorders*. Usual childhood diseases (UCHD) are included in the medical history section. The family history (FH) section asks for ages and status of health or age and cause of at death for immediate family members. Another area asks about the incidence of nine diseases among blood relatives, as well as providing a line to add any other condition. Notice some questions are gender specific, and others deal with serious illnesses and hospitalizations.

Two very important sections list current medications being taken and the listing of allergies. Drug reactions and interactions, both prescribed and over-the-counter, can cause significant symptoms. Some offices identify allergies with red ink or separate labels attached to the chart. Always question the patient about any allergies to drugs, food, or environmental factors, because true allergic reactions can be very serious, even life-threatening. If the patient indicates she does not have any allergies, enter "No known drug allergies" (NKDA) on the form and in the initial charting to indicate the question was addressed and not overlooked.

It is also necessary to determine the patient's personal habits. The excessive use of some prescribed drugs can lead to a dependency the same as with illegal drugs. Alcohol is a commonly abused substance and may require assistance to control. The use of tobacco in any amount or form has been determined to be unhealthy. If any habits are problematic, they may be addressed by the physician. You may be instructed to provide the patient with educational materials related to the problem and to make her aware of any community resources or office-sponsored meetings related to the habit.

OBTAINING A PATIENT HISTORY

Refer to Procedure 13-2, Obtain and Record a Patient History. This will help you practice interviewing a patient. With a copy of a history form or the one included in the Workbook, proceed through the form, asking clarifying questions and recording patient information. Include any significant additional remarks in your

13-2    Obtain and Record a Patient History

PURPOSE: To obtain and record the life medical history of a patient, including family, occupational, and social factors, to facilitate the diagnosis and health care plan for the patient.

EQUIPMENT: Medical history form, clipboard, and pens (black and red ink) or computer with appropriate software.

PERFORMANCE OBJECTIVE: Using the computer or copies of a medical history form and a pen, obtain and record a medical history by interviewing a person or reviewing a completed form. Allergies are identified or "NKDA" stated. All areas must be addressed and the form signed as appropriate.

1. Assemble the clipboard, medical history form, and pens.

2. Escort the patient to a private area where you can both sit comfortably.

3. Sit opposite patient. **RATIONALE: Facing the patients allow you to establish eye contact.**

4. Ask patient necessary questions, and record or enter answers neatly and accurately.

   NOTE:

   - Speak in a clear and distinct voice so that the patient can easily understand you.

   - Give the patient **adequate** time to answer before going on to the next question.

   - Explain any terms that the patient may not understand. **RATIONALE: A patient cannot give correct answers to inquiries he does not understand.**

   - Avoid getting off the subject and discussing **irrelevant** topics. **RATIONALE: This is inappropriate, unprofessional, and wastes time unless it is obvious that the patient needs to vent feelings.**

   - Use an additional sheet of paper to record pertinent information if necessary.

   - Ensure allergies are identified, recorded, and labeled on the chart as instructed.

5. When finished with the form, thank the patient and explain the next step in the examination. Ensure the patient is comfortable and explain whether there will be a wait.

6. Chart a summary of the findings on the patient's chart or in the EHR. Highlight significant information as instructed.

7. Gather all necessary forms into the patient's chart or EHR, and have it ready for the physician to use during the examination.

CHARTING EXAMPLE

04/10/XX

11:30 A.M.

CC: "I feel terrible, I think I have the flu." × 3 days, throat sore (6), aching, chills, and fever (102.8) 2 days ago. Coughing, becoming productive, (thick, green/yellow), OTC: Tylenol Flu (some relief), NKDA

S. Rose, MA

notes on the patient's chart. If you have access to a computer with office practice software, proceed through the form and enter the patient's responses directly into the EHR.

PATIENT EDUCATION

The medical assistant is often involved in patient education, which may include supplying information about diseases and disorders, explaining diagnostic tests, and providing instruction in health care procedures. Recording the patient's health history may identify areas where educational materials may be helpful. Your office policy may make it appropriate for you to mention these resources. Refer to the "Patient Education" box for general guidelines regarding this aspect of patient care.

AFTER THE HISTORY IS COMPLETED

After the history is completed and appropriate notations are made on the form and on the chart or in the EHR, the patient is weighed and measured and the vital signs obtained and recorded. This completes the baseline data, and the patient is ready for the physician's examination. With the areas of concern identified, you may have an indication of what type of examination the physician will need to do. According to the office policy, you might begin preparing the pa-

PATIENT EDUCATION

Patient education is a primary function of the medical assistant. Most patients are not trained health professionals and are somewhat confused by medical terminology, tests, procedures, and medications they encounter. Therefore, patient education becomes an important part of their medical care.

Whenever possible, the patient should be involved in making decisions about treatment or care. This will encourage the patient to participate more fully in the procedure. Patients will be more willing to cooperate if they understand the necessity for a particular procedure or treatment. Your careful and clear explanations of these procedures will encourage the patient to be more cooperative. If patients sense that you are truly concerned about their well-being, this will motivate them to comply. Always offer encouragement and praise where appropriate, even for the smallest accomplishment.

To properly instruct a patient, the medical assistant must know the material. Be prepared to answer any questions from the patient. If you cannot answer one of the patient's questions, tell the patient that you do not know the answer but will ask the physician. Never try to answer a question that you are not prepared to discuss. You could give incorrect information that could harm the patient's well-being. Never give information that is beyond your scope of practice.

In teaching a patient about health care and all that is involved in medical well-being, the primary goal of the medical assistant should be good communication. This means that each patient must be treated as an individual with particular needs. As the patient educator, you will have to meet these needs. You must communicate in the most efficient and effective manner for each individual. Listening is vital to this education. Patients may be shy or embarrassed by their problems or questions and may not ask direct questions. Therefore, you must listen carefully to the patient's comments and questions. Be familiar with information about the patient before proceeding with an explanation. This will help determine how to communicate best with each individual.

Never assume that a patient already knows the information you are conveying. Sometimes a patient will state that he understands something to keep from being embarrassed. If you sense that this is the situation, you should briefly repeat the information and provide printed material for the patient to take home to read. Printed materials, such as one-page handouts, brochures, pamphlets, and booklets on various procedures, examinations, diseases, conditions, and treatment plans, should be clear and concise in content. These informative materials should be appropriately distributed routinely to patients.

One very important aspect of patient teaching is your attitude toward the patient. The medical assistant must be open when approaching patients. This means that you must accept each patient as an individual who needs your help. There is no room in the medical office for prejudice. All patients should be treated with respect regardless of their financial status, race, religion, age, or station in life. Remember, your job is to provide assistance. Calling patients by pet names (e.g., Honey, Hon, and Dear) may be taken as **patronizing**, especially if your attitude is questionable. It is more respectful to patients if you call them by their titles (i.e., Mr. or Ms.) or their full names. The patient will let you know if a first-name basis is all right with her. If the patients sense any negative feelings on your part, then they will be less likely to pay attention to your instructions and suggestions.

Most patients are interested in getting better and staying healthy. Patient education involves not only instructing those who are sick but helping healthy patients stay well. By following current trends in wellness and prevention of medical problems, you can help patients help themselves to a healthier life.

The following are some general guidelines for patient education:

1. Become familiar with your office's or clinic's policy concerning patient education.
2. Thoroughly read all handout information given to patients that explains procedures, examinations, or treatment plans so that you can intelligently answer patients' questions.
3. Make yourself available to patients for answering questions. Always remember to ask patients if they have any questions about their treatment or diagnosis.
4. Always take the opportunity to explain procedures to patients and offer additional information when appropriate.
5. Post charts, posters, and other information that will benefit the patient. Be sure that this information is kept current and is posted in areas where patients may spend time waiting.
6. Have current health-related magazines available in the reception area.
7. Post meeting times and information for patient support groups (weight control groups, stop smoking groups, tough love meetings) and encourage their participation. Keep this information current.

tient. This could include partial or complete disrobing and putting on a gown, obtaining a urine specimen, or having the female patient empty her bladder in preparation for a pelvic exam. However, some physicians feel it is preferable to meet the patient initially while she is still clothed. They will review the history form and notations on the chart or in the EHR and conduct a brief screening conversation, then indicate what examination they will be performing.

Whichever procedure is followed, after the history is completed and the baseline measurements and vital signs recorded, express your appreciation to patients for their cooperation and indicate to them what follows next. Be sure to ask if they have any questions. If there is apt to be a waiting period, try to estimate the time involved and offer reading materials to occupy their time.

ACHIEVE UNIT OBJECTIVES

- ■ Complete the Workbook activities to meet the learning objectives.
- ■ Practice the procedure in this unit to meet the performance objectives.
- ■ Apply your knowledge at the end of this chapter in completing the Critical Thinking Challenge and Activities, as well as the StudyWARE on your Student CD-ROM.

UNIT 3
BODY MEASUREMENTS AND VITAL SIGNS

OBJECTIVES

Upon completion of this unit, you will be able to achieve the following:

LEARNING Objectives

1. Spell and define, using the glossary at the back of the text, all the Words to Know in this unit.
2. Explain why a patient's height and weight is measured at the initial and follow-up visits.
3. Identify the four vital signs and the body functions they measure.

4. Explain how the body controls temperature.
5. Explain situations in which oral measurement is contraindicated.
6. Identify the average normal temperature and the relative accuracy for oral, axillary, and rectal measurement.
7. Describe what causes pulse and why it can be felt; name and locate five pulse points.
8. Identify normal pulse rates and describe five factors that affect the rate.
9. Name two pulse characteristics besides rate and give descriptive words that define their meanings.
10. Name at least five indications for apical pulse measurement.
11. Define pulse deficit, explaining its significance and how it is measured.
12. Describe normal respiration, and explain four abnormal breathing patterns.
13. List the five circulatory factors reflected by the measurement of blood pressure.
14. Explain how the body maintains blood pressure.
15. Identify the phases of blood pressure, comparing them to the action of the heart.
16. Name six terms used to define types of hypertension.
17. Explain how pulse pressure is determined.
18. Explain an auscultatory gap.

PERFORMANCE Objectives

1. Measure and record height.
2. Measure and record weight.
3. Measure and record oral, axillary, and rectal temperature with an electronic thermometer.
4. Measure and record oral temperature with a disposable thermometer.
5. Measure and record core body temperature with an infrared tympanic thermometer.
6. Measure and record temperature with a temporal artery thermometer.

7. **Measure and record radial and apical pulse rates.**

8. **Measure and record respirations.**

9. **Measure and record blood pressure.**

WORDS TO KNOW

afebrile	essential	pulse deficit
aneroid	exhale	pulse pressure
antecubital	fatal	pyrogen
apex	febrile	radial
apical	femoral point	rales
apnea	groin	rectal
arrhythmia	height	respiration
aural	hyperventilation	rhythm
auscultate	idiopathic	sphygmomanom-
axillary	infrared	eter
blood pressure	inhale	stethoscope
brachial	mensuration	temperature
cardinal signs	oral	thermometer
carotid	orthostatic	thready
Cheyne-Stokes	palpate	vital
dorsalis pedis	popliteal	volume
dyspnea	pulse	weight

 CERTIFICATION CONNECTION

CMA
Vital signs
Principles of operation
(scales, stethoscope,
sphygmomanometers,
thermometers)

CMAS
Vital signs and
measurements

RMA
Vital signs and
mensurations

BODY MEASUREMENTS

Body measurements are sometimes referred to as **mensuration**, meaning the process of measuring. When used in connection with patient care, it refers to body measurements such as height and **weight**; vital signs; length of extremities; and the circumference of head, chest, or abdomen with infants. The initial measurements taken become the baseline for all that follow. This is extremely important with infants and children to ensure there is proper growth and development.

With adults, height reduction could indicate the presence of osteoporosis. A rapid weight gain could signal fluid retention.

Measurement of vital signs provides essential information regarding the function of the circulatory and respiratory systems. Monitoring while treatment and medication are being given for diseases and disorders of these systems is very important. The goal of treatment is to maintain the patient within as normal limits as possible.

Mensuration will usually follow the completion of recording the patient history with new patients in order to complete the initial base information. Follow-up visit measurement policy will be determined by the physician. Blood pressure may be measured at each visit and weight taken frequently. Height for adults may be monitored only occasionally unless a disease condition warrants more frequent measurement. Temperature may be measured only if an infectious condition is suspected. The measurement performed and the frequency of that measurement will largely be determined by the patient's condition.

HEIGHT AND WEIGHT

The young adult may be very interested in his height. It is especially important to those who wish to play certain sports. At the other end of life, the elderly are concerned about the loss of height. Most individuals know their approximate heights and subsequent measurements are of interest to them. The same is true of weight measurement. Athletes may have to gain or lose a certain amount of weight to meet regulations or goals. Many people of all ages are struggling to lose excess pounds and achieve a healthier weight range. Some fight eating disorders and struggle to gain a pound or two. Measurement of height and weight are very familiar to patients, and most understand their implications. Many patients monitor their weight at home, but the accurate measurement of height and weight is best done on a balance beam scale, which few have (Figure 13-6A). Scales should be balanced frequently and properly maintained to ensure accuracy. The scale should also sit on a firm surface. Figure 13-6B shows an electronic scale. Note the unit is plugged into the electric outlet. The patient stands on the platform and the weight is displayed in the window of the unit.

Reading the Scale

If you have never used a balance beam scale before, you may not be familiar with how to adjust the weights or how to read the height and weight scales. The height bar is calibrated in inches, by quarter-inch markings. When the height bar is lowered to touch the patient's head, the extension bar will indicate the height in

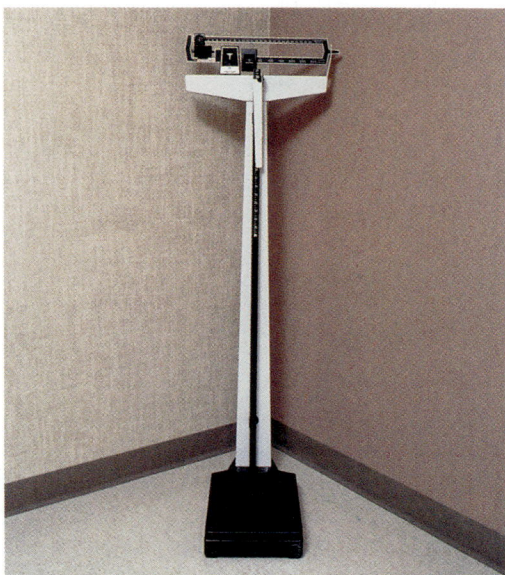

FIGURE 13-6A   The traditional balance beam scales with measuring bar

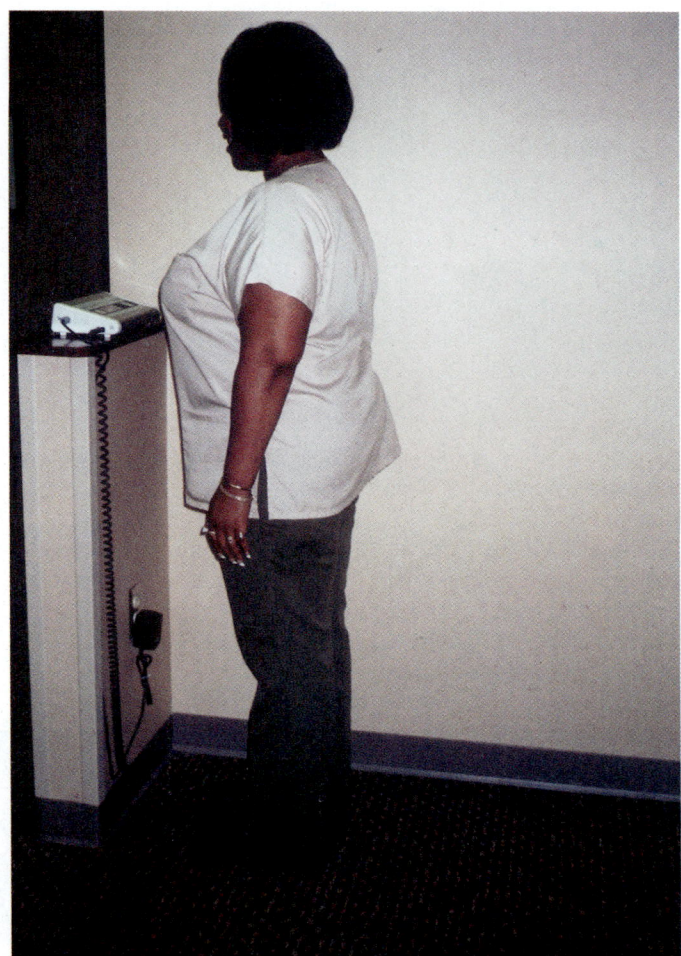

FIGURE 13-6B   An electronic scale

inches on the calibrated height bar. Height is usually recorded in total inches. If the reading is wanted in feet and inches, of course you will have to divide the number by 12. The height bar in Figure 13-7A indicates where the height is read.

Obtaining the patient's weight requires you to manipulate the two weights on the balance bar until the pointer rests in the middle of the rectangle at the end of the frame. The bottom large weight slides along the balance bar that is calibrated in 50-pound increments. Place the large weight into the groove you feel closest to the weight of the patient without going over it. The balance beam should indicate an inadequate weight amount by the pointer being above the center of the rectangle. Move the smaller weight, on the top of the balance beam, until you have added enough weight that the beam balances in the center of the rectangle. Note the top calibration is in full pounds divided into quarters (Figure 13-7B). If your large weight guess was too low, you will need to move that weight to the next higher 50-pound increment and readjust the smaller weight to balance. If you guessed too high, move the large weight one groove lower and then adjust the top. When the beam balances, add the two measurements together and record the patient's weight.

Measuring and Weighing the Patient

Tell the patient you are going to measure his height and weight and instruct him to remove his shoes. Remind patients that items in pockets, such as keys and coin purses, and handbags should be put aside. While they are getting ready, check the balance of the scale by

PATIENT EDUCATION

Patients may be asked to monitor their weight at home when they have certain conditions that can cause fluid retention, such as cardiac or kidney diseases. They may also be monitoring for a weight gain or loss program. Be sure to remind them that the usual home scale will be more accurate if placed on a surface other than carpet. However, the important thing is that it sit in the same location for all measurements. It is also important to remind them to weigh at about the same time each day, since weight will vary throughout the day. For example, weighing before breakfast one day and after the next will not provide an accurate assessment. The weight of clothing and shoes is another variable to mention. It would be best to weigh in clothing of about the same weight each day. A suggestion to weigh each morning while still in night clothing or underwear and before eating would provide consistent variables for a more accurate assessment of weight trends.

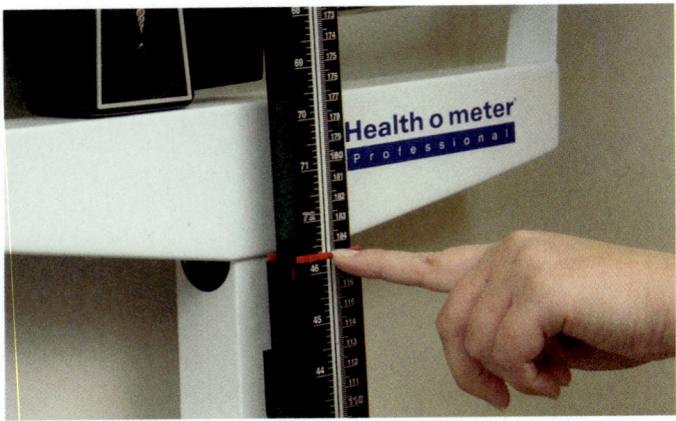

FIGURE 13-7A The height is read on the top section where the two sections of the height bar meet.

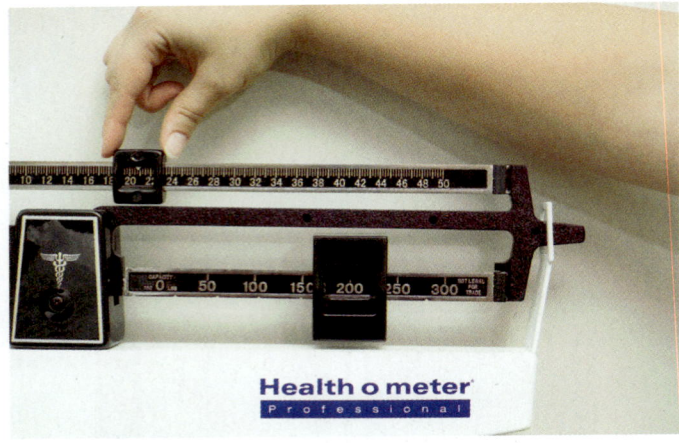

FIGURE 13-7B The balance bar reads 220¾ pounds.

placing both weights at "0" to determine if the weight bar pointer balances in the center of the rectangular opening. If not, make a slight adjustment of the scale until it does. (This will have to be demonstrated to you by an instructor or another employee.)

Raise the height bar *above* the patient's estimated height and extend the measuring bar. Most patients know approximately how tall they are if you ask. Place a paper towel on the scale base to provide a clean surface. Follow the steps in Procedure 13-3,

---

PROCEDURE PROCEDURE PROCEDURE PROCEDURE PROCEDURE PROCEDURE PROCEDURE PROCEDURE

13-3 Measure Height on a Balance Beam Scale

PURPOSE: To obtain an accurate measurement of a patient's height.

EQUIPMENT: Balance beam scale with extension measuring bar, patient's chart, pen (a measuring scale may be fixed to the wall).

PERFORMANCE OBJECTIVE: Having access to a balance beam scale and a patient, follow the steps in the procedure to accurately measure and record a patient's height. The reading must be within ¼" of the instructor's measurement.

1. Identify the patient.
2. Explain the procedure.
3. Instruct the patient to remove shoes. **RATIONALE: Accurate measurement cannot be obtained if shoes are worn.**
4. Place a paper towel on the scale platform. **RATIONALE: The paper towel provides a clean surface for the shoeless foot.**
5. Raise the measuring bar beyond the patient's height and lift the extension. **RATIONALE: Avoids the possibility of striking the patient if the bar is raised after the patient steps on the scale.**

6. Help the patient onto the scale as needed, facing you with his back to the measuring device. Advise the patient to stand erect.
7. Slide the measuring bar down slowly and carefully to rest on top of the patient's head, gently compressing hair. **NOTE: Measurement of height is from the top of the head, not the hair.**
8. Read the measurement in inches, and tell the patient what it is.
9. Help the patient from the scale. Tell the patient to put his shoes back on unless ready for a physical exam.
10. Place the measuring extension bar back in place, and discard the paper towel.
11. Record the height measurement on the patient's chart.

CHARTING EXAMPLE

5-12-XX

Ht. 68"

B. Hale, CMA

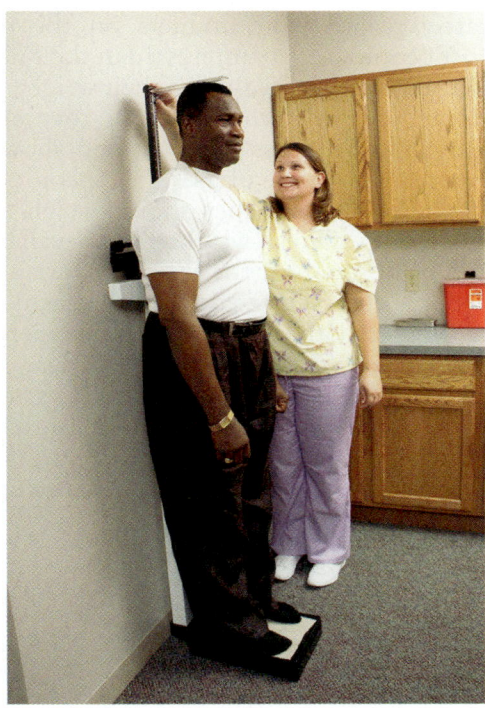

FIGURE 13-8   Measuring height

Measure Height on a Balance Beam Scale, to obtain the patient's height (Figure 13-8).

Please note the procedure indicates that the patient should face away from the scale with her back to the height bar. However, if you are measuring both height and weight, many patients want to face the bar so they can watch you balancing the scale to get their accurate weight. Facing the height bar initially eliminates the need to get off, turn, and get back on or prevents them from trying to turn around on the narrow scale base, which could result in a fall. It is also more difficult for elderly patients to get on the scale backward. They normally grasp the scale base to aid them when stepping on. Check with your employer to see which position is used in your office.

While the patient is still on the scale, proceed with Procedure 13-4, Weigh a Patient on a Balance Beam Scale, to obtain the weight. Figure 13-9 shows that you can adjust the weight from either side of the scale to obtain the reading. If there is room to position the scale away from the wall, it is often easier from the other side, where the patient is not in the way. Note that the height bar can remain lowered when you are only measuring the patient's weight.

PROCEDURE PROCEDURE PROCEDURE PROCEDURE PROCEDURE PROCEDURE PROCEDURE

13-4  Weigh Patient on Balance Beam Scale

PURPOSE: To obtain an accurate measure of the patient's weight.

EQUIPMENT: Balance beam scale, patient's chart, pen.

PERFORMANCE OBJECTIVE: Having access to a balance beam scale and a patient, follow the steps in the procedure to accurately read and record a patient's weight to within $\frac{1}{4}$ pound of the instructor's measurement.

1. Identify the patient.
2. Explain the procedure.
3. Instruct the patient to remove her shoes and items from pockets.
4. Balance the scales.
5. Place a paper towel on the base of the scale. **RATIONALE: Provides a clean surface for the shoeless foot.**
6. Help the patient onto the scale as needed.
7. Make sure the patient is in the center of the platform. Ask the patient to stand still while you the adjust the balance and read the weight. Remind the patient not to hold on to the scale. **RATIONALE: Holding on to any part of the scale will cause a lighter, inaccurate measurement.**
8. Help the patient from the scale and discard the paper towel.
9. Record the weight on the patient's chart. Be sure to record whether the patient was wearing street clothing or a gown.
10. Return the scale to balance at zero.

CHARTING EXAMPLE

5-12-XX

Wt. 147# (147 lbs) without shoes, in street clothing

B. Hale, CMA

NOTE: If patients are weighed with their clothes on, it is common to allow at least 3 pounds for women's clothing and 5 pounds for men's (according to office policy).

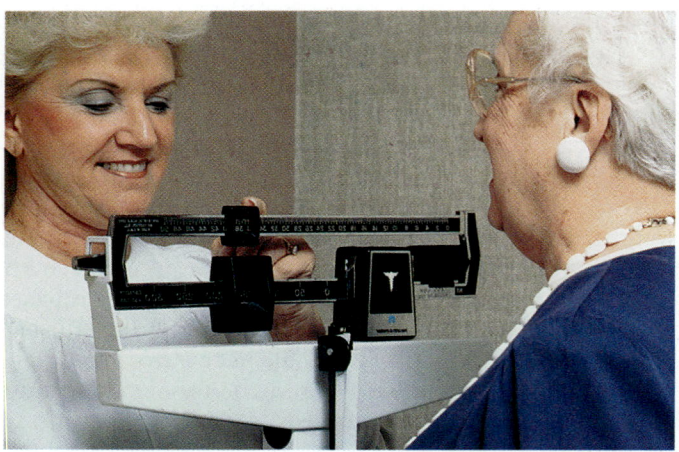

FIGURE 13-9   The weight of the patient may be read on either side of the scale.

Accurately record your findings on the patient's chart. Most people are very interested in their numbers. Since some may be sensitive about their weight, be careful about any remarks you make. If they are on a weight-gain or weight-loss program and show even a small change, give them praise and encouragement. Some may question what they should weigh for their height. There are different weight charts available, and one should be posted near the scale as a patient education tool. Some charts differentiate by age, while others will use gender or both. Figure 13-10 is gender-specific and also considers relative frame size. These are only guidelines, as the composition of the body tissue has an effect on the weight. Most people realize muscle tissue weighs more than fat, so a muscular person may look trim and yet weigh more than the same-size, not-so-fit person.

MEN			
Height	Small	Medium	Large
5' 2"	128–134	131–141	138–150
5' 3"	130–136	133–143	140–153
5' 4"	132–138	135–145	142–156
5' 5"	134–140	137–148	144–160
5' 6"	136–142	139–151	146–164
5' 7"	138–146	142–154	149–168
5' 8"	140–148	145–157	152–172
5' 9"	142–151	148–160	155–176
5'10"	144–154	151–163	158–180
5'11"	146–157	154–166	161–184
6' 0"	149–160	157–170	164–188
6' 1"	152–164	160–174	168–192
6' 2"	155–168	164–178	172–197
6' 3"	158–172	167–182	176–202
6' 4"	162–176	171–187	181–207

WOMEN			
Height	Small	Medium	Large
4'10"	102–111	109–121	118–131
4'11"	103–113	111–123	120–134
5' 0"	104–115	113–126	122–137
5' 1"	106–118	115–129	125–140
5' 2"	108–121	118–132	128–143
5' 3"	111–124	121–135	131–147
5' 4"	114–127	124–138	134–151
5' 5"	117–130	127–141	137–155
5' 6"	120–133	130–144	140–159
5' 7"	123–136	133–147	143–163
5' 8"	128–139	138–150	146–167
5' 9"	129–142	139–153	149–170
5'10"	132–146	142–156	152–173
5'11"	135–148	145–159	155–176
6' 0"	138–151	148–162	158–179

FIGURE 13-10   Chart of desirable weight for men and women

With the height and weight completed, it is time to measure the vital signs to complete the initial mensuration.

VITAL SIGNS

The terms **cardinal signs** or **vital** signs are used by health care personnel to identify the measurement of body functions that are essential to life. The four vital indicators are **temperature**, **pulse**, **respiration**, and **blood pressure**, commonly referred to as TPR and B/P. They indicate the body's ability to control heat; the rate, volume, and rhythm of the heart; the rate and quality of breathing; and the force of the heart and condition of the blood vessels. The vital signs give the physician an assessment of the status of the brain, the autonomic nervous system, the heart, and the lungs.

The correct measurement of vital signs is extremely important. Proper technique and attention to details are essential. Findings should be recorded immediately following measurement to avoid a memory error. Always repeat the procedure if you think you may have made a mistake in measuring or recording. Occasionally, you may have a problem measuring a vital sign because a patient's unusual physical condition makes measurement difficult. Inform the physician of your problem and follow the course of action advised. Avoid alarming the patient. *Never* estimate the measurement. The physician's choice of treatment and medication is often based on the findings; therefore, they must be accurate.

TEMPERATURE

The temperature of the body indicates the amount of heat produced by the activity of changing food into energy. The body loses heat through perspiration, breathing, and the elimination of body wastes. The balance between heat production and heat loss determines the body's temperature.

Conditions affecting body heat include metabolic rate, time of day, and amount of activity. Body temperature is usually lower in the morning following a period of rest. In the afternoon and evening, body temperature rises because of the heat produced by activity and the metabolism of food. These activities warm the blood that circulates through the body. "Normal" body temperature for an individual is that temperature at which his body systems function most effectively. Not all people have the same normal oral temperature. Refer to Table 13-1. An *average* normal oral temperature is 98.6°F (Fahrenheit) or 37°C (centigrade). Normal oral temperature of patients may vary from 97.6° to 99.6°F. A person with a temperature above normal is said to be

TABLE 13-1　Temperature Variations Considered "Normal"			
	Oral	**Axillary**	**Rectal**
Average normal temperature	98.6°F (37°C)	97.6°F (36.5°C)	99.6°F (37.5°C)
Range	97.6–99.6°F (36.5–37.5°C)	96.6–98.6°F (36–37°C)	98.6–100.6°F (37–38.1°C)

febrile or to have a temperature elevation. A person with a temperature that is normal or subnormal is said to be **afebrile**.

Controlling Body Temperature

The temperature-regulating center in the body is located in the hypothalamus of the brain. The action of the hypothalamus can be compared with a thermostat that turns the furnace in your home off and on to keep the room temperature at the set number of degrees. As discussed previously, the brain, autonomic nervous system, blood vessels, and skin cooperate to regulate temperature. This is achieved through a feedback mechanism from temperature receptors. In the body, the hot and cold peripheral receptors in the skin send messages to the hypothalamus about the environment surrounding the body. Temperature receptors in the spinal cord, abdomen, and other internal structures send messages about the internal body temperature. One section of the hypothalamus also has many heat-sensitive neurons, which increase their output of impulses when temperature rises and decrease their output when it drops. The signals from this section of the hypothalamus merge with those received in another section, along with the internal and skin receptors, to evaluate the situation and send signals to control heat loss or heat production. Therefore, this central center is referred to as the *hypothalamic thermostat.*

The hypothalamic thermostat is very effective. When receptors sense the body is too warm, they send a message to the brain, which in turn acts on the sweat glands of the skin to produce moisture. The moisture evaporates from the skin's surface and cools the body. At the same time, nerve impulses are sent to the surface blood vessels to dilate, which brings more blood in contact with the surface of the skin. The blood gives up heat, which cools the blood within the vessels and therefore cools the body.

PATIENT EDUCATION

The accurate measurement of temperature can help the physician make a diagnosis. Instruct the patient to inform the physician of any significant changes in temperature. Advise the patient at what point an oral temperature should be reported to the physician. Caution the patient that a fever should not be "watched" to see how high it will go. Prolonged high fever can cause brain damage and ultimately death.

The accurate measurement of other vital signs (pulse, blood pressure, and respirations) also helps the physician make a diagnosis. If there are significant health problems, the patient is instructed to monitor changes. For example, a patient with high blood pressure should be instructed to take and record blood pressure at home. This will help determine whether the treatment is effective. The patient will inform the physician of important changes that could affect the treatment.

TABLE 13-2	Classification of Fevers	
	Fahrenheit	**Celsius**
Slight	99.6°–101.0°	37.5°–38.3°
Moderate	101.0°–102.0°	38.3°–38.8°
Severe	102.0°–104.0°	38.8°–40.0°
Dangerous	104.0°–105.0°	40.0°–40.5
Fatal	over 106.0°	41.1°

When the body senses coolness, the opposite activities occur. Surface blood vessels constrict to keep the blood away from the surface of the skin and prevent the loss of heat. Impulses to the sweat glands are stopped when temperature falls below normal. The small papillary muscles around the hair follicles contract, causing gooseflesh. Heat is produced by the activity of the papillary muscles, thereby helping to warm the body. In addition, a portion of the hypothalamus becomes active when cold signals are received. Now hypothalamic messages are sent to skeletal muscles throughout the body, causing increased muscle tone that produces heat. When the muscle tone rises above a certain level, shivering results, and heat production is raised dramatically. This is evident with an infectious process, such as influenza. Microorganisms cause the patient to experience chills and shivering until the temperature rises to warm the body and a fever develops.

During an infectious process, the presence of microorganisms cause **pyrogens** to be secreted, which raise the "set point" of the hypothalamic thermostat. Pyrogens are toxins from bacteria or a by-product of degenerating tissues. When the set point is higher than normal, the body's heat production and conservation processes are activated. Surface blood vessels constrict, causing the person to feel cold even though the temperature is above normal. No sweat is secreted. Increased white blood cell activity from fighting bacterial invasion also produces heat. Chills and shivering begin and continue until the temperature reaches the higher set point, where the hypothalamus will continue to operate until the infectious process is reversed. Once this

occurs, the hypothalamic thermostat is reset to a lower or normal value, and the body's temperature reduction process results in profuse sweating and a hot, red skin from general vasodilation. After this onset reaction, the temperature will begin to fall.

The extent of the infection determines the amount of heat (fever) generated. A mild infection may cause the temperature to rise to 100°F. A moderate infection may elevate the temperature to 102°F. Fevers are categorized by the degree of body heat as slight, moderate, severe, dangerous, or **fatal** (Table 13-2). Fatality-associated elevated temperature depends on the extent of time the fever is present. Fevers of short duration well above 106.0°F have not proved fatal, but immediate measures to reduce body temperature must be administered. Temperatures below normal are called subnormal. Collapse will occur at about 96.0°F, and death follows if temperature goes below 93.0°F more than briefly.

Thermometer Types and Designs

Body temperature is measured by means of a **thermometer** in scales of Fahrenheit or the metric system equivalent, Celsius. Thermometers are of the following main types: disposable, in the form of plastic strips; self-contained digital; battery-operated electronic; a tympanic **infrared**; and a temporal artery thermometer. The mouth (**oral**), underarm (**axillary**), rectum (**rectal**), ear (**aural** or tympanic membrane), or the temporal area of the forehead may be used to measure body temperature. The large variety of thermometers, each with its own advantages and disadvantages, allow for personal preference in equipment selection for the physician's office. Table 13-3 briefly outlines the main features for each type.

Measuring Oral Temperature

Measuring body temperature by mouth is convenient, quick, fairly accurate, and relatively inexpensive. Remember that oral temperature requires contact with mucous membranes, so a thermometer either must be

TABLE 13-3	Comparison of Thermometer Types	
Type	**Advantage**	**Disadvantage**
Plastic disposable	Single use avoids cross-contamination, no cleaning, relatively fast	Must protect from heat, somewhat unpleasant for patient, storage and inventory costs
Digital	Quick, signals when registered, easily read, self-contained	Moderate initial cost, plastic cover, and battery expenses
Electronic probe	Quick, signals when registered, easily read, self-contained	Fairly expensive, cumbersome cord, requires recharging, probe cover costs, may cause inaccurate readings if patient bites too hard on probe
Tympanic infrared	Instant results, easily read, core temperature, individualized probe cover, eliminates mucous membrane concerns.	Expensive, probe cover costs, replacement battery costs. An improper seal in the ear canal, the presence of cerumen, or an infection of the middle ear may cause inaccurate readings
Temporal artery	Instant results, easily read, as accurate as rectal, noninvasive, no mucous membrane concerns	Expensive, requires probe cover or cleaning when used, requires environmental acclimation, somewhat delicate

disposable or requires a barrier cover. There are also factors that influence the accurate measurement:

- The thermometer must be place sublingually into the heat pocket.
- Patients must not have smoked or had anything hot or cold by mouth for at least 15 minutes prior to measuring.
- Patients must be able to appropriately maintain the thermometer in place for the required period of time.

Contraindications to Oral Measurement

Oral temperature measurement is not always the method of choice. Temperature must be measured by an axillary, rectal, tympanic, or temporal method in the following situations:

- Infants and children under age 6
- Patients with respiratory complications that result in mouth breathing or use of supplemental oxygen
- Confused, disoriented, or emotionally unstable patients
- Patients with oral injuries
- Patients with recent oral surgery
- Patients with facial paralysis
- Patients with nasal obstruction

Disposable Thermometers

Disposable plastic oral thermometers may be used in some offices, urgent care centers, and hospital emergency rooms. Because they are used only once and discarded, they are free from cross-contamination, and no time or equipment is required for cleaning. One disad-

vantage is the cost factor. The patient's reaction may also be less than enthusiastic. The plastic is thin and almost sharp. Also, care must be taken to avoid touching the dot matrix portion, which is placed in the patient's mouth. The dots can be placed up or down. The thermometer must be held under the tongue as far back as possible in the heat pocket, with the tongue pressed against the end and the mouth closed on the stem (Figure 13-11). Wait 60 seconds, then remove the thermometer. Allow 10 seconds for the dots to stabilize,

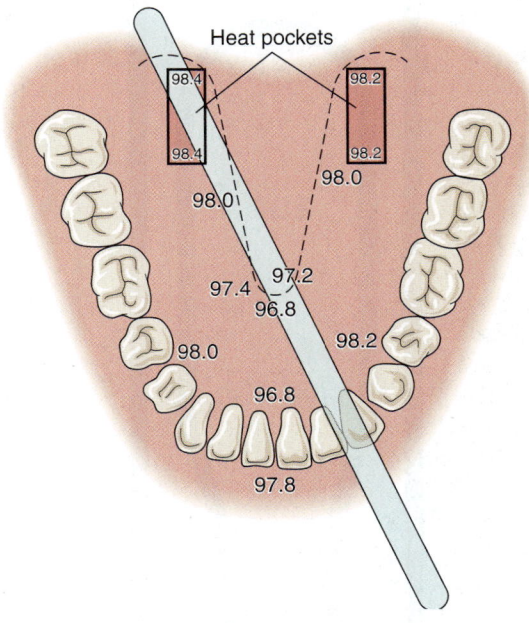

FIGURE 13-11 Dot matrix portion of the disposable thermometer must be placed sublingually into a heat pocket. *(Courtesy of 3M Health Care)*

then read and record the temperature. The heat in the mouth causes a reaction on the heat-sensitive dots printed on the surface of the plastic strip. Readings are calculated by counting the number of dots that change color within a degree grouping (Figures 13-12A and B). The last changed dot on the matrix indicates the correct temperature. Discard the thermometer in a biohazardous waste container. Plastic thermometers are not considered to be precisely accurate; however, for usual temperature determination, their single use and freedom from cross-contamination concerns may outweigh any minor disadvantages. (See Procedure 13-5.)

The disposable plastic thermometer can also be used to measure axillary temperature. The dot matrix portion is placed next to the body, deep in the axillary space, with the handle extending straight down the patient's side. The arm must be held tightly at the

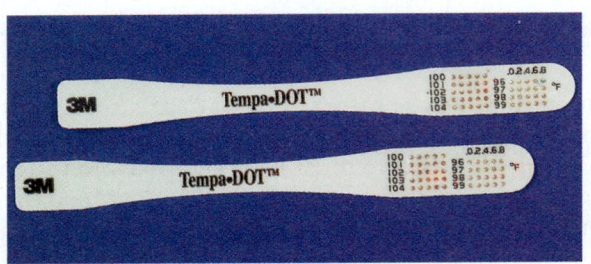

FIGURE 13-12A Disposable plastic thermometer

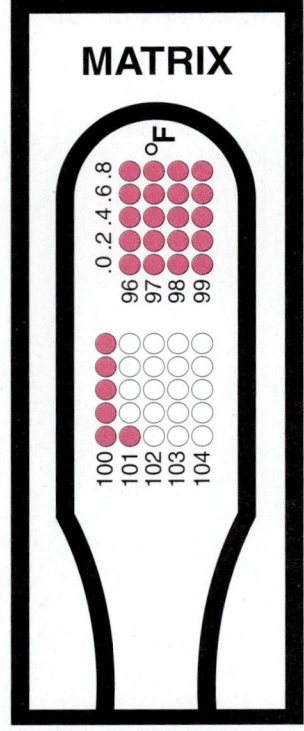

FIGURE 13-12B The matrix reads 101°F. *(Courtesy of 3M Health Care)*

side. After three minutes, remove the thermometer; wait 10 seconds, then read and record the temperature.

When disposable thermometers are exposed to high temperatures in their environment, the matrix dots will change color. If this should occur, place them in a freezer for 1 hour for each box of 100 thermometers. Then let them stand at room temperature for 1 day. The thermometers will then be ready for use, and their accuracy should not be affected.

Electronic Thermometers

The use of electronic thermometers is very common. They are quick, sanitary, and easily read and do not require cleaning. A small, battery-operated unit with a digital read-out window is very accurate and capable of measuring a temperature within a few seconds (Figure 13-13A). A metal probe, blue for oral, red for rectal, is attached by a cord to the battery unit. A disposable cover slips over the probe to provide each patient with an individual thermometer. The covered probe is inserted in the patient's mouth. It is usually held in place by the medical assistant because the time involved is short, and the probe, with its cord, is heavy and somewhat cumbersome (Figure 13-13B). As soon as the temperature level has been reached, the unit will sound a signal and the final reading will appear in the window of the unit. The probe cover is then discarded into a biohazardous waste container (Figure 13-13C) (Procedure 13-6).

Electronic thermometers are time saving and convenient, but they are somewhat expensive. Care must also be taken to adjust the unit frequently and correctly. It is critical that the dial be observed from a direct view at eye level while making adjustments. The unit must be returned to its charging stand after use to maintain the battery.

Some units have built-in operator prompts to signal when technique or other problems exist. If the phrase OPER ERR 9 (or something similar) shows on the readout window, it means the probe is not in contact with tissue. A readjustment of the thermometer will erase the message and allow the continued measurement of the temperature. A BAT LO (or similar) message indicates the unit's batteries do not have enough charge to take a temperature. The unit must be returned to the charger base for 6 to 8 hours to be fully charged or 45 minutes to permit a limited number of measurements. A PROB BAD (or similar) message indicates the probe is damaged and will not sense temperature properly. This can be corrected only by installing a new probe.

Another electronic thermometer is simple and self-contained. It is also a digital thermometer and is excellent for home use (Figure 13-14). The thermometer will register the temperature in about 60 seconds on an easy-to-read LCD panel that shows the temperature in tenths of degrees. The thermometer can be cleaned

13-5  Measure Oral Temperature with a Disposable Plastic Thermometer

PURPOSE: To determine a patient's oral temperature using a disposable plastic thermometer.

OSHA GUIDELINES: Standard Precautions require gloves to be worn if there is any possibility of coming into contact with blood, body fluids, or wound drainage. Biohazardous waste containers are required for discarding gloves and plastic thermometers.

EQUIPMENT: Disposable plastic thermometer, watch or timer, latex or vinyl gloves, biohazardous waste container, paper, pen or pencil.

PERFORMANCE OBJECTIVE: In a simulated or actual situation and given access to all necessary equipment and supplies, measure and record oral temperature within 4 minutes, following steps in the procedure and observing aseptic and safety precautions. Recorded findings must agree with the instructor's reading.

1. Wash hands and put on gloves.

2. Identify the patient. **RATIONALE: Speaking to the patient by name and checking the chart ensures that you are performing the procedure on the correct patient.**

3. Explain the procedure and what you are going to do.

4. Determine whether the patient has recently had a hot or cold drink or smoked. **NOTE: If so, allow 15 minutes before measuring. RATIONALE: Hot or cold substances in the mouth prevent accurate temperature measurement.**

5. Open the package by peeling back the top of the wrapper to expose the handle end of the thermometer.

6. Grasp the handle and remove from the wrapper. **NOTE: Do NOT touch the dot matrix portion,** which will be placed in the patient's mouth. **RATIONALE: Your hands would contaminate the thermometer and may interfere with the chemical reaction of the dots.**

7. Insert the thermometer into the patient's mouth as far back as possible into one of the heat pockets (see Figure 13-11).

8. Instruct the patient to press his tongue down on the thermometer and keep his mouth closed. **RATIONALE: Firm, direct contact is necessary for accurate measurement. Breathing through the mouth admits air, which may affect accuracy.**

9. Maintain this position for 60 seconds. **NOTE: Time by a watch.**

10. Remove the thermometer and wait 10 seconds for the dots to stabilize. **NOTE: Take special care to avoid touching the portion that has been in the patient's mouth.**

11. Read the thermometer. Discard it in the biohazardous waste container.

12. Remove gloves and discard them in the biohazardous waste container.

13. Wash hands.

14. Record the temperature.

CHARTING EXAMPLE

3-6-XX

T. 97.8

B. Davis (RMA)

---

with soap and water and sanitized with a disinfectant. Probe covers are available for clinic or office use. It may be used for oral, axillary, or rectal measurement. Some models have a beeper that sounds when the maximum temperature is reached. This feature is especially appealing to children.

Measuring Rectal Temperature

Rectal temperature is a very accurate measurement, simply because it is taken internally. Rectal measurement is appropriate with babies and young children who have not yet learned how to keep an oral thermometer in place. Often children complain bitterly about having a rectal temperature taken when they think they are "too big." The physician usually has a policy concerning the age limit for rectal temperatures, which you must follow.

Electronic thermometers may be used to measure rectal temperature. Use the rectal (red) probe to take a rectal temperature. Remove the rectal probe from its holder and attach a probe cover. The probe is inserted into the rectum $\frac{1}{2}$ inch for adults and $\frac{1}{4}$ inch for children. The use of lubricant is optional. The probe

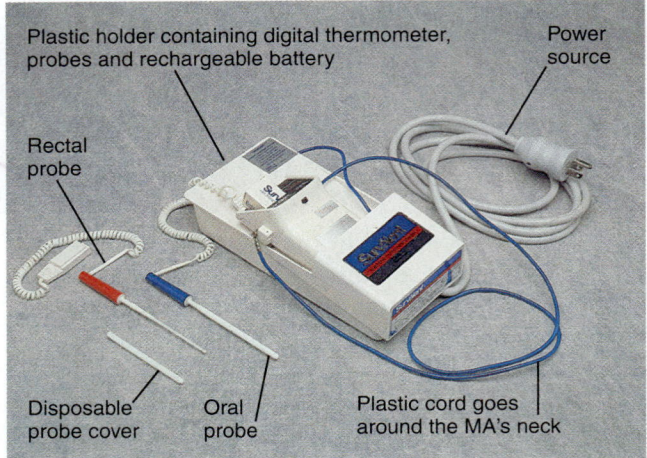

Plastic holder containing digital thermometer, probes and rechargeable battery

Power source

Rectal probe

Disposable probe cover

Oral probe

Plastic cord goes around the MA's neck

FIGURE 13-13A Electronic thermometer

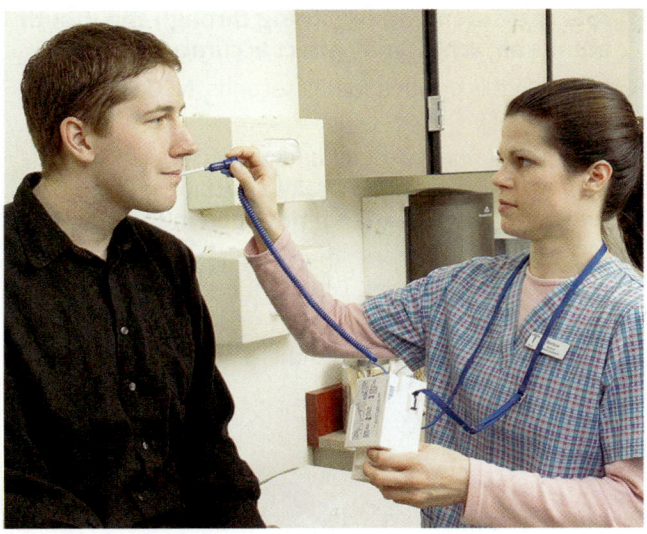

FIGURE 13-13B The medical assistant holds the probe of an electronic thermometer in the patient's mouth until it signals completion.

should be angled slightly to ensure contact with the rectal mucosa. After the reading is registered, remove the probe, and discard the cover in a biohazardous waste container.

When measuring the temperature of infants, they may be positioned on the stomach or the back. If positioning on the back, unfasten the diaper to expose the anus. Grasp the ankles securely with one hand, flexing the knees to the abdomen. With the other hand, insert the thermometer into the anal canal. Hold the thermometer securely in place. Maintain your grasp on the ankles so the infant cannot turn over. Be prepared for the procedure to initiate urination or expelling of stool. It would be wise to cover the male infant's penis with a diaper to absorb the urine stream. If positioning prone on a table, be certain to maintain control of the infant or

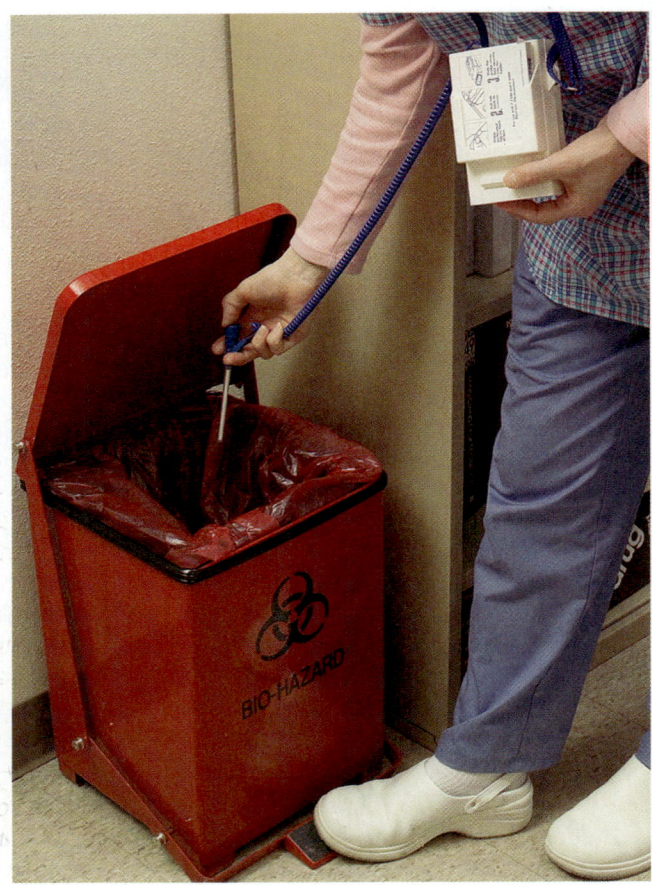

FIGURE 13-13C The probe cover is discarded into a hazardous waste container.

child's position to prevent turning over and causing injury to the rectum from the inserted thermometer probe.

Older children can be positioned either on their abdomen or side, whichever is preferred. Adults would be positioned on their side and draped with a sheet for privacy.

When recording a rectal measurement, place the letter *R* in parentheses following the reading. Normal rectal temperature is 99.6°F or 37.5°C, one full degree above normal oral temperature. Temperature must never be measured rectally if the patient has had recent rectal surgery. It is possible to damage the operative site or perforate newly sutured lines. (See Procedure 13-7.)

Measuring Axillary Temperature

Temperature can be measured by placing the electronic thermometer in the axilla (armpit). This method is the least accurate. Axillary measurement is appropriate when oral is contraindicated and rectal is inconvenient, undesirable, or contraindicated. Normal axillary temperature is 97.6°F or 36.4°C, one full degree *below* normal oral temperature. When recording axillary find-

PROCEDURE

13-6  Measure Oral Temperature with an Electronic Thermometer

PURPOSE: To determine a patient's oral temperature with an electronic thermometer.

OSHA GUIDELINES: Standard Precautions require a biohazardous waste container for discarding probe covers.

EQUIPMENT: Electronic thermometer unit, oral probe, probe cover, biohazardous waste container, paper, pen or pencil.

PERFORMANCE OBJECTIVE: In a simulated or actual situation and given access to all necessary equipment and supplies, measure the patient's oral temperature. The temperature will be read and recorded in 2 minutes, following correct procedural technique and observing aseptic and safety precautions. Recorded findings must agree the with the instructor's reading.

1. Wash hands; assemble equipment.
2. Identify the patient. **RATIONALE: Speaking to the patient by name and checking the chart ensures that you are performing the procedure on the correct patient.**
3. Explain the procedure and what you are going to do.
4. Ensure the patient has not smoked or consumed anything hot or cold in past 15 minutes.
5. Place the blue probe connector into the receptacle of the unit base and check to make sure it is properly seated.
6. Holding the blue probe by the collar, remove it from the stored position.
7. Insert the probe firmly into the probe cover to ensure that it is properly seated.

8. Insert the covered probe into the patient's mouth. **NOTE: The probe and connecting cord are rather heavy and cumbersome. It may be necessary to hold the thermometer steady in place.**
9. Maintain the covered probe in position the until the unit signals, approximately 10 to 15 seconds. **RATIONALE: Early removal results in inaccurate measurement.**
10. Remove the probe from the patient. Do not touch the probe cover. **RATIONALE: Probe is contaminated with patient's saliva.**
11. Read and record the temperature measurement. **NOTE: Temperature is displayed digitally in the window of the unit.**
12. Recheck your reading and recording.
13. Press the eject button to discard the used probe cover into the biohazardous waste container. **RATIONALE: All materials coming into contact with bodily secretions are deposited in a biohazardous waste container.**
14. Return the probe to the stored position in the unit. The thermometer display will read zero and shut off.
15. Store the unit in the charging stand. **NOTE: A red light in the upper left hand area of the display indicates that the thermometer is charging. RATIONALE: The unit should remain in the stand so it is fully charged and ready for use.**

CHARTING EXAMPLE

5/10/XX

T. 99.8

B. Davis (RMA)

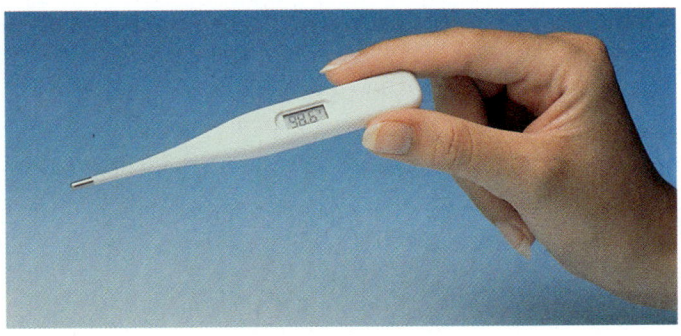

FIGURE 13-14 Electronic digital thermometer *(Courtesy of Omron Healthcare, Inc.)*

ings, place the letters *Ax* in parentheses following the reading. (See Procedure 13-8.)

Some manufacturers recommend using the rectal probe for taking an axillary temperature; others recommend the oral probe. Consult the instructional booklet with your equipment to determine which to use. Apply a probe cover, and insert the tip well into the axillary space with the probe extending down and slightly forward along the patient's side. Press gently into the space to establish good tissue contact. Have the patient lower his arm over the probe. Hold the probe in position to maintain good contact. Remove and read after the unit signals completion.

13-7  Measure Rectal Temperature with an Electronic Thermometer

PURPOSE: To determine a patient's axillary temperature using a clinical thermometer.

OSHA GUIDELINES: Standard Precautions require gloves to be worn if there is any possibility of coming into contact with blood, body fluids, or wound drainage. Biohazardous waste containers are required for discarding gloves and sheaths.

EQUIPMENT: Mannequin (if simulated), electronic thermometer, rectal probe, probe cover, drape (if adult), latex or vinyl gloves, lubricant, tissues, biohazardous waste container, paper, and pen or pencil..

PERFORMANCE OBJECTIVE: In a simulated or actual situation and given access to all necessary equipment and supplies, measure and record a patient's rectal temperature, following the steps in the procedure, and observing aseptic and safety precautions. The recorded findings must agree with the instructor's reading.

1. Wash hands and put on gloves.

2. Identify the patient. **RATIONALE: Speaking to the patient by name and checking the chart ensures that you are performing the procedure on the correct patient.**

3. Explain the procedure and what you are going to do to the child and parent or to adult patient.

4. Instruct the patient to remove appropriate clothing, assisting as needed. **NOTE: Provide privacy.**

5. Assist the adult patient onto the examining table and cover her with a drape. Avoid overexposure. Position the patient on her side. Ensure the patient's comfort and safety.

6. Place a small amount of lubricant onto a tissue and place it within reach.

7. Place the red probe connector into the receptacle of the unit base and check to make sure it is properly seated.

8. Holding the red probe by the collar, remove it from the stored position.

9. Insert the red probe firmly into the probe cover; ensure it is properly seated.

10. Remove the probe with cover.

11. Apply lubricant to the end of the probe cover.

12. Arrange the drape to expose the buttocks.

13. With one hand, raise the upper buttock to expose the anus.

14. With the other hand, carefully insert the lubricated thermometer probe into the anal canal approximately $\frac{1}{2}$ inch.

NOTES:
- **Angle the probe slightly to ensure contact with mucosa.**
- **Do not force the thermometer. Rotating will often facilitate insertion.**
- **If opening is not apparent, ask the patient to bear down slightly; this will usually expose the opening.**

NOTES:
- **When performing the procedure on infants or small children, ask the parent or accompanying adult to prepare the child while you prepare the thermometer.**
- **Position the infant as to the parent's or physician's preference.**
- **Ensure safety during the procedure by maintaining control of the infant's or child's position. (A parent can be instructed to assist you, especially if it comforts the child.)**

11. Hold the thermometer in place until the unit signals.

12. Withdraw the thermometer. Eject the probe cover into the biohazardous waste container.

13. Read the thermometer. Reread to check temperature and record the results.

14. Replace the probe in the unit.

15. Remove any excess lubricant from the anal area with a tissue. Wipe from front to back.

16. Ask the parent or accompanying adult to dress an infant or child.

17. Assist the adult patient from the examining table and instruct her to redress. **NOTE: Provide privacy as appropriate.**

18. Remove and discard gloves in the biohazardous waste container.

19. Record the temperature, placing (R) after the finding.

20. Return the thermometer to the charging stand.

CHARTING EXAMPLE

3-6-XX

T. 100.2 (R)

B. Davis, RMA

13-8    Measure Axillary Temperature with an Electronic Thermometer

PURPOSE: To determine a patient's axillary temperature with an electronic thermometer.

EQUIPMENT: Electronic thermometer, probe, probe cover, tissues, biohazardous waste container, paper, pen or pencil

PERFORMANCE OBJECTIVE: In a simulated or actual situation and given access to all necessary equipment and supplies, measure and record axillary temperature, following the steps in the procedure and observing aseptic and safety precautions. Recorded findings must agree with the instructor's reading.

1. Wash hands.

2. Identify the patient. **RATIONALE: Speaking to the patient by name and checking the chart ensure that you are performing the procedure on the correct patient.**

3. Explain the procedure and what you are going to do.

4. Assist the patient, as necessary, to expose the axilla. **NOTE: Provide privacy.**

5. Pat the axillary space with a tissue to remove perspiration. **RATIONALE: Perspiration prevents the probe from coming into direct contact with skin.**

6. Place the appropriate probe connector into the receptacle of the unit base and check to make sure it is properly seated.

7. Holding it by the collar, remove the appropriate probe from the stored position.

8. Insert the probe firmly into the probe cover to ensure that it is properly seated.

9. Place the probe deep in the axillary space. Position so that it is in direct contact with the top of the axillary space, with the probe extending down and slightly forward.

10. Hold the arm tightly against the body. Have the patient maintain this position until the thermometer emits its signal.

   NOTES: ■ **Help weak or confused patients maintain the position.**

   ■ **Be certain the thermometer remains deep in the axillary space. Children will require close attention and assistance.**

11. Remove the probe and eject the cover into the biohazardous waste container.

12. Read and record the findings. **NOTE: Place (Ax) after the reading.**

13. Reread and check the recording.

14. Return the thermometer to the charging stand.

15. Help the patient replace his clothing.

16. Wash hands.

CHARTING EXAMPLE

3-6-XX

T. 97.2 (Ax)

B. Davis, RMA

Axillary temperature can also be taken using the digital thermometer (Figure 13-15). The tip of the thermometer is placed into the axillary space and supported in place. The arm is held tight against the body until the signal is heard.

Tympanic Membrane Thermometer

Another method for temperature measurement is the instantaneous tympanic membrane (aural) thermometer. The thermometer operates by the principle of measuring the strength of the infrared heat waves generated by the tympanic membrane and digitally displays that temperature in less than 2 seconds. Because the tympanic membrane shares the same blood supply as the hypothalamus, it is believed the auditory canal is

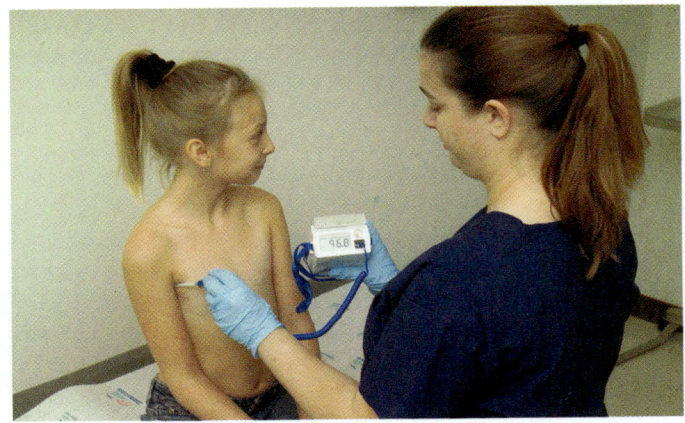

FIGURE 13-15 Measuring axillary temperature with a digital thermometer

an ideal site for obtaining an accurate assessment of the body's core temperature. Studies conducted with temperature-sensing devices placed internally in a large blood vessel have shown strong correlation in results.

Although its greatest asset is the instant result, it has become a real benefit to health care professionals in hospital emergency rooms, labor and delivery rooms, and pediatric units because it does not involve contact with mucous membranes and the site is so easily accessible. Another advantage is the readings are not affected by hot or cold liquids or smoking, as are oral methods. In addition, the patient does not even need to be conscious. There are a few instances, however, when inaccurate readings may be obtained, for instance if the probe is not properly sealed in the ear canal, if the beam is not directed toward the eardrum, if cerumen is present, or if there is an infection of the middle ear.

The thermometer is extremely easy to use. You simply position the covered plastic tip properly inside the auditory canal and press the scan button, and an infrared beam measures the heat waves (Figure 13-16). The results are displayed digitally on the screen. A release button ejects the probe cover, and in 10 seconds another temperature can be taken. The method is acceptable to patients and is a time saver to the health care worker. The units operate on three AAA alkaline batteries and will measure at least 10,000 temperatures before the batteries need to be replaced. Many clinics, urgent care centers, and private practices use aural thermometers. (See Procedure 13-9.)

Temporal Artery Thermometer

The latest thermometer to be developed is the temporal *scanner* or, as it is commonly called, the temporal artery thermometer (TAT) (Figure 13-17A). There are both home and clinical models available. The TAT determines body temperature by measuring the temperature of the skin over the temporal artery (TA) of the forehead where the artery is less than 2 mm below the surface of the skin. The probe of the thermometer has a sensor that assesses the infrared heat in the artery. Temperature is measured by scanning (gently sliding) the probe of the hand-held thermometer across the forehead, halfway between the eyebrow and the hairline, from the midline to the side hairline (Figure 13-17B). As long as the button is depressed and the scanner is moved slowly, it continually samples and records to measure the highest temperature. Multiple readings can cool the skin, so another immediate measurement may be slightly lower.

Clinical studies have shown TA measurement provides results more closely related to the true internal body temperature measured in a major artery than any other method. The normal TA measurement is equivalent to a rectal temperature, so therefore it is approximately one degree higher than oral measurement. *Note:* When recording on the chart, put (TA) after the temperature to indicate the method used. (See Procedure 13-10.)

Measuring temperature using a TAT has several advantages:

- Appropriate for all ages, infants through elderly
- Convenient, easily accessible, and fast
- Comfortable and safe for the patient
- Proven highly accurate
- No danger from contact with mucous membranes

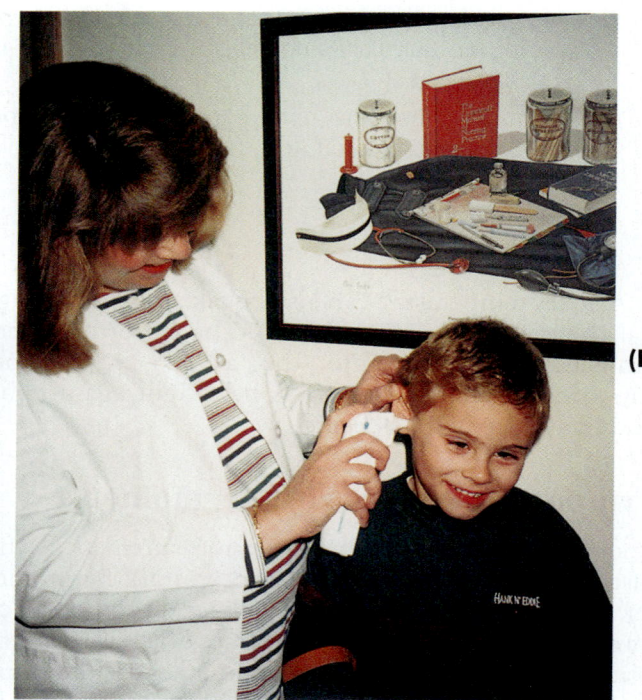

(D)

FIGURE 13-16 Tympanic (aural) thermometer; (A) holder; (B) tympanic thermometer; (C) cover; (D) measuring core body temperature with an aural thermometer.

13-9  Measure Core Body Temperature with an Infrared Tympanic Thermometer

PURPOSE: To determine a patient's core body temperature using an infrared tympanic thermometer.

EQUIPMENT: Tympanic thermometer unit, probe cover, waste container, paper, and pen or pencil.

PERFORMANCE OBJECTIVE: In a simulated or actual situation and given access to all necessary equipment and supplies, measure and record core body temperature within 3 minutes, following the steps in the procedure and observing aseptic and safety precautions. Recorded findings must agree with the instructor's reading.

1. Wash hands.
2. Identify the patient. **RATIONALE: Speaking to the patient by name and checking the chart ensures that you are performing the procedure on the correct patient.**
3. Explain the procedure and what you are going to do.
4. Remove the thermometer from the base.
5. Attach a disposable probe cover to the ear piece. **NOTE: The display should read "ready."**

6. Insert the covered probe into the ear canal, sealing the opening.
7. Press the scan button to activate the thermometer.
8. Withdraw the thermometer.
9. Observe the display window, noting the temperature.
10. Press the release button on the thermometer to eject the probe cover into a waste container.
11. Record the temperature using (T) or (Tc) to indicate tympanic or tympanic core temperature.
12. Return the thermometer to the base. **NOTE: Thermometers can be set to correlate with an oral or rectal reading. Usually, the oral mode is used, and a reading of 98.6°F is considered "normal."**

CHARTING EXAMPLE

5-10-XX

T. 100.3 (Tc)

J. Cook, CMA

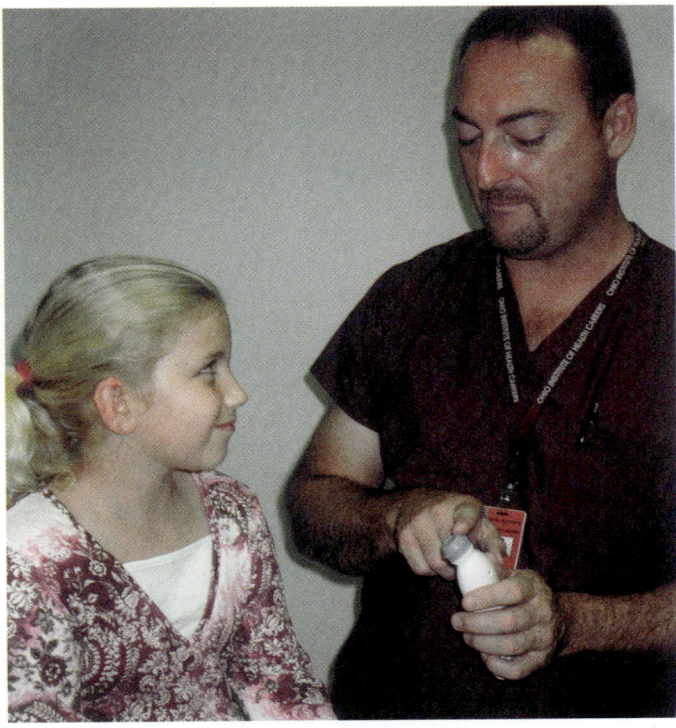

FIGURE 13-17A Temporal artery thermometer

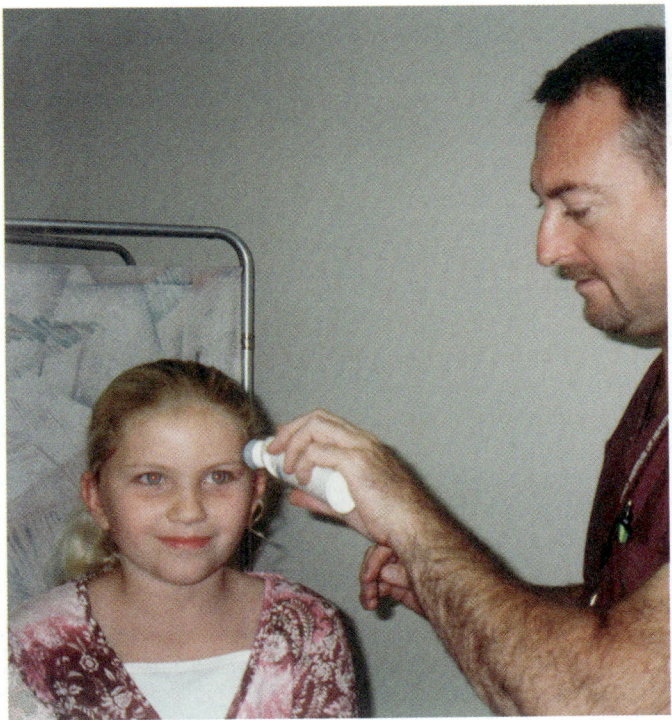

FIGURE 13-17B Slide thermometer across forehead.

13-10  Measure Temperature with a Temporal Artery Thermometer

PURPOSE: Measure a patient's temperature with a temporal artery thermometer.

EQUIPMENT: Temporal artery thermometer, pen, paper, alcohol wipe or cover.

PERFORMANCE OBJECTIVE: With access to all equipment, follow the steps in the procedure to measure and accurately record a patient's temperature using a temporal artery thermometer. Recorded findings must be within $1/10°$ of instructor's findings.

1. Wash hands.
2. Clean the probe with alcohol or attach a cover.
3. Identify the patient. **RATIONALE: Speaking to the patient by name and checking the chart ensures that you are performing the procedure on the correct patient.**
4. Explain the procedure.
5. Observe the forehead for perspiration and exposure to the environment; adjust as necessary (e.g., remove hat, hold back hair).
6. Position the probe at the midline of the forehead.

7. Keeping the probe flush on the skin, press and hold the scan button while slowly sliding the thermometer across the forehead until reaching the hairline. If perspiration is present, continue to hold button, lift probe from forehead, and position on neck behind ear lobe. **NOTE: You will hear clicking indicating a rise to a higher temperature until the maximum is measured.**
8. When scanning is completed, release the button and lift the probe from the forehead or neck. Read the temperature on the display. **NOTE: The reading will remain on the display until 15 to 30 seconds after the button is released, depending on the model. To turn off the thermometer immediately, depress and quickly release the button.**
9. Accurately record the measurement on the chart.

CHARTING EXAMPLE

4-10-xx

T. 99.5 (TA)

J. Cole, CMA

- Reading is not affected by oral factors such as hot and cold fluids, mouth breathing, oral surgery, or injury.
- Can be sanitized between patients like a stethoscope, with an antiseptic wipe, or clinical models have covers, caps, and sheaths if desired

Temperature of the skin is affected by the temperature of the surroundings. The sensor in the probe performs two processes when temperature is measured. At 1,000 times per second it reads the infrared heat within the artery and also measures the temperature in the immediate environment. The interior software performs calculations to determine the patient's temperature in relation to the surroundings. There are, however, a few factors that affect the accurate measurement:

- Do not glide the probe over burns, open sores, abrasions, or scars.
- The forehead side measured must have been exposed to the environment with, no hats, bangs, or bandages to trap heat.
- If there is perspiration on the forehead, measurement will be inaccurate. You must follow TA mea-

surement with placing the probe against the neck behind the earlobe to obtain accurate assessment (Figure 13-17C).

- The TAT must be in the same ambient temperature as the patient. It must be acclimated to the room temperature before it is use if it is moved from a hot to cold area or vice versa (e.g., window ledge exposed to hot sun or in line of air conditioning). Each 10° degree difference can cause a 1° error.
- Some models cannot be used near aerosol products or when oxygen is being administered.
- Do not drop or expose the unit to electric shocks.
- Do not try to sterilize except in gas sterilizer (follow manufacturer's directions).

It is important that the probe lens and cone be very clean so the thermometer can "see" the heat clearly. It can be cleaned with an alcohol swab or wiped with an alcohol preparation between patients. Hold the thermometer upside-down to prevent excess moisture from entering the sensor area. Occasionally follow with a damp water wipe to remove alcohol residue. If it does become wet, it will not damage the sensor but you cannot use the TAT until it dries. A variety of disposable

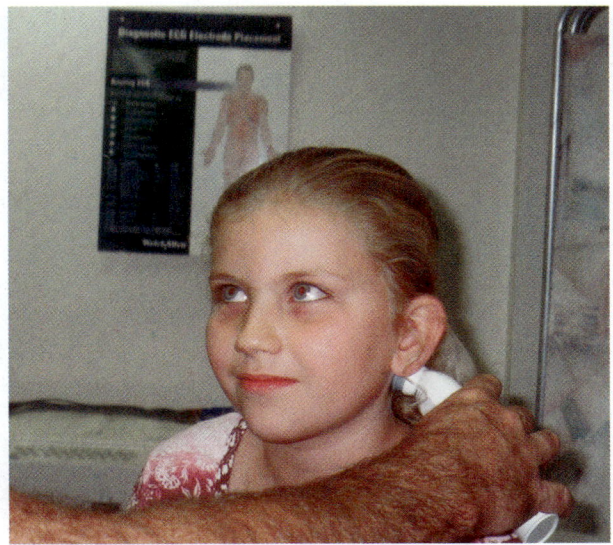

FIGURE 13-17C Touch neck behind ear lobe.

probe covers, caps, or sheaths can be used instead of alcohol cleaning if desired.

Head Injury and Diaphoresis   There will be perspiration on the forehead when an elevated temperature is resolving, which results in cooling the skin and causing a lower reading. During fever, the area of the artery behind the ear lobe is usually not affected and experiences a higher flow of blood, making it a good site for measurement. Perform the following technique to ensure accurate results:

1. Scan the temperature, keeping the button depressed.
2. Gently place the probe on the neck directly behind the ear lobe.
3. Release the button and read the temperature.

With head trauma and dressings, the scanner is placed behind the ear only. Head trauma results in increased blood flow behind the ear, as does diaphoresis.

False Readings   False low readings can be caused by:

- Multiple readings cooling the skin
- Allowing the probe to angle from the skin
- Scanning too rapidly
- Forehead in direct draft from fan or air-conditioning

False high readings can be caused by:

- Skin being covered (remove a hat or hold back hair for designated time; see instructional manual)
- Sunburn

The TAT has another unique feature. If the forehead is not an appropriate site for measurement, tempera-

ture can be measured in alternative sites. Temperatures can be taken over the femoral artery, lateral thoracic, or axillary areas.

Home Measurement

Often the physician will suggest a patient monitor his temperature at home. It may be the medical assistant's responsibility to instruct the patient about using a thermometer and how to record his temperature. The physician will have a certain elevated temperature level that is considered appropriate for an office visit. This should be made known to the patient, and he should be instructed to call the office if that level is reached.

Many different types of temperature measuring devices are available for home use in addition to the ones discussed in this unit. Usually exact measurement is not too critical, and so less expensive but easy-to-use models are appropriate. For children, the FeverScan ultra forehead thermometer (Figure 13-18A) provides an inexpensive method for identifying the presence of elevated temperature or a temperature trend, but it only measures in full degrees. A liquid crystal plastic strip is held against the forehead until the colors stop changing, about 15 seconds. The temperature is read *before* the strip is removed from the forehead. This simple thermometer is available at most pharmacies and children's stores.

Another type of thermometer is the mercury-free oral model. It resembles the former glass mercury style except it is filled with an environmentally safe mercury substitute (Figure 13-18B). It is used like the glass mercury thermometer in that it must be shaken down to about 95° before use and requires at least 3 minutes to register. It is more accurate than the plastic strip in that it is calibrated in tenths of degrees. The thermometer should be sanitized with soap and water and alcohol after use. It is not appropriate for infants and small chil-

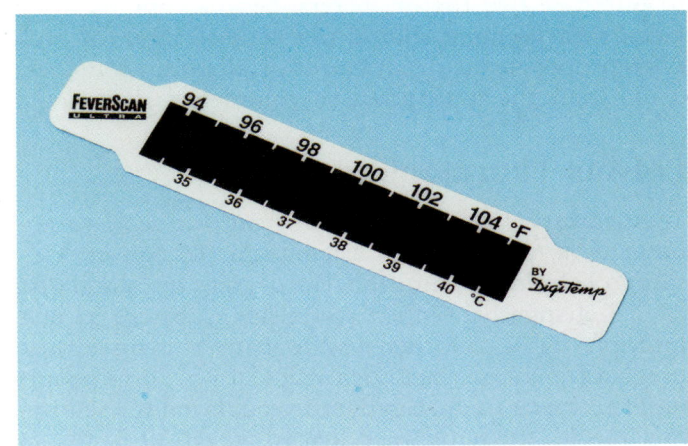

FIGURE 13-18A Thermometers for home use: FeverScan forehead thermometer

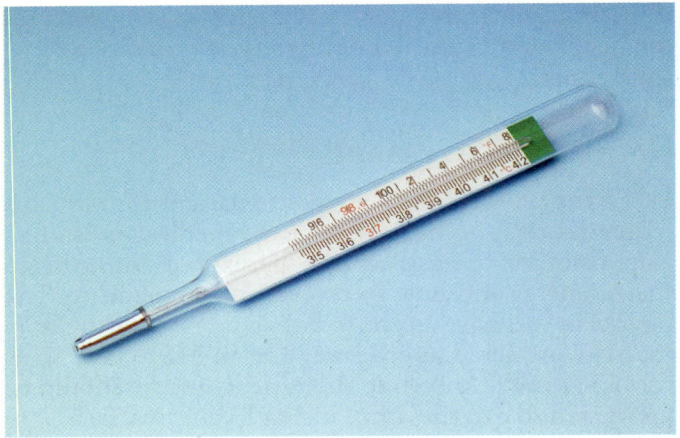

FIGURE 13-18B Mercury-free oral thermometer.

dren. This model is also inexpensive and available at most pharmacies. The home model of the temporal thermometer would provide excellent temperature assessment, but at present it is quite expensive. It is used very similarly to the clinical model and is available at large chain pharmacies and children's stores.

The ear thermometer has been used in the home for quite some time; however, false readings are common because of improper technique. Also, if the person has an ear infection or excessive cerumen in the canal, the reading will not be accurate. It is easy to use and is appropriate for infants and small children.

The digital thermometer is probably one of the best options for home because it is relatively inexpensive; is easy to use; has a digital readout; and can be used for oral, axillary, and rectal measurement. It registers temperature rather quickly and beeps when the maximum is reached. Children like to listen for the beep. If the family has very young children, and might be taking rectal temperatures, remind them that it would be best to purchase two thermometers, because one used for rectal measurement should not be used later for oral. With proper cleansing and alcohol, all family members could share the appropriate thermometers.

Celsius Thermometers

Temperature can be converted from one scale to another by a mathematical calculation. To convert Celsius to Fahrenheit, multiply the degrees by $\frac{9}{5}$ and add 32. To change Fahrenheit to Celsius, subtract 32 and multiply by $\frac{5}{9}$. Another way to convert temperature uses a different mathematical calculation. Some people find this easier to do. Centigrade equals Fahrenheit minus 32 with the remainder divided by 1.8.

$$C = \frac{F - 32}{1.8}$$

TABLE 13-4 Temperature Conversion and Comparison

To convert Celsius to Fahrenheit:

$$37°C \times \frac{9}{5}\left(\frac{333}{5}\right) = 66.6 + 32 = 98.6°F$$

$$C = \frac{F - 32}{1.8} \quad (C = 98.6 - 32 = \frac{66.6}{1.8} = 37)$$

To convert Fahrenheit to Celsius:

$$98.6°F - 32 = 66.6 \times \frac{5}{9}\left(\frac{333}{9}\right) = 37°C$$

$$F = (C \times 1.8) + 32 \quad (F = 37 \times 1.8 = 66.6 + 32 = 98.6)$$

Comparison	Celsius (C)	Fahrenheit (F)
Freezing	0°	32°
Body temperature	37°	98.6°
Pasteurization	63°	145°
Boiling	100°	212°
Sterilizing (autoclave)	121°	250.0°

To convert Fahrenheit to centigrade the equation is:

$$F = (C \times 1.8) + 32.$$

Table 13-4 shows examples of temperature conversions and compares some common temperatures.

PULSE

Each time the heart beats, blood is forced into the aorta, temporarily expanding its walls and initiating a wavelike effect. This wave continues through all the body's arteries, causing the alternating expansion and recoil of the arterial walls (Figure 13-19). This effect

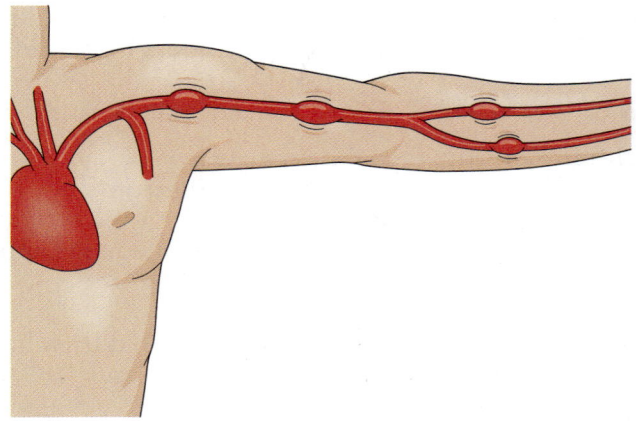

FIGURE 13-19 Blood pumped from the heart causes a wavelike effect in the arteries.

can be **palpated** (felt) in the arteries that are close to the body surface and that lie over bone or firm structures. When the artery is pressed against the underlying structure, it is possible to feel the rhythmic pulsation, known as the pulse.

Pulse Points

The pulse can be felt in several locations on the body (Figure 13-20). The **radial** pulse point is on the thumb side of the inner surface of the wrist, lying over the ra-

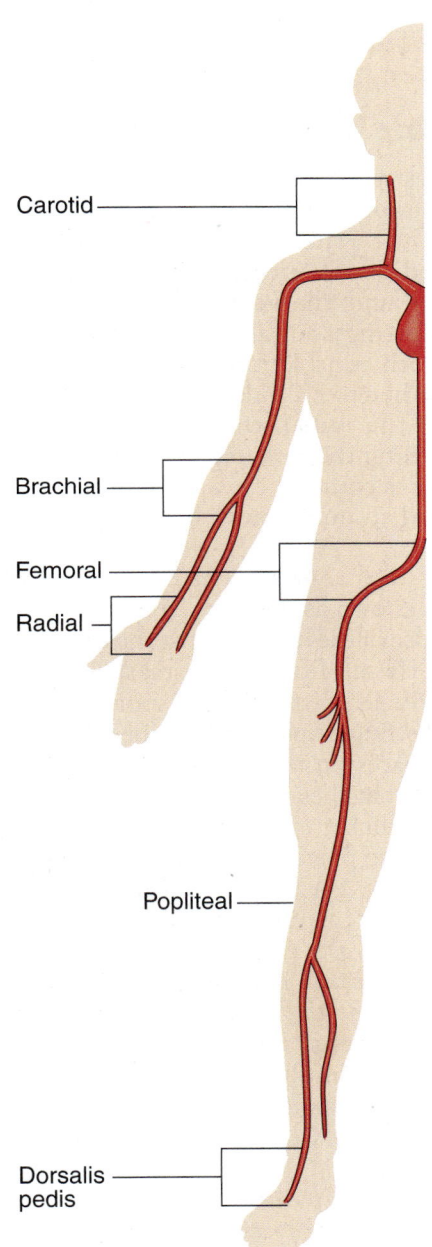

dius bone. The radial pulse point is used most frequently when measuring pulse rate.

The **brachial** artery pulse point is on the inner medial surface of the elbow, at the **antecubital** space (crease of elbow). This point is used to palpate and **auscultate** (listen to) blood pressure.

The **carotid** pulse can be felt in the carotid artery of the neck when pressure is applied to the area at either side of the trachea. It is the carotid pulse that is palpated during the cardiopulmonary resuscitation (CPR) life-saving maneuver.

The **femoral point**, located midway in the **groin** where the artery begins its descent down the femur; the **dorsalis pedis**, on the instep of the foot; and the **popliteal**, at the back of the knee, are other points palpated to evaluate circulation in the lower extremities.

Pulse Rate

The number of times the heart beats per minute is typically measured by counting the pulse in the radial artery. The average adult pulse rate is 72 beats per minute. The pulse rate is recorded as beats per minute preceded by a capital *P* (i.e., P. 72).

The rate of the pulse is influenced by several factors. The most obvious is exercise or activity. With increased activity, the heartbeat increases 20 to 30 beats per minute to meet the body's needs. It should return to normal within 3 minutes after activity has stopped. Of course, the rate of increase will be in proportion to the level of activity.

Pulse rate is directly related to age. The younger the person, the faster the heartbeat. A sample of age-related average pulse rates is shown in Table 13-5.

Pulse rate is also related to the gender of the patient. A female's pulse is approximately 10 beats per minute more rapid than a male's of the same age. Pulse rate is also related to size; therefore a larger person will have a slower rate than a smaller person. The relationship of size is particularly evident in animals. The heart rate of

Pulse points labeled (from top): Carotid, Brachial, Femoral, Radial, Popliteal, Dorsalis pedis

FIGURE 13-20 Pulse points of the upper and lower extremities and the neck

TABLE 13-5 Pulse–Age Relationship	
Age	**Pulse Rate**
Less than 1 year	100–170
2–6 years	90–115
6–10 years	80–110
11–16 years	70–95
Midlife adult	65–80
Older adult	50–65

a bird may be well over 200 beats per minute, while an elephant has a rate of about 30.

The physical condition of the body is another factor. Athletes, especially those who run or engage in strenuous sports, have a considerably slower pulse rate as a result of a more efficient circulatory system.

In general, the heart rate increases when the sympathetic nervous system is stimulated by feelings such as fear, anxiety, pain, or anger. The rate also increases with certain other conditions, such as thyroid disease, anemia, shock, or fever. A consistent rate of more than 100 beats per minute is known as *tachycardia*.

When the parasympathetic nervous system affects the heart, it causes the rate to be much slower. A consistent rate below 60 beats per minute is known as *bradycardia*. This may also occur with the use of certain medications, heart disease, emotional depression, and drugs. A rate below 60 beats per minute is also normal for many athletes.

Pulse Characteristics

When measuring pulse rate, two other characteristics must also be observed and recorded. The force or strength of the pulse is referred to as its **volume**. Words used to describe this quality are normal, full or bounding, weak, and **thready** (scarcely perceivable).

The quality of **rhythm** of the pulse refers to its regularity, or the equal spacing of the beats. The term **arrhythmia** refers to a pulse that lacks a regular rhythm. The pulse can be irregular (without a consistent pattern) or regularly irregular (unequally spaced but consistently the same beating pattern). A pulse can also be intermittent and occasionally skip or insert beats. Often caffeine or nicotine react on the heart to cause irregularity and increased rate.

Measuring the Radial Pulse

The patient should be completely relaxed and sitting comfortably or lying down when the pulse is measured and evaluated. Ideally the arm should be well supported, with the wrist near the level of the heart. Place the tips of your fingers at the wrist area, about an inch above the base of the thumb (Figure 13-21). Never use your thumb to measure pulse rate; there is a chance you may feel and record your own heart rate in your thumb's artery.

An appropriate amount of pressure applied to the artery will permit the pulsations to be felt. Too much pressure will shut off the circulation and therefore eliminate the pulse beat. Too little pressure will not compress the artery sufficiently against the radius. With practice, applying the correct amount of pressure will become routine. (See Procedure 13-11.)

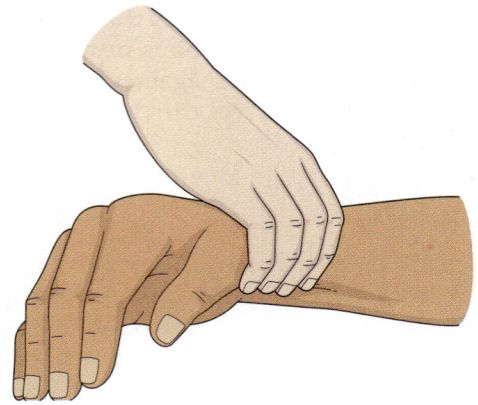

FIGURE 13-21   Measuring the radial pulse

Measuring the Apical Pulse

In instances when measuring heart rate by the radial pulse is not appropriate, it is necessary to listen to the heart at its **apex** with a **stethoscope**. This is a very accurate method of measuring pulse rate. The contraction of the atria and the ventricles will be heard as two closely occurring sounds, known as the "lubb dupp"; however, both contraction phases are counted as only one beat. Whenever a pulse rate is measured at a point other than the radial, the location should be noted when recording the rate (e.g., P. 97 [Ap]). Note that an **apical** pulse is counted for a full minute, so it is possible to record an uneven number.

Locating the Apex   The bottom or lower edge of the heart is known as the apex. This is the point of maximum impulse of the heart against the chest wall. It can be palpated at the left fifth intercostal space in line with the middle of the left clavicle. This spot may be located by pressing the fingertips between the ribs and counting down five spaces on the left chest wall (Figure 13-22A). Often the beat at the apex can be felt with the fingertips.

Another, quicker method for estimating the location of the apex is to place the outstretched *left* hand on the chest wall with the tip of the middle finger in the suprasternal notch and the thumb at a 45-degree angle (Figure 13-22B). The end of the thumb will be approximately over the apex. This is only an approximate measurement because the size of the chest and the hand will vary. For a ready reference point, the apex should be just below the left breast. Again, this is variable, particularly in the female, because of the size and placement of the breast. Refer to Procedure 13-12.

Apical Indications   Apical pulse measurement is indicated for infants and small children because of their normally rapid rate, which is easier to hear and count than to palpate. Patients with heart conditions,

PROCEDURE PROCEDURE PROCEDURE PROCEDURE PROCEDURE PROCEDURE PROCEDURE PROCEDURE

13-11  Measure the Radial Pulse

PURPOSE: To determine the rate, rhythm, and quality of a patient's radial pulse.

EQUIPMENT: Watch with sweep second hand, paper, and pen or pencil.

PERFORMANCE OBJECTIVE: In a simulated or actual situation and given access to all necessary equipment and supplies, within 4 minutes assess and record the quality and measure and record the rate of a patient's radial pulse following the steps in the procedure. Recorded rate findings must be within two beats per minute of the instructor's measurement and agree as to rhythm and quality characteristics.

1. Wash hands; assemble equipment.
2. Identify the patient. **RATIONALE: Speaking to the patient by name and checking the chart ensures that you are performing the procedure on the correct patient.**
3. Explain the procedure. Identify what you are going to do.
4. Determine the patient's recent activity. **RATIONALE: Exertion within the past 3 to 5 minutes will cause a temporary increase in pulse rate.**
5. Have the patient assume a comfortable position with the arm supported, palm of hand down, wrist near level of heart or placed across upper abdomen if lying down.
6. Locate the radial artery on the thumb side of the wrist. **NOTE: Do not use your thumb. Place the tips of your fingers lightly over the artery.**

7. Observe the quality of the pulse before beginning to count. Determine whether it is regular, strong, weak, or thready. **RATIONALE: Concentration on the quality prior to measurement assists in accurate evaluation.**
8. Check your watch. Begin counting beats when the second hand is at 3, 6, 9, or 12. **(NOTE: This makes 30 seconds easier to observe).**
9. Count a *regular* pulse for 30 seconds and multiply the results by two. This will always be an even number. If *irregular,* count for full minute. Do not multiply by 2. **RATIONALE: The pulse rate is recorded in beats per minute; you have already determined the total beats per minute.**
10. Record the pulse in beats per minute. **NOTE: Immediate recording helps eliminate errors.**
11. Describe the quality characteristics. **RATIONALE: In certain disease conditions the presence or absence of quality characteristics is a significant finding.**
12. Wash hands.

CHARTING EXAMPLE

5-10-XX

P. 96, weak but regular

J. Cook, CMA

especially if being medicated with cardiac drugs, will require apical measurement for greater accuracy. Apical measurement is always indicated if you have difficulty feeling a radial pulse and believe you may be missing beats. Other indications are an excessively rapid or slow rate, a thready or irregular quality, or with an existing or suspected pulse deficit.

Measuring an Apical-Radial Pulse

Certain heart conditions cause a symptom known as **pulse deficit**. A patient with a pulse deficit will have a higher apical than radial pulse rate. This difference indicates that some heart contractions are not strong

enough to produce a palpable radial pulse. It is important to determine the extent of the deficit by measuring the apical and radial rate at the same time.

A procedure called *apical-radial pulse* requires one person to measure the pulse rate radially while another auscultates the apical rate with a stethoscope (Figure 13-23). The radial rate is then subtracted from the apical, the difference being the pulse deficit. Ideally, two people measure the rate at the same time. If this is not possible, then the apical rate is measured and recorded, followed immediately by the radial. Apical-radial rates are always measured for 1 full minute. The physician may have a preferred method for recording this procedure. It will probably include

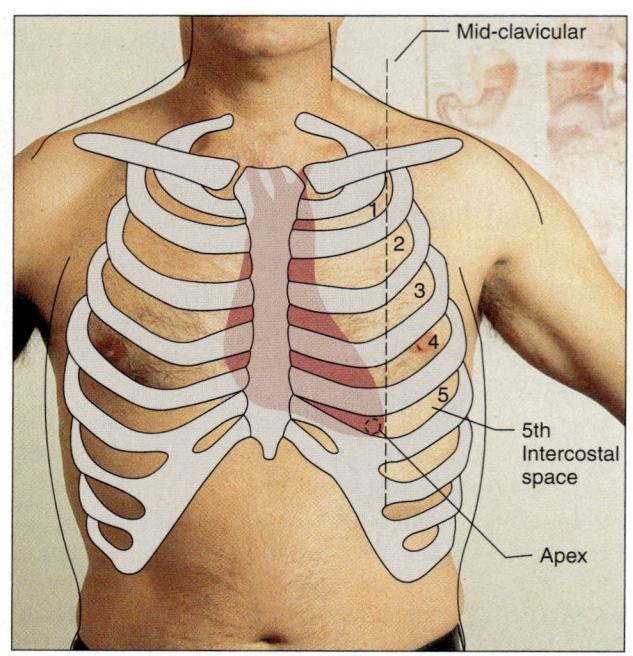

FIGURE 13-22A Locate the apical pulse by counting inter-costal spaces

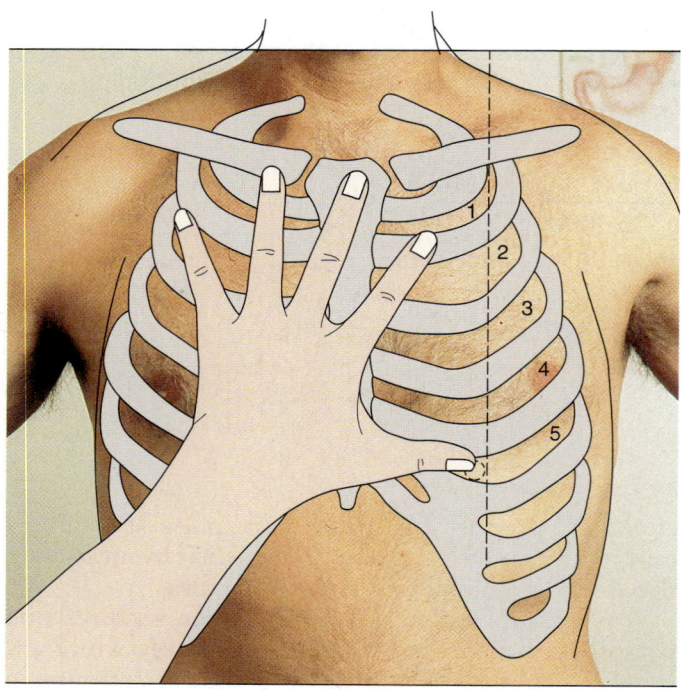

FIGURE 13-22B Alternative method for locating the apex of the heart

both apical and radial pulse rates and the deficit. Examples of a format that can be used are:

P. 97 (Ap) 75 (R), 22 deficit

or, written as a fraction: P. $\dfrac{97\,(Ap)}{75\,(R)}$ = 22 deficit

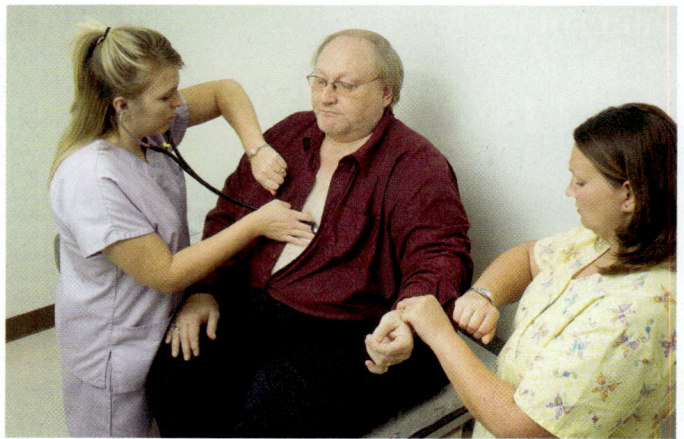

FIGURE 13-23 Measuring apical-radial pulse

RESPIRATION

The third vital sign to be measured is respiration. One respiration is the combination of total inspiration (breathing in) and total expiration (breathing out). Other frequently used terms are **inhale** and **exhale**.

Respirations are usually measured as one part of total vital signs assessment. Because patients can voluntarily control the depth, rate, and regularity of their breathing to some extent, it is important that they not be aware the procedure is being done. To accomplish this, it is common practice to observe and measure respiration immediately after assessing the pulse, while maintaining your fingers at the radial pulse or auscultating the apex. Using this method, the patient assumes you are still measuring pulse rate.

Quality of Respiration

Respirations should be quiet, effortless, and regularly spaced. Breathing should be through the nose with the mouth closed. Excessively fast and deep breathing, commonly associated with hysteria, is called **hyperventilation**. Difficult or labored breathing is called **dyspnea**. Frequently dyspnea is accompanied by discomfort and an anxious expression, caused by the fear of being unable to breathe. This patient will use the accessory respiratory muscles of the rib cage, neck, shoulders, and back to assist the breathing process.

The presence of **rales** (noisy breathing) usually indicates constricted bronchial passageways or the collection of fluid or exudate. Rales may be present with pneumonia, bronchitis, asthma, and other pulmonary diseases.

Respirations should be observed for the depth of inhalation. Three words are used to describe this quality: normal, shallow, or deep. Depth of inhalation can

PROCEDURE PROCEDURE PROCEDURE PROCEDURE PROCEDURE PROCEDURE PROCEDURE PROCEDURE

13-12  Measure the Apical Pulse

PURPOSE: To determine the rate, rhythm, and quality of a patient's apical pulse.

EQUIPMENT: Watch with sweep second hand, stethoscope, alcohol wipe, paper, and pen or pencil.

PERFORMANCE OBJECTIVE: In a simulated or actual situation and given access to all necessary equipment and supplies, within 5 minutes locate the apex of the heart, assess and record the quality, and measure and record the rate of a patient's apical pulse, following the steps in the procedure and observing aseptic precautions. Recorded rate findings must be within one beat per minute of the instructor's measurement and agree as to rhythm and quality characteristics.

1. Wash hands.

2. Prepare the stethoscope by wiping earpieces and chestpiece with germicidal solution to prevent transfer of organisms.

3. Identify the patient. **RATIONALE: Speaking to the patient by name and checking the chart ensures that you are performing the procedure on the correct patient.**

4. Tell the patient what you are going to do. If the patient is an infant or small child, explain the procedure to the parent.

5. Provide privacy and a gown or drape if indicated.

6. Uncover the left side of the chest. **RATIONALE: Auscultation must be done directly against the skin surface.**

7. Place the earpieces in your ears. The openings in the tips should be forward, entering the auditory canal.

8. Locate the apex by palpating to the left fifth intercostal space at the midclavicular line. **NOTE: If the chestpiece does not have a chill ring, warm it in the palm of one hand while locating the apex. This also prevents accidental striking against a hard surface and the resulting noise in your ears.**

9. Place the chestpiece of the stethoscope at the apex.

10. Determine the quality of the heart sounds. **NOTE: Concentrate on rhythm and volume. RATIONALE: The quality of the beat is significant in evaluation of the heart action.**

11. Concentrate on rate of beats. **NOTE: Be certain of sounds and pattern.**

12. Observe watch and begin counting rate when second hand is at 3, 6, 9, or 12. **RATIONALE: It is easier to measure 1 minute when beginning at one of these four numbers.**

13. Count the beats for a full minute. **NOTE: Both pulse phases count as one beat. RATIONALE: Apical rates are indicated when quality or rhythm irregularities are present or possible; therefore, full-minute measurement is essential.**

14. Remove the earpieces from your ears.

15. Record the rate and quality of the heart sounds.

    NOTE: ■ Immediate recording aids in eliminating errors.
    ■ Indicate it is apical measurement.

16. Assist or instruct the patient to dress unless the physician also wishes to assess heart action. Determine this by asking the physician prior to measurement or if your findings indicate the need.

17. Wipe the earpieces and chestpiece of the stethoscope with disinfectant. Return it to storage.

18. Wash hands.

CHARTING EXAMPLE

5-10-XX

P. 103 (Ap), full but irregular with an extra beat every four beats

J. Cook, CMA

---

be determined by watching the rise and fall of the chest. The rhythm of the respirations must also be assessed. This quality can be described as regular or irregular. Absence of breathing is known as **apnea**. A breathing pattern called **Cheyne-Stokes** occurs with acute brain, heart, or lung damage or disease and with intoxicants. It is characterized by slow, shallow breaths that increase in depth and frequency, followed by a few shallow breaths, and then a period of apnea for 10 to 20 seconds and often more (Figure 13-24). This type of breathing pattern frequently precedes death.

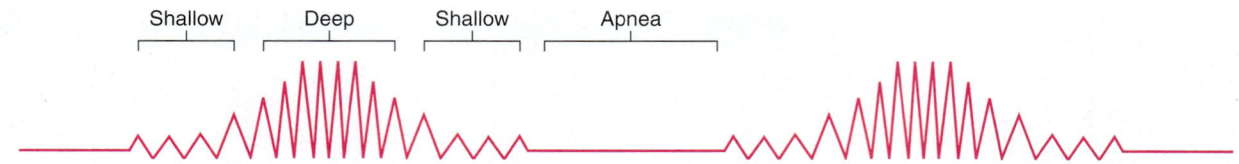

Shallow   Deep   Shallow   Apnea

FIGURE 13-24 Cheyne-Stokes breathing pattern

Respiration Rate

The normal respiration rate for adults is 16 to 20 times per minute. The respiration rate in infants and children has a greater range and fluctuates more during illness, exercise, and emotion than adult rates do. In the newborn, the rate per minute may range from 30 to 80; in early childhood, from 20 to 40; and during late childhood from 16 to 26. The rate will reach an adult normal range of 16 to 20 by age 15. An abnormally slow rate of respiration is known as *bradypnea*. A faster than normal rate of respiration is known as *tachypnea*.

Counting Respirations

It is necessary to observe the patient carefully while measuring respiration rate. If the patient is lying on the examination table, position the patient's arm across the upper abdominal area, placing your fingers over the radial pulse point. In this position you can visualize and feel respiration. With the patient in a sitting position, you will need to observe more carefully as you count the respirations (Figure 13-25). Remember, it is also necessary to keep your watch in view as you observe. With a little practice, you will be able to manage both at the same time.

When counting respirations as part of the TPR assessment, it is very important that you remember the number of heartbeats you have just counted. It may help you to use the following method:

1. Assume the pulse measuring position.
2. Observe, determine the characteristics, and describe to yourself the qualities of both the pulse and the respirations.
3. Count the number of heartbeats during the first 30 seconds of the minute.
4. Repeat the pulse rate to yourself as you count the number of respirations during the second 30 seconds. (*Note:* You *must* use the word "and" between each respiration so you do not accidentally add counts to the pulse rate.)

For example, if your patient's pulse rate after 30 seconds is 40, repeat this number as you count the respirations: "40 and 1, 40 and 2, 40 and 3," and so on, until the second 30-second period is past. At the end of a minute, you will have both rates counted. Multiply the rates by two and record. (Refer to Procedure 13-13.)

TEMPERATURE-PULSE-RESPIRATION RATIO

Respiration rate, like pulse, will increase with activity, excitement, fear, other strong emotions, and certain disease conditions. Whenever a patient, either child or adult, has been upset and crying, a time must pass before an accurate measurement of either pulse or respirations can be made. Strong emotions elevate the vital signs and may make a true measurement impossible. Respirations and the pulse are also affected by the degree of fever present. Table 13-6 demonstrates the relationship of the first three vital signs.

BLOOD PRESSURE

The fourth vital sign is blood pressure. Learning to assess blood pressure accurately requires attention to details, careful listening, and correct technique. The term *blood pressure* means the fluctuating pressure that the blood exerts against the arterial walls as the heart alternately contracts and relaxes. The blood pressure reflects the condition of the heart, the amount of blood forced from the heart at contraction, the condition of the arteries, and to some extent the volume and viscosity (stickiness) of the blood.

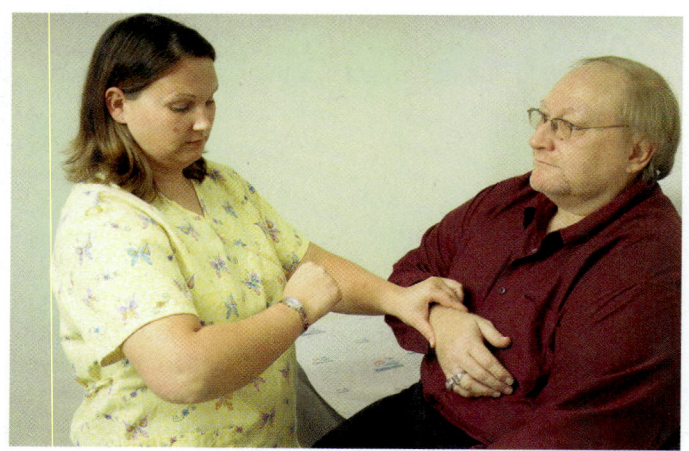

FIGURE 13-25 Measuring respirations

13-13  Measure Respirations

PURPOSE: To determine the rate, rhythm, sound, and depth of a patient's respirations.

EQUIPMENT: Watch with sweep second hand, paper, and pen or pencil.

PERFORMANCE OBJECTIVE: In a simulated or actual situation and given access to all necessary equipment and supplies, assess and record the quality and rate of a patient's respirations within 3 minutes, following the steps in the procedure. Recorded rate findings must be within two breaths per minute of instructor's measurement and agree as to rhythm, sound, and depth quality characteristics.

1. Wash hands.

2. Identify the patient. **RATIONALE: Speaking to the patient by name and checking the chart ensures that you are performing the procedure on the correct patient. NOTE: In this procedure, it is preferable *not* to explain to the patient what you are about to do. If the patient knows that you will be counting respirations, control of breathing is possible, resulting in an inaccurate measurement.**

3. Ask about recent activity level. **RATIONALE: Patient should have been relatively quiet for the past 2 to 5 minutes to obtain an accurate assessment.**

4. Place the patient in a comfortable position, sitting or lying down.

5. Assume the pulse measurement position. **RATIONALE: Respirations are more easily counted if patient's arm is across upper abdomen.**

6. Assess respiration quality. **NOTE: Determine depth, rhythm, and sound.**

7. Count respirations for 30 seconds. **NOTE: One rise and fall of the chest equals one respiration. Maintain the radial pulse position. RATIONALE: Patients must be unaware you are measuring respirations so they do not unintentionally or purposely alter the rate or rhythm.**

8. Multiply results by two and record. **NOTE: If respirations are irregular, count for a full minute and do *not* multiply results by two. RATIONALE: The rate per minute has already been determined.**

9. Record quality characteristics. **RATIONALE: In certain disease conditions, the presence or absence of quality characteristics is a significant finding.**

10. Wash hands.

CHARTING EXAMPLE

5-10-XX

R. 24, shallow, regular, and somewhat noisy

B. Cole, CMA

TABLE 13-6 Temperature–Pulse–Respiration Ratio		
Respiration	**Pulse**	**Temperature (F°)**
18	80	99
19 (plus)	88	100
21	96	101
23	104	102
25 (minus)	112	103
27	120	104
28 (minus)	128	105
30	136	106

* Plus and minus refer to a halfway point between two numbers.

Blood pressure is measured in the brachial artery of the arm at the antecubital space (Figure 13-26). It should be measured in both arms, at least initially. There is normally a 5- to 10-mm difference. Subsequent readings should be made on the arm with the higher pressure.

Maintaining Blood Pressure

Two main factors cooperate to maintain a fairly constant blood pressure. The first is the heart or pump, which exerts pressure on the blood. About 100,000 times a day the heart contracts, forcing blood into the aorta and throughout the blood vessels of the body. Without a strong, effective pump, the blood will not flow and the pressure will drop.

The second factor is the brain, which controls, through the autonomic nervous system, the rate of the heart and the size of the opening or caliber of the ar-

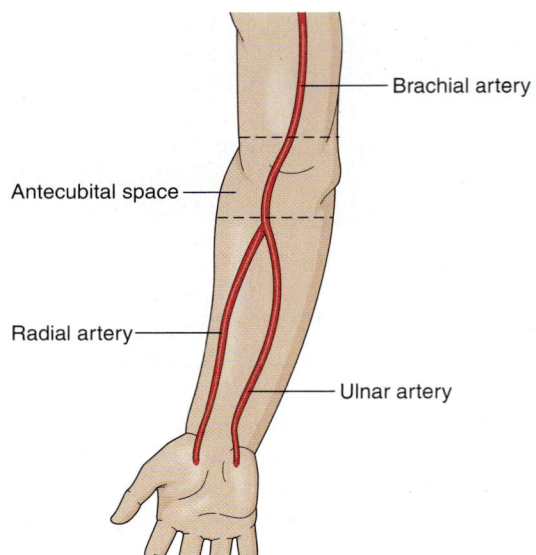

FIGURE 13-26   Blood pressure is measured in the brachial artery at the antecubital space.

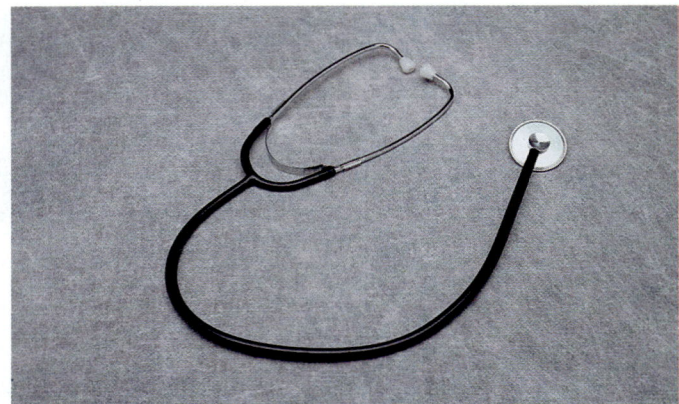

FIGURE 13-27A   Blood pressure measuring equipment: stethoscope.

teries. When sensors in the arteries detect an increase in arterial pressure, a message is sent to the brain, which in turn directs the arteries to dilate slightly (reducing resistance to the flow of blood) and directs the heart to slow down (reducing the amount of blood being forced out). When the pressure drops too far, the message to the brain results in slightly increased heart action and constriction of the arteries, which cause the pressure to rise. Both actions are needed to maintain homeostasis.

Blood Pressure Phases

The phases of blood pressure are identical to those of the pulse. A contraction phase, known as *systole*, corresponds to the beat phase of the heart and is the period of greatest pressure. The relaxation phase, known as *diastole*, corresponds to the resting or filling action of the heart and is the period of least pressure.

Normal Blood Pressure

Blood pressure is measured using a stethoscope and a **sphygmomanometer** (Figures 13-27A and B). Blood pressure readings are measurements of systolic and diastolic pressure written as a fraction; for example, B/P 120/80, where 120 is systolic and 80 is diastolic pressure.

An adult should have a systolic pressure less than 120 mm Hg and a diastolic pressure less than 80. Blood pressure readings persistently above 140/90 indicate stage 1 *hypertension* (high blood pressure).

Hypertension can result from things such as stress, obesity, high salt intake, sedentary lifestyle, and aging. Physical conditions that cause hypertension are kidney disease; thyroid dysfunction; neurologic disorders; and

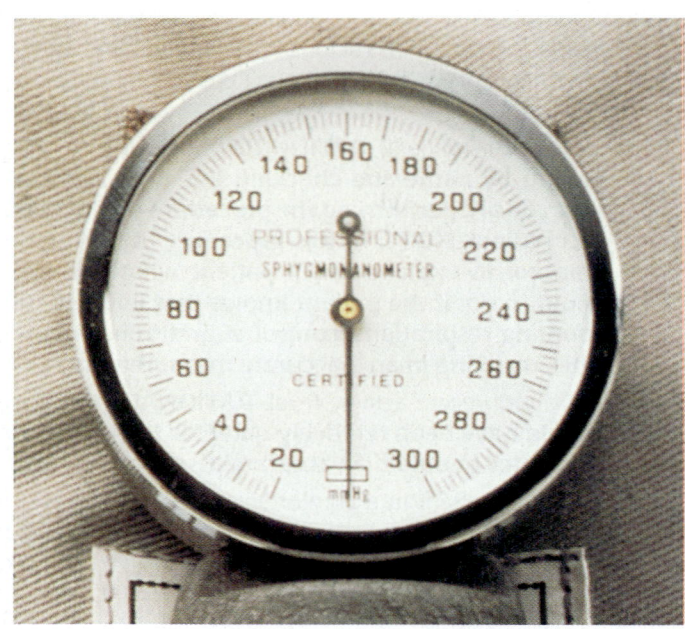

FIGURE 13-27B   Aneroid sphygmomanometer dial

vascular conditions (such as atherosclerosis and arteriosclerosis), which make circulation more difficult, therefore requiring a greater pressure to circulate the blood. An elevated pressure without apparent cause is said to be **idiopathic** or **essential** stage 1 hypertension. Other terms used to identify types of hypertension include:

- Primary—without another identifiable cause
- Secondary—results from renal disease or another identifiable cause
- Malignant—severe, difficult, or impossible to control

Hypertension can also be defined by stages as they relate to blood pressure findings. Table 13-7 contains information from the *Seventh Report of the Joint National Committee on Detection, Evaluation, and Treatment of High Blood Pressure.*

Table 13-7 classifies blood pressure for adults older than 18 years. It is based on the average of two or more properly measured B/P readings on each of two or more office visits. The *Seventh Report* added a new category, "prehypertension," and lowered the "normal" range to 120/80. It has been determined that people with prehypertension are twice as likely to develop hypertension as those with lower findings. The higher the blood pressure, the greater the chance for heart attack, heart failure, stroke, and kidney disease.

A blood pressure consistently below 90/60 indicates *hypotension* (low blood pressure), which may be normal for some persons. Hypotension will be present with heart failure, severe burns, dehydration, deep depression, hemorrhage, and shock.

A drop in blood pressure may occur when a patient changes from sitting to a standing position. This is known as **orthostatic** hypotension and occurs commonly in elderly patients because of decreased circulation efficiency. It often results in dizziness and sometimes syncope. Certain medications can also be the cause. Typically, if blood pressure is measured, it will show a drop of at least 20 mm Hg systolic and 10 mm Hg diastolic. Some physicians routinely assess orthostatic pressure on all older patients as part of the physical assessment.

Pulse Pressure

Pulse pressure refers to the difference between the systolic and diastolic reading and is an indicator of the tone of the arterial walls. For example, when the pressure is 120/80, the pulse pressure is 40, which is a normal finding. A pulse pressure over 50 or less than 30 mm Hg may be considered abnormal. A general rule of thumb is that the pulse pressure should be approximately a third of the systolic measurement. If less, the patient may have an auscultatory gap (absence of sound), and the pressure may have been incorrectly measured. This disorder will be described later.

Equipment Factors

It is important that sphygmomanometers be in proper working order and correctly calibrated. Figure 13-28 shows an **aneroid** sphygmomanometer.

Aneroid models must be checked regularly over the entire pressure range.

Studies have shown many sphygmomanometers used in family practice to be faulty. There are two primary areas of failure. The control valves of the cuffs often result in leakage, and a greater problem with accuracy occurs as a result of dial errors because they are rarely calibrated.

It is important that sphygmomanometers be serviced regularly. Faults in aneroid models have to be corrected by service technicians or the manufacturer.

The office should have a maintenance policy whereby all sphygmomanometers are on a scheduled service plan. This is normally a requirement for practices receiving reimbursement from third-party payers.

Blood pressure cuffs are critical to correct measurement. They are available in different sizes to measure blood pressure in neonates (infants), children, adults,

				Initial Drug Therapy	
Blood Pressure Classification	**Systolic Blood Pressure (mm Hg)**	**Diastolic Blood Pressure (mm Hg)**	**Lifestyle Modification**	**Without Compelling Indication**	**With Compelling Indications**
Normal	<120	and <80	Encourage	No antihypertensive drug indicated	Drugs for compelling indications
Prehypertension	120–139	or 80–89	Yes	No antihypertensive drug indicated	Drugs for compelling indications; other antihypertenive drugs as needed (diuretics, ACEI, ARB, BB, CCB)
Stage 1 hypertension	140–159	or 90–99	Yes	Thiazide-type diuretics for most; may consider ACEI, ARB, BB, CCB, or combination	
Stage 2 hyptertension	≥160	or ≥100	Yes	Two-drug combination for most usually (thiazide-type diuretic and ACEI, ARB, BB, CCB)	

TABLE 13-7   Classification and Management of Blood Pressure for Adults

ACEI, *angiotensin-converting enzyme inhibitor;* ARB, *angiotensin receptor blocker;* BB, *beta blocker;* CCB, *calcium-channel blocker.*
Source: *Seventh Report of the Joint National Committee on Detection, Evaluation, and Treatment of High Blood Pressure (JNC 7).*

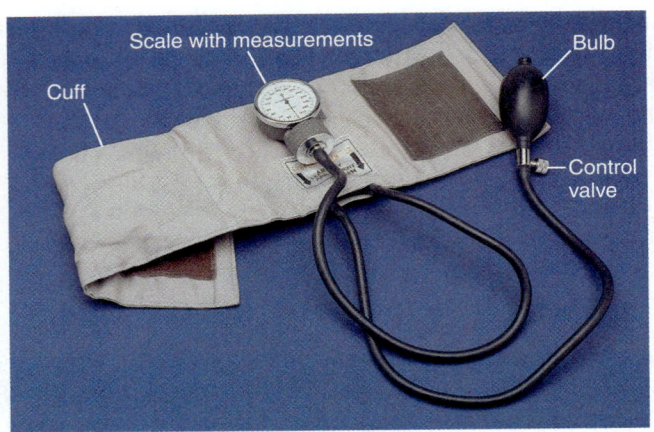

FIGURE 13-28 Aneroid sphygmomanometer

obese adults, and adult thighs (Figure 13-29). If the reading is to be accurate, the cuff must be the appropriate size. If it is too small for the upper arm, the reading will be falsely high; if too large, falsely low. To determine the proper size, compare the cuff width to the width of the upper arm. The cuff should be about 20% wider than the arm. When a cuff is too small and you do not have access to a wide adult cuff, measure to the width of the forearm. If the cuff is of adequate size, take the blood pressure reading in the forearm by placing the stethoscope over the radial artery.

An electronic sphygmomanometer is totally automatic and facilitates blood pressure measurement by providing a digital readout in the display window (Figure 13-30). It does not require the use of a stethoscope and should eliminate errors from improper technique or hearing difficulties. Once the cuff is applied, the operator presses a button (Figure 13-30A) and the cuff automatically inflates, releases pressure slowly, and records the results. The results in the readout window (Figure 11-30B) show a blood pressure of 128/78. The units are quite expensive and are more likely to be used in a cardi-

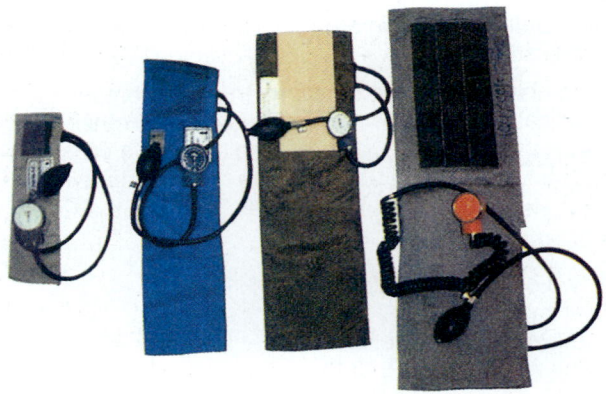

FIGURE 13-29 Blood pressure cuffs in different sizes to fit the arm of a small child to an adult thigh

ologist's office or a hospital setting. The equipment also has a pulse oximeter feature, which measures pulse rate and oxygen concentration when the sensor is attached to the finger. (Note white clip on patient's finger.) In the readout window (Figure 13-30B), note the pulse oximeter read an oxygen concentration of 97% and a pulse rate of 85. As with any piece of mechanical equipment, if the reading seems unlikely it should be repeated or checked with another piece of equipment.

Measuring Techniques

Because blood pressure readings are so critical to the determination of hypertension and consequently to the medication given for managing it, strict procedure techniques must be followed when using manual equipment. Several factors affect the accuracy of results.

1. The cuff must be completely deflated when applied.
2. The patient must be comfortable, with the arm slightly flexed at the elbow and the brachial artery on a level with the heart. The arm must be free of a constricting sleeve (Figure 13-31). *Note:* A study at Duke University, reported in the Harvard Medical School's *Heart Letter,* stated that researchers had taken blood pressure measurements through clothing on 36 volunteers to determine if readings would be inaccurate. One arm was bare, whereas the other was covered with clothing, either a shirt or a shirt with a light sweater. Simultaneous automated blood pressure measurements revealed that findings through light clothing were within 2 mm Hg of the results on bare skin. It was felt that based on this data, patients visiting a physician for a simple blood pressure reading may not need to change into a gown if the clothing covering the arm is light. This decision, however, needs to be made by the employing physician.
3. The center of the bladder in the cuff must be placed over the brachial artery. Fold the bladder area of the cuff in half to locate the center. Many cuffs have improper artery markings.
4. The manometer must be viewed directly from a distance of not more than 3 feet.
5. A palpatory reading should be taken first to determine proper inflation. Afterward, deflate the cuff completely by compressing with your hands before reinflation.
6. A minimum of 15 seconds should elapse between inflations (30 is better) to allow blood pressure to normalize.
7. The cuff should be inflated rapidly to 30 mm Hg above the palpatory reading.

To obtain a baseline reading for new patients it may be desirable to measure the pressure twice in each arm, once while the patient is sitting and once while lying down.

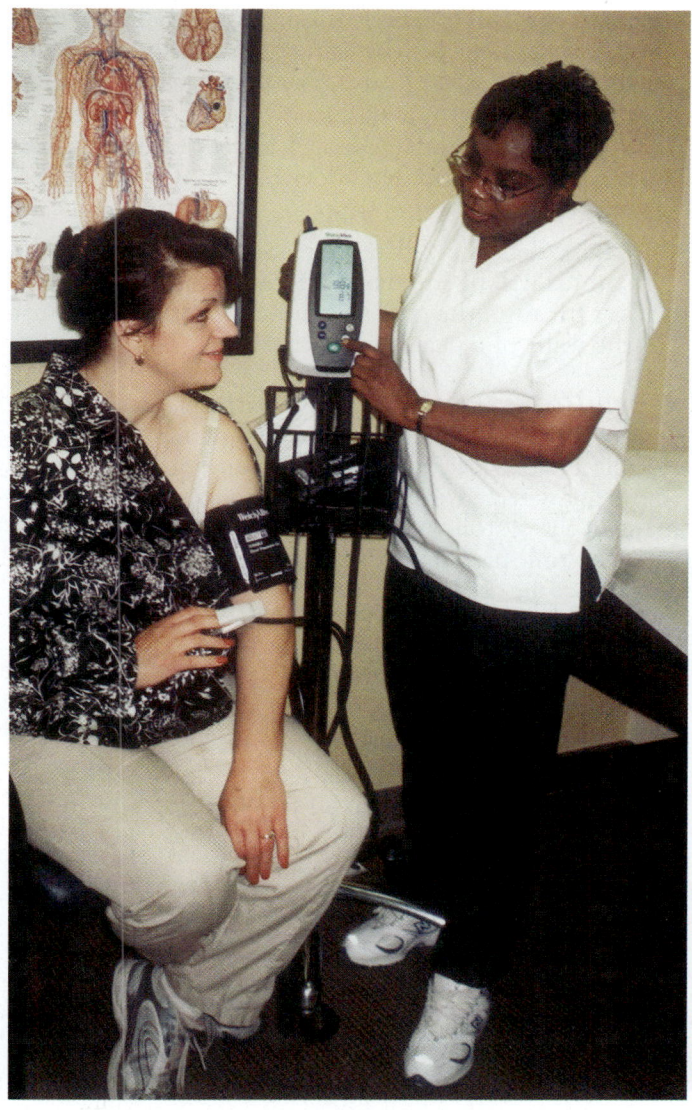

(A)

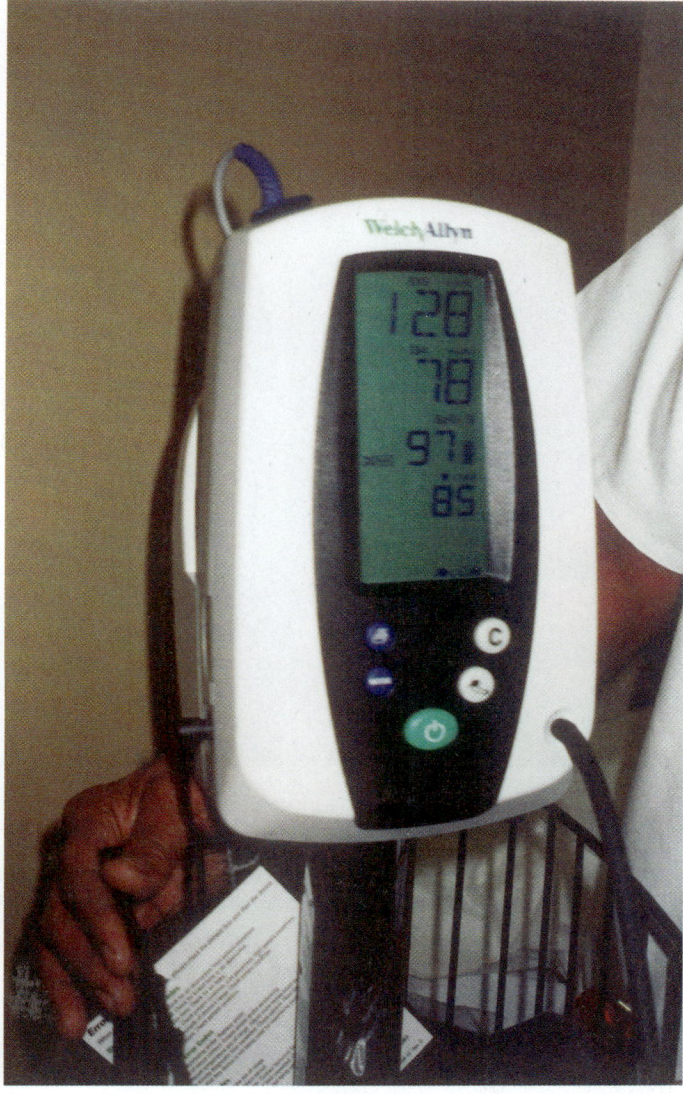

(B)

FIGURE 13-30   Measuring blood pressure with an electronic sphygmomanometer

As stated earlier, in certain situations, it may be necessary to obtain orthostatic blood pressure measurement in addition to the general measurement. If this is desired, simply follow the regular sitting or prone measurement by having the patient stand and immediately measure and record the results. Observe the patient for signs of dizziness or syncope.

Blood pressure has two phases, both of which must be determined. When the cuff is properly inflated, the valve must be opened carefully to allow deflation at a rate of 2 to 3 mm per beat. Listen for the first sounds of heartbeat, and note the reading as the systolic pressure once you have heard at least two consecutive beats. Continue to listen and observe as the cuff is deflated until you hear a sudden change in sound to a softer, muffled tone. Note this reading as the diastolic pressure. Continue to observe the manometer until the sound disappears. Note this reading also, even if 0. To record, for example, you would write: B/P 140/90/70. You should ask the physician which sound, the change or the absence, you are to record as the diastolic measurement. There are reasons to support either method.

Probably the mistake made most often in measuring blood pressure is reinflating the cuff after only partial deflation or too soon after complete deflation. Either error may cause a false reading and will also cause difficulty in hearing the sound changes because of venous congestion in the forearm. (Refer to Procedure 13-14.)

Augmenting Sound   To augment heartbeat sounds when they are difficult to hear, use the following technique:

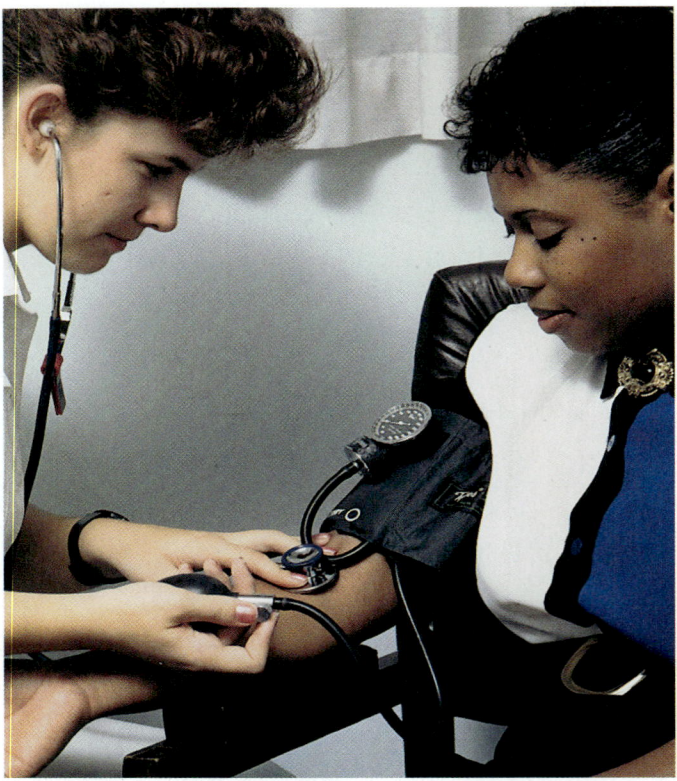

FIGURE 13-31 Measuring blood pressure

1. With the cuff properly applied and deflated, have the patient elevate the arm above the shoulder and make and release a fist a few times to aid in emptying forearm veins (Figure 13-32).
2. With the patient's arm still raised, rapidly inflate the cuff to 30 mm Hg above palpated pulse.
3. Have the patient lower his arm.
4. Begin deflation, listening for initial beats. The sounds will be intensified because the blood spurting through the cuff tourniquet is striking against the walls of a near empty artery.

Auscultatory Gap In some patients, usually those who are hypertensive, there is a silent interval between systolic and diastolic pressure, called an *auscultatory gap*. If this is not detected, it may lead to serious undermeasurement of the systolic pressure. For example, the patient's actual systolic pressure is 200, with a gap from 170 to 140 and a diastolic of 120/110. You inflate the cuff to 170 and hear nothing until the manometer reaches 140, which you presume is the systolic pressure. You would continue deflation and record 120/110 as the diastolic; therefore, you would have a pulse pressure of only 20 or 30 mm Hg. Keeping in mind the normal range for pulse pressure, however, you would view 20/30 as suspicious. Taking one third of 140 would give you about 47. To be certain you

---

PROCEDURE PROCEDURE PROCEDURE PROCEDURE PROCEDURE PROCEDURE PROCEDURE PROCEDURE

13-14  Measure Blood Pressure

PURPOSE: To determine a patient's palpatory and auscultatory blood pressure measurements.

EQUIPMENT: Stethoscope, aneroid manometer, alcohol wipe, paper, and pen or pencil.

PERFORMANCE OBJECTIVE: In a simulated or actual situation and given access to all equipment and supplies, within a 4-minute period of time, measure palpatory and auscultatory blood pressure and record findings following the steps in the procedure and observing safety and aseptic precautions. Recorded findings must be within 2 mm Hg of instructor's measurement. **(NOTE: Accurate procedure evaluation requires the use of a dual teaching stethoscope.)**

1. Wash hands.
2. Assemble the equipment.
3. Clean the earpieces and head of the stethoscope with antiseptic. **RATIONALE: This prevents the transference of microorganisms.**

4. Identify the patient. **RATIONALE: Speaking to the patient by name and checking the chart ensures that you are performing the procedure on the correct patient.**
5. Explain the procedure. **RATIONALE: If it is new to a patient, especially if a child, explain that the cuff will squeeze but that she must not move.**
6. Place the patient in a relaxed and comfortable sitting or lying position.
7. Expose the patient's upper arm well above the elbow, extending the arm with the palm up. The arm may be either bare or covered with light clothing. (See note regarding clothing on page 668) Remove the arm from a constricting sleeve. **NOTE: Arm must be relaxed, on a supporting surface, slightly flexed at the elbow, with the brachial artery approximately at the level of the heart.**
8. With the valve of the inflation bulb open, squeeze all air from the bladder, fold to identify the center, and

(continues)

PROCEDURE PROCEDURE PROCEDURE PROCEDURE PROCEDURE PROCEDURE PROCEDURE

13-14 Measure Blood Pressure (Continued)

place it over the brachial artery, with the bottom edge of the cuff 1 to 2 inches above the elbow. Wrap the cuff smoothly and snugly around the arm, with the deflated bladder centered over the brachial artery. Be certain the dial can be easily viewed and the end of the cuff does not interfere.

9. Take a position with the aneroid dial in direct view.

10. With *one hand,* close the valve on the bulb, turning clockwise. **NOTE: Do not overtighten, or it will be hard to open.**

11. Position your other hand to palpate the radial pulse.

12. Observing the manometer, rapidly inflate the cuff to 30 mm above the level where radial pulse disappears.

13. Open the valve, slowly releasing the air until the radial pulse is detected. **NOTE: This provides information for auscultatory measurement.**

14. Observe the dial reading. **NOTE: This is palpatory systolic pressure, which may be recorded, for example, as B/P 120 (P).**

15. Deflate the cuff rapidly and completely. Squeeze the cuff with hands to empty. **RATIONALE: All the air must be expressed between inflations to obtain accurate results. Adjust the position if necessary.**

16. Position the earpieces of the stethoscope in your ears with the openings entering the ear canals.

17. Palpate the brachial artery at the medial antecubital space with your fingertips.

18. Place the head of the stethoscope directly over the palpated pulse. **NOTE: The stethoscope head should not touch the cuff (creates static).**

19. Close the valve on the bulb and rapidly inflate the cuff to 30 mm above the palpated systolic pressure. **NOTE: A minimum of 15 seconds must have elapsed since the previous inflation. RATIONALE: This is the minimum time required for the normalizing of blood flow through the artery.**

20. Open the valve, slowly deflating the cuff. **NOTE: Pressure should drop 2 to 3 mm Hg per second.**

21. With your eyes directly in line with the dial, note the reading at which you hear systolic pressure. **NOTE: This must be at least two consecutive beats. Remember the systolic measurement.**

22. Allow the pressure to lower steadily until you note a change in sound to a softer, more muffled sound. Note this as diastolic pressure (if so instructed).

23. Continue to release pressure until all sound disappears. Note this point as diastolic pressure (if so instructed).

24. Release the remaining air. Squeeze the cuff between your hands. **RATIONALE: This removes all the remaining air to make the patient more comfortable and ensures accurate results if reevaluation is necessary.**

25. Record the systolic and whichever diastolic reading the physician prefers.

26. Reevaluate if indicated after a minimum of 15 seconds.

27. Remove the stethoscope from your ears.

28. Remove the cuff from the patient's arm.

29. Assist the patient with clothing, if necessary.

30. Clean the tips and head of the stethoscope with alcohol to disinfect. Fold the cuff properly, and place it with the manometer and stethoscope in storage.

31. Wash hands.

CHARTING EXAMPLE

6-30-XX

B/P 186/94 or B/P 186/94/56

B. Davis, CMA

had not missed a portion of the pressure, you would remeasure, palpating the systolic and then inflating the cuff 30 mm above. If sounds were still audible at that point, you would reinflate it higher *after complete deflation* until you hear the first sounds of systolic pressure.

When recording a blood pressure with an auscultatory gap, list your complete findings (e.g., B/P 200/120/110 with the auscultatory gap from 170 to 140).

Blood Pressure in Children

The blood pressure of infants and children is often omitted from the physical examination because it is so difficult to obtain. Variation in blood pressure caused by anxiety and emotional upset make accurate readings very challenging. Basically, the procedure is the same as with adults. Often physicians prefer to do the measurement last after having established some rapport with the child.

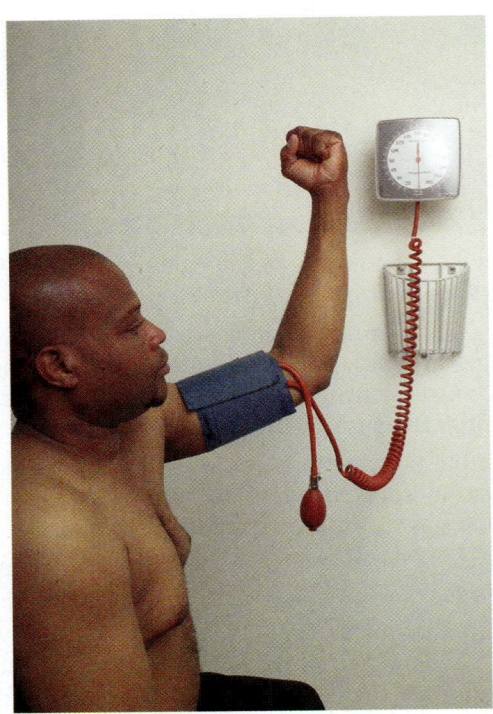

FIGURE 13-32   A technique to augment heart sounds in blood pressure measurement

The cuff size is important in measuring a child's pressure. It should be appropriate to the size of the arm. The inflatable bag must entirely encircle the extremity.

The level of systolic pressure gradually rises throughout childhood. Normal pressure for a 6-month-old is 70; at 1 year it is 95, and it rises to 100 at 6 years. By age 16, the systolic pressure will be 120, the adult average. The diastolic pressure reaches 65 by age 1 and does not change appreciably during childhood.

ACHIEVE UNIT OBJECTIVES

- ■ Complete the Workbook activities to meet the learning objectives.

- ■ Practice the procedures in this unit to meet the performance objectives.

- ■ Apply your knowledge at the end of this Chapter in completing the Critical Thinking Challenge and Activities, as well as the StudyWARE on your Student CD-ROM.

CRITICAL THINKING CHALLENGE

Susan was in to see Dr. Morrison a week ago. She had been experiencing a lot of fatigue, a loss of appetite and consequently weight, and elevated temperature along with night sweats. For some time her lifestyle had been rather carefree, and she had not been very responsible with her sexual behavior. She was frightened and felt she needed to rule out any chance of an HIV infection. Her work outlook was very promising. She was being considered for a new position with her company and would gain a nice salary increase if she was chosen. She would also be eligible for a higher level package of health and life insurance benefits.

The appropriate blood tests were done, and when the results were available, Blair Smith, the medical assistant, called her office. Because she did not answer, he left a message on her voice mail.

Susan returned to her office late in the day after a sales appointment. She thought she would finish up a few details before she went home. It seemed like everyone else had gone. While she was cleaning off her desk, she activated her phone to listen to see if there were any messages. She was shocked when she heard Mr. Smith's message saying her results were positive and she needed to call for an appointment to start treatment. It was then that she realized her boss had just gone past her cubicle to retrieve his forgotten briefcase. She wondered if he too had heard this very personal message. As she sat there, she became very angry. Early the next morning she phoned the physician's office and demanded to talk with the doctor. She wanted to know how this type of call could have happened and why anyone would be so inconsiderate and unprofessional as to leave such a message.

QUESTIONS

1. How does Mr. Smith's action impact the patient? (Consider her personal privacy, her job, and future insurance benefits.)

2. How could this error in judgment affect the practice?

3. How might this action affect Mr. Smith's career?

ACTIVITIES

1. Pair up with a classmate to practice recording a history. The one who is the patient can identify a disease and pretend to have the symptoms. (Check Chapter 11 for ideas). The medical assistant can conduct the interview and obtain the chief complaint and other secondary concerns. See if you can anticipate what type of examination and testing the physician may need to do.

2. Prepare a 3 × 5 card with all your personal health information. Keep this card in your purse or folded in your wallet. It will be very useful to have the information handy if you have to visit a new physician or the emergency department or are admitted to a hospital. The card should include:

   - Family physician's name, address, phone
   - Family member's age or age at death, health state, or cause of death
   - Your past serious illnesses, diagnoses, dates
   - Your past surgical procedures, dates
   - Dates of hospitalizations
   - Your current list of prescription and OTC drugs and dosage
   - If female, your age at first and last menstrual period
   - If female, dates of all births

StudyWARE™ CHALLENGE

- Study with the flash cards for Chapter 13 to review the key terms in this chapter.
- Solve the hangman activities for Chapter 13.
- Complete the true/false quiz in test mode for Chapter 13.

RESOURCES

Exergen Corporation. (2005). *Temporal scanner reference manual*. Watertown, MA.

Harvard Medical School. (1993, November). *Harvard Heart Letter, 4* (3).

Hegner, B., Caldwell, E., and Needham, J. (1999). *Nursing assistant: A nursing process approach* (8th ed.). Clifton Park, NY: Thomson Delmar Learning.

Scott, A., and Fong, E. (1998). *Body structures and functions* (9th ed.). Clifton Park, NY: Thomson Delmar Learning.

U.S. Department Health and Human Services. (2003, December) NIH Publication No 03-5233. Bethesda, MD: National Institutes of Health.

WEB LINKS

www.ama-assn.org (American Medical Association)
Web site maintained by AMA that contains information about the importance of a family medical history, especially when dealing with a condition that may have hereditary tendencies. Also contains an in-depth adult family history form that can be printed and completed.

www.lifeclinic.com (LifeClinic)
Maintained by physicians and educators, this site provides information about several medical conditions that can be positively affected by lifestyle and the close monitoring of changes in vital signs.

Physical Examinations and Assessment Procedures

The medical assistant is responsible for the preparation of patients for examinations and procedures performed by the physician. To gain full cooperation, patients need to be fully informed about what to expect. Keep in mind that just because these procedures and exams are routine for the health care team, they are not for the patient. Patients come to see the physician for many health concerns. Part of your duties is to answer any questions of the patient. Patients commonly ask:

- What exactly is the exam or procedure (brief definition)
- Why it has to be done
- Whether it hurts
- How long it lasts
- Whether there will be additional exams or procedures
- When results and reports will be available

Even if the physician has already explained all this to the patient, you may have to review it and answer questions. In addition to preparing the patient, the medical assistant must also prepare the examination instruments, the table, and the room. The physician may also want the medical assistant to assist directly with the examination by handing instruments, altering the patient's position, or recording his verbal remarks.

In this chapter, the medical assistant's role in the patient examination process is stressed. We discuss the performance of several evaluation tests for the eye and ear as well as preparation of the patient for procedures and examinations. This is followed by instruction for preparing, positioning, and draping the patient and assisting with or serving as writer for the physical examination. Many of the common specialty examinations and procedures as well as the specific examinations and procedures for assessing the pediatric patient are also discussed.

An important and continuing role for the medical assistant is educating the patient in healthful activities and disease or disorder management. Often opportunities for patient teaching occur before, during, and after the examination process. The medical assistant can make note of these and provide instructional sheets, pamphlets, community resources, and personal instruction following the physician's examination. There are many topics appropriate for discussion within "Patient Education" boxes throughout the chapter.

UNIT 1
PROCEDURES OF THE EYE AND EAR

OBJECTIVES

Upon completion of this unit, you will be able to achieve the following:

LEARNING Objectives

1. Spell and define, using the glossary at the back of the text, all the Words to Know in this unit.

2. Describe six patient education topics concerning the eye.

3. Explain why irrigation of the eye or ear is performed.

4. Explain why caution is indicated when administering eye drops or ointment.

5. Identify four vision screening tests and explain what they determine.

6. List five behaviors that indicate the child or adult may be having difficulty reading a vision chart.

7. Name three pieces of equipment used to assess hearing acuity.

PERFORMANCE Objectives

1. Irrigate the eye.
2. Irrigate the ear.
3. Instill ear medication.
4. Instill eye medication.
5. Measure distant vision acuity with a Snellen chart.
6. Measure near vision acuity with a Jaeger chart.
7. Determine color vision acuity using Ishihara plates.

WORDS TO KNOW

achromatic	deuteranopia	ophthalmic
acuity	instill	otic
anesthetize	irrigate	protanopia
audiometer	Ishihara	Snellen chart
auditory	Jaeger	tritanopia
cerumen	lavage	vertex
daltonism	occluder	wick
decibel		

CERTIFICATION CONNECTION

CMA
Treatment area (equipment preparation and operation)
Patient preparation and assisting the physician (examinations, procedures, instruments, supplies, and equipment)

Collection and processing specimens: diagnostic testing (vision testing, hearing testing)

CMAS
Examination preparation

RMA
Visual acuity

EYE AND EAR EXAMINATION

In assisting with eye and ear examinations, you may be expected to hand instruments to the physician as needed. Assembling the instruments in the order of use will be most helpful. You will be responsible for making sure that the instruments are clean and in working order. Otoscopes and ophthalmoscopes should be checked to be sure that the light bulbs and batteries are providing strong enough light (Figures 14-1A and B).

These tiny light bulbs (shown in Figure 14-2) must be changed from time to time because they eventually

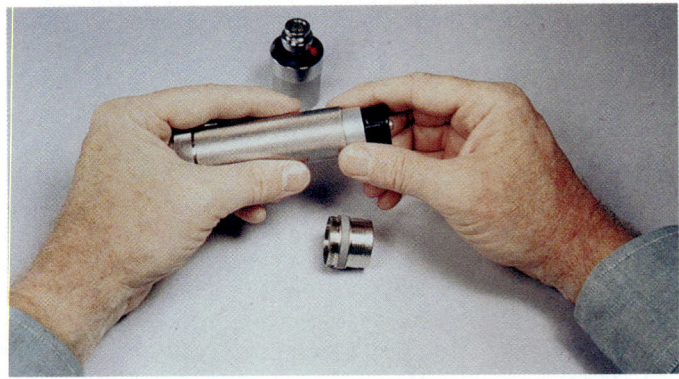

FIGURE 14-1A Power source and recharging methods for hand-held ophthalmoscopes and otoscopes. For C-cell conversion, remove the recharging module and rechargeable battery and replace with two C-cell batteries and converter. *(Courtesy of Welch Allyn, Inc.)*

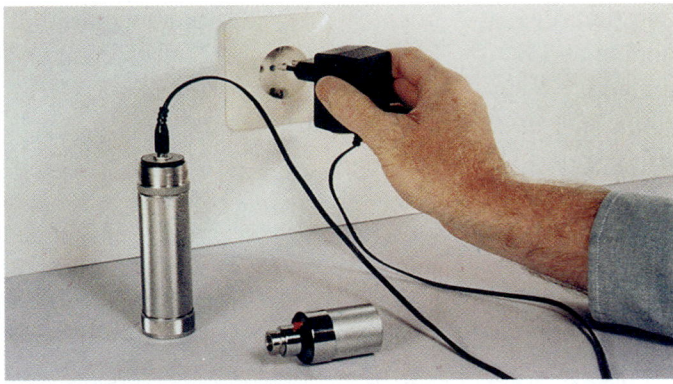

FIGURE 14-1B For rechargeable batteries, place transformer on handle and plug into outlet for easy overnight recharging. *(Courtesy of Welch Allyn, Inc.)*

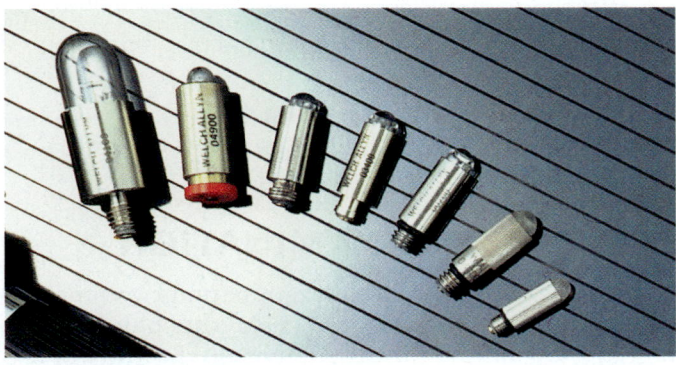

FIGURE 14-2 These tiny lamps are used in instruments requiring a light source and should be checked regularly for power availability. *(Courtesy of Welch Allyn, Inc.)*

burn out, as do any other kind of bulbs. If these instruments are the hand-held portable type, the batteries must also be changed or charged periodically. The medical assistant is usually responsible for these minor but important tasks. More often used in most medical offices are the wall-mounted units with both otoscope and ophthalmoscope instruments (Figure 14-3), which have an electrically powered light source.

The clinical medical assistant should check all exam and procedure rooms daily to make sure there are adequate supplies and lighting. A large part of the examination by the physician is by visual inspection. Lighting is also important to you and patients. You are constantly reading and recording information.

Some patients will need reassurance during the examination because of apprehension caused by an earlier experience or for other reasons. Usually a kind word and a reassuring smile will help them feel at ease, and their cooperation will follow. Remembering their comfort is vital.

Most physicians use the disposable plastic ear speculum, which eliminates the worry of disease transmission. If nondisposable speculums are used, they must be washed after every use with a mild detergent and placed in a disinfectant solution for at least 20 minutes before they can safely be reused to examine another patient. If the patient has an infected ear that has a discharge containing blood, a disposable ear speculum must be used, and protective gloves must be worn.

Patients with discharge of the ear or the eye may require **irrigation** (also known as **lavage**) to remove the drainage. The physician can then examine the ear or eye to determine the extent of injury or disease condition. Perform irrigations of the eye and ear following the steps in Procedures 14-1 and 14-2.

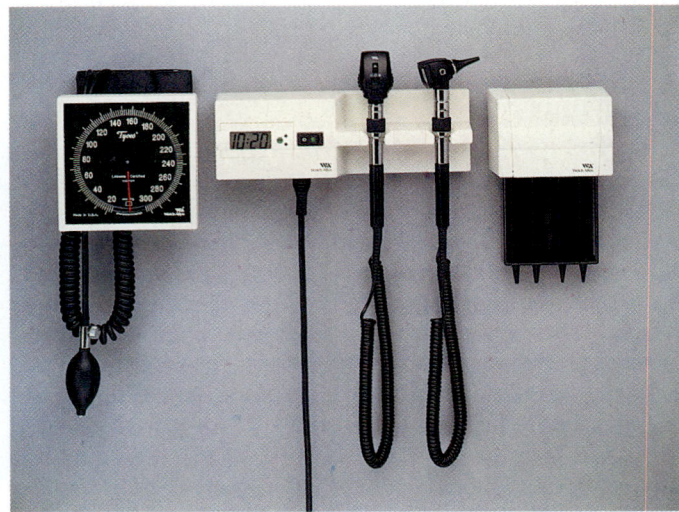

FIGURE 14-3 Wall-mounted set of scopes affords attractive and efficient access. *(Courtesy of Welch Allyn, Inc.)*

PROCEDURE PROCEDURE PROCEDURE PROCEDURE PROCEDURE PROCEDURE PROCEDURE

14-1  Irrigate the Eye

PURPOSE: To irrigate the patient's eye(s) to soothe tissues, relieve inflammation, and remove foreign objects and discharge.

OSHA GUIDELINES: To comply with Standard Precautions, gloves must be worn if there is any possibility of coming into contact with blood or any body fluids.

EQUIPMENT: Latex or vinyl gloves, small basin of lukewarm irrigation solution, towel, emesis basin, irrigation syringe or bottle of solution, gauze squares, patient's chart, and a pen.

PERFORMANCE OBJECTIVE: Provided with a patient or mannequin and all necessary equipment, irrigate the eye(s) following the steps of the procedure. The syringe must not touch the eye, and the patient must remain dry.

1. Wash hands. Assemble the items needed for the procedure; prepare lukewarm solution.

2. Identify the patient. **RATIONALE: Speaking to the patient by name and checking the chart ensures that you are performing the procedure on the correct patient.**

3. Explain the procedure to the patient and assist onto the examination table if desired.

4. Ask the patient which position would be more comfortable, sitting or lying down. Drape the patient with a towel to protect clothing.

5. Put on gloves.

6. Ask the patient to tilt her head back and to the side. Place the emesis basin against her head. Instruct the patient to hold the basin to catch the solution during irrigation. **NOTE: Placing a couple of tissues, gauze squares, or a towel between the face and the basin will help prevent the patient from getting wet during the procedure.** You may have to hold the basin yourself (Figure 14-4).

7. Gently wipe eye with a gauze square from the inner to outer canthus to remove any particles before proceeding with irrigation.

8. Fill a bulb or metal syringe with ordered solution.

9. Hold the affected eye open with the thumb and index finger of one hand or with the little finger of the hand in which you are holding the bottle of solution and slowly release the solution over the eye gently and steadily. **RATIONALE: This must be done from inner canthus to outer canthus to prevent any solu-**

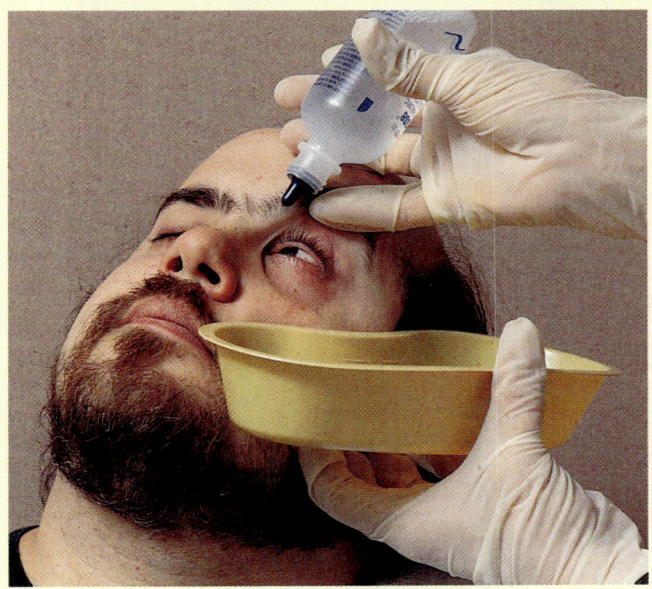

FIGURE 14-4 Direct the flow of irrigation solution from the inner canthus to the outer canthus.

tion from entering the other eye, which may not be affected, and for ease of catching solution.

10. When irrigation is completed, use gauze squares or tissues to blot the area dry.

11. Record the procedure in the patient's chart and initial. **NOTE: Be sure to record the type of solution that was used, which eye was irrigated, results, and any other important information you may have observed while performing the procedure.**

12. Wash the items and return them to the proper storage area.

13. Remove gloves and wash hands. **NOTE: Deposit gloves in an appropriate container based upon the conditions under which irrigation was performed.**

CHARTING EXAMPLE

3-30-XX

Right eye irrig w/ H$_2$O to remove sand, per Dr. White; tolerated well. Pt. states, "eyes less scratchy."

T. Edwards, CMA

PROCEDURE PROCEDURE PROCEDURE PROCEDURE PROCEDURE PROCEDURE PROCEDURE

14-2  Irrigate the Ear

PURPOSE: To irrigate the ear canal to remove foreign objects, impacted cerumen, or drainage.

OSHA GUIDELINES: To comply with Standard Precautions, gloves must be worn if there is any possibility of coming into contact with blood or any body fluids.

EQUIPMENT: Latex or vinyl gloves, small basin, ordered lukewarm irrigation solution, towel, ear basin, Pomeroy or bulb syringe, gauze squares, otoscope, ear speculum, and tissues.

PERFORMANCE OBJECTIVE: Provided with a patient, an anatomical model of the ear, or a mannequin and all necessary equipment, irrigate the ear following the steps of the procedure. The canal must be clean and the tympanic membrane visible for examination.

1. Wash hands. Prepare the solution as ordered, and assemble the necessary items for the procedure. **NOTE: Solution is usually between 100°F and 105°F for patient comfort.**

2. Identify the patient. **RATIONALE: Speaking to the patient by name and checking the chart ensures that you are performing the procedure on the correct patient.**

3. Explain the procedure.

4. Assist the patient onto the examination table or to a chair.

5. Put on gloves.

6. View the affected ear with an otoscope to see where cerumen or the foreign object is located so that the flow of solution can be directed properly. **RATIONALE: The flow should be directed upward and to one side.** To use the otoscope, place one hand gently against the patient's head, and grasp the auricle with your thumb and index finger, pulling up and back for adults and older children and down and back for babies up to 36 months. Avoid using too much pressure as you insert the speculum into the ear canal (Figure 14-5).

7. Ask the patient to turn her head to the affected side and back. Place a towel over the patient's shoulder to protect her clothing (Figure 14-6). For pediatric patients, ask a parent to hold the child on his or her lap and assist you during the procedure.

8. Position the ear basin under the ear for the patient to hold to catch the solution.

9. Use a gauze square to wipe away any particles from the outer ear before proceeding.

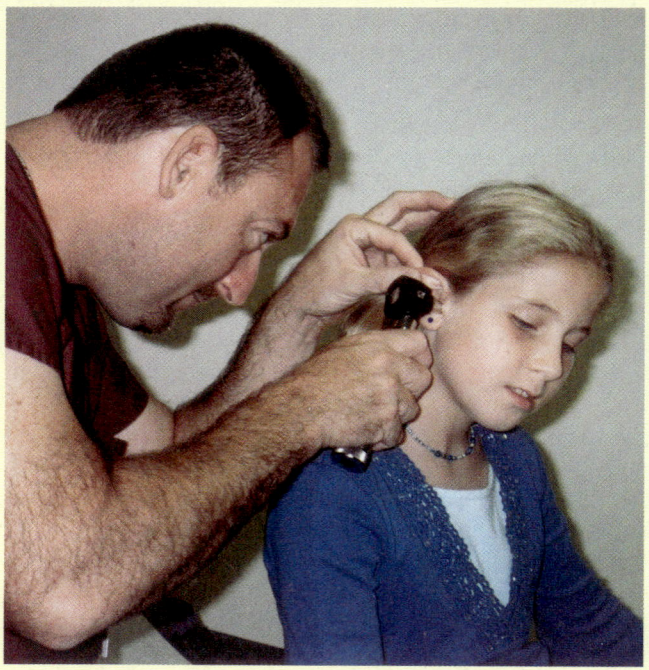

FIGURE 14-5 The otoscope enables viewing of the ear canal and tympanic membrane. The instrument has a light source and a magnifying lens to assist inspection.

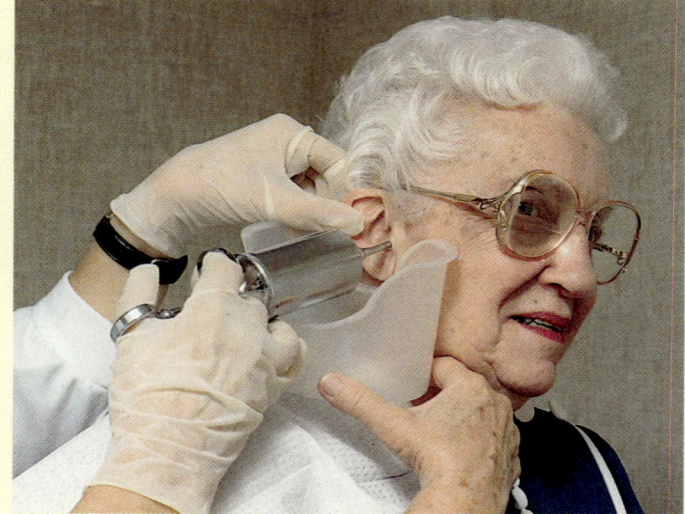

FIGURE 14-6 Drape the patient's shoulder and position the basin under the ear. Ask the patient to hold the basin as you straighten the ear canal and position the syringe for irrigation.

(continues)

PROCEDURE PROCEDURE PROCEDURE PROCEDURE PROCEDURE PROCEDURE PROCEDURE PROCEDURE

14-2  Irrigate the Ear (Continued)

10. Fill the syringe with the ordered solution.

11. With one hand, gently pull the auricle up and back for an adult (down and back for an infant or small child). **RATIONALE: To straighten ear canal.** With the other hand, place the tip of the syringe into the canal, and aim the flow of solution upward so the entire ear canal will be irrigated. DO NOT direct the flow of the solution straight into the ear or use force, or the result will be quite painful for the patient and may damage the tympanic membrane.

12. Use a gauze square to wipe the excess solution from the outside of the patient's ear.

13. Give the patient several gauze squares or tissues, and have the patient tilt his head to the side to allow drainage of excess solution from the canal.

14. Inspect the ear canal with an otoscope to determine if the desired results have been obtained. Repeat irrigation if necessary. **RATIONALE: All material must be removed to adequately inspect the ear canal and tympanic membrane. Patients sometimes feel a little dizzy following this procedure. Allow the patient time to gain balance; assist the patient from the examination table or call the physician to examine.**

15. Record the procedure on the patient's chart and initial, including which ear was irrigated, the solution used, the results of the procedure, and any other important observations.

16. Wash equipment and return it to the proper storage area.

17. Remove gloves and wash hands.

CHARTING EXAMPLE

5-20-XX

Irrigated pt's right ear with water @ 102°F, per Dr. Long; returned three pieces of cerumen (1.25 cm each). Pt states, "I can hear again!"—eardrum is shiny with a pearl-gray color.

T. Edwards, CMA

P PATIENT EDUCATION

1. While performing procedures involving the eye, the medical assistant may want to remind patients to use eye protection when indicated. You might suggest the use of safety glasses or goggles when working with tools that often make particles of material fly into the eye, causing injury. These safety measures are required at the workplace. Your reinforcement may possibly save someone's sight.

2. Remind patients to wear protective sunglasses whenever they are out in direct sun for extended periods because the eyes can become damaged as well as the skin.

3. Patients need to be reminded to have routine eye examinations, especially when the family medical history includes glaucoma, cataracts, or diabetes. Tonometry and funduscopy are recommended examinations of the eye that should be performed every 4 years for patients past 40 years old.

4. Explain to patients that over-the-counter eyedrops should be used carefully and only as directed. The extended use of some preparations may cause tissue damage. They should be used only when necessary and with the advice of the physician.

5. Advise patients not to rub their eyes, because further irritation and possibly tissue damage could result. Itching, burning, or watering eyes can be signs of infection. Rubbing the eyes can transmit additional infection and transmit germs to others, thereby spreading disease.

6. Tell patients that in the event of a chemical splash in the eye, flush the eye with clear (room temperature) water for 20 minutes (nonstop) and seek medical attention immediately.

Medicating the Eye and Ear

You may also have the responsibility of **instilling** drops into a patient's eye or ear. This simply means dropping a solution into the patient's eye or ear to medicate the tissue or to soothe an irritation. Sterile technique must be used when medicating the eye. Recording the name and amount of medication instilled and the organ to which it was administered is a must.

Instillation of the ear is also performed to soften cerumen (ear wax). **Cerumen** is a secretion of the ear. Patients sometimes try to remove it by using a cotton-tipped swab, but this often pushes it farther into the ear canal, where it becomes lodged and hardens. This buildup can become very uncomfortable and eventually impair hearing.

Sometimes it is necessary to instill medication into the ear to soften ear wax before an irrigation procedure can be performed. Follow the steps in Procedure 14-3 to instill ear drops.

Patients should have impacted cerumen removed by a member of the health care team to avoid further discomfort or possible injury to the ear. Many offices and clinics have adopted the water pic for this purpose because of the gentle flow it produces and its convenience for irrigation procedures. A bulb, metal, or plastic sy-

---

PROCEDURE PROCEDURE PROCEDURE PROCEDURE PROCEDURE PROCEDURE PROCEDURE PROCEDURE

14-3  Instill Ear Medication

PURPOSE: To treat infections, relieve pain, and soften ear wax.

OSHA GUIDELINES: To comply with Standard Precautions, gloves must be worn if there is any possibility of coming into contact with blood or any body fluids.

EQUIPMENT: Latex or vinyl gloves, gauze squares, sterile cotton-tipped applicators and cotton balls, sterile dropper, ordered medication (may be in the form of drops or ointment), tissues.

PERFORMANCE OBJECTIVE: Provided with an anatomical model of the ear or a mannequin and all necessary equipment, perform the ear instillation following the steps of the procedure. The dropper must not touch the ear, nor the tip of the ointment tube touch anything except the sterile applicator.

1. Verify the medication ordered by the physician in the patient's chart, and check expiration date.

2. Assemble the necessary items for the procedure. **NOTE: Otic medications are often kept in the refrigerator after they have been opened, so it is necessary to bring them to room temperature by letting the container sit out for a while or by running warm water over the bottle before using it. This is for the comfort of the patient.**

3. Wash hands and put on gloves.

4. Identify the patient. **RATIONALE: Speaking to the patient by name and checking the chart ensures that you are performing the procedure on the correct patient.**

5. Explain the procedure to the patient.

6. a. Open the bottle of otic medication and draw the medication into the dropper. **NOTE: Many prepared ear medications have their own dropper. It is vital that this dropper be used very carefully to keep it sterile. DO NOT touch the tip of the dropper to the ear! Place the bottle cap on a tissue or gauze square with the inside up. If the dropper touches anything OTHER THAN the solution INSIDE the bottle, it is considered contaminated.**

   b. If the medication ordered is an ointment, you should open the tube by removing the cap, being very careful not to touch the tip of the tube. **RATIONALE: If the tip of the tube is touched, it is considered contaminated.** Medication should be instilled by placing a small amount on the tip of a sterile cotton applicator and applying it gently into the ear canal. Use extreme caution to avoid puncturing the tympanic membrane.

7. Ask the patient to sit up straight and tilt the head slightly to the left for instilling the right ear and to the right for the left ear (some patients may prefer to lie down). If the patient is very young or uncooperative, you may need to have another's help with holding the patient during the procedure.

8. Hand a couple of tissues to the patient before you begin. Hold the auricle of the ear *gently* with one hand while you hold the dropper in the other. To straighten the ear canal to allow the medication to enter, pull up and back for adults, and down and back for infants and children up to 36 months.

(continues)

PROCEDURE PROCEDURE PROCEDURE PROCEDURE PROCEDURE PROCEDURE PROCEDURE

14-3  Instill Ear Medication (Continued)

9. Position the dropper with the medication into (but not touching) the ear canal (Figure 14-7). Depress the bulb to release the prescribed amount of drops into the ear. **NOTE: Advise the patient to remain in this position for a minute or so to allow the medication to set-**tle. Any excess may be wiped away with the tissues or gauze squares.

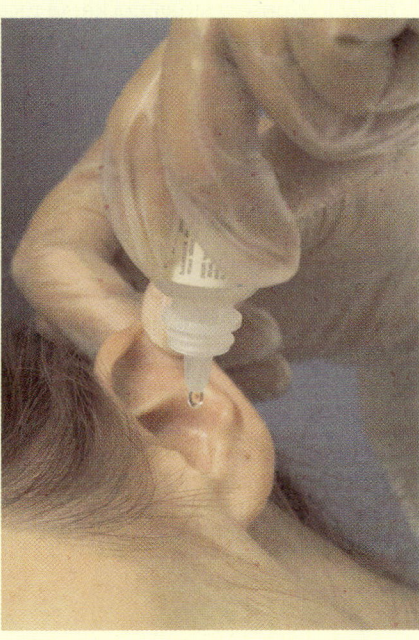

FIGURE 14-7 Ask the patient to tilt his head to the unaffected side as you instill the medication drops carefully into the affected ear canal.

10. Close the bottle or tube of medication. Avoid touching the dropper to the outside of the bottle. **NOTE: If you have touched the patient's ear or anything else, the dropper must be either sterilized or replaced before any other doses of medication can be taken from the bottle.**

11. Remove gloves and wash hands. (This is an ideal time to go over patient education material concerning the ears.) Sometimes physicians will request that sterile cotton be inserted into the ear canal to hold the medication in. Simply place a small portion of the sterile cotton ball gently into the canal after instilling the medication; this is sometimes referred to as a **wick**. It is often saturated with the medication before being placed in the ear canal.

12. Record the procedure on the patient's chart and initial. Be sure to note any complaints of the patient while performing the procedure (e.g., stinging or other discomfort).

13. Return the items to the proper storage area.

CHARTING EXAMPLE

6-13-XX

Instilled 2 gtt of Auralgan into left ear per Dr. Long. Given instruction for home care.

T. Edwards, CMA

ringe is also used to perform the ear irrigation procedure. Some patients will need both irrigation and instillation procedures. A softening solution may be instilled into a severely impacted ear, followed by irrigation to remove the excess ear wax.

After having irrigation procedures performed, even with gentle care, many patients feel a little dizziness. You must be sure that patients are completely stable before permitting them to leave.

A simple method of medicating the eye is accomplished by placing a small amount of ointment just inside the lower eyelid. The tip of the ointment tube must not touch the eyelid, or its contents would be considered contaminated. Care must also be taken when in-stilling eyedrops so that the tip of the dropper does not come in contact with eye tissue. Follow the steps in Procedure 14-4 to instill eye medication.

VISUAL ACUITY

Measuring visual **acuity** is a diagnostic screening procedure most often done by the medical assistant on the patient's initial visit prior to the physical examination. It should be performed in a well-lighted room with no interruptions. Observation of the patient for any conditions or behaviors that may indicate visual disturbances is an essential part of the overall examination.

14-4  Instill Eye Medication

PURPOSE: To instill medication (in the form of drops or ointment) into the eye(s) to relieve irritation; treat infection; dilate the pupil; or **anesthetize** the eye in preparation for an examination or for a surgical procedure.

OSHA GUIDELINES: To comply with Standard Precautions, gloves must be worn if there is any possibility of coming into contact with blood or any body fluids.

EQUIPMENT: Latex or vinyl gloves, ordered medication, sterile eye-dropper, sterile gauze squares, tissues.

PERFORMANCE OBJECTIVES: Provided with a patient, an anatomical model of the eye, or a mannequin and all necessary equipment, instill drops into the eyes following the steps of the procedure without contaminating the dropper or ointment tip.

1. Verify the medication ordered by the physician in the patient's chart (check the expiration date), and assemble necessary items for the procedure. **NOTE: Ophthalmic medications are often kept in the refrigerator after they have been opened, so it is necessary to bring them to room temperature by allowing the drops to sit out for a while or by running warm water over the bottle before using. This is for the comfort of the patient.**

2. Wash hands. Identify the patient. **RATIONALE: Speaking to the patient by name and checking the chart ensures that you are performing the procedure on the correct patient.**

3. Explain the procedure to the patient and assist her onto the examination table or chair.

4. Put on gloves.

5. a. Open the bottle of ophthalmic medication and draw the medication into the dropper. (Many prepared eye medications have their own dropper. It is vital that this dropper be used very carefully to keep it sterile. DO NOT touch the tip of the dropper to the eye!) **RATIONALE: If the dropper touches anything OTHER THAN the solution INSIDE the bottle, it is considered contaminated.**

   b. If the medication ordered is an ointment, you should open the tube by removing the cap, being very careful not to touch the tip of the tube or it will become contaminated.

6. Ask the patient to sit up straight and tilt the head back slightly (some patients may prefer to lie down). If the patient is very young or uncooperative, you may need to have another's help with holding the patient during the procedure.

7. Hand a couple of tissues to the patient before you begin. With one hand, use a sterile gauze square to touch the patient's skin just under the eye and gently pull down. This will expose a small pocket (a recessed area below the eye just inside the lower lid) (Figure 14-8).

8. Hold the dropper steadily approximately $1/4$ inch from the area, being careful NOT to touch the tissue of the eye. Tell the patient to look up while you gently drop the prescribed amount of drops into the pocket of the patient's eye. Ask the patient to blink to further distribute the medication. Ointment medication should be placed carefully and sparingly just inside the lower eye lid without touching the eye tissue. **RATIONALE: The tip can be contaminated if it is touched or touches any surface. NOTE: Advise the patient NOT to rub the eye and not to squeeze out the medications from the eyes. Remind the patient to use the tissues to gently blot excess medication from eyes and not to touch the eyes with bare hands.** (This is an ideal time to go over patient education material concerning the eyes.) Repeat for the other eye if ordered.

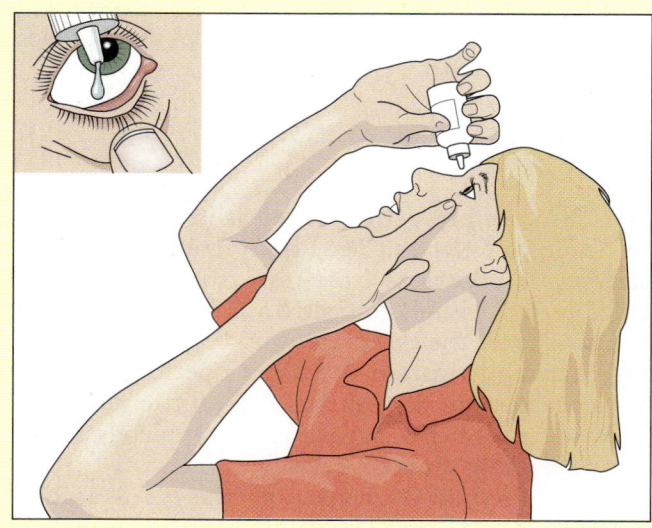

FIGURE 14-8 When instructing patients to use eye drops at home, tell them to tilt their head back and look up. Then gently pull down the skin under the eye to form a small pocket into which the drops are instilled.

(continues)

PROCEDURE PROCEDURE PROCEDURE PROCEDURE PROCEDURE PROCEDURE PROCEDURE

14-4 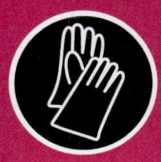 Instill Eye Medication (Continued)

9. Close the bottle or tube of medication. Avoid touching the dropper to the outside of the bottle. **NOTE: If you have touched the patient's eye or anything else with the dropper, it must either be sterilized or replaced before any other doses of medication can be taken from the bottle; otherwise the contents will become contaminated.**

10. Remove gloves and wash hands.

11. Record the procedure on the patient's chart and initial. Be sure to note any complaints of the patient while performing the procedure (e.g., burning or other eye discomfort).

12. Return the items to the proper storage area.

CHARTING EXAMPLE

3-06-XX

1 gtt of Lumigan instilled in each eye per Dr. White; c/o stinging sensation left eye only. Given instruction for daily home instillation.

T. Edwards, CMA

The following are examples of what to look for when performing visual acuity tests:

- Tilting the head to the side or forward
- Blinking or watering of the eyes
- Frowning or puckering of the face
- Closing of one eye when testing both eyes
- Any sign of straining to see

The most common screening device for *distance* vision is a **Snellen chart**, which shows at what distance the chart can be read by the patient. The regular chart has letters arranged in rows from largest to smallest (Figure 14-9).

Those who may have difficulty with reading or are non-English speakers should be tested with the chart or cards of the letter *E* arranged in different directions. Figure 14-9 shows two Snellen vision screening charts, which are made to standard specifications. These charts are hung on the wall with a mark 20 feet away to show where the patient should stand or sit to read the chart. The chart should be at the patient's eye level. Charts are available on a lighted view box to increase the visibility of the letters.

Distance visual acuity is written as a fraction. The numerator is the number of feet, or the distance from the chart; the denominator is the numbered line the patient can read. If one's distant visual acuity results are 20/100, it means that the person stood 20 feet from the chart and read the line that should be read at 100 feet. One who has 20/10 acuity can see at 20 feet what should be seen at a distance of 10 feet. A finding of 20/20 is average.

Common complaints that may indicate vision problems are listed in Table 14-1. These complaints pertain to both children and adults.

Patients should be screened with and without their corrective lenses and the results recorded as such on their charts. Note that if visual acuity is 20/200 or less in the better eye with corrective lenses, the patient is considered legally blind. Perform Procedure 14-5 to measure distance vision.

The **Jaeger** system is a common method of screening for *near* vision acuity. The screening procedure should be conducted in a well-lighted room without interruptions. The patient should be tested with and without wearing corrective lenses, and each eye is tested separately for a complete assessment to be made by the physician. The chart used for this procedure is a card held by the patient between 14 inches and 16 inches from the eye. You should measure with a yard-

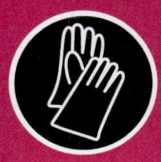

FIGURE 14-9 Snellen vision acuity screening charts. On the left, the letters appear in descending sizes; on the right, the letter E appears in various directions and in descending sizes.

TABLE 14-1 Possible Indications of Visual Disturbance

During Activities That Require Reading	Condition	Behaviors	Complaints
1. Exhibits difficulty with near or distance vision 2. Avoids reading, writing, and other related activities	1. Redness of the eye(s) or eyelid(s) 2. Crusting/swelling of eyelid(s) or styes 3. Poor eye coordination 4. Watering or discharge 5. Accident/injury to the eye	1. Looks cross-eyed 2. Rubbing eyes frequently 3. Confuses letters (e.g., *a* and *c, f* and *t, m* and *n*) 4. Turns head or leans forward to see better 5. Blinks continually 6. Irritable at attempting close work	1. Blurriness of vision 2. Nausea 3. Headaches often 4. Dizziness 5. Eyes sensitive to light 6. Feels like something in the eye(s)

If a patient has a past history or a current complaint of any of the areas listed above, a visual disturbance is suggested.

PROCEDURE

14-5  Screen Visual Acuity with a Snellen Chart

PURPOSE: To measure the distant visual acuity of a patient.

EQUIPMENT: Patient's chart, pen, Snellen chart, pointer, occular eye **occluder**, card or paper cup.

PERFORMANCE OBJECTIVE: Provided with a patient and the necessary vision-screening equipment, measure visual acuity following the steps in the procedure and accurately record the findings on the chart.

1. Identify the patient. **RATIONALE: Speaking to the patient by name and checking the chart ensures that you are performing the procedure on the correct patient.**

2. Explain the procedure to the patient—that patient is to read each line from the chart as you point to it with a pointer.

3. Ask the patient to read the chart with both eyes (OU) first, standing 20 feet from the chart.

4. To test acuity of the right eye, have the patient cover the left eye with an occluder, a card, or a paper cup. If patient wears corrective lenses, the procedure should be performed first wearing lenses and then without and recorded as such.

NOTE:

- **The chart should be at the patient's eye level.**
- **Tell the patient to keep both eyes open when covering one eye. This prevents squinting and blurring.**
- **Record any observations of individual accommodations made to read chart, such as squinting or turning the head.**
- **Follow office policy in giving the test. Asking patients to read only certain lines of the chart is less time consuming (e.g., begin at line 6).**

5. Record the smallest line that the patient can read without making a mistake. **NOTE: Some physicians allow up to 2 errors on the smallest line read.**

6. Have the patient cover his right eye and test acuity of the left, following the same procedure.

7. Record the number of the smallest line that the patient can read.

CHARTING EXAMPLE

2-14-XX

Snellen findings: Vision screening per Dr. White, right eye 25/30, left eye 20/40, no squinting observed

T. Edwards, CMA

No. 1.
.37M

In the second century of the Christian era, the empire of Rome comprehended the fairest part of the earth, and the most civilized portion of mankind. The frontiers of that extensive monarchy were guarded by ancient renown and disciplined valor. The gentle but powerful influence of laws and manners had gradually cemented the union of the provinces. Their peaceful inhabitants enjoyed and abused the advantages of wealth.

No. 2.
.50M

fourscore years, the public administration was conducted by the virtue and abilities of Nerva, Trajan, Hadrian, and the two Antonines. It is the design of this, and of the two succeeding chapters, to describe the prosperous condition of their empire; and afterwards, from the death of Marcus Antoninus, to deduce the most important circumstances of its decline and fall; a revolution which will ever be remembered, and is still felt by

No. 3.
.62M

the nations of the earth. The principal conquests of the Romans were achieved under the republic; and the emperors, for the most part, were satisfied with preserving those dominions which had been acquired by the policy of the senate, the active emulations of the consuls, and the martial enthusiasm of the people. The seven first centuries were filled with a rapid succession of triumphs; but it was

No. 4.
.75M

reserved for Augustus to relinquish the ambitious design of subduing the whole earth, and to introduce a spirit of moderation into the public councils. Inclined to peace by his temper and situation, it was very easy for him to discover that Rome, in her present exalted situation, had much less to hope than to fear from the chance of arms; and that, in the prosecution of

No. 5.
1.00M

the undertaking became every day more difficult, the event more doubtful, and the possession more precarious, and less beneficial. The experience of Augustus added weight to these salutary reflections, and effectually convinced him that, by the prudent vigor of

No. 6.
1.25M

his counsels, it would be easy to secure every concession which the safety or the dignity of Rome might require from the most formidable barbarians. Instead of exposing his person or his legions to the arrows of the Parthinians, he obtained, by an honor-

No. 7.
1.50M

able treaty, the restitution of the standards and prisoners which had been taken in the defeat of Crassus. His generals, in the early part of his reign, attempted the reduction of Ethiopia and Arabia Felix. They marched near a thou-

No. 8.
1.75M

sand miles to the south of the tropic; but the heat of the climate soon repelled the invaders, and protected the unwarlike natives of those sequestered regions

No. 9.
2.00M

The northern countries of Europe scarcely deserved the expense and labor of conquest. The forests and morasses of Germany were

No. 10.
2.25M

filled with a hardy race of barbarians who despised life when it was separated from freedom; and though, on the first

No. 11.
2.50M

attack, they seemed to yield to the weight of the Roman power, they soon, by a signal

FIGURE 14-10 Jaeger near vision acuity screening chart, which is held by the patient at a distance of approximately 14 to 16 inches from the eyes.

stick, a meterstick, or a tape measure for accuracy. This is the distance at which one with normal vision is able to read printed material (a newspaper) or work on something that requires close attention (sewing). The Jaeger screening test consists of reading material that has ascending sizes of type ranging from .37 mm to 2.5 mm (Figure 14-10). The test contains excerpts from a manuscript sectioned into short paragraphs, none of which are the same. The medical assistant should observe for any difficulty the patient exhibits (e.g., holding the chart right in front of the face, squinting, or blinking) while trying to read the card. The medical assistant records the section number that the patient can read easily. (Refer to Procedure 14-6.)

PROCEDURE

14-6  Screen Visual Acuity with the Jaeger System

PURPOSE: To determine near distance visual acuity of a patient using the Jaeger system.

EQUIPMENT: Jaeger near vision acuity chart, pen, patient's chart.

PERFORMANCE OBJECTIVES: Using the Jaeger near vision acuity chart, in a well-lighted area, determine the near distance visual acuity following the steps in the procedure. Accurately record results on the patient's chart.

1. After identifying the patient, explain the procedure.
   RATIONALE: Speaking to the patient by name and checking the chart ensures that you are performing the procedure on the correct patient.

2. Have the patient sit up straight but comfortably in a well-lighted area.

(continues)

PROCEDURE PROCEDURE PROCEDURE PROCEDURE PROCEDURE PROCEDURE PROCEDURE

14-6 Screen Visual Acuity with the Jaeger System (Continued)

3. Hand the Jaeger chart to the patient to hold, between 14 inches and 16 inches from the eyes. Figure 14-11 shows proper positioning of the card.

4. Instruct the patient to read (out loud to you) the various paragraphs of the card with both eyes open, first without wearing corrective lenses and then with.

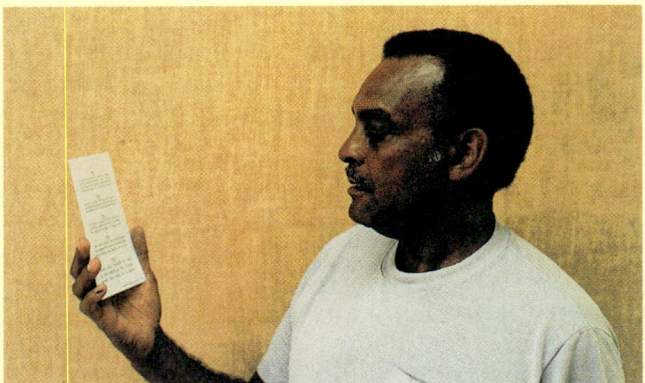

FIGURE 14-11 Patient reading the Jaeger near vision acuity chart at a distance of 14 to 16 inches from the eyes.

NOTE: Each eye should be tested individually having the person cover the left eye first while reading the card and then the right. Observe carefully for any difficulty the patient has in reading any of the lines on the card. Listen also to any remarks made by the patient and note them on the chart.

5. Record the results and problems, if any, on the patient's chart to assist the physician in determining the visual acuity of the patient. The smallest line of print that the patient can read should be recorded and initialed.

6. Thank the patient for cooperation and answer any questions.

7. Return the Jaeger chart to proper storage.

CHARTING EXAMPLE

8-17-XX

Screened vision w/Jaeger per Dr. White; read No 3 (62M) both eyes w/corrective lenses; No 11 (2.5) right eye (squinting); No 10 (2.2) left eye

T. Edwards, CMA

Many devices for screening visual acuity are available besides the methods already discussed. One compact instrument is the Titmus Vision Tester (Figure 14-12). In this system of screening, the patient looks into the instrument to view eight different specialized fields designed to detect all common vision problems. While administering this test, the medical assistant sits or stands next to the patient to operate the selection of visual fields. A vision occluder is built within the device for testing each eye individually as the patient reads the various lines. Again, the medical assistant must be alert in observing and listening while the patient completes this test. All complaints and observations should be recorded on the patient's chart along with the results of the test. The instrument comes with forms for recording the results of the test.

Color vision acuity means that one can accurately recognize colors. The inability to perceive colors of the spectrum distinctly is commonly termed *color blindness* or the technically correct and preferred term, color deficient. This is caused by changes that happen in the pigments of the cones in the retina of the eyes as they react to red, green, and blue light wavelengths.

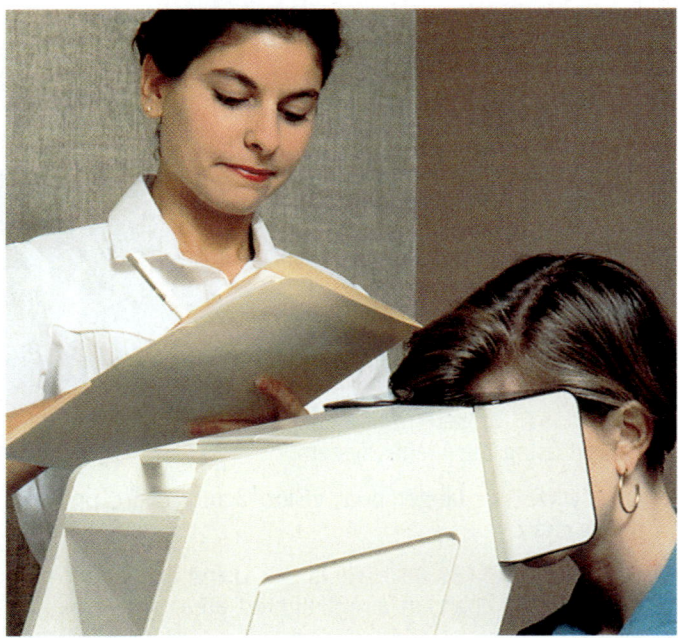

FIGURE 14-12 The medical assistant records the vision acuity as the patient is being tested on the Titmus Vision Tester.

There are two primary types of color deficiency: **Daltonism**, which is the most common, is a visual disorder in which the person cannot tell the difference between red and green. It is a hereditary disorder. **Achromatic** vision is total color blindness and very rare, where the person cannot recognize any color at all. These people see everything in white, gray, and black. The probable cause for this condition is that the cones in the retina are defective, or there may be none at all.

Several other conditions involve one's inability or weakness in distinguishing certain colors. In **deuteranopia**, the person has trouble telling any difference between varying shades of green and also of bluish reds and neutral shades. **Protanopia** is partial color blindness. These people have trouble with the perception of reds, and sometimes yellows and greens are confused. This condition is often referred to as red blindness. **Tritanopia**, which is the rarest, means that the person cannot distinguish blue color.

A method for screening patients for defects in distinguishing color vision acuity is with the **Ishihara** color plates book. A sample of the series of multicolored charts in the test book is shown in Figure 14-13. In these pictures of the color plates, a person with normal color vision acuity can see a pink-red number 8 against a blue-green background and a blue-green number 5 against a pink-red background.

Patients may be asked to trace the patterns of color with their finger as you observe them. There are letters and numbers (and curved lines and shapes for non-

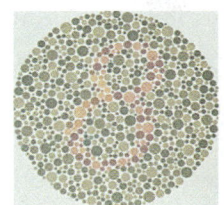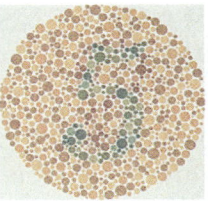

FIGURE 14-13 Sample color plates from the Ishihara's Test for color deficiency

readers) that are one color within another. When administering this procedure, make sure that the room is well-lighted, preferably with natural daylight (not direct sunlight), so that the patient is able to follow your instructions without straining to see. Whatever method of color vision assessment is used where you are employed, it is vital that you are accurate in reporting the results. Medical assistants should first be tested to determine if they have normal color vision to administer the test to patients. Perform Procedure 14-7 to measure color vision acuity.

All patients with thyroid conditions should routinely be screened for color vision acuity during their scheduled visits. The procedure should include testing with both eyes first and then each eye separately to see if there is any difference in the perception of color in either eye. The eye not used should be covered and not held shut. Grave's disease patients especially need frequent assessment of their color vision acuity changes. The color vision test results may lead to earlier diagnosis and treatment of Grave's ophthalmopathy.

PROCEDURE PROCEDURE PROCEDURE PROCEDURE PROCEDURE PROCEDURE PROCEDURE PROCEDURE

14-7 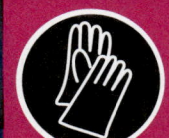 Determine Color Vision Acuity by the Ishihara Method

PURPOSE: To determine color vision acuity of a patient using the Ishihara method.

EQUIPMENT: Ishihara book, pen, patient's chart, proper lighting.

PERFORMANCE OBJECTIVE: Using the Ishihara book in a well-lighted area, determine the color vision acuity of a patient by following the steps of the procedure. The results will be accurately recorded on the patient's chart.

1. Obtain the chart from the back of the book. **NOTE: Before administering this screening test, you should first be tested.**

2. Explain the procedure to the patient.

3. Ask the patient first to read the plates with both eyes (if the patient wears corrective lenses, with them on).

4. Have the patient cover the left eye to test the right eye, and then cover the right to test the left. **NOTE: Make sure to note any difficulty or complaint of the patient during the screening process.**

5. Compare answers given with those on chart. Record those frames the patient misses and write down what the patient reports so that the degree of color deficiency may be determined by the physician.

CHARTING EXAMPLE

9-24-XX

Color vision screening per Dr. White; Ishihara color plates—accurately read.

J. Baker, RMA

CONTRAST SENSITIVITY SCREENING

A recent advance in the measurement of visual acuity is the development of the Pelli–Robson *contrast sensitivity* chart (Figure 14-14). This chart measures contrast sensitivity by determining the faintest contrast that an observer can see. Recent clinical evidence shows that contrast sensitivity is affected by all of the major eye diseases—diabetic retinopathy, macular degeneration, glaucoma, and cataract. Therefore, measuring contrast sensitivity provides a sensitive screening test for eye disease to provide earlier diagnosis and treatment.

Another contrast sensitivity screening method has been developed by Vectorvision. All patients can be tested with this method, but it is especially useful in screening small children, internationals, and people who are illiterate. This test has a series of four groups of circles. In these rows of circles, some are solid gray in color and some have vertical lines. The patient is instructed to look at the first group and tell you which circles have lines within them. The last correctly identified circle in each group is charted on a graph. The results of this test are interpreted by the physician.

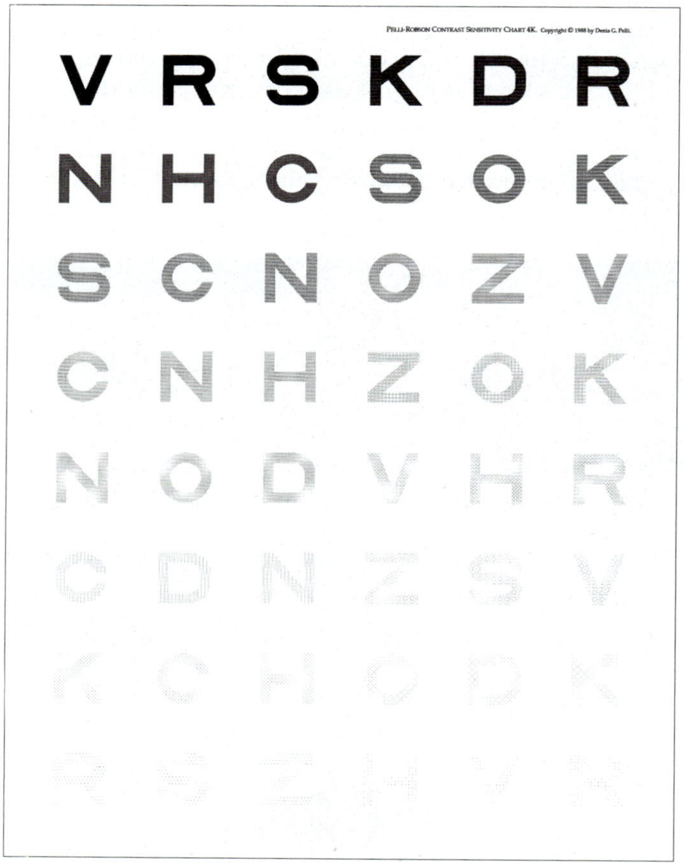

FIGURE 14-14 The Pelli-Robson contrast sensitivity chart. The faintest letters that can be read on the chart determine the patient's contrast sensitivity. The chart can aid the early diagnosis of certain eye diseases. *(Courtesy of Dr. Denis Pelli, NYU)*

AUDITORY ACUITY

The function of the ear is to enable sound to be perceived. If this process is impaired, hearing loss results. Diseases or conditions of the ear, if not treated, can cause damage to nerves and tissues, which may result in mild to profound deafness. Often patients try to hide a problem such as hearing loss because it is an embarrassment to them. They are sometimes afraid they may have to wear a hearing aid or worry that they may need surgery. Often the patient will try to compensate for the hearing loss by:

- Learning to read lips
- Always turning the best ear toward the sound source
- Pretending that they heard
- Increasingly turning up the volume on audio equipment
- Standing very close during conversation
- Sometimes withdrawing

The family members of the patient may relate this information to you. You should advise the person to have the patient schedule a time to have a doctor examine the ears and have a hearing test. You should note the information on the patient's chart and bring it to the physician's attention. The physician will discuss the problem with the patient during the scheduled appointment.

Sometimes the problem may be as simple as the patient having impacted cerumen, and after an irrigation, the person's hearing returns to normal. Sometimes it is not that simple, and further measures are necessary. The medical assistant is in contact with the patient usually more than the physician. It is the assistant's responsibility to act in the best interest of the patient in conveying important information observed. You can watch for any behaviors as you are getting patients ready for their scheduled appointments or when you talk to them over the phone. Often, it is a family member who makes the appointment for the one who has an obvious hearing problem. One of your most important duties is relaying information to the physician about patients.

Common behaviors of patients that indicate the loss of hearing ability are:

1. Frequently asking someone to repeat what was said during conversation
2. Talking in an inappropriately loud voice
3. Not responding when spoken to if out of sight range
4. Not pronouncing words well
5. Responding only when you speak very loudly
6. Playing radio, TV, and other audio devices at increased volume

Certain complaints may suggest hearing loss or **auditory** nerve damage. When patients disclose any of the following symptoms you should bring it to the attention of the physician for further assessment:

- Ringing in the ears
- Decreased hearing in one ear (or both), sometimes caused by impacted cerumen
- Infection or injury to the ear
- Bleeding or discharge from the ear(s)
- Any unusual noise or feeling inside the ears

These signs and any others that patients tell you should be written on the chart during in-person screening. Further examination by the physician is necessary to determine the extent of the problem and its treatment.

HEARING TESTS

An **audiometer** is an instrument used to measure one's hearing. The audiometer determines the hearing thresholds of pure tones of frequencies that are normally audible by an individual. Tone frequency refers to the sound vibrations per second. Tone intensity refers to the loudness. Some also measure bone and air conduction. The threshold of hearing is the point where a sound can barely be heard. Figure 14-15 illustrates the decibels of common environmental noise levels.

Audiometric devices are powered either by batteries or electricity. Whatever type is used in the facility where you are employed should be checked periodically for proper performance and accuracy. If the batteries need to be changed or if a wire is frayed, it should be taken care of before being used with patients, not only for their safety, but to make sure that it works efficiently. Several types of audiometers are available for use in determining hearing acuity. Many are still used that require the operator to manually turn a dial to emit the various frequencies for the patient to hear during the test. Companies that manufacture audiometers offer in-service demonstrations to make sure their equipment is used properly. Operational manuals should be kept with the instrument for handy reference.

The procedure for most audiometers is basically the same. The patient is instructed to place the earphones (marked red for the right ear and blue for the left ear) over the ears. The medical assistant tells the patient in the soundproof booth how the earphones are to be placed and how to work the control signal (Figure 14-16). The printer on the table next to the booth records the results of the hearing test. The printout is called an audiogram and is filed in the patient's chart after the physician reads the results of the test and makes an evaluation.

During the procedure the sound is automatically blocked by the machine in the ear that is not being tested. In the ear that is being tested, the machine provides a series of tones. The patient listens and signals (either by raising a finger or by using a hand-held control) as the various sounds are heard. The tones range in frequencies from very low to very high with a varied level of decibel intensity. After the right ear has been tested, the machine switches automatically to test the left ear. The medical assistant should report any complaints and any unusual behavior that the patient may

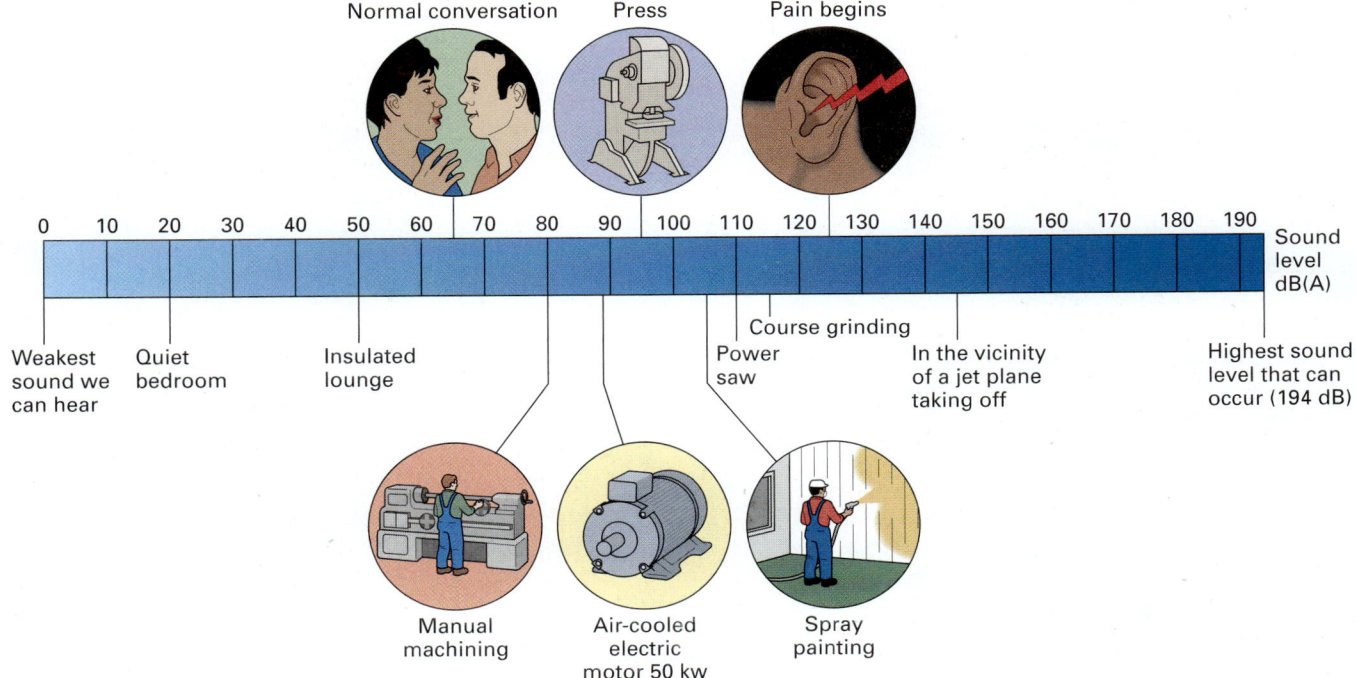

FIGURE 14-15   Noise levels associated with selected environments and machinery

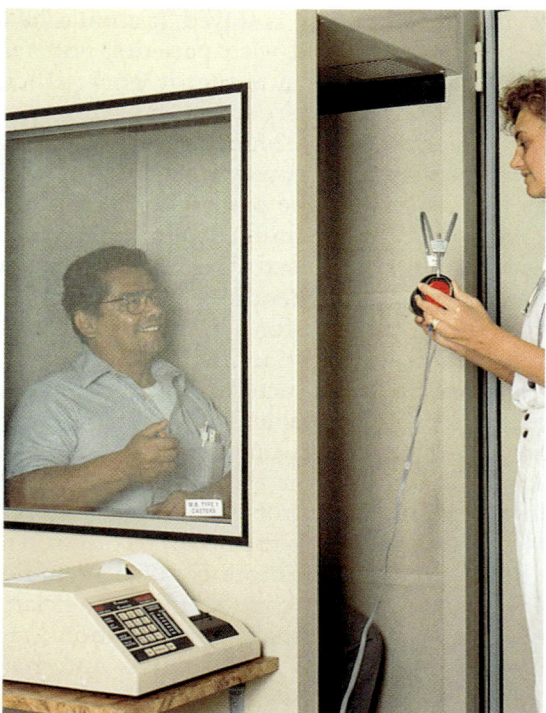

FIGURE 14-16   The patient, in a soundproof booth, is instructed to press the hand-held control button each time a sound is heard through the earphones. The signals are transmitted to a computer outside the booth and printed out as an audiogram.

have before or during the hearing test to the physician. You should note this on the patient's chart along with the results of the test and place your initials indicating that you have completed the test.

Hearing Assessment

Physicians use several audiometric assessment procedures to determine the cause of the patient's hearing loss, some of which are a part of the complete or routine physical examination.

During the physical examination, the physician will use a tuning fork to test the patient's hearing. A two-pronged metal tuning fork is used, its frequency varying with the size of the instrument. The common tests done are the Rinne and the Weber.

In the Rinne test, the examiner strikes the fork and then holds the shank (stem) against the patient's mastoid bone until the patient no longer hears the sound (Figure 14-17A). The prongs of the tuning fork are then placed about 1 inch from the auditory meatus (opening to the ear) and then next to it (Figure 14-17B). In a

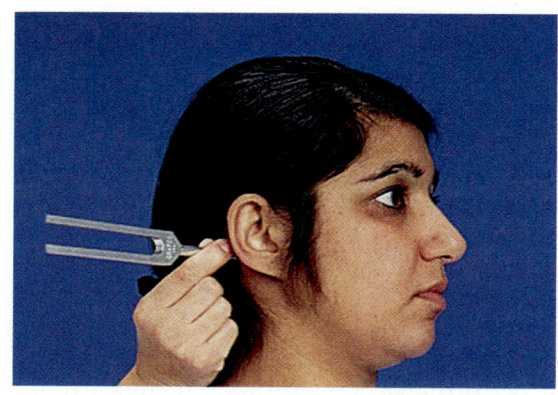

FIGURE 14-17A   The Rinne test is performed by striking the tuning fork and placing it on the mastoid bone behind the ear until sound is no longer heard (bone conduction).

PATIENT EDUCATION

1. Advise patients not to put anything into their ears to avoid damaging the tympanic membrane. The cerumen (ear wax) produced by the body has a purpose. It is to protect and moisten the membrane of the ear canal. Many people feel that they must completely remove this daily with a swab, which often results in it being packed down into the ear canal, where it hardens. This impacted ear wax (cerumen) must be removed by a qualified medical team member.

2. Instruct patients that ear drops and other ear medications should be used only with the advice of their physician. Earache, pain, or discharge should be reported to and examined by the physician as soon as possible.

3. Discuss the possibility of permanent hearing loss with patients who work around extremely loud noise or who have gotten into a habit of turning the volume way up when listening to audio systems, radios, or TVs. Explain to these patients that protective ear coverings should be worn while on the job (it is a safety requirement) and warn those who attend loud concerts or listen to loud music to wear protective ear plugs and turn down the volume before their hearing is lost from damage to nerves.

4. Urge patients to have regular hearing tests to detect loss of hearing or other related problems. It is recommended that this be done annually unless otherwise instructed by the physician or if there is a noticeable difference or problem with hearing. Patients who have a history of ear infections should have periodic hearing tests.

normal ear, the sound is heard about twice as long by air conduction as by bone conduction. If hearing by bone conduction is greater, the result is spoken of as a negative Rinne.

In the Weber test, the vibrating tuning fork is held against the **vertex** (crown of the head) or against the skull or forehead in the midline (Figure 14-17C). The sound is heard best by the unaffected ear if deafness is caused by disease of the auditory apparatus or by the affected ear if deafness is caused by obstruction of the air passages.

A small amount of hearing loss may be temporary because of a patient's physical condition, and a recheck in 1 or 2 weeks may be advisable.

A very useful diagnostic instrument that affords both audiogram and tympanogram, as well as acoustic reflex results, is shown in Figures 14-18A, B, and C. This device, the TM 262 Auto Tymp, is useful in providing objective data in determining complete diagnoses and documentation of diseases and disorders of the ear. It is additionally helpful in evaluation of follow-up treatment.

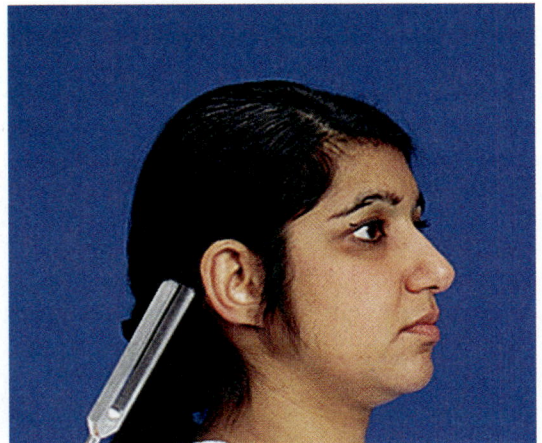

FIGURE 14-17B   Then the fork is immediately placed next to the ear to determine whether the vibrations can still be heard through the air (air conduction).

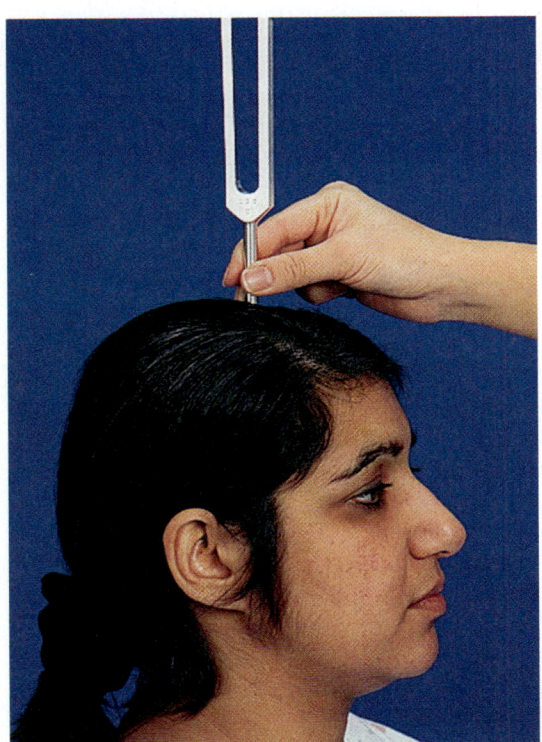

FIGURE 14-17C   The Weber test is performed by striking the tuning fork and placing it on the forehead or the vertex of the head to determine whether sound is heard equally by each ear.

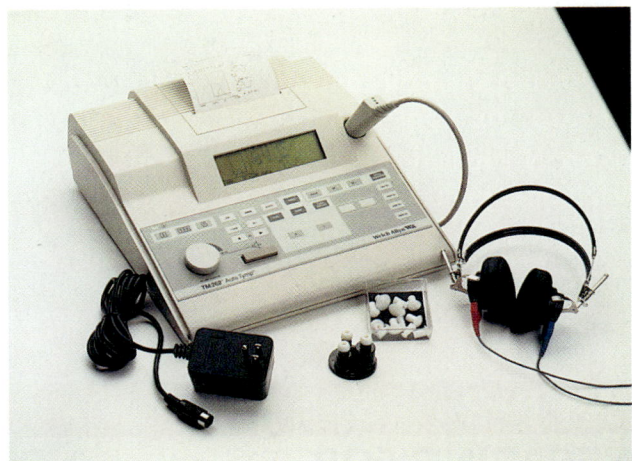

FIGURE 14-18A   The Auto Tymp diagnostic machine with transformer, eartips, and headset to evaluate hearing. It is easy to use for both operator and patient and requires only a few minutes to complete. *(Courtesy of Welch Allyn, Inc.)*

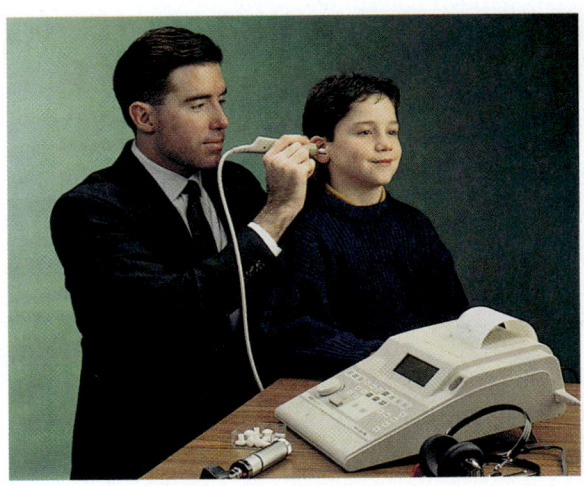

FIGURE 14-18B   Testing a child *(Courtesy of Welch Allyn, Inc.)*

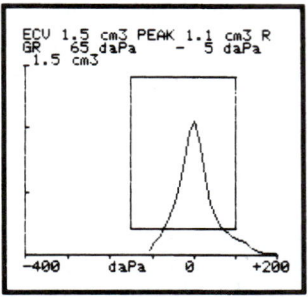
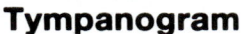

Tympanogram

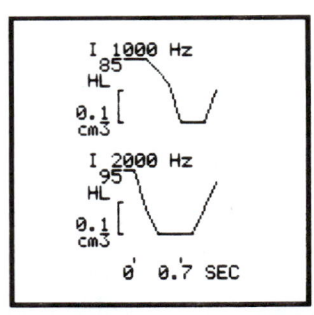

Acoustic Reflex Results

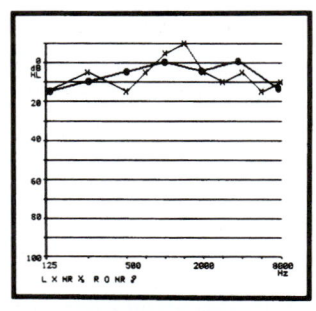

Audiogram

FIGURE 14-18C   Samples of printed test results *(Courtesy of Welch Allyn, Inc.)*

ACHIEVE UNIT OBJECTIVES

- Complete the Workbook activities to meet the learning objectives.
- Practice the procedures in this unit to meet the performance objectives.
- Apply your knowledge at the end of this chapter in completing the Critical Thinking Challenge and Activities, as well as the StudyWARE on your Student CD-ROM.

UNIT 2
PREPARING FOR EXAMINATIONS

OBJECTIVES

Upon completion of this unit, you will be able to achieve the following:

LEARNING Objectives

1. Spell and define, using the glossary at the back of the text, all the Words to Know in this unit.
2. Name the 12 examination positions and explain the purpose of each.
3. Identify examination room equipment that may need to be disinfected following a patient examination.
4. List the supplies that should be available in an examination room.

PERFORMANCE Objectives

1. Prepare and maintain the examination area.
2. Demonstrate positioning and draping a patient in recumbent position.
3. Demonstrate positioning and draping a patient in prone position.
4. Demonstrate positioning and draping a patient in Sims' position.
5. Demonstrate positioning and draping a patient in knee-chest position.
6. Demonstrate positioning and draping a patient in Fowler's position.
7. Demonstrate positioning and draping a patient in lithotomy position.

WORDS TO KNOW

anatomical position	flexed	prone
anterior	Fowler's	recumbent
dorsal	genucubital	shock
dowel	genupectoral	Sims'
dyspneic	horizontal	supine
fenestrated	incompetent	Trendelenburg
	lithotomy	

CERTIFICATION CONNECTION

CMA
Patient preparation and assisting the physician (examinations [body positions])

CMAS
Examination preparation

RMA
Patient positions

BEFORE THE EXAMINATION

The medical assistant must know how to operate the examination table in order to ensure the examination process goes smoothly and efficiently. The physician may require the patient to assume certain positions during the examination. Some of these necessitate changing the table structure. The exam table in Figure 14-19A is limited to changing the angle of the top half, pulling out the leg rest, and extending the hidden stirrups. The power table in Figure 14-19B can be

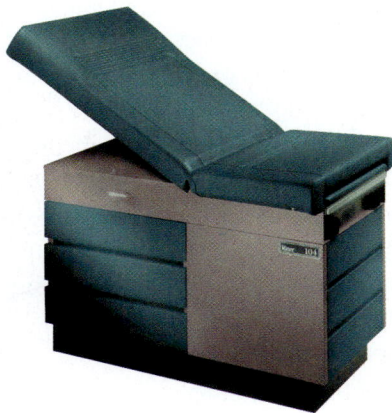

FIGURE 14-19A   A manual medical examination table commonly used in medical offices *(Courtesy of Midmark Corp.)*

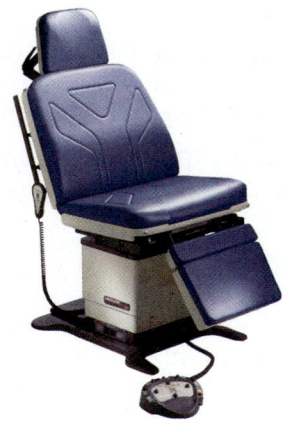

FIGURE 14-19B   A power table that can be adjusted by hand or foot controls *(Courtesy of Midmark Corp.)*

P PATIENT EDUCATION

Instruct the patient about the need for a specific position for the examination to be performed. This information should be included with the instructions on preparing for the examination. The patient must understand that the physician needs to examine certain parts of the body or perform certain procedures and tests, and the patient must be positioned in the most accessible manner.

---

adjusted for the height of the physician as well as for many examination positions. The desired position can be achieved by pressing a button on the programmed hand control or using the optional plug-in foot control.

Preparation of the room for an examination is also the responsibility of the medical assistant. The MA must ensure the room is clean and tidy and at a comfortable temperature. All surfaces within the room that may be potentially contaminated should be cleaned with a disinfectant between patient examinations. This would include cabinet and table surfaces where used supplies and instruments may be discarded and the examination table that may have soiled table paper.

After the examination table is cleaned, new table paper the proper width to appropriately cover the table, is pulled down. The paper is supplied in a roll that is inserted on a **dowel** under the head of the table. The jagged torn edge of the paper is folded and tucked under the seat section of the table for a neat appearance. It is important to check the amount of paper left on the roll periodically. Some tables accommodate two rolls so a replacement one would be immediately available if you ran out; otherwise you would need to make a trip to the supply cabinet. The table pillow is covered by a disposable cover or towel that is discarded after each use and replaced with a fresh one.

Preparation also includes checking for all the supplies needed within the room such as a hand-washing product; biohazardous waste containers; face guards; latex gloves; patient gowns; drapes; paper towels; tissues; a working light source; and standard examination equipment such as tongue blades, disposable speculums, gauze squares, and applicators. Gowns and drapes are usually stored in the table drawers, while other supplies are kept in examination cabinet drawers. Hand-washing products, paper towels, and biohazard bags will probably be kept under the sink cabinet. You will also need to prepare a tray of routine examination instruments used during the physical examination (see Unit 3). Follow Procedure 14-8 as an example of how to prepare and maintain an examination room.

A female medical assistant should be prepared to remain in the room when a female patient is being examined by a male physician. The patient should feel more relaxed, and the physician is protected from lawsuits that could result from patients claiming the physician acted improperly during the examination. Patient gowns and drapes are made of cloth or disposable paper. The patient is instructed how to wear the gown to facilitate examination. If the examination table is too high for the patient to get on it comfortably, a foot stool should be provided. A very ill patient or a small child should never be left alone on a table; a member of the family should be asked to sit with them if you must leave the room.

PROCEDURE PROCEDURE PROCEDURE PROCEDURE PROCEDURE PROCEDURE PROCEDURE

14-8  Prepare and Maintain Examination and Treatment Areas

PURPOSE: To provide an examination room that is comfortable, clean, and has the usual equipment and supplies necessary ready for an examination.

OSHA GUIDELINES: Standard Precautions recommend that proper hand washing, gloving, disinfection, and the disposal of contaminated items in a biohazard container be performed to avoid the transfer of microorganisms to other patients, yourself, and the environment.

EQUIPMENT: Latex gloves, disinfectant, disposable cloth, examination room furniture, pillow, table paper, patient gowns, drapes, hand-washing liquid, paper towels, tissues, gauze squares, tongue blades, applicators, disposable speculums, floor light, and biohazard waste container.

PERFORMANCE OBJECTIVE: Following an examination, given all necessary equipment and supplies, dispose of used materials appropriately and disinfect surfaces. Prepare the room for next examination by applying clean table paper, checking and replacing supplies and equipment, following the steps in the procedure.

1. Assess the room condition, temperature, and furniture.
2. Put on disposable gloves.
3. Place used supplies and disposable examination equipment in the biohazard container.
4. Tear the table paper near the top and roll it up with the pillow cover. Dispose of it in the waste basket unless contaminated with body fluid; then place it in the biohazard container.
5. Wipe permanent examination equipment with gauze squares and disinfectant.
6. Wipe the examination room table tops with disposable cloth and disinfectant if contaminated from discarded examination supplies.
7. Wipe any other equipment contaminated by the physician, such as a stool or floor lamp.
8. Disinfect the examination table and dispose of the cloth and gloves in the appropriate container.
9. Check the biohazard container for space; replace it if the bag is full.
10. Pull down clean table paper, fold the ragged edge, and place it under the table seat.
11. Place a clean cover on the pillow.
12. Check the table paper supply, gowns, and drapes.
13. Check the hand-washing dispenser and stock the supply.
14. Check the paper towel dispenser and supply more if needed.
15. Check the supplies in the cabinet and the examination table drawers and replace as needed.
16. Make a final visual check of the room.
17. Recheck periodically for cleanliness and examination readiness.

ASSISTING THE PATIENT

Never try to lift a patient who obviously weighs more than you can safely handle; have someone help you. If a patient needs help in moving on the table, reach under the arm at the shoulder and help the person move up. You should move with the patient. If it is necessary to help a patient out of a wheelchair, position the chair and lock the wheels before trying to help the patient move from the chair to the table. A procedure for assisting a patient from wheelchair is located in Chapter 19.

EXAMINATION POSITIONS

A patient will be asked to assume certain positions in order to facilitate examination of the body. During a comprehensive physical examination, several of the standard 12 positions may be utilized. The medical assistant must know the names and be able to assist the patient into the positions. The following is a list of examination positions that will be discussed:

Anatomical	Sims'	Lithotomy
Horizontal recumbent	Knee-chest	Trendelenburg
Dorsal recumbent	Fowler's	Jacknife
Prone	High Fowler's	Proctological

Procedures 14-8 through 14-13 have step-by-step instructions for assisting patients to assume most of the examination positions. Perform these procedures to become familiar with their names, the patient's position, and the relationship between the examination and the position. This information and skills are necessary before you begin to assist the physician to perform a partial or complete physician examination.

The physician may begin the examination by asking the patient to assume the **anatomical position**, which means to stand erect, arms at sides with palms pointed forward. This allows a visual inspection of posture and is usually followed by requests to perform several movements (see Unit 3). Next the patient will be asked to sit at the end of the examination table, with the legs hanging down. The medical assistant should assist the patient as needed. If the patient is short it may be necessary to pull out the step from the bottom of the table or use a small stepping stool. Be careful to be sure the patient does not fall. Once seated on the table, a drape should be placed over the legs for privacy and warmth. Again, several inspections and examinations are done with the patient in this position.

Next the patient will be asked to lie down on the table. The medical assistant should assist the patient to lie back and pull out the leg rest at the bottom of the table to support the patient's legs. A small pillow can be placed under the head for comfort. If a power table is used, and it is in the sitting position, press the appropriate button and reassure the patient as the table levels. Patients often feel like their head is lower than their body after being in an upright position. Readjust the drape as needed.

The **horizontal** recumbent or **supine** position is used for examination and treatment of the **anterior** portion of the body, including the breasts and abdominal organs (Procedure 14-9 and Figures 14-20A and B). The term **dorsal recumbent** is used to indicate that the legs

PROCEDURE PROCEDURE PROCEDURE PROCEDURE PROCEDURE PROCEDURE PROCEDURE PROCEDURE

14-9  Assist the Patient to the Horizontal Recumbent Position

PURPOSE: To assist the patient into a horizontal recumbent position for an examination.

OSHA GUIDELINES: Standard Precautions recommend that proper hand washing and gloving is performed to avoid the transfer of microorganisms to other patients, yourself, and the environment.

EQUIPMENT: Examination table, table paper, gown drape sheet, pillow, disposable pillow cover, or towel.

PERFORMANCE OBJECTIVE: In a simulated situation, with access to equipment, assist the patient to assume the horizontal recumbent position while providing for safety and privacy following the steps in the procedure.

1. Check the examination room for cleanliness. **NOTE: Always have clean paper on the table and a clean pillow cover or clean towel over the pillow. RATIONALE: Every precaution must be maintained to prevent any possible cross-contamination of disease.**

2. Identify the patient. **RATIONALE: Speaking to the patient by name and checking the chart ensures that you are performing the procedure on the correct patient.**

3. Give clear instructions to the patient regarding the amount of clothing to be removed and where it is to be placed.

4. Instruct the patient on use of the gown. **RATIONALE: The procedure to be performed dictates whether the front or back should be open.**

5. Assist the patient if help is needed. Otherwise respect the privacy and modesty of the patient by leaving the room while the patient changes.

6. Instruct the patient to sit on the end of the table and cover her legs with a drape. Assist as needed.

7. Instruct the patient to lie flat on the table with legs together.

8. Pull out the end extension on the table for leg support if needed.

9. The patient may rest her head on a small pillow if desired.

10. Instruct the patient to cross her arms on her chest or put them at the sides of her body.

11. Drape the sheet evenly over the patient but leave loose on all sides.

12. To position for dorsal recumbent, ask the patient to put the bottoms of both feet flat on the table with knees flexed.

13. For vaginal or rectal examination, drape the patient with one corner of the sheet over the chest, a corner wrapped around each leg, and the fourth corner over the pubic area. Physician will turn back the sheet at the pubic area.

14. Assist the physician as necessary with the examination.

15. Assist the patient from the table when the examination is completed. **NOTE: Patients may be dizzy from the change in position. Allow them to sit upright before standing.** Clean the room and replace the supplies. **NOTE: The examination table surface and base must be thoroughly cleaned with disinfecting cleanser at regular intervals and following any contact with body fluids that may contain bloodborne pathogens.**

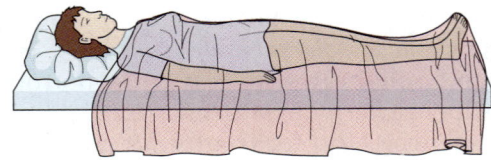

FIGURE 14-20A Horizontal recumbent or supine position

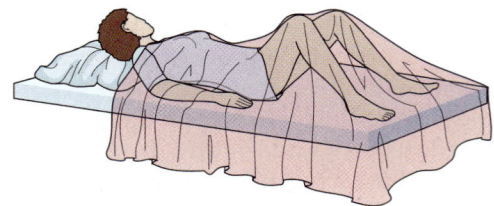

FIGURE 14-20B Dorsal recumbent position

are **flexed**. This position allows for relaxation of the abdominal muscles and thus easier examination of the abdominal area. This position may also be used for digital vaginal or rectal examination. The gown is open in the front, and a drape sheet of cloth or paper is used to cover the patient.

During a complete physical, the physician may request that the patient turn over so the ventral surface may be examined. This is called the **prone** position and is used to examine the spine and structures of the back. Assist the patient as necessary to turn over, instructing him to turn toward you. Watch to be certain the patient does not get too close to the edge when turning and fall off the table. Instruct the patient to lie face down with his arms folded to make a place to rest his head. Since the gown was originally put on with the opening in the front, it will be necessary to pull the gown up to expose the back. Reposition the drape to cover the exposed area. When the ventral surface is being examined alone, the patient is instructed to put on the gown with the opening in the back. Some patients may experience back discomfort lying in this position. Often placing a pillow under the abdomen will relieve the discomfort long enough to permit the examination. Perform Procedure 14-10 and refer to Figure 14-21.

The **Sims'** position is used in examination and treatment of the rectal area and for enemas, rectal tempera-

14-10  Assist the Patient to the Prone Position

PURPOSE: To assist the patient into a prone position for a examination.

OSHA GUIDELINES: Standard Precautions recommend that proper hand washing and gloving is performed to avoid the transfer of microorganisms to other patients, yourself, and the environment.

EQUIPMENT: Table, gown, table paper, drape sheet, pillow, and disposable pillow and cover or towel.

PERFORMANCE OBJECTIVE: In a simulated situation, with access to equipment, assist the patient to assume the prone position while providing for safety and privacy following the steps in the procedure.

1. Check the examination room for cleanliness. **NOTE: Always have clean paper on the table and a clean cover or clean towel over the pillow.**

2. Identify the patient. **RATIONALE: Speaking to the patient by name ensures that you are performing the procedure on the correct patient.**

3. Give clear instructions to the patient regarding the amount of clothing to remove and where it is to be placed.

4. Instruct the patient on use of the gown—to be open in back. Some offices furnish a modesty gown with a rectangular piece of material to be put on diaper fashion and tied on the sides. If necessary, instruct in its use.

5. Assist the patient if necessary. Otherwise respect the privacy of the patient by leaving the room while the patient undresses.

6. Instruct the patient to sit on the end of the table.

7. Instruct the patient to lie flat on the table with his legs together.

8. Pull out the end extension on the table for leg support if needed.

9. Cover the patient with a drape sheet and instruct the patient to turn toward you onto his stomach, being careful to stay in the center of the table to avoid a fall. **NOTE: Always instruct the patient to turn toward your body to prevent a fall. You can grasp the cover drape and keep it smoothly in place as patient turns over.**

10. Instruct the patient to turn the head to the side.

(continues)

PROCEDURE PROCEDURE PROCEDURE PROCEDURE PROCEDURE PROCEDURE PROCEDURE

14-10  Assist the Patient to the Prone Position (Continued)

11. Instruct the patient to flex his arms at the elbows with his hands at the side of his head.

12. Drape the sheet evenly and loosely on all sides.

13. Assist the physician as necessary with the examination.

14. Instruct the patient to turn onto his back, being careful to stay in the middle of the table to avoid a fall.

15. Instruct the patient to sit up for a moment to regain balance before trying to leave the table.

16. Clean the room and replace the supplies. **NOTE: The examination table surface and base must be thoroughly cleaned with disinfecting cleanser at regular intervals and following any contact with body fluids that may contain bloodborne pathogens.**

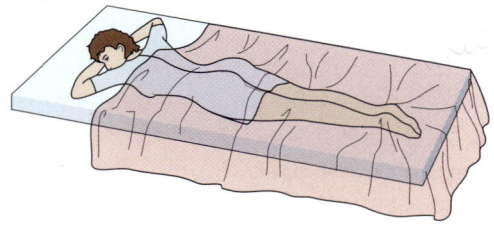

FIGURE 14-21   Prone position

ture, and instilling rectal medications (Procedure 14-11 and Figure 14-22). This position may also be used for perineal and some pelvic examinations. This is also called the lateral recumbent position.

The patient is positioned on her left side with the left arm extended behind the body and the right arm flexed upward. A pillow under the head adds to the comfort of this position. The left leg may be slightly flexed, but the right leg is sharply flexed upward. The

PROCEDURE PROCEDURE PROCEDURE PROCEDURE PROCEDURE PROCEDURE PROCEDURE

14-11  Assist the Patient to a Sims' Position

PURPOSE: To assist the patient into a Sims' position for an examination.

OSHA GUIDELINES: Standard Precautions recommend that proper hand washing and gloving is performed to avoid the transfer of microorganisms to other patients, yourself, and the environment.

EQUIPMENT: Table, table paper, gown, drape sheet, pillow, and disposable pillow cover or towel.

PERFORMANCE OBJECTIVE: In a simulated situation, with access to equipment, assist the patient to assume the Sims' position while providing for safety and privacy following the steps in the procedure.

1. Check the examination room for cleanliness. **NOTE: Always have clean paper on the table and a clean cover or clean towel over the pillow.**

2. Identify the patient. **RATIONALE: Speaking to the patient by name ensures that you are performing the procedure on the correct patient.**

3. Give clear instructions to the patient regarding the amount of clothing to remove and where it is to be placed.

4. Instruct the patient on use of the gown, to be open in the back. **RATIONALE: The procedure to be performed dictates whether the front or back should be open.**

5. Assist the patient if needed. Otherwise respect the privacy and modesty of the patient by leaving the room while the patient undresses.

6. Instruct the patient to sit on the end of the table.

7. Instruct the patient to lie back and turn on her left side. A pillow may be placed under her head. Pull out the leg rest from the table to support the left leg.

(continues)

PROCEDURE PROCEDURE PROCEDURE PROCEDURE PROCEDURE PROCEDURE PROCEDURE

14-11 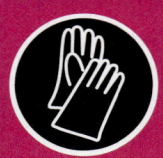 Assist the Patient to a Sims' Position (Continued)

8. Instruct the patient to place her left arm and shoulder behind her body. This places the weight of body on the chest.

9. Instruct the patient to flex her right arm with the hand toward the head in front of her body.

10. Instruct the patient to flex her left leg slightly with the buttocks near the edge of the table, being sure the patient does not fall.

11. Instruct the patient to flex her right leg sharply toward her chest.

12. Cover the patient with a **fenestrated** drape. If a regular sheet is used, hang the drape free from under the

arms to below the knees. The edge will be turned back for the procedure.

13. Assist the physician as necessary with the examination.

14. Instruct the patient to turn to her back, sit up, wait a moment for return of balance, and then move from the table. Assist the patient as necessary.

15. Clean the room and replace the supplies. **NOTE: The examination table surface and base must be thoroughly cleaned with disinfecting cleanser at regular intervals and following any contact with body fluids that may contain bloodborne pathogens.**

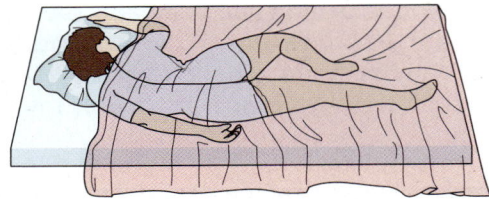

FIGURE 14-22 Sims' position

drape should cover at least from the axillary area to below the knees. The drape is raised to permit examination or treatment of the rectal area.

The *knee-chest* or **genupectoral** position is difficult for patients to assume. The chest and knees are placed flat against the table with the knees separated. The arms can be crossed under the head or flexed to each side, with the head turned to the side. The buttocks ex-

tend upward with the back straight. Patients will need assistance in assuming and maintaining this position. The medical assistant must remain with the patient for support and assistance while the patient is in this position. The patient should not be placed in the position until the physician is ready to do the examination. If the patient cannot get into the knee-chest position, it can be modified to a knee-elbow position, which is easier to assume and maintain. This position is called **genucubital**.

The knee-chest position is used for rectal or proctological examinations and occasionally a sigmoidoscopy if a proctological table is not available. The position causes the intestinal organs to move toward the chest, thereby straightening somewhat the sigmoid colon to facilitate insertion of instruments. (See Procedure 14-12 and Figure 14-23.)

PROCEDURE PROCEDURE PROCEDURE PROCEDURE PROCEDURE PROCEDURE PROCEDURE

14-12  Assist the Patient to a Knee-Chest Position

PURPOSE: To assist the patient into a knee-chest position for an examination.

OSHA GUIDELINES: Standard Precautions recommend that proper hand washing and gloving is performed to avoid the transfer of microorganisms to other patients, yourself, and the environment.

EQUIPMENT: Table, table paper, gown, drape sheet, pillow, and disposable pillow cover or towel.

PERFORMANCE OBJECTIVE: In a simulated situation, with access to equipment, assist the patient to assume the knee-chest position while providing for safety and privacy following the steps in the procedure.

(continues)

PROCEDURE PROCEDURE PROCEDURE PROCEDURE PROCEDURE PROCEDURE PROCEDURE

14-12 Assist the Patient to a Knee-Chest Position (Continued)

1. Check the examination room for cleanliness. **NOTE: Always have clean paper on the table and a clean pillow cover or clean towel over the pillow.**

2. Identify the patient. **RATIONALE: Speaking to the patient by name ensures that you are performing the procedure on the correct patient.**

3. Give clear instructions to the patient regarding which clothing to remove and where it is to be placed.

4. Instruct the patient on use of the gown to be open in the back. **RATIONALE: The procedure to be performed dictates whether the front or back should be open.**

5. Assist the patient if needed. Otherwise respect the privacy and modesty of the patient by leaving the room while the patient undresses. **NOTE: The equipment needed for the examination may be assembled while the patient is undressing if not done before. Everything must be prepared, covered, and ready for the physician's use before the patient is put into the knee-chest position.**

6. Instruct the patient to sit on the end of the table.

7. Instruct the patient to lie down on the table.

8. Cover the patient with drape.

9. Instruct the patient to turn toward you onto his stomach, being careful to stay in the middle of table.

10. Instruct the patient to get on his hands and knees.

11. Instruct the patient to flex his arms and fold them under his head, bringing the chest down to the table. If this is too difficult, have the patient rest on his elbows (genucubital position).

12. Instruct the patient to separate the knees and keep the thighs at a right angle to the table.

13. A fenestrated drape is usually used, but two small sheets may be draped to meet at the rectal area. A diamond drape may also be used.

14. Call the physician immediately to complete the examination.

15. Assist the physician as necessary with the examination.

16. Instruct the patient to lie flat on his stomach and then turn over on his back (while lying in middle of table) and sit up until balance returns before moving from the table.

17. Clean the room and replace the supplies. **NOTE: The examination table surface and base must be thoroughly cleaned with disinfecting cleanser at regular intervals and following any contact with body fluids that may contain bloodborne pathogens.**

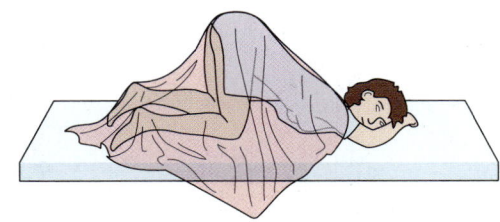

FIGURE 14-23   Knee-chest position

The **Fowler's** position is used for patients with respiratory or cardiovascular problems (Procedure 14-13 and Figures 14-24A and B). The patient who is **dyspneic** must be in a sitting or semisitting position to breathe comfortably. This position is also used to examine the trunk of the body (head, neck, and chest area). The patient may simply sit upright at the foot of the table or be supported by the back of the examination table. When the patient's upper body is at a 90-degree angle to the table it is known as a high Fowler's position

(refer to Figure 14-24A). If the patient is resting against the back of the table and it is lowered to a 30- to 45-degree angle, it is known as the semi-Fowler's position (refer to Figure 14-24B). *Taber's Cyclopedic Medical Dictionary* defines a third position of 45 to 60 degrees as Fowler's. The patient gown should open in the front, and the drape should cover from the axillary area down. When the high Fowler's position is used, the drape will naturally fall to cover from the top of the legs to over the feet.

The **lithotomy** position is used for vaginal or rectal examination (Procedure 14-14 and Figure 14-25). This position can also be used for examination of the male genital area and for catheterization of a female patient. The primary use of the position is for vaginal examinations of the female patient when a speculum is inserted, as when obtaining Pap smears.

Assisting a patient into lithotomy position requires that she first sit at the end of the table and then lie back. The leg support may be extended temporarily. A

PROCEDURE PROCEDURE PROCEDURE PROCEDURE PROCEDURE PROCEDURE PROCEDURE

14-13 Assist the Patient to a Fowler's Position

PURPOSE: To assist the patient into a Fowler's position for an examination.

OSHA GUIDELINES: Standard Precautions recommend that proper hand washing and gloving be performed to avoid the transfer of microorganisms to other patients, yourself, and the environment.

EQUIPMENT: Table, table paper, gown, drape sheet, pillow, and disposable pillow cover or towel.

PERFORMANCE OBJECTIVE: In a simulated situation, with access to equipment, assist the patient to assume the Fowler's position while providing for safety and privacy according to the steps in the procedure.

1. Check the examination room for cleanliness. **NOTE: Always have clean paper on the table and a clean pillow cover or clean towel over the pillow.**

2. Identify the patient. **RATIONALE: Speaking to the patient by name and checking the chart ensures that you are performing the procedure on the correct patient.**

3. Give clear instructions to the patient if clothing is to be removed.

4. Instruct the patient on use of the gown. **RATIONALE: The procedure to be performed dictates whether the front or back should be open.**

5. Assist the patient if needed or leave room while the patient undresses.

6. Ask the patient to sit at the end of the table.

7. Raise the head of table to the desired height for comfort of the patient, usually a 45-degree angle for semi-Fowler's and completely upright for high Fowler's.

8. Ask the patient to lean back on the rest.

9. Support the legs with the extension rest at the end of the table.

10. Drape the patient from the underarms to below the knees.

11. Assist with the examination as necessary.

12. Assist the patient to sit upright after Semi-Fowler's before moving from the table.

13. Lower the head of the table. **NOTE: Some tables have a release lever, and it is necessary to support the head of the table with one hand while releasing the lever so that the head of the table will not fall with a crash.**

14. Clean the room and replace the supplies. **NOTE: The examination table surface and base must be thoroughly cleaned with disinfecting cleanser at regular intervals and following any contact with body fluids that may contain bloodborne pathogens.**

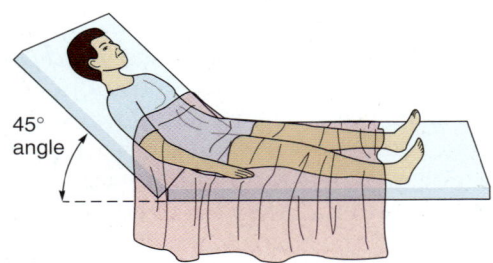

FIGURE 14-24A Semi-Fowler's position

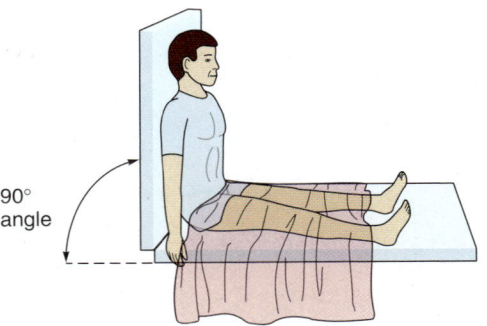

FIGURE 14-24B High Fowler's position

drape is placed over the patient from the chest to the feet. The stirrups are extended from the table and tightened or secured into position. The stirrups should be extended far enough to allow the patient to be comfortable in order to facilitate abdominal relaxation and prevent leg cramps. The legs are flexed, and the heel of each foot is placed in a stirrup. The patient

is instructed to slide down so that the hips are at the edge of the table. A pillow under the head will make the patient more comfortable. The arms may be crossed over the abdomen or placed at the sides. The medical assistant should ensure the patient is as comfortable as possible and provide support for the anxious patient.

14-14  Assist the Patient to a Lithotomy Position

PURPOSE: To assist the patient into a lithotomy position for an examination.

OSHA GUIDELINES: Standard Precautions recommend that proper hand washing and gloving is performed to avoid the transfer of microorganisms to other patients, yourself, and the environment.

EQUIPMENT: Table, table paper, gown, drape sheet, pillow, and disposable pillow cover or towel.

PERFORMANCE OBJECTIVE: In a simulated situation, with access to equipment, assist the patient to assume the lithotomy position while providing for safety and privacy following the steps in the procedure.

1. Check the examination room for cleanliness. **NOTE: Always have clean paper on the table and a clean pillow cover or clean towel over the pillow.**

2. Identify the patient. **RATIONALE: Speaking to the patient by name and checking the chart ensures that you are performing the procedure on the correct patient.**

3. Give clear instructions to the patient to remove clothing from the waist down. Ask patient to put on a gown, opening in the back.

4. Assist the patient if needed or leave the room while the patient is undressing. **NOTE: The equipment needed for the examination may be assembled while the patient is undressing if not done before. Everything must be prepared, covered, and ready for the physician's use before the patient is put into the lithotomy position.**

5. Ask the patient to sit at the end of the table.

6. Instruct the patient to lie back on the table.

7. Cover with a drape from chest to feet.

8. Support the legs with the extension on the table. (If there is no extension, be sure the patient moves back on the table before lying down.) **NOTE: Newer power examination tables allow the patient to sit while the table is tilted back, leg supports come up under the legs, and the end of table is lowered automatically.**

9. Position stirrups at a comfortable distance from the table and adjust the height if necessary. **RATIONALE: If the heels are too close to the table and buttocks, the patient may get leg cramps.**

10. Stabilize the stirrups so they will remain in position during the examination. **NOTE: Some tables are designed so that you must turn a knob at the side of the table. Some tables have several locking positions for stirrups as they swing outward.**

11. Assist the patient to put her heels into the stirrups; adjust as needed.

12. Ask the patient to move toward the end of the table. **NOTE: Place the back of your hand against the drape sheet at the end of the table. Ask the patient to move until she touches your hand.**

13. Check the patient's position to be sure her buttocks are at the end of the table and her legs are as comfortable as possible.

14. Push in the table extension, position a stool for the physician, and position the light.

15. Assist the physician as necessary.

16. When the examination is complete, ask the patient to slide back up on table.

17. Instruct the patient to sit up to regain balance before moving from table.

18. If examination was performed, offer tissues to remove excess lubricant before dressing.

19. Clean the room and replace the supplies. **NOTE: The examination table surface and base must be thoroughly cleaned with disinfecting cleanser at regular intervals and following any contact with body fluids that may contain bloodborne pathogens.**

Three additional body positions need mentioning but are used infrequently in most physicians' offices: the Trendelenburg, the jackknife, and the proctologic.

In the **Trendelenburg** or **shock** position, the patient is supine with the feet elevated slightly (Figure 14-26A). This position may easily be accomplished with a power table.

The controls would automatically lower the head of the table while keeping the patient in supine or horizontal recumbent position. With a manual table, the top section can be raised to elevate the thighs and hips, thereby achieving a lower position for the head and a modified Trendelenburg position. The lower legs are bent over the end of the table to maintain the position

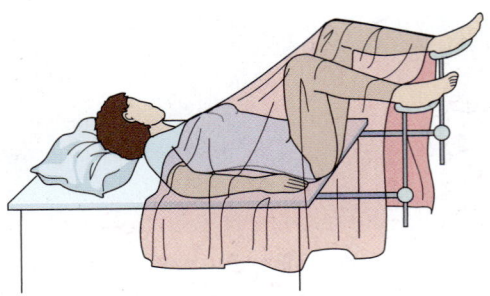

FIGURE 14-25 Lithotomy position

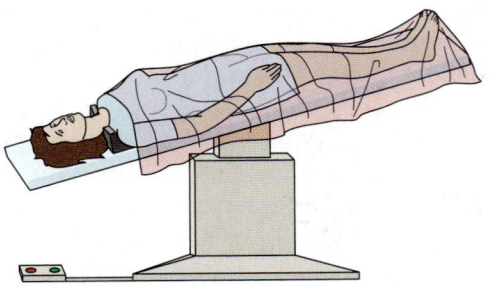

FIGURE 14-26A Trendelenburg or shock position with power table

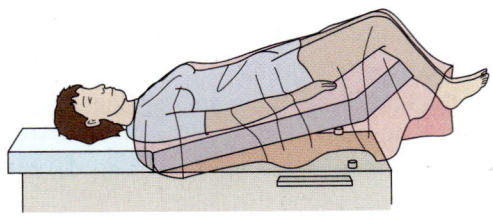

FIGURE 14-26B Modified Trendelenburg with manual table

(Figure 14-26B). This position would be used if a patient experiences or has symptoms of syncope. Patients may experience difficulty when blood samples are drawn, intravenous therapy is given, or with some examinations.

Trendelenburg positioning is frequently used in a critical care facility and by EMS personnel with trauma, hemorrhage, and dangerously low blood pressure. It is also beneficial in certain abdominal and pelvic surgical procedures to displace organs upward.

The position can also be used as a simple test for **incompetent** valves in persons with varicose veins. After being placed in straight-line Trendelenburg, the patient is asked to stand, and the physician observes whether the veins fill from above or below.

A special table would be needed for the jackknife position to be comfortable (Figure 14-27). The patient is in a semisitting position with the shoulders elevated and the thighs flexed at right angles to the abdomen. This position is especially useful for examination and instrumentation of the male urethra.

The proctologic position (Figure 14-28), requires a power table (Figure 14-29) or a special manual table that has an attachable kneeling extension and can be upended by a hand cranking mechanism. The top half of the table is flat, while the leg portion, with the extender, is at a right angle. The patient would be asked to disrobe from the waist down and kneel on the extension, flexing his upper body to lie on the table. If clothing is one piece, a gown open in the back is indicated. A drape is positioned over the patient from the mid-back down. The arms are usually

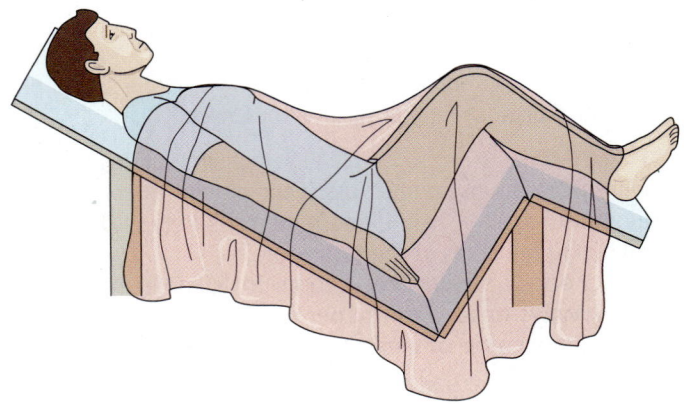

FIGURE 14-27 Jackknife position

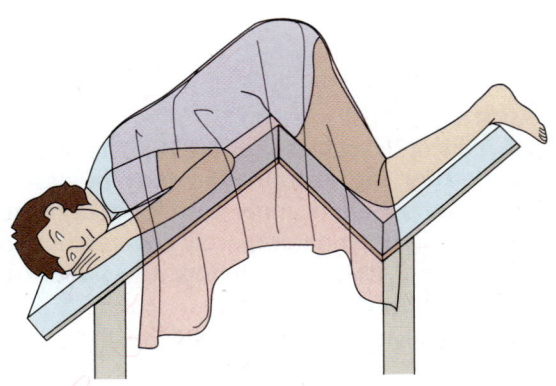

FIGURE 14-28 Proctologic position

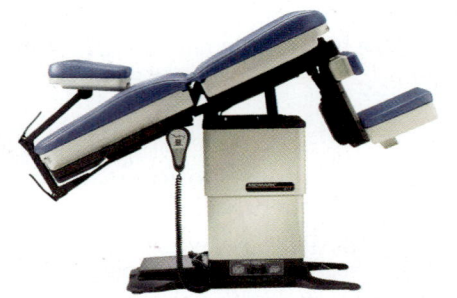

FIGURE 14-29 The Midmark power table in position for specialty exams (*Courtesy of Midmark Corp.*)

flexed at the side or under the head. The medical assistant operates the controls or cranks the table over until the buttocks are elevated. The head is lower than the body, and the internal abdominal organs move toward the chest. This helps to straighten the "S" curve of the sigmoid colon to facilitate sigmoidoscope insertion during a sigmoidoscopy. The position is also used for examination and treatment of rectal and anal conditions such as thrombosed and internal hemorrhoids.

Now that you have learned the patient positions used for physical examination, we will continue in the next unit with the examination process as we proceed through a complete physical examination.

ACHIEVE UNIT OBJECTIVES

■ **Complete the Workbook activities to meet the learning objectives.**

■ **Practice the procedures in this unit to meet the performance objectives.**

■ **Apply your knowledge at the end of this chapter in completing the Critical Thinking Challenge and Activities, as well as the StudyWARE on your Student CD-ROM.**

UNIT 3
THE PHYSICAL EXAMINATION

OBJECTIVES

Upon completion of this unit, you will be able to achieve the following:

LEARNING Objectives

1. **Spell and define, using the glossary at the back of the text, all the Words to Know in this unit.**
2. **Name the six examination techniques used by physicians and give examples of each.**
3. **Name the instruments, equipment, and supplies used in the CPE, and state the function of each.**
4. **Explain the role of the medical assistant in the examination process.**

5. **Discuss patient education as it relates to why physical examinations are done, general information regarding disease and injury prevention and breast and testicular self-examination.**
6. **Identify the nine sections of the abdominal cavity, and name the visceral organs therein.**
7. **Explain the POMR and SOAP methods of charting patient information.**
8. **Explain subjective and objective symptoms, and give five examples of each.**
9. **Discuss the physical examination schedules for adults.**

PERFORMANCE Objectives

1. **Prepare a patient for and assist with routine and specialty examinations.**

WORDS TO KNOW

acute	heart murmur	progress report
anxiety	hernia	prolapse
auscultation	initial	resonance
bimanual	inspection	R/O (rule/out)
bruit	laxative	sphincter
caustic	manipulation	sterile gauze
chronic	mensuration	square
coordination	nasal speculum	subjective
digitally	objective	subsequent
dimpling	occult	symmetry
douche	palpation	tongue depressor
duration	percussion	tuning fork
enema	percussion	turgor
explicit	hammer	vaginal
fast	peripheral	speculum
gait	PERRLA	visceral
gooseneck lamp	physical	writer
guaiac test paper	pitch	

CERTIFICATION CONNECTION

CMA
Patient preparation and assisting the physician (examinations; procedures; explanation and instructions; Instruments, supplies, and equipment)

THE COMPLETE PHYSICAL EXAMINATION

The primary reason for performing a complete physical examination (CPE) is to determine the general state of health and well-being of the patient. The CPE can be performed for various reasons such as an insurance examination before issuing a policy, as a requirement with a patient's employment, as a request by a patient, or to assess a patient's state of health. The exam will cover all major organs and systems of the body. The physician's findings enable her to establish an opinion as to the patient's condition and establish either a tentative or definitive diagnosis when there are abnormal signs and symptoms. Often laboratory tests or diagnostic procedures are ordered to provide additional information upon which to base the diagnosis. Once all data is obtained, the diagnosis is defined and the treatment plan, if indicated, can be established.

The Medical Assistant's Role

Preparation of the room is the first step in the examination process. The room should be clean and tidy and at a comfortable temperature. The medical assistant must be certain the examination table is clean and covered with new table paper or a cloth cover. There should be an adequate amount of supplies conveniently arranged for efficient use.

Preparation of the examination equipment is the next step. The equipment should be checked to be sure it is operating appropriately (e.g., light sources for scopes). It is especially embarrassing and time consuming to make adjustments because equipment will not work. The items commonly used for examinations are shown

---

P **PATIENT EDUCATION**

The patient needs to know why the physical examination is being performed. Explain that the data collected form a database against which all future examinations and observations will be compared. The patient must understand what is taking place and why. It is very important for the patient to be relaxed while being examined. Some examinations can be embarrassing to a patient, but a clear explanation of each procedure can help relax the patient. You can assist the patient greatly by giving empathy and support.

---

and numbered for identification in Figure 14-30. It is important for you to know the name and function of each item, as well as the examination routine, so you can anticipate the need and assist the physician if asked.

Preparation of the patient is a very important step. Often this begins at midnight the night before the exam and is called non-per-os (NPO), meaning nothing by mouth. Usually patients are asked to **fast** so that specific diagnostic blood tests may be drawn. It may also be more comfortable when other procedures are performed if nothing has been eaten before the examination.

The medical assistant will probably be the main person with whom the patient interacts prior to the examination. It is important for the patient to feel comfortable in his surroundings and with the anticipated medical exam. Remember, before the examination is done, the in-person interview has occurred and the chief complaint, if any, has been identified. The vital signs and other mensurations have been completed, and it is time to proceed.

Instruct the patient to go to the bathroom so she will be more comfortable during the exam. If the patient did not bring the morning's first voided specimen with her, provide a specimen container and instruct her to catch a sample for you to test. It is time consuming and embarrassing for the patient if the physician has to interrupt the examination for the patient to use the bathroom. Unnecessary interruptions are annoying and hinder the patient flow schedule.

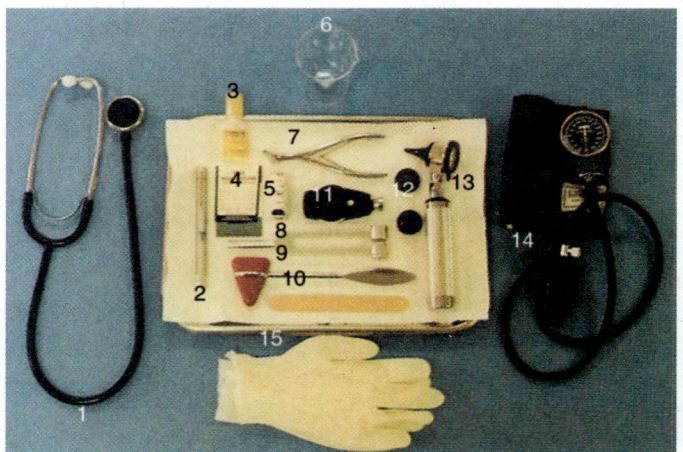

1. stethoscope	9. percussion hammer
2. penlight	10. tongue depressor
3. guaiac/occult blood test developer	11. ophthalmoscope (head)
4. guaiac/occult blood test	12. ear and nose speculum
5. flexible tape measure	13. otoscope head attached to
6. urine specimen container	base handle
7. metal nasal speculum	14. sphygmomanometer
8. tuning fork	15. latex or vinyl gloves

FIGURE 14-30 Example of instruments and supplies used in the physical examination

The next step is to ask the patient to disrobe and put on the examination gown. Explain whether it is to be opened in the front or back and offer assistance if needed. Show the patient where to place clothing after it is removed. It is usually considered appropriate to leave the room while the patient is disrobing. If the patient is capable of self-care, pull out the step at the end of the exam table (or provide a portable step) and instruct her to sit on the table after putting on the gown and cover her legs with the drape sheet, which provides privacy as well as warmth. After a brief time, knock on the door and enter the room. If assistance is needed, help the patient to disrobe and put on the gown. Assist her onto the table, being careful as she uses the step or stool so she does not fall. Do not try to assist patients by yourself if they are very large or need a lot of help. Get someone to help you so you do not injure yourself or the patient.

There may be a period of time before the physician enters the room. If the patient is anxious, you can describe the general format of the physical and answer any questions she may have. Reassure her that there may be momentary discomfort with some parts of the examination, but there should not be any pain. Explain that the patient should inform the physician if unusual discomfort or pain is experienced or any other symptom is felt that was not previously present.

This may also be an excellent opportunity for patient education if you have observed something or the patient has mentioned a concern. Knowing about the pamphlets and other resources available in your office, you can talk with the patient and indicate you will supply the material after the exam. There are some patient education boxes within this unit and throughout the text that have general information that is appropriate for discussion. This may give you some ideas upon which to build a conversation. This skill will become easier after you gain more knowledge and have more experience. Even if you feel inadequate, remember you are still probably more knowledgeable than the patient.

Assisting the physician with the examination is the last step in the examination process. The medical assistant positions the patient, hands examination instruments and supplies to the physician, and provides comfort to the patient as needed.

Assisting with the complete physical examination (CPE), the general physical exam, history and physical (H & P), physical exam (PE), or just plain **physical** (as it is often termed) is not difficult but is complex in that it is a *set* of procedures. You may also assist with the exam or write the findings.

In many facilities, the medical assistant accompanies the physician in the examination room and records the findings. The term **writer** is given to the medical assistant who writes what the physician dictates during the exam. The MA who performs this duty must have sound knowledge in medical terminology, anatomy, and physiology, and of course, good spelling and writing skills. Because the physician bases the diagnosis on these findings, accuracy is vital. Many physicians prefer to write their own findings on plain sheets of lined paper (a common practice is to use a rubber stamp that outlines a particular exam format), or on specially printed forms in the outlined order of their choice. Still other physicians prefer to dictate the findings of an examination into a recorder for transcription later by the medical assistant. With EHR, the findings could be entered directly into the software as the examination is conducted.

There is no absolute pattern of examination to follow as long as the examiner is consistent and forms a personal habit so as to be thorough and complete with each patient. The complete examination should include the whole body, from head to toe, front to back, and inside and out. In your career as a medical assistant, you will work with physicians who may be quite different in their systematic approach to patient examination.

An example of the review of systems and physical examination portion of a history and physical examination form used in a family practice office is shown in Figure 14-31. Note it is concise and requires listing only abnormal findings to conserve time and writing. There are many abbreviations, some of which are facility specific.

EXAMINATION TECHNIQUES

Physicians are skilled in a variety of techniques used in evaluating patients in the examination process. In assisting with an H & P, the medical assistant is expected to have a basic knowledge of these terms. There are basically six techniques used to evaluate patients during physical examinations. Each technique provides specific information regarding the condition of the patient's body.

1. **Inspection** is evaluation by the use of sight. This is usually the **initial** part of the exam when the physician looks at the patient to observe the skin's color and condition (rashes and discoloration), the general appearance (grooming, apparent state of health, posture), the level of **anxiety**, and **gait**. Awareness of person, place, and time as well as any visible injuries or deformities are noted.

2. **Palpation** is evaluation using the sense of touch. The body can be felt using one hand, two hands (**bimanual** as in vaginal examinations), or one finger (**digitally** as in rectal examination). Examination of the breasts is done with the flat surfaces of the fingers of both hands. Palpation can determine skin temperature, size and shape of organs, the position and presence of abnormal structures, as well as the degree of abdominal rigidity and aortic pulsations.

ROS: negative except—

☐ Hair loss	☐ Skin moles/ rash	☐ Chest pain/ discomfort	☐ Blood BM/ urine	☐ Weakness
☐ Change in vision	☐ Difficulty swallowing	☐ Stomach pain	☐ Difficulty w/ urination	☐ Foot problems
☐ Change in hearing	☐ Difficulty breathing	☐ Constipation	☐ Joint pain	☐ Blackouts
☐ Swollen glands	☐ Heart palpitations	☐ Diarrhea	☐ Numbness	☐ _____

PE: **NORMS:**   **ABNORMALS   TESTS**

☐ General:	Healthy & appears stated age.	_____
☐ Skin:	Without rashes, lesions, or malignant appearing nevi.	_____
☐ H&N:	NC/AT, no thyromegaly, no adenopathy, no carotid bruit.	_____
☐ EENT:	PERRLA, EOMI, TM's normal, Nares patent, Pharnyx clear.	_____
☐ Heart:	RRR, Nl. Heart tones, no murmurs, rubs, gallops.	_____
☐ Lungs:	Clear to auscultation bilaterally.	_____
☐ Breasts:	Symmetrical, no retraction, no discharge, no masses.	_____
☐ ABD:	Soft, NT/ND, no HSM, Nl.Bs, no bruits, no masses.	_____
☐ Back:	No scoliosis, no CVAT.	_____
☐ GU: ☐	_Un/circumcised, Nl. Male genitalia, no testicular lumps, no hernia.	_____
	Nl. Rectal tone, prostate not enlarged, no lumps.	_____
☐	_Nl. Exernal female genitalia, Nl. Cervix, no CMT, no adenexal masses.	_____
	Nl. Rectal tone, no masses.	_____
☐ Extrem:	No CC or E, FROM x 4, Nl. Pulses x 4, 5/5 strength x 4.	_____
☐ Neuro:	MSE appropriate, CN II-XII intact, Nl. DTR's, Nl. Motor/sensory/CB exam.	_____
☐ Feet:	Normal arches, No bunions, No hammer toes, No hallux varus.	_____

IMPRESSIONS / PLAN:

_____

_____

_____

_____

_____

_____

FIGURE 14-31   Review of systems and physical examination portion of an H&P form

---

PATIENT EDUCATION

A. To prevent injuries of the face and head:
  1. In work and recreational environments, wear protective head gear: hard hat at work (construction sites), helmet for sports (motorcycle riding, football).
    a. Wear protective face mask or goggles for sports such as football, basketball, and wrestling to prevent possible eye injuries.
    b. Use ear plugs to protect ears from exposure to loud noises that can lead to possible damage to auditory nerves resulting in hearing loss (machinery, band concerts) and from water when swimming.

B. To protect the skin:
  1. Keep skin clean and soft by using mild soap and water for bathing and a moisturizing lotion as necessary.
    a. Discourage sun worship. Encourage keeping covered in the sun or the use of a sun blocker to prevent damage of ultraviolet rays if one must be in the sun for prolonged periods. Discourage use of tanning beds.
    b. Wash hands of (chemical) irritants immediately to prevent caustic burns.

C. To prevent diseases of the respiratory system and other contagious diseases:
  1. Discourage eating or drinking after another person to keep from transmitting viruses and diseases.

  2. Wash hands after handling items in or from public places, which probably have been handled by multitudes of others (money, doorknobs, etc.).
  3. Discourage smoking or tobacco use of any kind (post antismoking pamphlets or meetings for patients to read).
  4. Remind patients of the dangers of drug and alcohol use and abuse (display information about Alcoholics Anonymous meetings).
  5. Encourage exercise and physical fitness programs with the advice of the physician.
  6. Promote proper nutrition and weight control by reminding patients to eat well-balanced meals regularly, and help them plan their diets.
  7. Encourage *safe sex* by providing explicit information to teach patients about the dangers of sexually transmitted diseases and AIDS.
  8. Discourage patients from using laxatives and enemas unless specifically ordered by the physician.
  9. Remind patients about immunizations and encourage their compliance.
  10. Encourage patients to read labels for contents of the products they buy and use for their safety.
  11. Remind patients to use seat belts.
  12. Promote regular medical and dental checkups.

3. **Percussion** is a means of producing sounds by tapping various parts of the body. The physician listens to the sounds to determine the size, density, and location of underlying **visceral** organs. **Pitch**, quality, **duration**, and **resonance** are terms used by physicians when referring to percussion. Direct percussion is termed *immediate* and is done by striking the finger against the patient's body. The type of percussion most often used is *indirect* or *mediate*. With indirect percussion, the examiner's finger is placed on the area and struck with a finger of the other hand.

4. **Auscultation** is listening to sounds made by the patient's body. Indirect or mediate auscultation is done with the stethoscope to amplify sounds that arise from the lungs, heart, and visceral organs. Sounds heard by this method of examination include **bruits**, murmurs, rales, rhythms, and bowel sounds. Direct or immediate auscultation is done by placing the ear directly over the bare surface area. Auscultation skill is acquired with experience. The physician must be able to determine normal from abnormal sounds. Some, such as the heart valve sounds, last only a fraction of a second and demand concentrated listening.

5. **Mensuration** means measurement. In this part of the examination, the patient's chest and extremities are measured and recorded. Usually a standard flexible tape measure is used. Mensuration includes all of the following measurements: height, weight, head, chest, other parts of the body as appropriate, temperature, pulse, respirations, and blood pressure. All measurements should be recorded in inches, feet, and pounds or kilograms and centimeters. Being consistent is especially necessary in keeping track of the pediatric patient's growth and development or in assessment and evaluation of any patient's change in readings that may contribute to a diagnosis.

Manipulation is the passive movement of a joint to determine the range of extension and flexion. This evaluation is especially important when patients have had joint injuries or have arthritis. Orthopedic physicians evaluate range of motion following surgical procedures such as knee and hip replacements. Insurance companies and state Industrial Commissions may request evaluation to determine continuation of coverage following trauma injuries and industrial accidents.

PHYSICAL EXAMINATION FORMAT

In reviewing the medical examination form in Figure 14-31, you will notice that the section immediately following "review of systems" has the areas outlined for recording the findings of the complete physical examination.

The format of the examination section of this form has been expanded in the following pages with an explanation of each of the body areas examined. Hopefully this will help you become familiar with what the doctor does in each section of the physical examination. Even though H & P forms vary in appearance, the contents will basically be the same. Notice the form has small boxes to check to be sure nothing is omitted. Each exam area has conditions to be observed and a line to note any abnormalities. If an additional diagnostic test is needed, it can also be noted after the abnormal finding.

Remember that the very first part of the physical includes measurement, vital signs, and vision screening, which the medical assistant normally completes. You may want to refer to appropriate units to review these procedures.

To make the physical examination format easier to read and understand, it is presented in a modified outline format.

1. First the examination area is listed in **bold print**.
2. Next, [enclosed in brackets] is the patient's position, the examination technique(s), and the equipment or supplies needed. The patient is gowned throughout the examination, positioned and draped as explained in Unit 2. The gown will probably be opened in the back and simply raised by the medical assistant or the physician for examining the chest and abdomen. The drape will also be repositioned throughout the examination to allow inspection and examination of the patient while providing as much coverage as possible.
3. There is a brief description of how the physician may conduct this portion of the examination.
4. Within each examination area are listed characteristics the physician may be observing and *in italics,* some applicable descriptive terms. Physicians each have their own style and depth of examination, which may not include all the areas and characteristics mentioned. The following will help you understand the components of a complete physical examination.

General Appearance

[Anatomical/ambulate/sitting; inspection; physician's senses]

The physician may ask the patient to stand in front of him in the anatomical position while he observes the patient's general appearance. A few questions may be asked to judge speech and appropriate responses. The patient is asked to walk across the room to observe the manner of walking and body movements and then instructed to sit on the table.

- Appearance—*grooming, state of health, body stature, nourished, appears stated age*
- Awareness—*to person, place, and time; confused; distressed*

- Gait—manner of walking, *shuffle, limp, balance, evidence of stiffness or pain*
- Speech—*slurring, stutter, loss of voice, impediment*
- Hearing—response to sound, volume of speech
- Breath—odors: *sweet and fruity with diabetes, acetone with acidosis, oral hygiene*

Skin

[Sitting/standing; inspection/palpation; physician's senses]

The physician will inspect anterior and posterior skin surfaces while the patient stands in front of him and as he progresses through the examination.

- Color—*redness, bruising, birth marks, darker areas or sock-like redness of lower legs* (may indicate poor circulation)
- Condition—*dry, flaky, soft, calloused fingers/hands, skin cracks,* **turgor** (measured by pinching back of hand and observing the length of time for return to normal; provides estimate of hydration)
- Blemishes—*moles, warts, scars, acne, rashes*
- Lumps—*palpable masses under the skin*
- Nails—*cuticles, groomed, brittle, peeling, grooved, spooning, clubbing, white lines*

Head and Neck

[Sitting; inspection/palpation/auscultation/manipulation; stethoscope]

The physician observes the patient in a sitting position, palpating and auscultating structures and giving instructions for movement to evaluate range of motion.

- Head—**symmetry**, *nodules, hair texture and distribution, scalp*
- Face—*skin condition, presence of facial hair, facial paralysis, eye symmetry*
- Neck—range of motion; palpation of thyroid gland for *size, nodules, and symmetry;* lymph nodes and parotid glands palpated, observation of swallowing, auscultation of carotid arteries (Figure 14-32). (Blockage of the artery causes a sound known as a *bruit*.)

EENT (eye, ear, nose, and throat)

[Sitting; inspection; ophthalmoscope, otoscope, **tuning fork**, **nasal speculum**, **tongue depressor**, **sterile gauze square**]

The physician will visually observe each area as well as use the ophthalmoscope and otoscope to view internal structures. The medical assistant will turn off and on lights as needed. Eye musculature is observed by requesting patient movement. Hearing is evaluated using the tuning fork, and the nasal passages will be examined with a speculum. The mouth, throat, and tongue are checked for lesions, and oral hygiene is evaluated.

- Eyes—observed for *protrusion, lashes, symmetry,* general condition

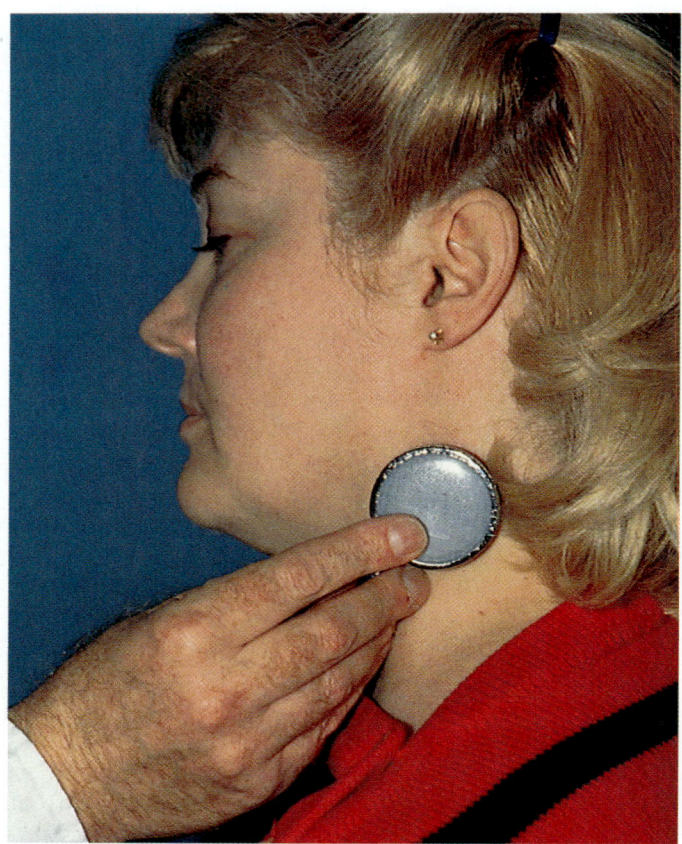

FIGURE 14-32 The physician auscultates the neck for the sounds made by blood flowing through the carotid artery.

Vision—The results of the Snellen, Jaeger, and Ishihara screening procedures previously completed following mensuration are charted at the top of the form by the medical assistant.

Pupils—(in darkened room with light source) checked for reaction to light and accommodation (L&A); if *equal*, is recorded as **PERRLA** (*pupils equal, round, and respond to light and accommodation*)

Sclera—*color, clearness, scarring*

Musculature—extraocular movements (EOM): movement up, down, right, and left while following physician's finger

Peripheral—side vision while looking straight forward

Internal structures—with ophthalmoscope views retina, optic disc, blood vessels (Figure 14-33)

- Ears—inspection, visual and otoscope

External—*size, symmetry, lobes, structure*

Middle—with otoscope; *external auditory canal, cerumen, drainage,* tympanic membrane (should be *pearly gray*), *scars* from perforations and infection

Hearing—tuning fork to test air, nerve conduction (see Unit 1)

- Nose—Inspection, visual and nasal speculum

Exterior—structure, *straight, curved, bulbous,* color

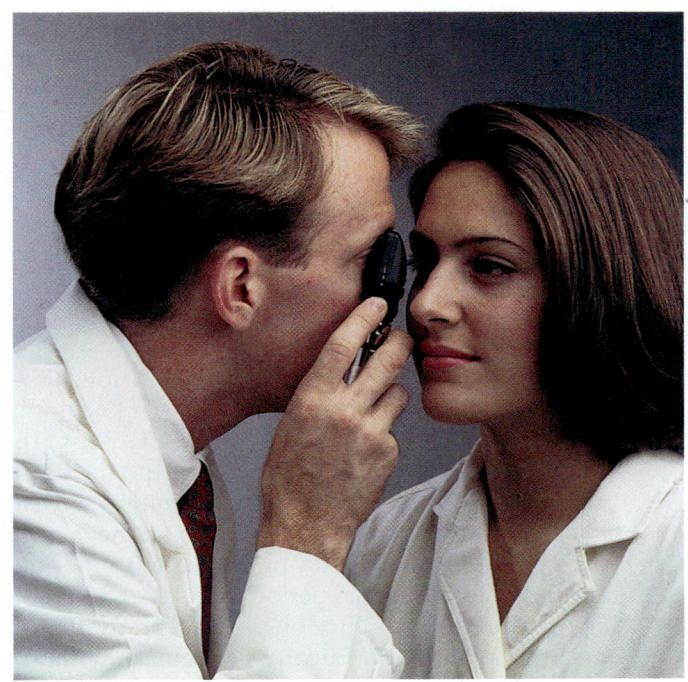

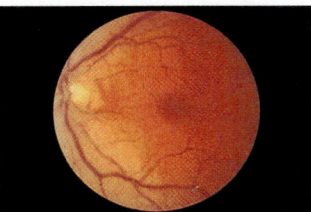

Normal Fundus—Structures are defined clearly: a normal red-orange color distinguishes the retina from the darker area, which is the fundus; arteries are red, veins are light purple.

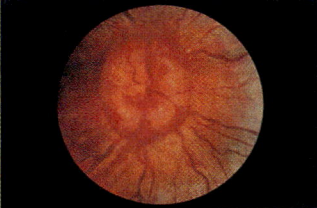

Papilledema—Shows swelling of the vessels with a small hemorrhage close to the optic papilla (optic disc) caused from head injury.

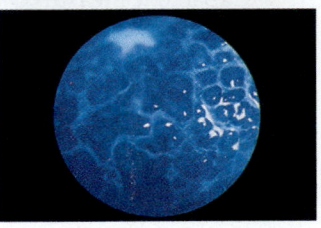

Giant Papillary Conjunctivitis (GPC)—An inflammation of the conjunctiva may occur as a reaction to contact lenses. A fluorescein dye is used to help in the identification of the microorganism.

FIGURE 14-33　Samples of what the physician may see when examining the patient's eye with the ophthalmoscope. *(Courtesy of Welch Allyn, Inc.)*

Interior—with nasal speculum and light checks mucosa, septum, *polyps*
- Throat—inspection with light source
  Mouth—with light and tongue depressor, checks inside surface of cheeks and jaw alignment; with gauze to hold tongue, check under tongue and mouth floor, frenulum
  Tongue—surface, mobility, depress while patient says "ah" to view tonsils, posterior pharynx
  Teeth—oral hygiene, condition of teeth, gums, bite, dentures (*Note:* if poor oral hygiene, following examination provide patient education and instructional materials and encourage dental visit.)

Chest
[Sitting; inspection/palpation; physician's senses]
The physician observes the seated patient as the chest is palpated for underlying nodes or masses. The chest structure is noted and the movement in response to breathing is observed.
- Inspection—for symmetry of sides, shape deformities *(barrel, pidgeon, funnel)*, intercostal spaces when breathing *(retract or bulge)*, posterior spine alignment, scapula levels
- Palpation—lymph nodes, *nodules, tenderness* (Figure 14-34)

Heart
[Sitting; auscultation; stethoscope]
The physician will auscultate the heart from both anterior and posterior chest wall. The medical assistant

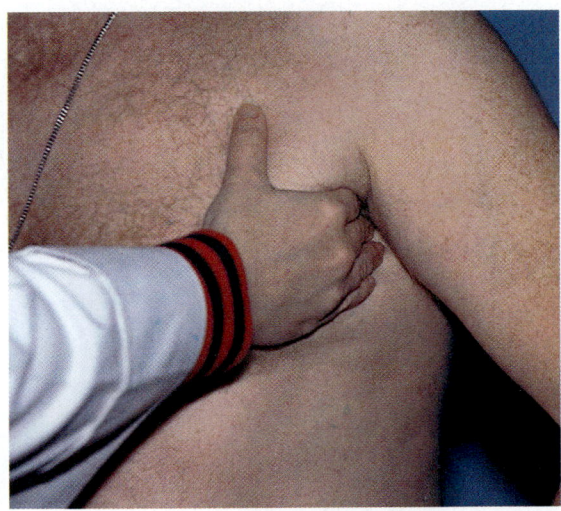

FIGURE 14-34　Palpation of the patient's axillary region

and patient must maintain silence during the examination in order for the physician to hear the heart sounds. Abnormalities may indicate the need for blood chemistries and an ECG for diagnosis. Referral to a cardiologist for stress and echocardiogram procedures may be necessary.
- Rate/rhythm—*beats per minute, regularity, volume, premature contractions*
- Sounds—auscultate valves (S_1, S_2,), **heart murmurs**, *ventricular gallop* (S_3), *atrial gallop* (S_4)
- Pericardium—*friction rub*

Lungs

[Sitting; auscultation/percussion; stethoscope]

The physician will auscultate the lungs on posterior and anterior chest wall. Again the medical assistant and patient must maintain silence except for the patient making speech sounds the physician may request. Percussion may be used if fluid, excess air, or a mass is suspected within the chest cavity.

- Rate/rhythm—*breaths per minute, regularity, volume, depth*
- Sounds—posterior auscultation (breathe with open mouth), *wheeze, rales, rhonchi, crackling, pleural friction rubs, bronchial constriction;* percussion for lung *consolidation, hyperinflation, pleural fluid* (Figure 14-35)
- Capacity—measured by the spirometer (Figure 14-36); different tests can be done: forced vital capacity involves forced inhalation followed by quick

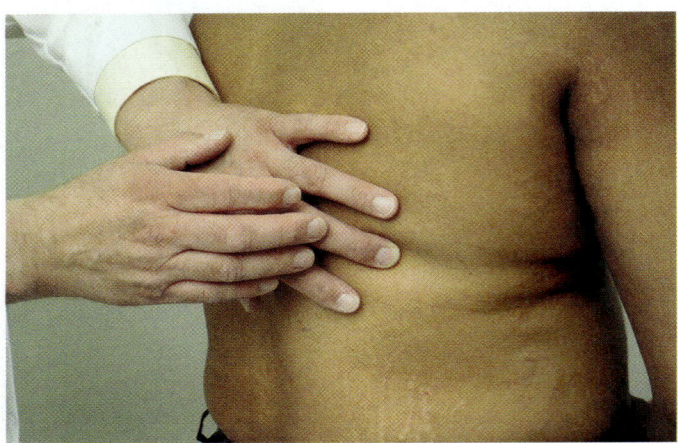

FIGURE 14-35 Using blunt percussion to examine the base of the lung

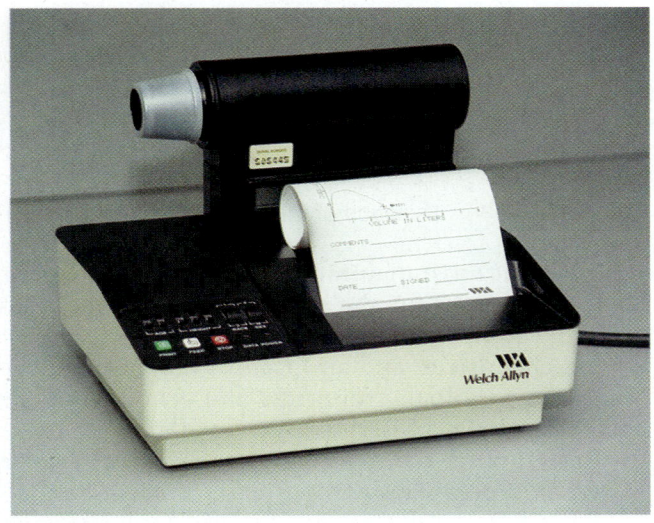

FIGURE 14-36 The spirometer is used to test pulmonary function.

and complete exhalation to determine the capacity of lungs. (Refer to Chapter 16 to review the procedure for performing spirometry.)

Breasts

[Sitting/recumbent; inspection/palpation; physician's senses]

The physician will inspect and palpate the breasts with the patient in sitting and lying positions. The physician may provide breast self-examination instruction to the patient or defer the responsibility to the medical assistant.

- Inspection—size, shape, symmetry, position, nipples, **dimpling**, *orange-peel skin*
- Palpate—*lumps, nodules, tenderness, mass,* in both supine and sitting position
- Patient education—Men can also develop breast cancer and should be examined. Instruct the female patient to perform monthly breast self-examination following her menstrual period (Figure 14-37). (See the Patient Education Box on p. 717.) Provide visual educational handout. Encourage regular mammograms as appropriate for her age-group.

Abdomen

[Supine/dorsal recumbent; auscultation/inspection/palpation/percussion; stethoscope]

Refer to Figures 14-38A, B, and C to review the sections of the abdomen and the location of the underlying organs.

The physician will stand at the side to inspect, auscultate, palpate, and percuss the abdomen with the patient in the supine and dorsal recumbent positions. A pillow under the patient's head and relaxing the abdominal muscles will facilitate deep palpation of the abdominal organs. Auscultating for bowel sounds requires the medical assistant and patient to maintain silence.

- Auscultation—(should be done first as palpation and percussion my alter bowel sounds); bowel sounds character and frequency, *bruits, organ friction rubs*
- Inspection—symmetry, *operative scars, protrusions (hernias), striae, umbilicus*

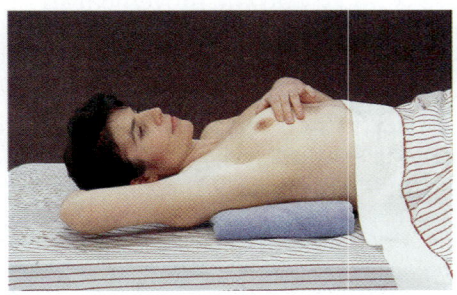

FIGURE 14-37 Breast self-examination, lying down (See the Patient Education box on page 717.)

Right hypochondriac	Epigastric	Left hypochondriac

Right lobe of liver
Gallbladder
Part of duodenum
Hepatic flexure of colon
Part of right kidney
Suprarenal gland
	Pyloric end of stomach
	Duodenum
	Pancreas
	Aorta
	Portion of liver
		Stomach
		Spleen
		  Tail of pancreas
		  Splenic flexure of colon
		Upper pole of left kidney

Right lumbar	**Umbilical**	**Left lumbar**
Ascending colon Lower half of right kidney Part of duodenum and jejunum	Omentum Mesentery Transverse colon Lower part of duodenum Jejunum and ileum	Descending colon Lower half of left kidney Parts of jejunum and ileum
Right inguinal	**Hypogastric**	**Left inguinal**
Cecum Appendix Lower end of ileum Right ureter Right spermatic cord in male Right ovary in female	Ileum Bladder Pregnant uterus	Sigmoid colon Left ureter Left spermatic cord in male Left ovary in female

FIGURE 14-38A   The nine regions of the abdominal cavity with underlying visceral organs

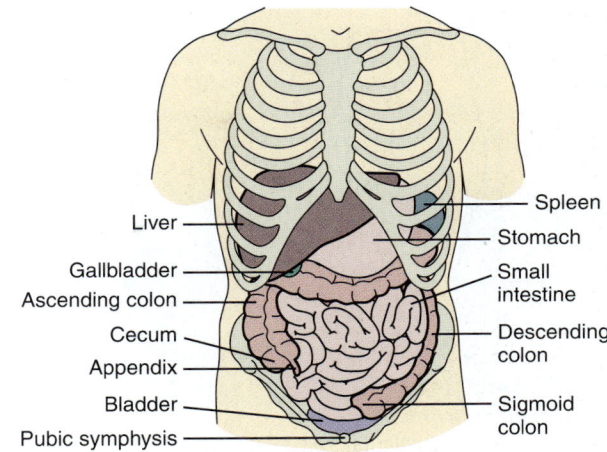

FIGURE 14-38B   Position of abdominal organs in the nine abdominal regions

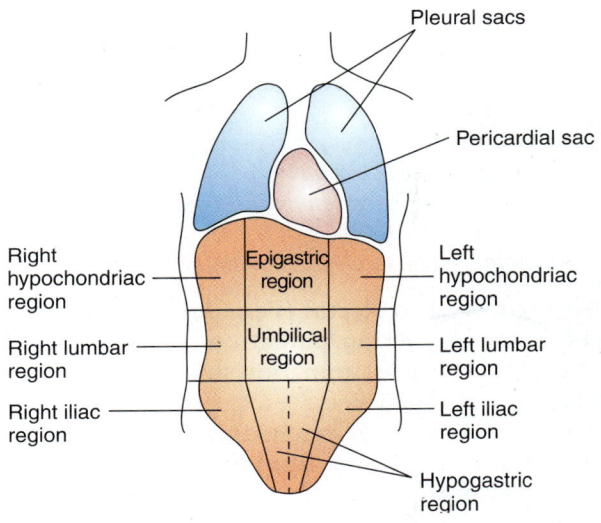

FIGURE 14-38C   Position of the nine abdominal regions

- Palpation—abdominal aorta pulse, *masses,* **hernias,** *tenderness, organs, muscular tension*
- Percussion—liver, spleen, and stomach size; *presence of air*

Back
[Standing; inspection/palpation/manipulation; physician's senses]
The physician will inspect the posterior surface to observe the spine and symmetry of bony prominences. A lateral view will detect excessive curvatures anteriorly and posteriorly. The patient may be asked to twist and bend over to evaluate curvatures and flexibility.
- Spine—*straight, concave and convex curvatures, kyphosis, lordosis, scoliosis,* manipulation to sides, twist, bend over, front and back, cervical manipulation and head all directions
- Symmetry—sides *equal,* pelvis and scapula *even*

Genitourinary and Rectal (Male)
[Standing; inspection/palpation; physician's senses, glove, lubricant, **guaiac test paper** (Hemoccult test kit), tissues]

The physician will wear gloves to inspect the external genitalia of the standing male patient. When the testes are palpated, males past puberty should be instructed in testicular self-examination (TSE). Printed instructions should be provided following the examination (Figures 14-39A and B). (See the Patient Education Box on p. 717.) The patient is asked to bear down and cough while the physician checks for hernias in the scrotum and inguinal ring. The patient is then instructed to turn around and bend over the table. The physician inspects the anus and then inserts the gloved and lubricated index finger into the anal canal to evaluate **sphincter** tone and internal hemorrhoids. The prostate is palpated through the anterior wall of the rectum. A test for **occult** blood is taken from a small amount of stool on the withdrawn index finger placed on the guaiac test paper. Tissues are used to remove the excess lubricant.

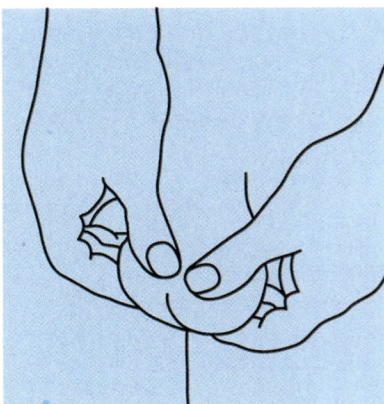

FIGURE 14-39A Testicular self-examination. Stand in front of the mirror. Look for swelling on the skin of the scrotum. (See the Patient Education box on page 717.)

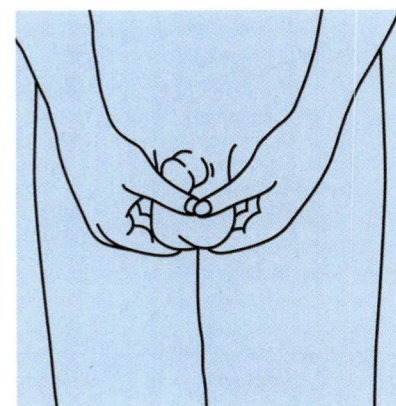

FIGURE 14-39B Examine each testicle with both hands. Position your index and middle fingers under the testicle with the thumbs on top. Gently roll the testicle between your thumbs and fingers. (Having one testicle larger than the other is normal.) Men should be advised to be examined by a physician as soon as possible if there are any abnormal findings, such as lumps or nodules, when doing TSE.

- Pubis—*lesions, infestation, distribution* of hair
- Penis—*lesions, scars, deformity, discharge, circumcision,* urinary meatus
- Scrotum—symmetry, *swelling, varicosities, fluid, masses, presence of hernia*
- Anus—*hemorrhoids, lesions, fissures,* **prolapse**, sphincter tone
- Prostate—size, *tenderness, nodules*

Genitourinary and Rectal (Female)

[Lithotomy; inspection/palpation; gloves, lubricant, **vaginal speculum**, examination stool, **gooseneck lamp**, guaiac paper (Hemoccult test kit), tissues]

When the appointment is scheduled, the patient must be instructed to refrain from using a **douche** or vaginal medications for 24 hours and from sexual intercourse for 48 hours prior to the examination. It is also preferred to schedule the examination the week following a menstrual period. The medical assistant assists the patient into lithotomy position. The physician puts on gloves or is assisted into gloves by the medical assistant. The physician usually sits on a stool at the foot of the table, with the light coming over his shoulder. First the perineal and anal areas are inspected. Then the speculum, which the medical assistant has warmed in running water, is inserted into the vagina to view internal structures. If a Pap test is to be done, it would be taken now (see Unit 4). If not, lubricant can be applied to the speculum. A bimanual examination follows. The physician inserts two fingers of the well-lubricated gloved hand into the vagina and examines internal structures by deep palpation with the other hand. Following the bimanual exam the index finger is inserted into the anus to examine the anal and rectal area. A test for occult blood is taken from a small amount of stool on the withdrawn index finger placed on the guaiac test paper. Tissues are used to

remove the excess lubricant. Additional tissues are offered to remove any residual lubricant.

- Pubis—*lesions, infestation, distribution* of hair
- Labia—*edema, redness, cysts, masses, varicosities*
- Vaginal orifice—*hymen, inflammation, bleeding, discharge, lesions*
- Vagina—*discharge, redness, lesions, mass, cervix*

Bimanual examination by palpation

- Uterus—size, *masses,* symmetry, *tenderness,* position
- Ovaries—size, *masses,* symmetry, *tenderness*

Rectal examination

- Anus: Inspection—*hemorrhoids, lesions, fissures, prolapse* Palpation—sphincter *tone, internal hemorrhoids, masses*

Extremities

[Recumbent; mensuration/manipulation; tape measure]

The physician will sometimes measure different parts of the body; however, the lower extremities are probably the most frequently measured, especially if the patient complains of back problems. It is very common to find one leg slightly longer than the other, but when the difference is too great, the pelvis and back are of out of alignment and therefore muscles may react with spasms.

- Leg—*medial surface is measured bilaterally from the anterior superior iliac spine to the bony prominence of the tibia at the ankle*
- Feet—*arches, toes, deformities, toenails, bunions*

All extremity joints are observed for range of motion by the physician either requesting the patient to move extremities or by passively flexing, extending, and rotating the arms and legs to evaluate the shoulders,

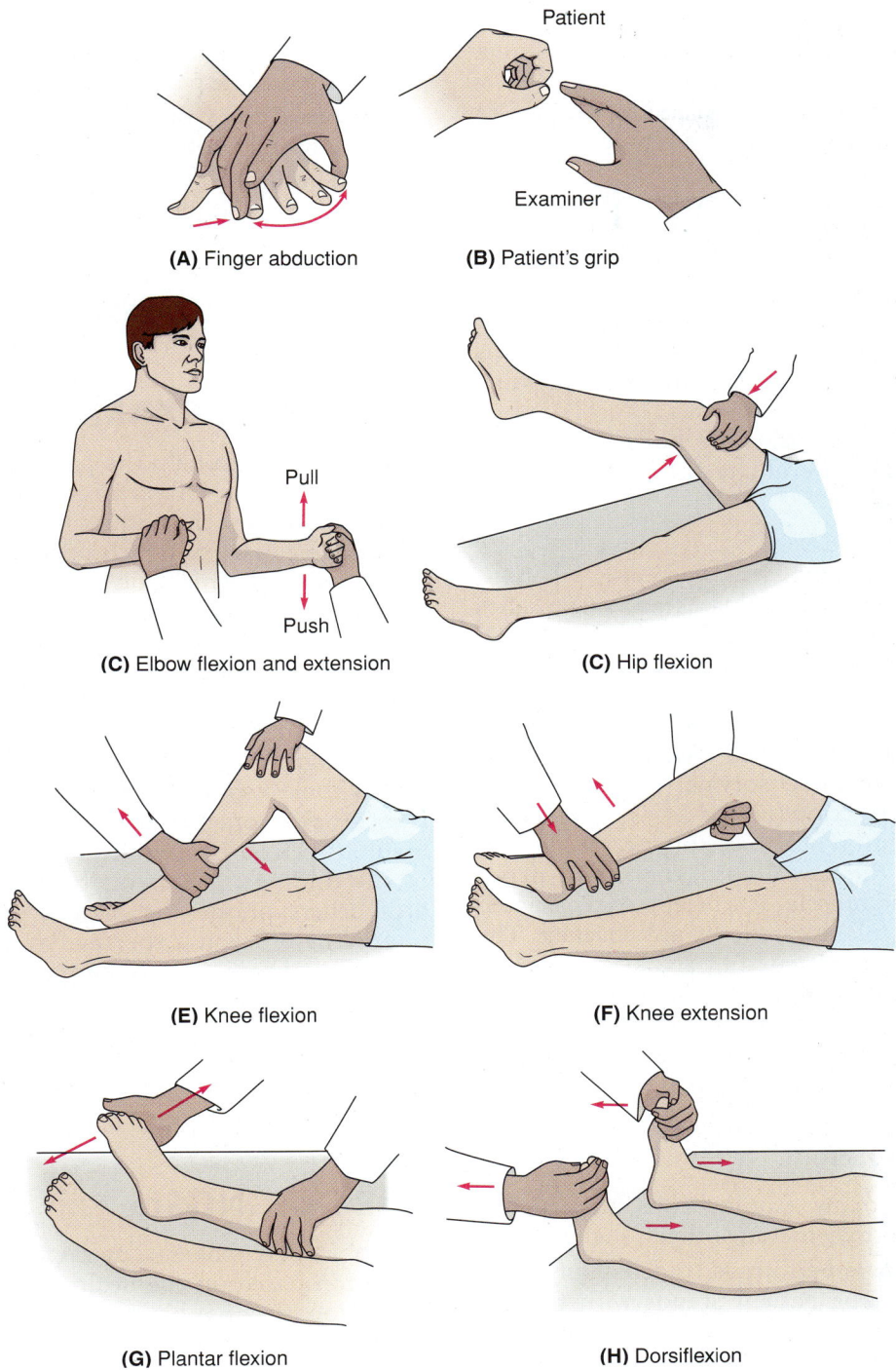

(A) Finger abduction

(B) Patient's grip

Patient

Examiner

Pull

Push

(C) Elbow flexion and extension

(C) Hip flexion

(E) Knee flexion

(F) Knee extension

(G) Plantar flexion

(H) Dorsiflexion

FIGURE 14-40   Testing muscle strength

hips, elbows, knees, wrists, and ankles. This can be combined with evaluating muscle strength.

Muscle Strength

Muscle strength is sometimes observed by asking the patient to perform a set of movements that the physician counteracts with resistance. Figure 14-40 shows some examples.

- Fingers—the patient is asked to spread his fingers (abduction) then the physician tries to force them together; measures ulnar nerve function
- Grip—the patient is asked to squeeze the index and middle finger of the physician as the physician tries to remove them to evaluate forearm muscles and condition of the hands.

- Elbow—the patient pushes and pulls against the physician's resistance to check flexion and extension strength of the arms.
- Hip—flexion of the hip is evaluated by the patient trying to raise his leg while the physician pushes down on the thigh.
- Knee—flexion of the knee is evaluated by the patient flexing the leg with the foot on the table and maintaining the position as the physician tries to straighten the leg.
- Knee—extension of the knee is evaluated by the patient trying to straighten the leg while the physician holds the leg flexed and exerts pressure at the ankle.
- Ankle—the patient pushes or pulls against the physician's hand to evaluate the plantar flexion and dorsiflexion.

Reflexes

[Sitting/supine; percussion; **percussion hammer**]

The physician systematically evaluates *involuntary* reflex action at several locations on the body with the patient in a sitting or lying position. The patient is instructed to relax the muscle. The physician positions the extremity so that the muscle is mildly stretched. Then the partially stretched tendon is tapped sharply to stimulate the sensory nerve endings in the muscle to cause a reaction (Figure 14-41). These tests evaluate the condition of the sensory nerve, the *automatic* synapse in the spinal cord, the motor nerve, and the innervated muscle. The biceps, triceps, patellar, Achilles, and plantar reflexes are checked. The plantar reaction is stimulated by stroking the plantar surface with the handle of the hammer or an object such as a key. Note on the physical exam form in Figure 14-31 the neuro area, the examination of CN II–XII, and the motor/sensory nerves.

Other Evaluations

In addition to the many examinations already discussed, the physician may include others, such as:

1. *Romberg balance test*—performed to detect any muscle abnormality. The patient stands with feet together and eyes open; if the balance seems all right, the examiner asks the patient to close the eyes. If there is any muscle abnormality, the patient possibly will fall. You should assist by standing close to help prevent this from happening.
2. Other tests for **coordination** may include:
   a. The patient sits up, spreads the arms out wide, and touches the fingertip to the nose, first the right and then the left quickly, with eyes open and then closed (Figure 14-42).
   b. The heel-to-shin test is performed by the patient while lying in the supine position: first the right

heel traces the left leg down from the knee, and then the left heel down right leg; may also be done while patient stands.
   c. Alternating motion is a test that may involve tapping the foot or clapping.
   d. The heel-to-toe test of coordination is having the patient touch the right heel to the left great toe and then the left heel to the right great toe; it can be done while the patient is standing or lying down. The patient is observed and evaluated by the examiner.

AFTER THE EXAMINATION

Always be sure to help the patient down from the examination table. Often after sitting there for some time, especially if the patient has been lying down, she can become dizzy or lightheaded, and there is the possibility of a fall, which you could prevent. You may also offer the courtesy of assisting her to get dressed when appropriate, especially with the elderly. Answer any questions about the follow-up appointment or further studies. Always let the patient know how long to expect to wait for reports from the lab, radiology, or other diagnostic procedures. Tell her when to call and with whom to speak when she phones for the report. It is a common practice to give the patient an appointment 1 week to 10 days after the physical for a report of the findings; others mail a report (Figure 14-43). Still others phone the patient or have the patient phone the office at a specific day and time. Whatever the policy where you are employed, you must realize that the patient is usually very concerned about what the physician will find, and waiting makes the anxiety far worse. Letting patients know about their health status as soon as possible in a professional manner will be appreciated.

THE DIAGNOSIS

The physician makes a decision about the patient's condition based on the health history, symptoms, examination findings, and any other procedures and laboratory tests thought necessary to confirm the decision. The term **R/O**, or **rule/out**, may be used to indicate that there is not yet conclusive evidence in the decision concerning a patient's condition or in confirming a diagnosis (e.g., R/O gallbladder disease—awaiting diagnostic x-ray studies).

Plan—This section of the form is where *all* measures for management of the care of the patient are listed, including diet, exercise, physical therapy, medication, surgery, and any others.

Following the completion of the physical examination, the physician will usually leave the patient's chart

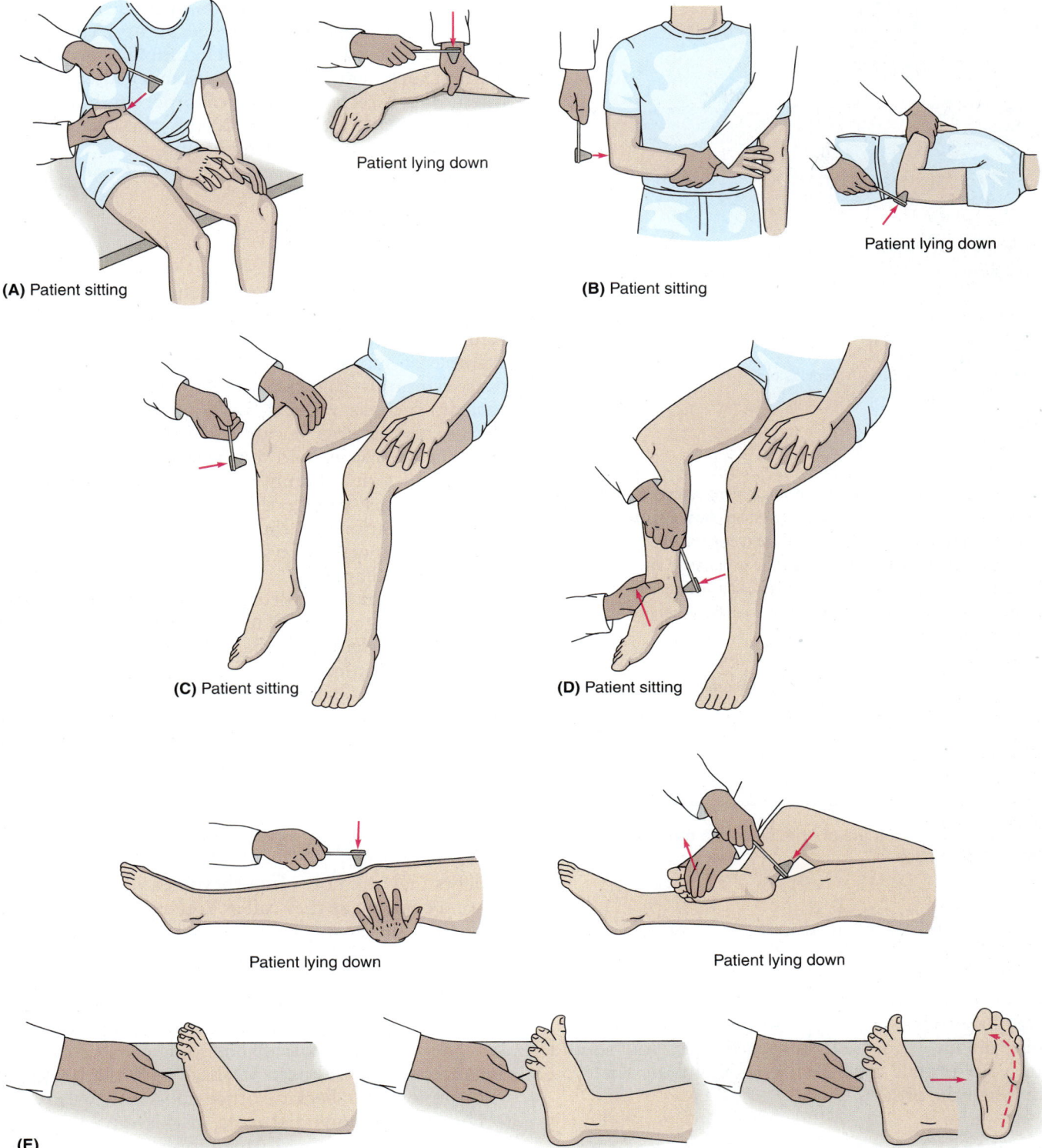

FIGURE 14-41   A percussion hammer is used by the physician to test (A) biceps, (B) triceps, (C) patellar, (D) Achilles, and (E) plantar reflexes.

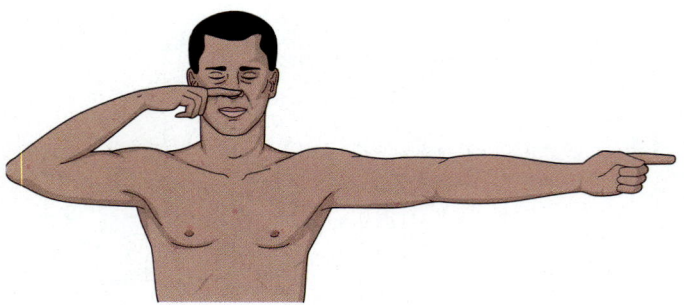

FIGURE 14-42 The physician observes the patient as the finger is touched to the nose to determine normal coordination.

From the desk of Dr. H. N. Finklestein
(Today's date)

Dear Mr. G.:

    We are pleased to inform you that the results of your physical examination, lab tests, EKG, and chest x-ray were normal. Your next physical exam should be scheduled within the next two to three years unless you experience any medical problems. Please feel free to call if you have any further questions or concerns or if we can be of service to you.

                Sincerely,

                H N Finklestein MD

                H.N. Finklestein, M.D.

FIGURE 14-43 Example of brief note as a report of the physical examination

in the chart holder on the door or in some other designated area for the medical assistant. You should then check the chart for orders to perform any additional procedures for the patient, such as ECG, lab tests, scheduling x-rays, or an appointment with a specialist. After you have finished the procedures, you should write your initials after each one, signifying that you completed the orders.

DOCUMENTATION OF THE EXAM

In documenting the physical examination, many physicians use the Problem Oriented Medical Record (POMR) method. It is sometimes referred to as POS, or problem-oriented system. This system is used for a new patient workup and for patients with serious or **chronic** illnesses. It is also used to document specific multiple complaints of patients. For **acute** or single minor complaints (such as a sore throat or a splinter), this system may not be used, for the chief complaint would not warrant such detail. Using this system ensures that pertinent data is recorded in logical order on the patient's chart with each return visit to the physician. Data is recorded under the following headings:

S   Subjective findings
O   Objective findings
A   Assessment of problems
P   Plan for treatment

    Under **subjecive** findings are those symptoms that the patient feels but that cannot be seen by another. Nausea, joint pain, headache, and abdominal pain are example of subjective findings. **Objective** findings are those symptoms that can be seen by another and by the patient, such as redness, rash, swelling, watery discharge, or bleeding. It can also include the patient's past health history and any information concerning the patient that a family member or friend has conveyed to either you or the doctor. Assesment documents evaluation of the symptoms. This includes laboratory reports, x-rays, vital sign recordings, and other aids to diagnosis.

    All action taken in the course of the patient's treatment generates additional information that continually modifies the original data base. **Subsequent** visits of the patient are recorded in the same manner (SOAP) as was the initial visit on sheets termed *progress notes*, sometimes referred to as **progress reports** or chart notes. Following each entry on the patient's chart should be the signature or initials of the health care provider or the person who performed the procedure.

PATIENT FOLLOW-UP

Patients may ask how often they need to have a physical, or a checkup as they call it. You may use Table 14-2 as a guide in giving advice to adult patients about examination and specialty procedures routinely performed on patients. Some physicians recommend annual physicals for their patients, others every 2 to 3 years unless a specific or chronic medical problem exists. The age of the patient has some consideration in this matter. You will need to check with the physician who employs you, because office policies may vary.

    The examinations discussed in this unit are by no means the only ones performed in medical offices and clinics. You will learn many others as you gain experience and knowledge in assisting. To learn other instruments used in medical offices or clinics, refer to the appendix of this text.

    Procedure 14-15 provides step-by-step instruction for getting a patient ready for and assisting with a general physical examination.

P PATIENT EDUCATION

Following the physician's examination is an ideal time to stress upon patients the importance of monitoring their health status as the physician has indicated. They may need to do regular home measurement of blood pressure, weight, or pulse rate, for example, or perform routine breast and testicular self-examinations as discussed in the examination format. You may have to so some patient education to help patients assume this responsibility. There will probably be pamphlets available for you to give to your patients about performing the self-examinations. You should be able to discuss the procedure with them and answer any questions they may have. The content will be similar to what is included in this patient education box.

Breast Self-Examination

Breasts should be examined on a specific day every month, 7 to 10 days following the beginning of a period for women that still menstrutate. Learn what your breasts feel like so you can identify a change. A firm ridge along the bottom is normal.

1. Lie on your back with a pillow or a large folded towel under the shoulder.
2. For the right breast, use the ends of the three middle fingers of the left hand to press the breast tissue against the chest wall to feel for lumps or thickening.

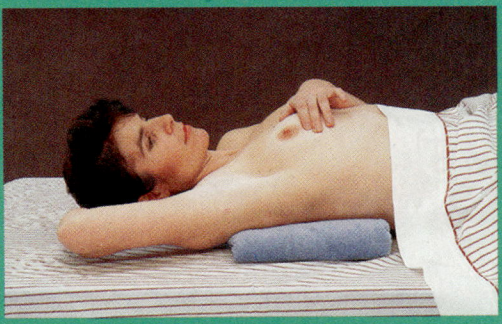

3. Move the fingers in a pattern: Start at the nipple and move around the breast in circles toward the chest wall or move up and down or in a wedge pattern. Use the same pattern each month. Cover the entire breast area.
4. Repeat for the left breast.
5. Stand in front of a mirror. Look at the breasts for symmetry; observe for any area that appears to be attached or falls differently. Observe with arms at sides and with arms raised.

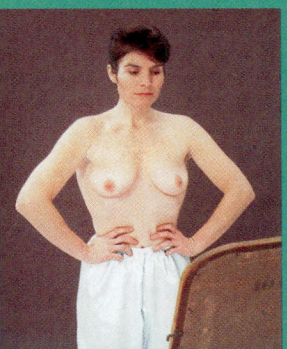

6. Do an extra breast exam while showering. Wet, soapy hands glide over the skin, making feeling the tissue easier.
7. Report any abnormal findings to your physician as soon as possible.

Testicular Self-Examination

It is recommended that men begin routine testicular self-examination at about 15 years of age. The testes should be carefully palpated after a warm shower or bath when the scrotal skin is relaxed.

1. Manually examine each testis. It is normal for one testis to be larger than the other.

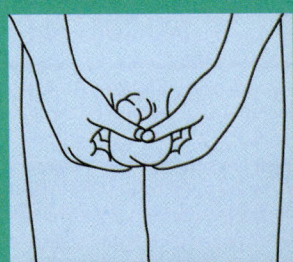

2. Gently roll the testes between the fingers and thumbs of both hands. Become familiar with the structure and feel of the testes.
3. Feel for lumps or nodules.
4. See the illustration to identify the structures.

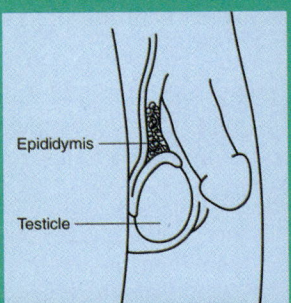

Epididymis

Testicle

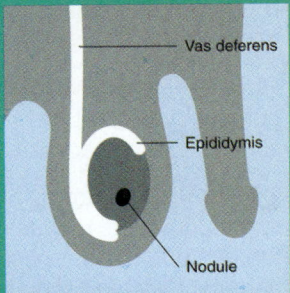

Vas deferens

Epididymis

Nodule

5. Report any abnormal findings to your physician as soon as possible.

Procedure/Screening	Age
TABLE 14-2 **Physical Examination Table**	
Hearing	65 years+ or as necessitated by symptoms
Vision	65 years+ or as necessitated by symptoms
	Tonometry/fundoscopy at 40, then every 4 years
Urinalysis	65 years+ or as necessitated by symptoms
Skin/melanoma	Begin at 40, then annually
Fecal occult blood test	Begin at 40, then annually
Digital rectal exam	Begin at 40, then annually
Sigmoidoscopy (flexible fiberoptic)	Begin at 50, then annually
Double contrast barium enema	Every 5 years as directed by physician
Colonoscopy	Every 10 years or as directed by physician
Pulmonary function tests	As needed for high-risk patients (COPD/smokers)
Total blood cholesterol	19–65+ as directed by physician
Thyroid testing	As needed for symptoms; baseline for females at menopause, then every 2 years
H & P	20–39 every 3 years, then annually after 40
Height/weight	Annually 13–65+, then as directed by physician
Blood pressure	Annually 13–65+, then as directed by physician if over 140/90
Males: self-testicular exam	Monthly (13–65+ as needed for symptoms) by physician
Females: mammogram	Baseline at 35, every 1–2 years, then annually at 50
Breast self-exam	Monthly, 35 annually (by physician)
Pap test and pelvic exam	Annually beginning at 18 or when sexually active

This physical exam schedule is meant to serve as a guide. The medical needs of patients will vary, as will physicians' recommendations.

PROCEDURE PROCEDURE PROCEDURE PROCEDURE PROCEDURE PROCEDURE PROCEDURE PROCEDURE

14-15  Prepare a Patient for and Assist with a Routine Physical Examination

PURPOSE: To have the patient, the room, and the examination equipment prepared for the physician to complete a physical examination as you assist with the process as needed.

OSHA GUIDELINES: To comply with Standard Precautions, gloves must be worn if there is any possibility of coming into contact with blood or any body fluids.

EQUIPMENT: Gown, drape, stethoscope, ophthalmoscope, otoscope, tongue depressors, sterile gauze squares, tuning fork, nasal speculum, tape measure, percussion hammer, vaginal speculum, guaiac test kit, disposable gloves, lubricant, tissues, towel, Mayo tray, examination stool, gooseneck lamp, and biohazardous waste container.

PERFORMANCE OBJECTIVE: In a simulated situation, with access to all equipment, check room for readiness, instruct the patient to prepare for the exam, assemble all equipment onto the Mayo stand, and assist the physician by positioning and draping the patient for each exam area and handing equipment as needed.

1. Prepare the examination room as in Procedure 14-8.
2. Review the patient's chart for completed history and the physical examination form. Have a pen ready if you are to write for the physician.
3. Wash hands.
4. Prepare the examination equipment on the Mayo tray in order of use and cover with a towel. Place it in a convenient location in the room.

(continues)

14-15    Prepare a Patient for and Assist with a Routine Physical Examination (Continued)

5. Pull out the step from the table. Place a gown and drape on the table.

6. Request that the patient follow you to the room.

7. Check the chart and explain the procedure to the patient. **RATIONALE: To ensure you have the correct patient and that they understand the examination process.**

8. Measure and record vital signs, height, and weight. **NOTE: If the physical follows the in-person interview and history, the mensuration would have been completed and recorded.**

9. Instruct the patient to go to bathroom to empty the bladder. Provide a labeled specimen bottle for a urine sample to be tested later.

10. Instruct the patient to remove clothing and place it on a chair, to put on the gown with the opening in back, to sit at the end of table, and to cover the legs with the drape. **NOTE: Evaluate ability to undress and to get onto the table unassisted. Assist the patient as needed, especially the elderly, weak, or disabled. Do not leave disoriented, weak, dizzy, or ill patients alone. Request temporary family assistance if you must leave the room.**

11. Ensure the patient is ready, and summon the physician.

12. Assist the physician as needed with the examination. Position and drape the patient, adjust lights, and hand equipment.

13. General appearance and skin inspection—when instructed, remove the drape, help the patient from the table for inspecting posterior surface and gait evaluation, and assist to re-sit.

14. Head and neck—stand by.

15. EENT—turn off lights for pupil and ophthalmoscope evaluation. (If physician desires, hand ophthalmoscope, then otoscope, nasal speculum, tongue blade, gauze squares, and tuning fork.)

16. Chest—may need to raise gown

17. Heart—ensure silence. May need to raise the gown. Note if ECG is requested.

18. Lungs—ensure silence. May need to raise the gown. Note if vital capacity is requested.

19. Breasts—raise gown for sitting exam, then assist the patient to lie back. Expose the breasts and cover with the drape.

20. Abdomen—raise gown to the breasts, then cover with the drape. Stand away from the side of the table.

21. Back—Physician's preference; may be done while the patient is standing for general inspection. If not, assist the patient to sit then stand in front of the physician.

22. Extremities—position the patient in supine position, and cover with the drape. Hand tape measure.

23. Reflexes—position patient in sitting position (most common). Hand percussion hammer.

24. Muscle strength—begin with sitting patient then assist to supine and drape.

25. Genitourinary and rectal (female)—assist the patient into lithotomy position and drape. Assist the physician to glove, and adjust lamp. Warm the speculum; hand when ready. Apply lubricant to a gloved finger. Prepare the guaiac paper.

26. When the exam is completed, allow the patient to relax a moment, then help to sitting position. Ensure she is stable, then assist from the table.

27. Provide tissues to remove excess lubricant and instruct the patient to dress.

28. Take specimens from the room to the laboratory for testing.

29. Return to the room and determine whether the patient has any questions.

30. Provide instructions and schedule any additional procedures requested by the physician.

31. Provide information for receiving the examination results. See the patient out.

32. Put on gloves to wrap up the table paper and dispose of used supplies in appropriate waste containers.

33. Disinfect table tops, gooseneck lamp, and examination table.

34. Remove and discard gloves in the biohazardous waste container.

35. Replace used supplies and cover the table and pillow with clean paper.

36. Give the room a visual check for completeness.

ACHIEVE UNIT OBJECTIVES

- Complete the Workbook activities to meet the learning objectives.
- Practice the procedures in this unit to meet the performance objectives.
- Apply your knowledge at the end of this chapter in completing the Critical Thinking Challenge and Activities, as well as the StudyWARE on your Student CD-ROM.

UNIT 4
SPECIAL EXAMINATIONS

OBJECTIVES

Upon completion of this unit, you will be able to achieve the following:

LEARNING Objectives

1. Spell and define, using the glossary at the back of the text, all the Words to Know in this unit.
2. Identify five reasons the liquid-based Pap test is preferred.
3. Name two ways the AutoPap test is utilized.
4. Interpret the American Cancer Society (ACS) guidelines for frequency of Pap tests.
5. Identify four specific ACS patient preparation instructions for more accurate Pap results.
6. Give two reasons the female patient should empty her bladder prior to a pelvic examination.
7. Stress why breast self-examination is necessary even when the physician performs an annual exam.
8. Give two reasons why the medical assistant should accompany the physician when a pelvic exam is performed.
9. List the three main Pap test reporting categories.

10. Name three types of gynecological instruments in addition to the speculum and explain their purpose.
11. Identify three processes or procedures done to confirm a diagnosis of pregnancy.
12. List five general responsibilities of the medical assistant in prenatal care.
13. Explain how to determine the estimated due date using Nagele's Rule.
14. List seven assessment responsibilities of the MA before the physician performs the prenatal examination.
15. Identify five conditions that may be diagnosed with a sigmoidoscopic examination.
16. Advise a patient as to what five types of persistent intestinal symptoms may indicate an abnormal condition that should be reported to the doctor, as identified in the patient education information.

PERFORMANCE Objectives

1. Prepare a patient for and assist with a gynecological examination and Pap test.
2. Assist with a sigmoidoscopy.
3. Administer a disposable cleansing enema.

WORDS TO KNOW

atypical	flexible	proctology
cervical	formaldehyde	proctoscope
constipation	fundus	risk
cytology	gestation	sigmoidoscopy
diagnostic	heartburn	stool
disclose	Lamaze	suction
douche	lumen	tarry
endocervical	mucosa	ThinPrep
endoscope	Nagele's rule	trimester
enema	obturator	trivial
evacuants	occult	tumor
evacuate	Papanicolaou	ulceration
exfoliated	pregnancy	vaginitis
fecal	prenatal	

CERTIFICATION CONNECTION

CMA
Treatment area
Patient preparation and
　assisting the physician
Collecting and processing
　specimens; diagnostic
　testing (processing
　specimens)

CMAS
Examination preparation

RMA
Health education
Physical examination
　(specialty examinations)

Many special examinations are performed on patients in various medical practices. Specialties often require additional staff training in assisting with particular procedures.

It is important to stay within your area of training until you have been properly instructed and evaluated in specific areas.

This unit addresses examinations that are specialized or for a specific purpose. In assisting with the CPE (Unit 3), the examination of the vagina and genitalia was described as a part of the total exam; the Pap test is not necessarily done at that time. Frequently women schedule appointments with their general/family practitioners for the Pap test. Many women prefer to see a gynecologist for this type of examination, especially after they have established a relationship with one during pregnancy and childbirth. When a patient calls for an appointment, be sure to make a distinction between a physical exam and a gynecologic (GYN) exam with a Pap test, so that the appropriate amount of time is allotted and the proper instructions are given. The CPE is a review of systems (ROS) of the total body. The gynecologic exam is that of the female reproductive organs only.

THE PAP TEST

The **Papanicolaou** (Pap) technique is a cytologic screening test to detect cancer of the cervix. This method of detection was developed by an American physician, George N. Papanicolaou, in 1883. This simple smear technique used samples taken from the vagina, the cervix, and the endocervix to look for **atypical cytology**. The samples were "smeared" onto slides and then sprayed with a fixative or placed in an alcohol solution and sent to a lab. Studies have shown that the technique produced many inadequate specimens, sometimes requiring repeating the procedure. Up to two thirds of the false negative reports were caused by the limitations of the sampling technique and the slide preparation. Often cells on the slide were piled up so those underneath could not be seen. Also, cervical cells were hidden by pus cells from infection, yeast cells, bacteria, and increased mucus. Therefore precancerous cells were not seen and the results were incorrectly reported negative. Furthermore, if the slide was not treated immediately after the smear was done, the cells dried out and became distorted, leading to possible reading errors.

In May 1996, after 50 years of conventional Pap testing, the U.S. Food and Drug Administration (FDA) ap-

PATIENT EDUCATION

When patients come in for their scheduled appointments, here are a few informative topics you might want to discuss with them.

1. Remind the patient at the time she schedules the appointment for a Pap test that she should not douche or engage in sexual intercourse for 48 hours before the examination. Because the specimen analysis could be misinterpreted during the menstrual flow, the patient should be advised to schedule the test about 5 days after her period.
2. Explain to female patients that they should *not* douche routinely, because it washes away natural protective vaginal secretions that aid in the resistance of possible invading microorganisms. Douching should be done only with the physician's orders.
3. Those female patients who are sexually active and not in a committed, monogamous relationship should be instructed to use condoms when engaging in sexual intercourse for protection against both sexually transmitted diseases and unwanted pregnancies.
4. Educate all females to perform breast self-examination at home routinely after their menstrual period. Pamphlets for distribution can be obtained from the American Cancer Society to help patients with the procedure.
5. Remind all female patients over age 35 to schedule a routine mammography for early detection of breast cancer.
6. Explain to female patients that any of the following symptoms could mean that infection or disease are present and that they should call for an appointment: foul vaginal odor; vaginal discharge that is other than clear; unusual bleeding; vaginal itching or soreness; or any other **vaginitis**, pain, or discomfort.
7. Advise female patients to refrain from using perfumed toilet articles such as soaps or bubble baths, vaginal sprays, tampons, toilet tissue, or feminine napkins because they may be irritating to the delicate vaginal tissues. Chronic irritation can lead to infection.

proved a new liquid-based method known by the brand names of **ThinPrep** and AutoCyte. This improved technique involves collecting the sample with a plastic **endocervical** "broom" and immediately placing it into a bottle of preservative solution. The broom is swished 10 times in the solution to remove the collected cells. The solution prevents the cells from drying out and significantly reduces the presence of mucus, bacteria, yeast, and pus cells on the slide prepared from the diluted cell samples in the solution. This technique slightly improves the detection of cancers but greatly improves the detection of precancers. This method also provides the ability to do additional studies from the same sample, such as tests for the presence of HPV, chlamydia, and gonorrhea.

Another method of screening called the AutoPap has been approved by the FDA and promises to improve the recognition of abnormal cells. Computerized instruments will retest Pap samples interpreted normal by technologists. These instruments can sometimes detect abnormal cells that are missed by humans. The AutoPap has also been approved to perform initial screenings instead of a technologist, but in this case, anything identified as abnormal would still be examined by a technologist. All these new innovations are an attempt to increase the degree of accuracy of the Pap test.

Female patients usually have the Pap test done routinely either as a part of the CPE with their family doctor or by their gynecologist. Patients who have complaints of severe menstrual pain or discomfort, unusual vaginal discharge, or lower abdominal pain (or any other problems) may have a Pap smear taken during the pelvic examination to rule out gynecological problems.

Some physicians recommend that females older than 35 have a Pap smear done every 6 months. Others feel that in healthy women one test every 1 to 3 years is sufficient. The American Cancer Society recommends the following guidelines for early detection of cervical cancer:

- All women should begin screening tests about 3 years after they begin having vaginal intercourse but no later than 21 years old. Screening should be done every year with a regular Pap test or every 2 years with a liquid-based Pap test.
- At age 30, women with three normal Pap tests in a row may have a screening every 2 to 3 years with either test method. Women with risk factors such as diethylstilbestrol exposure before birth; HIV infection; or a weakened immune system due to organ transplant, chemotherapy, or chronic steroid use should continue with annual testing.
- An option for women older than 30 is screening every 3 years plus the HPV DNA test. Human papil-

lomavirus (HPV) is a known risk factor for developing cervical cancer. The virus causes changes in the cervical cells that can be observed from the Pap test. Sexually active women younger than 30 are more likely to have an HPV infection, so screening results in this age-group are less diagnostic and the virus will probably go away on its own.

- Women 70 or older who have had at least three normal Pap tests in a row and no abnormal findings in the past 10 years may choose to stop cervical cancer screening. Women with the risk factors named above should continue as long as they are in good health.
- Women who have had a total hysterectomy (cervix and uterus removed) may choose to stop screening unless surgery was performed as a treatment for precancerous cells or cervical cancer. Women who have had a hysterectomy without removal of the cervix should still follow the guidelines.

Women should be especially conscientious in scheduling Pap tests if they have a family history of uterine or **cervical** cancer. As a medical assistant, you should check with your physician employer for his preference and advise patients accordingly.

Patient Preparation for the Pap Test

When the patient is scheduled for a Pap test, she must be given clear instructions to follow in preparation for the test. The following are recommended by the American Cancer Society for accurate results.

- Do not use tampons, birth control foams, jellies, or other vaginal creams for 48 hours before the test. (They alter the cervical and vaginal environment.)
- Do not **douche** for 48 hours prior to the test. (Douching could wash away **exfoliated** cancer cells and cause the test to be falsely reported as negative.)
- Do not have sexual intercourse for 48 hours before the test. (This adds extra cells and fluid to the environment, making reading more difficult.)
- Try to schedule the Pap test at least 5 days after the menstrual period. Avoid scheduling during the period. (Red blood cells make the test more difficult to read.)

Medical Assistant's Preparation for the Pap Test

Prior to bringing the patient into the examination room for the pelvic exam and Pap, the medical assistant should make the necessary preparations. You should wash your hands before you begin. The exam table should have a clean protective covering, either table paper or a cloth sheet. Place a gown and drape sheet on the end of the table for the patient (either cloth or disposable paper).

Prepare the Mayo tray with the instruments and supplies the physician will need to perform the pelvic exam and obtain the Pap test. Place the tray in a convenient location near the end of the exam table. Cover the equipment with a towel to help allay the patient's anxiety from seeing the equipment. The most commonly used items for this GYN procedure are pictured in Figure 14-44. After the patient is questioned to complete the requisition form, attach the label to the ThinPrep collection bottle and place it on the stand. (Note in Figure 14-45, the requisition form is prenumbered and has six matching prenumbered labels to attach to specimens. This helps eliminate errors from mismatching requisitions to specimens.) To aid in the inspection part of the pelvic exam, a gooseneck lamp should also be placed within reach of the examiner's stool at the end of the table.

Call the patient from the reception room to prepare her for the exam. Instruct her to go to the bathroom to empty her bladder before the test. If a specimen is to be obtained, instruct her as to the method of collection. A pelvic examination is uncomfortable for the patient if the bladder is full, besides making the examination difficult for the physician to perform. Examinations that have to be delayed while the patient goes to the bathroom disrupt the schedule and should be avoided. Certainly there are exceptions. Some patients may have trouble with bladder control or some other condition that requires frequent trips to the bathroom. Help these patients feel at ease, because they will most likely feel embarrassed.

When the patient comes back to the examination room, try to determine her level of anxiety regarding the examination. Take time to explain the procedure, letting her know what to expect, especially if it is her first time having a pelvic exam. *Never* assume that a patient knows about a procedure. Some patients are both afraid and embarrassed to ask questions because they believe they should already know about procedures. Try to make patients feel comfortable and at ease to help them relax for the exam. Complete the cytology request form (see Figure 14-45), making sure that you ask the patient all necessary questions, including complaints she may have and the date of the last menstrual period (LMP, the first day of her last period). Then instruct the patient to undress completely, tell her where to put her belongings, and explain how to put on the exam gown, opened in front. Politely offer your assistance. Ask her to slightly open the door when she is gowned. Allow the patient privacy for a couple of minutes to change.

Enter the room when the patient lets you know she is ready. Pull out the foot step at the end of the exam table and help her step up onto the exam table and sit at the end. Place the drape sheet over the top of her legs. This will give her privacy and warmth. Remember to

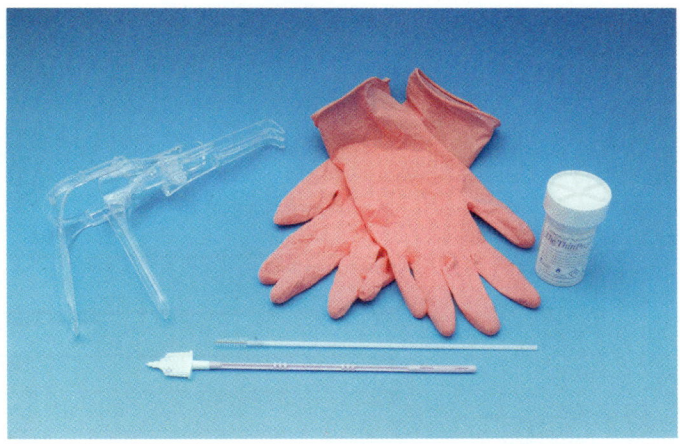

FIGURE 14-44   Equipment and supplies for a Pap test

push the foot step back in after the patient has been seated to avoid injury to you or the physician.

Alert the physician that the patient is ready to be examined. Most physicians prefer that the medical assistant (or nurse) accompany them into the exam room, not only to assist with the procedure, but also to verify their behavior in case of patient accusations.

Because of the importance of early detection of breast cancer, physicians include the breast exam during the patient's annual appointment for the Pap test and pelvic exam. Patients should be reminded to do a breast self-examination each month following their menstrual period (see the Patient Education box on page 717). Giving them a pamphlet of instructions to take with them for this procedure is recommended (Figure 14-46). Explain to the patient that the exam conducted by the physician with the annual Pap test is important but insufficient in detecting abnormal breast tissue between visits to the physician. Most women discover a lump or mass in their breasts themselves and report it to the physician. This leads to early detection and treatment, which greatly increases the survival rate.

Conducting the Examination

The physician usually listens to the heart and lungs and does a brief general check of the patient first. Then the patient's gown is lowered to the waist while the patient is still sitting up for the inspection part of the breast exam and palpation for lumps and masses. When this part is completed, pull the table extension out to support the lower legs and feet and help the patient lie down to assist the doctor in further palpation for any abnormalities of the breast tissue (often a towel is placed over the chest to provide a sense of privacy for the patient). Next, the physician will inspect and palpate the abdominal and pelvic areas. Remind patients to breathe slowly through the mouth to help relax abdominal muscles during the exam.

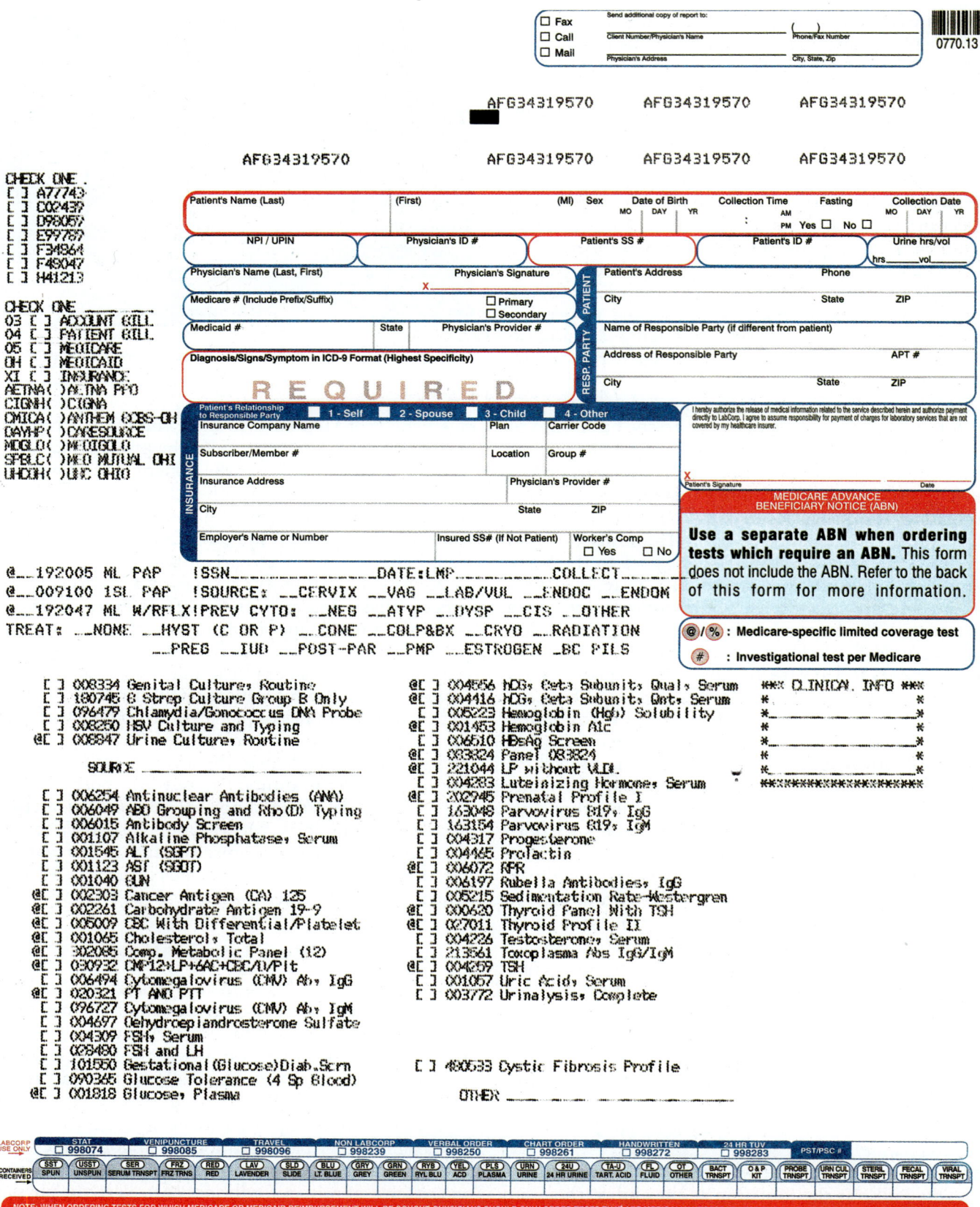

FIGURE 14-45 Laboratory requisition for OB/GYN practice

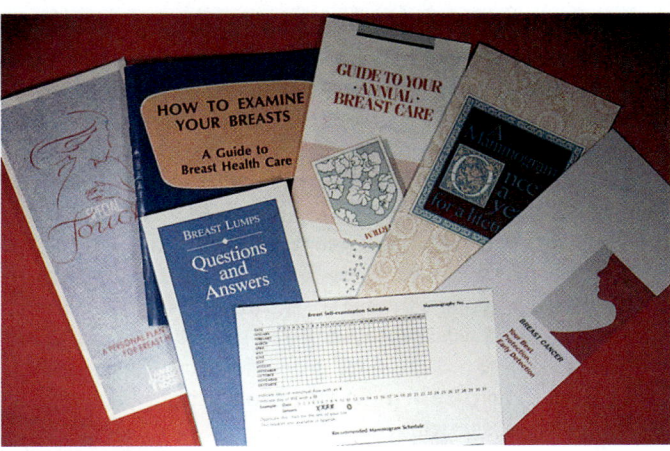

FIGURE 14-46   Breast self-examination (BSE) pamphlets and schedule

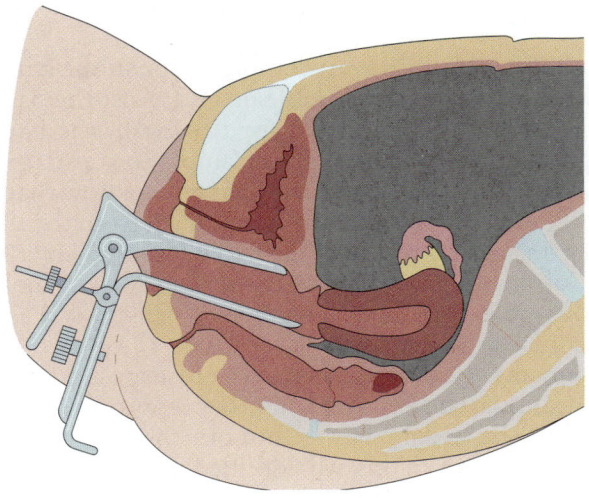

FIGURE 14-47   Lateral view of vaginal speculum in place for inspection and for obtaining specimens

Following this portion of the exam, help the patient into the lithotomy position. Assist her in getting her feet in the stirrups, adjusting them as necessary, and place the drape sheet over her knees. Ask her to scoot down to the end of the table until the buttocks are just at the edge (place your hand at the edge of the table and ask her to keep moving down until she feels the back of your hand). Be careful in assisting patients into positions, because the exam tables are usually rather narrow, and there *is* the possibility of a patient falling *off* of the table. The gooseneck lamp should be adjusted at the end of the table and the stool positioned comfortably for the physician. The medical assistant should put on latex or vinyl gloves and hand the physician gloves.

Adjust the gooseneck lamp if necessary, to the physician's preference, so that the external perineal structures can be observed. When ready, hand the warmed speculum, handles first, to the physician. Some physicians may want a plastic speculum run under water to facilitate insertion. After it is inserted, it may be necessary to again adjust the light so that the cervix can be seen clearly within the blades of the speculum (Figure 14-47). Hand the endocervical broom to the physician. The broom is inserted slightly into the cervical opening and twisted to obtain sample cells within and on the surface of the cervix. The broom is withdrawn and immediately placed in the ThinPrep bottle. It is swished 10 times through the solution, withdrawn to the top of the bottle, tapped a couple times to knock off any remaining solution and cells, and discarded on the Mayo stand. The labeled bottle is promptly capped.

The bimanual exam is performed following the collection of specimens (Pap smear, cultures, and so on) so that the lubricant will not interfere in the lab analysis. The examiner inserts two fingers (with a small amount of water-soluble lubricant) into the vagina

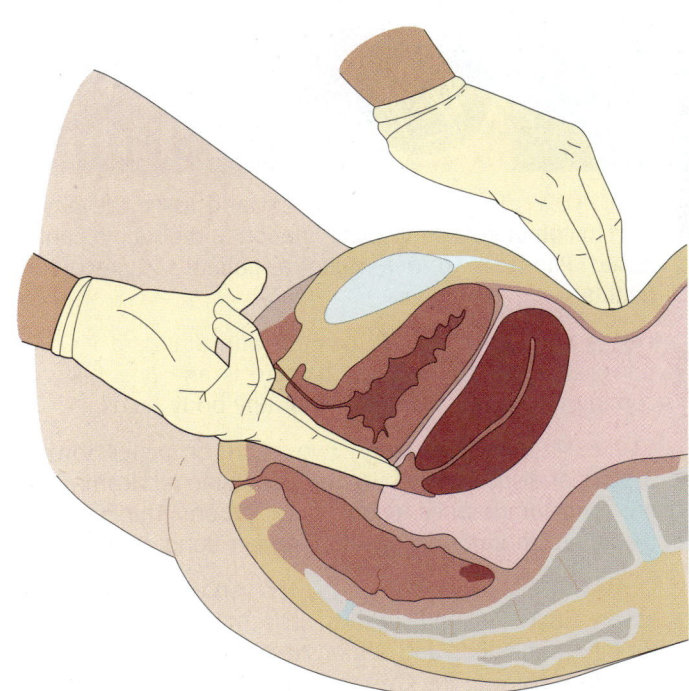

FIGURE 14-48   Bimanual pelvic examination

and palpates the pelvic area with the other hand (Figure 14-48). Normally, the physician does a rectal examination next. You should hand the doctor another latex or vinyl glove and lubricant to prevent cross-contamination between the vaginal and rectal tissues.

Instead of assisting, the medical assistant may be asked to write the findings of this examination while the physician conducts the exam. Whichever is your role, you will be a valuable assistant to both physician and patient.

AFTER THE EXAMINATION

When this exam has been completed, push the stirrups and the extension of the table in, and assist the patient to sit up. After lying down for the exam, the patient may feel faint or dizzy; if she attempts to stand up too quickly she may fall. After she has let you know that she has regained her balance, help her down from the table, and offer tissues to the patient to wipe away any residual lubricant. Discard the used tissues in a biohazardous waste container. Ask her to get dressed. Offer assistance to the patient.

Remember to advise her when to expect to receive the results of the Pap test and other reports in the mail, or when she should call to find out the report(s). Giving these instructions will decidedly reduce unnecessary phone calls to the office. If the physician requests a return appointment for the patient, politely assist her in scheduling it or direct her to the administrative area. As time permits, you may discuss patient education topics either before or after the exam as appropriate to the age and needs of the patient.

The medical assistant should return to the examination room to clean up the exam area. Wear gloves to protect yourself from disease transmission. Discard all disposables in biohazardous and appropriate containers, remove gloves, and wash hands. Restock the supplies as necessary, making the room ready for another patient to be seen. Place the labeled specimen(s) and attached requisition form in the proper area for pick-up by the lab representative.

Follow the steps in Procedure 14-16 to assist the physician with a gynecologic examination and a Thin-Prep Pap test.

PROCEDURE PROCEDURE PROCEDURE PROCEDURE PROCEDURE PROCEDURE PROCEDURE

14-16  Prepare the Patient for and Assist with a Gynecologic Examination and ThinPrep Pap Test

PURPOSE: To prepare the patient and assist the physician to complete a pelvic examination and obtain a liquid-based Pap test to determine a patient's gynecologic health.

OSHA GUIDELINES: To comply with Standard Precautions, gloves must be worn if there is any possibility of coming into contact with blood or any body fluids.

EQUIPMENT: Mayo tray, two cloth or paper towels, 3 pairs of disposable gloves, water-soluble lubricant, vaginal speculum, tissues, endocervical broom, ThinPrep bottle, label, laboratory requisition, rubber band, and pen.

PERFORMANCE OBJECTIVE: Given access to all necessary equipment and supplies, assist the patient to prepare for the examination and demonstrate the steps in the procedure to assist with the GYN exam and ThinPrep Pap test. All needed materials must be preassembled on the Mayo tray and covered; the patient properly prepared, draped, and positioned; and the equipment handed to the physician as needed. The specimen bottle must be labeled and have an accurately completed laboratory requisition attached.

1. Wash hands

2. Place a towel on the Mayo tray, assemble all necessary equipment, and cover. Place the requisition form on a nearby table.

3. Place the gown and drape on the exam table.

4. Call the patient from the reception room; check the chart to ensure you have the correct patient.

5. Instruct the patient to go to the bathroom to empty the bladder. Provide instructions and a specimen container if a urine specimen is needed. **RATIONALE: Urine in the bladder makes the examination uncomfortable for the patient and more difficult for the physician. Emptying the bladder now eliminates the need to interrupt the examination for a trip to the bathroom later.**

6. Explain the procedure and answer any questions.

7. Obtain the necessary information to complete the cytology requisition form.

8. Attach a label to the ThinPrep bottle and place it under the cover on the Mayo tray.

9. Instruct the patient to remove all clothing and put on the examination gown with the opening in front. Show her where to put her clothing.

10. Leave the room to allow for privacy unless assistance is needed.

11. When the patient is gowned, enter the room and pull out the step from the end of the table. Ask the patient to step on the step and sit on the table. **NOTE: Provide assistance as needed. The step is small, and the patient may step off the edge when trying to turn around to sit down.**

12. Cover the patient's legs with the drape. Push in the table step.

13. Notify the physician that the patient is ready. **NOTE: If the patient is apprehensive, stay with her if possi-**

(continues)

14-16

Prepare the Patient for and Assist with a Gynecologic Examination and ThinPrep Pap Test (Continued)

ble and provide reassurance and support. **Answer any questions she may have.**

14. Accompany the physician into the room and provide assistance as needed. **NOTE: A medical assistant or nurse should be in the room at all times during the examination and while obtaining the test to protect a male physician from being accused of improper behavior during the exam.**

15. Position the patient in a sitting position for basic assessment and initial breast examination.

16. Assist the patient to a supine position for a continued breast exam. Put the pillow under her head. Uncover her chest, and cover her breasts with the towel covering the Mayo tray if desired.

17. When the breast exam is completed, assist the patient to re-cover her chest with the gown and drape and prepare for the pelvic exam.

18. Assist the patient into a lithotomy position, helping her to place her feet into the stirrups, and adjust as needed. Push in the table extension.

19. Place the drape over the patient from the chest to the feet. Push the drape down between her legs until it touches the table. Place the back of your hand against the drape at the end of the table and instruct the patient to move her buttocks down until she touches your hand. **RATIONALE: The patient's buttocks must be at the end of the table so that the vaginal speculum can be inserted without the handle hitting the table.**

20. The physician will take his position on the exam stool at the end of the table.

21. Remove the cover from the Mayo tray, if not previously done. Hand gloves to the physician.

22. Adjust the gooseneck lamp so that the light facilitates inspection of the perineal and anal areas.

23. Put on gloves and run warm water over a metal speculum.

24. Hand the speculum, handle first, to the physician.

25. Hand the endocervical broom, handle first, to the physician.

26. Open the labeled specimen bottle and be ready to accept the endocervical broom. Hold the bottle secure while physician swishes the broom, or take the handle of the broom and swish thoroughly in the solution 10 times. Withdraw it from bottle, tap it against the

bottle edge to dislodge any cells and excess fluid, and place it on the Mayo tray. Cap the bottle securely and place it on the Mayo tray.

27. The physician will stand to perform the bimanual pelvic exam. Apply lubricant to the gloved index and middle fingers of the examining hand.

28. After the bimanual is completed, hand the physician a fresh glove and apply lubricant to perform the rectal examination. **RATIONALE: Prevents transferring vaginal organisms to the rectal area.**

29. When the physician has finished the exam, have the patient push back up the table, help her get her feet out of the stirrups, and push them in.

30. Assist the patient to sit up. Pull out the table step. When the patient's sense of balance has returned, assist her down from the table.

31. Hand tissues to the patient to remove any residual lubricant.

32. Instruct the patient to dress. Provide assistance as needed.

33. Advise the patient when results will be available and schedule a follow-up appointment if indicated.

34. Provide any patient teaching information pamphlets that are appropriate and dismiss the patient.

35. Discard all disposable items in the biohazardous waste container. Wrap up the table paper and towels and discard. If a metal speculum was used, place it in cool water, then wash, wrap, and autoclave.

36. Disinfect table surfaces and the exam room furniture.

37. Remove and discard gloves.

38. Place the labeled specimen bottle with the attached requisition in the lab pick-up area.

39. Restock supplies. Pull down fresh table paper on the exam table.

40. Record examination and Pap test on the chart.

CHARTING EXAMPLE

8/28/xx, 2:30 p.m.

Annual pelvic exam and ThinPrep Pap test. Last Pap 6/14/XX (normal), no breast concerns, last mammo 3/9/XX (normal) LMP 8/15/XX, no children, D&C 4/23/XX.

G. Talbert, CMA

REPORTING PAP TEST RESULTS

The system most widely used to describe Pap test findings is the Bethesda System. It was developed in 1988 and revised in 1991 and 2001. There are three general categories:

1. Negative for intraepithelial lesion or malignancy
   (Means there is no signs of cancer or precancerous changes. Other findings may be reported such as yeast, herpes, Trichomonas, or cellular changes caused by irritation or infection.)

2. Epithelial cell abnormalities
   (Means the cells of the lining layer of the cervix show changes that might be cancer or a precancerous condition. The cells are divided into (a) atypical squamous cells, (b) low-grade squamous intraepithelial lesions (SILs), (c) high-grade SILs, and (4) squamous cell carcinoma. These findings require repeat Pap tests and other interventions such as colposcopy (examining the cervix with a magnifying lens instrument) and biopsy.)

3. Other malignant neoplasms
   (Means there is likely an invasive squamous cell cancer. Additional diagnostic tests will be done followed by radiation, chemotherapy, or radical surgery.)

Figure 14-49 lists and defines some terms used in the cytology reports of Pap tests.

OTHER PROCEDURES

Other procedures may be done to make decisions regarding the condition of the uterus and cervix. Figures 14-50A through E picture gynecological instruments used in some of these procedures. The uterine sounds (A and B) are inserted into the uterus to ex-

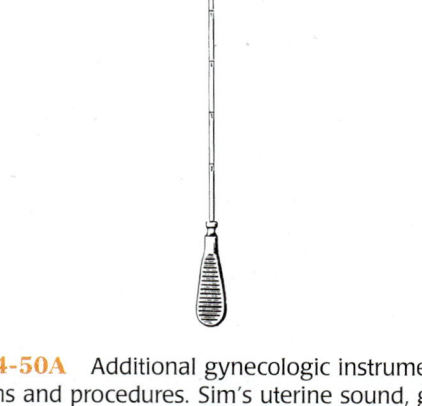

FIGURE 14-50A Additional gynecologic instruments used in examinations and procedures. Sim's uterine sound, graduated in inches *(Courtesy of JARIT Surgical Instruments)*

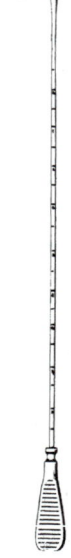

FIGURE 14-50B Sims' uterine sound, graduated in centimeters *(Courtesy of JARIT Surgical Instruments)*

plore the cavity and measure the depth. Note they are graduated in inches or centimeters. The curettes (C and D) are used to scrape the lining of the uterus for a specimen and to remove growths or remnants of an abortion. The biopsy forceps (E) permits taking a small piece of tissue for diagnostic examination. These instruments are most often used when performing surgical procedures.

atypical—not typical
CIN—cervical intraepithelial neoplasia
CIS—carcinoma in situ
condyloma—a lesion caused by human papillomavirus
dysplasia—precancerous lesion
epithelial—pertaining to epithelium
epithelium—cellular tissue that covers the surface of a body or that lines a body cavity
glandular—the cell making up the epithelium of a body cavity
HPV—human papillomavirus
lesion—a change in the tissue cells or a wound
malignant—a lesion that spreads out of the epithelium into underlying tissues
reactive changes—changes in cells caused by their reaction to infectious agents or a foreign body
reparative changes—changes in cells as they divide rapidly in an attempt to repair damaged tissue
SIL—squamous intraepithelial lesion (that lies within the squamous epithelium)
squamous—a type of cell that makes up the epithelium, the purpose of which is to protect underlying tissues

FIGURE 14-49 Terms and abbreviations used in cytology/Pap test reports

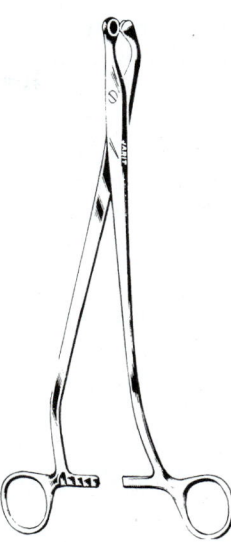

FIGURE 14-50E   Toms-Gaylor uterine punch biopsy forceps *(Courtesy of JARIT Surgical Instruments)*

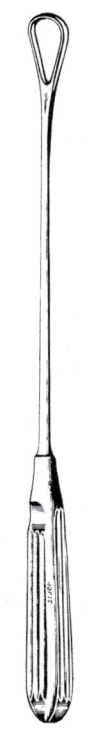

FIGURE 14-50C   Sims' uterine curette *(Courtesy of JARIT Surgical Instruments)*

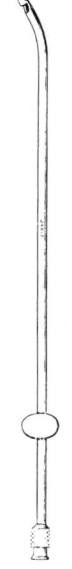

FIGURE 14-50D   Randall uterine curette *(Courtesy of JARIT Surgical Instruments)*

OBSTETRICS PATIENTS

The same principles apply in assisting with obstetrics patients as apply in assisting with the complete physical examination. You must be complete and efficient in documenting all information regarding patients. This enables the physician to provide quality care to patients.

Of primary concern with obstetrics patients is gaining their compliance with regular checkups. Some of your major responsibilities will be to provide patient education (both verbal and in printed form) and to give emotional support and encouragement. Refer to Chapter 11, Unit 13, for review of the reproductive system and information regarding **pregnancy**, labor, and childbirth. You should be familiar with the terminology for explanation to the parents.

Because convenient home pregnancy tests are available to the public, many women in their childbearing years have already tested their urine at home. Often, even after having performed the home test, they still may not be certain of the results. When patients suspect that they are pregnant, their visit to the doctor is to confirm pregnancy. Usually the patient has missed one or two menstrual periods. The diagnosis is made only after the patient has been given a complete evaluation. This is generally done by (1) interviewing the patient and obtaining a complete **prenatal** health assessment and history; (2) doing a complete physical examination; (3) ordering laboratory tests, such as urinalysis and pregnancy tests, blood tests, and cultures; and (4) performing any other diagnostic test indicated by the patient's condition.

ESTIMATING THE DATE OF DELIVERY

Probably the question of most interest to the expectant couple is when the baby will be born. This is medically known as the estimated day or date of delivery (EDD) or the estimated date of confinement (EDC). This can be determined, with a fair amount of accuracy, by using a formula known as **Nagele's rule**. The method was devised by Franz Nagele, a German obstetrician, in the early 18th century. The period of gestation (conception to birth) is determined by using the first day of the last menstrual period (LMP), subtracting 3 months, and then adding 7 days plus 1 year.

NAGELE'S RULE	
Last menstrual period	August 10, 2006
Minus 3 months	May 10, 2006
Plus 7 days, 1 year	May 17, 2007

A normal pregnancy can range from 37 to 41 weeks, so exact dates are not possible. An infant born before the 37th week is called premature, is considerably underweight, and presents challenges due to lack of development.

MEDICAL ASSISTANT'S ROLE

The medical assistant's role in prenatal evaluation and care of patients is to instill the importance of keeping regular appointments, encourage patients to eat a sensible well-balanced diet, alert the doctor of any problems or concerns, and provide patient education materials with explanations. Follow the office policy regarding prenatal and childbirth classes to provide information about times and places of such programs as **Lamaze** classes.

A medical history form (Figure 14-51) and a risk assessment form (Figure 14-52) are used in assessing the health status of pregnant women. Subsequent findings during prenatal visits are recorded on progress notes. Careful attention should be given to sections regarding (1) medications, drugs, alcohol, and smoking (consumption and use); (2) preexisting **risk** factors; and (3) past menstrual and obstetrical health history.

The effects on the fetus are well documented from certain medications, smoking, and alcohol as well as illicit drug use. Risks are also associated with certain systemic disease conditions, sexually transmitted diseases, age, physical stature, and mental factors. Examine Figure 14-52 to identify risks of preterm births and poor pregnancy outcomes.

PRENATAL VISITS

Routine prenatal visits to the physician's office usually follow the same format. It is very important to maintain continual evaluation of the mother's condition as well as that of the developing baby. Part of that responsibility belongs to the medical assistant. Each time before the patient is seen by the physician, the medical assistant will:

- Interview the patient to determine if any problems are being experienced and record any remarks and symptoms. (Early treatment of problems can keep them under control and avoid later serious situations.)
- Request her first morning urine specimen, which she brought with her, or have her give you one now. (Some complications of pregnancy can be identified by urine tests.)
- Measure the patient's weight and record the findings. (Weight reflects the mother's nutrition and the related health of the fetus. Excess as well as insufficient weight gain is undesirable. Excess gain could indicate fluid retention.)
- Measure and record her vital signs. (Monitoring blood pressure is extremely important. Hypertension is indicative of complications.)
- Check the chart to be sure all lab reports from tests ordered since the last visit are in the chart. Also check that any other studies or referral letters are included.
- Prepare the patient for the physician's examination by having her remove her clothes, from the waist down unless the breasts are also to be examined, and put on a gown with the opening in the front.
- Assist the patient onto the examination table and to sit at the end with a drape over her legs.
- Notify the physician that the patient is ready for the examination.

After the physician reviews any returned reports and your chart notes, the patient's current general condition will be discussed and the reported problems or findings will be further explored. Then it is time to proceed with the examination.

- Assist the patient into supine position for the prenatal examination.
- Provide assistance to the physician as appropriate for the **trimester** (3 month period) of the patient's **gestation** (nine [ten lunar] months or 38 to 42 weeks).
- Ultrasonography may be performed the first trimester to confirm pregnancy and later to monitor its progress (Figure 14-53). One of the most exciting times for the expectant parents is when the physician or technician locates the fetus using ultrasound technology. The equipment is capable of displaying the image on the screen and printing out the baby's first "picture" for the proud parents to show to family and friends.
- A fetoscope (special stethoscope) or a Doppler fetal pulse monitor and gel are applied to the abdomen to determine the developing fetus's heart rate.

PLEASE USE BALL POINT PEN

NAME_____

ADDRESS_____

PHONE _____ RELIGION_____

AGE _____ GR_____ PARA _____ AB_____

BLOOD TYPE _____ RH_____ SEROLOGY_____

HUSB. BL. TYPE _____ RH_____ GENOTYPE_____

_____

_____

_____

PAP SMEAR _____

SEND TOP (WHITE) COPY TO DEL. ROOM TERM _____

LMP_____ LIFE _____ EDC_____

NURSING_____ PEDIATRICIAN _____

ANESTHESIA_____

REFERRING M.D._____

PRENATAL PREPARATION _____

HUSBAND IN DELIVERY ROOM?_____

_____ RUBELLA TITER _____

MENSTRUAL CYCLE _____

G.C. CULTURE _____

PP AR SE T G.		DATE	WHERE CONFINED	WEEKS GESTATION	LENGTH OF LABOR	INFANT WT.	COMPLICATIONS
	1						
	2						
	3						
	4						

HISTORY AND PHYSICAL

CHILDHOOD_____

FAMILY _____

TRAUMATIC _____

ADULT _____

BLOOD TRANSFUSIONS _____

ALLERGIES_____

SURGERY_____

COMMENTS: _____

_____

MEDICATIONS _____

RH TITERS DATES: _____

HT. _____ NORMAL WT. _____ NORMAL B.P. _____

HEENT_____

HEART & LUNGS _____

BACK & BREASTS _____

ABDOMEN _____

SKIN & EXTREMITIES _____

PELVIC CAPACITY _____

PERIODIC VISITS		DATE	WEIGHT	BP	URINE	FHT	FUNDUS	PELVIC	COMMENTS
	1								
	2								
	3								
	4								
	5								
	6								
	7								
	8								
	9								
	10								
	11								
	12								
	13								
	14								

DELIVERY ROOM - TERM   SIGNATURE: _____ M.D.

FIGURE 14-51   Example of an obstetrics/prenatal history form

- The physician may palpate the abdomen to evaluate fundal height as a means of estimating the duration of the pregnancy. If it is not as expected, it could be an indication of multiple fetuses, excess amniotic fluid, poor development of the fetus, or even fetal death.

- A flexible centimeter tape is used to measure the height of the **fundus** (top of the uterus) from the

PRENATAL RISK ASSESSMENT FORM

Please print or type:

Patient Name	Case Number	ADC Number	E.D.D. month	day	year

| Physician Name | Physician Telephone | | | | |

Please check all that apply:

AT RISK OF PRETERM BIRTH

ABSOLUTE FACTORS *(one factor puts patient at risk)*

OBSTETRICAL HISTORY
- ❏ 1. PRETERM DELIVERY
- ❏ 2. DES EXPOSURE
- ❏ 3. CONE BIOPSY
- ❏ 4. SECOND TRIMESTER ABORTION
- ❏ 5. 1st TRIMESTER SPONTANEOUS ABORTIONS, more than 2

CURRENT PREGNANCY
- ❏ 6. UTERINE ANOMALY OR FIBROIDS
- ❏ 7. MULTIPLE GESTATION
- ❏ 8. ABDOMINAL SURGERY

- ❏ 9. CERVIX DILATED, more than 1.5 cm before 29 weeks
- ❏ 10. CERVIX EFFACED, less than 1 cm before 29 weeks
- ❏ 11. IRRITABLE UTERUS, more than 6 contractions per hr. confirmed
- ❏ 12. POLYHYDRAMNIOS
- ❏ 13. BLEEDING, if significant after 12 weeks
- ❏ 14. PYELONEPHRITIS
- ❏ 15. PRETERM LABOR
- ❏ 16. SMOKING, more than 10 cigarettes per day
- ❏ 17. PROM, confirmed

❏ YES ❏ NO   At least ONE of the above conditions has been checked. Patient is at risk of preterm birth.

AT RISK OF POOR PREGNANCY OUTCOME

ABSOLUTE FACTORS *(one factor puts patient at risk)*

OBSTETRICAL HISTORY
- ❏ 18. INFANT DEATH, stillborn, neonatal, post neonatal
- ❏ 19. CONGENITAL ANOMALY, major
- ❏ 20. LOW BIRTH WEIGHT, less than 2500g.
- ❏ 21. ECLAMPSIA or severe preeclampsia
- ❏ 22. INCOMPETENT CERVIX

CURRENT PREGNANCY
- ❏ 23. HEART DISEASE, class III or IV
- ❏ 24. DIABETES, insulin dependent
- ❏ 25. SICKLE CELL ANEMIA or other hemoglobinopathy
- ❏ 26. MALIGNANCY or leukemia
- ❏ 27. THYROID DISEASE, confirmed
- ❏ 28. EPILEPSY or on anticonvulsant
- ❏ 29. HEPATITIS or chronic liver disease
- ❏ 30. ASTHMA, on medication
- ❏ 31. TUBERCULOSIS, active
- ❏ 32. PNEUMONIA

- ❏ 33. HYPERTENSION, on medication
- ❏ 34. DEEP VENOUS THROMBOSIS
- ❏ 35. PLACENTA PREVIA, 3rd trimester
- ❏ 36. OLIGOHYDRAMNIOS
- ❏ 37. ECLAMPSIA or preeclampsia
- ❏ 38. ALLOIMMUNIZATION associated with fetal disease
- ❏ 39. RUBELLA EXPOSURE with rising titer
- ❏ 40. POSITIVE SEROLOGY
- ❏ 41. ACTIVE HERPES or positive culture, 3rd trimester
- ❏ 42. PRIMIGRAVIDA, less than 17 years or more than 35 years
- ❏ 43. FAMILIAL GENETIC DISORDER, confirmed
- ❏ 44. PSYCHOSIS
- ❏ 45. MENTAL RETARDATION
- ❏ 46. DRUG OR ALCOHOL ABUSE
- ❏ 47. OTHER_____

❏ YES ❏ NO   At least ONE of the above conditions has been checked. Patient is at risk of poor pregnancy outcome.

RELATIVE FACTORS *(two factors put patient at risk)*

- ❏ 48. PRIOR C-SECTION
- ❏ 49. PRENATAL CARE NON-COMPLIANCE, most recent pregnancy
- ❏ 50. GRAND MULTIPARA, more than 5 of 20 weeks or more
- ❏ 51. RECENT DELIVERY, less than 1 yr.
- ❏ 52. LATE INITIAL VISIT, after 14 weeks of pregnancy
- ❏ 53. MISSED PRENATAL APPOINTMENTS, 2 consecutive
- ❏ 54. AGE, less than 17 years or more than 35 years
- ❏ 55. Height, less than 5 ft.
- ❏ 56. OBESITY, more than 20% weight for height
- ❏ 57. UNDERWEIGHT, more than 10% weight for height
- ❏ 58. WEIGHT LOSS, continuing after 14 weeks

- ❏ 59. ANEMIA, less than 10 Hgb, or less than 30% Hct.
- ❏ 60. GONORRHEA, positive culture
- ❏ 61. DIABETES, gestational, diet controlled
- ❏ 62. CHRONIC BRONCHITIS
- ❏ 63. TRAUMA, requiring hospitalization
- ❏ 64. ILLITERACY or language barrier
- ❏ 65. DOMESTIC VIOLENCE
- ❏ 66. OTHER_____

❏ YES ❏ NO   At least TWO of the above conditions have been checked. Patient is at risk of poor pregnancy outcome.

Physician's Signature	Date

FIGURE 14-52   Example of a prenatal risk assessment form

symphysis pubis to evaluate the growth of the fetus after approximately the 3rd month.
- Upon completion of the examination, assist the patient to a sitting position and instruct her to dress.
- Record the appropriate information such as fundal height, fetal heart rate, procedures performed, and other pertinent patient or physician observations and remarks.

After the physician has completed the examination and talked with the patient, you should offer to answer any questions the patient may have. Encourage the patient to make her next appointment before leaving the facility. Give support and assistance by reminding her to call if there are any questions or problems.

As previously stated, it is very important that prenatal patients receive regular systematic evaluation. You

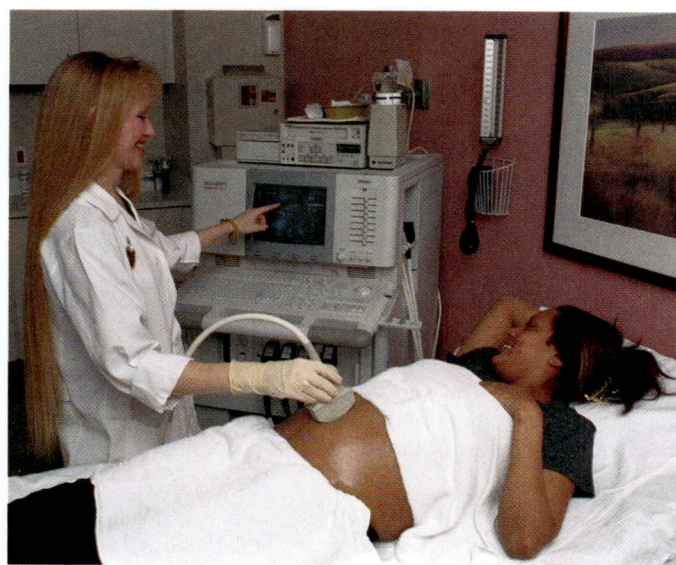

FIGURE 14-53 The patient may watch the monitor as the technician uses the ultrasound wand to assess the fetus, whose image is shown on the monitor.

GENERAL SCHEDULE FOR PRENATAL OR OBSTETRICAL APPOINTMENTS

FIRST AND SECOND TRIMESTER:
Monthly or every four weeks through the 28th week.

THIRD TRIMESTER:
Every two weeks in the 30th–36th weeks. Every week in the 36th+ week up to delivery.

FIGURE 14-54 Prenatal appointment schedule example

must stress the importance of keeping scheduled appointments so that the mother and baby may be closely monitored. Figure 14-54 illustrates the frequency for a normal pregnancy. Persons experiencing difficulties or at high risk will require more frequent evaluation.

The medical assistant should return to the exam room to clean up the area. Wear gloves (vinyl or latex) to protect yourself from disease transmission. Note: Especially in an OB-GYN practice, there is the possibility of patients who may be bleeding or who have an infection that can be transmitted by body fluids and therefore could be a threat to others. Discard all disposables in biohazardous or appropriate waste containers, remove gloves and dispose of them properly, and wash hands. Restock supplies as necessary, making the exam

room ready for the next patient. Place any specimens in the area for pick up by the lab representative.

To be of further assistance to both physician and patient, you may want to check all patients' charts to make sure that findings are documented in the SOAP method in a neat and legible manner and signed by the physician. Records may be requested at any time by insurance providers to verify the diagnosis and coding. This will lead to more efficient and expedient payment.

SIGMOIDOSCOPY

Sigmoidoscopy is a **diagnostic** examination of the interior of the sigmoid colon. It is a useful aid in the diagnosis of cancer of the colon, **ulcerations**, polyps, **tumors**, bleeding, and other lower intestinal disorders. The sigmoidoscope is a rigid metal or plastic (disposable) instrument with a light source and a magnifying lens, which permits viewing the mucous membranes of the sigmoid colon.

The metal and plastic types of scopes are still used to examine patients; however, another instrument has gained in popularity with physicians. It is a **flexible** sigmoidoscope, which is shown assembled with items necessary for the procedure to be perfomed in Figures 14-55 and 14-56A and B. Because it is flexible, it can be inserted much father into the colon with less discomfort. This instrument makes it possible to view more of the interior of the colon.

An **obturator** (a tool with a solid, rounded end) is inserted into the sigmoidoscope. The tip of the obturator and scope are lubricated and carefully inserted into the rectum and sigmoid. Then the obturator is removed so that the S shape of the colon can be seen. Patients find this an uncomfortable and unpleasant procedure.

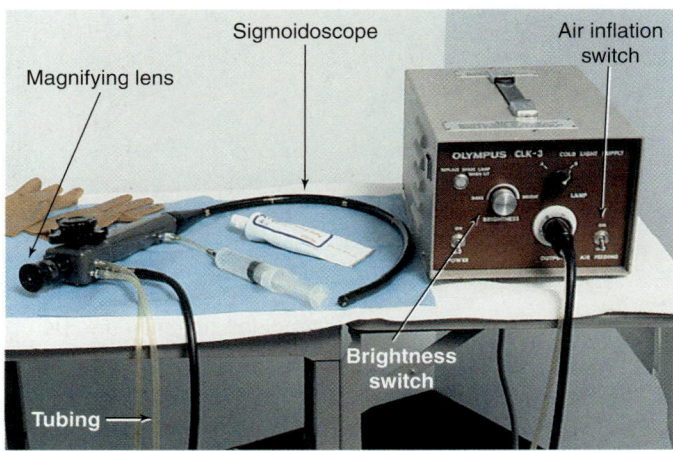

FIGURE 14-55 Parts of the flexible sigmoidoscope are labeled in the photo of a procedure setup. The examiner should wear PPE during this procedure.

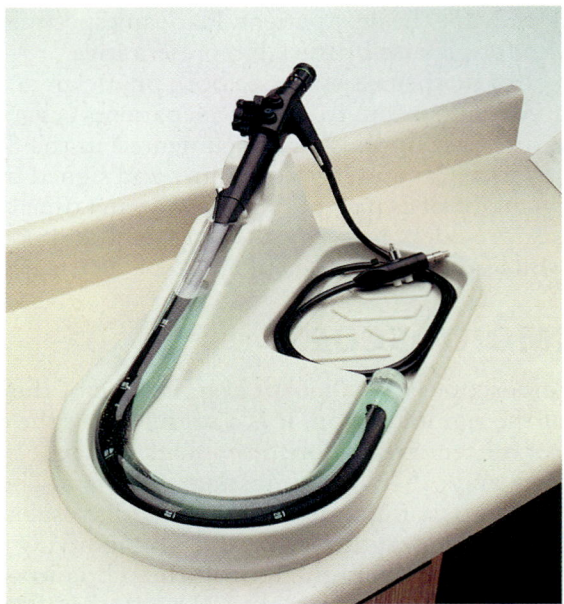

FIGURE 14-56A The flexible sigmoidoscope may be used with a video camera and the exam viewed on a monitor. The instrument can be stored and transported in the disinfection tray. *(Courtesy of Welch Allyn, Inc.)*

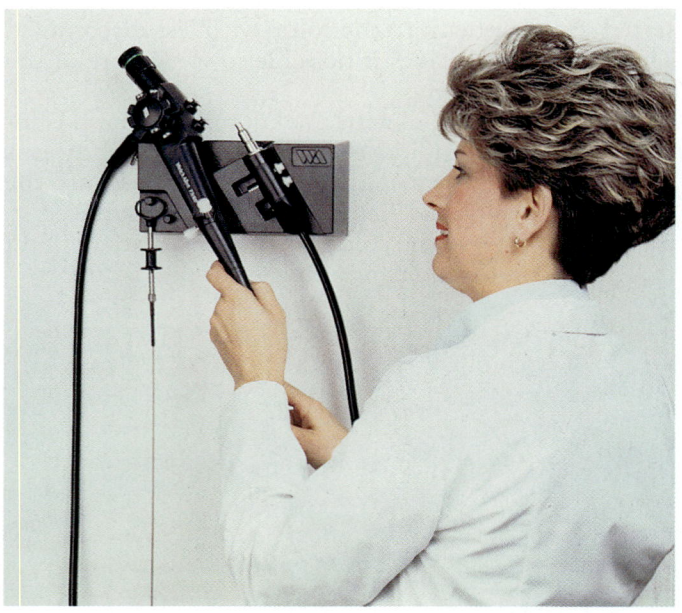

FIGURE 14-56B The flexible sigmoidoscope may also be stored on the wall hanger after being disinfected. *(Courtesy of Welch Allyn, Inc.)*

As with any examination of the abdomen, you should advise the patient to empty the bladder and evacuate the bowel before the procedure begins. This will make the exam easier for both the patient and the examiner. During the procedure, the patient should be instructed to breathe through the mouth deeply and

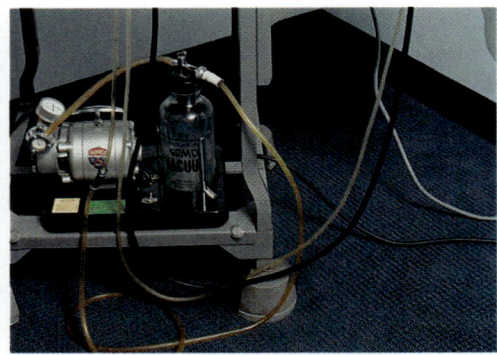

FIGURE 14-57 This suction machine is used when performing a sigmoidoscopy to remove any fecal or enema material to provide a better view of the tissues of the colon.

slowly to relax abdominal muscles. Patients may feel the urge to defecate during any colon examination because of the stretching of the inestinal wall from the instrument passing through and air being introduced with it. If patients use the breathing technique mentioned, this discomfort can be decreased. The procedure should last only a minute or two, especially if patients have followed preparation instructions.

Air is sometimes introduced into the colon (by the examiner's use of the inflation bulb attached to the rigid scope with tubing) to distend the wall of the colon for easier insertion of the **lumen** of the **endoscope**. The flexible scope provides for inflation by instilling air through a length of attached small tubing. It is controlled by a switch on the box that also controls the light source (see Figure 14-55). Patients find this to be uncomfortable and sometimes painful. The physician may need to use a suction pump to remove mucus, blood, or **fecal** material that is obstructing the view of the colon (Figure 14-57).

Assistance in handing necessary items to the physician and giving support to the patient are your roles during these exams. Refer to Procedure 14-17 for assisting with a sigmoidoscopy.

CLEANSING ENEMA

It is not a common procedure to administer an enema to a patient in the medical office or clinic, but it is sometimes a necessity for the successful completion of a sigmoidoscopy, or other rectal examination. Even though a patient may have received proper instructions and carried them out before the scheduled appointment, there is no guarantee that the patient was successful. In the event that the patient comes in for the appointment and is not sufficiently cleaned out for a sigmoidoscopy, the physician may order a cleansing enema so that the exam can be completed. It is generally best to proceed with the planned procedure, even with the delay of the enema. Usually this works out best for

14-17 Assist with a Sigmoidoscopy

PURPOSE: To assist in examination of the sigmoid colon.

OSHA GUIDELINES: To comply with Standard Precautions, gloves must be worn if there is any possibility of coming into contact with blood or any body fluids.

EQUIPMENT: Disposable latex or vinyl gloves, water-soluble lubricant, gauze squares, sigmoidoscope, long cotton-tipped swabs, drape sheet (fenestrated optional), suction machine (container with room temperature water), tissues, (if ordered by physician: biopsy forceps, specimen container for transport to lab, lab request form), pen, and patient's chart.

PERFORMANCE OBJECTIVE: With access to all equipment and supplies, demonstrate (insofar as feasible) each of the steps required to assist with the sigmoidoscopy procedure. The specimen must be labeled with the completed requisition attached. Record and sign the procedure including the date, time, patient's reaction, specimen obtained and sent to lab, and physician's comments.

1. Explain the procedure to the identified patient. **RATIONALE: Speaking to the patient by name and checking the chart ensures that you are performing the procedure on the correct patient.** Ask the patient to empty the bladder and bowel.

2. Assemble all needed items on a Mayo table near the end of the examination table (Figure 14-58). Plug in cord of light source to make sure it works properly, then turn off. **RATIONALE: If left on it will be uncomfortably warm for the patient and may cause a burn. NOTE: If a biopsy is scheduled, complete the lab request form and label the specimen container.**

3. Instruct the patient to disrobe from the waist down and let you know when he is ready. Assist the patient to sit at the end of the table and cover him with the drape sheet.

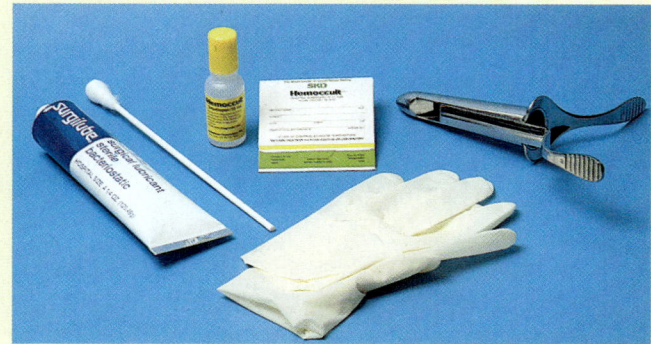

FIGURE 14-58 Equipment and supplies for a rectal examination

4. Both the medical assistant and the physician should wash their hands and put on latex or vinyl gloves.

5. Just before the physician is ready to begin the exam, assist the patient into a knee-chest or Sims' position, whichever the physician prefers. **NOTE: Many physicians have an examining table that permits the patient to kneel on a pad and then be placed in a jackknife position to facilitate the procedure.**

6. Assist the physician by applying about two tablespoons of lubricant on a gauze square for the tip of the obturator and the tip of gloved fingers. **NOTE: The physician makes a digital examination of the anus and rectum prior to insertion of the endoscope.**

7. As the physician finishes the digital exam, plug the sigmoidoscope into the light source. Secure the air-inflation tubing and have it ready to hand to the physician. When using a flexible sigmoidoscope, activate the switches for air inflation and light.

8. As the physician inserts the sigmoidoscope, be ready to hand items as needed. **NOTE: Have the suction machine plugged in and suction tip secured. RATIONALE: Often fecal material or unexpelled enema fluid is present and must be removed before adequate viewing can be accomplished.**

9. Be prepared to rinse the suction tip in water if it becomes clogged. (Note that flexible scopes aspirate through the attached tubing when suction is activated.)

10. If biopsy is indicated, hand biopsy forceps to the physician, and have a specimen container open so the physician can place tissue in it. Place the cap on the container securely.

11. Use tissues to clean lubricant and waste from the patient's anal area, and discard it into the biohazardous waste container.

12. Place a small pad or dressing over the anal area in case of light bleeding.

13. Assist the patient to resting prone position (or return table to starting position).

14. Assist the patient to a sitting position, allowing time for balance to return before helping him down from the table. Instruct the patient to dress (unless the patient has an appointment for additional examinations, such as x-rays, in the same office).

15. Disease transmission must be prevented. Wear gloves to clean the exam table and instruments. The metal scope and suction tip should be cleaned with detergent and

(continues)

PROCEDURE PROCEDURE PROCEDURE PROCEDURE PROCEDURE PROCEDURE PROCEDURE PROCEDURE

14-17  Assist with a Sigmoidoscopy (Continued)

water and placed in a disinfectant or boiled in a water sanitizer to be sanitized. **NOTE: The flexible sigmoidoscope is an expensive, complicated instrument. Follow the manufacturer's instructions for cleaning and sanitizing.**

16. Remove gloves and wash hands.

17. Attach a label and the completed requisition form to the specimen container.

18. Place the specimen container in the area for laboratory pick-up.

19. Restock the room and return the instruments to storage.

20. Record the procedure on the patient's chart and sign.

CHARTING EXAMPLE

4/19/XX, 10:00 a.m.

Sigmoidoscopic exam tolerated well by patient; biopsy of lesion on anterior wall at 10 inches. Pad placed over anal area in case of light bleeding. Specimen sent to lab. Follow-up when results received.

B. Jeffers, RMA

P PATIENT EDUCATION

It will most often be the medical assistant who tells the patient how to prepare for the sigmoidoscopy and explains how the test is performed. For successful examination, proper preparation is essential. In addition to having the patient restrict dairy products, raw fruits and vegetables, and grains and cereals from their diet, they should be encouraged to drink plenty of clear liquids and eat lightly the day before the scheduled appointment for the sigmoid colon exam. A plain Fleet's enema should be self-administered at home approximately 2 hours before the exam. Physicians may vary the instructions according to the patient's condition. It is best to ask before proceeding with instructions. If patients are not completely informed about preparations and the exam is attempted with unsatisfactory results, it will have to be repeated, which is both costly and inconvenient. Satisfactory results are obtained by giving patients both oral and written instructions. This practice will also be helpful in reducing phone calls with trivial questions.

Some exams, such as diagnostic sigmoidoscopy and x-rays, require the use of evacuants by the patient before the exam. This may present a problem in the patient's personal or employment schedule if instructions are not made clear before the appointment is scheduled. Most patients are fearful of what the diagnostic examination will disclose. Helping them choose a convenient appointment time and explaining the reasons for the preparations they must undergo will usually be appreciated.

When patients come in for rectal or sigmoidoscopy examinations, here are a few informative topics that you may discuss with them.

1. Remind them that laxatives and enemas should only be used by direction of the physician.

2. Constipation may be avoided/relieved by including fresh fruits and vegetables and cereals and grains in their diet, drinking plenty of liquids (water), and getting regular exercise.

3. Instruct them that if they have any of the following symptoms persistently, it could mean that a disease or an abnormal condition is present, and consulting the physician is strongly advised: heartburn or indigestion, nausea and/or vomiting, constipation or diarrhea, excessive gas or bloating, or stool that is tarry (black) or other than a normal brown color.

4. Inform patients who are age 40 and over that they should routinely test their stool for occult blood every 2 years for detection of cancer of the colon, or more often if advised by the physician (if family history indicates). All patients over age 50 should test annually.

5. Advise patients to include high-fiber foods in their diets, avoid too much fat (and saturated fats) and cholesterol, and eat red meats sparingly.

6. Urge patients to eat from a variety of foods (from the food pyramid in Chapter 20) and to eat four to six small meals rather than one or two large meals daily to promote better use of nutrients and more energy.

7. Suggest to patients that it is better to select snacks and beverages wisely; for example, choose fruits, vegetables, and juices over coffee, tea, soda pop, and high-calorie sweets or chips.

patient and staff, for rescheduling presents difficulties for everyone.

Often the patient did follow the list of instructions but just did not retain the enema solution long enough for it to work. You will likely be able to encourage the patient to hold the contents of the enema longer. You may want to explain that the longer the contents are held, the more successful the results will be. Often encouraging deep breathing and placing a couple of tissues over the anal opening and applying gentle pres-sure will aid in retaining the fluid. Otherwise, it may have to be repeated or the exam rescheduled.

For the patient's convenience, make sure that you use an examination room that is close to the restroom when you administer an enema. The enema is a simple procedure, one that patients can do at home when advised by the physician. Your patience and under-standing are needed here, because most patients are embarrassed to have this done. Procedure 14-18 pro-vides the information you need to carry out this duty.

PROCEDURE PROCEDURE PROCEDURE PROCEDURE PROCEDURE PROCEDURE PROCEDURE

14-18  Administer a Disposable Cleansing Enema

PURPOSE: To stimulate elimination of fecal matter from the lower intestinal tract.

OSHA GUIDELINES: To comply with Standard Precautions, gloves must be worn if there is any possibility of coming into contact with blood or any body fluids.

EQUIPMENT: Prepackaged disposable enema (plain Fleet's), water-soluble lubricant, Mayo tray, towel, latex or vinyl gloves, tissues, drape sheet, pen, and patient's chart.

PERFORMANCE OBJECTIVE: Provided with an anatomical model of the lower abdominopelvic cavity or a mannequin, and access to all equipment and supplies required, demonstrate administering a cleansing enema following the steps of the procedure.

1. Explain the procedure to the patient. **RATIONALE: Speaking to the patient by name and checking the chart ensures that you are performing the procedure on the correct patient.**

2. Instruct the patient to disrobe from the waist down. Provide a drape sheet and assist the patient onto the exam table.

3. Help the patient into a Sims' position, asking the patient to lie on the left side and to bring the right knee up to the waist.

4. Wash hands and put on latex or vinyl gloves.

5. Remove the protective covering from the tip of the enema container, and apply a small amount of lubricant if necessary to the tip; tip *is* prelubricated. **NOTE: It is easier to retain the solution if it is near body temperature. Warm the enema solution in *warm* water if it feels cold to the touch.**

6. Adjust the drape sheet to expose the buttocks.

7. With one hand, separate the buttocks to expose the anus; with the other hold the enema bottle, and gently insert the tip into the rectum, making sure that the tip points in the direction of the patient's navel. **NOTE: Advise the patient to breathe deeply and slowly through the mouth. RATIONALE: This aids patient to relax and makes instillation easier.**

8. Express the entire contents from the bottle slowly (squeeze from bottom to top of bottle).

9. Withdraw the enema tip slowly and provide the patient with tissues. Ask the patient to retain the liquid for as long as possible. **NOTE: Wait 5 to 10 minutes so that the solution will have time to work. NOTE: Tissues may be used to remove any lubricant or placed against the anus with pressure to aid in maintaining the enema. Discard in a biohazardous waste container if the tissues are left in the room.**

10. Direct the patient to the restroom as necessary; ask the patient to let you check the results before flushing. Report to the physician. If results seem inadequate, ask physician if procedure should be repeated.

11. If a proctologic exam is to follow, proceed to prepare the patient as appropriate.

12. Clean the room; discard disposables in the appropriate waste containers.

13. Remove gloves and wash hands.

14. Record the procedure.

CHARTING EXAMPLE

10-14-XX

Administered plain Fleet enema; tolerated well, good results, no remaining abdominal discomfort.

S. Long, RMA

PROCTOLOGIC POSITIONING, INSTRUMENTS, AND PROCEDURES

Proper positioning of patients during the exam is important for both the physician's viewing of the rectum and sigmoid colon and the patient's comfort. **Proctology** tables are designed especially for this procedure. They provide support of the patient's chest and head with the arm resting against the headboard as the table is tilted to the knee-chest position. Those who cannot tolerate this position are assisted into a Sims' position for the exam. Many physicians find this acceptable. You should ask about the physician's preference in patient position, because there are variations.

The physician may wish to view the intestinal **mucosa** following a normal bowel movement. More often, the patient is instructed to eat a light diet containing plenty of clear liquids and avoiding dairy products for 24 hours before the exam, and to have a plain cleansing enema the morning of, or 2 hours before, the exam. Still other physicians may wish patients to use laxatives the day before and an enema the night before and also the morning of the exam. Patients have usually eaten little within the past few days because of their abdominal distress.

In the diagnosis of hemorrhoids, fissures, and ulcerations, the physician usually begins investigative procedures by examining the anus and the interior of the rectum with a **proctoscope**. Figure 14-58 shows the items necessary for a basic rectal exam and occult blood test. The proctoscope permits viewing of the anal canal and lower rectal area when sigmoidoscopy is not necessary. It is a much better-tolerated examination.

During the sigmoidoscopy, the physician may want to take a biopsy of questionable tissue from the sigmoid colon to aid in confirming the diagnosis. It is a good rule to have all possibly necessary items available. When the patient has been prepared and the examiner is ready to begin the exam, the medical assistant hands the necessary instruments and supplies to the physician as needed.

Remember to advise patients to report any problems, such as bleeding, discharge, swelling, or any other unusual discomfort, following any procedure. A biopsy lab request form must be completed and accompany the tissue to the lab. Containers for biopsy specimens have a **formaldehyde** solution to preserve the tissue until the analysis is done.

There are other proctologic procedures that may need to be performed by the physician for patients in the office setting. Some of the instruments used in these procedures are shown in Figure 14-59A through C. The proctoscope (A) allows viewing of the anal canal and rectum, the biopsy forceps (B) permit removing a tissue sample for examination, and the snare (C) is used to detach polyps or other pendulous growths from the mucosa to be examined. All instru-

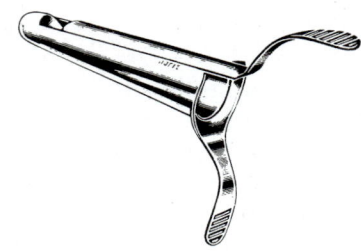

FIGURE 14-59A Additional instruments used in rectal examinations and procedures—Brinkerhoff rectal speculum *(Courtesy of JARIT Surgical Instruments)*

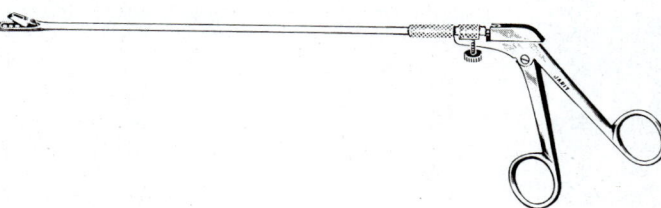

FIGURE 14-59B Turrell rotating shaft rectal biopsy forceps *(Courtesy of JARIT Surgical Instruments)*

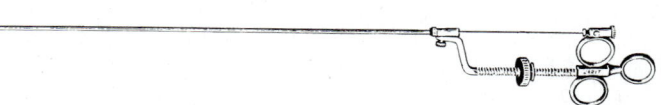

FIGURE 14-59C Norwood rectal snare *(Courtesy of JARIT Surgical Instruments)*

ments and items that come in contact with a body cavity must be free from microorganisms. The medical assistant is generally responsible for this task. Some instruments can be cleaned and then autoclaved. Others can be placed in a water sterilizer. Delicate instruments and those with plastic or rubber parts will require processing in a germicidal solution (see Chapter 12).

ACHIEVE UNIT OBJECTIVES

- **Complete the Workbook activities to meet the learning objectives.**
- **Practice the procedures in this unit to meet the performance objectives.**
- **Apply your knowledge at the end of this chapter in completing the Critical Thinking Challenge and Activities, as well as the StudyWARE on your Student CD-ROM.**

UNIT 5
PEDIATRIC EXAMINATIONS AND PROCEDURES

OBJECTIVES

Upon completion of this unit, you will be able to achieve the following:

LEARNING Objectives

1. Spell and define, using the glossary at the back of the text, all the Words to Know in this unit.

2. Refer to childhood growth and development tables to identify gross motor activities that are appropriate for 6-month-, 1-year-, and 18-month-old children.

3. Identify immunizations given to 2- and 12-month-old children according to the Childhood and Adolescent Immunization Schedule.

4. Determine the recommended screenings and procedures for an at-risk 2 year old as identified on the Preventive Pediatric Health Care chart.

5. Explain the difference between neglect and abuse, citing five examples of each.

6. Explain well and sick child office visits.

7. Explain the Healthcheck program.

8. List five responsibilities of the medical assistant when assisting with pediatric examinations.

9. Explain how to plot height and weight measurements on a National Center for Health Statistics growth chart.

PERFORMANCE Objectives

1. Perform pediatric vision screening.

2. Measure recumbent length of an infant.

3. Measure a child's height.

4. Weigh an infant.

5. Measure head circumference.

6. Measure an infant's chest.

WORDS TO KNOW

abuse	confidentiality	malnutrition
Apgar	development	neglect
attachment	Healthcheck	pediatric
bonding	immunization	percentile
caregiver	intercede	preventive
chronologic	lethargic	suspicion
circumference	listlessness	thrive

CERTIFICATION CONNECTION

CMA

Patient preparation and assisting the physician

Patient history interview

Collection and processing specimens; diagnostic testing (vision testing, hearing testing)

Preparing and administering medications (maintaining medication and immunization records)

CMAS

Basic health history interview

Vital signs and measurements

Examination preparation

THE PEDIATRIC PATIENT

Pediatrics is a specialty of medicine that cares for children from birth until essentially adulthood. Some practices limit care at 16 years of age, while others may continue until 18 or high school graduation. Usually teenagers will resist seeing a pediatrician when they perceive they are too "old." The initial pediatrician's examination will often be done in the hospital a few hours after birth, but the state of health of the newborn actually began many months before with the prenatal care of the mother. Almost immediately after birth, the infant is evaluated by the **Apgar** scoring system, as described in Unit 13 of Chapter 11. This score, from 0-10, determines the infant's first individual experience with medical care. The lower the score, the more intense the necessary medical intervention. Fortunately, most infants arrive in good condition.

Pediatric patients are examined much more frequently than adults and must be monitored carefully because of their rapid growth and **development**, especially in the 1st year. Growth refers to the changes in height and weight that can be measured as the infant begins to mature. Development refers to the infant's ability to control his body and use verbal and mental skills. These areas of assessment, as well as the apparent intellectual and social status of the developing child, are closely observed and compared with acceptable national standards. This comparison determines whether the child is at the appropriate level of development for the **chronologic** age. Children will vary in individual development due perhaps to inherited tendencies, but when characteristics are beyond acceptable levels, intervention will be initiated to identify the reason.

The infant begins its journey through the pediatrician's office at 3 to 4 weeks old. At this visit, the infant's height and weight will be measured, diet and eating concerns discussed, and any lab tests or other procedures deemed necessary will be performed. By 2 months, the baby will return for another examination and evaluation and begin the **immunization** schedule. The Department of Health and Human Services, Centers for Disease Control and Prevention releases a Recommended Childhood and Adolescent Immunization Schedule for children in the United States. It is approved by the Academies of both Pediatricians and family practice physicians (Figure 14-60).

The baby will continue to be examined at 2- to 3-month intervals throughout the first 18 months, and immunizations should be completed. A great deal of physical, mental, and social development occurs within a relatively short period of 2 years. The ability to sit, stand, and walk; to hold and use toys and utensils; and progress from babbling sounds to words. The child has developed her own personality and exhibits a degree of independence (Figure 14-61)

The child will continue to be examined on a yearly basis to monitor his development toward maturity. The American Academy of Pediatrics has established a schedule of recommended frequency of examinations in order to provide **preventive** care for normally developing, healthy children. Obviously, if health or development problems occur, a more frequent schedule will be necessary.

FAILURE TO THRIVE (FTT)

An infant or young child who is below the 3rd percentile on standardized growth charts is said to be failing to **thrive**. The cause may be from a physical problem such as unrepaired cleft palate or a disease condition. However, the cause may also be associated with the child's poor physical and emotional environment. Normally when a baby is born, a great deal of examining, touching, cuddling, and expressions of love are directed toward it. The infant is known to respond to this behavior, and this parent-child relationship is called "**attachment**" and "**bonding**." When this does not occur, there is a lack of emotional support for the baby. Often care is not provided on a consistent basis.

If food is offered, the baby may be too **lethargic** to eat. Parents may lack knowledge about infant care, have anxiety about being a parent, or just be unconcerned. Parental illness, drug abuse, an unwanted or ill infant, and other factors may cause difficulty. With irregular and often absent care, the infant will show physical, emotional, and social delays in development.

If the neglected baby is brought in for examination, there is a chance to identify the problem and provide encouragement and parental skill assistance to the parents. When conducting the interview and performing the procedures prior to the physician's examination, the medical assistant has an opportunity to observe the parental behavior as well as the baby's condition. Some symptoms of a FTT baby are **listlessness** and avoidance of eye contact. It will not seem concerned about you, a stranger. There may be no cooing or crying. Older infants may not be interested in toys or playing. Parents may exhibit a lack of concern, not ask questions, and express negative comments about the baby. Inform the physician of any behaviors you observe that seem "different" to you so that an awareness can be established and further examined.

CHILD ABUSE

Another area of awareness concerns the suspicion of child **neglect** or **abuse**. Neglect refers to the lack of or withholding of care. Abuse refers to inflicting emotional, physical, or sexual injury. The federal government enacted legislation called the Child Abuse Prevention and Treatment Act, that states that all threats or acts that might cause physical or mental harm to a child *must be* reported. This refers to **suspicion** of neglect of care as well as abuse. Anyone, whether a teacher, neighbor, social worker, family member, or health care worker, is obligated to report neglect or abuse to the proper authorities. The law protects the person who makes the report under a **confidentiality** provision. It should be mentioned that although parents are responsible for their child's care, that responsibility is often given to other **caregivers** such as grandparents, babysitters, or boyfriends or girlfriends of the single parent. This act applies to all caregivers.

As a medical assistant, you should be aware of neglect and abuse symptoms, some of which are not too obvious. During your interview and performance of routine procedures, you may feel there is a possibility of inadequate care. You should alert the physician before the examination so your suspicions can be evaluated. The appropriate authorities to whom the physician, or you, should make a report in your community should be identified in the office manual. Table 14-3 lists some of the more obvious examples of neglect and abuse for your information.

Recommended Childhood and Adolescent Immunization Schedule UNITED STATES • 2006

Vaccine ▼ / Age ▶	Birth	1 month	2 months	4 months	6 months	12 months	15 months	18 months	24 months	4–6 years	11–12 years	13–14 years	15 years	16–18 years
Hepatitis B[1]	HepB	HepB		HepB[1]	HepB						HepB Series			
Diphtheria, Tetanus, Pertussis[2]			DTaP	DTaP	DTaP		DTaP			DTaP	Tdap	Tdap		
Haemophilus influenzae type b[3]			Hib	Hib	Hib[3]	Hib								
Inactivated Poliovirus			IPV	IPV		IPV				IPV				
Measles, Mumps, Rubella[4]						MMR				MMR		MMR		
Varicella[5]						Varicella					Varicella			
Meningococcal[6]										MPSV4	MCV4	MCV4	MCV4	MCV4
Pneumococcal[7]			PCV	PCV	PCV	PCV				PCV	PPV			
Influenza[8]					Influenza (Yearly)					Influenza (Yearly)				
Hepatitis A[9]						HepA Series								

Vaccines within broken line are for selected populations

This schedule indicates the recommended ages for routine administration of currently licensed childhood vaccines, as of December 1, 2005, for children through age 18 years. Any dose not administered at the recommended age should be administered at any subsequent visit when indicated and feasible. ▨ Indicates age groups that warrant special effort to administer those vaccines not previously administered. Additional vaccines may be licensed and recommended during the year. Licensed combination vaccines may be used whenever any components of the combination are indicated and other components of the vaccine are not contraindicated and if approved by the Food and Drug Administration for that dose of the series. Providers should consult the respective ACIP statement for detailed recommendations. Clinically significant adverse events that follow immunization should be reported to the Vaccine Adverse Event Reporting System (VAERS). Guidance about how to obtain and complete a VAERS form is available at www.vaers.hhs.gov or by telephone, 800-822-7967.

▨ **Range of recommended ages** ▨ **Catch-up immunization** ▨ **11–12 year old assessment**

1. Hepatitis B vaccine (HepB). *AT BIRTH:* **All newborns** should receive monovalent HepB soon after birth and before hospital discharge. **Infants born to mothers who are HBsAg-positive** should receive HepB and 0.5 mL of hepatitis B immune globulin (HBIG) within 12 hours of birth. **Infants born to mothers whose HBsAg status is unknown** should receive HepB within 12 hours of birth. The mother should have blood drawn as soon as possible to determine her HBsAg status; if HBsAg-positive, the infant should receive HBIG as soon as possible (no later than age 1 week). **For infants born to HBsAg-negative mothers,** the birth dose can be delayed in rare circumstances but only if a physician's order to withhold the vaccine and a copy of the mother's original HBsAg-negative laboratory report are documented in the infant's medical record. *FOLLOWING THE BIRTHDOSE:* The HepB series should be completed with either monovalent HepB or a combination vaccine containing HepB. The second dose should be administered at age 1–2 months. The final dose should be administered at age ≥24 weeks. It is permissible to administer 4 doses of HepB (e.g., when combination vaccines are given after the birth dose); however, if monovalent HepB is used, a dose at age 4 months is not needed. **Infants born to HBsAg-positive mothers** should be tested for HBsAg and antibody to HBsAg after completion of the HepB series, at age 9–18 months (generally at the next well-child visit after completion of the vaccine series).

2. Diphtheria and tetanus toxoids and acellular pertussis vaccine (DTaP). The fourth dose of DTaP may be administered as early as age 12 months, provided 6 months have elapsed since the third dose and the child is unlikely to return at age 15–18 months. The final dose in the series should be given at age ≥4 years.

Tetanus and diphtheria toxoids and acellular pertussis vaccine (Tdap – adolescent preparation) is recommended at age 11–12 years for those who have completed the recommended childhood DTP/DTaP vaccination series and have not received a Td booster dose. Adolescents 13–18 years who missed the 11–12-year Td/Tdap booster dose should also receive a single dose of Tdap if they have completed the recommended childhood DTP/DTaP vaccination series. Subsequent **tetanus and diphtheria toxoids (Td)** are recommended every 10 years.

3. Haemophilus influenzae type b conjugate vaccine (Hib). Three Hib conjugate vaccines are licensed for infant use. If PRP-OMP (PedvaxHIB® or ComVax® [Merck]) is administered at ages 2 and 4 months, a dose at age 6 months is not required. DTaP/Hib combination products should not be used for primary immunization in infants at ages 2, 4 or 6 months but can be used as boosters after any Hib vaccine. The final dose in the series should be administered at age ≥12 months.

4. Measles, mumps, and rubella vaccine (MMR). The second dose of MMR is recommended routinely at age 4–6 years but may be administered during any visit, provided at least 4 weeks have elapsed since the first dose and both doses are administered beginning at or after age 12 months. Those who have not previously received the second dose should complete the schedule by age 11–12 years.

5. Varicella vaccine. Varicella vaccine is recommended at any visit at or after age 12 months for susceptible children (i.e., those who lack a reliable history of chickenpox). Susceptible persons aged ≥13 years should receive 2 doses administered at least 4 weeks apart.

6. Meningococcal vaccine (MCV4). Meningococcal conjugate vaccine (MCV4) should be given to all children at the 11–12 year old visit as well as to unvaccinated adolescents at high school entry (15 years of age). Other adolescents who wish to decrease their risk for meningococcal disease may also be vaccinated. All college freshmen living in dormitories should also be vaccinated, preferably with MCV4, although meningococcal polysaccharide vaccine (MPSV4) is an acceptable alternative. Vaccination against invasive meningococcal disease is recommended for children and adolescents aged ≥2 years with terminal complement deficiencies or anatomic or functional asplenia and certain other high risk groups (see *MMWR* 2005;54 [RR-7]:1-21); use MPSV4 for children aged 2–10 years and MCV4 for older children, although MPSV4 is an acceptable alternative.

7. Pneumococcal vaccine. The heptavalent **pneumococcal conjugate vaccine (PCV)** is recommended for all children aged 2–23 months and for certain children aged 24–59 months. The final dose in the series should be given at age ≥12 months. **Pneumococcal polysaccharide vaccine (PPV)** is recommended in addition to PCV for certain high-risk groups. See *MMWR* 2000; 49(RR-9):1-35.

8. Influenza vaccine. Influenza vaccine is recommended annually for children aged ≥6 months with certain risk factors (including, but not limited to, asthma, cardiac disease, sickle cell disease, human immunodeficiency virus [HIV], diabetes, and conditions that can compromise respiratory function or handling of respiratory secretions or that can increase the risk for aspiration), healthcare workers, and other persons (including household members) in close contact with persons in groups at high risk (see *MMWR* 2005;54[RR-8]:1-55). In addition, healthy children aged 6–23 months and close contacts of healthy children aged 0–5 months are recommended to receive influenza vaccine because children in this age group are at substantially increased risk for influenza-related hospitalizations. For healthy persons aged 5–49 years, the intranasally administered, live, attenuated influenza vaccine (LAIV) is an acceptable alternative to the intramuscular trivalent inactivated influenza vaccine (TIV). See *MMWR* 2005;54(RR-8):1-55. Children receiving TIV should be administered a dosage appropriate for their age (0.25 mL if aged 6–35 months or 0.5 mL if aged ≥3 years). Children aged ≤8 years who are receiving influenza vaccine for the first time should receive 2 doses (separated by at least 4 weeks for TIV and at least 6 weeks for LAIV).

9. Hepatitis A vaccine (HepA). HepA is recommended for all children at 1 year of age (i.e., 12–23 months). The 2 doses in the series should be administered at least 6 months apart. States, counties, and communities with existing HepA vaccination programs for children 2–18 years of age are encouraged to maintain these programs. In these areas, new efforts focused on routine vaccination of 1-year-old children should enhance, not replace, ongoing programs directed at a broader population of children. HepA is also recommended for certain high risk groups (see *MMWR* 1999; 48[RR-12]1-37).

The Childhood and Adolescent Immunization Schedule is approved by:
Advisory Committee on Immunization Practices www.cdc.gov/nip/acip • **American Academy of Pediatrics** www.aap.org • **American Academy of Family Physicians** www.aafp.org

FIGURE 14-60 Recommended Immunization Schedule

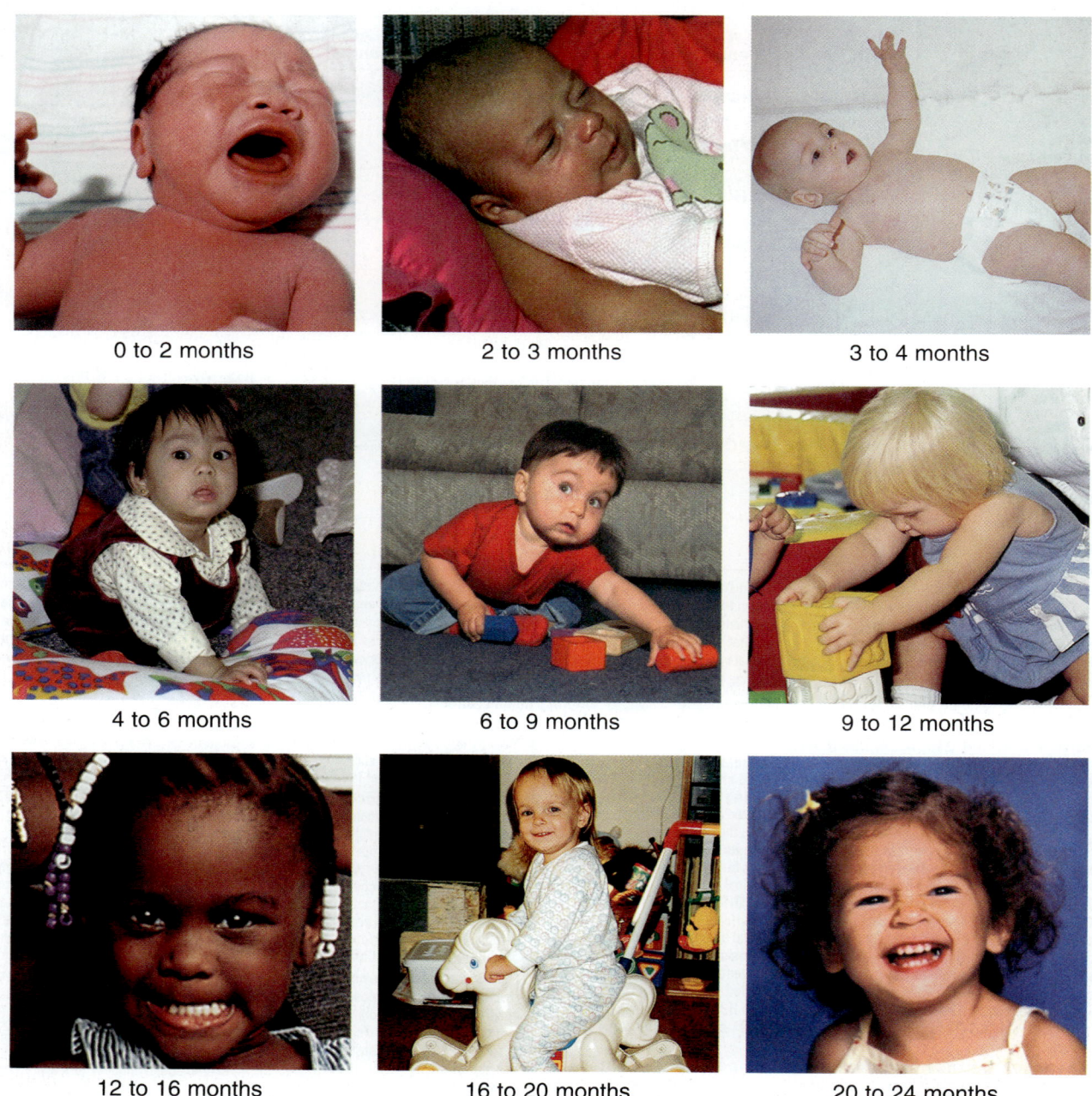

0 to 2 months

2 to 3 months

3 to 4 months

4 to 6 months

6 to 9 months

9 to 12 months

12 to 16 months

16 to 20 months

20 to 24 months

FIGURE 14-61 Growth and developmental stages of infants and toddlers

WELL OR SICK CHILD APPOINTMENTS

The pediatric practice will probably establish a different method of handling well and sick patients. When a parent calls for an appointment, it will be determined whether the visit is for a routine well-child examination or whether the child has symptoms of an illness. Specific well child hours are set aside in each day's schedule to care for the routine examinations and procedures as identified on the charts you have seen. However, when a child is ill, most pediatricians will attempt to see the child within a few hours of a parent's call. Parents can usually phone the pediatrician's office at all hours of the day or night and someone who is on call will respond. Some practices utilize an answering device to receive parental messages and then respond to those relatively soon. Practices may also set aside early office hours to see children who have become ill overnight.

TABLE 14-3 Symptoms of Neglect and Abuse	
Neglect	**Abuse**
Excessive length of time before seeking medical attention for illness or injury	Discoloration/bruises on the back, buttocks, or any other area
Apparent **malnutrition**	Evidence of burns in unusual places
Obvious lack of dental care	Internal abdominal pain
Immunizations neglected or incomplete	Dislocation of joints, such as shoulder and wrist
Poor personal hygiene	Frequent injuries requiring medical attention
Inadequate clothing for season or size; unclean	An x-ray of current injury showing evidence of untreated previous fractures
Developmental delay	Suspicious story about the injury; difference between description by child and parent or caregiver
Parental comments indicating lack of concern or not wanting child	Reports by the child of sexual or physical abuse

Reception Rooms

Every attempt is made to provide for the separation of well and sick children in the office. Pediatricians, in addition to scheduling times, will also provide separate reception areas. When an ill child is brought to the office, she immediately goes or is taken to the sick child room. At the very least, a separate area with its own toys should be set aside so that the office play area and toys are not available to the sick child.

When young patients come in to see the doctor, your attitude may be the deciding factor in their cooperation during the visit. Greeting them with a smile and speaking to them on their developmental level will help to gain their trust and cooperation. Patients of all ages are much more cooperative when they feel welcome. Some youngsters have had traumatic experiences in emergency care centers because of serious illness or injury. This leaves them fearful of health care providers in general. Unfortunately, some parents may even cause this fear by using threats of medical care and shots when disciplining children. If you take time, showing interest and patience, you can establish a rapport with the patients and help eliminate this potential problem.

The play area in the reception area helps the children feel welcome and provides a comfortable environment. A variety of safe, durable, washable, and educational toys should be provided. Toys that have many or tiny parts are not appropriate because many small objects all over the floor creates an unsafe walkway and could cause others to fall and possibly be hurt. It could also be a potential choking hazard for babies who put everything in their mouths. Keeping the toys clean and contained in one area will be one of your duties. Often a child will find an interesting toy while waiting to be called in to the examination room. Obviously the child's cooperation will be greater if the little patient is permitted to bring the toy with him to help keep him occupied while awaiting the doctor. It will also help you in performing any necessary procedures for the child in preparation for the doctor's examination.

You must make sure that when the child is finished with the toy that it is sanitized properly before returning it to the play area for other children. Remember, the play area should ideally be used only for well children who are waiting for annual physical examinations or other well visits, checkups, allergy injections, or immunizations. Sick children should be taken to a separate room as soon as they arrive to prevent the transmission of their disease to others who are present. The receptionist should be notified that an ill child is expected so she can be aware and act promptly.

Because you can never be sure of the health status of anyone, you must be vigilant in the practice of Standard Precautions. Sanitizing and disinfecting items and surfaces in the medical facility as needed is a vital part of your work day. Even when you are frantically busy with an overbooked schedule, remember to follow Standard Precautions. It should become a habit that is second nature to you for your protection and for the protection of patients and coworkers. A commercial disinfectant spray can help in the effort to cut down on disease transmission. You can use it quickly between patients when you are hurried. The best way to eliminate a potential disease transmission is to remove the contaminated item when possible until it can be properly sanitized.

Children (and patients of any age) becoming sick and vomiting is a concern in any medical facility. The administrative medical assistant should keep a disposable emesis basin near the window for this potential situation. You should also keep a commercial preparation accessible for use in cleaning up this type of waste.

Latex and vinyl gloves, paper towels, facial tissues, and biohazardous plastic waste bags should also be easily accessible. A covered waste receptacle lined with a biohazardous plastic bag for disposal of contaminated items should be available.

There may be occasions when a parent or caregiver brings a seriously ill or injured child into the facility unannounced. You must act quickly to provide immediate care to the patient and protect others from the possible transmission of the disease.

THE EXAMINATION

When you are assisting with the examination of a child, a very important responsibility is relaying information to the doctor from the parent or caregiver, and from the doctor to the patient and parent or caregiver. Your careful observation of the child and the parent or caregiver–child relationship could be critical information to the physician in the care and treatment of the child. Make note of any unusual observations, and advise the physician before the child is seen.

Cooperation with youngsters is generally obtained by explaining, in a calm, simple manner appropriate to their stage of development, what you and the doctor are going to do and why. If you sense behavior that is not cooperative, then you must ask the parent or caregiver to **intercede**. A child who is uncooperative for a procedure that is necessary will have to be restrained safely by you and the parent or another health care worker. Doing what has to be done as quickly as possible is the best way to handle the situation.

Young children are often amused with items that are not ordinary toys during an examination, such as a plastic drinking cup or tongue depressor (with supervision, of course). Giving children nonsharp instruments, such as a percussion hammer, stethoscope, or penlight, to examine may help them to overcome the fear of their use by the doctor during the exam (Figure 14-62). Be sure to clean these items properly when the examination is completed.

Pediatric patients should be regarded as individuals and given the kindness and respect you give to all patients. You may want to make a "poncho"-type covering for a little one by folding a disposable drape sheet in four sections and cutting the point off to make an opening to go over the child's head. Young boys and girls are often embarrassed and chilled sitting on the examination table in their underwear, awaiting the doctor. This is an easy way to help them feel more comfortable and keep them warm. They like the special treatment.

Another common practice to help little ones feel special is to provide them with bandages in colorful prints

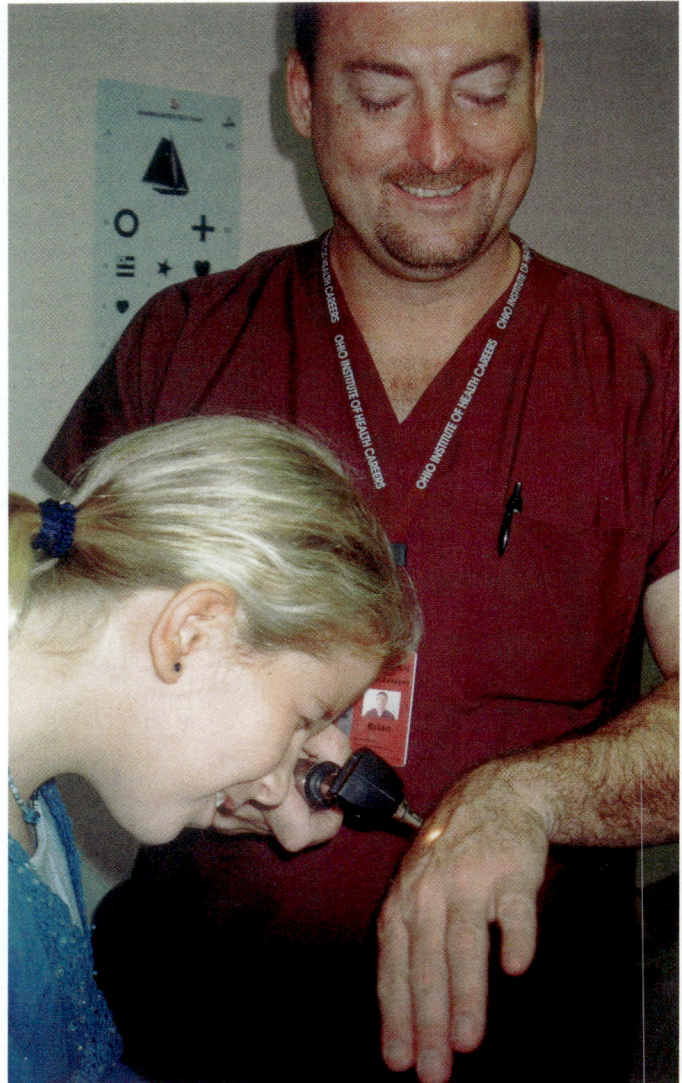

FIGURE 14-62 The medical assistant explains to the child how the doctor uses the otoscope to look in her ears.

or cartoon characters for their minor cuts and abrasions or for injection sites following immunizations. Most health care providers in medical facilities that treat pediatric patients offer a small token reward, such as stickers, balloons, or trinkets, after their treatment or exam is completed. (Ask the parent or caregiver for approval first.) This gives the child positive reinforcement and helps to establish and keep a good rapport between the medical team and the child.

HEALTH CARE DOCUMENTATION

You will also be required to complete many types of forms requesting information derived from health checkups for various facilities, such as schools or day care centers. An example of a comprehensive health care program that requires careful documentation of examination findings is the federally mandated program called **Healthcheck**. This is for eligible Medicaid patients who are between birth and 21 years of age. This program requires regular routine health maintenance checkups to detect and treat medical problems. The parent or primary caregiver must accompany the child at each visit. The recommended schedule for examinations is as follows:

Age	Examinations per year
Birth–12 months	6
1–2 years	2
2–21 years	1

The earlier a medical problem can be detected and treated, the better the prognosis for the child. Health care officials have developed this program for periodic intervals of examinations so that potential problems can be found before they become serious or beyond treatment stages. The screening procedures are simplified and relatively quick for determining abnormalities or illnesses (the results of these tests determine whether further testing is required). You should stress the importance of compliance with this program to the adult who is responsible for the child.

There are 13 areas that constitute the program:

1. Health
2. Developmental history from parent or primary caregiver
3. Complete physical exam (unclothed) (including vital signs ages 3–21 years) and height, weight, and head and chest measurements—plot results on growth charts
4. Nutritional assessment
5. Vision (include color vision acuity)
6. Hearing screening appropriate for the child's age
7. Immunization needs using standard schedule
8. Laboratory testing as indicated
9. Anemia or sickle cell tests as indicated
10. Urinalysis
11. Lead poisoning absorption annually for ages 1 to 4 years and as needed
12. Tuberculin test annually—Mantoux test on all individuals who have been or are suspected of having been exposed
13. Dental assessment—refer to dentist

Any other laboratory tests, x-rays, or cultures should be performed as indicated from findings in the health history or during the examination.

MEDICAL ASSISTANT RESPONSIBILITY

As a medical assistant, you will have certain routine responsibilities to perform with each pediatric examination. Generally you will:

- Assist in gathering data
- Document information
- Perform screening tests within your skill and ability level
- Assist the patient
- Assist the physician
- Provide patient education

Accuracy in the documentation of each of these components is essential to quality care for these young patients. Use the time with parents or caregivers and children to provide patient education as appropriate to the child's age and developmental stage.

ASSISTING WITH THE PEDIATRIC EXAM

The examination of a pediatric patient is basically the same format of the CPE for adults. The physician examines the patient from head to toe. Because little ones may be uncooperative at times, you should assist the doctor by holding the child still until the exam is completed. Often the physician will ask the caregiver to hold the baby while listening to the heart and lungs. The physician will ask the caregiver about the baby's eating and sleeping schedule and how the development is progressing (e.g., at 2 to 3 months, is the baby playing with his own hands?; at 6 months, is she crawling?). The doctor also observes the parent or caregiver relationship. Part of the examination of toddlers and children is to observe their gait. This is accomplished by placing the child across the room and observing her from behind as she walks to the caregiver.

There are some physicians who require that all patients from age 2 to 100 years have vital signs taken and recorded at every visit regardless of the reason for the appointment. Others feel it is only necessary periodically or when indicated by symptoms.

In Chapter 18, you will learn about medications, injections, and immunizations. Refer to this information and the immunization schedule for children. As a part of the pediatric exam, babies and children receive their immunizations. You will be required to have the proper immunizations ready for the physician to administer, or you may be asked to administer them. Office policies and physicians differ regarding this procedure. You will be required to record this information on the patient's chart and in the booklet that parents or caregivers keep. Make sure before the immunizations are given that you give the consent form to the parent or caregiver to sign after you have explained and they have read the possible side effects that are in printed form for them to keep. Instruct them to contact the doctor immediately if a serious reaction should occur from the immunization. If the child has a fever the day of the scheduled appointment, have the physician check the child before giving any immunizations. Be sure to have the physician outline exactly what needs to be done as a routine so you will be efficient in getting pediatric patients ready for the physician to examine.

EXAMINATION PREPARATION

The initial part of the pediatric check up and examination is the preparation of the baby or child. Remember to establish a good rapport with the child and the caregiver by being friendly and relaxed. Ask the caregiver about the child and how everything has been regarding the child's behavior and health, and whether there are any problems or questions. Refer to Table 14-4, which highlights growth and development during infancy and toddlerhood. The table shows the age at which the average child should be able to perform the activities listed.

Many caregivers or parents are unaware of developmental stages and what to expect from their children. Posting a chart regarding these growth and developmental stages of infants and children is most helpful for patient education. While preparing the child for the physician to come into the examination room, it is an ideal time to discuss patient education topics with the caregiver, such as the child's eating habits, sleep and daily activities, immunization schedules, toilet-training, and taking and recording a temperature. This is a great help to parents and caregivers in caring for their children. Printed booklets and pamphlets on a wide variety of topics should be offered to parents as appropriate to their children's ages. Your medical facility will have this kind of information in a more elaborate and expanded form. Patient education materials for patients to take with them about specific topics, such as sleep disturbances, nutrition for toddlers, and toilet training, should be available.

PEDIATRIC MEASUREMENTS

Growth Charts

It is essential in the course of the child's examination, diagnosis, and treatment to accurately record the growth and development of the child on his chart, in the caregiver's record booklet, and on the growth graph. This graph is a valuable visual for the physi-

cian because it allows the doctor to easily look at a glance at the child's growth and development pattern. All babies grow at different rates. The growth graph shows the normal growth of infants and children up to 20 years of age. The physician can then compare the child's measurements in relation to the **percentile**, that of other children the same age (this percentile is to the far right of the graph; see Figure 14-63A). There is a white curved line section, the one that is closest to the top of the page, where the height, length, and stature are recorded. The white curved line section below that is for plotting the weight of children. If the measurements of a baby or child fall above or below the normal height or weight areas and the family history does not warrant it, further examination and diagnostic testing is usually scheduled.

The National Center for Health Statistics (NCHS) growth charts become a permanent record of the child's development and are to be filed in the chart. At each subsequent visit, the child's growth should be recorded. These growth graphs aid in the diagnosis of growth abnormalities, nutritional disorders, and diseases of children from birth to 20 years of age. Of course, hereditary factors also influence growth patterns, hence the importance of having a complete family health history in the medical record.

Figures 14-63A through D show growth graphs for boys and girls. Two graphs record growth patterns of infant males and females from birth to 36 months, and two record growth patterns of boys and girls from 2 to 20 years of age. This information is printed across the top and bottom of the graph. Each of the squares across the page represents 1 month for the birth to 36-month graph and 1 year for the 2- to 20-year graph. Be sure you use the appropriate chart for the patient, as the normal development and growth patterns are different for males and females. On the front of each of the graphs is a ruled section to record the date, age, length/height/stature, and weight of the child at each appointment. The line for comments is for you to record a brief chief complaint that the caregiver (or the child, if old enough to speak) tells you. By looking at the line provided for the comments, you can see it is vital that you print small and neatly so that it can easily be read. The complaint or problem should also be neatly recorded on the chart.

MEASURING HEIGHT

Measuring the height of a baby from infancy to 36 months by recumbent length is recommended as the most accurate method of measurement (Figure 14-64). The baby should be placed on a pediatric or other examination table with the placement of the

TABLE 14-4   Growth and Development During Infancy

Age	Gross Motor	Fine Motor	Language	Sensory
Birth to 1 month	• Assumes tonic neck posture • When prone, lifts and turns head	• Holds hands in fist • Draws arms and legs to body	• Cries	• Comforts with holding and touch • Looks at faces • Follows objects when in line of vision • Alert to high-pitched voices • Smiles
2 to 4 months	• Can raise head and shoulders when prone to 45–90 degrees; supports self on forearms • Rolls from back to side	• Hands mostly open • Looks at and plays with fingers • Grasps and tries to reach objects	• Vocalizes when talked to; coos, babbles • Laughs aloud • Squeals	• Smiles • Follows objects 180 degrees • Turns head when hears voices or sounds
4 to 6 months	• Turns from stomach to back and then back to stomach • When pulled to sitting almost no head lag • By 6 months can sit on floor with hands forward for support	• Can hold feet and put in mouth • Can hold bottle • Can grasp rattle and other small objects • Puts objects in mouth	• Squeals	• Watches a falling object • Responds to sounds
6 to 8 months	• Puts full weight on legs when held in standing position • Can sit without support • Bounces when held in a standing position	• Transfers objects from one hand to the other • Can feed self a cookie • Can bang two objects together	• Babbles vowel-like sounds, "ooh" or "aah" • Imitation of speech sounds ("mama," "dada") beginning • Laughs aloud	• Responds by looking and smiling • Recognizes own name
8 to 10 months	• Crawls on all fours or uses arms to pull body along floor • Can pull self to sitting • Can pull self to standing	• Beginning to use thumb-finger grasp • Dominant hand use • Has good hand-mouth coordination	• Responds to verbal commands • May say one word in addition to "mama" and "dada"	• Recognizes sounds
10 to 12 months	• Can sit down from standing • Walks around room holding onto objects • Can stand alone	• Picks up and drops objects • Can put small objects into toys or containers through holes • Turns many pages in a book at one time • Picks up small objects	• Understands "no" and other simple commands • Learns one or two other words • Imitates speech sounds • Speaks gibberish	• Follows fast-moving objects • Indicates wants • Likes to play imitative games such as patty cake and peek-a-boo

(continues)

TABLE 14-4 Growth and Development During Toddlerhood (Continued)				
Age	Gross Motor	Fine Motor	Language	Sensory
12 to 15 months	• Can walk alone well • Can crawl up stairs	• Can feed self with cup and spoon • Puts raisins into a bottle • May hold crayon or pencil and scribble • Builds a tower of two cubes	• Says four to six words	• Binocular vision developed
18 months	• Runs, falling often • Can jump in place • Can walk up stairs holding on • Plays with push and pull toys	• Can build a tower of three to four cubes • Can use a spoon	• Says 10 or more words • Points to objects or body parts when asked	• Visual acuity 20/40
24 months	• Can walk up and down stairs • Can kick a ball • Can ride a tricycle	• Can draw a circle • Tries to dress self	• Talks a lot • Approximately 300-word vocabulary • Understands commands • Knows first name, refers to self • Verbalizes toilet needs	
30 months	• Throws a ball • Jumps with both feet • Can stand on one foot for a few minutes	• Can build a tower of eight blocks • Can use crayons • Learning to use scissors	• Knows first and last name • Knows the name of one color • Can sing • Expresses needs • Uses pronouns appropriately	

baby's head at the headboard. If necessary, someone holds the head in position while you stretch the legs out straight (infants tend to flex their legs). Measure from the vertex of the head to the heel of the baby. Refer to Figure 14-64 and Procedure 14-19 regarding how to place the baby on the exam table for measuring the recumbent length.

This procedure is written for measuring with a table that has a headboard and a measuring scale or using a portable measuring chart, as in Figure 14-64. If this is not available, recumbent length can be measured with a little improvising. Enlist the parent or another medical assistant to help position the infant. With the infant lying on an examination surface that is covered with paper, make a mark on the paper at the top of the infants head. With the parent holding the infant in position, straighten out one leg and mark on the paper at the bottom of the heel. Ask the parent to pick up the infant. Using a flexible tape or ruled measuring device, measure the distance between your two markings on the paper to obtain the recumbent length of the infant.

When the child is older and will cooperate, you can begin to measure the height and weight on the upright scales, or the adult scales as they are sometimes called. The shoes should be removed in order to get an accurate measurement. The child must stand still in the center of the platform until the height measurement is obtained. To reduce the amount of time the child is in place on the platform of the scales,

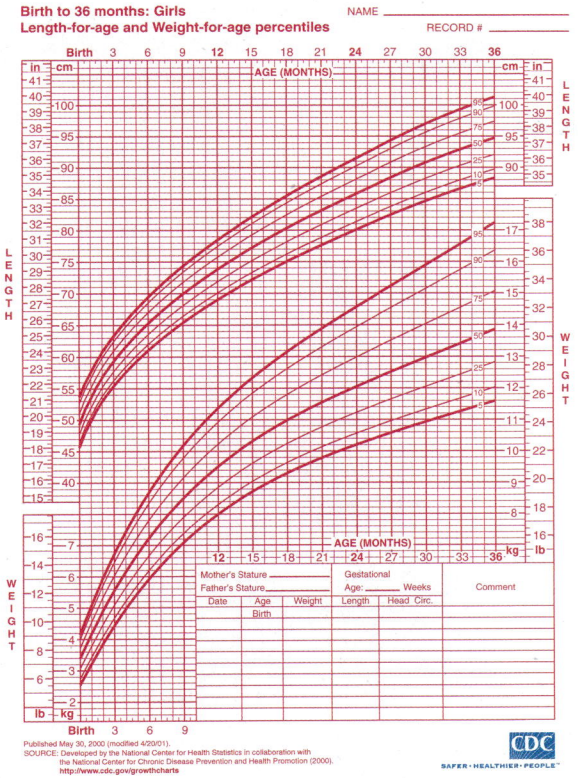

FIGURE 14-63A Growth graph for girls to record height and weight, ages birth to 36 months

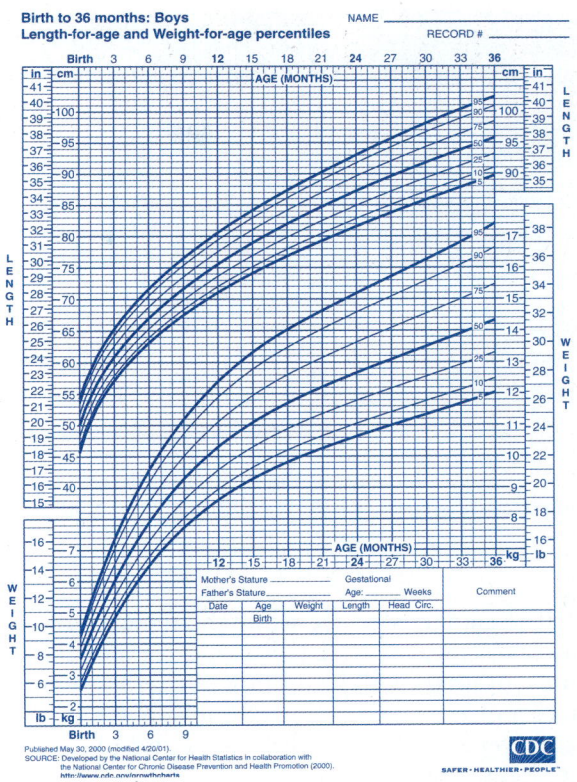

FIGURE 14-63B Growth graph for boys to record height and weight, ages birth to 36 months

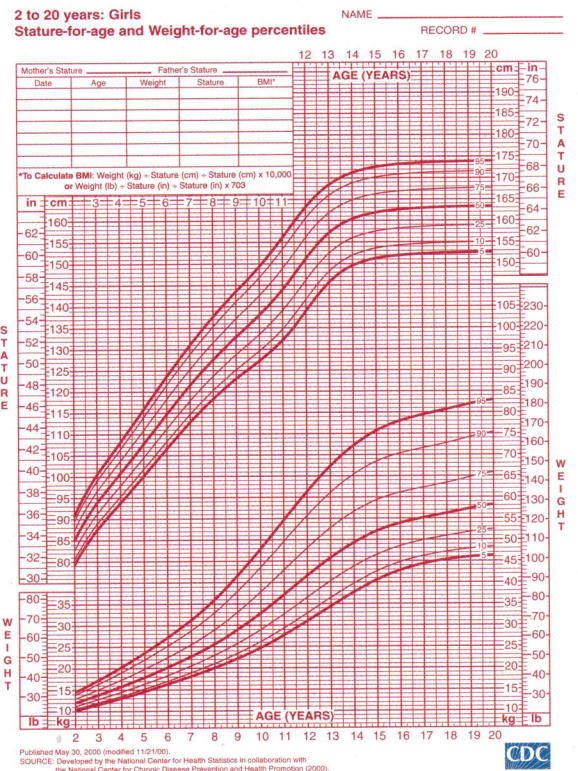

FIGURE 14-63C Growth graphs for girls to record height and weight, ages 2 to 20 years

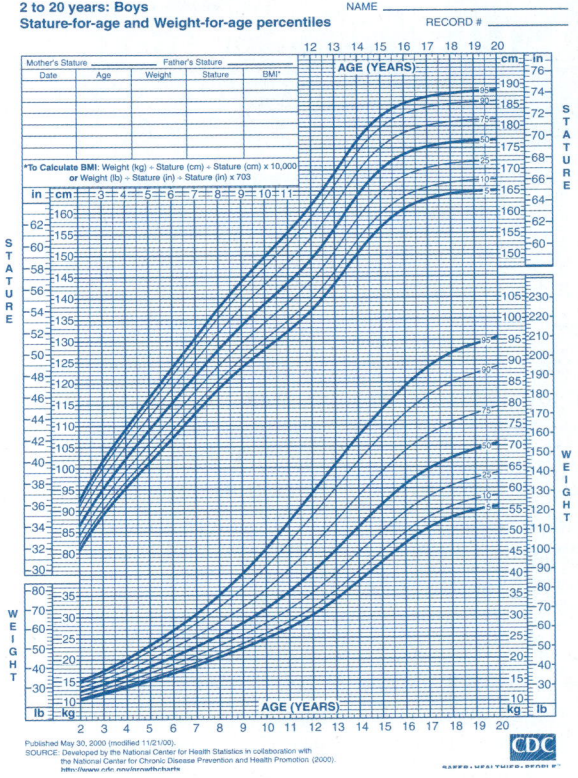

FIGURE 14-63D Growth graphs for boys to record height and weight, ages 2 to 20 years

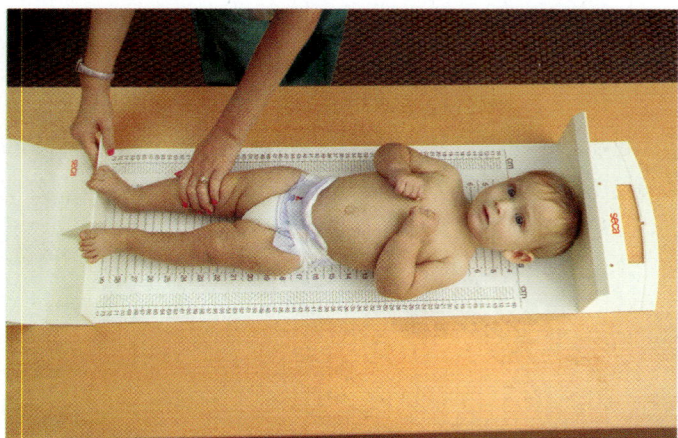

FIGURE 14-64 Measuring the recumbent length of an infant, measuring from the vertex of the child's head to the heel

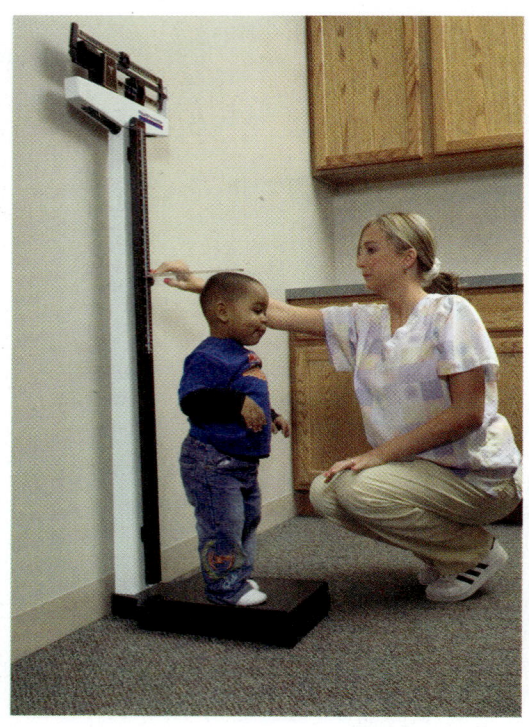

FIGURE 14-65 Place the measuring bar at the vertex of the child's head to obtain an accurate measurement of his height.

look at the chart and see what the measurement was at the last exam so that you can have an idea where the measurement will be. Follow Procedure 14-20 and refer to Figure 14-65 to place the measuring bar on the top (vertex) of the child's head and obtain an accurate height measurement.

PROCEDURE PROCEDURE PROCEDURE PROCEDURE PROCEDURE PROCEDURE PROCEDURE PROCEDURE

14-19  Measure Recumbent Length of an Infant

PURPOSE: To obtain an accurate measurement of recumbent length of an infant.

EQUIPMENT: Table with measuring device, ruled measuring tape, yardstick, or meterstick; patient's chart; parents' record booklet; growth graph; and pen.

PERFORMANCE OBJECTIVE: Provided with a clinical or toy doll (or an infant or small child under the close supervision of the parent, guardian, or instructor) and a pediatric table or examining table with a ruled measuring device, demonstrate each step of the procedure to measure recumbent length of an infant or small child. The measurement must be within $\frac{1}{4}$ inch of the actual length as determined by the instructor.

1. Wash hands and ask the parent to remove the infant's shoes and socks or booties.
2. Ask the parent to place the infant on the examination table with the head against the table headboard at the zero mark of the ruler. Gently straighten the infant's back and legs to line up along the ruler. Ask the parent

to hold the infant's head against the headboard of the table while you place the infant's heels against the footboard. If there is no footboard (to place the infant's feet against), use your right hand (see Figure 14-64). Place your left hand over the child's leg at the knee to secure the child in place and straighten the leg so you can read the recumbent length from the head (vertex) to the heel. **NOTE: Place your fingers behind the child's knee with your thumb over the kneecap; apply gentle pressure to help the straighten the leg.**

3. Read the length in inches or centimeters on the ruler. **NOTE: There may be discrepancies with measurement of newborns because they are so used to the fetal position that it is difficult to straighten the legs.**
4. Return the infant to the parent to re-dress.
5. Record the measurement on the patient's chart and in the parent's booklet of the child's growth and development. Plot the finding on the growth chart graph.

14-20  Measure Height

PURPOSE: To obtain an accurate measurement of a pediatric patient's height.

EQUIPMENT: Upright scale with extension measuring bar, patient's chart, and pen (a measuring scale may be fixed to the wall).

PERFORMANCE OBJECTIVE: With access to an upright scale with a height bar and a child to be measured, assist the child onto the scale and obtain and record a height measurement. Findings must be within ¼ inch of the instructor's measurement.

1. Raise the measuring bar and extension higher than the apparent height of the patient. **RATIONALE: Avoids the possibility of striking the patient with the extension when it is raised.**

2. Ask the parent to remove the young child's shoes. (Patients ready for physical exams will not have on shoes.) Place a paper towel on the platform of the scale. **RATIONALE: Accurate measurement cannot**

be obtained if shoes are worn. **The paper towel provides a clean surface for the shoeless foot.**

3. Help the child onto the scale facing you with his back to the measuring device. Tell him to stand straight (Figure 14-65).

4. Slide the measuring bar down slowly and carefully to rest on the top of the child's head, gently compressing the hair. **NOTE: Measurement of height is from the top of the head, not the hair. This can cause a discrepancy in the reading.**

5. Read the measurement in inches or centimeters, and tell the child and parent what it is.

6. Help the child down from scale. Ask the parent to put a young child's shoes back on unless scheduled for a physical exam.

7. Place the measuring extension bar back in place, and discard the paper towel.

8. Record the height measurement on the patient's chart.

WEIGHING THE PEDIATRIC PATIENT

It is customary to weigh infants unclothed for greater accuracy. Remember, a wet diaper may weigh several ounces, which would lead to an inaccurate measurement of the infant's true weight. Because you cannot control an infant's elimination, a dry diaper may be placed over the genital area in case urination occurs. It is possible to adjust the weight to accommodate for the diaper if the infant's weight is of great concern. Simply place it on the scale with the towel used to cover the base and adjust the balance weight to zero *before* the infant is place on the scale. If an infant gains or loses weight too quickly, it could be a signal of a disease or disorder and should be brought to the physician's attention. It is also important to ask the caregiver about the feeding schedule and appetite of the infant or child.

In some offices and clinics, the pediatric scales is kept on a stainless steel cart and simply wheeled to the patient's room. Other facilities may have a pediatric room in a family or general practice office where all infants and children are examined. In the specialty of pediatrics, every patient room may have an infant scale or the scale is kept in a specific location and the little one is carried there. It is best for you to ask the caregiver to transport the baby to the scales and place her on the scales for you. This reduces the possibility of a potential risk of accidental injury to the child on your part. Figures 14-66 and 14-67 show the proper positioning of the baby on the scales. Follow Procedure 14-21 to weigh an infant or baby up to 36 months or 38 pounds.

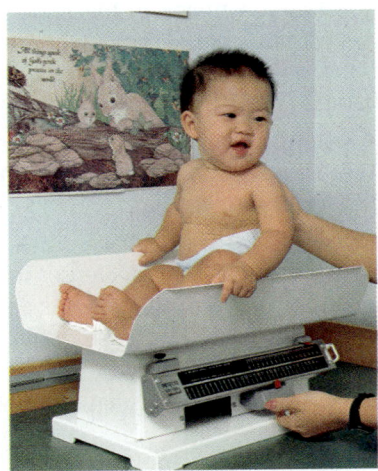

FIGURE 14-66 A baby is weighed in a sitting position on the scales; carefully place your hand close to the child for safety.

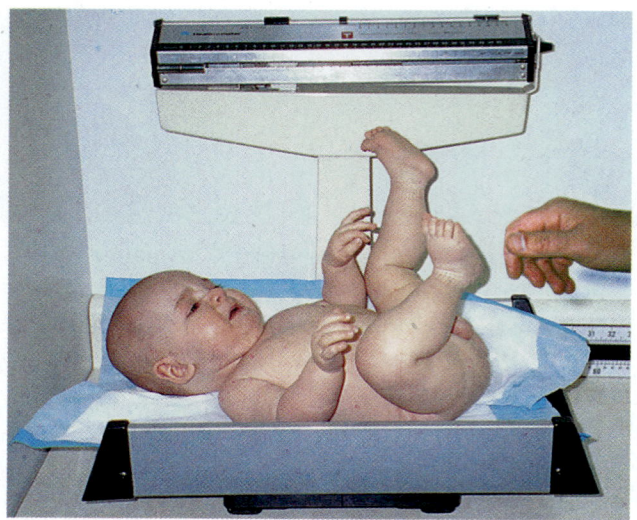

FIGURE 14-67   Infants who are too young to sit erect can be weighed lying on the infant platform scale. A hand should be held closely over the infant for safety.

As the infant grows into the toddler stage and on to a preschooler and passes the weight limit of the infant scale, the weight can be measured on the regular balance beam scale used for older children and adults. Follow Procedure 13-4, Weigh a Patient on a Balance Beam Scale, to measure the weight of these patients. Often the physician will ask for the weight to be taken with the child unclothed except for the underwear. This is a good time for you to make the poncho out of a drape sheet, as mentioned earlier, for while they are waiting for the physician. Remember that children have feelings and may be embarrassed without their clothes.

HEAD CIRCUMFERENCE

At the bottom of the growth graph for infants is a section to record the head **circumference** measurement. This is important for alerting the physician of abnormal development. This should be performed and recorded routinely at each office visit until the child is

---

PROCEDURE PROCEDURE PROCEDURE PROCEDURE PROCEDURE PROCEDURE PROCEDURE PROCEDURE

14-21   Weigh an Infant

PURPOSE: To obtain an accurate weight measurement of an infant.

EQUIPMENT: Infant balance scales, towel, dry diaper, patient's chart, growth graph, parent's record booklet, and pen.

PERFORMANCE OBJECTIVE: Provided with a clinical or toy doll (or an infant or small child under the close supervision of the parent, guardian, or instructor) and infant scales, demonstrate each step in the procedure to weigh infant or very small child. The weight must be within ¼ pound of the weight determined by the instructor.
1. Wash hands.
2. Ask the parent to remove the infant's clothing. **RATIONALE: This alleviates the infant's apprehension and conserves your time.**
3. Place a clean towel on the scale cradle to avoid disease transmission and to decrease shock from the cold metal for the infant. This will decrease the chance that the infant will move because of being uncomfortable or afraid.
4. Balance the scale at zero with the towel and dry draper in place.
5. Place the infant on the scale, holding one hand over the infant (almost touching) to give a sense of security.

Keep the dry diaper over the infant's genital area in case of an elimination. Talking in a quiet tone will also help keep infant still until the reading has been taken. **NOTE: The age of the baby may determine how the child is placed on the scales. Small infants will be easier to weigh lying down; those who can sit up on their own will most likely be more cooperative sitting on the scales (see Figures 14-66 and 14-67). In either case, the safety of the baby is primary.**
6. Slide the weight until the scale balances to determine the weight of the infant. Read the scale in pounds and ounces or kilograms and tell the parent the result.
7. Return the infant and diaper to the parent to dress.
8. Remove the towel from the scale, place it in proper receptacle, and balance the scale at the zero mark.
9. Record the weight on the growth chart, the patient's chart, and the parent's booklet. **NOTE: If the infant is restless when the weight is attempted, a notation should be made on the chart that the weight is approximate. Other attempts can be made at the same visit. If weight is needed to determine nutritional needs or medication dosage, you may have to weigh the parent holding the infant, then weigh the parent, and subtract to get the approximate weight of the child.**

36 months of age. A flexible measuring tape is required. It is often necessary to ask for assistance in keeping the child from pulling on the tape while you are measuring the head. Place the tape under the head if lying down, about an inch above the ears, and around to the forehead to get an accurate measurement. Refer to Figure 14-68 to see the correct placement of the measuring tape. Procedure 14-22 will help you to perform this measurement.

CHEST CIRCUMFERENCE

The chest circumference is measured by placing the flexible measuring tape around the child's chest just above the nipples (Figure 14-69). Often, it is difficult to keep the baby from moving. As said before, you should ask for assistance from the caregiver or another medical assistant. Place the measuring tape under the child and bring it around the baby's back to the chest to meet the zero mark. This measurement is not required on the growth graph but should be recorded on the chart. Refer to Procedure 14-23 for measuring an infant's chest circumference.

RECORDING MEASUREMENTS

After the measurements of height, weight, and head circumference have been obtained, they are plotted on the graph where the age and the measurement intersect. Refer to Figure 14-70. In this photo, the medical assistant is plotting the weight measurement on the

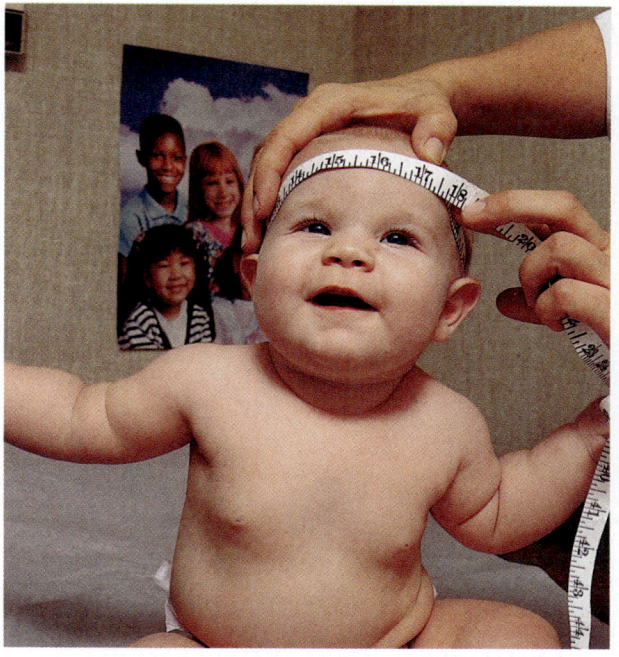

FIGURE 14-68   Measuring the head circumference of an infant

birth to 36 months graph. To record the height measurement, simply follow the age line (vertically) to the child's length measurement (horizontally) on the left, follow the horizontal line to the point at which the two intersect, and place a dot there with your pen. For recording the weight of the infant or child, stay on the vertical (age) line, and look to the right side of the

---

PROCEDURE PROCEDURE PROCEDURE PROCEDURE PROCEDURE PROCEDURE PROCEDURE PROCEDURE

14-22  Measure Head Circumference

PURPOSE: To obtain an accurate measurement of infants' and small children's head circumference in screening for head growth abnormalities.

EQUIPMENT: Flexible tape measure without elasticity, growth graph, patient's chart, and pen.

PERFORMANCE OBJECTIVE: Provided with a clinical or toy doll and a flexible tape measure, demonstrate each step in the procedure to measure the head circumference of an infant or small child. The circumference measurement must be within 1/4 inch (0.6 cm) of the doll's actual head circumference as determined by the instructor.

1. Wash hands.

2. Talk to the infant to gain cooperation. The infant may be held by a parent or may lie on the examination

table for the procedure. Older children of 2 or 3 years may stand or sit if they will remain still.

3. Use one thumb or finger to hold the tape measure with the zero mark against the infant's forehead (above the eyebrows). With your other hand, bring the tape around the infant's head just above his ears to meet in front. **NOTE: Pull the tape snugly to compress any hair (Figure 14-68).**

4. Read to the nearest 0.1 cm or 1/8 inch.

5. Record the measurement on the growth chart, parent's record booklet, and patient record.

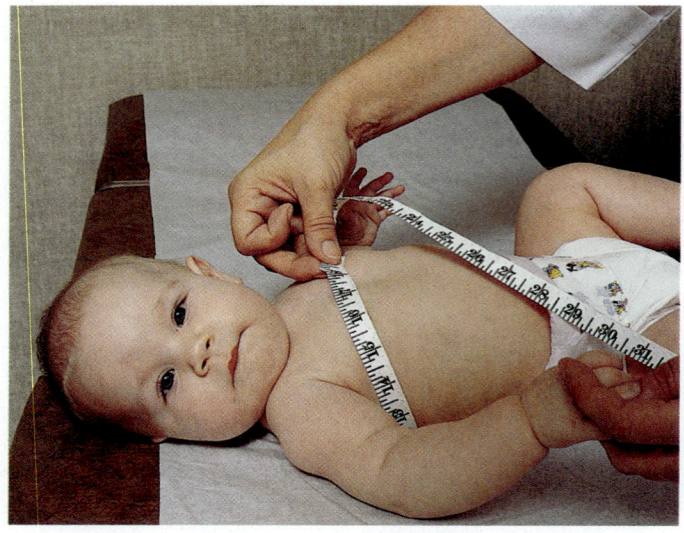

FIGURE 14-69 Measuring the chest circumference of an infant

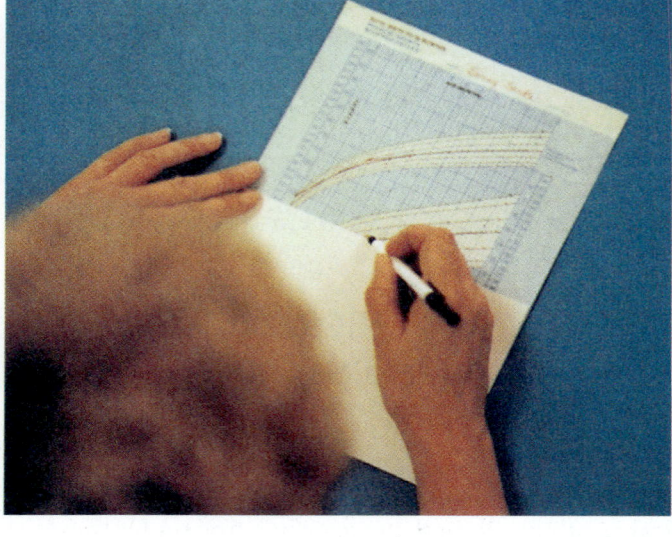

FIGURE 14-70 Plots weight measurements on a growth graph.

graph if over 16 pounds or on the left if under. Following the horizontal line from right to left, place a dot at the intersection of the weight and age lines.

The recumbent length of the child is recorded in inches or centimeters and the weight in either pounds or kilograms. Be consistent when measuring the child to avoid confusion.

VISION SCREENING

Vision and hearing screenings are identified on the Preventive Pediatric Health Care schedule as recommended by the American Academy of Pediatrics. You will notice that for the first 36 months vision screening is considered to be subjective or evaluated by his-

---

PROCEDURE PROCEDURE PROCEDURE PROCEDURE PROCEDURE PROCEDURE PROCEDURE PROCEDURE

14-23  Measure an Infant's Chest Circumference

PURPOSE: To obtain an accurate measurement of an infant's or small child's chest in screening for growth abnormalities.

EQUIPMENT: Flexible tape measure without elasticity, patient's chart, and pen

PERFORMANCE OBJECTIVE: Provided with a clinical or toy doll and a flexible tape measure, demonstrate each step in the procedure to obtain the chest measurement of an infant or small child. The chest measurement must be within ¼ inch (0.6 cm) of the doll's chest measurement as determined by the instructor.

1. Wash hands.

2. Talk to the infant or child to gain cooperation. The infant or child may lie down on the examination table or be held by a parent or guardian for the procedure. Children of 2 or 3 years and older may sit or stand on their own if they will cooperate and remain still for the procedure. **NOTE: Accurate measurement cannot be achieved if the child is crying.**

3. Take the measurement of the chest just above the nipples with the tape fitting around the child's chest under the axillary region.

4. Use one thumb to hold the tape measure with the zero mark against the infant's chest at the midsternal area. With the other hand, bring the tape around (under) the back to meet the zero mark of the tape in front. If you need assistance in holding the child still, ask the parent or another assistant. **NOTE: The measurement should be taken when the child is breathing normally, not with forced inspiration or expiration (see Figure 14-69). RATIONALE: Measurement would be inaccurate.**

5. Read the measurement to the nearest 0.2 cm or ⅛ inch.

6. Record on the patient's chart and in the parent's record booklet. **NOTE: This procedure can be used for obtaining the chest measurement of patients of all ages.**

tory. At age 3, the child is old enough to identify items on a vision screening chart and can be more easily evaluated.

Unless the vision is considerably impaired, deficiencies may not be too obvious. Usually the parent or caregiver will indicate that the child holds books too close to the face or that the child rubs the eyes frequently. Other observations may include excessive blinking, looking cross-eyed, or turning and tilting the head forward to see better. The subspecialty area of Pediatric Ophthalmology is able to evaluate the vision of very small children and should be consulted if indicated. However, the routine screening can be done in general at pediatric offices using the modified Snellen charts.

The Snellen big "E" chart (Figure 14-71A) requires that the child indicate with his fingers which way the E is facing. The Es become smaller and less bold as the acuity gets more difficult. Results are recorded on the last line correctly identified, the same as with adults on the regular screening chart. The kindergarten version of the chart (Figure 14-71B) uses various shapes and symbols in descending size to evaluate vision. When using either of these, review the charts up close with the child to be sure they know what they are supposed to do and that they can name the symbols. This will determine whether the child is actually having trouble seeing the chart or simply does not know what to call the letter or symbol you are pointing to. You can make the screening fun by taking your turn first. This also helps the child to understand what she is to do. Remember to praise the child as she proceeds through the screening to encourage cooperation. Most preschoolers have a short attention span, so you may need some assistance. The parent or caregiver can help by restating

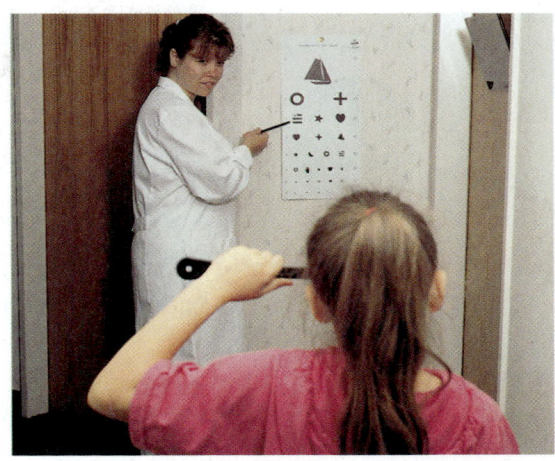

FIGURE 14-71B   The kindergarten vision screening chart with shapes and symbols in descending sizes

your instructions and maintaining the child's position. They can also monitor the covering of one eye as you proceed through the test. Watch the child for signs of visual difficulty such as tilting the head and frowning or straining to see as she reads the chart. Procedure 14-24 provides instruction to screen a child's vision.

HEARING SCREENING

Hearing in infants and small children is usually observed by their reaction to surrounding sounds. Infants will respond by turning their head toward the ticking of a watch held near their ear. Older infants respond to verbal and environmental sounds. The parents or caregiver will probably be the first ones to notice a hearing deficit. The child will not respond to voice cues and will not react to surrounding noise below a certain intensity. Again a pediatric specialist has the instruments and skills to evaluate hearing. As the child matures, an audiometer test can be given to more accurately screen hearing levels.

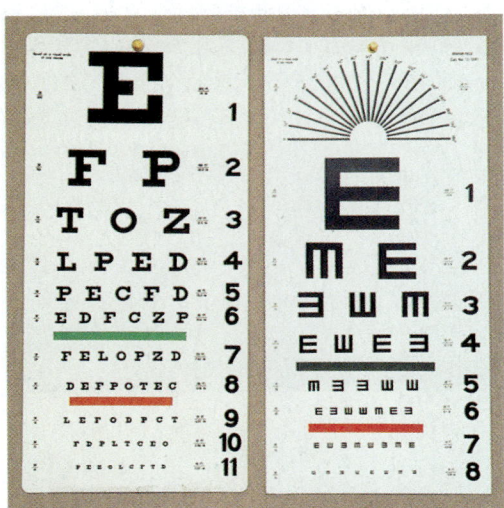

FIGURE 14-71A   Snellen visual acuity screening chart. The letter E chart on the right shows the letter in different directions and in descending sizes.

ACHIEVE UNIT OBJECTIVES

- Complete the Workbook activities to meet the learning objectives.
- Practice the procedures in this unit to meet the performance objectives.
- Apply your knowledge at the end of this chapter in completing the Critical Thinking Challenge and Activities, as well as the StudyWARE on your Student CD-ROM.

PROCEDURE PROCEDURE PROCEDURE PROCEDURE PROCEDURE PROCEDURE PROCEDURE PROCEDURE

14-24  Screen Pediatric Visual Acuity with a Modified Snellen Chart

PURPOSE: To measure distant visual acuity of a child

EQUIPMENT: Modified Snellen chart, pointer, eye occluder, patient's chart, and pen.

PERFORMANCE OBJECTIVE: Given access to all equipment and a child as a patient, measure and record visual acuity following the steps in the procedure.

1. Identify the patient. **RATIONALE: Calling the patient by name and checking the chart ensures that you are performing the procedure on the correct patient.**

2. Explain the procedure to the patient. Ensure the child understands what he is to do.

3. Ask the patient to read the chart with both eyes at a distance of 20 feet from the chart.

4. Have the patient cover his left eye (OS) with the occluder to test the acuity of the right eye.

5. Record the smallest line the patient read without making a mistake. **NOTE: Some physicians allow up to two errors on the smallest line read.**

6. Have the patient cover the right eye (OD) with the occluder to test the acuity of the left eye.

7. Record the smallest line read.

CHARTING EXAMPLE

4/17/XX

Vision screening with kindergarten screening chart per Dr. White, findings OD 20/35, OS 20/40; appeared to understand chart. Noticed some squinting during screening.

B. James, CMA

CRITICAL THINKING CHALLENGE

IMPACTING THE PATIENT, THE PRACTICE, AND YOUR CAREER

Ellen, the medical assistant, had just finished the in-person screening and examination preparation procedures on Dora, a middle-aged, poorly groomed female. She had instructed her to remove her clothing and put on the gown. She had also told her to open the examination room door slightly when she was ready. Ellen was having a hard time being enclosed in the room because Dora had pretty strong body odor due to her lack of personal hygiene. She had gone to look for the doctor and finally noticed him reviewing Dora's chart before entering the room. She told the doctor that Dora smelled pretty bad and doing a pelvic exam on her was not going to be pleasant. When they went to enter the room, Ellen noticed the door was already open, and she was sure Dora had heard her unkind remarks.

QUESTIONS

1. How might her remarks affect the patient?
2. How do her remarks reflect on the practice?
3. Could her remarks affect her career? (Could anything positive result from the remark?)

ACTIVITIES

1. Go to the American Cancer Society's web site at www.cancer.org and review the "Cancer Prevention and Early Detection Worksheets." You will need to go through a couple steps to get there. First select "Health Information Seekers," then click on "Men's and Women's Health." Then select the appropriate worksheet male or female.

2. Role play preparing a person for a CPE. Have a classmate act as if she were hearing impaired. See if you can explain what you want done without using language.

3. Practice identifying all the different examination instruments. Work with a classmate to set out instruments to be named. You might choose to make up trays for different types of examination procedures.

StudyWARE™ CHALLENGE

- Study with the flash cards for Chapter 14 to review the key terms in this chapter.
- Solve the crossword puzzle for Chapter 14.
- Complete the multiple choice quiz in test mode for Chapter 14.

RESOURCES

A guide for eye inspection and testing visual acuity. (1991). National Society for the Prevention of Blindness, Inc.

Bates, B. (1974). *A guide to physical examination.* Philadelphia: Lippincott.

Corning Metpath Laboratories. (1996). Patient education [Pamphlet]. Columbus, OH: Author.

Diagnostic tests, nurse's ready reference. (1991). Springhouse, PA: Springhouse Corporation.

Shapiro, P. (1995). *Basic maternal/pediatric nursing.* Clifton Park, NY: Thomson Delmar Learning.

WEB LINKS

www.aap.org (American Academy of Pediatrics)
Provides information on a wide range of subjects concerning child health and welfare.

www.cancer.org (American Cancer Society)
Provides information on cancer and breast and testicular self-exams.

www.cdc.gov/nip (Centers for Disease Control and Prevention)
Provides information about immunization schedules for American children and adolescents.

www.hearinglossweb.com (Hearing Loss Web)
Provides information for people who are hearing impaired, hard of hearing, late deafened, and oral deaf, including events, issues, support, and technology related to hearing loss.

The safety of all patients and health care providers is foremost regarding the collection of specimens. As you learned in Chapter 12, prevention of disease is of vital importance in preparation for these clinical tasks. You must be alert and conscientious in the performance of your duties to avoid disease transmission. Remember to practice Standard Precautions with each patient when you collect or handle a specimen.

In addition to following safety precautions, you should check with your family physician and find out if you need any updating on your own immunizations. Staying current with immunizations is essential. Also, for those who have respiratory conditions, having protection against pneumonia and influenza is generally recommended. Of course, you should have been administered the series of three HBV (hepatitis B virus) injections if you are going to be working directly with patients and there is a potential risk of your coming into contact with blood or other body fluids. The permanent record of this vaccine should be kept in your employee file. If you have not received the HBV, you are hired in to a new position in which you supposedly will not be in contact with patients, and your new employer states that it is not necessary for you to have the vaccine, the employer must sign a **waiver** regarding this. This signed document should also be kept in your employee file. There are individuals who are allergic to the contents of the culture media of certain vaccines. If you are allergic, this should be documented also in your employee file. Refer to Figure 15-1 for an example statement to decline the administration of the HBV immunization. When working with patients in the medical field, it makes good sense to be protected from every possible disease, because no one knows what will be encountered next with patients.

Further guidelines should be noted regarding safe and efficient practice of procedures in the physician's office laboratory (POL) and in dealing with patients. Pay attention to proper fit when wearing protective barriers. If a gown is too large or too small, the purpose of the gown will be defeated. Latex or vinyl gloves should also fit snugly but not too tight or too loose. These simple problems may seem to be trivial points but could pose a problem situation and a safety risk. Gloves that are too small will most likely tear. Loose clothing or gloves could catch on something and be ripped or snagged, which could present a possible exposure to potentially infectious materials.

When working with specimens and recording information, you must be careful not to touch items that you would normally touch without gloves, such as light switches, door and drawer handles and pulls, phones, charts, and equipment. Develop the habit of completing one task at a time when possible. Complete the procedure that requires gloving and other personal protective equipment (PPE), and then record the results after you have removed the protective barriers. For example, if you are assisting with a sigmoidoscopy wearing PPE, you should complete the assisting, clean up, remove the contaminated barriers, and then perform the charting of the procedure. If you write in the patient's chart with the contaminated gloves still on, you will be contaminating everything you touch and possibly exposing others to biohazardous residue.

Professionalism was discussed in the beginning of the text in Chapter 2. A reminder about jewelry and hair styles must be discussed here for safety reasons. Excessive jewelry is not only inappropriate, but it could also present a dangerous situation; for example, it could get caught on a piece of equipment or harbor pathogens in the crevices of the metal. When you are dealing with babies for their check-ups and often when

---

Statement of Refusal

I have been given complete information (oral and written) regarding the HBV immunization and the opportunity to receive it at no charge to me. At this time, I have decided not to have it administered. I understand the risk I am taking with possible exposure to hepatitis B, and I realize the seriousness of the disease. I may, at a later date, receive the HBV immunization if I so choose.

_____   _____
Signature of employee   Date

FIGURE 15-1   An example of the form that must be signed by employees who decline the HBV immunization. A copy must be filed in their employee record. The employee must have been given complete information both verbally and in printed form regarding the vaccine and may choose to receive it at a later date.

they are ill, they may be tempted to pull at dangling earrings, necklaces, and bracelets. This is a danger for many reasons: the jewelry could break, which could result in an injury to both you and the child, the pathogens that are on the jewelry could be transmitted to you or the child, or you could transmit the microorganisms from one patient to another. Remember that you cannot see microorganisms without a microscope, but they are everywhere. Another safety consideration is how you wear your hair. Both male and female health care providers who have long hair must keep their hair worn back and secured since there is a chance that a patient could grab onto your hair. Hair jewelry and ribbons should be conservative and, if worn, cleaned periodically to reduce the possibility of disease transmission. These seem to be remote possibilities but could actually happen, and it only takes one exposure to transmit diseases that are opportunistic. Remember: The health statuses of the patients are unknown in most cases. A patient may be susceptible and become infected with a microbe from the medical facility during a routine office call.

The laboratory director in the POL is responsible for the management of the laboratory and for making sure that quality control and quality assurance are provided. The cooperation of the entire staff is necessary for this to be accomplished. **Quality control** is defined as a process that validates final test results and determines any variations. Every laboratory, including the physician office laboratory, is required by law to have in place a carefully performed, documented, and on-going quality control program. This program ensures both the physician and patient that test results are accurate and is designed to discover and eliminate error.

The quality control program is designed to monitor all aspects of laboratory activity, including specimen collection and processing and the actual testing and reporting of results. It not only monitors the test procedure itself, but it also monitors reagents used in testing, the instruments, and personnel technique in performing tests.

Thorough and accurate records must be maintained on all equipment used to test patient samples. Temperatures must be checked daily and recorded in a log book on any refrigerators or freezers used to store reagents and patient samples and incubators used for cultures. Automated equipment must be maintained according to the manufacturer's recommendations.

Each test kit used comes with a "control," which is a sample with a known value range to be tested along with the patient specimen. The value range of the control can be a range of numbers or simply a positive or negative result. Controls are tested at specific intervals, usually according to manufacturer's directions. For example, a positive and negative control must be performed with each patient sample when using test kits, such as rapid strep and pregnancy tests. Urine reagent strips should be checked daily and each time a new bottle is opened. Manufacturer's directions should be followed when performing control samples on all automated analyzers.

Carefully maintained records showing consistent and accurate control sample results ensure that test conditions, procedures, and results are accurate.

The credibility of each individual is challenged in compliance of standards and guidelines set by regulatory bodies. In most situations, you are the only one who will know if you did or did not follow Standard Precautions and quality assurance recommendations. You must keep your mind on your work and pay attention to detail to protect yourself and others from possible contamination, and you must focus on accuracy and efficiency of the procedures and charting of information. Expedient and efficient work practices do not mean that you should hurry and make patients feel the brunt of it. Using a methodical and steady pace will help you in accomplishing a great deal of work in a reasonable amount of time. Further guidelines are listed in addition to those in Chapter 12, which all health care providers should follow to ensure that quality and safety in the lab are upheld.

Guidelines for a well-managed and efficient POL include:

1. Follow current state and federal regulations, and keep them on file.
2. Retain files of correspondences and all other documents regarding the lab up to date and accessible.
3. Maintain all material safety data sheets (MSDS) regarding all chemicals, reagents, and solutions (such as isopropyl alcohol, disinfectants, and even correction fluid) in a notebook that is readily accessible to all employees.
4. Have a "biohazard communications" manual that includes:
   - A "chemical hygiene plan" (the employer's plan) to prevent employees from being exposed to dangerous chemicals
   - A "biohazard safety" section that includes universal precaution techniques that conform to OSHA and CLIA regulations
5. Retain copies of all biohazard box or bag pick ups per state regulation.
6. Keep a log of all accidents and what was done for the person (i.e., who used the eye wash station and for what reason). The designated person will enter this data on the OSHA log.
7. Place all sharps, including intact needles and syringes (do not recap), into biohazard sharps container.
8. Keep long hair tied back securely and wear only a minimum amount of jewelry.
9. Keep a 10% bleach solution (made fresh daily) ready for cleanup of infectious wastes.
10. Record all lab work performed in a log with the date, time, name of test, who performed it, the results, and when it was sent to the reference lab and when the results were received.
11. Clearly post Standard Precautions for employees as a safety reminder.
12. Provide adequate lighting in all work areas.
13. Have a properly maintained fire extinguisher readily available and the directions for use clearly posted with it.
14. Keep hallways and walking paths free of clutter.
15. Have fire/evacuation routes clearly posted.

UNIT 1
THE MICROSCOPE

OBJECTIVES

Upon completion of this unit, you will be able to achieve the following:

LEARNING Objectives

1. **Spell and define, using the glossary at the back of the text, all the Words to Know in this unit.**
2. **Identify the parts of the microscope and the purpose of each.**
3. **Describe the proper way to adjust and focus the objectives and state their magnification powers.**

4. Explain how to properly maintain the microscope.

5. Explain the general purpose of the microscope in a medical office.

PERFORMANCE Objective

1. Properly use a microscope.

WORDS TO KNOW

binocular	magnify	quality control
compensate	minute	specimen
condenser	monocular	technical
high-power field (hpf)	objectives	waiver
low-power field (lpf)	proficient	

CERTIFICATION CONNECTION

CMA

Treatment area—principles of operation—microscope

Treatment area—preparing/ maintaining treatment area

Treatment area—safety precautions

RMA

Clinical medical assisting— instruments

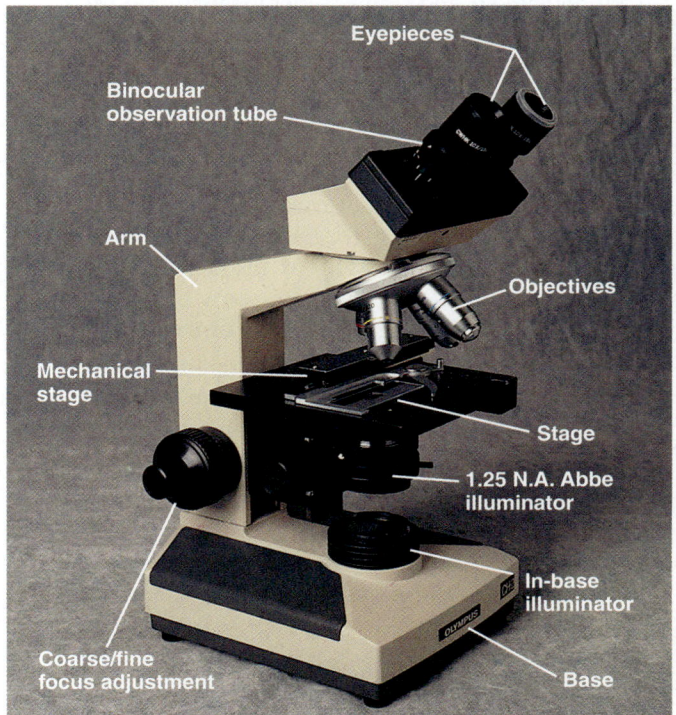

FIGURE 15-2 The parts of the microscope

PATIENT EDUCATION

Many patients may be frightened or confused about some of the laboratory procedures requested by the health care provider to aid in diagnosis. You may perform some of these in the office or clinic setting or send the patient to the lab for tests. If you send patients elsewhere, make sure you give accurate directions on how to get there.

Each test or procedure must be explained clearly and concisely to relieve patients' anxiety. Use language that patients will understand. Most people have little or no knowledge of medical terminology.

Certain lab tests require preparation by patients prior to arrival (e.g., fasting, taking or omitting certain medications). Be sure to instruct patients in these preparations and have clear, concise, written instructions available. Do not presume that patients know all about a procedure even if they have had the test before. Often, new techniques require additional or different instructions for preparation. Medical technology is constantly changing. It is important for health care providers (including medical assistants) to keep abreast of new developments in medicine. Inform patients that some procedures can cause temporary discomfort and how it may be relieved.

Give patients enough time to look over the printed instruction sheet or pamphlet, and make certain you answer all of their questions thoroughly before they leave.

The microscope is an essential piece of equipment in the laboratory. It is used to examine and identify **minute** objects that cannot be seen with the naked eye. Microscopes are fine and expensive **technical** instruments that must be handled with great respect. The operation and care manual should be kept handy for reference, because each microscope is slightly different. The amount of routine maintenance required will vary with the amount of use. Each POL must keep a maintenance log of all equipment. Routine inspection and maintenance should be recorded in this maintenance log with information regarding what was done, the date, and the agency that did the required labor to fix it. All maintenance forms or documents should be kept on file.

The part of the microscope that supports the eyepiece is called the arm. Figure 15-2 shows the labeled parts of a **binocular** microscope. The proper way to carry the microscope is to grasp the arm with one hand and place the other hand under the base, holding it at waist level. To secure a microscope while transporting it, the electrical cord for the light source should be loosely wrapped and secured with a twist tie or a rubber band. Wrapping the cord too tightly may cause the enclosed wires to break and lead to a short that could cause an electrical fire. The cord of the microscope should be kept loosely wrapped and out of the work area when not in use. It should always be unplugged by grasping the plug, never by pulling the cord. As when using any electrical appliance, all surrounding surfaces and hands should be dry. Wet hands or floors can lead to electric shock.

PARTS OF THE MICROSCOPE

A binocular microscope has two eyepieces. The **monocular** microscope has only one eyepiece or ocular lens. The eyepiece or ocular lens is in the upper part of the

---

PROCEDURE PROCEDURE PROCEDURE PROCEDURE PROCEDURE PROCEDURE PROCEDURE

15-1   Use a Microscope

PURPOSE: To gain skill in the use of the microscope.

OSHA GUIDELINES: To comply with Standard Precautions, gloves must be worn if there is any possibility of coming into contact with blood or any body fluids.

EQUIPMENT: Microscope, electrical outlet for light source of microscope, specimen on disposable glass slide with frosted end, cover glass (used usually for wet specimens only), lens cleaning tissues, latex or vinyl gloves.

PERFORMANCE OBJECTIVE: Provided with all necessary equipment and supplies, demonstrate the use of the microscope following the steps in the procedure with the instructor observing each step.

1. Wash hands and put on latex or vinyl gloves.

2. Assemble the necessary equipment.

3. Clean the ocular lens with lens cleaning tissues. **RATIONALE: Removal of makeup, oil, and eye secretions is necessary to ensure clear viewing and eliminate transmission of disease among office personnel. NOTE: Use only lens tissue paper to prevent damaging the surface of the lens.**

4. Plug the microscope light source into an electrical outlet, and turn on the light switch at the front base of the microscope.

5. Place the specimen slide on the stage with the frosted end up between the clips, and secure it over the opening of the stage. **NOTE: The frosted end is used for labeling the specimen in pencil.**

6. Watch carefully as you raise the substage so that it does not come into direct contact with the slide.

7. Turn the revolving nosepiece to low-power objective (10×) and begin to focus the coarse-adjustment dial until a wide shaft can be seen. **NOTE: Regarding microscope lighting—When you switch from a lower to a higher power objective (or vice-versa), the light will need to be turned up. The light source should be kept at a fairly low level for each objective to improve the clarity of the objects being viewed. Too much light may have a bleaching or glaring effect, and the object may not be seen at all or at least may not be seen well.**

8. When the outline of the specimen is in view, turn the fine-adjustment dial until the specimen can be seen in detail.

9. Adjust the substage diaphragm level or adjust the mirror to obtain proper lighting.

10. If sharper detail is needed, carefully turn the revolving nosepiece to the intermediate-power objective, and adjust fine-focus dial.

11. When using the oil-immersion lens objective or hpf, oil should be used very sparingly. **NOTE: A disposable cover slide should be used, and the lens must be cleaned after each use. Adjustment must be made for the amount of light needed by adjusting the diaphragm lever under the stage.**

12. When the specimen has been identified, turn off the light and return all items to the proper storage area. **NOTE: The microscope stage should be cleaned and recorded in the maintenance log.**

13. Remove gloves and wash hands. **NOTE: Results of the actual examination should be read and recorded in the laboratory test log by the physician. The medical assistant is responsible for assisting with the preparation of the specimen for microscopic examination unless otherwise instructed by the physician.**

tube of the microscope. The eyepiece contains a lens to **magnify** what is being seen.

The body tube leads to the revolving nosepiece. Attached to the revolving nosepiece are three (sometimes four) small lenses called **objectives**, each of which has a different magnifying power. The shortest has the lowest power. It is called the **low-power field (lpf)**. On most microscopes, it will magnify the object to be viewed 10 times, or make it 10× larger than when viewed by the naked eye. The low-power field is the lens used to scan the field of interest and to focus in on the specimen. To position each objective, you simply rotate the nosepiece until you hear a click.

For greater detail in viewing the specimen, turn the nosepiece to the next longer objective, the **high-power field (hpf)**. It will magnify the object approximately 40 times, or 40×. The longest objective is the oil-immersion objective. This high-power lens, when used with oil, magnifies objects about 100 times, or 100×. Using the fine-focus dial will bring the specimen into good definition.

The stage of the microscope has two clips that hold the **specimen** slide to be viewed. Just underneath the stage is a substage where a **condenser** is held that regulates the amount of light directed on the magnified specimen. It has a shutter or diaphragm to control the amount of light desired. The substage may be raised or lowered in focusing on the specimen.

A supply of lens paper should be kept nearby to clean the lenses after each use. Makeup, oil, secretions from the eyes, and dust can make it difficult to see through the lens, besides being a possible means of transmitting disease among office personnel. Because there may be several individuals in a medical office who use the microscope, it is advised to wipe the eyepieces with a disinfectant after each use to avoid the transmission of diseases. Eyeglasses are not necessary when performing microscopic work because the microscope may be focused to **compensate** for all visual defects except astigmatism.

It will take time and patience to learn how to operate the microscope. The supervision of an experienced operator is essential to becoming **proficient** in its use and care. (Refer to Procedure 15-1).

ACHIEVE UNIT OBJECTIVES

- ■ **Complete the Workbook activities to meet the learning objectives.**
- ■ **Practice the procedure in this unit to meet the performance objectives.**
- ■ **Apply your knowledge at the end of this Chapter in completing the Critical Thinking Challenge and Activities, as well as the StudyWARE on your Student CD-ROM.**

UNIT 2
CAPILLARY BLOOD COLLECTION

OBJECTIVES

Upon completion of this unit, you will be able to achieve the following:

LEARNING Objectives

1. **Spell and define, using the glossary at the back of the text, all the Words to Know in this unit.**
2. **State the purpose of wearing gloves when performing capillary blood collection procedures.**
3. **Explain the reasons for performing capillary blood collection in the medical office.**

PERFORMANCE Objective

1. **Perform capillary blood collection procedures for obtaining specimens.**

WORDS TO KNOW

diffuse	reagent
lancet	sterile
puncture	

 CERTIFICATION CONNECTION

CMA
Collecting and processing
   specimens and
   diagnostic testing
Methods of collection
Blood—capillary

RMA
Laboratory procedures

SKIN PUNCTURE

Capillary blood tests are frequently performed in the medical office or clinic because of the small amount of blood required, usually one to a few drops. Because most patients are extremely apprehensive, you must develop skill not only in performing the procedures but in conveying reassurance to the patient. When skin **puncture** procedures, commonly referred to as "finger sticks," are done correctly, the patient should feel minimal discomfort. Displaying confidence in carrying out the procedures competently will ensure patient safety and comfort.

Capillaries are minute blood vessels that convey blood from the arterioles to the venules. At this level, blood and oxygen **diffuse** to the tissues, and products of metabolic activity enter the bloodstream. For this reason, capillary blood is an ideal sample for many screening tests that require a very small amount of blood. (Refer to Procedure 15-2.)

Capillary blood is just under the surface of the skin. The most practical sites to use are the ring and great finger, rarely the earlobe, and in infants the lateral sides of the heel (Figure 15-3). Skin punctures should be made across fingerprints, not parallel to them (Figure 15-4).

The sterile lancet is widely used for simple blood tests that require capillary blood. You may be given the duty of instructing patients in use of one of the skin puncturing devices shown in Figure 15-5. Patients who use this technique daily should simply wash the puncture site thoroughly with soap and water. Alcohol tends to break down the skin if used for extended periods. Patients should be provided with a sharps container to keep at home to dispose of the lancets after use. Encourage them to dispose of the three-fourths full container appropriately.

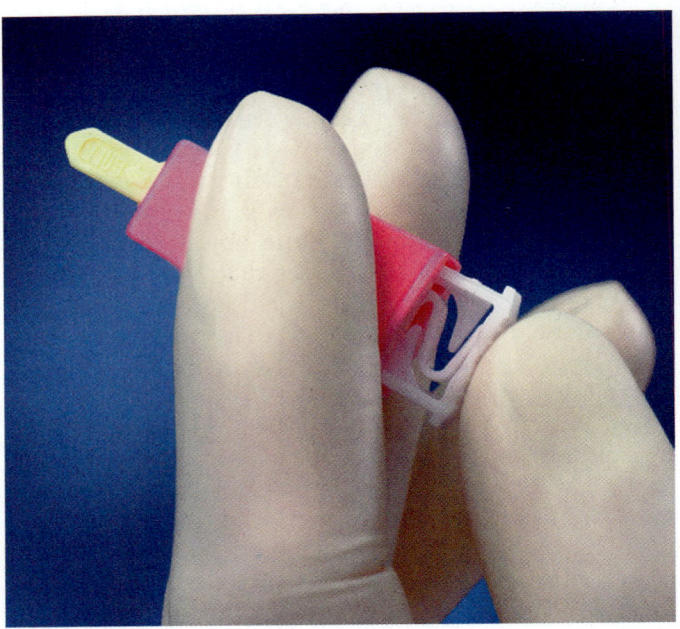

FIGURE 15-5 BD Microtainer™ brand lancets are available in different types for various purposes. *(Courtesy BD Vacutainer Systems)*

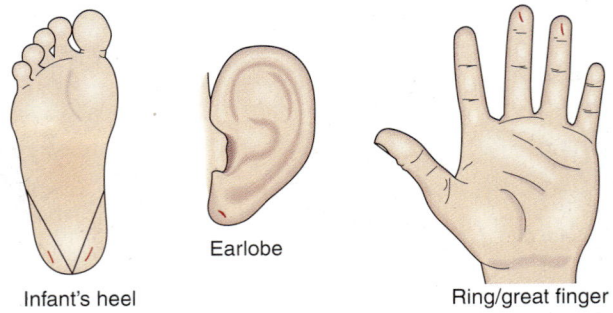

Infant's heel Earlobe Ring/great finger

FIGURE 15-3 These skin puncture sites are recommended because of abundant capillary flow for obtaining a specimen, besides being a convenient site for patients.

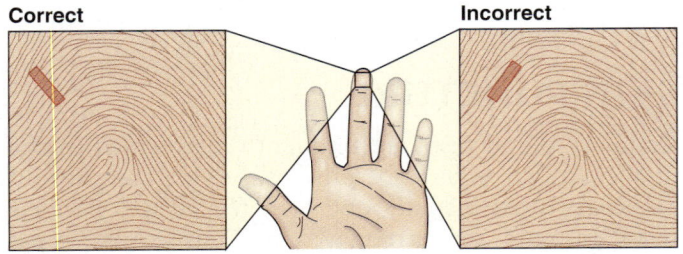

Correct Incorrect

FIGURE 15-4 Correct and incorrect capillary punctures (finger sticks). The correct puncture is made with a sterile lancet with the capillary puncture device across the fingerprints.

P PATIENT EDUCATION

Most patients, especially youngsters, are apprehensive about having blood taken. The medical assistant must calmly explain to each patient that screening tests, such as a hemoglobin or a blood glucose, are performed with a small amount of blood taken from the finger, earlobe, or infant's heel. Let the patient know ahead of time what you are going to do to gain cooperation. You should tell the patient that there will be a little pain or discomfort during the initial skin puncture, but it will not last long. Reassure the patient that this procedure is short-lived and necessary for the physician to aid in making a diagnosis or evaluating the condition.

With strict regulations regarding quality control and quality assurance, you are required to keep a log book to record all specimens and the results of the tests performed. The log should include:

1. Date
2. Patient's name
3. Test performed
4. Results of the test
5. Your initials
6. Any kit, reagent strip, or **reagent** lot numbers and expiration dates
7. Quality control results

15-2  Puncture Skin with a Sterile Lancet

PURPOSE: To obtain a few drops of capillary blood for screening tests.

OSHA GUIDELINES: To comply with Standard Precautions, gloves must be worn if there is any possibility of coming into contact with blood or any body fluids.

EQUIPMENT: Latex or vinyl gloves; sterile **lancet**; alcohol; cotton balls; sharps container; flat, stable surface.

PERFORMANCE OBJECTIVE: Provided with all necessary equipment and supplies, and using other students as patients, demonstrate the skin puncture procedure following all steps to obtain capillary blood for test(s) specified by the physician or instructor. The instructor will observe each step.

1. Identify the patient. **RATIONALE: Speaking to the patient by name and checking chart ensures that you are performing the procedure on the correct patient.**

2. Explain the procedure to the patient.

3. Inspect the patient's fingers (or other puncture site) and select the most desirable site.

   NOTE:

   - **The main sites are the ring or great finger, earlobe, or infant's lateral areas of heel.**

   - **Some patients have a preference for a particular site.**

   - **The earlobe is less sensitive to pain than fingers.**

   - **Do not use areas that are bruised, calloused, or injured.**

4. Wash hands, put on latex or vinyl gloves, and assemble the needed items on the flat surface.

5. Wipe the desired site with an alcohol-saturated cotton ball and let dry (Figure 15-6A). Do not blow the skin to expedite drying. **RATIONALE: You may contaminate the skin with microorganisms in the exhaled air.**

6. Take the **sterile** lancet out of the package without contaminating the point. **NOTE: Another must be used if the point is touched.**

7. Hold the patient's finger (or other site) securely between your thumb and great finger. In your other hand hold the lancet, pointed downward, with your thumb and index or great finger. Puncture the site quickly with a firm, steady, down-and-up motion to approximately a 2-mm depth (Figure 15-6B). **NOTE: Control entry and exit of lancet in same path to avoid ripping skin. To obtain a better blood sample, puncture across fingerprints, not parallel to them.**

8. Discard the first drop of blood by blotting it away with a dry gauze square. **RATIONALE: The first drop may contain traces of alcohol or tissue fluid that would dilute the sample and make the test inaccurate.**

FIGURE 15-6A Clean the site with alcohol and let it dry.

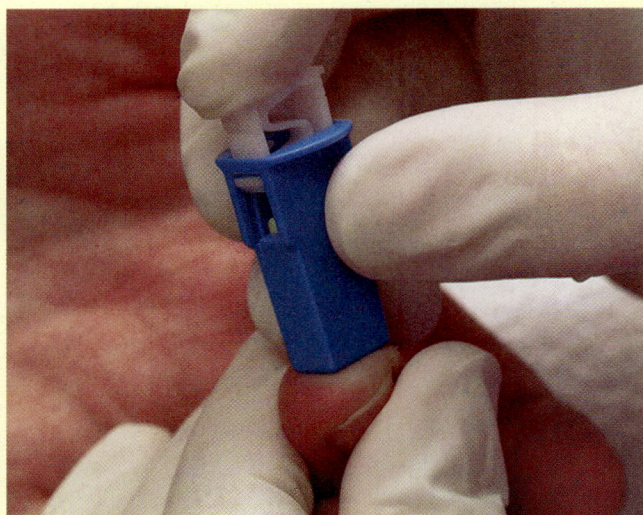

FIGURE 15-6B Position the lancet firmly against the puncture site. Hold the lancet between the fingers and place the thumb on the white activation button. Press the white button to activate the lancet. Do not pull the lancet away from the puncture site until after activation.

(continues)

15-2  Puncture Skin with a Sterile Lancet (Continued)

9. Keep applying gentle pressure on either side of the puncture site until the necessary amount of blood has been obtained. **NOTE: Too much pressure will cause tissue fluid to mix with blood resulting in a diluted sample and incorrect test results.**

10. Wipe the site with a cotton ball and ask the patient to gently hold it for a minute or two. **NOTE: Check the site to be sure the bleeding has stopped. Determine whether the patient is allergic to adhesive before applying a bandage to the puncture site (use a gauze square and hypoallergenic tape if patient is allergic).**

11. Remove gloves, wash hands, and discard used items in the proper receptacle (Figure 15-6C).

12. Record the procedure on the patient's chart. **NOTE: A solution of approximately ¼-cup bleach per gallon of tap water (a 1:100 dilution of common household bleach) should be made fresh daily and kept readily available for clean up of accidental spills of blood or body fluids.**

CHARTING EXAMPLE

8-5-XX

Rt. ring finger punctured, filled two microhematocrit tubes with capillary blood; Hct 37%; Hgb 12.4.

J. Watkins, CMA (CL)

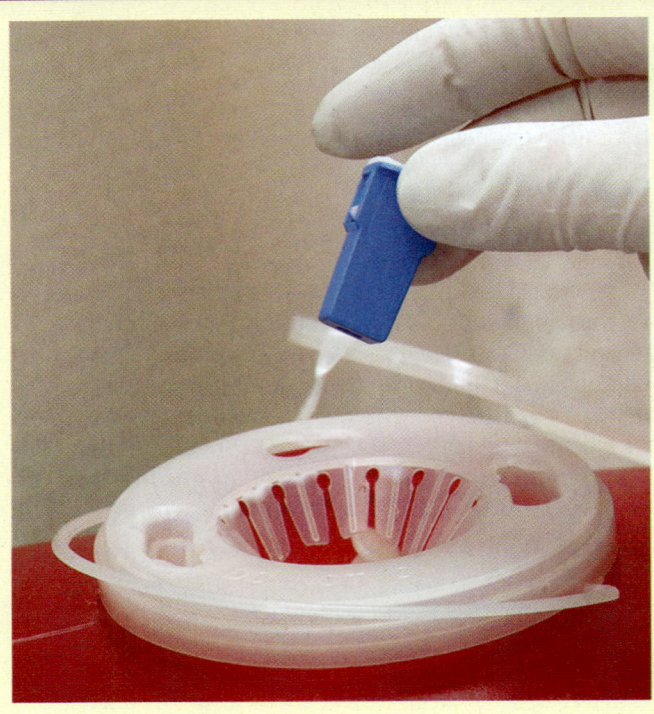

FIGURE 15-6C Dispose of the used lancet in the appropriate sharps container.

ACHIEVE UNIT OBJECTIVES

- Complete the Workbook activities to meet the learning objectives.

- Practice the procedure in this unit to meet the performance objectives.

- Apply your knowledge at the end of this chapter in completing the Critical Thinking Challenge and Activities, as well as the StudyWARE on your Student CD-ROM.

UNIT 3
VENOUS BLOOD COLLECTION

OBJECTIVES

Upon completion of this unit, you will be able to achieve the following:

LEARNING Objectives

1. Spell and define, using the glossary at the back of the text, all of the Words to Know in this unit.

2. Explain how to obtain serum from whole blood.

3. List the different colors used to code blood specimen tubes.

4. List the correct order of draw for blood specimen tubes.

5. Identify by the colors of the tubes what additives are contained in the tubes.

PERFORMANCE Objectives

1. Perform a venipuncture using a syringe and needle.

2. Perform a venipuncture using a vacuum tube and multiple sample needle and adapter.

WORDS TO KNOW

elasticity	heparin	tourniquet
gauge	meniscus	venipuncture
hematoma	oxygenate	venous
hemolysis		

 CERTIFICATION CONNECTION

CMA

Methods of collection—
    blood—vein

RMA

Laboratory procedures

Venous means pertaining to the veins. As veins return blood to the heart and lungs to be **oxygenated** and recirculated, they carry the waste products of the body. Venous blood tests permit measurement of the kind and amount of those waste products.

VENIPUNCTURE

When more than a few drops of blood are required to perform tests, a venipuncture is performed. **Venipuncture** is the surgical puncture of a vein.

Usually, the patient is seated in a chair with the arm supported for the venipuncture procedure. In the event that a patient faints from this position, first remove the **tourniquet**, withdraw the needle, and hold a bandage over the puncture site. Then the patient must be helped carefully to the floor. Spirits of ammonia (ammonia in-

halant) may be used to help revive the patient. The physician should check the patient before you proceed further. Patients who say they feel faint should put their head down between their knees. Usually this will help within a few minutes, and the procedure can be accomplished with no further interruptions. Often, following a complete physical examination, the patient may still be lying on the examination table. This makes an ideal work area for the medical assistant, and the position for the patient is most comfortable. In case the patient feels faint, there is no worry of accidental falling when the patient is lying down. The law regarding who performs venipuncture varies from state to state. Usually the health care provider is aware of it and will not ask you to perform the procedure unless it is lawful.

Applying the Tourniquet

The area of choice for venipuncture is most often the inner arm at the bend of the elbow (Figure 15-7). The veins in this area are the median basilic and the median cephalic (commonly referred to as antecubital veins). A means of promoting better palpation and sometimes visual position of the veins is a tourniquet. Tourniquets are available in many materials. Soft, flat bands are probably the most popular and economical. Some medical facilities use a tourniquet only once and then discard it with the gloves they remove after drawing blood samples. It comes in widths of 1 to 2 inches and can be cut into any length desired, usually from 12 to 16 inches. If the hair on the patient's arm is especially thick, it may be wise to apply the tourniquet over the patient's sleeve. This will keep the tourniquet from pinching and pulling the hair, and the patient will most likely be more cooperative with your thoughtfulness. Tourniquets are is easily washed with a detergent solution and quickly cleaned with alcohol and a cotton ball. Velcro tourniquets are cloth strips, approximately 1½ to 2 inches wide. They are not so easily cleaned and cannot be used on patients with larger than average

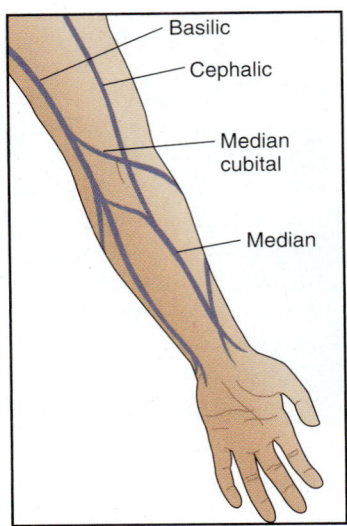

FIGURE 15-7 The veins of the arm. The median cephalic vein is the one most often used for venipuncture.

- Basilic
- Cephalic
- Median cubital
- Median

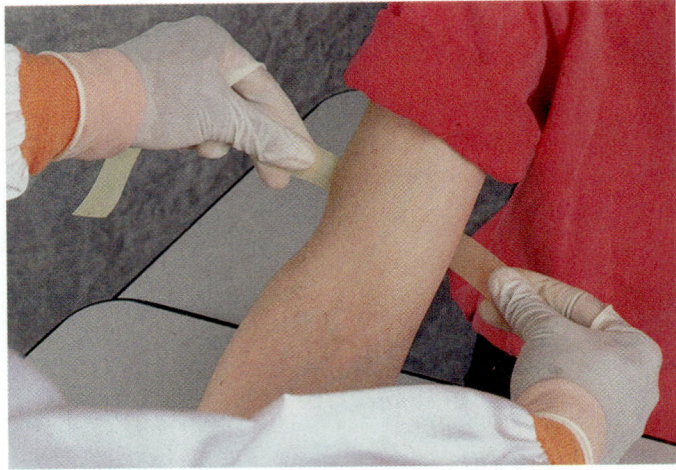

FIGURE 15-8A Wrap the tourniquet around the arm no more than 3 inches above the venipuncture site.

arms. Wiping them off with alcohol will help prevent most of the staining problems. In very difficult to draw patients, you may try using a blood pressure cuff as a tourniquet. Be careful not to inflate it too tightly on the patient's arm, or you may cut off the circulation completely and cause unnecessary discomfort to the patient. Be sure that the cuff size is appropriate for the size of the arm. Care also must be taken to avoid getting blood on the cuff. It must be discarded (or sanitized and sterilized before reuse) if it does become contaminated. Tourniquets that are very worn or permanently visibly soiled (even after washing) should be discarded.

The tourniquet is placed on the patient's upper arm, about 3 inches above the elbow (Figure 15-8A through D).

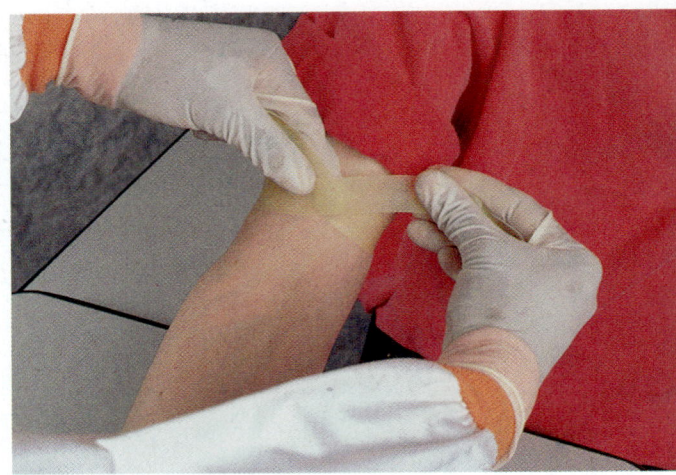

FIGURE 15-8B Stretch the tourniquet tight and cross the ends.

P PATIENT EDUCATION

Explain to the patient that there will be minimal pain or discomfort, similar to how as it feels when you stick yourself with a pin accidentally. Normally this slight pain lasts only momentarily.

Explain to the patient that relaxing will help speed up the procedure. Occasionally there will be some bruising at the venipuncture site, but this will not last long. Even if the patient has had previous venipunctures, explain the procedure and answer questions. The patient will feel more relaxed if you display confidence in your ability.

If the patient expresses concern about contracting an infection from the needle puncture, reassure the patient that the needle is sterile, is used once, and then is discarded.

If the patient has questions concerning the diagnosis, answer in general terms, unless you are instructed otherwise. The physician should answer questions about a diagnosis.

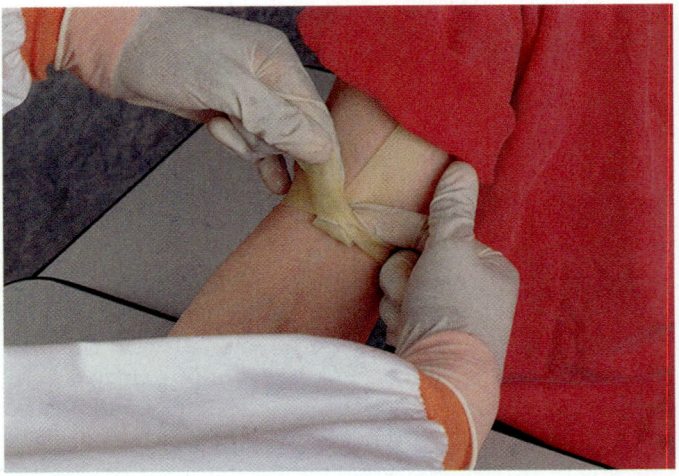

FIGURE 15-8C While holding the ends tight, tuck one portion of the tourniquet under the other.

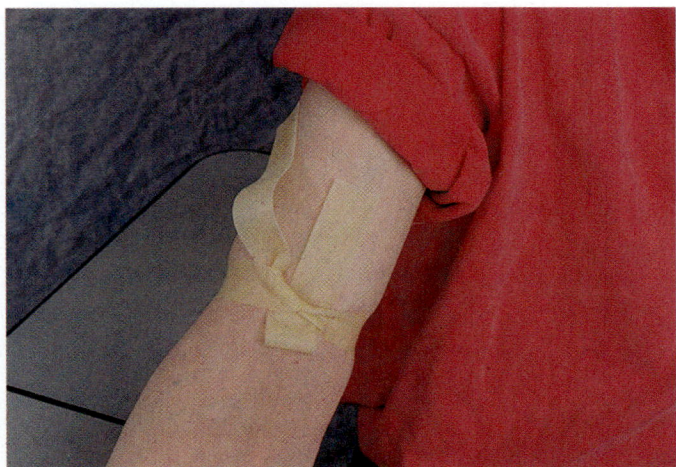

FIGURE 15-8D   Check that the tourniquet will not come loose. The ends of the tourniquet should be pointed upward and not hanging into the intended venipuncture site.

Before applying the tourniquet, it is a good idea to check both arms of the patient or simply ask which arm is better for this procedure. Many patients have had the procedure performed and know that one arm is better. Some patients will have a preferred arm because of their work or planned activities.

Butterfly Needle Method

Some patients are extremely difficult to obtain blood from, so may be necessary in these cases to draw the sample from a vein on the back of the hand using a smaller gauge needle. These veins are small, and the procedure is painful. The tourniquet should be applied just above the wrist in this case. A method that may be used in this type of situation is called the butterfly needle method (Figure 15-9). A skilled phlebotomist can

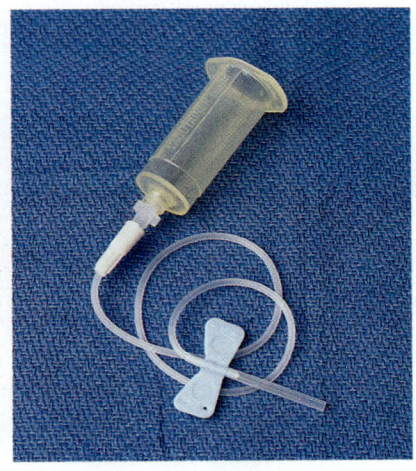

FIGURE 15-9   Butterfly needle assembly

perform this procedure successfully alone. (Refer to Procedure 15-3).

Venipuncture must always be done carefully to avoid causing a **hematoma** (collection of blood just under the skin). When the needle is inserted into the vein, it punctures the wall of the vein and blood can then leak out into surrounding tissues. This bleeding causes discoloration and sometimes swelling. If the vein has been punctured from the needle going completely through the vein (in one side and out the other) then the chances of a hematoma are even greater. Consult with the physician about applying ice, which can be helpful in reducing discomfort and swelling. Gentle pressure applied immediately on withdrawing the needle will help prevent this problem.

Use a cotton ball saturated with alcohol or an alcohol presaturated pad to swab the entire area. The alcohol will help make the skin more sensitive to your touch and disinfects the area. Slowly move your fingertip across the patient's arm at the bend of the elbow. Veins have **elasticity** and will give somewhat when depressed. Feeling the subtle spring-back movement will help you find a suitable vein for the procedure. You should ask the patient to clench the fist only if the vein does not stand out. This pressure of the clenched fist may interfere with some chemistry tests. A few gentle taps to the antecubital area with two of your fingers will also help the vein stand out for better view and access. Another method to encourage blood flow in difficult to draw patients is to place a warm compress on the antecubital area for a few minutes before you begin the procedure. This will help make the veins stand out to the touch if not to the sight.

Methods of Performing a Venipuncture

There are two methods of performing this procedure: the syringe or sterile needle method and the vacuum tube or sterile needle method. Sterile technique must be used because a foreign object is introduced directly into the vein.

A 21–23 **gauge** needle is generally used. The gauge must be large enough to allow blood to flow through the needle without causing **hemolysis** (breakdown of blood cells).

Needle and Syringe Method   The needle and syringe method is often used when very small veins are involved because it is less damaging to the tissues than the vacuum method. The size of the syringe will vary according to the amount of blood needed. Usually a 10- to 20-mL syringe is used when drawing several tubes, each 5 to 15 mL (refer to Procedure 15-4).

PROCEDURE PROCEDURE PROCEDURE PROCEDURE PROCEDURE PROCEDURE PROCEDURE

15-3  Obtain Venous Blood with the Butterfly Needle Method

PURPOSE: To obtain venous blood specimen(s) of infants, of children, or of patients with veins that are difficult to draw (veins are not easily seen or felt). Suggested sites to obtain blood are the antecubital or lower arm and the back of the hand.

OSHA GUIDELINES: To comply with Standard Precautions, gloves must be worn if there is any possibility of coming into contact with blood or any body fluids.

EQUIPMENT: Sterile butterfly needle (22 G), syringe (or vacuum tubes and needle adaptor), appropriate specimen tube(s), pen, patient's chart, lab request form, spirits of ammonia, emesis basin, tourniquet, latex or vinyl gloves, alcohol prep, cotton balls or gauze squares, bandage, Mayo tray table, and biohazard sharp's container.

PERFORMANCE OBJECTIVE: Provided with all necessary equipment, and using a training model, demonstrate the steps necessary for obtaining blood specimen(s) using the butterfly method. The student must achieve a satisfactory score on the evaluation checklist. (Often, this procedure is performed by two persons: one can insert the needle, and the other can pull back on the plunger of the syringe or change vacuum tubes using the adaptor as the other person secures the needle.)

1. Wash hands.
2. Identify the patient, and complete the appropriate lab request form.
3. Assemble all necessary equipment on the Mayo tray table next to the patient.
4. Securely attach the butterfly needle to the syringe.
5. Put gloves on.

6. Palpate the vein and clean the venipuncture site of the arm or hand with alcohol prep, and dry with cotton or gauze.
7. Apply the tourniquet approximately 3 inches above the needle insertion site.
8. Ask the patient to make a fist and hold it until you say to release it.
9. Remove the needle guard and quickly insert the butterfly needle into the vein.
10. Push any air out of syringe before using it to draw a blood specimen.
11. Pull back on the plunger of the syringe slowly until an adequate amount of blood is obtained, and then ask the patient to release his fist. (Fill the appropriate vacuum tube[s] without physically forcing the blood into the tube[s]; be certain to fill tubes in the correct order.)
12. Release the tourniquet and withdraw the needle quickly.
13. Apply the gentle pressure over the site with cotton or gauze, and ask the patient to hold his arm slightly up for a few minutes to help prevent a hematoma.
14. Attend to the patient and apply a bandage to the site. **NOTE: Ask if the patient has an allergy to adhesive.**
15. Place the used needle and all other contaminated supplies in a biohazard sharps container or bag.
16. Place specimens in the appropriate lab transport container.
17. Remove gloves and discard them in a biohazard container or bag.
18. Wash hands.
19. Record the procedure on the patient's chart and initial.

PROCEDURE PROCEDURE PROCEDURE PROCEDURE PROCEDURE PROCEDURE PROCEDURE

15-4 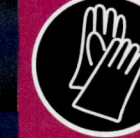 Obtain Venous Blood with a Sterile Needle and Syringe

PURPOSE: To obtain venous blood specimens when the amount needed is more than a few drops.

OSHA GUIDELINES: To comply with Standard Precautions, gloves must be worn if there is any possibility of coming into contact with blood or any body fluids.

EQUIPMENT: Sterile needle (19–23 G, 1 to 1½ inches in length), 10–20 mL syringe for specimen tubes, laboratory specimen packaging materials, pen, patient's chart, alcohol, latex or vinyl gloves, cotton balls, tourniquet, lab request form (labeled appropriately with the vacuum blood specimen tubes that were

(continues)

PROCEDURE PROCEDURE PROCEDURE PROCEDURE PROCEDURE PROCEDURE PROCEDURE

15-4   Obtain Venous Blood with a Sterile Needle and Syringe (Continued)

ordered), gauze squares, adhesive bandage, spirits of ammonia, emesis basin, biohazardous waste container (should be within reach), and sharps container. **NOTE: A tray is a convenient way to carry all necessary items for venipuncture procedures. It should be stocked with lab request forms, specimen tubes, cotton balls, alcohol dispenser, syringes, sterile needles, sharps container, latex or vinyl gloves, tourniquet, frosted-end slides, adapter for vacuum tube method, pen and pencil, gauze squares, spirits of ammonia, and bandages. This handy carrier may be set next to the patient. It should be restocked daily during routine checking of supplies.**

PERFORMANCE OBJECTIVE: Provided with all necessary equipment and supplies and using a training arm model, demonstrate the steps necessary for obtaining venous blood using the sterile needle and syringe method. The instructor will observe each step.

1. Identify the patient. **RATIONALE: Speaking to the patient by name and checking the chart ensures that you are performing the procedure on the correct patient.**

2. Wash hands and put on latex or vinyl gloves. Assemble all needed items on a flat, stable surface next to the patient. **NOTE: Label all required specimen tubes and complete a lab request form.**

3. Explain the procedure to the patient, and ask if there is a preferred venipuncture site. If the patient has no preference, visually check both arms and select a vein that can be palpated (felt) easily with your fingertip after application of alcohol. Ask a patient who is eating or chewing gum to remove the contents from his mouth before you begin to eliminate any possibility of the patient choking in the event that he faints or becomes ill during the procedure. **NOTE: Ask the patient to lie down if there is any sign of apprehension. Most often, the patient will be sitting down with one arm extended and supported on the arm rest of the chair or on a table. Providing a comfortable position will relax the patient and elicit better cooperation.**

4. Secure a needle onto a syringe by holding the needle guard in one hand and turning the syringe barrel clockwise. Push in the plunger of the syringe all the way to release any air from the barrel. It is a good practice to pull back one half to one third of the way and then push forward to push out all of the air. This makes it easier to start pulling back once you are in the vein. It is also less traumatic to the patient.

5. Apply a tourniquet to the patient's upper arm, about 3 inches above the bend in the elbow (Figure 15-10A). **RATIONALE: The tourniquet slows down blood flow, increasing volume within the vein and thereby aiding palpation and visualization of the blood vessel.**

   a. Bring the ends of the tourniquet up evenly and cross them.

   b. Switch so that you are holding an end in each hand comfortably.

   c. Stretch the end in your right hand to apply gentle pressure over the area of the arm while you hold the other end against the patient's arm.

   d. Tuck any excess stretched end under the section that is held against the arm so that there is nothing in the way of the puncture site. **NOTE: Proceed quickly, as a tourniquet should not be left on longer than 1 minute. If a tourniquet is applied too tightly, it will prevent blood flow, and the patient will be most uncomfortable.**

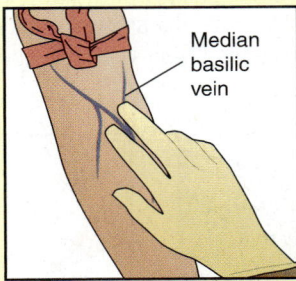

Median basilic vein

FIGURE 15-10A   Find the vein and apply a tourniquet.

6. Clean the site lightly with an alcohol-saturated cotton ball, and let it air dry (Figure 15-10B). **RATIONALE: Blowing on the site to dry it will contaminate the tissue.** You should ask the patient to clench the fist only if the vein does not stand out. This pressure of the clenched fist may interfere with some chemistry tests. A few gentle taps to the antecubital area with two of your fingers will also help the vein stand out for better view and access. Another method to encourage blood flow in difficult to draw patients is to place a warm compress on the antecubital area for a few minutes before you begin the procedure. **RATIONALE: This will assist further in making the vein stand out.** Take off the needle guard and, with the bevel of the needle up, insert the needle tip into the vein with a

(continues)

PROCEDURE PROCEDURE PROCEDURE PROCEDURE PROCEDURE PROCEDURE PROCEDURE

15-4  Obtain Venous Blood with a Sterile Needle and Syringe (Continued)

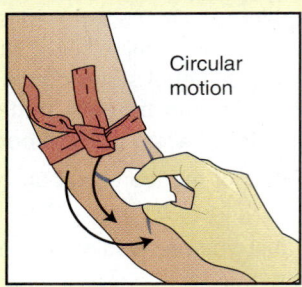

FIGURE 15-10B Apply alcohol and allow the site to dry.

quick and steady motion, following the path of the vein at approximately a 15-degree angle. **NOTE: Holding the skin at the site to stretch it slightly will help keep the vein from moving as the puncture takes place. The needle should be inserted no more than ¼ to ½ inch, or it may pass through the vein. RATIONALE: This helps maintain the position of the vein.**

7. Hold the barrel of the syringe in one hand, and with the other hand pull the plunger back slowly and steadily until the barrel is filled with the amount of blood needed to fill the specimen tubes (Figures 15-10C and D). As you ob-

serve the blood flow into the syringe, ask the patient to slowly open the fist, and then release the tourniquet. Release the tourniquet by quickly pulling up on the end of the portion that is tucked in (Figure 15-10E).

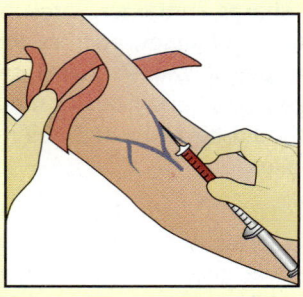

FIGURE 15-10E Release the tourniquet.

8. Pull the needle out in the same path as it was inserted and place a gauze square over the site as the needle is withdrawn (Figure 15-10F). **NOTE: Have the patient apply gentle pressure and slightly elevate the arm.**

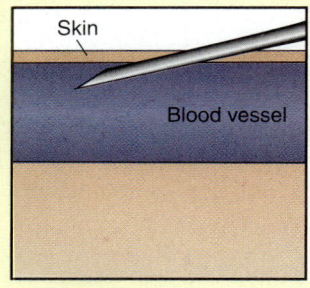

FIGURE 15-10C The needle enters the blood vessel.

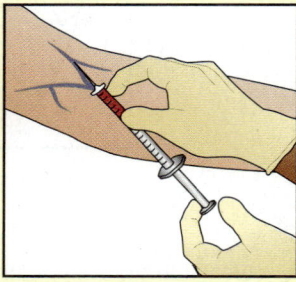

FIGURE 15-10D Withdraw blood slowly.

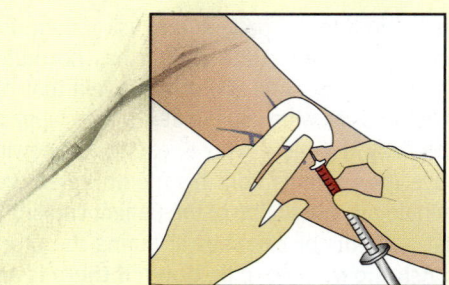

FIGURE 15-10F Apply a sterile pad before withdrawing the needle.

(continues)

15-4  Obtain Venous Blood with a Sterile Needle and Syringe (Continued)

9. Blood tubes that are to be filled from the syringe should be placed in a secure holder. Quickly fill the required specimen tubes by inserting the needle into the rubber-stoppered end. Gently push the plunger of the syringe to fill. Angle the needle toward the top of the tube so that blood runs down the side to prevent hemolysis. **RATIONALE: Forcing blood into tubes will cause hemolysis. Vacuum tubes fill easily because the vacuum draws in blood. NOTE: Specimen tubes must be filled quickly, because clotting will begin within minutes in the syringe and needle.** Fill the tubes with blood from the syringe in the following order: red, blue, green, lavender, and gray. **RATIONALE: Blood in the syringe contains no anticoagulant.** Blood smears should be made at this time if needed. **NOTE: Before filling the tubes containing powdered additives, you should tap the tube(s) gently to allow any of the contents that may have collected around the top to fall to the bottom of the tube. Check with the laboratory manual regarding the required amount of blood for test(s) ordered by the physician that contain additives. Test results may be false or inaccurate if there is a ratio imbalance of blood and additive.**

10. Stand red-stoppered tubes vertically to clot so that serum can be drawn after centrifugation. **NOTE: Do not shake blood, or hemolysis will occur.** In tubes that contain an anticoagulant, use a figure-eight motion to gently mix the blood.

11. Deposit the needle and syringe intact in the sharps biohazardous waste container. DO NOT RECAP the needle. Wrap labeled specimen tubes together with the lab request form and secure them with a rubber band. **NOTE: Keep them near the centrifuge so that serum-only transfer tube(s) may be added when completed.** The completed lab request form is usually placed in one side of the lab-provided biobag and the specimens in the other protected (sealed and leak-proof) side to be sent to a reference lab for analysis.

12. Attend to the patient's needs; apply a bandage over the puncture site (Figure 15-10G).

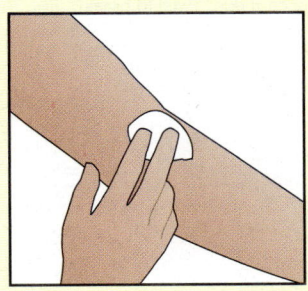

FIGURE 15-10G Have the patient apply pressure to the site until a clot forms.

13. Discard disposables in the proper receptacle. Remove gloves, wash hands, and return items to the proper storage area.

14. Record the procedure in the log book and on the patient's chart and initial. Refer to the charting example.

LOG BOOK EXAMPLE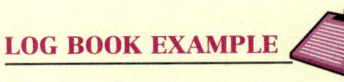

Date	Patient's Name	Number	Test	Sent	Results	Filed by
4-18-XX	Bernie L. Mitchell BD 7-18-61	7843	CBC	4-18-XX		

CHARTING EXAMPLE

4-18-XX

One CBC tube drawn from Mr. Mitchell's L arm: packaged for reference lab pick-up.

J. Watkins, CMA

Saf-T Clik Shielded Blood Needle Adapter

Instructions For Use
PREPARATION

1. Before attaching needle, push ends of Saf-T Clik® together to ensure outer sleeve is seated.

"CLICK"

2. Open needle cartridge. Twist to break the tamperproof seal. Remove cartridge cap to expose rear needle with threaded hub. Do not remove front needle cover. Use up to 1½" blood collection needle.

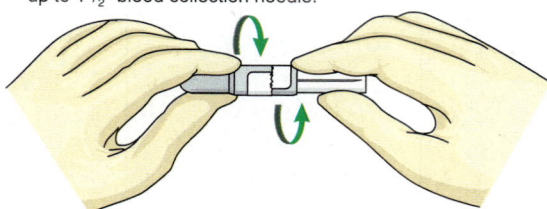

3. Attach needle to Safety Adapter. Screw needle into Safety Adapter until firmly seated.

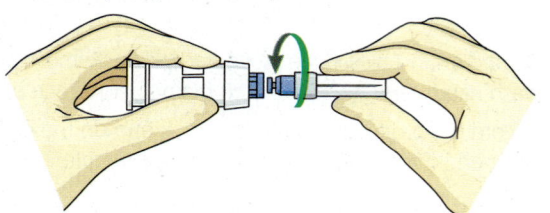

AFTER VENIPUNCTURE

4. When sampling is complete, grasp the Safety Adapter's outer sheath sliding it forward over the exposed contaminated needle until a distinctive "CLICK" is heard. "LOCKED, LOCKED" is visible when Adapter is locked. The contaminated needle is now safely covered.

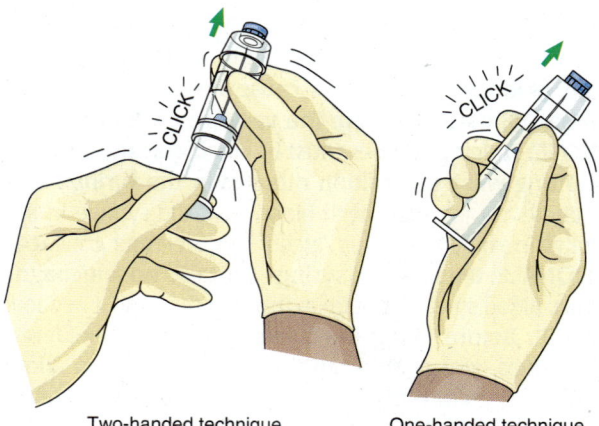

Two-handed technique   One-handed technique

5. Discard the Safety Adapter or Contaminated Needle Assembly according to hospital procedures. Do not reuse needle or Safety Adapter.

FIGURE 15-11 Instructions for using the Saf-T Click® shielded blood needle adapter *(Courtesy of MPS Acacia).*

Vacuum Method The vacuum method is probably the most popular because it is so convenient. Blood specimens enter directly into the tubes for the desired tests rather than having to be transferred. It is vital that the correct tubes be used, however.

Figure 15-11 shows instructions for use of the Saf-T Click® shielded blood needle adapter. It was designed to protect the phlebotomist from accidental needle injury, thereby reducing possible disease transmission.

This adapter may be used with all standard blood collection needles and does not change the procedure for venipuncture. After its use, the phlebotomist simply slides the protective sheath forward until the "click" is heard, and the needle is safely covered and locked so that there is no danger of injury to the phlebotomist or patient.

Figure 15-12 shows a blood needle adapter covered and locked after use. Both types of needle adapters are completely disposable and must be discarded in the biohazardous sharps waste receptacle. Procedure 15-5 describes the Vacuum Method for venipuncture.

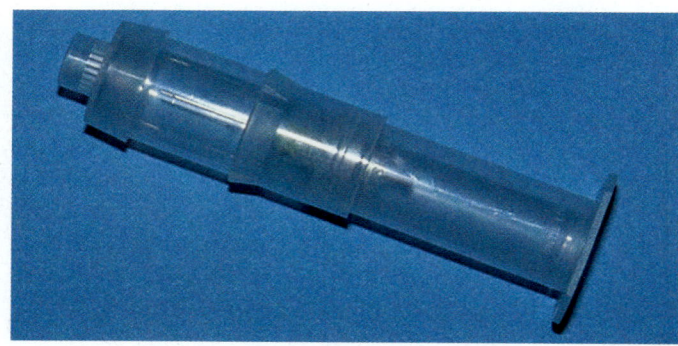

FIGURE 15-12 The Eclipse™ Safety Shielding Blood Collection needle helps protect the user from accidental injury. The shield is activated immediately after the needle with withdrawn from the vein. *(Courtesy of MPS Acacia)*

Specimen Collection

Specimen test tubes are color coded for the various departments in the lab. Red-stoppered tubes come in sizes ranging from 3 to 15 mL. They are used to collect

PROCEDURE PROCEDURE PROCEDURE PROCEDURE PROCEDURE PROCEDURE PROCEDURE

15-5  Obtain Venous Blood with a Vacuum Tube

PURPOSE: To obtain venous blood specimens when the amount needed is more than a few drops.

OSHA GUIDELINES: To comply with Standard Precautions, gloves must be worn if there is any possibility of coming into contact with blood or any body fluids.

EQUIPMENT: Multiple sample sterile needles (19–23 G, 1 to 1½ inch in length), plastic adapter (a shielded blood needle adapter is recommended for safety), labeled specimen tubes (vacuum), alcohol, latex or vinyl gloves, sharps container, cotton balls, gauze squares, tourniquet, lab request forms, pen, patient's chart, bandages, biohazardous waste container, and laboratory specimen packaging material.

PERFORMANCE OBJECTIVE: Provided with all necessary equipment and supplies and using a training arm model, demonstrate the steps necessary for obtaining venous blood using the vacuum tube method. The instructor will observe each step. **NOTE: The instructor will determine the student's skill in the performance of this procedure on other students as patients.**

1. Identify the patient.

2. Wash hands and assemble all needed items on a Mayo table next to the patient. **Note: Label all required specimen tubes and complete a lab request form before gloving. Put on latex or vinyl gloves.**

3. Secure a needle onto the adapter by screwing the grooved end of the needle into the grooved tip of the adapter, holding the needle guard and turning the adapter in a clockwise motion. Set aside.

4. Explain the procedure to the patient, and ask if there is a preferred venipuncture site. Ask the patient if he has any questions before you proceed. If there is no site preference, visually check both arms, and select a vein that can be palpated (felt) easily with your fingertip after applying alcohol. **NOTE: Ask the patient to lie down if there is any sign of apprehension. Generally the patient will be sitting down the with the arm extended and supported on the arm rest of chair or on a table. Providing a comfortable position will help to relax the patient and elicit better cooperation.** If the patient is eating or chewing gum, ask him to remove the contents from his mouth before you begin to eliminate any possibility of the patient choking in the event that he faints or becomes ill during the procedure.

5. Clean the site with a lightly alcohol-saturated cotton ball, and let it air dry. (Blowing on the site to dry it will contaminate the skin.)

   a. Push the rubber-stoppered end of the vacuum tube into the adapter until the needle is inserted just into the rubber to hold the tube in place.

   b. Apply a tourniquet to the patient's upper arm, about 3 inches above the bend in the elbow. **RATIONALE: The tourniquet slows down blood flow, increasing volume within the vein and thereby aiding palpation and visualization of the blood vessel.**

   c. You should ask the patient to clench the fist only if the vein does not stand out. This pressure of the clenched fist may interfere with some chemistry tests. A few gentle taps to the antecubital area with two of your fingers will also help the vein stand out for better view and access. Another method to encourage blood flow in difficult to draw patients is to place a warm compress on the antecubital area for a few minutes before you begin the procedure. This will assist further in making the vein stand out.

6. Take off the needle guard and, with the bevel of the needle up, insert the tip of the needle into the vein with a quick and steady motion, following the path of the vein at approximately a 15-degree angle (Figure 15-13A). **NOTE: Holding the skin at the site to stretch it slightly will help keep the vein from**

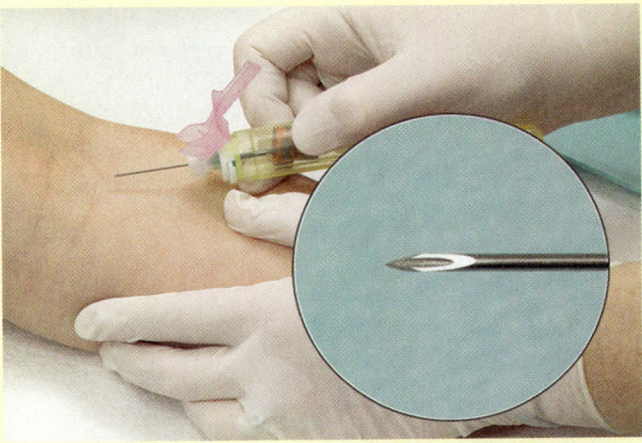

FIGURE 15-13A While holding the skin taut, hold the needle with the bevel up and penetrate the vein with a smooth rapid movement.

(continues)

15-5  Obtain Venous Blood with a Vacuum Tube (Continued)

moving as the puncture takes place. The needle should be inserted no more than ¼ to ½ inch, or it may pass through the vein.

7. Hold the adapter with one hand, and with the other hand place your index and great fingers on either side of the protruding edges of the adapter. Push the vacuum tube completely into the adapter with your thumb, allowing the needle to puncture the stopper (Figure 15-13B). Blood will flow into the tube by vacuum force if the other end of the needle is in the vein properly. As you observe blood flow into the syringe, ask the patient to slowly open the fist, and then release the tourniquet. When the tube is filled, pull it out of the adapter by holding it between your thumb and great finger and pushing against the adapter with your index finger (Figure 15-13C). **NOTE: Fill the required number of tubes for the tests ordered by the physician.** Begin with blood culture tubes first, then red, red/black, green, lavender, gray, and blue, in that order. **NOTE: Before filling the tubes containing powdered additives, you should tap the tube(s) gently to allow any of the contents that may have collected around the rubber stopper to fall to the bottom of the tube. Check with the laboratory manual regarding the required amount of blood for test(s) ordered by the physician that contain additives. Test results may be false or inaccurate if there is a ratio imbalance of blood and additive. RATIONALE: This order will prevent any possible**

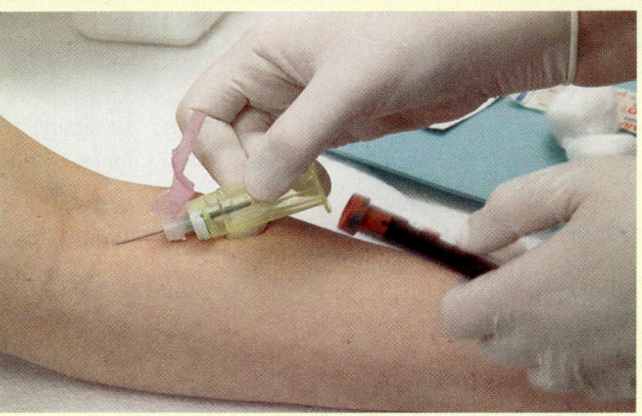

FIGURE 15-13C   When the tube has stopped filling, remove it gently from the needle and holder. Invert it several times to mix the additives. Fill the required number of tubes for the tests ordered by the physician.

traces of additive from entering the "serum-only" specimen tube. Remember to mix blood with additive gently using a figure-eight motion. **NOTE: Do not shake blood or hemolysis will occur.**

8. Remove the tourniquet by pulling on the end that was tucked under, then pull the needle out of the vein in the path of insertion and place a gauze square over the site as the needle is withdrawn. Ask the patient to elevate his arm slightly to help stop bleeding, and apply gentle pressure. **NOTE: If a blood smear is needed for a differential, turn the CBC (lavender) tube (if still attached to adapter) upside down and gently press tube down to release a drop of blood onto the glass slide.** Make blood smear (or as many as have been ordered), label the frosted end with a pencil, air-dry quickly, and send with other specimens. If using a blood analyzer system, you should place the lavender stopper tube in the closed vial to run the test.

9. Set red tubes vertically to clot so that serum can be obtained by centrifugation for serum-only tests.

10. Same as steps 10–14 for needle and syringe procedure except for disposing of needle from plastic adapter carefully into biohazardous waste or sharps container. If Saf-T Clik® is used, dispose of the entire locked unit in the biohazardous waste or sharps container.

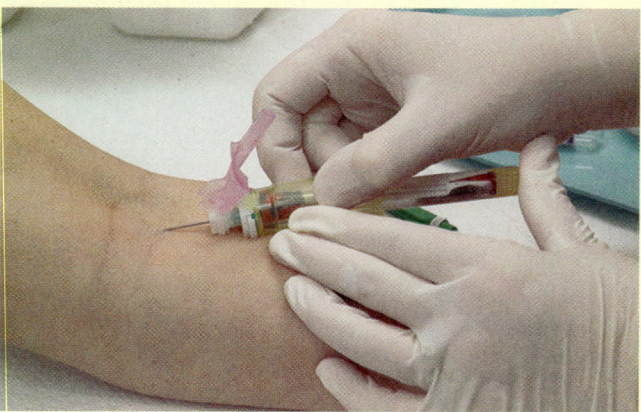

FIGURE 15-13B   Grasp the flange of the vacuum tube holder and push the tube forward until the needle has completely entered the tube.

(continues)

15-5  Obtain Venous Blood with a Vacuum Tube (Continued)

11. Deposit the needle in the sharps biohazardous waste container (Figure 15-13D). Place labeled specimen tubes with the lab request form securely in the appropriate specimen container for safe transport to the lab (Figure 15-13E). **NOTE: Keep near centrifuge so that serum-only transfer tube(s) may be added when completed.** The completed lab request form is usually placed in one side of the lab-provided biobag and the specimens in the other protected (sealed and leak-proof) side to be sent to a reference lab for analysis (Figure 15-13F).

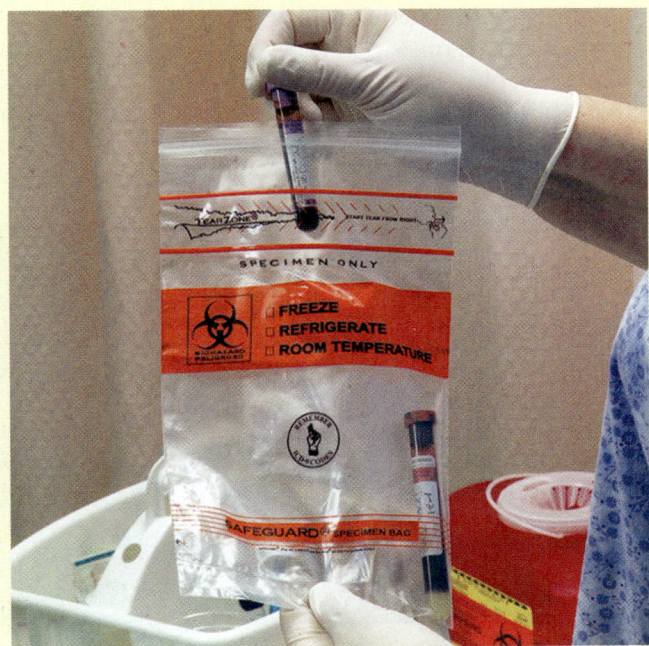

FIGURE 15-13D After removing the needle from the vein, activate the safety device immediately and dispose of the needle into the sharps container.

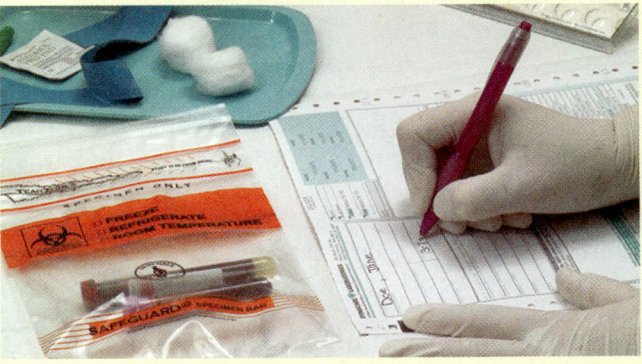

FIGURE 15-13F Complete the lab request form.

12. Attend to the patient's needs; apply a bandage over the puncture site (Figure 15-13G).

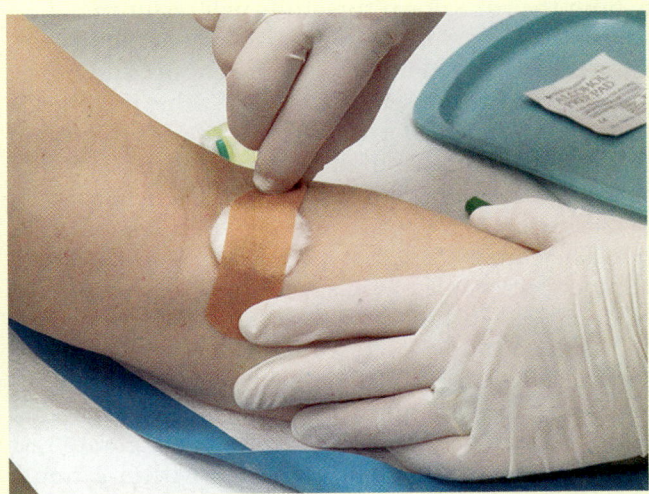

FIGURE 15-13G Check the patient, and apply a bandage over the puncture site.

13. Discard disposables in the proper receptacle. Remove gloves and wash hands. Return items to the proper storage area.

14. Record the procedure in the log book and on the patient's chart. Refer to the charting example.

FIGURE 15-13E Label the tubes and package the specimens for transport.

(continues)

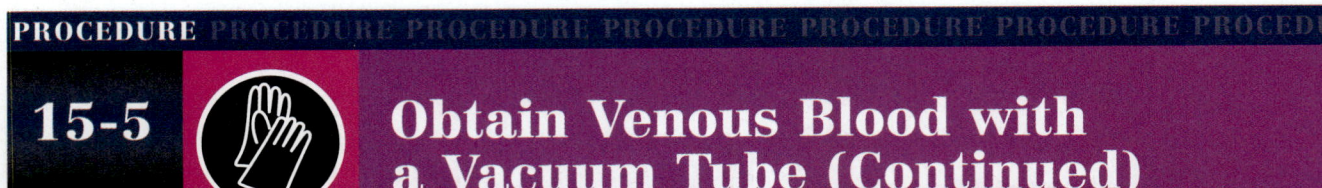

PROCEDURE PROCEDURE PROCEDURE PROCEDURE PROCEDURE PROCEDURE PROCEDURE PROCEDURE

15-5   Obtain Venous Blood with a Vacuum Tube (Continued)

LOG BOOK EXAMPLE

Date	Patient's Name	Number	Test	Sent	Results	Filed by
5-28-XX	Bernie L. Mitchell BD 7-18-61	7843	CBC	5-28-XX		

CHARTING EXAMPLE

5-28-XX

One CBC tube drawn from Mr. Mitchell's L arm: packaged for reference lab pick-up.

J. Watkins, CMA (CL)

whole blood that is allowed to clot so that the serum can be drawn off by centrifugation. The serum can be drawn out by a disposable pipette and deposited into a transfer tube, which is labeled for the particular test to be done. There are other methods to easily transfer serum from the centrifuged tube. The most efficient way is to use the red/black stoppered tube, which has a gel in the bottom. During centrifugation, the gel liquifies and travels to the center of the tube, separating the red cells from the serum. You can then carefully pour the serum into a transfer tube and label for analysis. Another method is to place a slender rubber-tipped tube down carefully into the centrifuged tube (pushing the tube down forcefully will result in hemolysis) just to the **meniscus** of the packed red blood cells. The screened filtered opening at the rubber end of the inner tube allows the serum to fill the tube, leaving the red blood cells at the bottom. Then, pour off the serum into a transfer tube and label for analysis. Lavender-stoppered tubes contain ethylenediamienetetraacetic acid additive (EDTA) and are generally called CBC tubes. They are usually 5 or 10 mL in size and are also used to collect whole blood specimens. Gray-stoppered tubes are used in blood glucose tests and are usually 5 mL. They contain oxalate. Blue-stoppered tubes must be completely full because of the large amount of citrate. These tubes are most often the 5-mL size and are used for testing pro-thrombin times. For accurate test results, the test should be performed within 2 hours from the time it is drawn. The green-stoppered tubes generally are the 5-mL-sized tubes that contain **heparin** and are used to determine several chemical constituents. The blood specimen vacuum tubes that are used for pediatric patients are the same as the tubes used for adults, except for the sizes, which are between 2 mL and 3 mL. Tests drawn in the blue tubes should be performed within 2 hours for accurate results or centrifuge. Freeze the plasma until testing may be performed.

Order of Draw

When several blood specimens are ordered, they should be drawn into the color-coded stoppered tubes in the following order: yellow (for blood cultures), red or red/black (red-gray), blue, green, lavender, and gray (Figure 15-14). The red or red/black tubes do not contain additives and should be drawn first in multiple sample draws to prevent possible contamination from the additives in the other tubes (Figure 15-15). In cases that require only one blue stoppered tube, a 5-mL red-stoppered tube should be drawn first and discarded. This will prevent thromboplastin from the site of the draw from interfering with the results of coagulation testing.

Blood in specimen tubes that contain an anticoagulant must be mixed immediately in a figure-eight motion 8 to 10 times. Gentle mixing will prevent hemolysis. The tubes with red stoppers must be allowed to stand vertically and undisturbed for at least 20 to 30 minutes to allow clotting to occur. The tube(s) must then be properly balanced in a centrifuge and spun for varying lengths of time, depend-

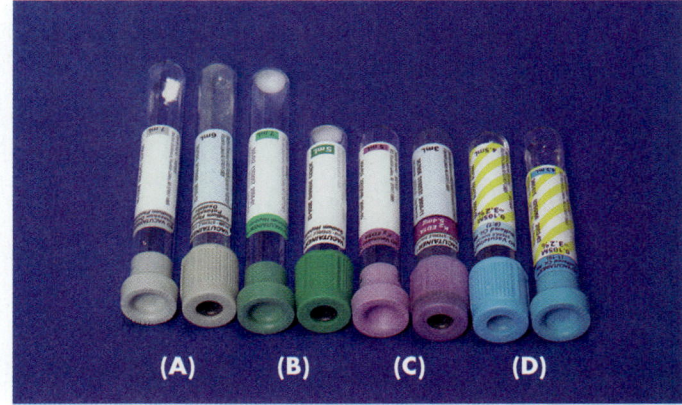

FIGURE 15-14 Vacuum tubes come in several sizes and are color-coded for a variety of uses. (A) Gray top: antiglycocytic agent. (B) Green top: heparin. (C) Lavender top: EDTA. (D) Light blue top: citrate.

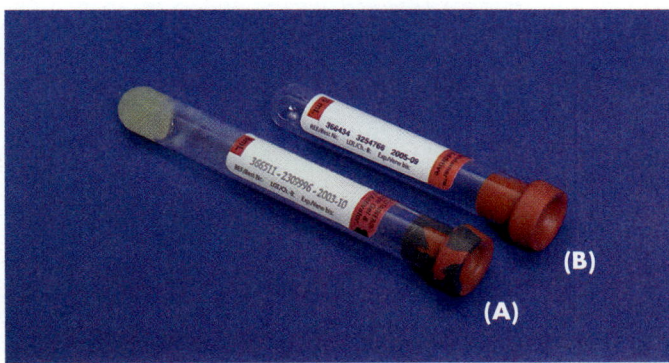

FIGURE 15-15 Standard vacuum tubes. (A) Red/gray-top tube contains clot activators and thixotrophic gel. (B) Plain red-top tube contains no anticoagulant or additives.

ing on the centrifuge speed. The serum, which is a clear, light yellow liquid, is then carefully drawn off with a pipette (usually disposable ones provided by the laboratory) or by using one of the methods discussed earlier.

Blood collection tubes and supplies must be checked for the expiration date, and if out of date, not used. This is in compliance with quality control and quality assurance regulations. A log book must be kept of all specimens collected and sent for analysis. The log book must contain the following information:

1. Date collected
2. Patient's full name, DOB, Social Security number, or records number
3. Date sent to lab
4. Test requested
5. Date results received
6. Test results—may not be kept in specimen log book unless the test is being performed "in house." Generally, a copy is filed in the patient's chart and a copy in the lab file in order of the date collected.

A lab request form, such as the one in Figure 15-16, must be completed and sent with the specimen(s) and listed in the log book.

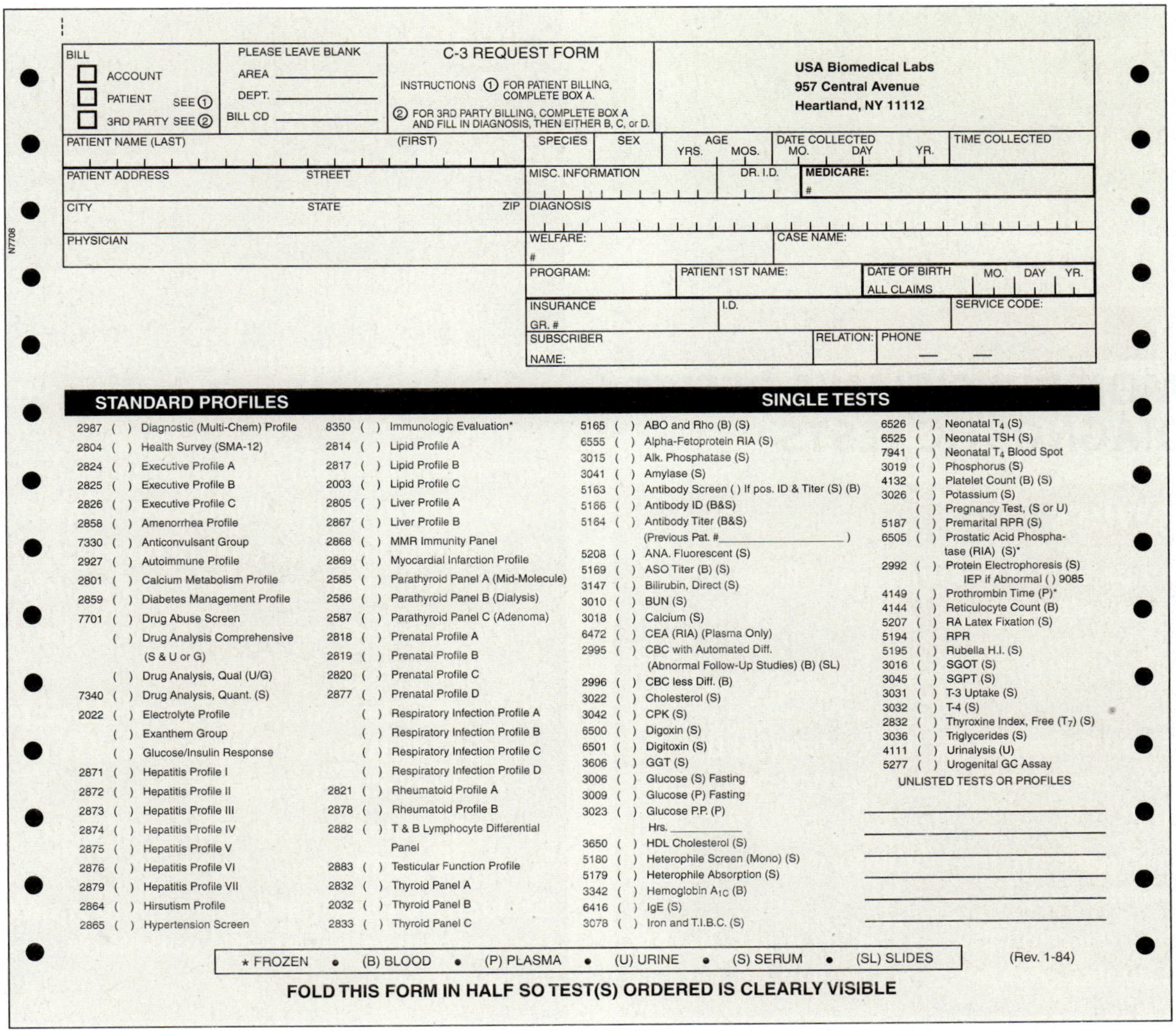

C-3 REQUEST FORM

BILL
☐ ACCOUNT
☐ PATIENT   SEE ①
☐ 3RD PARTY SEE ②

PLEASE LEAVE BLANK
AREA _____
DEPT. _____
BILL CD _____

INSTRUCTIONS ① FOR PATIENT BILLING, COMPLETE BOX A.
② FOR 3RD PARTY BILLING, COMPLETE BOX A AND FILL IN DIAGNOSIS, THEN EITHER B, C, or D.

USA Biomedical Labs
957 Central Avenue
Heartland, NY 11112

PATIENT NAME (LAST)   (FIRST)   SPECIES   SEX   AGE YRS. MOS.   DATE COLLECTED MO. DAY YR.   TIME COLLECTED

PATIENT ADDRESS   STREET   MISC. INFORMATION   DR. I.D.   MEDICARE: #

CITY   STATE   ZIP   DIAGNOSIS

PHYSICIAN   WELFARE: #   CASE NAME:

PROGRAM: PATIENT 1ST NAME: DATE OF BIRTH MO. DAY YR. ALL CLAIMS

INSURANCE GR. #   I.D.   SERVICE CODE:

SUBSCRIBER NAME: RELATION: PHONE

N708

STANDARD PROFILES   **SINGLE TESTS**

2987 ( ) Diagnostic (Multi-Chem) Profile	8350 ( ) Immunologic Evaluation*	5165 ( ) ABO and Rho (B) (S)	6526 ( ) Neonatal T$_4$ (S)
2804 ( ) Health Survey (SMA-12)	2814 ( ) Lipid Profile A	6555 ( ) Alpha-Fetoprotein RIA (S)	6525 ( ) Neonatal TSH (S)
2824 ( ) Executive Profile A	2817 ( ) Lipid Profile B	3015 ( ) Alk. Phosphatase (S)	7941 ( ) Neonatal T$_4$ Blood Spot
2825 ( ) Executive Profile B	2003 ( ) Lipid Profile C	3041 ( ) Amylase (S)	3019 ( ) Phosphorus (S)
2826 ( ) Executive Profile C	2805 ( ) Liver Profile A	5163 ( ) Antibody Screen ( ) If pos. ID & Titer (S) (B)	4132 ( ) Platelet Count (B) (S)
2858 ( ) Amenorrhea Profile	2867 ( ) Liver Profile B	5166 ( ) Antibody ID (B&S)	3026 ( ) Potassium (S)
7330 ( ) Anticonvulsant Group	2868 ( ) MMR Immunity Panel	5164 ( ) Antibody Titer (B&S)	( ) Pregnancy Test, (S or U)
2927 ( ) Autoimmune Profile	2869 ( ) Myocardial Infarction Profile	(Previous Pat. #_____)	5187 ( ) Premarital RPR (S)
2801 ( ) Calcium Metabolism Profile	2585 ( ) Parathyroid Panel A (Mid-Molecule)	5208 ( ) ANA. Fluorescent (S)	6505 ( ) Prostatic Acid Phospha-tase (RIA) (S)*
2859 ( ) Diabetes Management Profile	2586 ( ) Parathyroid Panel B (Dialysis)	5169 ( ) ASO Titer (B) (S)	2992 ( ) Protein Electrophoresis (S) IEP if Abnormal ( ) 9085
7701 ( ) Drug Abuse Screen	2587 ( ) Parathyroid Panel C (Adenoma)	3147 ( ) Bilirubin, Direct (S)	4149 ( ) Prothrombin Time (P)*
( ) Drug Analysis Comprehensive (S & U or G)	2818 ( ) Prenatal Profile A	3010 ( ) BUN (S)	4144 ( ) Reticulocyte Count (B)
	2819 ( ) Prenatal Profile B	3018 ( ) Calcium (S)	5207 ( ) RA Latex Fixation (S)
( ) Drug Analysis, Qual (U/G)	2820 ( ) Prenatal Profile C	6472 ( ) CEA (RIA) (Plasma Only)	5194 ( ) RPR
7340 ( ) Drug Analysis, Quant. (S)	2877 ( ) Prenatal Profile D	2995 ( ) CBC with Automated Diff. (Abnormal Follow-Up Studies) (B) (SL)	5195 ( ) Rubella H.I. (S)
2022 ( ) Electrolyte Profile	( ) Respiratory Infection Profile A	2996 ( ) CBC less Diff. (B)	3016 ( ) SGOT (S)
( ) Exanthem Group	( ) Respiratory Infection Profile B	3022 ( ) Cholesterol (S)	3045 ( ) SGPT (S)
( ) Glucose/Insulin Response	( ) Respiratory Infection Profile C	3042 ( ) CPK (S)	3031 ( ) T-3 Uptake (S)
2871 ( ) Hepatitis Profile I	( ) Respiratory Infection Profile D	6500 ( ) Digoxin (S)	3032 ( ) T-4 (S)
2872 ( ) Hepatitis Profile II		6501 ( ) Digitoxin (S)	2832 ( ) Thyroxine Index, Free (T$_7$) (S)
2873 ( ) Hepatitis Profile III	2821 ( ) Rheumatoid Profile A	3606 ( ) GGT (S)	3036 ( ) Triglycerides (S)
2874 ( ) Hepatitis Profile IV	2878 ( ) Rheumatoid Profile B	3006 ( ) Glucose (S) Fasting	4111 ( ) Urinalysis (U)
2875 ( ) Hepatitis Profile V	2882 ( ) T & B Lymphocyte Differential Panel	3009 ( ) Glucose (P) Fasting	5277 ( ) Urogenital GC Assay
2876 ( ) Hepatitis Profile VI	2883 ( ) Testicular Function Profile	3023 ( ) Glucose P.P. (P) Hrs.	UNLISTED TESTS OR PROFILES
2879 ( ) Hepatitis Profile VII	2832 ( ) Thyroid Panel A	3650 ( ) HDL Cholesterol (S)	_____
2864 ( ) Hirsutism Profile	2032 ( ) Thyroid Panel B	5180 ( ) Heterophile Screen (Mono) (S)	_____
2865 ( ) Hypertension Screen	2833 ( ) Thyroid Panel C	5179 ( ) Heterophile Absorption (S)	_____
		3342 ( ) Hemoglobin A$_{1C}$ (B)	_____
		6416 ( ) IgE (S)	_____
		3078 ( ) Iron and T.I.B.C. (S)	_____

★ FROZEN   (B) BLOOD   (P) PLASMA   (U) URINE   (S) SERUM   (SL) SLIDES   (Rev. 1-84)

FOLD THIS FORM IN HALF SO TEST(S) ORDERED IS CLEARLY VISIBLE

FIGURE 15-16 A laboratory request form for diagnostic tests

Often, specimens are picked up by couriers for delivery to out-of-town or out-of-state laboratories for analysis. The federal government requires that specimens are shipped or transported in securely closed, watertight containers. Blood tubes should be enclosed in a second durable watertight container. The doubly secured specimens are then placed in a shipping container with a label stating it is biohazardous. It is then ready for safe transport to the reference laboratory. A second label should read: In case of breakage, send to this address: Centers for Disease Control and Prevention, Attention: Biohazards Control Office, 1600 Clifton Road, Atlanta, GA 30333.

ACHIEVE UNIT OBJECTIVES

- Complete the Workbook activities to meet the learning objectives.
- Practice the procedures in this unit to meet the performance objectives.
- Apply your knowledge at the end of this chapter in completing the Critical Thinking Challenge and Activities, as well as the StudyWARE on your Student CD-ROM.

UNIT 4

COMMON PHYSICIAN'S OFFICE LAB DIAGNOSTIC TESTS

OBJECTIVES

Upon completion of this unit, you will be able to achieve the following:

LEARNING Objectives

1. Spell and define, using the glossary at the back of the text, all of the Words to Know in this unit.
2. List and describe the regulatory bodies that govern the POL.
3. List and describe the laboratory practices that yield quality assurance in the POL.
4. Define the terms quality control and quality assurance.
5. Differentiate between normal and abnormal results for common diagnostic tests performed in the POL.
6. Identify panic values for diagnostic test results.
7. List normal values for RBC for males and females.
8. List normal values for WBC overall and identify the various WBCs by function and normal counts.
9. List normal values for platelet counts.
10. Define the purpose of the WBC differential.
11. Describe how the erythrocyte sedimentation rate is useful in diagnoses.
12. Explain the purpose of the glucose tolerance test (GTT).
13. Define and describe the indications for the hemoglobin A1C test.
14. Identify common immunology tests ordered by health care providers and how they are used in diagnoses.
15. Identify the implications of an infant who has a positive PKU result.
16. Explain the need for collecting a PKU test and describe the proper collection procedure for the specimen.
17. Differentiate between a properly collected and improperly collected blood specimen.
18. Identify different types of urine specimens and why they are ordered for testing.
19. Define the three components of the routine urinalysis.
20. Explain the procedure for collecting urine specimens for substance analysis and the chain-of-custody procedure.
21. Understand various collection techniques for fecal specimens.
22. Identify tests that require sputum specimens and properly instruct a patient on collecting a specimen.

PERFORMANCE Objectives

1. **Perform a hemoglobin test on a blood specimen and document the quality control(s) for the test.**

2. **Perform a hematocrit test on a blood specimen.**

3. **Perform an erythrocyte sedimentation rate (ESR).**

4. **Perform a glucose test on a blood specimen and document the quality control(s) for the test.**

5. **Perform a pregnancy test and document the quality control(s) for the test.**

6. **Perform the physical and chemical parts of a urinalysis.**

7. **Prepare a urine specimen for examination of urine sediment.**

8. **Instruct a male and a female patient on the proper procedure for obtaining a midstream, clean-catch urine specimen.**

9. **Instruct a patient on the proper procedure for collecting a fecal specimen for occult blood screening.**

10. **Instruct a patient on collecting a sputum specimen.**

phenylketonuria
  (PKU)
physical
physician's office
  laboratory
  (POL)
polycythemia

protein
  (albumin)
provider-
  performed
  microscopy
  (PPM)
specific gravity

sputum
stability
STAT
supernatant
urinalysis
urobilinogen
waived

CERTIFICATION CONNECTION

CMA
Instruments, supplies, and
  equipment
Collecting and processing
  specimens; diagnostic
  testing
Processing specimens
Quality control
Performing selected tests:
  urinalysis; hematology;
  blood chemistry;
  immunology;
  pregnancy testing;
  guaiac testing

RMA
Allergy testing
Laboratory procedures:
  safety, CLIA '88;
  quality control
  program
Laboratory equipment
Laboratory testing: urine,
  blood, throat culture,
  stool for occult blood,
  sputum; perform waived
  laboratory procedures;
  know training
  requirements for
  moderate and complex
  laboratory procedures;
  recognize normal and
  abnormal values of
  common laboratory
  tests

WORDS TO KNOW

acquired
  immuno-
  deficiency
  syndrome
  (AIDS)
allergy
allosteric
  protein
bilirubin
cancer
catheterization
chemical
cholesterol
complete blood
  count

differential
gestational
  diabetes
glucose
glycohemoglobin
glycosylation
guaiac
hematuria
human chorionic
  gonadotropin
human immuno-
  deficiency
  virus (HIV)
immunology
immunoassays

infectious
  mononucleosis
in vivo
ketone
  (acetone)
leukocyte
  esterase
metabolism
microhematocrit
morphology
nitrite
panic value
pediatric
percentage
phenylalanine

LABORATORY CLASSIFICATION AND REGULATION

The **physician's office laboratory (POL)** falls under many regulatory bodies. The complexity of the laboratory tests performed determines the classification of the POL and under which body it will be regulated. The three laboratory classifications under the Clinical Laboratory Improvement Amendments of 1988 (CLIA '88) are **waived**, moderately complex, and highly complex. **Provider-performed microscopy (PPM)** has several criteria for allowing testing to be performed by trained individuals other than laboratory personnel such as physicians, midlevel practitioners under the supervision of a physician, or a dentist. The primary instrument, as you should be able to identify from the category of testing, is the microscope, limited to bright-field or phase-contrast microscopy.

A certificate of waiver allows only those tests to be performed in a POL that are on the list of waived tests. The *waived* status is granted according to the difficulty in performing the diagnostic tests. Waived tests that can be performed in a medical office following package insert directions are basically those that have been manufactured for patient home testing and cleared by the FDA. The thought behind this category of tests is that the tests employ methodology that is so simple and accurate that an error in the interpretation of the results will not cause harm to the patient, and that if the test is performed incorrectly, there also would be no harm to the patient. Due to technology, this category of testing changes frequently, so consulting the CDC web site for governmental regulations is advisable. Generally speaking, nonautomated tests such as visual color comparison tests fall into the waived category.

The application for the certificate of waiver is obtained from the Centers for Medicare and Medicaid Services (CMS), formerly the Health Care Financing Administration (HCFA), when the facility registers with this organization. Laboratory tests on the certificate of waiver list may be billed to Medicare and Medicaid for reimbursement. The certification must be renewed every 2 years for a published fee, and all tests performed by the medical assistant in the POL must be restricted to this list. CMS does not stipulate any specific staff requirements or proficiency tests, although it is stipulated that the laboratory must follow good laboratory practices, including quality assurance and quality control.

Moderately complex laboratory tests must be performed under more stringent regulations and with a more expanded requirement of personnel. For instance, CLIA mandates that there must be a personnel director such as a physician who oversees the non-waived laboratory; testing personnel who are responsible for processing the specimens, monitoring the testing process for reliability, and reporting the results; a technical consultant who oversees all of the testing performed in the facility; and a clinical consultant with a minimum of a doctoral degree. An error in the testing or reporting of tests in this category could endanger a patient's life—thus the additional requirements for patient safety.

Highly complex laboratory tests go beyond the requirements listed above in that the testing personnel must have very specific and specialized training to perform those tests. Testing of this nature would not typically be performed in a POL and is usually found in hospital laboratory settings and reference laboratories.

Quality Assurance and Quality Control

Regulatory bodies periodically inspect laboratories and medical offices to ensure quality assurance and quality control. Quality assurance (QA) in the health care field refers to all evaluative services and the results compared with accepted standards. Quality control (QC) is a process that assesses testing procedures, reagents, and technique of the person performing the tests. Quality control feeds directly into quality assurance in the laboratory setting, because before any patient tests are performed and reported, the instruments and reagents are first tested with the QC material, with the results compared against standard results for these manufactured products. Results from the QC that do not fall within the prescribed parameters must be investigated and rectified to protect patients from receiving erroneous lab results and subsequent treatment.

All laboratories are required to follow quality assurance programs. The purposes of quality assurance programs are to evaluate the quality and effectiveness of health care according to accepted standards and to ensure accuracy and validity in testing procedures. When required, POLs must also participate in proficiency testing programs for those procedures they perform; additionally, strict records of quality control results, temperature readings, and maintenance logs are required.

Other bodies that provide regulation inspections of a POL are CMS and OSHA. Private agencies also issue accreditation and state licensing for approved operation of the POL. The laboratory may be operated under a provisional certificate, which is issued until the Department of Health and Human Services (HHS) inspects the facility. Inspections of laboratory facilities may be made unannounced at any time. If OSHA, a separate entity from CMS, finds a POL in noncompliance of regulations during a visit, a monetary fine per item, per employee is applied.

In the POL, no matter what the classification, the following practices must be followed to ensure reliable and accurate data and to ensure quality health care to the patients being served.

Quality assurance involves *proper*:

1. Patient identification
2. Patient preparation and specimen collection
3. Specimen processing and transportation
4. Instrumental and technical performance
5. Safety
6. In-service training and education of all health care personnel

All state and federal health and safety regulations and laws apply to the POL according to the three lab categorizations. It is important to stay abreast of current regulations applicable to the facility with which you are employed.

HEMOGLOBIN AND HEMATOCRIT

Hemoglobin and hematocrit screening tests require a small amount of blood, most often capillary blood. Usually the ring or great finger is used for the reasons described in Unit 2.

Hemoglobin

Hemoglobin (Hgb or Hb) is an **allosteric protein** found in erythrocytes, which transports molecular oxygen in the blood to the cells of the body. The red blood cells circulate to deposit the oxygen and carry away carbon dioxide as a waste product. One quick and easy method for measuring a patient's hemoglobin is the use of a hemoglobinometer (Figure 15-17). Older technologies made this procedure a more tedious process, but today, instrumentation is advanced to the point that a drop of blood is applied to a card, and in a short period of time (usually less than 1 minute), a result is displayed (Figure 15-18). Refer to Procedure 15-6 for performing this important screening test.

Because hemoglobin is essential to circulate oxygen in the body, it is important for you to be familiar with the normal ranges for hemoglobin for males and females in the event you need to contact the health care provider immediately. Anemia is the medical term given when a patient's circulating erythrocytes are deficient. The normal range of hemoglobin for males is 14 to 18 g/dL; for females the range is 12 to 16 g/dL. Once a patient's hemoglobin falls below 10 g/dL, the patient may experience shortness of breath and tiredness and have a pale appearance to her skin. It is generally accepted that a hemoglobin result of less than

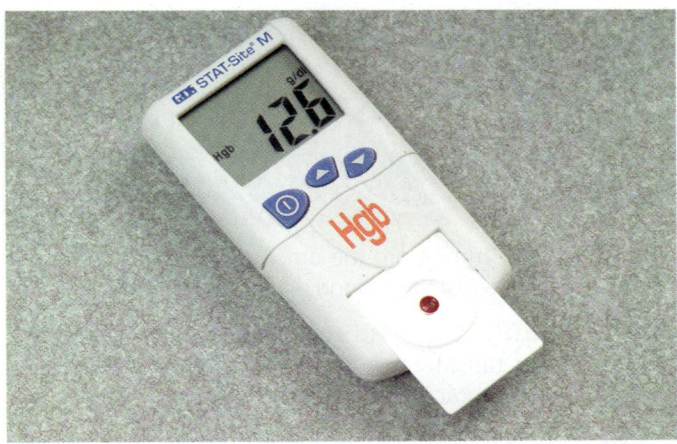

FIGURE 15-18   Results from performing a hemoglobin test on capillary blood

5 g/dL is not compatible with life; it is doubtful you would come across a result such as this in the ambulatory health care setting.

However, when taking results by phone from other laboratory facilities, a report of a very low hemoglobin could be reported, so you should be aware that this result would be considered a **panic value** requiring immediate intervention by the health care provider. While most attention is given when a patient's hemoglobin is low, another condition needs to be considered in patient screening; in conditions of **polycythemia**, the bone marrow produces too many red blood cells, with the most common patient complaints being weakness and fatigue. Other symptoms include redness of the skin, pain in the extremities, and what appears to be bruising. When a patient has profound anemia, a blood transfusion may be indicated to increase the circulating red blood cells; a patient with polycythemia may need to have a unit of blood withdrawn to provide relief of the symptoms.

Hematocrit

The hematocrit (Hct) is another hematology test that screens patients for anemia that is not used as commonly now as it was in recent years. Very small glass or plastic tubes are used for the testing procedure; the hematocrit performed in this manner is referred to as a **microhematocrit** (Figure 15-19). Either capillary blood or venous blood may be used for this test. Most of the tubes are marked approximately three fourths of the way up the tube to prevent overfilling of the tube; the tubes are designed to draw by capillary action so that no additional equipment is needed for aspirating the blood into the tubes. Once the tubes are filled, a small amount of clay sealant is used to close one end of the tube so the blood does not leak out during the

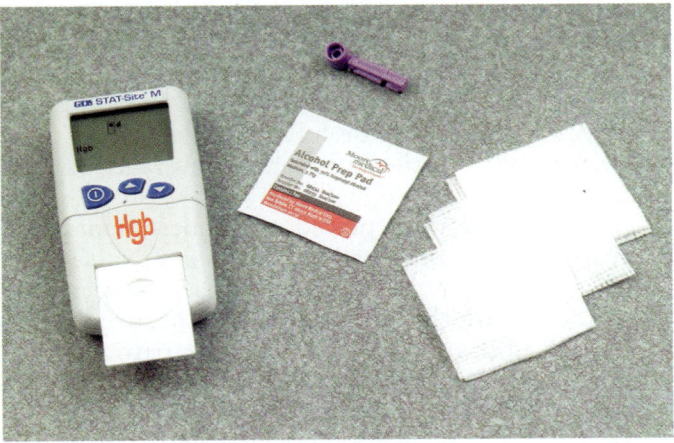

FIGURE 15-17   A hand-held hemoglobinometer commonly found in a POL

PROCEDURE PROCEDURE PROCEDURE PROCEDURE PROCEDURE PROCEDURE PROCEDURE

15-6  Hemoglobin Determination Using a Hemoglobinometer

PURPOSE: To measure the amount of hemoglobin (Hbg or Hb) in the circulating blood.

OSHA GUIDELINES: To comply with Standard Precautions, gloves must be worn when there is any possibility of coming into contact with blood or body fluids.

EQUIPMENT: Hemoglobinometer, reagent card, sterile lancet, cottom balls or gauze, alcohol, gloves, work surface, patient's chart, and blue or black pen.

PERFORMANCE OBJECTIVE: With the equipment and supplies listed above, and using another student as a patient, demonstrate the steps required to perform a hemoglobin determination using the instrument, with the instructor observing each step.

1. Assemble all supplies and the hemoglobinometer; place them on a secure work surface.

2. Explain the procedure to the patient. **RATIONALE: Speaking to the patient by name as well as checking the chart ensures you are performing the proper procedure on the correct patient.**

3. Wash hands and don gloves. Follow the desired capillary puncture procedure as outlined in Unit 2.

4. Place a large, beaded drop of blood on the reagent card while making sure the instrument is on. Wipe the patient's finger with a cotton ball or dry gauze and have the patient apply pressure to the site of the puncture.

5. Once the instrument displays the results, chart this on the patient's medical record expressed as (the number) g/dL.

6. Dispose of the lancet in the biohazard sharps containers. The remaining soiled articles are to be disposed of in the biohazard trash container.

7. Record the results as well as the quality control sample results, in the log book. Refer to the package insert to ascertain the controls are within the prescribed range set by the manufacturer.

LOG BOOK EXAMPLE

Date	Patient's Name	Test	Results	Performed by:
10/9/XX	Melody C. Jones	Hbg	14.3 g/dL	CKA
10/9/XX	High control	Hbg	19.8 g/dL	CKA
10/9/XX	Low control	Hbg	7.6 g/dL	CKA

CHARTING EXAMPLE

10/9/XX

Capillary puncture of Lt. middle finger performed for Hbg.

Results: 14.3 g/dL

CKA

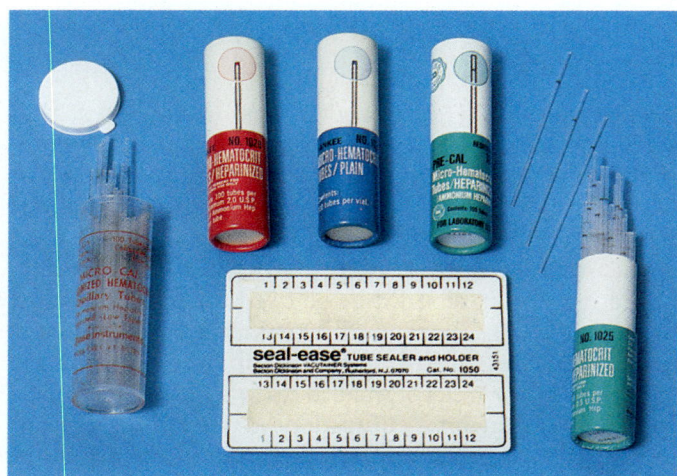

FIGURE 15-19 Microhematocrit (capillary blood) tubes with clay sealant

centrifugation, process (Figure 15-20). Be sure that you have adequately sealed the tube prior to centrifuging, or the blood can be spun out of the tube, resulting in no measurement of the hematocrit value. Microhematocrits should always be collected in duplicate, with the results between the two readings averaged for the result.

The tubes are then placed in a microhematocrit centrifuge, commonly called a *microfuge*, as seen in Figure 15-21. The tubes are centrifuged at a very high speed for a relatively short period of time, usually not more than 5 minutes; the process of centrifuging separates the cell components, with the erythrocytes going to the bottom of the tube because they are heaviest and the plasma migrating to the top. In the middle of the tube is a very thin layer known as the *buffy coat* that contains the leukocytes and platelets (Figure 15-22).

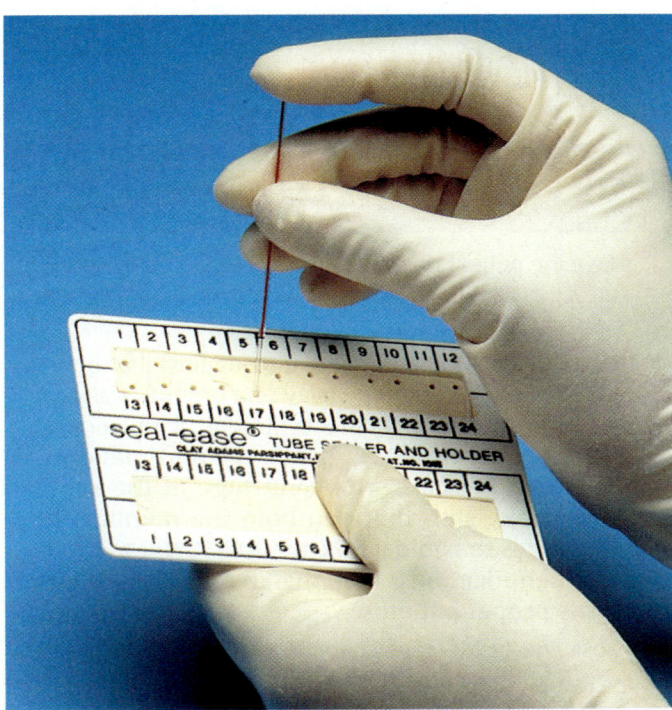

FIGURE 15-20   Carefully push the glass tube (filled to the fill line with capillary blood) into clay to seal one end before placing it in the microhematocrit centrifuge.

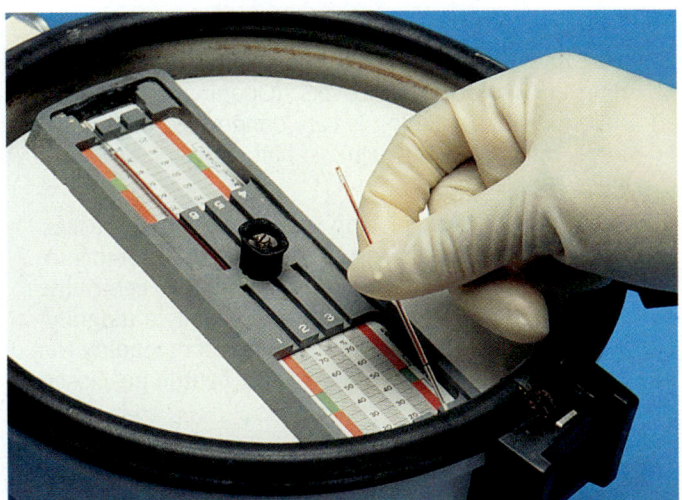

FIGURE 15-21   There are grooved slots for up to six microhematocrit tubes to be centrifuged at once. Be sure to note the space number for each patient's hematocrit tube, and write it down to avoid confusion and erroneously reporting patient results. Carefully place the sealed end of tube against the padding of the centrifuge wall (toward you).

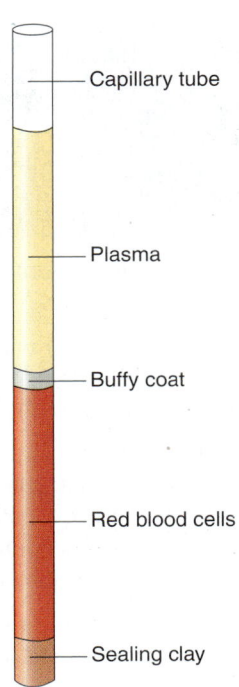

FIGURE 15-22   A blood-filled microhematocrit tube after centrifugation

for adult males is 40% to 54%; the adult female range is 37% to 47%. (Refer to Procedure 15-7).

Hematocrits are read by looking down onto the tube against the values chart within the centrifuge. Refer to Figure 15-23 for a closer look into the centrifuge to understand how the measurement may be read. Once the tubes have been centrifuged, the readings are performed by placing the sealed end of the tube against the

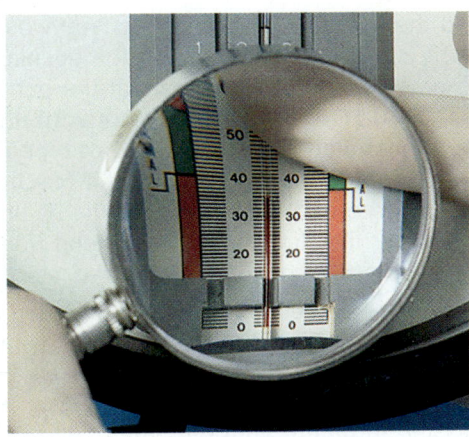

FIGURE 15-23   Obtain a hematocrit reading by looking down onto the tube against the values chart within the centrifuge. After centrifugation, the hematocrit reading is obtained by placing the sealed end of the tube against the padding, making sure that the line between the packed red blood cells and the clay is at "0" (zero). Read the hematocrit at the bottom of the meniscus. The reading in this photo is 35%.

The hematocrit is always expressed as a **percentage** of the total blood volume, and what you are measuring and recording is the percentage of packed red blood cells in the microhematocrit tube as compared with the rest of the blood sample. The normal hematocrit range

PROCEDURE PROCEDURE PROCEDURE PROCEDURE PROCEDURE PROCEDURE PROCEDURE

15-7  Determine Hematocrit (Hct) Using a Microhematocrit Centrifuge

PURPOSE: To determine the volume of packed erythrocytes in whole blood.

OSHA GUIDELINES: To comply with Standard Precautions, gloves must be worn if there is any possibility of coming into contact with blood or any body fluids.

EQUIPMENT: Autolet or sterile lancet, microhematocrit tube(s), sealing clay, microhematocrit centrifuge, latex or vinyl gloves, cotton balls, alcohol, patient's chart, pen (if hemoglobin is done by this procedure, conversion chart will also be needed to determine Hb), and Table 15-1.

PERFORMANCE OBJECTIVE: Provided with all necessary equipment and supplies, and using other students as patients, demonstrate the steps in the procedure for determining hematocrit (Hct) readings using the microhematocrit centrifuge. The instructor will observe each step.

1. Assemble the needed items on a Mayo table. Check to see that the centrifuge is plugged into the electrical outlet.

2. Identify the patient and explain the procedure. **RATIONALE: Speaking to the patient by name and checking the chart ensures that you are performing the procedure on the correct patient.**

3. Wash and dry hands, and put on latex or vinyl gloves.

4. Follow the desired skin puncture procedure.

5. Hold the microhematocrit tube as you would hold a pencil or pen, horizontally with the opening next to the drop of blood that appears at the puncture site. **RATIONALE: Holding the tube horizontally slightly tilted downward assists the flow of blood to enter the tube by capillary action until it reaches the fill line or three-quarter point.** Hold the tip of a gloved finger over the Hct tube to keep blood from flowing out. Obtain as many tubes as ordered, usually one or two. Avoid bubbles in the capillary tube.

6. Wipe the outside end of the glass tube with a gauze square while still holding it horizontally. Carefully seal *only one end* of the tube by placing it into the clay and turning it until the entire end is solid clay. **NOTE: Do not apply too much pressure or the glass tube will break.** Only a very small amount of clay is needed. You may leave the tube standing up in the tray until you are finished tending to the needs of the patient.

7. Have the patient hold a dry gauze square on the puncture site. **NOTE: Check to make sure bleeding has stopped.** Offer the patient a bandage.

8. Secure the sealed end of the tube against the rubber padding in the centrifuge (clay end of tube is always toward you). Balance the centrifuge with another tube opposite it. **NOTE: If two or more patients' tubes are placed in the centrifuge at the same time, make sure that you note the numbers of the spaces to avoid a mix-up. RATIONALE: Accurate identification is essential to assigning results to the proper patients.**

9. Close the inside cover carefully over the tubes, and lock it into place by turning the dial clockwise. Then close and lock the outside cover. Listen for it to click into place.

10. Turn the timer switch to 3 to 5 minutes. (Most timing switches indicate that you turn past the desired time and then back to the time you want set.) It will automatically turn off.

11. Wait until the centrifuge has completely stopped spinning and unlock both covers. (Opening a centrifuge before it stops spinning is very dangerous—centrifugal force pulls objects, such as hair, jewelry, or loose sleeves of lab coats, into it.)

12. Read the results by placing the bottom line of packed RBCs (red blood cells) (up to buffy coat but not including it) the against calibrated chart in the centrifuge where the tube is resting. (There is usually a magnifying glass attached to centrifuge to assist in reading Hct accurately.) Keep the cover of the centrifuge closed when not in use.

13. Discard used items in the proper waste receptacles, remove gloves, and wash hands.

14. Record the reading in the patient's chart and on the log sheet as a percentage.

15. Return items to the proper storage areas.

CHARTING EXAMPLE

4-21-XX

Finger stick of L ring finger for capillary blood for Hct— reading is 47%

S. Davis, RMA

padding or gasket, making certain that where the clay ends is at the "0" point of the reader. Read the hematocrit at the bottom end of the meniscus, although with most microhematocrit tubes, the meniscus is not obvious. Use of a magnifying lens to read the hematocrit is advised for accuracy in reporting the results. There are also microhematocrit readers that are not built within the centrifuge, but these are more complicated to use. Remember to measure both tubes and average the re-

sults for reporting. You can also roughly calculate what the hemoglobin for that patient may be by dividing the hematocrit value by 3; for example, a patient with a hematocrit value of 45% would have a hemoglobin of approximately 15 g/dL. Conversely you could take the hemoglobin value for a patient and multiply it by three for an estimate of the hematocrit value—for example, a hemoglobin of 12 g/dL should yield a result of 36% plus or minus 3% (refer to Table 15-1).

TABLE 15-1   Approximate Relationship Between Hematocrit, Red Blood Cell Count, and Hemoglobin in Adults

For Red Blood Cells of Normal Size—To Be Used for Checking Purposes Only*			For Red Blood Cells of Normal Size—To Be Used for Checking Purposes Only		
Hematocrit (%)	Red Blood Cell Count (×1 million per millimeter of blood)	Hemoglobin (in grams per 100 mL)	Hematocrit (%)	Red Blood Cell Count (×1 million per millimeter of blood)	Hemoglobin (in grams per 100 mL)
30	3.4	9.8	53	6.1	17.7
31	3.6	10.4	54	6.2	18.0
32	3.7	10.7	55	6.3	18.3
33	3.8	11.0	56	6.4	18.6
34	3.9	11.3	57	6.6	19.1
35	4.0	11.6	58	6.7	19.4
36	4.1	11.9	59	6.8	19.7
37	4.3	12.4	60	6.9	20.1
38	4.4	12.8	61	7.0	20.3
39	4.5	13.1	NORMAL HEMATOCRITS	NORMAL RED BLOOD CELL COUNTS	NORMAL HEMOGLOBINS
40	4.6	13.3	Men:	Men:	Men:
41	4.7	13.6	Range	Range	Range
42	4.8	13.9	40–54%	4,600,000–6,200,000	14.0–18.0 grams
43	4.9	14.2			
44	5.1	14.8	Aver. 47%	Aver. 5,400,000	Aver. 15.8 grams
45	5.2	15.1			
46	5.3	15.4	Women:	Women:	Women:
47	5.4	15.7	Range	Range	Range
48	5.5	16.0	37–47%	4,200,000–5,400,000	11.5–16.0 grams
49	5.6	16.2			
50	5.7	16.5	Aver. 42%	Aver. 4,800,000	Aver. 13.9 grams
51	5.9	17.1			
52	6.0	17.4			

*The relationship shown between hematocrit and red blood cell count is based on normal cells (which have an average mean corpuscular volume of 0.87). The relationship between hemoglobin and red blood cell count is based on normal cells (with a mean corpuscular hemoglobin of 29). These relationships do not hold true in cases of microcytic or macrocytic anemias, which probably will not be more than 5% to 10% of blood examined by clinical laboratories and blood banks.

AUTOMATION FOR HEMATOLOGY TESTING

There are several automated instruments on the market that are relatively inexpensive and easy to operate. These instruments have the capability of measuring more than simply the hemoglobin and hematocrit values; some of the parameters these instruments measure include:

- Total red blood cell count
- Total white blood cell count
- Total platelet count
- Hemoglobin
- Hematocrit
- Total granulocyte count
- Total lymphocyte and monocyte count
- Percentage of granulocytes
- Percentage of lymphocytes and monocytes
- Red blood cell indices

Many factors go into interpreting results from what is commonly known as the **complete blood count,** or CBC, one of the more common tests ordered in health care provider's offices. Refer to Figures 15-24 and 15-25, which show examples of automated hematology instruments. When a health care provider looks at the total red blood cell count, the hemoglobin, hematocrit, and indices are also considered for the big picture. Although the total white blood cell count is reviewed, the ratios or percentages of the granulocytes to the lymphocytes or monocytes is considered, since these cells protect the body in different

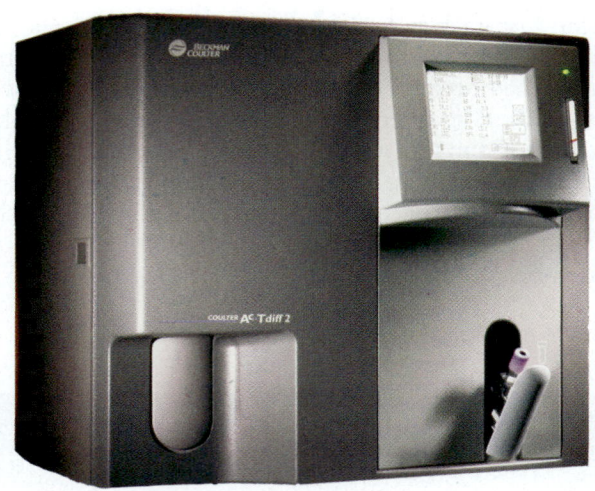

FIGURE 15-25 The COULTER ACT diff 2 uses a closed vial system with results of tests in less than a minute. A printed document is generated with a list of tests and results. *(Courtesy of Beckman Coulter)*

ways. Generally speaking, consider the following when reviewing a CBC:

- The normal total red blood cell count for an adult male is 4.5 to 6.0 million per millimeter. A decrease in the total number of red blood cells constitutes a type of anemia.
- The normal total red blood cell count for an adult female is 4.0 to 5.5 million per millimeter. A decrease in the total number of red blood cells constitutes a type of anemia.
- The normal total platelet count for males and females is 150,000 to 400,000 per millimeter.
- The normal total white blood cell count for males and females is 3,500 to 11,000 per millimeter. When the WBC count is elevated, it indicates a disease process of some type, whether it is an infection or precursor to leukemia. When the WBC is decreased, the patient could be immunocompromised due to HIV or AIDS infection or current cancer therapy in the form of chemotherapy or radiation treatments. When the WBC count is decreased, the patient is more prone to opportunistic infections since immunity is compromised.
- The granulocyte ratio should be larger than the lymphocyte/monocyte ratio. The normal percentage range for granulocytes is 50% to 70% with the lymphocyte/monocyte percentage generally in the 20% to 40% range.

Recall Chapter 11, Unit 8, on the Circulatory System and the blood. Remember that:

- The red blood cells are filled with hemoglobin, making their primary function delivering oxygen to the cells and picking up carbon dioxide to be exhaled.

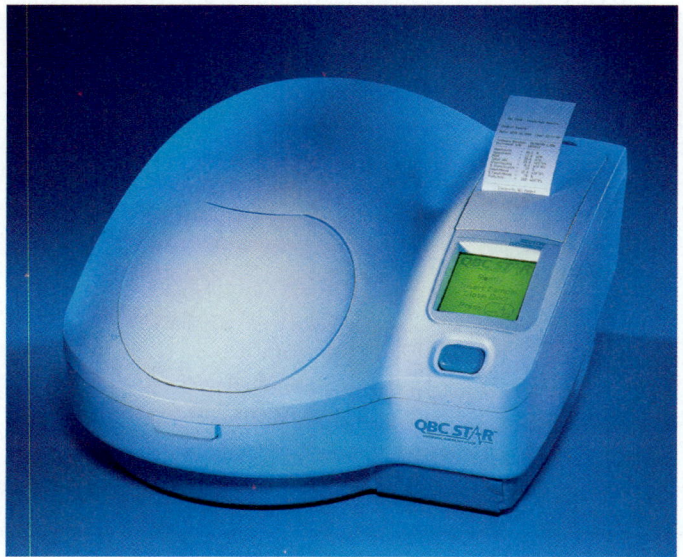

FIGURE 15-24 The QBC STAR offers efficient and accurate point-of-care testing in hematology. *(Courtesy of Becton, Dickinson, and Company)*

- The chief function of the white blood cells is to protect the body against invaders such as bacteria and viruses. The granulocytes engulf bacteria and debris, as do the monocytes. The lymphocytes produce antibodies against specific antigens, usually viruses.
- The platelets, with other clotting factors, stop bleeding when an injury occurs.

THE WBC DIFFERENTIAL

The WBC **differential** is a count that is performed on 100 white blood cells and differentiates the various types seen in that representative sample. The numbers of neutrophils, eosinophils, basophils, monocytes, and lymphocytes are counted, and during this screening, the technician will review the slide for abnormalities of the red blood cells such as size and shape, referred to as **morphology**. Often there are premature white or red blood cells that will be seen on the differential slide that indicate disease processes, such as leukemia. Medical assistants are not trained to perform these counts, but it is useful for you to have an idea of what such a report entails. Refer to Figure 15-26 for an illustration of how cells become mature and how they appear upon maturity. Table 15-2 provides a specific description of the function of each of the cells counted in a WBC differential. In order for the differential count to be performed, a slide must be prepared and stained for examination under the microscope. Many laboratories use an automated slide preparer as well as an automated staining apparatus. Because the cells cannot be differentiated into their different categories without staining, laboratories will use either the Wright's stain or the Giemsa stain prior to reviewing the slides under the oil immersion lens of the microscope.

ERYTHROCYTE SEDIMENTATION RATE

The erythrocyte **sedimentation** rate is also known as the ESR or the sed rate. It is the rate at which red blood cells settle in a calibrated tube within a given time, ranging from 1 to 2 hours, depending on the method used. This test is not a true diagnostic test, but instead gives the health care provider an idea of how much inflammation is occurring in a patient's body in response to another disease condition. The basis of the test is that certain proteins in the blood become altered in disease processes that in turn allows for the red blood cells to stick together and thus become heavier, settling at a higher rate of speed than would normally occur.

Some of the indications in which the ESR would be helpful in the assessment of the patient's condition include:

- Acute infections
- Acute inflammatory processes
- Chronic infections
- Rheumatoid arthritis or autoimmune disorders
- Temporal arteritis and polymyalgia rheumatica
- Monitoring inflammatory and malignant diseases

There are also conditions in which there is inflammation but the ESR does not increase. An example of one of these conditions is *sickle cell anemia*; the red blood

TABLE 15-2 Categories of White Blood Cells and Their Functions

White Cell Type	Percent in Normal WBC	Function
Granulocytes		
Neutrophils		Phagocytosis and killing of bacteria; release of pyrogen that produces fever
Segmented	56 ± 10	
Band	3 ± 2	
Eosinophils	2.7 ± 2	Phagocytosis of antigen-antibody complexes; killing of parasites
Basophils	0.3 ± 1	Release of chemical mediators of immediate hypersensitivity
Lymphocytes	34 ± 10	
B lymphocytes		Humoral immunity; production of specific antibodies against viruses, bacteria, and other proteins
T lymphocytes		Cell-mediated immunity including delayed hypersensitivity and graft rejection; regulation of immune response
Monocytes	4 ± 3	Phagocytosis of microorganisms and cell debris; cooperation in immune response

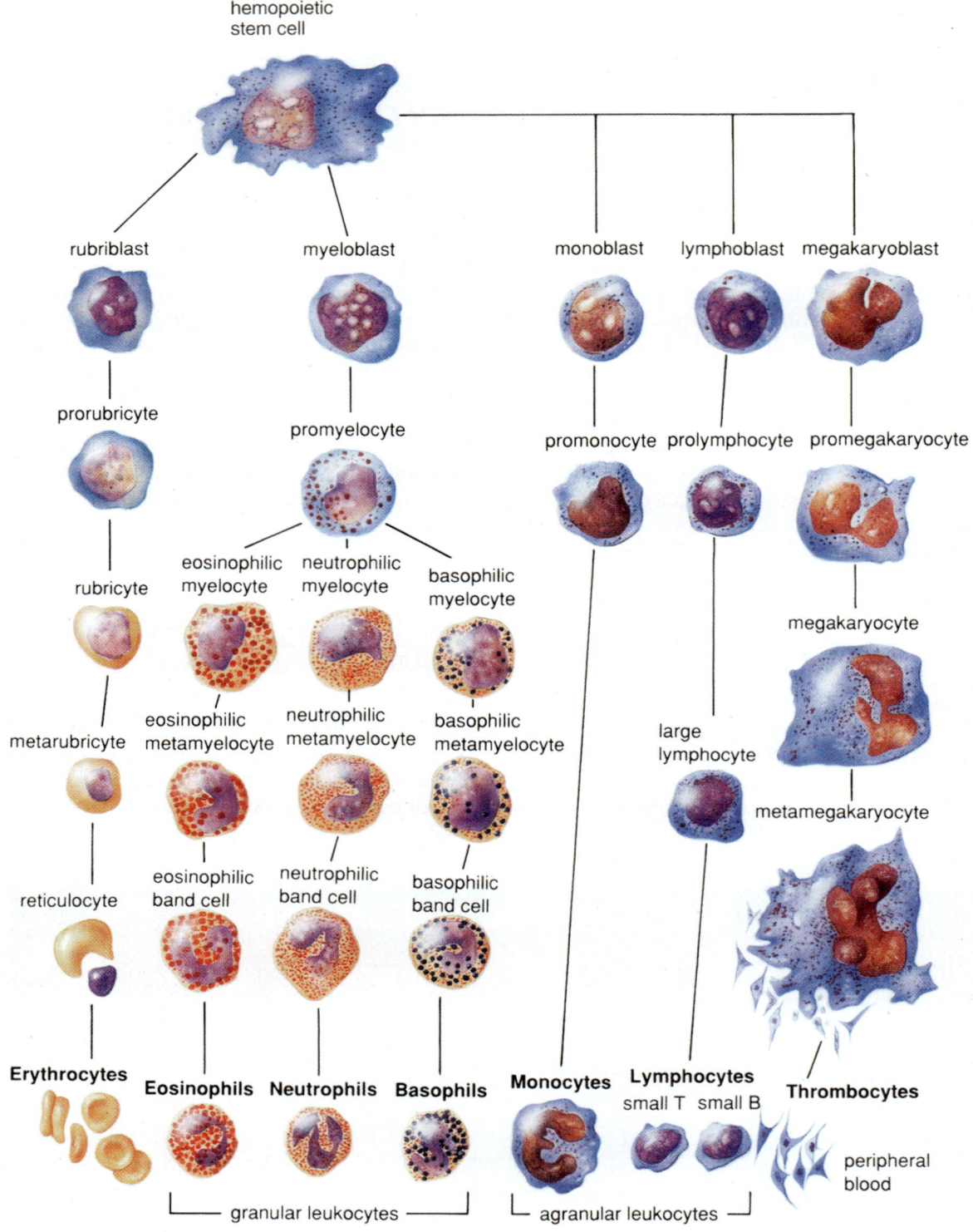

FIGURE 15-26   Blood cells and platelets from stem cell to maturity

cells are not shaped in their normal biconcave disk shape but are abnormally formed in such a way that they appear curved. Because of this shape, the red blood cells cannot form the *rouleaux* pattern where the cells stack upon one another, thus resulting in a low ESR value. Another example is *polycythemia vera* or *secondary,* in which the body produces too many cells, leaving little plasma for the red blood cells to fall through within the designated period of time for the test.

The two most common methods used for performance of the ESR are the Westergren (modified Westergren) and the Wintrobe methods. Figures 15-27 and 15-28 show the waived ESR test. The normal rate at which red blood cells fall is 1 millimeter every 5 minutes (1 mm/ 5 min). Depending on the method used for the testing, it is imperative that when recording the results, the method of testing is denoted when charting the results. It is also very important that the results be read at precisely the time at which the test is timed for conclusion. Reading the test before the designated time can yield a false negative result, and reading the test after the designated time could yield a false positive result. Commonly, female patients have higher ESR rate readings than males; a normal ESR rate value for a female is 0 to 20 mm/hr, while for men the normal is 0 to 10 mm/hr. Review Procedure 15-8 for performing an erythrocyte sedimentation rate.

GLUCOSE TESTING

Typically, capillary blood samples are used in medical practices to screen the blood glucose level of diabetic patients. These tests are simple to perform, relatively painless, and provide quick results. This type of testing utilizes a hand-held meter with specially designed reagent strips to which the blood sample is directly applied. There are many types of meters, known as *glucometers* or glucose meters (Figure 15-29), that are available for use that give reliable results.

SEDIPLAST® **ESR SYSTEM** is easy to use:

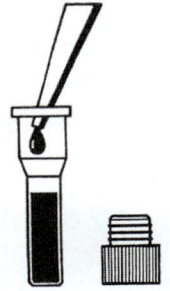

1 - Remove the stopper on the pre-filled vial, and fill to the indicated line with blood. Replace stopper and invert several times to mix.

2 - Insert the pipette through the pierceable stopper, and push down until the pipette touches the bottom of the vial. The pipette will autozero the blood, and any excess will flow into the closed reservoir compartment.

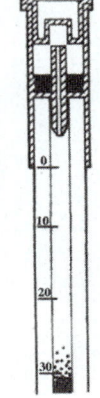

3 - Let the pipette stand for one hour, and then read the numerical results of the ESR.

Normal values		Specifications	
Male (under 50)	0–15 mm/hr	Overall length	200 mm
Male (over 50)	0–20 mm/hr	Graduations	0–150 mm
Female (under 50)	0–20 mm/hr	Bore Size (I.D.)	2.55 mm
Female (over 50)	0–30 mm/hr	Uniformity of Bore	± 0.05 mm

FIGURE 15-27 SEDIPLAST ESR System instructions *(Courtesy of Polymedco, Inc.)*

PROCEDURE PROCEDURE PROCEDURE PROCEDURE PROCEDURE PROCEDURE PROCEDURE

15-8  Perform an Erythrocyte Sedimentation Rate (ESR)

PURPOSE: To measure the rate of fall of red blood cells within a prescribed time.

OSHA GUIDELINES: To comply with Standard Precautions, gloves must be worn when there is a possibility of coming into contact with blood or body fluids.

EQUIPMENT: Goggles or face shield, gloves, prefilled vial, calibrated sed rate pipette, EDTA tube with patient's blood, sed rate stand, flat work surface, timer, patient's chart or laboratory report form, and blue or black pen.

PERFORMANCE OBJECTIVE: Provided with all of the necessary supplies as listed above, demonstrate the steps required in the procedure for performing a sed rate with the instructor observing each step.

1. Assemble all supplies at the flat work surface.

2. Don gloves and goggles or face shield before uncapping the EDTA sample.

3. Remove the stopper on the prefilled vial; fill to the indicated line with blood. Replace the stopper on the prefilled vial and invert several times to mix.

4. Insert the pipette through the pierceable stopper, pushing down until the pipette touches the bottom of the prefilled vial.

5. Set the timer for exactly 1 hour if performing the Wintrobe method of testing; 2 hours if performing the Westergren method.

6. At the end of the 60 minutes, read the numerical results of the test, using the designation of mm/hr after the numerical reading.

7. Dispose of the testing materials in a biohazardous waste container.

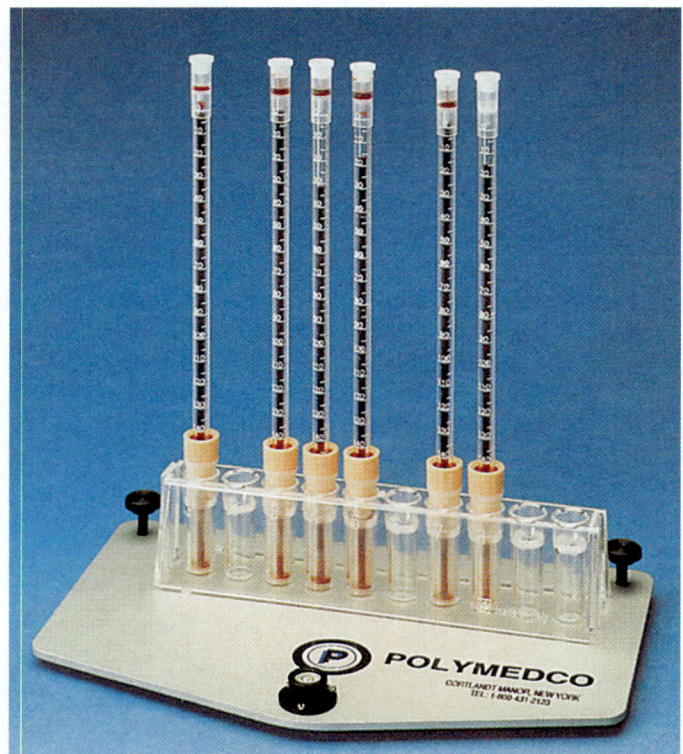

FIGURE 15-28 The SEDIPLAST Westergren sedimentation method is a completely closed system that provides safety for the user and reliable results *(Courtesy of Polymedco, Inc.)*

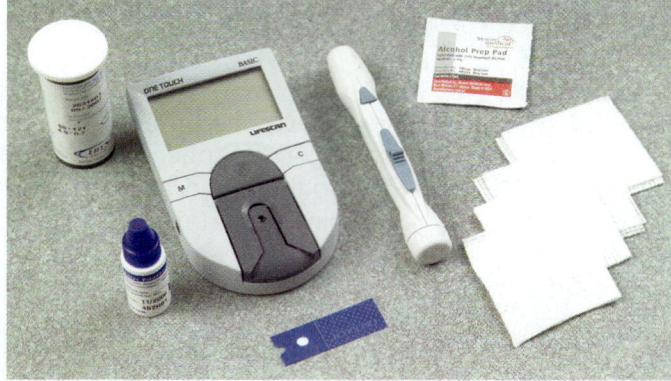

FIGURE 15-29 An example of a commonly available glucometer and supplies for glucose testing

Performing Quality Controls

Very important to the integrity of the results is for you to perform the quality controls at the beginning of each day and log the results prior to reporting any patient results. Also, if you have to open a new bottle of reagent strips during the day, you may need to calibrate the instrument, change the code to agree with what is printed on the bottle, and repeat the quality controls.

This helps to ensure that both the meter and the reagents are working properly so that you do not provide inaccurate results. You will find that many patients perform this testing at home to assist them in monitoring their blood sugars in case insulin adjustment is needed. Patients frequently bring their meters to the office for a printed report of the last 30 days, as shown in Figure 15-30. Some of the meters use a blood sample so small that instead of puncturing the finger, the patient punctures the forearm to obtain the specimen, and technology has accelerated to make these instruments much more common and affordable for home use. Procedure 15-9 provides general instructions for perfor-

---

PROCEDURE PROCEDURE PROCEDURE PROCEDURE PROCEDURE PROCEDURE PROCEDURE

15-9  Screen Blood Sugar (Glucose) Level

PURPOSE: To determine the sugar (glucose) level of the blood.

OSHA GUIDELINES: To comply with Standard Precautions, gloves must be worn if there is any possibility of coming into contact with blood or any body fluids.

EQUIPMENT: Sterile lancet, reagent strips, bottle (for color chart), glucometer, latex or vinyl gloves, cotton balls, alcohol, gauze squares, watch or clock, and facial tissue.

PERFORMANCE OBJECTIVE: Provided with all necessary equipment and supplies, and using other students as patients, demonstrate the steps required in the procedure for determining blood glucose levels. The instructor will observe each step.

1. Assemble all needed items on a Mayo table or comparable flat, steady surface. **NOTE: If a glucometer is to be used, make sure it has been turned on for the required time and has been calibrated for accuracy (follow instruction manual).**

2. Identify the patient and explain the procedure. **RATIONALE: Speaking to the patient by name and checking the chart ensures that you are performing the procedure on the correct patient. NOTE: If test is to be for a fasting blood sugar level, be certain the patient has not had anything by mouth for the past 8 to 12 hours.**

3. Wash hands and put on latex or vinyl gloves. **NOTE: As you converse with the patient during his scheduled appointment, be sure to inquire about medications (both prescription and OTC), any home remedy that has been taken, and his diet, and record all information on the patient's chart. Most diabetics are encouraged to keep a record (or diary) of their daily routine of medicines, blood glucose readings, nutritional intake, and exercise, especially if one's condition has been unruly. Reporting this information to the physician is valuable in assessing the patient's condition and plan of treatment because there are substances that can affect the accuracy of the readings of some blood glucose monitors.**

4. Follow the desired skin puncture procedure.

5. Open the reagent strip bottle and take one of the plastic strips out without touching the chemically treated pads. **RATIONALE: Touching the reagent strip may alter the results.** Reclose the bottle.

6. Apply a large drop of blood from the patient's finger so that pad is completely covered.

7. Begin timing *immediately* (**STAT**) for *exactly* the amount of time specified by the manufacturer. Give the patient a dry gauze square to hold over the puncture site after wiping it with an alcohol-saturated cotton ball.

8. Wait for instrument to display the results. The number displayed is the blood glucose level.

9. Discard all used items in the proper receptacle, remove gloves, and wash hands. You should perform a capillary puncture for a glucose reagent strip from an FBS (fasting blood sugar) sample, unless otherwise ordered by the health care provider.

10. Record the result in the patient's chart (e.g., 98 mg/dL of blood, initial). Refer to charting example.

11. Record in the log book the lot number and the expiration date of the reagent test strips.

LOG BOOK EXAMPLE

Date	Patient's Name	Test	Results	Obtained by
6-12-XX	Mark J. Stanford	FBS	98 mg/dL	S. Davis, RMA

glucose reagent strips Lot #875913-42 Exp 9/30/XX

CHARTING EXAMPLE

6-12-XX

Finger stick of L great finger for capillary blood for FBS—reading is 98 mg/dL of blood.

S. Davis, RMA

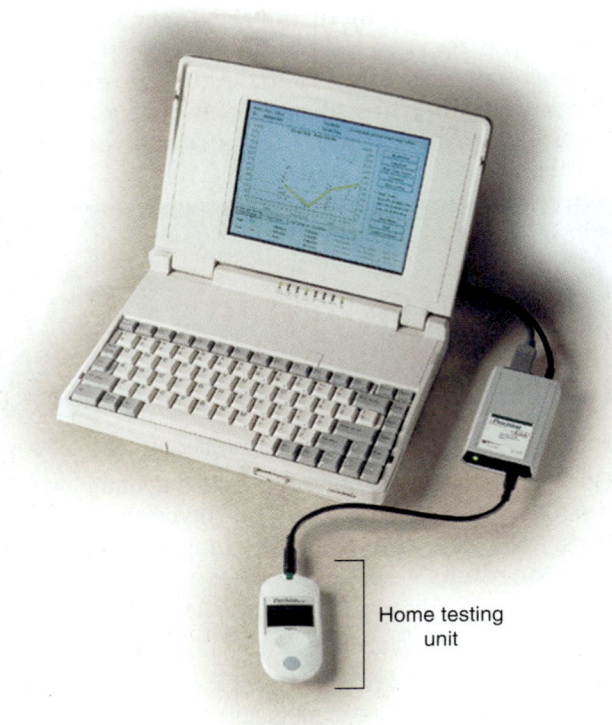

FIGURE 15-30 The Precision Link Blood Glucose Data Management System provides the patient with a simple glucose meter that stores up to 125 readings. At the patient's next office visit, it is attached to the computer for a graph of those results to be displayed on the monitor as well as being printed for the patient's chart. *(Courtesy of Abbott Diagnostics)*

mance of a blood sugar test. Remember, there are many different types of meters on the market, so you will need to check the manufacturer's instructions prior to testing.

Glucose Tolerance Test

The reported normal fasting blood glucose range varies; however, if you learn that 70 to 126 mg/dL is an average range for a fasting specimen, you will be able to determine the correct range on an examination. Remember what the term *fasting* means that the patient has had nothing to eat or drink for at least 12 hours prior to having the test drawn. Patients frequently ask about the term fasting; it should be emphasized that they should not eat mints, chew gum, drink coffee or juices, or smoke. However, many providers will permit their patients to sip a small amount of water to take their medications. Always be sure to ask the patient if they have adhered to the requirement prior to taking the sample.

When a patient has a consistently high fasting blood sugar (FBS), the next test usually ordered is the *glucose tolerance test,* or GTT. There are basically two reasons for this test to be ordered: diagnosis of diabetes mellitus or

hypoglycemia. This test determines the patient's ability to metabolize a glucose (carbohydrate) load within a prescribed amount of time. Figure 15-31 displays various types of readings and their indications.

If you are administering this test, check with the health care provider and policy and procedure manual to see if urine specimens are to be collected with the blood samples; this used to be common practice, but the stress of the test and the timing has led many providers to believe that the urine tests do not have to collected. Before you begin the test, it is essential that you collect the fasting specimen. If the patient's fasting blood sugar is 150 mg/dL or above, do not administer the glucose load to the patient. Immediately inform the provider of the results and await further instructions; administering the glucose load could be very dangerous to the patient when the blood sugar is already this high. Timing for the collection of subsequent samples is critical; usually, 30 minutes after the glucose load has been ingested, a blood sample is collected. Following that ini-

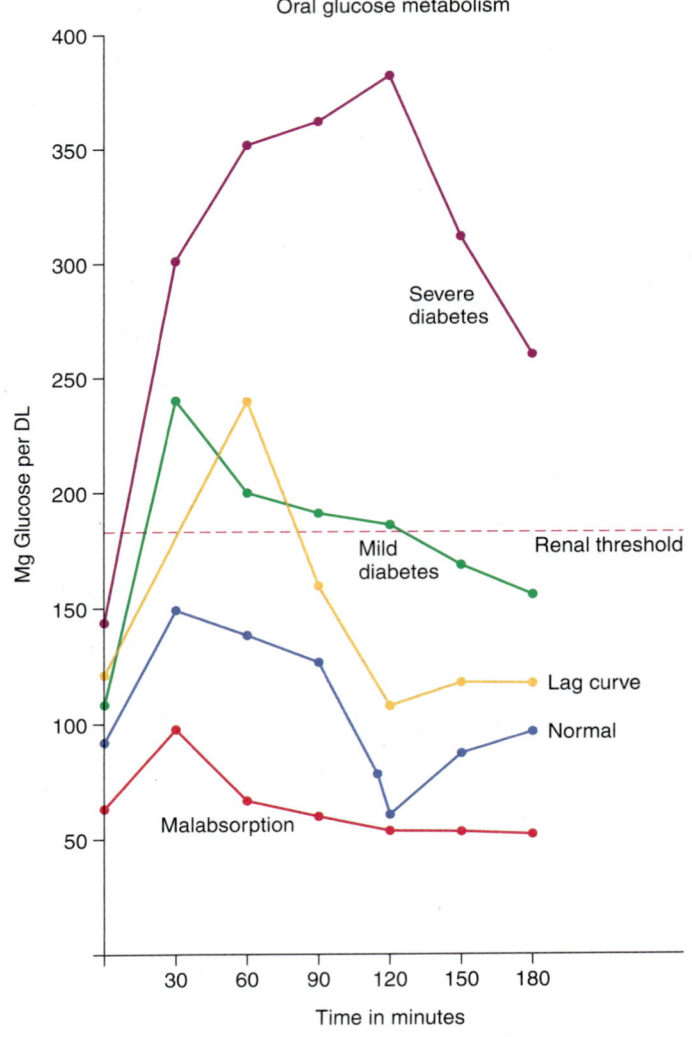

FIGURE 15-31   Graph of a 3 hour glucose metabolism

tial collection, another will be collected 30 minutes later, and then once every 60 minutes for the duration of the test. Figure 15-32 shows a typical GTT report form. If the patient becomes nauseated and vomits, the test must be discontinued and the provider informed.

A GTT is performed on many pregnant women to determine whether they have **gestational diabetes**. This test may be ordered at any time during pregnancy when there are symptoms that might be associated with dia-betes such as extreme thirst, visual difficulties, fatigue, weight loss, dehydration, and a high glucose reading. Women who have miscarried or have delivered very large babies are most at risk for having gestational diabetes. If the patient is a known diabetic, regular home glucose screenings will be ordered by the provider; in addition, frequent office exams and in-office glucose screening will be used to monitor the patient's condition to help prevent complications during the pregnancy.

DATE		PATIENT		ADDRESS	
GLUCOSE TOLERANCE TEST			HOURS		
TIME	BLOOD SUGAR	URINE SUGAR	ACETONE	PATIENT S CONDITION (SYMPTOMS)	
FASTING	mg/dL				
1/2 HR	mg/dL				
1 HR	mg/dL				
2 HR	mg/dL				
3 HR	mg/dL				
4 HR	mg/dL				
5 HR	mg/dL				
6 HR	mg/dL				
PHYSICIAN		PHONE		TECHNOLOGIST	

FIGURE 15-32 Laboratory report form for glucose tolerance test (GTT)

Hemoglobin A1C

Glycohemoglobin, or hemoglobin A1C (HbA1c), is a modified form of hemoglobin that is elevated when the blood glucose remains high. A capillary puncture helps to determine how the diabetic patient has been controlling the blood sugar during the last 2 or 3 months since the last office visit. This test is important in assessing the level of control the patient has had since the office visit. Hemoglobin A1C is the stable molecule that is formed when sugar and hemoglobin bond together, a process known as **glycosylation**. Very commonly, the provider will request a random blood sugar level with the HbA1C to fully assess the patient's compliance with the diabetic regimen.

PROCEDURE PROCEDURE PROCEDURE PROCEDURE PROCEDURE PROCEDURE PROCEDURE

15-10 Perform Hemoglobin A1C (Glycosylated Hemoglobin) Screening

PURPOSE: Evaluate diabetic patients' overall compliance with diet regimen for management of blood glucose levels.

EQUIPMENT: Sterile lancet, disposable gloves, other personal protective equipment (PPE) per laboratory policies, alcohol wipe, clean gauze or cotton balls, testing instrument, reagents, black or blue pen, biohazard waste container, and sharps container.

PERFORMANCE OBJECTIVE: Provided with the supplies listed above and a simulated patient chart, the student will perform a Hemoglobin A1C screening on a blood sample. The student must complete the procedure within 25 minutes, with the instructor observing each step, at a competency level pre-established by the instructor.

1. Assemble the necessary equipment and supplies; wash hands.

2. Identify the patient.

3. Provide an explanation of the procedure and equipment to the patient.

4. Don disposable gloves and other PPE as required.

5. Perform the capillary puncture and collect the blood sample per the manufacturer's directions for the instrument.

6. Record the results of the test on the patient's health record.

7. Check the patient's finger for excessive bleeding and provide a clean gauze or cotton ball, instructing the patient to apply pressure to the site.

8. Dispose of contaminated sharps in the sharps container and other contaminated materials in the biohazardous waste container.

9. Remove gloves and wash hands.

CHARTING EXAMPLE

Lafferty, Jerry B.
ID# 143896LA

07/27/XX	0855	Hemoglobin A1C	5%

Brooke Bourne, RMA

As a medical assistant, you are vital in reminding the diabetic patient to have regular eye examinations as well as paying specific attention to nutritional needs. It is also important for diabetics to report sores that do not heal and nerve pain since high glucose levels can exacerbate these problems. Nonhealing sores can lead to *necrosis* or *gangrene*, which may require amputation of the affected body part, so it is urgent for the patient to call in to report such a condition.

CHOLESTEROL TESTING

Cholesterol is a steroid normally found in the body; however, when cholesterol levels are over 200 mg/dL, this can cause *atherosclerosis* or *arteriosclerosis*, a hardening of the arteries. Also, if cholesterol levels stay elevated for an extended period of time, *plaque* can build up on the inside of the arteries, narrowing the size of the artery and not allowing blood to flow through normally. You have probably heard of *angioplasty*, a surgical procedure that allows a cardiac surgeon to go into an affected artery or arteries through the use of special instruments and remove the plaque by inflating a small balloon on the tip of the scope and dragging it along the arterial walls. There are several CLIA waived tests available on the market for screening cholesterol levels in the POL; one is a card that does not provide a specific number for the cho-

---

PROCEDURE PROCEDURE PROCEDURE PROCEDURE PROCEDURE PROCEDURE PROCEDURE

15-11  Perform a Cholesterol Screening

PURPOSE: Screen a cholesterol level for hypercholesterolemia.

EQUIPMENT: Sterile lancet, disposable gloves, other personal protective equipment (PPE) per laboratory policies, alcohol wipe, clean gauze or cotton balls, testing instrument (if indicated—some tests are done without an instrument), reagents, black or blue pen, biohazardous waste container, and sharps container.

PERFORMANCE OBJECTIVE: Provided with the supplies listed above and a simulated patient chart, the student will perform a cholesterol screening on a blood sample. The student must complete the procedure within 25 minutes, with the instructor observing each step, at a competency level pre-established by the instructor.

1. Assemble the necessary equipment and supplies; wash hands.
2. Identify the patient.
3. Provide an explanation of the procedure and equipment to the patient.
4. Don disposable gloves and other PPE as required.
5. Perform the capillary puncture and collect the blood sample per the manufacturer's directions for the instrument or the reagent card.
6. Record the results of the test on the patient's health record.
7. Check the patient's finger for excessive bleeding and provide a clean gauze or cotton ball, instructing the patient to apply pressure to the site.
8. Dispose of contaminated sharps in the sharps container and other contaminated materials in the biohazardous waste container.
9. Remove gloves and wash hands.

CHARTING EXAMPLE

Bennett, Anna
ID# 145709

1/7/XX	1050	Fasting cholesterol	156 mg/dL

Mary Adams, MA

PROCEDURE PROCEDURE PROCEDURE PROCEDURE PROCEDURE PROCEDURE PROCEDURE PROCEDURE

PROCEDURE

15-12  Screen and Follow Up Blood Test Results

PURPOSE: Screen and follow lab results for normal, abnormal, and panic values to relay information to the health care provider.

EQUIPMENT: Scenarios of simulated lab reports for examination and analysis, and reference materials supplied by the instructor (e.g., Internet, laboratory reference manuals, textbook, etc.)

PERFORMANCE OBJECTIVE: Provided with the supplies listed above and simulated laboratory reports for blood studies, the student will review the results and make notations as to whether the results are normal, abnormal, or panic value and follow up. The student must complete the procedure within 50 minutes, with the instructor observing each step, at a competency level pre-established by the instructor.

1. Screen the test results to determine whether they are normal, abnormal, or panic value.

2. Screen the test results to determine whether laboratory reports are missing any key elements.

3. Identify panic values, the disease state that may be a result of them, or the disease state that may be caused if left untreated.

4. Identify the appropriate action for panic values with the health care provider.

5. Identify the appropriate action for the abnormal values with the health care provider.

6. Identify the appropriate action for the normal values with the health care provider.

CHARTING EXAMPLE

Amick, Deborah Ann

ID# 27456123

08/03/XX   1802   Spoke with patient regarding low Hgb level per Dr.'s instructions. Phoned Rx into pharmacy for her to start immediately. Return 4 weeks for repeat hgb check.

Laura Treolo, RMA

---

lesterol level but a range. There are also instruments available that utilize the same technology as many of the glucometers for testing and provide a specific number for the cholesterol level. Cholesterol tests should be collected as a fasting specimen, so patients should be instructed to refrain from eating or drinking anything for 12 to 16 hours prior to the test. The cholesterol numbers considered "ideal" varies, ranging from 180 to 200 mg/dL. Your health care provider will establish the ideal level for the particular office and patients.

IMMUNOLOGY

Immunology is the study of the body's ability to prevent and fight off infection. While this sounds like a very detailed science, and indeed it is, tests have been developed that can be performed at the waived level to diagnose common diseases and illnesses. **Immunoassays** are the diagnostic tests that use techniques for measuring the amount of antigens and antibodies present relative to a specific illness.

Mononucleosis Testing

Infectious mononucleosis is an illness caused by the Epstein Barr virus (EBV); you may have heard it referred to as the "kissing disease" or "mono." This virus can be transmitted in other ways, but all transmissions involve contact with saliva. It is considered an extremely contagious disease, and it is most commonly found individuals between the ages of 10 and 25 years. EBV is related to the herpes virus and can be spread for a period of up to 6 months after initial contact and infection. The symptoms are similar to those of the flu, and the infection can affect the lymph nodes, throat, salivary glands, liver, and spleen; bed rest, good nutrition, and plenty of fluids are indicated for treatment of the viral infection. The presence of the virus remains throughout a patient's life, although the symptoms associated with mononucleosis usually do not recur. Testing for infection and subsequent antibody production is performed by a "monotest," a type of immunoassay that detects the presence or absence of the antibodies to EBV for diagnosis.

15-13  Perform a Screening for Infectious Mononucleosis

PURPOSE: To determine the presence (or absence) of antibodies to the Epstein-Barr Virus (EBV).

EQUIPMENT: Sterile lancet, disposable gloves, other personal protective equipment (PPE) per laboratory policies, alcohol wipe, clean gauze or cotton balls, quality control materials, reagents, black or blue pen, biohazardous waste container, and sharps container.

PERFORMANCE OBJECTIVE: Provided with the supplies listed above and a simulated patient chart, the student will perform an infectious mononucleosis screening on a blood sample. The student must complete the procedure within 25 minutes, with the instructor observing each step, at a competency level pre-established by the instructor.

1. Assemble the necessary equipment and supplies; wash hands.

2. Identify the patient.

3. Provide an explanation of the procedure and equipment to the patient.

4. Don disposable gloves and other PPE as required.

5. Perform the capillary puncture and collect the blood sample per the manufacturer's directions.

6. Perform quality control testing on two additional cards, one negative and one positive, while performing testing on the patient's sample. **NOTE: Control samples must only be run once per day or any time a new box of reagents has been opened.**

7. Records the results of the quality control analyses in the quality control log; do not report patient results if quality control results are not in the acceptable range.

8. Record the results of the test on the patient's health record.

9. Check the patient's finger for excessive bleeding and provide a clean gauze or cotton ball, instructing the patient to apply pressure to the site.

10. Dispose of contaminated sharps in the sharps container and other contaminated materials in the biohazardous waste container.

11. Remove gloves and wash hands.

CHARTING EXAMPLE

Thomas, Ronald
ID# TH09321-07
09/12/XX   1448   Monotest   Positive
                                    Kristina Frye, CMA

LOG BOOK EXAMPLE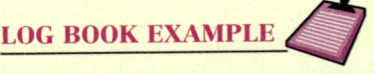

Date	Control Level	Control Lot #	Expiration Date	Reagent Lot #	Expiration Date	Results	Initials
09/12/XX	Positive	40589J	02/28/11	32159	04/25/09	Positive	dlr
09/12/XX	Negative	40593J	02/28/11	32159	04/25/09	Negative	dlr

Pregnancy Testing

Pregnancy tests are performed to measure the amount of **human chorionic gonadotropin** (hCG) in the urine or blood. Occasionally, testing may be ordered for hCG in the diagnosis of certain tumors, such as germ cell tumors originating in the ovaries or male testes, since hCG or a similar substance may be produced by these tumors. Normally, hCG is produced by the placenta during pregnancy, which helps to maintain the pregnancy and normal development of the fetus. Levels of hCG show a steady increase in the first 14 to 16 weeks following fertilization.

Home pregnancy tests and screening tests in most POLs are performed on a urine specimen, ideally a first morning specimen since that specimen will be the most concentrated. Although the quantity of hCG cannot be determined, the test will indicate if hCG levels have exceeded the nonpregnant levels. The simple urine tests commonly employ either a "plus" (+) mark that displays upon completion of the test or two lines that are similar to an "equals" (=) sign. A single line (−) indicates the patient is not pregnant or that the level of hCG is undetectable (Figure 15-33). When obtaining a specimen from a patient in the provider's

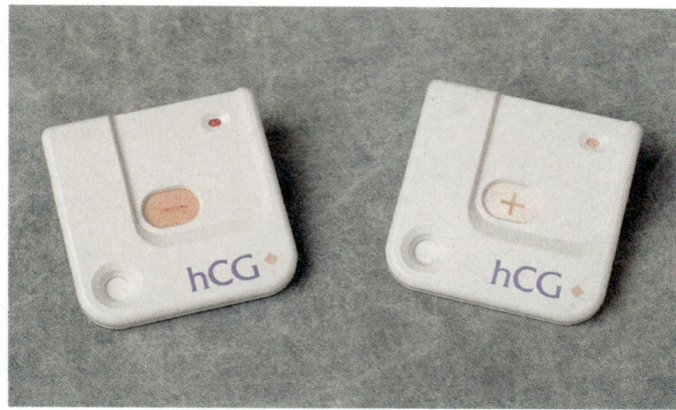

FIGURE 15-33   In simple urine tests, a plus sign or equals sign commonly signifies a patient is pregnant, while a single line or minus sign signifies the patient is not pregnant or the level of hCG is undetectable.

office, ask when the last menstrual period (LMP) occurred and document this on the patient's chart. The blood test is a more accurate test than the urine test and will provide a quantitative result that indicates how long the woman has been pregnant and give an idea of when the fetus will be due for delivery. This test also is tracked to make sure the fetus is developing at a normal rate for those women who have had problem pregnancies or miscarriages in the past and can be used to assist in the determination of ectopic pregnancies.

Allergy Testing

Allergy tests are another type of immunology testing found in certain offices such as otorhinolaryngologists' (ENT) offices or allergy specialists. There are basically three types of direct allergy tests performed:

1. *Skin prick test.* The allergen (the substance to which the patient is suspected for allergy) is applied directly to the patient's skin and scratched or pricked into the epidermis. The areas of application are observed for reaction from antibodies, usually as a reddening of the area with itching.

2. *Intradermal injections.* This test is more sensitive than the skin prick test. A small amount of the allergen is injected between the epidermis and dermis with an observation of the area for a reaction. Usually reactions occur immediately, although patients may be instructed to return 24 to 72 hours later for delayed responses to the allergen.

3. *Skin patch test.* An allergen-soaked pad is placed on the surface of skin for 24 to 72 hours to observe for a reaction.

In certain cases, the *radioallergosorbent test* (RAST) is indicated, as some individuals cannot tolerate the skin tests; this test determines the presence of immunoglobulins (IgE among others) that are present in greater amounts in those with allergies. This test is not as specific as the specific allergen applications.

Testing for HIV

Another type of immunology testing includes testing for **human immunodeficiency virus** (HIV), which can result in **acquired immunodeficiency syndrome** (AIDS), a tragic disease in which the body can no longer fight off any type of infection. The first stages of the infection mimic the flu or mononucleosis with fatigue, slight fever, aching, lymph node swelling (lymphedema) and tenderness, and weight loss. There are rapid tests available for home use that detect the antibody to HIV; the results are generally available in 30 minutes. The standard screening tests are *enzyme immunoassays* (EIA), which take approximately a week for reporting of the results. Depending on the office in which you are assigned for your externship or employed, you may be drawing blood specimens for this screening. Always remember to follow policy and procedure for collection and follow Standard Precautions—treat all patients as if they are or could be infected with HIV or hepatitis to protect yourself and others.

PKU TESTING

A screening test done with capillary blood from in infant's heel is the **phenylketonuria** (PKU). Phenylketonuria is a congenital disease caused by a defect in the **metabolism** of the amino acid **phenylalanine**. This unmetabolized protein accumulates in the bloodstream and can prevent the brain from developing normally. If this condition goes undetected and untreated, the result is mental retardation. This screening is required in all states and Canadian provinces, most commonly by the blood test but occasionally with a urine specimen. The blood test requires that a few drops of the infant's blood be soaked through the outlined circles (from the back of the card) of the treated paper attached to health department's requisition (Figure 15-34). The requisition is a multi-part form that must be completed accurately and fully; usually the parents bring the form with them when they return with the infant for the testing. Upon completion of the requisition form and collection of the specimen, the form and the PKU testing card is to be mailed to the state health department for processing. Most often this test is done in a hospital or larger clinic facility setting, but you may be requested to perform this test in a pediatrician's office. Refer to Figure 15-35 for correct and incorrect specimen samples.

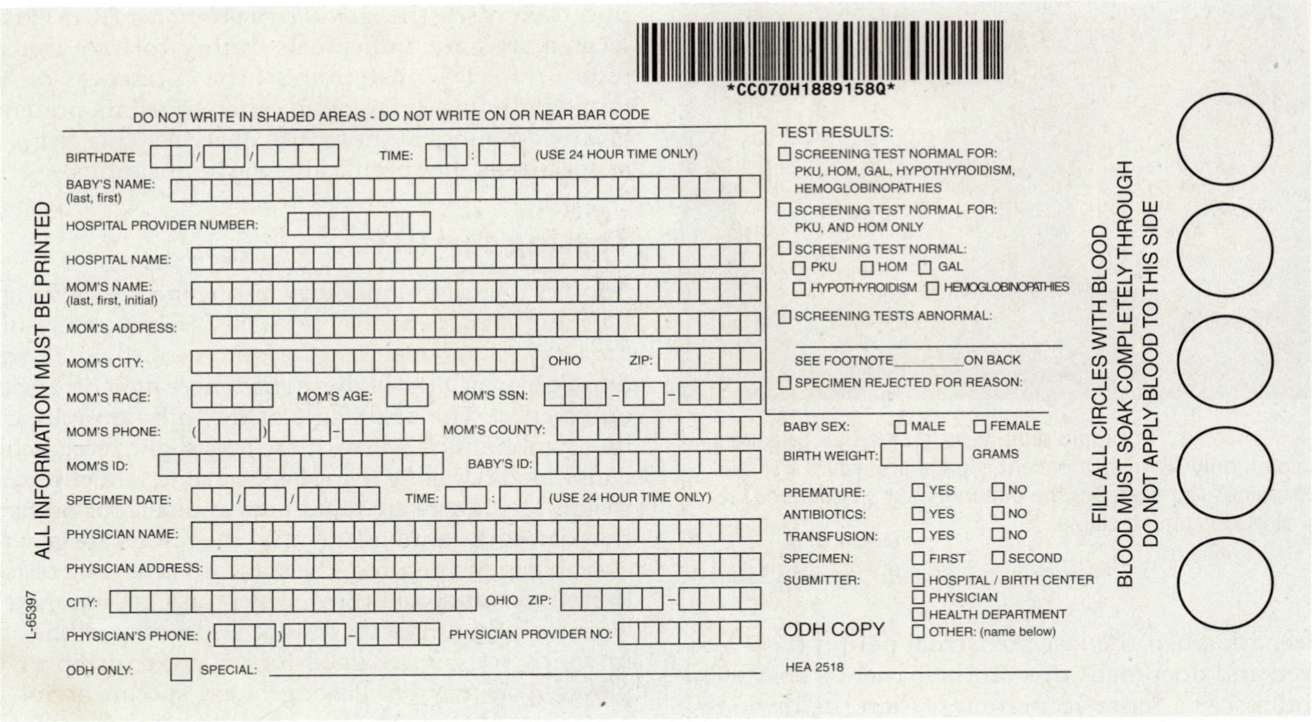

FIGURE 15-34 PKU blood test form

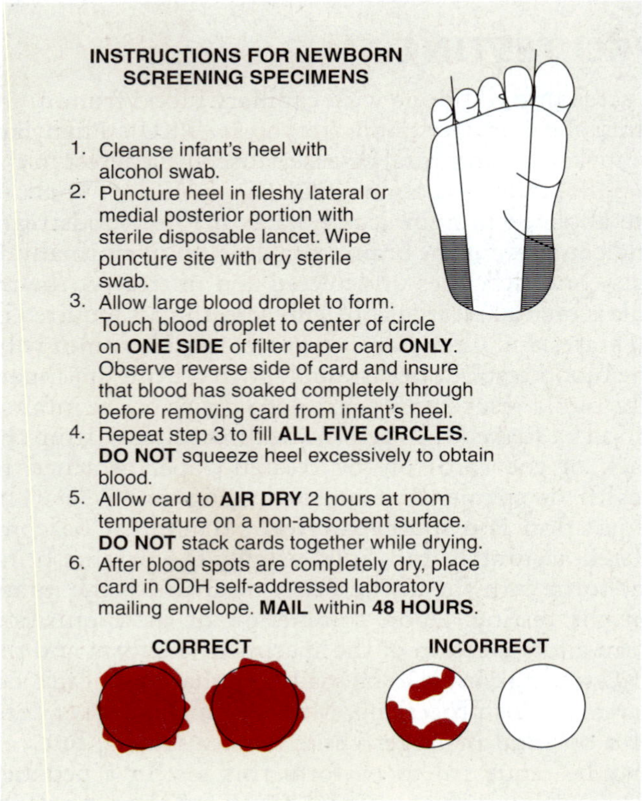

FIGURE 15-35 Instructions for completion of information and examples of properly and improperly completed slides

URINE SPECIMENS

Urinalysis is probably the most frequently performed test in the medical office. Examination of the urine consists of the major areas of testing: **physical**, **chemical**, and microscopic (Figure 15-36).

Specimens for urinalysis are usually collected in plastic disposable containers, either nonsterile or sterile, depending on the type of specimen indicated for testing (Figure 15-37). The following should be

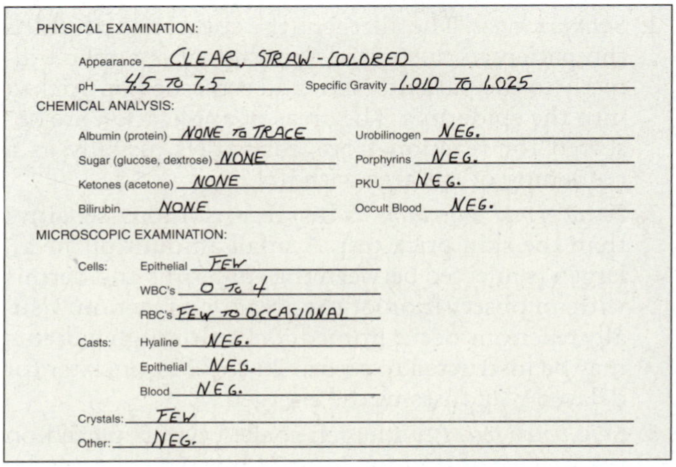

FIGURE 15-36 Lab report form showing normal values for a routine urinalysis.

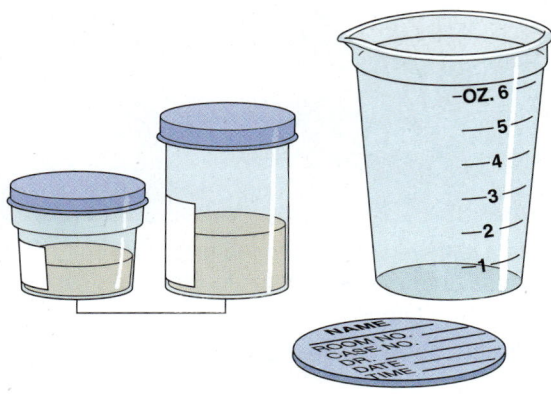

FIGURE 15-37 Plastic disposable urine specimen containers with identification labels and lids

noted on the container: patient's name, date of collection, time of collection, and test(s) to be performed on the specimen. Ideally any testing should be performed within 1 hour of collection to prevent decomposition of the specimen due to bacterial overgrowth and cellular breakdown. If the specimen cannot be tested within the 1-hour time frame, the specimen must be refrigerated to preserve its integrity; just as important is that when testing is to be performed on the refrigerated specimen, the specimen must be allowed to return to room temperature and stirred well prior to any analysis, whether it is physical, chemical, or microscopic.

First Morning Urine Sample

The first morning urine sample is the best for testing because it is the most concentrated specimen since the urine has been in the bladder overnight. However, most often health care providers order random specimens that most patients have little difficulty in providing; random means that the specimen is not scheduled and requires no advance preparation. Many providers prefer for the specimens be collected as midstream clean-catch specimens, and for this type of specimen you must be able to provide adequate instructions for compliance. Patients should be instructed to use the provided antiseptic wipes to cleanse the genital area from front to back in a single motion and discard, whether they are male or female. Women need to be instructed to gently spread the labia during the cleansing and during the collection of the specimen. In the case of the male patient, instructions need to be provided to those who are not circumsized that the foreskin must be retracted prior to the area being cleansed. If the male is circumsized, the antiseptic wipes are to be used as described above, in a single front to back motion and discarded, for three wipes.

After this step of the procedure, the patient should be instructed to:

- Not touch the inside of the sterile specimen container nor the inside of the lid
- Void partially into the commode and stop
- Collect the middle portion of the specimen in the cup and stop (usually about three ounces)
- Finish voiding into the commode
- Replace the lid on the container, wipe any residual urine from the outside of the container, and either return the container to you or place it in a designated spot

The partial voiding before collection of the specimen clears the urethra of contaminants such as bacteria, mucus, cells, or other debris that could adversely affect the results. This step helps to provide a more sterile specimen so that if a culture of the urine is indicated, the specimen will be less likely to be contaminated. (Refer to Procedure 15-14).

24-Hour Urine Specimen

On occasion, a 24-hour urine specimen will be ordered. A written laboratory order will be given to the patient, and either you or a laboratory technician will be responsible for providing the instructions for collection to the patient. It is essential that you provide instructions that the patient can understand for proper collection of this specimen, and printed instruction sheets are most helpful for this. The patient will be provided with a container in which to collect the sequential specimens over the 24-hour period; it is up to you to check the lab manual to see if a preservative needs to be added to the container or other special instructions need to be provided. In some cases, the patient simply needs to refrigerate the specimen the entire length of the 24-hours prior to submitting the specimen to the laboratory for testing. A difficult concept for patients to grasp is the timing of the specimen; the patient begins the timing of the 24-hour period at the first void of urine on the first day, although this specimen is not collected as part of the total specimen.

Following this void (of which the patient needs to document the time), the patient collects all urine specimens and places those in the collection container until the 24-hour period is over. Any specimen voided after the 24 hours is over should *not* be collected; as soon as convenient for the patient, the container should be returned to the laboratory or hospital for testing. Depending on the test being performed, the health care provider may receive results in as little as a day or results may take several days before being reported.

PROCEDURE PROCEDURE PROCEDURE PROCEDURE PROCEDURE PROCEDURE PROCEDURE

15-14

Instruct a Patient on the Collection of a Clean-Catch Midstream Urine Specimen

PURPOSE: To instruct a male or female patient in the proper collection of a clean-catch midstream urine specimen to prevent contamination of the urine sample.

EQUIPMENT AND SUPPLIES: Computer, printer, paper, sterile container, antiseptic wipes, disposable gloves, pen, and label for container.

PERFORMANCE OBJECTIVE: Provided with the supplies listed above, the student will prepare a written brochure for instructing both a male and female patient in the collection of a clean-catch, midstream urine specimen. After instructing the patient in the collection of the specimen, the student will provide the container to the patient for collecting the specimen, following Standard Precautions. The student will have 25 minutes for completion of the collection (not including preparation of the brochures).

1. Student will prepare the printed brochures for instructing male and female patients in the proper collection of urine specimens.

2. The instructor will review the brochures for accuracy in instruction, grammar, spelling, and punctuation prior to the student giving to the patient.

3. Assemble supplies to provide to the patient.

4. Instruct the patient for the collection as outlined in the brochure. See if the patient has any questions prior to the collection.

5. Provide the patient with the sterile cup labeled with the patient's name, identification number, the date, and the time, as well as the antiseptic wipes. Direct the patient to the restroom.

6. Collect the specimen from the patient upon exit from the restroom, observing Standard Precautions in handling the specimen.

Pediatric Urine Specimens

Pediatric urine specimens are another type of specimen collection that may be encountered in pediatrician or family practice offices. Special urine collection bags fit over the genital area of the baby and are secured with adhesive (Figure 15-38). The infant's skin should be washed and dried thoroughly, usually by the parent, prior to the bag being affixed to the skin; otherwise, the bag will not remain in place for the collection of the specimen. Once the pediatric bag is returned to the office, it is necessary to transfer the contents to a container. The parent(s) need to provide the baby's name as well as date and time of collection before processing; parents should also be advised that if the specimen cannot be returned to the facility prior to 1 hour following collection, the specimen should be refrigerated to protect its integrity and accuracy of results.

Urinary Catheterization

Catheterization is a specialized type of urine collection that is indicated in the following instances:

- A sterile specimen is indicated for testing
- The patient is unable to void
- Medication needs to be instilled into the bladder

When catheterization is ordered, the procedure includes the introduction of a sterile plastic tube into the bladder; catheters can be straight, which means they are used only for a short-term basis, or in-dwelling when they remain for a longer period of time (e.g., Foley catheters). This procedure is not performed routinely in most offices, although you may encounter it in urology offices and even sometimes in obstetrics and gynecology offices. Generally the urologist will perform the catheterization. Many times a culture and sensitivity (discussed later in the chapter) will be ordered on the specimen because there may be an infection causing the patient to be unable to void. If you are in an office where catheterization is performed often, your primary role will probably be one of assisting the health care provider. Remember that catheterization is a *sterile* technique, and contamination of any part of the catheterization kit is unacceptable. Severe bladder infections can occur with compromise of the sterile technique required for this procedure.

PHYSICAL URINALYSIS

Included in the physical testing of the specimen are the following:

- Color
- Clarity

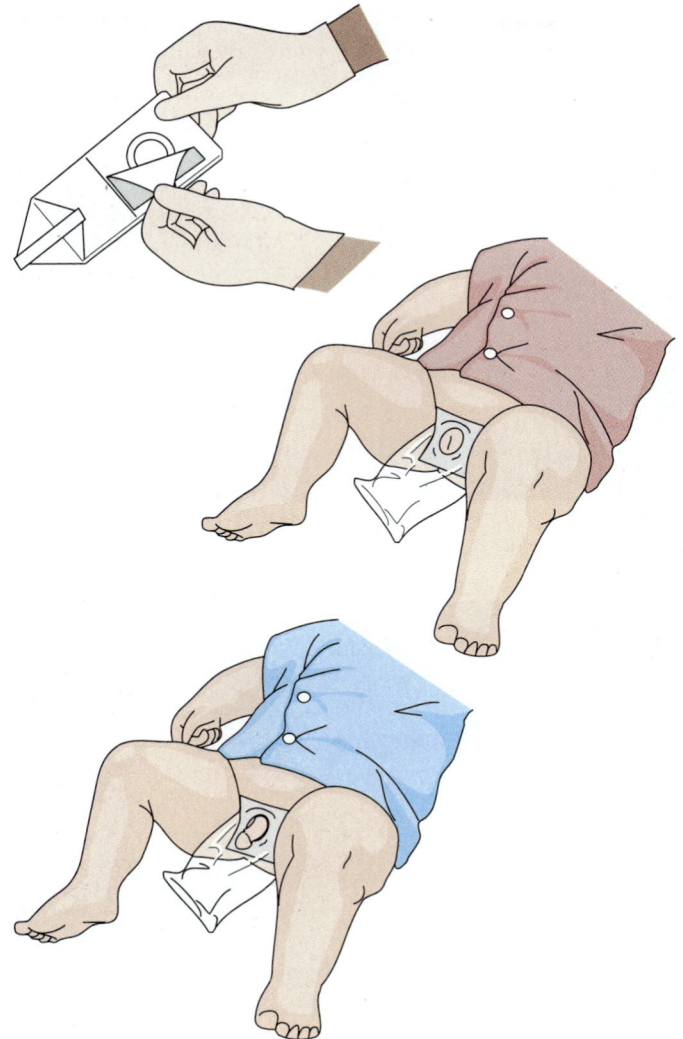

FIGURE 15-38 Example of a pediatric urine collection unit in the proper position

- Volume (in certain specimens)
- Odor (although not reported on lab report form)
- Specific gravity

Color and Clarity

Standard color descriptions include yellow, and straw, dark straw, light straw, light yellow, and dark yellow; occasionally colors will be described as red (blood), brown (old blood), orange (pyridium), green (jaundice), and blue (certain medications). The clarity of a specimen refers to how clear it is; therefore, standard clarity descriptions include clear, slightly hazy, hazy, cloudy, and turbid. The most accurate way to describe color and clarity is to decant (pour) the specimen into a clear tube so that the opaqueness of the collection container does not adversely affect your analysis of these properties. If you can easily read print through the tube containing the specimen, the description would be clear; a few particles floating around in the specimen would be slightly hazy. If the print is fuzzy, the specimen would be described as hazy, and if you cannot see the print at all, the specimen will be described as cloudy or turbid, with turbid being the worst description.

Volume

Twenty-four hour urine specimens must have the volume assessed, although only a representative sample is submitted to the laboratory for testing; it is unnecessary to assess the volume of a routine urine specimen for testing.

Odor

The odor of a specimen can provide you with insight as to what abnormal condition the patient may have; for instance, if you notice a very strong ammonia-like smell, it probably indicates a urinary tract infection (UTI) from the presence of bacteria. A mousy or musty odor is associated with phenylketonuria, while a fruity smell is linked to diabetes from the presence of ketones. Although you will not record the odor of a specimen on the report form, these particular odors are helpful in confirming findings as you perform the testing. Keep in mind that certain foods, garlic in particular, may emit a strong odor that will not indicate a pathologic condition.

Specific Gravity

Specific gravity, defined as the weight of substances dissolved in a substance as compared with those found in distilled water, once were assessed as a physical process, either through the use of a urinometer or a refractometer. However, the chemical reagent strips now include this parameter, resulting in offices no longer assessing the specific gravity as a physical property but rather as a chemical property. You should keep in mind that the specific gravity of water is 1.000 to 1.003, and the normal range of the specific gravity of urine is 1.005 to 1.030, with most urine results falling in the 1.015 number. The more dilute the specimen (the more water and less dissolved substances in the specimen), the lower the specific gravity will be. Conversely, more substances in the specimen with less water results in a higher specific gravity. Remember we are comparing the specimen with distilled water, a substance that should not have anything dissolved in it and that is considered relatively pure and without any solutes.

CHEMICAL URINALYSIS

Urine specimens should be analyzed as soon as possible after collection; in the event that more than an hour has transpired and the specimen has been refrigerated, be sure to allow the specimen to return to room temperature and gently mix it before testing as constituents will settle to the bottom. Also, because specimens with bilirubin can become degraded due to exposure to light, it is important that all specimens be collected in an opaque container so that false negative results for this are not reported.

Reagent strips are convenient, relatively inexpensive, reliable, and quick and serve to reveal the presence of abnormal substances in the urine as well as assess other numerical values such as pH, urobilinogen, and specific gravity. The reagent strips provide both qualitative and quantitative assessments. Qualitatively, the strips will reveal the presence of an abnormal result, and quantitatively, they determine how much of a substance is actually present in the specimen. The specially treated pads on the reagent strip are designed in such a way that the specific pad will react chemically with the urine to produce a color change. After the color change, the strip is compared with known values on the bottle for reporting (Figures 15-39A and B). These reagent strips can be used in a manual method where the per-

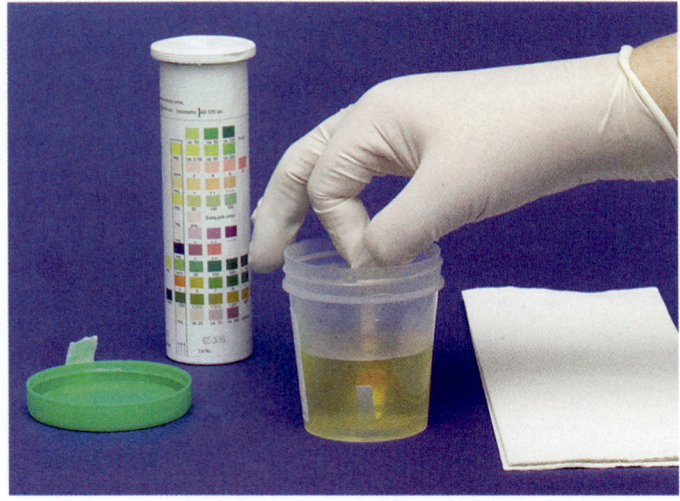

FIGURE 15-39A The reagent strip is immersed into the urine.

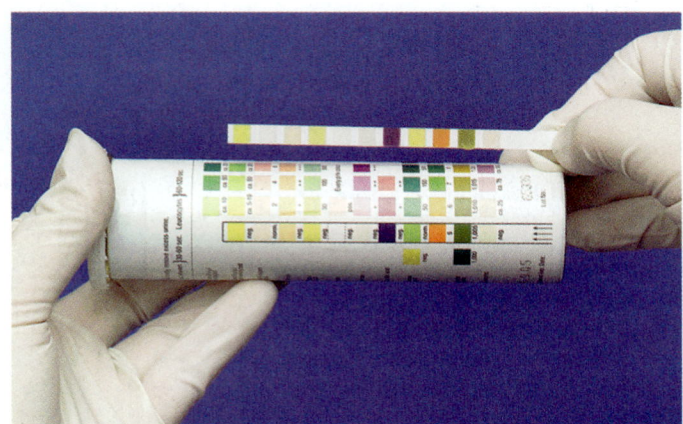

FIGURE 15-39B Compare the reagent strip with the color chart of known values on the bottle.

son performing the test views the strip and reports the color change as a result at the appropriate time, or instruments are available that will read and print out the results when the strip is inserted into the instrument (Figure 15-40). The instruments must be checked daily with quality control and trends that show the instrument may need calibration, cleaning, or new reagent strips. These results must be recorded in a log each time they are checked as part of the quality assurance program. The following indicates some or all of the analytes that may be checked either manually or with the use of an instrument: glucose, protein, ketone, bilirubin, urobilinogen, blood, nitrate, pH, leukocyte esterase, and specific gravity.

Fresh urine specimens should be used, and when testing manually, it is imperative that exact timing of each of the analytes be employed. You should have adequate lighting for reading the color changes on the

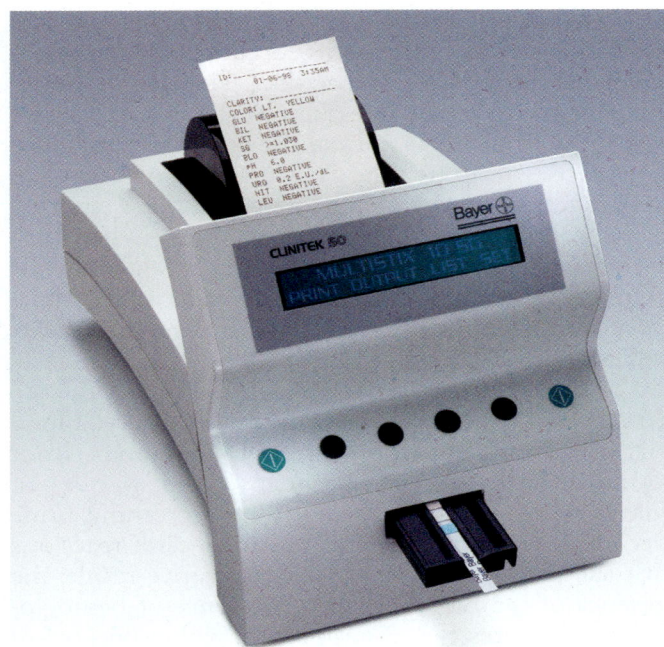

FIGURE 15-40   The Clinitek 50 urine chemistry analyzer
(Courtesy of Bayer Diagnostics)

strips as well as color vision to allow you to differentiate color changes on the pads. If no change is seen after the pads have been dipped in the specimen and the appropriate time has elapsed, the result is reported as negative. However, remember that specific gravity, pH, and urobilinogen always have number designations associated with them; for those other pads that change, you must compare the pads to the strip bottle and consult with your supervisor or policy and procedure manual to see how abnormal results are reported.

Proper handling of the reagent strips includes protecting them from light, capping them tightly once a strip has been removed, and protecting them from exposure to moisture. Unless manufacturers' instructions state otherwise, reagent strips should be stored at room temperature, not in the refrigerator. Be certain to check the expiration date on the bottle; when testing patient specimens, it is unacceptable procedure to use expired strips for reporting results. Additionally, many reagent strip bottles indicate that they should not be used 60 days after the bottle is opened; it is imperative that the person opening the strips record that date, and the date needs to be monitored. Using the strips after 60 days will exceed the open vial **stability**, which can affect the accuracy of the testing.

There are many companies that manufacture urine test strips, as well as those that manufacture the strips to be used with instruments to read the results. Many of the instruments provide standardized readings of reflectance photometry with a printout for the patient's record.

Normal and Abnormal Values

pH   The normal pH for urine is 5.0 to 7.0; remember the pH scale: anything less than 7.0 is acid in nature, 7.0 is neutral, and readings above 7.0 are alkaline. Urine should be slightly acidic to combat bacteria, since bacteria do not like acidic environments; therefore, the majority of urine specimens analyzed should be in the 5.0 to 6.5 range (Figure 15-41).

Protein   **Protein (albumin)** is a substance that should not be normally found in urine specimens; one of the functions of the tubules in the nephrons of the kidneys is to reabsorb the protein for the body. In cases of kidney disease or infection, protein may be found in the specimen; depending on the circumstances, this can be a very important indicator of kidney disease or failure. Most laboratories require that a *confirmatory* test be done so that a result is not reported erroneously; in this case, the confirmatory test is the sulfosalicylic acid (SSA) test. The SSA test *precipitates* albumin (a protein) in a measurable visual state for reporting purposes; if the SSA is negative, this confirmatory test will override the results of the reagent test. If the confirmatory test shows the presence of albumin, consult the practice's policy and procedure manual for reporting the results. Protein may be found in specimens of renal failure as well as specimens in which urinary tract infection (UTI) is found (bacteria are protein-based, thus resulting in the increased levels of protein). Also, increased protein levels can be found in cases of blood in the urine from injury, infection, or menstruation since red blood cells are composed of protein. Thus, there are many causes of protein presence in the urine, and it is up to you to be discriminating in reporting the results and their follow up.

Ketone   **Ketone (acetone)** bodies are not normally present in urine specimens; ketonuria indicates that fat has been broken down and metabolized in the digestive

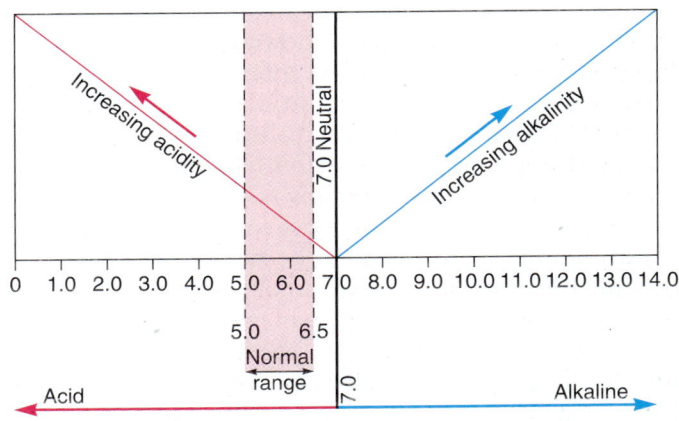

FIGURE 15-41   Scale of pH for urine

tract. Urine specimens with ketone bodies present are described as having a fruity odor, something you may notice when you uncap the specimen for testing. Ketones may be found in the following conditions: uncontrolled diabetes mellitus; diet high in fat; starvation (anorexia); and wasting of the body from other disease conditions. Patients that are restricted in their caloric intake for weight loss may have ketone bodies in their urine, but in this particular instance, this is a desirable presence because it indicates that their bodies are burning fats, resulting in weight loss. Many POLs and hospital laboratories require a confirmatory test for this result on the chemical reagent strip; the most common confirmatory test utilized is the Acetest®, in which a drop of urine is applied directly to a tablet, the test is timed, and the results are reported according to comparison with a color chart included with the reagent tablets. Follow the policies and procedures of the office or laboratory for performing and reporting the confirmatory test. When elevated levels of ketones are found in the urine specimen, it is termed ketonuria.

Bilirubin

Bilirubin is a pigment that is yellow to orange in color and is the result of the liver's degradation of hemoglobin. Part of the liver's function within the circulatory system is to "recycle" red blood cells by removing them from circulation after approximately 120 days (unless they are damaged, in which case they are removed sooner) and using parts of these cells to build new blood cells. However, in patients who have liver damage or disease such as tumors, hepatitis, or cirrhosis, bilirubin may be found in the urine. Many times, bilirubin can be detected in a urine sample before the patient exhibits traits such as jaundice and ascites.

Characteristically, a urine specimen from a patient with hepatitis will have an orange to greenish coloration, and if the specimen is shaken, it will have a green foam. Besides taking care to protect yourself from this virus, *all* urine specimens need to be protected from light, as this will cause bilirubin to break down and go undetected. Consider babies who are born with or develop jaundice immediately following birth—how is the bilirubin broken down in the infant? The baby is exposed to an ultraviolet light in order to degrade the bilirubin so that the body will reabsorb it. In most laboratories the presence of bilirubin is confirmed by another diagnostic test since many false positives are seen with the reagent strips. The most common test used for confirmation is the *Ictotest®*; the test is performed by placing 10 drops of urine on an absorbent mat, applying a tablet to the top of the pad, adding two drops of water, and timing the test to report the results. If the mat shows a bluish to purple color, the results are positive; if the mat shows a pink to red color, there is no bilirubin in the specimen and these results will override the results of the reagent strip.

Urobilinogen

Urobilinogen is a normal by-product of hemoglobin degradation that occurs in the intestines by normal intestinal flora (bacteria). The chemical reaction that occurs in the intestines by the normal flora is what gives stools their normal brown color. Urobilinogen is excreted through the intestines, and most laboratories require that when reporting, a number is reported with the units expressed in *Ehrlich* units. When urobilinogen is found excreted in the urine in high levels, it often indicates that the liver or gallbladder are dysfunctional as well as being indicative of spleen and heart problems.

Hematuria

Hematuria is the presence of red blood cells or hemoglobin in the urine. Hemoglobin is not normally found in urine specimens except in cases of women who are menstruating. When screening urine specimens, there are three different types of reactions with the reagent strip that yield a positive result: the presence of red blood cells; the presence of hemoglobin; and, the presence of *myoglobin*, a globin released in cases of extensive muscle injury. If the reagent strip detects any of these substances as a positive result, the confirmation of results is done by way of a microscopic examination of the specimen. Even then there could be a positive blood result but no red blood cells seen in the urine because the tested substance is hemoglobin released from the red blood cells; also, if myoglobin is present from muscle injury, nothing will be seen on microscopic examination. This is why microscopic examinations are designated for those specifically trained for making these types of distinctions.

Nitrite

Nitrite is present in urine samples that have increased numbers of microorganisms, namely bacteria. Normally, urine is considered a sterile fluid excreted from the body; however, in cases in which bacteria have invaded, nitrates are reduced to nitrites **in vivo**. Urine specimens that have a high number of bacteria will have a characteristic smell of ammonia; remember that urine specimens that are left out at room temperature for longer than an hour encourage bacterial growth, so it is imperative that if a urine specimen cannot be tested within an hour that the specimen be refrigerated to prevent this overgrowth of bacteria from occurring and giving a false positive result. As bacteria change nitrate to nitrite, these microorganisms will also ingest glucose and cellular elements and excrete protein, all of which could be misinterpreted in diagnosing and treating the patient. Confirmation of bacteria, *bacteriuria*, in the urine is achieved by microscopic examination as well as culture and sensitivity, discussed later in this chapter.

Leukocyte Esterase

Leukocyte esterase is commonly checked with other analytes on the reagent strip. This test detects esterase, an enzyme released by white blood cells when significant numbers of these cells are present in a fluid. When a health care provider reviews symptoms of the patient as well as the results of the chemical analysis, particularly if nitrites are positive also, a diagnosis of a urinary tract infection may be made. Confirmation of the presence of white blood cells (leukocytes) is done by microscopic examination. *Pyuria* is the term used when white blood cells are found in the urine specimen in increased numbers.

Glucose

Glucose is a substance that is not normally found in urine samples. The reagent strip that tests for the presence of glucose is specific to that sugar specifically; bear in mind that other sugars exist and can be excreted by the body, such as fructose (fruit sugar), lactose (milk sugar), and galactose (also a milk sugar). Glucose in a urine specimen indicates that the *renal threshold* has been exceeded. Think back to Chapter 11 on the urinary system and recall that the nephrons are responsible for reabsorbing glucose (sugar), as this is the body's major nutrient. When the glucose level in the blood is greater than what the nephrons can reabsorb, the result is for glucose to "spill over" into the urine, a condition known as *glycosuria* or *glucosuria*. Different patients will have different renal thresholds; some may have low thresholds in which glucosuria will result if the blood sugar exceeds 130 mg/dL. In other patients, the renal threshold may be as high as 200 mg/dL before glucose will be detected in the urine. Normally, the renal threshold is established at 180 mg/dL, meaning that if the blood glucose level exceeds 180 mg/dL, the overage of glucose will be secreted in the urine. At one time, it was common practice for diabetic patients to check their urine specimens for glucose; however, this practice is no longer commonly used for controlling diabetes. Also, remember that technologic advances with home blood glucose meters make it very easy and relatively painless for patients to check their blood sugars, thus providing more accurate results and interpretation of their results. The only confirmatory test for the presence of urine glucose is checking the blood glucose due to variances in renal thresholds.

Specific Gravity

Specific gravity is a complex concept for many people to grasp. When specific gravity was first measured as part of the urinalysis, it was considered a physical examination, as the measurement was made through the use of a refractometer or a urinometer. However, with scientific advances, reagent strips now measure this. Specific gravity gives us an indication of how concentrated or how dilute a specimen is. Let us examine once again how specific gravity is based—distilled water provides the basis. Distilled water should have no particles dissolved in it; it should be pure. The specific gravity of distilled water is 1.000 + 0.003 (you should memorize this value for certification/registration exams). Since urine should have some dissolved substances in it, the specific gravity of urine will be higher than the value established for distilled water. Values for the specific gravity of urine range from 1.005 to 1.030, with most specimens falling in the range of 1.010 to 1.025. The higher the specific gravity reading, the more dissolved substances are present, and the lower the reading, the less dissolved substances are present, with more fluid. This can be very important in patients with dehydration as well as those patients suspected to have diabetes insipidus, a condition in which large amounts of very dilute urine are excreted by the body. A good indicator of specific gravity can be the color of the urine: If the specimen is a very light yellow or straw, chances are that the specific gravity will be low. Conversely, if the specimen has more of a medium straw to darker straw or yellow color, there will probably be more dissolved substances and a higher specific gravity. Review the steps of Procedure 15-15 for chemical testing of urine specimens using a reagent strip.

MICROSCOPIC EXAMINATION OF URINE

According to CLIA '88, medical assistants may not read or interpret results of microscopic urine sediments; however, preparation of the urine specimen may be requested of the medical assistant for another to view the slide and report the results. Refer to Procedure 15-16 for proper preparation of urine sediment for microscopic analysis.

You should be familiar with some of the microscopic require that may be reported in the sediment of a urine specimen; some of these elements require immediate attention for pathologic conditions. Figure 15-42 displays common microscopic elements found and reported in urine sediment. Usually, red blood and white blood cells are reported in increments of five; bacteria and epithelial cells are quantitated as rare, few, moderate, or many or slight, 1+, 2+, 3+, 4+; mucus is identified as slight, moderate, or much.

Remember that each laboratory has its own reporting system, so familiarize yourself with each lab. Following are guidelines for normal values:

- *WBCs:* females, 10 to 20/hpf; males, 0 to 10/hpf
- *RBCs:* females, 5 to 10/hpf (unless on menstrual period); males 0
- *Epithelial cells:* few to moderate (epithelial cells are not seen as often in male patients)
- *Bacteria:* none to slight (remember urine is considered a sterile body fluid)

PROCEDURE PROCEDURE PROCEDURE PROCEDURE PROCEDURE PROCEDURE PROCEDURE

15-15  Test Urine with Multistix® 10 SG

PURPOSE: To detect *p*H, protein, glucose, ketones, blood, bilirubin, urobilinogen, leukocytes, and specific gravity in urine.

OSHA GUIDELINES: To comply with Standard Precautions, gloves must be worn if there is any possibility of coming into contact with blood or any body fluids.

EQUIPMENT: Multistix® 10 SG reagent strips, fresh urine specimen, disposable gloves, watch or other timepiece, tongue depressor, patient's chart, pen, and adequate lighting to read color chart on reagent bottle (for accurate test results, use strips before the expiration date on the bottle).

PERFORMANCE OBJECTIVE: Provided with all necessary equipment and supplies, demonstrate the steps required to perform the procedure for using Multistix® 10 SG. The instructor will observe each step.

1. Wash hands, put on gloves, and assemble all needed items on a cleared counter.

2. Stir the urine with a tongue depressor to evenly distribute solutes throughout the specimen.

3. Remove the cap from the bottle, and take out one reagent strip without touching the test paper end. Place the cap securely back on bottle. **Note: Study times are given on the bottle for reading each test section.**

4. Dip the test paper end of the reagent strip into the urine specimen. With the reagent side of the strip down, pull it across the inside of the specimen container opening to remove excess urine. **Rationale: If the strip is too saturated, treated test paper chemicals will run together and make results inaccurate.**

5. a. Place the reagent strip next to the color chart on the bottle by holding the bottom of the bottle in your left hand and the strip by your right thumb and index finger.

   b. Read the results by comparing the color of the reacted reagent strips with the color chart on the bottle.

   c. Place the bottle on its side, and hold it at the bottom with your left hand.

   d. Hold the reagent strip in your right hand with your thumb and index finger, and line it up with the color chart on the bottle.

   e. Read the test results from the bottom to the top in order of shorter to longer timings. Proper timing is essential for accurate results.

6. Begin timing tests immediately. **Note: The scale below is in the same order as the reagents on the strip and on the color chart on the bottle when properly aligned and observed from left to right.**

   2 minutes—leukocytes
   60 seconds—nitrite
   60 seconds—urobilinogen
   60 seconds—protein (albumin)
   60 seconds—pH
   50 seconds—blood
   45 seconds—specific gravity
   40 seconds—ketone
   30 seconds—bilirubin
   30 seconds—glucose (quantitative)
   10 seconds—glucose (qualitative)

7. Discard the used reagent strip, gloves, and other disposables into the proper receptacle. Wash hands. Return Multistix® 10 SG to the proper storage area.

8. Record the results as indicated for each section on the patient's chart and in the log book. Refer to the charting example.

LOG BOOK EXAMPLE

Date	Patient's Name	Number	Test	Sent	Results	Filed by
7-17-XX	Marcene Mitchell BD 8-8-63	7539	UA Clinitek	7-17-XX	large amount of leukocytes	J. Watkins, CMA

CHARTING EXAMPLE

7-17-XX

Clean-catch urine specimen from Marcene Mitchell tested with Clinitek 50 shows clear yellow urine positive for leukocytes, all other tests negative.

J. Watkins, CMA

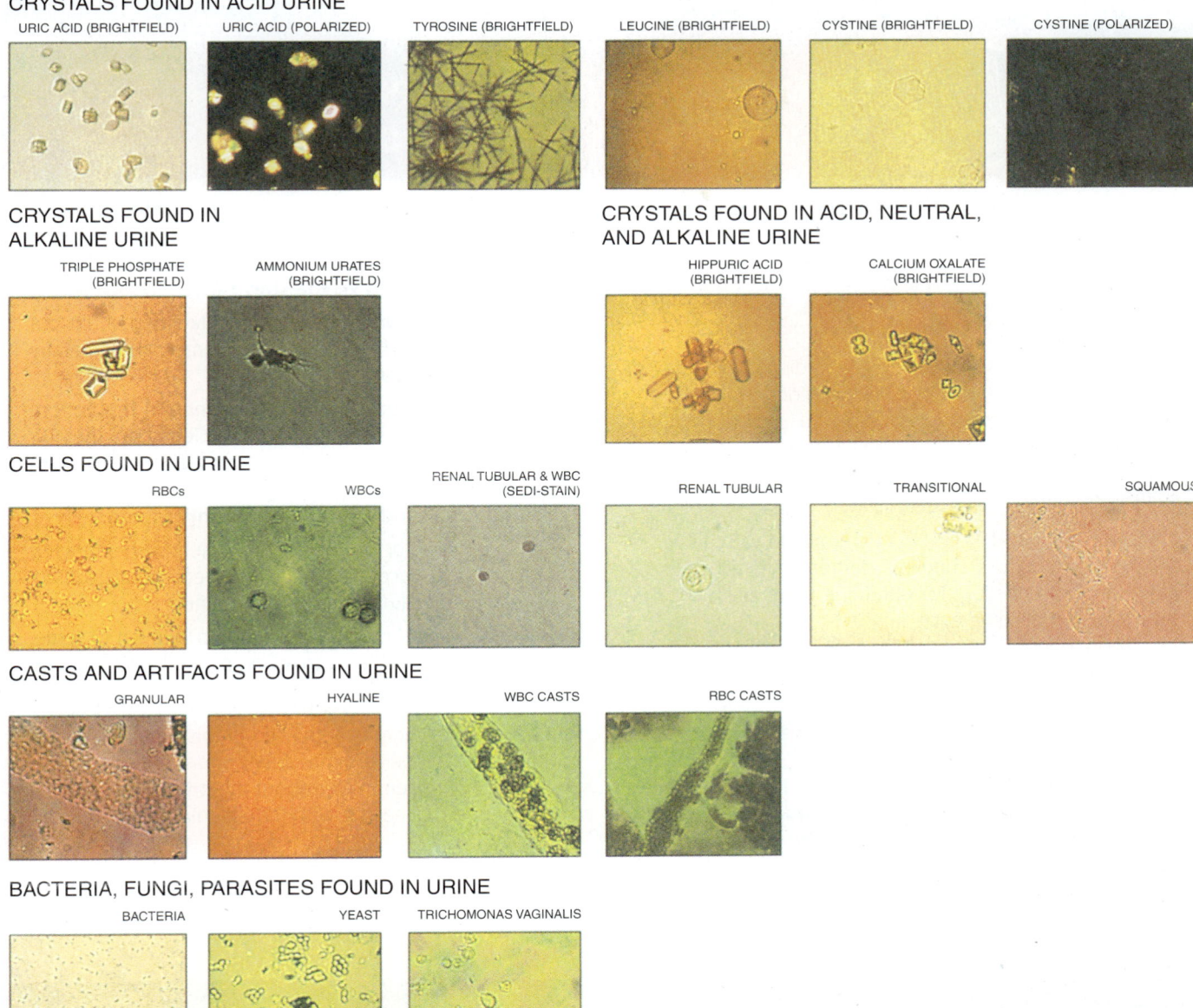

CRYSTALS FOUND IN ACID URINE
URIC ACID (BRIGHTFIELD) URIC ACID (POLARIZED) TYROSINE (BRIGHTFIELD) LEUCINE (BRIGHTFIELD) CYSTINE (BRIGHTFIELD) CYSTINE (POLARIZED)

CRYSTALS FOUND IN ALKALINE URINE
TRIPLE PHOSPHATE (BRIGHTFIELD) AMMONIUM URATES (BRIGHTFIELD)

CRYSTALS FOUND IN ACID, NEUTRAL, AND ALKALINE URINE
HIPPURIC ACID (BRIGHTFIELD) CALCIUM OXALATE (BRIGHTFIELD)

CELLS FOUND IN URINE
RBCs WBCs RENAL TUBULAR & WBC (SEDI-STAIN) RENAL TUBULAR TRANSITIONAL SQUAMOUS

CASTS AND ARTIFACTS FOUND IN URINE
GRANULAR HYALINE WBC CASTS RBC CASTS

BACTERIA, FUNGI, PARASITES FOUND IN URINE
BACTERIA YEAST TRICHOMONAS VAGINALIS

FIGURE 15-42 Crystals, cells, and casts found in urine sediment *(Courtesy of Bayer Diagnostics)*

- *Mucus:* slight
- *Spermatozoa:* indicative of pathologic state in men; should not be reported in females except in rape cases, and then only under legal authority, as it could be perceived as an invasion of privacy
- *Trichomonas:* indicative of infection, not seen in males as often as females
- *Yeast:* presence of budding yeast indicates infection with *Candida albicans*
- *Crystals:* certain crystals may appear in urine specimens without indication of disease, as they are formed as a result of diet. For instance, calcium ox-

alate crystals may seen in those individuals that have high caffeine intake. Other crystals identified in specimens without pathology include triple phosphate, amorphous urate or phosphate, and uric acid. Crystals that indicate disease include cholesterol, tyrosine, cystine, leukocine, and sulfa.

- *Casts:* hyaline casts may be seen in specimens without indication of disease. However, casts reported as finely granular, coarsely granular, WBC casts, RBC casts, mixed cell casts, waxy, or fatty casts are indicative of a serious kidney (renal) problem and require immediate attention by the health care provider.

PROCEDURE PROCEDURE PROCEDURE PROCEDURE PROCEDURE PROCEDURE PROCEDURE PROCEDURE

15-16  Obtain Urine Sediment for Microscopic Examination

PURPOSE: To obtain urine sediment to determine microscopic contents of urine.

OSHA GUIDELINES: To comply with Standard Precautions, gloves must be worn if there is any possibility of coming into contact with blood or any body fluids.

EQUIPMENT: Fresh urine specimen, disposable latex or vinyl gloves, two centrifuge tubes, centrifuge, frosted-end glass slides with cover glass, tapered pipette, patient's chart, pen, pencil, tongue depressor, microscope with light source, urine sediment chart, timer or timepiece, and sharps container.

PERFORMANCE OBJECTIVE: Provided with all necessary equipment and supplies, demonstrate all steps required in the procedure for obtaining urine sediment. The instructor will observe each step.

1. Wash hands, put on gloves, and assemble all the needed items on a cleared counter surface near the centrifuge.

2. Stir the urine specimen with tongue depressor, and pour equal amounts (approximately 10 mL) into each of two test tubes, or use plain water in one of the test tubes. **NOTE: Remember that equal weight is required for proper operation of the centrifuge.**

3. To balance the centrifuge, place the centrifuge tubes on opposite sides. Urine should be spun at 1,500 revolutions per minute for 3 to 5 minutes. **NOTE: Set the timer or write down the start time.**

4. When the centrifuge has completely stopped, lift out the tube containing the urine specimen and carefully pour off the urine (**supernatant**).

5. There will still be a few drops of urine in the bottom of the test tube with the sediment. Gently tap the bottom of the tube on the counter or against your palm to mix the urine and sediment together. **NOTE: Make sure that all sediment is thoroughly mixed.**

6. Obtain a drop or two of urine sediment with a tapered pipette and place it on a clean frosted-end glass slide, or calibrated slide for urine sediment.

7. Place a cover slip over the specimen, allow it to settle, and place it on the microscope stage. If using a calibrated slide, this step is omitted.

Unless you are highly experienced in this area, the health care provider will perform provider-performed microscopy. Consult with your employer about the office policy in this matter before proceeding with the examination.

PROCEDURE PROCEDURE PROCEDURE PROCEDURE PROCEDURE PROCEDURE PROCEDURE PROCEDURE

15-17  Perform Screening for Pregnancy

PURPOSE: To determine the presence (or absence) of human chorionic gonadotropin (HCG).

EQUIPMENT: Disposable gloves, other personal protective equipment (PPE) per laboratory policies, urine specimen, quality control materials, reagents, black or blue pen, and biohazardous waste container.

PERFORMANCE OBJECTIVE: Provided with the supplies listed above and a simulated patient chart, the student will perform a pregnancy screening on a urine

sample. The student must complete the procedure within 25 minutes, with the instructor observing each step, at a competency level pre-established by the instructor.

1. Assemble the necessary equipment and supplies; wash hands.

2. Don disposable gloves and other PPE as required.

3. Perform quality control testing on two reagent cards, one negative and one positive. **NOTE: Control samples must only be run once per day or any time a new box of reagents has been opened.**

(continues)

PROCEDURE PROCEDURE PROCEDURE PROCEDURE PROCEDURE PROCEDURE PROCEDURE PROCEDURE

15-17    Perform Screening for Pregnancy (Continued)

4. Record the results of the quality control analyses in the quality control log; do not report patient results if quality control results are not in the acceptable range.

5. Prepare the reagent for patient testing and process it according to the manufacturer's directions.

6. Record the results of the test on the patient's health record.

7. Dispose of contaminated waste in the biohazardous waste container.

8. Remove gloves and wash hands.

CHARTING EXAMPLE

Jones, Sally Mae

ID# 098762

1/10/XX	1347	Pregnancy test	Negative
			Bryan Riffe, CMA

QUALITY CONTROL LOG

Date	Control Level	Control Lot #	Expiration Date	Reagent Lot #	Expiration Date	Results	Initials
1/10/XX	Positive	15962V	12/31/09	454590	6/7/10	Positive	jva
1/10/XX	Negative	15963V	12/31/09	454590	6/7/10	Negative	jva

PROCEDURE PROCEDURE PROCEDURE PROCEDURE PROCEDURE PROCEDURE PROCEDURE PROCEDURE

15-18    Screen and Follow Up Urine Test Results

PURPOSE: Screen and follow up lab results for normal, abnormal, and panic values to relay information to the health care provider.

EQUIPMENT: Scenarios of simulated lab reports for examination and analysis and reference materials supplied by the instructor (e.g., Internet, laboratory reference manuals, textbook, etc.)

PERFORMANCE OBJECTIVE: Provided with the supplies listed above and simulated laboratory reports for urine studies, the student will review the results and make notations as to whether the results are normal, abnormal, or panic value and follow up. The student must complete the procedure within 50 minutes, with the instructor observing each step, at a competency level pre-established by the instructor.

1. Screen the test results to determine whether they are normal, abnormal, or panic value.

2. Screen the test results to determine whether laboratory reports are missing any key elements.

3. Identify panic values, the disease state that may be a result of them, or the disease state that may be caused if left untreated.

4. Identify the appropriate action for panic values with the health care provider.

5. Identify the appropriate action for the abnormal values with the health care provider.

6. Identify the appropriate action for the normal values with the health care provider.

CHARTING EXAMPLE

Denson, Anita

ID# DEN0345678

6/7/XX 1725 Called patient to inform her that her urinalysis results were normal

Judy Adams, MA

COLLECTION OF SPECIMENS FOR SUBSTANCE ABUSE ANALYSIS AND CHAIN OF CUSTODY

It is essential that the procedure be explained to the patient in its entirety before you ask the patient to sign the consent and release form for testing of this sort. Many times this type of collection is performed by the medical assistant, so it is important that you understand the implications of this procedure. The purpose of this test is to detect the presence of illegal or illicit drugs or chemical substances and may prevent a person from obtaining or retaining a job. Most commonly, urine specimens are collected for this testing; if alcohol abuse is detected, it is most often tested by blood testing, although breath tests are commonly employed. Patients should be informed that all drugs that have been consumed within the 30 days prior to testing are likely to be revealed by the test, even including over-the-counter (OTC) medications. Explain that concealing information is inadvisable, as the testing procedure is very sensitive; advise patients that there is a section of the form that allows the patient to list all substances consumed in the last month. Ask the patient to be as accurate and honest as possible when completing this form to be fair to them in interpretation of their results.

After you explain the procedure to the patient, before you proceed with collection of the specimen, you must have the patient to sign the *chain-of-custody* form that further informs the patient regarding the reason for the test. Once the patient signs the chain-of-custody form, it releases you to collect the specimen, prepare it for transport to the testing facility, and release the results to the agency requesting the testing.

Although different testing facilities have different requirements, the following are usually followed for collection:

- Prior to the patient entering the bathroom facility, either bluing is added to the toilet or the handle for flushing is taped down.
- If you are the same sex as the patient, it may be required for you to be present in the bathroom facility for monitoring purposes.
- The temperature of the specimen is immediately checked following collection and recorded with the patient observing you.
- The lid of the container is taped closed and the patient is asked to initial as verification that this is her specimen and that she has observed you closing the specimen.
- Most often, after specimen collection, the patient will again sign or initial the form to indicate she has seen the processing of her specimen.

A sample chain-of-custody form is found in Figure 15-43. Persons who require Department of Transportation (DOT) physicals have this type of testing on a routine or random basis, and you will find this type of testing often in pre-employment screening.

Once the specimen has been collected, verified as valid by you, and initialed by the patient and signatures have been obtained for the chain-of-custody form, the form will accompany the specimen to the testing facility. It is important that you press down hard when completing the form for all carbon copies to be legible. Copies of the form are then routed as follows:

- Medical review officer
- Laboratory (testing facility)
- Patient
- Collector
- Employer

FECAL (STOOL) SPECIMENS

It is not unusual to find that fecal specimens are hard for patients to collect properly, and it can be difficult for you to instruct proper collection of these specimens. Fecal specimens can provide a great deal of diagnostic insight into a patient's condition, and it is essential that you properly instruct the patient on collection of the specimen. Stool (fecal) specimens may be ordered to check for occult (hidden) blood, ova and parasites, or bacterial or viral infections. There is also a collection for pinworm screening in which ordinary office transparent tape is affixed to a tongue depressor (sticky side out)

P PATIENT EDUCATION

Instructing patients in the collection of stool specimens is a good opportunity to give helpful advice in regard to bowel problems. The following is a list of suggestions for discussion with patients.

1. Advise patients to drink plenty of fluids to help reduce the incidence of constipation.
2. Urge patients to refrain from using laxatives, enemas, or suppositories unless specifically ordered by the physician.
3. Instruct patients regarding straining during a bowel movement, which could cause hemorrhoids (and other problems). Sitting or standing for prolonged periods can also be a factor in the development of hemorrhoids.
4. Remind patients that a change in bowel habits should be reported to the physician.
5. Advise patients that a proper well-balanced diet (from the food pyramid guide), consistent meal times, and exercise are the best way toward regularity regarding bowel habits.
6. Remind patients to wash hands with soap and water before *and* after using the bathroom every time to avoid spreading germs.

USA LABS
ID#

Referred by

Health Care Provider
Address
Phone

**DO NOT WRITE
IN THIS AREA**

CHAIN OF CUSTODY

STEP 1 — TO BE COMPLETED BY EMPLOYER/COLLECTOR.
DONOR IDENTIFICATION—PLEASE PRINT

LAST NAME

FIRST NAME   M.I.

SOC. SEC. NO. _____ — _____ — _____

EMPLOYEE NO. _____

DONOR I.D. VERIFIED   ☐ PHOTO I.D.

☐ EMPLOYER REPRESENTATIVE

SIGNATURE OF EMPLOYER REP.

REASON FOR TEST (CHECK ONE)

☐ (1) PRE-EMPLOYMENT   ☐ (2) POST ACCIDENT   ☐ (3) RANDOM

☐ (4) PERIODIC   ☐ (5) REASONABLE SUSPICION/CAUSE

☐ (6) RETURN TO DUTY

☐ (99) OTHER (SPECIFY)

TESTS REQUESTED: TOTAL TESTS ORDERED

SPECIMEN   ☐ Urine   ☐ Blood   (SUBMIT ONLY ONE SPECIMEN WITH EACH REQUISITION)

STEP 2—COLLECTOR, FOR URINE SPECIMENS, READ TEMPERATURE WITHIN FOUR MINUTES OF COLLECTION.
CHECK THE BOX IF TEMPERATURE IS WITHIN THE SPECIFIED RANGE ☐ 90°–100°F / 32°–38°C

OR RECORD ACTUAL TEMPERATURE HERE: _____

STEP 3—TO BE COMPLETED BY COLLECTOR.   COLLECTION SITE

COLLECTION DATE _____ TIME _____ ☐ AM PM _____
                                                          ADDRESS

REMARKS _____
                                                          CITY   STATE   ZIP

_____   (   )
                                                          PHONE

I certify that the specimen identified on this form is the specimen presented to me by the employee identified in Step 1 above, and was collected, labeled and sealed in the donor's presence.

COLLECTOR'S NAME PRINT (FIRST, M.I., LAST)   SIGNATUE OF COLLECTOR

STEP 4—TO BE INITIATED BY THE DONOR AND COMPLETED AS NECESSARY THEREAFTER.

PURPOSE OF CHANGE	RELEASED BY SIGNATURE	RECEIVED BY SIGNATURE	DATE
A. PROVIDE SPECIMEN FOR TESTING			
B. SHIPMENT TO LABORATORY			
C.			

COMMENTS:

Self-stick   identification
Labels for sealing specimen:

(123)   (123)   (123)   (123)

SPECIMEN PACKAGE INTEGRITY WAS ☐ ACCEPTABLE ☐ UNACCEPTABLE WHEN RECEIVED IN LAB.

RECEIVER'S INITIALS

FOR OFFICE USE

FIGURE 15-43 Sample chain-of-custody form

and used while a child is asleep to check for eggs being laid outside the rectum during the nighttime hours.

Normal practice is for patients to be instructed to obtain a stool specimen at home and bring it to the laboratory for testing. Depending on the type of testing being performed, refrigeration may or may not be required. Testing for occult blood will be discussed in a subsequent section, as the instructions to the patient are more detailed than for other specimens. Fecal specimens are not considered sterile, so a patient may collect the specimen in a clean container. It used to be customary practice for the patient to bring only a small amount of the specimen for testing; however, in testing for bacterial or viral infections and ova and parasites, the entire specimen should be collected and transported for testing. The patient should be advised not to contaminate the stool specimen with urine, because constituents of urine destroy microorganisms in the stool specimen; this can present a challenge for many female patients.

Laboratory personnel will observe the specimen for abnormalities such as obvious discoloration, pus, or other such things and test those areas specifically. It is not unusual for a health care provider to order fecal specimens in sequences of three consecutive specimens; that is, for three consecutive days that a patient has a bowel movement, the specimen should be collected. Many patients misinterpret these directions, so you need to take caution when instructing patients for this collection. Patients may not void on consecutive days, and if this is the case, then they simply collect the specimens on three days that they have had a bowel movement. For instance, if a patient has a bowel movement on Monday, Thursday, and Saturday, this is three consecutive days for that particular patient. On the other hand, if a patient has more than one bowel movement per day, only one specimen should be collected for that given day. Refer to Procedure 15-19, Instruct a Patient to Collect a Stool Specimen, as well as Figure 15-44 for an example of a collection container.

Occult Blood Specimens

Occult blood specimens from stools are common screening tools for early detection of the possibility of colon cancer, particularly in those patients older than 50 years. These tests are based on the **guaiac** reagent that turns blue when oxidized in the presence of blood. The test may detect bleeding in the digestive tract that is invisible to the naked eye but is enough to follow up with

---

PROCEDURE PROCEDURE PROCEDURE PROCEDURE PROCEDURE PROCEDURE PROCEDURE

15-19 Instruct a Patient to Collect a Stool Specimen

PURPOSE: To instruct patients to obtain an adequate stool specimen for laboratory analysis.

EQUIPMENT: Specimen container with lid, lab request form, pen, patient's chart, label, rubber band, printed instructions (optional), tongue depressors, and note pad.

PERFORMANCE OBJECTIVE: With all necessary equipment and supplies and using other students as patients, demonstrate the steps of the procedure for instructing a patient in collecting an adequate stool specimen for laboratory analysis. The instructor will observe each step.

1. Assemble the items next to the patient.

2. Write identifying information on the request form and label (usually on the cover), and affix the label to specimen cup.

3. Identify the patient and explain the physician's orders. **RATIONALE: Speaking to the patient by name and checking the chart ensures that you are performing the procedure on the correct patient.** Give printed instructions or write out if necessary.

4. Instruct the patient to obtain a small amount of stool (about 3 or 4 tablespoons) from the next bowel movement, within next few days. Explain that nothing else should be placed in the cup besides stool (no tissue paper, urine, and so on). Patients may defecate onto a paper plate and obtain a small specimen from the plate, which is then discarded. Or, they may use a tongue depressor to obtain the specimen from the toilet bowl.

5. Instruct the patient to place the specimen in the cup, secure the cover tightly, and write the date and time the specimen was obtained on the cover of the cup; then bring the specimen to the lab or medical office with the request form as soon as possible. **NOTE: To prevent bacterial growth, the specimen should be refrigerated if it cannot be received by the lab within 2 hours.**

6. Record that the patient was given instructions.

CHARTING EXAMPLE

5-30-XX

verbal and printed instructions to collect stool specimen given to Sarah

J. Watkins, CMA

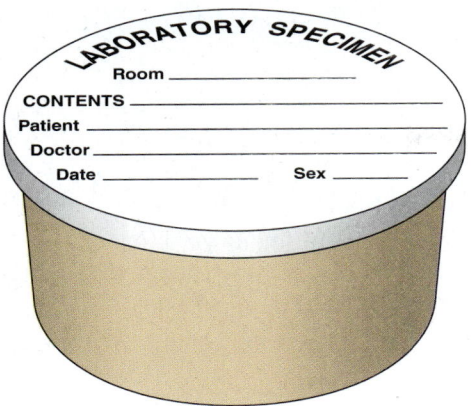

FIGURE 15-44   Laboratory stool specimen container with identification lid

other diagnostic testing such as colonoscopy. When the patient collects the specimen at home, he should be instructed to collect only a very small amount for the test. A tongue depressor or disposable stick is used to collect a minute amount to be applied to the reagent packet; usually, there are two areas upon which the specimen should be applied, and these "windows" should come from different parts of the fecal specimen. If the specimen is returned to the office, you may have the responsibility of applying the specimen to the appropriate areas of the reagent slide and processing it by applying the color developer for observation of either the blue (positive) or brown-green (negative) reaction. Be certain to observe the control area to ascertain that the control reactions are correct prior to reporting any patient results. Refer to Figure 15-45 for instructions regarding collection of the specimen and interpretation of results.

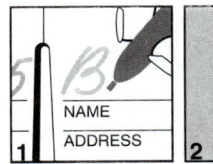 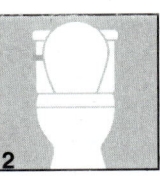 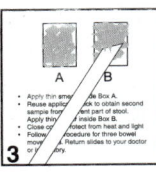 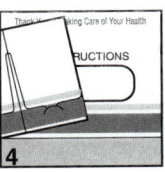 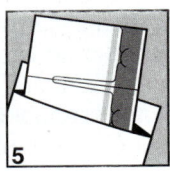

1. Remove slide from paper dispensing envelope. Using a ball-point pen, write your name, age, and address on the front of the slide. **Do not tear the sections apart.**
2. Fill in sample collection date on section 1 before a bowel movement. Flush toilet and allow to refill. You may use any clean, dry container to collect your sample. Collect sample before it contacts the toilet bowl water. Let stool fall into collection container.
3. Open front of section 1. Use one stick to collect a small sample. Apply a thin smear covering Box A. Collect second sample from different part of stool with same stick. Apply a thin smear covering Box B. Discard stick in a waste container. **DO NOT FLUSH STICK.**
4. Close and secure front flap of section 1 by inserting it under tab. Store slide in any paper envelope until the next day. **Important: This allows the sample to "air dry."**
5. Repeat steps 2-4 for the next two days, using sections 2 and 3. After completing the last section, store the slide overnight in any paper envelope to air dry.
   The next day, remove slide from the paper envelope and place in the Mailing Pouch, if provided. Seal pouch carefully and **immediately return to your doctor or laboratory.**
   Note: Current U.S. Postal Regulations prohibit mailing completed slides in any standard paper envelope.

IMPORTANT NOTE: Follow the procedure exactly as outlined above. Always develop the test, read the results, interpret them and make a decision as to whether the fecal specimen is positive or negative for occult blood BEFORE you develop the Performance Monitors®. Do not apply Developer to Performance Monitors® before interpreting test results. Any blue originating from the Performance Monitors® should be ignored in the reading of the specimen test results.

READING AND INTERPRETATION OF THE HEMOCCULT® TEST
the world's leading test for fecal occult blood

Negative Smears*

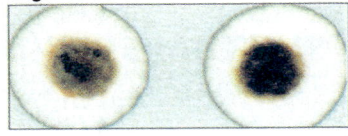

Sample report: negative
No detectable blue on or at the edge of the smears indicates the test is negative for occult blood.
(See **LIMITATIONS OF PROCEDURE**.)

Negative and Positive Smears*   **Positive Smears***

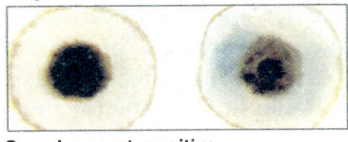   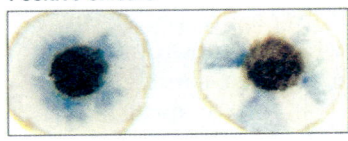

Sample report: positive
Any trace of blue on or at the edge of one or more of the smears indicates the test is positive for occult blood.

FIGURE 15-45   Hemoccult test *(Courtesy of Beckman Coulter, Inc.)*

15-20  Perform a Hemoccult Test

PURPOSE: To determine the presence of occult blood in the stool.

OSHA GUIDELINES: To comply with Standard Precautions, gloves must be worn if there is any possibility of coming into contact with blood or any body fluids.

EQUIPMENT: Hemoccult slide(s) prepared by patient, developer, timer or timepiece, patient's chart, pen, biohazard bag, and latex or vinyl gloves.

PERFORMANCE OBJECTIVE: Provided with all necessary equipment and supplies and using samples obtained from own stool, demonstrate each step in the Hemoccult testing procedure.

1. a. Wash hands and assemble items needed for testing on counter.

    b. Put on gloves.

2. Open the test side of the Hemoccult paper slide.

3. Remove the cap from the bottle of developer.

4. Place two drops of developer on each of the sections of the reagent paper slide: A, B.

5. Immediately begin timing for 1 minute. At 30 seconds, watch closely for any change of color that may be developing. Read at 60 seconds.

6. Compare the test with the control color and read the results.

7. Place one drop of developer between the positive and negative control. Read within 10 seconds.

8. a. Discard the test in a biohazardous waste bag.

    b. Remove gloves and wash hands.

9. Record test results on the patient's chart and log sheet as either positive or negative and sign. **NOTE: A positive reading means that there is occult blood in the stool. Negative means that no occult blood is present. If the first slide is negative and the second and third are positive, record as:**

CHARTING EXAMPLE

7-24-XX

Hemoccult slides: 1. neg
2. pos
3. pos

J. Watkins, CMA

This test is also indicated in patients with a personal or family history of colorectal cancer, rectal polyps, or ulcerative colitis. Remember that bleeding hemorrhoids can also give a positive result for occult blood, although this condition is not serious besides being uncomfortable for the patient. The test was designed to help detect hidden, invisible (occult) blood in the stool early enough to take corrective measures to avoid the spread of cancer. Cancer of the colon is one of the leading cancer killers in the country, so it makes sense to periodically check fecal specimens to protect patients' health. The test is painless to complete, and the results are quick; it is advisable that a patient collect a minimum of three consecutive specimens in the event that bleeding is present on one day but perhaps not on others. It is common practice for many providers to perform this test while examining patients; therefore, it may be your responsibility to develop the test once the provider has collected the specimen by digital swab. If the patient is provided with slide(s) to take home and mail in at a later time, special envelopes that protect the mail carriers are provided. There are many different types of slide tests for this type of analysis. Procedure 15-20 explains the proper method for developing and interpreting a hemoccult slide.

SPUTUM SPECIMENS

Sputum specimens are indicated for diagnostic analysis when a patient has an unresolved cough with mucus production. Although the upper respiratory tract is not considered sterile, the lower respiratory tract is, and when infection occurs in the lower respiratory tract, it can be serious for the patient. Instructing patients in the proper collection of a sputum specimen can be difficult since it is vital that a specimen representative of the lower respiratory tract is obtained for the diagnos-

PROCEDURE PROCEDURE PROCEDURE PROCEDURE PROCEDURE PROCEDURE PROCEDURE

15-21  Instruct a Patient to Collect a Sputum Specimen

PURPOSE: To instruct patients in collection of an adequate sputum specimen for laboratory analysis.

EQUIPMENT: Sputum specimen container and lid, label, pen, patient's chart, label request form, note pad, rubber band, and printed instruction sheet (optional).

PERFORMANCE OBJECTIVE: Provided with all necessary equipment and supplies and using other students as patients, demonstrate the steps of the procedure for instructing a patient in the collection of a sputum specimen for analysis. The instructor will observe each step.

1. Assemble the items next to the patient.

2. Write the patient's name on a specimen cup label, and complete the lab request form.

3. Explain the physician's orders to the identified patient. Give printed instructions, or write them out if you feel the patient has a difficult time understanding you.

4. Instruct the patient to remove the lid from the sterile specimen container and to expel secretions from a first morning coughing episode into the center of the cup, being careful not to touch the inside of the cup. The container should not be more than half full.

5. Instruct the patient not to allow saliva, tears, sweat, mucus from the nose or mouth, or any other sub-

stance to enter the cup. **NOTE: Secretions must be coughed up (expectorated) from the lower respiratory tract (lungs, bronchial tubes, and trachea), or the test will not be acceptable.**

6. When secretions have been obtained and the cup sealed with its cover, the patient should write the time and date that it was obtained on the label and the lab request form and bring them to the lab or medical office as soon as possible. **NOTE: If the patient cannot bring the specimen in within 2 hours after collection, it should be refrigerated.**

7. Secure the completed lab request form to the specimen container with a rubber band or tape. Send it to the lab. **NOTE: If the patient prepares the specimen at home, show the patient how to do this.**

8. Record that instruction was given to the patient in sputum collecting.

CHARTING EXAMPLE

5-30-XX

Verbal and printed instructions for collection of sputum specimen given to Jaren.

J. Watkins, CMA

---

tic testing (refer to Procedure 15-21). When instructing a patient on collecting such a specimen, provide the following directions:

- The first morning specimen is the best specimen for testing; the most productive cough with the most concentrated specimen occurs upon waking.
- Rinse the mouth with water and expel the water. This action washes the superficial cells from the oral (mouth) cavity. Saliva and mucus from the mouth and nasal passages are *not* the desired secretions for the analysis and may interfere with the test results, with a false positive for infection.
- Uncap the sterile container without touching the inside of the container or the lid.
- Cough deeply from down deep in the lungs and expel the specimen into the cup. The container should not be more than half full.

- Securely recap the container, indicate the date and time of the collection of the specimen, and store the container according to which specimen testing has been ordered.

Occasionally, the health care provider will induce coughing in a patient to produce the specimen; however, this is rarely done. More commonly if a provider needs a more specific sample, the patient is scheduled for an outpatient procedure for a bronchial washing or brushing to obtain a lower respiratory tract specimen. Emphasize to the patient how important it is to follow the directions provided in order to obtain an accurate diagnosis.

Sputum specimens are used to diagnose several conditions, including cancer, viral infections, bacterial infections, fungal infections, and tuberculosis. Each of these conditions is different from the others and dif-

When you are giving instructions to patients concerning the collection of sputum specimens, you may also want to advise them about health habits regarding the respiratory tract. Some of the areas you may want to remind them of are:

- Advise patients not to smoke; give advice about stop-smoking programs.
- Instruct patients to drink plenty of fluids, especially if they have a respiratory ailment.
- Remind patients to help diminish the transmission of viruses and other germs by using disposable paper products at home when a family member is sick.
- Advise patients to wash hands often, especially when they are infected or when another family member is sick.
- Urge them to take all the prescribed medication, as directed, for infections to avoid a recurrence of the illness.
- Advise patients to get proper rest and diet to help them regain strength and resistance to disease.

ferent testing is utilized for the diagnoses. Tuberculosis is a unique type of bacterial infection most commonly found in the lungs with extremely contagious implications. Bacterial cultures will be discussed later in this unit. **Cancer** is detected in the sputum specimen through the use of the Papanicolaou stain, the same stain that is used for the detection of cancer of the cervix in women. The sputum specimen is processed, centrifuged, and applied to a microscopic slide, then stained and examined by either a cytologist or pathologist to confirm or refute the presence of cancerous cells.

A **ACHIEVE UNIT OBJECTIVES**

- ☐ Complete the Workbook activities to meet the learning objectives.
- ☐ Practice the procedures in this unit to meet the performance objectives.
- ☐ Apply your knowledge at the end of this chapter in completing the Critical Thinking Challenge and Activities, as well as the StudyWARE on your Student CD-ROM.

UNIT 5
BACTERIAL SPECIMEN COLLECTION, CULTURES, AND DIAGNOSTIC TESTS

OBJECTIVES

Upon completion of this unit, you will be able to achieve the following:

L **LEARNING Objectives**

1. Spell and define, using the glossary at the back of the text, all the Words to Know in this unit.
2. Explain the need for bacterial specimen collection.
3. Identify various types of microbiologic collection techniques and diagnostic tests that would be ordered on such specimens.
4. Differentiate between culture and sensitivity.
5. Explain the proper procedure for performing the Gram's stain and identify each of the components of the stain.
6. Differentiate between Gram-positive and Gram-negative reactions on a Gram's stain.
7. Identify the basic morphologic shapes for various types of microorganisms.
8. Differentiate between some common gram positive and gram negative descriptions for bacterial identification.
9. Describe various media for cultures; differentiate between primary media, selective media, and enrichment media.
10. Describe how to properly label specimens.
11. Appropriately document information regarding specimens on the patient's chart.

P **PERFORMANCE Objectives**

1. Obtain a throat culture.
2. Test a throat swab for group A strep with a rapid diagnostic test and interpret the results.
3. Obtain a wound culture.

WORDS TO KNOW

agar	Gram negative	sensitivity
culture	Gram positive	tuberculosis
exudate	hemolysis	

 CERTIFICATION CONNECTION

CMA

Collecting and processing specimens; diagnostic testing

Cultures: throat, vaginal, wound, urine, blood

Performing selected tests

Microbiology: theory/ terminology; cultures—blood, urine, vaginal, wound, throat, stool; Gram staining; tuberculosis testing

RMA

Laboratory testing—throat culture swabs; prepare culture plates for incubation

There is always a possibility of transmitting diseases when handling any type of specimens, including those being tested for microorganisms. Today, disposable items are used nearly exclusively to help to eliminate transmission of disease from these types of specimens. However, you should always be cognizant of breaking the cycle of infection through the use of proper hand-washing and aseptic technique; avoidance of eating, drinking, and other hand-to-mouth gestures that increase the risk of cross-contamination; and not wearing garments outside of the laboratory setting. Items used that are not disposable need to be properly disinfected or sterilized to protect others from contamination.

BACTERIAL SPECIMEN COLLECTION

While it is typical for us to think of bacteria as being the primary cause of infections, you need to keep in mind that there are several types of microorganisms that can and do cause infections in susceptible individuals. Bacteria, viruses, and fungi can all be extracted from specimens for identification and providing medication to eliminate the infection from the patient (Figure 15-46). Most commonly, a **culture** is obtained from a patient from the part of the body that appears to be infected. Cultures are performed by a qualified individual by swabbing a sample of the **exudate** (drainage) from the throat, mouth, ear, eye, nose, vagina, anus, or infected wounds (Procedure 15-22). The cultures are collected in

---

PROCEDURE PROCEDURE PROCEDURE PROCEDURE PROCEDURE PROCEDURE PROCEDURE

15-22  Perform a Wound Collection for Microbiologic Testing

PURPOSE: Obtain a wound culture from a patient utilizing sterile technique.

EQUIPMENT: Sterile culturette, gloves, other personal protective equipment as required by the collection procedure, pen, and simulated patient chart.

PERFORMANCE OBJECTIVE: Using the equipment above, the student will obtain a wound culture from a patient that protects the integrity of the specimen. The student must complete the skill at a minimum level of competency assigned in advance by the instructor.

1. Assemble necessary supplies for collection of the specimen and ascertain that the culturette is not expired.
2. Identify the patient.
3. Explain the procedure.
4. Verify the health care provider's order.
5. Remove the sterile swab from the sleeve.

6. Collect an adequate specimen without touching any other area except for the exudate and gently rolling the swab in the affected area.
7. Reinsert the sterile swab into the sleeve and break the ampule.
8. Record the patient information on the culturette (not the wrapper); if required, complete a lab requisition form for an outside laboratory.
9. Correctly document the procedure in the patient's medical record.

CHARTING EXAMPLE

Burress, Donald

ID# 222558-07

05/15/XX 0830 Infected appendectomy surgical site (LLQ) swabbed per provider's orders; C&S sent to Ace Reference Laboratories for processing.

Joni Purcell, MA

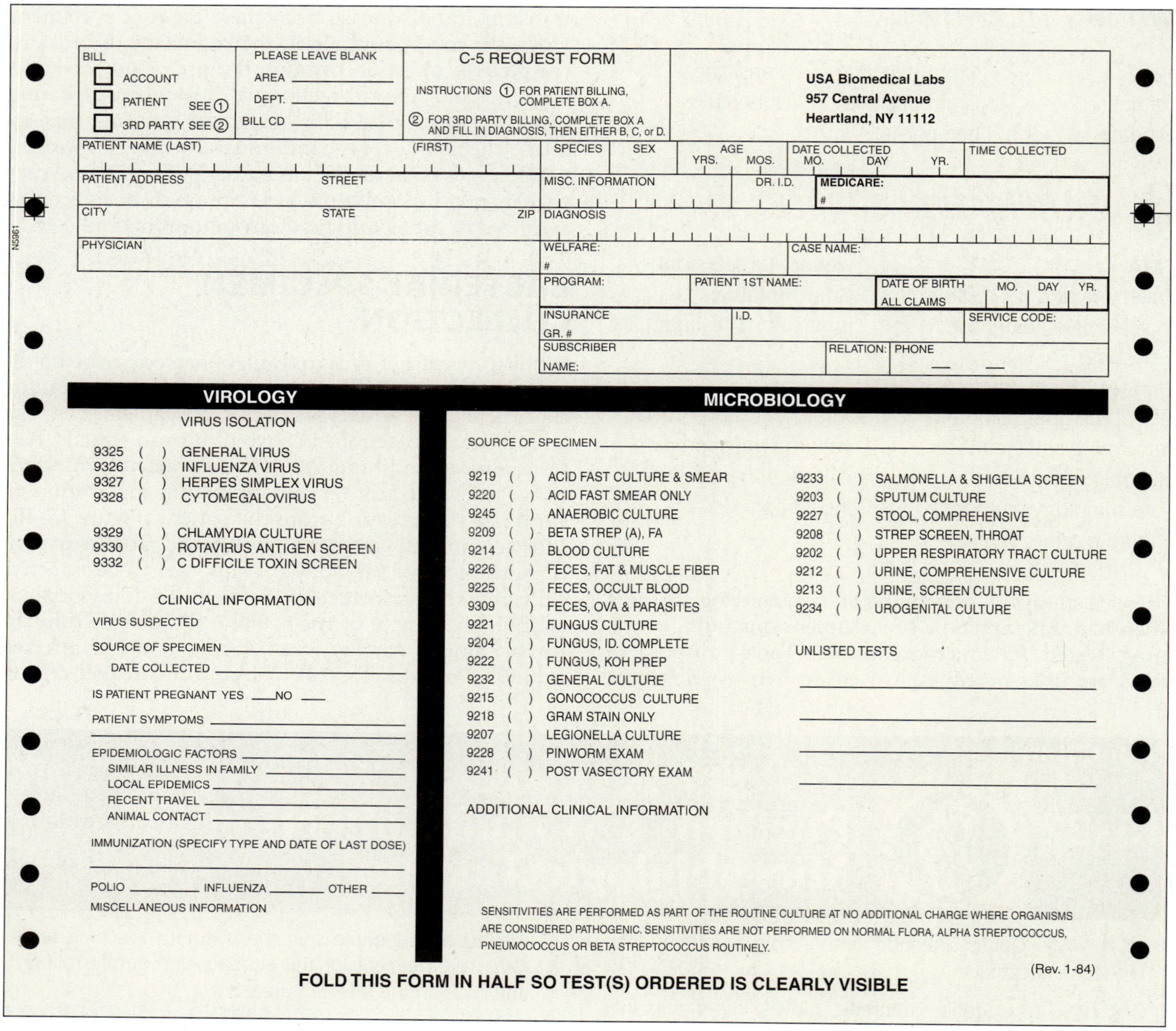

BILL
☐ ACCOUNT
☐ PATIENT SEE ①
☐ 3RD PARTY SEE ②

PLEASE LEAVE BLANK
AREA
DEPT.
BILL CD

C-5 REQUEST FORM
INSTRUCTIONS ① FOR PATIENT BILLING, COMPLETE BOX A.
② FOR 3RD PARTY BILLING, COMPLETE BOX A AND FILL IN DIAGNOSIS, THEN EITHER B, C, or D.

USA Biomedical Labs
957 Central Avenue
Heartland, NY 11112

PATIENT NAME (LAST) (FIRST) | SPECIES | SEX | AGE YRS. MOS. | DATE COLLECTED MO. DAY YR. | TIME COLLECTED
PATIENT ADDRESS STREET | MISC. INFORMATION | DR. I.D. | **MEDICARE:** #
CITY STATE ZIP | DIAGNOSIS
PHYSICIAN | WELFARE: # | CASE NAME:
PROGRAM: | PATIENT 1ST NAME: | DATE OF BIRTH ALL CLAIMS MO. DAY YR.
INSURANCE GR. # | I.D. | SERVICE CODE:
SUBSCRIBER NAME: | RELATION: | PHONE

N5961

VIROLOGY

VIRUS ISOLATION

9325 ( ) GENERAL VIRUS
9326 ( ) INFLUENZA VIRUS
9327 ( ) HERPES SIMPLEX VIRUS
9328 ( ) CYTOMEGALOVIRUS

9329 ( ) CHLAMYDIA CULTURE
9330 ( ) ROTAVIRUS ANTIGEN SCREEN
9332 ( ) C DIFFICILE TOXIN SCREEN

CLINICAL INFORMATION

VIRUS SUSPECTED
SOURCE OF SPECIMEN
DATE COLLECTED
IS PATIENT PREGNANT YES ___ NO ___
PATIENT SYMPTOMS
EPIDEMIOLOGIC FACTORS
SIMILAR ILLNESS IN FAMILY
LOCAL EPIDEMICS
RECENT TRAVEL
ANIMAL CONTACT
IMMUNIZATION (SPECIFY TYPE AND DATE OF LAST DOSE)
POLIO ___ INFLUENZA ___ OTHER ___
MISCELLANEOUS INFORMATION

MICROBIOLOGY

SOURCE OF SPECIMEN

9219 ( ) ACID FAST CULTURE & SMEAR
9220 ( ) ACID FAST SMEAR ONLY
9245 ( ) ANAEROBIC CULTURE
9209 ( ) BETA STREP (A), FA
9214 ( ) BLOOD CULTURE
9226 ( ) FECES, FAT & MUSCLE FIBER
9225 ( ) FECES, OCCULT BLOOD
9309 ( ) FECES, OVA & PARASITES
9221 ( ) FUNGUS CULTURE
9204 ( ) FUNGUS, ID. COMPLETE
9222 ( ) FUNGUS, KOH PREP
9232 ( ) GENERAL CULTURE
9215 ( ) GONOCOCCUS CULTURE
9218 ( ) GRAM STAIN ONLY
9207 ( ) LEGIONELLA CULTURE
9228 ( ) PINWORM EXAM
9241 ( ) POST VASECTORY EXAM

9233 ( ) SALMONELLA & SHIGELLA SCREEN
9203 ( ) SPUTUM CULTURE
9227 ( ) STOOL, COMPREHENSIVE
9208 ( ) STREP SCREEN, THROAT
9202 ( ) UPPER RESPIRATORY TRACT CULTURE
9212 ( ) URINE, COMPREHENSIVE CULTURE
9213 ( ) URINE, SCREEN CULTURE
9234 ( ) UROGENITAL CULTURE

UNLISTED TESTS

ADDITIONAL CLINICAL INFORMATION

SENSITIVITIES ARE PERFORMED AS PART OF THE ROUTINE CULTURE AT NO ADDITIONAL CHARGE WHERE ORGANISMS ARE CONSIDERED PATHOGENIC. SENSITIVITIES ARE NOT PERFORMED ON NORMAL FLORA, ALPHA STREPTOCOCCUS, PNEUMOCOCCUS OR BETA STREPTOCOCCUS ROUTINELY.

(Rev. 1-84)

FOLD THIS FORM IN HALF SO TEST(S) ORDERED IS CLEARLY VISIBLE

FIGURE 15-46 Example of a laboratory request form for a study to determine different types of microorganisms

a specialized container usually referred to as a *culturette*; the culturette is a sterile swab with a soft tip that is used to brush against the infected area and replaced in the sleeve of the collection device (Figures 15-47 and 15-48). There is an ampule in the culturette that must be crushed after collection that serves to keep the specimen moist and nourished until the specimen can be processed. In cases of the rapid group A strep test, a sterile swab, *not* cotton-tipped, is used for collection of the specimen and immediately processed; this is discussed later in this unit. Keep in mind that culturing is the means of *isolating* a disease-causing microorganism, a process that takes longer than a bacteriologic smear.

Blood Culture

One specialized type of culture is a *blood culture*; blood is drawn from the patient, usually directly into a particular formulated broth in a vacuum bottle. Blood is considered a sterile fluid, and when a blood culture is positive for infection, this is indicative of a systemic infection. This is a very important finding that requires

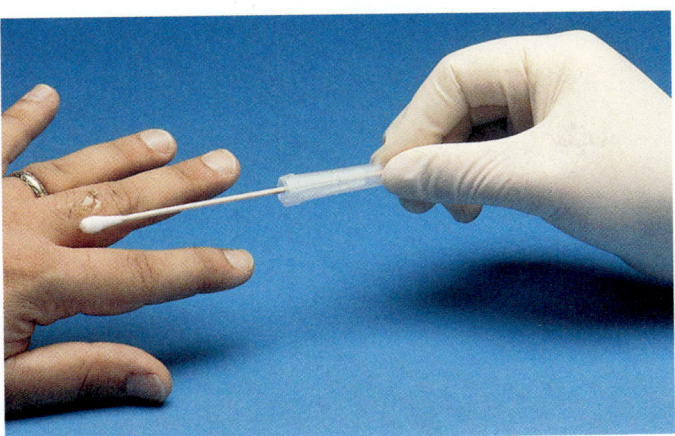

FIGURE 15-47   Demonstration of using a culturette to obtain a wound culture

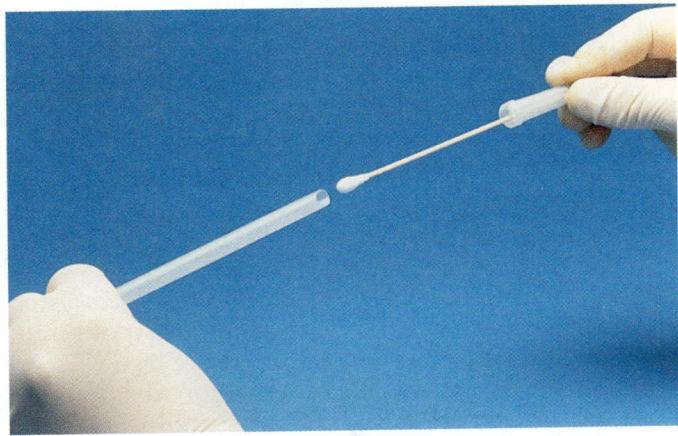

FIGURE 15-48   After collection, the swab is returned to the protective sheath, the ampule is crushed, and it is transported to the lab for analysis.

immediate attention. Of the utmost importance in collecting such a specimen is protection of the sterile environment; there are specific procedures for collecting the specimen from the preparation of the patient's skin to placement of the collected specimen into a microbiologic incubator designed for such specimens.

Usually when a health care provider orders a test for analysis for detection of a microorganism, the order calls for a culture and **sensitivity**. In order for a sensitivity to be performed, there must first be an organism present. The first step of this type of order is the collection of the specimen and inoculation of special media, or **agar**, to encourage the growth of present microorganisms in the specimen. If after 48 hours no growth is observed by the microbiologist, a sensitivity will not need to be performed. However, when growth of a microorganism is identified in a specimen, the next step of the procedure is for the microbiologist to test the organism against different types of antibiotics for sensitivity to the antibiotics. If an organism is sensitive to an antibiotic, growth of that organism is prohibited; conversely, if an organism is resistant to an antibiotic, that organism will grow up to the antibiotic with no inhibition. Some POLs still perform testing in this manner for primarily urine specimens; however, the latest methodology employs *minimum inhibitory concentration (MIC)*, a specialized test performed only in a microbiology lab, that not only identifies the microorganisms but also identifies the most appropriate antibiotic to be used as well as the lowest dose that is effective in combating the infection. Most instruments can also identify the cost of the indicated medications for the health care provider for making the decision in prescribing the most appropriate medication. This saves on health care costs when the least expensive medication indicated for use as well as the dose is identified for the patient.

GRAM STAINING AND MICROBIOLOGIC SMEARS

Although, as a medical assistant, you probably will not perform either Gram staining or preparation of microbiologic smears, it is important that you understand the reasons for this type of testing and indications of various results.

Hans Christian Gram, a Danish scientist, developed the staining technique in 1884 for identification of various microorganisms that caused pneumonia. With this technique, there are several distinctive steps and elements of the stain with which you should be familiar:

- Apply the specimen to the microscopic slide and affix the necessary, required identification (Figure 15-49).
- Heat fix the slide by placing it on a slide warmer for the facility's prescribed amount of time.

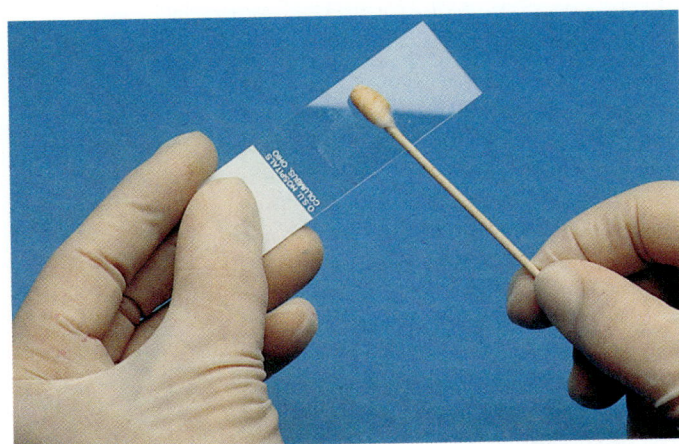

FIGURE 15-49   The proper method for applying a specimen to a slide for bacteriologic staining

- First apply of the *primary dye*, which is the crystal violet (purple-colored dye). Usually this stain is left on the slide for 30 seconds.
- Wash the slide with distilled water.
- Apply Gram's iodine, the *mordant*, to the slide for 30 seconds. The iodine helps the bacterial cell walls that are Gram positive to retain the crystal violet or purple part of the stain.
- Flood the slide with distilled water.
- Apply ethanol or acetone, which is the *decolorizer*. This ensures that a microorganism does not retain the crystal violet to give a false positive result. Flood the slide with the decolorizer until you no longer see the purple color, but be careful not to rinse too long.
- Flood the slide with distilled water.
- Apply safranin (red stain) to the slide for 30 seconds.
- Flood the slide with distilled water.
- Drain the slide and blot with bibulous paper; a qualified individual will examine microscopically to interpret the results of the staining procedure.

If the microorganisms on the slide are identified as **Gram positive**, the color of those organisms will be dark blue to violet, because the bacterial cell walls retained the crystal violet color even after the decolorizer was applied. If the microorganisms are **Gram negative**, their color characteristics will be red or pink; these organisms do not have the same cell wall characteristics and thus will absorb the counterstain (safranin) in their cell walls. Characteristically, Gram-negative microorganisms have a more dangerous connotation than Gram-positive organisms.

MORPHOLOGIC SHAPES

Also significant when taking certification examinations as well as for laboratory reports is a basic understanding of the description of the shape of the organisms. There are three basic morphologic shapes when describing bacteria: *coccus, bacillus,* and *spiral.* Coccus-shaped organisms are very round; the Latin term coccus means "berry-shaped." Bacillus-shaped organisms are rod shaped (think of a fat hyphen; this is how they appear under the microscope). Spiral-shaped organisms, also referred to as *spirochetes,* are corkscrew-shaped. Figure 15-50 illustrates these shapes.

Make a note of the following shapes:

- Gram-positive cocci in clusters: *Staphylococci*
- Gram-positive cocci in chains: *Streptococci*
- Gram-negative cocci in pairs (*diplococci*): *Neiserria gonorroeae*
- Gram-negative bacilli (rods): *Escherichia coli*

Remember that the bacteriologic smear is not definitive for diagnosing the type of microorganism present in the specimen; the staining characteristics

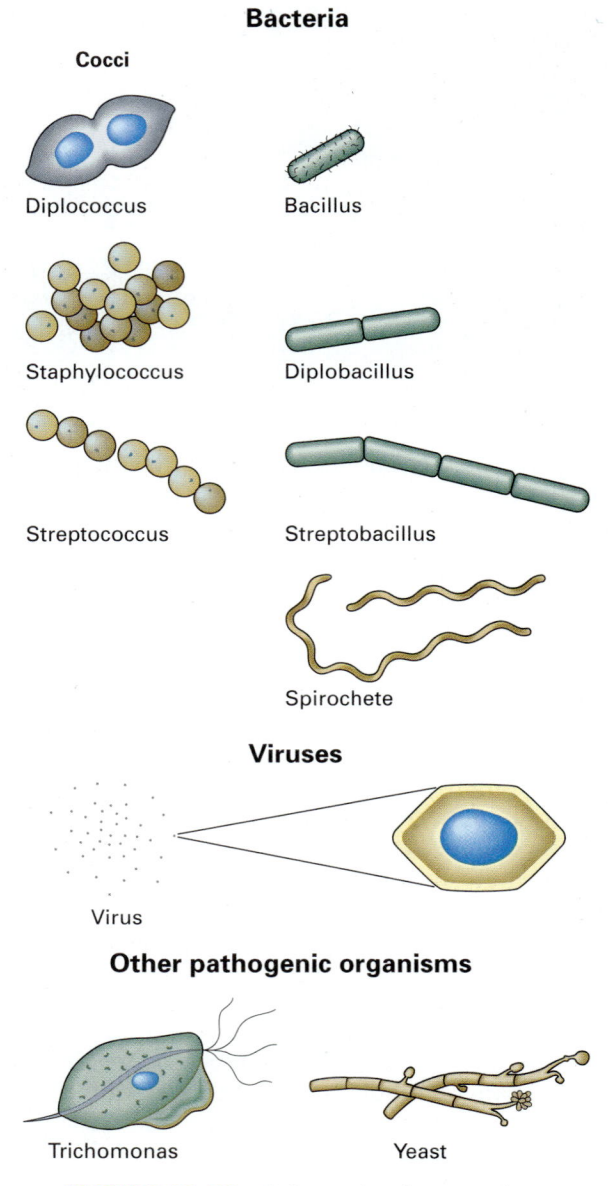

FIGURE 15-50 Pathogenic microorganisms

are helpful for the health care provider to get an early start on treating the infection, but the identification of the microorganism is the final definite step for appropriate treatment. Refer to Table 15-3 for staining characteristics of certain bacteria and the diseases that they cause.

A different type of stain is used when a patient is suspected of having **tuberculosis**, a very contagious airborne disease. The stain is called an *acid-fast* stain; tuberculosis will not appear definitively on the Gram stain, so this stain must be used. If microorganisms stain pinkish to red, there is a good possibility that the patient has a type of a *Mycobacterium,* but until the culture is completed, it will not be known if it is tuberculosis or another type of *Mycobacterium* infection.

TABLE 15-3　Some Important Pathogenic Bacteria and Their Reaction to the Gram's Stain

Gram-Positive Reaction (+) (Reaction of Purple Stain)		Gram-Negative Reaction (−) (Loss of Purple Stain)		Gram-Variable Reaction (+/−)	
Bacterium	Disease It Causes	Bacterium	Disease It Causes	Bacterium	Disease It Causes
Bacillus anthracis	Anthrax	*Bordetella pertussis*	Whooping cough	*Mycobacterium leprae*	Leprosy
Clostridium botulinum	Botulism (food poisoning)	*Brucella abortus* (bovine strain)	Infectious abortion in cattle and undulant fever in humans	*Mycobacterium tuberculosis*	Tuberculosis
Clostridum perfringens	Gas gangrene, wound infection	*Brucella melitensis* (goat strain)			
Clostridium tetani	Tetanus (lockjaw)	*Brudella suis* (porcine strain)			
Corynebacterium diphtheriae	Diphtheria	*Escherichia coli*	Urinary infections		
Staphylococcus aureus	Carbuncles, furunculosis (boils), pneumonia, septicemia	*Haemophilus influenzae*	Meningitis, pneumonia		
Streptococcus pyogenes	Erysipelas, rheumatic fever, scarlet fever, septicemia, strep throat, tonsillitis	*Neisseria gonorrhoeae*	Gonorrhea		
		Neisseria meningitidis	Nasopharyngitis, meningitis		
Streptococcus pneumoniae	Pneumonia	*Pseudomonas aeruginosa*	Respiratory and urogenital infections		
		Rickettsia rickettsii	Rocky mountain spotted fever		
		Salmonella paratyphi	Food poisoning, paratyphoid fever		
		Salmonella typhi	Typhoid fever		
		Shigella dysenteriae	Dysentery		
		Treponema pallidum	Syphilis		
		Vibrio cholerae	Cholera		
		Yersinia pestis	Plague		

Culture Media

Media, or agar, is a substance used to grow the microorganisms for identification and sensitivity. Media comes in Petri dishes, tubes, and broths, to name a few. Depending on the type of specimen, there are a multitude of media that may be used to encourage the growth of the organism for health providers to prescribe the most appropriate medication for the infection.

Primary media is a media that encourages the growth of all microorganisms; typically, tryptic soy agar with 5% sheep blood is utilized as a primary media. Blood agar is used for the colony count for urine specimens, and the plate is streaked in a distinctive fashion. As a rule, greater than 100,000 colonies will indicate an urinary tract infection (UTI), particularly if the organism is identified as Gram negative. *Selective* media is an agar that discourages the growth of certain organisms; examples of selective media include EMB (eosin-methylene-blue) and MacConkey, which are formulated to encourage only the growth of Gram-negative organisms and inhibit the growth of any Gram-positive organisms.

Selective media is commonly used for urine specimens to control the growth of Gram-positive organisms and encourage the growth of Gram-negative ones; Gram-negative organisms are found in the intestinal tract and are commonly a source of infection in the urinary tract due to improper wiping of the anus. Another commonly used selective media is the Thayer-Martin plate, which is used to isolate gonorrhea from vaginal or penile excretions. Enrichment medium is an agar that has additional nutrients to encourage the growth of more *fastidious* organisms, such as an agar commonly called a "chocolate" agar from the color of the media in the Petri dish. Throat cultures are usually inoculated to blood agar and chocolate agar; if strep is present in the specimen, the blood agar will show **hemolysis**, which assists the microbiologist in determining the strain of *Streptococci*. Stool specimens are "planted" on several types of agar plates to isolate a pathogenic organism; remember that stool is not considered sterile, so extra steps need to be taken to isolate a disease-causing organism in this type of sample.

Some of the more common pathogens found in stool specimens are *Shigella*, *Salmonella*, and *Campylobacter*, all of which produce intense gastrointestinal symptoms such as intense diarrhea and are considered extremely contagious if hands are not adequately washed. Many times an infection will break out in a day care center and spread quickly, because the young children do not wash their hands properly. To control such an outbreak, it is important that everyone involved is instructed in proper handwashing technique to control the spread of the pathogen.

If culturing for tuberculosis, the media used is commonly referred to as an L-J (Lowenstein-Jensen) slant, a media that is a sea green color. Tuberculosis is a "slow" grower, so these slants are maintained for a minimum of 4 weeks to observe for growth on the slants. If growth is observed, the slant is sent to a state health laboratory for confirmation of the results. Even slower growers are fungi; the agar plates are maintained for up to 8 weeks, and to prevent the agar from drying out during this lengthy time, *parafilm* is used to "seal" the plates.

Although it is doubtful that a medical assistant would inoculate the media with a collected specimen, you should know what is involved, because you could be hired as a specimen processor. Refer to Figures 15-51, 15-52, and 15-53 for proper inoculation of an agar plate.

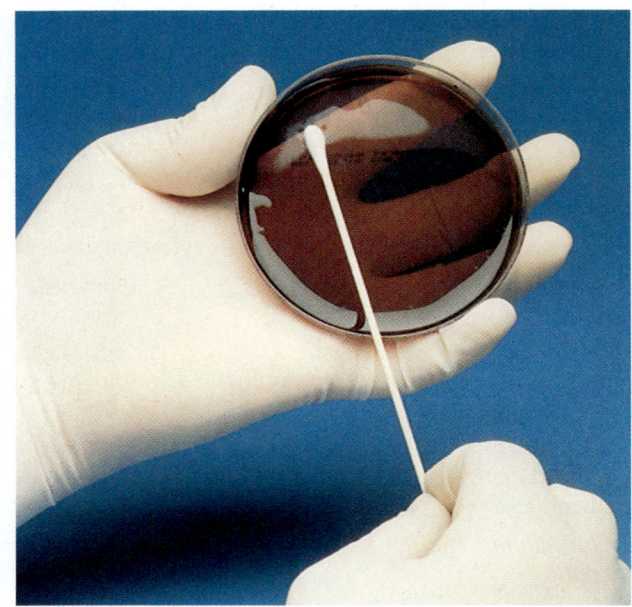

FIGURE 15-51 Smear the culture plate with the specimen from a swab.

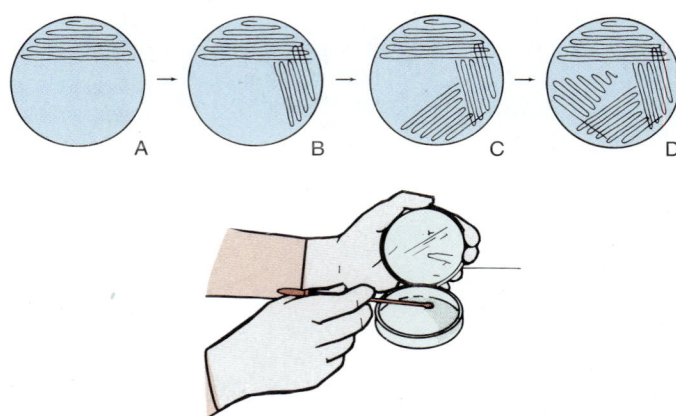

FIGURE 15-52 Pattern for streaking an agar plate. Notice the rotation of the plate to isolate the microorganism.

The basic steps for inoculation of a plate follow:

- Check the patient's identification on the swab as well as the type of culture ordered.
- Collect the appropriate agar for inoculation.
- Label the agar with the patient's name, identification number, the source of the specimen, the date and time of inoculation, and your initials. This identification is placed on the bottom side of the Petri dish with either a marker, wax pencil, crayon, or adhesive label.

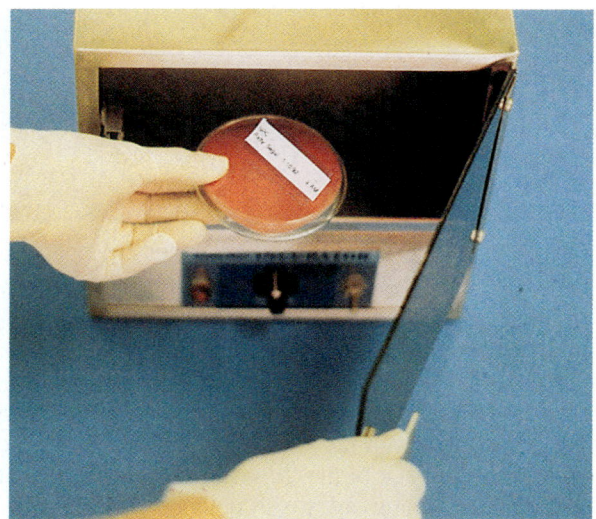

FIGURE 15-53   Place the culture plate in the incubator, agar side up. For proper identification of the plate, the label should be placed on the agar side.

- Remove the swab from the culturette and gently roll it on approximately one fourth of the plate(s). After inoculation, dispose of the culturette in the biohazard waste container.
- Most commonly in microbiology labs, a disposable plastic loop is used for *streaking* the plates, although some labs use a fine-wire loop that must be *flamed* between inoculations. Refer once again to Figure 15-50 for an idea of a properly streaked plate. The idea is to isolate the organism for identification, so as the plate is turned, smaller amounts of the original specimen are streaked out by the fourth turn of the plate. There is a definite art to proper inoculation of plates.
- After the plates have been streaked, place them in an incubator. Usually, incubators are maintained at 37° C (normal body temperature); however, depending on the microorganism suspected, incubators may also be set at 25° C (fungal isolation and identification) and 42° C (*Campylobacter*). Recall also that there are anaerobic microorganisms that grow better with increased carbon dioxide (CO_2) and decreased oxygen, so there are special packages for incubating these types of organisms. Temperatures are monitored and recorded on a daily basis as part of the quality control and quality assurance for the lab.
- This would end your part of the processing; from here a specially trained microbiologist is responsible for looking at the plates at 24 and 48 hours for the presence of a pathogenic microorganism, isolation identification of that organism, and drugs that will inhibit the growth or kill the organism.

Throat Cultures

In most practices and clinics, throat swabs are obtained from patients complaining of sore throats, fever, swollen glands, and cough. Common practice in the past was to obtain the culture to send to the laboratory for the traditional performance of the culture, isolation of the microorganism, and susceptibility testing. However, now there are many rapid group A strep kits available that will provide results of the swab in just a few minutes' time, so waiting 24 to 48 hours is no longer necessary. Some health care providers will order a traditional throat culture if the group A strep test comes back as negative, as this test is specific for only this group of strep; keep in mind that there are more groups of strep than just group A. Whether you are collecting a throat swab from a patient for the rapid test or routine culture, remember that you should swab the peritonsillar area in the back of the oral cavity, taking care not to touch the swab to the lips, cheeks, gums, teeth, or tongue. Inform your patient that there may some momentary discomfort while obtaining the specimen, and be certain to have the patient to open his mouth wide with the head tilted back for better visualization and access to the oral cavity. If obtaining a specimen from a small child, it is easier for you and less traumatic for the child if the parent, or guardian holds the child in the lap. Refer to Procedure 15-23 for the proper collection of a throat culture and to Procedure 15-24 for performance of a rapid group A strep test.

PATIENT EDUCATION

As you obtain throat cultures from patients, you may want to give them some helpful advice concerning their condition. Generally, when a person has a sore throat, it is associated with other respiratory symptoms as well. The following suggestions may provide some relief from discomfort and help them toward better health:

1. Advise patients to drink plenty of liquids (fruit juices) and to eat sensibly from the basic food groups.
2. Urge patients to get extra rest and dress comfortably (according to the weather and temperature outside).
3. Suggest use of gargles or throat lozenges (or both) to relieve a painful sore throat.
4. Remind them to avoid tobacco and smoking.
5. Instruct them to cough or sneeze into a tissue and discard it into the proper waste container to prevent the spread of germs.
6. Remind them to wash their hands frequently.
7. Remind them not to eat or drink after others and to use disposables at home when there is illness.

15-23  Obtain a Throat Culture

PURPOSE: To isolate a disease-causing organism to determine effective treatment of the patient.

OSHA GUIDELINES: To comply with Standard Precautions, gloves must be worn if there is any possibility of coming into contact with blood or any body fluids.

EQUIPMENT: Sterile swabs, sterile tongue depressor, disposable gloves, pen, patient's chart, penlight (optional), and wax crayon or label.

PERFORMANCE OBJECTIVE: Provided with all necessary equipment and supplies, and using a lifelike clinical doll, infant or small child under close supervision, or other students as patients, demonstrate the steps required to perform the procedure for obtaining a throat culture. The instructor will observe each step.

1. Assemble the needed items near the identified patient. Label the culture plate and complete a request form if required. Wash hands and put on gloves.

2. Identify the patient. **RATIONALE: Speaking to the patient by name and checking the chart ensures that you are performing the procedure on the correct patient.**

3. Explain the procedure to the patient, and assist the patient to a comfortable position. Sitting is the usual position for adults. It may be easier to work with children if they are lying down. Assistance may be necessary.

4. Open a sterile swab, and ask the patient to open his mouth as wide as possible.

5. Depress the tongue with a sterile tongue depressor held in one hand. Hold the sterile swab in the other. Ask the patient to say "ah" to assist depression of the tongue (this also prevents the patient from feeling a gag reflex by diverting attention). Quickly insert the swab into the back of the throat and roll over at least two areas, touching areas with obvious exudate.

6. Remove the swab and depressor from the patient's mouth. Attend to the patient and offer tissues. Tearing may result from the procedure.

7. Place the swab into the container for transportation to the lab. Tape the request form securely.

8. Discard all disposable items in the proper receptacle.

9. Remove gloves and wash hands.

10. Record the procedure on the patient's chart and initial.

CHARTING EXAMPLE

5/4/XX

1150 Throat culture obtained and sent to reference laboratory.

E. O'Nan, RMA

15-24  Perform a Rapid Strep Screening Test for Group A Strep

PURPOSE: To screen a patient specimen for the presence of group A strep.

OSHA GUIDELINES: To comply with Standard Precautions, gloves must be worn when there is any possibility of coming into contact with blood or body fluids.

EQUIPMENT: Gloves, sterile throat swab, tongue blade, commercial test kit for group A strep with positive and negative controls, patient's chart or laboratory report form, biohazard container.

PERFORMANCE OBJECTIVE: With the supplies listed above, and with another student as the patient, demon-

strate the steps of the procedure for performing the rapid strep test with the instructor observing each step.

1. Assemble supplies.

2. Identify the patient, introduce yourself, and explain the procedure.

3. Wash your hands and don gloves.

4. Using the tongue blade to keep the tongue out of the way, insert the sterile swab into the back of the oral cavity to collect the specimen from the peritonsillar crypts. Do not touch the swab to the lips, gums, cheeks, teeth, or tongue.

(continues)

15-24  Perform Rapid Strep Screening Test for Group A Strep (Continued)

5. Label the reagent chamber for the test with the patient's name.

6. Following the manufacturer's instructions exactly, perform the test on the patient's specimen.

7. Perform the positive and negative controls, recording the results in the laboratory log record, knowing what action must be taken if the results of the quality control are not within the manufacturer's prescribed range.

8. Dispose of waste in a biohazardous waste container.

9. Properly complete the lab report form or accurately enter the results on the patient's chart.

CHARTING EXAMPLE

7/6/XX

1435 Group A Strep positive.

J. Hart, CMA

QUALITY CONTROL LOG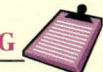

Date	Control Level	Control Lot #	Expiration Date	Reagent Lot #	Expiration Date	Results	Initials
7/6/XX	Positive	14567	9/12/2015	19865	12/10/2010	Positive	JH
7/6/XX	Negative	14568	9/12/2015	19865	12/10/2010	Negative	JH

ACHIEVE UNIT OBJECTIVES

■ Complete the Workbook activities to meet the learning objectives.

■ Practice the procedures in this unit to meet the performance objectives.

■ Apply your knowledge at the end of this chapter in completing the Critical Thinking Challenge and Activities, as well as the StudyWARE on your Student CD-ROM.

2. Have the ability to identify panic values for commonly ordered laboratory tests.

3. Discuss various types of blood tests frequently ordered by health care providers.

4. Differentiate between normal and abnormal results for common diagnostic tests performed in reference and hospital laboratories.

PERFORMANCE Objective

1. Screen and follow up test results appropriately.

UNIT 6
OTHER FREQUENTLY ORDERED LABORATORY TESTS AND NORMAL VALUES

OBJECTIVES

Upon completion of this unit, you will be able to achieve the following:

LEARNING Objectives

1. Spell and define, using the glossary at the back of the text, all the Words to Know in this unit.

WORDS TO KNOW

centrifuge   plasma   serum

CERTIFICATION CONNECTION

CMA

Collecting and processing specimens; diagnostic testing

Blood chemistry: kidney function tests; liver function tests; lipid profile

RMA

Laboratory testing—recognize normal and abnormal values of common laboratory results

SCREENING TEST RESULTS

While many tests are not performed in the health care provider's office, it may be your responsibility to screen the test results as they are returned to the provider's office, either in hard copy, over the Internet, or via the telephone. Most laboratory reports will come with flagged results for abnormalities, but you should have an idea of what a *panic* value is as well as how to follow up on the results as the provider instructs.

When processing specimens for transport by a reference laboratory, you will be provided a laboratory manual that specifies the collection procedure for accurate specimen reporting. A piece of equipment that is essential to processing specimens is a **centrifuge**, an instrument that rotates at variable rates of speed to separate components of the blood.

For **serum** specimens, blood in the evacuated tube must be allowed to clot for 15 to 30 minutes prior to being loaded in the centrifuge. Serum is then extracted from the specimen and sent for testing in a properly labeled tube with a laboratory requisition form.

Plasma specimens result from an anticoagulant present in the evacuated tube; care needs to be taken when removing the specimen from the centrifuge to not mix the cells and the plasma together. It is also imperative that you load the centrifuge properly; a centrifuge must be properly balanced to function as intended. An improperly loaded centrifuge can vibrate and literally "walk off" a countertop, resulting in instrument damage and possible injury to workers present. If you have never used a centrifuge, be sure to have someone demonstrate the proper balancing procedure for loading tubes for centrifugation to prevent this accident from occurring.

COMMON TESTS AND NORMAL VALUES

Refer to Table 15-4 for commonly ordered tests, their indications, and normal value ranges. Figure 15-54 is an example of a typical laboratory requisition form for outside testing.

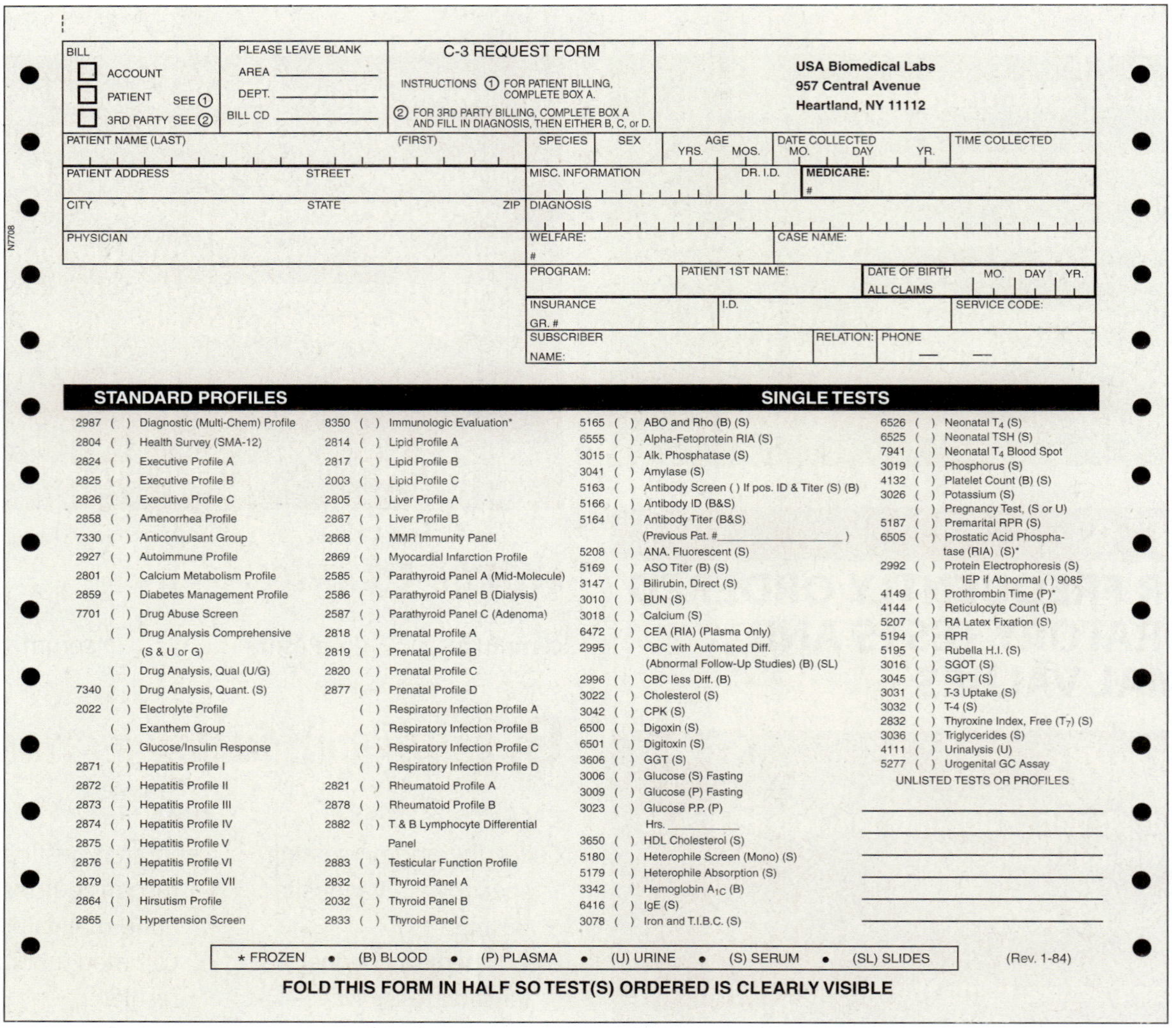
BILL
ACCOUNT
PATIENT SEE ①
3RD PARTY SEE ②
PLEASE LEAVE BLANK
AREA
DEPT.
BILL CD
C-3 REQUEST FORM
INSTRUCTIONS ① FOR PATIENT BILLING, COMPLETE BOX A.
② FOR 3RD PARTY BILLING, COMPLETE BOX A AND FILL IN DIAGNOSIS, THEN EITHER B, C, or D.
USA Biomedical Labs
957 Central Avenue
Heartland, NY 11112
PATIENT NAME (LAST) (FIRST)
SPECIES
SEX
AGE YRS. MOS.
DATE COLLECTED MO. DAY YR.
TIME COLLECTED
PATIENT ADDRESS STREET
MISC. INFORMATION
DR. I.D.
MEDICARE: #
CITY STATE ZIP
DIAGNOSIS
PHYSICIAN
WELFARE: #
CASE NAME:
N7708
PROGRAM:
PATIENT 1ST NAME:
DATE OF BIRTH ALL CLAIMS MO. DAY YR.
INSURANCE GR. #
I.D.
SERVICE CODE:
SUBSCRIBER NAME:
RELATION:
PHONE

STANDARD PROFILES

2987 ( ) Diagnostic (Multi-Chem) Profile
2804 ( ) Health Survey (SMA-12)
2824 ( ) Executive Profile A
2825 ( ) Executive Profile B
2826 ( ) Executive Profile C
2858 ( ) Amenorrhea Profile
7330 ( ) Anticonvulsant Group
2927 ( ) Autoimmune Profile
2801 ( ) Calcium Metabolism Profile
2859 ( ) Diabetes Management Profile
7701 ( ) Drug Abuse Screen
( ) Drug Analysis Comprehensive (S & U or G)
( ) Drug Analysis, Qual (U/G)
7340 ( ) Drug Analysis, Quant. (S)
2022 ( ) Electrolyte Profile
( ) Exanthem Group
( ) Glucose/Insulin Response
2871 ( ) Hepatitis Profile I
2872 ( ) Hepatitis Profile II
2873 ( ) Hepatitis Profile III
2874 ( ) Hepatitis Profile IV
2875 ( ) Hepatitis Profile V
2876 ( ) Hepatitis Profile VI
2879 ( ) Hepatitis Profile VII
2864 ( ) Hirsutism Profile
2865 ( ) Hypertension Screen
8350 ( ) Immunologic Evaluation*
2814 ( ) Lipid Profile A
2817 ( ) Lipid Profile B
2003 ( ) Lipid Profile C
2805 ( ) Liver Profile A
2867 ( ) Liver Profile B
2868 ( ) MMR Immunity Panel
2869 ( ) Myocardial Infarction Profile
2585 ( ) Parathyroid Panel A (Mid-Molecule)
2586 ( ) Parathyroid Panel B (Dialysis)
2587 ( ) Parathyroid Panel C (Adenoma)
2818 ( ) Prenatal Profile A
2819 ( ) Prenatal Profile B
2820 ( ) Prenatal Profile C
2877 ( ) Prenatal Profile D
( ) Respiratory Infection Profile A
( ) Respiratory Infection Profile B
( ) Respiratory Infection Profile C
( ) Respiratory Infection Profile D
2821 ( ) Rheumatoid Profile A
2878 ( ) Rheumatoid Profile B
2882 ( ) T & B Lymphocyte Differential Panel
2883 ( ) Testicular Function Profile
2832 ( ) Thyroid Panel A
2032 ( ) Thyroid Panel B
2833 ( ) Thyroid Panel C

SINGLE TESTS

5165 ( ) ABO and Rho (B) (S)
6555 ( ) Alpha-Fetoprotein RIA (S)
3015 ( ) Alk. Phosphatase (S)
3041 ( ) Amylase (S)
5163 ( ) Antibody Screen ( ) If pos. ID & Titer (S) (B)
5166 ( ) Antibody ID (B&S)
5164 ( ) Antibody Titer (B&S) (Previous Pat. #________)
5208 ( ) ANA. Fluorescent (S)
5169 ( ) ASO Titer (B) (S)
3147 ( ) Bilirubin, Direct (S)
3010 ( ) BUN (S)
3018 ( ) Calcium (S)
6472 ( ) CEA (RIA) (Plasma Only)
2995 ( ) CBC with Automated Diff. (Abnormal Follow-Up Studies) (B) (SL)
2996 ( ) CBC less Diff. (B)
3022 ( ) Cholesterol (S)
3042 ( ) CPK (S)
6500 ( ) Digoxin (S)
6501 ( ) Digitoxin (S)
3606 ( ) GGT (S)
3006 ( ) Glucose (S) Fasting
3009 ( ) Glucose (P) Fasting
3023 ( ) Glucose P.P. (P) Hrs. ______
3650 ( ) HDL Cholesterol (S)
5180 ( ) Heterophile Screen (Mono) (S)
5179 ( ) Heterophile Absorption (S)
3342 ( ) Hemoglobin A_{1C} (B)
6416 ( ) IgE (S)
3078 ( ) Iron and T.I.B.C. (S)
6526 ( ) Neonatal T_4 (S)
6525 ( ) Neonatal TSH (S)
7941 ( ) Neonatal T_4 Blood Spot
3019 ( ) Phosphorus (S)
4132 ( ) Platelet Count (B) (S)
3026 ( ) Potassium (S)
( ) Pregnancy Test, (S or U)
5187 ( ) Premarital RPR (S)
6505 ( ) Prostatic Acid Phosphatase (RIA) (S)*
2992 ( ) Protein Electrophoresis (S) IEP if Abnormal ( ) 9085
4149 ( ) Prothrombin Time (P)*
4144 ( ) Reticulocyte Count (B)
5207 ( ) RA Latex Fixation (S)
5194 ( ) RPR
5195 ( ) Rubella H.I. (S)
3016 ( ) SGOT (S)
3045 ( ) SGPT (S)
3031 ( ) T-3 Uptake (S)
3032 ( ) T-4 (S)
2832 ( ) Thyroxine Index, Free (T_7) (S)
3036 ( ) Triglycerides (S)
4111 ( ) Urinalysis (U)
5277 ( ) Urogenital GC Assay
UNLISTED TESTS OR PROFILES

* FROZEN • (B) BLOOD • (P) PLASMA • (U) URINE • (S) SERUM • (SL) SLIDES
(Rev. 1-84)
FOLD THIS FORM IN HALF SO TEST(S) ORDERED IS CLEARLY VISIBLE

FIGURE 15-54 Laboratory request form

TABLE 15-4   Normal Values of Commonly Performed Laboratory Tests and Their Indications

Chemistry	Normal Range	Indication if Abnormal
Total cholesterol	130–200 mg/dL (fasting)	Atherosclerosis, arteriosclerosis
HDL cholesterol	>45 mg/dL (fasting)	This is the "good" cholesterol; when levels are less than 45 mg/dL, the patient is more apt to have deposits of plaque in the arteries. The function of this type of cholesterol is to transport the "bad" cholesterol out of the vessels and to the liver.
LDL cholesterol	<100 mg/dL (fasting)	This is the "bad" cholesterol, primarily responsible for depositing on the interior of arterial walls. If the LDL cholesterol cannot be controlled through diet, medication is used to help lower it, as well as the total cholesterol.
Triglycerides	40–150 mg/dL (fasting)	This is a lipid but is not as structurally complex as cholesterol molecules. High levels of triglycerides can contribute to heart disease and hardening of the arteries. Lipid panels usually consist of the total cholesterol, HDL cholesterol, LDL cholesterol, and triglycerides.
Creatinine	0.7–1.4 mg/dL	Creatinine with BUN are indicators of renal (kidney) function; when levels of creatinine become elevated, it may indicate there is a problem with renal function.
Uric acid	3.5–7.5 mg/dL	Uric acid is the responsible agent for gouty arthritis when levels exceed 7.5 mg/dL. Keeping the uric acid level down helps to prevent attacks of gout.
BUN (blood urea nitrogen)	8–20 mg/dL	Urea is one of the waste products found in urine; when the kidneys are not functioning properly, urea will build up in the bloodstream. Since this is a waste product, elevation of the BUN indicates a problem with the nephron units in the kidneys. BUN and creatinine are frequently ordered tests for those patients who have renal problems as well as those on dialysis to monitor the effectiveness of the treatment.
Sodium (Na)	132–145 mEq/L	Sodium can be a good indicator of a patient's hydration; when sodium levels are above 145 mEq/L, it indicates a level of dehydration.
Potassium (K)	3.5–5.2 mEq/L	Potassium is essential for proper muscle functioning, particularly the heart muscle. If potassium becomes depleted due to diuretics, the most common complaint is leg cramps and heart palpitations. Conversely, if potassium exceeds 5.2 mEq/L, it can result in heart palpitations as well. Elevated potassium is also an indicator of renal disease or dysfunction.
CK (creatine kinase)	10–200 IU/L	CK is an enzyme found in muscles that is released if a muscle is damaged. This enzyme is especially helpful in diagnosing a myocardial infarction (MI) in patients with chest pain.
Prothrombin time (PT)	Normal 10–13 seconds International normalized ratio (INR): 1.0–1.4	This is a coagulation test commonly used to assess the therapeutic range of warfarin therapy, an anticoagulant used in patients with a history of blood clots (thrombosis). The INR is used as the reference; if the INR is less than 1.0, it indicates that the patient needs an increased dose of warfarin to prevent additional formation of clots. If the INR is greater than 1.4, it indicates that the blood is becoming too thin, and a decreased dose should be advised.

PANELS

Typically, when a series of related tests are ordered for outside testing, the tests will be compiled into a panel or a profile. For instance, a liver panel would include enzymes and chemistries related to liver function and dysfunction: LDH, alkaline phosphatase, AST, ALT, and total bilirubin may be included in such a panel or profile. Another example of a profile would be a kidney function test that might include electrolytes (sodium, potassium, chloride, carbon dioxide), BUN (blood urea nitrogen), and creatinine. Many times when individual tests are ordered on a laboratory requisition form, the reference or testing laboratory will combine them into a profile for better reimbursement by insurance providers. Panels are usually less expensive than the individual tests based on how insurance companies reimburse for health care. Health insurance carriers constantly change their methods for reimbursement, so it is vital that you stay abreast of insurance developments when completing the requisitions for maximum reimbursement.

ACHIEVE UNIT OBJECTIVES

- ☐ **Complete the Workbook activities to meet the learning objectives.**
- ☐ **Apply your knowledge at the end of this chapter in completing the Critical Thinking Challenge and Activities, as well as the StudyWARE on your Student CD-ROM.**

CRITICAL THINKING CHALLENGE

IMPACTING THE PATIENT, THE PRACTICE, AND YOUR CAREER

You work as a medical assistant in a busy multi-physician practice with Inez and Cheryl, and there are other practitioners as well, such as nurse practitioners and physician assistants. The office manager has a schedule worked out for different medical assistants to take calls regarding laboratory results for screening of results and follow up with the individual provider. Cheryl, recently graduated from a reputable medical assisting program and new to the practice, is taking laboratory results today, and when you ask her at 3:30 PM whether she wants to take a break, you happen to notice that she took a report from a hospital laboratory for a hemoglobin of 4.8 g/dL at 9:18 AM. Nothing else is noted on the result as to whether the result has been reported to the provider or whether any action was indicated.

QUESTIONS

1. Is there an impact for the patient with this particular result? If you think there is, expand on what the indication for the patient might be.
2. What impact, if any, is indicated for the practice (and the specific health care provider)?
3. Does this result have any impact on your career? On Cheryl's?

ACTIVITIES

1. Go to the Internet and research at least five different CLIA waived tests as well as what the tests check.
2. Have your instructor arrange a field trip to an office that sends out laboratory specimens to a reference laboratory or hospital laboratory. Review the manual for ordering the tests as well as proper completion of the requisition forms. While there, ask the office person responsible for completing these forms to allow each member of the class to complete one properly.
3. Ask your instructor if a field trip to a hospital or clinic laboratory could be arranged for your class to see automated instruments such as hematology, chemistry, and coagulation equipment.
4. Ask your instructor if a field trip to a hospital microbiology laboratory might be feasible for your class to observe how cultures are set up and read by the microbiologists; also, take a look at the automated blood culture instrument that alarms if a bottle turns positive for infection.
5. Research commonly ordered laboratory tests not specified in this chapter either through the Internet or by going to a health care provider's office. List the name of the tests, their indications, normal values, and panic values, if any.

StudyWARE™ CHALLENGE

- Study with the flash cards for Chapter 15 to review the key terms in this chapter.
- Solve the hangman activities for Chapter 15.
- Complete the multiple choice quiz in test mode for Chapter 15.

RESOURCES

Heller, M., & Krebs, C. (2002). *Clinical handbook for health care professionals* (2nd ed.). Clifton Park, NY: Thomson Delmar Learning.

WEB LINKS

www.cdc.gov (Centers for Disease Control and Prevention)
Promotes health and quality of life by preventing and controlling disease, injury, and disability.

www.fda.gov/cdrh/clia (Clinical Laboratory Improvements Amendments)
Provides information on quality standards for all laboratory testing.

16 Diagnostic Tests, X-Rays, and Procedures

Diagnostic tests, x-rays, and procedures will be discussed in this chapter. The medical assistant has a multiple role in these diagnostic aids. You will be responsible for instructing and preparing patients for procedures, tests, and x-rays. In some cases, you will either carry out the test(s) or procedure(s) or assist the health care provider. After completion, you will alert the physician of the results and, with order of the doctor, notify the patient. Then you will file the report of the results in the patient's chart.

Often, as a part of the complete physical examination, the physician may order certain tests or other procedures (e.g., chest x-ray, mammography, intravenous pyelogram). If these diagnostic tests are performed on site, the results may often be determined while the patient is still present. If referrals must be made for diagnostic tests and so on, patients may be asked to return within a week to 10 days for a final report of the findings. This gives the medical assistant and the physician time to gather reports in the patient's chart to screen and follow up. You may want to advise patients to bring a list of concerns so they will not forget to ask necessary questions. This practice may reduce the number of phone consultations required.

UNIT 1
DIAGNOSTIC TESTS

OBJECTIVES

Upon completion of this unit, you will be able to achieve the following:

LEARNING Objectives

1. Spell and define, using the glossary at the back of the text, all the Words to Know in this unit.
2. Describe scratch, patch, and intradermal skin tests and state their purpose.
3. Describe the schedule and instructions for administering allergy injections.
4. Describe patient education concerning allergies and treatment.

PERFORMANCE Objectives

1. Perform a scratch skin test.
2. Perform a patch skin test.

WORDS TO KNOW

adrenalin	desensitizing	interpret
adverse	eosinophil	obsolete
anaphylactic	epinephrine	RAST
antibody	extract	systemic
antigen	histamine	venom
contact	hypersensitive	wheal
dermatitis	immune	

CERTIFICATION CONNECTION

CMA

Principles of asepsis
Aseptic technique
Disposal of biohazardous material
Practice Standard Precautions

Patient preparation—procedures, explanation, and instructions
Identify and respond to (anaphylactic) shock

RMA

Asepsis—terminology, bloodborne pathogens and Universal Precautions, and medical asepsis
Allergy testing—scratch test, intradermal skin testing, RAST testing
Recognize emergencies and provide appropriate response

CMAS

Asepsis in the medical office
Prepare patients for clinical examination
Recognize and respond to medical emergencies

SKIN TESTS

Three procedures are commonly used to determine allergic reactions in patients. They are the scratch, intradermal, and patch tests. The physician determines the diagnosis by evaluating the results of the tests along with the patient's medical history, physical exam, and other laboratory tests. The medical assistant may assist the physician in performing these tests or may perform them by order of the physician. Tests should always be performed under the direct supervision of the physician.

The tests involve introducing an **antigen** directly into the patient's skin to induce a reaction. If the reaction is negative (normal), there will be no change in the appearance of the skin following testing. A normal **immune** reaction occurs in the body when an antigen and **antibody** unite and the foreign substance is excreted by the body.

A positive allergic reaction to a test is shown by a raised area on the skin, much like a mosquito bite, called a **wheal** (hive). This is caused by interaction of the antigen and antibody, which releases **histamine** and is termed a **hypersensitive** reaction. Histamine is naturally produced by the body to attach itself to certain cells to cause dilation of blood vessels and contraction of smooth muscles. Most cells release histamine during allergic reactions. As a part of the normal inflammatory response of the body, histamine protects tissue against injury (the scratch test), and it is the reason that redness and a wheal are produced. The inflammatory response of the body is specific in that it is the whole body's defense against infection, chemicals, or other physical factors.

Besides histamine, researchers are finding other chemicals released during the allergic response. Many have allergies to a variety of substances, including certain foods, pollens, dust, drugs (medications), chemicals, **venom** of stinging insects, animal dander, molds, pollutants, and other allergens. There are also some that are not so well known. It is very important to realize that cockroaches and their egg casing and fecal matter are major sources of allergens in large cities. The extermination of these roaches is of concern, because the chemicals used to eliminate them can cause serious problems for those who have allergies and respiratory diseases. Asthma patients are most sensitive to these sprays and other methods of getting rid of the roaches. The allergen remains even after the roaches are killed. Thorough cleaning is necessary to rid the home of the allergen as much as possible after extermination has been completed. Advising patients of the risks is extremely important.

Certain irritants can make allergies worse. These irritants can be caused by smoke, paint fumes, perfumes, insect sprays, gasoline, cleaning materials, and personal grooming products (hair sprays, soaps, lotions, etc.). Sensitivity to these irritants is most likely in those who have allergies. The best advice for such patients is to avoid being around these substances. Reaction to these substances ranges from slight to severe. Severe reactions can be life-threatening. A life-threatening reaction must be counteracted with an injection of **adrenalin** immediately to prevent **anaphylactic** shock. Symptoms of anaphylactic shock initially include intense anxiety, weakness, sweating, and shortness of breath. These may be follwed by hypotension, shock, arrhythmia, respiratory congestion, laryngeal edema, nausea, and diarrhea.

For example, those who have known allergies to the venom of stinging insects or to certain foods that produce intense life-threatening allergic reactions are instructed to carry an anaphylactic shock kit with them at all times. The kit contains a self-injecting dose of adrenalin for emergency use. Instruct patients with food allergies to read the contents (ingredients) on all labels of foods and over-the-counter medications to avoid adverse reactions. Herbal remedies, when combined with prescribed medications and foods, can produce health risks. Check with the pharmacist before taking such combinations of over-the-counter medicines and prescriptions from your physician. It is also a good practice to advise patients to ask the server or the dinner host about the contents of some foods on restaurant menu, such as soups, breads, and desserts. Some of these foods may contain ingredients that may result in an allergic reaction for those who are sensitive to these substances. You may also want to inform these patients, if they do not already wear them, to get a medic alert bracelet or necklace. These are very helpful in the event that a medical emergency occurs; the medic alert tag informs others of their condition if they are not able to speak or if they are found unconscious.

Treatment for many allergy patients consists of an allergy immunotherapy program. Over a considerable period, which can be indefinite, this therapy gradually provides immunization against the substance to which the person is allergic. Increasing amounts of the allergen are injected as long as the patient can tolerate each dose. Treatment generally takes a few years. It is usually effective in reducing symptoms of most allergies. Often patients bring their serum from the allergy specialist to the family doctor's office or clinic for administration. All allergy serum should be refrigerated unless otherwise specified. These **desensitizing** injections of allergy serum (which patients refer to as "allergy shots") should always be administered under the direct supervision of a physician because anaphylactic shock can occur within seconds. Following any injection, the patient must be observed for 20 minutes for possible reaction. Any reaction or unusual symptom must be reported to the physician and noted on the patient's chart and on the schedule sheet accompanying the allergy serum. An example of this schedule is shown in Figure 16-1.

Because patients generally continue this therapy once a week (or even more frequently) over a few years, it is vital to rotate the injection sites frequently. A practical method of keeping a record of where the allergy serum is injected each time is by alternating arms and numbering the injection sites. This pattern allows up to 18 injection sites, and then it can be repeated. This may help in preventing tissue damage from recurring frequent injections of the same area. Keep track of the pattern on the schedule that comes with the allergy serum, or in the patient's chart, by recording which arm, the number of the injection site, and, of course, the date and your initials.

Figure 16-2A shows an illustration of a suggested clockwise pattern; Figure 16-2B shows a charting method. Refer to Chapter 18 for the procedure for administering injections.

Allergy injections are administered to patients who have demonstrated a reaction to one or more allergens. One method of testing is administration of an intradermal injection; a minute amount of allergen is introduced just below the epidermis of the skin and the site is observed for a reaction. A positive reaction to the allergen is the appearance of a wheal.

The size of the wheal is **interpreted** by the physician after a timed 20- to 30-minute period. Wheals are measured in centimeters by using a tape measure or by comparison (Figure 16-3). A trained skin tester may observe the reaction and make an interpretation by inspection alone.

Extracts of substances that are commonly the cause of allergy in patients are manufactured in applicator bottles. These should be refrigerated and the expiration date noted for accurate test results. Many of the skin testing extracts vary in strength from one company to another. Because specific allergens may also differ geographically, skin tests are sometimes unreliable. Standardization would be helpful. New methods are being

Company's Name
(maker of serum)

Physician's Name/Allergist
Address and Phone Number

Patient's Name　　　　　　　　　　　　　　　　　　　　　　　　　　　Lot Number of Serum
Account Number　　　　　　　　　　　　　　　　　　　　　　　　　　Expiration Date

INSTRUCTIONS FOR ADMINISTRATION

—Preparations should always be made for physician to treat anaphylaxis should it occur.
—Patients who are being treated with beta-blocker medications should not be given allergy serum.
—Use 27G $\frac{1}{2}$-inch needle.
—Administer $\frac{3}{8}$ to $\frac{1}{2}$ inch into subcutaneous tissue between deltoid and biceps muscle (but not into the muscle).
—Aspirate plunger of syringe to ensure needle is not in a blood vessel.
—Reschedule patient for injection if he or she is feverish or is wheezing.
—Observe patient for possible reaction for 20 minutes following injection.
—Administer cold packs on site if local redness, itching, or wheal develops—alert physician for administration of antihistamine PRN.
—If a systemic or general reaction occurs, such as hives, sneezing, or wheezing, alert physician for dosage and administration
of epinephrine (subcutaneous).
—**Contact allergist for rescheduling instructions if systemic reaction occurs.**

SCHEDULE

Administer allergy serum injections every _____ days. If no adverse reaction occurs, resume scheduled dose.
If adverse local reaction occurs, resume schedule with the last well-tolerated dose. Proceed with the following schedule until
maximum dose is reached and well-tolerated. Then repeat maximum dose tolerated until vial is empty.

Dose	Date Administered	Adverse Reaction
0.10 mL	Month/day/year	Type of reaction,
0.15 mL	Initials of one who	if any (note the
0.20 mL	administered the	severity and
0.30 mL	injection	symptoms of
0.40 mL	and which arm	the patient)
0.50 mL	was injected	
*0.50 mL	Rt or L	

*Reorder before last dose is administered. Allow 2 weeks for delivery.

FIGURE 16-1　　Example of schedule and instructions for allergy serum injections

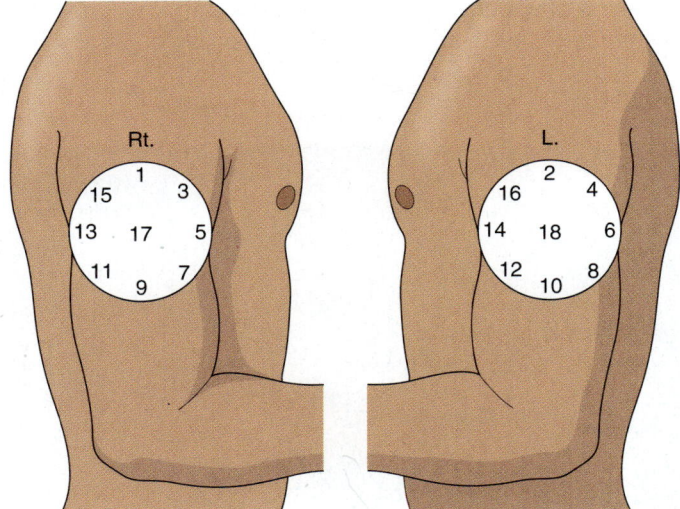

FIGURE 16-2A　　This alternating pattern allows 18 sites to help prevent tissue damage.

Progress Notes _____

Patient's Name _____

Date _____

Page _____

4-16---	0.10 mL	Rt arm #1, JY
4-24---	0.15 mL	L arm #2, JY
5-1---	0.20 mL	Rt arm #3, JY
5-8---	0.30 mL	L arm #4, JY

FIGURE 16-2B　　Example of charting an allergy serum injection on a patient's chart

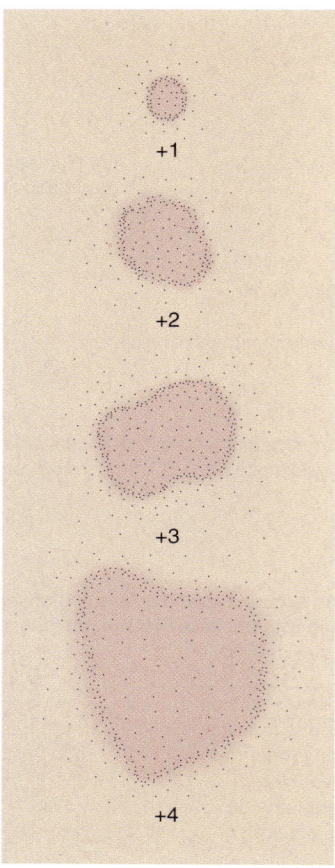

FIGURE 16-3 Sizes of wheals (welts) from +1 to +4 in reaction to scratch testing of allergens

researched, and skin testing may one day become an **obsolete** procedure.

Scratch Test/Skin Prick Test

Desirable sites for the scratch test/skin prick test are the arms and the back, depending on the number of tests to be performed and, in some cases, the preference of the patient. Small children are easier to restrain if they are lying face down while the test is being administered. The area to be tested should be comfortably accessible to both patient and physician or assistant. The patient must stay in the same position for at least 20 minutes, so comfort is essential for compliance.

The tests should be numbered in a pattern with washable ink on the surface of the skin. Explain to the patient that there will be some discomfort when administering either the scratch test or the intradermal test, but it will not last long. Instruct the patient to inform you of any itching, redness, or swelling at the site of injection. Advise the patient to avoid scratching the area to allow for accurate interpretation following the prescribed timing of the test(s). Several extracts may be applied to the patient's skin in rows from evenly spaced applicators that have

been dipped into various bottles of allergen substances. The applicator provides a small drop of the substance on the skin in preparation for the scratch test. Figure 16-4 shows a medical assistant applying seven different extracts on the patient's skin. Usually, the skin is prepared with alcohol and allowed to air dry. Alcohol may also be used to remove the ink after the test is completed. A sterile needle or lancet is used to tear the surface of the skin in a scratch of about 1/8 inch or less to allow a drop of the antigen to enter the epidermis (Figure 16-5). Some test materials are packaged in sealed glass capillary tubes, the contents of which are shaken onto the skin after the tube is snapped. Only a small drop should be used. Otherwise,

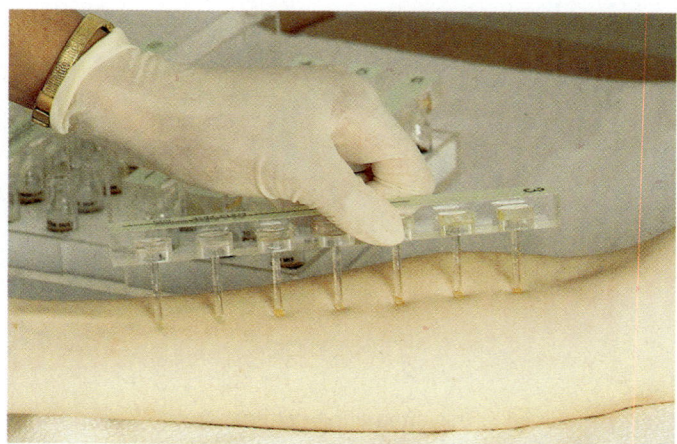

FIGURE 16-4 Allergy extracts are placed on the skin with a multiple applicator.

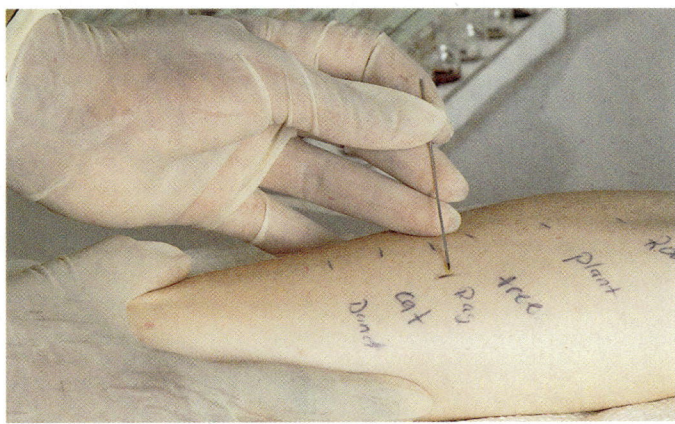

FIGURE 16-5 Each extract is labeled with ink for identification. The medical assistant uses a sterile fine-point needle or lancet to scratch the surface of the skin to allow the extract to enter the epidermis.

antigens may run together, and test results will be inaccurate. The scratches should be from 1½ to 2 inches apart, allowing possible reactions to spread without interfering with each other. A nonallergy-producing plain base fluid control is used for comparison in interpreting the results. (See Procedure 16-1.)

Reactions usually occur within the first 20 minutes. (Itching at the test site may be relieved by application of cold or ice packs after the test site has been evaluated by the physician. Look at the examples in Figure 16-6 of graduated sizes of reactions to allergy testing.) Many physicians wish to recheck the test sites in 24 hours for delayed reactions. If the physician's interpretation of the skin tests is consistent with the patient's history and physical examination findings, more advanced studies will not be necessary. It is not advisable to perform intradermal tests on patients who have had positive scratch tests.

PROCEDURE PROCEDURE PROCEDURE PROCEDURE PROCEDURE PROCEDURE PROCEDURE PROCEDURE

16-1  Perform a Scratch Test

PURPOSE: To determine an allergy-causing substance.

OSHA GUIDELINES: To comply with Standard Precautions, gloves must be worn if there is any possibility of coming into contact with blood or any body fluids.

EQUIPMENT: Sterile needle(s) or lancet(s), allergen (extract), cotton balls, alcohol, pen, patient's chart, timer or timepiece, control, biohazard sharps container and bag, and disposable latex or vinyl gloves.

PERFORMANCE OBJECTIVE: Provided with all necessary instruments and supplies and a suitable simulated skin surface (such as an orange), demonstrate each of the steps required in the scratch test procedure within 45 minutes. Each step will be observed by the instructor.

1. Assemble all needed items on a Mayo table or other suitable flat work area near the patient, wash hands, and put on gloves.

2. Explain the procedure to the identified patient as you prepare the test site with an alcohol-saturated cotton ball. Sites most commonly used are the upper arm and back. Help the patient into a comfortable position.

3. Apply a small drop of one extract onto the site, and continue until all extracts are applied.

4. Mark the site(s) with an initial abbreviation or the number of the extract in pen if more than one test is to be administered. Leave about 1½ to 2 inches between test sites. **RATIONALE: An adequate area for possible reaction must be allowed. Accurate assessment requires measurement of individual reaction areas, which might come together if placed too close.**

5. Remove a sterile needle or lancet from its package without contaminating it. Make a ⅛-inch scratch in the surface of the skin.

6. Begin timing a 20-minute period.

7. Discard disposables and gloves in the proper receptacle, return the items to the proper storage area, and wash hands.

8. As soon as the 20-minute period is up, reglove and check each site after cleansing with an alcohol-saturated cotton ball. **NOTE: Be careful not to wipe off the identification of the extract until after interpretation of the reaction has been made by the tester or physician.**

9. Compare the reaction of the site with the package insert drawings or measure in centimeters. **NOTE: This step cannot be realistically carried out when a simulated surface is used. However, until the new medical assistant gains experience on the job, the physician will probably make this comparison personally.** Cold packs or an ice bag may be applied to the site to relieve itching. Repeat step 7 and then proceed to step 10.

10. Record the test results on the patient's chart.

CHARTING EXAMPLE

5-12-XX

Patricia Marie Stevens tested +3 reaction 10 minutes after application of ragweed extract, L forearm.

S. Davis, RMA

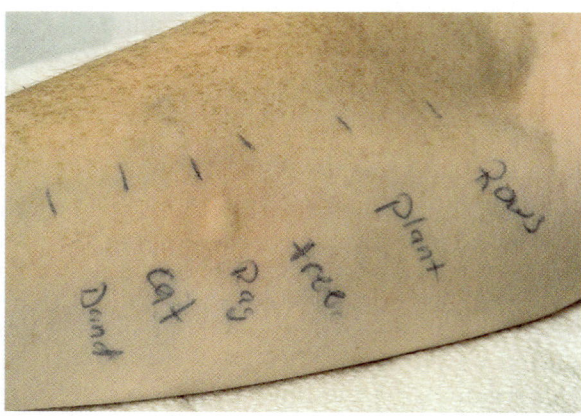

FIGURE 16-6   After timing the skin tests for 20 minutes, observe the reaction and record it on the patient's chart. Pictured here is a +3 reaction to ragweed.

Intradermal Test

The intradermal test, thought to be more accurate, is often performed if the scratch test is negative or unclear. Although the solutions used for intradermal tests are about 100 times more dilute than those used for scratch tests, they are still potentially dangerous. Severe reactions may occur, however, with either method. Generally, the diluted solutions used prevent **systemic** reactions. Intradermal test sites are performed at spaced intervals on the forearm (Figure 16-7) or scapular area. In the event of a severe **adverse** reaction, a tourniquet can be applied proximal to the site when the arm is used. Serum or vaccine is sometimes used in intradermal testing. If the initial test is negative, it is often repeated with a stronger solution. Usually, the reaction time is 15 to 30 minutes. **Epinephrine** should be administered

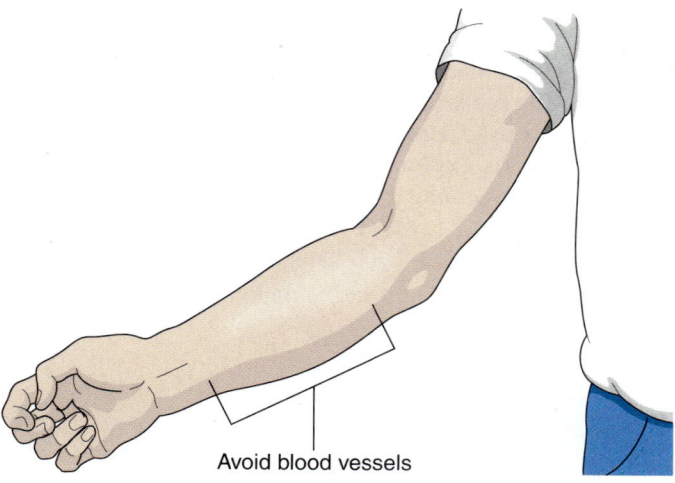

FIGURE 16-7   The forearm is the most common area for and provides up to 14 sites for intradermal skin tests.

about an inch above the site by order of the physician if severe reaction occurs.

In performing an intradermal test, a fine-gauge needle (usually 26 G and $\frac{3}{8}$ to $\frac{5}{8}$ inches long) is used. The antigen is introduced into the dermal layer of the skin in minute dosages of 0.01 to 0.02 mL by sterile technique. The area will appear as a small blister from the fluid raising the skin. The reaction period is up to 30 minutes, and the interpretation of the results is the same as in the scratch tests. Some antigens such as fungi and bacteria produce delayed reactions 24 to 48 hours after administration. Be sure to impress upon the patient the importance of comparing the reaction to something well known (e.g., size of welt [size of a dime], redness, itching), and record all symptoms of the reaction with the date and time, especially if it is at a time when the office is closed. Provide an emergency phone number or instructions to call EMS (911 where applicable) in case a severe or life-threatening reaction should occur.

Intradermal tests are sometimes used by physicians to determine medication sensitivity or immunization needs. Follow the procedure for intradermal injections in Chapter 18.

Patch Test

The patch test is done to determine the cause of **contact dermatitis**. A patch consisting of a gauze square saturated with the suspected allergy-causing substance is placed on the surface of the skin and secured with non-allergenic tape (Figure 16-8). The arm is the usual site of choice for convenience. The results are read after a 24-hour period and then repeated after a 48-hour period. A control is necessary and should be placed on the arm near the patch if the substance of the patch test is not a known skin irritant. Redness or swelling of the area indicates a reaction, and its interpretation is based on grading as for scratch and intradermal tests. Refer to Procedure 16-2.

RAST Testing

The radioallergosorbent test (**RAST**) is a blood test that may be done with a skin test or instead of one. Individual allergens or allergen groups can be identified by the measurement of serum antibodies (an example of an allergen group could be a food panel). The antibody tested is immunoglobulin E (IgE), which may be produced in response to exposure to certain allergens;

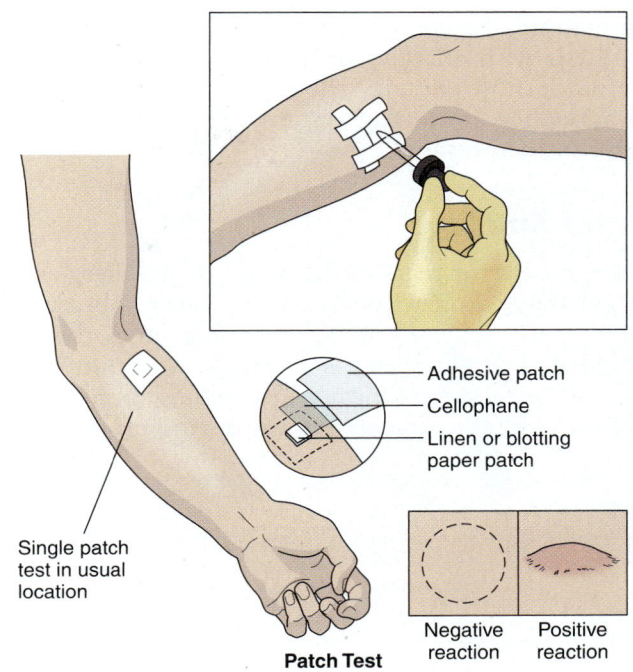

Adhesive patch
Cellophane
Linen or blotting paper patch

Single patch test in usual location

Negative reaction   Positive reaction

Patch Test

FIGURE 16-8   As the patch test is applied, instruct the patient to keep the patch clean and dry and to keep it intact until the results are read by the health care provider.

PROCEDURE PROCEDURE PROCEDURE PROCEDURE PROCEDURE PROCEDURE PROCEDURE

16-2   Perfom a Patch Test

PURPOSE: To determine the causative substance of suspected contact dermatitis.

OSHA GUIDELINES: To comply with Standard Precautions, gloves must be worn if there is any possibility of coming into contact with blood or any body fluids.

EQUIPMENT: Commercially prepared paper with suspected substance or gauze saturated with substance and mock control substance, latex or vinyl gloves, alcohol, cotton balls, gauze squares, biohazardous waste bag, nonallergenic tape, pen, and patient's chart.

PERFORMANCE OBJECTIVE: After practicing with water in lieu of the suspected substance, students will be provided with all necessary supplies, including the suspected substance. Using another student as a patient, demonstrate each of the steps required in carrying out the skin patch test, including the 48-hour recheck. The instructor will observe each step.

1. Assemble the items on a Mayo table or other suitable flat work area next to the patient, wash hands, and put on gloves.
2. Explain the procedure while assisting the identified patient to a comfortable sitting position.
3. Clean the test site with an alcohol-saturated cotton ball, and let it air dry.
4. Apply the suspected substance to the test site, and the mock control substance next to it, and secure them with nonallergenic tape. **NOTE: Usually the test patch is placed near an unaffected area in patients with contact dermatitis. Remove gloves and wash hands.**
5. Record the date, time, substance, and area tested on the patient's chart.
6. Schedule the patient to return in 48 hours.
7. Instruct the patient to keep the area clean and dry until the return appointment.
8. Remove the patch with gloved hands; read the results and record them. **NOTE: Discard gloves and the patch in a biohazardous waste bag.**

CHARTING EXAMPLE

7-21-XX

Verita Joan Stevens—patch test for adhesive applied on L forearm; Verita was instructed to return for evaluation in 24 hours.

S. Davis, RMA

many times, the IgE levels are found to be higher in individuals with allergies or asthma. The RAST test is useful for those patients who cannot have the skin tests because they are taking certain medications, such as some antidepressants.

Nasal Smear

A helpful aid for years in the diagnosis of allergies has been a smear done with nasal secretions to observe the eosinophil count. If there are many and they are clumped together, there is a strong indication of allergy. This is a simple means of screening for an allergy and is usually the first step in the testing program.

ACHIEVE UNIT OBJECTIVES

- ■ Complete the Workbook activities to meet the learning objectives.
- ■ Practice the procedures in this unit to meet the performance objectives.
- ■ Apply your knowledge at the end of this chapter in completing the Critical Thinking Challenge and Activities, as well as the StudyWARE on your Student CD-ROM.

UNIT 2
CARDIOLOGY PROCEDURES

OBJECTIVES

Upon completion of this unit, you will be able to achieve the following:

LEARNING Objectives

1. Spell and define, using the glossary at the back of the text, all the Words to Know in this unit.
2. Explain the reasons for performing an ECG.
3. Describe the electrical conduction system of the heart.
4. Describe methods of a routine 12-lead ECG.
5. Define *artifacts* and list their causes on an ECG.
6. Describe the reason for mounting an ECG tracing.

7. State the purpose of a Holter monitor, and explain the procedure to a patient.
8. State the purpose of defibrillation.
9. Describe cardiac stress testing, and discuss the proper placement of the electrodes.
10. State the purpose of cardiac stress testing.
11. Describe patient education regarding the heart.

PERFORMANCE Objectives

1. Apply limb and chest electrodes properly.
2. Perform a routine 12-lead ECG.
3. Demonstrate the procedure for proper hook-up of a Holter monitor.

WORDS TO KNOW

amplifier	electrocardio-	precordial
arrhythmia	graph	Purkinje
artifacts	electrode	reliable
atrial	galvanometer	repolarization
depolarization	Holter monitor	sedentary
augmented	impulse	segment
cardiology	interference	simultaneous
computerized	intermittent	somatic
countershock	interpretive	standardization
current	interval	stylus
defibrillator	limbs	trace
electrocardio-	mechanical	treadmill
gram	multichannel	voltage

 ## CERTIFICATION CONNECTION

CMA
Treatment area—equipment preparation and operation; principle of operation of electrocardiograph
Performing selected tests—electrocardiography (EKG/ECG)

RMA
Electrocardiography—standard, 12-lead ECG; mounting techniques; other electrocardiographic procedures

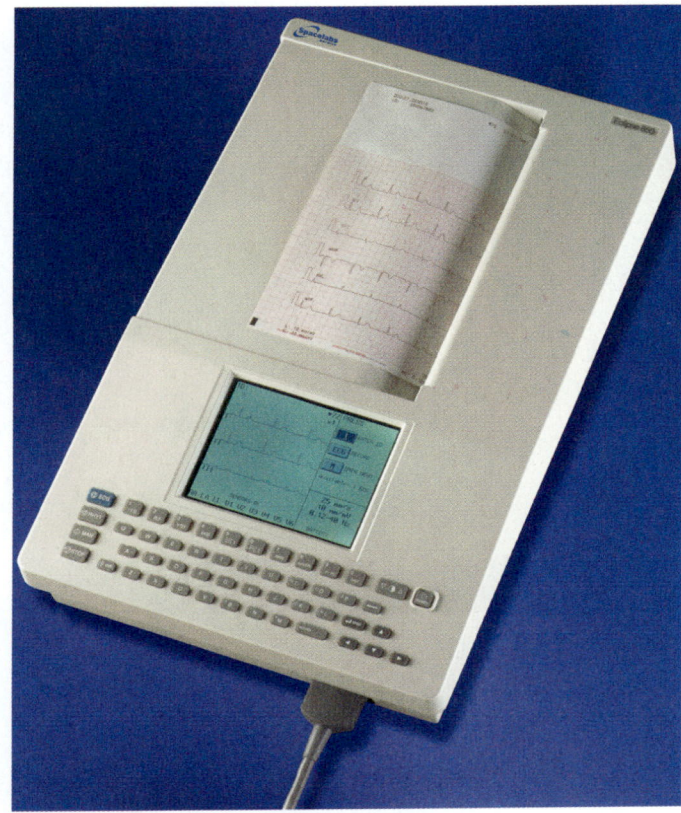

FIGURE 16-9   The portable Eclipse 850 electrocardiograph *(Courtesy of Spacelabs Medical, Inc.)*

In family and general practice, internal medicine, and **cardiology**, a procedure frequently used in the diagnosis of heart disease and dysfunction is the **electrocardiogram**. This procedure is painless and safe, and patients should be told so to eliminate apprehension.

You will obtain the electrocardiogram (EKG/ECG) (recording) by operating the **electrocardiograph** (machine). Figures 16-9 and 16-10 show three widely used models of ECGs.

Through a process of electrical transmission, this machine **traces impulses** of the heart on paper to create a permanent record of its activity.

All muscle movement produces electrical impulses. The ECG is a recording of the electrical impulses of the heart muscle. To accomplish this, **electrodes** are placed on the patient's **limbs** and chest and pick up the electrical **current** produced by the contractions of the heart. Some electrodes are pictured in Figures 16-11 and 16-12. The minute impulses are transmitted to the electrocardiograph by metal tips (or clips) on the patient cables (wires) that are attached to the electrodes. Figure 16-13 displays AstroTraceClips, sometimes referred to as the "universal clip" because they can be used with most types of electrodes. The current enters the electrocardiograph through the wires to reach the **amplifier**, which enlarges the impulses. They are transformed into **mechanical** motion by the **galvanometer**. The **stylus** produces a printed representation on ECG paper. ECG paper is made for the different types of machines, standard, single, and **multichannel** (Figure 16-14). As the heated stylus moves against the tracing paper, the impulses given off by the

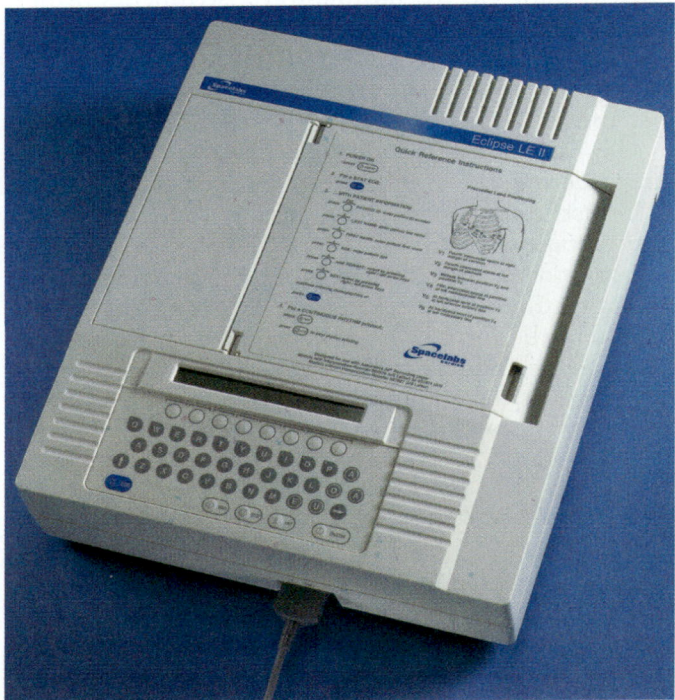

FIGURE 16-10   The multichannel Eclipse LE II electrocardiograph *(Courtesy of Spacelabs Medical, Inc.)*

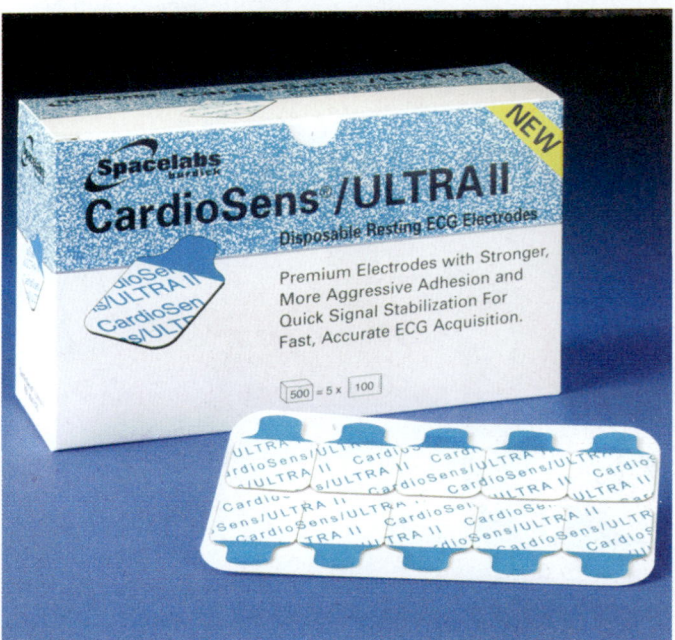

FIGURE 16-11   Cardio-Sens Ultra II disposable sensors and others that are similar are commonly used in obtaining electrocardiograms. *(Courtesy of Spacelabs Medical, Inc.)*

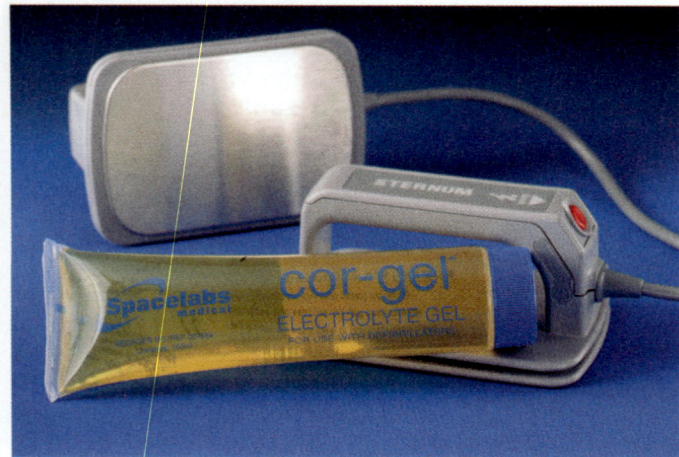

FIGURE 16-12 Electrolyte gel is applied to the paddles of the defibrillator shown in Figure 16-31. *(Courtesy of Spacelabs Medical, Inc.)*

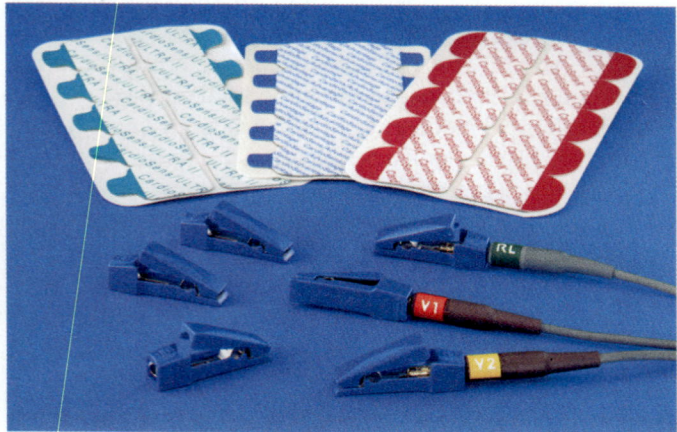

FIGURE 16-13 AstroTrace clips *(Courtesy of Spacelabs Medical, Inc.)*

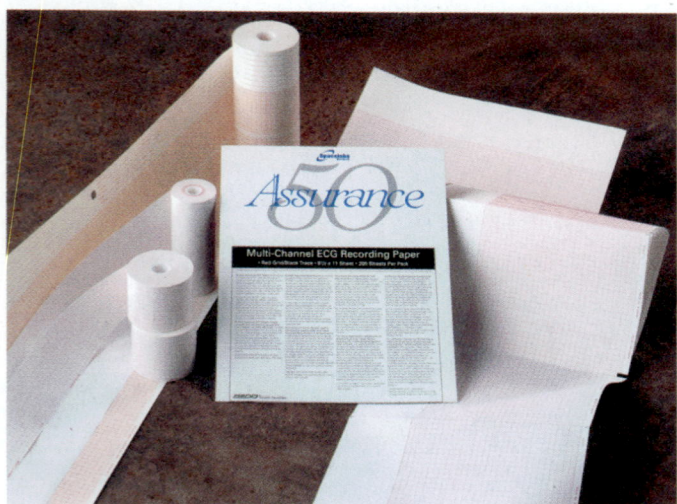

FIGURE 16-14 ECG blush coat paper *(Courtesy of Spacelabs Medical, Inc.)*

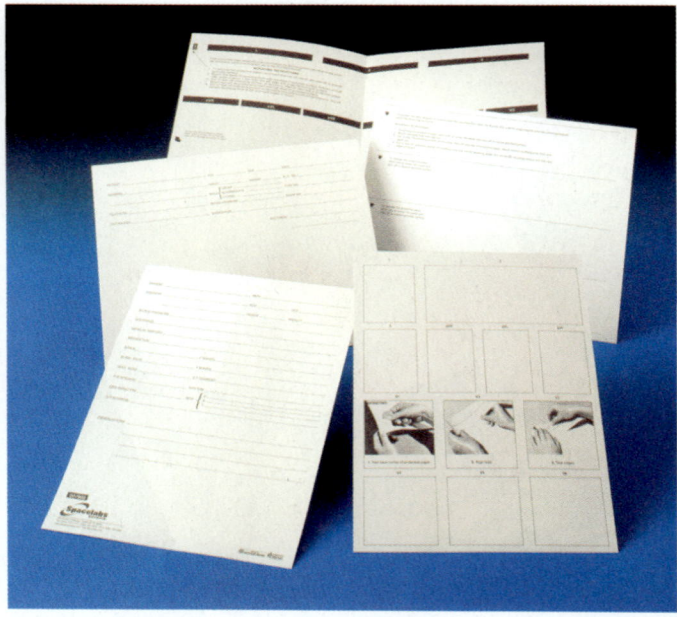

FIGURE 16-15 Various types of mounts for ECG tracing paper for patients' permanent records *(Courtesy of Spacelabs Medical, Inc.)*

heart are recorded. The tracing paper should be handled carefully to protect it from being accidentally marked. Dot matrix paper makes tracings easy to read and copy because they are clear and legible.

Some ECGs are mounted onto permanent folders for filing (Figure 16-15); however, as technology advances, many electrocardiograph instruments print a tracing that does not need to be mounted. Many of the instruments have advanced to the point that the patient data is entered through a keypad on the instrument.

The ECG is interpreted by a physician, usually the one ordering the procedure. Newer, more expensive ECG instruments have the capability to perform basic interpretations of the tracings, although a physician will still review the tracings. Some physicians prefer to have a cardiologist interpret the ECG and submit the results in the form of a written report. The physician interpreting the ECG will compare the measurement, rate, rhythm, duration of the electrical waves, **intervals**, and **segments** with known normal ECG readings.

PATH OF ELECTRICAL IMPULSES

The heart is a four-chambered pump that produces a minute electrical current by muscular contraction (Figure 16-16). An electrical impulse originates in the modified myocardial tissue of the sinoatrial (SA) node, causing the atria to contract (Figure 16-17). This contraction is the beginning of **atrial depolarization**, which is the first part of the cardiac cycle. The first impulse as

muscles of the ventricles to contract and produce the QRS complex of waves on the ECG paper. The T wave on the graph paper follows, representing the **repolarization** of the ventricles, or the time of recovery before another contraction.

ROUTINE ELECTROCARDIOGRAPH LEADS

The routine ECG consists of 12 leads, or recordings of the electrical activity of the heart from different angles. The first three leads are called standard or bipolar leads and are labeled with Roman numerals I, II, and III. These leads are obtained by placing limb electrodes on the fleshy part of the upper outer arms (refer to Figure 16-12) and the inner lower calves (Figure 16-18). Lead I records the electrical voltage difference between the right arm and left arm. Lead II records the difference between the right arm and the left leg. Lead III records the **voltage** difference between the left arm and left leg (Figure 16-19).

The **augmented** leads are the next three in the standard 12-lead ECG. They are aVR, aVL, and aVF. aVR is the recording of the heart's voltage difference between the right arm electrode and a central point between the left arm and the left leg (augmented voltage right arm). aVL is the recording of the heart's voltage difference between the left arm electrode and a central point between the right arm and the left leg (augmented voltage left arm). aVF is the recording of the heart's voltage dif-

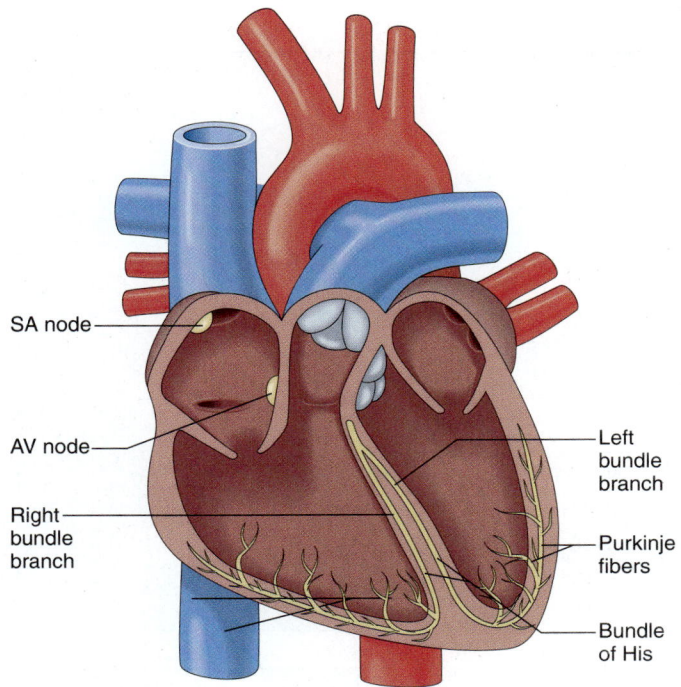

FIGURE 16-16   Anatomy of the heart

recorded on the graph paper is termed the P wave. The impulse continues through the heart tissue to the atrioventricular (AV) node, to the bundle of His, and spreads to the **Purkinje** fibers. These fibers cause the

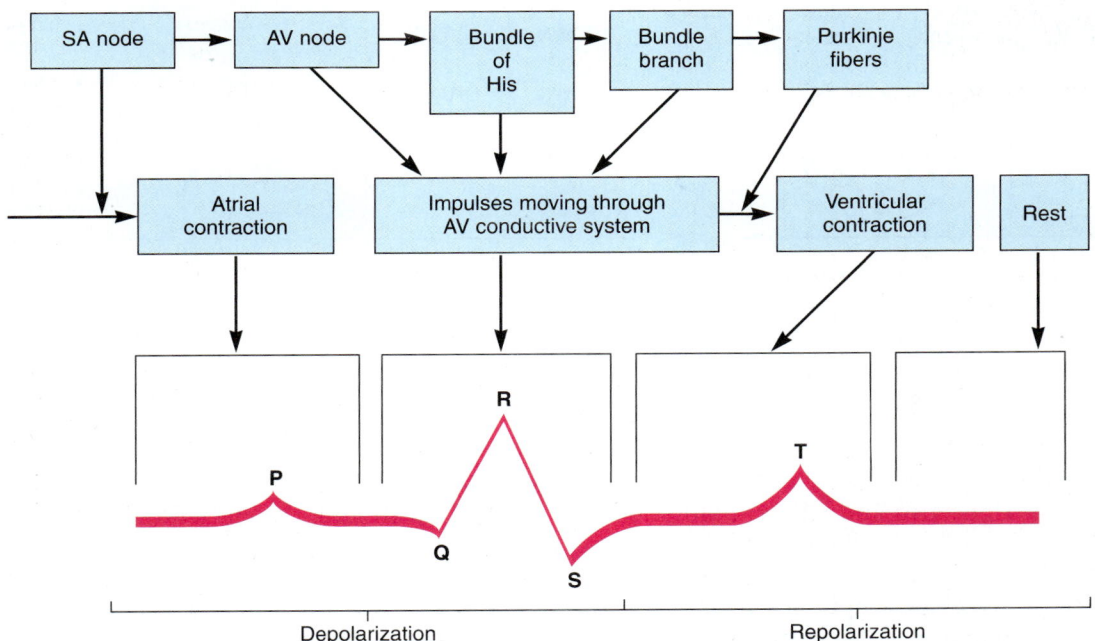

FIGURE 16-17   Cardiac impulses on an ECG tracing: (A) course of electrical impulses; (B) cardiac muscle reaction to impulses; (C) ECG tracing of impulse waves; (D) phases of the cardiac cycle *(Courtesy of Spacelabs Medical, Inc.)*

LEAD ARRANGEMENT AND CODING

STANDARD LIMB LEADS

LEAD MARKING CODE	LEAD	ELECTRODES CONNECTED	COLOR CODE		
				BODY	INSERT
●	LEAD 1	LA and RA	RL	GREEN	GREEN
	LEAD 2	LL and RA	LL	RED	RED
			RA	WHITE	GRAY
	LEAD 3	LL and LA	LA	BLACK	GRAY

AUGMENTED LIMB LEADS

LEAD MARKING CODE	LEAD	ELECTRODES CONNECTED	COLOR CODE		
				BODY	INSERT
● ●	aVR	RA and (LA-LL)	RL	GREEN	GREEN
	aVL	LA and (RA-LL)	LL	RED	RED
			RA	WHITE	GRAY
	aVF	LL and (RA-LA)	LA	BLACK	GRAY

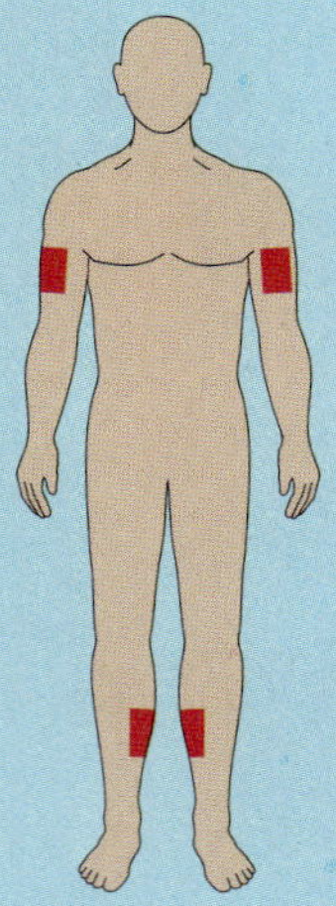

CHEST LEADS

LEAD MARKING CODE	LEAD	ELECTRODES CONNECTED	COLOR CODE		
				BODY	INSERT
● ● ●	V_1	V_1 and (LA-RA-LL)	V_1	BROWN	RED
	V_2	V_2 and (LA-RA-LL)	V_2	BROWN	YELLOW
	V_3	V_3 and (LA-RA-LL)	V_3	BROWN	GREEN
● ● ● ●	V_4	V_4 and (LA-RA-LL)	V_4	BROWN	BLUE
	V_5	V_5 and (LA-RA-LL)	V_5	BROWN	ORANGE
	V_6	V_6 and (LA-RA-LL)	V_6	BROWN	VIOLET

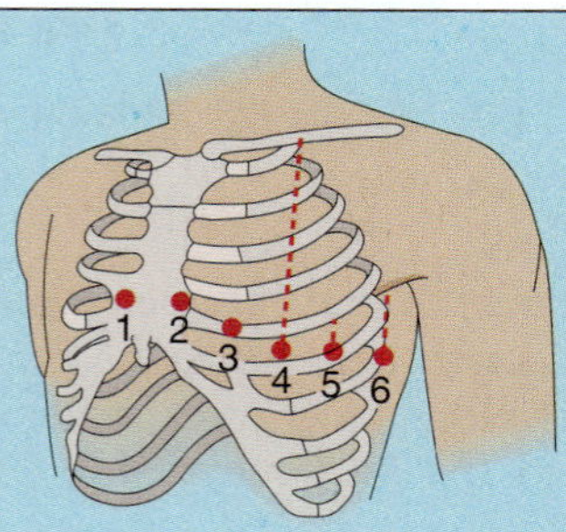

V_1 Fourth intercostal space at right margin of sternum

V_2 Fourth intercostal space at left margin of sternum

V_3 Midway between position 2 and position 4

V_4 Fifth intercostal space at junction of left midclavicular line

V_5 At horizontal level of position 4 at left anterior axillary line

V_6 At horizontal level of position 4 at left midaxillary line

FIGURE 16-18 Proper placement of electrodes for the standard 12-lead ECG and lead markings *(Courtesy of Spacelabs Medical, Inc.)*

ference between the left leg electrode and a central point between the right arm and left arm (augmented voltage left leg or foot). The term *augmented* means "to become larger." Because these three leads are produced by such small impulses, the amplifier of the ECG machine augments their size sufficiently for recording them on the graph paper.

The six standard chest or **precordial** leads are obtained by affixing the electrodes to the anatomical positions shown in Figure 16-20.

Most electrocardiographs have an automatic lead marker to identify each of the 12 standard leads. A standard marking code is used with the automatic method. (Refer to Procedure 16-3.)

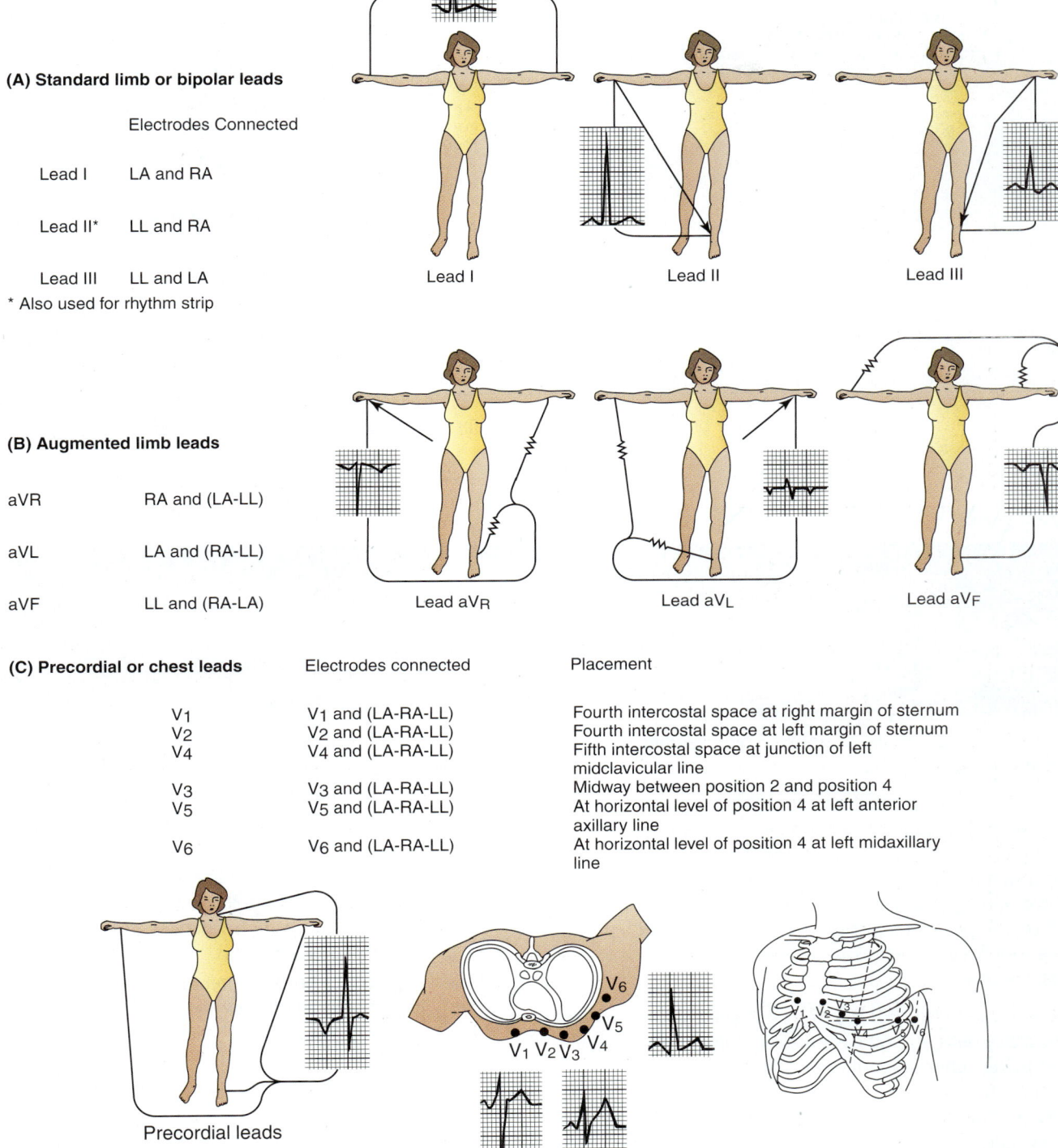

(A) Standard limb or bipolar leads

Electrodes Connected

Lead I   LA and RA

Lead II*   LL and RA

Lead III   LL and LA

* Also used for rhythm strip

Lead I   Lead II   Lead III

(B) Augmented limb leads

aVR   RA and (LA-LL)

aVL   LA and (RA-LL)

aVF   LL and (RA-LA)

Lead aV$_R$ Lead aV$_L$ Lead aV$_F$

(C) Precordial or chest leads

	Electrodes connected	Placement
V$_1$	V$_1$ and (LA-RA-LL)	Fourth intercostal space at right margin of sternum
V$_2$	V$_2$ and (LA-RA-LL)	Fourth intercostal space at left margin of sternum
V$_4$	V$_4$ and (LA-RA-LL)	Fifth intercostal space at junction of left midclavicular line
V$_3$	V$_3$ and (LA-RA-LL)	Midway between position 2 and position 4
V$_5$	V$_5$ and (LA-RA-LL)	At horizontal level of position 4 at left anterior axillary line
V$_6$	V$_6$ and (LA-RA-LL)	At horizontal level of position 4 at left midaxillary line

Precordial leads

FIGURE 16-19   Lead types, connections, and placement: (A) standard limb or bipolar leads; (B) augmented or unipolar limb leads; (C) precordial or chest leads *(Courtesy of Spacelabs Medical, Inc.)*

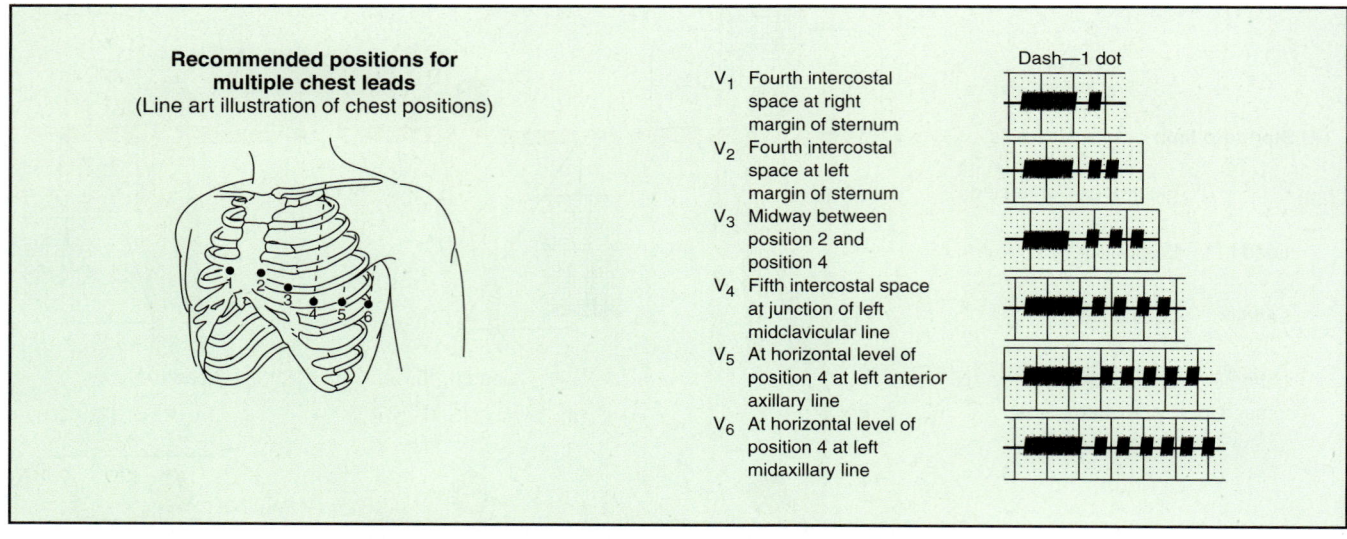

Recommended positions for multiple chest leads
(Line art illustration of chest positions)

V₁ Fourth intercostal space at right margin of sternum

V₂ Fourth intercostal space at left margin of sternum

V₃ Midway between position 2 and position 4

V₄ Fifth intercostal space at junction of left midclavicular line

V₅ At horizontal level of position 4 at left anterior axillary line

V₆ At horizontal level of position 4 at left midaxillary line

Dash—1 dot

FIGURE 16-20 Example of common coding system for ECG leads *(Courtesy of Spacelabs Medical, Inc.)*

PROCEDURE PROCEDURE PROCEDURE PROCEDURE PROCEDURE PROCEDURE PROCEDURE

16-3 Obtain a Standard 12-Lead Electrocardiogram

PURPOSE: To obtain a graphic representation of the electrical activity of the patient's heart.

EQUIPMENT: Electrocardiograph; ECG paper; disposable pregelled adhesive electrodes as appropriate for use with patient cable of ECG machine; lead wires with snaps, clips, or tips to attach to electrodes; patient cable; electrolyte (pads, cream, or gel); chest strap; treatment table; pillow; drape sheet; tissues; paper towels; ECG mount; footstool; tongue depressor; patient's chart; pen; and disposable razor.

PERFORMANCE OBJECTIVE: Provided with an electrocardiograph and all essential equipment and supplies and using other students as patients, demonstrate each of the steps required in obtaining a standard 12-lead ECG reading within 30 minutes. The instructor will observe each step. **NOTE: The specified disrobing may be simulated.**

1. Plug in the ECG machine to an outlet away from known electrical interference. Plug in the patient cable wire to the machine. Assemble the electrodes and attach them to the straps. Apply electrolyte pads and set them aside. Turn the machine on. Wash hands.

2. Ask the identified patient to disrobe from the waist up and remove clothing from the lower legs. Provide privacy and show the patient where to put her belongings. Explain the procedure.

3. Assist the patient onto the treatment table and cover her with a drape sheet. Ask the patient to lie down. Pull out the leg rest. Adjust a pillow under the patient's head for comfort.

4. Place the arm electrodes (with electrolyte) on the fleshy outer area of the upper arm, with the connectors pointing toward the shoulders. Leg electrodes should be placed on the fleshy inner area of the lower leg near the calf, with connectors pointing toward the

(continues)

16-3  Obtain a Standard 12-Lead Electrocardiogram (Continued)

upper body. **RATIONALE: This placement of electrodes the eliminates friction from examining table and body movement. NOTE: Especially when disposable electrodes are used, it is very important to use a gauze square to rub sites vigorously to increase circulation and promote better contact of the electrodes.**

5. Connect the lead wire tips to the appropriate electrodes by snapping or clipping the electrodes securely in place. **NOTE: The power cord and patient cable must not be allowed to touch.**

6. Attach all six pregelled disposable adhesive chest electrodes, V_1 through V_6 (shaving dense chest hair as necessary for placement of electrodes) (Figure 16-21). Figures 16-22A and B show male and female patients with electrodes properly placed for a 12-lead ECG.

7. Performing an ECG on a female patient who has larger breasts may present a problem when attaching the leads. Because the left breast may extend down over the location of the 3rd, 4th, and 5th leads, it may be necessary to elevate the breast tissue before they can be correctly applied. You should elevate the breast using the back of the hand instead of touching the breast with your fingers (Figure 16-22C). After all the leads are attached, the chest can be covered with the gown to provide for minimum exposure and for warmth while the ECG is ob-

tained. Figure 16-22D shows the chest wall with the leads attached and the breast tissue extended over a portion of the leads.

8. Turn the lead selector switch to STD, and adjust the stylus to the center of the graph paper.

9. Move the record switch to the 25 mm/second position, and run it for a few seconds to adjust the centering of the stylus. Make a standardization mark 2 mm wide and 10 mm high. Press "auto" and run the 12-lead ECG.

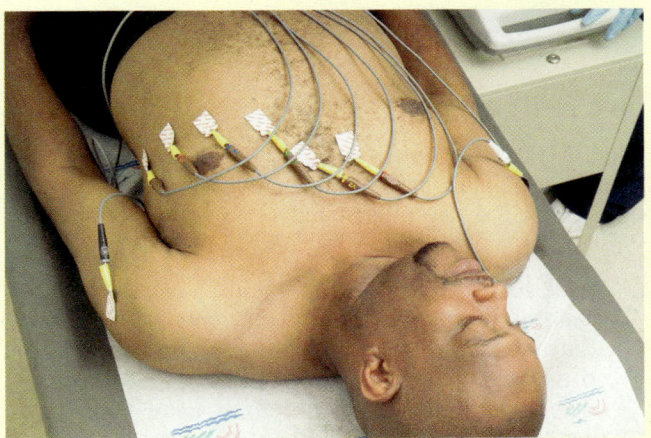

FIGURE 16-22A A male patient with electrodes placed properly for a standard 12-lead ECG

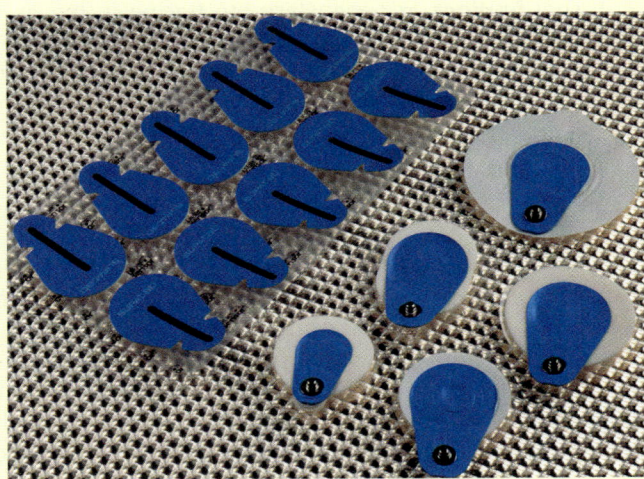

FIGURE 16-21 Adhesive pregelled disposable electrodes *(Courtesy of Spacelabs Medical, Inc.)*

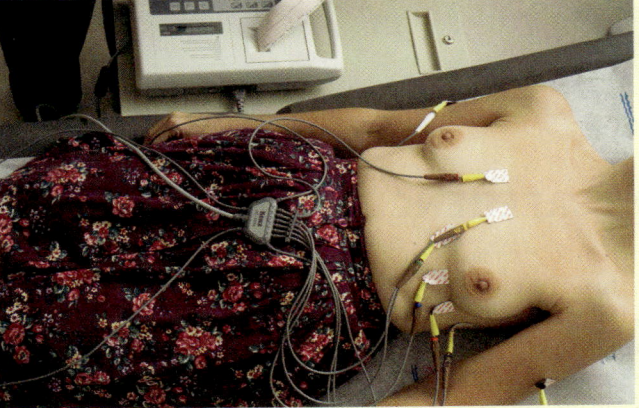

FIGURE 16-22B A female patient with electrodes placed properly for a standard 12-lead ECG

(continues)

16-3  Obtain a Standard 12-Lead Electrocardiogram (Continued)

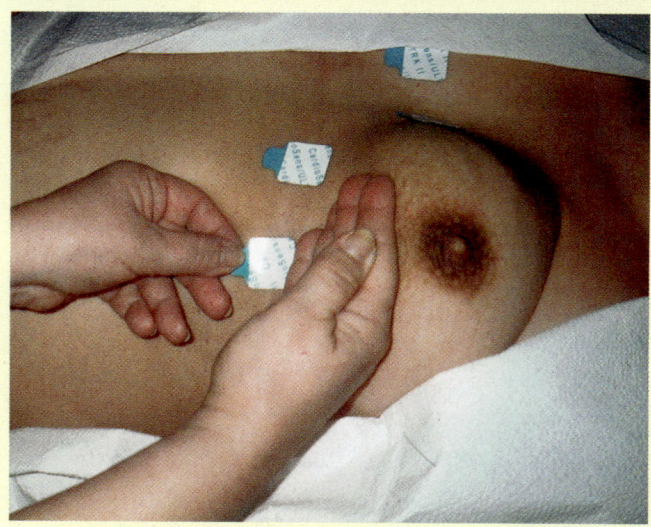

FIGURE 16-22C When placing electrodes for a standard 12-lead ECG on a female with larger breast, elevate the breast using the back of the hand.

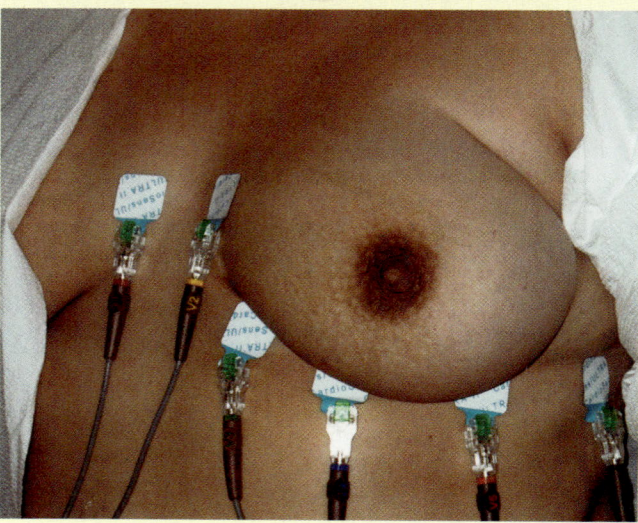

FIGURE 16-22D A female patient with larger breast with electrodes placed properly for a standard 12-lead ECG

10. Tear the off tracing from the machine. **NOTE: Immediately mark it with the patient's name and age, the current date, and your initials.** Roll or loosely overlap the tracing back and forth, carefully secure it with a paper clip, and set it aside. **NOTE: This is not required with a computerized ECG printout.**

11. Remove the tips of the lead wires from the limb electrodes. Remove the electrodes from the patient. Clean sites with a warm, wet paper towel and dry. Discard used towels in the proper receptacle.

12. Assist the patient to a sitting position and then down from the table when ready. Assist the patient in dressing if necessary.

13. Change the table paper and pillow cover, and discard used disposables. Wash hands.

14. **NOTE: Alert the physician of any complaints or unusual findings at once.** Place the tracing in the patient's chart for the physician to interpret. Record the appropriate entry on the patient's chart (e.g., pt experienced SOB while lying flat).

INTERFERENCE

As with any procedure, a full explanation must be given to the patient to gain cooperation. Providing privacy and adequate draping of the patient during the procedure will ease patient apprehension and avoid chills. The patient must be relaxed for a good tracing to be obtained, as any movement of the patient may cause **interference** on the tracing. Shivering from nervousness or cold can produce muscle voltage artifacts, for example. This additional activity is called **somatic** tremor. Arm electrodes should be placed close to the shoulders of the upper outer arms to decrease the possibility of muscle voltage **artifacts** and arrhythmias (Figure 16-23).

Other artifacts that may appear on the ECG, called AC interference, are caused by electrical activity. The latest models of electrocardiographs have sensitive filtering devices that eliminate most of the interference. All power cords should be kept away from the patient, and the patient table should be away from the wall to eliminate the possibility of interference from electrical wiring within the wall. The patient must be properly connected with the electrodes and properly grounded

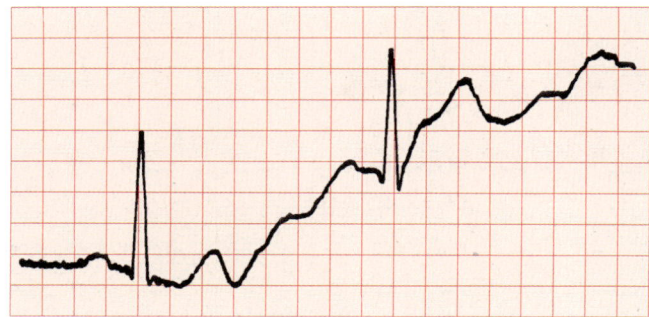

FIGURE 16-23A   ECG interference artifacts and arrhythmias: somatic tremor or involuntary muscle movement *(Courtesy of Quinton Cardiology, Inc.)*

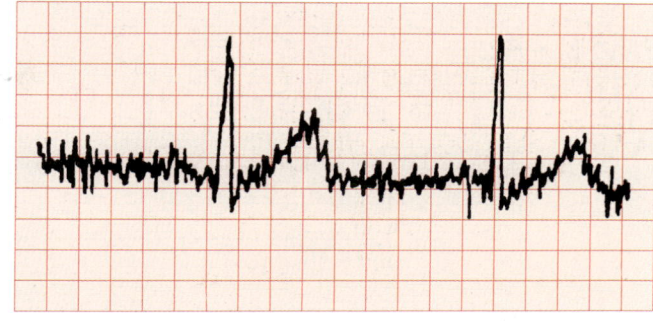

FIGURE 16-23B   AC (alternating current) *(Courtesy of Quinton Cardiology, Inc.)*

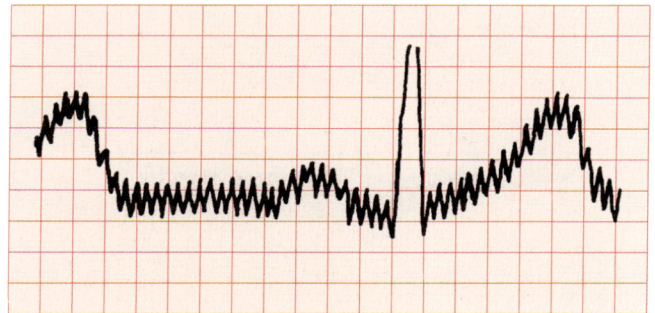

FIGURE 16-23C   Wandering baseline *(Courtesy of Quinton Cardiology, Inc.)*

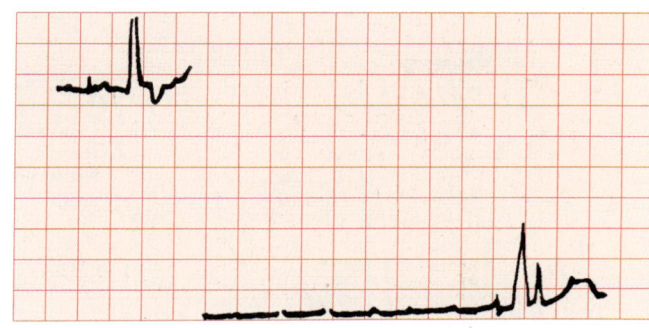

FIGURE 16-23D   Interrupted baseline *(Courtesy of Quinton Cardiology, Inc.)*

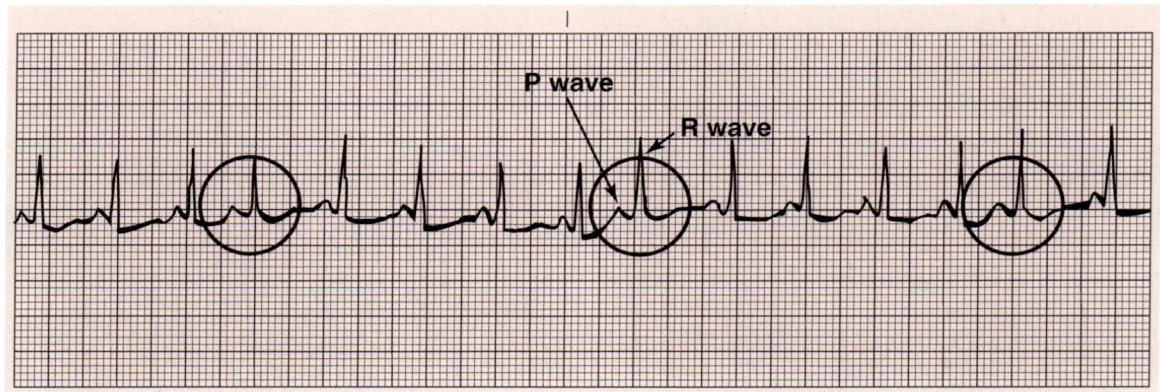

FIGURE 16-23E   Premature atrial contractions (PAC)

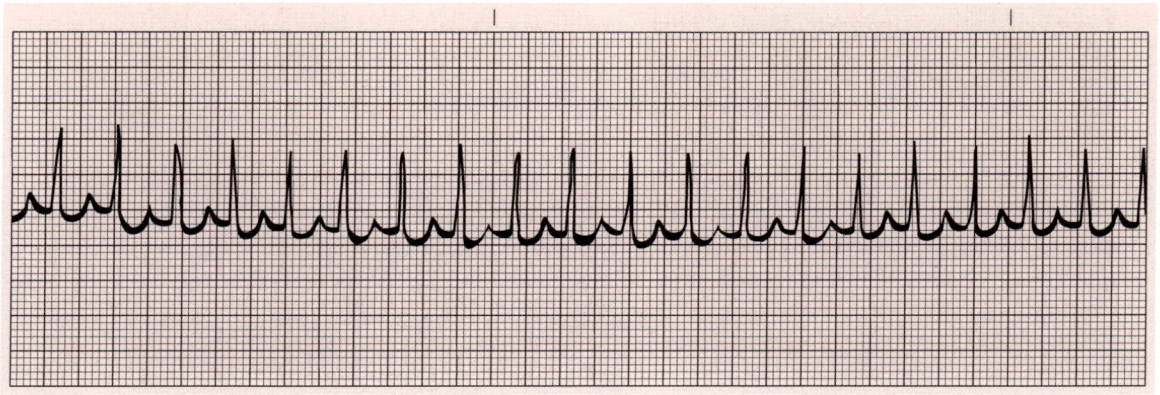

FIGURE 16-23F   Paroxysmal atrial tachycardia (PAT)

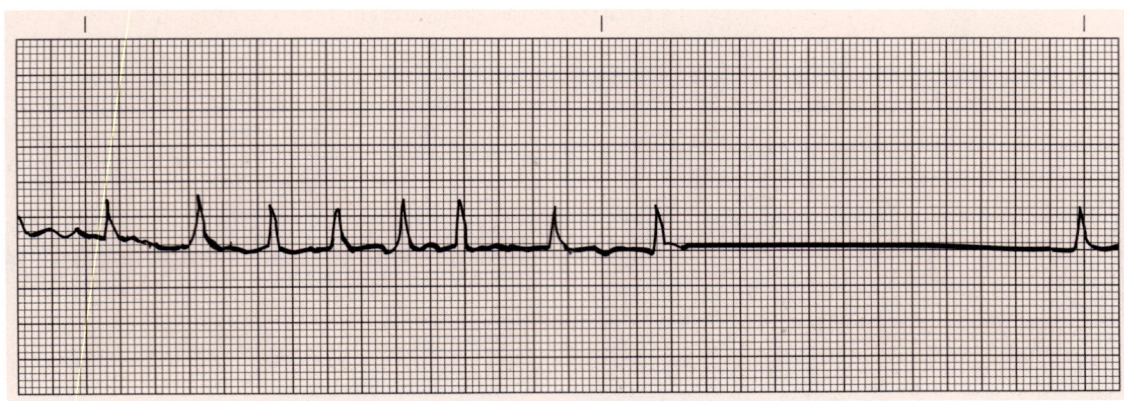

FIGURE 16-23G   Atrial fibrillation

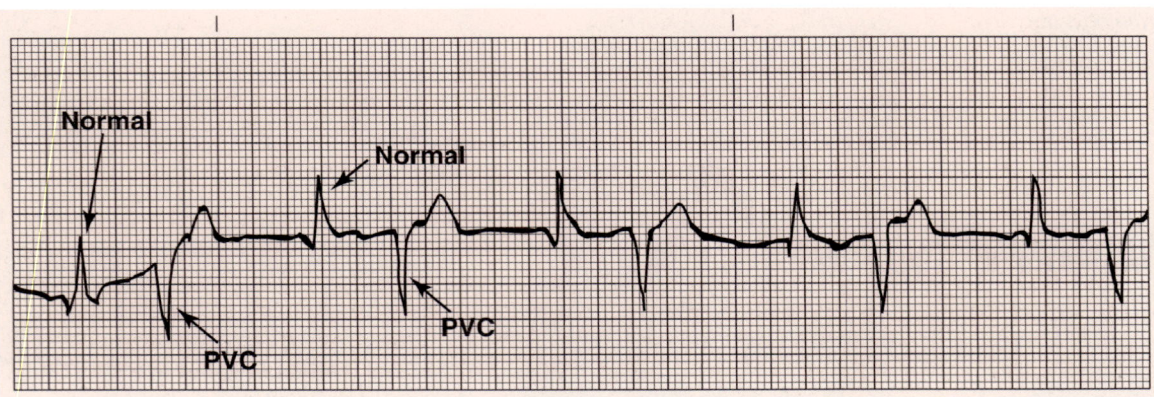

FIGURE 16-23H   Premature ventricular contractions

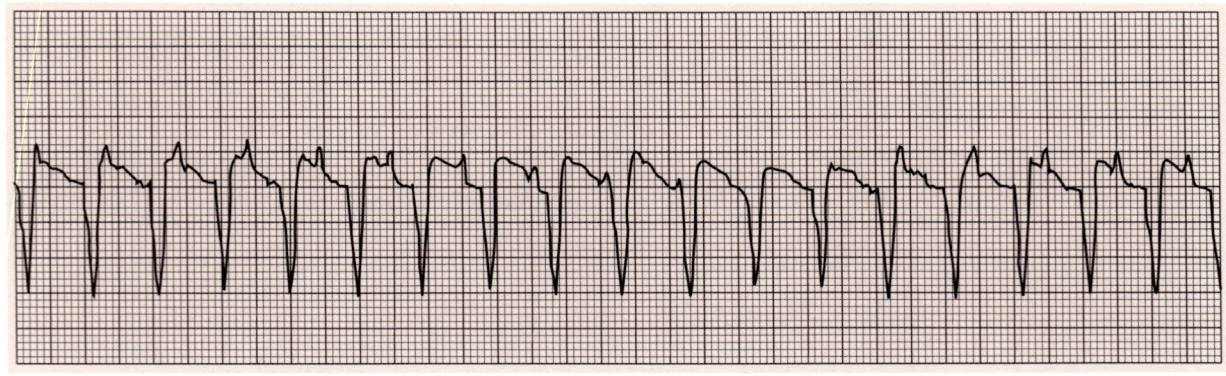

FIGURE 16-23I   Ventricular tachycardia

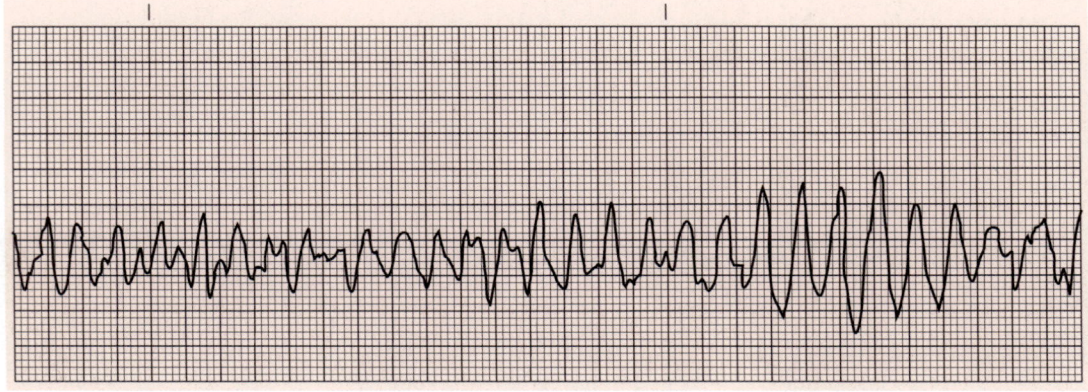

FIGURE 16-23J   Ventricular fibrillation

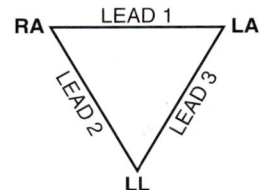

LOCATION OF SOURCE OF ARTIFACTS

Leads 1, 2, and 3 can be helpful in locating the source of interference. Refer to the triangle. Notice that each limb electrode is involved in recording two of the three leads. This means that if an artifact is observed in two leads but not in the third, the artifact is probably caused by a condition at or near the electrode that is common to the two leads. Examples: tremor on leads 1 and 3 and not on lead 2 indicates that the left arm is the probable source since it is common to leads 1 and 3. Similarly, a large amount of AC interference appearing in leads 1 and 2 and a smaller amount in lead 3 would most likely indicate that the AC source is near the right arm. If interference problems cannot be readily solved, contact your Burdick dealer or the Burdick Corporation for the name of your nearest Burdick field representative. They have equipment to help you find the interference source and can offer suggestions to eliminate or reduce the problem.

FIGURE 16-24 Sources of artifacts from leads *(Courtesy of Spacelabs Medical, Inc.)*

(see Figure 16-22). Using good technique will also reduce AC interference. The sources of artifacts from different leads is shown in Figure 16-24.

Wandering baseline can be caused by improperly applied electrodes. Another cause is improperly cleaned skin. Oils, creams, and lotions should be removed from the patient's skin with alcohol, or the conduction of electrical impulses will be impaired. Interrupted baseline is caused by an electrode becoming separated from the wire or by a broken lead wire. Follow the manufacturer's instructions for repairing the electrocardiograph.

All of the **computerized** channel ECG machines require the disposable electrodes and electrolyte pads. These are widely used because of their convenience. Because they are more expensive, you should use them wisely and avoid unnecessary waste.

STANDARDIZATION

The **standardization** of the ECG is necessary to enable a physician to judge deviations from the standard. The usual standardization mark is 2 mm wide and 10 mm

high. This mark should begin each lead to provide a **reliable** reading. If the tracing is too large, the sensitivity dial should be turned down to ½ to produce a standardization mark 5 mm high and 2 mm wide. If the tracing is too small, the sensitivity dial can be turned up to 2, making the impulse 20 mm high and 2 mm wide. You must pay close attention to the tracing as it is being run to make adjustments as needed. Figure 16-25 shows the standardization marking from an electrocardiograph with the sensitivity dial set at ½, 1, and 2.

The stylus should be centered in the middle of the paper. The baseline will allow you to observe the centering and make adjustments as necessary. The temperature of the stylus can be adjusted to control the thickness of the line.

The tracing paper is normally run at a speed of 25 mm per second. If the ECG cycles are too close together, the speed can be changed to 50 mm per second (Figure 16-26). This adjustment should be noted in pen on the tracing.

Any obvious abnormality should be brought to the physician's attention immediately if the patient is experiencing pain or discomfort at the time it is observed.

The ECG is an extremely important procedure. Every detail must be performed accurately.

It is extremely important that the patient be relaxed and comfortable during the ECG procedure. Reassure the patient by answering any questions. Explain that the machine does not "put electricity" into the body. Your calm, efficient manner will help the patient relax.

Computerized electrocardiographs have many time-saving features. They have **simultaneous** 12-lead **interpretive** analysis. Data are not only printed out but also stored in their memory. The entire ECG tracing is generated in about 1 minute. There is no time involved in mounting. A manual mode provides additional leads, such as the rhythm strip of lead II. These machines are relatively lightweight and can be easily moved if necessary.

The ECG can detect damage from previous heart attacks, enlargement of the heart muscle, disturbances in the rhythm, and other abnormal conditions. Three examples of the heart's electrical activity are shown in Figure 16-26. This may give you a better understanding

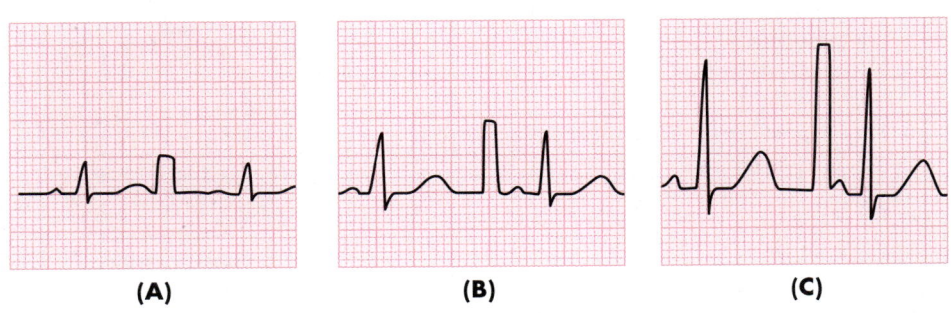

(A)   **(B)**   **(C)**

FIGURE 16-25 Standardization markings with sensitivity dial set on (A) ½, (B) 1, and (C) 2 *(Courtesy of Spacelabs Medical, Inc.)*

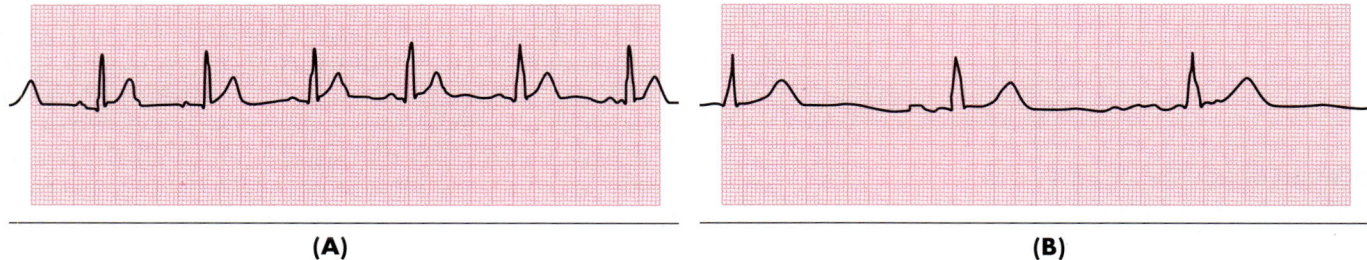

(A)   **(B)**

Illustrated below are a normal ECG and a normal artery.

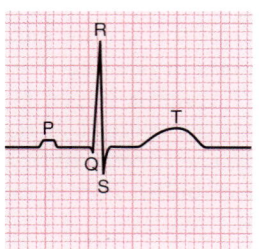

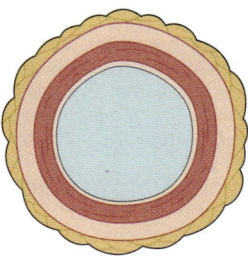

The artery narrows as the atheroma, fatty deposits, (atherosclerosis) becomes larger and hardens, causing a decrease in circulation (arteriosclerosis) in the heart. This condition causes heart pain (angina pectoris).

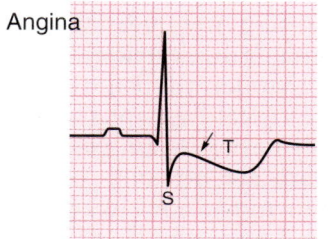

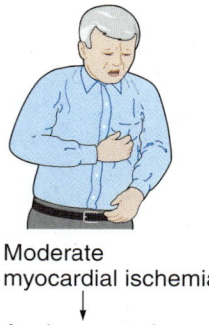

Moderate
myocardial ischemia
↓
Angina pectoris

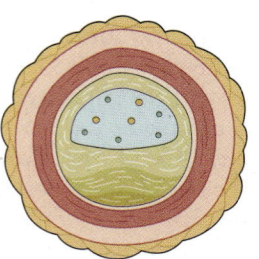

Moderate atherosclerotic
narrowing of lumen

The ECG shows what happens during an MI (myocardial infarction), or heart attack, caused by a coronary occlusion (blockage) from deposits of calcium in the arteries.

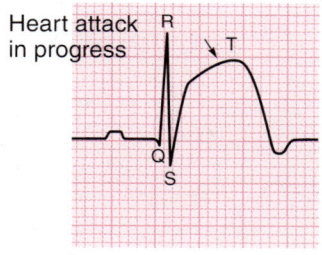

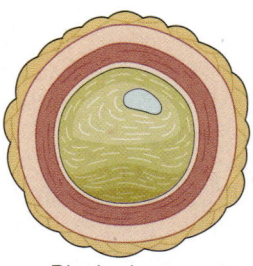

Blocked artery

(C)

FIGURE 16-26   ECG paper: (A) lead II run at 25 mm/sec; (B) lead II run at 50 mm/sec (lead II is also known as a rhythm strip); (C) ECG examples and progression of coronary artery disease

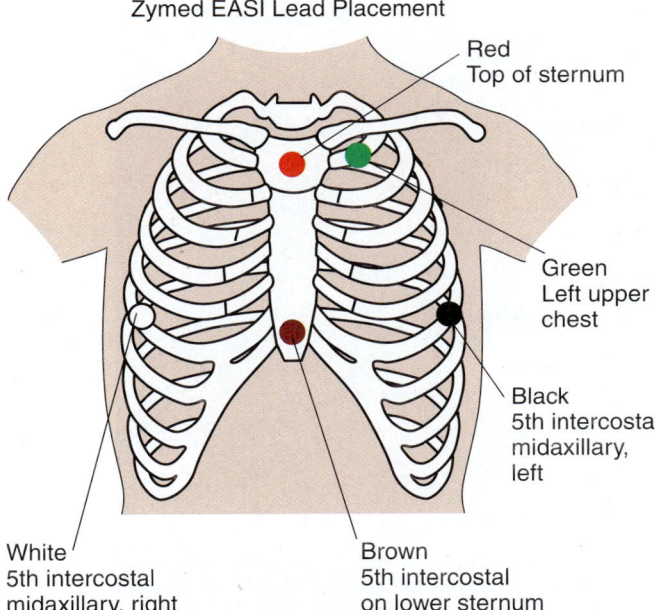

Zymed EASI Lead Placement

Red
Top of sternum

Green
Left upper
chest

Black
5th intercostal
midaxillary,
left

White
5th intercostal
midaxillary, right

Brown
5th intercostal
on lower sternum

FIGURE 16-27A   Zymed five-lead ECG: electrode placement

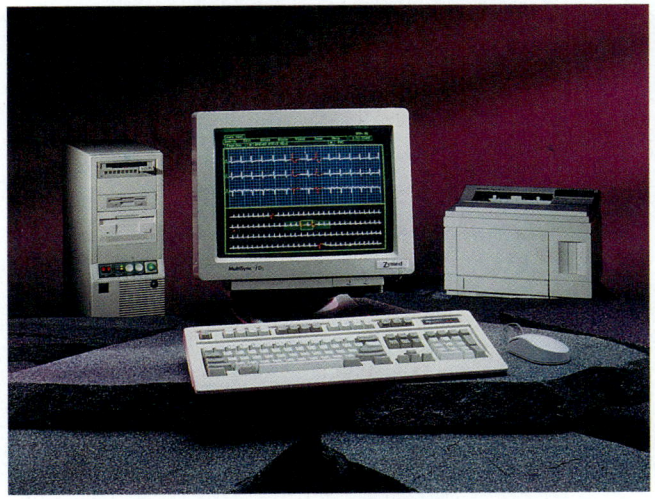

FIGURE 16-27B   Zymed five-lead ECG: computed tracing

obese, or have a high serum cholesterol level. Another factor in heart problems is a **sedentary** lifestyle, which is usually accompanied by obesity.

Zymed Medical Instrumentation provides a computerized ECG with only five leads. The electrodes are placed only on the patient's chest. This ultra-efficient electrocardiogram provides the same information as the standard 12-lead. Figure 16-27 shows the electrocardiograph and the placement of the electrodes. This technology offers a multichannel tracing that can be viewed on a monitor to assess the heart's activity. This method also keeps a memory of ECGs for review of the patient's condition and the progress of treatment.

STRESS TESTS

ECG stress tests are done by some physicians on a routine basis for patients with a high risk of developing heart disease. They are more often done in a limited manner for patients interested in starting a strenuous exercise program or those who continue to have chest pain even after a routine ECG has been read as normal. Figure 16-28 illustrates the BaseLine prep kit and instructions for cardiac stress testing. The stress test ECG is done while a patient is exercising on a **treadmill** under careful supervision. Figure 16-29 shows a physician reading the computerized printout of a stress test in progress. The medical assistant monitors the patient's blood pressure while he exercises on the treadmill. The purpose of this test is to detect the unknown cause of a patient's heart trouble. (Refer to Chapter 11, Unit 8, for discussion regarding additional cardiovascular testing.) Even with ECGs and other diagnostic tests, the physician cannot predict future heart attacks.

of what happens during normal beating of the heart and when it is in crisis. As you can see, the changes in the normal pattern can aid the physician in detecting many heart conditions. Before the physician can confirm a diagnosis, an examination that considers the patient's symptoms, medical history, and other diagnostic tests are necessary. It is usually recommended for patients between the ages of 35 and 40 to establish a base reading. Physicians may then refer to this ECG in the event of later problems. Most often an ECG is performed along with the routine annual physical examination every 5 to 10 years after a baseline normal reading has been established. Some physicians prefer to have a tracing more often, even annually, for patients who have a history of hypertension, are smokers, are

PATIENT EDUCATION

During the time you spend with patients in performing electrocardiographic testing and its instruction, you will have ample opportunity to give patients some of the following suggestions:

1. Remind them to eat a low-fat, low-cholesterol diet and keep their salt/sodium intake at a minimum.
2. Advise them to get proper rest and exercise and keep their weight at an acceptable level.
3. Instruct cardiac patients to take their prescribed medication regularly and to report any problems they may experience to the physician immediately.
4. Remind them to keep their scheduled appointments and make a list of questions for the doctor to review with them at that time.
5. Advise them not to take OTC medications.
6. Urge them not to use tobacco and to avoid alcoholic beverages.

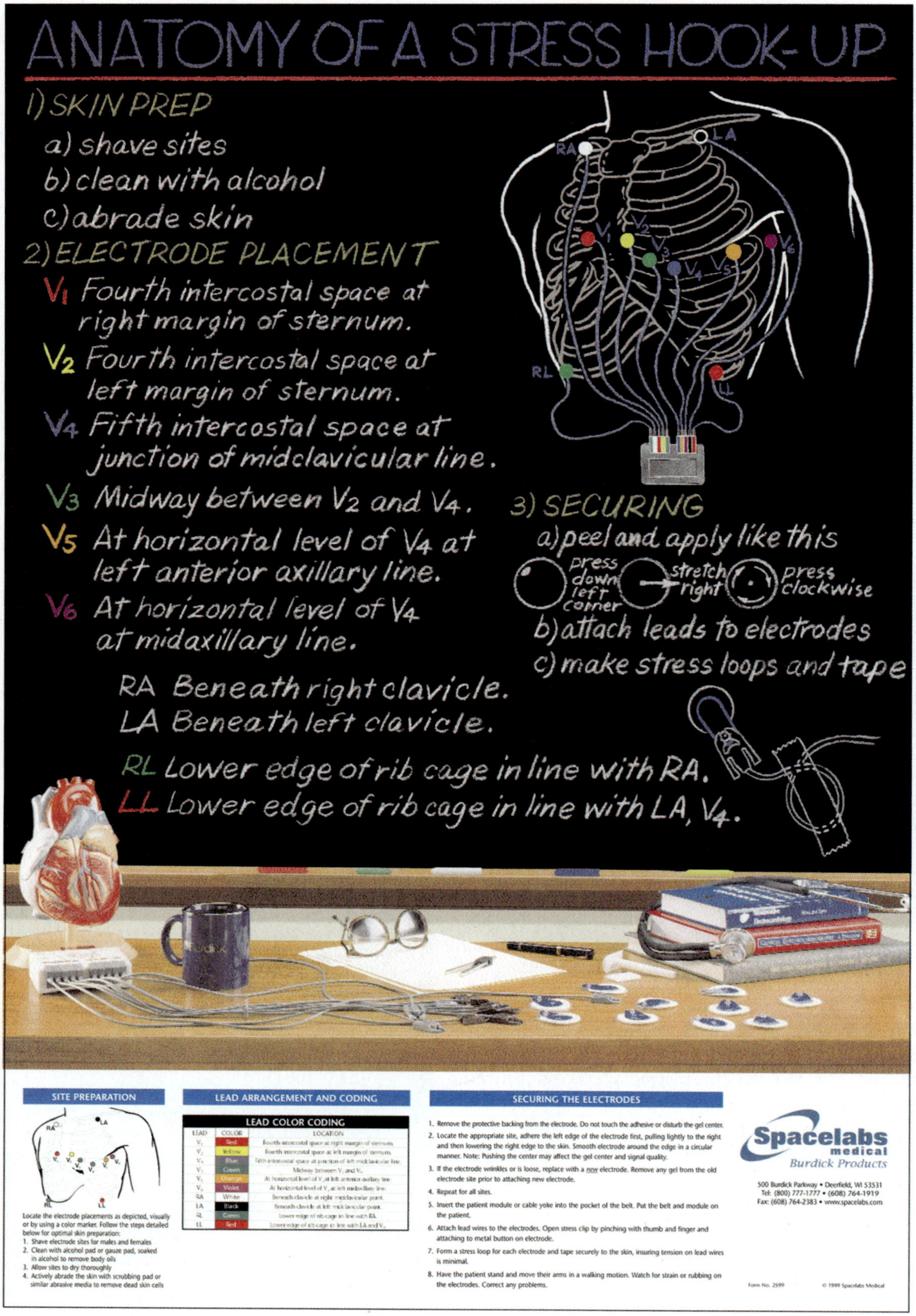

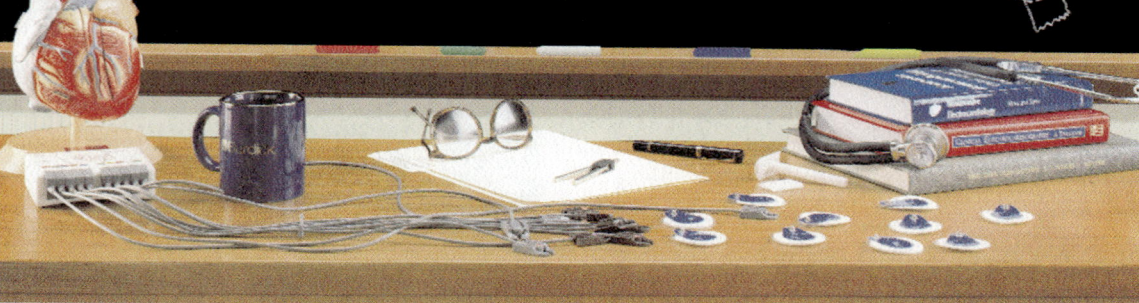

FIGURE 16-28 Instructions for stress ECG hook-up *(Courtesy of Spacelabs Medical, Inc.)*

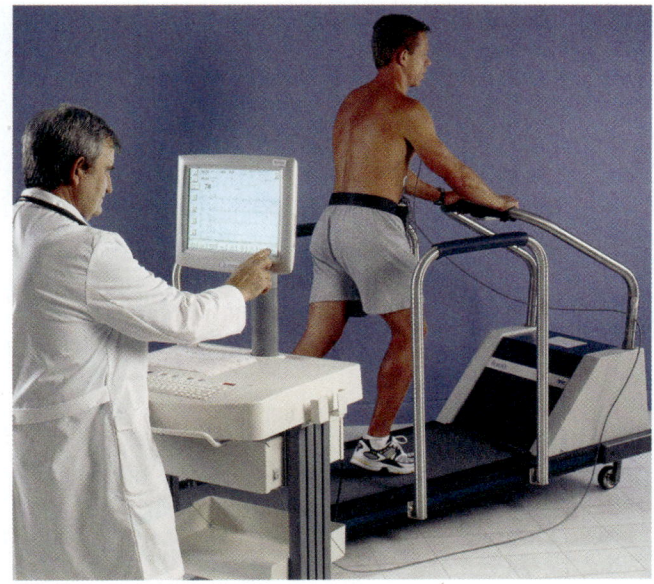

FIGURE 16-29 The Quest Exercise Stress System *(Courtesy of Quinton Cardiology, Inc.)*

asked to keep a diary of all activities and note any pain or discomfort experienced during this monitoring. The patient is instructed to press the "event button" when any cardiac symptoms are experienced. At the end of the test period, the patient returns to have the electrodes and monitor removed. The cassette is then placed in a computerized analyzer for a permanent printout of the results (or sent to a laboratory for interpretation). Evaluation of the 24 hour tracing reveals any cardiac **arrhythmias**, chest pain, and effectiveness of cardiac medications and correlates any symptoms with the patient's activity at the time it occurred. You should instruct patients to carry on with all routine daily activities during this test. Advise patients to take a "sponge bath" and not to get into a tub or shower while conducting this test. Ask patients to avoid using electric blankets or being around metal detectors, magnets, and high-voltage areas, because these might interfere with the recording. This method of monitoring is also used in evaluating the status of recovering cardiac patients. (See Procedure 16-4.)

HOLTER MONITOR

Patients who have normal routine ECGs but still have **intermittent** or irregular chest pain or discomfort are often tested over a period of 24 hours or more by a device known as a **Holter monitor**. This method of recording the electrical activities of a patient's heart for a time is also referred to as an ambulatory (walking) or "24-hour ECG." The ECG electrodes are attached to the patient's chest wall. A portable cassette recorder (monitor) is attached to a belt worn around the patient's waist (Figure 16-30). During the prescribed time, usually 24 hours, the patient's heart action is recorded. The patient is

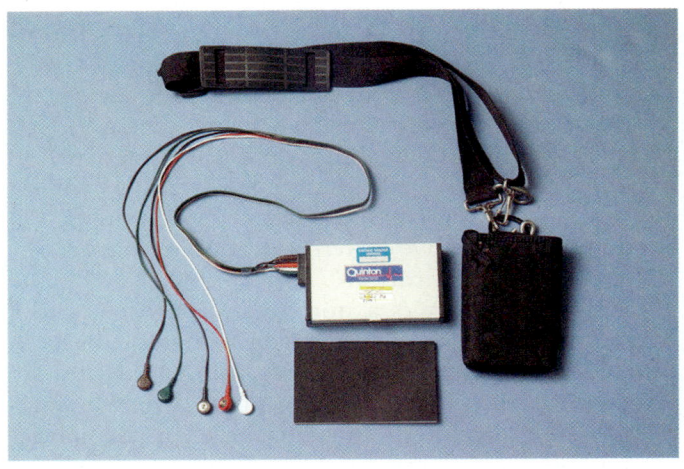

FIGURE 16-30A Holter Monitor and supplies.

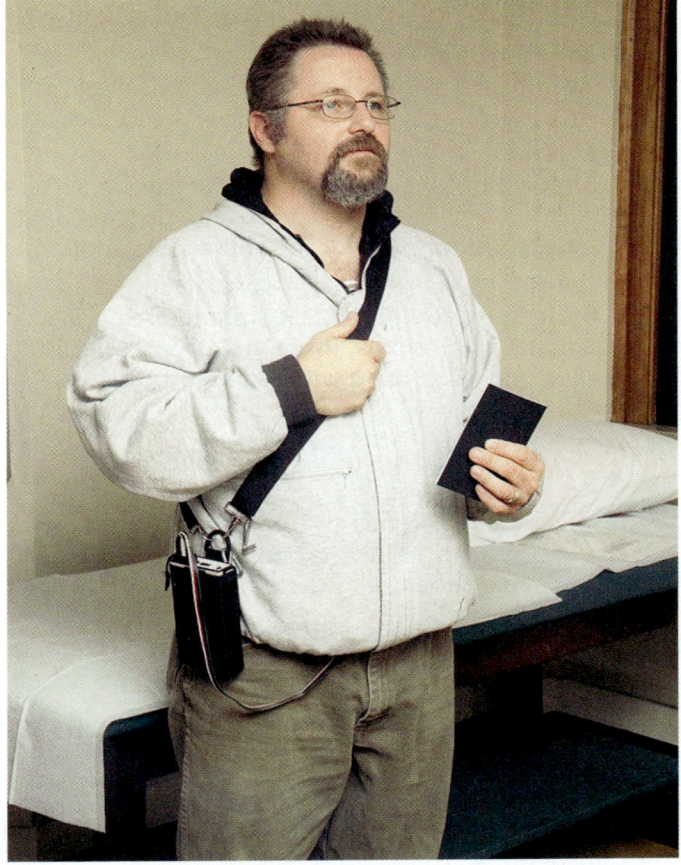

FIGURE 16-30B Correct placement of the Holter monitor on a patient

PROCEDURE PROCEDURE PROCEDURE PROCEDURE PROCEDURE PROCEDURE PROCEDURE PROCEDURE

16-4 Holter Monitoring

PURPOSE: To detect chest pain and cardiac arrhythmias, to evaluate chest pain and cardiac status following pacemaker implantation or after an acute myocardial infarction, and to determine correlation of symptoms and activity.

EQUIPMENT: Disposable razor and shaving cream, alcohol and swabs, pregelled adhesive electrodes, lead wires, appropriate batteries and tape recorder, standard ECG, diary for patient, belt for recorder, nonallergenic adhesive tape to secure electrodes as needed, drape sheet, patient's chart, and pen.

PERFORMANCE OBJECTIVE: With all equipment and supplies provided, demonstrate the steps of the procedure for hooking up a patient for the Holter monitor within 60 minutes. The instructor will observe each step.

1. Explain the procedure to the identified patient. Ask the patient to remove his clothing from the waist up (provide a drape sheet). Assist the patient to sit at the end of the examination table.

2. Wash hands and assemble the equipment and supplies on a Mayo table or other suitable work area near the patient.

3. Test the Holter monitor for proper working order, and replace the batteries if indicated. **RATIONALE: Batteries must function for the entire test period.**

4. Use the shaving cream and razor to remove chest hair if necessary. **RATIONALE: A smooth area provides optimal skin contact. Rinse and dry the electrode sites, and clean them with alcohol swabs.**

5. Rub each site vigorously with a gauze square or skin rasp, and apply the electrodes and lead wires carefully, making sure there is good skin contact. Use extra tape to secure the electrodes and wires. Refer to Figure 16-30B.

6. Place the belt around the patient's waist, and advise the patient about proper care of the recorder and precautions (refer to text). Assist the patient in dressing to help avoid disturbing the wires and electrodes. Remind the patient not to take a tub bath or shower during the 24-hour period.

7. Instruct the patient to go about his routine daily activities but to be sure to note in the diary any symptoms or problems experienced (include the time it occurred and how long it lasted). **RATIONALE: Accurate reporting and recording is essential for correct interpretation of ECG findings when compared with activity taking place when symptoms occurred.**

8. Record the date and time that the monitor began on the patient's chart and in the patient's diary, and initial.

9. Give the patient the diary to take for completion, and arrange a return appointment time.

10. When the patient comes in for the appointment the next day, assist in disrobing. Remove the electrodes and wires, clean the electrode sites, and place the cassette from the recorder in the computerized ECG for a printout of the tracing. Place the diary and recording of the ECG in the patient's chart for evaluation by the physician and initial.

Another version of this test permits the patient to activate the recording device only when experiencing symptoms. This patient-activated monitor can be worn for several days.

OTHER CARDIOVASCULAR EQUIPMENT

Many medical offices, clinics, and emergency centers are equipped with a **defibrillator** (Figure 16-31). These units are designed to provide **countershock** by a trained individual to convert cardiac arrhythmias into regular sinus rhythm. Part of your routine duties may be to

check this, and other equipment and supplies, to ensure that they are in proper working order and that everything is ready in case of a cardiac emergency. Employers offer in-service training periodically to all employees in assisting with emergency procedures. All employees should have current cardiopulmonary resuscitation (CPR) certification.

Echocardiography is a noninvasive diagnostic tool that records sound waves reflected through the heart. A transducer (similar to a microphone) sends and receives these sound waves and records them. Measurements are calculated to determine abnormalities within the heart. See Figure 16-32 for an example of this diagnostic technology.

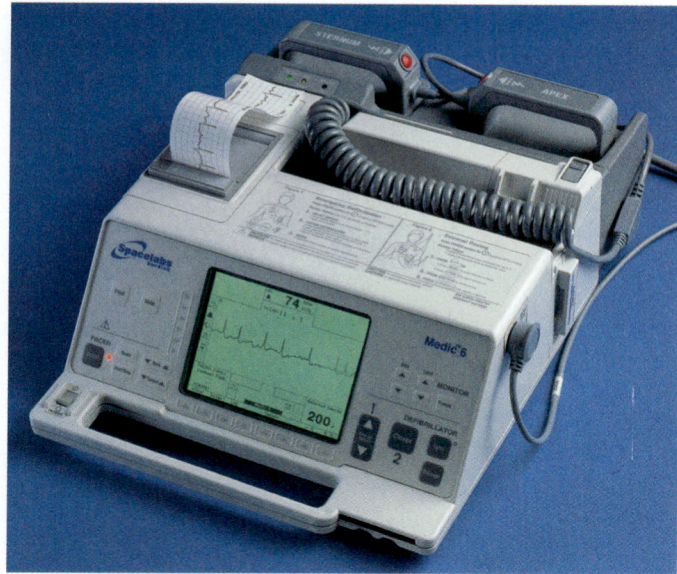

FIGURE 16-31   The Medic 6 defibrillator *(Courtesy of Space-labs Medical, Inc.)*

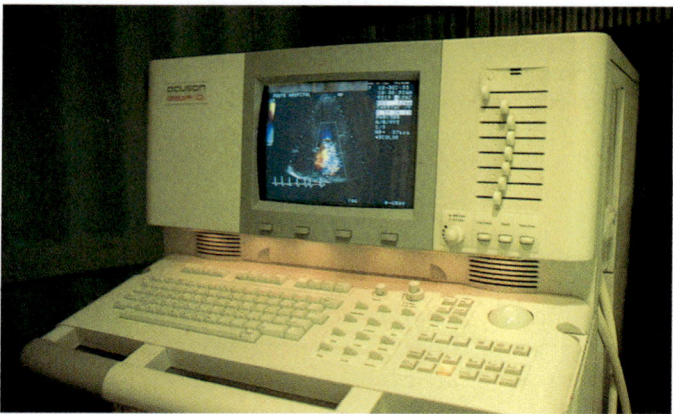

FIGURE 16-32   Echocardiograph *(Photo by Marcia Butterfield, courtesy of W.A. Foote Memorial Hospital, Jackson, Michigan)*

ACHIEVE UNIT OBJECTIVES

■ **Complete the Workbook activities to meet the learning objectives.**

■ **Practice the procedures in this unit to meet the performance objectives.**

■ **Apply your knowledge at the end of this chapter in completing the Critical Thinking Challenge and Activities, as well as the StudyWARE on your Student CD-ROM.**

UNIT 3
DIAGNOSTIC PROCEDURES

OBJECTIVES

Upon completion of this unit, you will be able to achieve the following:

LEARNING Objectives

1. **Spell and define, using the glossary at the back of the text, all the Words to Know in this unit.**
2. **Describe a spirometry test, and state the purpose of it.**
3. **Explain what magnetic resonance imaging (MRI) is.**
4. **List the contraindications for an MRI.**
5. **Describe ultrasound and state the purpose of it.**
6. **Explain the patient preparation for ultrasound procedures.**
7. **Describe patient education concerning the Procedures in this unit.**

PERFORMANCE Objectives

1. **Instruct a patient about the spirometer and perform a spirometry test.**

WORDS TO KNOW

claustrophobia	magnetic	sonogram
diagnostic	resonance	sophisticated
echocardiography	imaging	spirometer
echoes	maturity	transducer
electromagnetic	noninvasive	ultrasonic
implants	oscilloscope	scanning

CERTIFICATION CONNECTION

CMA
Treatment area—principles of operation—spirometer
Patient preparation— procedures; explanation and instructions;

instruments, supplies, and equipment
Diagnostic testing— respiratory testing; medical imaging

VITAL CAPACITY TESTS

Vital capacity is defined as the greatest volume of air that can be expelled during a complete, slow, unforced expiration following a maximum inspiration. Vital capacity should equal inspiratory capacity plus expiratory reserve. Vital capacity is usually reported in both absolute values and statistically derived values based on the age, sex, and height of the patient. The statistical value is reported as a percentage.

Several devices are used to measure the capacity of the lungs. Many physicians prefer to use the hand-held **spirometer**, which comes with vital capacity charts.

Vital capacity testing is performed to evaluate patients who are suspected to have pulmonary insufficiency. The spirometer is an instrument used to test the capacity of the lungs. Vital capacity testing aids in the diagnosis of and degree of functional or obstructive abnormalities. It also helps the physician find the cause of dyspnea and evaluate the effectiveness of medication and therapy.

When scheduling patients for tests of vital capacity, it is important to advise them to eat lightly and not to smoke for at least 6 hours before the appointment. Patients should refrain from routine treatment, and medication should not be taken until after the test is completed.

In preparing to perform this diagnostic procedure, instruct the patient regarding the necessary steps and demonstrate the use of the spirometer. Routine procedures, such as height, weight, and vital signs, should be taken and recorded on the patient's chart. Showing the patient how to hold the instrument and what is expected will yield a more accurate test result. Disposable mouthpieces are used to prevent disease transmission. Most spirometers are computerized and have a printout of the results within minutes of administering the test. You should type in the patient's name, age, height, race, gender, account number, and any other information, if applicable, before you start the test.

Figure 16-33 pictures a medical assistant coaching a patient through the procedure. A clip is placed on the patient's nose to force the expired air out of the lungs directly into the mouthpiece (make sure patient's mouth is sealed around the mouthpiece) and into the spirometer. Instruct the patient to stand up straight and to take in a slow deep breath. Coach the patient to expel all the air from the lungs quickly until he cannot exhale any more, within approximately 15 seconds. Give the patient a couple of practice runs before beginning the official test, because it is an awkward procedure for most people. Follow each of the expirations with a few seconds of resting for the patient. Watch for signs of stress, dizziness, coughing, or other problems the patient may have during the test. Generally three to five expirations are tested. The results are analyzed by the computerized instrument, and the diagnostic data

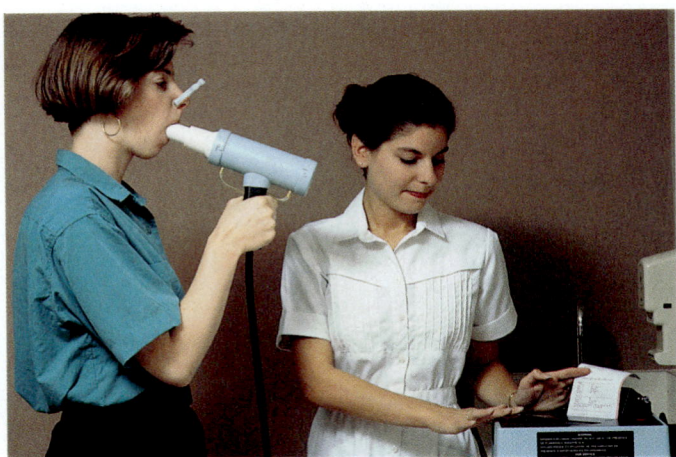

FIGURE 16-33   The medical assistant operates the computerized spirometer while the patient blows exhaled air from the lungs into the disposable mouthpiece.

are printed for evaluation by the physician. Test results below 80% are usually considered abnormal. This spirometry reading is placed in the patient's chart, along with a notation of any symptoms or problems the patient may have had during the test and your initials. Spirometry tests should not be performed when the patient has been diagnosed with angina, acute coronary insufficiency, or recent myocardial infarction. Allow the patient to sit and relax to wait for consultation with the physician. Instruct the patient to resume medication and therapy routine as directed by the physician. (Refer to Procedure 16-5.)

You may be instructed to schedule patients for further pulmonary function studies to be performed by a pulmonary and thoracic specialist. More **sophisticated** equipment may be necessary to evaluate a patient's condition.

SONOGRAPHIC STUDIES

Sonograms are records obtained by **ultrasonic scanning**. Ultrasonography is a technique in which internal structures are made visible by recording the reflections, or **echoes**, of ultrasonic sound waves directed into the tissues. These high-frequency sound waves are conducted through the use of a **transducer** (a hand-held instrument resembling a microphone). While the transducer is held against the body area to be tested, it sends sound waves through the skin to various organs. As the echoes are sent back, the transducer picks them up and changes them into electrical energy. This energy is transmitted into an image on a monitor or printed out on paper in wavy lines. The picture formed on the screen represents a cross section of the organ. Photos of these images are taken for permanent records. The physician interprets these images to aid in the diagno-

PROCEDURE PROCEDURE PROCEDURE PROCEDURE PROCEDURE PROCEDURE PROCEDURE PROCEDURE

16-5  Perform Spirometry Testing

PURPOSE: Evaluate patients suspected of having pulmonary insufficiency.

EQUIPMENT AND SUPPLIES: Spirometer and disposable mouthpieces.

PERFORMANCE OBJECTIVE: Provided with the spirometer, disposable mouthpiece, and simulated patient chart, the student will prepare a patient for spirometry testing and perform the procedure within 25 minutes, with the instructor observing each step.

1. Assemble the necessary equipment and supplies; wash hands.

2. Identify the patient.

3. Provide an explanation of the procedure and equipment to the patient; let the patient become familiar with the equipment by having the patient breathe into the machine.

4. Be sure the patient is in a comfortable position and any restrictive clothing (such as a tie or collar) is loosened before initiating the procedure.

5. Instruct the patient to sit or stand as straight as possible and not bend at the waist while blowing into the disposable mouthpiece. Also instruct the patient to make a tight seal around the mouthpiece with the lips.

6. After telling the patient to take deep breaths in (inhalation), coach the patient to breathe all of the air out of the lungs until unable to expire any longer, usually about 15 seconds.

7. Allow the patient to have a practice run before performing the actual test.

8. Support the patient during the test and have the patient keep blowing into the mouthpiece until told to stop. Watch for signs of stress, dizziness, coughing, or other problems during the test.

9. Chart the procedure in the patient's record and place the results in the chart for the provider's review.

---

sis and treatment of the patient. **Echocardiography** is a technique used to examine the heart: echoes are converted into electrical impulses, which create a picture of the tissues being examined on an **oscilloscope**.

Ultrasonography is useful in examination of the abdominopelvic cavity to locate aneurysms of the aorta and other blood vessel abnormalities. The size and shape of internal organs can also be determined with ultrasound. It can be of value in the identification of cysts and tumors of the eye and in the detection of pelvic masses and obstructions of the urinary tract. In obstetrics and gynecology, where the radiation of x-ray examination is avoided, ultrasound is useful in the diagnosis of multiple pregnancies and in determining the size, **maturity**, and position of the fetus. Patient preparation may vary, but usually the patient is instructed to drink a large amount of water, up to a quart. This will distend the bladder, help to push the uterus into place, and increase the conduction of the sound waves. Sonograms are not useful in viewing the lungs, for echoes are not created by structures containing air.

When scheduling patients for this type of study, you should give them a few important instructions. They should avoid eating foods that produce gas and drink plenty of fluids (specific amounts are required

for certain tests) as mentioned earlier (Figure 16-34). Check with the radiology facility regarding what the patient may drink. Some facilities allow other liquids besides water. However, no alcoholic beverages are permitted. Further instruct the patient *not* to void following drinking the water (or other liquids). Explain to the patient that the procedure involves lying on an examination table for 45 minutes to an hour. It is an accurate and painless diagnostic tool. A gel or lotion is used to produce better sound wave conduction and to allow the transducer to glide more easily across the skin.

Besides being a diagnostic procedure, ultrasound is used in the treatment of diseased or injured muscle tis-

---

(1) ABDOMINAL ULTRASOUND: Take nothing by mouth after midnight. No breakfast on the morning of the examination.

(2) PELVIC ULTRASOUND: Drink 24–30 ounces of fluid 1 hour before the examination. Do not urinate after drinking the fluid.

(3) FETAL ULTRASOUND: Drink 24–30 ounces of fluid 1 hour before the examination. Do not urinate after drinking the fluid.

FIGURE 16-34 Preparation for ultrasound procedure

sue. Sound waves vibrate into the tissues, producing heat, which helps to relieve inflammation and pain. It also increases circulation, which speeds up healing of injured muscle tissues. Another common use of ultrasound is in dentistry. Sound vibrations make it possible for tartar to be painlessly removed from the teeth.

Specific in-service training is necessary before using this instrument, because the patient can be burned if precautions are not followed precisely.

MAGNETIC RESONANCE IMAGING (MRI)

A technique to view the structures inside the human body is called **magnetic resonance imaging** (MRI). This method allows physicians to examine a particular area of the body without exposing the patient to x-rays or surgery. This **noninvasive** procedure, which may range from 30 to 60 minutes, requires that the patient lie on a padded table that is moved into a tunnel-like structure (Figure 16-35).

There is no advance patient preparation required for this examination. The MRI procedure becomes an *invasive* procedure only when an intravenous contrast media is administered to the patient under certain conditions. This *contrast enhanced* technique is done during the last series of images of the examination to detect certain pathologies. The patient may resume normal activity following the procedure. There are no known harmful effects to the patient from this imaging technique.

The magnetic resonance machine scans all planes of a body structure to produce an image processed by a computer, without moving the patient. Radio signals are sent from the scanner that are influenced by strong magnetic fields to which the body responds. Figure 16-36 shows an image of the lumbar spine in the sagittal plane. Note the herniated disc and the clarity of the image. The MRI has reduced a great number of diagnostic exploratory surgeries. It is most useful in helping to diagnose brain and nervous system disorders, cardiovascular disease, cancer, and diseases of the visceral organs. Magnetic resonance imaging can be performed for particular areas of the body, such as the hip, shoulder, or neck. This specific imaging of small areas takes less time, approximately a half hour. Explain the time requirement to the patient as a courtesy. The patient may better plan transportation if the time of the appointment and the length of time the test takes is known. MRI is also used to help monitor the effectiveness of treatment. Since the MRI uses a strong **electromagnetic** field, it is extremely important that any metal objects be removed before the procedure is performed. The technician will request that the patient remove all metallic objects, including jewelry, hairpins, and nonpermanent dentures before being placed in the tunnel for the MRI. Patients should be interviewed thoroughly regarding their health history. Inform patients that at the facility where the MRI will be performed, they will generally be asked to sign a consent form prior to the procedure. Female patients should refrain from even wearing mascara, since tiny metallic flakes may be present in it. During the procedure, these minute pieces of metal may become hot and burn the patient.

During the process the many repetitive noises sound like clanging and banging, humming, and whirring. This is just the sound of the electromagnetic field. There are no sensations of pain and no known side effects. The patient must be still and relax for the test to be properly completed. The technician observes the patient during the entire time. Patients may speak

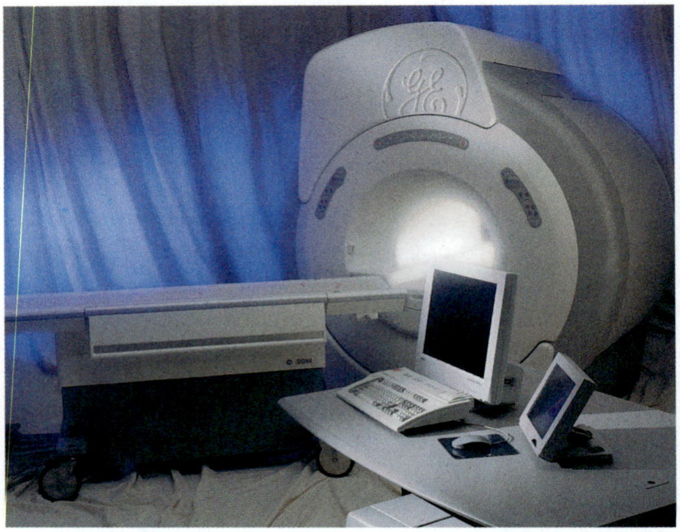

FIGURE 16-35 Magnetic resonance imaging (MRI) system which shows up on a computer screen *(Courtesy of GE Medical Systems.)*

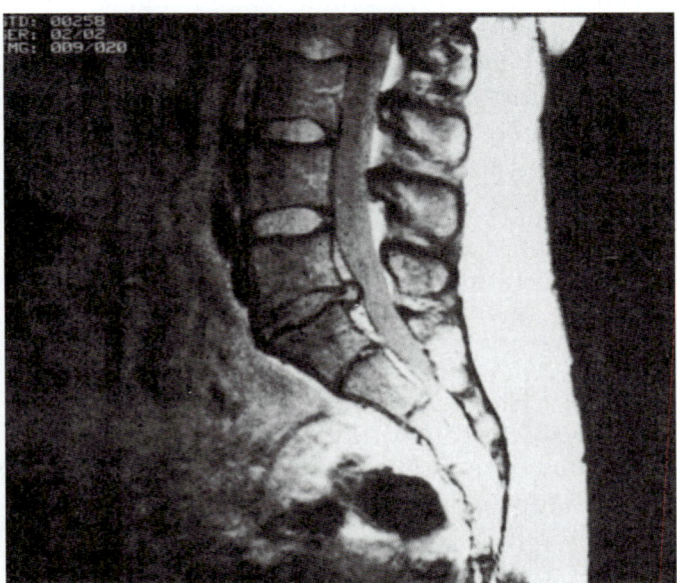

FIGURE 16-36 MRI showing a herniated disc in the lumbar spine *(Courtesy of GE Medical Systems.)*

PATIENT EDUCATION

Assure the patient that the studies are done in a controlled environment. Always provide clear and concise oral *and* written instructions for examinations that require advance preparation. Be sure that the patient understands the necessary preparations. Answer all questions. Emphasize the importance of being on time for the radiologic appointment to avoid unnecessary delays, because some examinations are very long.

If the patient is not familiar with the facility where the x-ray studies are scheduled, give specific instructions (and a map) of how to get there and where to park. Patients appreciate this courtesy. Often, this information is printed on the appointment or information sheet the facility provides to medical offices and clinics for referral appointments.

If x-rays are considered as a part of the assessment of their condition, it is of vital importance that you advise all female patients who are of childbearing age to inform you if they are pregnant, or could possibly be. X-rays are contraindicated in pregnant females, especially in the first trimester, because radiation is damaging to the fetus. During screening, you should always ask females for the date of the first day of menstrual flow of their last menstrual period (LMP) for documentation in their chart. This will help in preventing any misunderstanding concerning a possible pregnancy. Other diagnostic exams can be performed that are safe for the fetus during this time as necessary.

to the technician by the use of a microphone inside the tunnel.

The MRI procedure is contraindicated in patients who have pacemakers, have metallic implants, are in the first trimester of pregnancy, are severely claustrophobic, or are obese. The claustrophobia can be handled by counseling or the use of a sedative administered by a physician before the procedure is begun.

ACHIEVE UNIT OBJECTIVES

- Complete the Workbook activities to meet the learning objectives.
- Practice the procedures in this unit to meet the performance objectives.
- Apply your knowledge at the end of this chapter in completing the Critical Thinking Challenge and Activities, as well as the StudyWARE on your Student CD-ROM.

UNIT 4
DIAGNOSTIC RADIOLOGIC EXAMINATIONS

OBJECTIVES

Upon completion of this unit, you will be able to achieve the following:

LEARNING Objectives

1. Spell and define, using the glossary at the back of the text, all the Words to Know in this unit.
2. Instruct patients in preparation for radiologic studies.
3. Explain the importance of diet in preparation for x-rays.
4. Explain why pregnant women should not have x-rays.
5. Describe x-rays that require no preparation.
6. Explain the importance of patient education in scheduling a mammography.

WORDS TO KNOW

absorb	electron	lesion
artifact	enema	mammography
compression	evacuate	planes
computed trans-	flatus	radioactive
axial tomog-	flexible	radiograph
raphy (CTAT)	fluoroscope	radiologist
conjunction	intravenous	radiopaque
contract	pyelogram	residual
contrast	(IVP)	barium
cystoscope	iodine	retrograde
distends	KUB (kidneys,	Roentgen
electromagnetic	ureters,	therapeutic
radiation	bladder)	

CERTIFICATION CONNECTION

CMA
Patient preparation—
  procedures, explanation,
  and instructions

Diagnostic testing—medical
  imaging

RADIOLOGIC STUDIES

Radiology is a mysterious realm to most patients. The perceptive medical assistant can sense that patients exhibit a fear of what is going to happen to them during the radiology procedure(s), and even more frightening is what the radiologist may find. Generally, patients know if there is something seriously wrong with them. These patients and all others need to feel a comforting touch. The medical assistant should show genuine caring and compassion to patients who are in pain and discomfort. When they are in your care and you can see that they are confused and unsure of what will happen next, you can offer them support and reassurance. Often, just talking to them for a few minutes can ease their fears and uncertainties. Asking the patient if they have ever had an x-ray before is certainly the first question you should pose. If you can give the patient an idea of what to expect and describe what it is like, you can decrease the stress and anxiety of the patient. Figure 16-37 shows a technologist getting a patient positioned and adjusting the angle of the beam of the x-ray tube. When the physician orders x-rays to aid in the diagnosis of a condition, it could be the patient's first encounter with this process. Children especially can be apprehensive about what is going to happen to them. You can explain to a child that having x-rays taken is just like having pictures taken with a camera; the x-ray machine is really a great big metal camera taking a picture of the inside of their body. Explain that you have to be very still when having an x-ray taken just like when you have a photograph taken so that the picture does not get blurred and out of focus. The child will be more cooperative when given an explanation of what to expect. Generally, the radiology tech-

nologist will be very understanding with children and will show the child the x-ray film when it is processed. Explain to adults that a big lead apron will be put over the patient to protect the reproductive organs from the x-rays. Visual aides are helpful to show patients what radiologic equipment looks like. The x-ray the physician has ordered will determine the extent of what patient education is indicated. Some radiologic studies require preparation before they can be performed. You must make sure that the patient understands all instructions clearly to avoid misunderstandings and time delays. Often the explanation will be quite simple because the patient already knows there is an obvious problem, such as an injury. For example, Figure 16-38 shows a severe fracture of the femur.

All radiology departments have signs prominently displayed in several areas of their facility that tell female patients to inform the radiology technologist or radiologist physician if they are pregnant or if they possibly could be pregnant. X-rays can be damaging to an unborn child, especially in the first 3 months of pregnancy (first trimester), sometimes before the patient is

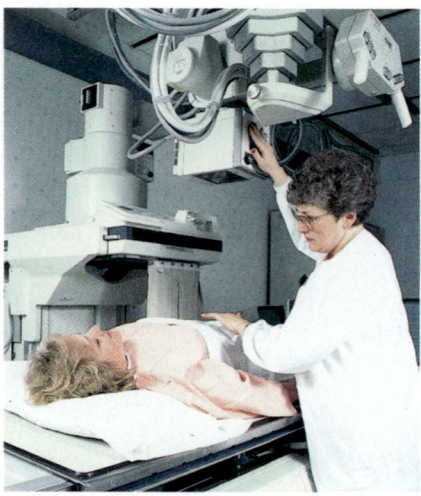

FIGURE 16-37 The radiology technician positions the patient and adjusts the x-ray tube over the patient. *(Photo by Marcia Butterfield, courtesy of W.A. Foote Memorial Hospital, Jackson, Michigan)*

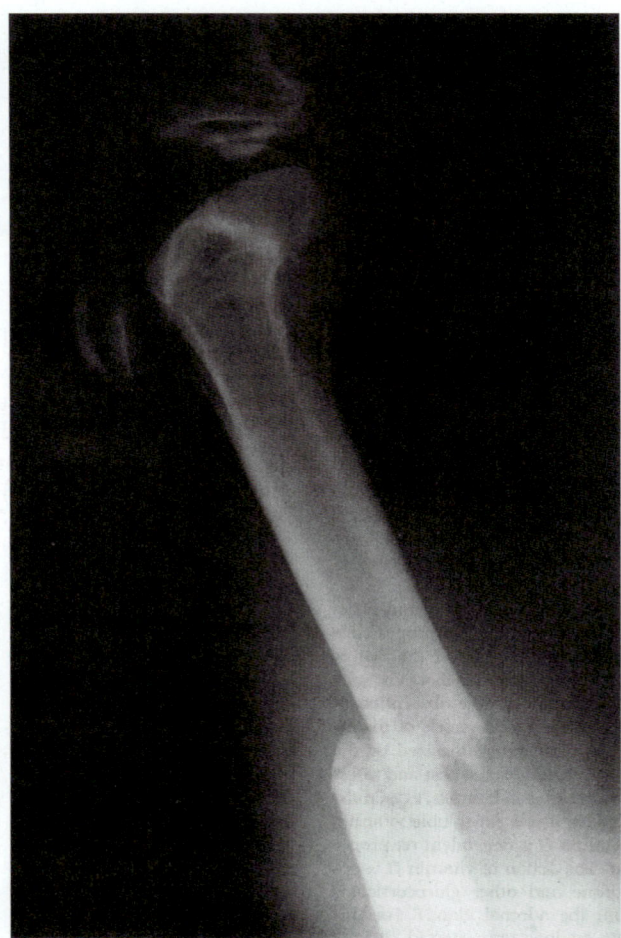

FIGURE 16-38 X-ray showing a severe fracture of the femur

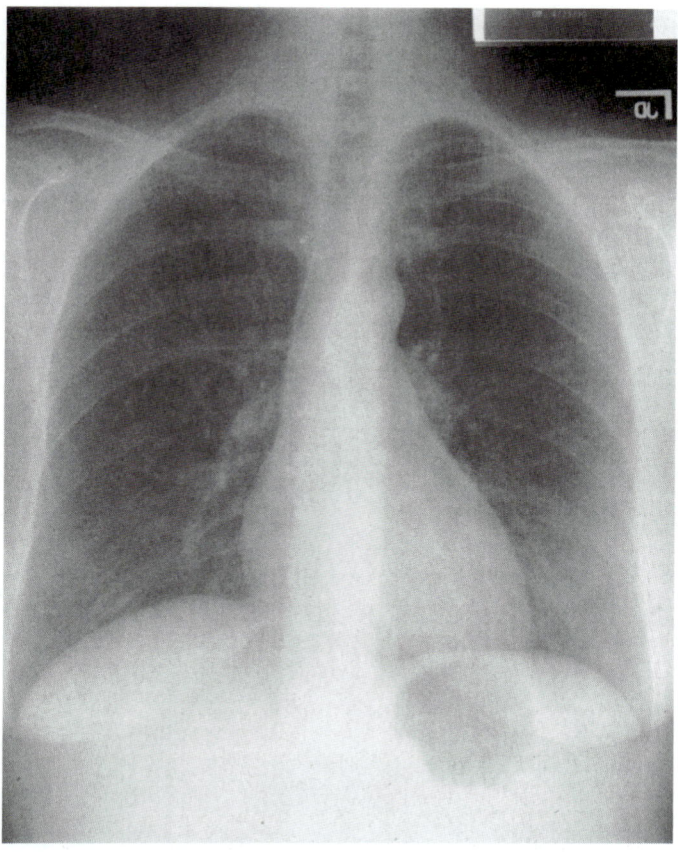

FIGURE 16-39   Chest x-ray—anterior posterior (AP) view of the chest

even aware she is pregnant. Before scheduling any female patient whose age indicates that she is within the childbearing years, you must always ask if she could be pregnant.

Radiologic studies are made by the use of x-rays (**roentgen** rays), which are high-energy **electromagnetic radiation** produced by the collision of a beam of **electrons** with a metal target in an x-ray tube. An x-ray photograph is taken of the requested part of the patient's body, and a permanent film picture is made. Patients must follow preparation instructions for certain radiologic studies. Bone studies do not require preparation and are performed to aid in the diagnosis of tumors, fractures, and other disorders and diseases. Chest x-rays do not normally need advance preparation. When the physician orders an x-ray of the chest (Figure 16-39), the patient is asked to hold still in the positions shown in Figure 16-40 so that a permanent film (upon inspiration of breath) can be taken and evaluated by the radiologist. A report of the radiologic studies is sent to the primary physician. The physician may request to view the films. **Therapeutic** radiation is used in the treatment of cancer. Following are the most commonly ordered radiologic studies for which you may be responsible in scheduling and preparing patients. It is very important to review the preparation instructions for various radiologic and sonographic studies when you schedule the patient's appointment, because techniques and preps can vary from one facility to another and are also subject to change with technology.

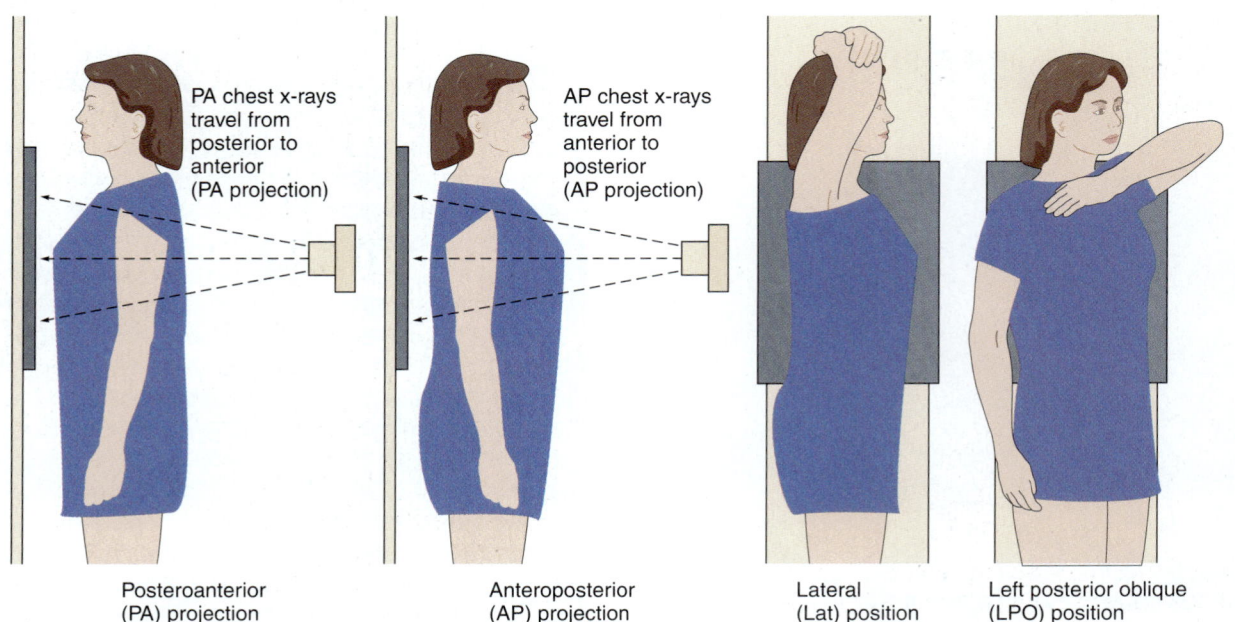

PA chest x-rays travel from posterior to anterior (PA projection)

AP chest x-rays travel from anterior to posterior (AP projection)

Posteroanterior (PA) projection

Anteroposterior (AP) projection

Lateral (Lat) position

Left posterior oblique (LPO) position

FIGURE 16-40   Radiographic projection positions to obtain different views of the chest

Gallbladder Imaging

The gallbladder stores bile that is produced in the liver to break down fat in the digestive process. When the gallbladder malfunctions, the patient experiences abdominal discomfort (nausea) and pain. The cholecystogram enables the physician to diagnose the cause of the patient's distress; however, this procedure is rarely performed. The oral cholecystogram is also referred to as a gallbladder series and a double dose gallbladder. Refer to Figure 16-41, which shows gallstones present on the permanent film of the cholecystogram.

An imaging technique that has replaced the cholecystogram is the abdominal ultrasound. Ultrasound, or sonography, is a process of using sound waves with a frequency of over 20,000 vibrations per second to produce images of the internal structures of the body. An image is produced when continuous sound waves are projected toward the desired area to measure and record the reflected image. This procedure requires a 12-hour fast for a morning appointment. This generally means that the patient should have nothing to eat or drink past midnight the night before the scheduled ultrasound and no breakfast the morning of the appoint-ment. Some radiology facilities offer afternoon appointments for abdominal ultrasounds. To prepare for this, the patient is instructed to have a fat-free liquid breakfast before 9:00 AM the day of the appointment with nothing to eat or drink until after the ultrasound. The abdominal ultrasound includes gallbladder, pancreas, liver, and other visceral organs. Sonograms are very useful in aiding in the diagnosis of gallstones, tumors, heart defects, and fetal abnormalities.

In addition to abdominal ultrasound examinations, you may be required to give patients necessary information about pelvic and fetal ultrasound procedures. In the procedure for a pelvic ultrasound, a vaginal probe is used to aid in visualizing internal structures. It is helpful for patients to be aware of this before it is done so that they will be prepared. Refer to Unit 3 of this chapter for review.

In preparation for this study of the gallbladder, the patient must follow a prescribed diet and take prescribed medications (a **contrast** medium) to make the gallbladder visible on the x-ray film (Figures 16-41 and 16-42). Generally, the patient is advised to avoid drinking alco-

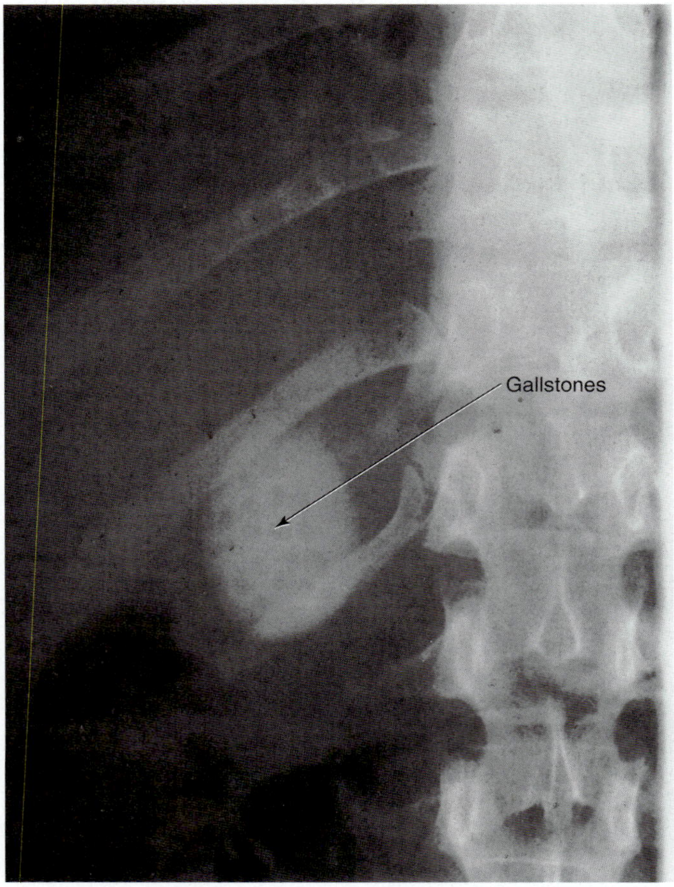

Gallstones

FIGURE 16-41 Gallbladder x-ray showing several gallstones

PATIENT EDUCATION

Most patients with gallbladder trouble already know they should avoid fatty foods. The usual preparation for a cholecystogram is a nonfatty evening meal the night before the scheduled appointment. Foods that are permitted are fresh fruits and vegetables, lean meat (broiled), toast, bread, jelly, and coffee or tea. Fatty foods will cause the gallbladder to **contract** and empty the contrast medium, which the patient usually takes following the evening meal.

The medication is usually in pill form, with directions to swallow one tablet every 5 minutes with a minimum amount of water until all are consumed. Repeating this a second night is necessary to define the gallbladder sufficiently. This takes approximately half an hour. Spreading the consumption of the contrast medium out over this time allows the gallbladder to **absorb** the substance. The patient is instructed to eat or drink nothing after midnight the night before the cholecystogram is performed. In addition to these preparations, many physicians request an **enema**, laxative, or both to help remove fecal material and gas, which could cause shadows, blockages, or other **artifacts**.

Often, when the series of **radiographs** is completed, patients are given a drink called "fatty meal" or are instructed to return after a meal containing fats to observe radiographs that show how the gallbladder functions during digestion of fats.

1. Two days prior to exam, starting at 6 PM, take one tablet of Oragrafin every 5 minutes until six tablets have been taken.

2. On day prior to exam, repeat step 1.

3. Day prior to exam, take 4 oz. of Neoloid or three Dulcolax 5 mg tablets from 2–4 PM.

4. Evening before exam, eat a fat-free meal—dry toast, tea, fruit, jello.

5. Nothing by mouth after midnight.

6. No breakfast.

FIGURE 16-42   Diet preparation for gallbladder (x-ray) series

ESOPHAGUS, UPPER GI SERIES

1. Nothing by mouth after midnight.

2. No breakfast.

IF SMALL BOWEL

1. Day prior to exam—take 4 oz. of Neoloid or three Dulcolax 5 mg tablets from 2–4 PM.

2. Nothing by mouth after midnight.

3. No breakfast.

FIGURE 16-43   Preparation for upper gastrointestinal (UGI) series

holic and carbonated beverages the day before the exam, because these drinks may produce **flatus** (gas). Unless otherwise specified by the physician, you should remind patients to take their regularly prescribed medication(s).

The preparation for the gallbladder ultrasound is minimal in comparison with the cholecystogram. The preparation for the sonogram is much easier for the patient because it only requires preparation on the same day as the appointment. You should still advise patients regarding their diet and what to expect during the visit to the radiology facility.

Upper GI Series—Barium Swallow

For this study, the patient must drink the contrast medium during the examination while the **radiologist** observes the flow of the substance directly by means of a **fluoroscope**. The contrast medium is a mixture of bar-

ium and water, usually flavored to increase palatability. In radiology, it is now a custom to use "Fizzy's," crystals similar to Alka-Seltzer combined with a small amount of water to add air to the stomach. This is called a "double contrast." Next, a thickened barium mixture is ingested by mouth. Then, to further examine the esophagus and duodenal bulb, a thin barium mixture is given to the patient. Radiologic films are taken for a permanent record of the upper digestive tract. During the study, the patient is positioned so that different angles of the digestive organs can be seen.

The physician observes the functioning of the esophagus, stomach, duodenum, and small intestine as the barium passes. Such disorders or diseases as hiatal hernias, peptic or duodenal ulcers, and tumors may be diagnosed as a result of the upper GI series. Adherence to a restricted diet the day before and on the day of the exam is also necessary (Figure 16-43).

Lower GI Series—Barium Enema

Patients who are scheduled for this radiologic study should follow the preparation listed in Figure 16-44 very strictly. Stress the avoidance of milk and all dairy

PATIENT EDUCATION

UGI preparation requires that the patient eat a light evening meal of only clear liquids (see Figure 16-43). The patient should have nothing to eat or drink from midnight until after the x-ray series the next day. Prescribed medications must not be consumed until after the films have been taken, or the view of the structures could be impaired. Dairy products, carbonated beverages, and alcohol are not permitted. The digestive tract should be clear of all foods to avoid blockage of or shadows on the anatomical structures to be observed.

Constipation may result from the barium, and patients should be advised to drink plenty of clear liquids to help relieve it. You should also mention that their stool may appear lighter than usual from the white barium, and that this should not be a cause for concern. Laxatives are ordered only by the physician. Patients should phone the medical office if any problem arises.

PATIENT EDUCATION

Patients must prepare for a barium enema by precisely following instructions, usually beginning the day before the appointment. The instructions generally include laxatives and enemas to clear the bowel of fecal matter and gas. The patient should eat lightly, avoid dairy products, and drink plenty of clear liquids to encourage more comfortable **evacuation**. Patients should have nothing to eat or drink past midnight the night before the x-ray (see Figure 16-44). On the day of the appointment, the patient should have an enema 2 hours before the scheduled appointment.

BARIUM ENEMA OR COLON EXAMINATION

a. Beginning the morning of the day before the examination, change to an all liquid diet,* as outlined below. Do not take any more solid food until after the examinations.

b. At 12:30 PM, or half an hour after lunch on the day before the examination, drink entire contents of a bottle of Citrate of Magnesia (10 oz.).

c. At 1:00 PM, drink one glass of fluid.

d. At 3:00 PM, take two Dulcolax tablets with a large glass of water.

e. At 4:00 PM, drink one large glass of fluid.

f. At 5:00 PM, or as close as possible, have a liquid dinner.

g. At 6:00 PM, drink one large glass of fluid.

h. Bedtime—drink one large glass of fluid.

i. You may have one cup of coffee, tea, or water on the morning of the examination.

*ALL LIQUID DIET

You may have any of the following: coffee, tea, carbonated beverages, clear gelatin desserts, strained fruit juice, bouillon, clear broths, tomato juice. Do not drink milk of any kind.

Please call the office if you have any questions regarding the above instructions.

FIGURE 16-44 Preparation for barium enema

products for better visualization of the colon. Be sure to explain the importance of adequate preparation for these studies. Improper preparation could result in the need to repeat the tests.

In this examination, barium sulfate is the contrast medium. It is introduced into the colon by an enema tube, and the radiologist observes the flow into the lower bowel. Many physicians order a barium enema with air-contrast. This procedure **distends** the barium-filled colon with air to make the structures more visible by fluoroscopy. Permanent radiographs are taken periodically during the procedure. This study is helpful in diagnosing diseases of the colon, tumors, and **lesions**.

The barium enema procedure generally takes several minutes and produces discomfort and some pain. Patients should be told to breathe through the mouth slowly and deeply to help relax the abdominal muscles. A strong urge to defecate is normal, and patients often cannot resist the urge. After several films have been taken and the study of the lower bowel is completed, the patient is allowed to use the toilet.

Patients should be encouraged to drink plenty of liquids for the next few days to help evacuate the **residual barium** sulfate in the lower colon.

Intravenous Pyelogram

In studies of the genitourinary system, the **intravenous pyelogram (IVP)** (Figure 16-45) requires that the patient prepare with laxatives, enemas, and fasting (Figure 16-46). The IVP consists of an intravenous injection of **iodine**, the contrast medium, to define the structures of the urinary system. **CAUTION:** Patients who have a known iodine allergy should alert the radiology department personnel so that a noniodine preparation may be used in their x-ray studies. Patients who are suspected of having an allergy to iodine should be tested by order of the physician. This information should be obtained during the medical history interview and documented accurately. Allergies should be recorded or circled in red ink so that attention is brought to this vital information. A **retrograde** pyelogram is a study of the urinary tract done by inserting a sterile catheter into the urinary meatus, through the bladder, and up into the ureters. The **radiopaque** contrast medium then flows upward into the kidneys. This diagnostic test is usually done in **conjunction** with **cystoscopy**. Patients should have iodine-sensitive tests prior to the examination to determine the possibility of an allergic reaction. A voiding cystogram may be ordered in conjunction with an IVP. In this case, the contrast medium is injected into the bladder by catheter, and no special patient preparation is needed.

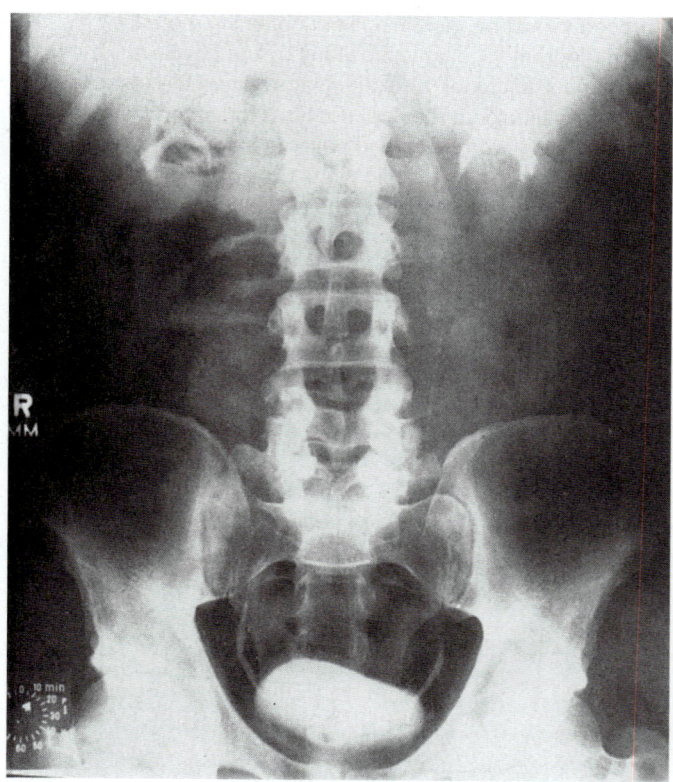

FIGURE 16-45 Radiologic x-rays of kidneys, ureters, and bladder (KUB)

ALL LIQUID DIET

You may have any of the following: coffee, tea, carbonated beverages, clear gelatin desserts, strained fruit juice, bouillon, clear broths, tomato juice. Do not drink milk of any kind.

1. Day prior to exam—three Dulcolax 5 mg tablets from 2–4 PM.

2. You may drink only one glass of liquid on the morning of the exam.

FIGURE 16-46   Preparation for intravenous pyelogram (IVP)

KUB

The **KUB (kidneys, ureters, bladder)** is an x-ray of the patient's abdomen, sometimes termed "flat plate of abdomen." This requires no patient preparation and is used in the diagnosis of urinary system diseases and disorders. It may also be useful in determining the position of an intrauterine device (IUD) or in locating foreign bodies in the digestive tract. In some cases, surgery is indicated to remove an object that may block the normal digestive flow, but many small objects are easily passed with solid foods, especially in young children whose internal structures are more **flexible**. The physician ultimately makes this decision in patient care.

Mammography

Mammography aids in the diagnosis of breast masses, some of which may be as small as 1 cm in size or less. Women who practice self-examinations regularly each month and find lumps in breast tissue early have a much better cure rate if a malignancy is found. Breast self-examination (see Chapter 14, Unit 3) and regular examinations by the physician should be strongly reinforced to female patients in addition to their scheduled mammography. The American Cancer Society recommends a baseline mammography at the age of 35 for all women. After age 40, women are urged to have a mammography every year. Some insurance companies will not pay for this exam before a woman is 40 without a written order from the patient's physician. However, most insurance providers will pay for a mammography at any age if it is diagnostic.

At any time a lump is found, patients should be advised to see the physician at once for examination. This procedure requires the patient to move into various positions so that different angles of the breast tissue may be x-rayed (Figure 16-47). The x-ray pictures are called mammograms. Patients are usually advised to wear slacks or a skirt for ease in preparation for the procedure (Figure 16-48), because it is necessary to undress to the waist for the examination. The only preparation required is that the patient wash

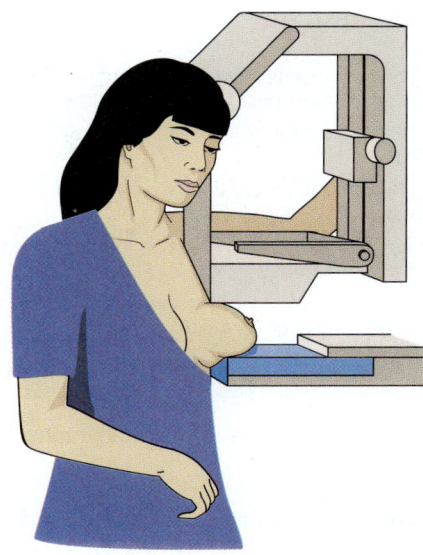

FIGURE 16-47   Breasts are compressed by plates during mammography to produce a clearer image of the mammary structures.

PATIENT EDUCATION

Because this procedure is often very uncomfortable and even sometimes painful in many women, there are suggestions that may be helpful in reducing the discomfort the medical assistant should schedule the mammography during the first week following the patient's menstrual cycle, because the breasts must be compressed firmly during the procedure to obtain a satisfactory image for diagnostic purposes (see Figure 16-47), and during this time, the patient would experience less discomfort. It is advisable to tell patients to omit caffeine from their diets for 7 to 10 days prior to this examination to reduce the possible effects of swelling and soreness that caffeine often produces. Compression of the breasts during this procedure requires less radiation to be used. It also allows a much clearer picture to be taken of the breast tissue. Following this exam, some areas of the breast(s) may become temporarily discolored. However, it does not damage the breast tissue and should not be alarming. At the advice of the physician, a mild analgesic may be taken to relieve any discomfort or aching that may be experienced by the patient.

Explaining these details to patients and requesting their cooperation with the radiology technician during this procedure will be helpful in obtaining a quality mammogram for diagnostic study by the physician. It is also important to let patients know when the results will be available so that they will not worry unnecessarily. Remind patients again of the importance of breast self-examinations on a continuing basis. The mammography is not a substitute for this important means of detection.

To ensure the best results for your mammogram, please follow these procedures prior to your appointment:

a. BE SURE TO NOTIFY OUR PERSONNEL IF YOU ARE PREGNANT.

b. Please shower or bathe as close to your appointment time as possible.

c. Do not use deodorants, powders, perfumes, etc. on the breast or underarm areas.

d. You will only have to undress to the waist, so wear an easily removable top such as a blouse.

FIGURE 16-48 Instructions for mammography preparation.

the chest and underarms and rinse and dry thoroughly. No deodorants, perfumes, or powders are to be used on the day of the mammography, because the film on the skin from these substances could interfere with the radiograph.

Body Scans

Rapid scanning of single-tissue **planes** is performed by a process that generates images of the tissue in "slices" about 1 cm thick. Figure 16-49 illustrates how different parts of the body are sectioned for the image. This method of radiology is called the computed tomography (CT) scan or **computed transaxial tomography (CTAT)**. These procedures can be performed in seconds and aid in diagnosis of diseases and disorders of the breast or other internal organs (Figure 16-50).

The branch of medicine that uses radionuclides in the diagnosis and treatment of disease is nuclear medicine. Almost any organ of the body may be viewed and

PATIENT EDUCATION

It is very important for the medical assistant and other health care providers to realize that in some cultures and religions, women are to keep themselves covered at all times when they are in public and in the presence of men. A breast examination and mammography would be especially problematic for the patient unless a female physician or technologist conducted the exam or the mammography. Be sure that you explain to the patient or ask an interpreter to explain the preparation, examination, and the imaging to prepare the patient for this experience. Relieving anxiety about this matter will help the patient understand and not be afraid of what to expect.

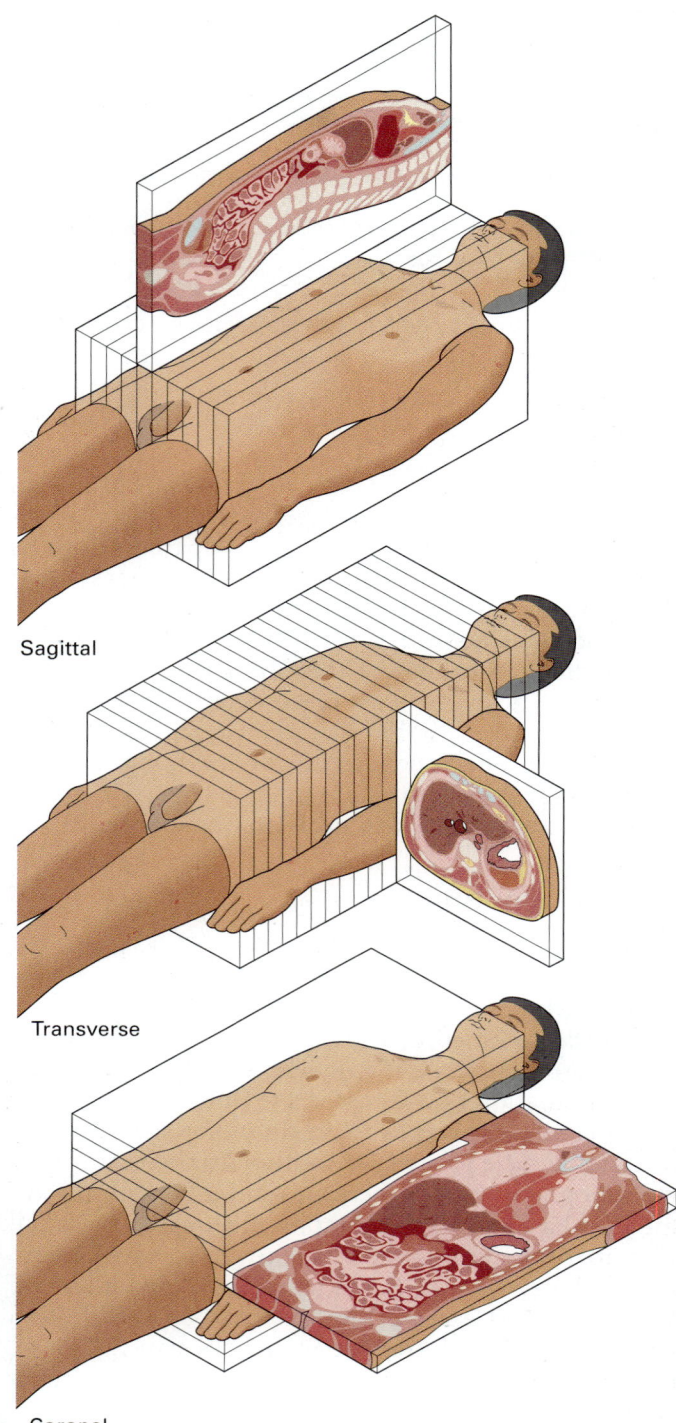

Sagittal

Transverse

Coronal

FIGURE 16-49 Computed tomography provides a three-dimensional view of the internal structures of the body.

recorded by having the patient ingest, or be injected with, radioactive material.

Uptake studies refer to procedures in which patients ingest a **radioactive** substance under careful supervi-

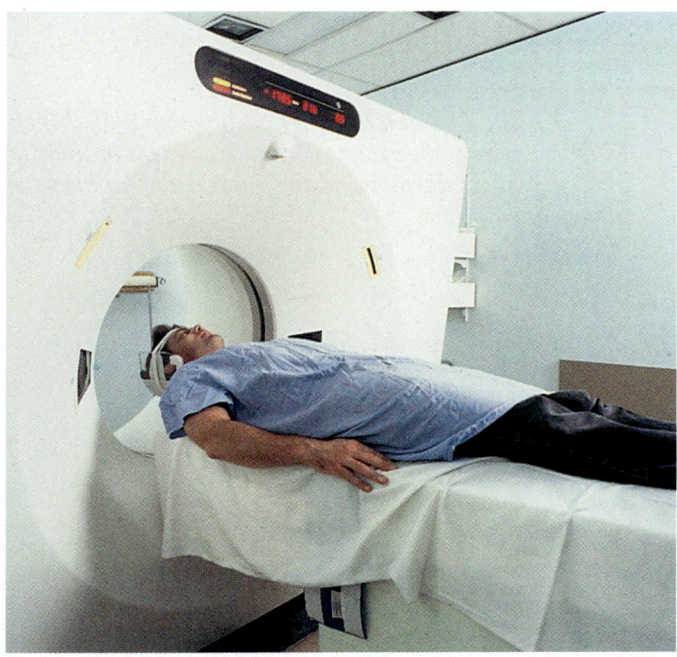

FIGURE 16-50　Patient in position for a CT scan

sion and return within 24 hours to have the amount of radioactive substance in a particular organ measured. For example, the radioactive thyroid uptake determines the function of the thyroid gland. Tumors of the thyroid may also be determined by this method. In female patients, pregnancy should be determined prior to the radioactive thyroid uptake, for it is seriously damaging to the fetus, especially within the first trimester of pregnancy.

ACHIEVE UNIT OBJECTIVES

- ■ Complete the Workbook activities to meet the learning objectives.
- ■ Apply your knowledge at the end of this chapter in completing the Critical Thinking Challenge and Activities, as well as the StudyWARE on your Student CD-ROM.

CRITICAL THINKING CHALLENGE

IMPACTING THE PATIENT, THE PRACTICE, AND YOUR CAREER

Jamie was working with patients one busy afternoon when her clinical supervisor requested that she schedule a patient for a barium enema. Since Jamie was preparing a 6-month-old baby for an examination at the time, she replied that she would schedule the appointment as soon as she was finished in the exam room. When Jamie came out of the exam room, the physician asked her to perform an ECG on a patient; immediately following completion of this task, she was asked to explain a prep for an IVP. The afternoon continued in this fashion, and at the end of the day, Jamie inadvertently placed the chart of the patient needing the barium enema with the others to be filed.

The next day the patient called Jamie inquiring as to the appointment for the test; realizing her mistake in not making the appointment, Jamie informed the patient she would call immediately and make the appointment. However, when Jamie contacted the radiology department, she was told that it would be 2 weeks before there was an open appointment slot. Jamie also saw that the physician had ordered the barium enema *stat*, another mistake on her part. She asked the radiology department if there was any chance they could squeeze this patient in, but it was not possible for them to do so. Jamie contacted the patient with the date and time in 2 weeks and did not inform the physician of the exchange between her, the patient, and the radiology department.

QUESTIONS

1. What impact could Jamie's actions have on the patient?
2. What impact could Jamie's actions have on the practice?
3. What impact could Jamie's actions have on her career?

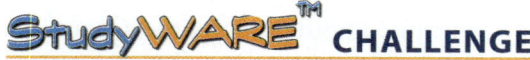 **CHALLENGE**

- Study with the flash cards for Chapter 16 to review the key terms in this chapter.
- Solve the hangman activities for Chapter 16.
- Complete the multiple choice quiz in test mode for Chapter 16.

RESOURCES

Carlton, R., & Adler, A. (2006). *Principles of radiographic imaging* (4th ed.). Clifton Park, NY: Thomson Delmar Learning.

Lazo, D. (2005). *Fundamentals of sectional anatomy: An imaging approach*. Clifton Park, NY: Thomson Delmar Learning.

WEB LINKS

www.sinuses.com (Sinusitis)
This web site is maintained by Wellington S. Tichenor, M.D. It explores the symptoms and treatment of sinusitis and other sinus diseases and the interrelated problems of allergy and asthma.

As a clinical medical assistant, you may assist with a variety of sterile procedures, including in-office surgery. Maintaining medical asepsis is vital to prevent the transmission of diseases *before, during,* and *following* any of the invasive procedures performed in the medical office or clinic. In compliance with Standard Precautions, proper barriers, such as latex or vinyl gloves, gown, and face mask or shield, must be worn to protect the health care staff from possible **contamination** while performing these procedures. All disposable waste must be placed in a plastic biohazard bag or in a sharps container and discarded properly to prevent disease transmission.

The medical assistant must have a good working knowledge of the care and function of basic instruments used in the medical office to perform minor surgical procedures.

Setup for various procedures can vary slightly according to the physician's preference. However, sterile technique will always remain the same for any invasive procedure. Basic information for assisting the physician and preparing the patient is covered in this chapter, along with a description of the specialized instruments used in the performance of minor in-office surgery.

UNIT 1
Instruments

UNIT 2
Preoperative Preparations

UNIT 3
Assisting with Minor Surgical Procedures

UNIT 1
INSTRUMENTS

OBJECTIVES

Upon completion of this unit, you will be able to achieve the following:

LEARNING Objectives

1. **Spell and define, using the glossary at the back of the text, all of the Words to Know in this unit.**
2. **Discuss the different parts of the instruments and the function of each part.**
3. **Describe the proper care of surgical instruments.**
4. **List the function of all instruments discussed in this unit.**

WORDS TO KNOW

contamination   needle holder   serrations
forceps   ratchet   speculum
hemostat   retractor

CERTIFICATION CONNECTION

CMA
Preparing equipment
Instruments, supplies,
  and equipment

CMAS
Asepsis in the medical
  office

RMA
Surgical supplies

Each instrument used in the performance of minor surgical procedures has a specific function.

Many times, its function can be determined simply by a visual inspection of the instrument. Surgical instruments used in the medical office are very costly and must be carefully maintained for longevity and maximum function. Always follow manufacturer's recommendations for cleaning, sterilization, and storage of all instruments.

INSTRUMENT CARE

Most instruments should be cared for in the same manner. The following is a list of general rules to follow when cleaning and caring for instruments.

1. Blood, tissue, and other body fluids must not be allowed to dry on an instrument.
2. Instruments should be soaked in a room-temperature solution containing a detergent and a solvent immediately after each use.
3. The detergent in the soaking solution should be of a neutral pH, which will help to prevent corrosion of the surfaces of the instrument.
4. The soaking solution should contain a special protein that breaks down blood and body fluids on the surface of the instrument.
5. Instruments should be placed in a plastic container for soaking to prevent damage to their points and cutting edges.
6. Separate delicate instruments from heavier ones to prevent damage.
7. Separate sharp instruments from others when cleaning and storing.
8. All surfaces and crevices must be scrubbed with a brush to remove any foreign material.
9. A careful visual inspection should be conducted during each cleaning to check for any nicks, dullness, or warping of the surfaces.
10. Damaged instruments should not be used and should be either repaired or replaced.

INSTRUMENT COMPONENTS

Each part of an instrument's structure has a specific function. Figures 17-1A through C illustrate the different key components of an instrument; an explanation of their function follows.

- *Ring handle* (Figure 17-1A): designed so that the thumb and finger can be inserted into the rings
- *Thumb handle*: a handle similar to that of a tweezer that is squeezed between the thumb and finger
- *Ratchet* (Figure 17-1A): locking mechanism designed to close in varying degrees to hold the instrument closed, used to clamp tissue and vessels
- *Serrations* (Figure 17-1B): little fissures that are engraved into the surface of the blades of hemostats and forceps designed to prevent slippage, providing a firm grip, when clamping a tissue
- *Teeth* (Figure 17-1C): very sharp projections designed to hold the tissue when grasping. Teeth can be heavy or delicate, and some are classified as nontraumatic.

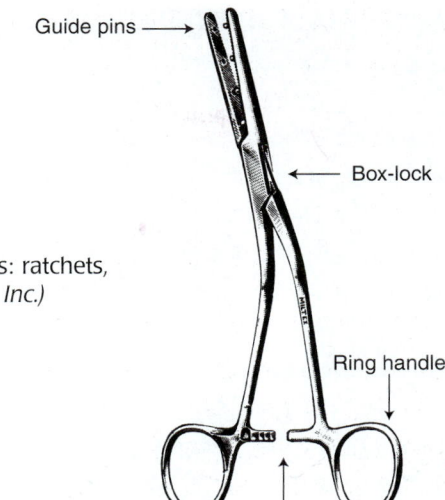

FIGURE 17-1A   Structural features of instruments: ratchets, box-locks, pins, and ring handle *(Courtesy of Miltex, Inc.)*

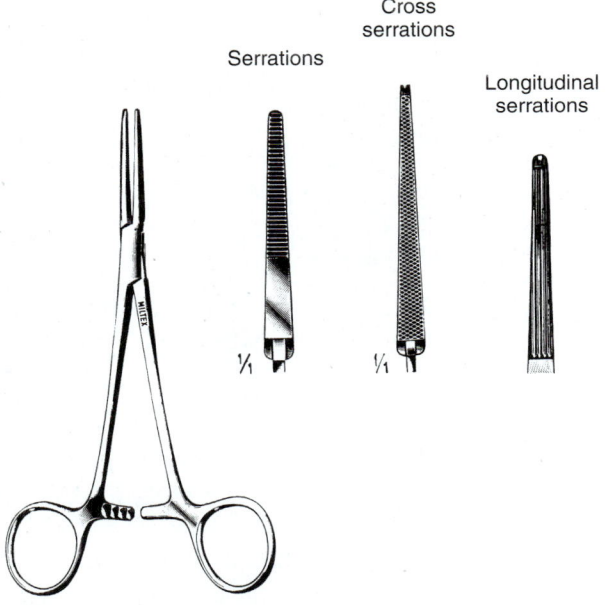

FIGURE 17-1B   Serrations *(Courtesy of Miltex, Inc.)*

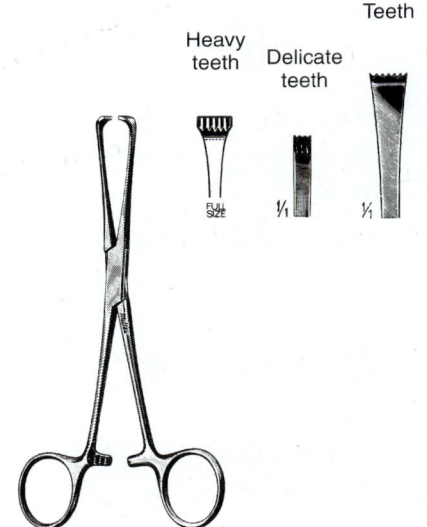

FIGURE 17-1C   Teeth *(Courtesy of Miltex, Inc.)*

INSTRUMENT CLASSIFICATION

Most instruments are classified according to their function as follows:

- *Cutting*: includes scissors and scalpels
- *Clamping or grasping*: includes **hemostats**, clamps, **forceps**, and **needle holders**
- *Dilating/probing*: **retractors**, scopes, **specula**, probes, and dilators

Table 17-1 lists some common instruments, along with their use.

TABLE 17-1 Instruments Used in Minor Office Surgical Procedures

Figure Number	Category: Description	Use
	Operating Scissors:	
A	*Deaver* 5½″ (14 cm) straight, sharp-sharp	Cut tissue and suture
B	*Sistrunk* 5½″ (14 cm) slightly curved, blunt-blunt	Same
C	*Deaver* 5½″ (14 cm) straight, sharp-blunt, and curved, sharp-blunt	Same
	Bandage Scissors:	
D	*Lester* 5½″ (14 cm) side curved	Cut dressings, tape
E	*Knowles* finger 5½″ (14 cm)	Same
F	*Spencer suture* 3½″ (8.75 cm)	Cut suture
G	*Littauer stitch* 5½″ (14 cm)	Same
	Petit-Point Hemostats:	
H	*Mosquito* 4¾″ straights, curved	Grasp tissue to hold, clamp, or pull out of the way
I	*Mosquito* 3½″ straight, curved	Same
	Towel Forceps:	
J	*Backhaus* (clip) 3½″ (8.75 cm)	Grasp towels, dressing; hold drape towels in place (use caution—will puncture skin)
K	*Jones* (clip) 3″	Same
L	*Knife handle* #3 5″ (12.5 cm) holds blades 10, 11, 12, 15	Accept blades
M	*Blades*	Cut tissue
	Sponge-Holding Forceps:	
N	*Forrester* 7″ (18 cm) straight, smooth jaws or serrated	Pick up and hold dressings
	Needle Holders:	
O	*Brown* 5¼″ (13.5 cm)	Grasp suture needle
P	*Collier* 5″ (13 cm)	Same
	Dressing and Tissue Forceps:	
Q	*Thumb* 4″ (10 cm) serrated	Pick up dressings, delicate tissue
R	*Tissue* 4½″ (11 cm) 1 × 2 teeth	Grasp tissue securely for control during dissection or suturing
S	*Adson serrated,* extra delicate, 0.8-mm-wide tip	Pick up delicate tissue
T	*Semken* dressing 4¾″ (12 cm) serrated	Pick up dressings
U	*Cushing* 7¼″ (18.5 cm) serrated handle, scraper end, bayonet, 1 × 2 teeth	Close skin
V	*Plain splinter* 3½″ (8.75 cm)	Remove splinters
W	*Judd-Allis tissue* 6″ (15 cm)	Grasp tissue
X	Grave's vaginal speculum	Enlarge vaginal cavity
Y	Vienna nasal speculum	Enlarge nasal cavity

(continues)

TABLE 17-1   Instruments Used in Minor Office Surgical Procedures (Continued)

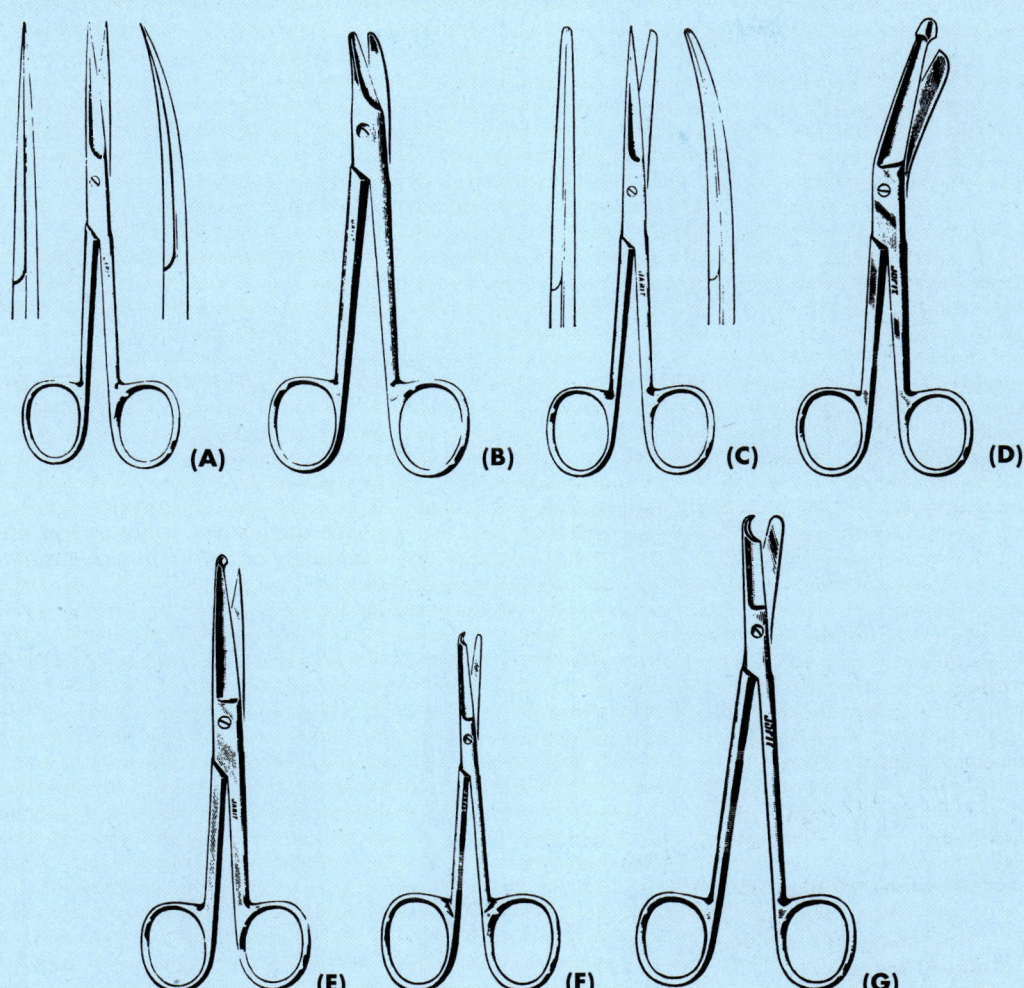

Operating scissors: (A) Deaver, (B) Sistrunk, (C) Deaver.
Bandage scissors: (D) Lester, (E) Knowles finger, (F) Spencer suture, (G) Littauer stitch
(Courtesy of JARIT® Surgical Instruments)

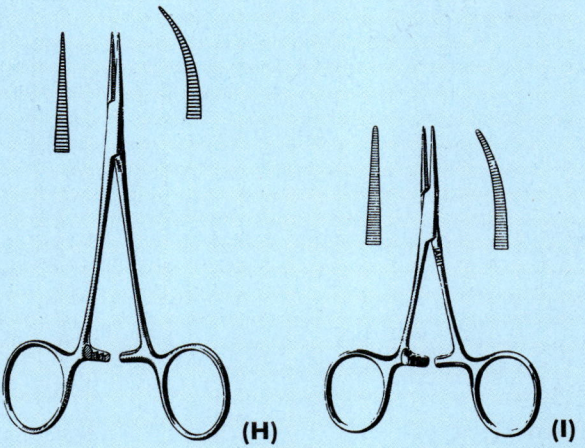

Petit-point hemostats: (H) and (I) mosquito *(Courtesy of JARIT® Surgical Instruments)*

TABLE 17-1   Instruments Used in Minor Office Surgical Procedures (Continued)

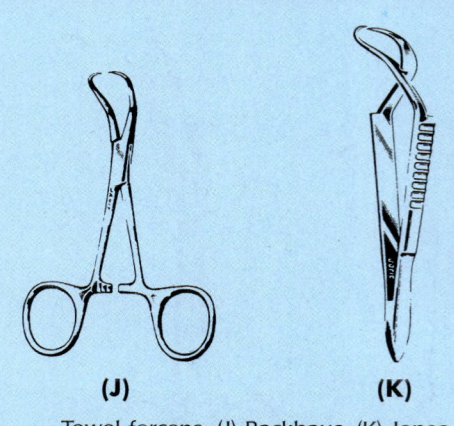

Towel forceps: (J) Backhaus, (K) Jones
(Courtesy of JARIT® Surgical Instruments)

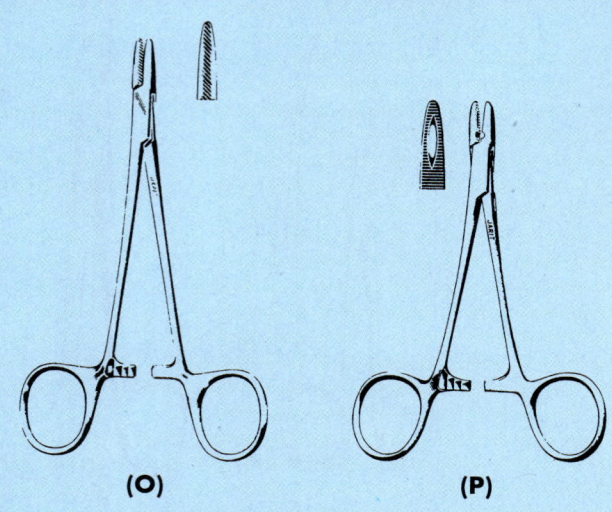

Needle holders: (O) Brown, (P) Collier
(Courtesy of JARIT® Surgical Instruments)

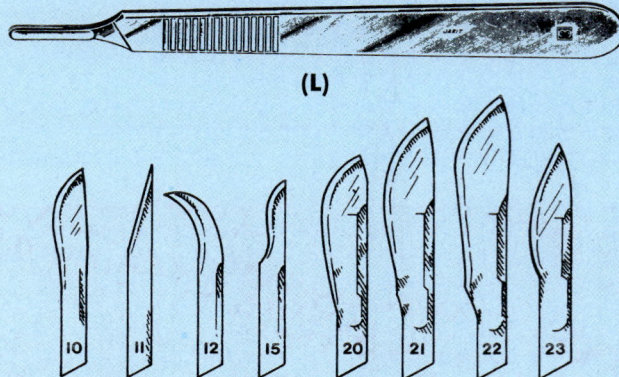

(L) Knife handle, (M) Blades
(Courtesy of JARIT® Surgical Instruments)

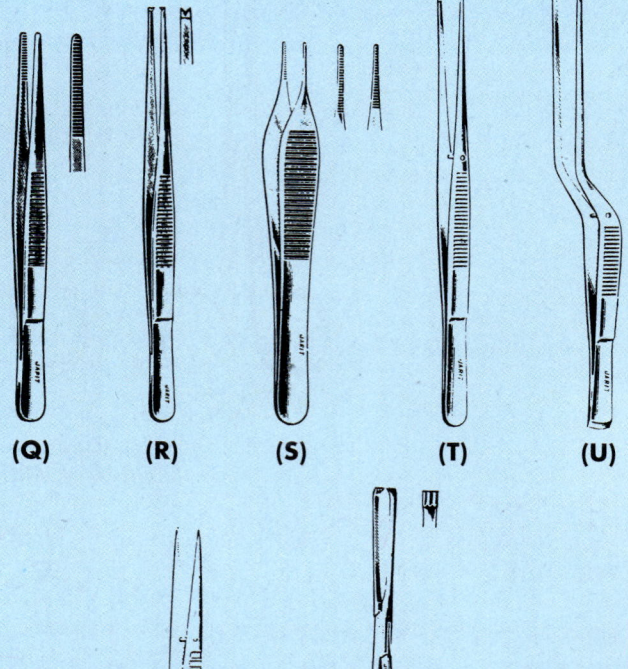

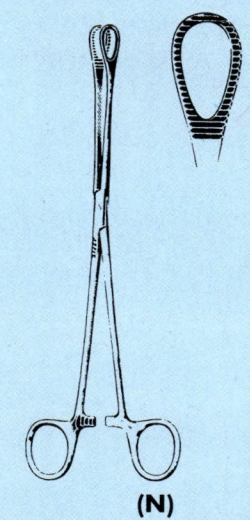

(N) Foersfer sponge-holding forceps
(Courtesy of JARIT® Surgical Instruments)

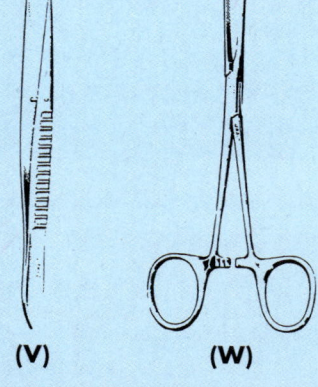

Dressing and tissue forceps: (Q) thumb, (R) tissue, (S) Adson,
(T) Semken dressing, (U) Cushing, (V) plain splinter,
(W) Judd-Allis tissue *(Courtesy of JARIT® Surgical Instruments)*

(continues)

TABLE 17-1   Instruments Used in Minor Office Surgical Procedures (Continued)

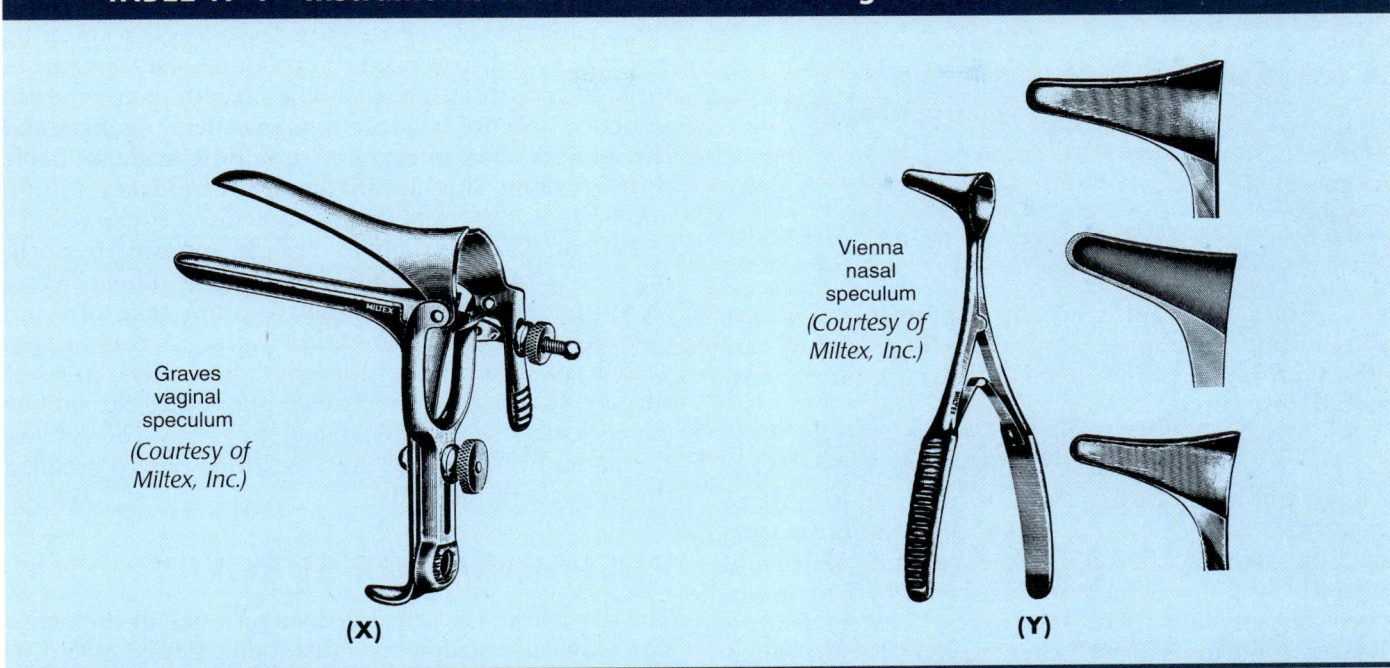

Graves
vaginal
speculum
*(Courtesy of
Miltex, Inc.)*

(X)

Vienna
nasal
speculum
*(Courtesy of
Miltex, Inc.)*

(Y)

ACHIEVE UNIT OBJECTIVES

- ■ Complete the Workbook activities to meet the learning objectives.
- ■ Apply your knowledge at the end of this chapter in completing the Critical Thinking Challenge and Activities, as well as the StudyWARE on your Student CD-ROM.

UNIT 2
PREOPERATIVE PREPARATIONS

OBJECTIVES

Upon completion of this unit, you will be able to achive the following:

LEARNING Objectives

1. Spell and define, using the glossary at the back of the text, all the Words to Know in this unit.
2. Explain scheduling and preop and postop instructions for patients for minor office surgery.

3. Explain the importance of obtaining the consent form for the surgical procedure.
4. Describe various procedures that require sterile technique.
5. Describe important information that should be recorded on patient's chart.
6. Explain the importance of proper skin preparation before an invasive procedure.
7. Discuss the importance of maintaining the sterile field.

PERFORMANCE Objectives

1. Prepare skin for a minor surgical procedure.
2. Set up a sterile tray.

WORDS TO KNOW

adverse	authorize	microbial
anesthesia	contaminate	preoperative
anesthesiologist	fenestrated	(preop)
anesthetic	hemophilia	scheduling
antiseptic	invasive	

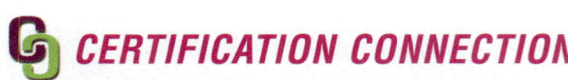

CERTIFICATION CONNECTION

CMA
Surgical asepsis

CMAS
Asepsis in the medical
    office

RMA
Surgical supplies
Surgical procedures

The medical assistant is usually responsible for **scheduling** minor office surgery. A number of procedures are now performed in the medical office or outpatient/ambulatory surgery center.

You may be asked to schedule an appointment for a patient to have a surgical procedure as an outpatient at a large ambulatory care center or hospital. Be sure to check with the person who makes the appointment regarding the preparation for the patient. When you write the appointment date and time for the patient, make certain the patient has directions to the facility. The assistant in the hospital or surgeon's office generally phones the patient the day before the surgery to confirm the appointment. Be sure to cover all points listed in the patient education box when scheduling a patient for a minor surgical procedure.

Be sure the patient understands the procedure and the instructions regarding **preoperative** (**preop**) and

---

postoperative (postop) care. Most medical facilities have printed instructions for patients. Remember that some patients you see are either non-English speaking or cannot read. You need to explain as well as you can verbally and observe the patient's reactions to your instructions. Printed instructions in other languages and the services of an interpreter should be made available to the patient. This eliminates any misunderstandings, and patients feel more at ease knowing they can refer to it. Patients should be advised of the appropriate clothing to be worn on the day of the surgery. Loose-fitting clothing, clothing easy to put on and take off, and clothing that is not their "Sunday best" should be suggested as appropriate for the anatomical area of surgery. It is a good practice to phone the patient the day prior to the appointment, not only to reassure the patient and answer any questions but to confirm the physician's schedule.

PREPARING FOR SURGERY

The day before the scheduled surgery, get all the necessary surgical instruments and supplies ready. A routine inventory of all supplies and sterile items is vital so that a sterile tray setup can be made for any surgical procedure.

All surgical instruments must be properly labeled and autoclaved. Most of the instruments will already be sterilized (as they should be after each use). The basic setup for most minor surgical procedures includes the following sterile items:

- Scalpel handle and blades or disposable scalpel
- Hemostats
- Needle holder
- Needles and suture material (absorbable or nonabsorbable)
- Suture scissors
- Thumb forceps
- Probe
- Gauze squares
- Vial of **anesthetic** medication
- Syringes
- Towels
- Bandages

Some of these supplies may be wrapped and sterilized together. All sterile packages must be labeled with the contents, date the package was sterilized, and the signature of the person who prepared and sterilized it. Autoclaved items remain sterile if they have been properly processed and have been protected from moisture for 30 days. Packages should be checked before use for any tears or other signs of tampering to ensure sterility.

Most items used today are disposable and come already sterile in the manufacturer's packaging. You

---

PATIENT EDUCATION

Preop
In scheduling, advise patient of:

1. Approximate length of time for procedure
2. Appropriate clothing to wear at appointment
3. Amount of time to fast as instructed by physician
4. Arranging for someone to accompany him if necessary
5. Anticipated time off work or arranging for home care
6. The surgical procedure by providing printed education materials

When patient arrives for appointment:

1. Provide written instructions regarding the surgical procedure and follow-up care.
2. Explain surgical consent form, and obtain patient's signature.
3. Answer any questions concerning procedure.
4. Ascertain if the patient has any allergies to any medications, including topical preparations, latex products, and adhesive tapes.

must make sure that the package has not been torn or punctured to ensure sterility. The sterilization of the product is guaranteed only to a certain date marked on the package, and this date must be checked.

A variety of minor **invasive** surgical procedures are performed in the medical office, and each requires several instruments. Figure 17-2 shows an example of a specific surgical instrument tray setup and supplies commonly used in minor office procedures. You must become familiar with the physician's preference for particular items and the way they are to be arranged for use. Until you are certain about the details of a particular procedure, you may want to keep a notebook handy for reference.

The room where the surgery will take place and the sterile tray should be set up before the patient is escorted to the area to be prepared for the procedure. Procedure 17-1 lists the steps involved in setting up a sterile tray.

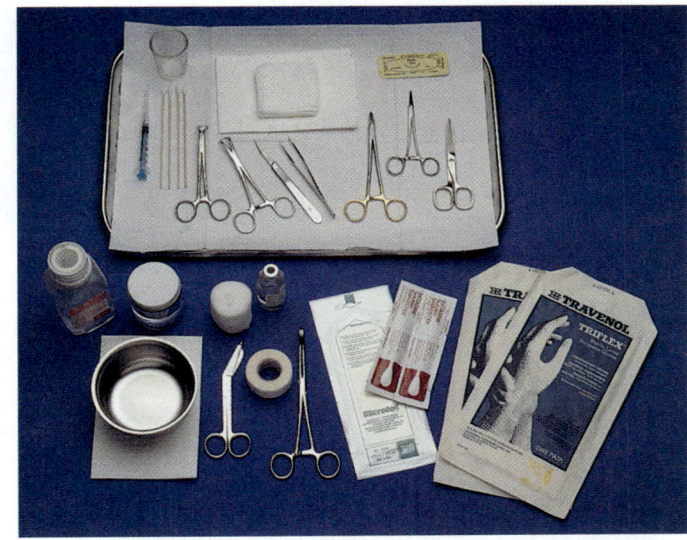

FIGURE 17-2   An example of a surgical setup tray

PROCEDURE PROCEDURE PROCEDURE PROCEDURE PROCEDURE PROCEDURE PROCEDURE PROCEDURE

17-1   📋 Sterile Tray Set-up

PURPOSE: Set up a sterile tray with the equipment required to perform a minor surgical procedure.

EQUIPMENT: Mayo stand, disposable sterile field drapes, and instruments and equipment required for the procedure.

PERFORMANCE OBJECTIVE: With access to all equipment and supplies, set up a sterile tray for a minor surgical procedure, according to the physician's preference.

1. Wash hands.

2. Sanitize and disinfect the Mayo tray and adjust the stand so that the tray is at waist level.

3. Place a sterile drape package on a clean, dry surface (Figure 17-3A).

4. Open the pack to expose the sterile drape with the corners facing toward you. **NOTE: You may turn the package to properly position its contents.**

5. Grasp the sterile drape between the thumb and finger and lift the drape up enough that it unfolds but does not touch anything (Figure 17-3B). **NOTE: Be sure the drape does not brush up against your uniform or the counter.**

6. Grasp the opposite corner (Figure 17-3C) and allow the drape to completely unfold.

7. Place the drape over the Mayo tray without reaching over the drape (Figure 17-3D). **NOTE: Reaching over the sterile drape will contaminate it.**

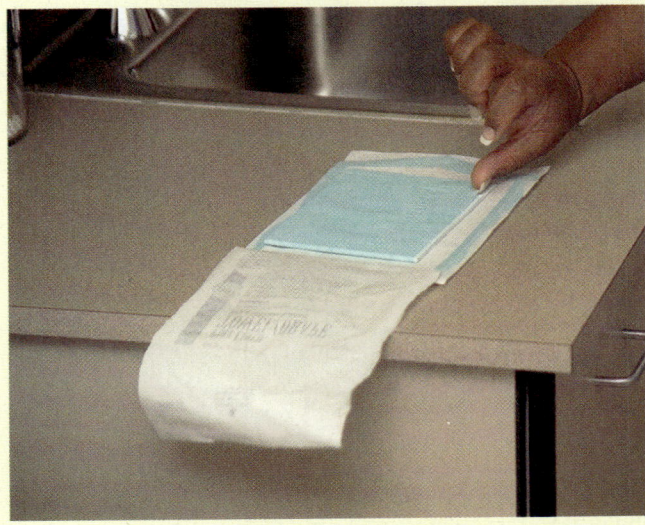

FIGURE 17-3A   Place the sterile drape package onto a flat, dry surface and pull the pack open. Carefully pick up the sterile drape by the corner.

(continues)

17-1  Sterile Tray Set-up (Continued)

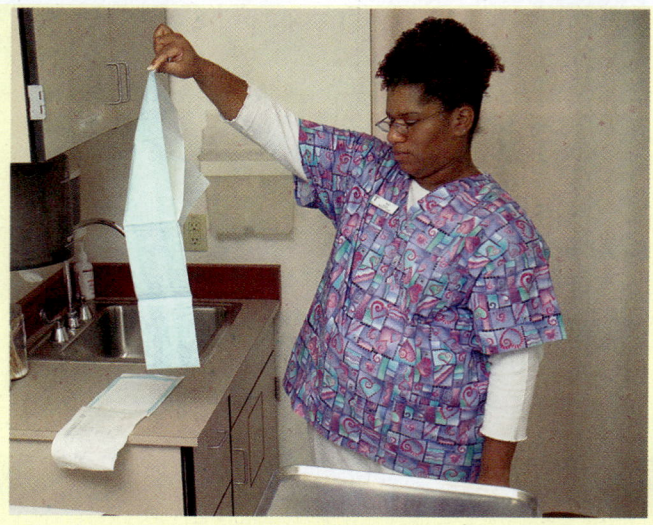

FIGURE 17-3B Lift the drape straight up and allow it to unfold. Make sure the drape does not brush up against your uniform, the tray, or the countertop.

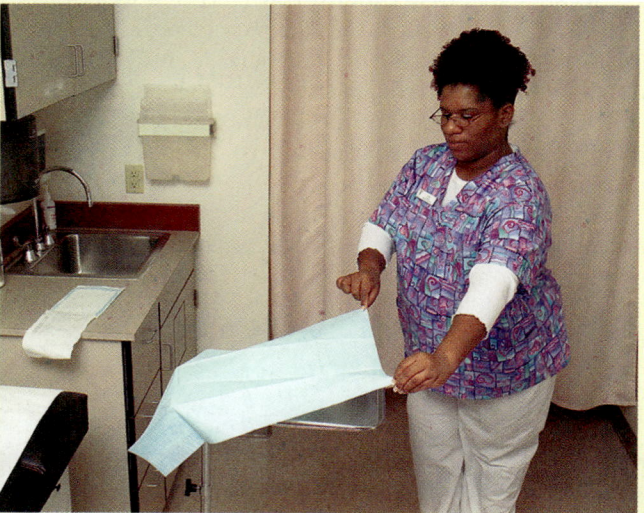

FIGURE 17-3D Adjust the position of the drape until it covers the tray.

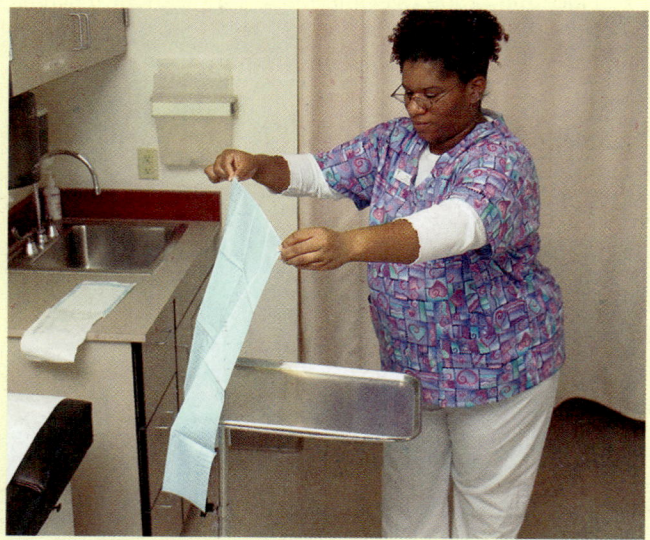

FIGURE 17-3C Grasp the opposite corner of the unfolded drape and place it on the Mayo stand without leaning over the drape.

8. Properly open the fan-folded sterile pack or prepack-aged sterile pack (Figures 17-4A through F) and allow the instrument to drop onto the sterile field (Figures 17-4G through L). **NOTE: Never reach over the sterile field, as it could become contaminated.**

9. Apply sterile gloves or use sterile transfer forceps to arrange the instruments on the sterile field according to the physician's preference.

10. Place a sterile drape over the field to protect sterility until the procedure begins.

(continues)

17-1  Sterile Tray Set-up (Continued)

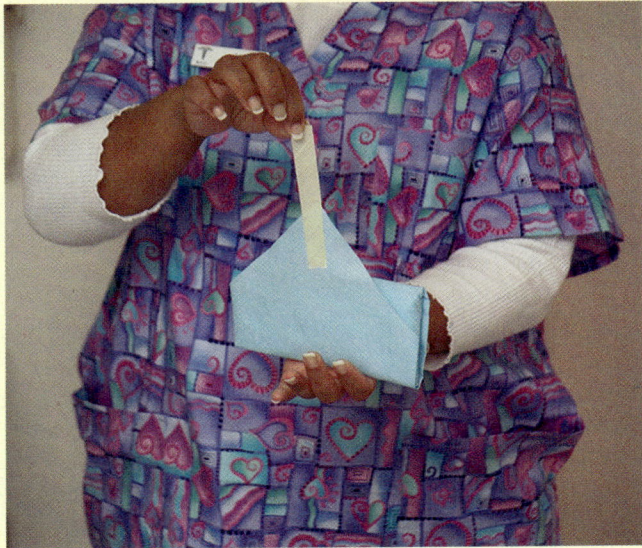

FIGURE 17-4A Grasp the tape on the top flap and open the flap away from you.

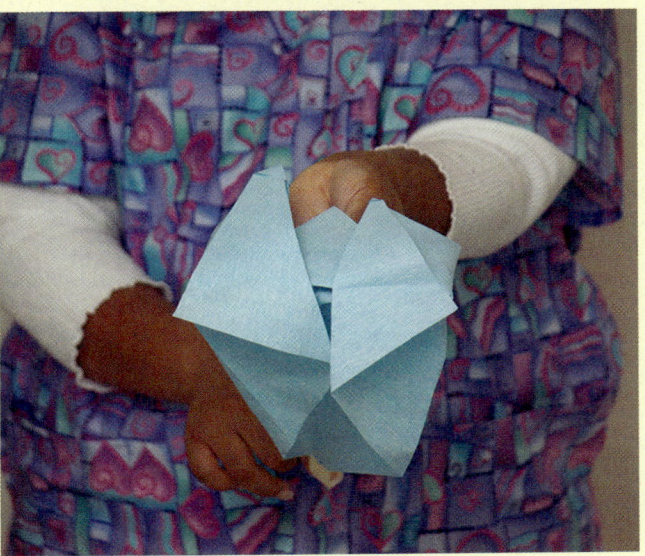

FIGURE 17-4B Gently unroll the pack in the palm of your hand, being careful not to touch the inside of the pack.

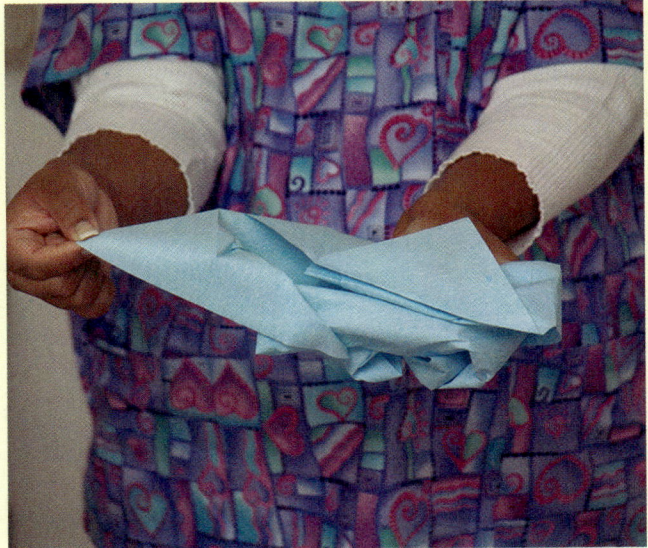

FIGURE 17-4C Grasp the tips of the side flaps and unfold them by reaching around the side or under the pack. DO NOT reach over the pack.

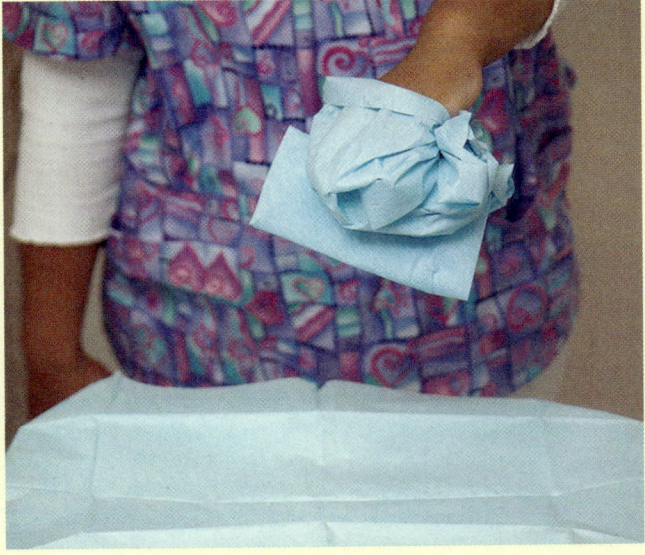

FIGURE 17-4D Gather all the flaps together in the palm of your hand so they are back out of the way when the item is dropped onto the field.

(continues)

PROCEDURE PROCEDURE PROCEDURE PROCEDURE PROCEDURE PROCEDURE PROCEDURE

17-1   Sterile Tray Set-up (Continued)

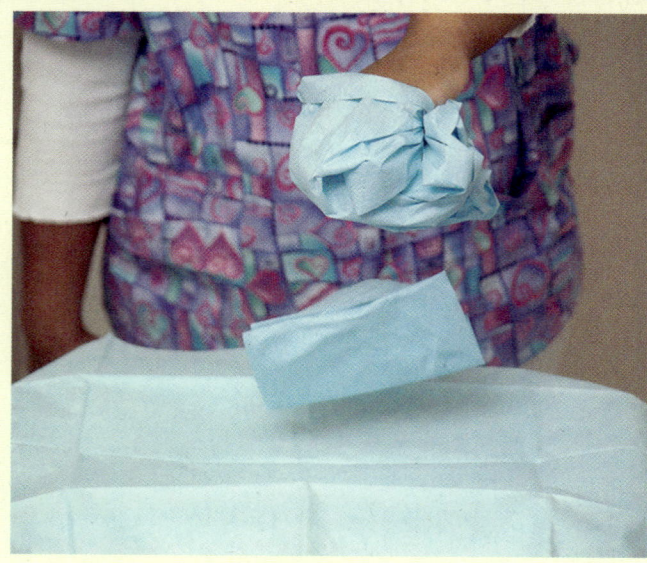

FIGURE 17-4E   Drop the instrument onto the sterile field.

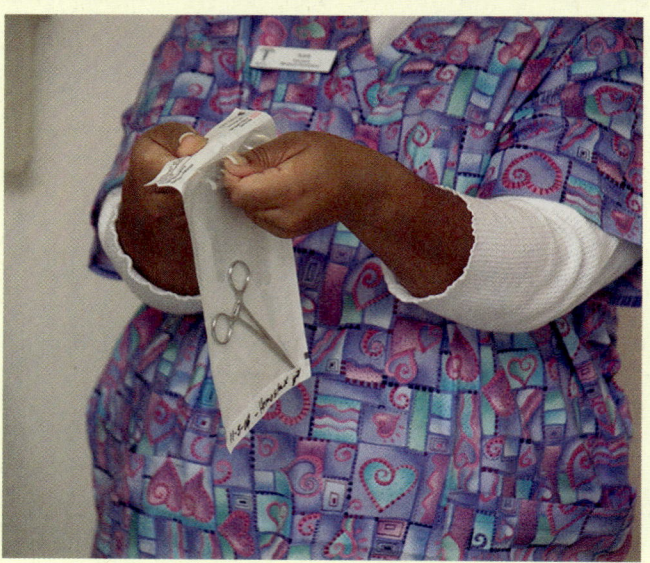

FIGURE 17-4F   Grasp the flaps on the sterile peel-apart pack and open the pack.

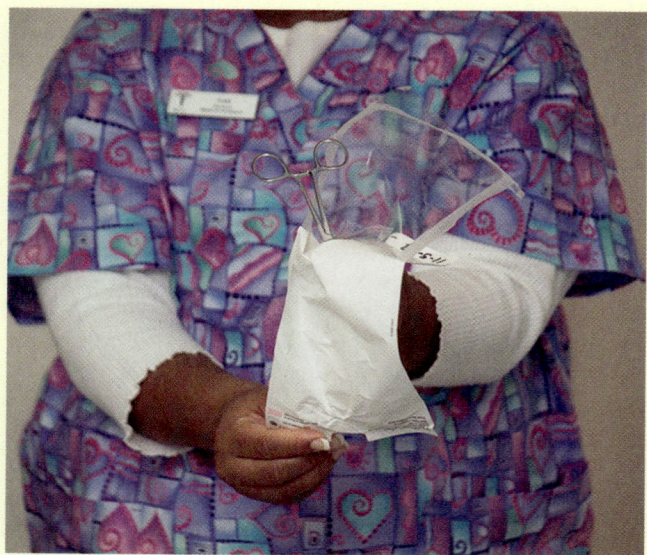

FIGURE 17-4G   Pull the bottom flap back and grasp the flap and the instrument inside the pack simultaneously.

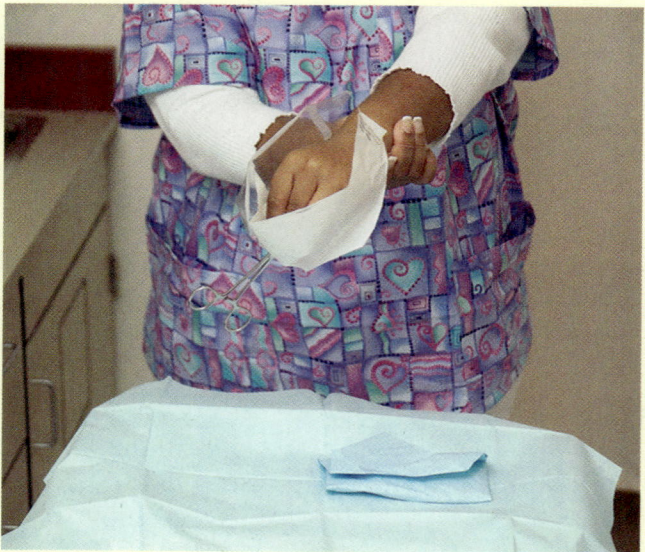

FIGURE 17-4H   Turn the pack so that the instrument will easily fall onto the sterile field when released.

(continues)

PROCEDURE PROCEDURE PROCEDURE PROCEDURE PROCEDURE PROCEDURE PROCEDURE

17-1  Sterile Tray Set-up (Continued)

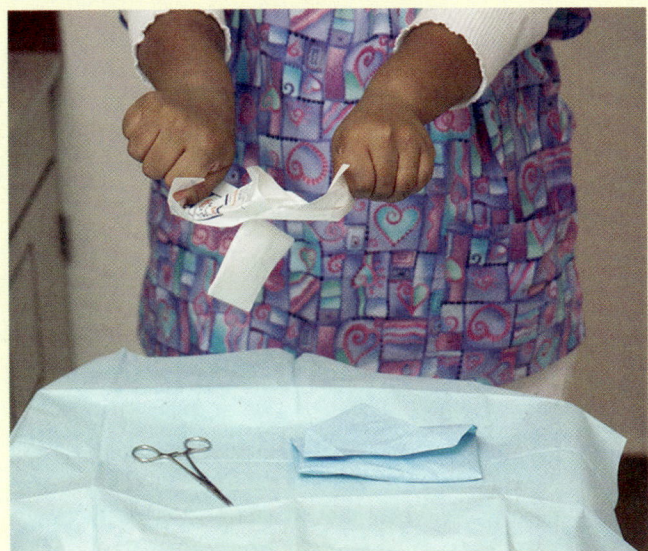

FIGURE 17-4I   Drop the instrument onto the sterile field.

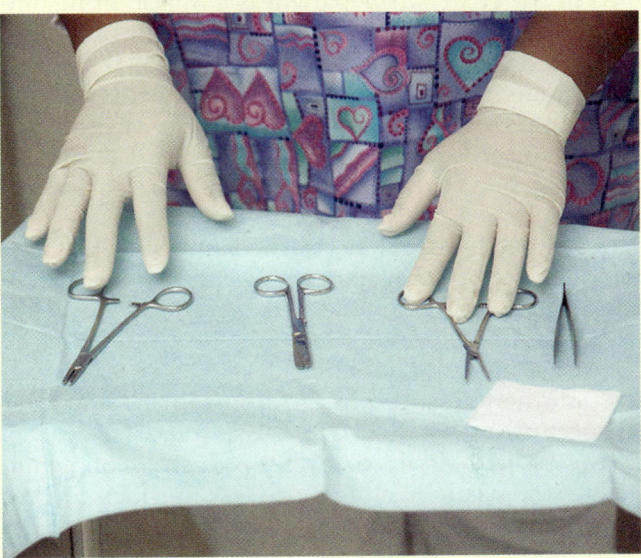

FIGURE 17-4J   Apply sterile gloves and arrange the instruments on the tray in the proper order.

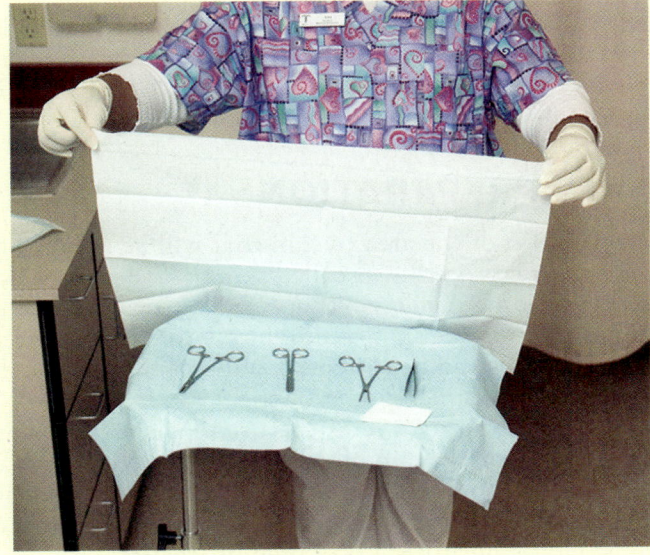

FIGURE 17-4K   Grasp another sterile drape by the corners.

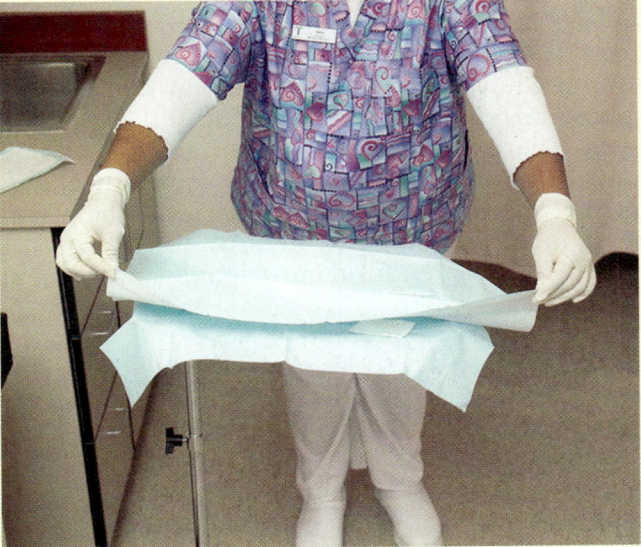

FIGURE 17-4L   Cover the sterile tray until the procedure begins.

PREPARING THE PATIENT

When the patient arrives for surgery, a consent form must be completed. An example is shown in Figure 17-5. You should allow the patient time to ask any questions about the procedure and answer them adequately. The patient's signature must be on the consent form, which is filed in the chart. If the patient is a minor, or incompetent, the person **authorized** to give consent must sign for the patient following an explanation of the procedure and answering any questions. The patient's vital signs should be taken, and any complaints or problems should be recorded on the patient's chart. The patient should then empty the bladder before being positioned and draped for the procedure.

Most procedures are performed under local **anesthesia**, which the physician administers. Large group practices may have a qualified **anesthesiologist** on staff. A careful medical history must be taken from the patient to determine possible allergic or **adverse** reactions. This helps avoid complications during and after the procedure.

If the patient discloses a family history of **hemophilia**, (a serious blood clotting disease in which there is the absence of one of the necessary blood clotting factors for blood to coagulate) or is himself a hemophiliac, you should bring it to the physician's attention immediately. This information should be marked in red ink on the patient's chart. Hemophilia is a sex-linked hereditary trait that occurs mostly in males. Patients who have this diagnosis must have surgery of any type *only* at a completely equipped, well-staffed medical-surgical hospital to protect their safety and well-being.

In procedures requiring that a biopsy be taken for analysis, careful labeling and handling of the specimen is vital. The laboratory provides a formalin solution container for preservation of the tissue specimen. This container is sterile, and the specimen must be placed directly in the solution with sterile transfer forceps. A completed lab request form must accompany the specimen for analysis.

In certain surgical procedures, such as the removal of warts or polyps, an electrocautery device may be used. Often this is used to control bleeding of the surgical site by electrocoagulation. Controlled high-frequency current is applied by the physician to the surgical area to coagulate the blood to close the incision. If the reusable tips are preferred by the physician for surgical procedures, they must be autoclaved to prevent possible cross-contamination. Disposable tips are available.

Another method used in removing skin tags, warts, and other skin disorders and growths is by cryosurgery. Often, certain gynecologic treatments and surgical procedures are performed with this instrument. This process uses subfreezing temperature to destroy or remove tissue. Generally, the substances used are solid carbon dioxide or liquid nitrogen. It is sometimes referred to as cold cautery. Refer to Procedure 17-2 for preparing a patient's skin for minor surgery.

CONSENT TO OPERATE

Date ________ Time ________ A.M. P.M.

1. I authorize the performance upon ________
   of the following operation ________
   to be performed under the direction of Dr. ________
2. The following have been explained to me by Dr. ________
   A. The nature of the operation ________
   B. The purpose of the operation ________
   C. The possible alternative methods of treatment ________
   D. The possible consequences of the operation ________
   E. The risks involved ________
   F. The possibility of complications ________
3. I have been advised of the serious nature of the operation and have been advised that if I desire a further and more detailed explanation of any of the foregoing or further information about the possible risks or complications of the above listed operation it will be given to me.
4. I do not request a further and more detailed listing and explanation of any of the items listed in paragraph 2.

Signed ________
(Patient or person authorized to consent for patient)

Witness ________

FIGURE 17-5 A sample consent form for surgical procedures.

SKIN PREPARATION

Preparation of the area of skin that will be affected by the surgical procedure is called skin prep. Because body hair encourages **microbial** accumulation, it is sometimes shaved. The skin cannot be completely sterilized, or the cells would be destroyed, but an **antiseptic** can be used to reduce microbial growth.

Many physicians prefer the use of disposable skin-prep kits that contain all the necessary items for this procedure. To protect yourself and the patient from possible disease transmission, you should wear latex or vinyl gloves during the skin prep procedure.

You must be extremely careful to avoid nicking the patient's skin (see Figure 17-6.) Microorganisms can enter the body through a break in the skin, and an infection could develop from carelessness. If this should happen, the physician must be notified immediately. Practice in the procedure for this skill is necessary to become proficient.

17-2      Prepare Skin for Minor Surgery

PURPOSE: To remove hair from the surgery site to prevent infection and to clean the skin and apply antiseptic solution to reduce microbial growth.

OSHA GUIDELINES: To comply with Standard Precautions, gloves and other protective barriers must be worn if there is any possibility of coming into contact with blood, or any body fluids.

EQUIPMENT: Small basin for soap solution, 4 × 4-inch gauze squares (sponges), disposable razor, scissors, antiseptic soap solution, emesis basin for disposables, gooseneck lamp, sterile drape sheet or towels (or **fenestrated** drape sheet), latex or vinyl gloves, and skin antiseptic.

PERFORMANCE OBJECTIVE: Provided with all necessary equipment and supplies and other students to act as patients, demonstrate each of the steps required in the skin prep procedure. **NOTE: In the institutional setting, preparing the forearm may be sufficient; moreover, the shaving process may be demonstrated by using a razor with no blade.**

1. Wash and glove hands, and assemble all the needed items.

2. Identify the patient. **RATIONALE: Speaking to the patient by name and checking the chart ensures that you are performing the procedure on the correct patient.**

3. Explain the procedure to the patient. Ask the patient to remove necessary clothing. Explain where the patient should put her belongings. Assist the patient if necessary.

4. Assist the patient into the proper position on the treatment table and drape her with a sheet or light bath blanket as directed by the physician.

5. Adjust the gooseneck lamp to light the area to be shaved.

6. Place gauze squares in the soapy solution and use one at a time to soap the area to be shaved. After use, discard each into an emesis basin.

7. When the skin prep site is covered by scalp hair, beard, or pubic hair, use scissors to clip hair in preparation for shaving. **NOTE: Use caution when clipping hair with scissors and in shaving with a razor to avoid both self-injury and harm to the patient.** Shave hair by placing the razor against the skin at about a 30-degree angle (Figure 17-6). Hold the skin taut for easier shaving. Shave in the direction hair grows. Wipe soap and hair from the razor with a tissue. Swish the razor through soapy water, shake excess water from it, and shave the next area.

8. Remove all soap and hair from the area by wetting a sterile gauze square with sterile water and wiping the area. Dry the area with sterile gauze squares.

9. Apply antiseptic solution to the surgery site with a gauze square held by transfer forceps. **NOTE: Begin application in the center of the site and move outward in a circular motion (Figure 17-7H). RATIONALE: This pattern of continuous movement ensures total coverage without contamination from untreated areas.**

10. Cover the prepared area with a sterile drape sheet or towel until the physician is ready to begin. **NOTE: Instruct the patient not to touch the sterile field (either the sterile field of the surgical site or the instrument tray setup).**

11. Discard disposable items and return other items to the proper storage area. Remove gloves and wash hands.

12. Attend to the patient's comfort. Patients are usually apprehensive about even minor surgical procedures. Reassurance at this time is most important.

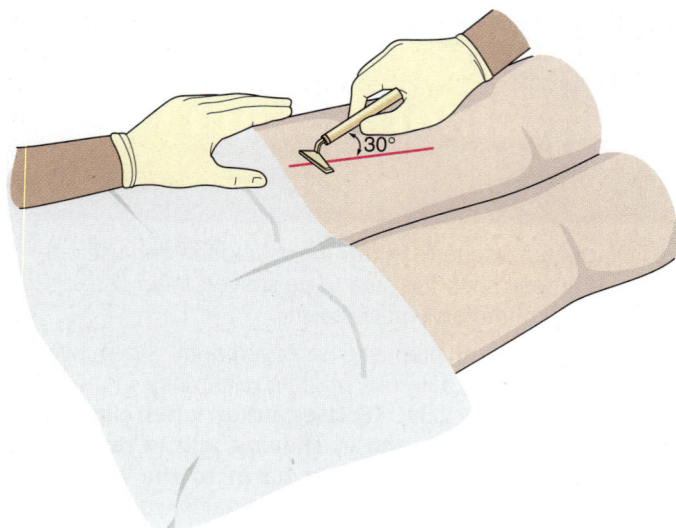

FIGURE 17-6 Angle for shaving a surgery site (or for suture insertion)

The patient's skin must also be prepped with an antiseptic, such as iodine, prior to surgery. The antiseptic is applied after the skin has been shaved and properly cleansed. The solution is applied in a circular motion (see Figure 17-7), using care not to contaminate the area during the application.

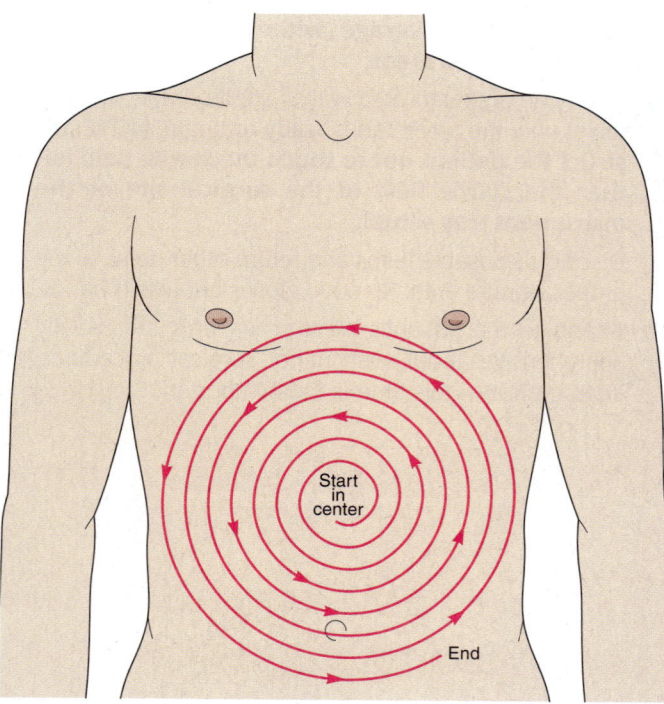

FIGURE 17-7 Apply all solutions to the skin in this circular pattern. Prepping the skin with an antiseptic solution should begin at the center of the incision site and proceed outward in one continuous circular motion as shown.

When assisting with acupuncture procedures, preparation of the skin is simply to use an antiseptic, such as alcohol (if the skin is obviously dirty, you should wash the area with soap and water and dry it before proceeding).

ACHIEVE UNIT OBJECTIVES

- ■ **Complete the Workbook activities to meet the learning objectives.**
- ■ **Practice the procedures in this unit to meet the performance objectives.**
- ■ **Apply your knowledge at the end of this chapter in completing the Critical Thinking Challenge and Activities, as well as the StudyWARE on your Student CD-ROM.**

UNIT 3
ASSISTING WITH MINOR SURGICAL PROCEDURES

OBJECTIVES

Upon completion of this unit, you will be able to achieve the following:

LEARNING Objectives

1. Describe the minor surgical procedures discussed in this unit.
2. Explain the tray setup for suture removal.
3. Explain the clean-up process following a minor surgery.
4. Describe the different types of anesthetics used in minor surgical procedures.
5. List the medical assistant's duties in minor surgery.

PERFORMANCE Objectives

1. Demonstrate the medical assistant's role in assisting with a minor surgical procedure.
2. Apply sterile gloves.
3. Demonstrate suture removal.

WORDS TO KNOW

biopsy
coagulation
cryosurgery
dominant
electrocautery
expiration

histology
hypoallergenic
incision and
    drainage
    (I & D)

postoperative
stress
suture

CERTIFICATION CONNECTION

CMA

Aseptic technique
Disposal of biohazardous
    material
Practice standard
    precautions

CMAS

Asepsis in the medical
    office

RMA

Surgical supplies
Surgical procedures

Many minor surgical procedures are now performed in the medical office, clinic, and ambulatory care center. It is usually the medical assistant's duty to schedule the surgery, educate the patient about preoperative and **postoperative** care, prepare the room and equipment for the surgery, and assist the physician, as needed. Medical assistants should have a general knowledge of the procedures performed in their place of employment and be able to assist the physician with little or no direction. When assisting with a surgical procedure, it is critical to maintain strict sterile technique. A break in sterile technique or a breech of the sterile field can result in an infection for the patient. Table 17-2 lists some of the common surgical procedures performed in the medical office along with some general information about each.

GENERAL INFORMATION

Many physicians prefer to perform minor surgical procedures first on the day's schedule. The doctor may require that patients fast for a certain time before the

TABLE 17-2 In-office Minor Surgical Procedures	
Procedure	**General Description**
Laceration repair	Closing a wound or laceration by placing **sutures** or stitches or staples in the skin to hold the edges of the wound together for proper healing
Sebaceous cyst removal	Excision of a small, painless sac containing a build-up of sebum, the secretion from a sebaceous gland
Incision and drainage (I & D)	Incision into a localized infection, such as an abscess, to drain the exudates from the area
Biopsy	Excision of a small amount of tissue for microscopic examination. Specimen must be preserved in a solution of 10% formalin until transported to the laboratory and prepared for examination.
Needle biopsy	Fluid or tissue cells are aspirated through a needle into a syringe for microscopic examination. This specimen must also be properly preserved.
Cryosurgery	Destruction of tissue and skin lesions using extremely cold temperatures
Electrosurgery and cautery	Removal of benign skin lesions, such as warts and skin tags, by use of electric current. Figure 17-8 illustrates an **electrocautery** unit. This procedure is performed when a biopsy is not required and also to control bleeding during a procedure.
Chemical destruction	Tissue is destroyed by applying silver nitrate to the area.
Laser surgery	A concentrated laser beam (intense light beam) is used to destroy a target area without harming the surrounding tissue.

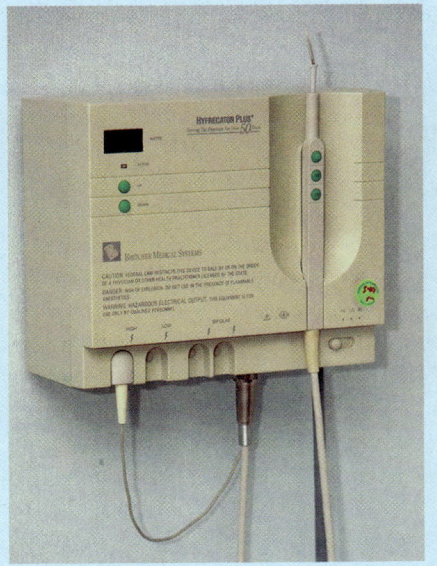

FIGURE 17-8 An electrocautery unit

procedure. Fasting lessens the possibility of nausea and vomiting, which some patients may experience during and following any type of surgery. It is best to check with the doctor regarding preference in preop instructions.

Outpatient, or ambulatory, surgery in recent years has become more acceptable than ever before for a number of reasons. Anesthesia has been significantly improved and causes fewer side effects in patients following surgical procedures. This allows them to awaken faster and easier. Also, the required time for many surgeries has decreased because of advances in instruments, such as the "scopes" used in laparoscopic surgeries. For example, the abdominal laparoscopy requires two to three very small incisions for insertion of the scope, a suction, and possibly a 3rd instrument. The gallbladder, growths, and tumors can be removed with this advanced technology. Because patients naturally feel more comfortable at home, following the "same-day surgery," most patients of all ages are sent home to recover and do so more rapidly than when in the hospital. Postsurgery infection rate has also declined in those patients who go home immediately following surgery. All of this is highlighted by the reduced cost from the elimination of a hospital stay. Printed instructions should be given to the patient and explained to him and his family. The patient should, of course, be given the physician's phone number and urged to phone if there are any complications or concerns. You should have a standard set of printed instructions readily available for telephone triage of those outpatient surgery patients who may call in with questions or concerns. Any calls that suggest a serious problem or condition should be referred to the physician immediately. Refer to the patient education box regarding what you should caution patients about following any surgery.

STERILE GLOVES

If the physician wishes you to assist directly with the surgical procedure, sterile gloves must be worn (Figure 17-9). Dressing changes should also be performed wearing sterile gloves to protect both yourself and the patient. In addition, you may assist with needle biopsies, intrauterine device (IUD) insertions, and lacerations resulting from injuries. All of these procedures require sterile techniques.

Before you put sterile gloves on, you must perform a complete and careful hand washing to remove as many microorganisms as possible. Refer to the procedure and figures for proper hand washing in Chapter 12. Routine hand washing should take 20 seconds. There are a few ways to make sure you have spent the whole 20 seconds actually washing your hands. You can sing the popular "Happy Birthday" song or one of your choosing at a normal pace. Watch the sweep hand and sing at the pace it

---

PATIENT EDUCATION

Usual care of patient:

1. Keep site clean and dry
2. Place no stress on the area
3. Drink plenty of fluids
4. Get proper rest
5. Eat a sensible, well-balanced diet
6. Return for follow-up appointment

Patients should report to the physician any of the following:

1. Unusual pain, burning, or other uncomfortable sensation
2. Swelling, redness, or other discoloration
3. Bleeding or other discharge
4. Fever above 100°F (37.7°C)
5. Nausea and vomiting
6. Any other problem or symptom

Following suture removal, patients should be advised to:

1. Keep the site dry for at least 24 hours
2. Cover the area to keep it clean
3. Apply supportive bandaging as needed
4. Report any sign of infection immediately to the physician

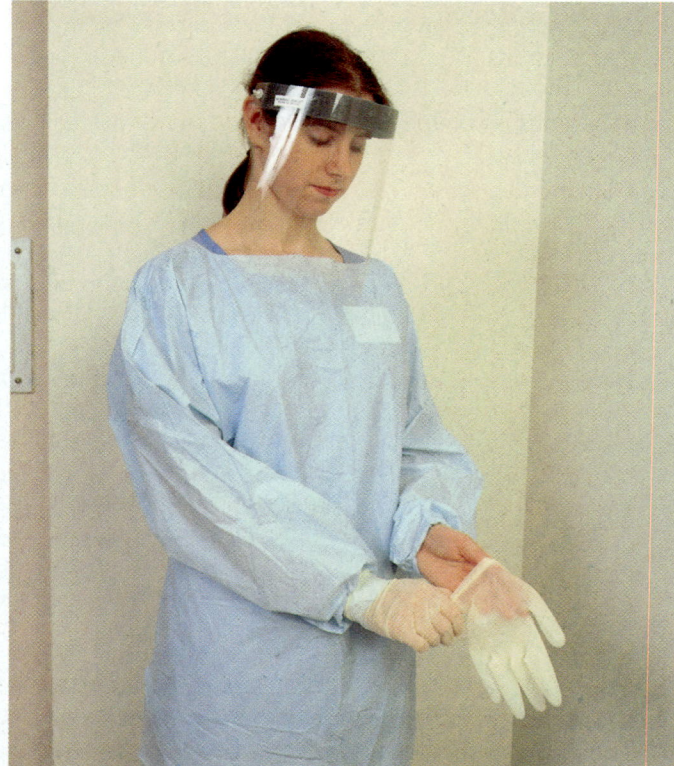

FIGURE 17-9 The medical assistant shown in this picture is wearing PPE (face shield, gown, and gloves) in preparation for assisting with a procedure that may involve contact with blood or body fluids.

will fill for 20 seconds. Timers are nice, but if your hands are soiled you should not touch them to set the time for 20 seconds. Do not just rinse your hands: Always remember to use soap. Your initial hand washing before you begin to work each day, and in between handling obviously contaminated materials, should last for approximately 1 minute. Keeping a timer and setting it for the amount of time for the appropriate hand washing procedure will be of great help to you, because it is easy to misjudge how long you take in performing this procedure. A thorough surgical scrub should be performed for 6 minutes. If it

has been within 48 hours since the last surgical scrub was performed, 3 minutes is sufficient. Just before you begin to assist with surgery, after you have properly washed your hands and before putting on sterile gloves, you should put on the appropriate personal protective equipment (PPE). This may include face shield or face mask, eye protectors (goggles), and gown (Figure 17-9). Additional pairs of sterile latex or vinyl gloves should be kept nearby during the surgical procedure in case of an accidental tear or puncture. Refer to Procedure 17-3 for instructions for properly putting on sterile gloves.

PROCEDURE PROCEDURE PROCEDURE PROCEDURE PROCEDURE PROCEDURE PROCEDURE PROCEDURE

17-3  Put on Sterile Gloves

PURPOSE: To protect both patient and medical assistant from contamination.

OSHA GUIDELINES: To comply with Standard Precautions, gloves and other protective barriers must be worn if there is any possibility of coming into contact with blood or any body fluids.

EQUIPMENT: Package of sterile latex or vinyl gloves of proper size and biohazardous waste bag.

PERFORMANCE OBJECTIVE: After practicing with clean gloves, each student will be provided with a package of sterile gloves. Standing in front of a clean, clear counter surface, demonstrate the correct method of putting on sterile gloves. The instructor will observe each step.

1. Remove your wristwatch, rings, and other jewelry from your hands and wrists, and perform a surgical

scrub using a nail brush. Thoroughly dry your hands with, sterile towels. **NOTE: Hands are now clean but unsterile.**

2. Tear the seal and open the package of sterile gloves as you would open a book (Figure 17-10A). Place them on a clean counter surface with the cuff end toward your body. **NOTE: Do not touch the inside of the package. RATIONALE: Hands would contaminate the inside of the sterile package.**

3. Grasp the glove for your **dominant** hand by the fold of the cuff with the finger and thumb of your nondominant hand (Figure 17-10B). Insert your dominant hand, carefully pulling the glove on with the other hand, keeping the cuff turned back. **NOTE: Dominant hand is now gloved and sterile (Figure 17-10C).**

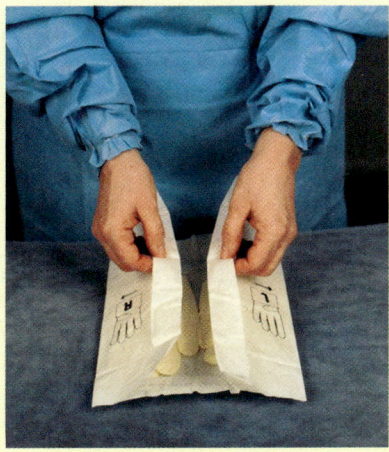

FIGURE 17-10A Open the package by pulling on the center paper folds.

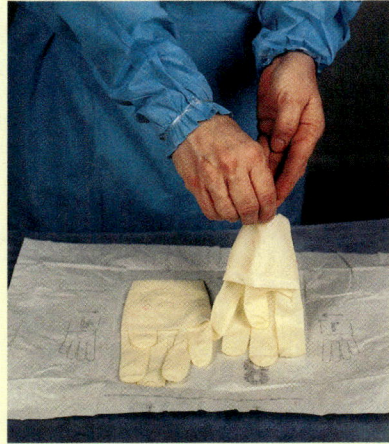

FIGURE 17-10B Grasp the fold of the inside cuff of the gloves with the thumb and fingers of your dominant hand.

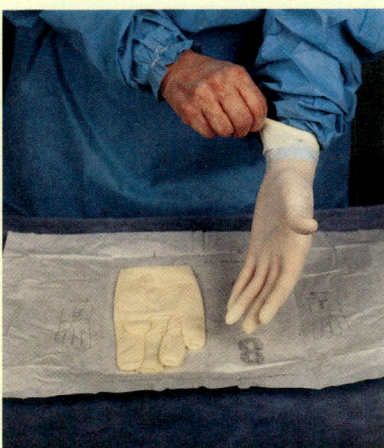

FIGURE 17-10C Insert your nondominant hand into the glove, and pull the glove on with your dominant hand by the turned-down cuff.

(continues)

17-3  Put on Sterile Gloves (Continued)

4. Place gloved fingers under the cuff of the other glove and insert your nondominant hand (Figure 17-10D). Put the glove on by pulling on the inside fold of the cuff (Figure 17-10E). Avoid touching the thumb of your dominant hand to the outside cuff of the other glove where it has been contaminated.

5. Now both hands are gloved and sterile. Place your fingers under the cuffs to smooth the gloves over the wrists (Figure 17-10F) and smooth out the fingers for better fit. **NOTE: Check for tears and holes (Figure 17-10G). RATIONALE: Any break in the integrity of the glove would not maintain sterility.**

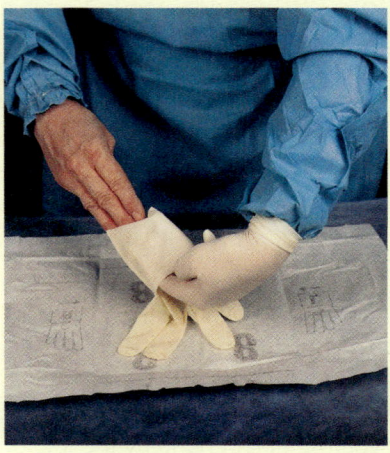

FIGURE 17-10D   Insert the fingers of your gloved nondominant hand under the folded-down cuff of the glove, and insert your dominant hand.

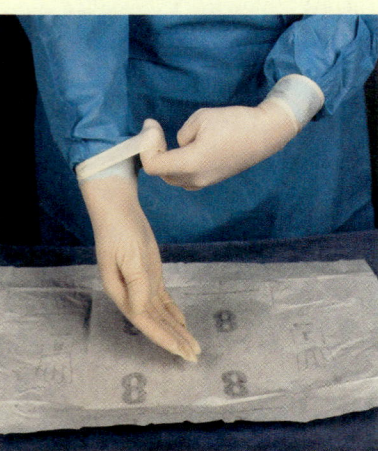

FIGURE 17-10E   Place the gloved fingers of your nondominant hand under the folded-down cuff of the glove to pull the glove on your dominant hand up over the cuff of the gown.

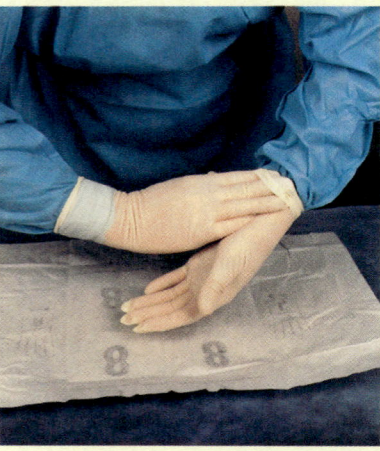

FIGURE 17-10F   Place the gloved fingers of your dominant hand (palm down) under the cuff of your gloved nondominant hand to push over the cuff of the gown.

(continues)

17-3  Put on Sterile Gloves (Continued)

6. Keep your hands above waist level. Do not touch anything other than items in the sterile field. **NOTE: Contact with any nonsterile object or surface will contaminate gloved hand(s), requiring removal and regloving.**

7. Remove the gloves by pulling the glove off your dominant hand with your thumb and fingers (Figure 17-10H).

Hold the outside cuff and pull the glove off inside-out. Slip your ungloved hand into the palm of the gloved hand, and slip the glove off inside-out (Figure 17-10I). **NOTE: Be careful not to touch the contaminated side of the gloves when removing.**

8. Deposit the gloves in a biohazardous waste bag.

9. Wash hands.

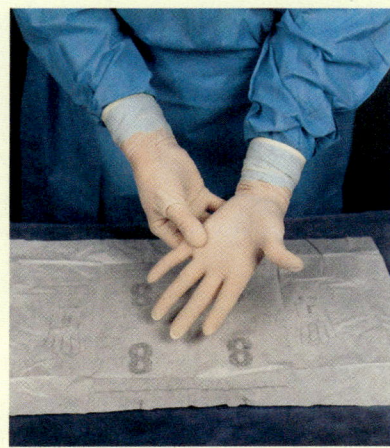

FIGURE 17-10G   Check the gloves for tears, holes, and imperfections. Inspect both, palm sides up and down, for proper fit.

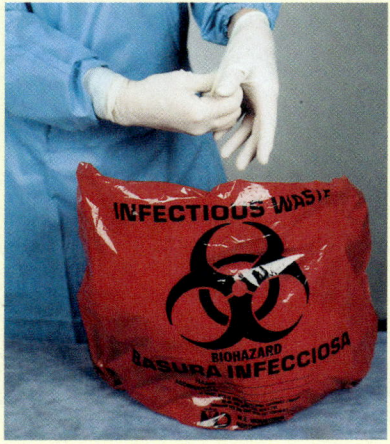

FIGURE 17-10H   To remove the gloves, pull the glove off from your nondominant hand by grasping the outside of the glove, and hold it with your gloved dominant hand.

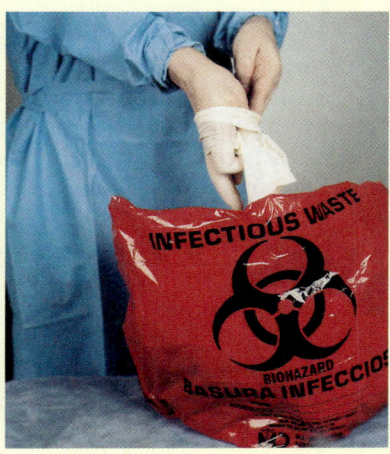

FIGURE 17-10I   Slip the fingers of your ungloved hand under your gloved hand (at the base of the palm), fold over the glove held in your hand, and slip it off the hands into the biohazard bag. Wash hands with antibacterial soap, and dry thoroughly.

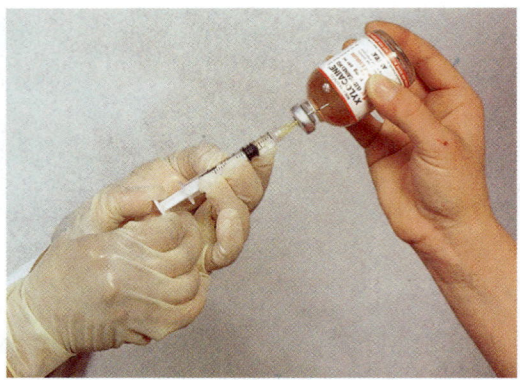

FIGURE 17-11 Hold the anesthetic solution in a convenient position so that the physician can fill the syringe without contamination.

ANESTHETICS

Before any minor surgical procedure begins, the area is usually anesthetized using a local anesthetic. The most common local anesthetic agents used are Xylocaine (lidocaine hydrochloride) and Novocaine (procaine hydrochloride). The physician is the one to actually inject the anesthetic into the area, but you may be asked to hold the vial while the physician draws up the medication (Figure 17-11). The anesthetic usually begins to numb the area within approximately 5 to 15 minutes and will keep the area anesthetized for up to 3 hours. Some physicians prefer to use an anesthetic with the additive epinephrine. This helps to constrict the blood vessels in the area, which prolongs the effect of the anesthetic.

ASSISTING THE PHYSICIAN

Some physicians prefer to perform minor surgical procedures themselves and have the medical assistant prepare the patient, the room, and the equipment only. However, there are those physicians who like to have the medical assistant directly involved in assisting with the procedure, and those physicians usually have their own preference as to how the instruments are set up and what duties the medical assistant will be expected to perform. Procedure 17-4 lists the general steps involved when assisting with a minor surgical procedure.

SUTURE MATERIAL

The term *suture* means a type of thread that is used to join skin of a wound, either an accidental laceration or a surgical incision, together. A type of suture called catgut is eventually absorbed by the body and does not need to be removed (generally used in major surgeries). It is made from the intestines of sheep. Suture is also made of a material such as silk, nylon, or other man-made substances that must be removed in a matter of days depending on the area of the body where they are inserted.

For convenience, most physicians prefer to use suture that has a needle already attached. Figures 17-12A and B shows examples of different types of suture materials and needles used in closing wounds.

Most offices have a policy regarding the treatment of lacerations. If the injury is severe and may result in serious blood loss, it is usually treated in the emergency room or trauma center. However, many patients will come to their primary care physician to have a laceration sutured.

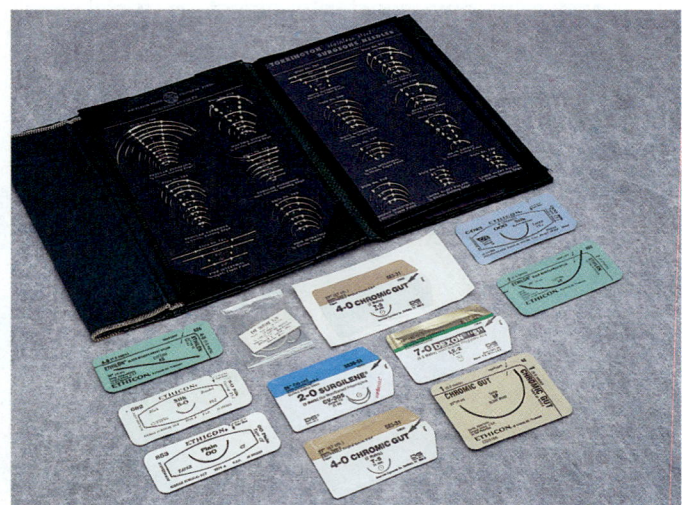

FIGURE 17-12A A variety of suture packs and curved and straight surgical needles

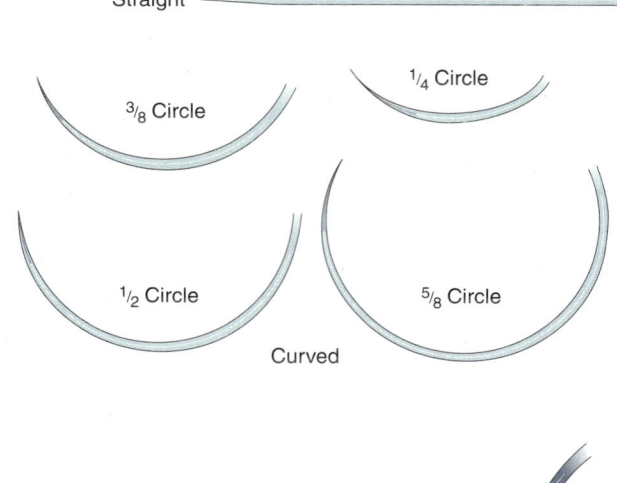

Straight

¾ Circle   ¼ Circle

½ Circle   ⅝ Circle

Curved

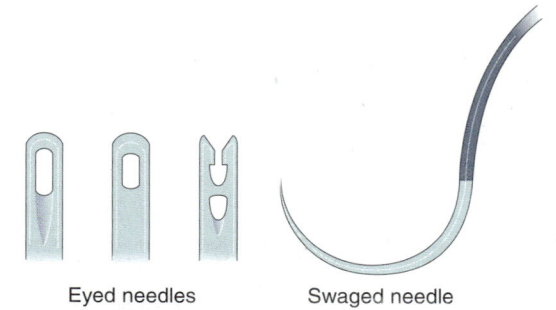

Eyed needles   Swaged needle

FIGURE 17-12B Various needle shapes used in the insertion of sutures to close wounds

PROCEDURE PROCEDURE PROCEDURE PROCEDURE PROCEDURE PROCEDURE PROCEDURE

17-4  Assisting with Minor Surgery

PURPOSE: To assist a physician in the performance of a surgical procedure and to provide support for the patient.

OSHA GUIDELINES: To comply with Standard Precautions, gloves and other protective barriers must be worn if there is any possibility of coming into contact with blood or any body fluids.

EQUIPMENT: Basic sterile setup: needle and syringe, needle holder, appropriate suture, scalpel handle and blade, thumb forceps, surgical scissors, hemostats, retractor, three or four pairs of latex or vinyl gloves, gauze squares, cotton-tipped applicators, alcohol pad, fenestrated sheet or towels, towel clamps, bandages, bandage scissors, tape, ordered anesthetic, antiseptic (small glass container for antiseptic solution), plastic biohazardous sharps container and waste bag (and waste receptacle), patient's chart, pen, **histology** request form for laboratory analysis if a biopsy is indicated, Mayo tray table, and proper lighting (extra back-up sterile setup). **NOTE: Some of the equipment may differ, according to the procedure performed.**

PERFORMANCE OBJECTIVE: Provided with all necessary equipment and supplies, demonstrate (insofar as possible) each of the steps required in assisting with minor surgery. The instructor will observe each step. **NOTE: Some steps will need to be simulated in the instructional setting.**

1. Wash hands.

2. Assemble the appropriate equipment and supplies on a counter or table near a Mayo tray. Position the Mayo tray table next to the treatment table, and check the condition and **expiration** dates of sterile items. **RATIONALE: If an item is expired or the package shows signs of improper conditions, items may no longer be sterile.**

3. Set up a sterile tray and cover it with a sterile drape.

4. Bring the scheduled patient into the treatment room. Advise the patient to empty his bladder. **RATIONALE: This ensures the patient's comfort during the procedure. Anxiety often results from the urge to void.** When the patient returns, take vital signs and record. **RATIONALE: Vital signs must be within acceptable limits to proceed with the procedure.** Explain the procedure to the patient and obtain a signature on the consent form. **RATIONALE: A signature on the consent form is absolutely essential before any invasive procedure is performed. If a biopsy is to be taken, complete a lab request form for histology analysis.**

5. Instruct the patient to disrobe as necessary for the procedure, and advise him where to place his belongings. Assist the patient if needed. Allow privacy and ask the patient to let you know when he is ready for positioning.

6. Assist the patient to the treatment table and into the desired position for surgery. Perform a skin prep procedure. Give the patient support and understanding, and answer any questions at this time. Drape the patient appropriately.

7. When the physician is ready to begin the surgical procedure, remove the sterile towel from the prepared sterile setup. Assist the physician by handing sterile gloves, use alcohol prep to wipe the top of the anesthetic vial, and hold it for the physician to draw out the amount needed.

8. If you are to assist with the surgical procedure, wash hands and put on sterile latex or vinyl gloves. Hand instruments and other sterile items to the physician as needed; mop excessive blood with gauze sponges as needed. **NOTE: If a biopsy is to be performed, special care must be taken to preserve the specimen. According to the physician's preference, the tissue may be placed on a gauze square to be handled later or deposited directly into an open specimen container. Label and attach a completed laboratory requisition when the procedure is completed.** You may assist the physician in suturing the incision by clipping each individual suture after the knot is tied by the physician. You should perform any other assistance as directed by physician during the procedure. If additional sterile items are needed during the procedure, open the package and hand it to the physician for removal, or drop it onto the center of the sterile field.

9. When the surgery is completed, assist in (or perform) cleaning and bandaging the surgery site, remove gloves, and wash hands. Tend to the patient by helping him into a sitting position to regain balance, and when stable, from the table. Assist in dressing if necessary. Give the patient education regarding any return visit, care of surgery site, and any other orders from the physician. Ask the patient if he is allergic to adhesive; if so, use **hypoallergenic** tape to secure the bandage.

10. Put on gloves to clean up the treatment table, discard disposable items in a biohazardous waste bag, place the instruments in a detergent solution to soak after rinsing with cold water, remove gloves and wash hands, and restock the room.

17-5  Assisting with Suturing a Laceration

PURPOSE: To close a wound (laceration or incision) with a sterile material until it is healed.

OSHA GUIDELINES: To comply with Standard Precautions, gloves and other personal protective barriers must be worn if there is any possibility of coming into contact with blood or any body fluids.

EQUIPMENT: Items needed for skin prep (refer to Procedure 17-1): alcohol, cotton balls, PPE, biohazard bag, gauze squares, bandages and tape, bandage scissors, antiseptic, ordered anesthetic, tetanus toxoid, patient's chart, pen; sterile items: swabs, needle and syringe, latex or vinyl gloves, fenestrated drape, ordered suture material, gauze squares, hemostats, needle holder, scissors. **NOTE: Suture packs containing all necessary items except suture material are generally already made and kept readily available for emergency use. NOTE: Check the expiration date of items. (Restraints may be necessary for a child. A cloth sheet may be used to wrap around the child's arms and legs to immobilize him during the procedure; a papoose [restraining] board can also be used for small children.)**

PERFORMANCE OBJECTIVE: Provided with all necessary equipment and supplies and other students to act as patients, demonstrate each of the steps required in the procedure to assist with suturing a laceration. **NOTE: In the instructional setting, the instructor will pose as physician and simulate the procedure with a mannequin to check the steps of the procedure.**

1. Wash hands and assemble all needed items, using sterile technique.

2. Identify the patient. **RATIONALE: Speaking to the patient by name and checking the chart ensures that you are performing the procedure on the correct patient.**

3. Explain the procedure to the patient. Advise the patient to empty her bladder.

4. When the patient returns, take and record vital signs. **RATIONALE: The patient may have lost a considerable amount of blood, which could alter vital signs. The patient may experience weakness and may not feel well enough to be left alone.**

5. Ask the patient to remove necessary clothing. Explain where the patient should place her belongings.

6. Assist the patient into the appropriate position for skin prep of the wound. Proceed with the steps for preparing skin for minor surgery, because the area for suture insertion must be prepared the same way. Drape the patient appropriately.

7. Put on PPE and sterile latex or vinyl gloves. Arrange the instruments and other sterile items in the order that the physician will use them. **NOTE: Do not reach, cough, sneeze, wave, talk, or cross over the sterile field, or it can become contaminated. Carefully cover the sterile field with a sterile towel until the physician is ready to begin.** Remove gloves and wash hands.

8. When the physician is ready to begin the suturing procedure, remove the sterile towel from the prepared setup. Hand sterile gloves to physician and use an alcohol prep to wipe the top of the anesthetic vial. Hold the vial for the physician to draw out the desired amount. If you assist with the suturing procedure, wash hands and put on sterile gloves. Hand instruments and other sterile items to the physician as needed; mop excessive blood from the wound with sterile gauze as needed. Assist the physician by clipping each individual suture as directed by the physician.

9. When the wound has been closed with sutures, assist with or perform cleaning and bandaging the site as the physician orders (you may need to reglove to keep from getting the dressing and bandage soiled), remove gloves, dispose of them in biohazardous waste bag, and wash hands. **NOTE: Some individuals are allergic to adhesive. Be sure to ask the patient before applying tape. Hypoallergenic tape may be preferred.**

10. Administer tetanous toxoid if ordered. Tend to the patient. Assist with sitting up, getting dressed, helping from the treatment table, and so on. **NOTE: Allow the patient sufficient time to regain balance before standing alone, because dizziness may occur.**

11. Instruct the patient in the care of sutures and provide a return appointment for their removal. Refer to the patient education box: Patients can develop infections following a wound sustained in an accident.

12. Put on latex or vinyl gloves to clean up the treatment table, discard disposables in a biohazard bag/sharps container, place instruments in detergent solution after rinsing with cool water, remove gloves and PPE, and dispose of them in the biohazard bag. Wash hands and restock treatment room.

13. Record the procedure on the patient's chart and initial.

Working cases into an already full schedule can present delays for other patients waiting for scheduled appointments. Prepare the patient for the physician and assist as needed. After the suturing is complete, the physician can see other patients while you take care of the laceration patient and clean up the work area.

Your efficiency and expedient preparation of setting up the treatment room will be appreciated by both the physician and the patient in this situation. Follow the steps in Procedure 17-5 for assisting with suturing a laceration. Always make sure that you record the number of sutures (stitches) that the physician inserts and the anatomical location. Go over patient education and any additional instructions from the physician with the patient before she leaves the office. If the patient is given instructions by the physician to redress and bandage the wound at home, show the patient how to do this. Alert patients to call with any questions or concerns.

POSTOPERATIVE INSTRUCTIONS

Make sure that return appointment visits are confirmed and reminder cards are given to patients before they leave the office. Phoning patients the next day is an excellent way to follow up and reassures them that you and the physician are genuinely concerned about their progress. It will also bring to the physician's attention any problems that could be eliminated early. If patients do have complaints, it is best to have the physician check the problem as soon as possible.

Follow-up visits are essential so that assessment of progress can be made by the physician and for the removal of sutures. In general, you should advise all patients who have had any minor surgical procedure to limit their activity for at least a couple of weeks, or however long the physician has ordered according to the procedure performed.

Specific instructions, such as soaking or applying topical medications, will be given by the physician for certain individual cases. Physicians generally instruct patients (or teach you how to instruct patients) about packing or special bandaging procedures, such as with ingrown toenail removals. Physicians may prescribe an analgesic for minor pain and discomfort the patient may experience following the procedure.

SUTURE REMOVAL

Patients usually see the family or general practitioner for suture removal following laceration repair from an injury. In many offices, it is the medical assistant's responsibility to remove the sutures. It is vital that you check the emergency center's report regarding the number of sutures put in, so you can be sure to remove all of them.

Be sure to remove the same number of sutures as were inserted by the primary care physician. Suture that is not removed will become infected, so care in removing all of the material is vital. Patients sometimes report that one or two stitches have already come out during a bandage change at home. This should also be noted on the patient's chart. Follow the steps in the procedure for suture removal. Removal of staples is performed with a staple extractor as described in Procedure 17-6 for suture removal. Check the report also for a tetanus booster and record on the patient's chart to bring the immunization record up to date. Before you remove the sutures, check the number of days that the physician who put them in recommended as the time to wait before removal. Ask the physician to inspect the healing wound. After the sutures or staples have been removed, physicians may order additional closure materials to cover healing incisions or lacerations (Figures 17-13A through D). A support skin closure may be necessary to keep the skin together until the wound is completely healed. The type of supportive closure should be noted on the patient's chart. New advances in skin closures offer a sutureless substance applied to small lacerations. This type of closure is an adhesive material and is used frequently with children who may be frightened and thus uncooperative. A sutureless procedure is much quicker and less traumatic for the child and staff as well.

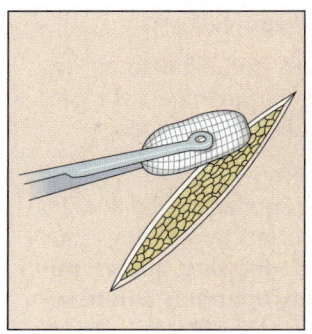

FIGURE 17-13A Care of an incision/wound with a closure applications: Use transfer forceps with sterile gauze to apply antiseptic.

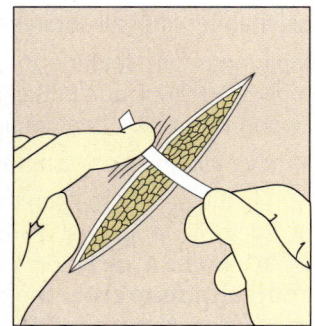

FIGURE 17-13B Apply Steri-Strip closure to the center of the incision.

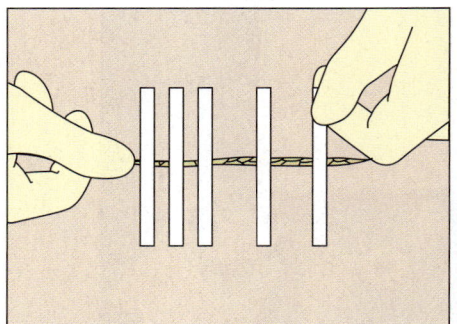

FIGURE 17-13C Apply closures to each side for evenness, then fill in and cover the full wound area. If ordered, apply a topical medication and a sterile bandage.

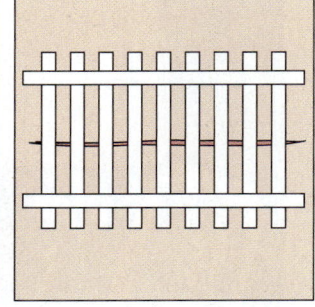

FIGURE 17-13D For additional support, closures may also be applied parallel to the incision or wound.

17-6  Remove Sutures

PURPOSE: To remove suture(s) from a healing laceration or incision.

OSHA GUIDELINES: To comply with Standard Precautions, gloves and other protective barriers must be worn if there is any possibility of coming into contact with blood or any body fluids.

EQUIPMENT: Sterile: thumb forceps, suture-removal scissors (or staple extractor), gauze squares, latex or vinyl gloves, cotton-tipped applicators, butterfly or Steri-Strip closures; antiseptic solution, hydrogen peroxide, basin with warm soapy water, bandages, tape, towels, biohazardous waste bag, bandage scissors, patient's chart, and pen.

PERFORMANCE OBJECTIVE: Provided with all necessary equipment and supplies, and using a mannequin or model as the patient, demonstrate the steps required to remove sutures. The instructor will observe each step. Simulation should be made by the instructor.

1. Wash hands and move a Mayo table next to the treatment table, or to where the patient will be during the procedure.

2. Assemble all necessary items on the Mayo table tray (Figure 17-14). Ask if patient is allergic to adhesive. If so, use hypoallergenic tape to secure the bandage (ask also about allergies to topical preparations, such as povidone-iodine mixture, or any medications).

3. Bring the scheduled patient to the treatment room. Ask the patient about the healing condition of the incision or laceration, take vital signs, and record on the patient's chart. (If sutures resulted from a laceration injury, ask appropriate questions regarding where and when injury occurred and when a tetanus booster was administered [file ER report in chart].) Record.

4. Ask the patient to remove appropriate clothing for inspection of the healing incision (offer to help if needed).

5. Assist the patient to the treatment table and into the required position and drape appropriately. Explain the procedure and answer any questions.

6. Put on gloves and remove the bandage. Clean the incision with antiseptic solution using cotton-tipped applicators. **NOTE: If the bandage has stuck to the incision (record condition of site on chart [i.e., excessive blood or drainage]), apply gauze squares that have been soaked with soapy warm water solution, or hydrogen peroxide, to the area for a few minutes to loosen the bandage from the sutures and scab.** This will make removal of the bandage easier. (Pulling off a stuck bandage may reopen the wound or pull out sutures.) Either result would be very painful. Advise the physician that the incision site is ready to be checked.

7. After the physician orders suture removal, open a sterile package containing the necessary instruments on the Mayo tray and proceed. Grasp the knot of the suture material with thumb forceps, and gently but firmly pull up, making just enough space to place the suture removal scissors to clip the suture as close to the skin as possible (Figures 17-15A and B). Pull the suture with the forceps (back) toward the healing incision so that no **stress** is put on it. **RATIONALE: Pulling the suture away from the site could possibly pull the incision open. CAUTION:** Do not pull a suture that has been on the surface of the skin (exposed to the outside) through the path of the suture being removed, or infection may develop. Continue in this manner until all sutures are removed.

8. Apply antiseptic solution to site, and allow to air dry. Apply Steri-Strips or a butterfly closure if necessary for support during the healing process, and bandage.

9. Remove gloves and wash hands.

10. Instruct the patient to keep the bandage clean and dry for 24 to 48 hours, or as directed by the physician. **RATIONALE: A dirty or wet dressing allows microorganisms to enter the tiny openings where sutures were removed until they are healed.** Advise the patient to avoid undue stress for the appropriate amount of time for the anatomical area. Give the patient education regarding home care and a follow-up appointment if ordered by the physician.

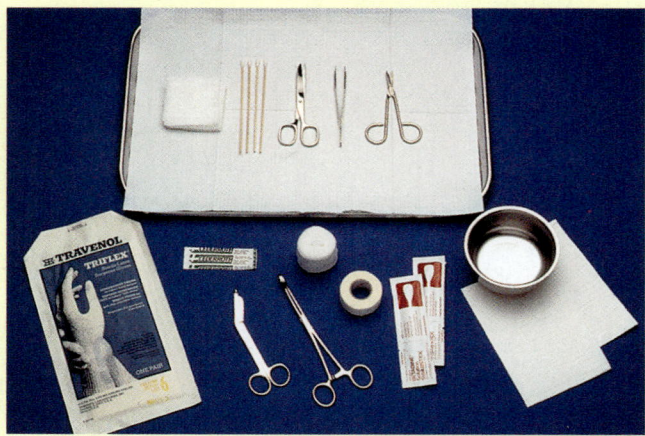

FIGURE 17-14 An example of a suture-removal tray setup

(continues)

17-6      Remove Sutures (Continued)

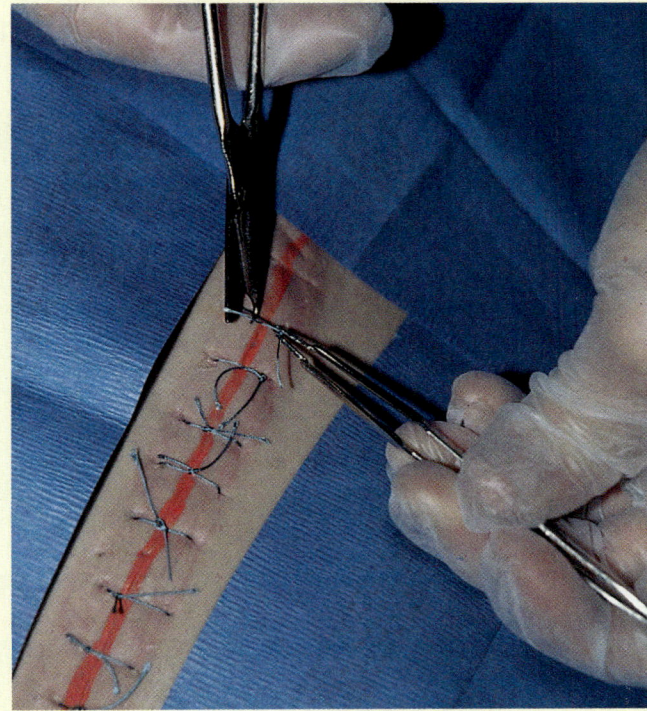

FIGURE 17-15A   Suture removal: Grasp the suture knot with thumb forceps, and place the curved tip of the suture-removal scissors just next to the skin under the suture and clip.

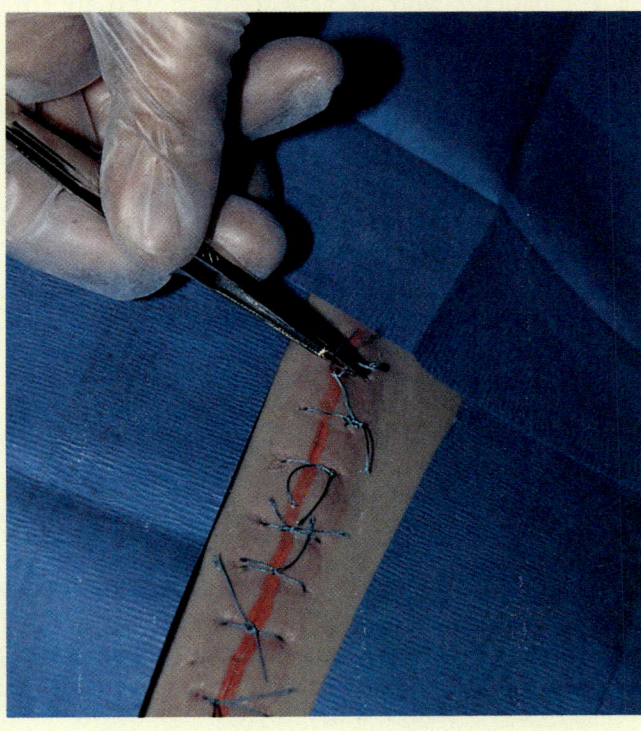

FIGURE 17-15B   Gently pull the suture up and toward the incision with the thumb forceps to remove (pulling the suture away from the incision may pull the incision open).

11. Record on progress notes in the patient's chart: (1) anatomical area of incision or laceration; (2) condition of site; (3) number of sutures removed; (4) type of antiseptic applied; (5) support closures applied; (6) type of bandage applied; and your signature. Be sure to include the ER report if sent from the facility where the injury was treated, and record the date of the tetanus booster if applicable.

NOTE: If skin staples (or clips) are to be removed, the physician may perform the procedure. However, you may be instructed to do so. Basically, skin staples are removed in the following manner: Follow steps 1 through 6 above.

Place the sterile staple extractor under a staple (one at a time), and squeeze the handles of the extractor completely closed (Figure 17-16). (Explain to the patient that a tugging sensation may be felt.) Lift the staple away from the skin and place it in a biohazardous waste container. Continue the process until all are removed. Resume the procedure above with step 8.

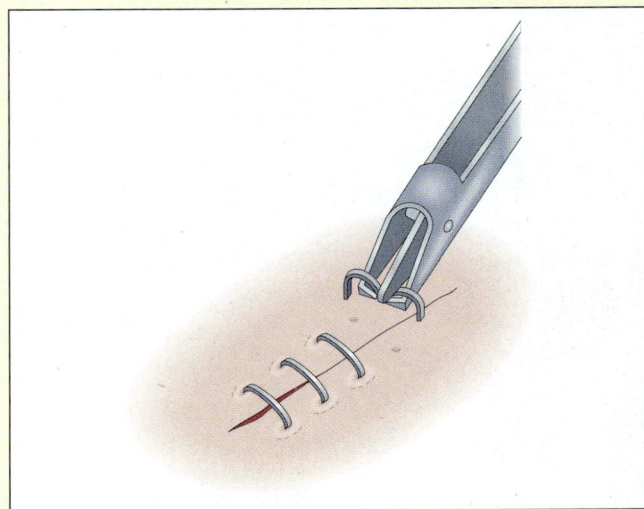

FIGURE 17-16   Removal of a staple. The staple extractor reforms the staple (clip). Then, the staple is lifted from the incision.

Skin closures give support to the wound and offer the patient more flexibility.

PROTECTIVE BANDAGES

The type of bandage that the physician orders will vary and should be appropriate for the wound and the patient. For patients who are very active or who are employed in activities that could further injure or cause the wound to become dirty or wet, the wound should be wrapped in a very thick dressing to cushion and protect it and to allow it to heal. Make sure you advise the patient to keep the dressing clean and dry. Remind the patient to place plastic bag over the extremity to keep it dry during showers or baths. If the wound is on the trunk of the body, taking a shower or bath should not be done unless the physician has approved it. Usually a sponge bath is preferred until the bandage comes off. This is important in minimizing the possibility of infection.

If an infection should occur, you may be asked to obtain a specimen for laboratory analysis and culture. Simply use a sterile cotton swab and insert the tip into the center of the infected area of the wound. Then transfer the swab with the specimen into the culture medium. Provide patient education regarding care of the site and when to return for a follow-up appointment. Additionally, physicians advise using an elastic bandage to offer more protection and support of surgical areas of the extremities, especially for pediatric and physically active patients. Application of an Ace wrap increases circulation of the area, which hastens the healing process.

Until you are confident in assisting with various office surgeries, it is suggested that you keep a notebook or file cards to help you learn the instruments and steps required for each procedure.

ACHIEVE UNIT OBJECTIVES

- Complete the Workbook activities to meet the learning objectives.
- Practice the procedures in this unit to meet the performance objectives.
- Apply your knowledge at the end of this chapter in completing the Critical Thinking Challenge and Activities, as well as the StudyWARE on your Student CD-ROM.

CRITICAL THINKING CHALLENGE

IMPACTING THE PATIENT, THE PRACTICE, AND YOUR CAREER

Barry was the medical assistant assigned to assist with a cyst removal scheduled immediately following the lunch break. Before Barry went to lunch, he asked Renita to set up the surgical room because he might be late getting back from running errands, and she was not leaving for lunch anyway. Renita reluctantly agreed and began setting up the room for the surgical procedure. As she removed the sterile packet from the drawer, she noticed that it was the last one. She placed all the instruments (still wrapped) on the Mayo stand next to the exam table. Barry returned late, just before the physician came out of her office. Barry quickly washed his hands, finished setting up the tray of instruments and supplies, and brought the patient in for the procedure. He asked Mr. Case to remove his shirt and lie on the exam table. Barry performed the skin prep and placed the fenestrated drape sheet over the patient just before the doctor came in to begin the procedure. During the surgery, the physician asked Barry to get another sterile pack from the drawer. Barry returned and reported that there were none in the drawer. The physician was upset about this and had to make do with what she had. After the patient was taken care of and left the room, the doctor spoke sternly to Barry about not being prepared for the procedure. Barry wanted to say that it was Renita's fault, but decided not to because she really did a favor for him.

QUESTIONS

1. Who was at fault here?
2. What was Barry's first mistake?
3. Was Renita responsible for any problems?
4. What should Barry have done?
5. Do you think Barry handled the reprimand from the doctor well?
6. Because Barry didn't know that there were no sterile packs in the drawer, should the doctor blame him?
7. Did Renita really do Barry a favor?

ACTIVITIES

1. Practice identifying the instruments and state their function with a group of your classmates.
2. Research information about some of the pioneers in modern medical surgery.

StudyWARE™ CHALLENGE

- Study with the flash cards for Chapter 17 to review the key terms in this chapter.
- Solve the hangman activities for Chapter 17.
- Complete the multiple choice quiz in test mode for Chapter 17

RESOURCES

JARIT Surgical Instruments, 9 Skyline Drive, Hawthorne, NY 10532.

Heller, M. E., & Krebs, C. (2004). *Delmar Learning's clinical handbook for the medical office*. (2nd ed.). Clifton Park, NY: Thomson Delmar Learning.

Lindh, W. Q., Pooler, M. S., Tamparo, C. D., & Dahl, B. M. (2006). *Comprehensive medical assisting*. (3rd ed.). Clifton Park, NY: Thomson Delmar Learning.

Outpatient surgery: A sign of progress, regarding women and health-care (1994). Columbus, OH: Mount Carmel Health.

WEB LINKS

www.jarit.com (JARIT Surgical Instruments)
  This site provides information about surgical instruments.

www.miltex.com (Miltex, Inc.)
  This site provides information about surgical instruments.

18 Assisting with Medications

Administering medications is one of the most sensitive and important duties that the medical assistant will perform.

You must first become familiar with the medications that are most frequently given to the patients treated in your office. Knowing the properties of the medications will help in answering patients' questions and recognizing common side effects that patients may exhibit. The *Physicians' Desk Reference,* or PDR, and the *Physicians' Desk Reference for Nonprescription Drugs* will become valuable resources. Because these resources are frequently referred to, they should be kept in a central, accessible location for use by all members of the health care team. You should also become familiar with the many terms and abbreviations used in administering medications. Some of the most common ones are included in this chapter and in the Appendix.

The laws may vary from state to state in regard to your administering medications. You should check with your employer about this matter. Some physicians prefer always to administer medications to patients themselves, thereby preventing a possible medical-legal concern.

A review of the basic math skills will be helpful in preparing medications. The areas in which to practice are addition, subtraction, multiplication, division, fractions, decimals, percentages, and ratio proportion. Refer to Table 18-6 for examples of these math problems. Accuracy and care must always be taken in assisting with and administering medications to patients. Although the medical assistant will not usually start an IV in the medical office, the AAMA now requires students to be familiar with the terminology associated with IV therapy and the theory behind it.

UNIT 1
PRESCRIPTION AND NONPRESCRIPTION MEDICATIONS

OBJECTIVES

Upon completion of this unit, you will be able to achieve the following:

LEARNING Objectives

1. **Spell and define, using the glossary at the back of the text, all the Words to Know in this unit.**

2. **Explain how to use PDRs for both prescription and nonprescription medications.**

3. **Explain how to properly phone in prescriptions to a pharmacist.**

4. **Describe how to write a prescription as ordered by the physician.**

5. **Describe the drugs that are under federal regulation according to category, or Schedules I through V.**

6. **Define abbreviations commonly used in regard to medications.**

7. **Explain how to record medications properly on the patient's chart.**

8. **Explain how to categorize medications used in the medical office.**

9. **Describe medical/legal/ethical concerns regarding medications.**

10. **List and discuss the necessary information required when recording medications.**

WORDS TO KNOW

accuracy	dispense	expertise
administer	Drug Enforcement	generic
auxiliary	Administration (DEA)	license

narcotic
over-the-counter (OTC)
pharmaceutical

Physicians' Desk Reference (PDR)
prescribe

prescription
reference
resource
vial

CERTIFICATION CONNECTION

CMA
Pharmacology
Maintaining medication records
Medication disposal

CMAS
Basic pharmacology

RMA
Drugs

COMMONLY PRESCRIBED MEDICATIONS

Depending on the type of medical practice, certain medications will be more commonly prescribed than others. It is a good idea to keep a list of these medications handy with the most often questioned information. This list should include the usual dosage and possible side effects. The entire staff should become knowledgeable about these medications.

The list in Table 18-1 is meant as an introduction. The common names of some types of drugs are listed. Consulting the **Physicians' Desk Reference (PDR)** or other resource for complete information is suggested.

PATIENT EDUCATION

Many patients are very anxious about receiving medication, whether by mouth, injection, or any other route of administration. Careful and complete explanation of the procedure or disease and the need for medications is essential for reassuring the patient. The patient must understand when and how to take prescribed medications to receive the full benefits of them. Some medications are to be taken before meals or after meals, with certain fluids or excluding certain fluids, or in the presence or absence of certain foods or other medications. Carefully explained verbal and written instructions are essential for the patient's compliance. The patient must understand that the medication dosage cannot be changed without first consulting the physician. Emphasize also that the medication should be continued or finished as directed, even if the patient begins to feel better.

TABLE 18-1 Selected Drug Classifications

Classification	Action	Examples
Analgesic	Relieves pain without causing loss of consciousness	acetaminophen (Tylenol), aspirin, morphine, ibuprofen (Advil, Motrin)
Anesthetic	Produces a lack of feeling. May be local or general depending on the type and how administered	lidocaine HCl (Xylocaine), procaine HCl (Novocaine)
Antacid	Neutralizes acid	Amphojel, Gelusil, Mylanta, Aludrox, Milk of Magnesia
Antianxiety	Relieves anxiety and muscle tension	benzodiazepines: diazepam (Valium) and chlordiazepox-ide HCl (Librium)
Antiarrhythmic	Controls cardiac arrhythmias	lidocaine HCl (Xylocaine), propranolol HCl (Inderal)
Antibiotic	Is destructive to or inhibits growth of microorganisms	penicillins (Pentids, Duracillin, Polycillin, Pipracil, Augmentin), cephalosporins (Keflin, Mandol, Rocephin)
Anticholinergic	Blocks parasympathetic nerve impulses	atropine, scopolamine, trihexyphenidyl HCl (Artane)
Anticoagulant	Prevents or delays blood clotting	heparin sodium, Dicumarol, warfarin sodium (Coumadin)
Anticonvulsant	Prevents or relieves convulsions	carbamazepine (Tegretol), phenytoin (Dilantin), ethosuximide (Zarotin)
Antidepressant	Prevents or relieves the symptoms of depression	monoamine oxidase (MAO) inhibitors: isocarboxazid (Marplan), phenelzine sulfate (Nardil), amitriptyline HCl (Elavil), imipramine HCl (Tofranil)
Antidiarrheal	Prevents or relieves diarrhea	Lomotil, Pepto-Bismol, Kaopectate
Antidote	Counteracts poisons and their effect	naloxone (Narcan)
Antiemetic	Prevents or relieves nausea and vomiting	Tigan, Dramamine, Phenergan, Reglan, Marinol
Antihistamine	Acts to counteract histamine	Dimetane, Benadryl, Seldane
Antihypertensive	Prevents or controls high blood pressure	methyldopa (Aldomet), clonidine HCl (Catapres), metoprolol tartrate (Lopressor)
Anti-inflammatory	Counteracts inflammation	naproxen (Naprosyn), aspirin, ibuprofen (Advil, Motrin)
Antimanic	Used for the treatment of the manic episode of manic-depressive disorder	lithium
Antineoplastic	Kills or destroys malignant cells	busulfan (Myleran), cyclophosphamide (Cytoxan)
Antipyretic	Reduces fever	aspirin, acetaminophen (Tylenol)
Antitussive	Prevents or relieves cough	codeine, dextromethorphan
Bronchodilator	Dilates the bronchi	isoproterenol HCl (Isuprel), albuterol (Proventil)
Contraceptive	Prevents conception	Enovid-E 21; Ortho-Novum 10/11-21, 10/11-28; Triphasil-21
Decongestant	Reduces nasal congestion and/or swelling	oxymetazoline (Afrin), epinephrine HCl (Adrenalin), phenylephrine HCl (Neo-Synephrine), pseudoephedrine HCl (Sudafed)
Diuretic	Increases the excretion of urine	chlorothiazide (Diuril), furosemide (Lasix), Mannitol (Osmitrol)
Expectorant	Facilitates removal of secretions from bronchopulmonary mucous membrane	guaifenesin (Robitussin)

(Adapted from Rice, Principles of Pharmacology for Medical Assistants, *4th ed., copyright 2006, Clifton Park, NY: Thomson Delmar Learning.)*

(continues)

TABLE 18-1   Selected Drug Classifications (Continued)

Classification	Action	Examples
Hemostatic	Controls or stops bleeding	Humafac, Amicar, vitamin K
Hypnotic	Produces sleep or hypnosis	secobarbital (Seconal); chloral hydrate ethchlorvynol (Placidyl), flurazepam (Dalmane)
Hypoglycemic	Lowers blood glucose level	insulin; chlorpropamide (Diabinese), glyburide (Micronase)
Laxative	Loosens and promotes normal bowel eliminations	Metamucil powder, Dulcolax
Muscle relaxant	Aids in relaxation of skeletal muscle	Robaxin, Norflex, Paraflex, Skelaxin, Valium
Sedative	Produces a calming effect without causing sleep	amobarbital (Amytal), butabarbital sodium (Buticaps), phenobarbital
Tranquilizer	Reduces mental tension and anxiety	Thorazine, Mellaril, Haldol
Vasodilator	Produces relaxation of blood vessels; lowers blood pressure	isorbide dinitrate (Isordil), nitroglycerin
Vasopressor	Produces contraction of muscles of capillaries and arteries; elevates blood pressure	metaraminol (Aramine), norepinephrine (Levophed)

PHARMACEUTICAL REFERENCES

The PDR is one valuable **resource** that the medical assistant should keep handy in the medical office. The purpose of the PDR is to provide accurate, reliable, and current information about most prescribed medications and related products. You may need to consult the PDR for the proper spelling, strength, or other information concerning medications that are not given frequently to assist the physician in accurately prescribing medications.

One of your responsibilities may be to order the current edition of the PDR so that the practice may keep abreast of the newest **pharmaceuticals** approved by the Food and Drug Administration (FDA). This reference book is published annually. A supplement with the latest information is sent to subscribers quarterly. There are six sections:

- Section 1: Manufacturers' Index (white pages)—includes an alphabetical listing of all manufacturers listed in the PDR along with their addresses, phone numbers, and emergency contacts. Also contains a listing of each manufacturer's products and the page number for each product in the PDR.
- Section 2: Brand and Generic Name Index (pink pages)—Lists the page number of each product by both brand and generic name.
- Section 3: Product Category Index (blue pages)—Lists all products by category.

- Section 4: Product Identification Guide (gray pages)—Displays full color pictures of the different forms of the products. This section is an alphabetic listing by manufacturer.
- Section 5: Product Information Section (white pages)—This section includes an alphabetic listing (by manufacturer) of products. The information is arranged into categories as follows:

Brand name: The name given to the drug by the manufacturer (e.g., Tylenol)

Generic name: The common name of the drug (e.g., acetaminophen)

Description: Lists the chemical composition of the drug and its origin

Clinical pharmacology: Explains the drug's effect on the body and how it works

Indications & Usage: Lists the different conditions for which the drug is prescribed

Contraindications: States reasons why the drug should not be given and why it should not be given to certain people

Warnings: States the potential dangers associated with the drug

Precautions: Lists possible undesirable effects that the drug may produce in a patient

Adverse Reactions: A listing of the possible side effects of the drug

Dosage & Administration: Lists the usual daily dosage for adults and children, including the time interval

How supplied: Lists the different forms of the drug

● Section 6: Diagnostic Product Information (green pages)—Lists usage guidelines for various common diagnostic agents. Other information included in this section is:
   a. Key to Controlled Substances Categories
   b. Key to FDA Use-in-Pregnancy Ratings
   c. U.S. Food and Drug Administration Telephone Directory
   d. Poison Control Centers
   e. Listing of Discontinued Products
   f. Adverse Event Report Form (MedWatch)

Guidelines for Using the PDR

1. Find the brand name of the drug (listed in alphabetic order) in the pink section of the PDR. There will two page numbers listed after the manufacturer's name (which is in parentheses). The first page number locates the product identification number, and the second page number is the location of the product information in the white section.
2. If you only know the classification of the drug, go to the blue section and look for the drug category.
3. Sometimes the drug you are looking for will not be listed in the PDR, and other reference sources should be consulted.

Note: The medical assistant should become familiar with the PDR's contents page with each new edition to become proficient in assisting the physician with needed information. The *Physicians' Desk Reference for Nonprescription Drugs* is also another valuable resource that can be of great assistance in identifying **over-the-counter (OTC)** medicines that patients use for self-medication. The format of this reference book is similar to the PDR for prescription products. Sections on patient education material, support groups, and diagnostic home use products are also included.

Getting familiar with the arrangement of both PDRs will prove its worth very quickly when a difficult situation is encountered in the medical practice.

Many other sources of information about pharmaceutical products are used by physicians. Most offices have more than one **reference** for this purpose. *The National Formulary,* the *Pharmacopoeia of the United States of America* (USP), and the *Pharmacopoeia Internationalis* are three reference books that contain facts and comparisons of a vast variety of pharmaceutical products.

An excellent information source about a drug is the package insert itself. It lists a wealth of information, including the clinical pharmacology of the drug, usage, warnings, precautions, drug interactions, usual dosage, and contraindications.

DRUG CATEGORIES AND CLASSIFICATIONS

Drugs are classified into different categories or groups:

● Those that prevent disease (vaccines and immunizations)
● Those that have a particular action on the body (analgesics)
● Those that have a target effect on organs and body systems (cardiac drugs)
● How they are prepared (liquid, suppository, tablet, etc.)

Table 18-1 lists selected drugs by their classification and action and gives some examples of each category.

DRUG ACTIONS

Drug actions are usually grouped in one of three ways:
1. Action that directly affects one or more body tissues
2. Effect on microorganisms
3. Replacement of a body chemical

Drug actions are classified as:

● Local—action takes place in the area where it was administered.
● Remote—action takes place in an area of the body that is away from the administration site.
● Systemic—action takes place throughout the body
● Synergistic—one drug works with or counteracts another drug.

DRUG FORMS

Drugs are manufactured in many different forms, including:

● Liquid: Drug is dissolved or suspended in a solvent (either water or alcohol)
● Solid and semisolid: Tablets, capsules, caplets, lozenges, suppositories, and ointments (Figure 18-1)

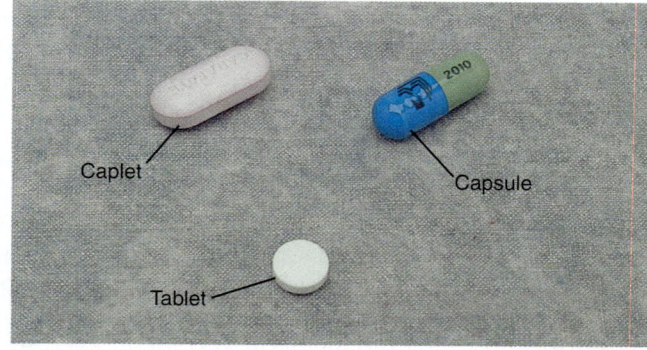

FIGURE 18-1 Difficult forms of oral medication: caplets, tablets, and capsules

- Transdermal: Small adhesive patch is placed directly on the skin. The patch consists of different layers, and the medication is contained in one of the layers and is absorbed through the skin (Figures 18-2A and B).
- Ocular: Drug is between two very thin membrane layers and is placed into the lower lid of the eye.
- Implantable: Positioned beneath the skin, such as an infusion pump. Some implantable devices contain a reservoir that can be refilled.

THE MEDICATION ORDER

Before a prescription is written, a medication order must be given by a physician or other authorized prescriber. Information for the prescription is obtained directly from the medication order. If the order is illegible, incomplete, or unclear, the order must not be carried out until it is rewritten or clarified. Many offices are now using electronic charting, which helps to eliminate error or illegible orders. A medication order should contain the following information:

- Full name of the patient
- Name of the medication (usually the **generic** name is used)
- Dosage and route of administration
- How often the medication is to be administered

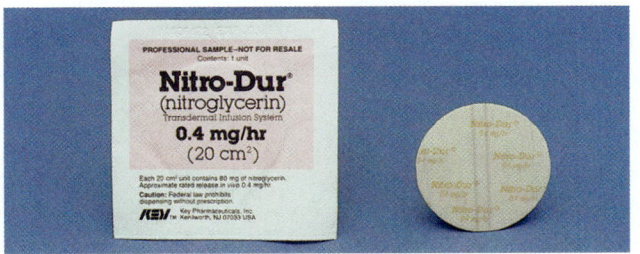

FIGURE 18-2A   The Nitro-Dur skin patch is a transdermal nitroglycerin patch, applied once a day. *(Courtesy of Novartis)*

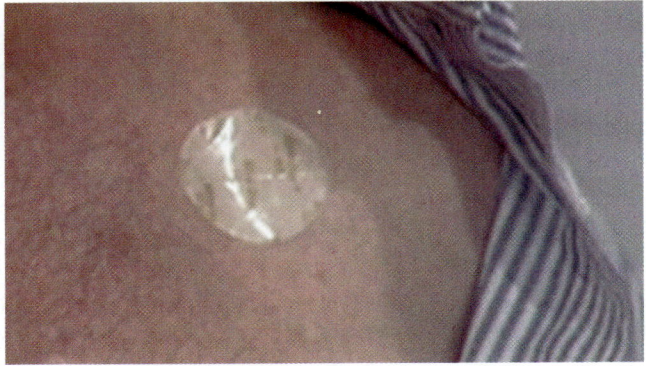

FIGURE 18-2B   Transdermal nitroglycerin patch, applied to the skin. *(Courtesy of Novartis)*

- Date and time order was written
- Any specific directions for administering the medication
- Signature of the prescriber

WRITING PRESCRIPTIONS

A **prescription** is a written order for a particular medication or treatment for a particular patient by a **licensed** physician. It is a legal document. Most prescriptions are hand written by the physician, especially those for **narcotics**. However, some physicians delegate the task of writing the information on the prescription blank to the medical assistant. The physician will then check the prescription and sign it. In many states, for instance, prescriptions for controlled substances can only have one drug, the controlled substance, written on it. It is now required that the quantity be in both numerical and written form. Any medication that is **prescribed** must be recorded on the patient's chart. Figure 18-3 shows an example of a prescription blank. When the physician prescribes only one medication for a patient, the single medication prescription pad is used. With the advancement

DEA NUMBER (MAY BE PRINTED)   TELEPHONE NUMBER

PHYSICIAN'S NAME
ADDRESS ZIP

PATIENT'S NAME _____ DATE _____
ADDRESS _____
Rx
Sig:
Refill _____ Times
Please label ( )

_____
PHYSICIAN'S SIGNATURE

DEA NUMBER (MAY BE PRINTED)   TELEPHONE NUMBER

PHYSICIAN'S NAME, ADDRESS, ZIP

PATIENT'S NAME _____ DATE _____
ADDRESS _____

Sig:	LABEL MEDICATION	mg/cc	Quantity	Refills
Rx 1.				
Rx 2.				
Rx 3.				
Rx 4.				
Rx 5.				

_____
PHYSICIAN'S SIGNATURE

FIGURE 18-3   Sample prescription blanks for single medication and multiple medications

Parts of a Prescription

1. The physician's name, address, telephone number and registration number.
2. The patient's name, address, and the date on which the prescription is written.
3. The *superscription* that includes the symbol Rx ("take thou")
4. The *inscription* that states the names and quantities of ingredients to be included in the medication.
5. The *subscription* that gives directions to the pharmacist for filling the prescription.
6. The *signature* (Sig) that gives the directions for the patient.
7. The physician's signature blanks. Where signed, indicates if a generic substitute is allowed or if the medication is to be dispensed as written.
8. REPETATUR 0 1 2 3 PRN. This is where the physician indicates whether or not the prescription can be refilled.
9. LABEL Direction to the pharmacist to label the medication appropriately.

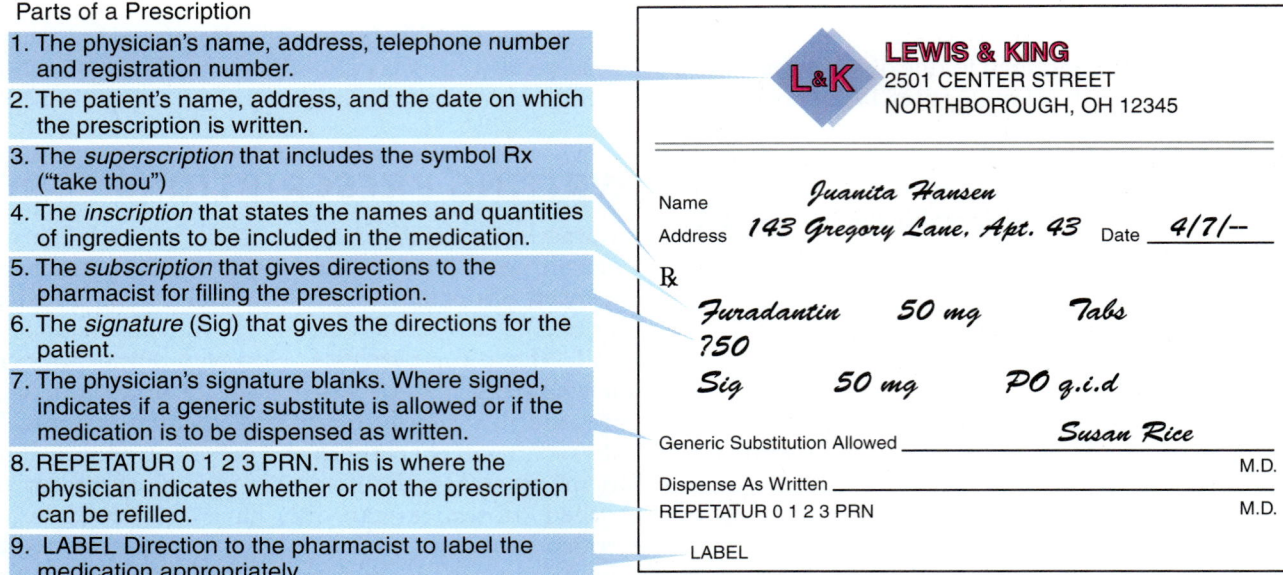

LEWIS & KING
L&K
2501 CENTER STREET
NORTHBOROUGH, OH 12345

Name   *Juanita Hansen*
Address   *143 Gregory Lane, Apt. 43*   Date ___*4/7/–*___

Rx

Furadantin   50 mg   Tabs
?50
Sig   50 mg   PO q.i.d

Susan Rice

Generic Substitution Allowed _____
                                                        M.D.

Dispense As Written _____
REPETATUR 0 1 2 3 PRN   M.D.

LABEL

FIGURE 18-4   Parts of a prescription

in health information software, prescriptions may now be printed by selecting a particular drug, its strength and dosage, and the amount ordered. Special prescription paper with tamper-proof watermark is used to print the document. Computer-generated prescriptions reduce the possibility of forgery and also help to eliminate errors from illegible handwriting. Physicians use the multiple medication prescription pads for those patients whose condition requires several medications to be prescribed at a time. This eliminates having to write in the patient's name, date, and other information on each single prescription order. It also saves the doctor from having to sign each individual sheet.

The prescription should contain the parts shown in Figure 18-4. This standard information helps the pharmacist fill the prescription. It is much easier for pharmacists today to fill prescriptions because of prepared and prepackaged medications. Although it is rare, some medications must still be prepared by the licensed pharmacist from the directions on the prescription. When phoning in prescriptions, you must give the pharmacist all the information that the prescription contains. To ensure **accuracy**, you should ask the pharmacist to repeat the information. This practice will help avoid dangerous misunderstandings.

When patients have their prescriptions filled by a pharmacist, the container often has an **auxiliary** label(s) on it. Pharmacists frequently use one or more of these labels to alert the patient of special instructions or warnings regarding a particular medication ordered by the doctor. Warning labels are made in a variety of bright colors to attract attention to their messages (Figure 18-5). Encourage patients to read and comply with the warning labels. Patients who take many med-

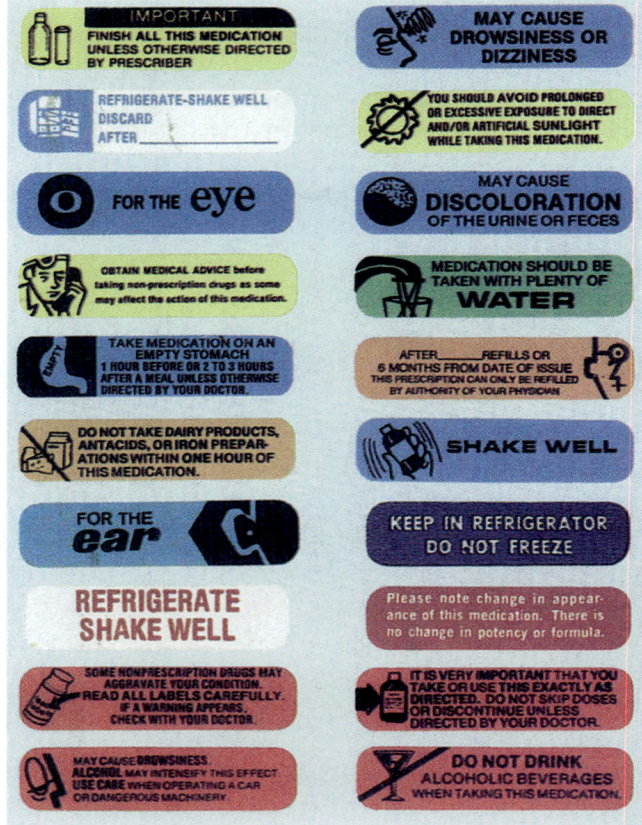

FIGURE 18-5   Examples of instruction and warning labels for prescription medications

ications every day can often become so used to seeing the warning labels that they may be ineffective. The instruction "DAW" written on a prescription means that the physician does not want the medication prescribed to be substituted—it should be exactly what was written for the patient.

CONTROLLED SUBSTANCES

All physicians who prescribe, **dispense**, or **administer** controlled substances in the United States must register with the United States Department of Justice **Drug Enforcement Administration (DEA)**, under the Controlled Substances Act of 1970. A form must be filled out with the physician's state license number and signature and be accompanied by a standard fee (Figure 18-6). If the physician moves the medical practice, this change of address must be reported in writing to the nearest DEA field office. Registration must be renewed every 3 years. The certificate must be filed at the registered location and be available for inspection by officials on request. If the physician practices medicine in more than one location, as long as they are within the same state, individual registration must be filed for each address only if controlled substances are administered or dispensed at each place. If prescriptions only are written at other locations, registration needs to be filed with the DEA just for the primary location. Physicians must be in compliance with the requirements of the 1984 Diversion Control Amendments to administer, dispense, or prescribe any controlled substance. A current printed schedule of controlled substances is enclosed with the application, and this should also be kept on file. Table 18-2 lists the drugs that are under federal control according to their actual or potential level for abuse or addiction in five categories or schedules.

A controlled substance is any drug that has the potential for abuse or addiction. Controlled substances include "street drugs" such as heroin, cocaine, stimulants, depressants, and narcotics and any drug derived from them. Controlled substances are categorized into five different schedules, base on their potential for abuse or addiction, as follows:

- Schedule I: These drugs have no recognized medicinal use in the United States, and prescriptions for such drugs are prohibited.
- Schedule II: These drugs must have a written or typed prescription order with the physician's personal signature and DEA registry number and may not be refilled. In an emergency, the doctor may phone in a limited amount of the medication to the pharmacist. However, a written, signed prescription order for the controlled substance must be presented to the pharmacist within 72 hours in compliance with DEA regulations.
- Schedule III: Prescriptions may be written or phoned for these drugs, and they may be refilled five times within 6 months.
- Schedule IV: Prescriptions may be refilled up to five times in 6 months.
- Schedule V: These drugs are subject to state and local regulations. A written prescription for Schedule V medications may not be required.

There are strict guidelines not only for the prescribing of controlled substances, but also for their storage in the medical office. They must be protected from misuse by storing them in a cabinet or compartment with a double lock. Controlled substances must not be kept with other pharmaceuticals in the office. A record must be maintained and kept for 3 years for any controlled substances dispensed. All controlled substances must be counted at the end of each day,

TABLE 18-2	Schedules of Controlled Substances			
Drug Category	**Potential for Abuse (Addiction)**	**Medical Use**	**Potential for Dependence**	**Example**
Schedule I	High	Unaccepted; limited to research	High	Heroin, LSD, marijuana, peyote
Schedule II	High	Accepted; tightly restricted	Severe psychic or physical	Amphetamines, morphine
Schedule III	Less than I or II Low to moderate	Acceptable	High psychological	Certain opioids, barbiturates, and some depressants
Schedule IV	Low	Acceptable	Limited physical and psychological	Phenobarbital propoxyphene
Schedule V	Low	Acceptable	Limited physical and psychological	Small amounts of codeine in cough preparations and analgesics

DEA Form 224
(Nov. 1999)

OMB NO.
1117-0014

APPLICATION FOR REGISTRATION
Under Controlled Substances Act of 1970

READ INSTRUCTIONS BEFORE COMPLETING

No registration will be issued unless a completed application form has been received (21 CFR 1301.13).

The Debt Collection Improvement Act of 1996 (PL 104-134) requires that you furnish your Federal Taxpayer Identifying Number to DEA. This number is required for debt collection procedures should your fee become uncollectable. If you do not have a Federal Taxpayer Identifying Number, use your Social Security Number.

USE BLACK INK

Name: Applicant or Business

(Last,

First, MI)

Taxpayer Identifying Number   and/or   Social Security Number

Proposed Business Address   (When using a P.O. Box you must also provide a street address)

City   State   Zip Code

Applicant's Business Phone Number   Applicant's Fax Number

REGISTRATION CLASSIFICATION:

1. BUSINESS ACTIVITY: (X only one)
- RETAIL PHARMACY
- HOSPITAL/ CLINIC
- PRACTITIONER- (Specify professional degree, e.g.) (DDS, DO, DVM, MD, etc.
- TEACHING INSTITUTION (Instructional purposes only)
- MID-LEVEL PRACTITIONER (MLP)- (Specify professional degree, e.g.) (PA, NP, OD, NH, AMB, AS, etc.

3. DRUG SCHEDULES: (X all that apply)
- SCHEDULE II NARCOTIC
- SCHEDULE II NON NARCOTIC
- SCHEDULE III NARCOTIC
- SCHEDULE III NON NARCOTIC
- SCHEDULE IV
- SCHEDULE V

2. INDICATE HERE IF YOU REQUIRE ORDER FORM BOOKS.

↓ATTACH CHECK HERE↓

4. ALL APPLICANTS MUST ANSWER THE FOLLOWING:

(a) Are you currently authorized to prescribe, distribute, dispense, conduct research, or otherwise handle the controlled substances in the schedules for which you are applying under the laws of the state or jurisdiction in which you are operating or propose to operate?

Yes - State License No.   Pending   N/A

Yes - State Controlled Substance No.   Pending   N/A

(b) **MLP only:** Applicant is authorized to engage in the following controlled substance activites by the **state** in which applicant practices.

	Prescribe	Administer	Dispense	Procure*		Prescribe	Administer	Dispense	Procure*
SCHEDULE II NARCOTIC					SCHEDULE III NON NARCOTIC				
SCHEDULE II NON NARCOTIC					SCHEDULE IV				
SCHEDULE III NARCOTIC					SCHEDULE V				

*Procure means to individually obtain controlled substances by purchase or receipt of samples from a manufacturer or distributor. It does not include receipt of controlled substances from, or pursuant to an order from a collaborating or supervising physician.

ATTENTION ▶ **FEE IS $210. FOR 3 YRS**

Continue on Reverse

FIGURE 18-6 Licensed physicians who prescribe, administer, or dispense controlled substances must register with the Drug Enforcement Agency of the U.S. Justice Department. *(continues)*

4. CONTINUED

(c) Has the applicant ever been convicted of a crime in connection with controlled substances under state or federal law?

☐ YES   ☐ NO

(d) Has the applicant ever surrendered or had a federal controlled substance registration revoked, suspended, restricted or denied?

☐ YES   ☐ NO

(e) Has the applicant ever had a state professional license or controlled substance registration revoked, suspended, denied, restricted, or placed on probation?

☐ YES   ☐ NO

(f) If the applicant is a corporation (other than and traded by the public), association, partner, stockholder or proprietor been controlled substances under state or federal controlled substance registration revocation whose stock is owned or ever had a state professional license or confiscated, has any officer, revoked, suspended, denied, restricted, or place of time in connection with a restricted or denied, registration

☐ NO

5. EXPLANATION FOR ANSWERING "YES" TO ITEM(S) 4(c), (d), (e), OR (f).
Applicants who have answered "yes" to item(s) 4(c), (d), (e), or (f) are required to submit a statement explaining such response(s). The space provided below should be used for this purpose. If additional space is needed, use a separate sheet and return with application.

6. PAYMENT METHOD (X only one)

☐ VISA   ☐ MASTER CARD   ☐ CHECK   ☐ U.S. MONEY ORDER

Credit Card Number

Expiration Date

SIGNATURE OF CARD HOLDER

FEES ARE NOT REFUNDABLE

7. CERTIFICATION FOR FEE EXEMPTION

☐ MARK THIS BLOCK IF APPLICANT NAMED HEREON IS A FEDERAL, STATE, OR LOCAL GOVERNMENT OPERATED HOSPITAL, INSTITUTION, OR OFFICIAL.
The undersigned hereby certifies that the applicant named hereon is a federal, state, or local government operated hospital, institution, or official, and is exempt from payment of the application fee.

Signature of Certifying Official (other than applicant)   Date

Print or Type Name of Certifying Official   Print or Type Title of Certifying Official

8. APPLICANT SIGNATURE (must be an original signature in ink)

Signature   Date

I hereby certify that the foregoing information furnished on this application is true and correct.

Print or Type Name

President, Dean, Procurement Officer, etc...)

MAKE A COPY FOR YOUR RECORDS.

RETURN COMPLETED APPLICATION WITH FEE IN ATTACHED ENVELOPE

MAKE CHECK OR MONEY ORDER PAYABLE TO
DRUG ENFORCEMENT ADMINISTRATION

UNITED STATES DEPARTMENT OF JUSTICE
DRUG ENFORCEMENT ADMINISTRATION
CENTRAL STATION
P.O. BOX 28083
WASHINGTON, D.C. 20038-8083

For information, call 1 (800) 882-9539

See "Privacy Act" Information on last page of application.

and a careful record of the count must be maintained. The count must be verified by two different people. A record of the counts must be submitted to the DEA every 2 years. Due to an increase in theft and substance abuse, many offices no longer keep controlled substances in the office.

Medical Assistant Duties

The medical assistant must be well informed about the regulations that encompass controlled substances. The medical assistant may be responsible for the following:

- Knowledge of federal and state laws that manage controlled substances, drugs, and pharmaceutical samples
- Keeping a thorough record and inventory of all drugs and samples
- Keeping all drugs, including controlled substances, in a secure location
- Reminding the physician concerning their DEA registration and renewal
- Keeping track of all prescription pads
- Properly disposing of expired drugs and keeping a record of their disposal

RECORDING MEDICATIONS

You will be expected to read and record many types of medications. Accurately recording the medication(s) administered to patients is absolutely necessary. When giving the physician's orders in giving medications to patients, you should always prepare, administer, and each one yourself. In situations where the physician present and giving the order while you are an injectable, each of you should check the name, the dose, the expiration date, and any details. The one who administers the record and sign the patient's chart. It ded that you document a medica- have anyone else do this for you. the medication on the chart is e action (of administering the ble reaction the patient may

luded in recording med-
t's chart. The follow-
ould be included in
the traditional ap-
here, when, and
ber all the in-

and who
's name
out.

What—What medication is given. The medication name should be recorded accurately and legibly; *how much*, meaning the strength and dose of the substance, should also be recorded.

When—The date and time the medication is administered should be recorded. This can also help you to check the expiration date of the medication before administered.

Where—Refers to the route of administration medication: oral, sublingual, topical, or enteral. If administered by injection of the must be noted.

Why—Answer this question for the patient verbally and with printed patient education material as necessary.

Memorizing the commonly used abbreviations and symbols given in Table 18-3 will prepare you to carry out this responsibility. Because medications can be prescribed in either metric or household measurements, it is important to know equivalents between the two to calculate the dose of the prescribed medication (Table 18-4).

Documenting Medication Side Effects

As with any medication given either at the medical facility or elsewhere, any reaction or side effect observed by a health care professional or reported by the patient must be documented on the patient's chart.

Immunizations require even further documentation. In addition to the aforementioned, the name of the medication and the name of the pharmaceutical company who manufactured it must be clearly written out. Companies that produce massive quantities of a particular immunization must assign a lot number to each batch of the product. The lot numbers can be used to keep track of and report to the manufacturer any unusual side effects or other problems experienced by a patient who received the medication. The manufacturer can then conduct an evaluation to find the cause of the patient's problem. The lot number provides the means of the trace. The expiration date is also very important. The manufacturer states that the medication or drug is guaranteed for its intended effect only until the expiration date printed on the container. Finally, the physician's name and complete address must be written on the chart and the form the patient provides for legal documentation. To reduce the time and effort of repeating this task, a name/address stamp is most practical. Figure 18-7 gives an example of a medication properly recorded on a patient's chart.

FIGURE 18-6 (Continued)

Print or Type The (e.g., DEA Form 224 (Nov. 1999)

4. CONTINUED

(c) Has the applicant ever been convicted of a crime in connection with controlled substances under state or federal law?

☐ YES   ☐ NO

(d) Has the applicant ever surrendered or had a federal controlled substance registration revoked, suspended, restricted or denied?

☐ YES   ☐ NO

(e) Has the applicant ever had a state professional license or controlled substance registration revoked, suspended, denied, restricted, or placed on probation?

☐ YES   ☐ NO

(f) If the applicant is a corporation (other than a corporation whose stock is owned and traded by the public), association, partnership, or pharmacy, has any officer, partner, stockholder or proprietor been convicted of a crime in connection with controlled substances under state or federal law, or ever surrendered or had a federal controlled substance registration revoked, suspended, restricted or denied, or ever had a state professional license or controlled substance registration revoked, suspended, denied, restricted, or place on probation?

☐ YES   ☐ NO

5. EXPLANATION FOR ANSWERING "YES" TO ITEM(S) 4(c), (d), (e), OR (f).
Applicants who have answered "yes" to item(s) 4(c), (d), (e), or (f) are required to submit a statement explaining such response(s). The space provided below should be used for this purpose. If additional space is needed, use a separate sheet and return with application.

6. PAYMENT METHOD (X only one)

☐ VISA   ☐ MASTER CARD   ☐ CHECK   ☐ U.S. MONEY ORDER

Credit Card Number

☐☐☐☐☐☐☐☐☐☐☐☐☐☐☐☐

Expiration Date
☐☐ ☐☐

SIGNATURE OF CARD HOLDER

FEES ARE NOT REFUNDABLE

7. CERTIFICATION FOR FEE EXEMPTION

☐ MARK THIS BLOCK IF APPLICANT NAMED HEREON IS A FEDERAL, STATE, OR LOCAL GOVERNMENT OPERATED HOSPITAL, INSTITUTION, OR OFFICIAL.
The undersigned hereby certifies that the applicant named hereon is a federal, state, or local government operated hospital, institution, or official, and is exempt from payment of the application fee.

Signature of Certifying Official (other than applicant)   Date

Print or Type Name of Certifying Official   Print or Type Title of Certifying Official

8. APPLICANT SIGNATURE (must be an original signature in ink)

Signature   Date

I hereby certify that the foregoing information furnished on this application is true and correct.

Print or Type Name

Print or Type Title (e.g., President, Dean, Procurement Officer, etc...)

RETURN COMPLETED APPLICATION WITH FEE IN ATTACHED ENVELOPE

MAKE CHECK OR MONEY ORDER PAYABLE TO
DRUG ENFORCEMENT ADMINISTRATION

UNITED STATES DEPARTMENT OF JUSTICE
DRUG ENFORCEMENT ADMINISTRATION
CENTRAL STATION
P.O. BOX 28083
WASHINGTON, D.C. 20038-8083

For information, call 1 (800) 882-9539

See "Privacy Act" Information on last page of application.

DEA Form 224 (Nov. 1999)   **MAKE A COPY FOR YOUR RECORDS.**

FIGURE 18-6 (Continued)

and a careful record of the count must be maintained. The count must be verified by two different people. A record of the counts must be submitted to the DEA every 2 years. Due to an increase in theft and substance abuse, many offices no longer keep controlled substances in the office.

Medical Assistant Duties

The medical assistant must be well informed about the regulations that encompass controlled substances. The medical assistant may be responsible for the following:

- Knowledge of federal and state laws that manage controlled substances, drugs, and pharmaceutical samples
- Keeping a thorough record and inventory of all drugs and samples
- Keeping all drugs, including controlled substances, in a secure location
- Reminding the physician concerning their DEA registration and renewal
- Keeping track of all prescription pads
- Properly disposing of expired drugs and keeping a record of their disposal

RECORDING MEDICATIONS

You will be expected to read and record many types of medications. Accurately recording the medication(s) administered to patients is absolutely necessary. When following the physician's orders in giving medications to patients, you should always prepare, administer, and record each one yourself. In situations where the physician is present and giving the order while you are preparing an injectable, each of you should check the specific medicine, the dose, the expiration date, and any other necessary details. The one who administers the injection should record and sign the patient's chart. It is never recommended that you document a medication for anyone else or have anyone else do this for you. The person who records the medication on the chart is the one responsible for the action (of administering the medication) and any possible reaction the patient may experience.

Many factors need to be included in recording medication information on the patient's chart. The following is a list of the details that should be included in recording medications. Ask yourself the traditional approach of who, what, how (much), where, when, and why, to make it easier for you to remember all the information every time.

> Who—Who ordered the medication and who should take it. Include the physician's name accurately and correctly spelled out.

> What—What medication is given. The medication name should be recorded accurately and legibly; *how* much, meaning the strength and dose of the substance, should also be recorded.

> When—The date and time the medication is administered should be recorded. This can also help you to check the expiration date of the medication before administering it.

> Where—Refers to the route of administration of the medication: oral, sublingual, topical, or parenteral. If administered by injection, the site must be noted.

> Why—Answer this question for the patient verbally and with printed patient education material as necessary.

Memorizing the commonly used abbreviations and symbols given in Table 18-3 will prepare you to carry out this responsibility. Because medications can be prescribed in either metric or household measurements, it is important to know equivalents between the two to calculate the dose of the prescribed medication (Table 18-4).

Documenting Medication Side Effects

As with any medication given either at the medical facility or elsewhere, any reaction or side effect observed by a health care professional or reported by the patient must be documented on the patient's chart.

Immunizations require even further documentation. In addition to the aforementioned, the name of the medication and the name of the pharmaceutical company who manufactured it must be clearly written out. Companies that produce massive quantities of a particular immunization must assign a lot number to each batch of the product. The lot numbers can be used to keep track of and report to the manufacturer any unusual side effects or other problems experienced by a patient who received the medication. The manufacturer can then conduct an evaluation to find the cause of the patient's problem. The lot number provides the means of the trace. The expiration date is also very important. The manufacturer states that the medication or drug is guaranteed for its intended effect only until the expiration date printed on the container. Finally, the physician's name and complete address must be written on the chart and the form the patient provides for legal documentation. To reduce the time and effort of repeating this task, a name/address stamp is most practical. Figure 18-7 gives an example of a medication properly recorded on a patient's chart.

TABLE 18-3   Abbreviations and Symbols Commonly Used in Administering Medications

Abbreviation	Meaning	Abbreviation	Meaning
aa	of each	kg	kilogram
ac	before meals	L	liter, left
ad	up to	lb, LB(S)	pound(s)
adde	add, let it be added	m, min	minim
ad lib	as much as needed, as desired	M	mix
agit	shake, stir	mcg	microgram
$AgNO_3$	silver nitrate	mg, MG	milligram
alt dieb	alternate days	mL, ML	milliliter
alt hor	alternate hours	noc	night
alt noc	alternate nights	non rep	do not repeat
am	morning	NPO	nothing by mouth
a, ante	before	OS	left eye
aq	water	OD	right eye
Ba	barium	OU	in each eye, both eyes
bid, BID	twice a day	oz, ℥	ounce
BSA	body surface area	p̄	after
/c, c	with	pc	after meals
CAP(S)	capsule(s)	pil	pill
comp	compound	po	by mouth
contra	against	prn, PRN	as necessary, whenever necessary
coq	boil	pt	patient
DAW	dispense as written	pulv	powder
DC, Disc	discontinue	qh	every hour
dil	dilute	q (2,3,4) h	every (2, 3, 4) hours
div	to be divided	qid, QID	four times a day
dos	doses	q m	every morning
dr, ʒ	dram	qns	quantity not sufficient
EENT	eye, ear, nose, and throat	qs	quantity sufficient
elix	elixir	rep	let it be repeated
emul	emulsion	R	right
et	and	Rx, ℞	take, recipe
ext	extract	s̄	without
Fe	iron	sat	saturated
fl	fluid	Sig, Sig, S	write on label, give directions
G	gauge	sol	solution
garg	gargle	ss	one-half
GI	gastrointestinal	stat, STAT	immediately
g, G, Gm, gm	gram	sub cu, Subc	subcutaneous (under the skin)
GR	grain	suppos	suppository
gt	drop	syr	syrup
gtt	drops	T, tbsp	tablespoon
GU	genitourinary	TAB	tablet
guttat	drop by drop	tid, TID	three times a day
H_2O_2	hydrogen peroxide	tinc	tincture
hr	hour	t, tsp	teaspoon
hs	bedtime, hour of sleep	ung	ointment
IM	intramuscular	w/o	without
inj	injection	i, ii, iii, etc.	1, 2, 3 capsules, tablets, pills, and so on
IV	intravenous		
K	potassium		

TABLE 18-4 Metric Measurements and Household Equivalents	
Metric	**Household**
1 Gm	1/4 tsp
15 Gm	1 tbsp (3 tsp)
30 Gm	1 oz (2 tbsp)
1 kg	2.2 lb
	1 gt
1 mL (1 cubic centimeter)	15 gtt
5 mL	1 tsp
15 mL	1 tbsp (3 tsp)
30 mL	1 fl oz (2 tbsp)
500 mL	(1 pt or 2 cups)
1000 mL	4 cups (1 qt)
2.5 cm	1 in
1 m	39.37 in

Steven C. James (patient)

9-23-XX:

Energix-B 0.5 ml IM L deltoid
per Dr. Elizabeth R. Evans, 100 E. Main St
Suite 205, Yourtown, US 98765-4321
SKB Lot #345 exp 1 yr. S. Markey (EE)

FIGURE 18-7 A sample recording of an immunization on a patient's chart

CALCULATIONS

Basic math skills should be among your many areas of **expertise**. These skills may mean monetary savings to your employer because there are competitive prices for everything, including medical supplies and medications. When ordering injectables, for instance, you may find that a multiple-dose **vial** is more economical for the needs of the practice than a single-dose vial. Determining what is cost effective for the practice and shopping for the best values will make you an asset to the practice. Table 18-5 provides examples of the common math problems you may encounter in determining

costs, dosages, and other mathematical calculations in the medical setting.

STORING MEDICATIONS

"A place for everything and everything in its place" is the rule for storing medications. Many necessary forms, prescription blanks, and records must be kept. Commonly used medications must be rotated according to their expiration dates. The most practical way to store medications is to categorize them by their classification as in Table 18-1. Medications may also be stored alphabetically. Labeling shelves increases efficiency, as do pull-out shelves. The medication storage cabinet, closet, or room must be locked and accessed only by a qualified member of the health care team.

Most pharmaceutical companies send their representatives to visit medical facilities on a regular basis. They will usually bring samples of new or frequently used medications along with information about the cost. Most representatives are more than willing to answer questions from the physician and medical assistant, providing them with the most up-to-date information.

Sample medicines are a very helpful way for the physician to introduce a new medication to a patient to determine whether the person can tolerate the substance, or as a consideration to give the patient a few complimentary doses. When samples are given to patients, they must be recorded on the patient's chart just as if it were a prescription. All information must be charted each time a sample medication is given for any reason. Keeping samples in order is an ongoing task. Storing them according to category, ailment, or alphabetically are some of the common ways to organize them. You should pay careful attention also to the product's expiration date and properly discard outdated substances. Check with local regulatory agencies on how to discard. A common practice is to flush old meds down the toilet or to place them in biohazard containers for waste removal.

Special attention needs to be given to the many medicines that require refrigeration, such as antibiotics and immunizations. Sometimes refrigeration is necessary only after the bottle or vial has been opened or after it has been reconstituted. There are also medications that must be stored in the freezer, such as the polio vaccine. Remember to check freezer and refrigerator temperatures daily to comply with MSDS (Material Safety Data Sheet) regulations. It is most important to check labels, directions, and package inserts to determine the proper method of storage for all products, as storage requirements may change.

TABLE 18-5 Review Examples of Math Problems

Addition

```
  876
  493
+ 521
 1890
```

Subtraction

```
  691          581
-  98        -  98
  593          483
```

Fractions $\dfrac{\text{numerator}}{\text{denominator}}$

Addition

$\dfrac{2}{5} + \dfrac{4}{5} = \dfrac{6}{5} = 1\dfrac{1}{5}$

$\dfrac{1}{5} = \dfrac{3}{15}$

$+ \dfrac{1}{3} = \dfrac{5}{15}$

$\dfrac{8}{15}$

$1\dfrac{7}{8} = 1\dfrac{35}{40}$

$+ 7\dfrac{7}{10} = 9\dfrac{28}{40}$

$10\dfrac{63}{40} = 11\dfrac{23}{40}$

Multiplication

```
   437
 ×  25
  2185
   874
 10925
```

To Prove
Divide your
answer by
437

```
         25
437)10925
     874
    2185
    2185
```

Division

```
        56.80
70)3976.00
   350
   476
   420
   560
   560
```

To Prove
Multiply
your answer
by 70

```
   56.80
 ×    70
 3976.00
```

Subtraction

$\dfrac{3}{5} - \dfrac{1}{3} = \dfrac{9}{15} - \dfrac{5}{15} = \dfrac{4}{15}$

$3\dfrac{7}{16} - 2\dfrac{1}{8} = 3\dfrac{14}{32} - 2\dfrac{4}{32} = 1\dfrac{10}{32} = 1\dfrac{5}{16}$

Multiplication

$\dfrac{1}{2} \times \dfrac{7}{16} = \dfrac{1}{5} \times \dfrac{7}{8} = \dfrac{7}{40}$

$\dfrac{1}{5} \times \dfrac{7}{10} = \dfrac{1}{5} \times \dfrac{7}{10} = \dfrac{7}{50}$

Division

$\dfrac{1}{12} \div \dfrac{2}{3} = \dfrac{1}{12} \times \dfrac{3}{2} = \dfrac{1}{8}$

$1\dfrac{1}{4} \div 3 = \dfrac{5}{4} \times \dfrac{1}{3} = \dfrac{5}{12}$

Decimals

Addition	Subtraction	Multiplication	Division
87.43	796.37	394.75	$272.52\tfrac{1}{5}$
+ 39.57	− 55.62	× 68.29	35)9538.27
127.00	740.75	3552.75	70
		7895	2538.27
		315800	2450.00
		236850	088.27
		26957.4775	70
			18.27
			17.5
			.77
			7

Percentages   To find out what percent (%) one number is of another, use the number following the word "of" as a denominator and make a fraction. Divide the numerator by the denominator—for example:

25 is what percent of 35?

$\dfrac{25}{35} = \dfrac{5}{7} =$

```
        .70 = 70%
7)5.00
  4 9
    10
```

Ratio   Ratios show how one quantity relates to another and are separated by a colon (:)—for example:

$20 : 100 = \dfrac{20}{100} = .20$ parts or 20%

Proportion   A set of two equal ratios is a proportion. In the equation, a double colon (::) separates each of the equal ratios—for example:

To mix a cleaning solution knowing the correct portions for a small amount, you can find out how much baking soda to use to make a larger amount, using x for the unknown amount.

$\dfrac{1}{2}$ cup baking soda : 16 oz. water :: x amount of baking soda : 32 oz. water

$\dfrac{1}{2} : 16 :: x : 32$

$.5 : 16 :: x : 32$

$16x = 32 \times .5$

$16x = 16$

$x = 1$ cup baking soda

UNIT 2
METHODS OF ADMINISTERING MEDICATIONS

OBJECTIVES

Upon completion of the unit, you will be able to achieve the following:

LEARNING Objectives

1. Spell and define, using the glossary at the back of the text, all the Words to Know in this unit.

2. List and describe the various methods of administering medications.

3. Explain how to apply a transdermal patch medication properly.

4. Describe precautions in applying a transdermal patch medication.

5. Explain the importance of checking medications prior to administration.

6. Explain patient education to females regarding vaginal medications.

7. List considerations regarding drug action in the body.

PERFORMANCE Objective

1. Obtain and administer oral medication.

WORDS TO KNOW

body surface area (BSA)	buccal	infusion
	douche	interaction

nomogram	salve	tolerance
ointment	sublingual	topical
parenteral	suppository	transdermal

 CERTIFICATION CONNECTION

CMA
Preparing and administering oral medication

CMAS
Basic pharmacology

RMA
Perform 6 "rights" when dispensing medications

Identify and describe routes of medication administration:
• Rectal
• Topical
• Sublingual
• Oral
• Inhalation
• Instillation

ADMINISTERING MEDICATION

There are many methods of medicating patients, and even though you may not administer every type, you should know something about each one. You will also assist in the preparation of different types of medications for patients and in the instruction of patients in specific directions for taking medications. The methods of administering medications are: oral, including **sublingual** and **buccal**; inhaled; **topical**; sprays, including **transdermal**; vaginal; rectal and urethral; and injected.

When administering any medication to a patient, you should follow a standard format checklist, commonly referred to as the "six rights" of medication administration, to make certain that you are accurate and efficient.

Before you administer the medication, always be sure that you have the right:

1. Patient
2. Medication
3. Dose/amount
4. Route/method
5. Technique
6. Time/schedule

It may seem unlikely that one would make a mistake and administer a medication to a patient in error. However, care must be taken in identifying the patient for whom the medication is intended before it is administered, or a mistake can happen. Many offices and clinics care for many patients in the course of the daily schedule, with multiple family members being seen in the same treatment room; therefore, if careful attention is not given, an error could result. Reading a med-

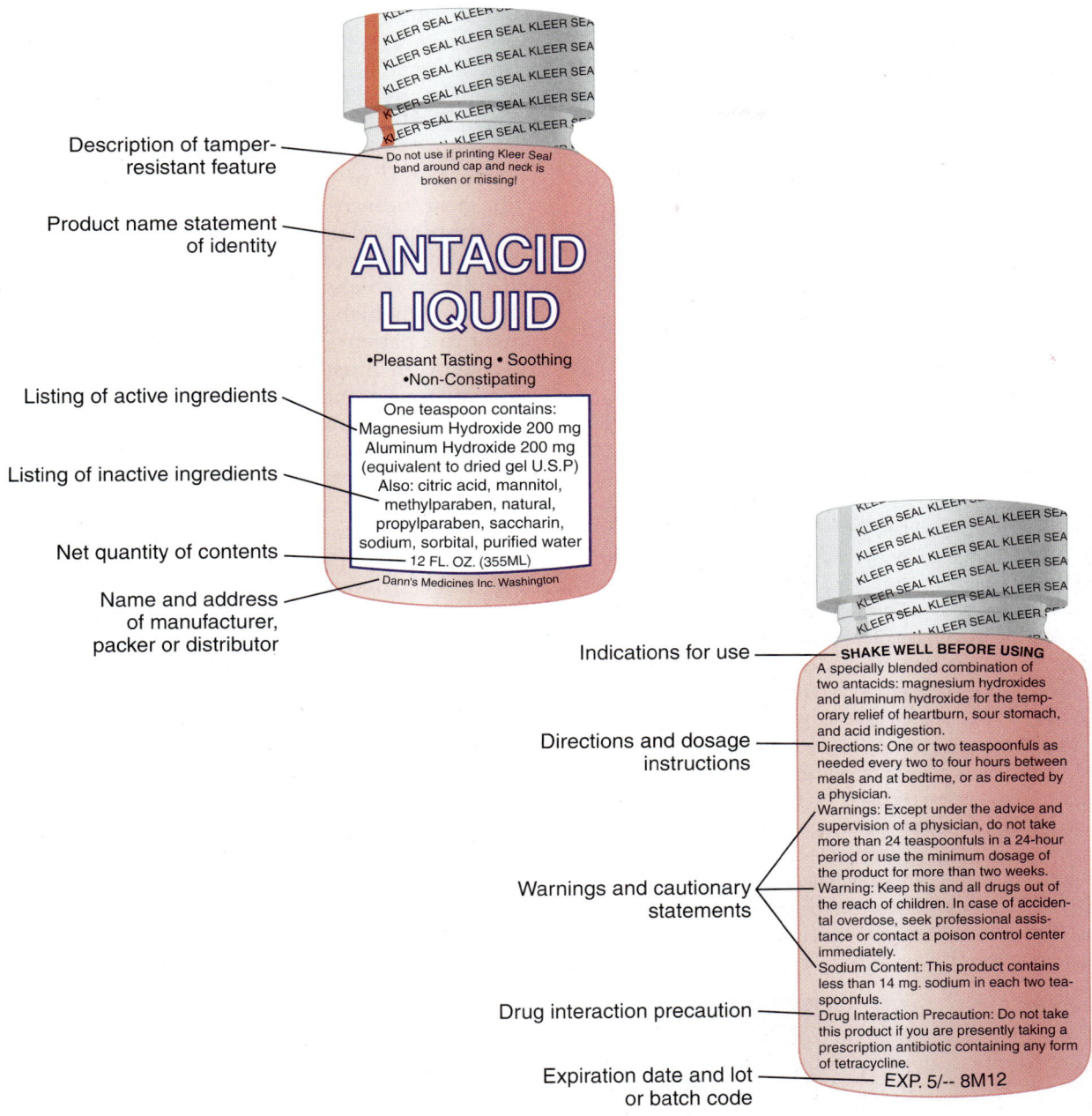

Description of tamper-resistant feature

Product name statement of identity

Listing of active ingredients

Listing of inactive ingredients

Net quantity of contents

Name and address of manufacturer, packer or distributor

Do not use if printing Kleer Seal band around cap and neck is broken or missing!

ANTACID LIQUID

•Pleasant Tasting • Soothing
•Non-Constipating

One teaspoon contains:
Magnesium Hydroxide 200 mg
Aluminum Hydroxide 200 mg
(equivalent to dried gel U.S.P)
Also: citric acid, mannitol,
methylparaben, natural,
propylparaben, saccharin,
sodium, sorbital, purified water
12 FL. OZ. (355ML)

Dann's Medicines Inc. Washington

Indications for use

Directions and dosage instructions

Warnings and cautionary statements

Drug interaction precaution

Expiration date and lot or batch code

SHAKE WELL BEFORE USING
A specially blended combination of two antacids: magnesium hydroxides and aluminum hydroxide for the temporary relief of heartburn, sour stomach, and acid indigestion.
Directions: One or two teaspoonfuls as needed every two to four hours between meals and at bedtime, or as directed by a physician.
Warnings: Except under the advice and supervision of a physician, do not take more than 24 teaspoonfuls in a 24-hour period or use the minimum dosage of the product for more than two weeks.
Warning: Keep this and all drugs out of the reach of children. In case of accidental overdose, seek professional assistance or contact a poison control center immediately.
Sodium Content: This product contains less than 14 mg. sodium in each two teaspoonfuls.
Drug Interaction Precaution: Do not take this product if you are presently taking a prescription antibiotic containing any form of tetracycline.
EXP. 5/-- 8M12

FIGURE 18-8 Medication labels provide a vast amount of information about a drug.

ication label can provide a lot of information about the medication about to be administered. Figure 18-8 illustrates the information that is printed on a medication label.

Reading the label of the ordered medication and the amount or dose when you obtain it from storage, as you prepare it, just before you administer it, and again after you have administered it will safeguard you from committing an error. If an error is made, necessary steps must be taken immediately to report it to the doc-

tor so emergency care can be given to the patient if necessary. A medication error can include:

- Drug given to wrong patient
- Wrong drug given to the correct patient
- Incorrect drug dosage administered
- Incorrect documentation placed in the patient's chart
- Drug given by an incorrect route
- Drug given at the wrong time

It is common practice and sound advice to follow these precautions when giving any medications:

Compare the medication order with the container when taking the container from storage (Figure 18-9).

Compare the medication order with the container when preparing the medication.

Compare the medication order with the container before administering the medication.

Compare the medication order with the container just after administering the medication to the patient.

This practice ensures accuracy in giving any medication.

If there is ever a chance that a medication was given in error, the necessary action must be taken immediately. Admitting such a mistake is not a pleasant experience, but it is necessary for the well-being of the patient. Reporting the error to the physician at once is essential.

Properly instructing the patient about how a medication should be taken is extremely important. If the patient does not understand the directions or the need for carrying out the physician's orders, then the medication will be virtually useless and may be dangerous because the patient may not take it or may take it incorrectly. Patients who are given medication that may induce drowsiness should be made aware of the dangers of driving or operating machinery while taking the medication. Even though the physician may give these instructions to patients, you should make sure the information is clearly understood before the patient leaves the office. You should be mindful of recording all medications given to patients, including sample packages. On the patient's chart, record the name of the medication, the strength, directions for use, and how many were dispensed. Writing the directions for use for the patient will eliminate possible confusion for the patient. Package inserts enclosed with all medication contain the necessary information. This same information is found in the PDR. If there is any further question, the PDR should be consulted.

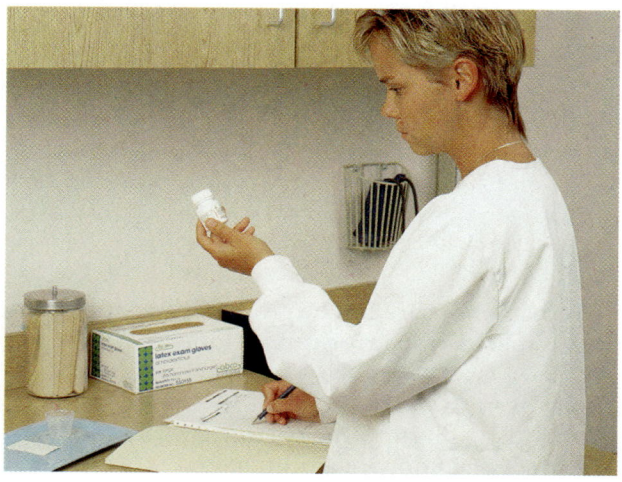

FIGURE 18-9   Check the medicine label as you take it from the shelf.

The route or method of administering medication is equally important. Carefully reading the order provides instruction in how the physician wants the medication to be administered (e.g., topical—applying a cream or other preparation to the skin; by injection—intramuscular, subcutaneous, intradermal; transdermal—skin patch; or orally—buccal or sublingual). All of these methods of administration are very different.

Technique refers to how the method is administered (e.g., skill in giving different types of injections, the manner in which you apply a topical preparation, or the way in which you administer an inhalation treatment to a patient).

Attention must be given to time and schedule in administering medicines. For example, immunizations must be given within a certain time frame for maximum effectiveness in the immunity process of the patient. The time a medication is administered is also important to the well-being of the patient. For instance, some medicines should not be taken when the stomach is full, and some should not be taken when the stomach is empty. Determining the time the patient has eaten last is important. Checking the time also should remind you to check the expiration date of the medication to be sure of its quality strength.

Other considerations for route of administration may include:

● Age of the patient
● Physical condition
● Body size or mass
● Gender

Most oral medications are intended for absorption in the small intestine. The remaining methods are **parenteral**, or intended for absorption outside the digestive system.

ROUTES OF ADMINISTRATION

Drugs may be administerd by many different routes depending on the rate of absorption desired, distribution, biotransformation, and elimination. Different routes of administration include:

● Applied to the skin: Transdermal patches, lotions, ointments, and creams
● Inhalation: Sprays, aerosols, inhalers
● Sublingual: Any tablet, liquid, drop, or spray that is placed under the tongue to dissolve
● Buccal: Placed between the cheek and gum (usually a tablet)
● Rectal: Inserted into the rectum (suppository, ointment)
● Vaginal: Inserted into the vagina (tablet, ointment, cream, suppository)

Oral Administration

One of the most common methods of administering medications is the oral method. These medicines are in the form of pills, tablets, capsules, caplets, lozenges, syrups, sprays, and other liquids, which are swallowed. These medications are usually given to patients as pre-scriptions, although they may be administered in the office (Procedure 18-1). For example, an analgesic may be given to a patient while in the office for relief of pain. The OPV (oral live polio vaccine) is given orally to infants and children in the medical office by the physician or the medical assistant.

PROCEDURE PROCEDURE PROCEDURE PROCEDURE PROCEDURE PROCEDURE PROCEDURE PROCEDURE

18-1　Obtain and Administer Oral Medication

PURPOSE: To obtain the ordered oral medication and administer it to the patient.

EQUIPMENT: Ordered oral medication, medicine cup (disposable), disposable paper cup filled with water, medicine tray.

PERFORMANCE OBJECTIVE: Provided with all necessary equipment and supplies, demonstrate the steps required to obtain the ordered oral medication, and administer it to the patient. The instructor will observe each step.

1. Obtain the medication from the storage area and read the label carefully, comparing it with the order. **NOTE: Work in a well-lighted area, and avoid distractions.**

2. Calculate the dosage, if necessary, and wash hands.

3. Take the bottle cap off, and place it inside-up on counter. **RATIONALE: The counter top is considered contaminated and must not come into contact with the inside of the cap. Likewise, touching the inside of the bottle or cap will result in contamination.** Read the label of the medication container.

4. If in pill or capsule form, pour the desired amount into the cap. Then pour the medication into a medicine cup. If it is liquid medicine, pour it directly into a measuring device to the calibrated line of the ordered amount. **NOTE: Hold the measuring device at eye level with your thumbnail placed at the desired amount (Figure 18-10).** Syrup or liquid medications may also be given in disposable plastic measuring spoons or droppers. Liquids should be poured from the opposite side of the bottle's label to prevent the contents from dripping and discoloring the label.

5. Place the medication container on a tray and the ordered dose in a medicine cup. Place a cup of water on the tray for the patient to drink with the medicine if allowed. Read the label of the container again.

6. Take the medication tray to the patient and confirm the patient's identification. Explain the procedure.

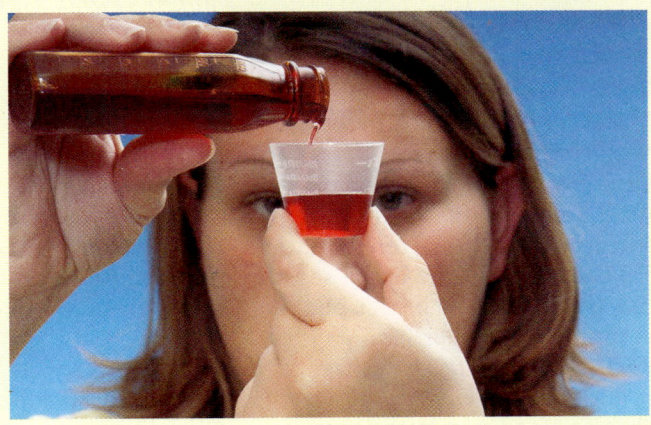

FIGURE 18-10 Hold the medicine cup at eye level when pouring for accurate measurement.

7. Give the patient the medication and offer the cup of water if allowed. Observe the patient taking the medicine and report any reaction or problem to the physician. **NOTE: Some liquid medications, such as a cough suppressant, should not be taken with water. Water can wash away the coating created by swallowing the liquid medication.**

8. Discard any disposables and return the medication container and tray to the proper storage area. **NOTE: Read the label of the medication container again.**

9. Record the information on the patient's chart.

CHARTING EXAMPLE

3-19-XX

Two tsp Robitussin administered orally at 2:35 PM for nasal congestion and cough; instructed to take two oz medicine bottle home and take two tsp q4hr

S. Davis, RMA

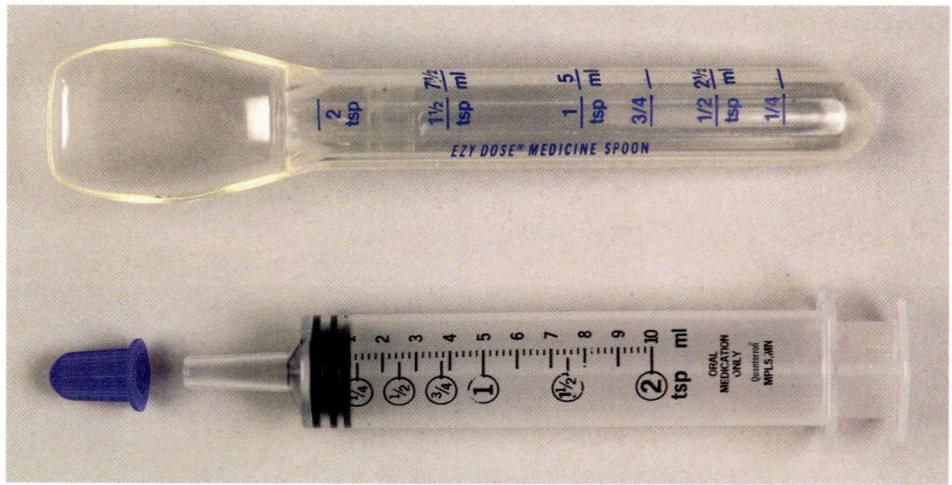

FIGURE 18-11   Calibrated medication spoon and syringe

Patient education is not only vitally important, it can be very helpful and practical as well. In the case of new parents who are uneasy about giving medicine to their infant, it is crucial that you give proper instruction for the child's well-being. Giving or dispensing medication to the parents (patients) to give to their child to take at home is the same as a prescription, because the physician prescribed it. Medication given in this manner is dispensed.

Oral medications have many advantages. An obvious one is their convenience. If a patient exhibits an intolerance or an adverse reaction to an oral medication, the remedy may be to just discontinue the medicine. The reaction to a single oral dose would certainly be much less dangerous than if the medication were given by injection. They are also easily stored and are economical for the medical practice and the patient.

If the medication to be given orally is a liquid, one of several devices are available for proper measurement of the dosage: medicine cups, calibrated medicine spoons or syringes (Figure 18-11), or calibrated medicine droppers (Figure 18-12).

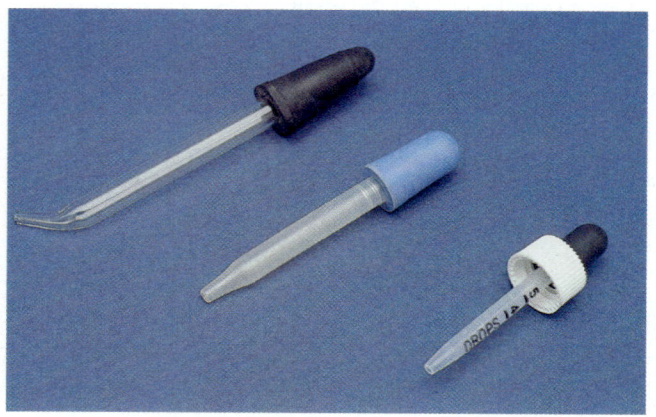

FIGURE 18-12   Examples of calibrated medicine droppers

Sublingual and Buccal Administration

The sublingual method of administering medication involves placing the medication, usually tiny tablets or spray, under the tongue. This introduces the medication immediately into the bloodstream. An example is nitroglycerine, which is usually prescribed for patients who suffer from angina. Tiny tablets or spray are also administered by the buccal method, that is, placed or sprayed in the mouth between the gum and the cheek. The medication is then absorbed through the mucous membranes. Patients should avoid eating, drinking, or chewing while the medication is in place. Instruct patients how to use these medications properly, because sublingual and buccal medications should not be swallowed whole, or their intended action may be delayed or ineffective.

Inhalation Administration

Medications given to patients by the inhalation method are in the form of gases, sprays, fluids, or powders to be mixed with liquid and used with equipment that will produce a mist or vapor. These are breathed into the respiratory tract. The patient usually self-administers the medication at home, often by using an inhaler. After being instructed properly, the patient should feel comfortable in doing so. Manufacturers prepare instruction material on the proper use and care of their equipment. You should keep a file of these for the most commonly prescribed medications.

A form of inhalation medication that should be kept in every medical practice is oxygen. Although it is not given often in most practices, it should be available for emergency use. Many companies offer instruction in the use and care of such equipment. They also offer various home oxygen treatment programs for patients who need this treatment daily. The physician will de-

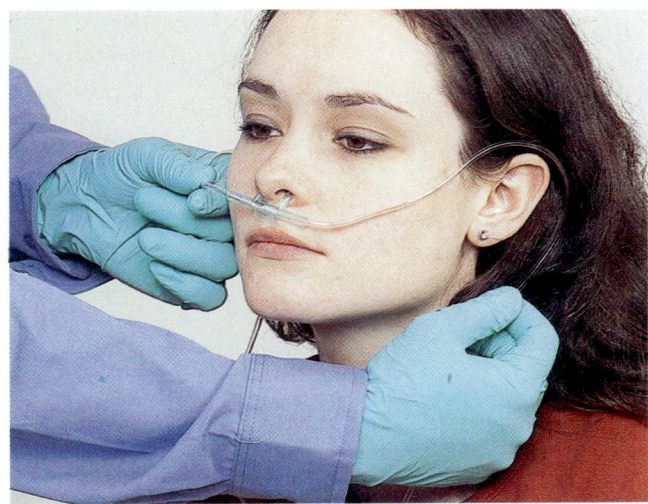

FIGURE 18-13A   Nasal cannula

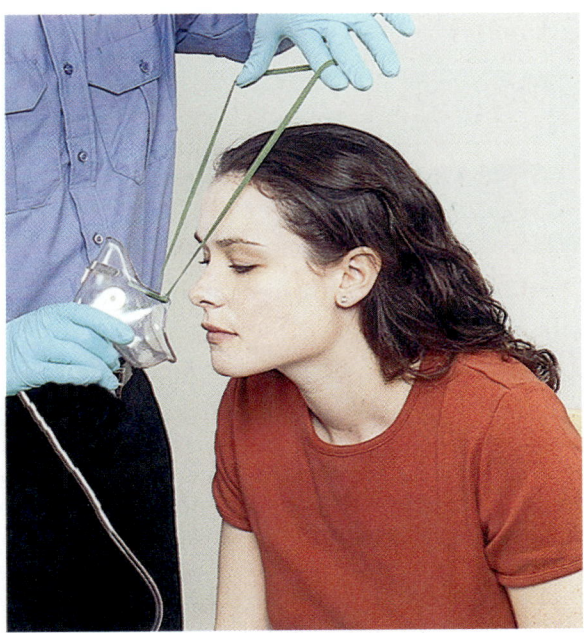

FIGURE 18-13B   Oxygen mask

Topical medications must be applied as instructed for maximum effect. For example, a patient should apply a medication to reduce itching with gentle single strokes. If the medication is rubbed into the skin vigorously, the itching will increase from the heat produced from the friction, which increases the circulation.

The patch type of medication, commonly called the *transdermal patch,* is a convenient method of choice for medicating patients for many medical conditions (Figure 18-14). It is painless and helps to ensure patient compliance. The patch is placed on the skin according to the directions of the pharmaceutical company. It then releases minute dosages of the desired medicine into the patient's tissues, which carry it into the circulatory system. The patient receives timed-release treatment without worrying about when to take medication. Patients return as scheduled or as indicated to have the effectiveness of the medication evaluated. Patients should be properly instructed to apply the transdermal patch themselves. When applying the transdermal patch, one must be extremely careful when handling it to avoid getting the medication on the fingers. A priming dose of medication is in the adhesive edge of the patch. The medication intended for the patient can also be absorbed by the person who applies it. If you are not careful to wash your hands with soap and water immediately after application of the transdermal medicating patch, the effects could be undesirable or even dangerous to the one who applied it. Traces could also be transferred to another person, which could also present problems. Wearing disposable gloves when applying transdermal patches is a suggested practice, especially when a potential adverse reaction is possible for the person who applies the patch.

Several commonly prescribed medications are available as transdermal systems. Figure 18-15 shows a once-a-day patch. Transdermal patches containing time-released amounts of nicotine have become popular as a means of quitting cigarette smoking. These are

termine the method of delivery (nasal cannula or mask) and the rate of delivery, prescribed in liters of oxygen per minute (LPM). Figures 18-13A and B illustrate the nasal cannula and the mask. Setting aside a time when this service could benefit the entire medical staff would be advantageous.

Topical Administration

Topical medications are used in treating diseases or disorders of the skin or mucous membranes. They come in sprays, lotions, creams, **ointments**, paints, **salves**, wet dressings, and transdermal patches.

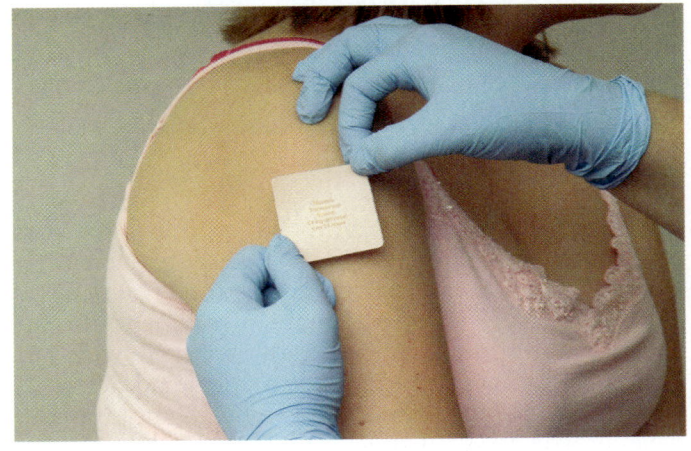

FIGURE 18-14   Placing a transdermal patch on a patient

You must make sure the patient understands the proper method of self-administration of vaginal medications, because many women are embarrassed about asking. For example, many women may not know that vaginal medications should be used during the menstrual flow because this is an ideal time for growth of microorganisms.

Vaginal medications may seem undesirable because they tend to be messy. Most vaginal medications are ordered for use at bedtime, so better patient compliance is gained. You may also advise patients to use disposable panty liners or, with the advice of the physician, to insert a tampon to hold the medication in the vaginal canal.

Stress to female patients the importance of completing the prescribed treatment plan that the doctor has ordered. Remind patients who have STDs (sexually transmitted diseases) to have their partners seek medical attention and follow treatment if necessary. Some infections can be harbored in the partner with no symptoms, and the patient may be reinfected if the partner is not treated. Often, patients stop using a medication after a few doses or a few days because the symptoms seem to clear up. Unless all of the prescribed medication is used, the condition or problem could return. Many self-medications are available for women with gynecological symptoms. You should urge patients to seek advice from the physician if their complaints do not improve with the use of these OTC products, because they may have a serious condition.

You may also want to instruct female patients about good personal hygiene. Advertising has made women believe that they should be clean "inside and out." However, frequent douching or bathing with perfumed soaps or other toilet articles may leave the body open to infection by washing the natural body secretions away or irritating the delicate vaginal tissues. Patients should be aware that vaginal sprays and douches are really not necessary. Daily showering or bathing should be sufficient. Excessive odor and vaginal discharge are symptoms of infection and should be brought to the attention of the physician.

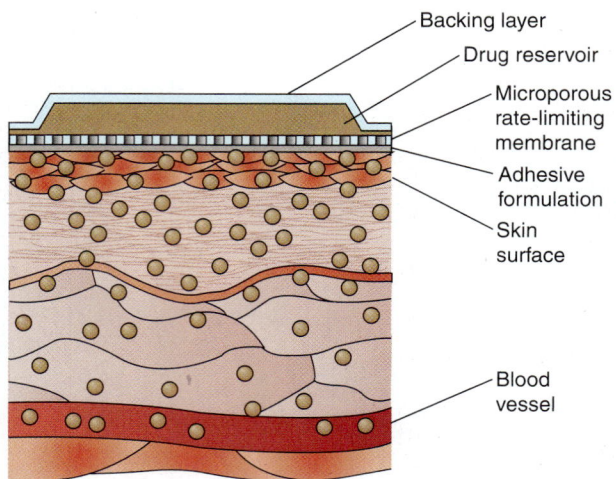

FIGURE 18-15 The Nitro-Dur is a multilayered unit. It consists of a blocking layer, a reservoir of nitroglycerin, a rate-controlling membrane, and an adhesive layer that has a priming dose of nitroglycerin. *(Courtesy of Novartis)*

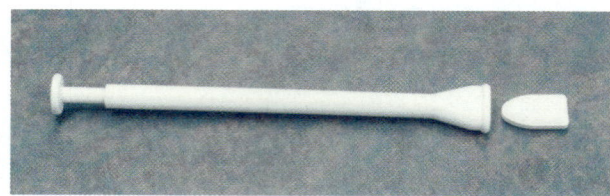

FIGURE 18-16 Vaginal medication and applicator

more nicotine than the patient is used to and will cause potentially serious side effects. Many patients also do not realize the serious effects of smoking while wearing the patches. A high dose of nicotine could produce dangerous consequences, such as elevated blood pressure and heart dysfunction. Some of the side effects experienced by patients include insomnia, racing and pounding heart, hyperactivity, and irritability. In discussing the dosage that is specific to each patient, be sure that you stress to the patient that adjusting the dosage in individual patient cases can control unnecessary problems.

Vaginal Administration

Vaginal medications can be applied in the form of creams, **suppositories**, tablets, **douches**, foams, ointments, tampons, sprays, and salves (Figure 18-16).

CONSIDERATIONS OF DRUG ACTION

Several considerations may affect how the body responds to a drug. These are age, weight, **body surface area (BSA)**, method of administration, **tolerance**, allergies, time, and

intended to curb the craving for nicotine. Patients may obtain the patches OTC; they supply decreasing doses of nicotine over a 3-month period. The patch is changed every 24 hours. Before recommending the transdermal patches, a thorough interview with the patient regarding the extent of nicotine addiction is vital. Many patients have tried to stop smoking and have already reduced their intake of nicotine. Often, the initial dose of the transdermal patches contains

interaction. Pediatric and geriatric patients and some other individuals usually require a smaller dose than an average adult. Special medications, such as chemotherapy drugs, are determined by the BSA, which is derived by plotting the patient's height and weight on a **nomogram**. To achieve a specific blood level of a medication, the dosage must be calculated according to the patient's weight. An example of figuring dosage calculation for children using the nomograms is in Figure 18-17.

> Child's ht, 42 inches; wt, 40 pounds—use to find the child's BSA on nomogram
> (Adult strength medication, 220 mg)
> child's dose = m (child's BSA) × (drug dose) mg
> child's dose = 0.7 × 220 mg
> child's dose = 0.49 × 220 mg
> child's dose = 107.8 mg

The different methods of administering medications and the rate at which the body uses them varies. Medications given by injection are circulated in the bloodstream rapidly; transdermal patch **infusion** systems deliver small amounts of medication in a sustained time-release manner; oral medicines take considerable time before they are absorbed by the small intestines. If a patient has to take a particular medication for a long time, a tolerance may develop requiring an increase in the amount or a change in medicine for the desired effect to take place. An allergy to a medication may occur at any time in an individual. Careful attention must be given to the medical history and to the patient's responses during the interview. Further, the medical assistant must be alert to checking any notations in red ink signifying allergies. If a patient phones you to let you know that a medication that was taken (prescribed the day before) gave her a reaction, it must be determined exactly what the reaction is (was) and the extent of it, and this must be carefully recorded on the patient's chart. Occasionally a patient may have an intolerance of a medication and not a reaction. A medication intolerance (e.g., vomiting it) should also be charted. Many patients take several medications daily. Helping patients determine what to take their medicine with and when to take it will encourage the desired result.

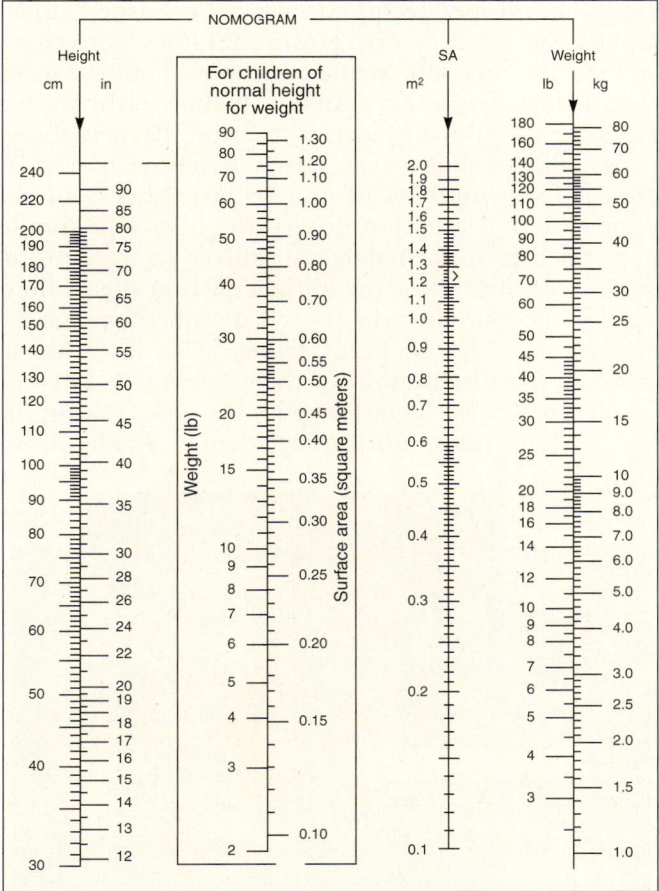

FIGURE 18-17   The information derived from the nomogram is useful in calculating dosage.

ACHIEVE UNIT OBJECTIVES

■ Complete the Workbook activities to meet the learning objectives.

■ Practice the procedure in this unit to meet the performance objectives.

■ Apply your knowledge at the end of this chapter in completing the Critical Thinking Challenge and Activities, as well as the StudyWARE on your Student CD-ROM.

UNIT 3
INJECTIONS AND IMMUNIZATIONS

OBJECTIVES

Upon completion of the unit, you will be able to achieve the following:

LEARNING Objectives

1. Spell and define, using the glossary at the back of the text, all the Words to Know in this unit.

2. Correctly identify the parts of a syringe and needle.

3. Name the tissue layers and sites of injection for intradermal, intramuscular, and subcutaneous injections.

4. List and explain the immunization schedule for normal infants, children, and adults.

5. Explain the importance of informing patients, or the responsible party for a minor, verbally and in writing, of both the benefits and the risks of immunizations before they are administered.

6. Discuss the importance of patient education regarding medications.

7. Identify the various sites for administering insulin injections.

8. Explain the theory of IV therapy.

PERFORMANCE Objectives

1. Withdraw medication from an ampule and a vial.

2. Demonstrate how to administer intradermal, intramuscular, and subcutaneous injections properly.

3. Demonstrate how to prepare and administer an insulin injection.

4. Demonstrate an intramuscular injection by the Z-track method.

5. Reconstitute a powder medication for injection.

WORDS TO KNOW

ampule	haemophilus	mumps
anaphylactic	hepatitis B	paroxysmal stage
antitoxin	immunization	pertussis
booster	incubation	photophobia
catarrhal stage	influenza	retardation
cholera	insulin	rubella
débridement	intradermal (ID)	rubeola
decline stage	intramuscular (IM)	sensitivity
diphtheria	intravenous (IV)	series
epiglottitis	lethal	subcutaneous
epinephrine	measles	(sub q)
flu	meningitis	tetanus

toxin	typhoid	vial
trimester	vaccine	Z-track IM

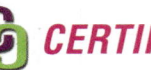 CERTIFICATION CONNECTION

CMA
Preparing and administering parenteral medications
Maintaining medication and immunization records
Principles of IV therapy

CMAS
Basic pharmacology

RMA
Parenteral medications

INJECTIONS

You will be helping to prepare and possibly to administer medications in the form of injections. Because this method of medication introduces the substance directly into the tissues, where it quickly enters the patient's bloodstream, extreme caution must be practiced. The proper technique must be learned under supervision. Latex or vinyl gloves should be worn to administer an injection. Medication should only be given to patients when a physician is available nearby should the patient exhibit any adverse reaction. There is always a possibility of **anaphylactic** shock. Refer to Chapter 16, Unit 1, for symptoms of anaphylactic shock. In the event that this situation occurs, the physician should be notified to immediately administer an injection of **epinephrine** just above the initial injection site. Following the injection into the muscle or subcutaneous tissue, the area should be massaged. This is to aid in speeding the distribution of the epinephrine into the circulatory system as fast as possible. Keep taking the patient's vital signs until the patient is stable. Provi-

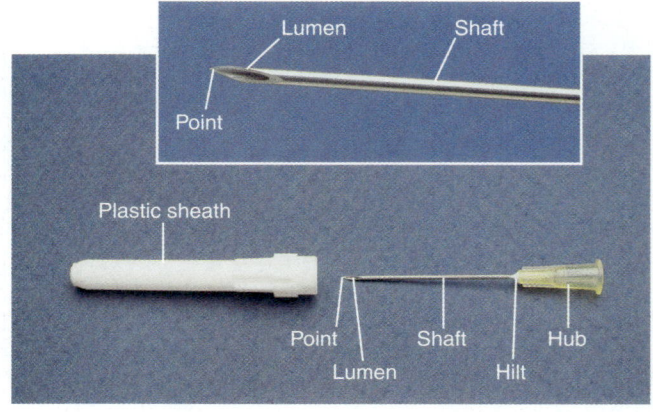

FIGURE 18-18A   Parts of a needle

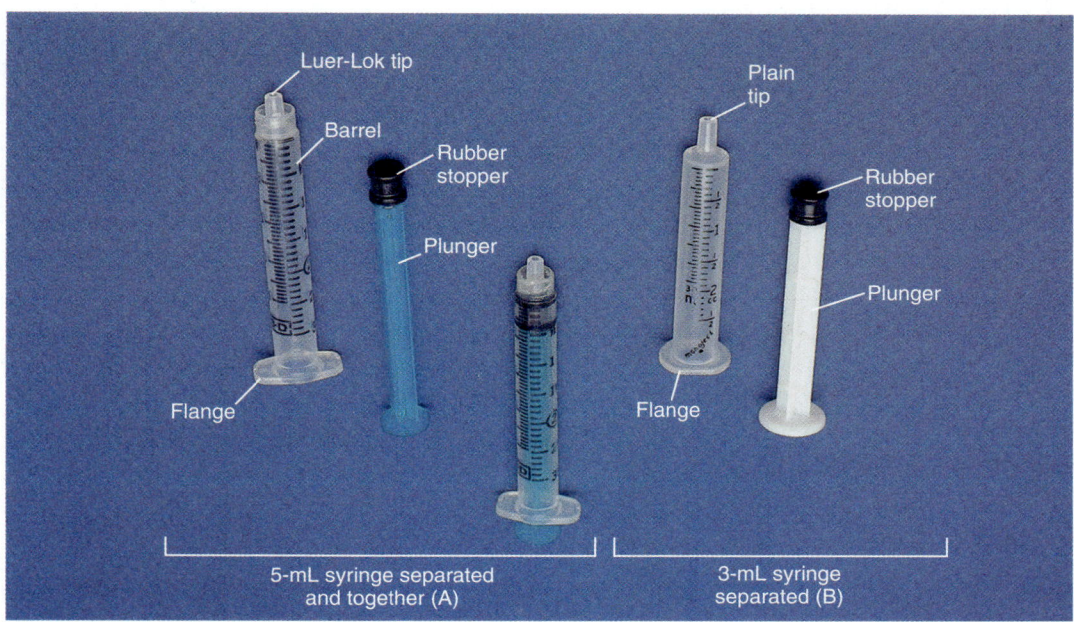

Luer-Lok tip

Barrel

Rubber stopper

Plunger

Flange

Plain tip

Rubber stopper

Plunger

Flange

5-mL syringe separated and together (A)

3-mL syringe separated (B)

FIGURE 18-18B   Parts of a syringe

sions should always be made for emergency situations. Even if the patient's past history reveals no **sensitivity** to a particular drug, there is no guarantee of what the next dose may do. Information regarding an allergic episode must be recorded on the patient's chart. There should also be a flag (sticker) of the medication allergy placed on the outside and inside of the patient's chart. Advise the patient to wear an identification bracelet containing information about the medication allergy.

The term *hypodermic* simply means under the skin. You must become familiar with the parts of the syringe and needle and proficient in handling them. Figures 18-18A and B picture a needle and syringe with labeled parts. Different syringes are calibrated in different measurements, so you must be careful to choose the correct syringe and to draw up the correct dosage according to the medication order (Figure 18-19). Syringes commonly used in the medical office to administer medication include:

- 3-mL syringe, which is calibrated in milliliters. Each small line represents 0.1 mL, and the longer lines represent 0.5, 1.0, 1.5, 2.0, 2.5, and 3.0 mL.
- Tuberculin syringe, calibrated in tenths of a milliliter. This syringe has only a 1.0-mL capacity. Each small line represents 0.1, 0.2, 0.3 mL, etc.
- Insulin syringe, calibrated in units. Capacity is 100 units.

You must also be able to properly read the amount of medication in the syringe. The plunger of the syringe has a black rubber tip at the end inside the barrel. This tip has a pointed projection in the center. You read the syringe by reading the calibration mark that lines up with the point on the black rubber tip of the plunger.

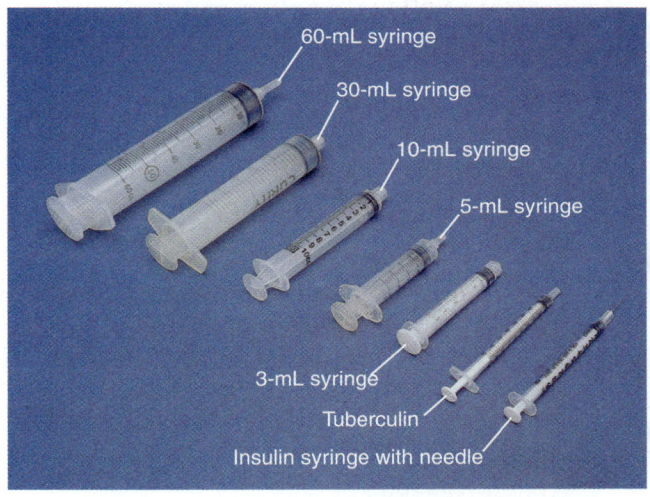

60-mL syringe

30-mL syringe

10-mL syringe

5-mL syringe

3-mL syringe

Tuberculin

Insulin syringe with needle

FIGURE 18-19   Various sizes of disposable syringes

Practice with different types of syringes and needles; filling the syringe with varying amounts of sterile water from a **vial** and **ampule** will give you confidence (see Procedures 18-2 and 18-3). While handling the syringe and needle, use caution to avoid dangerous needle sticks. It is recommended that to prevent injuries, needles should *never* be recapped after use. Used needles and syringes should be discarded intact in the biohazardous sharps waste container. Even though you are strongly urged to never recap needles, in reality it may be necessary in certain circumstances to do so. For your safety, you should recap a needle by placing your nondominant hand behind your back, and holding the syringe and needle intact, "scoop" the cap onto the

18-2 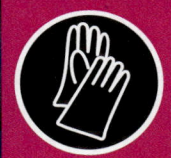 Withdraw Medication from an Ampule

PURPOSE: To withdraw from an ampule an ordered amount of medication into a syringe.

EQUIPMENT: Ampule of medication (sterile water for injection), medication tray, sterile gauze square, sterile needle and syringe, filter needle, disposable gloves, and needle resheather.

PERFORMANCE OBJECTIVE: Provided with all necessary equipment and supplies, demonstrate each of the steps required to withdraw medication (sterile water for instructional purposes) from an ampule; the procedure will be repeated three times, each time withdrawing a specific quantity of fluid as predetermined by the instructor. **NOTE: Injectables obtained from an ampule should be withdrawn with a filter needle to prevent minute particles of glass from entering the syringe and mixing with the injectable substance. The filter needle is then taken off (using a needle resheather) and the needle to be used during the injection attached. Avoid using the last few drops of the substance to further eliminate particles. Using a new needle also ensures a sharp point for swifter insertion, causing less pain for the patient.**

1. Disinfect the neck of the ampule with an alcohol swab.

2. Place a sterile gauze square over the middle of the ampule and hold the ampule between the thumb and index finger of one hand (Figure 18-20A). **RATIO-**

NALE: Sterile gauze will keep any fragments of glass from flying.

3. Flick the pointed end of the ampule with your index finger to release medication into the bottom of the ampule before opening it.

4. Grasp the tip of the ampule and snap it off. Discard the tip.

5. Make sure that the syringe and filter needle are secured by turning the barrel to the right while holding the needle guard. Remove the guard.

6. Expel the air from the syringe by pushing down on the plunger. Insert the tip of the needle into the solution while holding the ampule in an upright position. **NOTE: Do not touch the rim of the ampule to maintain sterile technique.**

7. Draw back the plunger quickly and steadily to fill the syringe with medication (Figure 18-20B). Keep the needle point below the meniscus level of the liquid to prevent air bubbles from entering the syringe. (**NOTE: If air bubbles do enter, turn the syringe pointing up and gently tap the barrel to free the bubbles to**

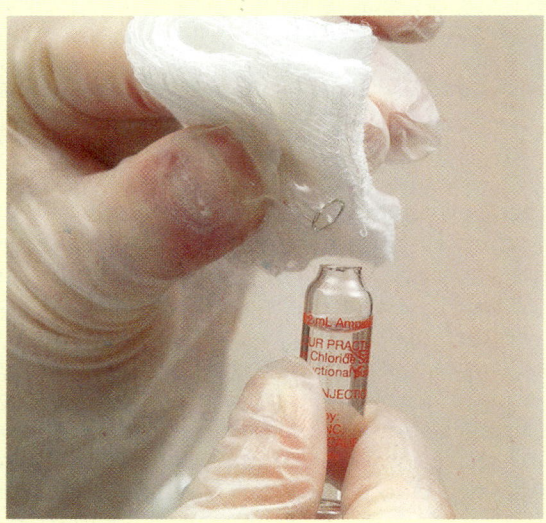

FIGURE 18-20A Remove top from ampule. Snap away from you by pulling top toward you.

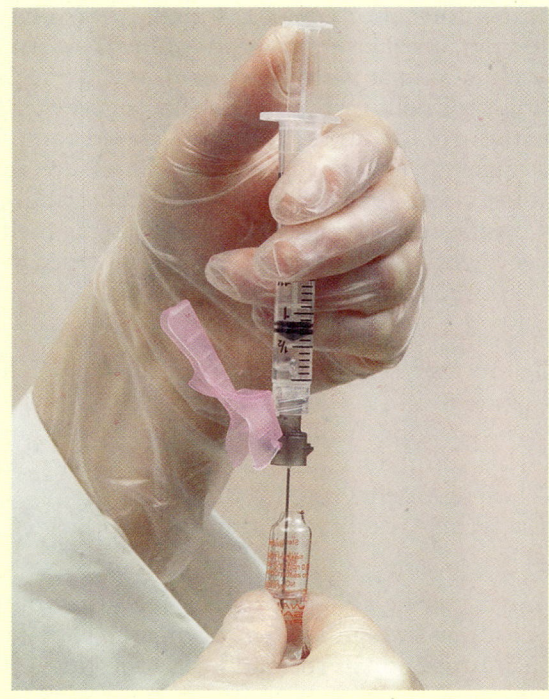

FIGURE 18-20B Draw the required dose into the syringe.

(continues)

18-2  Withdraw Medication from an Ampule (Continued)

the top. Gently push the plunger up to release the air bubbles.)

8. Place the filter needle of the syringe into the needle resheather and twist it off of the syringe. Place the original capped needle onto the syringe securely, and remove the cap just before administering the injection. Maintain sterility and safety. Place the filled syringe on the medication tray.

9. Discard the ampule and gauze in the proper receptacles.

18-3  Withdraw Medication from a Vial

PURPOSE: To withdraw an ordered amount of medication into a syringe from a vial.

EQUIPMENT: Multiple- and single-dose vials (sterile water for injection), alcohol-saturated cotton balls, sterile needle and syringe, medication tray.

PERFORMANCE OBJECTIVE: Provided with all necessary equipment and supplies, demonstrate each of the steps required to withdraw medication (sterile water for instructional purposes) from multiple- and single-dose vials. The procedure will be repeated three times, each time withdrawing a specific quantity of fluid as predetermined by the instructor.

1. Calculate the dosage if required and wash hands.

2. Use an alcohol-saturated cotton ball to clean the rubber-topped vial.

3. Secure a needle onto the syringe by holding the needle guard and turning the barrel of the syringe to the right.

4. Remove the needle guard, and pull back on the plunger to fill the syringe with the same amount of air as medication that has been ordered. **RATIONALE: This prevents a vacuum from forming in the vial and thus makes it easier to withdraw solution.** Some injectible medications should not have air injected into the vial. Refer to the package insert for direction in this step of the procedure.

5. Hold the syringe by the barrel between your thumb and fingers; hold the vial upside-down with your other hand (Figure 18-21A). Insert the needle into the rubber top and push the plunger in, expelling the air into the vial.

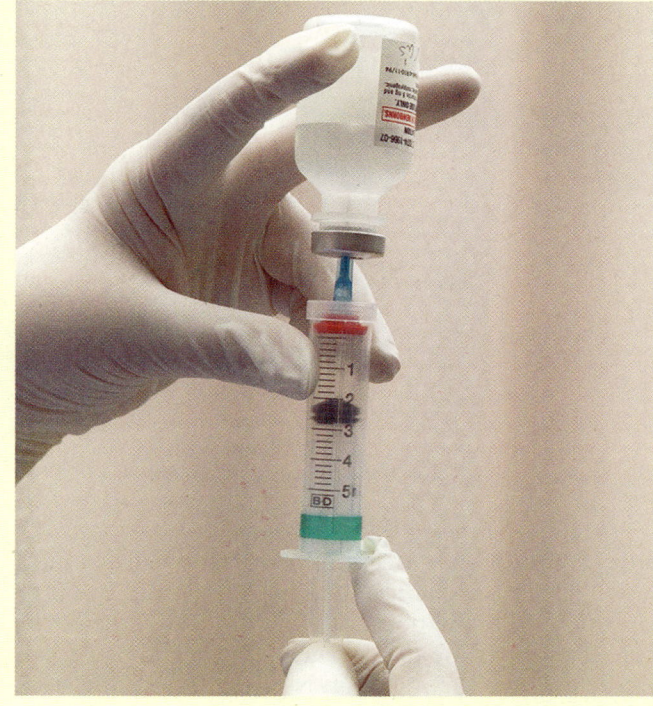

FIGURE 18-21A   Hold the syringe pointed upward at eye level and with the bevel of the needle in the medication. Pull back the plunger and aspirate the quantity of medication ordered.

6. Pull back on the plunger so the desired amount of medication will flow into the syringe, keeping the needle below the level of solution to prevent air bubbles. **NOTE: Air takes up space where medication**

(continues)

PROCEDURE PROCEDURE PROCEDURE PROCEDURE PROCEDURE PROCEDURE PROCEDURE PROCEDURE

18-3  Withdraw Medication from a Vial (Continued)

should be, and the dosage would not be correct if air remained. To release air bubbles if they appear, flick the barrel of the syringe with a finger in a quick, hard motion (Figure 18-21B). They will be released into the hub of the syringe. Push the plunger carefully to make sure they are out of the needle. Withdraw the needle from the vial.

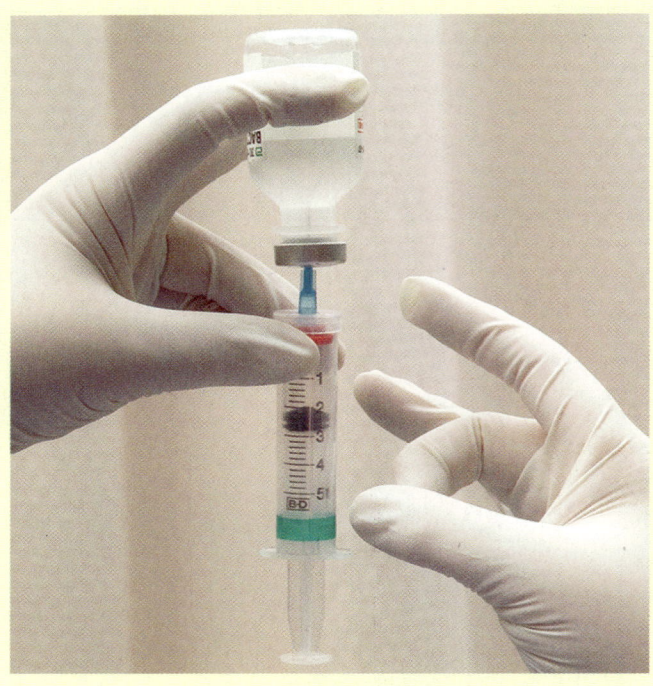

FIGURE 18-21B   Tap the syringe to eliminate air bubbles.

7. Let go of the plunger. Hold the barrel of the syringe and pull the needle out of the vial, keeping the syringe in a vertical position. Check for air bubbles. Replace the needle guard by carefully scooping it onto the needle, as shown in Figure 18-21C, to keep the needle sterile and for safety.

8. Keep the medication with the loaded syringe on the medication tray to ensure proper identification. Place an alcohol-saturated cotton ball with the syringe to administer the medication.

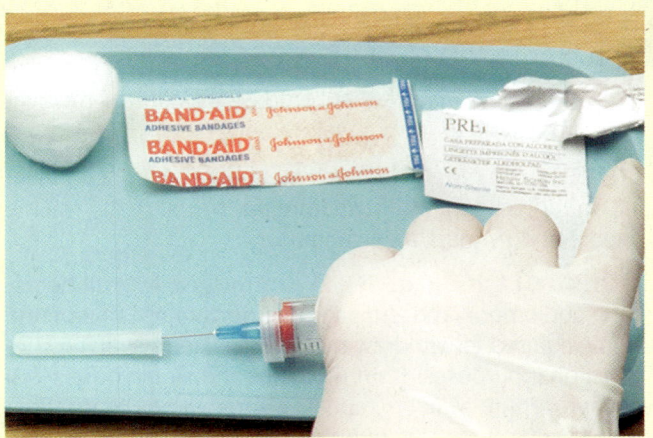

FIGURE 18-21C   After the correct dose has been withdrawn, recover the sterile needle. Place the medication on a tray along with the medication card and an alcohol wipe and safely transport to the patient.

needle (Figure 18-22). Keeping your other hand behind you will lessen the chance of being tempted to use it to recap the needle, the point at which most needle sticks occur. The only time it may even be necessary to recap a needle is *before* the injection is given. If a needle stick would occur before the injection were to be given, the needle and syringe should be discarded and the procedure repeated or the patient could become infected from the contaminated needle.

Some needle and syringe units have a shield that locks into place over the used needle to prevent injury to the user (Figure 18-23). There are also safety devices that activate by the touch of a finger to click a shield over the used needle or retract the needle into a sleeve on the syringe. Another safety device to protect health care team members from contaminated needle sticks is

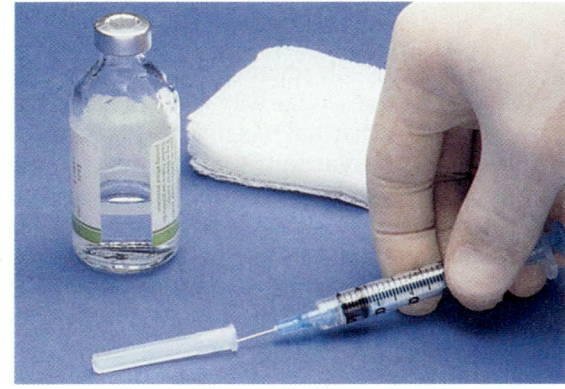

FIGURE 18-22   Keeping one hand behind your back, "scoop" the needle into the needle cover carefully so it does not become contaminated, and to prevent a needle stick.

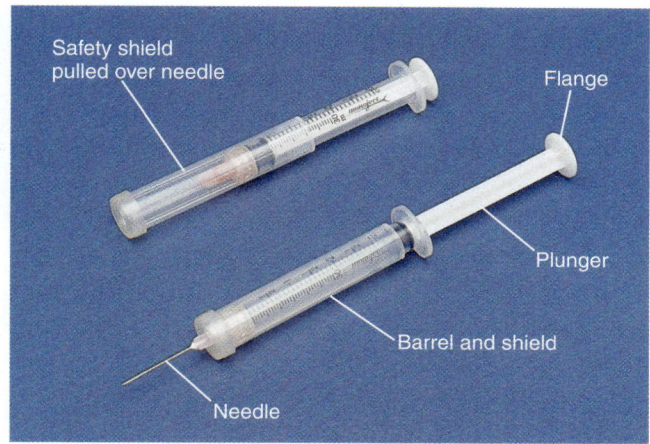

FIGURE 18-23   Syringe with a safety shield that pulls over the needle

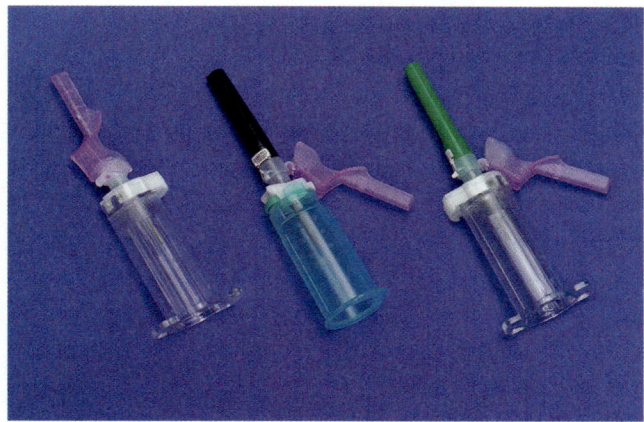

FIGURE 18-24   Syringe with locking safety cover

a sheath cover that clicks into place to completely cover the used needle (Figure 18-24).

ADMINISTERING INJECTIONS

Injectable medications also come in single-dose, pre-filled, disposable sterile syringes and cartridges. This method guarantees an accurate dosage and is also convenient and time-saving. The single-dose units are assembled by inserting the cartridge into a reusable injector (Figures 18-25A to C).

Some injectable medications come in powdered form and must be reconstituted before administration. Procedure 18-4 lists the steps necessary to reconstitute a powdered medication in a vial.

The administration techniques for injecting medications are extremely important. Improper injection techniques can result in infection and cause damage to nerves, blood vessels, and tissues and can lead to legal action. When proper technique is used, however, giving medications by injection can be a minimally painful experience for the patient.

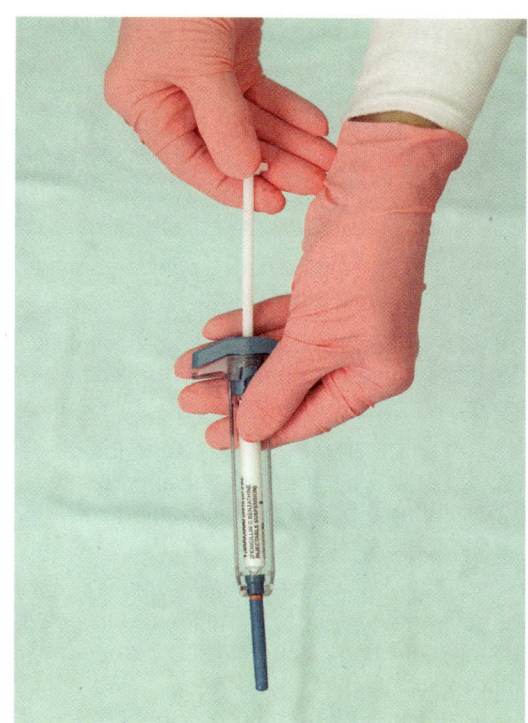

FIGURE 18-25A   Reusable injection system with cartridges

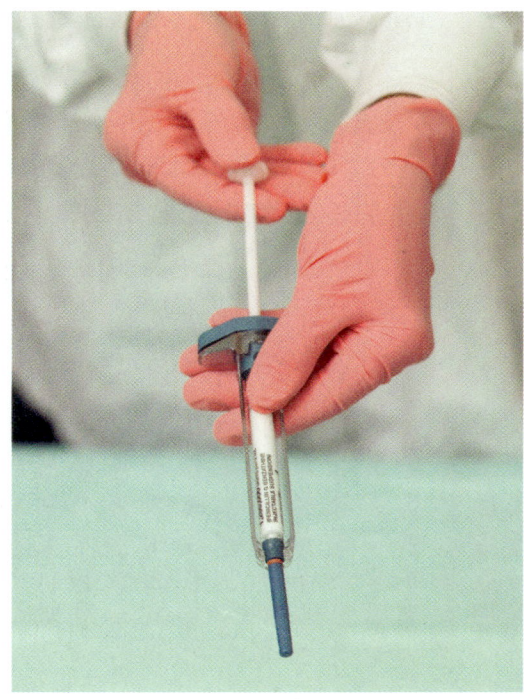

FIGURE 18-25B   Secure the needle by twisting it clockwise.

Each type of injection must be given at a specific angle in order for the medication to be absorbed properly. Figure 18-26 illustrates the proper angles used for the different types of injections.

18-4  Reconstitute a Powder Medication

PURPOSE: To add a diluent to a powdered medication in a vial, preparing it for administration.

EQUIPMENT: Powdered medication, diluent, two sterile needles and syringes, alcohol wipes, disposable gloves, and sharps container.

PERFORMANCE OBJECTIVE: Using the proper equipment and supplies, demonstrate the appropriate technique for reconstituting a powdered medication.

1. Wash hands.

2. Assemble the needle and syringe units.

3. Remove the tops from the diluent and powder medication vials, and clean the rubber stopper with an alcohol swab.

4. Insert the needle through the rubber stopper of the diluent and aspirate the proper amount.

5. Insert the needle into the rubber stopper of the powdered medication and inject the diluent.

6. Remove the needle from the top of the vial and discard it in a sharps container.

7. Gently roll the vial of medication between your hands to thoroughly mix it.

8. The vial of prepared medication must be labeled with the following information: strength, date and time of preparation, your initials, and the expiration date of the medication.

9. Use a second sterile needle to withdraw the medication for administration.

10. Wash hands.

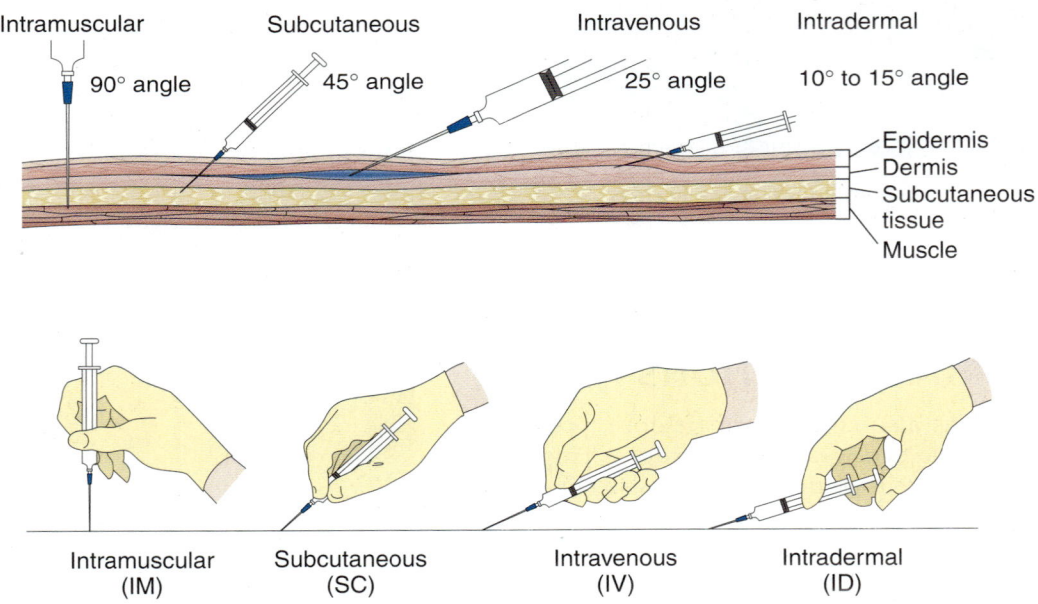

FIGURE 18-26 Angles of injection with appropriate needles for types of injection

You can relieve the patient's anxiety by explaining the procedure. Being honest with patients is most important. In the case of children's immunizations, for example, it is far better to explain that the injection will hurt for a minute than to say it will not. You may give the child a simplified explanation of the disease for which the immunization is meant. This may help the child understand how it is really better in the long run to hurt for a minute rather than suffer the dreaded disease. If the child shows extreme apprehension, it is advisable to have assistance in restraining the child before proceeding with the injection. Instructing parents in how they can explain injections to their children can be helpful. Some pharmaceutical companies provide badges of courage or other awards to pediatric patients who display bravery in receiving their immunization injections. This gives the child a sense of pride in good behavior and makes future visits much easier for all concerned.

Authorization forms should be in order before immunizations are administered to minors. You should allow sufficient time for parents (or those responsible for the child) to read the information regarding the vaccine and have all questions answered before obtaining the authorization signature. This form must be filed in the patient's chart.

The site to be injected should be free from restrictive clothing. Patients should be asked to remove these items of clothing while the medication is being prepared.

Follow correct gloving procedure before you begin to administer the injection. Proper preparation of the skin at the site of injection is necessary before and after injecting the medication, because microorganisms can enter the body through a break in the skin. Alcohol is the antiseptic usually used, because it is least irritating to the skin and is economical.

Proper disposal of used needles and syringes is also of vital importance in preventing possible accidents to the medical and custodial staff of the facility and avoiding transmission of disease. Disposable syringes and needles should be used only once and discarded properly. Keep the needle guard on the needle until just before you are ready to administer the injection. (Again, this is a situation where recapping a needle may be necessary. Remember to scoop the cap onto the needle; do not use your other hand, or you risk a needle stick, besides risking contamination of the needle before it is to be used for injecting the patient.) Afterward dispose of the entire syringe and needle intact in the biohazardous sharps container according to Standard Precautions recommendations. *Do not recap.* Remove latex or vinyl gloves before hand washing.

Intradermal Injections

Intradermal (ID) injections are used in allergy and tuberculin testing. The intradermal injection is administered just under the surface of the skin with a fine-gauge needle (26G or 27G). The bevel of the needle should be facing upward so that the substance will be expelled into the dermis. The needle is generally $\frac{3}{8}$ to $\frac{5}{8}$ inch in length, and the angle of the insertion into the skin is 10 to 15 degrees (Figure 18-27). The sites for this

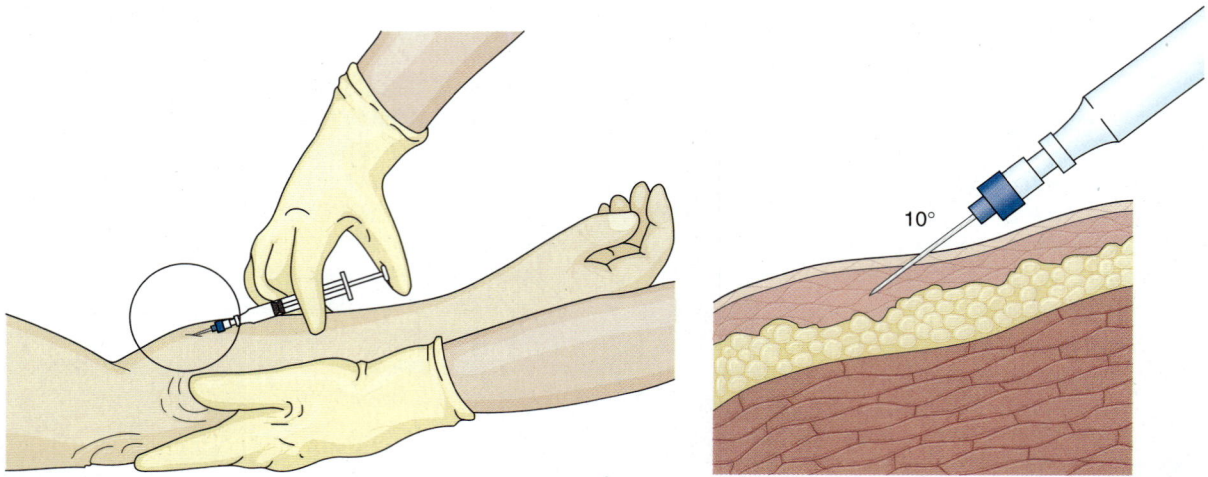

FIGURE 18-27 Intradermal injection

type of injection are usually the anterior forearm and the mid-back area. Proper positioning of patients is vital for accuracy of results and for the patient's comfort. Make sure the patient's forearm is supported on the treatment table and that the patient is sitting comfortably, or have the patient lie down on the treatment table.

A small wheal should develop at the site of the injection to give evidence that the medication is in the dermal layer of the skin. Very small amounts of medication, from 0.01 to 0.05 mL, are administered by this method of injection. The speed of the reaction and the size of the wheal should be recorded. The patient should be watched carefully and any reaction reported to the physician at once; however, most allergy testing is performed under the direct supervision of the physician. The patient must be observed for 20 minutes or more after the injection is administered. In the event of a hypersensitive reaction, a preparation of epinephrine may be injected by order of the physician. Refer to Procedure 18-5 for administering intradermal injections.

PROCEDURE PROCEDURE PROCEDURE PROCEDURE PROCEDURE PROCEDURE PROCEDURE

18-5  Administer an Intradermal Injection

PURPOSE: To inject liquid solutions of 0.01 mL and 0.05 mL into the dermal layer of tissue for allergy and immunity testing of patients.

EQUIPMENT: Medication (sterile water for injection in vial/ampule), cotton balls, adhesive bandage (or hypoallergenic tape), sterile needle and syringe (needle is usually ³⁄₈ to ⁵⁄₈ inch in length and 25G to 27G), medication tray, alcohol prep, patient's chart, pen, and latex or vinyl gloves.

PERFORMANCE OBJECTIVE: Provided with all necessary equipment and supplies, demonstrate each of the steps required in administering an intradermal injection; three injections will be administered to a latex training arm with the instructor observing each step. The dosage amount will be determined by the instructor each time.

1. Wash and glove hands. **CAUTION:** Be extremely careful when using the "scoop" method for recapping the needle by always placing the hand you are not using behind your back, so you will not be tempted to help with the procedure. Prepare the syringe with the ordered amount of medication. Replace the needle guard by carefully scooping it onto the needle. **NOTE: Read the label of the medication, and compare it with the order.**

2. Place the medication tray near the patient. Compare the medication order with the patient's chart, identify the patient, and explain the procedure.

3. Use an alcohol prep to clean the injection site (Figure 18-28A). Allow the alcohol to air dry. Do not blow on the area to dry it. **RATIONALE: The area may be contaminated by microorganisms in the exhaled air.**

(continues)

PROCEDURE PROCEDURE PROCEDURE PROCEDURE PROCEDURE PROCEDURE PROCEDURE PROCEDURE

18-5  Administer an Intradermal Injection (Continued)

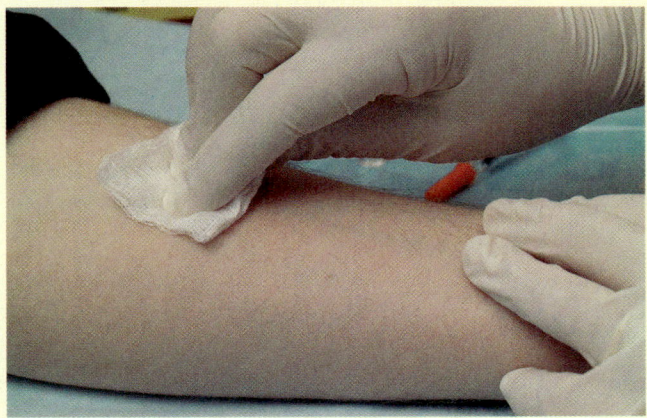

FIGURE 18-28A   Cleanse the site with an alcohol swab. Allow the area to air dry.

4. Remove the needle guard. Hold the patient's skin taut between your thumb and fingers to steady the area to be injected. With your other hand, insert the needle at a 10- to 15-degree angle of insertion and slowly expel the medication from the syringe by depressing the plunger (Figures 18-28B and C). **NOTE: Bevel of needle should be up; this allows the material to produce a wheal by infiltrating the dermal layer of the skin.**

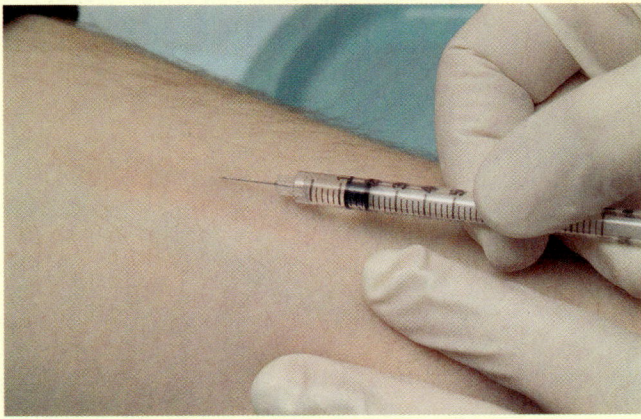

FIGURE 18-28B   Hold the patient's skin taut between your thumb and fingers and insert the needle at a 10- to 15-degree angle.

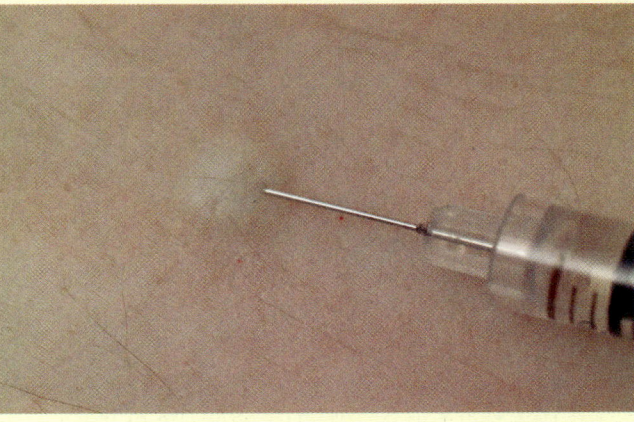

FIGURE 18-28C   Slowly inject the medication by depressing the plunger. A small wheal should develop at the site of the injection.

5. Remove the needle quickly by the same angle of insertion and wipe the site with a cotton ball. **NOTE: Do not massage the injection site. RATIONALE: Massaging distributes the material throughout the tissues.**

6. Observe the patient and time the reaction. Give the patient instructions as ordered, and answer any questions. Determine whether patient is allergic to adhesive before applying a bandage. Hypoallergenic tape is recommended if so.

7. Discard disposable items and gloves into a biohazardous waste bag. (Place the entire syringe and needle intact into the biohazardous sharps container according to Standard Precautions recommendations. If using a click-in-place shield/cover over the used needle, secure the cover and drop the entire needle and syringe intact into the biohazard sharps container. Wash hands. Return the medication and tray to the proper storage area.

8. Record information.

CHARTING EXAMPLE

7-21-XX

0.1 mL ID (intradermal) L forearm MSTA (Mumps Skin Test Antigen) Pt advised to have site evaluated within 48–72 hours

S. Davis, RMA

Subcutaneous Injections

Subcutaneous (sub q) injections are used to administer small doses of medication, usually not more than 2 mL. The injection is most often given in the upper outer part of the arm (deltoid area), abdominal area, or upper thigh (midvastus lateralis area) (Figure 18-29). The length of the needle ranges from ½ to ⅝ inch and the gauge from 25G to 27G. Subcutaneous injections are administered at a 45-degree angle of insertion. (See Procedure 18-6.) Many medications, including allergy injections, insulin, and immunizations are administered by the subcutaneous method. Refer to Chapter 16, Unit 1, for specific details in giving allergy injections. The patient should be asked to sit or lie on the treatment table for safety.

Intramuscular Injections

As the name suggests, **intramuscular (IM)** injections are placed into muscle tissue. The most common sites for this method of injection are the deltoid (up-

per outer arm), gluteus medius (upper outer portion of the hip), ventrogluteal (lateral outside portion of the hip), and vastus lateralis (midportion of the thigh) (Figures 18-30A to D).

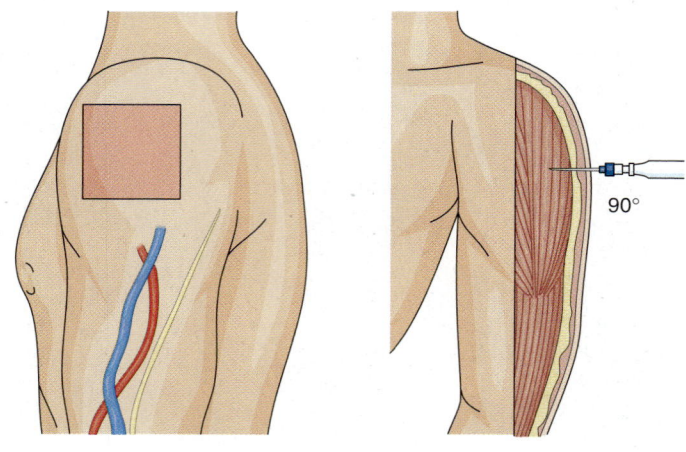

FIGURE 18-30A   IM site: Deltoid

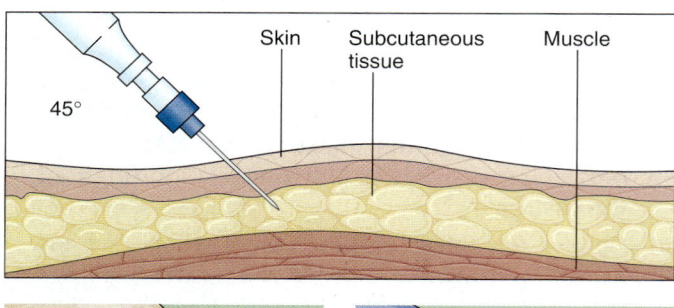

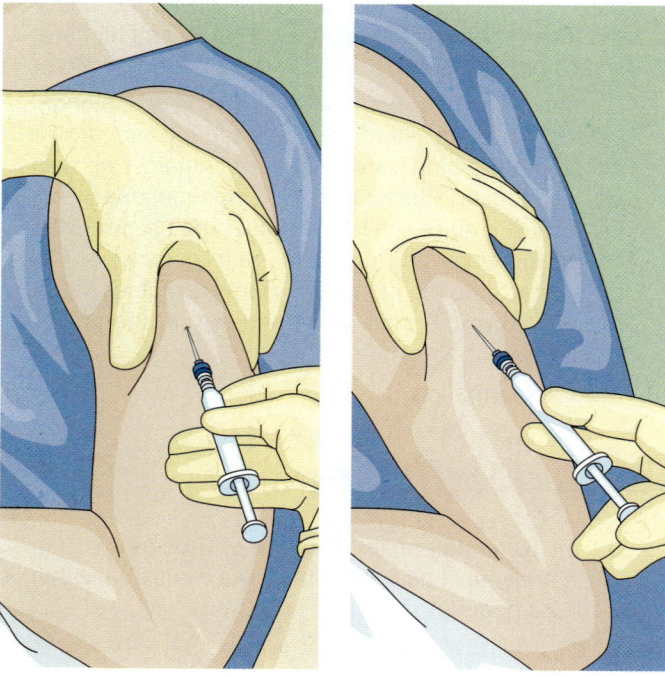

FIGURE 18-29   Subcutaneous injection

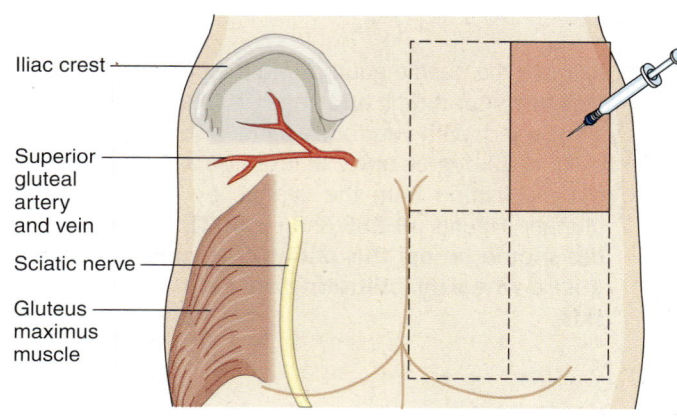

FIGURE 18-30B   IM site: Gluteus medius

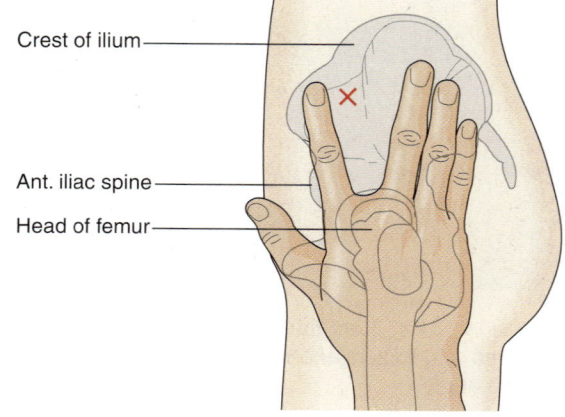

FIGURE 18-30C   IM site: Ventrogluteal

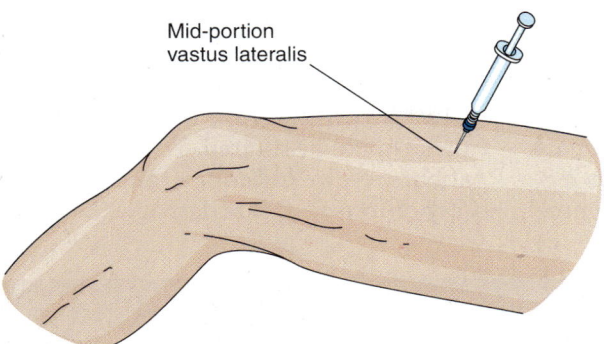

Mid-portion
vastus lateralis

FIGURE 18-30D   IM site: Vastus lateralis

PROCEDURE PROCEDURE PROCEDURE PROCEDURE PROCEDURE PROCEDURE PROCEDURE PROCEDURE

18-6  Administer a Subcutaneous Injection

PURPOSE: To inject aqueous solutions of 0.5 to 2.0 mL into the subcutaneous tissue.

EQUIPMENT: Medication (sterile water for injection in vial or ampule), alcohol preps, adhesive bandage (hypoallergenic tape), sterile needle and syringe (needle is usually $^1/_2$ to $^5/_8$ inch, 25G), and latex or vinyl gloves.

PERFORMANCE OBJECTIVE: Provided with all necessary equipment and supplies, demonstrate each of the steps required in administering a subcutaneous injection. Three injections will be administered to a latex training arm with the instructor observing each step. The dosage amount will be determined by the instructor each time.

1. Compare the medication with the physician's order and wash and glove hands. **CAUTION:** Prepare syringe and place it on the medication tray.

2. Compare the medication order with the patient's chart, identify the patient, explain the procedure, and ask the patient to remove clothing if necessary.

3. Use an alcohol prep to clean the injection site. Remove the needle guard.

4. Bunch the patient's skin between the thumb and finger of one hand, and with the other hand hold the syringe securely.

5. Insert the needle at a 45-degree angle with a steady penetration. Let go of the patient's skin.

6. With one hand, hold the barrel of the syringe while pulling back on the plunger slightly with the other hand to make sure a blood vessel has not been penetrated. If no blood appears in the syringe, proceed by slowly pushing down on the plunger to expel medication into tissues. **NOTE: If blood appears in the syringe, pull the needle out carefully at the angle of entry. Discard the medication, syringe, and needle. Replace with a new syringe and medication.**

RATIONALE: Blood in the needle indicates the possibility of the needle placement being within a blood vessel. Medication injected directly into the bloodstream causes rapid absorption and may cause undesirable as well as dangerous results.

7. Pull the needle out at the angle of insertion, wipe the injection site with a cotton ball, and gently massage the area. **RATIONALE: Massaging the site helps distribute medication throughout the tissue.**

8. Observe the patient for a possible reaction and report to the physician if a reaction occurs. Be sure that the patient is comfortable and can easily be observed by a member of the health care team in case of a reaction. Extra caution must be taken when giving desensitizing allergy injections. Reactions may take 15 to 20 minutes to develop. Instruct the patient to wait for a full 20 minutes in case of a possible reaction. Answer any questions. Determine whether the patient is allergic to adhesive before applying a bandage. Hypoallergenic tape is recommended if so.

9. Discard all used disposable items. (Place the entire syringe and needle in a sharps container. If using a click-in-place shield/cover over a used needle, secure the cover and drop the entire needle and syringe intact into the biohazard sharps container.) Remove gloves, and wash hands. Return the medication and tray to the proper storage area.

10. Record information.

CHARTING EXAMPLE

7-28-XX

0.6 mL sub q Rt arm Allergy serum advised to wait for 20 min to be evaluated before leaving

S. Davis, RMA

Proper positioning of patients is important. For injections in the deltoid area, the patient should be sitting. If the site is the gluteus muscle, ask the patient to lie in prone position on the treatment table with the toes pointed inward or to lean over the treatment table and stand on the non-injection-site leg. This will allow the muscle to relax and make the procedure much easier. For injection of the vastus lateralis site, the patient may be sitting or lying in the horizontal recumbent position.

The site of injection must be recorded so that injection sites can be rotated. This practice is necessary when patients receive injections routinely to reduce the possibility of muscle tissue damage. (See Procedure 18-7.)

PROCEDURE PROCEDURE PROCEDURE PROCEDURE PROCEDURE PROCEDURE PROCEDURE

18-7  Administer an Intramuscular Injection

PURPOSE: To inject large amounts of medication, 0.5 mL to 3.0 mL, and oil-based substances or irritating solutions that are more easily tolerated in the muscle tissue.

EQUIPMENT: Medication (sterile water for injection in vial or ampule), cotton balls, alcohol preps, adhesive bandage (or hypoallergenic tape), sterile needle and syringe (needle usually is 1 to 3 inches length, 18G to 23G), medication tray, patient's chart, pen, and latex or vinyl gloves.

PERFORMANCE OBJECTIVE: Provided with all necessary equipment and supplies, demonstrate each of the steps required in administering an intramuscular injection. Three injections will be administered to a latex training arm with the instructor observing each step. The dosage amount will be determined by the instructor each time.

1. Wash and glove hands. **CAUTION:** Prepare the syringe with the ordered amount of medication. Replace the needle guard by the scoop method. Place the medication on the tray. **NOTE: Read the label of the medication and compare it with the order.**

2. Compare the medication order with the patient's chart. Identify the patient and explain the procedure. Ask the patient to remove any clothing if necessary.

3. Use an alcohol prep to clean the injection site. **NOTE: Allow the alcohol to dry. Remove the needle guard.**

4. Secure a large area of skin (to accommodate the large amount of medication) between the thumb and fingers of one hand. With the other hand, grasp the syringe midway as you would a dart and hold it over the site at 90-degree angle. Insert the needle quickly with a firm and steady action. **NOTE: Avoid force when injecting to keep bruising to a minimum.** Pull back the plunger to make sure a blood vessel has not been penetrated. If no blood is seen in the barrel of the syringe, proceed by pushing down on the plunger and expelling the medication into the muscle. **NOTE: If blood appears in the syringe barrel, pull out the needle at the angle of insertion. Discard the syringe, needle, and medication and begin again with a new syringe and medication. RATIONALE: Blood in the needle indicates the possibility of the needle placement being within a blood vessel. Medication injected directly into the bloodstream causes rapid absorption and may cause undesirable and dangerous results.**

5. Pull the needle out at the angle of insertion carefully and quickly. Wipe the injection site with a cotton ball, and gently massage the area. **RATIONALE: Massaging the site helps distribute the medication throughout the tissue.**

6. Observe the patient for any reaction, and report to the physician if needed. Determine whether the patient is allergic to adhesive before applying a bandage. Hypoallergenic tape is recommended if so.

7. Discard disposable items. (Place the entire syringe and needle in a sharps container. If using a click-in-place shield/cover over the used needle, secure the cover and drop the entire needle and syringe intact into the biohazard sharps container.) Wash and sterilize reusable items, remove gloves, and wash hands. Return the medication and tray to the proper storage area.

8. Record information.

CHARTING EXAMPLE

12-4-XX

1,000 units/kg Sterile Bacitracin IM (intramuscular) Rt hip

Parent advised to wait with child for 20 min to be evaluated before leaving

J. Watkins, CMA

When administering IM injections, the needle is 1 to 3 inches in length or longer, in order to penetrate many layers of tissue. The angle of injection is 90 degrees. IM injections are indicated when large doses of medication or oil-based, non-water based, or thicker medications must be given. Dosage may vary from 0.5 to 3.0 mL. Medications given by the IM method are absorbed quickly by the rich blood supply of the muscle tissue.

The gauge of the needle ranges between 18G and 23G to accommodate the density of the substance. In giving injections intramuscularly to pediatric patients, the gauge and length of the needle may be smaller.

For injecting substances that may be irritating or may cause discoloration of the subcutaneous tissues, the **Z-track IM** method is used. Tissue is displaced by holding it to the side of the injection site. Following injection of the medication, the tissue is moved back over the site, blocking any residual substance. Using this technique prevents the medication from following the path of the needle and leaking out into the tissues. (Refer to Procedure 18-8.) After Z-track IM administration, the injection site should *not* be massaged, because this action would encourage the irritating substance to circulate into the subcutaneous tissues.

PROCEDURE PROCEDURE PROCEDURE PROCEDURE PROCEDURE PROCEDURE PROCEDURE PROCEDURE

18-8 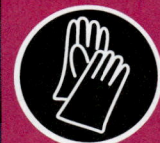 Administer an Intramuscular Injection by the Z-Track Method

PURPOSE: To inject substances (which may be irritating or discoloring to the tissues) deep into the muscle layer of tissue. Some substances would cause tissue discoloration and irritation if given in the subcutaneous tissues from leakage in following the path of the needle when administered. The site of injection is in the gluteal muscle of the buttocks (upper outer quadrant; for some medications the deltoid muscle may be used). Dose is from 0.5 mL to 3.0 mL.

EQUIPMENT: Medication (sterile water for injection in vial/ampule), cotton balls, alcohol preps, adhesive bandage (or hypoallergenic tape), sterile needle and syringe (needle usually is 2 to 3 inches, 19G to 21G), sterile gauze square, medication tray, patient's chart, pen, and latex or vinyl gloves.

PERFORMANCE OBJECTIVE: Provided with all necessary equipment and supplies, demonstrate each of the steps required in administering a Z-track intramuscular injection using a clinical mannequin. Three injections will be administered with the instructor observing each step. The dosage will be determined by the instructor.

1–3. Same as for intramuscular injection.

4. Use a gauze square to securely hold the patient's skin at the injection site to one side to displace skin and tissues until the injection is completed. Insert the needle into the gluteal muscle of the buttocks or deltoid at a 90-degree angle, holding the syringe as you would a dart. The first and second fingers may be used to aspirate while the thumb and ring finger hold the syringe near the needle end. If no blood is seen in the barrel of the syringe, proceed by expelling the medication into the muscle. Wait a few seconds before removing the needle. **NOTE: If blood is seen in the barrel of the syringe, pull the needle out quickly at angle of the insertion.** Discard the syringe, needle, and medication, and begin again with a new syringe and medication. **RATIONALE: Blood in the needle indicates the possibility of the needle placement being within a blood vessel. Medication injected directly into the bloodstream causes rapid absorption and may cause undesirable and dangerous results. NOTE: Read the package insert of the medication carefully. There may be additional instructions for certain medications.** Some Z-track injection instructions suggest that 0.5 mL of air be in the syringe to follow the medication to prevent leakage from the needle track.

5. Pull the needle out at the angle of insertion and let go of the skin quickly so that displaced tissue will cover the needle track and prevent it from leaking into the surrounding subcutaneous tissues. Cover the injection site with a cotton ball, and hold it in place for a few seconds. **NOTE: Do not massage the area. RATIONALE: Massage causes distribution of the medication, which is undesirable with Z-track injections because of the tissue-irritating properties of the medication.**

6–8. Same as for intramuscular injection.

ADMINISTERING INJECTIONS TO INFANTS AND SMALL CHILDREN

Injections that are given to infants and small children need special attention. The size of the child's arm or leg will help you decide the size of the underlying muscle, which determines the needle length appropriate for the muscle thickness. The gauge of the needle is determined by the viscosity of the medication. The vastus lateralis is the preferred injection site for infants and young children. You must be sure to aspirate between 5 and 10 seconds (tiny blood vessels take time to flow) before injecting the medication to prevent entering a blood vessel, which would be critical in a child. If you do enter a blood vessel while aspirating, you must withdraw the needle and start over. For injecting the left vastus lateralis, place your palm on the head of the femur (see Figure 18-30D) so that your index finger points to the crest of the ilium; then, spread your fingers so that your index finger and your great finger form a "V." Lightly prepare the tissue with an alcohol prep, and proceed with assistance in holding the child during the procedure. Administer the injection carefully in the center of the "V" by holding the tissue between your thumb and finger to secure the site to be injected.

You must tell the child what you are going to do and include that it may hurt for a few seconds. Explain to a child who can understand that holding still will help you do it quicker and more easily and will keep it from hurting as much. Always ask the parent or caregiver to help hold the child to prevent an undue injury during the injection procedure. Try to distract the baby or child with a story, a toy, or other amusement to keep them from feeling the discomfort. You can ask the parent or caregiver who is holding the child to reposition the child immediately after you are finished with the injection to further distract her from what just happened. You can quickly talk to the child in a pleasant tone and with a smiling face. When this tactic is orchestrated, tears are often very short-lived. Keeping the child's mind off the discomfort is the key. Offer the child a token of appreciation for the cooperation you received. For instance, tell the child "thank you" for helping give the medicine to keep him from getting sick. Many offices give stickers and other small rewards. For a child who is very apprehensive and unruly, you must ask for help in securing the child's position or possible injury could result to the child or others. Restraint is in the best interest of all to prevent a dangerous situation.

Discourage parents and other caregivers from threatening children who are misbehaving with "getting a shot from the doctor." Explain to those who use this threat that the child will be afraid of health care professionals and that it makes your job more difficult when children come in for immunizations and other

PATIENT EDUCATION

It is vitally important that all patients who self-administer injections are instructed properly in safety regarding storage, use, and disposal of used syringes and needles. The medical assistant must stress that all of these materials must be kept safely out of reach of children. The potential danger of used and discarded needles must be stressed to avoid possible accidents. Remind patients not to remove the needle from the barrel of the syringe after use. Provide patients with a sharps containers. Advise patients to keep these containers in a safe place at home and to return them to their medical facility when they return so the medical assistant can dispose of them properly. Having patients follow this safety procedure will help avoid unnecessary punctures to the skin. This is an especially important precaution for diabetics, who are prone to develop infections from such punctures.

It is also of vital importance to remind the diabetic patient to record daily blood glucose levels, ketone test results, and the dosage amount of insulin. Impress on the patient how important it is to bring this record to the next appointment for the physician to review. This daily information, along with an interview, examination, and laboratory findings, help the physician to make adjustments as necessary in the treatment plan for each patient.

procedures. Ask them to please refrain from this means of discipline.

Intravenous Injections

The **intravenous**, or **IV**, method of injection is used by the physician, usually in an emergency situation. You are not qualified to administer medications by this method but may prepare medications to be given intravenously. IV medications have an immediate effect on the patient because they are introduced directly into the bloodstream. Needles are 1 to 1½ inches in length and are usually 20G to 21G. Intravenous preparations vary in amount from a few mL to much larger doses, which are given by IV drip. The items needed are needle and syringe, medication, tourniquet, alcohol preps, an adhesive bandage, and IV stand if necessary.

Usually you will draw up medication in the syringe for an intravenous injection. After filling the syringe, be sure to carefully recap the needle by the scoop method to avoid contaminating the needle. Then place the vial or ampule on the medication tray so that the physician can check to be certain it is correct. You may be asked to stay with the patient while waiting for the emergency squad or ambulance to transport the patient to the hospital. Observing the patient for signs of distress and reactions to the administered medication is an important responsibility. The physician must be notified immediately of any complications. All information should be recorded on the patient's chart.

PRINCIPLES OF IV THERAPY

Since medical assistants are so versatile, they sometimes work in outpatient infusion centers. Whether the facility is an emergency room, a cancer center, a dialysis clinic, or a physician's office, the medical assistant must be familiar with the purpose and process of infusion therapy. Depending on the specific facility's protocols, medical assistants can insert, monitor, and remove intravenous supplies. It is therefore vitally important that the medical assistant understand the reasons for the infusion therapy, the advantages and disadvantages of intravenous therapy, the potential complications, the proper insertion and infusion techniques, the equipment and supplies to be used, and the appropriate delivery, care, maintenance, and discontinuation of infusion therapy.

The role of the medical assistant will vary depending on the facility. Always be sure to check what the laws of their state are, because they relate to whether medical assistants can participate in intravenous (IV) or infusion therapy. All facilities should have a policy manual delineating exactly what role medical assistants will play in IV therapy. Even if the facility will not allow medical assistants to insert or remove IV lines, the medical assistant should be familiar with how to assess the patient for adverse complications of IV therapy.

As with any invasive procedure, it is very important to practice Standard Precautions when working with patients on IV therapy, because there is increased opportunity for infection transmission. Since the IV equipment dwells in the patient for a while, the patient may develop allergies to latex, medical tape, or even the iodine preparations. The medical assistant must be careful to change the sites and equipment according to office protocols and to assess each patient on IV therapy for signs and symptoms of infection.

Indications for Infusion Therapy

Even though infusion therapy places the patient at risk for infection and other complications, sometimes the intravenous route is ordered because it gives good, long-term access for infusion of medications, fluids, electrolytes, blood and blood products, and nutritional supplements. Additionally, a dehydrated patient may need fluid volume replacement and maintenance. One other advantage to having an indwelling line in the patient is that it facilitates access for multiple purposes such as phlebotomy, medication administration, as well as hydration.

Advantages of Infusion Therapy

Intravenous (IV), or infusion, therapy is considered when other access methods are not as appropriate. Absorption is immediate. Distribution of medications is faster, which maximizes bioavailability. Medications can be injected immediately into the bloodstream, without waiting for gastrointestinal processing or absorption from muscle or fat. Fluids can be administered into the bloodstream for increased blood pressure, hydration, or electrolyte replenishment. Access to a vein in an emergency is immediate, as veins can sometimes collapse. Antidotes and medications to reduce the effects of other medications can be quickly administered. The unconscious patient or the patient who cannot swallow can benefit from the passive treatment through IV therapy. If the gastrointestinal system must be rested, as with inflammatory bowel disease, the patient can still be nourished. Intravenous therapy can maintain a tighter control of blood levels of electrolytes because it is not dependent on absorption through the gastrointestinal, integumentary, or musculoskeletal systems. The equipment dwells in the patient and does not have to be inserted several times, which saves time for the medical assistant and usually is more comfortable for the patient.

Disadvantages of Infusion Therapy

Although there is usually only slight local discomfort from the IV therapy equipment, there are some more serious disadvantages to IV therapy. The fluid can lead fluid outside the vein into the surrounding tissue, known as infiltration. The needle can dislodge or the catheter can displace. A clot or thrombus can form, creating thrombosis. A solid, liquid, or gas can travel into the circulatory system, which is called an embolism. The patient can have an allergic or hypersensitivity reaction. Improper technique can cause transmission of hepatitis, HIV, and other diseases. The IV therapy can introduce microbes that can cause a systemic infection, known as sepsis. Too much fluid administered can cause fluid overload. Although medications can be administered rapidly by IV, this increases the possibility of overdose. Deposits can separate from a solution and create precipitation. Some medications are incompatible to be mixed with each other.

Preparations for IV Therapy

A variety of preparations are available for IV therapy. The medical assistant must be very careful to select the preparation that the physician ordered. Infusates are classified as crystalloids, which form crystals, and colloids, which are glutinous and do not form true solutions. Crystalloids are usually electrolyte solutions that are isotonic, hypotonic, or hypertonic. Colloid infusions raise colloid osmotic pressure.

A variety of infusions are administered to patients to supplement caloric intake, provide water, promote renal output, and supply nutrients. Common hydrating solutions include sodium chloride 0.45%, dextrose 2.5% in 0.45% saline, dextrose 5% in water, dextrose 5% in 0.45% saline, and dextrose 5% in 0.2% saline. Isotonic infusates, those equal to the normal fluids in the body, are 0.9% sodium chloride (NaCl), also called normal saline solution (NSS), and 5% dextrose. Hypotonic solutions have less serum osmolality by causing fluid to shift out of the blood into the cells. These would be used to hydrate dehydrated cells. For example, 2.5% dextrose and 0.45% NSS are hypotonic solutions. Hypertonic solutions cause fluid to shift out of the cells and into the blood. Hypertonic solutions include 3.0% NaCl or 10% dextrose in water. These would reduce edema or introduce sugar into the cells.

Patient Preparation and Site Selection

If unsure of where to place the IV, the wise medical assistant will review anatomy and physiology before beginning IV therapy. If not comfortable starting an IV, the medical assistant should not do it; rather, another colleague should be asked to place the IV and further training should be requested from the facility. There is significant risk to the patient if an IV is not inserted, assessed, or removed properly. The medical assistant has a duty to the patient to perform the procedure properly.

Placement of an IV is not simply a technical skill. You are placing the cannula in a patient. Usually the patient will be anxious and may need to be comforted with information and professional behavior. Make sure the client is physically comfortable. Be sure that you safely follow the six rights (patient, drug, dose, route, time, procedure). Research any drugs with which you are not familiar before administrating them. Be careful not to mix incompatible drugs. Never give a medication or initiate IV therapy without consent from the patient or adult responsible for the patient, because to do so is assault and battery.

Place the IV in the best possible site for the patient. Use the distal veins in the upper extremities first. Palpate the veins prior to venipuncture, using the vein appropriate for the prescribed infusate. Use larger veins for irritating and hypertonic preparations. Place the IV in a site that will sustain the infusion for 48 to 72 hours. Remember that the arm may need to be stabilized with a board if the patient is active. Always use the smallest cannula that will deliver the prescribed infusate. Do not use irritated or sclerosed veins on locations of flexure. Do not use a tourniquet on fragile veins. Do not use an extremity that is on the side of the body where a radical mastectomy has been performed, that is impaired after a stroke, that is partially amputated, or that has third-degree burns. Never use an arteriovenous fistula, shunt, or graft for peripheral infusion therapy—they are only for hemodialysis.

Good sites include the metacarpals, cephalic, accessory cephalic, median cephalic (antecubital), basilic, median basilic, median cubital, or median antecubital.

Equipment and Supplies

Although some facilities still use glass containers for IV fluid, the most popular way to infuse intravenous infusates is from plastic containers, flexible or semirigid. These plastic containers are then spiked and attached to infusate administration sets. Do not spike the container until you are ready to infuse it to the patient. Store containers away from light if possible. Once you spike the container, you will need to infuse the fluid or dispose of it, because it cannot be reused once spiked.

Infusate is then administered through an administration set, which includes the following features: a piercing pin to spike the bag, a drip chamber to control the drip rate, a clamp to close or control the flow, an injection port to add medication, and a clamp to open or close the flow prior to the luer slip, which attaches to the cannula. The administration set is attached to the bag of infusate and the patient.

Squeeze the drip chamber to induce the fluid to begin passing through the tubing. Macrodrip tubing will allow larger drops at a slower rate, but microdrip tubing will allow smaller drops to flow at a faster rate. Be sure to have the clamp closed or the fluid will pass quickly through the set and out on the floor.

Controlling the fluid passage, allow a few drops of fluid to flow out of the line into a trash can and clamp the flow off. The set is then primed to attach to the cannula in the patient.

The drop factor is the number of drops needed to deliver 1 mL of fluid. It is based on the diameter of the administration tubing and is clearly marked on the administration set package. You will need to calculate the drop factor when determining the infusion rate, or a computerized pump may do it for you once you program the administration set's drop factor into the computer.

The medical assistant must be sure to document, not only in the patient chart, but also on the label, what the infusate is and what time it was started. Always be sure to write clearly and take care not to smear the information.

Delivery, Care, Maintenance, and Discontinuation

The medical assistant should not attempt to start an IV line without training. Some courses are available at local colleges, but usually the medical assistant is trained by a more experienced professional in the facility where the medical assistant is employed. Ideally, the medical assistant should practice first on a training device and then perform a number of supervised sticks before being allowed to attach an IV line alone. Sometimes the facility will permit a medical assistant to lay out supplies and prime the tubing, but not do the phlebotomy. Medical assistants should be sure to check with the state and the facility to see what medical assistants are permitted to do where they work.

As with the administration of any medication, always check to be sure that you have all the information you need from the physician. The order for any infusion must include that date and time of day, infusate name, route of administration, volume to be infused, dosage of infusate, rate of infusion, duration of infusion, name of patient, and physician's signature. Be sure all this information is documented correctly in the patient record. Do not use abbreviations because of the increased chance of errors.

Many infusate names look similar, so be sure to get the correct bag of medication. Remember not only to get the correct drug name, but also the correct dosage. For example, 5% dextrose is not the same as 10% dextrose.

Before any invasive procedure, you must wash your hands. This is especially true before inserting a venous access device. Many infections could be prevented if medical assistants were faithful in always washing hands before inserting IVs.

The tourniquet allows for pooling of blood distal to the strapping and this facilitates the location of veins. However, it increases the blood pressure distal to it—which gives the patient some discomfort if left on too long. The tourniquet can also provide a reservoir for microbes. If you are not using disposable tourniquets, be sure to disinfect them between patient use. Latex tourniquets can sensitize patients to latex allergies and should never be used with latex-allergic patients. Never apply a tourniquet so tightly that it obstructs arterial flow, nor leave it on longer than 4 to 6 minutes. Nerve damage can occur if you place the tourniquet on the patient for too long or wrap it too tightly. You should always be able to palpate a distal pulse.

To facilitate venous access, lower the extremity and allow gravity to aid in pulling the blood downward. Asking the patient to make a fist also distends the veins. You may also gently stroke the skin over the veins, especially if you rub with alcohol, to enhance friction. Some medical assistants tap the vein using the thumb and index finger to engorge the vein with blood. Applying warm compresses over the vein also increases blood flow. If applying one tourniquet does not distend the vein, try using several, placing them 2 to 3 inches apart. The transilluminator is also helpful.

Sometimes patient hair impedes the visualization of veins. Do not shave the hair, as this increases the chance of infection. Instead, gently cut it close to the skin.

Be especially cautious with patients who are receiving anticoagulation therapy. They are prone to bleed for extended periods of time. Avoid using tourniquets if possible, as these patients bruise easily. Also, be careful not to push as hard with antimicrobial preparations.

Patients with irritated, burned, or diseased skin are more vulnerable to trauma. Older patients and patients receiving corticosteroid therapy have delicate veins, so try not to use a tourniquet with these patients.

Patients with peripheral edema are sometimes difficult to obtain venous access on. Even if you are successful in inserting the cannula, the vessel may collapse from the oncotic pressure created by the edema. If an infiltration occurs, compartment syndrome can result. It is often difficult to visualize veins through the edema, but applying digital pressure can displace tissue pressure temporarily and allow for visualization.

Obese patients may have veins that are easy to see or deeply imbedded, depending on how the adipose tissue displaces them. Multiple tourniquets may be needed for successful venipuncture.

Always check for allergies to latex, tape, and iodine, and use caution with patients who may have been exposed repeatedly to these products. Latex reactions are more common in women, asthmatics, persons with histories of allergies, persons with occupational exposure to latex, persons with allergies to fruits and vegetables, patients who frequently are catheterized, and persons with histories of genitourinary or intra-abdominal surgeries. Use non-latex products, paper tape, and other antibacterial products on patients allergic to latex, tape, and iodine, respectively.

Before initiating infusion therapy, ensure that you have all the necessary equipment. Check the physician order for the correct infusate. Obtain the correct style of administration set for the patient's need. Ensure that you have the correct patient and that the patient is in a comfortable position.

Prepare for IV therapy as follows:

1. Wash your hands well.
2. Don gloves.
3. Select a vein.
4. Apply the tourniquet.
5. Clean the site.
6. The physician may apply anesthesia spray or cream, or give you an order to do so. Some patients prefer to have anesthesia on the site before phlebotomy.
7. Access the veins according to facility protocols.
8. Introduce the cannula further into the patient's vein and remove the needle.
9. Attach the primed line to the cannula.
10. Dispose of the needle in a sharps container.
11. Secure the IV site with dressings and tape.
12. Cover with a transparent dressing.
13. Ensure the patient's comfort.
14. Remove gloves.
15. Wash your hands.
16. Document the procedure.
17. Continue to observe the patient.

After placing the IV infusion, the medical assistant's commitment to the patient is not over. Besides documenting the start of the procedure, the medical assistant must continue to monitor the patient as long as the patient is in his or her care and document appropriately.

Document the date and time of insertion. Be specific about the location of the cannula. Include the brand name and style, gauge, and length of the device. Document the infusate administered. Record the method of infusion: gravity, electronic infusion device (list name brand and model number), and document the patient's response to the procedure. Always document according to the facility's policy.

Be familiar with the protocol for the equipment in the office. Read the instruction manual of the pumps. Keep current on trends in IV therapy. Be cautious when mixing any medications in IV lines.

When ordered to flush an indwelling IV port, ensure you have the correct patient. Wash your hands. Insert a syringe into the port and gently flush with saline, then the medication ordered, then the saline. Follow the facility's protocol for flushing lines.

Although the facility may not allow you to start IV therapy, they may encourage you to discontinue peripheral infusion lines. To do so, have gauze ready to apply pressure. Ensure you have the correct patient. Wash your hands and don gloves. Gently remove the cannula and apply pressure to the patient's site. When the patient's bleeding has stopped, apply a sterile bandage to the site. Dispose of the IV line according to the facility policy.

Rarely medical assistants are asked to give a bolus delivery of medication directly into the IV line. Use a straight needle and syringe and insert the needle into a port. Be sure that you are authorized to give an IV push. Always identify yourself to the physician ordering the IV push as a medical assistant, not a nurse. Once you have given a medication by IV push, you cannot retrieve it. Sometimes you cannot reverse it. For this reason, your facility may require a nurse to give an IV push or two medical assistants to check a medication before giving it IV push.

PREPARING AND INJECTING INSULIN

The medical assistant is often the one who will give instruction to the diabetic patient in the technique of self-administration of daily **insulin** injections. You may be of great help in demonstrating the proper method of filling a syringe, preparing the injection site, and acquiring skill in injecting the insulin. Generally, the physician teaches the patient initially about diet, dosage, and the different types of insulin. You may be delegated to do follow-up patient education in this area. Because the insulin-dependent diabetic patient must administer this injection at home to herself at least once each day, you should instruct the patient to follow a pattern of rotation of injection sites, an example of which is shown in Figure 18-31. Explain to the patient to number each area of the body that is injected each time in the boxes

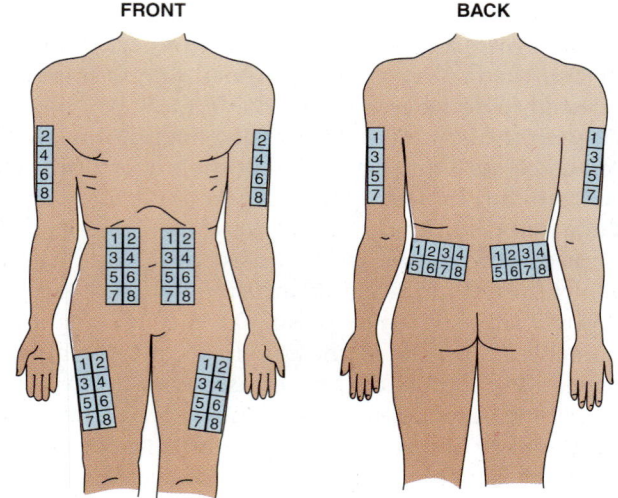

FIGURE 18-31   Possible sites and rotation for insulin administration

in an alternating rotation pattern. This method offers the patient the means to develop her own personal schedule. Printed patient education material for patients is available from most pharmaceutical companies to help patients gain an understanding of their diabetes. You may also want to refer patients to educational programs held at local hospitals or through the American Diabetes Association.

IMMUNITY

Our immune system responds immediately to the invasion of disease-causing microorganisms. If the exposure to the disease is slight and our susceptibility is low, our immune response may defend us from coming down with the disease itself. However, if we are susceptible to the disease, meaning our resistance is low, we develop the disease, experience the symptoms, and become sick. Antibodies are produced to protect us, making us resistant to further attacks of the specific pathogen that has made us sick. For instance, if you get mumps, the body produces antibodies to destroy the mumps-causing organisms. After recovery from the illness, antibodies against mumps will protect you from coming down with it again. This process is called *natural immunity*.

Artificial immunity is produced by administering **immunizations** or **vaccines** made from the dead or harmless infectious agents that trigger the immune response in the body to manufacture antibodies against the particular disease-causing agent.

TYPES OF VACCINES

Vaccines given to infants, children, and adults to protect against illnesses that can prove to be very serious are categorized according to the type of immune stimulation. The categories of vaccines include:

- Live attenuated (changed) pathogens: The pathogen itself is altered in some way by the manufacturer and then injected into the body, which stimulates the body to produce antibodies. Examples of this type of vaccine include varicella and measles.
- Pathogenic toxins: Some pathogenic organisms produce a poisonous substance known as a toxin, which will stimulate antibody production. Examples of this type of vaccine include diphtheria and tetanus.
- Killed pathogen: The pathogenic organism is rendered inactive and then injected into the body, which stimulates antibody production. This type of vaccine may require several doses to ensure lasting immunity. Examples of this type of vaccine include pertussis (whooping cough), rabies, and poliomyelitis.

IMMUNIZATION SCHEDULES

The recommended childhood and adolescent immunization schedule for the United States can be found in Figure 18-32. Immunization schedules may vary in other countries for infants, children, and adults. You should make sure before administering any immunization that the patient does not have an active illness or fever. If this is the case, the vaccine should be rescheduled for when the patient is well. Also, check the patient's health/medical history to be sure the patient has no past history of convulsions or allergies of any kind. If an allergy is known, bring it to the attention of the physician *before* the vaccine is administered. You may want to look the immunization up in a medications reference book for contraindications, precautions, and warnings. It is strongly advised that the parent/patient be made aware of the benefits and risks of all vaccines. Sufficient time should be given to the responsible person to read printed material after a verbal explanation is given regarding the vaccine(s). An opportunity must be provided for any questions of the parent/patient to be answered by the doctor before administration of immunization(s). When more than one dose of a vaccine is necessary to reach adequate immunization against a particular disease, such as the DPaT injections, it is referred to as a primary "**series**." Each of these should be given with at least 6 to 8 weeks between each dose within a reasonable period. The primary series requires a **booster** for the immunization to be most effective and complete.

DISEASE PROTECTION

In years past, diseases that people are now immunized against were dreadful illnesses that affected children and adults and often caused death. In the following text is a brief description of each of the diseases, the symptoms, the method of transmission, the **incubation** period, and its treatment. This is to help you in answering questions about the diseases in the immunization schedule when patients ask why they need to have

the vaccine. Certainly a few seconds or minutes (or even hours) of discomfort are well worth the minor suffering to gain protection from a potentially fatal disease.

The anatomy and physiology section of this text (Chapter 11) provides information regarding pneumonia and influenza, which are diseases affecting the respiratory system. A brief description follows.

Influenza   Commonly referred to as "the **flu**," **influenza** is a disease caused by a myxovirus that affects the respiratory tract. It is spread by direct contact, by droplet infection from the vapor of coughing and sneezing from an infected person, and by indirect contact from handling soiled items (such as used tissues) of the patient. The incubation period is between 1 and 4 days. Symptoms include sudden onset of fever, chills, sore throat, cough, muscle aches and pains, general malaise, and weakness. Treatment for the flu consists of bed rest, increased intake of fluids, antipyretics, and mild analgesics. Immunization against some strains of influenza is recommended for high-risk patients, such as the elderly and those with chronic illness, respiratory distress, or other conditions that warrant protection from infectious disease.

Pneumonia   Pneumonia is an acute inflammation of the lungs. Eighty-five percent of pneumonia cases are caused by the *pneumococcus* bacterium. Pneumonia may also be caused by other bacteria, a virus, rickettsiae, and fungi. The *pneumococcus* bacterium disease (pneumonitis) is spread by droplet infection and direct contact with an infected person. The incubation period is only a few hours after exposure to the bacteria. The symptoms are abrupt in onset and include severe chills, high fever, headache, chest pain, dyspnea, rapid pulse, cyanosis, and cough with blood-stained sputum. Bed rest; increased fluid intake; analgesics; antipyretics; and, in many cases, oxygen are necessary for successful treatment of the patient. Pneumovax is a vaccine to protect high-risk patients from contracting the disease generally. Only one immunization is required for life protection, although boosters may be considered after 10 years. Those age 65 and older are encouraged to get this vaccine.

Haemophilus Influenza Type B   Hemophilus or **haemophilus**, also known as **Hib** and **HIB**, is a disease caused by a small, gram-negative, nonmotile parasitic bacterium that leads to severe destructive inflammation of the larynx, trachea, and bronchi. The disease is transmitted by droplet airborne infection. Incubation is from 1 to 3 days. The symptoms are sudden onset of fever, sore throat, cough, muscle aches, weakness, and general malaise. General care is bed rest, increased fluid intake, antipyretics, antibiotics, and analgesics as necessary. Because this particular disease affects infants and small children, immunization is recommended to this population. Each year, this illness attacks one in every two hundred infants in the United States; the most at-risk

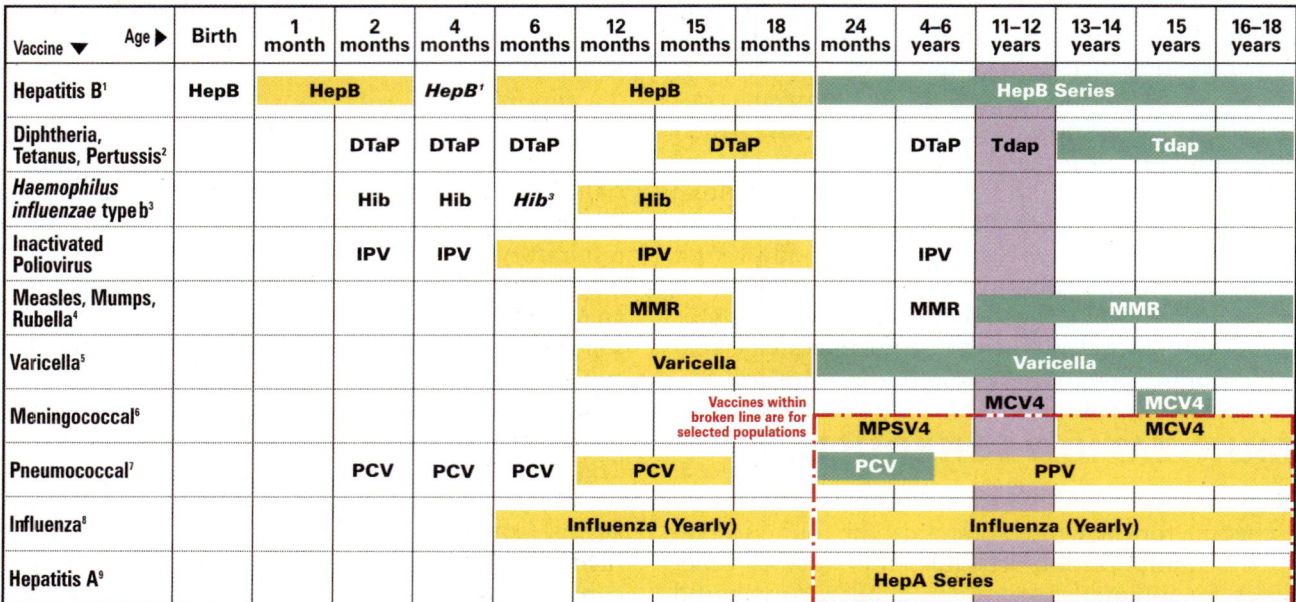

DEPARTMENT OF HEALTH AND HUMAN SERVICES • CENTERS FOR DISEASE CONTROL AND PREVENTION

Recommended Childhood and Adolescent Immunization Schedule UNITED STATES • 2006

Vaccine ▼ Age ►	Birth	1 month	2 months	4 months	6 months	12 months	15 months	18 months	24 months	4–6 years	11–12 years	13–14 years	15 years	16–18 years
Hepatitis B[1]	HepB	HepB		HepB[1]		HepB					HepB Series			
Diphtheria, Tetanus, Pertussis[2]			DTaP	DTaP	DTaP		DTaP			DTaP	Tdap	Tdap		
Haemophilus influenzae type b[3]			Hib	Hib	Hib[3]	Hib								
Inactivated Poliovirus			IPV	IPV		IPV				IPV				
Measles, Mumps, Rubella[4]						MMR				MMR		MMR		
Varicella[5]						Varicella					Varicella			
Meningococcal[6]											MCV4		MCV4	
									MPSV4			MCV4		
Pneumococcal[7]			PCV	PCV	PCV	PCV			PCV		PPV			
Influenza[8]					Influenza (Yearly)				Influenza (Yearly)					
Hepatitis A[9]						HepA Series								

Vaccines within broken line are for selected populations

This schedule indicates the recommended ages for routine administration of currently licensed childhood vaccines, as of December 1, 2005, for children through age 18 years. Any dose not administered at the recommended age should be administered at any subsequent visit when indicated and feasible. ▇ Indicates age groups that warrant special effort to administer those vaccines not previously administered. Additional vaccines may be licensed and recommended during the year. Licensed combination vaccines may be used whenever any components of the combination are indicated and other components of the vaccine are not contraindicated and if approved by the Food and Drug Administration for that dose of the series. Providers should consult the respective ACIP statement for detailed recommendations. Clinically significant adverse events that follow immunization should be reported to the Vaccine Adverse Event Reporting System (VAERS). Guidance about how to obtain and complete a VAERS form is available at www.vaers.hhs.gov or by telephone, 800-822-7967.

▇ Range of recommended ages   ▇ Catch-up immunization   ▇ 11–12 year old assessment

1. Hepatitis B vaccine (HepB). *AT BIRTH:* All newborns should receive monovalent HepB soon after birth and before hospital discharge. **Infants born to mothers who are HBsAg-positive** should receive HepB and 0.5 mL of hepatitis B immune globulin (HBIG) within 12 hours of birth. **Infants born to mothers whose HBsAg status is unknown** should receive HepB within 12 hours of birth. The mother should have blood drawn as soon as possible to determine her HBsAg status; if HBsAg-positive, the infant should receive HBIG as soon as possible (no later than age 1 week). **For infants born to HBsAg-negative mothers,** the birth dose can be delayed in rare circumstances but only if a physician's order to withhold the vaccine and a copy of the mother's original HBsAg-negative laboratory report are documented in the infant's medical record. *FOLLOWING THE BIRTHDOSE:* The HepB series should be completed with either monovalent HepB or a combination vaccine containing HepB. The second dose should be administered at age 1–2 months. The final dose should be administered at age ≥24 weeks. It is permissible to administer 4 doses of HepB (e.g., when combination vaccines are given after the birth dose); however, if monovalent HepB is used, a dose at age 4 months is not needed. **Infants born to HBsAg-positive mothers** should be tested for HBsAg and antibody to HBsAg after completion of the HepB series, at age 9–18 months (generally at the next well-child visit after completion of the vaccine series).

2. Diphtheria and tetanus toxoids and acellular pertussis vaccine (DTaP). The fourth dose of DTaP may be administered as early as age 12 months, provided 6 months have elapsed since the third dose and the child is unlikely to return at age 15–18 months. The final dose in the series should be given at age ≥4 years.

Tetanus and diphtheria toxoids and acellular pertussis vaccine (Tdap – adolescent preparation) is recommended at age 11–12 years for those who have completed the recommended childhood DTP/DTaP vaccination series and have not received a Td booster dose. Adolescents 13–18 years who missed the 11–12-year Td/Tdap booster dose should also receive a single dose of Tdap if they have completed the recommended childhood DTP/DTaP vaccination series. Subsequent **tetanus and diphtheria toxoids (Td)** are recommended every 10 years.

3. *Haemophilus influenzae* type b conjugate vaccine (Hib). Three Hib conjugate vaccines are licensed for infant use. If PRP-OMP (PedvaxHIB® or ComVax® [Merck]) is administered at ages 2 and 4 months, a dose at age 6 months is not required. DTaP/Hib combination products should not be used for primary immunization in infants at ages 2, 4 or 6 months but can be used as boosters after any Hib vaccine. The final dose in the series should be administered at age ≥12 months.

4. Measles, mumps, and rubella vaccine (MMR). The second dose of MMR is recommended routinely at age 4–6 years but may be administered during any visit, provided at least 4 weeks have elapsed since the first dose and both doses are administered beginning at or after age 12 months. Those who have not previously received the second dose should complete the schedule by age 11–12 years.

5. Varicella vaccine. Varicella vaccine is recommended at any visit at or after age 12 months for susceptible children (i.e., those who lack a reliable history of chickenpox). Susceptible persons aged ≥13 years should receive 2 doses administered at least 4 weeks apart.

6. Meningococcal vaccine (MCV4). Meningococcal conjugate vaccine (MCV4) should be given to all children at the 11–12 year old visit as well as to unvaccinated adolescents at high school entry (15 years of age). Other adolescents who wish to decrease their risk for meningococcal disease may also be vaccinated. All college freshmen living in dormitories should also be vaccinated, preferably with MCV4, although **meningococcal polysaccharide vaccine (MPSV4)** is an acceptable alternative. Vaccination against invasive meningococcal disease is recommended for children and adolescents aged ≥2 years with terminal complement deficiencies or anatomic or functional asplenia and certain other high risk groups (see *MMWR* 2005;54 [RR-7]:1-21); use MPSV4 for children aged 2–10 years and MCV4 for older children, although MPSV4 is an acceptable alternative.

7. Pneumococcal vaccine. The heptavalent **pneumococcal conjugate vaccine (PCV)** is recommended for all children aged 2–23 months and for certain children aged 24–59 months. The final dose in the series should be given at age ≥12 months. **Pneumococcal polysaccharide vaccine (PPV)** is recommended in addition to PCV for certain high-risk groups. See *MMWR* 2000; 49(RR-9):1-35.

8. Influenza vaccine. Influenza vaccine is recommended annually for children aged ≥6 months with certain risk factors (including, but not limited to, asthma, cardiac disease, sickle cell disease, human immunodeficiency virus [HIV], diabetes, and conditions that can compromise respiratory function or handling of respiratory secretions or that can increase the risk for aspiration), healthcare workers, and other persons (including household members) in close contact with persons in groups at high risk (see *MMWR* 2005;54[RR-8]:1-55). In addition, healthy children aged 6–23 months and close contacts of healthy children aged 0–5 months are recommended to receive influenza vaccine because children in this age group are at substantially increased risk for influenza-related hospitalizations. For healthy persons aged 5–49 years, the intranasally administered, live, attenuated influenza vaccine (LAIV) is an acceptable alternative to the intramuscular trivalent inactivated influenza vaccine (TIV). See *MMWR* 2005;54(RR-8):1-55. Children receiving TIV should be administered a dosage appropriate for their age (0.25 mL if aged 6–35 months or 0.5 mL if aged ≥3 years). Children aged ≤8 years who are receiving influenza vaccine for the first time should receive 2 doses (separated by at least 4 weeks for TIV and at least 6 weeks for LAIV).

9. Hepatitis A vaccine (HepA). HepA is recommended for all children at 1 year of age (i.e., 12–23 months). The 2 doses in the series should be administered at least 6 months apart. States, counties, and communities with existing HepA vaccination programs for children 2–18 years of age are encouraged to maintain these programs. In these areas, new efforts focused on routine vaccination of 1-year-old children should enhance, not replace, ongoing programs directed at a broader population of children. HepA is also recommended for certain high risk groups (see *MMWR* 1999; 48[RR-12]1-37).

The Childhood and Adolescent Immunization Schedule is approved by:
Advisory Committee on Immunization Practices www.cdc.gov/nip/acip • American Academy of Pediatrics www.aap.org • American Academy of Family Physicians www.aafp.org

FIGURE 18-32 Recommended childhood and adolescent immunization schedule—United States, 2006 *(National Immunization Program, Centers for Disease Control and Prevention)*

group is between the ages of 6 months and 5 years. With the rise in popularity of day care centers, immunization against the Hib bacterium is the most sensible way to prevent this often resistant-to-antibiotic disease from spreading through the very young population in the United States. Complications of this childhood disease include **meningitis**, which could result in damage to the nervous system or in mental **retardation**; **epiglottitis**, which could cause a child to choke to death if immediate treatment is not given; joint infections; and forms of crippling arthritis. The Hib vaccine is administered in a series of three subcutaneous or intramuscular injections at 2, 4, and 6 months. A booster is given at 18 months.

Measles, Mumps, and Rubella
The MMR vaccine protects children from all three childhood diseases. **Measles** is medically termed **rubeola**. It is also referred to as "old-fashioned" and 10-day measles. It is spread by direct contact, droplet infection, and indirect contact from infected items of a patient. It has a 10- to 21-day incubation period. In the prodromal (earliest) stage, the patient exhibits fever, malaise, runny nose, cough, and sometimes conjunctivitis; it progresses with loss of appetite, **photophobia**, sore throat, and eventually Koplik's spots (the red skin rash). The cause is the rubeola virus, which is an acute and highly contagious viral disease involving the respiratory tract. Complications of measles can result in deafness, brain damage, and pneumonia. Treatment for measles is bed rest, increased fluid intake, antipyretics, antibiotics, cough medicine, and calamine lotion. The patient should be kept in isolation to prevent transmission to others. Quiet activity is suggested for the patient during recovery time, usually a few days.

Mumps is an acute contagious febrile disease that causes inflammation of the parotid and salivary glands. Parotitis is transmitted by droplet infection or direct contact with an infected person. The usual incubation period is from 14 to 28 days. Symptoms include chills and fever, headache, and pain below and in front of the ear(s) for 5 to 7 days' duration. Another symptom is pain between the ear and the angle of the jaw with drinking or eating acidic substances. Bed rest and a soft diet, including increased fluid intake, is recommended. Application of cold packs to control swelling of the glands of the neck, and in males, of the testicles in orchitis, is advised.

Rubella, also called German measles or 3-day measles, is an acute contagious viral disease characterized by an upper respiratory infection. If a female acquires rubella during the first **trimester** of pregnancy, fetal abnormalities may result. You should remind female patients in childbearing years of this concern and to be tested for a rubella antibody titer and be vaccinated before becoming pregnant if needed. *Females should not be vaccinated during pregnancy.* Be sure to determine this before administering the vaccine. Rubella is transmitted by droplet infection and by direct contact. The incubation period is from 12 to 23 days. Symptoms include slight fever, sore throat, drowsiness, malaise, swollen glands and lymph nodes, arthralgia, and a diffuse fine red rash (Figure 18-33). Treatment is bed rest, liquids, antipyretics, and sponge baths. Complications of rubella can result in blindness, deafness, brain damage, heart defects, enlarged liver, and bone malformation.

Diphtheria
This acute infectious disease is caused by *Corynebacterium diphtheriae*, which is a gram-positive, nonmotile, nonspore-forming, club-shaped bacillus. **Diphtheria** diagnosis is confirmed by throat culture. Transmission is by direct and indirect contact. The incubation period is between 2 and 5 days. Symptoms include headache, malaise, fever, and sore throat with a yellowish white or gray membrane. Treatment consists of adequate liquids and a soft diet; antibiotics; bed rest; and, in some cases, a tracheostomy.

Pertussis
Whooping cough, or **pertussis**, is an acute infectious disease characterized by respiratory drainage, then a peculiar paroxysmal cough, and finally a whooping inspiration (sounds like a shrill trumpeting cry; the name comes from the whooping crane that makes this sound). This disease is most common in children younger than 4 years, although it can affect children of all ages if they have not been immunized against it. Pertussis is caused by the small, nonmotile,

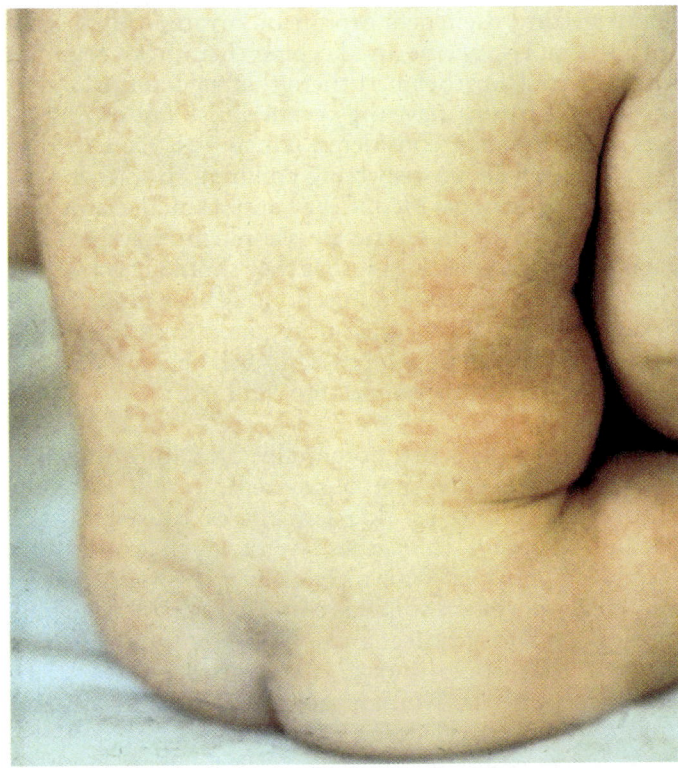

FIGURE 18-33 Eleven-month-old infant with rubella. This infant has typical discreet macupapular erythematous rash indistinguishable from that seen in other viral illnesses.

gram-negative bacillus *Bordetella pertussis*. It is transmitted by direct and indirect contact. The incubation period is from 7 to 14 days. Symptoms of whooping cough in the **catarrhal stage** include an increase in leukocyte count marked by lymphocytosis, respiratory drainage, sneezing, slight fever, dry cough, irritability, and loss of appetite; in the **paroxysmal stage** symptoms include a violent cough with whooping inspiration sounds and forceful vomiting that can evoke hemorrhaging from various portions of the body from the straining; and in the **decline stage** symptoms include a decline in coughing and return of appetite. A trace cough may last for several months to 2 years.

Rabies

Rubies is a viral disease transmitted in the saliva of infected animals (nonvaccinated animals, such as dogs, cats, bats, foxes, raccoons, and skunks in the wild) and through airborne transmission, which is possible in heavily infested bat caves. Human symptoms of the disease may include fever, pain, aggressive behavior, hallucinations, extreme weakness, and thirst. For the unfortunate victim who has been bitten by a rabid animal, a vaccine that consists of a series of five injections is very effective in combating the disease. There do not seem to be any side effects of this vaccine. If one is not treated with the vaccine until after the symptoms appear, it is always a fatal disease. The rabies vaccine for animals is still the best means of prevention. You may help in educating patients about this potential problem by reminding them about getting their pets protection against this disease with the rabies vaccine and keeping them from roaming unsupervised. Further alert them that wild animals, even the cute little ones, have the potential risk of carrying rabies and are to be considered dangerous. Explain that people, especially unsuspecting children, should not approach wild animals even if they appear mild-mannered. Another point for those who are planning to travel to rural areas of foreign countries is that they should check about getting pre-immunization injections against rabies in addition to the established list of required immunizations. Health officials are hopeful that this will help prevent serious illness and death around the world.

Tetanus

This acute, potentially fatal, infectious disease affects the central nervous system. **Tetanus** was commonly referred to as "lockjaw." It is caused by the bacillus *Clostridium tetani,* the **toxin** of which is one of the most **lethal** poisons known. The bacillus is found in superficial layers of the soil. It is a normal inhabitant of the intestinal tracts of horses and cows. Tetanus affects only wounds that contain dead tissue, transmitted commonly in puncture wounds, abrasions, lacerations, and burns. Immediate cleaning of the wound and **débridement** are necessary initially in treatment. There is a short incubation period of 3 to 21 days, and a longer one of 4 to 5 weeks. The symptoms of tetanus are stiffness of the jaw, esophageal muscles, and sometimes neck muscles.

Progressing rigidity follows soon with fixed jaw (thus lockjaw), altered voice, fever, painful spasms of all body muscles, irritability, and headache. Motor nerves transmit impulses from the infected central nervous system to muscle. Maintaining an airway and administering **antitoxin** are vital. Additionally, treatment consists of sedation, controlling muscle spasms, maintaining fluid balance, penicillin G, tracheostomy, and oxygen as necessary. The patient must be kept in a quiet room to prevent the triggering of muscle spasms.

Rotavirus

Rotavirus is a disease that affects infants and small children, causing diarrhea and vomiting in many cases. This virus strikes over 500,000 children under the age of 3 years in the United States each year. It also is cause to hospitalize approximately 50,000 each year because of dehydration from the effects of the disease. Every year, approximately 20 children die from rotavirus. A child or infant who has rotavirus should be given medical attention immediately, because dehydration can be a serious threat to the child's life. Maintaining the child's fluid levels is vital. The means of transmission is from an infected child. Often, children have no symptoms for a couple of days before they begin the diarrhea, and for a couple of days after the diarrhea stops, the child seems to be better. Even during these times when the child or infant does not seem to be sick, the virus can be passed on to other children. Child day care center workers should strive to prevent this virus by frequent hand washing of the children and of themselves.

There is a rotavirus vaccine that can be given to infants along with other immunizations at 2, 4, and 6 months of age. If an infant has not had the vaccine by the age of 7 months, it is thought to be unnecessary. The rotavirus vaccine has not yet been added to the recommended childhood immunization schedule but is available to physicians who recommend it for their patients.

Varicella Zoster

Better known as "chickenpox," this virus is highly contagious and is spread by direct contact and droplets from the respiratory tract in the prodromal stages or in the early stages of the rash. It is a member of the herpes virus family and is often called herpes zoster. It primarily affects young children. The rash develops into vesicular fluid eruptions that are infectious until they become dry scabs. Incubation is between 2 and 3 weeks. Symptoms include highly pruritic rash, fever, headache, loss of appetite, and general malaise, which last from a few days to 2 weeks. The treatment is baking soda paste for the itching eruptions, bed rest, liquids, antipyretics, and oral antihistamines if necessary for control of the itching. There is a relatively new vaccine for the prevention of this disease. The Varivax vaccine is given to children between 12 and 18 months by injection, with an additional dose given between 11 and 12 years. The most common complication of chickenpox is secondary infections. Many children are also affected with respiratory ailments and ear infections.

Hepatitis A

Hepatitis A is also referred to as infectious hepatitis. The symptoms of hepatitis A are much the same as hepatitis B. A vaccine consisting of two injections 6 months apart is available, but it is generally recommended only for those who travel to countries that are in distant continents. You can find further information about hepatitis A in Chapter 11, Unit 10.

Hepatitis B

This is a highly contagious, potentially fatal form of viral hepatitis. It is caused by the **hepatitis B** virus (HBV). It has been known as "serum hepatitis." Hepatitis B is transmitted by contaminated serum in blood transfusions or by using contaminated needles or instruments. It has an incubation period of 14 to 50 days. The symptoms are slow at onset with fever, malaise, loss of appetite, nausea, and vomiting, progressing to include jaundice, weakness, dark urine, and whitish stool. Bed rest and a forced-fluid diet are recommended. Alcohol and fats should be eliminated from the patient's diet. The hepatitis B vaccine is urged for all who may be at risk, especially *all health care workers*. It is thought to be in widespread proportions everywhere, and immunization is strongly urged to protect the country's population and to prevent a massive epidemic. The hepatitis B virus vaccine, Hep B, is given to neonates whose mothers have not had the disease before leaving the hospital. The second dose is given between 1 and 4 months of age, and the third dose between 6 and 18 months. A booster dose is recommended for children between 11 and 12 years. Protecting the very young from this often fatal disease is a sensible means of control of possible epidemics.

Meningitis (Bacterial)

In the 1990s, there was an increase in the number of cases of bacterial meningitis among young adults between the ages of 15 and 24 years. Bacterial meningitis is a highly contagious disease that can cause serious and long-lasting effects on the nervous system. Death within 24 to 48 hours after contracting the disease is a very real possibility. Fortunately, this type of meningitis can be prevented with a meningococcal vaccine. Persons who have an altered immune system or a serious health condition and women during pregnancy should not have this vaccine. For most people, the vaccine is safe and results in minor reactions, such as slight soreness at the injection site and mild fever. These reactions are common with most vaccines. Viral meningitis is not as serious an illness and has no vaccine at this time.

Inactivated Polio Vaccine

In addition to the oral polio vaccine, there is a higher-potency killed polio vaccine, IPV (inactivated polio vaccine), that is given by injection. Parents are to be given the informa-tion about each type of vaccine that their child may receive before it is administered. In this way, the parents can make a decision about what they want for their children based on facts presented them. Infants are given two injections in their 1st year, with 8 weeks between them. Children should have another injection at 18 months, when they begin school, and every 5 years until the child is 18 years old. IPV is recommended for those who have a low resistance to serious infections, for those in close daily contact with them, or for adults who have never been vaccinated against polio when their children are given the oral vaccine.

Other Vaccines

Remind patients to protect themselves and their families against all of these diseases to prevent the return of epidemics. There are other diseases, such as **cholera** and **typhoid**, for which there are vaccines to prevent dangerous epidemics that have the potential to wipe out entire populations. Many underdeveloped countries have such situations even today. Immunizations other than what appears in the schedule in Figure 18-32 are not recommended on a routine basis in most Western countries. It has been said that an ounce of prevention is worth a pound of cure. The prevention of disease often means saving lives and, in many cases, also improving the quality of life. Health officials advise immunizations as determined necessary. Check with your family physician to keep abreast with new recommendations of the CDC regarding vaccines. Refer to Figure 18-34 for vaccines that are recommended for adults. Travel to some countries requires immunizations against particular diseases before entry is permitted. To provide up-to-date immunization information by country, computer databases have been established. One such program containing health information for travelers in over 200 countries is available from Immunization Alert, Storrs, Connecticut. Current information may also be obtained at local and state health departments. You should provide the patient with a card or booklet to accurately record each immunization and the month, day, and year for each (Figure 18-35). Record each vaccine on the patient's chart, as was discussed earlier in this chapter. Any reaction to the vaccine, no matter how slight, must also be recorded on the patient's chart. Remind patients to make appointments and carry the immunization record (or a copy) with them at all times.

Because of the continuing research and advances in the production of vaccinations against many infectious diseases, these illnesses are rarely experienced in developed countries, except in severely poverty-stricken areas. Unfortunately, however, third-world nations are still constantly fighting a losing battle against communicable diseases. Deaths from them are staggering in number. This is mainly caused by inadequate education, poor living conditions, and lack of funding for vaccines.

Recommended Adult Immunization Schedule
United States, October 2006–September 2007

Recommended adult immunization schedule, by vaccine and age group

Age group (yrs) ▶ / Vaccine ▼	19–49 years	50–64 years	≥65 years
Tetanus, diphtheria, pertussis (Td/Tdap)[1]*	1-dose Td booster every 10 yrs / Substitute 1 dose of Tdap for Td		
Human papillomavirus (HPV)[2]*	3 doses (females)		
Measles, mumps, rubella (MMR)[3]*	1 or 2 doses	1 dose	
Varicella[4]*	2 doses (0, 4–8 wks)	2 doses (0, 4–8 wks)	
Influenza[5]*	1 dose annually	1 dose annually	
Pneumococcal (polysaccharide)[6,7]	1–2 doses		1 dose
Hepatitis A[8]*	2 doses (0, 6–12 mos, or 0, 6–18 mos)		
Hepatitis B[9]*	3 doses (0, 1–2, 4–6 mos)		
Meningococcal[10]	1 or more doses		

Recommended adult immunization schedule, by vaccine and medical and other indications

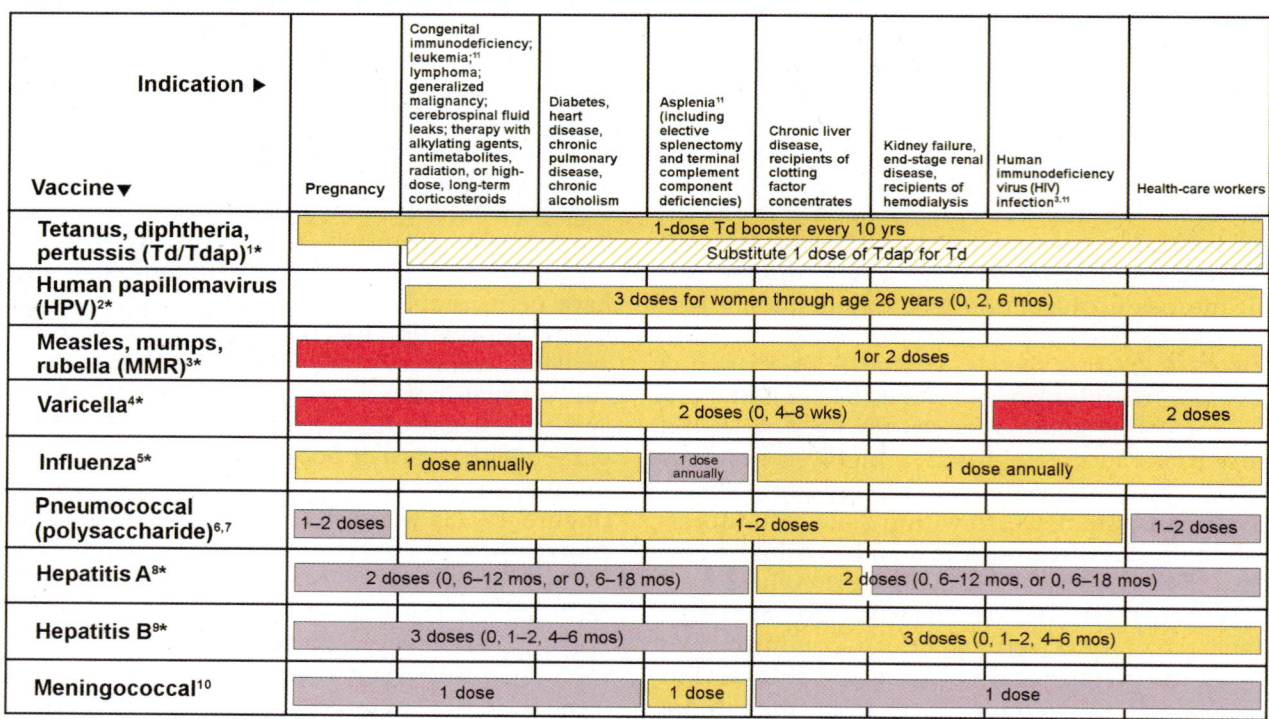

Indication ▶ / Vaccine ▼	Pregnancy	Congenital immunodeficiency; leukemia;[11] lymphoma; generalized malignancy; cerebrospinal fluid leaks; therapy with alkylating agents, antimetabolites, radiation, or high-dose, long-term corticosteroids	Diabetes, heart disease, chronic pulmonary disease, chronic alcoholism	Asplenia[11] (including elective splenectomy and terminal complement component deficiencies)	Chronic liver disease, recipients of clotting factor concentrates	Kidney failure, end-stage renal disease, recipients of hemodialysis	Human immunodeficiency virus (HIV) infection[3,11]	Health-care workers
Tetanus, diphtheria, pertussis (Td/Tdap)[1]*	1-dose Td booster every 10 yrs / Substitute 1 dose of Tdap for Td							
Human papillomavirus (HPV)[2]*		3 doses for women through age 26 years (0, 2, 6 mos)						
Measles, mumps, rubella (MMR)[3]*	*(Contraindicated)*	1 or 2 doses						
Varicella[4]*	*(Contraindicated)*	2 doses (0, 4–8 wks)					*(Contraindicated)*	2 doses
Influenza[5]*	1 dose annually			1 dose annually	1 dose annually			
Pneumococcal (polysaccharide)[6,7]	1–2 doses	1–2 doses						1–2 doses
Hepatitis A[8]*	2 doses (0, 6–12 mos, or 0, 6–18 mos)			2 doses (0, 6–12 mos, or 0, 6–18 mos)				
Hepatitis B[9]*	3 doses (0, 1–2, 4–6 mos)			3 doses (0, 1–2, 4–6 mos)				
Meningococcal[10]	1 dose		1 dose	1 dose				

* Covered by the Vaccine Injury Compensation Program

These recommendations must be read along with the footnotes, which can be found on the next 2 pages of this schedule.

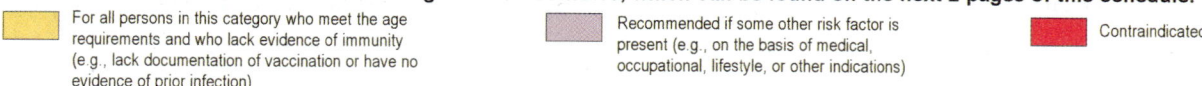

For all persons in this category who meet the age requirements and who lack evidence of immunity (e.g., lack documentation of vaccination or have no evidence of prior infection)

Recommended if some other risk factor is present (e.g., on the basis of medical, occupational, lifestyle, or other indications)

Contraindicated

FIGURE 18-34   Recommended adult immunization schedule by vaccine, age group, and indication—United States, October 2006–September 2007 *(Centers for Disease Control and Prevention. Retrieved October 30, 2007, from www.cdc.gov/nip/recs/adult-schedule.pdf)*

(continues)

Footnotes

1. Tetanus, diphtheria, and acellular pertussis (Td/Tdap) vaccination. Adults with uncertain histories of a complete primary vaccination series with diphtheria and tetanus toxoid–containing vaccines should begin or complete a primary vaccination series. A primary series for adults is 3 doses; administer the first 2 doses at least 4 weeks apart and the third dose 6–12 months after the second. Administer a booster dose to adults who have completed a primary series and if the last vaccination was received ≥10 years previously. Tdap or tetanus and diphtheria (Td) vaccine may be used; Tdap should replace a single dose of Td for adults aged <65 years who have not previously received a dose of Tdap (either in the primary series, as a booster, or for wound management). Only one of two Tdap products (Adacel® [sanofi pasteur, Swiftwater, Pennsylvania]) is licensed for use in adults. If the person is pregnant and received the last Td vaccination ≥10 years previously, administer Td during the second or third trimester; if the person received the last Td vaccination in <10 years, administer Tdap during the immediate postpartum period. A one-time administration of 1-dose of Tdap with an interval as short as 2 years from a previous Td vaccination is recommended for postpartum women, close contacts of infants aged <12 months, and all health-care workers with direct patient contact. In certain situations, Td can be deferred during pregnancy and Tdap substituted in the immediate postpartum period, or Tdap can be given instead of Td to a pregnant woman after an informed discussion with the woman (see http://www.cdc.gov/nip/publications/acip-list.htm). Consult the ACIP statement for recommendations for administering Td as prophylaxis in wound management (http://www.cdc.gov/mmwr/preview/mmwrhtml/00041645.htm).

2. Human Papillomavirus (HPV) vaccination. HPV vaccination is recommended for all women aged ≤26 years who have not completed the vaccine series. Ideally, vaccine should be administered before potential exposure to HPV through sexual activity; however, women who are sexually active should still be vaccinated. Sexually active women who have not been infected with any of the HPV vaccine types receive the full benefit of the vaccination. Vaccination is less beneficial for women who have already been infected with one or more of the four HPV vaccine types. A complete series consists of 3 doses. The second dose should be administered 2 months after the first dose; the third dose should be administered 6 months after the first dose. Vaccination is not recommended during pregnancy. If a woman is found to be pregnant after initiating the vaccination series, the remainder of the 3-dose regimen should be delayed until after completion of the pregnancy.

3. Measles, Mumps, Rubella (MMR) vaccination. *Measles component:* adults born before 1957 can be considered immune to measles. Adults born during or after 1957 should receive ≥1 dose of MMR unless they have a medical contraindication, documentation of ≥1 dose, history of measles based on health-care provider diagnosis, or laboratory evidence of immunity. A second dose of MMR is recommended for adults who 1) have been recently exposed to measles or in an outbreak setting; 2) were previously vaccinated with killed measles vaccine; 3) have been vaccinated with an unknown type of measles vaccine during 1963–1967; 4) are students in postsecondary educational institutions; 5) work in a health-care facility, or 6) plan to travel internationally. Withhold MMR or other measles-containing vaccines from HIV-infected persons with severe immunosuppression. *Mumps component:* adults born before 1957 can generally be considered immune to mumps. Adults born during or after 1957 should receive 1 dose of MMR unless they have a medical contraindication, history of mumps based on health-care provider diagnosis, or laboratory evidence of immunity. A second dose of MMR is recommended for adults who 1) are in an age group that is affected during a mumps outbreak; 2) are students in postsecondary educational institutions; 3) work in a health-care facility; or 4) plan to travel internationally. For unvaccinated health-care workers born before 1957 who do not have other evidence of mumps immunity, consider giving 1 dose on a routine basis and strongly consider giving a second dose during an outbreak. *Rubella component:* administer 1 dose of MMR vaccine to women whose rubella vaccination history is unreliable or who lack laboratory evidence of immunity. For women of childbearing age, regardless of birth year, routinely determine rubella immunity and counsel women regarding congenital rubella syndrome. Do not vaccinate women who are pregnant or who might become pregnant within 4 weeks of receiving vaccine. Women who do not have evidence of immunity should receive MMR vaccine upon completion or termination of pregnancy and before discharge from the health-care facility.

4. Varicella vaccination. All adults without evidence of immunity to varicella should receive 2 doses of varicella vaccine. Special consideration should be given to those who 1) have close contact with persons at high risk for severe disease (e.g., health-care workers and family contacts of immunocompromised persons) or 2) are at high risk for exposure or transmission (e.g., teachers of young children; child care employees; residents and staff members of institutional settings, including correctional institutions; college students; military personnel; adolescents and adults living in households with children; non-pregnant women of childbearing age; and international travelers). Evidence of immunity to varicella in adults includes any of the following: 1) documentation of 2 doses of varicella vaccine at least 4 weeks apart; 2) U.S.–born before 1980 (although for health-care workers and pregnant women, birth before 1980 should not be considered evidence of immunity); 3) history of varicella based on diagnosis or verification of varicella by a health-care provider (for a patient reporting a history of or presenting with an atypical case, a mild case, or both, health-care providers should seek either an epidemiologic link with a typical varicella case or evidence of laboratory confirmation, if it was performed at the time of acute disease); 4) history of herpes zoster based on health-care provider diagnosis; or 5) laboratory evidence of immunity or laboratory confirmation of disease. Do not vaccinate women who are pregnant or might become pregnant within 4 weeks of receiving the vaccine. Assess pregnant women for evidence of varicella immunity. Women who do not have evidence of immunity should receive dose 1 of varicella vaccine upon completion or termination of pregnancy and before discharge from the health-care facility. Dose 2 should be administered 4–8 weeks after dose 1.

5. Influenza vaccination: *Medical indications:* chronic disorders of the cardiovascular or pulmonary systems, including asthma; chronic metabolic diseases, including diabetes mellitus, renal dysfunction, hemoglobinopathies, or immunosuppression (including immunosuppression caused by medications or HIV); any condition that compromises respiratory function or the handling of respiratory secretions or that can increase the risk of aspiration (e.g., cognitive dysfunction, spinal cord injury, or seizure disorder or other neuromuscular disorder); and pregnancy during the influenza season. No data exist on the risk for severe or complicated influenza disease among persons with asplenia; however, influenza is a risk factor for secondary bacterial infections that can cause severe disease among persons with asplenia. *Occupational indications:* health-care workers and employees of long-term–care and assisted living facilities. *Other indications:* residents of nursing homes and other long-term–care and assisted living facilities; persons likely to transmit influenza to persons at high risk (i.e., in-home household contacts and caregivers of children aged 0–59 months, or persons of all ages with high-risk conditions); and anyone who would like to be vaccinated. Healthy, nonpregnant persons aged 5–49 years without high-risk medical conditions who are not contacts of severely immunocompromised persons in special care units can receive either intranasally administered influenza vaccine (FluMist®) or inactivated vaccine. Other persons should receive the inactivated vaccine.

FIGURE 18-34 (Continued)

Footnotes

6. Pneumococcal polysaccharide vaccination. *Medical indications:* chronic disorders of the pulmonary system (excluding asthma); cardiovascular diseases; diabetes mellitus; chronic liver diseases, including liver disease as a result of alcohol abuse (e.g.,cirrhosis); chronic renal failure or nephrotic syndrome; functional or anatomic asplenia (e.g., sickle cell disease or splenectomy [if elective splenectomy is planned, vaccinate at least 2 weeks before surgery]); immunosuppressive conditions (e.g., congenital immunodeficiency, HIV infection [vaccinate as close to diagnosis as possible when CD4 cell counts are highest], leukemia, lymphoma, multiple myeloma, Hodgkin disease, generalized malignancy, organ or bone marrow transplantation); chemotherapy with alkylating agents, antimetabolites, or high-dose, long-term corticosteroids; and cochlear implants. *Other indications:* Alaska Natives and certain American Indian populations and residents of nursing homes or other long-term–care facilities.

7. Revaccination with pneumococcal polysaccharide vaccine. One-time revaccination after 5 years for persons with chronic renal failure or nephrotic syndrome; functional or anatomic asplenia (e.g., sickle cell disease or splenectomy); immunosuppressive conditions (e.g., congenital immuno-deficiency, HIV infection, leukemia, lymphoma, multiple myeloma, Hodgkin disease, generalized malignancy, or organ or bone marrow transplantation); or chemotherapy with alkylating agents, antimetabolites, or high-dose, long-term corticosteroids. For persons aged ≥65 years, one-time revaccination if they were vaccinated ≥5 years previously and were aged <65 years at the time of primary vaccination.

8. Hepatitis A vaccination. *Medical indications:* persons with chronic liver disease and persons who receive clotting factor concentrates. *Behavioral indications:* men who have sex with men and persons who use illegal drugs. *Occupational indications:* persons working with hepatitis A virus (HAV)–infected primates or with HAV in a research laboratory setting. *Other indications:* persons traveling to or working in countries that have high or intermediate endemicity of hepatitis A (a list of countries is available at http://www.cdc.gov/travel/diseases.htm) and any person who would like to obtain immunity. Current vaccines should be administered in a 2-dose schedule at either 0 and 6–12 months, or 0 and 6–18 months. If the combined hepatitis A and hepatitis B vaccine is used, administer 3 doses at 0, 1, and 6 months .

9. Hepatitis B vaccination. *Medical indications:* Persons with end-stage renal disease, including patients receiving hemodialysis; persons seeking evaluation or treatment for a sexually transmitted disease (STD); persons with HIV infection; persons with chronic liver disease; and persons who receive clotting factor concentrates. *Occupational indications:* health-care workers and public-safety workers who are exposed to blood or other potentially infectious body fluids. *Behavioral indications:* sexually active persons who are not in a long-term, mutually monogamous relationship (i.e., persons with >1 sex partner during the previous 6 months); current or recent injection-drug users; and men who have sex with men. *Other indications:* household contacts and sex partners of persons with chronic hepatitis B virus (HBV) infection; clients and staff members of institutions for persons with developmental disabilities; all clients of STD clinics; international travelers to countries with high or intermediate prevalence of chronic HBV infection (a list of countries is available at http://www.cdc.gov/travel/diseases.htm); and any adult seeking protection from HBV infection. Settings where hepatitis B vaccination is recommended for all adults: STD treatment facilities; HIV testing and treatment facilities; facilities providing drug-abuse treatment and prevention services; health-care settings providing services for injection-drug users or men who have sex with men; correctional facilities; end-stage renal disease programs and facilities for chronic hemodialysis patients; and institutions and nonresidential daycare facilities for persons with developmental disabilities. *Special formulation indications:* for adult patients receiving hemodialysis and other immunocompromised adults, 1 dose of 40 μg/mL (Recombivax HB®) or 2 doses of 20 μg/mL (Engerix-B®).

10. Meningococcal vaccination. *Medical indications:* adults with anatomic or functional asplenia, or terminal complement component deficiencies. *Other indications:* first-year college students living in dormitories; microbiologists who are routinely exposed to isolates of *Neisseria meningitidis*; military recruits; and persons who travel to or live in countries in which meningococcal disease is hyperendemic or epidemic (e.g., the "meningitis belt" of Sub-Saharan Africa during the dry season [December–June]), particularly if contact with local populations will be prolonged. Vaccination is required by the government of Saudi Arabia for all travelers to Mecca during the annual Hajj. Meningococcal conjugate vaccine is preferred for adults with any of the preceeding indications who are aged ≤55 years, although meningococcal polysaccharide vaccine (MPSV4) is an acceptable alternative. Revaccination after 5 years might be indicated for adults previously vaccinated with MPSV4 who remain at high risk for infection (e.g., persons residing in areas in which disease is epidemic).

11. Selected conditions for which *Haemophilus influenzae* type b (Hib) vaccination may be used. Hib conjugate vaccines are licensed for children aged 6 weeks–71 months. No efficacy data are available on which to base a recommendation concerning use of Hib vaccine for older children and adults with the chronic conditions associated with an increased risk for Hib disease. However, studies suggest good immunogenicity in patients who have sickle cell disease, leukemia, or HIV infection or have had splenectomies; administering vaccine to these patients is not contraindicated.

This schedule indicates the recommended age groups and medical indications for routine administration of currently licensed vaccines for persons aged ≥19 years, as of October 1, 2006. Licensed combination vaccines may be used whenever any components of the combination are indicated and when the vaccine's other components are not contraindicated. For detailed recommendations on all vaccines, including those used primarily for travelers or that are issued during the year, consult the manufacturers' package inserts and the complete statements from the Advisory Committee on Immunization Practices (http://www.cdc.gov/nip/publications/acip-list.htm).

Report all clinically significant postvaccination reactions to the Vaccine Adverse Event Reporting System (VAERS). Reporting forms and instructions on filing a VAERS report are available at http://www.vaers.hhs.gov or by telephone, 800-822-7967.

Information on how to file a Vaccine Injury Compensation Program claim is available at http://www.hrsa.gov/vaccinecompensation or by telephone, 800-338-2382.To file a claim for vaccine injury, contact the U.S. Court of Federal Claims, 717 Madison Place, N.W., Washington, D.C. 20005; telephone, 202-357-6400.

Additional information about the vaccines in this schedule and contraindications for vaccination is also available at http://www.cdc.gov/nip or from the CDC-INFO Contact Center at 800-CDC-INFO (800-232-4636) in English and Spanish, 24 hours a day, 7 days a week.

Approved by the Advisory Committee on Immunization Practices, the American College of Obstetricians and Gynecologists, and the American Academy of Family Physicians

FIGURE 18-34 (Continued)

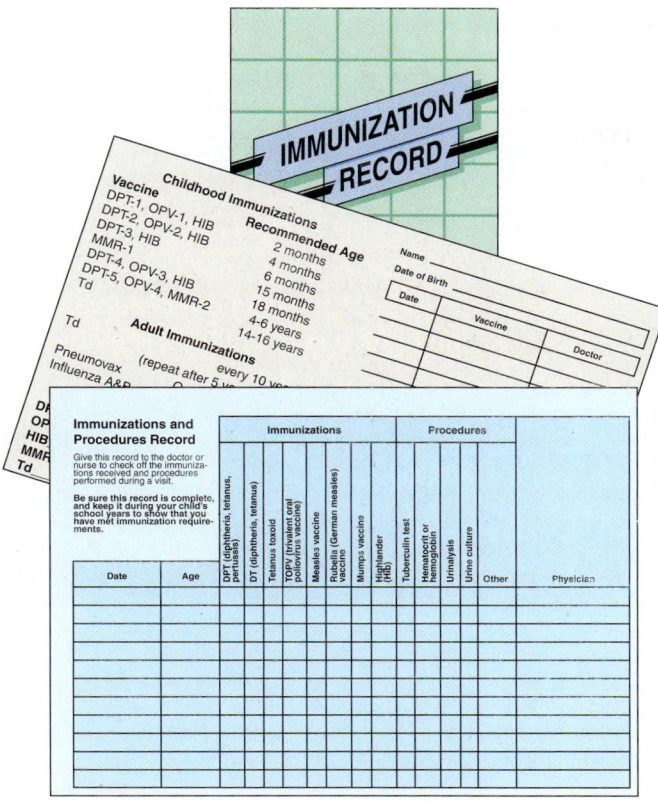

FIGURE 18-35 Sample immunization schedules and record booklets

- ■ **Complete the Workbook activities to meet the learning objectives.**
- ■ **Practice the procedures in this unit to meet the performance objectives.**
- ■ **Apply your knowledge at the end of this chapter in completing the Critical Thinking Challenge and Activities, as well as the StudyWARE on your Student CD-ROM.**

ACTIVITIES

1. Make flash cards with drug categories on one side and an example of each type of drug on the other side.
2. Practice calculating dosages.
3. Make a chart or table of the different types of injections, needle gauge and length, examples of medications given by each route, and the amount of medication given.

CRITICAL THINKING CHALLENGE

IMPACTING THE PATIENT, THE PRACTICE, AND YOUR CAREER

Darlene was the medical assistant assigned patients in the clinical area for the day. She was having a busy morning with many infants and children having exams and getting their immunizations. When Mrs. Jackson brought her baby, Kenya, for her 4-month check-up, she told Darlene that the baby had been coughing a lot. Darlene, wanting to go to lunch as soon as Kenya was ready for the doctor, said that the cough was probably from the dust in the house. Darlene weighed and measured Kenya and plotted the measurements on the growth graph. Darlene checked the immunization schedule and got out the DTP, Hib, and the OPV. Darlene gave the immunizations to the baby and told Mrs. Jackson that Dr. Lane would be in soon. Then she left for lunch. As Dr. Lane examined the baby, she noticed that Kenya felt warm. When she took an axillary temperature and it read 103.2°F, she explained to Mrs. Jackson that the baby was sick. She would have to bring Kenya back for her immunizations after she finished the antibiotic she was prescribing for bronchitis. Mrs. Jackson told the doctor that Darlene had already given the immunizations to Kenya just before she left the office to go to lunch. Darlene had not even recorded that she gave the immunizations. Dr. Lane looked quite concerned.

QUESTIONS

1. What do you think Mrs. Jackson will do?
2. Who is responsible if the baby has a serious reaction?
3. What might happen when Darlene returns from lunch? Will Darlene be fired for doing what she did?

CRITICAL THINKING CHALLENGE

IMPACTING THE PATIENT, THE PRACTICE, AND YOUR CAREER

It is a practice of some religious beliefs to fast for a period during the year. This situation may present itself to you in your career. Within the time of fasting, the patient tells you that he cannot take prescribed medication because taking anything during that time would be a sacrilege. Taking the medicine orally would bring a terrible anxiety for the patient about being disrespectful toward the holy day. No matter what you try, the patient says he cannot take the medicine. You realize that there is a language barrier besides the religious observance. You know how crucial it is that he take the antibiotic for his pneumonia and drink plenty of fluids. The observance of the holy days begins in 24 hours.

QUESTIONS

1. Is it that critical that a patient take a prescribed medication? What might be an option to his treatment?
2. Can you go to the physician and ask him to take this problem?
3. What would you do in this situation?

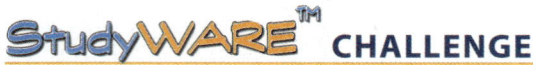 **CHALLENGE**

- Study with the flash cards for Chapter 18 to review the key terms in this chapter.
- Solve the crossword puzzle for Chapter 18.
- Complete the true/false quiz in test mode for Chapter 18.

RESOURCES

Heller, M., & Krebs, C. (1997). *Clinical handbook for health care professionals.* Clifton Park, NY: Thomson Delmar Learning.

Lindh, W. Q., Pooler, M. S., Tamparo, C. D., & Dahl, B. M. (2006). *Comprehensive medical assisting* (3rd ed.). Clifton Park, NY: Thomson Delmar Learning.

Miller, B. F., & Keane, C. B. (1997). *Encyclopedia and dictionary of medicine, nursing, and allied health* (6th ed.). Philadelphia: W.B. Saunders.

Physicians' desk reference (56th ed.). (2002). Monvrale, NJ: Medical Economics.

Physicians' desk reference for nonprescription drugs and dietary supplements (22nd ed.). (2001). Oradell, NJ: Medical Economics.

Protecting yourself against prescription errors (1996, January). *Health After 50.*

Rice, J. (2006). *Principles of pharmacology for medical assisting.* (4th ed.). Clifton Park, NY: Thomson Delmar Learning.

Venes, D. (2001). *Taber's cyclopedic medical dictionary* (19th ed.). Philadelphia: F.A. Davis.

WEB LINKS

www.cdc.gov/nip (The Centers for Disease Control and Prevention National Immunization Program) *Provides information on the importance of vaccines.*

Emergencies, Acute Illness, Accidents, and Recovery

Individuals working in health care can expect to be confronted with emergency or accident situations. Patients may be brought into the physician's office, you may be witness to an incident in your community or neighborhood, and almost certainly you will be responding to phone calls concerning injuries or sudden illness. When anything happens within your family or immediate neighborhood, your relatives and neighbors will probably expect you to be the "resident authority" just because you are a medical assistant. It is important for you to acquire first aid skills and have a working knowledge of appropriate actions to take in common accident or illness situations. It is your responsibility to maintain current certification to provide the basic life support measures involving **obstructed** airway, resuscitation, or CPR.

If you should happen upon a situation where an unknown person has become ill or lost **consciousness**, check for a universal emergency medical identification symbol (Figure 19-1). This symbol was designed by the American Medical Association as a means for individuals with certain medical conditions to alert health care workers of their conditions when they are unable to. The tag is worn around the neck, wrist, or ankle. Some may identify the particular problem the person has, others may not. If a tag is found, the person should have an information card on his person, usually inside a wallet, that identifies his condition and provides some directions to follow (Figure 19-2). All patients who

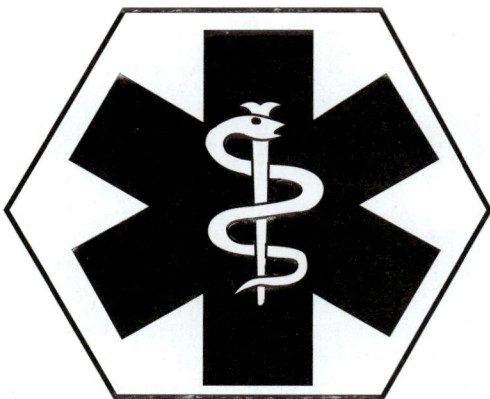

FIGURE 19-1   Universal emergency medical identification symbol

---

EMERGENCY

I am a laryngectomee (no vocal cords).

I breathe through an opening in the neck, not through the nose or mouth.

If artificial respiration is necessary:

1. Keep neck opening clear of all matter.
2. Don't twist head sidewise.
3. Apply oxygen only to neck opening.
4. Don't throw water on head.
5. Mouth-to-opening breathing is effective.

FIGURE 19-2   Emergency medical information card

have conditions that could cause emergency episodes, such as heart conditions, diabetes, epilepsy, allergies, or a laryngectomy, should be encouraged to wear a **universal emergency medical identification** tag.

This chapter deals with emergency care in cases of acute illness, accident, or injury. It also discusses care within the physician's office and first aid outside the health care setting. The last unit covers the use of exercise, supporting devices, and equipment to assist an individual to recover and regain mobility following illness or injury. This information will be of value not only in your professional life but also in your personal life.

UNIT 1
MANAGING EMERGENCIES IN THE MEDICAL OFFICE

OBJECTIVES

Upon completion of this unit, you will be able to achieve the following:

LEARNING Objectives

1. Spell and define, using the glossary at the back of the text, all the Words to Know in this unit.
2. Define a medical emergency.
3. Explain the purpose of the universal emergency medical identification symbol.
4. List items that might be found in an emergency kit.
5. Identify nine items of information to document on an incident report.
6. Explain the purpose of an AED and its three capabilities.

WORDS TO KNOW

bandage	incident report	trauma
certification	ipecac	universal
consciousness	obstructed	emergency
coroner	post mortem	medical
emergency	resuscitation	identification
emetic		

 CERTIFICATION CONNECTION

CMA
Emergencies
Principles of operation (oxygen)

CMAS
Medical office emergencies

RMA
Maintain emergency crash cart
Understand mandatory reporting guidelines and procedures

19-1  Perform an Abdominal Thrust on an Adult Victim With an Obstructed Airway (Continued)

21. Return to the victim's head, remove the mouthpiece, and check whether the object has dislodged; if so, remove it. If not, repeat the sequence until it is dislodged or assistance arrives.

22. If the object is removed, check for breathing. If the victim is breathing but has no pulse, begin CPR with chest compressions.

23. After the victim has resumed breathing and the heart is beating or EMS services have taken over the rescue, remove your gloves and the mouthpiece and dispose of them in the biohazard waste container.

24. Document the procedure.

CHARTING EXAMPLE

6/24/XX, 1:25 PM

Pt. sitting in reception room, began choking on piece of candy. Complete airway obstruction. Notified Dr. Green, EMS called. Given multiple abd. thrusts; became unconscious. Given 3 cycles unconscious choking procedure. Performed 3 minutes 2 person CPR with Dr. Green. EMS assumed rescue at 1:33 PM. Breathing and heart rate restored. Transported to Memorial Hospital.

J. Cole, CMA

An infant or toddler experiencing a blocked airway will have difficulty breathing, coughing, and crying and may display cyanosis. The recommended AHA and ARC course of action is:

1. Place the baby face down on your forearm, which is extended on your thigh (Figure 19-12).

2. The head should be lower than the body and supported by your hand.

3. With the heel of your other hand, give five quick, forceful blows between the infant's shoulder blades.

4. If this is unsuccessful, turn the infant face up; support the head.

5. Place two fingers on the midsternal area just below the nipple line.

6. Give five quick thrusts down, compressing the chest one third to one half the chest depth (Figure 19-13).

7. Continue with five back blows and five chest thrusts until the object is dislodged or the infant becomes unconscious.

8. If unsuccessful, call out for help to notify EMS.

9. If no help arrives, give the infant CPR for 1 minute, then call 911 yourself.

10. Continue CPR until assistance arrives.

Some additional information is:

● Even if the procedure is successful and infant seems fine, check with the physician for further instructions.

● If you can *see* the object, try to remove it with your finger.

● *Do not* try to grasp the object and pull it out if the infant is conscious.

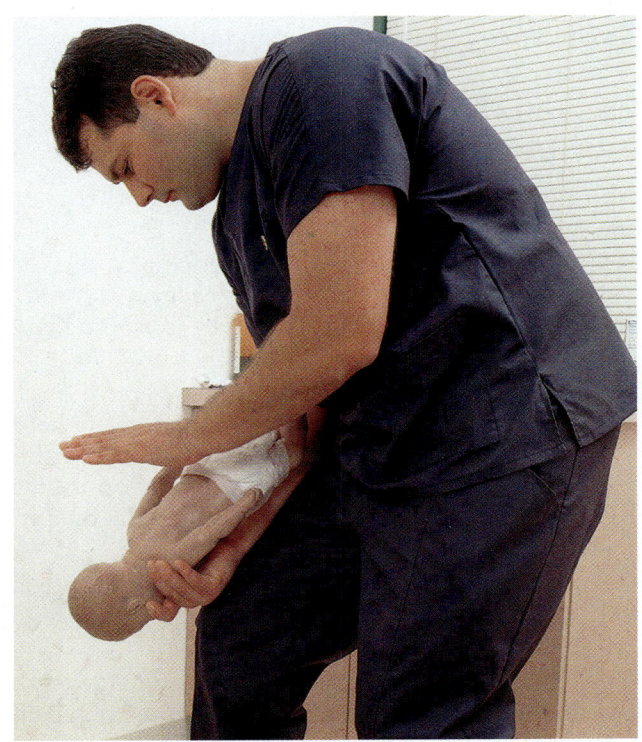

FIGURE 19-12 With the infant face down on your forearm, give five back blows.

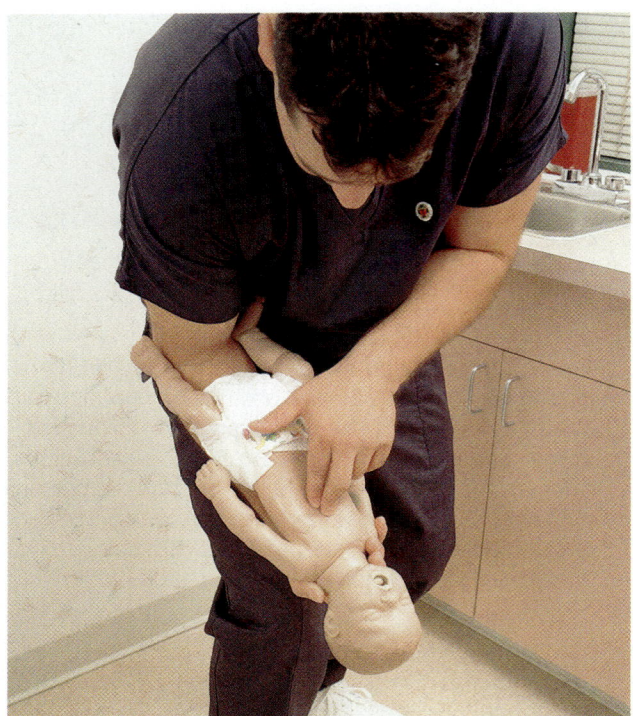

FIGURE 19-13   With the infant face up on your forearm, give five chest thrusts.

● *Do not* perform the procedure on an infant who stops breathing for other reasons, such as asthma, swelling in the throat, head injury, or an infectious process.

Accidental, Allergic, and Drug-Induced Distress

Respiratory problems can also arise from other conditions, such as:

1. A patient suffering from severe edema of the vocal cords as a result of an allergic reaction to food or stings of bees or wasps must be hospitalized as quickly as possible.

2. The victim of a drowning must receive rescue breathing immediately. This can be given before the patient is taken from the water if there is help to support the patient while resuscitation is given. A person surviving drowning needs to be hospitalized for follow-up observation.

3. Poisoning by toxic gases, such as carbon monoxide, or suffocation may also require immediate rescue breathing.

4. A person having an asthma attack may have great difficulty breathing. The physician must determine the treatment needed, but you can be helpful in attempting to calm the patient. Emotional upset often starts an asthma attack.

5. Some medications may cause a slowing or **cessation** of breathing.

6. Electric shock may cause respiratory paralysis. The victim must be moved away from the source of the electricity by indirect means (never touch the victim) and then be given rescue breathing and CPR if necessary.

CARDIOPULMONARY RESUSCITATION (CPR)

All medical assistants should take an approved CPR and a standard first aid course and participate in refresher courses periodically. The curriculum accrediting bodies of CAAHEP and ABHES require that students enrolled in their accredited programs attain Provider Level CPR certification and receive first aid training. This content must be taught by individuals holding instructor's certification with one of the four organizations recognized as qualified to instruct medical assistants. They are:

1. American Red Cross
2. American Heart Association
3. American Safety and Health Institute
4. National Safety Council

Procedures are constantly being refined, and the procedure you learn may be altered in the future. For example, there is now a recommendation that a one-way valve face piece be used in a health care environment as a guard against communicable diseases.

CPR AND DISEASE TRANSMISSION

Much concern has been voiced regarding the safety of the layperson rescuer. Statistics show that the most likely place of providing lay CPR is in the home, where 70% to 80% of respiratory and cardiac arrest occurs. The greatest concern over the risk of disease transmission should be directed to persons who perform CPR frequently, such as health care providers, prehospital emergency personnel, lifeguards, and others whose job-defined duties require them to perform first-response medical care. The layperson who responds to an emergency of an unknown victim should be guided by the moral and ethical values of preserving life and assisting those in distress balanced against the risk that may exist. It is realistic to believe that any emergency situation involves exposure to certain body fluids and has the potential for disease transmission. These can be minimized by using a face shield or face mask barrier device. They may provide a degree of protection. Masks without one-way valves, including the **S**-shaped devices, offer little if any protection and should not be considered for routine use. Obviously, **intubation** and bag compression by trained medical emergency personnel is more effective and highly desirable because it does not require personal contact.

The probability that a rescuer will become infected with HBV or HIV as a result of performing CPR is minimal. Although some incidents have been documented from blood exchange or penetration of the skin, infection during mouth-to-mouth has not been documented. HBVpositive saliva has not been shown to be infectious even to oral mucous membranes. Saliva has not been implicated in the transmission of HIV even after bites, percutaneous inoculation, or contamination of cuts and open wounds with HIV-infected saliva. The theoretical risk of infection is greater for salivary transmission of herpes simplex and airborne diseases, such as tuberculosis and other respiratory infections. Rare instances of herpes simplex transmission during CPR have been reported. Rescuers with impaired immune systems may be particularly at risk of acquiring tuberculosis and should be tested initially and about 12 weeks after a known exposure. Performance of mouth-to-mouth when blood is apt to be exchanged, such as in trauma cases, does pose a theoretical risk of HBV or HIV transmission. Because of this concern, public safety and health care personnel should follow the guidelines established by the CDC and OSHA. These involve the use of latex or vinyl gloves and mechanical ventilation equipment. Rescuers who themselves are ill should not perform the procedures if other methods of ventilation are available.

An alternative lay method of mouth-to-nose **resuscitation** is effective and is especially recommended when it is impossible to ventilate through the mouth because of serious injury or if a tight mouth-to-mouth seal cannot be achieved, such as with absence of teeth. To do this, the rescuer's mouth is sealed over the victim's nose, the head tilt is maintained, and the lower jaw is lifted to close the victim's mouth. After the breaths are given, the rescuer must remove the mouth from the victim to allow expiration.

The perceived risk of disease transmission during CPR has reduced the willingness of laypersons to provide mouth-to-mouth in unknown cardiac arrest victims. If a lone rescuer refuses to initiate mouth-to-mouth ventilation, he should at least access the EMS system, open the airway, and perform chest compressions until a rescuer arrives who is willing to provide ventilation or until EMT or paramedics can use the necessary barrier devices.

Responding to Cardiac Arrest

Sudden cardiac arrest (SCA) is the leading cause of death in the United States according to the American Heart Association. The Centers for Disease Control and Prevention estimates that approximately 330,000 people die annually, in out-of-hospital and emergency room settings. When an SCA occurs, it is imperative that immediate action take place. The majority of adults (80% to 90%) are in ventricular fibrillation when the initial ECG is obtained. The time from collapse to defibrillation is critical. The window of opportunity for survival of sudden cardiac arrest is very narrow. Resuscitation is most successful if defibrillation is performed within about the first 5 minutes after the victim has collapsed. CPR performed immediately after collapse can double or triple the victim's chance of survival according to American and European medical reports. CPR should be given until an AED is available. CPR is also necessary immediately after an AED shock, because most victims experience a period of no pulse after the shock. CPR is beneficial in restoring effective rhythm. The chain of survival involves the following sequence of events occurring as quickly as possible:

1. Recognition of early warning signs
2. Activation of the EMS system
3. Basic CPR
4. Early defibrillation
5. Intubation
6. Intravenous administration of medications

With infants and children, the prime concern is usually respiratory. A lone rescuer in this situation is currently advised to first give appropriate CPR for approximately 2 minutes and then break to summon the EMS system.

The provision of CPR first is indicated because arrest from asphyxia, as with drowning, is more common than cardiac arrest in children, and the child is much more likely to benefit from initial CPR.

CPR Procedure

The American Heart Association issued the following statement in the *Guidelines 2000 for CPR and Emergency Cardiovascular Care:* "All professional rescuers (BLS ambulance providers, health care providers, and appropriate laypersons, who have a duty or obligation to respond, such as lifeguards and police) should learn both the one- and two-rescuer techniques. When possible, airway adjunct methods, such as mouth-to-mouth devices, should be used." A variety of appliances are available, from the simple CPR mouth barriers and pocket masks to the CPR ventilating masks and Ambu-bag and masks. An extremely valuable additional piece of equipment is the AED. The use of this device has been incorporated into the resuscitation process for general health care providers.

Defibrillation

In addition to initial lifesaving methods of resuscitation and CPR, for the past several years, health care facilities and EMS providers have been using defibrillation equipment to respond to cardiac emergencies. This technology has now become practical for use by general health care workers and laypersons.

The AED consists of two large electrodes (pads that are placed on the patient's chest) and cables that connect to the machine. A battery package serves as the source of power so that the equipment can operate in any location (Figures 19-14A and B). (Some units have a self-contained battery.) The AED is indicated only when the victim is unresponsive, is not breathing, and has no pulse. There are four universal steps to follow. This description is not intended to be operating instructions, because some differences exist between different machines, and those must be followed. The AED is used in connection with CPR to restore cardiac function.

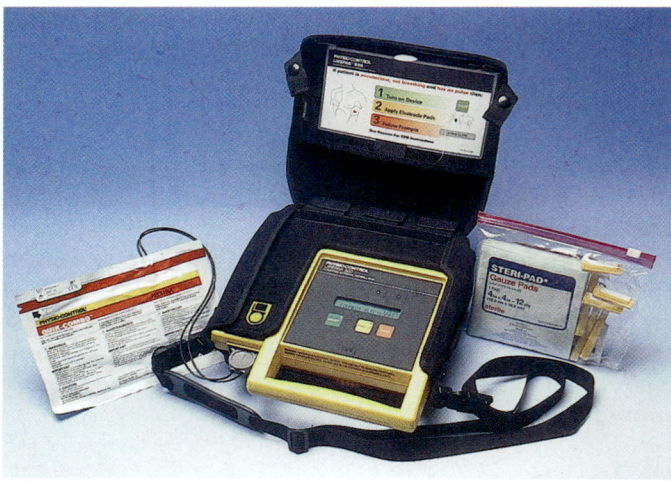

FIGURE 19-14A The automated external defibrillator (AED)

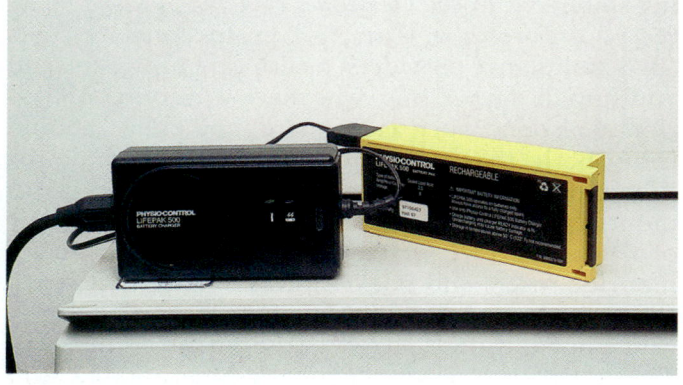

FIGURE 19-14B The rechargeable battery is the power source for the AED.

AED Universal Steps

- Turn on the power.
- Attach the electrode pads of the AED to the victim's chest (must be against dry bare skin and may require cutting or shaving of hair. Usually, a disposable razor is with the equipment).
- Analyze the rhythm. Some machines respond automatically; others require a button to be pushed. Stop CPR. It is critical that no one touches the victim while the rhythm is being analyzed.
- Charge the AED if so advised by the AED message; some charge automatically.
- Advise everyone to stay clear, and then push the shock button if the AED so indicates.
- If the victim responds, leave the electrodes in place in case of rearrest. If no response, repeat the analysis and shock sequence.
- Continue efforts until emergency medical services arrive.

Because of ease of operation, defibrillators are being placed in many public buildings, health clubs, recreational facilities, and airplanes. In a physician's office, designated personnel should be trained to operate the equipment to be prepared to respond to life threatening emergencies. Accurate recording of time, actions, and the use of the defibrillator is very important to document emergency response and provide for risk management. Equally important is the scheduled equipment check to ensure the battery is charged, the cables are intact, and the dated electrode package remains sealed and has not expired. Successful lawsuits have been awarded for unsuccessful resuscitation as the result of inoperable equipment. Each minute of ventricular fibrillation results in an approximate 10% decrease in survival. CPR provided within 4 minutes and defibrillation in less than 8 minutes still gives a patient only about a 43% chance of survival. Survival of cardiac arrest depends upon immediate response. With cardiac arrest, every minute is critical.

Caution is needed with the use of AED equipment in certain situations:

- It is not for children under 8 years of age because the electric energy setting is too high.
- The victim must not be in water; drag him from the area before using.
- If the victim has an implanted pacemaker or defibrillator, place the electrode at least 1 inch to the side.
- Remove and wipe dry any area with a transdermal patch that interferes with electrode placement.

The CPR procedure in this text (see Procedure 19-2) assumes the lone rescuer is a person with the benefit of devices to observe Standard Precautions. If you are in a situation where this procedure would be anticipated, such as in a physician's office, equipment should be

PROCEDURE PROCEDURE PROCEDURE PROCEDURE PROCEDURE PROCEDURE PROCEDURE

19-2 Perform Adult Cardiopulmonary Resuscitation (CPR)

PURPOSE: To provide the victim with adequate oxygen and circulation of the blood when respiratory collapse and/or cardiac arrest have occurred, until breathing and heart action can be restored.

OSHA GUIDELINES: To comply with Standard Precautions, gloves must be worn and a mouth barrier device used if there is any possibility of coming into contact with blood or any body fluids.

EQUIPMENT: (For simulation) Training mannequin, gauze squares, sanitizing material, CPR ventilation mask, disposable gloves, and AED.

PERFORMANCE OBJECTIVE: In the course taught by a certified instructor, using a training mannequin (Figure 19-15), demonstrate the procedure. Perform each step as instructed, using Standard Precautions at a competency established by the instructor.

1. Gently shake the victim and ask, "Are you OK?" Call for help. **NOTE: Call to another person, or phone 911 or the local emergency service before beginning resuscitation. RATIONALE: This summons assistance while you are attempting to revive the victim.**

2. Put on gloves and get a ventilation mask and the AED.

3. Position the mannequin on its back on the floor.

   NOTE:
   - The victim must always be in a recumbent position on a firm surface (floor or ground).
   - Never practice this procedure on a person.

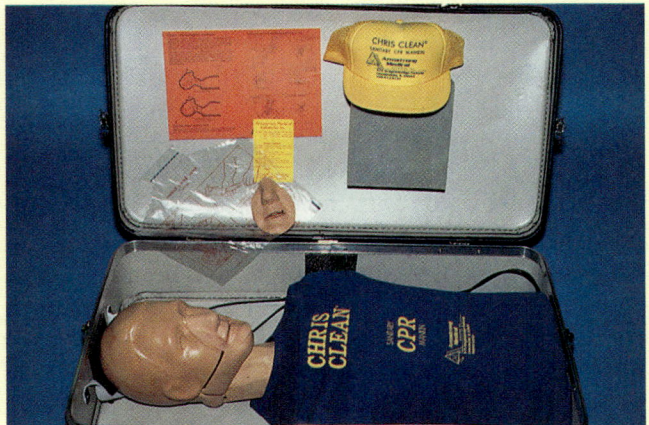

FIGURE 19-15   Chris Clean CPR training mannequin with disposable parts

4. The rescuer is positioned at the victim's side near her head and shoulders.

5. Open the airway. **NOTE: Use a head tilt, listen for air exchange at the mouth and nose, and sense for exhaled air on the rescuer's cheek** (Figure 19-16). **RATIONALE: Often, in the absence of muscle tone, the tongue may obstruct the airway; tilting the head is all that is required to permit breathing.** If this is not effective, continue with the procedure.

6. Position the victim to maintain an open airway. Place a ventilator mask over the victim's mouth; holding it tightly against the face, deliver two slow rescue breaths of 1-second duration each, producing a visible chest rise. **NOTE: If you are using a breathing device that does not cover the nose as well as the mouth, it will be necessary to pinch the nostrils together to prevent breaths from escaping out the nose.**

7. Check for a carotid pulse by placing your index and middle fingers into the natural groove at the side of the victim's neck. Check carefully, because the pulse will probably be weak (Figure 19-17). The pulse check should take no more than 10 seconds.

8. If the victim has a pulse, continue rescre breaths at a rate of one breath every 5 seconds (about 10 times per minute) until breathing returns.

9. If the victim does not have a pulse, chest compression must be started. Locate the lower margin of the victim's rib cage and follow it to the notch where the ribs meet the sternum in the center of the chest.

10. Place your index finger on the lower end of the sternum.

11. The heel of the hand closest to the head is then placed on the lower sternum next to the index finger of the first hand.

12. Place the heel of the hand that located the notch over the hand on the sternum and lock your fingers. Hold your fingers high, away from the body.

13. Rise on your knees so your shoulders are directly over your hands on the victim's sternum. Lock your elbows and keep your arms straight (Figure 19-18).

14. Use a smooth, even motion to push straight down on the chest and compress about 1½ to 2 inches for a count of 30 compressions. (The rate of compressions

(continues)

PROCEDURE PROCEDURE PROCEDURE PROCEDURE PROCEDURE PROCEDURE PROCEDURE

19-2  Perform Adult Cardiopulmonary Resuscitation (CPR) (Continued)

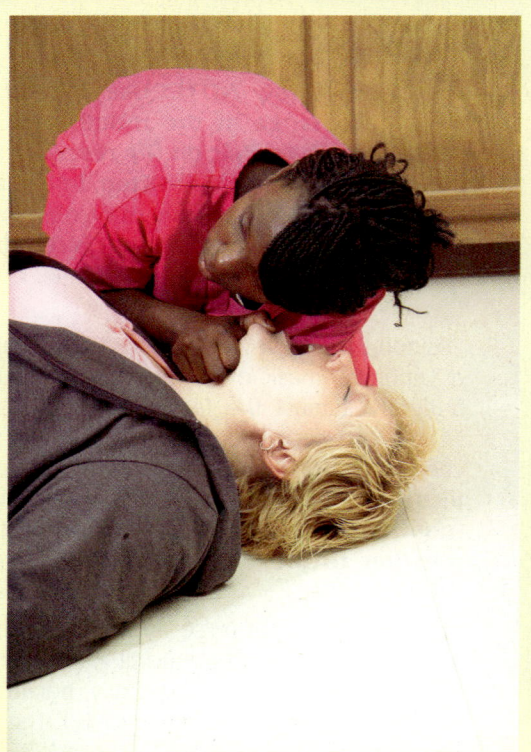
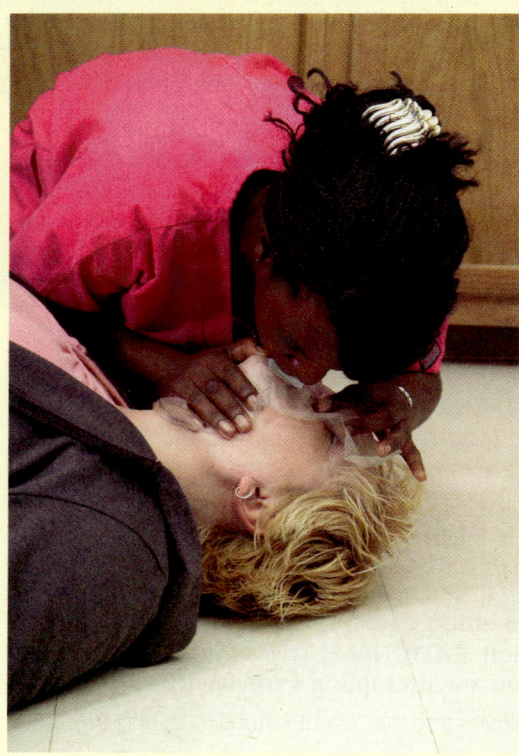

FIGURE 19-16 After opening the airway, look, listen, and feel for breathing; if the victim is not breathing, give two slow, full breaths.

is approximately 100 times per minute.) Release the pressure on the sternum briefly between compressions but do not move your hands.

15. After administering 30 compressions, give the victim two ventilations. **KEY POINT: Do this without moving from your position beside body.**

16. Repeat four cycles of compressions and ventilations before pausing to check for breathing, signs of circulation, and presence of a carotid pulse.

NOTE:

- If no pulse is felt, resume compressions and respirations.
- Check every few minutes.

When a second rescuer arrives, if an AED *is not* available.

17. Change to two-person CPR and give 15 compressions for every two ventilations until EMS arrives or an advanced airway is in place.

18. If an AED *is* available, the first rescuer continues one-person CPR while the second rescuer prepares the AED equipment by the victim's head.

19. Quickly prepare the patient for a shock: bare the chest and attach the electrode pads as instructed by the AED equipment.

20. Have all persons clear the victim's body, then press the ANALYZE button. **NOTE: The AED will determine the heart status and the need for a shock.**

21. If a shock is indicated, be sure the body is clear, then press the SHOCK button. **NOTE: Some machines are automatic; once the analysis is completed, the shock will be given if indicated. Stay clear of the victim until the analyze/shock sequence is completed.**

22. Analyze/shock cycles may be repeated once or twice. If the victim does not immediately respond, continue with CPR until the victim revives, EMS arrives, or a physician pronounces the victim dead.

(continues)

19-2  Perform Adult Cardiopulmonary Resuscitation (CPR) (Continued)

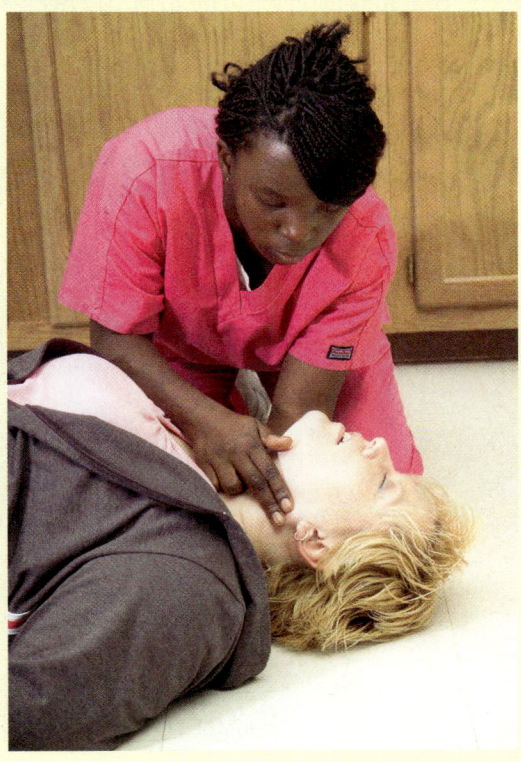

FIGURE 19-17　Palpate for the carotid pulse for no more than 10 seconds to determine whether the heart is beating.

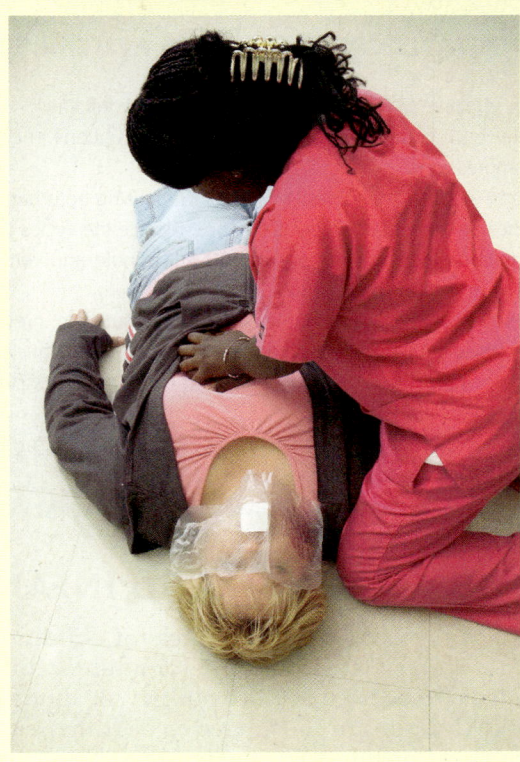

FIGURE 19-18　Chest compression position; use smooth, even motions to compress the chest straight down, about 1½ to 2 inches for an adult.

23. If a shock is *not* indicated by the AED (no fibrillation), then begin two-person CPR with a ratio of 15 compressions to two ventilations until the patient resumes breathing and cardiac function, EMS arrives, or the physician pronounces the victim dead.

24. Use alcohol or Zephiran to clean the mannequin. **NOTE: It is recommended that mannequins with disposable mouthpieces and air bags are used in training for CPR, as shown in** Figure 19-15, **to prevent disease transmission.** For those mannequins that have no disposable parts, they must be carefully and faithfully cleaned after each use with a clean gauze pad soaked in a liquid chlorine bleach and water solution, or with rubbing alcohol. The soaked

gauze pad should remain in contact with the area for at least 30 seconds and then wiped clean. It should be dried with a clean gauze pad.

CHARTING EXAMPLE

9-23-XX

Mohammed was reported collapsed on the sidewalk outside the office at 2:15 PM. Dr. Long was not in the office. Patient found without respiration or heartbeat. EMS summoned by Maria. Two-person CPR administered for six minutes by Maria and Sue. EMS arrived and took over resuscitation efforts. Stabilized and transported to First Hospital at 2:48 PM.

S. Seiple, CMA

available. A ventilation barrier device of some form should also be accessible to prevent acquiring organisms from the victim. A second rescuer should arrive, then the responsibility can be shared, with one person continuously giving the chest compressions while the second provides ventilation. Perform any variables to the procedure as may be indicated by a certified instructor of CPR.

Also, remember if the procedure is provided by the physician or an employee within the office, it must be recorded on a chart. If the victim is not a patient, a new chart must be established and the incident recorded. As soon as care is provided, a doctor-patient relationship is established, and there are legal responsibilities.

IMPORTANT CPR POINTS TO REMEMBER

- For effective CPR, push hard, push fast, allow full chest recoil after each compression, and minimize interruptions in chest compressions.
- Compress the adult chest $1\frac{1}{2}$ to 2 inches using both hands.
- Once an advanced airway is in place, replace the cycles with uninterrupted compressions at 100 per minute and ventilations at 8 to 10 per minute.
- Rescuers should switch roles every 2 minutes to prevent compression fatigue and to ensure the maintenance of effective compressions. The switch should be done in less than 5 seconds if possible.

This procedure is for information only. CPR must be taught and evaluated for competence by an approved instructor.

CPR FOR CHILDREN AND INFANTS

Health care provider CPR procedures for children and infants vary somewhat from those for adults. Children are considered to be from age 1 to puberty, or about 12 to 14 years old. Infants are considered to be from newborn discharge from hospital to 1 year old. The use of an AED that is dose-attenuated is recommended for children older than 1 year.

If a health care provider is treating a child *found* in cardiac arrest, she should initially provide five cycles of CPR before attaching an AED. If the collapse is *witnessed,* the AED should be used as soon as it is available. The AED device must be dose-attenuated for children 8 and younger. There is no recommendation for infants at this time.

It is very important for health care providers to be certain rescue breaths are effective, because arrest from asphyxia is more common than cardiac arrest. Opening the airway may need to be attempted a couple of times before ventilation is successful. Procedure 19-3 presents the steps for your information, but instruction and performance evaluation by an approved instructor is necessary for competence achievement.

Providing CPR for infants uses a slightly different technique than for children.

- When assessing the infant's consciousness, flick the bottom of the foot.
- Using a resuscitation mouthpiece, cover the infant's mouth and nose.

- Observe the infant's chest for evidence of effective breaths (see Figure 19-19).
- Give chest compressions one third to one half the depth of the infant's chest using the two-thumb, encircling hands technique, approximately 100 per minute.
- Use the two-person 15:2 ratio for infant CPR.
- Use the brachial artery in the arm to check for a return of the pulse (Figure 19-20).

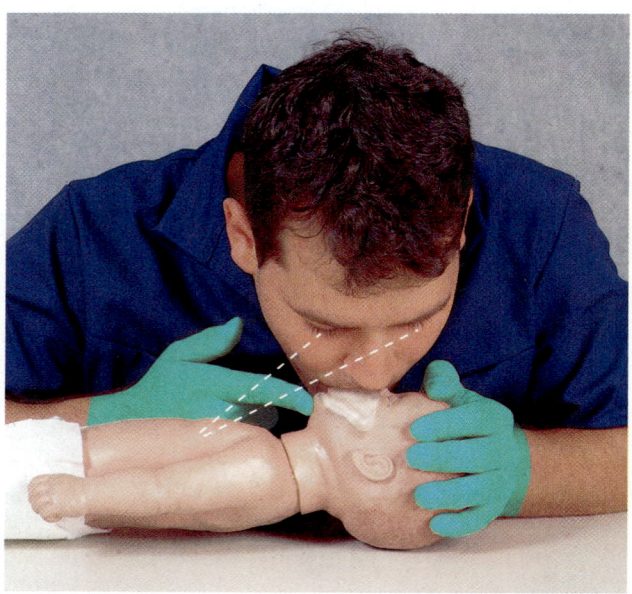

FIGURE 19-19   Observe the infant's chest for effectiveness of ventilations.

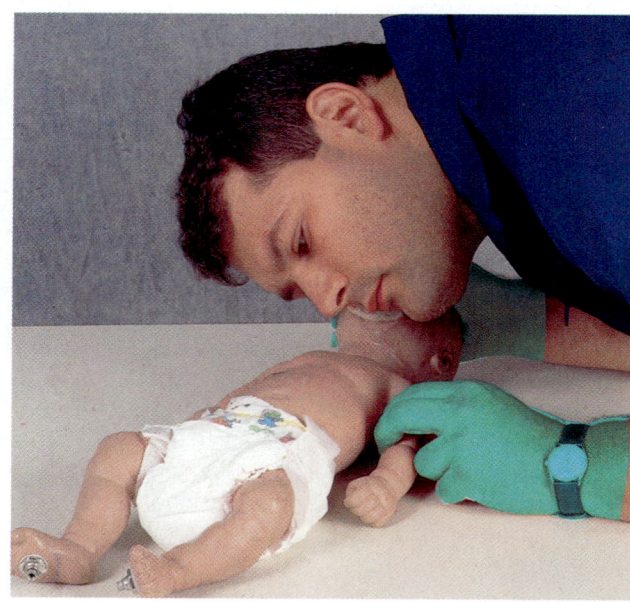

FIGURE 19-20   Check for a pulse in the brachial artery while observing for breaths.

19-3  Perform Cardiopulmonary Resuscitation (CPR) for Children

PURPOSE: To provide a child age 1 to 14, who is not breathing and has no cardiac function, with sufficient oxygen and circulating blood to maintain life untill breathing and cardiac function return.

OSHA GUIDELINES: To comply with Standard Precautions, gloves must be worn and a mouth barrier device used if there is any possibility of coming into contact with blood or any body fluids.

EQUIPMENT: (For simulation) Training mannequin, gauze squares, sanitizing material, dose-attenuated AED, gloves, and ventilation mask.

PERFORMANCE OBJECTIVE: In a course taught by a certified instructor, using a training mannequin, demonstrate the procedure using Standard Precautions at a competency established by the instructor.

1. Gently shake and call to the child to check for consciousness.

2. Call to another person to phone 911 or the local emergency service, and begin resuscitation. **RATIONALE: This summons assistance while you are attempting to revive the victim. If alone, and the sudden collapse is *witnessed*, call 911, get an AED, then begin CPR, and use the AED as appropriate. If an unresponsive victim is a likely asphyxiated, provide five cycles of CPR, then phone for EMS.**

3. Place the child on his back on a firm surface. Put on gloves.

4. Tip the victim's head back and lift his chin to open an airway.

5. Listen and watch for breathing. Place your ear by the child's mouth to listen. Also, sense if breath is felt on your cheek, and the watch the chest for breathing.

6. If no breathing is observed, use a mouth barrier and give two effective breaths, 1 second each (Figure 19-19).

   ■ If the barrier only covers the mouth, pinch the nostrils and give breaths.

7. Check the carotid pulse as for an adult. Check the pulse in conjunction with assessment for signs of circulation, which includes evaluating the victim for breathing, coughing, or movement. This assessment should take no more than 10 seconds. At the same time, keep the airway open.

8. If a pulse is present, continue 12 to 20 breaths per minute.

9. If no pulse is present, start cardiac compressions. A lone rescuer gives 30 compressions per two ventilations. Compressions should be one third to one half the depth of the child's chest.

10. Do five cycles of compressions and breaths, and then check for signs of pulse and breathing. **The second rescuer arrives with an AED with a pediatric dose-attenuating system for a child less than 8 years old or about 55 pounds and 50 inches tall. Do NOT use an adult AED for children, as the shock is too strong. Do not use the pediatric system for older children and adults, as the shock dose is likely to be inadequate.**

11. The second rescuer prepares the AED next to the child's head as the first rescuer continues with CPR. **NOTE: A minimum of five cycles of CPR should be given BEFORE the AED is used when the collapse is not witnessed.**

12. Attach the AED to the child as instructed by the equipment and clear the victim's body.

13. Press ANALYZE and wait for the evaluation.

14. Press SHOCK if indicated. **NOTE: Some AEDs are automatic and will proceed with a shock once the analysis is completed. Stay clear of the victim until the analyze/shock cycle is completed.**

15. If the victim does not respond, continue with ventilations and compressions at the two-person ratio of 15:2 until the victim revives or EMS arrives.

16. Sanitize the mannequins used in training for CPR. **NOTE: Use a solution of ¼-cup bleach to a gallon of water, or according to the manufacturer's instructions.**

CHARTING EXAMPLE

4-23-XX, 3:13 PM

Maria was carried into the office from the apartment next door because she was found not breathing in her bed. CPR was started by Sarah at 3:15 PM. Dr. Long was involved in a joint aspiration. The baby responded and started crying at 3:18 PM. After initial examination by Dr. Long at 3:20 and observation for 30 minutes, she was determined stable and taken by her parents to nearby Children's Hospital for further evaluation.

S. Mitchell, CMA

CPR for infants must also be taught and evaluated for competence by an approved instructor.

If you should ever happen to be in a remote location and CPR must be administered to someone, some guidelines have been identified. You should provide CPR as long as physically able. If there is no EMS help and none will be available, you will need to accept your situation.

If no signs of life have occured after 15 minutes, the chance that CPR alone can restore a heartbeat is very slim, the victim has for all purposes died, and there is no possibility of meaningful survival. The key to this evaluation is "no signs of life," which means no pulse, no gasping respirations, no maintenance of body temperature with progressive mottling (bluish spotting) of the skin, increased dependent livido (bluish-gray coloring), and persistently fixed and dilated pupils. As hard as it may be to accept, continuation of CPR will not change the outcome.

CPR When There Is Cervical Spine Injury

With injuries from falls, vehicles, gymnastic equipment, diving, and athletics, there is always the chance of cervical spine injury. A person who requires emergency ventilation or CPR following an injury needs to be in a supine position on a firm, flat surface to receive proper care. If the victim is lying face down or on his side, the rescuer must roll the victim in such a way that the head, shoulders, and torso move together as a unit, *without twisting*. This maneuver is also know as "logrolling." This is especially critical to help prevent any additional spinal injury. If two persons are available, one should move the head and neck as the other turns the rest of the body. The head should not be tilted to open the airway; instead, a procedure called "jaw thrust" is indicated. This can be accomplished by grasping the angles of the victim's lower jaw and lifting with both hands, one on each side, displacing the jaw forward without tilting the head. When efforts to provide resuscitation fail to ventilate the victim, try adjusting the hand positioning and jaw displacement airway opening maneuver.

Attempt to ventilate using a mouth barrier device if available. If not available, remember, if there is an inadequate seal over the victim's mouth, efforts to ventilate will not provide an adequate amount of air. This can occur when the victim has ill-fitting or dislodged dentures or a complete absence of teeth. Readjust or remove dentures and try again. If efforts are still inadequate, use the mouth-to-nose technique. If there is marked injury to the mouth or jaw, ventilation without an advance airway system may not be possible.

When there is a spinal injury and ventilation or CPR is not required, and when the person is not in any danger from his surroundings, it may be best to provide emotional support and not move him. As with any injury, always watch for signs of shock. When EMS personnel arrive, they will be able to attach a collar to support the neck and position the person on a board to prevent any additional back or neck injury when transporting to emergency care.

Shock

Shock may be associated with many different kinds of injuries and is a serious depressor of vital body functions. Symptoms include a rapid, thready, weak pulse; shallow, rapid respirations; dilated pupils; ashen color; and cool, clammy skin. All of these result from decreased blood volume because there is diminished cardiac output and the blood pressure drops. It is possible for shock to cause death even when the injury causing the shock is not life threatening. First aid measures include placing the patient in a recumbent position with feet elevated, unless there is a head injury, in which case the patient is kept flat. If the patient has difficulty breathing or has a chest injury, the head and shoulders should be elevated. It is best to place a blanket under and over the patient to maintain body warmth but not to overheat.

Shock can be caused by various circumstances. It can be associated with a heart attack or respiratory collapse. It frequently follows trauma or physical injury. Extensive burns, electrical shock, hemorrhage, near drownings, and severe infection can all result in shock. Another type, an anaphylactic shock, is an acute allergic reaction to a foreign substance, which may include certain foods, bee stings, or injections of therapeutic or **prophylactic** substances. The patient may have dyspnea, cyanosis, and seizures. Epinephrine and oxygen should be immediately available for use by the physician or by the medical assistant under the direction of the physician. No patient should be given an allergy injection and then be allowed to leave the office immediately, because anaphylactic shock may result from these injections. Patients may also have severe reactions to penicillin, aspirin, serums, vaccines, local anesthetics, salicylates, and x-ray contrast media.

Stroke

The common term for a cerebrovascular accident (CVA) is stroke. A CVA is the result of a ruptured blood vessel in the brain or an occlusion of a blood vessel. The patient may have a light stroke with very little damage or a more extensive one with immediate paralysis in the form of sagging muscles on one side of the face or the inability to use an arm or leg. One entire side of the body may be paralyzed. The patient may complain of numbness. The pupils of the eyes may be unequal in size. There may be mental confusion, slurred speech, nausea, vomiting, or difficulty in breathing and swallowing. Control of urine and bowels may also be lost. Avoid any unnecessary movement of the patient. Keep in mind that the patient who appears to be unconscious or is unable to speak may be able to hear what is being said. If a patient is experiencing a CVA, loosen the clothing and be sure the patient is positioned so as not to choke on excess saliva. Strokes are now called "brain attacks" and are considered to be emergency situations. (See Chapter 11, Unit 8.) The patient who exhibits any of the warning signs of stroke needs immediate emergency assistance to ensure optimal recovery. Remember, approximately one third of patients with a major stroke die as a result of the condition. Quick, appropriate intervention in many cases limits damage caused by blood vessel occlusion and helps restore patients to the prior state of health. The American Heart Association has adapted a series of actions to take for EMS and emergency personnel to evaluate and react to stroke similar to that of cardiac response. It involves initial field evaluation criteria, rapid transportation, medical evaluation, CT scan interpretation, and injection with fibrinolytics if it is an ischemic stroke and actions for acute hemorrhage if not.

ACHIEVE UNIT OBJECTIVES

- ■ Complete the Workbook activities to meet the learning objectives.
- ■ Practice the procedures in this unit to meet the performance objectives.
- ■ Apply your knowledge at the end of this chapter in completing the Critical Thinking Challenge and Activities, as well as the StudyWARE on your Student CD-ROM.

UNIT 3
FIRST AID IN ACCIDENTS AND INJURIES

OBJECTIVES

Upon completion of this unit, you will be able to achieve the following:

LEARNING Objectives

1. Spell and define, using the glossary at the back of the text, all the Words to Know in this unit.

2. Identify four pieces of information that can help you evaluate the severity of an illness or injury.

3. Describe the symptoms of an allergy to stings.

4. Explain the classifications of burns.

5. Describe how to remove a foreign body from the eye.

6. Describe how to remove a foreign body from the ear.

7. List three first aid measures to take when dealing with an open fracture.

8. Explain the effects of cold applications.

9. Explain the effects of heat applications.

10. Describe four types of wounds.

PERFORMANCE Objectives

1. Demonstrate the proper method of cleaning a wound.

2. Demonstrate application of dressing and recurrent turn bandages.

3. Demonstrate application of dressing and open spiral bandages.

4. Demonstrate application of dressing and closed spiral bandages.

5. Demonstrate application of dressing and figure-eight bandages to the hand.

6. Demonstrate application of cravat bandages to the head.

7. Demonstrate application of triangular bandages to the head.

WORDS TO KNOW

abrasion	immobilize	recurrent
anaphylactic	incision	shock
chemical	laceration	splinter
electrical	molten	superficial
foreign body	puncture	thermal
friction		

CERTIFICATION CONNECTION

CMA
Emergencies, assessment, and triage
First aid

CMAS
Recognize and respond to medical emergencies
Employ first aid

RMA
Identify procedure for heat treatments
Identify procedures for cold treatments
First aid procedures

SUDDEN ILLNESSES AND INJURIES

Knowing what to do when an accident or injury occurs is very helpful not only in your professional life but also in your personal life. When you have a basic understanding of first aid, you can quickly and efficiently respond to sudden incidents that may occur without becoming overly anxious or upset. As you come into contact with injury incidents, you will begin to learn when they can be handled with simple first aid and when they require the assistance of a physician or advanced emergency medical services. As stated in Unit 1, many illnesses and injuries can occur in varying degrees of severity. As an example, consider a burn. A burn confined just to the skin surface can probably be managed without medical assistance unless it covers extensive body surface, whereas a relatively small area of burn can require medical attention if it extends into underlying tissue. If you are ever called on to make a judgment, it is always better to "err" on the conservative side and seek medical or advanced emergency services than to underestimate the severity of an injury.

Keep in mind what you learned in Unit 2 regarding recognizing and responding to an emergency. When answering the office phone, you need specific information before you can decide if the situation warrants emergency medical care, an office visit, or management at home. You will need to ask the caller to give you a brief history of the victim's situation, the nature of the initial injury or illness, the time the accident occurred or the illness began, and a description of the victim's current condition. Unlike cardiac or respiratory arrest, which always requires emergency response, the sudden illnesses and injuries discussed in this unit may or may not. The decision depends upon the extent and severity of the condition and the reaction or response of the individual. After obtaining the facts, you can make an informed assessment and respond appropriately.

Bee, Wasp, and Hornet Stings

Bees, wasps, and hornets cause deaths every year. If the victim is not sensitive to the sting, the result may only be a painful swelling with redness and itching. When several stings are received at one time, the victim may become quite ill. The patient may develop severe hives or generalized edema.

When a patient is severely allergic to stings, they can cause acute illness. The patient may become restless, complain of headache, have shortness of breath, or have mottled blueness of the skin. In the cases where shortness of breath is not apparent, the victim may appear to be in shock and have severe nausea, vomiting, and bloody diarrhea. The severely allergic patient should always have a special emergency kit close at hand when there is a possibility of a sting. (Refer to Chapter 16, Unit 1, for a discussion about **anaphylactic** shock and stings.) If there is evidence of anaphylactic shock, epinephrine should be given as a lifesaving measure.

A honeybee leaves the stinger in the skin, and it should be immediately removed by scraping it out carefully with a sharp object. Never grasp the stinger with your fingers or a tweezers, as that would inject more of the venom. Wasps, hornets, and yellow jackets retain their stingers and can sting repeatedly.

Bites

An animal bite may tear skin and cause a bruise. The bite is dangerous because of the possibility of infection or rabies. The wound should be thoroughly cleansed with an antiseptic soap and rinsed well. The area should be bandaged and immobilized, and the victim should be examined by a physician as soon as possible. The animal should be held for observation for at least 15 days to see if it is rabid. The bite must be reported to the police or local health authorities, who will examine the animal for rabies. The decision must be made regarding the use of antirabies serum. If the skin is broken and the animal cannot be tested, antirabies serum should be used. When the animal can be observed and is found to be free of rabies, no serum is necessary.

There is also concern regarding human bites because of HIV and hepatitis B. The only way HIV could be transmitted in this manner is if the bite breaks the skin and the person doing the biting has bleeding gums. It is still necessary to cleanse the wound thoroughly, cover with a sterile bandage, and have a physician examine the area. Patients who have sustained such a bite from another person should be advised to have injections to be immunized against hepatitis B.

BURNS

Burns are terrible injuries. Extensive burns require painful treatment and a long period of rehabilitation. They often result in permanent disfigurement and physical and emotional problems. About two million people per year suffer burns. About 300,000 people are burned seriously; approximately 6,000 burn victims die.

Types of Burns

Burns are basically of three types: **thermal**, **chemical**, and **electrical**, with thermal being the most common.

Thermal—Caused by residential fires, automobile accidents, playing with matches, accidents with gasoline, space heaters, firecrackers, scalding water from the stove or tub), and coming into contact with curling irons, stoves, or clothing irons. Some childhood burns, such as from cigarettes, can be traced to deliberate abuse. Sunburn occurs when there is overexposure to the sun.

Chemical—From contact with, ingestion, inhalation, or injection of acids or alkalines.

Electrical—Occur after contact with faulty electrical wiring, a child chewing on an electrical cord, or from downed high-voltage power lines. Though rare, an electrical burn can also come from a lightning strike.

Classification of Burns

Burns are classified by three methods. One is by the percentage of body surface area (BSA) involved in the burn. The Rule of Nines illustrated in Figure 19-21A and the Lund and Browder chart in Figure 19-21B are methods used to estimate the size of the burn. These methods establish a standard by which all injuries can be estimated. Note that the Lund and Browder chart is more specific and has a way to estimate areas for different age groups, because body proportions are quite different for infants and small children as compared with adults.

A familiar classification reflects the extent of burn as a relationship to the layer of skin involved and is estimated from one to four degrees (Figure 19-22A). A first-degree burn is a **superficial** injury primarily to the epidermis, resulting in reddening of the skin and moderately severe pain. A sunburn or contact with boiling water or steam may cause this type of burn (Figure 19-22B). A second-degree burn involves the epidermis and part of the dermis. The leakage of plasma and electrolytes from the capillaries damaged by the burn into the surrounding tissues raises up the epidermis to form blisters and results in mild to moderate edema and pain (Figure 19-22C). A third-degree burn involves the epidermis, dermis, and subcutaneous skin layers. No blisters appear, but white, leathery tissue and

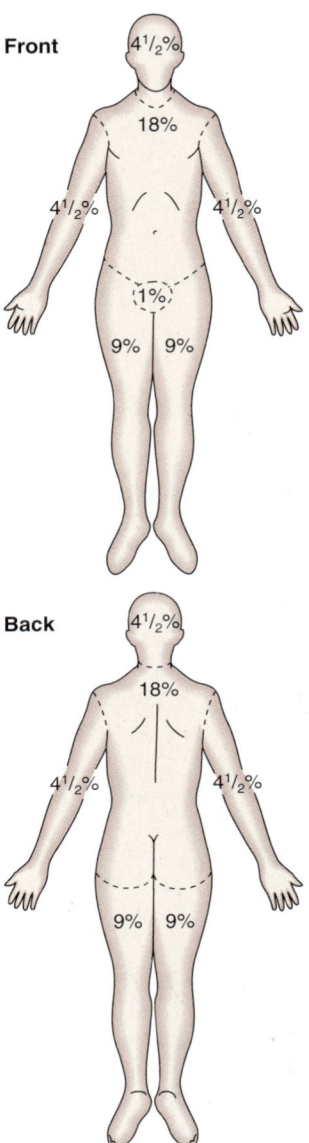

FIGURE 19-21A   Diagram for use in calculating the extent of burns or other injuries for an adult

thrombosed vessels are visible. A fourth-degree burn indicates that the damage extends through the subcutaneous tissue into muscle and bone. The tissue appears deeply charred (Figure 19-22D).

Another classification of burns measures the severity of a burn by a combination of two methods. It correlates the burn's depth with its size (BSA) to determine its severity, which is then classified as a minor, moderate, or major burn.

● A *minor* burn has less than 2% of BSA at the third-degree level and burns on less than 15% for adults and 10% for children at the second-degree level.

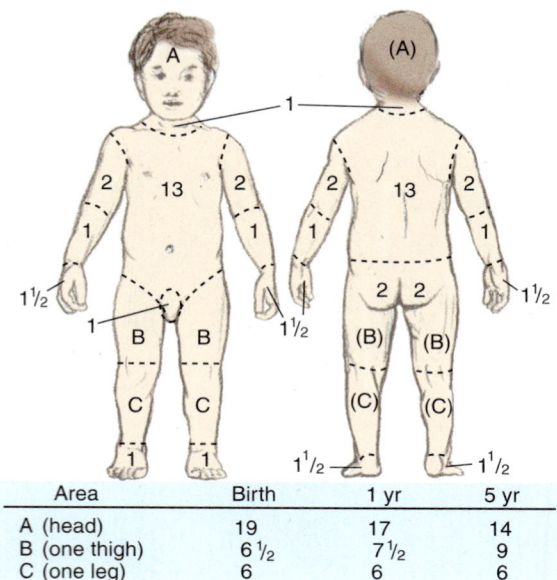

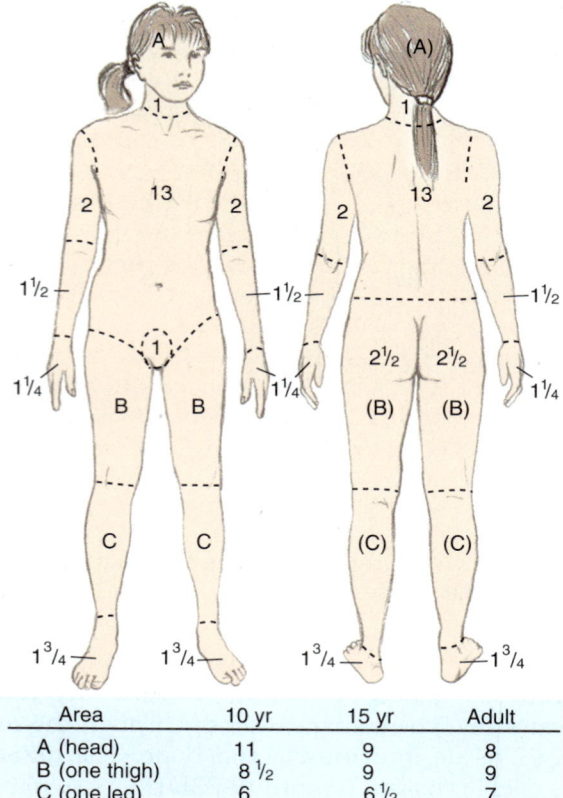

Area	Birth	1 yr	5 yr
A (head)	19	17	14
B (one thigh)	6 1/2	7 1/2	9
C (one leg)	6	6	6

Area	10 yr	15 yr	Adult
A (head)	11	9	8
B (one thigh)	8 1/2	9	9
C (one leg)	6	6 1/2	7

FIGURE 19-21B Lund and Browder chart for estimating the extent of burns. Because this chart takes proportional age-size differences into account, it can be used for infants and children as well as adults.

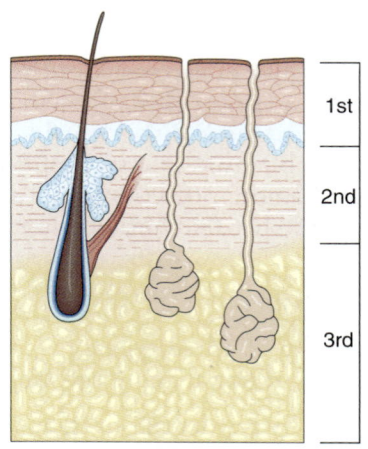

FIGURE 19-22A Layers of skin in relation to degree of burn

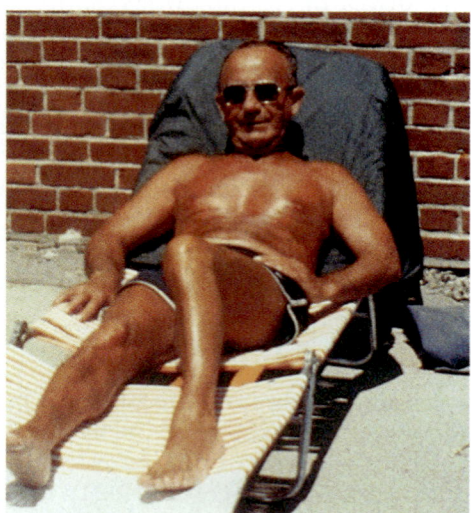

FIGURE 19-22B First-degree burns involve the top layer of skin. *(Courtesy of the Phoenix Society of Burn Survivors, Inc.)*

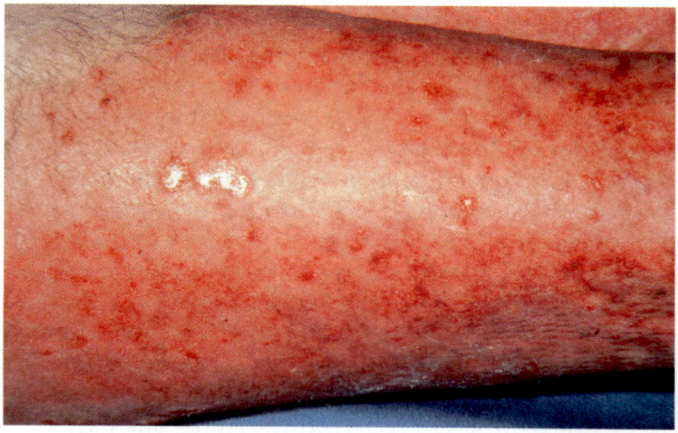

FIGURE 19-22C Second-degree or partial-thickness burns affect the top layers of skin. The healing process is slower, and scarring may occur. *(Courtesy of the Phoenix Society of Burn Survivors, Inc.)*

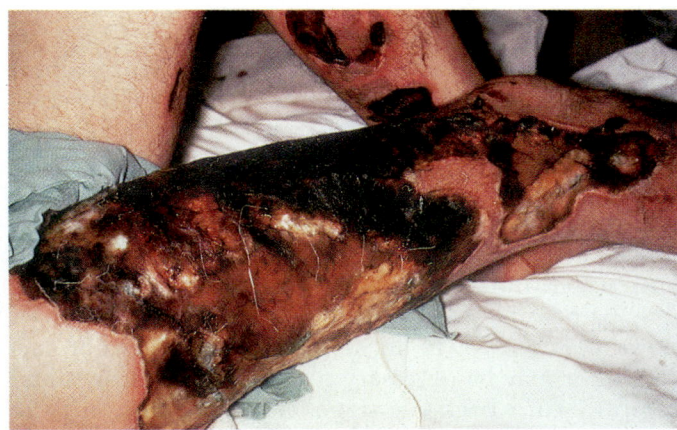

FIGURE 19-22D Fourth-degree or deep, full-thickness burns are the most serious, affecting or destroying all layers of skin plus the fat, muscle, bones, and nerves. *(Courtesy of the Phoenix Society of Burn Survivors, Inc.)*

- A *moderate* burn is one where third-degree burns cover 2% to 10% of BSA; second-degree burns cover from 15% to 25% on adults or over 10% on children.
- A *major* burn is one where a third-degree burn covers more than 10% of BSA or second-degree burns cover more than 25% in adults or 20% in children; burns of the hands, feet, or genitalia are also major burns; burns that are complicated by fractures, affect poor risk patients, or are electrical are also major burns.

The Phoenix Society of Burn Survivors, Inc., states that some professionals are no longer using the term "degree" to designate extent of burns. Instead, they refer to burns as:

Partial thickness burns = second-degree
Full thickness burns = third-degree
Deep full thickness burns = fourth-degree

The classification of burns used will probably be at the discretion of the physician or the treatment facility involved.

Treatment of Burns

The first priority in the treatment of burns is to "stop the burning process." If burns are minor, they will heal without special treatment. Applying cold water to the area should stop the pain and may even keep the burn from progressing into deeper tissue layers. The application of butter or ointments is contraindicated for two reasons: it will hold in the burn and cause more pain, and it will be painful to remove when the burn is evaluated and treated. In addition, butter contains salt, which would be very painful if the skin surface was broken. The use of ice is also contraindicated because of the chance of frostbite to the damaged tissue. Treat first-degree burns with cold water and a dressing to protect the area. A victim of severe sunburn would be

encouraged to soak in a tub of cool water and drink large amounts of fluids. Patients who are on photosensitive drugs need to be warned about their increased danger from exposure to the sun and the need to wear protective sunscreen and clothing. Pharmacists generally place a warning label on the prescription bottles containing these drugs.

In second-degree burns, first aid may include treatment for **shock**, removal of any jewelry because edema may be severe, providing ample amounts of liquid to drink, and covering the burned area with a sterile dressing. Healing may be facilitated if the blisters are opened by the physician under aseptic conditions and the area covered with a sterile dressing. Patients should be cautioned to refrain from breaking blisters and peeling the skin, because this leaves the area open to infection.

Third-degree burns should receive immediate medical treatment. If over 10% of the BSA is involved, it is considered a major burn and will require surgical intervention, IV fluids for fluid replacement, medication for pain, and probably tetanus antitoxin or a toxoid booster shot. The only first aid that is appropriate is to cover the burned area with sterile dressings and treat the patient for shock. Remember to avoid applying a dressing to second- and third-degree burns with any material that could adhere to the area, because it will cause pain and tissue damage when it has to be removed. No attempt should be made to remove clothing that is in contact with the burn. The patient will need surgical care to remove the burned fabric, clean the area, and dress the wound.

Some physicians use the term "fourth-degree burn" for burns involving all layers of the skin, muscle, and bone. This can result from an industrial injury, such as contact with **molten** metal. Of course, this is extremely severe and requires immediate treatment similar to third-degree burns.

Treating Electrical and Chemical Burns

When burns are caused by electricity or chemicals, other factors need to be considered before first aid can be given. An electrical burn results from contact with electrical wiring, power lines, or lightning. The first concern is to remove the victim from the source of electricity, but only *after* the electrical source has been turned off. This situation requires evaluation. If the electrical source is from the wiring within a home, the main electrical supply coming into the house can be shut off at the electrical box, thereby making rescue safe. If the electrical source is power lines, the electric company must be summoned. If the person and the electrical source are in a wet area, keep in mind that electricity conducts well through water. If you come into contact with the water, you could receive a severe shock or be electrocuted. EMS personnel have been electrocuted trying to rescue people from situations involving downed wires and water. Because of this potential for a lethal accident, policy states that they summon the electric company or the fire department to deal with the electrical source prior to any rescue attempt.

If the voltage is of a sufficient amount, it is possible for the victim to suffer circulatory and respiratory arrest, which will necessitate administering CPR and obtaining advanced medical care. The everyday electrical burn is treated like any other burn; however, the extent of the damage may not be readily observable. Electrical burns can cause extensive internal damage along the conduction pathway, which may take a few days to manifest itself. Persons struck by lightning will need CPR and immediate emergency treatment. They may have hallmark "ferning" markings on their body, which are characteristic of lightning burns. They too may have extensive internal damage, and if they were standing when struck, may have extensive burns to the soles of the feet where the lightning exits the body.

Chemical burns are treated by removing any clothing from the burn area and then immediately flooding the area with water for at least 15 minutes. A dry chemical should first be brushed off carefully before flushing the patient's skin because some chemicals, such as lime, are activated by water. Following the flooding of water, chemical burns, like all other burns, should be covered with a sterile dressing. A chemical burn of the eye should be flooded with water continuously for at least 20 minutes (refer to Figure 12-10). A physician should always examine eye burns immediately.

FIRST AID FOR COMMON INJURIES

Dislocations

At least half of all dislocations involve the shoulder, but dislocations are possible at any freely moving joint. When a bone end slips out of the socket or when the capsule surrounding a joint is stretched or torn, a dislocation is likely to occur. There is usually severe pain and obvious deformity of the joint area. There may be loss of function of the affected limb. There is also noticeable swelling. Dislocations are best treated by a physician. The only first aid measure is to **immobilize** the dislocation during the trip to the medical office or hospital. Treat all sprains, strains, and dislocations as if they are a fracture. The injured extremity should be carefully supported in the position in which it was found to avoid additional injury. This involves splinting from the joint above to the joint below the injury. With a shoulder involvement, this will probably involve immobilizing the affected arm by wrapping it to the body for support.

Foreign Bodies

Foreign bodies are substances or objects that become lodged in any part of the human body. It is fairly common for a speck of dirt, soot from a fire, or an eyelash to lodge in the eye, for example. Always wash your hands before touching the eyes. A foreign body under the lower lid can usually be seen easily and can be removed with a bit of cotton or a fold of tissue moistened with water. If a foreign body is under the upper lid, it may be possible to remove it by pulling the upper lid down over the lower lid. If this procedure is not successful, it may be necessary to grasp the eyelashes and carefully turn back the upper lid over a cotton swab (Figure 19-23). An object located under the upper lid may also be removed with a folded piece of moistened sterile gauze. If the material cannot be easily removed or is on the cornea, try flushing with large amounts of water to dislodge it (see Chapter 14). Any object imbedded on the cornea will require removal by a physician. Until the object can be removed, a sterile compress should be placed over both eyes to help keep the injured eye from moving, which will cause discomfort and additional irritation. The patient must be warned not to rub the affected eye, which would only imbed the object deeper into the cornea. When chemicals, either liquid or powder, get in the eyes, use a sterile eye irrigation solution to dilute and neutralize the chemical. This solution should be continuously dripped into the eye for 20 minutes. Prepacked solutions should be kept in the physician's office for emergency use. When in a situation where a sterile solution is not available, use any clean tap or bottled water to flush the eye. Eye injuries should be evaluated by a physician as soon as possible.

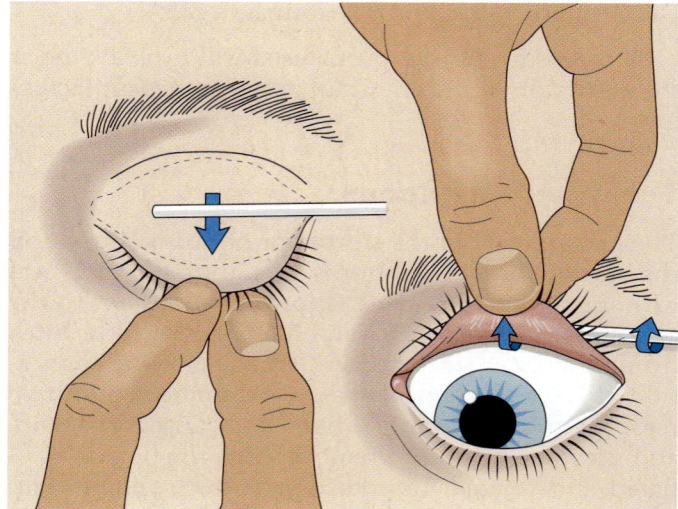

FIGURE 19-23 Remove a foreign object from the upper eyelid by turning the eyelid back over a cotton-tipped swab or the stem of a wooden kitchen match.

First aid for an object lodged in the ear consists of placing several drops of warm olive oil, mineral oil, or baby oil into the ear and pulling back on the earlobe to straighten the external canal while the head is tilted toward the unaffected side (Figure 19-24). Then let the oil run out and see if the object will come out with it. Never try to dig an object out of the ear; damage can be done to the external canal or tympanic membrane. If first aid measures are not successful, a physician should examine the patient.

Children are notorious for putting things, such as beans, pebbles, buttons, or marbles, in their ears or up their noses. Instilling oil in the ear when there are large, smooth objects to be removed may make them more difficult to grasp and retrieve. Often, these can be removed from the nose with forceps or irrigated out of an ear by directing water against the wall of the external canal. However, water should never be used with any object, such as beans or peas, that would swell, thereby causing pain and making removal much more difficult.

You may get a call from a parent who is frightened because a child has swallowed a small object. It is best for the physician to perform a fluoroscopic examination to see if the object is actually in the stomach. If the object is not sharp, it will probably pass on through the intestinal tract and be eliminated in the stool.

Splinters can generally be removed with a needle at home or with a splinter thumb forceps in the office (Figure 19-25). The skin should be washed with soap and water. The needle should be held over a flame until

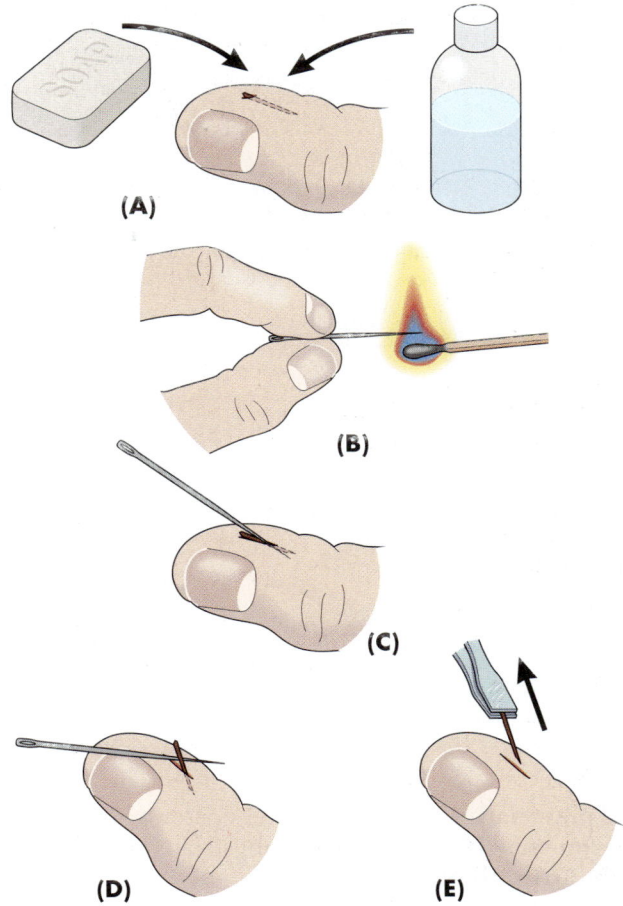

(A)

(B)

(C)

(D)   (E)

FIGURE 19-25   Removing a splinter: (A) Clean the area around the splinter, (B) heat the needle in a flame and let cool, (C) open the skin over the splinter, (D) lift the splinter from the skin, and (E) remove the splinter with tweezers.

it is thoroughly heated and then cooled before making a slit over the splinter. Lift the end of the exposed splinter with the needle, and it remove it by grasping with a pair of tweezers. If a splinter or thorn is under a fingernail, it is best to have a physician remove it. After the splinter or thorn is removed, the area should again be washed with soap and water and covered with an adhesive bandage.

One of the hazards of fishing, or of being around individuals who are casting for fish, is that hooks may become embedded in fingers, backs, scalps, or any part of the anatomy that is exposed. It is best for a physician to use a local anesthetic for such removal. If you do not have a physician nearby, push the barb on through the flesh and then cut if off with a pair of nipper pliers (Figure 19-26). After this is done, you can back out the remainder of the hook. The other possibility is to cut off the shank of the hook and pull out the barbed end. After the hook is removed, the area should be carefully cleaned and a dry dressing applied. If the removal is done away from the office, the patient should be seen

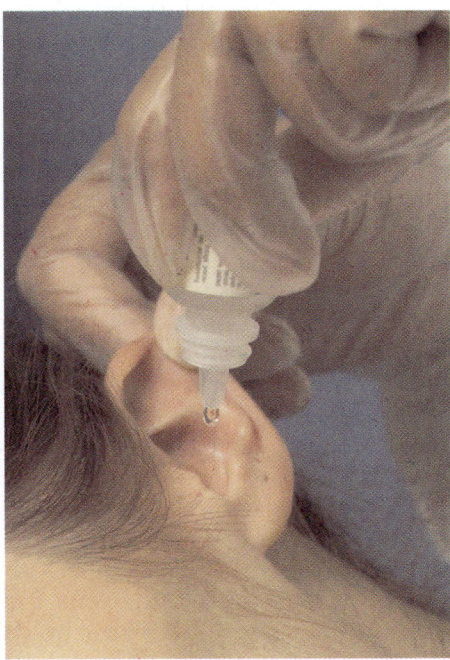

FIGURE 19-24   After the patient's head is tilted to the side, pull back on the ear to straighten the external canal and instill eardrops.

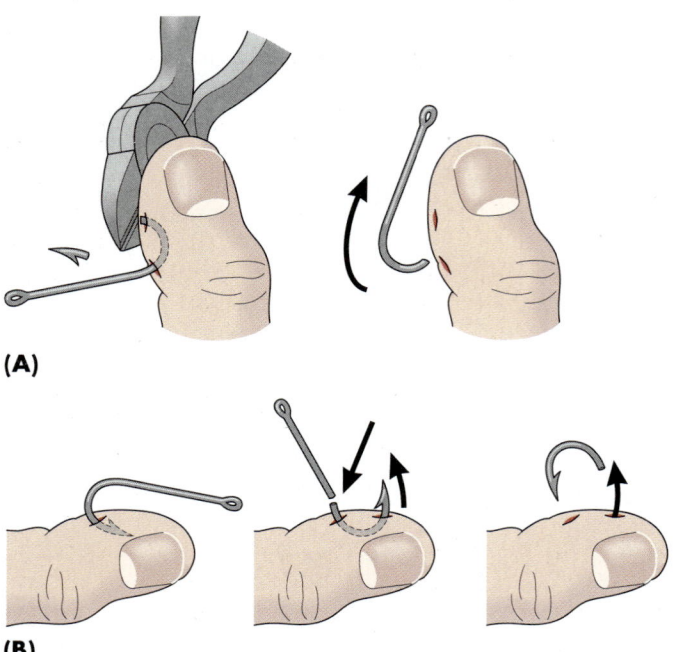

FIGURE 19-26 (A) Removing a fish hook by cutting the barb or (B) cutting the shank

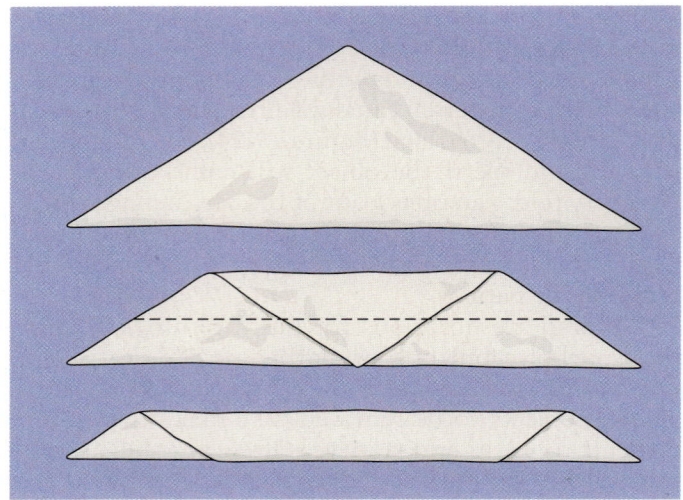

FIGURE 19-27 Folding a triangular bandage to make a cravat bandage

by a physician. A tetanus toxoid booster or tetanus antiserum may be needed. The physician may also prescribe an antibiotic.

Fractures

Fractures are breaks in a bone caused by trauma or bone disease. In a *closed* or *simple fracture,* there is no open wound. In an *open* or *compound fracture,* there is an open wound. First aid for an open fracture is to control bleeding and to splint without moving the bone ends. The patient may also need to be treated for shock. You should check the pulse and motor and sensory reflexes (PMS). Capillary refill of the distal area to all fracture sites on an injured limb will be impaired. To ensure good perfusion and nonimpaired neurological function, treatment must be administered as soon as possible. A fracture can be accurately diagnosed only by an x-ray unless bone ends can be seen in an open wound or a severe deformity is present. A physician is the only person who should attempt to straighten, or reduce, a fracture.

Strains and Sprains

Strains are the result of overuse of a muscle or group of muscles. They may be caused by improper lifting or by slipping while moving a heavy object. Muscle strain is common after engaging in any strenuous activity that you are not accustomed to doing. First aid is to rest the injured muscles in a comfortable position. Application of

ice and then heat will help to relieve muscle strain. The physician may prescribe an analgesic or muscle relaxant.

Sprains are injuries to ligaments surrounding a joint. They are usually the result of twisting the joint and are sometimes so severe that a fracture may also occur. A common site is the ankle. Treatment as soon as possible after the injury is to elevate the sprained area and apply ice for the first 24 hours. An elastic bandage is helpful for support but should not be put on too tightly. Temporary support may be given to an ankle by use of a cravat bandage, which may be applied over the shoe (Figure 19-27). (Note: A cravat is a folded, triangular bandage.)

Applying Heat and Cold Treatments

In the treatment of injuries, often physicians order the application of a heat or cold pack. The physician will give specific instructions concerning the length of time and where to apply the treatment.

Many offices and clinics today use disposable heat and cold packs because of their convenience (Figure 19-28). These plastic packs contain chemicals that are activated by either squeezing the bag or mixing the contents to produce cold or by bending a metal disc to initiate heat. Many of these disposable packs are reusable by boiling or freezing them, which is of further convenience to the patient. When using these packs, it is recommended that they be placed in a cloth covering or a disposable towel to protect the skin. If the physician requests moist heat or cold treatment, you should use a clean, moist cloth towel between the plastic pack and the skin. Moisture facilitates conduction to tissues. Moist heat is less likely to cause burns of the skin, and it also provides deeper penetration to tissues. Unless

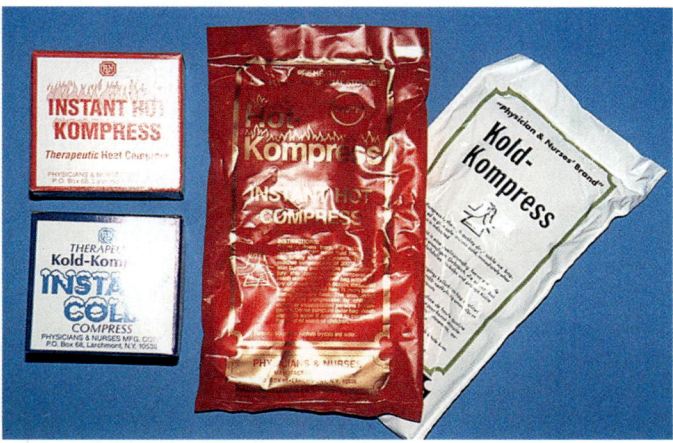

FIGURE 19-28 Examples of heat and cold disposable packs before activating the chemicals

otherwise ordered by the physician, the pack should be left in place for 20 minutes at a time. Generally, the standard instruction is on for 20 minutes and off for 10. This may be repeated to increase circulation, but constant hot or cold is never advised.

Application of cold decreases local circulation temporarily, bacterial growth, and body temperature. It also is a temporary anesthetic, relieves inflammation, helps control bleeding, and reduces swelling. The average temperature is between 50° and 80°F (10° to 26.7°C). Cold applications are used in burns, sprains, strains, and bruises and in the initial treatment of injuries to the eye.

Heat applications are used to increase tissue temperature, circulation, and rate of healing. When heat is applied to an injured area, pain decreases. The average temperature is between 105° and 120°F (40.6° to 49°C). Heat treatments are used to relieve congestion in deep muscle layers and visceral organs and muscle spasms. The heat dilates blood vessels, which helps to increase circulation and reduce localized swelling *after* the initial 24 to 48 hours of cold treatment following the injury.

WOUNDS

It is important to know the characteristics of and be able to identify and treat many types of wounds. **Abrasions** involve a scrape of the epidermis with dots of blood and possibly the presence of foreign material, such as dirt or gravel. First aid is to carefully clean the area with soap and water, apply an antiseptic solution or ointment, and cover with a dressing. If the abrasion resulted from contact with rusty metal or an unusually dirty object, an injection of tetanus toxoid or antitoxin may be required.

A wound caused by a sharp object that leaves a clean cut is called an **incision** and may need sutures to close. Some people prefer to use tape steristrips for closure rather than sutures if the wound is not too long and

not in an area that bends. The area must be carefully cleaned with soap and water, and an antiseptic may be applied before covering with a sterile dressing. A **laceration** is a tearing of body tissue and is more difficult to clean and suture properly. Special care must be taken to avoid infection. In the first aid care of an incision or laceration, the first concern must be control of bleeding. This is accomplished with direct pressure to the wound area and elevation of the extremity. If direct pressure is not effective, indirect pressure on the appropriate pressure point should be used.

A **puncture** wound is one made with a pointed object, such as an icepick, knife, or nail. First aid is to clean the wound area and if necessary enlarge the hole with a probe to allow for irrigation with antiseptic solutions. A puncture wound may also be the result of an animal or human bite. It is usually possible to identify the type of bite by looking at the shape of the wound. A human bite is identified by the shape of the denture and needs to be carefully cleaned. An animal bite may result in a laceration. A snake bite will show a two-fang wound. Treatment for snake bite has changed from past practices. Recommended first aid is:

Do not apply cold packs or ice.
Do not apply a tourniquet.
Do not cut into the wound or attempt to suck out venom.

These once-used practices do little good and may cause additional harm. Instead, cleanse the area to remove any surface venom, and immobilize the victim. If the bite is located on an extremity, try to maintain the extremity *below* the level of the heart.

Initially, all bites should be thoroughly cleansed with soap and water and covered with a dressing. Any human or animal bite where the skin is broken should be seen by a physician.

A gunshot wound entrance will be a small deep puncture site with evidence in some cases of powder burns. The exit area may be considerably larger and have irregular borders. This type of wound needs to be treated by a physician. First aid would be to keep the patient in shock position and carefully monitor vital signs while taking measures to control hemorrhage. Gunshot and stab wounds must be reported to the police. The location of either of these wounds would dictate the first aid measures to be taken. Stab wounds or impaling by any object that penetrates the chest cavity require prompt attention. If air can enter the pleural space, it will collapse the lung, since atmospheric air has greater pressure than that within the chest cavity. First aid involves covering the opening and the impaling object with an airtight dressing as soon as possible. Impaled objects to the chest, abdomen, or any other body area must be left alone until a physician or surgeon can remove them and repair the opening.

Cleaning and Bandaging Wounds

Human skin cannot be sterilized, but the microorganisms that may be harmful can be washed off the skin's surface with soap, water, and **friction**. Applying an antiseptic following the washing will make the skin essentially germ free. The procedure of cleaning a wound is usually the responsibility of the medical assistant and is presented in Procedure 19-4.

When the wound does not bleed excessively and does not involve tissues below the skin, the area can be thoroughly cleaned. If a wound is superficial and will heal well with simple cleaning and protection from contamination, there is no need for sutures. Some clean cuts may be closed with adhesive steristrips or butterfly closures.

When bleeding has been severe, no attempt should be made to clean the area because it may restart the bleeding. Because the patient will need additional medical care, it can be cleaned then. A pressure bandage should be applied securely and the patient taken for emergency medical care immediately. (A pressure bandage usually consists of multiples layers of gauze squares or pads tightly fastened to the skin with tape or bound with a roller bandage, ace bandage, or a cravat.) If such a patient comes to your office, wait for instructions from the physician before removing the pressure dressing. You will be responsible for having a suture set up for use when the physician is ready. You may question the patient or a relative to find out what caused the wound and how large and deep it is. You should also in-

---

PROCEDURE PROCEDURE PROCEDURE PROCEDURE PROCEDURE PROCEDURE PROCEDURE PROCEDURE

19-4   Clean Wound Areas

PURPOSE: To remove blood, debris, and surface microorganisms from the area of injury.

OSHA GUIDELINES: Standard Precautions require gloves to be worn if there is any possibility of coming into contact with blood, body fluids, or wound drainage. All contaminated materials are to be placed in a biohazardous waste container.

EQUIPMENT: Basin, mild detergent, warm water, sterile gauze sponges, sterile sponge forceps, latex or vinyl gloves, sterile water, irrigation syringe, a biohazardous waste bag, and bandage.

PERFORMANCE OBJECTIVE: Provided with all necessary equipment and supplies, demonstrate cleansing wounds following the procedure steps and Standard Precautions.

1. Assemble the equipment and materials.
2. Wash hands and put on latex or vinyl gloves.
3. Grasp several gauze sponges with sponge forceps.
4. Dip the sponges into warm detergent water. **NOTE: Make certain the water is at a comfortable temperature.**
5. Wash the wound and wound area to remove microorganisms and any foreign matter. **NOTE: Be careful not to injure the patient further with the instrument. Clean the wound area with sponges only, working from the inside to 2 to 3 inches around the wound as you would for a surgical prep. RATIONALE: This prevents bringing microorganisms from the surrounding skin into an open wound.**

6. Discard the sponges into a biohazardous waste bag or other disposable container.
7. Irrigate the wound thoroughly with sterile water.
8. Blot the wound dry with sterile gauze, and dispose of the gauze in the container with the cleansing sponges.
9. Cover with a dry sterile dressing.
10. Call the physician to inspect the wound and assist as needed with treatment.
11. Apply a sterile dressing and bandage it in place.
12. Advise the patient to call the physician immediately if evidence of infection develops. **NOTE: The patient should be told to watch for redness, swelling, and sensation of pain or fever. Typed instructions should be given to the patient for follow-up care.**
13. Clean up the work area. Place all used materials and gloves in the biohazardous waste bag and into the proper receptacle for safe disposal.
14. Wash hands.
15. Record and initial the procedure on the patient's chart.

CHARTING EXAMPLE

5-3-XX

Extensive wound over knee and lateral surface of right leg from fall off bicycle onto gravel area by road. Also jagged 10 cm laceration from broken glass fragment. Wound cleansed thoroughly, two glass fragments removed and wound closed with four sutures. Sterile dressing and bandage applied. Patient given follow-up instructions.

S. Davis, RMA

quire about the most recent tetanus immunization booster and record the information on the patient's chart. The physician will write the orders for the necessary immunization(s). You should not proceed with any medication or injection until the order has been written by the physician.

After the physician has treated the wound, it may become your responsibility to apply the dressing. The fol-

lowing illustrations and procedures will provide you with guidelines to satisfactorily care for the patient.

● An injury to fingers or toes or an amputation can be effectively covered with a nonstick dressing over the wound area, which is held in place with **recurrent** turns bandaging (as shown in Figure 19-29 and Procedure 19-5).

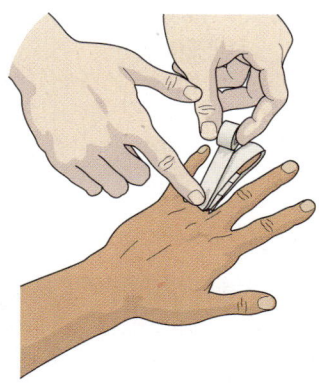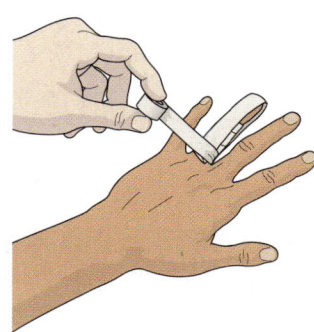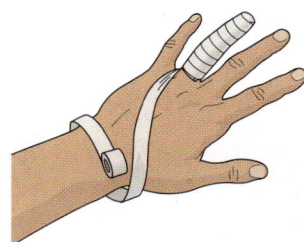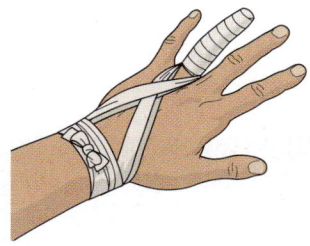

FIGURE 19-29   Recurrent turn bandage on a finger

PROCEDURE 19-5
Apply a Recurrent Turn Bandage to a Finger

PURPOSE: To hold a dressing on a finger in place.

OSHA GUIDELINES: To comply with Standard Precautions, gloves must be worn if there is any possibility of coming into contact with blood or any body fluids.

EQUIPMENT: Scissors, dressing, adhesive tape, bandage, latex or vinyl gloves, and a biohazardous waste bag.

PERFORMANCE OBJECTIVE: Provided with all necessary equipment and supplies, apply a recurrent turn bandage following the procedure steps and Standard Precautions. **NOTE: This procedure explains how to apply a dressing to a wound and then cover it with a bandage.***

1. Wash hands.
2. Assemble supplies.
3. Put on gloves.
4. Carefully open a dressing without contaminating it, and place it over the injury area.
5. Secure the dressing with a bandage of gauze. **NOTE: Start at the proximal end of the finger on the palm side and then directly over the finger to the proximal end on the back of the hand, and repeat several times.**

(*Omit step 4 to eliminate dressing application.)

6. Hold the recurrent turns in place with spiral turns.
7. Secure the bandage by tying off the gauze at the wrist. **NOTE: Tie off using a figure-eight turn.**
   a. From the finger, take the end of the bandage diagonally across the back of the hand to the wrist.
   b. Circle the wrist once or twice.
   c. From the opposite side of the wrist, continue back to the finger and loop.
   d. Repeat the figure-eight and tie off or tape it at the wrist, or tape it in place. **NOTE: It is difficult to tear and handle tape while wearing gloves.**
8. Discard the contaminated materials and gloves in a biohazardous waste bag.
9. Wash hands.
10. Record and initial the procedure on the patient's chart.

CHARTING EXAMPLE

1-12-XX

Recurrent turn bandage applied over dressing on left ring finger.

J. Finelli, RMA

● An injury on the arms or legs will require the dressing to be held in place with an open or closed spiral bandage (as shown in Figure 19-30 and Procedure 19-6).

● A wound on the palm or back of the hand may be protected with a dressing and a figure-eight bandage (as shown in Figure 19-32 and Procedure 19-7).

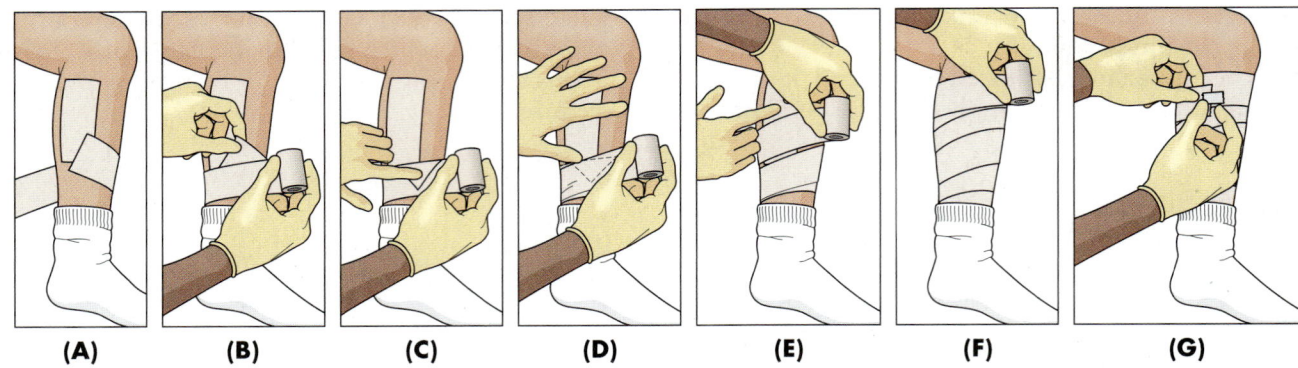

(A)   (B)   (C)   (D)   (E)   (F)   (G)

FIGURE 19-30   (A–E) Application of an open spiral bandage; (F and G) application of a closed spiral bandage

---

PROCEDURE PROCEDURE PROCEDURE PROCEDURE PROCEDURE PROCEDURE PROCEDURE

19-6  Apply a Bandage in an Open or Closed Spiral

PURPOSE: To support and cover a dressing. **NOTE: This procedure describes how to apply a dressing to a wound and then cover it with a bandage.***

OSHA GUIDELINES: To comply with Standard Precautions, gloves must be worn if there is any possibility of coming into contact with blood or any body fluids.

EQUIPMENT: Bandage, adhesive tape, scissors, sterile dressing, bandage, and a biohazardous waste bag.

PERFORMANCE OBJECTIVE: Provided with all necessary equipment and supplies, apply an open and closed spiral bandage, so that the dressing is secure, following procedure steps and Standard Precautions guidelines.

1. Wash hands.
2. Assemble needed supplies.
3. Put on gloves.
4. Carefully open a dressing, without contaminating it, and place it over the wound area.
5. Anchor the bandage by placing the end of the bandage on a bias at the starting point (see Figure 19-30A).
6. Encircle the part, allowing the corner of the bandage end to protrude (see Figure 19-30B). **CAUTION: Take care not to wrap extremities straight around, because it impedes circulation to the distal part of the extremity.**
7. Turn down the protruding tip of the bandage (see Figure 19-30C).
8. Encircle the part again (see Figure 19-30D).

(*Omit step 4 to eliminate dressing application.)

9. Continue to encircle the area to be covered with spiral turns spaced so that they do not overlap (see Figure 19-30E).
10. If a closed spiral bandage is desired, overlap spiral turns until the dressing is completely covered (see Figure 19-30F).
11. Complete the bandage by taping it in place (see Figure 19-30G).

NOTE:

■ Tape should be long enough to hold the bandage snugly in place and applied to run in the opposite direction from body movement.

■ Tearing adhesive tape is difficult while wearing gloves. You may find it necessary to first remove gloves and discard them into the proper container (see Figure 19-31).

12. If gloves are removed, reglove to clean the area.
13. Discard contaminated materials and gloves in a biohazardous waste bag.
14. Wash hands.
15. Record and initial the procedure on the patient's chart.

CHARTING EXAMPLE

4-18-XX

Open spiral bandage applied over dressing on left lower leg.

C. Spatz, CMA

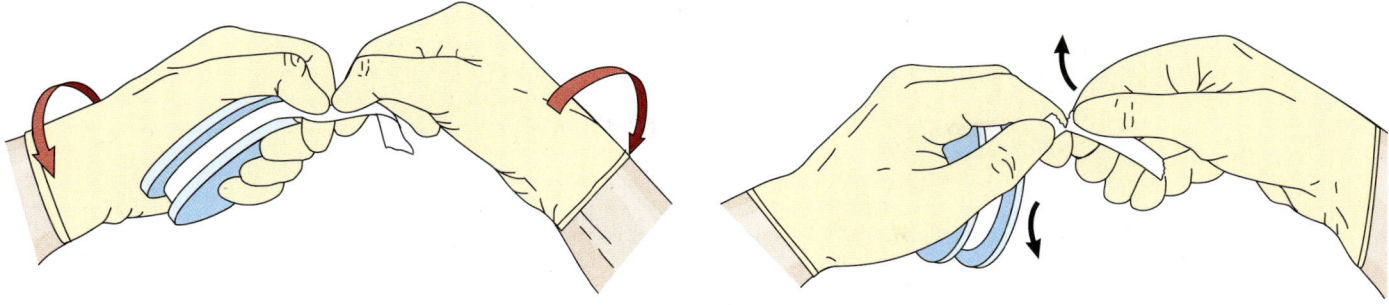

FIGURE 19-31   Tearing adhesive tape is simpler if you grasp the edge of the strip between the thumbnails and forefingers and using a quick rotary motion of the hands in the opposite directions.

PROCEDURE PROCEDURE PROCEDURE PROCEDURE PROCEDURE PROCEDURE PROCEDURE PROCEDURE

19-7  Apply a Figure-Eight Bandage to a Hand and Wrist

PURPOSE: To hold a dressing securely on a hand. **NOTE: This procedure describes how to apply a dressing to a wound and then cover it with a bandage.***

OSHA GUIDELINES: To comply with Standard Precautions, gloves must be worn if there is any possibility of coming into contact with blood or any body fluids.

EQUIPMENT: Sterile dressing, bandage, latex or vinyl gloves, bandage, scissors, and a biohazardous waste bag.

PERFORMANCE OBJECTIVE: Provided with all necessary equipment and supplies, apply a figure-eight bandage to a hand and wrist neatly to secure a dressing following the procedure steps and Standard Precautions.

1. Wash hands.
2. Assemble the needed supplies.
3. Put on gloves.
4. Apply a dressing over the wound.

(*Omit step 4 to eliminate dressing application.)

5. Anchor the bandage with one or two turns around the palm of the hand.
6. Roll the gauze diagonally across the front of the wrist and in a figure-eight pattern around the hand (see Figure 19-32).
7. Cut the gauze and tape at the wrist. **CAUTION: Do not impair circulation.**
8. Discard contaminated materials and gloves in a biohazardous waste bag.
9. Wash hands.
10. Record and initial the procedure on the patient's chart.

CHARTING EXAMPLE

6-14-XX

Figure-eight bandage applied to right hand.

M. Gomes, CMA

- When applying a dressing to the forehead, ears, or eyes, a cravat may be used to hold the dressing in place (Figure 19-33 and Procedure 19-8). A cravat can be made from a triangular bandage (see Figure 19-27 and Procedure 19-9).
- A bandage that is particularly useful in keeping a dressing in place over a large head wound or a burn is the triangular bandage (Figure 19-33).
- The easiest and probably quickest way to bandage arms, legs, fingers, and toes is with tubular gauze

bandage (Figure 19-34). This is accomplished with the use of an appropriately-sized cylindrical cage applicator. The amount of tube gauze you expect to use is stretched over the applicator and placed over the extremity. By manipulating the cylinder around the extremity, grasping the tube gauze, withdrawing the cylinder, twisting the gauze, and repeating the sequence, a snug gauze bandage can be placed over the dressing.

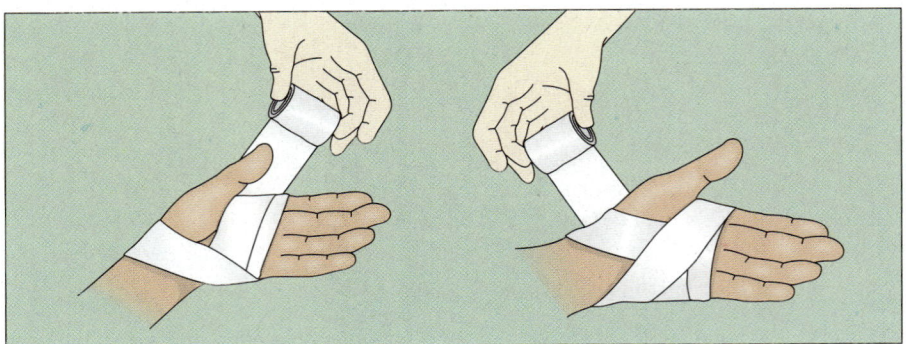

FIGURE 19-32   Figure-eight bandage to hand and wrist

PROCEDURE PROCEDURE PROCEDURE PROCEDURE PROCEDURE PROCEDURE PROCEDURE PROCEDURE

19-8

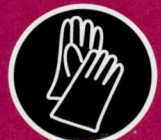

Apply a Cravat Bandage to Forehead, Ear, or Eyes

PURPOSE: To hold a dressing neatly and securely in place. **NOTE: This procedure explains how to apply a dressing to a wound and then cover it with a cravat bandage.***

OSHA GUIDELINES: To comply with Standard Precautions, gloves must be worn if there is any possibility of coming into contact with blood or any body fluids.

EQUIPMENT: Sterile dressing, cravat bandage, latex or vinyl gloves, and a biohazardous waste bag.

PERFORMANCE OBJECTIVE: Provided with all necessary equipment and supplies, apply a cravat bandage to the head following the procedure steps and Standard Precautions.

1. Wash hands.
2. Assemble the needed supplies.

(*Omit step 4 to eliminate dressing application.)

3. Put on gloves.
4. Carefully place a dressing over the wound.
5. Place the center of the cravat over the dressing.
6. Take the ends around to the opposite side of the head and cross them. Do not tie (see Figure 19-33).
7. Bring the ends back to the starting point and tie them.
8. Discard the contaminated materials and gloves in a biohazardous waste bag.
9. Wash hands.
10. Record and initial the procedure on the patient's chart.

CHARTING EXAMPLE

8-28-XX

Cravat bandage applied over dressing on head.

S. Cimenella, CMA

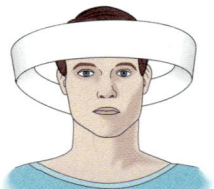
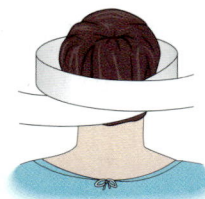
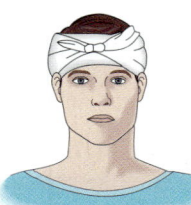

FIGURE 19-33   Applying a cravat bandage to the head

ACHIEVE UNIT OBJECTIVES

- ■ **Complete the Workbook activities to meet the learning objectives.**
- ■ **Practice the procedures in this unit to meet the performance objectives.**
- ■ **Apply your knowledge at the end of this chapter in completing the Critical Thinking Challenge and Activities, as well as the StudyWARE on your Student CD-ROM.**

19-9  Apply a Triangular Bandage to the Head

PURPOSE: To cover and support a dressing on the head. **NOTE: This procedure explains how to apply a dressing to a wound and then cover it with a triangular bandage.***

OSHA GUIDELINES: To comply with Standard Precautions, gloves must be worn if there is any possibility of coming into contact with blood or any body fluids.

EQUIPMENT: Triangle bandage, sterile dressing, latex or vinyl gloves, and a biohazardous waste bag.

PERFORMANCE OBJECTIVE: Provided with the necessary equipment, apply a triangular bandage to the head following the procedure steps and Standard Precautions so that the dressing is neat and secure.

1. Wash hands.
2. Assemble the needed supplies.
3. Put on gloves.
4. Carefully place a dressing over the wound area.
5. Fold a hem about 2 inches wide along the base of the bandage (see Figures 19-34A and B).
6. With the hem on the outside, place a bandage on the head so that the middle of the base is on the forehead

(*Omit step 4 to eliminate dressing application.)

close to the eyebrows and the point hangs down in back (see Figures 19-34C and D).

7. Bring the two ends around the head above the ears, and cross them just below the bump at the back of the head.
8. Draw the ends snugly around the head, and tie them in the center of the forehead.
9. Steady the head with one hand, and with the other hand, draw the point down firmly behind to hold the dressing securely against the head. Grasp the point, and tuck it into the area where the bandage ends cross (see Figures 19-34E to G).
10. Discard the contaminated materials and gloves in a biohazardous waste bag.
11. Wash hands.
12. Record and initial the procedure on the patient's chart.

CHARTING EXAMPLE

9-14-XX

Triangular bandage applied over dressing on head wound.

M. Jackson, RMA

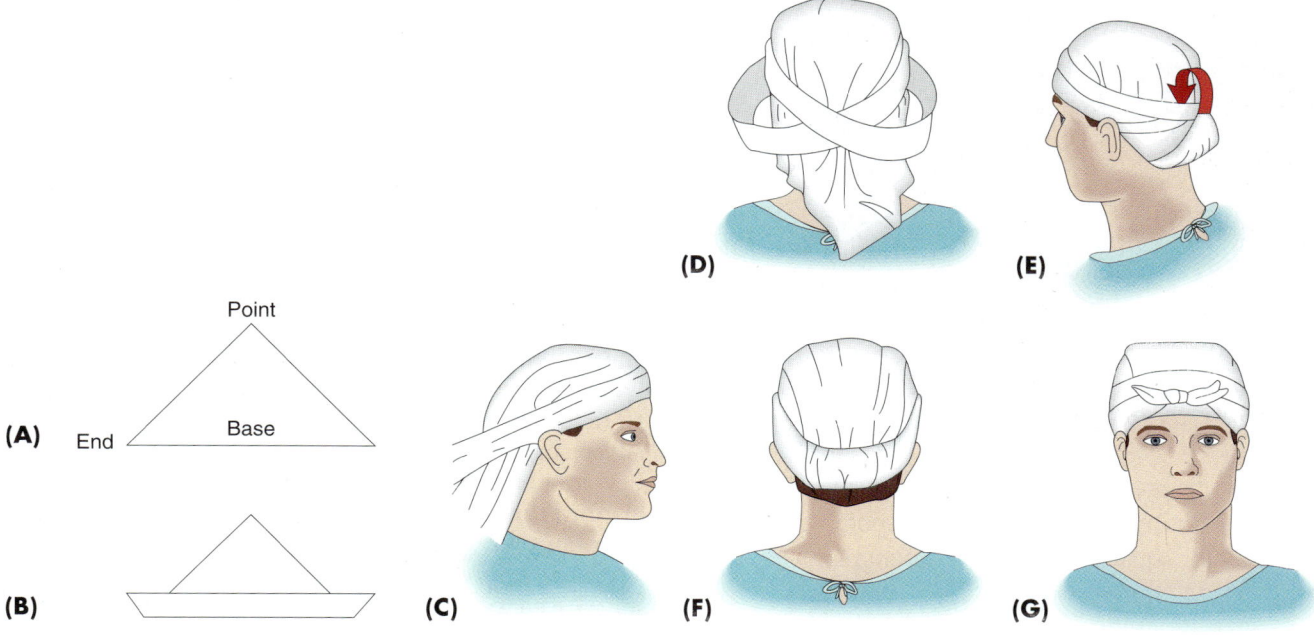

FIGURE 19-34 Applying a triangular bandage to the head

UNIT 4
RECOVERING FUNCTION AND MOBILITY

OBJECTIVES

Upon completion of this unit, you will be able to achieve the following:

LEARNING Objectives

1. Spell and define, using the glossary at the back of the text, all the Words to Know in this unit.
2. Explain why it is important to role-play being a patient.
3. Identify situations when the use of mobility equipment is indicated.
4. Role play instruction of range of motion exercises.
5. Describe how to make the home safer for people using mobility aids.

PERFORMANCE Objectives

1. Demonstrate application of a sling.
2. Demonstrate fitting and instruction in use of a cane.
3. Demonstrate fitting and instruction in use of crutches.
4. Demonstrate instruction in use of a walker.
5. Demonstrate movement of patient from a wheelchair to and from an examination table.

WORDS TO KNOW

ambulate	gait	stabilize
angle	mobility	support
axilla	quad-base	triangular
balance	range-of-motion	bandages
crutches	(ROM)	wheelchair
flexibility	sling	

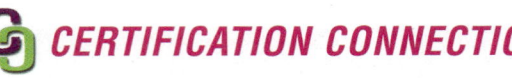

CERTIFICATION CONNECTION

CMA
Principles of operation (physical therapy modalities, wheelchair)
Patient instruction (instructing and demonstrating the use and care of patient equipment)

CMAS
Employ first aid and CPR appropriately

RMA
Therapeutic modalities (maintain familiarity with range of motion exercises)
Instruct patients in the use of assistive devices

This unit discusses the various devices that may be indicated in the process of recovering and gaining mobility and provides procedures covering the most common ones. Not only should you learn to instruct others in the proper use or application of the various pieces of equipment, but you should also participate in the patient's experience. Practice being the medical assistant and the patient so that you can appreciate the patient's dependence and understand the constraints involved. Few people realize the amount of strength and energy required to walk a long hallway or climb a flight of stairs using crutches. Spending a few hours in a wheelchair can also prove to be a very enlightening experience.

INDICATIONS FOR MOBILITY DEVICES

Many times, following a serious illness or an accident, some form of supporting device or equipment is needed to allow a person to have as much **mobility** as possible. This may take the form of only a splint or a **sling** to support extremities or it may be nearly complete reliance in the form of a **wheelchair**. Examples of situations when the use of some type of device may be needed are as follows:

- After an accident or injury—Sprains, fractures, and dislocations require temporary **support** and absence from use to permit healing.
- Following a stroke—If there has been a loss of use of the extremities or if the person has become somewhat unsteady on his feet, something may be needed to help him maintain **balance**.
- After surgery—When joints are replaced, supportive devices are necessary until muscles are strengthened around the new implant and the person is allowed to bear her own weight when she **ambulates**.
- With a severe medical condition—Patients with congestive heart failure, emphysema, or similar debilitating illnesses frequently use supportive devices to aid their mobility.

- Arthritis sufferers—The use of a cane or **crutches** to support a portion of the body weight reduces the discomfort in the knees, hips, and lower back.
- The aged—The elderly often become unsteady on their feet and, because of the fear of falling, use a cane or walker to help **stabilize** themselves while walking.
- Physically challenged—Persons with physical disabilities often require supportive devices to assist them with mobility.

Range-of-Motion Exercises

In addition to the use of mobility devices, patients can benefit greatly by improving their strength and **flexibility**. This can be accomplished with participation in a regular program of exercise. Regular exercise improves circulation and muscle tone and relieves tension. People who have followed an exercise routine regularly report that they experience a better outlook on life, have more energy, and feel healthier. The degree of exertion in any exercise routine will vary with individuals, and the physician's advice should be taken.

For patients who cannot engage in strenuous exercise, walking and **range-of-motion** exercises (**ROM**) are suggested to improve circulation and flexibility, and promote muscle tone (Figure 19-35).

ROM is defined as any body action involving muscles, joints, and natural directional movements, such as abduction, adduction, extension, flexion, pronation, and rotation. Such exercises are usually applied actively or passively in the treatment of orthopedic deformities, assessment of injuries and deformities, and athletic conditioning. These movements help to move each joint through its full range. Patients who have arthritis, bursitis, and other disabilities can be helped by these exercises.

Study the illustrations in Figure 19-35, and perform the motions yourself. Patients are frequently sent to a physical therapist for treatment and instruction, but the medical assistant may be responsible for reinforcing the therapist's instruction about how to perform the exercises.

Arm Sling

A sling is often used to support an arm after a fracture or injury to the shoulder or arm. This aids the patient by supporting and protecting the injured extremity so

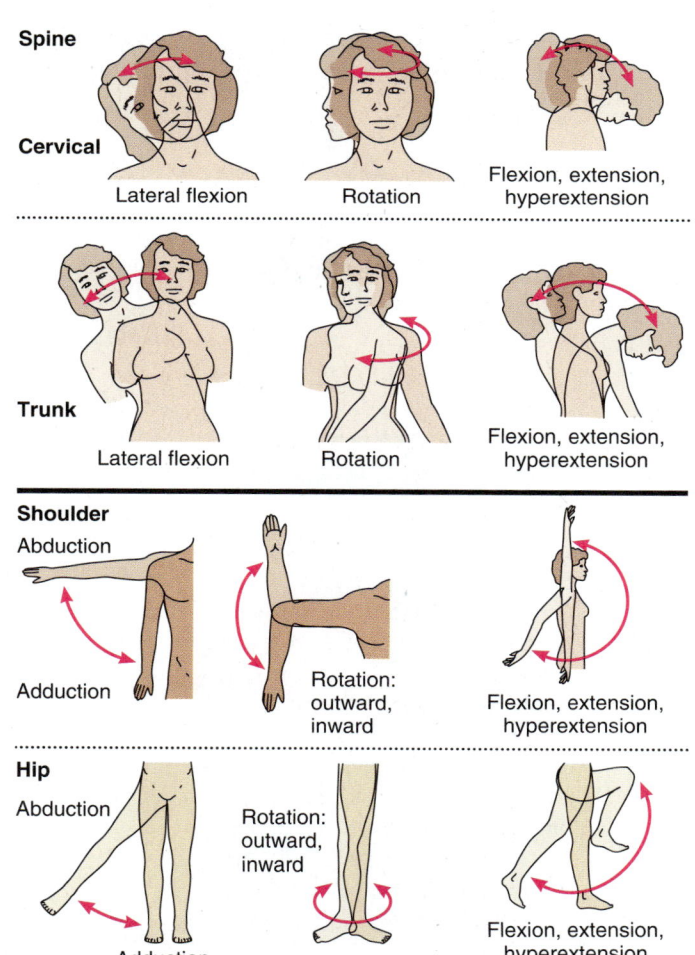

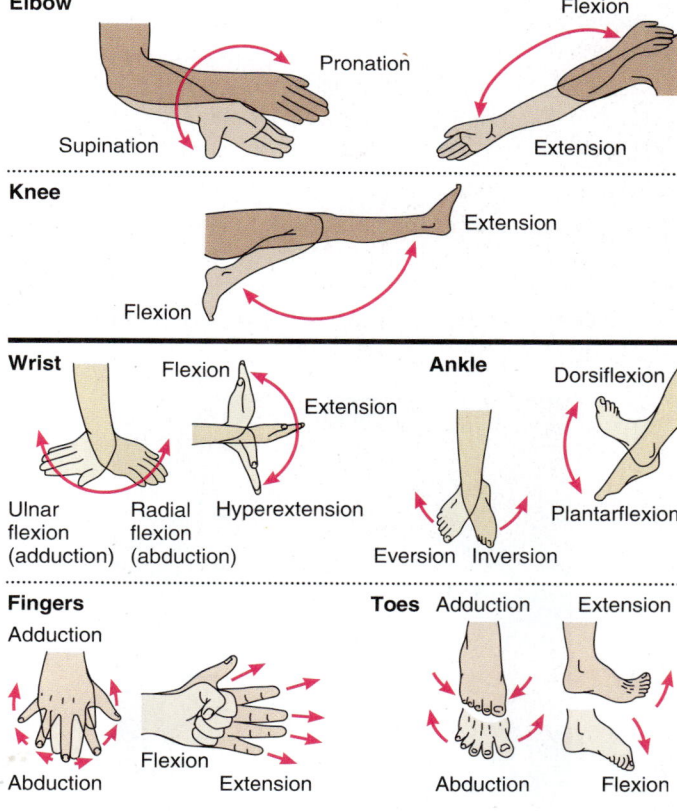

FIGURE 19-35 Range-of-motion exercises are helpful to patients who have limited physical activity. They improve circulation, increase flexibility, and promote improved muscle tone.

that most activities can be continued until it is healed. It is important to learn the correct way to apply a sling with the patient standing, sitting, or lying down. Care must be taken to elevate the hand properly to assist the return of circulation and avoid swelling. You must also be sure that the sling is tied to one side and never over the spine, where a knot becomes extremely uncomfortable.

Triangular bandages (Figure 19-36A) may be made from muslin or purchased in individual packages. Some physicians like to use a print material for children. The standard adult sling is about 55 inches across the base and 36 to 40 inches along the sides. (See Procedure 19-10.) Another type of sling, the buckle style (Figure 19-36B), is used for long-term support in instances such as supporting an arm affected by stroke.

PROCEDURE PROCEDURE PROCEDURE PROCEDURE PROCEDURE PROCEDURE PROCEDURE

19-10   Apply an Arm Sling

PURPOSE: To provide support for an injured arm or shoulder.

OSHA GUIDELINES: To comply with Standard Precautions, gloves must be worn if there is any possibility of coming into contact with blood or any body fluids.

EQUIPMENT: Triangle or buckle-type sling.

PERFORMANCE OBJECTIVE: Provided with the necessary equipment, demonstrate the steps in the procedure for applying an arm sling so that the arm is supported properly and the sling is correctly tied.

1. Wash hands.
2. Place one end of a triangle bandage over the shoulder on the uninjured side and let the other end hang down over the chest (see Figure 19-36A).
3. Pull the point behind the elbow of the injured arm.
4. Pull the end of the bandage that is hanging down up around the injured arm and over the shoulder. Elevate the hand 4 to 5 inches above the elbow. **RATIONALE: Elevation aids in the return of circulation, which**

reduces swelling and discomfort. Tie the ends together at the side of the neck (never over the spine).

5. Bring the point of the bandage at the elbow over the front of the sling, and pin it to the sling with a safety pin.

NOTE:

- If a pin is not available, twist the point until it is snug against the elbow, and tie it in a single knot.
- Be sure the ends of the fingers extend slightly beyond the edge of the sling. **RATIONALE: It is necessary to be able to observe the fingers for signs of impaired circulation, such as swelling or discoloration.**

CHARTING EXAMPLE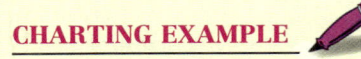

6-23-XX

Triangular sling applied to left arm for support following fall. Fingers elevated and extended from sling. No swelling observed, color normal.

P. Blair, RMA

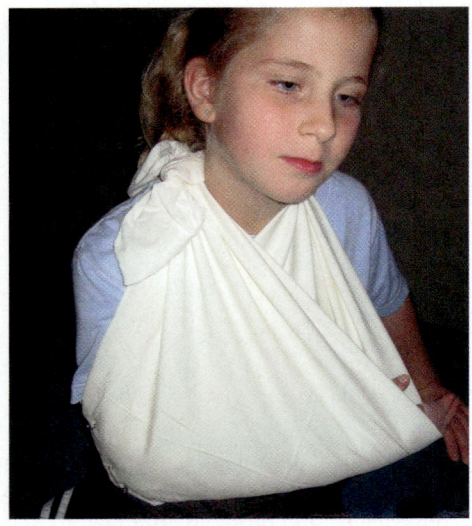

FIGURE 19-36A   Applying an arm sling

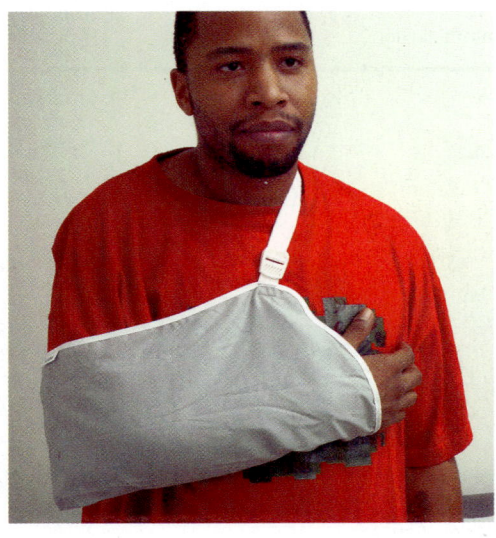

FIGURE 19-36B   Canvas and strap arm sling for support

Canes

The patient who needs only a cane for support should have one that is the proper length to fit comfortably in the hand with the arm hanging naturally at the side and the elbow flexed at about a 25- to 30-degree **angle**. The handle should be just below hip level. Many canes are adjustable; if not, they must be fitted to the correct length. Canes come in a variety of materials and types (Figure 19-37). An elderly patient usually has less trouble with a **quad-base** cane, because its four "feet" provide a stable base that gives better support. The patient should carry the cane on the strong or uninjured side. The cane should swing forward with the injured extremity. Part of the weight is carried by the cane being firmly placed on the floor simultaneously with the injured extremity. Refer to Procedure 19-11.

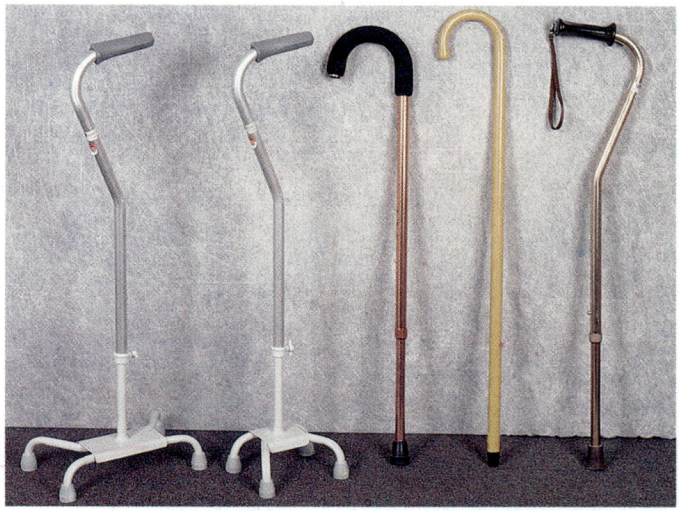

FIGURE 19-37   Types of standard canes: quad canes and single-tip canes

PROCEDURE PROCEDURE PROCEDURE PROCEDURE PROCEDURE PROCEDURE PROCEDURE PROCEDURE

19-11   Use a Cane

PURPOSE: To adjust a cane for proper height and teach a patient correct and safe use of a cane.

EQUIPMENT: Cane.

PERFORMANCE OBJECTIVE: Provided with a cane, demonstrate adjusting the length of a cane, and provide the patient with instruction to properly and safely use a cane. The cane will be the appropriate length, and the patient will demonstrate correct usage.

1. Identify the patient, and confirm the physician's orders. **RATIONALE: Speaking to the patient by name and checking the chart ensures that you are performing the procedure for the correct patient.**

2. Assemble the equipment. Check the cane for an intact rubber tip. **NOTE: The patient must be wearing nonskid shoes or foot coverings. RATIONALE: This helps prevent slipping or falling.**

3. Adjust the height of the cane so that the patient's elbow is flexed comfortably at approximately a 25- to 30-degree angle, and check that the handle of the cane is positioned just below the hip level of the uninjured or strong side.

4. Demonstrate for the patient the **gait** ordered for safe ambulation.
   a. Move the cane and injured extremity forward simultaneously.
   b. Then, move the strong or uninjured extremity forward.

5. Allow the patient to practice the procedure. **NOTE: Observe the patient, and be alert to assist the patient and rescue him in case of a fall.**

6. Demonstrate going up stairs. Move the uninjured extremity up first, then move the injured extremity up. Remind the patient to use the cane for support, and have the patient practice.

7. Demonstrate going down stairs. The move uninjured extremity down first. Then move the injured extremity down. Remind the patient to use the cane for support, and have patient practice.

8. Instruct the patient to take small, slow steps. **RATIONALE: This aids in maintaining balance. NOTE: Answer any questions the patient may have and give emotional support.**

9. Ensure that the cane height is correct and that the patient is using the cane correctly.

10. Record and initial on the patient's chart.

CHARTING EXAMPLE

7-23-XX

Cane adjusted for proper height. Rubber tip securely in place. Proper use of cane demonstrated to Julio, and he correctly returned the demonstration. Practiced on level floor and short flight of stairs. Advised him regarding selection of appropriate shoes to prevent slipping or falling.

B. Cox, CMA

Crutches

It is often necessary for a patient to walk with crutches to give a foot, ankle, knee, or leg injury or surgery an opportunity to heal. It is important for the crutches to be adjusted to the correct height (Figure 19-38A). This is accomplished by holding the crutches up to the side of the patient and adjusting them so that the undearm pad is 2 to 3 inches below the **axilla**. The handhold should be adjusted so that the hands fit comfortably with the arms extended. The axillary piece and the handhold should be foam padded for comfort. The patient should be instructed to stand on the uninjured foot while swinging the injured leg forward as the crutches are moved forward (Figure 19-38B). The weight of the body should be on the hands and never on the axillary area, because over time, prolonged pressure on the axillary nerves can cause nerve damage.

Crutches can be used in three different gait or step patterns (refer to Procedure 19-12). The four-point gait shows the right crutch being positioned first, followed by moving the left foot. Then, the left crutch is moved forward, followed by the right foot. This makes for good stability but requires practice to coordinate the movements. The three-point gait positions both crutches and the left foot forward, then brings up the right foot. (The foot moved with the crutches depends upon which extremity is injured.) The two-point gait matches the crutch to the opposite foot, moving them together. Practice all three gaits following the procedure until you are certain you could instruct a patient in the safe use of crutches.

Other varieties of crutches are designed for special situations. Lofstrand or forearm crutches (Figure 19-38C) eliminate axillary pressure, and with the forearm cuff is more stable. This type would be used for long-term rehabilitation. The platform crutch (Figure 19-38D) is used when a patient's hand or forearm is not able to bear her body's weight.

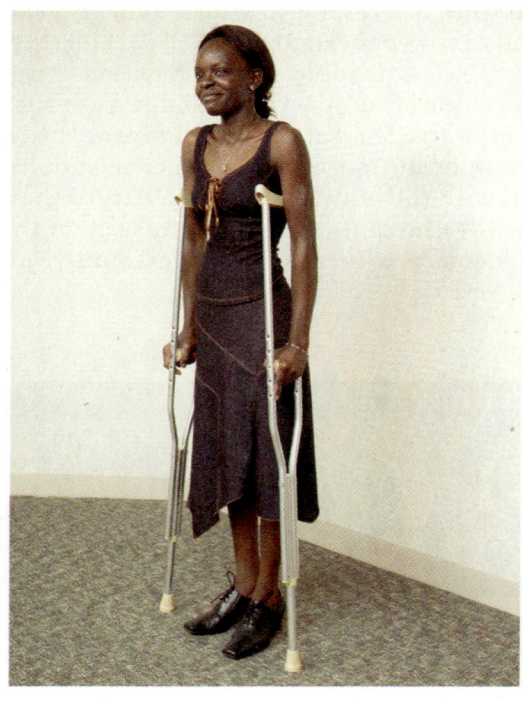

FIGURE 19-38B Axillary crutches

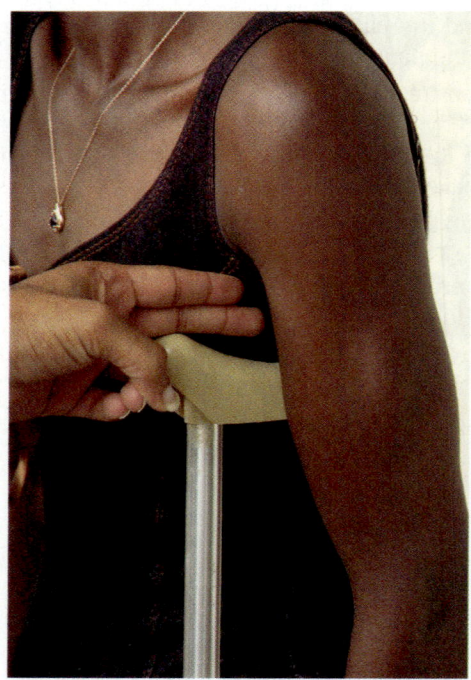

FIGURE 19-38A Measuring for axillary crutches. Note the height is about 2 to 3 inches below the patient's axilla.

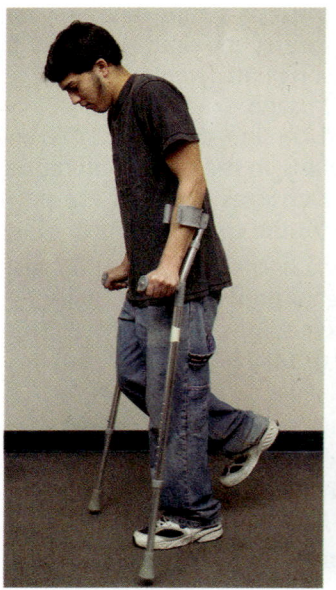

FIGURE 19-38C Lofstrand or forearm crutches

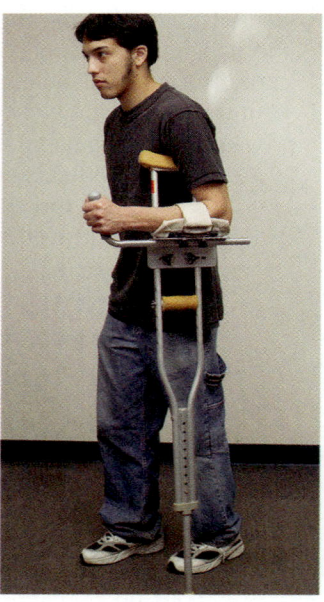

FIGURE 19-38D Platform crutch. This is an ideal substitute for a cane if the patient cannot bear weight on the forearm or hand.

PROCEDURE PROCEDURE PROCEDURE PROCEDURE PROCEDURE PROCEDURE PROCEDURE

19-12  Use Crutches

PURPOSE: To adjust crutches' length and teach a patient to correctly and safely use crutches.

EQUIPMENT: Crutches, hand pads, and rubber tips.

PERFORMANCE OBJECTIVE: Provided with all necessary equipment and supplies, adjust the length of the crutches, and demonstrate the steps of this procedure to instruct a patient in the correct use of crutches. The crutches will be the correct length, and the patient will be able to demonstrate the proper and safe use of crutches.

1. Identify the patient, and confirm the physician's orders. **RATIONALE: Speaking to the patient by name and checking the chart ensures that you are performing the procedure for the correct patient.**

2. Assemble the equipment. Make sure the crutches are intact (hand pads and rubber tips) and stable.

3. Stabilize the patient upright near a wall or chair for support. **NOTE: The patient must be wearing non-skid shoes or foot coverings. RATIONALE: This helps prevent slipping or falling.**

4. Adjust the length of the crutches for the patient so that the handles are comfortable, with a 30-degree angle bend of the elbows and 2 inches between the axilla and the top of the crutches.

   NOTE:

   ■ Explain to the patient to support her weight at the handles and not under the arm. **RATIONALE: Pressure in the axilla from upper body weight may damage nerves.**

   ■ Tell the patient to take small steps slowly to avoid losing balance and possibly falling.

   ■ Instruct the patient to stand on her uninjured foot while swinging the injured leg forward with crutches.

   Crutches should be placed approximately 4 to 5 inches in front and 4 to 5 inches to the side of the patient's heels. Use Figures 19-39A through C to show the ordered gait for walking safely with crutches.

5. Demonstrate the proper use of crutches.

6. Allow the patient to practice the procedure to ensure correct use.

7. Record the procedure on the patient's chart.

CHARTING EXAMPLE

2-16-XX

Jill's crutches were measured and adjusted for proper height. Hand pads and tips firmly attached. Demonstrated three-point gait, and had her return demonstration. Instructed not to bear weight on axillary area. Advised to select appropriate shoes to help prevent slipping or falling.

B. Cox, CMA

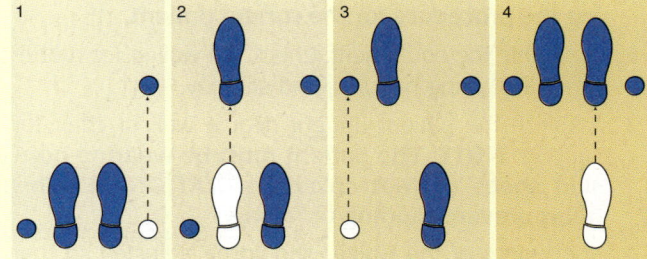

FIGURE 19-39A Four-point gait

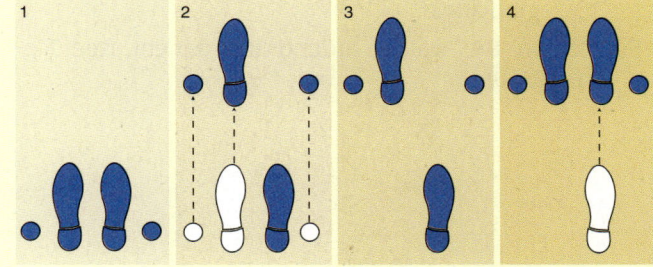

FIGURE 19-39B Three-point gait

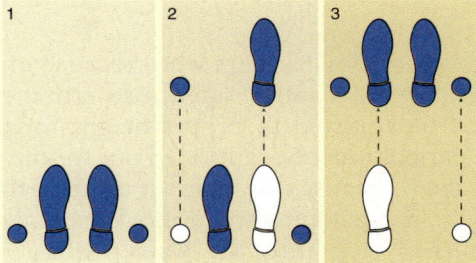

FIGURE 19-39C Two-point gait

PROCEDURE PROCEDURE PROCEDURE PROCEDURE PROCEDURE PROCEDURE PROCEDURE PROCEDURE

19-13  Use a Walker

PURPOSE: To adjust the walker's height and teach a patient the proper and safe use of a walker.

EQUIPMENT: Walker, handles, and rubber tips.

PERFORMANCE OBJECTIVE: Provided with a walker, adjust it to the appropriate height and demonstrate the steps in the procedure to instruct a patient in the proper use of a walker. The patient will be able to demonstrate the safe and correct use of a walker.

1. Identify the patient, and confirm the physician's orders. **RATIONALE: Speaking to the patient by name and checking the chart ensures that you are performing the procedure for the correct patient.**

2. Assemble the equipment. Check the walker for rubber tips, pads at the handles, and stability.

3. Stabilize the patient upright near a wall or chair for support. **NOTE: The patient must be wearing non-skid shoes or foot coverings. RATIONALE: This helps prevent slipping or falling.**

4. The height of the walker should be adjusted so that the handles are at the patient's hip level, and the bend of the patient's elbows is at a comfortable 25- to 30-degree angle.

5. Position the walker around the patient (see Figure 19-40).

6. Instruct the patient to pick up the walker, move it slightly forward, and walk into it.

   NOTE:

   ■ Instruct the patient to keep all four feet of the walker on the floor.

   ■ Explain to the patient not to slide the walker. **RATIONALE: It may slip or catch and cause a fall.**

   ■ Instruct the patient not to step too close to walker. **RATIONALE: This makes it difficult to maintain balance.**

7. Demonstrate the correct use of a walker.

8. Have the patient practice the procedure.

9. Observe the patient, and be ready to assist in case of a possible fall.

10. Record and initial on the patient's chart.

CHARTING EXAMPLE

1-29-XX

Walker adjusted to appropriate height, and hand grips and rubber tips examined. Demonstrated safe use of the walker, and reminded Sally to wear nonskid shoes or slippers when walking. We also discussed being aware of floor coverings and possible hazards. She returned the demonstration and talked about the presence of hazards at her residence.

S. Moore, CMA

Walker

A walker is useful for patients who, because of age or physical condition, cannot safely use crutches. The walker may be adjusted to proper height for the patient. The patient must be cautioned not to step too far into the walker, because this makes it difficult to maintain balance. The patient should move the walker forward and then step into the walker while leaning slightly foward (Figure 19-40 and Procedure 19-13).

Some walkers come with wheels so that patients can push them along as they walk and therefore can move a little quicker. This type of walker is less stable and may cause some patients to fall if it rolls away from them. Some more expensive wheeled walkers come with hand brakes that the patient can use to control the rolling, but this depends upon the response action and hand strength of the patient for control and safety. Some walkers even have a seating area so that the patient can stop and rest while walking. Many retirement and nursing home patients use walkers that they will bring to the physician's office. Become familiar with their use, and be able to instruct or correct a patient's usage.

Wheelchair

When a patient comes to your office in a wheelchair, you need to know how to help that patient from the wheelchair to the examination table and back to the

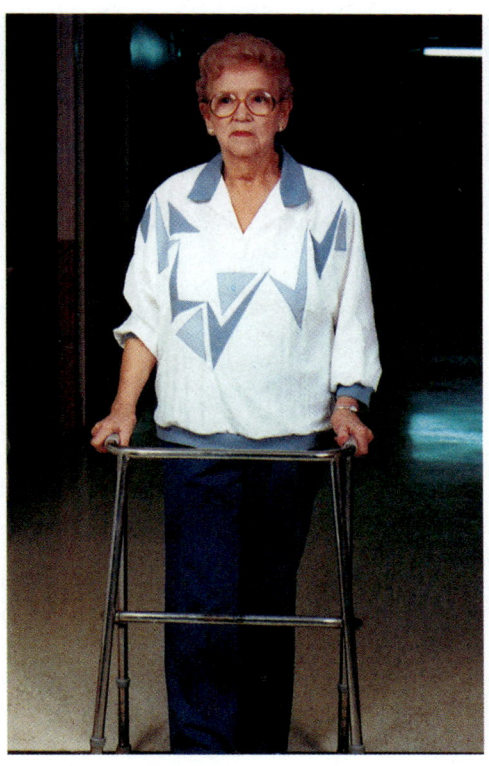

FIGURE 19-40   A walker provides stability and allows the patient to be mobile.

wheelchair. This is not an easy task to do alone if the patient is unable to support his own weight. Always take care to enlist help from coworkers in order to prevent injury to a patient and yourself. Usually, examination rooms are limited in size, which also adds to the difficulty of getting the patient to and from an examination table. Always remember to lock the

wheels to prevent the chair from rolling away when assisting the patient to stand. It might be necessary to return her to the chair and adjust your position or hold. (Refer to Procedures 19-14 and 19-15).

Patients who are residents of retirement or nursing facilities are often seen in the office. Many of them will arrive by wheelchair and may be accompanied by

PROCEDURE PROCEDURE PROCEDURE PROCEDURE PROCEDURE PROCEDURE PROCEDURE PROCEDURE

19-14  Assist a Patient from a Wheelchair to an Examination Table

PURPOSE: To safely move a patient from a wheelchair to an examination table.

EQUIPMENT: Examination table and wheelchair.

PERFORMANCE OBJECTIVE: Provided with necessary equipment, demonstate the steps in the procedure for assisting a patient from a wheelchair to an examination table in a safe manner.

1. Unlock the wheels of the chair, and wheel the patient to the examination room. **NOTE: Wheelchairs should always be locked in position when sitting still to prevent unexpected movement. This is accomplished by flipping the brake on each wheel.**

2. Position the chair as near as possible to the place you want the patient to sit on the table.

3. Lower the table to chair level. **NOTE: If this cannot be done, position a footstool beside the table, and determine if assistance will be needed.**

4. Lock the wheels on the chair.

5. Fold the footrests back. If necessary, assist the patient to move her feet.

6. Stand directly in front of the patient with your feet slightly apart. To give a good base, place one foot forward, between the patient's legs.

(continues)

PROCEDURE PROCEDURE PROCEDURE PROCEDURE PROCEDURE PROCEDURE PROCEDURE PROCEDURE

19-14    Assist a Patient from a Wheelchair to an Examination Table (Continued)

7. Bend your knees and have the patient place her hands on your shoulders while you place your hands under the patient's armpits; assist the patient to a standing position. Pause in this position for a moment before the next step (Figure 19-41A).

8. Maintaining the position of your hands, pivot or side step to a position beside the table (Figure 19-41B).

9. Place one foot slightly behind you for support, and help the patient to a sitting position on the table.

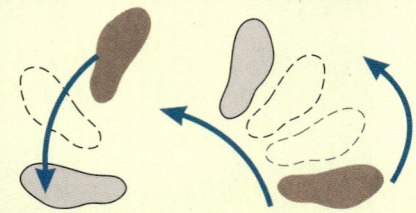

FIGURE 19-41B   Position of feet when turning to assist a patient from a wheelchair onto the examination table

10. If it is necessary to use a stool, determine the assistance required, and enlist the needed help *before* taking the patient from the wheelchair.

11. While supporting the patient, stabilize the stool by placing your feet on the outside next to the legs, and assist the patient to step onto the stool. **CAUTION: Be certain the patient steps onto the stool squarely to avoid tipping the stool.**

12. Assist the patient to sit on the table.

13. If the patient needs assistance to lie down, place one hand around the patient's back. Help the patient raise her legs to the table by placing your free arm under her legs and lifting them as the patient turns. **NOTE: If the patient needs to remove clothing, get someone to help you. One person balances the patient while the other removes necessary clothing.**

14. Place a pillow under the patient's head. Drape the patient appropriately. **NOTE: Never leave a very ill or weak patient alone on a table. There is danger of a fall.**

15. Unlock the chair wheels, and move the chair out of the way. **NOTE: If the room is small, it may be necessary to place the chair outside the examination room.**

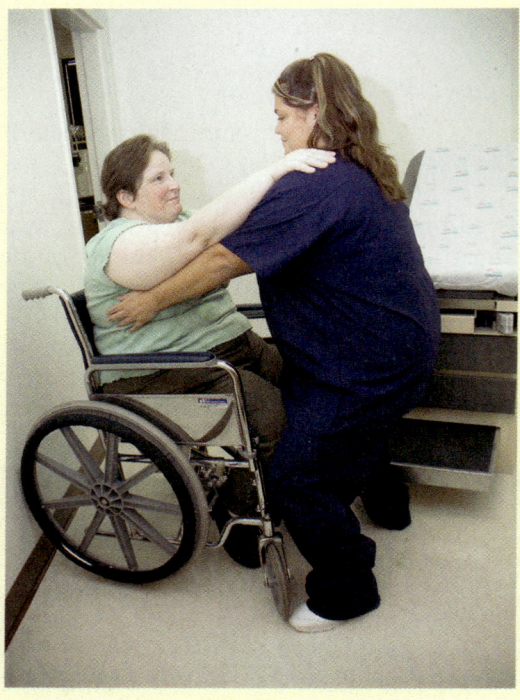

FIGURE 19-41A   Assisting a patient from a wheelchair

a nursing aide. To make it easier to assist these patients to stand or walk, a wide strap called a gait belt may be placed around their waist (Figure 19-42). The belt provides a way to hold and support the patient while she is trying to walk or being assisted in and out of chairs or wheelchairs. The belt is grasped in front to assist the patient to rise and stand from a sitting position. It is held in the back to support the patient while walking. Practice using the gait belt so that when a patient does arrive, you will have some experience with the device. All of the procedures in this chapter need to be practiced many times so that you feel comfortable and confident when the need arises to use them.

PROCEDURE

19-15 Assist a Patient from an Examination Table to a Wheelchair

PURPOSE: To safely move a patient from the examination table to a wheelchair.

EQUIPMENT: Wheelchair and examination table.

PERFORMANCE OBJECTIVE: Provided with a wheelchair and an examination table, demonstrate the steps in the procedure to assist the patient from the examination table to a wheelchair in a safe manner.

1. Reposition the chair and lock the wheels.

2. Assist the patient to a sitting position on the table. Support his back if necessary. Lift the patient's legs as the patient is the turned until his feet dangle over the of the table.

3. Enlist help if needed and assist the patient to dress.

4. Ask the patient to put his hands on your shoulders. Support the patient on his sides below the armpits. Assist the patient to step onto the floor, or have a step-

stool in place if the table cannot be lowered to chair height. **CAUTION: Take special care to ensure that the patient steps squarely on the stool when getting down from the examining table. Place your feet against the legs of the footstool, on the outside, to maintain its position.**

5. Support the patient into a standing position on the stool or floor.

6. Help the patient step down from the stool.

7. Side step or pivot the patient to a position in front of the chair.

8. Have the patient reach back to the arms of the chair as you help in lowering the patient into the chair.

9. Adjust the footrests.

10. Unlock the wheels, and return the patient to the reception room.

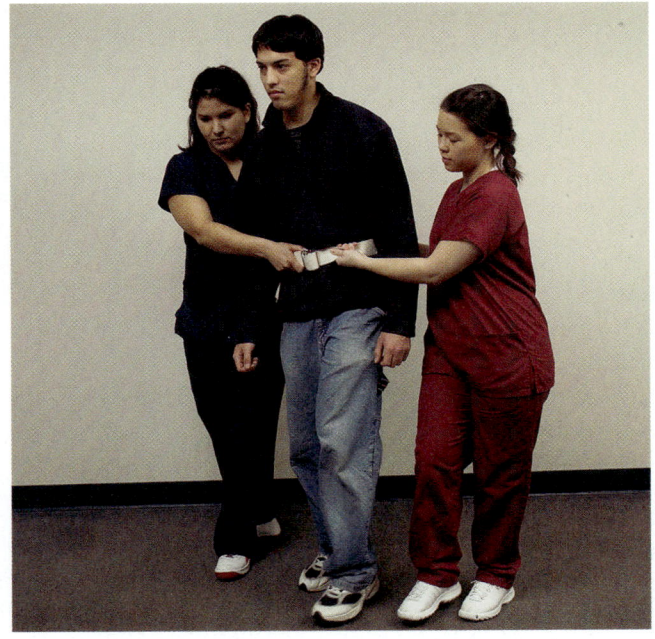

FIGURE 19-42   A gait belt makes it easier to support the patient when walking.

Physical therapists, therapy aids, and medical supply representatives are trained to fit and instruct people in how to use various pieces of equipment. When it is known that a disability will occur, as with planned surgery, this is done prior to the procedure so that the patient is prepared to function as soon as possible after it is performed.

Even being as careful as possible when assisting patients to walk or move about the office, you still may have one who becomes faint, slips, or suddenly becomes weak. Usually there is no way a single person can hold up someone who becomes "dead weight." The best option in this case is to ease the patient to the floor in such a way as to prevent injury. If you are supporting the patient from behind and he begins to fall backward, grasp him under the arms, put one leg back with the foot at a right angle, slide the other leg forward under the patient, and ease him to slide down your leg onto the floor (Figure 19-43A). If you are walking beside the patient and he begins to fall forward, grasp him around the waist, extend your leg farthest from the patient forward, bend at the knees, and slowly lower the patient to the floor (Figure 19-43B). You must be careful to avoid injuring your own back by trying to support too much

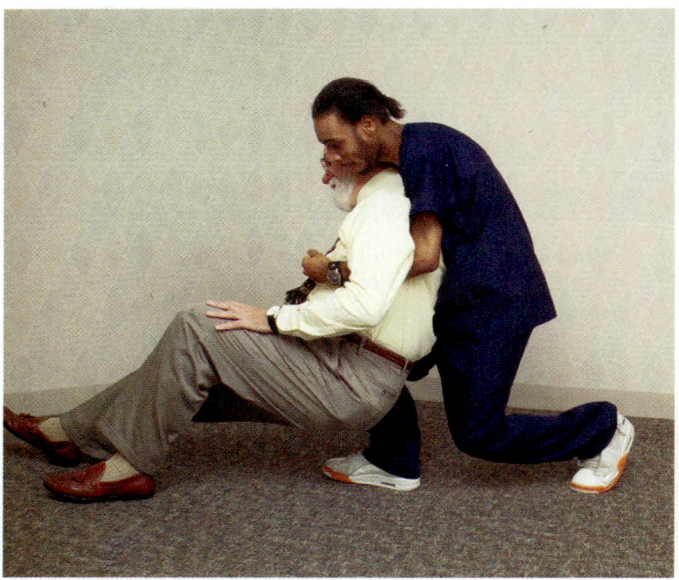

FIGURE 19-43A Easing a falling patient safely to the floor, from behind the patient

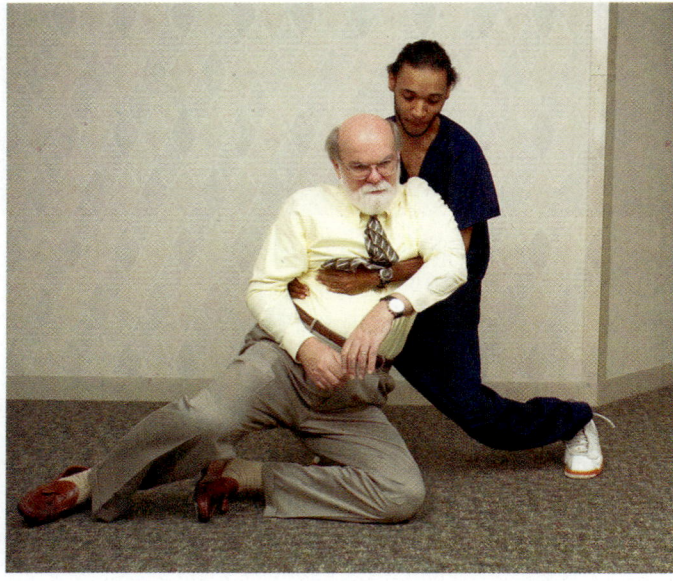

FIGURE 19-43B Easing a falling patient safely to the floor, from beside the patient

weight. Keep your back as straight as possible, bend from the knees, and use your large thigh muscles to handle the weight. Whenever a patient falls, have the physician examine him as soon as possible, and be sure to carefully document the incident on the chart and on an accident/incident form as indicated by the office policy manual.

SAFETY AT HOME

Patients and their families must be informed of the importance of maintaining a safe home environment for persons using ambulatory aids. Care must be taken to keep floors free of spills and clutter. It is especially important to remove all loose throw rugs or damaged floor coverings which might cause the patient to fall. Any bare floor care product, such as floor wax, that might cause the floor to be slippery must be avoided. It

is also important to ensure that appropriate footwear is worn. It should be well-fitting and have a nonslip walking surface.

ACHIEVE UNIT OBJECTIVES

- ☐ **Complete the Workbook activities to meet the learning objectives.**
- ☐ **Practice the procedures in this unit to meet the performance objectives.**
- ☐ **Apply your knowledge at the end of this chapter in completing the Critical Thinking Challenge and Activities, as well as the StudyWARE on your Student CD-ROM.**

CRITICAL THINKING CHALLENGE

IMPACTING THE PATIENT, THE PRACTICE, AND YOUR CAREER

Mary Santino was an 80-year-old Italian woman for whom English was a limited second language. She lived alone, but two of her children were only a few miles away. She was experiencing increased pain in her right hip, and it was becoming obvious that she was going to need a surgical procedure to correct her problem. Attempts to get her to take off her excess weight to reduce the stress on her hip had not been successful. Until an appointment could be arranged with an orthopedic surgeon and her surgery scheduled, Dr. Long suggested that she use a cane to take some of the weight-bearing load off her hip. Shelly, the medical assistant, retrieved an adjustable standard cane from the storage room for her to use temporarily. She had Mary stand up and shortened the cane for the proper height. Shelly explained to Mary to put the cane in her left hand and put weight on it at the same time she put weight on her right leg. She took Mary to the stairway to show her how to go up and down stairs because Mary lived in a two-story home. After watching Mary trying to use the cane, Shelly felt she was having a lot of difficulty. She didn't seem to have enough strength in her left arm to take much stress off her leg. She also seemed to have problems using the proper gait, often using the cane with the wrong leg. She was especially concerned about her not going up or down stairs correctly. But then she thought that maybe with a little more practice at home she would be more successful, because Mary indicated she understood what to do.

Shelly has assumed that Mary will improve because she said she understood. Shelly didn't stop to consider what factors might be causing Mary's problems with instruction or what other options she had to teach her. She didn't consider the risk factors of the home or what options might have been implemented.

QUESTIONS

1. How might this patient teaching effort affect the patient?
2. Could Shelly's inadequate teaching affect the practice?
3. Could Shelly's career be affected in any way?

ACTIVITIES

1. Role play using a gait belt to get a classmate up from a sitting position or to walk in the hall.
2. Practice easing "patients" to the floor while walking behind or beside them when they fall.
3. Develop an emergency scenario and phone in to the "office" for assistance.
4. Go online to read about the controversy between Dr. Heimlich and the United States Life Saving Association and the medical establishment over the use of the Heimlich maneuver instead of CPR as appropriate for drowning victims.

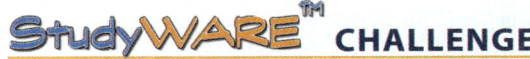 CHALLENGE

- Study with the flash cards for Chapter 19 to review the key terms in this chapter.
- Solve the hangman activities for Chapter 19.
- Complete the true/false quiz in test mode for Chapter 19.

RESOURCES

American Heart Association (2005). Guidelines for CPR and ECC. Dallas; Author.

Beebe, R., & Funk, D. (2001). *Fundamentals of emergency care.* Clifton Park, NY: Thomson Delmar Learning.

American College of Emergency Physicians. (1999). *EMT-Basic field care: A care-based approach.* St. Louis: Mosby.

Hegner, B. R., Caldwell E., & Needham J. F. (1999). *Nursing assistant: A nursing process approach* (8th ed.). Clifton Park, NY: Thomson Delmar Learning.

Lindh, W. Q., Pooler, M. S., Tamparo, C. D., & Dahl, B. M. (2006). *Comprehensive medical assisting: Administrative and clinical competencies* (3rd ed.). Clifton Park, NY: Thomson Delmar Learning.

Simmers, L. (2001). *Diversified health occupations* (5th ed.). Clifton Park, NY: Thomson Delmar Learning.

Wellness Letter. (2000). *Is it a heart attack? If you're woman, will you know?* University of California, Berkeley.

WEB LINKS

www.aaem.org (American Academy of Emergency Medicine)
Provides current resources and news.

www.americanheart.org (American Heart Association)
Find symptoms of heart attack and stroke and information on association services, managing your weight, and cholesterol. Locate the 2005 Guidelines for CPR and ECC and find centers where you can train.

www.redcross.org (American Red Cross)
Learn about health and safety services and classes in first aid, CPR, and AED. Take the CPR quiz.

www.ncemi.org (National Center for Emergency Medicine Informatics)
A collection of many items. Note clinical calculators and medical e-tools.

www.usla.org (United States Lifesaving Association)
Discussion regarding CPR versus the Heimlich manuever for victim of drowning. Go to page nine, article in Cleveland Scene, 2004 New Times, Inc.

SECTION 5
Behaviors and Health

As you gain experience in the field, it will soon become apparent that patients have a tendency to depend on you for advice. The physician prescribes a treatment plan for the patient to follow and usually discusses it with the patient. Generally, the patient's next step is to ask you to explain the details. Therefore, you must have a complete understanding of the policies of the health care facility. Personal opinions should be restrained. This chapter concerns the significance of diet, exercise, weight control, sleep, and the way personal behaviors influence health. In the second unit there is a discussion about the abuse of or addiction to substances such as tobacco, alcohol, and prescription and illegal drugs. Each substance is examined as to how it affects the user, how it affects an unborn child, the symptoms of withdrawal, and treatment options.

The third unit looks at various related therapy options as supplements to or in comparison with conventional medicine. A look at the use of alternative therapies provides you with information for making informed decisions about controversial treatments.

This chapter will provide you with the knowledge to adopt behaviors that positively influence your own and your patient's health. Hopefully, it will also enable you to recognize and provide assistance to individuals who need to change their behavior before their health is destroyed.

UNIT 1
NUTRITION, EXERCISE, AND WEIGHT CONTROL

OBJECTIVES

Upon completion of this unit, you will be able to achieve the following:

LEARNING Objectives

1. Spell and define, using the glossary at the back of the text, all of the Words to Know in this unit.

2. Discuss the do's and don'ts listed in the Guidelines for Good Health.

3. Discuss the food pyramids.

4. Name the fat- and water-soluble vitamins.

5. Name the essential minerals.

6. Describe the parts of a food label and how to interpret the amounts.

7. Describe and discuss dietary and health concerns of adolescents.

8. Explain the importance of sleep and a positive outlook in regard to health.

9. Provide instruction to patients for performing stretching exercises.

WORDS TO KNOW

additive	dietician	protein
amenorrhea	emaciation	purge
anorexia nervosa	health	REM (rapid eye
anorexic	infirmity	movement)
beriberi	malnutrition	rickets
binge	NREM (non-rapid	scurvy
bulimia nervosa	eye	sleep apnea
calorie	movement)	tactile
carbohydrate	nutrition	therapeutic
deprivation	obese	

CERTIFICATION CONNECTION

CMA
Providing instruction for health maintenance and disease prevention
Nutrition

RMA
Vitamins and calories
Patient instruction; health and wellness, nutrition

With today's attention to physical fitness, the medical assistant must be well informed to answer the inquiries patients make concerning diet and exercise programs. The physician will decide what is best for each patient after all data from the medical history, examination, laboratory findings, and other pertinent information have been evaluated. It is up to you to reinforce the physician's orders and help patients adapt those orders to their particular lifestyles.

As you begin to practice skills in communicating information to patients regarding treatment plans and their overall health, it is important for you to have a basic understanding of the meaning of health. **Health** is defined by the World Health Organization as a state of complete physical, mental, and social well-being. Health is not merely the absence of disease or **infirmity**. All things conducive to good health are referred to as healthful. Healthful living habits are essential for one to maintain good physical condition or to stay physically fit. There are simple guidelines that can help to keep us in good health, increase vitality, and possibly even increase life expectancy. Figure 20-1 outlines the

---

GUIDELINES FOR GOOD HEALTH

DO:
- Exercise regularly
- Eat a sensible, well-balanced diet including high-fiber, low-fat, cereal and grain foods
- Practice health and safety rules at home and work
- Use sunscreen with SPF 15+ as needed
- Get adequate rest and recreation
- Nurture your spirit daily

DON'T:
- Smoke or use tobacco (including chew and snuff)
- Drink alcohol in excess
- Expose skin to sun for prolonged periods
- Use drugs or medications unless prescribed for a specific purpose
- Overeat or gain too much weight
- Expose yourself to unnecessary x-rays

FIGURE 20-1 Guidelines for good health

TABLE 20-1		Examples of Nutrients and Calories in Common Foods				
Food	**Portion**	**Total Grams**	**Calories**	**Carbohydrates**	**Protein**	**Fats**
Green beans	1 cup	125	45	10	2	trace
Baked fish	3 oz.	85	80	trace	17	1
Butter	1 tablespoon	14	100	trace	trace	11
Apple	1 large	212	125	32	trace	1
Cheeseburger with bun	4 oz.	194	525	40	30	31
Pecan pie	1/8 pie	138	575	71	7	32

Adapted from Taber's Cyclopedic Medical Dictionary.

suggestions advised for the general population. Those who are in the health care professions are urged to set a good example to those patients we teach.

NUTRITION

Patient education in proper nutrition is one of your many responsibilities. **Nutrition** is defined in *Taber's Cyclopedic Medical Dictionary* as "all the processes involved in the taking in and utilization of food substances by which growth, repair, and maintenance of activities in the body as a whole or in any of its parts are accomplished; includes ingestion, digestion, absorption, and metabolism (assimilation)." This means what you put into your body is all that your body has available to use to keep you healthy. If you fail to give it the proper nutrients (ingredients), it can't keep you functioning at the optimum level.

You are probably familiar with the basic nutrients. The body gets energy from **carbohydrate**, fat, and **protein** nutrients. Other elements such as water, electrolytes, fiber, minerals, and vitamins are nutrients that are essential to the process of metabolism. An individual who consumes inadequate energy nutrients becomes malnourished; excessive amounts may cause obesity, diabetes, and certain cancers. Absence of or inadequate exercise may also lead to obesity and heart disease. With age, lack of exercise causes loss of strength and flexibility, bone loss, and an increased likelihood of falls. When one provides the body with adequate amounts of these essential nutrients, along with exercise and restful sleep, one can anticipate relatively good health and increased years of life. Being able to discuss these essential elements for healthy living with patients is a very valuable skill.

Calories

The energy nutrients of carbohydrates, proteins, and fats have calorie values. A calorie is a unit of heat. Technically, it is the amount of heat needed to raise the temperature of a kilogram of water one centigrade from 14.5° C to 15.5° C. Foods are a combination of nutri-

ents, and therefore calories, but not all nutrients have the same caloric value. For example, a gram of carbohydrate or protein will have *approximately* 4 calories, while a gram of fat has *approximately* 9 calories. It is very interesting to compare food calories in relation to their amount. For example, for 100 calories you could have 1 tablespoon of butter or more than 3 cups of green beans. Which will satisfy your hunger the best? If the physician puts a patient on a 1,200-calorie diet for weight loss, knowing the caloric content of food is necessary. Small inexpensive paperback booklets are available at grocery and book stores that list the most common food values in calories, carbohydrates, proteins, and fats. These are essential to anyone trying to select foods wisely. Table 20-1 shows a sample of widely diverse nutrient values and calories.

Another part of good health concerns the amount of exercise we get. Exercise burns calories as well as making us more flexible, strong, and healthy. The ideal balance would be to eat an amount of nutrients equal to what we use, but that is not easily done. Most people tend to believe they eat less than they do and exercise more than they actually do. The basic amount of calories required to maintain an average-sized adult expending a low level of energy is 1,500 to 1,800 per day, or about 70 calories per hour. This refers to the amount of energy it takes just for normal body functions. Theoretically, eat less and lose weight; eat more and you gain. This ratio can be affected by the amount of energy we expend. Unfortunately, if you are trying to lose weight, it takes a lot more effort to burn 100 calories that it does to consume them. Table 20-2 lists how many calories you would burn from engaging in 1 hour of various activities.

The Food Pyramid

The food guide pyramid (Figure 20-2) was originally introduced in the spring of 1992 by the United States Department of Agriculture. The pyramid concept replaced the "food wheel" and the old basic four food groups that had been used since 1946. The

TABLE 20-2 Calories Burned in 1 Hour of Activity or Exercise by an Average 160 Pound Person	
Activity or Exercise	**Calories Burned per Hour (approx.)**
Sitting, reading	80
Playing golf, not walking or carrying bag	200
Moderate speed walking or bicycling, housework	250
Swimming, tennis doubles, ballet exercises	350
Fast walking, singles tennis, water skiing	400
Running, climbing stairs, heavy manual work	660
Soccer, handball	700

Adapted from Taber's Cyclopedic Medical Dictionary *and* Life and Health; Targeting Wellness.

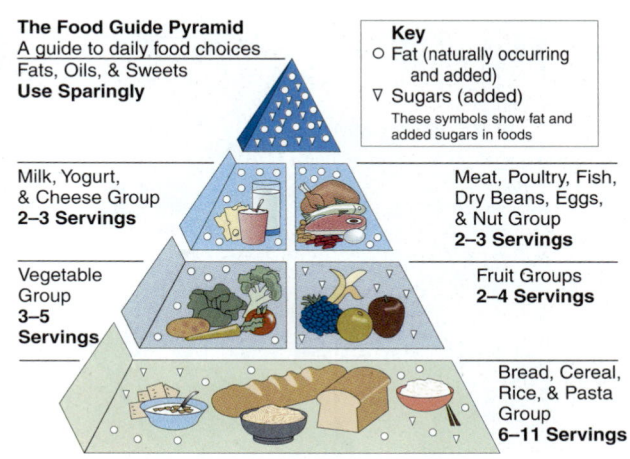

FIGURE 20-2   Former Food Guide Pyramid showing the recommended servings for daily nutritional needs (*From* How to Eat for Good Health, *courtesy of National Dairy Council*).

pyramid is divided into six sections; the foods listed in the largest sections are those foods that should be consumed in the greatest quantities. Notice that at the top of the triangle, for example, are fats, oils, and sweets; this indicates that foods such as butter, salad oil, candy, and other sweets should be used sparingly. Explaining the food pyramid to patients was relatively easy. However, apparently few people followed its guidelines, and there has been a steady fattening trend since 1992 when it was released. In 2003 a report was published that stated the pyramid might be upside down.

Dietary Guidelines for Americans

The United States Department of Agriculture (USDA), in cooperation with the Department of Health and Human Services (HHS), is charged to develop and release Dietary Guidelines for Americans (DGA) at 5-year intervals. In 2003, an appointed advisory committee of 13 prominent experts in nutrition and health began gathering science-based evidence and expert testimony. Then they summarized and synthesized the knowledge regarding nutrients and food components and came up with their recommendations, which are the 2005 Dietary Guidelines for Americans that were released in January of 2005. Their purpose was to develop advice about how good dietary habits can promote health and reduce risk for major chronic diseases. Some of the committee's findings are:

- Poor diet and sedentary lifestyle contribute to 400,000 deaths per year in the United States.

- Poor diet and sedentary lifestyle leads to:
    1. Cardiovascular disease
    2. Hypertension
    3. Dyslipedemia
    4. Type 2 diabetes
    5. Diverticular disease
    6. Osteoporosis
    7. Overweight and obesity
    8. Iron deficiency
    9. **Malnutrition**
    10. Certain cancers
- Adults need 30 minutes of moderate exercise most days of the week and may need up to 60 minutes per day to prevent gain. Children and adolescents need 60 minutes of moderate to vigorous exercise most days of the week. Individuals also need to reduce sedentary behaviors of television and video viewing to treat and prevent overweight conditions.
- The recommended percentage of daily intake of nutrients in any weight-loss program is carbohydrates, 45% to 65%; fats, 20% to 35%; and proteins, 10% to 35%.
- The relationship of transfatty acid intake to LDL cholesterol is direct and progressive, and increased amounts increase the risk of coronary heart disease (CHD). Daily intake of 1% or less is recommended.
- The relationship of cholesterol intake to LDL concentration is direct and progressive, and increased amounts increase risk of CHD. Adults with an LDL above 130 mg/dL should limit intake to less than 200 mg of dietary cholesterol daily.
- The amount of food offered influences the amount eaten; it is recommended that portions be limited, especially of energy-dense foods.
- Weight is maintained by a balance of energy intake to energy expenditure regardless of the proportions of fat, carbohydrate, and protein in the diet.

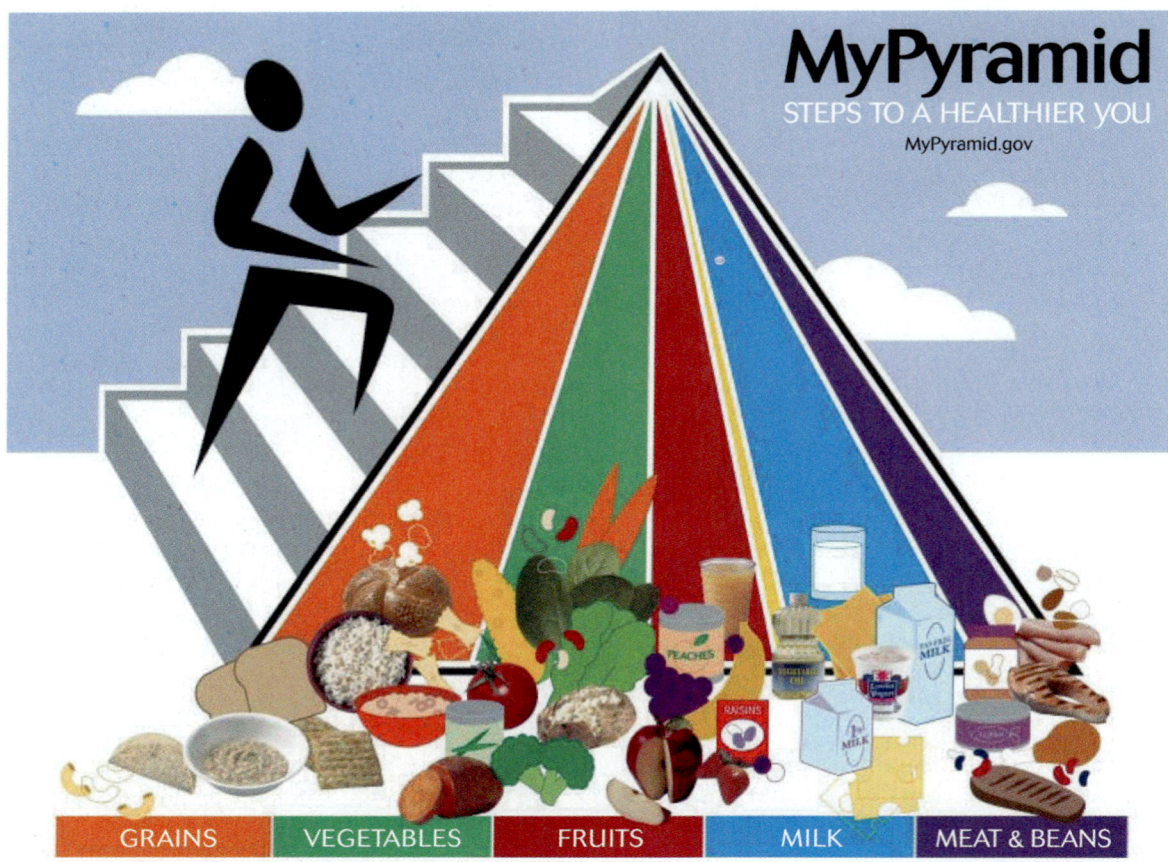

MyPyramid
STEPS TO A HEALTHIER YOU
MyPyramid.gov

GRAINS	VEGETABLES	FRUITS	MILK	MEAT & BEANS

GRAINS Make half your grains whole	**VEGETABLES** Vary your veggies	**FRUITS** Focus on fruits	**MILK** Get your calcium-rich foods	**MEAT & BEANS** Go lean with protein
Eat at least 3 oz. of whole-grain cereals, breads, crackers, rice, or pasta every day 1 oz. is about 1 slice of bread, about 1 cup of breakfast cereal, or 1/2 cup of cooked rice, cereal, or pasta	Eat more dark-green veggies like broccoli, spinach, and other dark leafy greens Eat more orange vegetables like carrots and sweetpotatoes Eat more dry beans and peas like pinto beans, kidney beans, and lentils	Eat a variety of fruit Choose fresh, frozen, canned, or dried fruit Go easy on fruit juices	Go low-fat or fat-free when you choose milk, yogurt, and other milk products If you don't or can't consume milk, choose lactose-free products or other calcium sources such as fortified foods and beverages	Choose low-fat or lean meats and poultry Bake it, broil it, or grill it Vary your protein routine — choose more fish, beans, peas, nuts, and seeds

For a 2,000-calorie diet, you need the amounts below from each food group. To find the amounts that are right for you, go to MyPyramid.gov.

Eat 6 oz. every day	Eat 2½ cups every day	Eat 2 cups every day	Get 3 cups every day; for kids aged 2 to 8, it's 2	Eat 5½ oz. every day

Find your balance between food and physical activity
- Be sure to stay within your daily calorie needs.
- Be physically active for at least 30 minutes most days of the week.
- About 60 minutes a day of physical activity may be needed to prevent weight gain.
- For sustaining weight loss, at least 60 to 90 minutes a day of physical activity may be required.
- Children and teenagers should be physically active for 60 minutes every day, or most days.

Know the limits on fats, sugars, and salt (sodium)
- Make most of your fat sources from fish, nuts, and vegetable oils.
- Limit solid fats like butter, margarine, shortening, and lard, as well as foods that contain these.
- Check the Nutrition Facts label to keep saturated fats, *trans* fats, and sodium low.
- Choose food and beverages low in added sugars. Added sugars contribute calories with few, if any, nutrients.

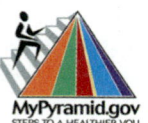

MyPyramid.gov
STEPS TO A HEALTHIER YOU

U.S. Department of Agriculture
Center for Nutrition Policy and Promotion
April 2005
CNPP-15

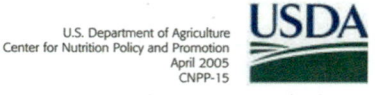

USDA is an equal opportunity provider and employer

FIGURE 20-3 MyPyramid *(U.S. Department of Agriculture)*

- Other conclusions include the recommended amounts of nutrients needed per day, special nutrients for specific people, a relationship between fat intake and health, the healthy effects of intake of fish with high levels of EPA and DHA, the health benefits of fiber, and others. (See the Activities at the end of this chapter for directions to the web site.)

The DGA serve as a base for all government programs related to nutrition, such as the National School Lunch Program and the WIC program (Supplemental Nutrition Program for Women, Infants, and Children). They also are the basis for the USDA's Food Pyramid.

The Department of Agriculture, who is responsible for the pyramid, undertook the task of revising it based upon the scientific findings of the DGA and released its new version in April 2005 (Figure 20-3). It is no longer a "pyramid for everyone." There are now 12 pyramids, each geared to different lifestyles and nutritional needs. It is hoped this new design will guide people to healthy eating. You can access the food pyramid information by going to www.mypyramid.gov on the Internet. Here you will be given the opportunity to enter your age, gender, height, weight, and level of exercise into the data. In return you will receive a calorie pattern (number of calories) estimated for your needs and your own personal modified pyramid. Also available on the site is a Meal Tracking Worksheet to write down your foods. The MyPyramid Tracker allows you to enter your daily intake and have it assessed against your entered daily activity to get your energy balance status score. You can track your progress for up to 1 year.

It is hoped the new pyramid will encourage Americans to make healthier food choices and be active every day. To make it easier, the new pyramid also uses household measures to give amounts to eat instead of the old "servings" number, which varied between foods. By looking at the pyramid, you can easily identify your daily amounts of each of the nutrients. Refer to the pyramid; you will note the recommended amounts are for a 2,000-calorie diet; when you obtain your own printout, the amounts may vary. You will need to explain to patients how to obtain their own pyramid or prepare it for them. Looking at Figure 20-3 you can make the following observations:

- The orange section refers to grains—eat 6 oz. a day.
- The green section refers to vegetables—eat 2½ cups a day.
- The red section refers to fruits—eat 2 cups a day.
- The yellow thin section refers to fats and oils—limit intake.
- The blue section refers to milk products—get 3 cups a day.
- The purple section refers to meat and beans—eat 5½ oz. a day.

Within each section are explanations about your selection options and portion sizes. This design is certainly more specific than the previous one, because you can modify it for individual needs and it is somewhat more confusing at first. Hopefully as it is used on food packaging and dietary literature, it will become more familiar and useful.

There are cooking magazines and cookbooks with recipes that can reinforce healthy eating habits. Helping patients to select materials that may benefit them is a way to keep them motivated to follow a diet plan. Patient education materials can be offered to patients in the reception area. Give patients support by letting them know that you are pleased that they are making progress in healthy choices in their diets.

Vitamins and Minerals

Vitamins are organic substances found in foods that are essential to good health and growth. Vitamins are called micronutrients. As the name implies, only a trace quantity is required for enzymatic reaction in the body. If the body does not receive adequate vitamins or does not absorb them sufficiently, deficiency diseases may result. The major ones are **rickets**, **scurvy**, and **beriberi**. Rickets is the result of a deficiency of vitamin D; scurvy, of vitamin C or ascorbic acid; and beriberi, of vitamin B or thiamine. Vitamins A, D, E, and K are fat-soluble vitamins. Vitamin C and the B-complex vitamins are water-soluble. With a well-balanced diet, there is little likelihood of vitamin-deficiency diseases.

Vitamins are added to many foods because of their loss in preparation. Patients will be advised by the physician if a vitamin or mineral supplement is necessary.

Minerals are naturally occurring, nonorganic, homogeneous, solid substances. Thirteen are said to be essential to good health. They are supplied by a variety of meats and vegetables (Figure 20-4). Minerals found to be lacking most often from the diet are calcium, iron, and iodine. Metabolic disturbances can be caused by insufficient amounts of zinc, copper, magnesium, and potassium.

The principal vitamins, minerals, and micronutrients are listed in Table 20-3, and a basic calorie chart is

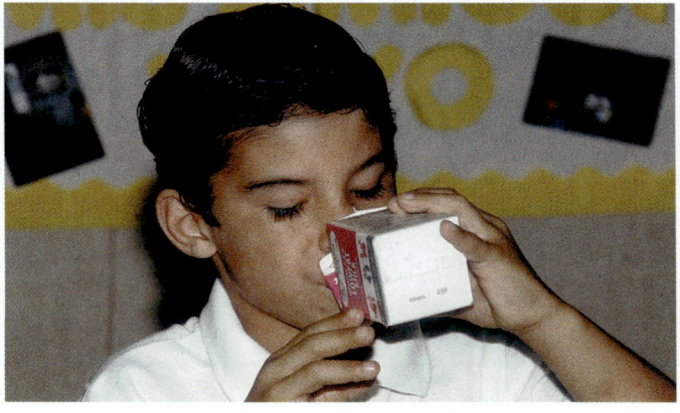

FIGURE 20-4 Milk is an important source of calcium and phosphorus.

TABLE 20-3 Principal Micronutrients

Micronutrient	Principal Sources	Functions	Effects of Deficiency and Toxicity	Usual Therapeutic Dosage
Vitamin A	Fish liver oils, liver, egg yolk, butter, cream, vitamin A-fortified margarine, green leafy or yellow vegetables	Photoreceptor mechanism of retina, integrity of epithelia, lysosome stability, glycoprotein synthesis	*Deficiency:* Night blindness, perifollicular hyperkeratosis, xerophthalmia, keratomalacia *Toxicity:* Headache, peeling of skin, hepatosplenomegaly, bone thickening	10,000–20,000 mcg (30,000–60,000 units/day)
Vitamin D	Fortified milk is main dietary source, fish liver oils, butter, egg yolk, liver, ultraviolet irradiation	Calcium and phosphorus absorption, resorption, mineralization, and collagen maturation of bone; tubular reabsorption of phosphorus (?)	*Deficiency:* Rickets (tetany sometimes associated), osteomalacia *Toxicity:* Anorexia, renal failure, metastatic calcification	*Primary Deficiency* 10–40 mcg (1,400–1,600 units)/day) *Metabolic Deficiency* 1–2 mcg/day 1.25–$(OH)_2D_3$ or 1α–$(OH)D_3$
Vitamin E group	Vegetable oil, wheat germ, leafy vegetables, egg yolk, margarine, legumes	Intracellular antioxidant, stability of biologic membranes	*Deficiency:* RBC hemolysis, creatinuria, ceroid deposition in muscle	30–100 mg/day
Vitamin K (activity) Vitamin K_1 (phytonadione) Vitamin K_2 (menaquinone)	Leafy vegetables, pork, liver, vegetable oils, intestinal flora after newborn period	Prothrombin formation, normal blood coagulation	*Deficiency:* Hemorrhage from deficient prothrombin *Toxicity:* Kernicterus	In situations conducive to neonatal hemorrhage, 2–5 mg during labor or daily for 1 wk prior; or 1–2 mg to newborn
Essential fatty acids (linoleic, arachidonic acids)	Vegetable seed oils (corn, sunflower, safflower); margarines blended with vegetable oils	Synthesis of prostaglandins, membrane structure	Growth cessation, dermatosis	Up to 10 g/day
Thiamine (vitamin B_1)	Dried yeast, whole grains, meat (especially pork, liver), enriched cereal products, nuts, legumes, potatoes	Carbohydrate metabolism, central and peripheral nerve cell function, myocardial function	Beriberi, infantile and adult (peripheral neuropathy, cardiac failure, Wernicke-Korsakoff syndrome)	30–100 mg/day
Riboflavin (vitamin B_2)	Milk, cheese, liver, meat, eggs, enriched cereal products	Many aspects of energy and protein metabolism integrity of mucous membranes	Cheilosis, angular stomatitis, corneal vascularization, amblyopia, sebaceous dermatosis	10–30 mg/day
Niacin (nicotinic acid, niacinamide)	Dried yeast, liver, meat, fish, legumes, whole-grain enriched cereal products	Oxidation-reduction reactions, carbohydrate metabolism	Pellagra (dermatosis, glossitis, GI and CNS dysfunction)	Niacinamide 100–1,000 mg/day

(continues)

	TABLE 20-3	Principal Micronutrients (Continued)		
Micronutrient	Principal Sources	Functions	Effects of Deficiency and Toxicity	Usual Therapeutic Dosage
Vitamin B$_6$ group (pyridoxine)	Dried yeast, liver, organ meats, whole-grain cereals, fish, legumes	Many aspects of nitrogen metabolism (e.g., transaminations, porphyrin and heme synthesis, tryptophan conversion to niacin), linoleic acid metabolism	Convulsions in infancy, anemias, neuropathy, seborrhea-like skin lesions Dependency states	25–100 mg/day
Folic acid	Fresh green leafy vegetables, fruit, organ meats, liver, dried yeast	Maturation of RBCs, synthesis of purines and pyrimidines	Pancytoperia, megaloblastosis (especially pregnancy, infancy, malabsorption)	1 mg/day
Vitamin B$_{12}$ (cobalamins)	Liver, meats (especially beef, pork, organ meats), eggs, milk and milk products	Maturation of RBCs; neural function; DNA synthesis, related to folate coenzymes; methionine and acetate synthesis	Pernicious anemia, fish tapeworm and vegan anemias, some psychiatric syndromes, nutritional amblyopia Dependency states	In pernicious anemia 50 mcg/day IM first 2 wk, 100 mcg twice/wk next 2 mo, thereafter 100 mcg/mo
Biotin	Liver, kidney, egg yolk, yeast, cauliflower, nuts, legumes	Carboxylation and decarboxylation of oxalocetic acid, amino acid and fatty acid metabolism	Dermatitis, glossitis Dependency states	150–300 mcg/day
Vitamin C (ascorbic acid)	Citrus fruits, tomatoes, potatoes, cabbage, green peppers	Essential to osteoid tissue, collagen formation, vascular function, tissue respiration and wound healing	Scurvy (hemorrhages, loose teeth, gingivitis)	100–1,000 mg/day
Sodium	Wide distribution—beef, pork, sardines, cheese, green olives, corn bread, potato chips, sauerkraut	Acid-base balance, osmotic pressure, pH of blood, muscle contractility, nerve transmission, sodium pumps	*Deficiency:* Hyponatremia *Toxicity:* Hypernatremia, confusion, coma	
Potassium	Wide distribution—whole and skim milk, bananas, prunes, raisins	Muscle activity, nerve transmission, intracellular acid-base balance and water retention	*Deficiency:* Hypokalemia, paralysis, cardiac disturbances *Toxicity:* Hyperkalemia, paralysis, cardiac disturbances	
Calcium	Milk and milk products, meat, fish, eggs, cereal products, beans, fruits, vegetables	Bone and tooth formation, blood coagulation, neuromuscular irritability, muscle contractility, myocardial conduction	*Deficiency:* Hypocalcemia and tetany, neuromuscular hyperexcitability *Toxicity:* Hypercalcemia, GI atony, renal failure, psychosis	10–30 ml 10% calcium gluconate soln IV in 24 h

(continues)

	TABLE 20-3	**Principal Micronutrients (Continued)**		
Micronutrient	**Principal Sources**	**Functions**	**Effects of Deficiency and Toxicity**	**Usual Therapeutic Dosage**
Phosphorus	Milk, cheese, meat, poultry, fish, cereals, nuts, legumes	Bone and tooth formation, acid-base balance, component of nucleic acids, energy production	*Deficiency:* Irritability, weakness, blood cell disorders, GI tract and renal dysfunction *Toxicity:* Hyperphosphatemia in renal failure	Potassium acid and di-basic phosphate parenteral 600 mg (18.8 mEq)/day
Magnesium	Green leaves, nuts, cereal grains, seafoods	Bone and tooth formation, nerve conduction, muscle contraction, enzyme activation	*Deficiency:* Hypomagnesemia, neuromuscular irritability *Toxicity:* Hypermagnesemia, hypotension, respiratory failure, cardiac disturbances	2–4 ml 50% magnesium sulfate soln/day IM
Iron	Wide distribution (except dairy products)—soybean flour, beef, kidney, liver, beans, clams, peaches Much unavailable (<20% absorbed)	Hemoglobin, myoglobin formation, enzymes	*Deficiency:* Anemia, dysphagia, koilonychia, enteropathy *Toxicity:* Hemochromatosis, cirrhosis, diabetes mellitus, skin pigmentation	Ferrous sulfate or gluconate 300 mg orally three times a day
Iodine	Seafoods, iodized salt, dairy products Water variable	Thyroxine (T_4) and triiodothyronine (T_3) formation and energy control mechanisms	*Deficiency:* Simple (colloid, endemic) goiter, cretinism, deaf-mutism *Toxicity:* Occasional myxedema	150 mcg iodine/day as potassium iodide added to salt 1:10–40,000 ppm
Fluorine	Wide distribution—tea, coffee Fluoridation of water supplies with sodium fluoride 1.0–2.0 ppm	Bone and tooth formation	*Deficiency:* Predisposition to dental caries, osteoporosis (?) *Toxicity:* Fluorosis, mottling, pitting of permanent teeth, exostoses of spine	Sodium fluoride 1.1–2.2 mg/day orally
Zinc	Wide distribution—vegetable sources Much unavailable	Component of enzymes and insulin, wound healing, growth	*Deficiency:* Growth retardation, hypogonadism, hypogeusia; cirrhosis, acrodermatitis enteropathica	30–150 mg zinc sulfate/day orally
Copper	Wide distribution—organ meat, oysters, nuts, dried legumes, whole-grain cereals	Enzyme component	*Deficiency:* Anemia in malnourished children; Menkes' kinky hair syndrome *Toxicity:* Hepatolenticular degeneration, some biliary cirrhosis (?)	0.3 mg/kg/day copper sulfate orally

(continues)

TABLE 20-3 Principal Micronutrients (Continued)

Micronutrient	Principal Sources	Functions	Effects of Deficiency and Toxicity	Usual Therapeutic Dosage
Cobalt	Green leafy vegetables	Part of vitamin B$_{12}$ molecule	*Deficiency:* Anemia in children (?) *Toxicity:* Beer-drinker's cardiomyopathy	20–30 mg/day cobaltous chloride orally
Chromium	Wide distribution— brewer's yeast	Part of glucose tolerance factor (GTF)	*Deficiency:* Impaired glucose tolerance in malnourished children, some diabetics (?)	

shown in Table 20-4. Careful study of these charts will give you an understanding of the food sources, the function of each in the body's growth and repair, the effects of deficiency and toxicity, and the dosages recommended for daily intake.

Several servings of fiber-rich foods (fruits, vegetables, peas and beans, whole grain cereals) should be included in the daily diet to promote a healthy digestive tract and prevent constipation. Notice that the sections of the food pyramid that list these nutrients are more than half the size of the entire pyramid to show their importance. Encourage patients to modify cooking techniques by using less fats, oils, and sugars and by baking, broiling, boiling, roasting, grilling, poaching, or steaming meats and other foods instead of frying. These modified cooking practices can also help to reduce the amount of calories, cholesterol, sodium, sugar, and saturated and total fat from the diet.

TABLE 20-4 Nutritional Content in a Single Serving of Common Foods

Food	Total Calories	Fat Grams	Calories from Fat	Carbohydrate Grams	Calories from Carbohydrate	Protein Grams	Calories from Protein
Breads and Cereals							
Whole wheat bread (1 slice)	65	1	9	11	44	3	12
Biscuit (2-inch diameter)	103	4.8	43.2	12.8	51.2	2	8
Spaghetti (1 cup)	190	1	9	39	156	7	28
Shredded wheat (²/₃ cup)	100	0.5	4.5	23	92	3	12
Bran flakes (1 cup)	106	0.6	5.4	28.2	112.8	4	16
Granola (¹/₃ cup)	125	5	45	19	76	3	12
Dairy Products							
Milk (1 cup)							
Whole	159	8.2	73.8	11.4	45.6	8	32
2% low-fat	121	4.7	42.3	11.7	46.8	8	32
Skim (non-fat)	86	0.44	4	11.8	47.2	8	32
Yogurt (1 cup), plain low-fat	144	3.5	31.5	16	64	12	48

(continues)

TABLE 20-4　Nutritional Content in a Single Serving of Common Foods (Continued)

Food	Total Calories	Fat Grams	Calories from Fat	Carbohydrate Grams	Calories from Carbohydrate	Protein Grams	Calories from Protein
Dairy Products (Continued)							
Cottage cheese (1 cup)							
Regular	217	9.4	84.6	5.6	22.4	27	108
Low-fat (2%)	203	4.4	39.6	8.2	32.8	31	124
Cheddar cheese (1 oz)	112	9.4	84.6	0.36	1.4	7	28
Swiss cheese (1 oz)	107	7.8	70.2	0.96	3.8	8	32
Egg (1 large, uncooked)	82	6.5	58.5	0.5	2	6	24
Fruits and Vegetables							
Apple (1 medium)	96	1	9	24	96	Trace	0
Avocado (1 medium)	334	32.8	295.2	12.6	50.4	5	20
Banana (1 medium)	127	0.3	2.7	33	120	1	4
Broccoli (1 stalk, raw)	40	1	9	8	32	4	16
Carrot (1 large, raw)	30	0.2	1.8	7	28	1	4
Orange (1 medium)	64	0.3	2.7	16	64	1	4
Potato (1 large, baked, no skin)	145	0.2	1.8	32.8	131.2	3	12
Tomato (1 medium, raw)	25	Trace	0	5	20	1	4
Meat, Poultry, Fish, and Legumes							
Beef							
Ground, lean (3 oz)	230	16	144	0	0	21	84
Roast, chuck (3 oz)	226	13	117	0	0	25	100
Lamb, chop (3 oz)	220	15	135	0	0	20	80
Pork, chop (3 oz, pan fried)	335	27	243	0	0	21	84
Chicken, breast (1/4 lb, roasted)	140	3	27	0	0	27	108
Turkey, light meat (3 oz)	135	3	27	0	0	25	100
Flounder (3 oz)	80	1	9	0	0	17	68
Shrimp, fresh (1/4 lb)	103	0.9	8.1	6.8	27	17	68
Kidney beans (1 cup cooked)	218	0.9	8.1	39.6	158.4	15	60
Lentils (1 cup cooked)	212	0	0	38.6	154.4	16	64
Split peas (1 cup cooked)	230	0.3	2.7	41.6	166.4	16	64
Miscellaneous							
Butter (1 tablespoon)	102	11.3	102	0	0	Trace	0
Margarine (1 tablespoon)	102	11.3	102	0	0	Trace	0
Mayonnaise (1 tablespoon)	102	11.3	102	0	0	Trace	0

FOOD LABELS

The federal Nutritional Labeling and Education Act requires manufacturers to put Nutrition Facts labels on all their food in order that consumers may know what they are eating. The labels contain a wealth of information about the food item. Figure 20-5 shows labels from four different foods. Label (A) is from a box of cereal, (B) is from a box of frozen breaded fish sticks, (C) is from a box of granola bars, and (D) is from a jar of crunchy peanut butter. Note that all labels have the same format. Starting at the top, the first item is:

- Serving Size: This indicates how much of the product the figures relate to; it is followed by the total grams.
- Servings Per Container: This indicates how many servings of the above size are in the box or package.

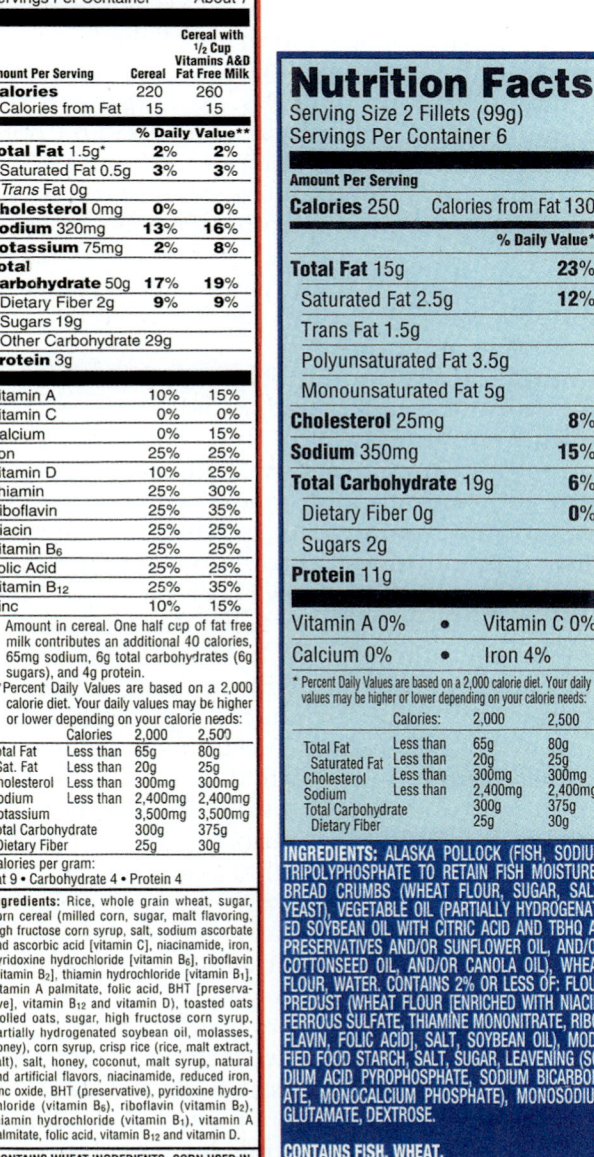

(A)

(B)

(C)

(D)

FIGURE 20-5 Food labels; (A) cereal, (B) fish sticks, (C) granola bars, and (D) peanut butter.

- Amount Per Serving: This indicates the number of calories per serving. These samples also list how many of those calories are from fat.
- Listing of the food nutrients with their respective gram amount. Notice the % Daily Value amounts. These percentages represent how much is in the serving of the total daily amount of the item that a person on a 2,000-calorie diet should consume. For example, 2 tablespoons of peanut butter contain almost one-fourth of the amount of fat allowed per day.
- Observe the fats section. It is broken down into several types. As of January 2005, manufacturers were required to list the amount of trans fat in their product, because it has been shown to have a direct relationship with elevated LDL cholesterol and heart disease. Manufacturers are expected to reformulate their products to avoid listing this fat. Some physicians believe that any margarine, vegetable shortening, or partially hydrogenated oils should be avoided. They are typically found in baked goods and packaged and fast foods.
- Other items listed that are important to patients are the amounts of cholesterol, fiber, sodium, and sugars.
- A list of vitamins and minerals in the serving are included next. Two of these samples have hardly any listed, but the box of cereal, label (A), lists a large amount; manufacturers add them to "fortify" their products.
- The list of ingredients follows the nutritional information and should include everything in the product. You will note many chemical **additives**: some enhance taste or color, while others prolong the shelf life of the product.

As stated before, labels have a lot of information if you understand how to use them. The information is helpful not only to dieters but also to those with chronic conditions such as diabetes and heart disease. Observe your food labels and become familiar with their contents so you can effectively explain them to patients.

Many physicians prefer not to deal with patients' diets and will refer them to a **dietician** to teach dietary basics and plan for their specific needs. It is rather time-consuming at first and requires frequent follow up until the patient is comfortable and achieving desired results. You still may be asked about something that gives you the opportunity to reinforce what the dietician has said and helps the patient to understand.

Encourage patients to read food labels at the grocery store before they buy any food. As patients are planning their daily menu, advise them to again read food labels and note the percentage of each of the nutrients. They should also pay attention to the serving size, which is usually not what is normally consumed). It is important to understand how the ingredients are listed. The ingredient with the highest content in the product is listed first. The last ingredient listed is the one with the least amount contained in the product. Remind patients about attractive wording, such as no cholesterol and low fat. Some food labels claim to be low in fat or salt, or to contain no (zero) cholesterol, but then they are generally high in sugar and calorie content. Table 20-4 lists single servings of some common foods with their total calorie content; carbohydrate, protein, and fat grams; and total calories from fats, proteins, and carbohydrates. This may be used as a guide in meal planning. Prepared foods and many of the fast foods we eat usually have more fat, sugar, and salt than those foods that we cook for ourselves. Advise patients that eating fast foods should be the exception and not a regular meal habit. Reduced-calorie food items can also have a high salt or sodium content. Manufacturers add increased amounts of salt and other flavor enhancers in order to make the lower-calorie food item taste better.

People who have food allergies will find the labels very helpful in avoiding those foods that could cause them problems.

Look again at the sample labels in Figure 20-5. At the end of the list of ingredients on each label some of the ingredients are listed again. This serves to identify quickly those items that may cause allergic reactions to sensitive people. Some of the most common food offenders are fish, wheat, milk, peanuts, sulfites, and shellfish. A peanut allergy is so serious that it may be life threatening. Note on the (C) label the words "This product is manufactured in a facility that uses peanuts and nuts." Even though this food item contains no peanuts, it is manufactured with equipment that also processes peanut items. Even traces of peanuts can be a problem to a person with a severe peanut allergy.

Another feature you will find on some labels is shown in label (A). At the bottom you will note the word "Exchange." This designation is to assist patients with diabetes to select food within a category, this time it is carbohydrates, to maintain their carbohydrate-fat-protein balance. Their dietary amounts are stated in exchanges, and they can select any foods up to their daily limit within that food category.

Explaining to patients how to count calories, carbohydrates, fat grams, and so on will help them realize the importance of planning meals that are well balanced and sensible. For those who are interested in eating a healthier diet, labels help eliminate the guesswork. Having the contents listed on packages also makes it easier for those who are on special diets and those watching their caloric intake, fat grams, cholesterol content, and so on. Food labels can also make menu planning a more pleasant and interesting project. Remind patients to read *all* labels carefully.

Meal Supplements

When patients suffer from loss or lack of appetite or they cannot tolerate a normal diet, it may be necessary for the physician to prescribe a protein-vitamin-mineral food supplement. Patients who might need this type of treatment include elderly, chronically ill, postoperative, underweight, anemic, and **anorexic** patients. This treatment should be conducted only under the supervision of a physician. Remind patients to take these supplements regularly as directed. The supplements generally come in at least vanilla and chocolate flavors and can be purchased in drug, health, and grocery stores. They are available in individual ready-to-drink cans or in powder form to be mixed with liquid. They can be ordered as a meal substitute or as between meal nourishment. They can be very beneficial for patients receiving chemotherapy to supply extra nourishment in an easy-to-use liquid format when eating regular food is not appealing.

Health Concerns in Adolescents

Special focus should be directed to a predominantly adolescent condition called **anorexia nervosa**. Anorexia nervosa is a psychoneurotic disorder in which the patient—usually a female, but not exclusively—refuses to eat over a period of time. Often, vigorous exercise is a part of the daily routine to help burn calories. Many problems can stem from the ongoing weight loss, including **emaciation** and **amenorrhea**. This disorder may be the result of emotional stress or conflict. The patient has a poor self-image and is obsessed with a fear of becoming obese. Signs of this disorder are a change in personality, irritability, refusal to eat, and weight loss. A similar disorder, also seen mainly in adolescent females, is **bulimia nervosa**. Unlike the patient with anorexia, the patient with bulimia eats a very large quantity of food at one time (as much as 5,000 calories), but uses **purging** (vomiting, laxatives, and diuretics) to rid the body of the calories. Usually, the patient eats normal meals with others to keep the disorder secretive. This is one of the reasons that this disorder is sometimes difficult to diagnose. The bulemic's **binge** eating and purge behaviors also originate from poor self-image and feelings of inadequacy. Symptoms of bulimia are dark circles under the eyes, muscle wasting, dental cavities, and damage to tooth enamel caused by the acid from the stomach from frequent vomiting. Problems with gastrointestinal and cardiovascular systems are a potential danger in this disorder. Referral for psychiatric therapy and nutritional counseling as soon as possible are necessary to arrest these potentially fatal disorders. Make a sincere effort to give positive reinforcement to patients in an area of their personal interest (e.g., hobby, school project or activity). Your patience and understanding is extremely important in making these patients feel accepted and supported.

The adolescent in general needs a little extra attention in regards to the promotion of or in possibly the initial establishing of good health habits. Give this patient a chance to ask questions and discuss problems in private. Often there are fears about many timely issues, such as sexual behavior, STDs and HIV, pregnancy and birth control, substance abuse (drugs and alcohol), depression and suicide, domestic issues and abuse (emotional, physical, and sexual), peer pressure, and a wealth of other topics that she may feel she cannot talk to anyone else about because of being embarrassed or intimidated. You may be the only one who will treat her as an individual and listen objectively to her problems. Sometimes just getting a chance to let it out is helpful. Offer your listening ear, and support and refer the patient to the physician or to an appropriate service agency as necessary (e.g., mental health center, teen pregnancy free clinic). Some teenagers are reluctant to speak to the school nurse or other authoritative figure because of the possibility of having a parent called.

Being a teenager is a very stressful time. Many pressures begin to surface, creating many demands that pile up rapidly on an already-confused and mood-swinging young pre-adult. One very common problem that you may be influential in curbing is the cigarette habit. Giving adolescents the facts about smoking and health may make all the difference in their decision to resist this temptation. Health care professionals have a responsibility to give this age group of patients their careful attention whenever the opportunity occurs, simply because they do not appear very often for health care services.

WEIGHT CONTROL

A good weight-control program should contain foods from the food pyramid to be nutritionally sound. Eating should be an enjoyable, relaxing experience. But in our fast-food society, people tend to eat more food with more calories more often. A **calorie** is a unit of heat, and all food substances have caloric value (see Table 20-4). All of the body's processes burn calories to provide energy and sustain life. If you overeat regularly, the unused calories are not wasted but stored as fat. If you reduce calorie intake, the stored fat will be used by the body for energy, and you will begin to shed the extra weight. You should make patients aware that they should eat their meals slowly, because it takes approximately 20 minutes for the brain to realize that the stomach is full. Those who follow this practice in a relaxed atmosphere eat *less* and digest their food better. It is now recommended that eating several (five to six) small meals daily not only allows for better use of nutrients by the body for more energy, but it is much easier on the digestive tract. This practice also helps in weight control.

A variety of magazines, books, and businesses offer weight-control plans that promise success for each individual. Over-the-counter drugs promise miraculous weight loss in a matter of weeks. You can be influential in helping patients avoid possible health hazards by warning them of the danger in these quick-weight-loss programs. Many people do lose weight in a short time, but they gain it right back as soon as the program ends. Others do permanent damage to their health.

One respected weight-loss program is Weight Watchers. Most people who have reached their weight-loss goals through this program have maintained a satisfactory weight because they have learned how to change their eating habits. Many support groups offer similar programs. Positive reinforcement is one of the keys to their success. Many physicians realize the frustration of trying to reduce weight and suggest these support groups to patients. You will want to encourage patients who are trying to follow a diet by showing a genuine interest as they work to reach their goals.

There is no "one list" that can be a low-calorie diet to follow for everyone who needs to lose weight. A list of foods with their calorie content or a basic diet as a guide can be helpful to those who wish or need to reduce their weight. Physicians want their patients to lose weight if they are either on the threshold of obesity or have already been diagnosed as **obese**. Weighing more that 30% above your ideal body weight (obese) puts you at risk for developing serious health problems such as heart disease, stroke, diabetes, cancer, and **sleep apnea**.

DIETS

The number of special diets is far too numerous to list in this book. A few therapeutic diets that may be helpful to you in providing education to patients are briefly discussed here. These are general guidelines to follow. You should follow the triage/patient education policy established by the physician(s) in your medical facility when advising patients either by phone or face-to-face. If you are uncertain or have any questions regarding what to tell patients about their treatment plan, you should ask the physician. Physicians usually have printed dietary information about the most common types of diets to which you can refer and also provide to patients.

- **Clear liquid diet:** Pedialyte for infants and children, Gatorade for adults, clear gelatin, decaffeinated coffee and tea, clear broth, no-caffeine sodas, artificially flavored drink mix, flavored frozen juice bars and treats, clear juice, and water as directed by physician—offered to patients at least every 2 hours the first 24 hours for patients with diarrhea.
- **BRAT diet:** Bananas, rice, applesauce, toast, and clear liquids/water (Pedialyte for infants) for 24 hours as tolerated by patients after diarrhea stops, or as directed by the physician.

- **Soft diet:** Creamed hot cereals, gelatin, pudding, ice cream, sherbet, mashed or baked potatoes, puréed vegetables, creamed soups, baked turkey/chicken/fish, meatloaf, milk, poached egg, macaroni and cheese, yogurt, applesauce, and graham crackers. These are suggestions for foods that may be more easily tolerated for patients who have gastrointestinal disorders, such as a duodenal ulcer or gastritis. This diet is also for those who are just getting over an intestinal virus.
- **Low-calorie diet:** Basically counting calories and adding up the total will help those who wish to shed a few pounds, especially if cardiovascular exercise is included at least three times a week for a minimum of 30 minutes. Eating no more than a total of 30% of calories from fat each day is recommended for a healthy heart, especially if there is a family history of heart disease.

There are low-fat, no-sugar, high-fiber, low- or no-salt, and low-residue diets, and the list continues with specialized therapeutic diet plans for individual needs. Therapeutic diets are used in the treatment of patients with a specific disease or disorder. Standard printed diet sheets, pamphlets, booklets, and other patient education topics can be displayed on a wall-mounted rack for convenience to patients and you. Post information about nutrition, heart-healthy cooking classes, and other topics on the bulletin board for patients to get involved in their health care. Patients who have a medical condition with dietary needs beyond the printed materials in your facility should be referred to a registered dietitian (RD). Reinforce the need for this referral and how important it is that they give their full cooperation. A patient's background and lifestyle will be considered and adjustments made as necessary. A dietician will work closely with other health care team members in individual **therapeutic** diet planning.

Popular Diets

There have been many popular or fad diets over the years. Ones promising weight loss seem to be the most common. Most will work initially, but long-term success requires good, old-fashioned less calories in, more exercise out to achieve and maintain a desirable weight. Some quick fix diets have been the Grapefruit Diet, in which you consume primarily grapefruit; the Cabbage Soup Diet, in which you eat a mixture of cabbage and other vegetables for a short period of time; and low-carb diets, which have become very popular and actually resulted in the manufacture of special low-carb foods and meals. Many books were published to promote the diets. The Adkins and the South Beach diets were two very popular versions. These too have faded somewhat from their original lofty place, and others will undoubtedly take their place.

Cultural Influence on Diet

Various cultures have a long history of dietary preferences and practices. Since so many different cultures have come to the United States, you will surely come into contact with many of them. It is interesting to learn about ethnic and religious practices that differ from your own; it can make your life experiences exciting. Some dietary practices of different cultural or religious groups will be familiar to you. To introduce you to the diversity, a brief listing follows:

- Asian: The main foods are rice, vegetables, fruits, and curries. Meat, fish, and chicken are used in small amounts. Most foods are prepared by sautéing in a wok.
- Catholic: Abstain from eating meat on Ash Wednesday and Fridays during Lent. Older Catholics may still adhere to the former restriction of no meat on any Fridays. They often choose something, such as a favorite food, to abstain from throughout the total Lenten season.
- Chinese: Rice is the main staple, along with soybean products. Pork, eggs, and vegetables are also favorites (Figure 20-6). Tea is the beverage of choice.
- Hindu: Followers believe life is sacred and animals are the dwelling places of ancestor's souls. Therefore they eat primarily vegetables.
- Islamic: Followers of this religion are called Muslims. They have dietary laws governing the method of killing animals for food. Eating pork or drinking alcohol is prohibited. During the daylight hours, the month of Ramadan, Muslims do not eat food or drink water but spend the day in reflection, intense worship, reading the Quran, and developing self-control.
- Italian: Pasta with various tomato sauces and cheese are popular foods. Southern Italy enjoys fish and highly seasoned food, while Northern Italy eats more meat and root vegetables.
- Japanese: Rice, soybean paste, vegetables, fruits, and fish. Food is frequently fried and topped with soy sauce. Sushi is rice combined with fish, eel, or squid, rolled in sheets of dry seaweed, and cut into small wheels. It is very popular in the United States.
- Jewish: Orthodox Jews have strict dietary laws, many dating to Biblical times. Foods prepared by these laws are called kosher (Figure 20-7). Meat and poultry must be killed and treated in a specific manner. Meat and milk products must not share the same preparation dishes and must be eaten 6 hours apart. The laws also forbid eating hindquarters of meat. Shellfish, pork, and many other items are on the forbidden list. No cooking is permitted on the Sabbath (Friday sundown to Saturday sundown), so things must be made ahead of time.
- Mexican: The favorite foods are rice, beans, chili peppers, tomatoes, and corn meal. The meat is usually

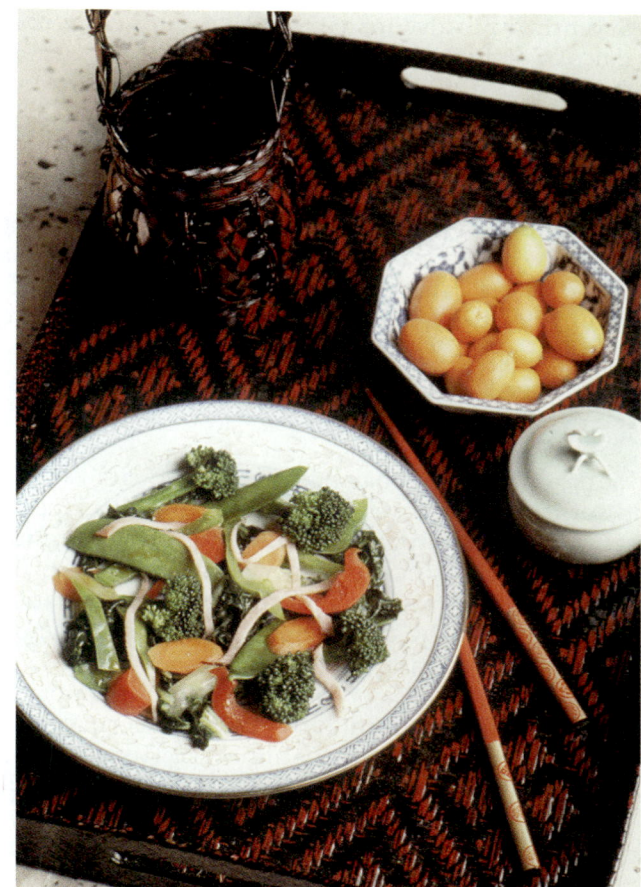

FIGURE 20-6   Traditional Chinese foods

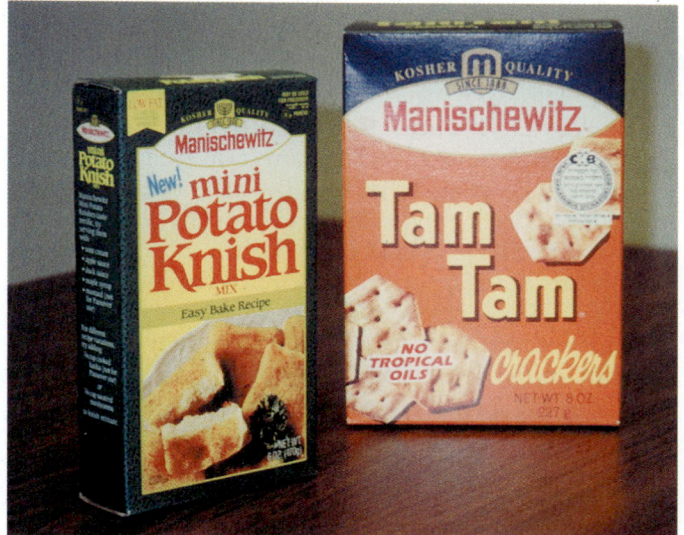

FIGURE 20-7   Kosher food

cooked with vegetables in a thick souplike chili. Tortillas and tamales are flat breads made from corn meal and are filled with meat and vegetable mixtures, then wrapped in corn husks and steamed.

- Seventh-Day Adventist: Observe Saturday as their day of worship. They abstainfrom coffee, tea, and alcohol, which they consider harmful. The diet consists of milk, eggs, and vegetables. No meat, fish, or poultry is eaten. Meat substitute from soybeans provides protein.

After this brief introduction to various dietary differences, it is easy to see how some cultural and religious practices could cause challenges to diet modifications that might be needed due to the lack of some nutrients in the diet.

EXERCISE

In addition to a well-balanced diet, adequate exercise and sufficient rest are essential to good health. Special diets and exercise programs must be approved for individuals by the physician, who will determine the patient's needs and tolerance from careful examination and medical history. This is done to safeguard the patient from overexertion and stress.

Exercise is defined as physical exertion for improvement of health or correction of physical deformity. The safest form of exercise, and one almost everyone can participate in, is walking. Often patients are reluctant to walk if they have to walk alone because they fear for their safety. You may suggest that they seek a walking partner and try to go in daylight hours. The purchase of a treadmill is a good investment (for those who can afford it), because it is available at any time and in any weather. You may suggest that patients inquire at a local enclosed shopping mall about walking clubs that meet before the mall opens. This way the patients will have a safe and comfortable environment in the company of others with the same interest. This idea could be quite helpful in motivating them to stick to a routine for their better health. There are so many different exercise programs available that people can choose according to their individual needs and goals. A combination of proper diet and proper exercise brings satisfying results in overall good health.

Regular exercise improves circulation and muscle tone and relieves tension. People who have followed an exercise routine regularly report that they experience a better outlook on life, have more energy, and feel healthier. The degree of exertion in any exercise routine will vary with individuals, and the physician's advice should be taken.

Protecting Muscles

It is very important to prepare your muscles for exercise in order to avoid discomfort and limited motion. This is especially true when you begin an exercise program. If you get sore aching muscles, you will not be able to participate in exercise and may become discouraged.

People who exercise regularly or participate in vigorous activity will go through simple exercises to gently warm up and stretch muscles.

Even before walking, proper stretching is recommended to keep from straining muscles and to help prevent other possible injuries. Table 20-5 illustrates the 10 basic stretching exercises to help prepare for exercise.

A period of time following exercise should be used to repeat the pre-exercise stretches and is known as the cool-down. This allows muscles to adjust to a nonexercise state and helps to eliminate soreness. Read the instructions and practice the different exercises. Even if you are not preparing to exercise, these will help you relax tense muscles from daily stress or long periods of sitting.

All of the behaviors that influence health are governed by one's mental (or social) health, and vice versa. A positive outlook is most helpful in coping with life in general. (Refer to Chapter 4.) Learning coping and problem-solving skills can help us deal with the everyday stress and the occasional crisis of routine living.

HEALTHY SPIRIT

Many physicians recognize the power of a patient's belief system. Nurturing the spirit (the soul) has overall benefits. Practicing a chosen religious belief can help the feelings of completeness and belonging. Being a member of an organization where there are others who offer their support and caring is essential to one's sense of worth. It helps with fulfillment of our basic needs. Self-esteem needs can also be met with activities that reinforce our significance and our independence of one another. Many meaningful religious ceremonies give us a sense of direction and remind us of purpose. Meditation and other relaxation exercises including reflection have a calming effect. These are excellent ways to unwind and relieve stress and help one in getting a good night's rest.

SLEEP

Getting sufficient rest is necessary for good health. Rest is usually thought of as another word for sleep and is defined as a time away from activity. Most people use the words rest and sleep interchangeably. Sleep is the natural way for the body to restore itself. Adequate rest/sleep equips us with strength to handle various daily activities. Winding down from strenuous or hectic activity is usually essential before one is able to rest and relax enough to go to sleep. Even though the number of hours of sleep needed varies from person to person, quality sleep should not be interrupted. The average number of hours of sleep is between 6 and 9 hours in a 24-hour period for most adults. Sleep patterns may change as we age. Each of us has a pattern of sleep and sleep needs specific to us.

TABLE 20-5   Ten Basic Stretching Exercises

Illustration	Area of the body	Description
	Neck muscles	Keep shoulders down while you tilt your head to the right. Place your right hand on the left side of your head, and pull gently toward your right shoulder for about 15–25 seconds. Repeat for the left side.
	Calf muscles	Place feet flat on the floor, 2–3 feet away from a wall. Lean your forearms flat against the wall, then step toward the wall with the left foot, bending the knee while keeping the heel of the right foot flat on the floor for about 15–25 seconds. Repeat with the right leg.
	Thigh muscles (quadriceps)	Lean into the wall with your left hand, and pull your right ankle up gently with your right hand for 15–25 seconds. Repeat for the left ankle.
	Outer thigh muscles	Stand next to and press your left hand against the wall as you place your right hand on your right hip. Bend the right knee slightly, rest the left foot on its side, and hold for 15–25 seconds. Repeat for the left leg.
	Hip muscles (hip flexor)	Get into a kneeling position with your right foot flat on the floor, and bend the right knee up to touch your chest. Keep your left leg on the floor behind you (arms at your sides) and stretch and hold for 15–25 seconds. Repeat; bring the left knee to your chest; keep your right leg on the floor behind you.

(continues)

TABLE 20-5   Ten Basic Stretching Exercises (Continued)

Illustration	Area of the body	Description
	Groin muscles	While sitting on the floor, bring your heels together, and hold them with your hands. Gently push your legs down with your elbows (or ask someone to do it for you), and hold for 5–10 seconds; use resistance to feel stretching (avoid straining) and then relax. Repeat 5–10 times. This is often called the butterfly stretch.
	Back and side muscles	Sit up straight on the floor with both legs straight out. Bring the left leg up with your knee bent, and place your foot on the floor to the right of the right knee. Then place your right elbow on the upper part of your left knee. Your left hand should be in back of you to help you look over your left shoulder. Take in a deep breath before you begin to twist your upper body and exhale slowly while you hold this posture for 10–25 seconds. Repeat for the right leg.
	Lower back	Lie flat on your back and bring your left knee up. Cross it over to your right hip (keep your arms stretched out to your sides). Keep your shoulders against the floor, and turn your head to the left, then press your left thigh with your right hand to the floor, and hold for 10–25 seconds. Repeat for the right leg.
	Hamstrings	Lie flat on your back and bend your knees, placing both feet flat on the floor. Raise your right leg up so that your heel is toward the ceiling. Hold your right leg behind the knee with both hands and pull into your chest. Relax your foot and keep straightening your leg until it becomes uncomfortable, and then hold the position for 10–20 seconds. Repeat for the left leg.
	Lumbar muscles (lower back)	Lie on your back with your knees bent up to your chest. Place your hands behind your knees, press into your chest, and hold for 10–25 seconds, then relax and repeat several times.

When a patient tells you he has not been getting any sleep at night, you must ask him how long he *does* sleep and *when* he sleeps. Often, there is sufficient sleep but not all at once at night when he thinks he should sleep. If the person is obviously not getting sufficient sleep, the physician needs to be alerted when the patient first mentions it. Often, the patient does not consider it a problem worth telling you because initially it is just annoying to him. Insomnia is a term used to describe not being able to sleep. There could be a serious physical or emotional (psychological) problem that is the reason for the insom-

nia. Generally, the physician will ask the patient to keep track of when and how long at a time he sleeps for a specific amount of time. Establishing a record of the sleep dysfunction helps the physician to make a decision about diagnostic and treatment plans. Being comfortable and ready to go to sleep should be stressed to those patients who have trouble sleeping. Patients who awaken once in a while, whether the reason is apparent or not, should not be alarmed. Those who wake up several times each night on a regular basis are at risk for health problems if sleep interruption continues. Sleep **deprivation** is a term that means lack of sleep. Many people experience times when sleep is not sufficient but manage to function. Within a day or so of getting sufficient rest and sleep, they are back to a normal sleep pattern.

Those who suffer from sleep deprivation on a long-term basis exhibit irritability, fatigue, poor concentration and remembering ability, clumsiness, and sometimes visual or **tactile** hallucinations. Research studies have shown that a person needs both **REM (rapid eye movement)** and **NREM (non-rapid eye movement)** stages of sleep. The NREM stage begins approximately 90 minutes after a person goes to sleep. Those who can sleep for at least 6 hours uninterrupted feel better and more rested. That is because they have benefited from the effects of the proper sequence of sleep. Explain to patients that their sleep schedule may need to be altered. Patients often get stuck in a pattern because they think they have to sleep at a certain time. It is possible that some try to change their biological clock. Most people know that it is not easy to do. Sometimes all a patient needs to do is talk to someone about their concerns. Just listening and a suggestion from you to read or play soft music or engage in a quiet activity can be helpful. One needs to realize that sleep is not a luxury, but it is necessary for the body to function well.

ACHIEVE UNIT OBJECTIVES

- ■ Complete the Workbook activities to meet the learning objectives.
- ■ Apply your knowledge at the end of this chapter in completing the Critical Thinking Challenge and Activities, as well as the StudyWARE on your Student CD-ROM.

UNIT 2
HABIT-FORMING SUBSTANCES

OBJECTIVES

Upon completion of this unit, you will be able to achieve the following:

LEARNING Objectives

1. **Spell and define, using the glossary at the back of the text, all of the Words to Know in this unit.**

2. **List the major groups of abused drugs and give an example of each.**
3. **List the nine indications of drug or alcohol abuse.**
4. **Identify the level of alcohol that is considered legal intoxication.**
5. **Explain the patterns of drinking necessary for a diagnosis of alcoholism.**
6. **Name seven characteristics of a child born with fetal alcohol syndrome.**
7. **List at least 10 diseases caused by the use of tobacco.**
8. **Name the symptoms of marijuana intoxication.**
9. **Identify the medical uses of marijuana.**
10. **Identify the seven initial effects of cocaine use.**
11. **Describe the meaning of the term "run."**
12. **Discuss the clinical use of methadone.**
13. **Identify signs of injection drug use.**
14. **Name the three date rape drugs and explain why they are effective.**

WORDS TO KNOW

abstinent	barbiturate	induction
addiction	binge	intervention
aggression	delirium tremens	intoxicated
Al-Anon	dependence	metabolized
Al-Ateen	depressant	nicotine
alcohol	euphoria	relapse
Alcoholics	fetal alcohol	sedate
Anonymous	syndrome	stimulant
alcoholism	hallucinogen	synthetic
amnesia	hangover	tar
amphetamine	illicit	tremulousness

CERTIFICATION CONNECTION

CMA
Resource and community services
Pharmacology, substance abuse

CMAS
Patient information and community resources

RMA
Patient instruction, health and wellness

A habit is a pattern of behavior that is acquired over a time by repetition. Habits can be either advantageous or disadvantageous depending on the effects they have. Many of our habits are so much a part of us that we do not even realize they exist. Changing a behavior that has become a habit is difficult. It takes a great deal of effort and commitment to repattern personal activities. Teaching good health habits to patients is an important duty of the medical assistant. The entire medical staff must strive to set a good example, because example can be the best teacher.

In times of stress, one may be inclined to relieve anxiety or depression by using chemical substances. Other persons turn to chemical substances to experiment with the feelings they produce. Often, this is a response to peer pressure, which can be very strong. Regardless of why persons turn to chemical substances, they need to know that abuse and dependency can follow and that the stakes can be very high. Even individuals under the supervision of a physician may become dependent.

Unfortunately, the influence of advertising has encouraged chemical substance use by promoting fast relief, quick weight-loss, instant sleep and wakefulness, and a variety of other "feel-good" promises from the makers of chemical products. Although a substance may well relieve symptoms temporarily, the cause of the problem will still exist. If undetermined or undetected physical or emotional problems are not diagnosed and treated, they may balloon into more complex problems that are only worsened by the abuse of chemical substances. You can play an important part in recognizing potential chemical abusers and helping them take steps toward treatment.

TYPES OF HABIT-FORMING SUBSTANCES

It is possible to abuse or become addicted to many substances when they are used on a regular and frequent basis. Common household products such as glue, solvents, electronic equipment cleaning products, aerosol can propellants, and the like have been used to achieve a degree of chemical "buzz." Alcohol, marijuana, and tobacco products are other substances that users can develop a dependency for with continued usage. Several drugs, both prescription and illegal, are highly addictive and can lead to life-threatening consequences. Drugs usually fall into certain categories based upon the effects they produce. The most common are:

- **Stimulants**—caffeine, cocaine, crack, **amphetamines**, methamphetamine
- Sedatives/**depressants**—alcohol, valium, librium, phenobarbital, seconal
- Opiates—morphine, codeine, heroin
- Synthetic opiates—demerol, dilaudid, methadone
- **Hallucinogens**—LSD, PCP, ketamine, ecstasy

The following pages contain an in-depth discussion of these drugs, how they work, the problems with their use, how they affect the unborn child, and what treatments are available. Most of the information in this unit was contributed by a Certified Addiction Registered Nurse who works with clients daily at a treatment facility in California. Hopefully this introduction will give you a basic understanding of the difficulties people experience dealing with this disease and help you to be supportive of their struggle to get free from their addiction.

THE DISEASE OF DEPENDENCY

The use of alcohol, tobacco, and other drugs often results in numerous health problems. The ability to recognize the symptoms of drug abuse or dependency is an important skill for any medical professional.

Addiction and alcoholism are now recognized as diseases, not behavioral weaknesses or just the result of bad judgment. Alcoholism is recognized as a major health problem by the American Medical Association, American Osteopathic Association, and the American Bar Association. Excessive long-term use can reduce resistance to infections and eventually lead to cirrhosis of the liver as well as complicate other diseases and conditions.

The terms **addiction** and **dependence** are both used to mean that the user cannot control the amount and frequency of use despite very negative consequences. A person who is addicted or dependent continues to use their drug of choice, knowing that they are ill, broke, in legal trouble, or that a loved one will leave them if they do not stop. Drug abuse indicates a less serious, although dangerous, problem.

Currently the most common drugs of abuse are tobacco; alcohol; marijuana; stimulants, including cocaine and methamphetamine; and opiates. Hallucinogens and depressants are also popular among certain populations. Each type of drug affects specific receptors in the brain, as well as various organs and systems of the body. Repeated use causes physical, psychological, emotional, and spiritual problems. Legal and financial consequences are also common. Figure 20-8 lists signs of possible drug and alcohol abuse that may cause you to confront an individual.

ALCOHOL

Alcohol is a sedative anesthetic. This means that it **sedates**, or has a calming effect, and it decreases sensation or relieves pain. It is absorbed in the small in-

INDICATIONS OF DRUG OR ALCOHOL ABUSE
• Abrupt change in mood/attitudes • Sharp decline in attendance/performance at school/work • Resistance to discipline/rules at home/school • Deterioration in relationships • Sudden, unusual temper outbursts • Increased frequency in borrowing money • Stealing from others • Increased intense secrecy about actions and belongings • Associating with new friends

FIGURE 20-8 Some of the common warning signs of possible drug or alcohol abuse. Be aware of these signs when dealing with patients and those in your personal life. Early intervention is critical.

testine and broken down, or **metabolized**, by the liver. In general, a person can metabolize one ounce of alcohol in a 90-minute period. This is roughly equivalent to one glass of wine, one beer, or one mixed drink. When the blood alcohol level reaches 0.08, a person is considered legally **intoxicated** or drunk. Physical symptoms of intoxication are slurred speech, lack of coordination, unsteady gait, dizziness, and blackouts. Psychological symptoms include irritability, mood swings, short attention span, decreased judgment and inhibitions, and memory problems. Intoxication lasts less than 12 hours after the last drink and is usually followed by a hangover. A **hangover** is the unpleasant group of symptoms that occur approximately 4 to 6 hours after alcohol consumption. The symptoms include nausea and vomiting, gastritis, headache, fatigue, sweating, and thirst. Hypoglycemia, or low blood-sugar, and the imbalance of lactic acid and other substances in the blood are the reasons for these symptoms.

Binge drinking is the consumption of five or more drinks within a few hours for the express purpose of getting drunk. This is a dangerous activity popular among teenagers and college students. High doses of alcohol can depress respirations, and toxic levels can cause death. Also, because of the effects of decreased judgment and inhibitions, binge drinkers can become involved in violent or illegal activities, as well as unplanned and unwanted sexual encounters resulting in sexually transmitted diseases (STDs) and pregnancy.

In order to be diagnosed with **alcoholism**, a person must engage in one of three patterns of behavior: regular, daily intake of large amounts of alcohol; regular heavy drinking limited to weekends; or long periods of sobriety interspersed with heavy binges that last weeks or months. There are numerous physical effects of excessive drinking, including alcoholic hepatitis, cirrhosis, esophagitis, ulcers, bleeding disorders, and malnutrition. In addition to the physical deterioration resulting from alcohol consumption, there are psychological and social consequences of equal importance. An alcoholic often faces relationship failures, loss of child custody, loss of employment, and financial and legal problems. Such events put these patients at high risk for depression and suicide.

Fetal Alcohol Syndrome

Studies have shown that any amount of alcohol during pregnancy can cause brain damage, growth retardation, and physical defects in the fetus. **Fetal alcohol syndrome** is an extreme example of the effects of alcohol during pregnancy. A child born with this diagnosis has observable facial characteristics including small head circumference, low-set ears, drooping eyelids, thin upper lip, and small chin. These children have behavioral and learning disabilities that require specialized professional **interventions** in order for them to lead happy, successful lives.

Current studies have also shown that the use of alcohol and other drugs by the father, even when the mother is **abstinent**, or drug-free, can have effects on the fetus. Researchers have reported low birth weight, abnormal EEGs, and greater likelihood of hyperactivity in sons of alcoholic fathers. You must teach patients about the harmful effects on unborn children from the consumption of alcohol.

Alcohol Withdrawal

Symptoms of alcohol withdrawal include anxiety, nausea and vomiting, sweating, irritability, and elevated blood pressure and heart rate. Tremors may begin 2 to 3 hours after withdrawal and persist for up to 5 or 6 days. Usually the hands are involved first, but often tremors include the arms, legs, feet, tongue, and eyelids. Seizures may occur within the first 48 to 72 hours of withdrawal. **Delirium tremens**, or DTs, is an acute complication of alcohol withdrawal. It often has a sudden onset about 3 to 4 days after drinking has stopped and usually lasts 2 to 7 days but can last as long as 5 weeks. Symptoms include confusion, fearfulness, increased tremors, irritability, fever, illusions, and hallucinations. This is a medical emergency.

Treatment

Initially a patient in acute withdrawal from alcohol is managed with sedatives and anticonvulsant medications. Librium (chlordiazepoxide), Valium (diazepam), and Ativan (lorazepam) are commonly prescribed for safe and effective detoxification. A diet high in vitamins and calories is recommended for those suffering from poor nutrition.

Recovery

The disease of alcoholism is incurable, progressive, and often fatal. Alcoholics who have stopped drinking are not considered "cured," but instead are in recovery. There are a variety of methods of recovery.

Alcoholics Anonymous, or AA, was founded in the mid-1930s. It is a group of self-acknowledged alcoholics whose goal is to stay sober and support others to achieve sobriety. They hold meetings regularly in most communities. AA members share their experience, strength, and hope and work the 12 Steps of a sobriety program as a means of dealing with their disease. Other support groups have branched off this initial organization. **Al-Anon** and **Al-Ateen** are for family members and close friends of the alcoholic to help them understand and cope with their loved one's illness.

Residential, outpatient, and day treatment centers also provide those in recovery with knowledge, support, behavior modification, and professional counseling. When social groups or rehabilitation centers are not sufficient in aiding a patient to remain abstinent, medications are sometimes prescribed. Antabuse (disulfiram) prevents the liver from metabolizing alcohol normally. When a person drinks after taking Antabuse, the result is nausea and vomiting. This drug does not affect the desire for alcohol, and it is difficult to persuade patients to continue taking it.

An increasingly popular medication is ReVia (naltrexone), which reduces the craving, or desire, to drink. The patient must be motivated to take the pills as prescribed and see their doctor or mental health professional regularly in order for this to be effective. To reduce the temptation to skip taking a pill, researchers are considering a once-a-month injection that would gradually release the drug over time.

Campral (acamprosate) works on the nerve circuitry of the brain to promote abstinence. The Federal Drug Administration (FDA) approved this medication in 2004, and several large studies have proven it to be effective. A number of other new medications are in the experimental stages for the treatment of alcohol dependence.

TOBACCO

According to a report by the Surgeon General in 2004, every organ of the body is harmed by smoking tobacco. Research caused the printing of the statement "The Surgeon General has determined that cigarette smoking is hazardous to your health" on every package of cigarettes in the United States, and many foreign countries did the same. The list of diseases caused by smoking includes abdominal aortic aneurysm; acute myeloid leukemia; cataract; pneumonia; periodontitis; chronic lung disease; coronary heart and cardiovascular diseases; cancer of the cervix, kidney, pancreas, stomach, bladder, esophagus, larynx, lung, mouth, and throat; effects on the reproductive organs, and sudden infant death syndrome (SIDS). Cigarette smoking contributes to approximately one of every five deaths in the United States.

Nicotine is the psychoactive drug in tobacco that produces addiction. It acts as a stimulant to the central nervous system and reaches the brain within seconds of inhaling a lit cigarette. Nicotine is also an appetite suppressant. In large doses it can produce tremors, decreased urine output, and rapid respiratory rate. Women older than 30 who smoke and take oral contraceptives are more prone to heart disease, strokes, and blood clots.

Secondhand smoke causes lung cancer and heart disease in adults and increases the risk of respiratory illnesses in children. Studies have shown children who are exposed to passive smoke may have poor development and reduced lung function, in addition to frequent respiratory illnesses. Community action in many areas has resulted in making most public places smoke-free. The symbol in Figure 20-9 is a common sight in buildings.

Smoking and Pregnancy

Smoking during pregnancy increases the risk of low birth weight, premature, and stillborn babies. Children of women who smoked during pregnancy have a higher rate of behavioral disorders.

Withdrawal

Withdrawal symptoms can occur within 1 hour of smoking cessation, or stopping, and can last for up to 2 weeks. This discomfort causes people to smoke more

FIGURE 20-9 This common symbol is displayed in most public places with the notation "No Smoking" or "Thank you for not smoking."

often, which reinforces the habit and produces rapid dependency. The symptoms include decreased heart rate, nervousness, anxiety, headache, fatigue, insomnia or inability to sleep, constipation, diarrhea, and weight gain. Tobacco craving may last an extended period of time after the withdrawal symptoms have subsided.

Treatment

Evidence suggests that many smokers successfully quit as a result of the suggestion and support of a health care professional. Their success is increased by the availability of self-help materials that give information about the symptoms of withdrawal and steps to take to deal with them effectively. It is a worthwhile task of a medical assistant to be sure the office has these materials and to offer them to patients who are identified smokers. These can be obtained from the American Lung Association, the American Cancer Society, and other such organizations.

Counseling and behavioral therapy programs exist to help people stop smoking. The statistics on the success rates of these are inconclusive, which means they have not proven to be either effective or ineffective.

Pharmacologic interventions are proving to be very effective. Nicotine gum and skin patches reduce the severity of withdrawal and eliminate the inhalation of the other toxins found in cigarettes while the smoker learns to change behaviors and habits that go along with lighting up. With time, the amount of gum or the dosage of the patch is decreased until they have tapered off of nicotine entirely.

Zyban (bupropion) is a medication that is prescribed as an effective aid to smoking cessation. It had twice the success rate as the nicotine patch in a study directly comparing the two methods. Originally prescribed as an antidepressant, it has been found to decrease the cravings for cigarettes and to actually make the experience of smoking unpleasant. Pamelor and Aventyl (nortriptylene) also appears to be a successful new therapy in the treatment of nicotine addiction and withdrawal.

Nonsmoking Tobacco

In an attempt to escape the harmful effects of smoking, many people, primarily young males, are using snuff or a chewing tobacco. They think they are avoiding the dangers, but they have only traded for different ones. This form of tobacco is very addictive and therefore results in ever-increasing usage to get the same effects. Blood pressure rises and heart rate increases. The material is placed between the cheek and gums and causes very unpleasant saliva production as well as damage to the teeth, gums, and mouth leading to stained teeth, bad breath, loss of taste, and oral and throat cancer.

MARIJUANA

The most commonly used illegal drug in the United States is marijuana. Marijuana comes from the hemp plant *Cannabis sativa*. The leaves, flowers, and stems are dried, crushed, and smoked in pipes or cigarettes (often called joints). Sometimes it is cooked into foods or brewed as a tea. When the resin is extracted from the plant and concentrated, it becomes hashish or the liquid form, hash oil.

The main psychoactive chemical in marijuana is THC (delta-9-tetrahydrocannabinol). When marijuana is smoked, THC passes from the lungs into the bloodstream and on to various organs of the body, including the brain. Certain brain cells have receptors that bind to THC, which causes the drug's effect or high. Symptoms of marijuana intoxication are increased physical sensation, time distortion, dry mouth and thirst, relaxation, increased visual stimulation, short-term memory loss, increased heart rate, **euphoria**, and loss of coordination. Effects of repeated, long-term abuse are problems with memory and learning and difficulty thinking and problem solving. One study showed that the risk of heart attack is significantly increased during the first hour after smoking marijuana due to its effect on blood pressure and heart rate.

Regular marijuana smokers have more frequent respiratory illnesses and chest infections, as well as a daily cough and phlegm production and obstructed airways. The risk of cancer of the lungs, head, and neck is increased in frequent users. Studies have also shown that THC damages immune cells in the body, making it more difficult for the user to fight off infections and disease.

There is an increase in depression, anxiety, and personality disturbance associated with the use of marijuana. Because of its effects on the brain, which result in memory and learning problems, marijuana smoking is hazardous for teenagers and students. Users receive lower grades and are less likely to graduate than students who do not use marijuana. Memory can be affected for up to 4 weeks after last using THC but does appear to return to normal if the person remains abstinent from the drug.

Marijuana and Pregnancy

Infants born of mothers who used marijuana while pregnant can have problems affecting their nervous system. Some of these symptoms are a high-pitched cry, increased **tremulousness** (shaking or trembling), and an abnormal response to visual stimulation. Older children of women who used marijuana show behavior, language, and attention disorders and poor decision making skills. The risk of birth defects greatly increases when marijuana is used in combination with alcohol during pregnancy.

Withdrawal

Users can become addicted or dependent on marijuana. They continue to use the drug despite of the major problems it causes in their social, family, school, or work situations. This usage, along with cravings for the drug throughout the day, are indications of drug dependence. Symptoms of withdrawal are irritability; restlessness; insomnia; decreased appetite; weight loss; tremors; anxiety; and increased **aggression**, or hostile behavior.

Treatment

Individual counseling and group therapy have been successful in treating marijuana dependence. Learning about the damaging effects of the drug, along with developing skills to get through the day without using, aid the person in their recovery. Residential or day treatment centers are also options for the person seeking treatment. Marijuana Anonymous groups are common in most communities and operate along the same principles as AA. No medications are presently marketed specifically for the treatment of marijuana dependency. Researchers are working on a drug that would block the effects of THC, which could be useful in preventing **relapse**, or return to abuse of the drug.

Medical Marijuana

THC is effective for the treatment of the nausea and vomiting caused by chemotherapy. Marinol (Dronabinol) is a prescribed THC medication that reduces these symptoms and often helps to stimulate the appetite of cancer and AIDS patients. Other medical uses may be developed in the treatment of glaucoma, head injuries, strokes, and Alzheimer's and Parkinson's diseases. THC also has been studied as effective for pain control.

Currently, some physicians in various locations throughout the United States have begun prescribing marijuana for relief of pain, nausea, weight loss, and other symptoms of AIDS and terminal cancer. Athough marijuana is not legalized, there are special arrangements made in certain communities to decriminalize its use by these patients under medical supervision.

STIMULANTS

Caffeine

The most commonly used stimulant is caffeine and is found in coffee, tea, and sodas or soft drinks. Caffeine is absorbed quickly into the bloodstream after ingestion and stimulates the central nervous system. The effects of caffeine are a feeling of alertness, nervousness, diuresis (sweating), increased heart rate, rambling thoughts, muscle twitches, insomnia, and tremors. These symptoms are uncommon among casual one- or two-cup-a-day coffee drinkers.

Caffeine is not considered addictive, but people can develop a physical tolerance or dependence on the drug. Many users experience headache and digestive problems when withdrawing from caffeine.

Cocaine

Cocaine is a fine powder that is derived from the leaves of the coca plant found in Peru, Columbia, and Bolivia. It is a short-acting central nervous system stimulant. It is the opinion of several experts in the field of drug abuse that cocaine is the most addicting of all **illicit**, or illegal, drugs.

When the powder is snorted (inhaled through the nostrils), it passes through the nasal epithelium into the bloodstream and to the brain within 3 minutes. When injected into a vein, the most common and effective route, the cocaine reaches the brain within 15 seconds. The effects of cocaine, or "coke," are euphoria, endless energy, and a sense of well-being and confidence. The drug also decreases tension, fatigue, and appetite. The high lasts from 15 minutes to 1 hour. There are numerous unpleasant physical effects as well. Increased and irregular heart rate; high blood pressure; headaches; abdominal pain and nausea; and increased risk of stroke, seizures, heart attack, and death are a few of the hazards of cocaine abuse.

Chronic users are often malnourished because of the loss of appetite. Those who snort the drug risk the loss of the sense of smell, nosebleeds, problems with swallowing, hoarseness, and a constant runny nose. Injection drug abusers face many other health risks, which will be addressed later in this unit.

Over time, continuous use of cocaine results in personality changes. The abuser becomes short-tempered and suspicious. They lose the ability to enjoy simple things that formerly brought them pleasure. They have difficulty concentrating and have an almost constant craving for the drug. Frequent high doses of cocaine can cause a psychotic state where the user experiences extreme paranoia and auditory and visual hallucinations. This severe disturbance can last from days to months.

Cocaine combined with alcohol produces a third chemical in the liver. This substance intensifies the effects of cocaine and increases the risk of sudden death.

Cocaine and Pregnancy Because the blood vessels are constricted, blood flow is decreased to the fetus when the mother uses cocaine. The decrease in oxygen is believed to be one of the reasons for the increased risk of abruptio placentae, or the premature separation of the placenta from the uterus; premature birth; and sometimes death of the fetus. Infants born to women who abuse cocaine during pregnancy are smaller, are often premature, have decreased head size, have difficulty sleeping and eating, and have central nervous system irritability including tremors. Children whose mothers used cocaine while pregnant have learning and behavioral problems and a higher incidence of hyperactivity disorders.

Withdrawal   As the drug wears off, the euphoria is followed by a deep depression called a "crash." Often the user is very emotional, sometimes crying uncontrollably for no apparent reason. They are often very tired and sleep for hours or even days after having used for a length of time. At the same time, they experience strong cravings for more cocaine, even though they know they are unhealthy or have other factors that indicate a need to stop using.

Treatment   Presently, research at the National Institute on Drug Abuse is focusing on trying to develop a drug that would block or reduce the effect of cocaine. They are also seeking a medication that would reduce or eliminate the strong craving for the drug that dependant patients experience. These would be a helpful addition to a treatment program. Some physicians prescribe an antidepressant for patients in treatment for cocaine dependence, to combat the long-term severe depression. This enables the patient to cope more effectively with other aspects of recovery. Counseling and residential or outpatient treatment are also of major importance for the support and skills needed to remain abstinent. There are also Cocaine Anonymous meetings in most locations.

Crack

Crack is cocaine that has been mixed with baking soda and water and heated. When it cools, the hardened substance is cracked into little pieces, which are then smoked. The high is intense and fast. The crash is dramatic, which intensifies the craving for more. This is the most addictive form of cocaine. In addition to all of the effects of cocaine, there are physical effects of the toxic chemical being smoked. These symptoms are wheezing, shortness of breath, black phlegm, coughing blood, parched throat and lips, and singed eyebrows and lashes.

Recovery from crack addiction is very difficult. Statistics in one study showed that 90% of people who had sought treatment for crack dependence had returned to using within 1 year.

Amphetamines

Amphetamines are potent stimulants with effects similar to cocaine, although longer lasting and less euphoric. The most common route of administration is pill form. It is also snorted, injected, and smoked.

A person on amphetamines can be irritable, talkative, elated, paranoid, aggressive, energetic, or disoriented and have increased sexual desire and decreased appetite. Physical symptoms are increased heart rate and blood pressure, dilated pupils, perspiration or chills, nausea, vomiting, diarrhea, and headache. Amphetamines may remain in the system for 7 to 34 hours. Repeated use causes cravings for increasingly higher doses. The crash is similar to that of cocaine, including the depression, which can last for several weeks. Users are at higher risk of suicide during this time.

Students trying to stay awake to study, truck drivers on long trips, and young women trying to lose weight make up the highest number of abusers of amphetamines. There are legitimate medical uses, most commonly in the treatment of attention-deficit hyperactivity disorder (ADHD). Ritalin, Adderall, and Concerta are in this category of medications.

Methamphetamine

Methamphetamine is a white, odorless, bitter-tasting powder. The chemical make-up is similar to amphetamine, but it has a more potent effect on the central nervous system. It is a powerfully addictive drug that is being abused by a rapidly increasing number of Americans. It is produced in private homes and secret locations referred to as "meth labs" using over-the-counter ingredients. The gases and leftover substances from the manufacture of methamphetamines are toxic and combustible, causing another whole area of health and safety concerns. Legislation is being passed in many states to control the sale of cold medications containing ingredients used in the making of this drug.

Methamphetamine can be smoked, snorted, taken orally, or injected. Users describe a "flash" immediately after injecting or smoking. This is an extremely pleasurable sensation that lasts only a few minutes. It takes 3 to 5 minutes to feel the effects of snorting, which produces a less intense euphoria. As with all stimulants, the user feels alert, wakeful, and energetic and has decreased appetite. With repeated use, dependence develops. The users increase the amount taken, use more often, and change to a different way of taking it to produce faster results. Often people binge on this drug, which is called a "run." They use large amounts frequently over several days until they are unable to continue. At this point they collapse from exhaustion and lack of nutrition.

Methamphetamine causes irreparable cell damage in the part of the brain that responds to pleasure. Chronic abuse can lead to a psychotic state, as described with cocaine abuse. Users can exhibit out-of-control rages and extremely violent behavior. The drug also causes body temperature to increase to dangerous levels, resulting in convulsions and life-threatening situations.

Yet another health hazard of methamphetamine is the increased sexual activity that occurs among many abusers. Because of heightened desire and sensation, increased impulsiveness, and decreased rational thought, users sometimes have unprotected sex with multiple partners during a run. This puts them at high risk for HIV and hepatitis A and B.

When methamphetamine use is stopped, the withdrawal symptoms are anxiety, fatigue, paranoia, aggression, and long-term depression. An intense craving for the drug persists, which increases the likelihood of relapse.

Methamphetamine and Pregnancy

Research shows an increase in premature births and other prenatal complications when methamphetamines are used during pregnancy. Babies show abnormal reflexes and are extremely irritable and difficult to comfort. Some birth defects have been linked to use during pregnancy.

OPIATES

Opiates are drugs that are made from the opium poppy plant and include morphine, codeine, and heroin. The term opioid includes opiates and **synthetic**, or man-made, drugs that are similar to morphine in their effects or chemical make-up. Demerol, Dilaudid, and Methadone fall into this category.

People have been using opiates for 6,000 years for the treatment of pain, cough, nervousness, diarrhea, and depression. One hundred years ago there was no regulation of opiates, so they were used in a variety of potions and tonics available to anyone. This lead to a huge number of people becoming addicted because they did not know what was in the medicines they were buying. In 1906, the U.S. government became concerned about the increasing rate of addiction and began passing laws to limit the availability of opiates.

Opioids are powerful pain relievers. They actually reduce the response to pain, so that the patient realizes the pain is still present but it does not bother them or cause them to suffer with it. Morphine is widely used in hospitals after surgeries and injuries. When opioids are used for pain, there is decreased risk of addiction. However, when a patient continues to use the prescription pain medicine after the need for pain relief is gone, addiction can occur. There is an ever-increasing number of patients who "doctor shop," or go from one office to another with complaints of pain in order to collect prescriptions for opioids. It is important to coordinate care by requesting records from previous doctors and pharmacies to prevent participation in a patient's drug-seeking behavior. In 2001, over 2 million Americans were abusing prescription pain medicine. This is the fastest growing population of opiate dependants.

Opioids can be taken orally, smoked, snorted, or injected. They enter the bloodstream quickly and have an effect on the central nervous system and the brain. Symptoms include a decrease in pulse, respirations, temperature, and reflexes. Users have constricted pupils; slow, slurred speech; poor memory; and inability to pay attention. They appear sleepy or "nod off" easily. New users often experience nausea and vomiting. An overdose can cause coma or death due to decreased respiration.

Heroin

Heroin is the most widely abused drug of the illicit opiates. Heroin is usually a white or brown powder or a thick, dark, sticky substance called black **tar**. Usually it is smoked or injected. The effects of heroin are euphoria, a warm flushing of the skin, dry mouth, drowsiness, and a heavy feeling of the arms and legs lasting up to 2 to 3 hours. Tolerance to the drug occurs over a short period of time, so the user needs to use more in order to feel the effects. Users report that they rarely get the same good feeling that they got the first time they used but they feel compelled to keep trying. When the dose wears off, the user has nausea, stomach and muscle cramps, runny nose, restlessness, and diarrhea. The user needs more heroin to get the desired high and uses more often to keep from feeling "dope sick." Addiction occurs very quickly.

Heroin itself does not damage any organs of the body. The lifestyle of the heroin addict is the cause of the health problems seen in this population. Impurities are mixed with street drugs and can be extremely toxic. The user spends time using and seeking the drug and does not attend to other needs of daily life. They do not eat, do not brush their teeth, and do not take care of daily hygiene. Heroin users become malnourished, have dental problems, and encounter the hazards of injection drug use. In addition, legal, emotional, financial, and spiritual problems multiply when individuals become consumed by their addiction.

Heroin and Pregnancy

The most harmful aspect of heroin abuse during pregnancy is the repeated withdrawal from the drug. Every time the drug wears off, the fetus goes into withdrawal along with the mother. During the first trimester of pregnancy, miscarriage is often the result. During the last trimester, the mother often goes into premature labor as a result of heroin withdrawal. In addition, the drug-chasing lifestyle does not include proper prenatal care or nutrition. Women who become involved in prostitution to earn money to buy their drugs expose themselves and their unborn babies to risks of sexually transmitted infections, including HIV and hepatitis C. Babies born to heroin-addicted women are often low birth weight with a small head circumference. Some studies are showing that babies who underwent repeated withdrawal while in the uterus are difficult to stabilize at birth. Of course the risks of injection drug use are many and are especially dangerous to a developing fetus. Table 20-6 shows the effects of different drugs on prenatal development. Alcohol is clearly the most destructive.

Withdrawal   Some symptoms of withdrawal start within a few hours after the last dose wears off. The symptoms are described as similar to a bad case of the flu, with aching, runny nose, stomach cramps, nausea, and diarrhea. The symptoms build up over 48 to 72 hours after the last dose and become severely uncomfortable but rarely life-threatening. One symptom is a jerking spasm in the legs that led to the term "kicking" the drug. The term "cold turkey" comes from the description of goose bumps and chills during withdrawal.

Treatment   Clonidine is sometimes prescribed for relief of withdrawal symptoms. Clonidine reduces some of the nervous system discomfort and anxiety and lowers the blood pressure. Often, doctors prescribe an antianxiety medication like Ativan or Valium along with an antidiarrheal. The major physical symptoms are relieved within 5 to 14 days, but the craving persists. Acupuncture has been proven to help alleviate both withdrawal symptoms and cravings.

Recovery   Self-help groups such as Narcotics Anonymous and Heroin Anonymous, residential and day treatment centers, and counseling have aided thou-

sands of heroin addicts in becoming abstinent. However, because of the area of the brain affected by opiates, many people find it impossible to stop using. The craving is too intense for them to be able to overcome it and feel normal without the drug.

Methadone has been used since the late 1960s to treat heroin addiction. It is a synthetic opiate that stops the craving, eliminates withdrawal symptoms, and allows the patient to maintain a more normal lifestyle. Methadone, when dosed correctly, does not cause the patient to feel high and blocks the effects of heroin if the patient uses. Methadone is dispensed in liquid or tablet form and is prescribed in clinics that are regulated by state and federal laws; it cannot be prescribed for addiction by private physicians. Patients need to be in early withdrawal when they first enter methadone maintenance programs. They are prescribed a daily dose that is adjusted individually to a point where the patient is comfortable and does not feel the urge to use. Patients are monitored by urine drug screens to test for illicit drug use and receive counseling and support from the program staff. Figure 20-10 is an example of an evaluation sheet used by a drug treatment clinic to determine the severity of a patient's withdrawal.

Although a percentage of patients do continue to use drugs while in these programs, they still maintain a healthier way of life than when they were using daily. The concept of reducing harmful behaviors instead of enforcing abstinence is referred to as harm reduction. Many patients stay on methadone for the rest of their lives. Others decide to repair the problems that have been created due to their drug use while they stabilize on methadone. Many go back to school, find jobs, im-

TABLE 20-6   Comparison of the Effects of Drugs on Prenatal Development

Effect	Alcohol	Marijuana	Cocaine	Heroin	Tobacco
Low birth weight	X		X	X	X
Impaired growth	X				
Facial malformation	X				
Small head size	X			X	
Intellectual and development delays	X	X			
Hyperactivity, inattention	X	X		X	X
Sleeping problems	X	X	X	X	
Poor feeding	X		X		
Excessive crying	X	X	X	X	
Higher risk of SIDS				X	X
Organ damage, birth defects	X				
Respiratory problems	X			X	X

Source: U.S. Department of Health and Human Services

Clinical Opiate Withdrawal Scale

For each item, circle the number that best describes the patient's signs or symptoms.
Rate on just the apparent relationship to opiate withdrawal. For example, if heart rate is increased because
the patient was jogging just prior to assessment, the increased pulse rate would not add to the score.

Patient's Name: _____   Date and Time   /   /   :

Reason for this assessment: _____

Resting Pulse Rate: _____ beats/minute
Measured after patient is sitting or lying for one minute
- 0 pulse rate 80 or below
- 1 pulse rate 81-100
- 2 pulse rate 101-120
- 4 pulse rate greater than 120

Sweating: *Over past 1/2 hour not accounted for by room temperature or patient activity*
- 0 no report of chills or flushing
- 1 subjective report of chills or flushing
- 2 flushed or observable moistness on face
- 3 beads of sweat on brow or face
- 4 sweat streaming off face

Restlessness: *Observation during assessment*
- 0 able to sit still
- 1 reports difficulty sitting still, but is able to do so
- 3 frequent shifting or extraneous movements of legs/arms
- 5 Unable to sit still for more than a few seconds

Pupil size
- 0 pupils pinned or normal size for room light
- 1 pupils possibly larger than normal for room light
- 2 pupils moderately dilated
- 5 pupils so dilated that only the rim of the iris is visible

Bone or Joint aches *If patient was having pain previously, only the additional component attributed to opiates withdrawal is scored*
- 0 not present
- 1 mild diffuse discomfort
- 2 patient reports severe diffuse aching of joints/ muscles
- 4 patient is rubbing joints or muscles and is unable to sit still because of discomfort

Runny nose or tearing *Not accounted for by cold symptoms or allergies*
- 0 not present
- 1 nasal stuffiness or unusually moist eyes
- 2 nose running or tearing
- 4 nose constantly running or tears streaming down cheeks

GI Upset: *Over last 1/2 hour*
- 0 no GI symptoms
- 1 stomach cramps
- 2 nausea or loose stool
- 3 vomiting or diarrhea
- 5 Multiple episodes of diarrhea or vomiting

Tremor *Observation of outstretched hands*
- 0 No tremor
- 1 tremor can be felt, but not observed
- 2 slight tremor observable
- 4 gross tremor or muscle twitching

Yawning *Observation during assessment*
- 0 no yawning
- 1 yawning once or twice during assessment
- 2 yawning three or more times during assessment
- 4 yawning several times/minute

Anxiety or Irritability
- 0 none
- 1 patient reports increasing irritability or anxiousness
- 2 patient obviously irritable or anxious
- 4 patient so irritable or anxious that participation in the assessment is difficult

Gooseflesh skin
- 0 skin is smooth
- 3 piloerection of skin can be felt or hairs standing up on arms
- 5 prominent piloerection

Total Score _____
The total score is the sum of all 11 items

_____

Initials of person
completing Assessment: _____

_____

Score:

5-12 = *mild*

13-24 = *moderate*

25-36 = *moderately severe*

more than 36 = *severe withdrawal*

FIGURE 20-10 Scale used to score the severity of withdrawal symptoms

prove their relationships, find a spiritual community, and seek medical and dental care over a period of time. Then, when things are more manageable, they slowly taper their dose down and eventually stop taking methadone. This is a very successful plan for many patients.

Methadone is the treatment of choice for pregnant, opioid-dependent women. Because the women receive a steady, measured dose of medication, it reduces the ups and downs of drug use. Also, it introduces the women to a safe, medical environment where they can access prenatal care and other services for a healthier pregnancy and outcome.

A baby born to a woman who has been on methadone during her pregnancy is dependent on methadone. The infant must be monitored for signs and symptoms of withdrawal. This is usually done in the neonatal intensive care unit at the hospital using the Finnegan scale. The baby is commonly treated with morphine drops, which are adjusted according to symptoms. The baby is stabilized and then slowly weaned off of the morphine. The parents are taught how to recognize symptoms of withdrawal or sedation and to medicate the baby accordingly. In some cases, Phenobarbital is also needed for the baby's comfort. The need for medication varies greatly and does not seem to be associated with the mother's dose of methadone during pregnancy. Some infants don't need any medication, and some babies are very difficult to stabilize and comfort.

The newest treatment for opiate addiction is Buprenorphine. This medication is prescribed in tablets that are taken sublingually and dissolve in about 10 minutes. Buprenorphine has a greater ability to block the effects of other opiates and eliminate the cravings. Physicians who have been trained and received special certification can prescribe this medication from their offices. This allows more convenient and confidential treatment. OBAT (office-based opiate therapy) is a fast-growing field in the treatment of addiction.

Patients usually reveal their addiction to the staff or physician during a visit. Often these are patients who are addicted to prescription pain medicines, but some are also heroin or methadone dependant. They are evaluated, and the doctor determines whether they are appropriate for Buprenorphine. If they are motivated to stop abusing their drug of choice, they are given an appointment to come in for **induction**, or to begin Buprenorphine treatment. The patient must be in full withdrawal in order to take their first dose. The first dose is administered, and the patient remains in the office for observation. If relief is not achieved in a specified amount of time, a second dose is administered. The patient is given instruction and education about the medication and returns daily for the first several days to stabilize the dose and deal with any side effects or questions. It is recommended that the patient receive counseling and routine urine drug screens to support her recovery. The safety of Buprenorphine during pregnancy is being studied.

INJECTION DRUG USE

A patient who always presents to the office in long sleeves, long pants, and even high-necked shirts is suspicious for injection drug use (IDU). When a person has been shooting drugs into their veins (IV), into the muscle (muscling), or under the skin (skin-popping), they develop scarring; discoloration; and hard, tough patches of skin. Often a medical assistant or nurse will be the first to note this when they attempt to give an injection or draw blood for lab work. Sometimes it is almost impossible to find a vein due to scarring or because the veins are collapsed, and the patient will offer advice on where there is one that might work.

Patients also develop abcesses at the injection sites. These are caused by impurities in the drugs and by using dirty needles. Some abcesses can be treated with warm compresses and sterile dressings. Some need to be opened and drained, while others require antibiotics. Left untreated, they sometimes develop into cellulitis, which can require hospitalization. The additives and particles that do not dissolve in the injected solution can clog blood vessels that lead to the heart, lungs, liver, kidneys, and brain. This can lead to internal infections and necrosis, or death of the cells in these organs.

HIV/AIDS continues to infect and kill thousands of people worldwide daily. It is transmitted through unprotected homosexual and heterosexual intercourse and injection drug use. When people are taught to use new needles or to clean their needles with bleach and only use their own, the risk of transmitting disease is reduced drastically. Some communities, in an effort at harm reduction, offer new syringes to users in exchange for their used ones. Studies show a decrease in the spread of diseases in these locations.

More than two thirds of new cases of hepatitis C each year are from injection drug use. Hepatitis C is the most common blood-borne infection in the United States. It enters the liver and progresses slowly over a period of 10 to 30 years. Patients experience extreme tiredness, weakness, loss of appetite, and jaundice. Some people with chronic hepatitis C develop liver failure due to cirrhosis. Many people are never significantly affected by the disease as long as they abstain from alcohol and any other liver toxins. There are drugs available that are effective in the treatment of hepatitis C. They are usually administered over a 6- or 12-month period and have side effects similar to those of chemotherapy. There is currently no vaccine against hepatitis C.

Reports of pneumonia and tuberculosis are higher in drug abusers. In opiate users this is because of the depressed respiratory system. Damaged tissues in the airways of smokers of various drugs cause them to be more prone to airborne infections. Also, both groups generally suffer from overall poor health along with a high incidence of tobacco abuse. Endocarditis, an infection of the lining of the heart, is another infection reported among injection drug users.

HALLUCINOGENS, DISSOCIATIVE DRUGS, AND CLUB DRUGS

LSD

Lysergic acid diethylamide (LSD), also known as acid, is the strongest mood- and perception-altering drug known. It is a chemical compound made from a rye fungus. A dose as small as 30 mcg can cause effects that last 12 or more hours. It is usually taken orally in pill form or small pieces of paper that have been soaked in the drug (called "blotter acid").

Physical effects are increased blood pressure and heart rate, dizziness, loss of appetite, dry mouth, sweating, nausea, numbness, and tremors. The major effects are on the emotions and senses. The user's emotions may range from extreme joy to terror in a matter of minutes. Some people report feeling multiple emotions at the same time. Colors, sounds, smells, and other sensations are intensified. Users experience hallucinations in which items, people, and even their own bodies change shape. Time moves at a different pace. LSD is unpredictable and can cause enjoyable or nightmare-like episodes. Sometimes a feeling of loss of control or insanity can occur with an increase in anxiety and despair.

Tolerance develops with repeated, frequent use, and the user needs larger doses to achieve the desired effect. There are no physical withdrawal symptoms. There are reports of severe depression and mood swings following the use of LSD. Some users experience a psychosis in which they are unable to recognize reality and communicate normally for an extended period of time after the drug has worn off. This mental state has been known to last for years in some users. Other hallucinogens are mescaline, psilocybin, and ibogaine.

PCP and Ketamine

PCP and Ketamine are known as dissociative anesthetics because they cause the user to feel disconnected with his environment and experience insensitivity to pain. PCP was developed as a veterinary anesthetic. It was never approved for use on humans because of the extreme agitation it caused during clinical studies. It is snorted, smoked, or taken in pill form. Physical effects are shallow, rapid breathing and increased blood pressure, heart rate, and body temperature. High doses cause a dangerous rise in these functions along with nausea, slurred or garbled speech, blurred vision, dizziness, and decreased awareness of pain. Muscle contractions cause uncontrolled and uncoordinated movements. Users display unpredictable and often violent behavior on PCP. High doses put users at risk for convulsions, coma, hyperthermia, and suicide. Repeated use can lead to addiction. Memory loss, depression, and psychotic episodes are reported to follow the use of PCP and can last for up to a year.

Ketamine is also classified as a dissociative anesthetic and is used in veterinary as well as human surgical procedures. It is snorted or taken orally as a tablet or an odorless, tasteless liquid. It is similar to PCP but has a more rapid onset, is less potent, and is shorter acting. It causes a feeling of floating or being separated from the body. Alternately, some users report feeling terrified and fearing that they were going to die while on Ketamine. Judgment and coordination are affected while on the drug and for up to 2 days after use. Memory problems and psychotic symptoms can last up to 3 days following one dose.

Amnesia, or loss of memory, is also an effect of Ketamine. Because of this, it has been used on unsuspecting victims by sexual predators. The drug is added to a beverage that is drunk by the unsuspecting victim, and the victim is then sexually assaulted while under the influence of the drug. This is referred to as a "date rape" drug.

Ecstasy

Ecstasy, also known as MDMA, is a combination stimulant and hallucinogen. It causes distorted time perception and increased sensory stimulation, combined with an increase in energy similar to amphetamines. Ecstasy is popular in clubs and at raves, or all-night dance parties. When taken orally it becomes effective within an hour and lasts from 3 to 6 hours. The drug is also snorted, which causes a more rapid onset of effect.

Symptoms of MDMA intoxication are increased heart rate and blood pressure. The drug affects temperature regulation and causes a severe rise in body temperature. Because it is used at parties where people are dancing for hours at a time, the increase in physical activity combined with the rise in body temperature leads to severe dehydration. Hyperthermia and occasionally heart and kidney failure can result. Use of Ecstasy damages brain cells and affects the chemical balance, causing mood swings and depression following use.

DEPRESSANTS

Depressants are drugs that relieve anxiety, cause relaxation or sleep, and generally cause the patient to calm down. **Barbiturates** and benzodiazepines fall into this category of medications.

GHB

GHB was sold over the counter in the United States until 1992. It was popular with bodybuilders because it stimulates increased levels of growth hormone, which aids in fat reduction and muscle building. It is also a central nervous system depressant. At low doses, GHB relieves anxiety and causes relaxation. It is a colorless, tasteless, and odorless liquid. The effects are felt 10 to 20 minutes after it is taken and last up to 4 hours. Increased doses result in vomiting, a dreamlike state, decreased muscle tone, dizziness, decreased respirations, sleep, and tremors. An overdose can cause seizures, loss of consciousness, coma, and death. Tolerance and physical dependence can result from repeated use. Withdrawal symptoms include insomnia, muscle cramps, tremor, and anxiety.

Rohypnol

Rohypnol is a powerful benzodiazepine. This category of drug is used to treat anxiety, to relax muscles, and as a sedative-hypnotic. This drug is not prescribed in the United States but is used in other countries to treat seizure disorders. It is sold in tablet form and is colorless, odorless, and tasteless when mixed into a beverage. Rohypnol causes sedation and **amnesia**. Because of these effects, it is not widely abused intentionally. It is, however, classified with Ketamine and GHB as a "date rape" drug. These three drugs can each be dissolved in drinks without the victim realizing their presence. The effects leave the person without the ability to resist or to even understand what is happening to them. Victims are susceptible to emotional and psychological as well as physical harm as a result of sexual assault while under the influence of these drugs. They are also at higher risk of contracting sexually transmitted diseases, and female victims can unknowingly and unintentionally become pregnant. Women and men alike are cautioned to keep track of their drinks when they are out among people they do not know and trust and to not drink anything that has been left unattended.

Phenobarbital, pentobarbital, and Seconal are commonly prescribed barbiturates used in the treatment of insomnia or, in some cases, high blood pressure and epilepsy. They are also used to sedate patients before and during surgery. They are produced in capsule, injectable, and suppository form. They produce a feeling of euphoria, relief from anxiety, and drowsiness. A person who is intoxicated from barbiturates acts very much the same as someone intoxicated from alcohol. They exhibit slurred speech, unsteady gait, mood swings, and impaired attention and memory. Alcohol increases the effects of these drugs and can lead to an overdose and death.

Dependence develops with continued use of barbiturates. Withdrawal symptoms can begin within 24 hours of discontinuing use. Symptoms of withdrawal are restlessness; elevated blood pressure and heart rate; irritability; anxiety and sleeplessness; and tremors of the hands, tongue, and eyelids. Severe withdrawal can follow long-term dependence and can be life threatening.

Benzodiazepines were developed in the 1950s to treat anxiety without the dangerous effects on the central nervous system caused by barbiturates. Ativan, Valium, Librium, and Xanax are commonly prescribed benzodiazepines. They are administered in tablet, liquid, and injectable forms. These drugs reduce anxiety and relax muscles and produce a feeling of well-being. However, when the effects of the drug wear off, users often feel increased anxiety. It is not uncommon for people who have a legitimate disorder requiring this drug to begin overusing it and to become dependent. Benzodiazepines are often used by people involved in abusing other substances because they help reduce the effects of withdrawal from the other drugs.

Symptoms of withdrawal from benzodiazepines are much the same as those from alcohol and barbiturates. Users should discontinue these drugs slowly over a period of time with medical supervision. Withdrawal symptoms can occur between 24 and 72 hours after discontinuing the drug. Convulsions and extremely high blood pressure can result and become a medical emergency.

PATIENT CARE

When working with patients who are chemically dependent, it is important to remember that they are suffering from a disease. They are, most likely, in need of medical attention for a variety of problems. Like any other patients, they deserve to be treated with respect and dignity. These patients often enter a medical office with fear of being judged and looked down upon. Compassionate care by the medical assistant, who is often the first person a patient encounters, can make a significant difference in the life of a person in need.

ACHIEVE UNIT OBJECTIVES

- Complete the Workbook activities to meet the learning objectives.
- Apply your knowledge at the end of this chapter in completing the Critical Thinking Challenge and Activities, as well as the StudyWARE on your Student CD-ROM.

UNIT 3
RELATED THERAPIES

OBJECTIVES

Upon completion of this unit, you will be able to achieve the following:

LEARNING Objectives

1. **Spell and define, using the glossary at the back of the text, all the Words to Know in this unit.**

2. **Differentiate between complementary and alternative therapies.**

3. **Explain the placebo effect.**

4. **List six guidelines to use when considering a related therapy.**

5. **List the four requirements for FDA (the Food and Drug Administration) approval.**

6. **Describe what is required for a therapy to be accepted as effective.**

7. **Briefly describe the related therapies discussed.**

WORDS TO KNOW

acupuncture	herbal	placebo
alternative	homeopathy	reflexology
aromatherapy	humor	shiatsu
ayurvedic	hypnosis	therapeutic
biofeedback	massage	visualization
complementary	naturopathy	yoga
faith		

 CERTIFICATION CONNECTION

CMA
Resource information and community services
Providing instruction for health maintenance and disease prevention
Identifying community resources

CMAS
Patient information and community resources

RMA
Therapeutic modalities, alternative therapies

ALTERNATIVES TO THE TRADITIONAL MEDICAL MODEL

A great deal of interest has arisen lately in methods of health care other than the traditional medical model with which we are familiar. Some of this interest comes from dissatisfaction with current, at times impersonal, care and the lack of "face time" with physicians. The impact of the HMO and the limiting coverage from insurance companies for certain procedures has also caused concern. Another factor may be expectations for "cures." When conventional medicine fails to improve or correct our problems, we are willing to resort to other possibilities, no matter how unconventional or expensive. We have heard about celebrities who are choosing **alternative** methods to treat their serious illnesses and people who travel to other countries to obtain treatment and medications that are not approved in the United States. Many of these people will testify to the effectiveness of their nonconventional treatment.

Interest in related therapies may also come from learning about health care methods from other cultures. The United States is a true "melting pot" of people from around the world. We live together and learn about the cultures of our neighbors and friends. We see and hear about the different approaches to disease and disorders used in their cultures. We see on television and read in our newspapers about the effectiveness of treatments not offered by conventional medicine. And of course, we are constantly bombarded with the documented "healed" testimonies from gravely ill people in sensational advertisements in magazines, "junk" mail, and gossip news.

Some authorities make a distinction between the various types of related therapies. One type is called **complementary** therapies. These are treatments that are considered to supplement or add to the conventional form of medicine. Some examples are the use of **massage**, acupressure, **acupuncture**, and **hypnosis**. Another type of therapy is called alternative. This is interpreted by some as meaning a method that is used instead of conventional medicine, such as the use of laetrile, shark cartilage, and other products made from various animal parts. Often alternative therapies are not validated by research, and no scientific evidence exists that they are or can be **therapeutic**. Some people have claimed cures from these and other remedies, but without scientific study, the **placebo** effect or spontaneous healing can not be ruled out. (A placebo effect refers to the fact that some people respond favorably to a known ineffective treatment because they believe it is working. This occurs in about 30% to 40% of patients.) In this unit, the word "related" will also be used to mean any treatment, either complementary or alternative, because the therapies may not be "labeled" by their practitioners, and to our knowledge, no authority has developed a classification standard.

The National Center for Complementary and Alternative Medicine defines these therapies as "medical practices that are not commonly used, accepted, or available in conventional medicine." In the booklet *Alternative Medicine* by Harvard Medical School, another definition states "those interventions not taught widely in U.S. medical schools nor generally available in U.S. hospitals." Currently, an effort is being made by medical science to become more knowledgeable of therapies from other cultures and those of previous generations in this country. They are trying to distinguish which ones are safe and effective, which are effective but may carry health risks, which are ineffective, and which ones are both ineffective and unsafe. Some medical schools are introducing courses on alternative therapies to provide physicians with a knowledge of nonconventional choices for their own evaluation and to be able to provide care and advice to patients who may select adjunct (added to) treatments.

INCREASED POPULARITY OF RELATED MEDICAL THERAPIES

There has been a dramatic increase in the use of alternatives to traditional medicine. Researchers from Harvard Medical School discovered that 42% of adults in the United States (82 million people) routinely use complementary medical therapies for treating common medical situations. It was estimated that Americans made 629 million office visits and spent an estimated 27 billion of their own dollars on complementary care. It was also documented that most of these therapies are used in addition to, not as a replacement for, their conventional medical care. In another study, it was determined that 60% of the related therapy users discuss their use with their medical doctor, which was a favorable and positive finding.

When selecting a related therapy, it is a good idea to use some guidelines. There are so many **herbal** therapies, healing techniques, and therapeutic approaches that it is difficult to know which ones might provide some benefit and which are a waste of money and time or even a risk to one's health. It is essential that the traditional medical provider be informed of a patient's related therapy treatments, especially when there are major health problems involved. Many herbal formulas contain compounds that react with prescription medications. In addition, products classified as "dietary supplements" are not under regulatory guidelines, so action or side effects have not been scientifically established. A good example is the interaction with the common herb St. John's Wort. It affects the action of drugs such as Coumadin (an anticlotting drug) and Crixivan (an AIDS drug). It can reduce the level of cyclosporine (an immunosuppressant) in the blood, which has caused organ rejection in several transplant patients. It also reduces the effectiveness of birth control pills. Other drug interactions are known to be potentially dangerous. Remember, there is no regulatory agency governing the purity, stated strength, or method of production of herbal compounds.

There are two prime questions that need to be considered when choosing a related therapy approach: "Is it safe?" and "Does it work?" Some safety factors to think through before trying a therapy are:

- Are there any published studies on the effectiveness of this treatment in reputable medical journals or publications from known medical institutions or organizations?
- Is the treatment a "secret" that only certain providers can offer?
- Is it necessary to travel to another country to take advantage of the treatment?
- Does the provider oppose the person continuing to see their conventional medical doctor? (This is a reason to be skeptical, because conventional medicine should not be abandoned while pursuing a complementary therapy.)

There are a growing number of studies on the effectiveness of related therapies. Information is available on the Internet, but reliable sources with evidence of careful analyses are difficult to find. The National Institute of Health and the National Library of Medicine have information available on their web sites but may be difficult to evaluate (see resources at the end of this chapter).

If someone is thinking about trying unorthodox or related therapy treatments that are untested, they need to think twice and follow some specific guidelines.

- *Read up*—Read labels, look for research information, and talk to a doctor and a pharmacist about the ingredients before taking the medication or treatment. Also, consider the cost, especially if there is no medical evidence that the treatment works. Realize that insurance probably will *not* cover the therapy.
- *Be skeptical*—If it sounds too good to be true, it probably is. The more spectacular the claim and the more it costs, the more one needs to be skeptical.
- *Tell your doctor*—Physicians have become more aware of other therapies because of the increase in their popularity. The doctor needs to know if a patient is visiting a related therapist or taking any herbal remedy to watch for possible signs of drug interactions or adverse effects from the treatment.
- *Combine related and conventional therapies carefully*—Related therapies can be beneficial in some situations. For example, the American Cancer Society reports that options such as aromatherapy, medita-

tion, massage, and biofeedback appear to help patients deal with pain and improve their quality of life. However, there are no proven related cures for cancer, and conventional treatment offers the best option and must be continued.

● *Choose a professional who has appropriate training and credentials*—Some of the major related therapy providers are licensed or at least credentialed by their respective professions. This does not guarantee that the treatment will be effective, however; it just means that the person is trained in that specialty.

● *Put safety first*—A label that reads "all natural" or "organic" does not necessarily mean it is safe, because there is probably no regulation controlling the product. The same is true for some treatments. For example, body manipulations may be helpful for one person's condition but very harmful for an other. Read about and understand the therapy. Discuss the option with the physician for medical insight before beginning treatment.

FOODS

There are volumes written about the claims of certain foods. There is a strong body of evidence showing that *fruits and vegetables* promote good general health. Some foods may even protect against heart disease and certain cancers. Eating a diet with 9 servings of fruits and vegetables a day lowers the risk of ischemic stroke by 31%. Folates in the diet reduce homocysteine in the blood—a substance that is linked to the risk of heart disease, stroke, and Alzheimer's. Fruits and vegetables also reduce obesity because they contain fewer calories and are filled with fiber to help people feel full. The most benefit comes from eating a variety of fruits and vegetables so that you consume a greater number of vitamins and minerals and benefit from the interaction between the nutrients. A general rule is the brighter the color, the greater the amount of protective phytochemicals (compounds that are known to be beneficial). Strawberries, blueberries, spinach, and kale are very colorful and have high antioxidant activity. Spinach, for example, not only has a lot of folate but also contains vitamin C, which helps the body to absorb the iron in the spinach. This natural combination of elements is much more beneficial than taking isolated nutrients in supplements.

The benefit from *whole grains* is well documented in its ability to lower the risk for heart disease, adult-onset diabetes, hypertension, and some types of cancer. Whole grains contain complex carbohydrates, minerals, and antioxidants. There is also growing evidence that drinking *tea* may lower the rate of heart disease and cancer. This is based upon three areas of research. Tea has an antioxidant property that my help prevent the artery damage that can lead to heart attacks. Sec-

ond, studies show tea drinkers have lower cholesterol levels, which also lowers heart disease risk. Third, when comparing sets of tea drinkers to nondrinkers, the drinkers have lower rates of heart attack. Tea has also been associated with lowering the risk of developing cancer. Green tea may help protect against breast, colon, rectal, lung, and pancreatic cancer; however, there are contradicting studies showing increased rates in other cancers. Apparently, only regular tea is beneficial, because herbal, instant iced tea mixes, or bottled teas contain undetectable levels of healthful substances.

Ginger is a food substance that can settle the stomach in certain instances. It has been studied for use in motion sickness, chemotherapy nausea, postsurgical nausea, and morning sickness with mixed results. The research did show taking a 1-gram dose 30 minutes before travel could be recommended. *Garlic* is another food item that has been promoted as healthful. It does seem to have some ability to lower cholesterol and blood pressure, thereby preventing heart disease. It has been used for centuries to treat many conditions from tuberculosis to hemorrhoids and to ward off vampires. Laboratory studies have suggested that garlic might help fight cancer, but *human studies* have not determined it lowers cancer risk. However, dietary histories of 564 Chinese people with stomach cancer were compared with 1,131 individuals without the disease. It was concluded the risk of developing stomach cancer was 60% lower among people who ate the most alliums (garlic, onions, leeks, and shallots), which seems to infer some protective benefit. Its cousin, the onion, was used for a poultice (a hot mashed mass inside a cloth) to treat chest congestion in the past.

Walnuts and other nuts in general have been identified as being able to reduce the risk of heart disease. Even though they are loaded with calories and fat, researchers believe that because they are rich in monounsaturated and polyunsaturated fats, they lower the LDL and raise the HDL cholesterol levels. However, this is possible only when these types of fat *replace* the saturated fats in meats and dairy products.

Our ancestors have used many other food-type substances over the years. Native Americans used many wild berries, roots, and other things growing in their environment to make medicinal products. Early pioneers dug sassafras and ginseng root and used many herbs and compounds to treat their families. People still use these roots today. A hundred years ago, women used a product called Lydia E. Pinkham's Vegetable Compound to ease "all those painful complaints and weaknesses so common to our best female population." One component of the product that did some of the "easing" was alcohol, which of course "ladies" did not consume in its other form. Its main ingredient was a woodland plant called black cohosh, which is still used today. Many of these former compounds have been studied and have been determined to contain beneficial properties.

Some other food items have been promoted as medicinal. Perhaps the most famous is Laetrile (the chemical compound anygdalin), a product of the kernels of fruit pits from peaches, almonds, and apricots. It is an alternative therapy for the treatment of cancer that was used in Russia in the 1840s and in the United States in the 1920s. The theory behind its effectiveness is that the bacteria in the intestinal tract react to the compound and produce cyanide, which in turn increases the acid content of tumors, which then destroys lysosomes and kills the cancer cells. Scientific clinical trials were conducted that proved the treatment was not effective. Because of this finding and the fact that some patients even developed cyanide poisoning, the drug was banned from the United States. It is still available in some foreign countries, including Mexico, where U.S. citizens who think it might provide them a cure most often obtain the drug.

Interesting information regarding many unusual treatments can be found on the Internet, but care must be taken to evaluate the content. You can read about the benefits of blue-green algae and vitamins you have never heard of, like B_{15}. Two reliable sites operated by the National Cancer Institute of the National Institutes of Health (NIH) are in the resource information at the end of this chapter.

HERBAL PRODUCTS AND DIETARY SUPPLEMENTS

There has been a 380% increase in the use of herbal products since 1990, with an estimated 17% of people using herbal medicines regularly. In the past few years, the dietary supplement business has skyrocketed into a $12-billion industry in the United States alone. In 1999, Congress appropriated funds for the Office of Dietary Supplements as part of the NIH to investigate the safety and effectiveness of herbal medicines. Scientific study is underway, and some results are beginning to be published. The most important thing to understand about dietary supplements is that there is a big difference in these products and conventional over-the-counter (OTC) drugs, even though they may be displayed on the same shelves in drug and grocery stores. The Food and Drug Administration (FDA) closely regulates OTC drugs but has virtually no responsibility over supplements. The FDA requires that OTC drugs be tested for stated effectiveness and that they meet standards for purity of their contents. With supplements you do not know for sure what you are buying. Substances passing OTC regulations require clinical trials, designated dosage establishment, documentation of side effects, and characteristics of people who

had adverse reactions. Manufacturers are also required to show the product is at least as good as any previously approved product for the same purpose. These reports are published in scientific journals for professional and public review. This whole process requires about 15 years from lab to consumer and costs about $500 million per item. It is no wonder that the manufacturers of supplements fight being brought under FDA control. At present, they have an exempt FDA status category of "dietary supplements" established by Congress in 1994. Untested products can be sold as supplements and direct claims as to the effectiveness or health benefit cannot be made; however, indirect claims are allowed and have been stretched to the limit. Labels on dietary supplements should contain a list of ingredients and their strength, a suggested dosage, and any warning to its use. There should also be the standard statement, "These statements have not been evaluated by the Food and Drug Administration. This product is not intended to diagnose, treat, cure or prevent any disease." A few of the most common products that may have some benefit are:

St. John's wort—Is widely used for herbal treatment for depression. A clinical trial in 1996 showed it worked as well as older antidepressant drugs for mild to moderate depression with few side effects. No standards for dosage, its preparation, or its long-term safety have been developed. Even though classified as a supplement, it has druglike actions.

Black cohosh—Is a large woodland plant found in eastern North America that is used for menopause relief as an alternative to traditional hormone therapy. It is effective in controlling hot flashes, night sweats, headaches, heart palpitations, and mood changes. Its effect seems to suggest that it contains a natural estrogen-like substance and the known salicylates found in aspirin. There are no recognized major studies on the compound, and there is a lack of scientific trials common to all supplements. It appears the side effects are mild when taken in moderate amounts, but it can include vomiting, dizziness, and headaches in larger doses. Because it is not standardized, each manufacturer indicates the dosage. It is recommended that black cohosh should not be taken for more than 6 months, because no long-term studies have be done on its safety.

Melatonin—Is a hormone produced naturally in the pineal gland within the brain. It plays a part in regulating sleep patterns. As a supplement, it is used to regulate sleep and prevent jet lag. It has also been promoted as an anti-aging agent. Evidence does seem to support its effect on sleep, and laboratory studies indicate it has antioxidant properties at much larger concentrations than in the body. No evidence exists that it slows the aging process or reduces the risk of developing cancer. A potential risk from melatonin is the resulting drowsiness that impairs function and may cause morning-after headaches. It has also been reported to interfere with conception.

Willow bark—Has been used to relieve pain for more than 2,400 years. Hippocrates prescribed chewing on willow leaves to relieve childbirth pain. In the second century, it was used to reduce fever and inflammation. In 1897, a Bayer chemist determined that acetylsalicylic acid (aspirin) could be extracted from a willow-bark-related compound. Now, willow bark is being sold as a natural pain relief medication. Double-blind trials of 210 people with chronic low back pain determined willow bark extract to be a useful and safe treatment, at least for low back pain. Again, remember, it is not controlled or standardized. The recommended maximum daily dose is 240 mg, but it should not be used by people who have problems tolerating aspirin.

Echinacea—Is an herb reported to stimulate the immune system to help prevent developing a cold or the flu. It has been used for centuries by Native Americans to treat everything from coughs to burns and snakebites. Trials have reported milder symptoms and fewer sick days among echinacea users, but the studies were not totally scientific. It is difficult to recommend the product, because it grows in three forms, each with a different concentration of ingredients. It also depends upon which part of the plant is used: the leaf, roots, or flowers. Analysis in 1999 of a dozen brands found great variety in concentrations. It is apparently more effective in liquid than tablet or capsule form. Potential side effects include severe allergic reactions, which indicates all people with asthma or allergic rhinitis should avoid usage. Echinacea can also be toxic to the liver if taken longer than 8 weeks; therefore anyone using other drugs known to affect the liver are at potential risk.

Saw palmetto—Is a plant that produces berries containing phytosterol compounds that scientists think might slow down the production of male testosterone, which stimulates prostate growth. The compound is used to treat symptoms of benign prostate hypertrophy. Several traditional medications are available but are sometimes not effective and may cause a decline in sexual desire or erectile dysfunction. Little research has been done in the United States, but European investigation suggests it is safe and effective for the symptoms but can upset the gastrointestinal system and cause nausea in some. It is again noted that, without regulation, there is no guarantee of the purity or content of the product.

Glucosamine—Is a substance promoted as a product to relieve the pain of osteoarthritis. It reportedly promotes healthy cartilage formation to maintain or replace that which is worn away by age and use. European studies did confirm that it provides pain relief and increases mobility. It is widely used in the United States. No side effects have been noted.

Ginseng—Is the root of a Chinese shrub and has been studied primarily in Asia. Varieties of ginseng come from other places, such as Siberia, Japan, and even the United States. Scientific investigation has failed to support its claims as an aphrodisiac. There is evidence it improves circulation and elevates mood.

Gingko biloba—Is a product from the leaves of the ginkgo tree and is promoted as an agent to improve memory and mental function by increasing blood flow to the brain. European studies suggest that it may slow the progress of or even prevent Alzheimer's disease. It also appears to be an antioxidant and might help prevent atherosclerotic plaque. Side effects of nausea, vomiting, and diarrhea occur at extremely high doses.

This discussion of common herbs and supplements only scratches the surface of products that are available in grocery and health food stores. Remember, there is no industry control, so you are never sure of what you purchase. If the word "standardized" is used on the label, it is probably what it says it is. The use of supplements requires reading and careful consideration. Look for quality of evidence in reports, how many people are using the product, and their experiences. Discuss it with a physician; many are now familiar with supplements and can provide advice. Choose a brand tested in published studies if possible. For a database of medical literature, refer to the National Library of Medicine through a library, or find abstracts on their web site listed at the end of this chapter. Learn as much as you can to make the wisest selection.

RELATED THERAPIES

The following is a brief look at several therapies that promote some form of medical intervention or treatment. If you find it interesting, there are many resources on alternative and complementary therapies for additional study.

Acupuncture

Acupuncture is a form of traditional Chinese medicine that is also practiced by the Japanese, Koreans, and the French. It consists of using extremely thin, sterilized needles, sometimes electrified with low-voltage, that are inserted on points along the network of 12 body meridians (channels) to connect the different levels from the organs to the skin. It is used as an anesthetic or to treat pain. Chinese medicine addresses the whole person when diagnosing or treating an illness. They have a fundamental philosophical idea of Qi (pronounced Chee); they believe the presence of this vital energy flows through the body and divides the living from the dead. Maintaining Qi is essential for good health. Illness results from disturbances in the flow of Qi, either too much or too little through the meridians. Qi is actually the balance of two opposing energies, yin and yang. Yin organs are those which are solid, such as the heart, spleen, lungs, kidney, and liver. There is an interacting corresponding hollow yang organ. These are the small intestine (heart), stomach (spleen), large intestine (lungs), bladder (kidney), and gallbladder (liver). (The organs do not necessarily correspond to Western anatomical organs. The spleen, for example, includes the entire digestive tract, while the heart is where one's conscious is, not the brain.) When yin and yang are in harmony, they work to achieve and maintain health. Acupuncture acts on Qi flowing through the meridians to help the body redirect the energy.

Acupuncture has a long history, but studies have not validated its effects. Western hypothesis is that acupuncture triggers the release of pain-killing molecules in the brain and central nervous system to provide relief from pain. Care needs to be taken in selecting a practitioner. Licensing requirements vary from state to state, and some have no requirements. A safe alternative is to find one who is certified from the National Certification Commission for Acupuncture and Oriental Medicine.

Aromatherapy

Aromatherapy is a treatment that uses essential oils extracted from plants for a therapeutic effect. Different oils are used for specific conditions, such as lavender for first aid of burns, neroli for anxiety, and tea tree for antibacterial and antifungal action. Use of oils goes back thousands of years. In 4500 BC, a Chinese emperor recorded therapeutic properties of plants that match those assigned properties today. Some of the oils have an estrogen-like effect; others are sedative or anti-infectious. There are a wide variety of chemical properties in the oils and their associated function. The issue of safety with using the oils has been discussed, but no definitive answers have been established. The quality and chemical content of the product changes because of conditions during growth, such as weather and altitude. Maintaining their composition is important. They must be stored in amber glass bottles to provide protection from light. Bottles must be sealed tightly and stored away from heat. They can be diffused through the air, inhaled, or absorbed through the skin with massage. Oils can also be used as a compress, in wound care, or as a mouth-rinse.

There is therapeutic value in using oils for stress and anxiety; insomnia and restlessness; common colds and flu; muscular and neuralgic pain; arthritis; headaches and migraines; and digestive disorders and constipation. Many oils are sold in department, beauty, and drug stores that are supposed to affect your mood, but these are not the same as the medicinal therapeutic oils use by practitioners.

Ayurvedic Medicine

Ayurvedic medicine is the traditional healing system of India and is perhaps the oldest formal medical system in the world. It addresses mental and spiritual well-being and physical health. Treatment is tailored to the individual's need with a strong emphasis on preventive self-care. Ayurveda identifies three types of energies that are present in all things: vata, pitta, and kapha. Vata energy is associated with movement. Pitta relates to metabolism and those types that tend to be intense, quick to anger, and have a medium build. Kapha is linked to structure and the types that are slow moving, calm, and have a larger body frame. Each person has a unique combination but is dominant in one. The practitioner tries to assess the proportion of the energies and customize a health program to bring them into a health balance.

Sickness results from the energies being out of balance. The practitioner asks questions to determine the diet, sleep, and elimination habits; emotional temperament; and personal and family history. He takes a pulse in both wrists and examines the tongue, eyes, and general appearance. He listens to the heart, lungs, and even the tone of the voice. Based on his opinion, he outlines a program of diet, herbal formulas, yoga postures, aerobic exercise, breathing techniques, meditation, and a variety of massages. In some cases, when cleansing is needed, he will order steam baths, laxatives, and herbal enemas and even induce vomiting. Practitioners are difficult to find in the United States, but Indian communities, restaurants, and grocery stores might know of someone. There is an Ayurvedic Institute in Albuquerque, New Mexico, that might know whether there is a graduate in your area. They can be contacted at 505-291-9698. Herbal preparations from India are not recommended because of the lack of sanitary conditions in production.

Biofeedback

Biofeedback is a method that enables a person, usually with the help of electronic equipment, to learn to control otherwise involuntary bodily functions. It is also defined as any technique that increases the ability of a person to voluntarily control physiological activities by being provided with information about those activities.

An example of this is learning to control heart rate by seeing or hearing its activity. The yogis of India have been reported to slow their heartbeat, increase their body temperature, and survive with little oxygen to influence bodily functions. Some methods of feedback involve skin response monitors to register autonomic tension or relaxation and skin temperature. Other monitors can indicate muscle activity or register brain waves. Therapeutic uses can be helpful with asthma, cardiovascular disorders, headaches, insomnia, controlling stress, and neuromuscular problems. Biofeedback has also been helpful in treating incontinence, migraines, and irritable bowel syndrome. Remarkable results have been attained with the electroencephalogram (EEG) application. Persons with learning difficulties, addiction, attention deficit, hyperactivity, and identity syndrome have reported benefits. The technique has been taught to persons with brainstem stroke or motor neuron disease who are totally paralyzed. By learning to control brain wave patterns, they can activate an alphabet board to communicate. It is believed this technique may some day be used to operate machines and vehicles.

Faith

One of the fastest-growing areas of study in medical schools is the healing power of prayer. Seventy-nine of the nation's 125 medical schools offer courses on prayer and spirituality; there were only three 10 years ago. There have been studies conducted that showed positive results with patients who have chest pains, heart attack, and AIDS. One study gave emergency room heart patients the opportunity to receive prayer. Those who agreed were divided into prayed-for and not-prayed-for groups. The names of the prayer group were sent to prayer gatherings around the world in every major religion. The prayed-for group experienced half as many and some times no side effects or complications from catheterization and angioplasty as did the other group. It was felt that prayer has a positive effect on recovery. Some skeptics believed it was a placebo effect, so the researcher repeated the study, except this time they used mice and test tube microbes. It also showed the same type of outcome: the prayed-for mice made uneventful recovery, and the microbes flourished. A study of cardiac patients in 1995 reported those who lacked social support were much more likely to die within 6 months after cardiac surgery. Another group of older patients who had open heart surgery and who had no social support or received no comfort from religion were three times more likely to die within 6 months of surgery than those who received such support. Studies show that you don't have to believe in God or another higher being to benefit from intercessionary prayer. The empathy, love, and compassion of the prayer influence the effectiveness of prayer. If you think it is a sham, it will not work. Even though some physicians and health care providers do not accept the power of **faith** and prayer, many do recognize something or someone else was responsible for a patient's unexpected recovery.

Homeopathy

Homeopathy is a 200-year-old system of medicine based on the Law of Similars. This means that if a dose of a substance can cause a symptom, that same substance in minuscule amounts can cure the symptom. It is a highly controversial form of medicine and lacks any scientific explanation as to why it might work. Homeopathic medicines are produced from various natural sources, such as plants, metals, minerals, venoms and stings, and bacteria or human tissue. The materials are diluted many times in a base of water and alcohol. With each dilution, it is shaken vigorously, which practitioners believe gives the final product its power to heal. Sometimes, they are diluted to the point that no molecules of the ingredient remain. Practitioners contend that molecules leave a "memory" in the solution, to which the body responds. Because the medicines are so dilute, it may take weeks before any therapeutic effect is seen. Critics believe any response is a placebo effect. Studies have shown insufficient evidence to arrive at any conclusion as to its effectiveness on any clinical condition. Homeopathic medicines are classified and regulated by the FDA as OTC drugs. Holistic healers, such as naturopaths, herbalists, chiropractors, acupuncturists, midwives, and even some medical doctors, also use the drugs. Because they are so dilute, they cause few safety concerns. But patients should be cautioned to not rely on homeopathy or substitute it for conventional medicine, especially if they have a potentially life-threatening condition. Also, beware of the practitioner who says conventional medications will interfere with the homeopathic treatment and want them to be discontinued. Some also discourage immunization of children, which can be dangerous to the child and the community.

Humor

Humorous intervention by the health care professional or patient is used to produce a beneficial response. The physical response to **humor** and laughter affects most of the major systems of the body, increasing heart rate and blood pressure and improving muscle tone. In addition, following the viewing of a humorous video, IgA concentration in the blood and spontaneous lymphocyte multiplication increased, while adrenalin and cortisol secretion decreased. Clinical significance of this reaction is unclear, but research has shown that humor can play a part in reducing anxiety. There is some evidence to indicate that humor can be used by patients to cope with cancer. One patient discovered that watching Candid Camera films would give him 10 minutes of "belly laughs" and resulted in 2 hours of painfree sleep. Dr. Hunter "Patch" Adams is one of this country's leading proponents of humor in medicine, as portrayed in the movie bearing his name. There are Laugh Mobiles and Humor Carts used in clinical settings to lift patient's spirits. They may contain Play Doh, finger paint, water guns, coloring books, bubbles, humorous books, funny costumes, and video and audio tapes.

The patient must be assessed to determine if humor is appropriate. The criteria are:

- Timing—The patient might not think it is appropriate at present.
- Receptiveness—What might be funny one time may not be at another.
- Content—Be sure the content is not offensive in any way.
- Patient's beliefs—Determine whether the patient feels humor has a place in patient care.
- Relationship with patient—If a "joking relationship" has been established, it may be appropriate; if not, it may not be.

More research is needed to understand the role of humor in recovery or coping with illness. It is known that laughter increases NK cell activity, lymphocyte proliferation, monocyte migration, and the production of IL-2 and IgA, which are positive effects in the immune system.

Hypnosis and Self-Hypnosis

Hypnosis can be a very beneficial therapy to improve health and well-being. Most of us think of it as some theatrical trick that causes people to do funny things, but it can be a powerful therapeutic tool. It is effective against skin conditions, insomnia, stage fright, shyness, a habit such as smoking, weight gain, and pain, and it promotes rapid surgical recovery. It is something that a person can learn to do. The ability to achieve a "trance state" is inborn in about 90% of all people. Psychologist Dr. Fisher defines a trance as "a state of heightened attention in which your concentration is so focused that you are completely unaware of what's going on around you." In this state, both mind and body are very receptive to suggestions, and the right suggestions can change the way we act. He says it is possible to induce this state of trance yourself with self-hypnosis, so that you can give yourself specific instructions to make any changes you want. There are two essential steps to self-hypnosis:

1. Learn how to induce a trance whenever you want.
2. Use mental imagery to talk to your body and mind.

Dr. Fisher describes the steps to take to enter a trance and claims it should take less than a minute to achieve. A highly hypnotized person may feel totally detached, whereas a lesser state may only produce deep relaxation and alertness. The depth of the trance doesn't matter as much as the motivation to achieve the changes desired. He describes the steps to a trance as follows:

Step 1.   Sit or lie down with your head in a relaxed position. Focus your gaze upward as if you are trying to see your eyebrows. Close your eyes. Continue looking upward. Take a deep breath, and hold it for a count of three.

Step 2.   Exhale. Relax your eyes. Envision yourself gently floating downward, as if entering a safe and comfortable place.

Step 3.   When you are ready to come out of the trance, count backward slowly from three to one. Look upward. Open your eyes and slowly bring the world back into focus.

Dr. Fisher goes on to say that it is important to make your hypnotic suggestions concrete and very specific and express them to yourself in mental imagery. You need to see and feel yourself being the way you would like. The suggestions must be repeated 8 to 10 times each day for 90 seconds at a time. As an example, you want to lose weight, but you eat without really savoring the food or sensing when you are full. While in the trance, visualize yourself on a "TV screen" as you now appear. On an adjacent "screen," picture how you want to look after reaching your target weight. Twist the imaginary knob to turn the image on the first screen into the image on the second. (This will help keep you motivated.) Now, picture yourself eating slowly and consciously enjoying every bite. Picture pausing after each bite and asking yourself if you want more.

Obviously, this "treatment" will need to continue until you reach your goal. The format can be transferred to address other changes that are desired. Remember, hypnotherapy works only if the client wants it to.

Hypnotherapy provided by a therapist is actually supported by more scientific research than many other complementary therapies. Trance induction can be achieved by different techniques and may be adapted to the client. Often, the client is asked to focus on a point or concentrate on his breathing until his eyelids become heavy and he closes them and relaxes. The client controls the depth of his trance by his state of relaxation. In the trance, the therapist uses guided imagery to direct the client to address his concerns. The state is ended slowly by allowing the client to control the speed of return by counting from three to one or by the therapist slowly counting.

Clinically, hypnotherapy has been used in childbirth; to provide acute or chronic pain relief; for stress management; to control certain phobias; for postamputation phantom limb pain, nausea, and hypertension; and in irritable bowel syndrome. It has even proved useful as a "numbing agent" in simple injuries that required suturing. Some physicians have incorporated hypnosis as a supplemental therapy in their practice. As with any therapy, it is important to choose a qualified professional practitioner. Hypnosis is not a substitute for treating a psychological condition, such as depression or a psychosis.

Magnet Therapy

Americans spend $500 million a year on magnetic devices to relieve headache, arthritis, tendonitis, foot pain, and other ailments. A neurologist, Dr. Michael Weintraub, recently completed a large study on the effectiveness of magnets. For 30 years, he had participated in many scientific studies using medications for treating headache and spinal pain. Relief was often inadequate, and side effects were common. He became interested in nondrug therapies like acupuncture and massage. He later was introduced to the use of magnets by one of his patients who had a cervical herniated disk. His recommendation of steroids helped until the patient returned to work, which worsened the pain. After consulting a neurosurgeon, the patient began using magnets instead of opting for surgery and had become pain-free. Dr. Weintraub's skepticism prompted him to investigate the use of magnets as a therapeutic device. He studied patients with unmanageable peripheral neuropathy common to patients with diabetes, with alcoholism, or receiving chemotherapy.

- His first small study used magnets in the shoes of 14 people and resulted in a 64% reduction in symptoms, a much higher rate than with conventional therapy.
- A second study used a real magnet in one shoe and a worthless device in the other. The results showed a 90% improvement in the magnetic-treated foot after 4 months of therapy.
- A recent study followed NIH protocol and involved 375 patients in 27 states, with 95% having moderate to severe neuropathy pain. With 98% of the data in, results indicate a significant improvement in pain, numbness, and tingling.
- A small study was also conducted on 15 patients with carpal tunnel syndrome, with a finding of 50% reduction in pain, numbness, and tingling. He also has had success in treating patients with arthritis and heel spurs.

It is theorized that magnets interrupt the action of small nerve fibers that cause pain and numbness and improve oxygen flow into the tissue. Further research is needed to explain why they work, but evidence shows they do in many instances.

Massage

Therapeutic massage is the second most popular related therapy in the United States. It encompasses a wide range of approaches using hands to manipulate muscles and soft tissue. It is a powerful means to treat stress-related conditions, such as insomnia, headaches, and irritable bowel syndrome, and health conditions such as sciatica and depression. There are different types of massage:

- *Swedish* is the most common type of Western massage, using kneading and long strokes to reduce pain, relieve insomnia, reduce stress, and promote relaxation.
- *Sports* massage is a vigorous, deep-tissue manipulation to promote greater flexibility, loosen muscles, relieve muscle swelling, and treat injuries to tendons and ligaments.
- *Trigger-point* massage applies concentrated pressure to "trigger points," the areas of irritability in a muscle that are palpable as lumps or knots and may be painful or cause referred pain. This therapy attempts to apply enough pressure to release the chronic contraction of the muscle and stretch the surrounding muscles to prevent recurrence.
- **Shiatsu** massage comes from Japan and makes use of firm finger pressure applied to specific points on the body to balance the flow of chi (vital energy). The massage is done on the lightly clothed patient who lies on a pad on the floor. It has been used to treat low back pain, constipation, and nervous disorders.
- *Thai* massage is also performed through light clothing and on a floor pad. It combines stretches with hand pressure in a meditative, dancelike movement.

There are many other variations of massage. One that is strictly therapeutic is manual lymph drainage massage. This is particularly beneficial for correcting lymph fluid buildup in the arm following mastectomy and lymph node removal. This and some other forms are considered to be medically related and are being used with terminally ill and cancer patients. Insurance companies may cover them, especially if ordered by the physician.

It is recommended that care be taking in selecting a therapist. They are licensed in 25 states. Credentials from a training program accredited by the Commission on Massage Training Accreditation and a certificate from the National Certification Board of Therapeutic Massage and Bodywork are signs of the highest credential in the field.

Other Therapies

If this view into related therapies has been of interest to you, you may want to explore some others.

Hand **reflexology**—This practice claims there is a map on the hands that matches a corresponding body part. Stimulating these points on the hand sends impulses to help the muscles in the corresponding body part relax and blood vessels open to increase circulation, therefore allowing more oxygen and nutrients to enter and promote healing.

Naturopathy—This is a multidisciplinary approach to health care based on the belief that the body has power to heal itself. Treatment is based on assessment of the correct diet, rest, relaxation, exercise, fresh air, clean water, and sunlight the patient is receiving. Herbal products, detoxification procedures, massage, hydrotherapy, counseling, and advice on lifestyle may be used. They may also use homeopathy and acupuncture.

Tai chi—This is a Chinese movement discipline that improves strength, flexibility, and sense of balance. It can help reduce frailty and falls in elderly patients. It involves a series of fluid movements performed while relaxed but maintaining focus on a pattern of movements. Proper breathing with the exercises helps to integrate the body and mind and enhance the flow of qi and overall health.

Visualization *and guided imagery*—Visualization refers to what you see in your mind's eye, whereas imagery involves all the senses. It can be effective in controlling heart rate, blood pressure, breathing, blood levels of stress hormones, and many other areas. It is a good adjunct therapy for cancer, heart disease, and chronic pain. There is good evidence that it reduces nausea with chemotherapy, reduces postoperative pain, shortens hospital stays, and reduces anxiety. The therapy works when patients visualize some activity affecting their problem. An example might be a patient with cancer visualizing immune cells attacking the malignant cells and destroying them. The more senses that are used, the more "real" it will seem to the brain. Scientists believe that the brain activity may influence the autonomic nervous system that controls important bodily processes.

Yoga—This is a discipline of breath control, meditation, and stretching and strengthening exercises that is thought to promote mental, physical, and spiritual well-being. It has been practiced for thousands of years. There are many types of yoga, such as bhaktri, jnana, karma, laya, raja, and hatha yoga. It places great emphasis on mental and physical fitness. It increases strength; balance; flexibility; and, some claim, energy and calmness. It consists of breathing exercises, assuming a number of positions, and meditation.

This introduction to the use of specific foods, herbs, supplements, and complementary and alternative therapies may give you a basic understanding of the vast amount of options that are available to patients who are searching for nontraditional methods of health care. Many have been proven to be beneficial when provided by a trained professional and are complementary to traditional medicine.

ACHIEVE UNIT OBJECTIVES

- Complete the Workbook activities to meet the learning objectives.
- Apply your knowledge at the end of this chapter in completing the Critical Thinking Challenge and Activities, as well as the StudyWARE on your Student CD-ROM.

CRITICAL THINKING CHALLENGE

IMPACTING THE PATIENT, THE PRACTICE, AND YOUR CAREER

Lisa, a 16-year-old girl, is in the office today because her mother wants Dr. Long to give her a check-up. Dr. Long and Lisa's family have been friends for several years. She said she is worried because Lisa seems to be having trouble at school. Her grades have gone down and she seems to be depressed. Lisa says she just can't remember everything because her classes are hard. She has also had two colds lately, which is unusual for Lisa. Her mother is also concerned because she seems to have stopped hanging around with her old friends. Carla, the medical assistant, began her in-person interview and took vital signs. Lisa's blood pressure and pulse were elevated, even though she had been sitting in the reception room for about 20 minutes. Carla also thought she could detect an odor around Lisa that might be from smoking. When she asked Lisa if she had just smoked before she came into the office, she at first denied it, but when Carla stated that she detected an odor, Lisa admitted she had. In fact, with further discussion and Carla's suspicion that she had really smoked marijuana, Lisa admitted she had been experimenting a few times, but she promised she wouldn't do it again. She begged Carla not to tell the doctor or say anything to her mother. She told Carla she would stop back in another month to see her privately and prove she wasn't using anymore. Carla wants to honor Lisa's request and maintain the patient's confidentiality, but she also knows she should inform the doctor.

QUESTIONS

1. How would Carla's reporting or not reporting impact the patient?
2. How could the practice be impacted?
3. How could Carla's career be affected?

ACTIVITIES

1. Go online at www.mypyramid.gov to obtain your personal food pyramid guide.
2. After obtaining your recommended daily calorie amount, plan a day's meals to include all the recommended nutrients and still stay within your limit. You can get calorie values from a good medical dictionary or nutrition text.
3. Go to www.health.gov/dietaryguidelines to read about how the government establishes its dietary recommendations. Find the 2005 Dietary Guidelines Advisory Committee Report, then click on D. Science Base. Section 10 lists the major conclusions from their research.

StudyWARE™ CHALLENGE

- Study with the flash cards for Chapter 20 to review the key terms in this chapter.
- Solve the crossword puzzle for Chapter 20.
- Complete the multiple choice quiz in test mode for Chapter 20.

RESOURCES

Alternative medicine: A selection of articles on complementary and integrative therapies (2001, March). Boston: Harvard Health Publications.

American Heart Association. An eating plan for healthy Americans [brochure]. Dallas: Author.

Are you obese? (1999, October 27). *Journal of the American Medical Association, 282*(16).

Can spirituality improve your health? (2001, July). *Bottom Line Health Poll*, p. 11.

Complementary medicine. (1996, January). *Harvard Women's Health Watch*, p. 3.

Diet, glycemic index, and the food pyramid. (2000, December). *Harvard Women's Health Watch*.

Hand reflexology. (2000, November). *Bottom Line Health*, p. 7.

Lindh, W.Q., Pooler, M.S., Tamparo, C.D., & Dahl, B.M. (2006). *Thomson Delmar Learning's comprehensive medical assisting: Administrative and clinical competencies* (3rd ed.). Clifton Park, NY: Thomson Delmar Learning.

Magnet therapy does work. (2001, September). *Bottom Line Health*, p. 3.

National Clearinghouse for Alcohol and Drug Information, P.O. Box 2345, Rockville, MD, 20847-2345.

NIDA National Institute on Drug Abuse, U.S. Department of Health and Human Services, National Institute of Health, P.O. Box 30652, Bethesda, MD, 20824-052.

Royal College of Nursing. (2001). *The nurses' handbook of complementary therapies* (2nd ed.). London: Harcourt Publishers Limited.

Tai chi: meditative movement for health. (2000, December). *Harvard Women's Health Watch,* p. 6.

Weil, A. (2001, September). Ayurvedic medicine: living in balance. *Dr. Andrew Weil's Self Healing,* pp. 2-3.

Weil, A. (1999, August). The healing power of massage. *Dr. Andrew Weil's Self Healing,* pp. 2-3.

Weil, A. (2001, March). Visualization and guided imagery explained. *Dr. Andrew Weil's Self Healing,* p. 2.

U.S. Department of Agriculture and Health and Human Services. (2005). *Dietary Guidelines for Americans.* Dietary Guidelines Advisory Committee Report. Retrieved January 15, 2006, from www.health.gov/dietaryguidelines.

U.S. Department of Agriculture, Center for Nutritional Policy and Promotion. Retrieved January 15, 2006, from www.mypyramid.gov.

WEB LINKS

www.acupuncturealliance.org (The Acupuncture and Oriental Medicine Alliance)
Provides general information on acupuncture and oriental medicine.

www.aaom.org (The American Association of Oriental Medicine)
A professional organization of practitioners of oriental medicine. Provides information, promotes professionalism and legislative activities, and works to protect access to herbs.

www.eatright.org (American Dietetic Association)
Provides information on nutritional health.

www.americanyogaassociation.org (American Yoga Association)
Provides general information about yoga and choosing a qualified teacher and information about the association's activities.

www.health.org (Department of Health and Human Services SAMHSA's National Clearinghouse for Alcohol and Drug Information)
Provides alcohol and drug facts.

www.health.gov/dietaryguidelines (Department of Health and Human Services' Office of Disease Prevention and Health Promotion)
Provides information from Dietary Guidelines Advisory Committee.

www.niam.com (National Institute of Ayurvedic Medicine)
The largest and most authentic resource of information on Ayurvedic medicine in the United States.

www.niddk.nih.gov (National Institute of Diabetes & Digestive & Kidney Diseases)
Provides information on weight control.

www.drugabuse.gov (National Institute on Drug Abuse)
Provides information on drug abuse.

www.nccam.nih.gov (National Institutes of Health—Center for Complementary and Alternative Medicine)
Provides information on various health topics, research, clinical trials, and training for complementary and alternative medicine.

www.nlm.nih.gov (National Library of Medicine)
Provides health information for the public, health care professional researchers, librarians, and publishers.

www.sram.org (The Scientific Review of Alternative Medicine)
A journal devoted exclusively to objectively analyzing claims of "alternative medicine."

www.mypyramid.gov (U.S. Department of Agriculture)
Provides dietary information and personal pyramid of requirements.

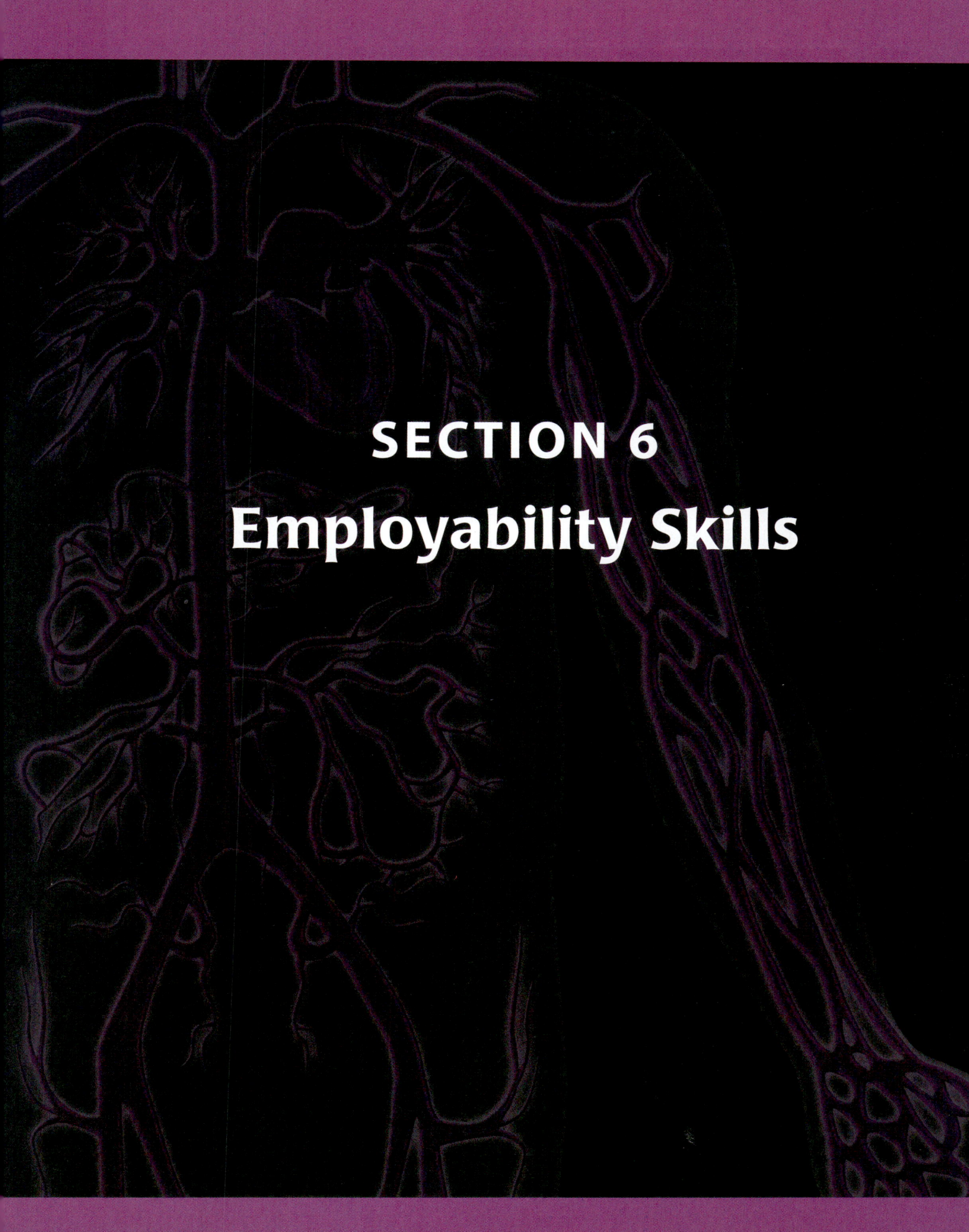

SECTION 6
Employability Skills

21

Explore, Enter, and Succeed in Employment

UNIT 1
Externship

UNIT 2
The Job Search

UNIT 3
Career Entry and Success

Medical assistant employment requires either administrative or clinical skills or a combination of both. Physicians in private practice usually have an average of three employees. In group practice, there may be from five to as many as forty or more, depending on the number of physicians and the size of the facility.

In seeking employment, you will be aware of the different opportunities and decide which area of medical assisting you would prefer. Many medical assistants prefer general or family practice because of its variety and challenge; others enjoy the specialty fields with their new developments and rapid change. There are many health care facilities whose job descriptions specify particular duties, such as medical secretary, clinical office assistant, transcriptionist, insurance clerk, or receptionist. The generally trained medical assistant should be able to perform in the dual role of administrative and clinical assistant and will therefore be a valuable asset to any medical practice.

Participating in an externship program, as discussed in Unit 1, will not only help you to become more competent in medical assisting skills, but also help you to decide which area of practice you enjoy the most. The externship also helps you to develop good work habits in preparation for full time employment.

Unit 2 will discuss the job search and application techniques you can use to obtain your desired position. Once employment is obtained, your success and satisfaction depends upon the effort you make to be a part of the team. In Unit 3 we discuss the significance of performance evaluation and continuing education as components of your advancement in your career.

UNIT 1
EXTERNSHIP

OBJECTIVES

Upon completion of this unit, you will be able to achieve the following:

LEARNING Objectives

1. Spell and define, using the glossary at the back of the text, all the Words to Know in this unit.

2. Explain the purpose of an externship experience.

3. Discuss the 11 criteria for an externship site.

4. List the five main areas that should be included an a externship agreement policy.

5. Explain how an externship differs from an employed position.

6. Discuss how externship experiences and hours can be validated.

7. List areas that might be included on an evaluation instrument.

8. Describe how student evaluation of classroom and externship experiences can be used by the school.

WORDS TO KNOW

accredited	of Allied	externship
Accrediting	Health	initiative
Bureau of	Education	interpersonal
Health	Programs	objective
Education	(CAAHEP)	obligation
Schools	competencies	on-site
(ABHES)	coordinator	performance
administrative	curriculum	objectives
clinical	evaluation	policy
Commission on	experience	supervisor
Accreditation		

DEFINING THE PURPOSE

Two professional accrediting organizations, the **Accrediting Bureau of Health Education Schools (ABHES)** and the **Commision on Accreditation of Allied Health Education Programs (CAAHEP)** have said that an **externship**

experience must be part of the school's curriculum for preparing students to practice as medical assistants if the school desires to be **accredited** by their organizations. An externship has been defined as "An integral part of the **curriculum** which must be scheduled prior to graduation." An externship is a period of time when a student is placed in an actual health care setting, under the supervision of a practicing health care provider, to apply the skills learned in the classroom. The **experience** is an important part of a student's total training and is to include an opportunity to perform various **clinical** and **administrative** procedures. The externship sites can be in a physician's offices (preferably family practice), internal medicine, OB/GYN, or general surgery, or at an accredited hospital or clinic. The guidelines also say that a student's externship performance should be evaluated, and the **evaluation** should be part of the student's record. A minimum of 160 hours is recommended for the externship.

EXTERNSHIP POLICY

The school will draft a statement of policy regarding the externship. The statement will indicate how the externship should be established. It will include such things as:

- Philosophy and goals of the externship experience
- The role of the school
- The role of the health facility
- The **on-site** supervisor's role
- The student's **obligation**

The externship must be understood to be a learning, not a working, experience. You are not to replace any employee or assume anyone's job responsibilities. There are to be no financial benefits paid. Many facilities cooperate with externship programs as a way to identify a future employee. If you do well in your externship, you may get the opportunity for full-time employment after completing your training program.

SELECTING EXTERNSHIP SITES

Someone from the school will be designated as the individual responsible for identifying externship sites, probably the curriculum director. The site must understand their role is to provide students with a supervised rotation through administrative and clinical duties. The on-site supervisor is to provide assistance and evaluate the student's performance. The school must keep records of each student's experience, including the site, the dates of externship, and the evaluations by the site.

It is very important to establish a good relationship with sites so that the facility is willing to continue to serve as an extension of the school's program. It requires a lot of time and often persuasion to establish a site. All parties involved—the school, the student, and the site personnel—must work together to maintain the relationship for future students. If expectations are clearly defined and provided in writing, many misunderstandings can be avoided. Some things to be defined are as follows:

- The site will provide an educational experience rather than a work experience.
- The site will provide a variety of direct experiences, not just repetitive routine duties.
- The site has a good reputation for ethical practice.
- The site must use up-to-date equipment and methods of practice.
- The philosophy, goals, and objectives of the externship are thoroughly explained to the facility.
- An on-site person must willingly agree to supervise the student.
- The on-site person accepts responsibility for ensuring that opportunities are provided for performance of a wide variety of tasks.
- The on-site person accepts the responsibility for documenting experiences and evaluating performance.
- The length of the externship and the approximate number of hours per day are defined.
- The role of the school coordinator is defined and observation of the student and consultation with the on-site supervisor must be ensured.
- A formal written contract or agreement should be signed.

EXTERNSHIP OBJECTIVES

In order for your externship experience to achieve its purpose, a list of **performance objectives** will be compiled by the school. These will be like the ones you have already accomplished in the classroom. You and your on-site **supervisor** must be aware of these goals, and both of you should work to achieve them. Probably the supervisor will be expected to observe your performance of each procedure and approve your competence before you are to perform without supervision. As the opportunity arises for you to perform a procedure, take the initiative to request the supervisor's observation so you can achieve another **objective**. At the same time, the supervisor should alert you to new opportunities as they arise. Soon you will have met many of your objectives and will be working on your own.

EXTERNSHIP AGREEMENTS

The school will probably draft an externship agreement that puts into writing many of the elements we have discussed. It makes it a matter of record that you are participating in an educational experience provided by a clinical facility. It is similar to a contract and may list

at least five main areas concerning the externship: the length of the externship, the obligations of all parties involved, the requirement of the education experience, the necessity for supervision, and the responsibility for evaluation. It might also establish a procedure for addressing any problems that might occur. The following is some specific information that might be included within those five areas:

1. School name, address, and phone number
2. Student's name (address and phone number optional)
3. Date the externship begins and ends
4. Number of hours per week the student is due at the site; may even specify specific time frames
5. Student's responsibility for personal appearance, conduct, punctual attendance, and adhering to facility's policies
6. The requirement of an on-site supervisor and his role
7. The school coordinator's role
8. The school's plan for the externship experience
9. Places for dates and signatures of the persons involved, such as:
    1. Facility's representative
    2. On-site supervisor
    3. Student
    4. School coordinator
    5. School representative
10. Procedure for addressing any problem that might arise during the externship

PLANNING FOR EXTERNSHIP EXPERIENCES

In order to ensure that an educational experience occurs, the school coordinator will develop a training plan. The plan specifies that the list of administrative, clinical, and general **competencies** should be experienced during the externship. The plan's record sheets should identify the competencies that have been taught and evaluated in the classroom and as well as indicate those that need to be experienced during the externship. The sheets can also serve as a format for documenting all competencies demonstrated during the externship that are observed by the on-site supervisor. This record will become an important document to verify competence in performance of various procedures when applying for employment. Figure 21-1 is an example of a partial list of competencies with checks to indicate those deemed competent during the school program. The form contains a column for the on-site supervisor to initial when the competency is observed and deemed competent during the externship. The goal of an ex-

SAMPLE EXTERNSHIP TRAINING RECORD

Student _____　　Facility _____

Coordinator _____　　Supervisor _____

Competency	In school	Externship	Date
Answer office phone	✓	LK	1/10
Receive phone messages	✓	LK	1/10
Obtain/record messages	✓		
Schedule appointments	✓		
Obtain patient information	✓		
Initiate charge slip	✓		
Calculate charge slip	✓		
Process payment	✓		
File alphabetically	✓		
File numerically	✓		
Pull numerical file	✓		
Operate transcriber	✓		
Prepare letter from machine	✓		
Make corrections	✓		
Compose correspondence	✓	LK	1/15
Total charges	✓		
Use copy machine	✓	LK	1/25
Operate office computer		LK	1/27
Prepare ledger card	✓	N/A	
Record charges	✓		
Collection letter	✓		
Write check	✓		
Deposit slip	✓		
Balance bank statement	✓		
ETC.			

Competency	In school	Externship	Date
Handwashing	✓		
Measure infant length	✓		
Weigh infant	✓		
Head circumference	✓		
Snellen chart	✓		
Ishihara method	✓		
Oral temperature	✓		
Rectal temperature	✓		
Axillary temperature	✓		
Electronic thermometer		LK	2/6
Radial pulse	✓	LK	2/6
Apical pulse	✓		
Respirations	✓	LK	2/6
Blood pressure	✓	LK	2/6
Irrigate eye	✓		
Irrigate ear	✓		
Horizontal recumbent	✓		
Prone position	✓		
Sims' position	✓		
Knee-chest position	✓		
Semi-Fowler's	✓		
Lithotomy	✓		
Use microscope	✓		
ETC.			

FIGURE 21-1　Competency documentation

ternship is to gain experience in as many of the areas as possible. In order to facilitate the goal, the plan may indicate specific periods of time rotating through various areas of practice, for example, 2 weeks in clinical, 1 week billing, 1 week filing insurance claims, 1 week as a receptionist, 1 week with the manager, and so on.

It is also important to validate that the total number of hours have been experienced during the externship. Some form of recording time spent at the facility must be developed. One example is shown in Figure 21-2. Blank calendars can be filled in with the name of the month and the calendar days. The essential information is completed at the top. The number of hours spent at the facility are listed on the calendar days and totaled at the end of the week. On this sample, the on-site supervisor has made some notes regarding the student. When the school coordinator visits the site and talks with the supervisor, this record of attendance and remarks will serve as a basis for discussion with the student.

The school coordinator may also make and record observations while visiting the student on-site. This may include such things as appearance, attitude, apparent relationship with the staff, remarks of the supervisor and other facility employees, student remarks, and personal observation of performance. The recording of these pertinent observations provide a means of measuring progress or will indicate the need for intervention to assist the student to succeed.

SAMPLE EXTERNSHIP EXPERIENCE RECORD

Student ___ Connie Krebs ___

Address ___ 100 E. Main St. ___

Phone ___ 123-4567 ___

___ Barbara Wise ___
(School Coordinator)

Facility ___ Kerry Peoples, M.D. ___

Address ___ 101 Fitness Lane ___

Phone ___ 614-800-9110 ___

___ Lucille Keir ___
(On-Site Coordinator)

JANUARY 20XX						WEEK TOTAL
MON	TUE	WED	THU	FRI	SAT	
			1	2	3	
4	5 6	6 6	7 3	8 6	9 3	10 24
11	12 6	13 ill	14 ill	15 6	16 3	17 15
18	19 6	20 3	21 6	22 6	23 3	24 24
25	26 6	27 6	28	29	30	31

MONTH TOTAL HOURS ___

						WEEK TOTAL
MON	TUE	WED	THU	FRI	SAT	

MONTH TOTAL HOURS ___

–NOTES–

1/5/XX Arrived on time, oriented to office, to work with B. Harris – (L. Keir)

1/9/XX Appears eager to learn, is performing satisfactorily, has been filing, typing correspondence, scheduling appointments. Handling mail and posting payments this a.m. Observed receiving payment from patient, handled appropriately (L. Keir)

1/13/XX Called in sick (LK)

1/14/XX " " "

1/15/XX Returned to office, T. 98.2, no symptoms, permitted to work (LK)

FIGURE 21-2 Recording externship hours

EXTERNSHIP EVALUATION

Another means of determining student success is evaluation by the on-site supervisor. Periodically the school coordinator should provide the on-site supervisor with some type of an evaluation form on which to record observations, remarks, and suggestions. The evaluation instrument should reflect the objectives and competencies for the externship experience. It is also beneficial if the instrument is easily completed so that the on-site supervisor does not need to spend an excessive amount of time to provide the evaluation. Some areas that might be considered as appropriate for evaluation could include:

- Appearance—personal grooming, uniform cleanliness, shoes
- Attitude—courteous, confident, cooperative, interested

- Maturity—accepts supervision, adapts to change, accepts assignments, maintains composure
- Dependability—punctual, completes tasks, accepts responsibility
- **Initiative**—seeks new learning opportunities, seeks work to do, performs extra duties
- Administrative tasks—performs receptionist, secretarial, and managerial duties
- Clinical tasks—collects database, measures vital signs, assists physician, performs lab and diagnostic procedures
- **Interpersonal** relationships—patient relations; works well with physician, coworkers, supervisor

The evaluation instrument designed could contain a simple "never" to "always" or "unsatisfactory" to "excellent" rating scales for several identified criteria, but the criteria statements often do not lend themselves to such easy evaluation. Perhaps the most desirable form lists the areas to be evaluated with descriptors within each area to be addressed. By leaving a space for remarks, the supervisor can use her own words to describe the level of performance. Figure 21-3 is an example of this type of evaluation form.

Externship facilities may be willing to go through all the on-site requirements to cooperate with a school because they feel the responsibility to assist in preparing

---

SAMPLE CLINICAL EVALUATION

_____   _____
            (Student)   (Facility)

Please enter your observations that best describe the knowledge and performance of the above named student in the spaces below.

_____

APPEARANCE (personal grooming, uniform, etc.)

_____

ATTITUDE (interested, courteous, confident, cooperative)

_____

MATURITY (accepts supervision, adapts to situation, accepts assignments)

_____

DEPENDABILITY (punctual, completes tasks, accepts responsibility)

_____

INITIATIVE (seeks new learning opportunities, performs extra duties)

_____

ADMINISTRATIVE TASKS (performs receptionist, secretarial, and managerial tasks)

_____

CLINICAL TASKS (completes database, performs lab and diagnostic skills)

_____

INTERPERSONAL (cooperates with co-workers, supervisor, physician)

Evaluated By _____   Please complete by _____
              (On-Site Supervisor)   (Date)

Date _____   Thank you, _____
                                                      (Coordinator)

FIGURE 21-3 Externship evaluation form

medical assistants. Others, as stated before, may do so as a means of "trying out" a prospective employee. As long as everything goes along well, the arrangement will be good. However, unfortunately this does not always occur. If the student is not reliable, either in attendance or being on time or in following through with assignments, then a problem will arise. At times there may be legitimate personal conflicts with existing employees, especially if someone suspects the student may be hired into her position. This may result in an unfriendly environment.

At times, a student may have great difficulty transferring classroom performance into actual patient care for some reason. Because the externship is a learning and not an employment situation, the facility may allow the student to complete his hours, but they may not be willing to cooperate in the future since the experience was not a benefit for them. It is extremely important for all students to perform to the best of their ability, not only to have a rewarding learning experience for themselves but also to protect the site for future students.

When all attempts to solve problems fail, and the externship simply cannot continue, a method needs to be provided so the facility can discontinue their cooperation. The school should remove the student and make the exit as favorable as possible. School **policy** will perhaps place the student at another site until the number of hours are achieved, or some other solution may need to be designed.

It is also recommended that externship experiences be evaluated by the students. Students should indicate whether their classroom instruction provided them with adequate skills to allow them to feel comfortable in the on-site facility. Another area concerns the equipment used in the classroom; was it current and similar to what is used in the workplace? Did they feel their presence was welcomed in the facility, or did the employees act as if they were in the way? Was the supervisor helpful and willing to provide instruction and assistance? Did they have the opportunity to rotate through many different areas, or were they allowed to do just the simpler, repetitious tasks? Were the school **coordinator** visits helpful? Did they feel they got enough support from the school? The student's remarks can be utilized to adjust the externship so that it is a better learning experience for the student and more beneficial for the facility.

ACHIEVE UNIT OBJECTIVES

- Complete the Workbook activities to meet the learning objectives.
- Apply your knowledge at the end of this chapter in completing the Critical Thinking Challenge and Activities, as well as the StudyWARE on your Student CD-ROM.

UNIT 2
THE JOB SEARCH

OBJECTIVES

Upon completion of this unit, you will be able to achieve the following:

LEARNING Objectives

1. Spell and define, using the glossary at the back of the text, all the Words to Know in this unit.
2. Describe the purpose of each style of resumé.
3. Explain the purpose of a cover letter to accompany a resumé.
4. Describe employment agency services.
5. Explain when it might be appropriate to pay an employment fee.
6. List six places to assist you in your job search.
7. Define the common abbreviations used in the newspaper "Help Wanted" section.

PERFORMANCE Objectives

1. Prepare a resumé.

WORDS TO KNOW

categorize	experience	resumé
chronological	functional	specifications
classified	negotiable	targeted
dual	qualifications	transcript
elaborate		

CERTIFICATION CONNECTION

CMA
Resume and cover letter
Methods of job searching

The job search begins with the desire to work. A medical assistant with skills in communication, medical office procedures, and clinical skills should discover excellent opportunities for employment.

Preparing yourself for your first employment in your chosen career is an exciting time. A personal review of your strengths and weaknesses will help you uncover some of your best qualities and remind you of what might need extra attention. Ask family and friends to help you sort out ideas. Often, good advice may come from those who know you well.

It might be helpful for you to think about your personal characteristics. Think about the regular things in your life. For example:

- Are you outgoing, friendly, and like having people around or are you more reserved, have just a few good friends, and enjoy being alone?
- Are you usually on time or a little early or just in time and sometimes a little late?
- Can you work with very little direction or do you like to have things spelled out clearly so you feel you won't make a mistake?
- In your spare time, do you want to engage in some group activity or sport or would you rather attend a cultural event or read?

Everyone has personal characteristics that affect their way of doing things. When evaluating yours, you might want to make two lists; one for what you feel are your strong points and another for your weaker ones. Later when a prospective employer asks you a question about what you think are your strong and weaker areas, you will have already thought it through and can answer with responses that will have a positive impact. Even negative traits can be expressed in a positive format. For example, if you have an employer reference or school notation about frequent tardiness, you might respond by saying you are taking steps to change your behavior. You are getting up 15 minutes earlier and are rewarding yourself with dinner out on Friday nights for being on time all week.

Another area to gain insight into your qualifications is to review the evaluations you had during your school program and especially during your externship. These should indicate your strong and weaker areas that are specific to medical assisting. Again this helps you realize what you have to offer as a prospective employee in addition to your educational background and any other past employment experiences. Getting a good idea about who you are will help you write your resume and cover letter and prepare you for your in-person interview.

THE RESUMÉ

The first steps before you can present yourself for employment is to develop a personal **resumé**. A resumé is an outlined summary of your abilities and **experiences**.

The goal of a resumé is to make a favorable impression so you will obtain an interview for a position. It should be complete, accurate, and neatly organized. The resume will describe to prospective employers your employment objectives, educational background, previous work experience, professional affiliations, com-

munity service, personal interests, honors, and whatever else you feel is important for them to know. It need not contain personal information about your marital status, race, religion, age, or any other facts that may be used to illegally discriminate against you. The purpose of the resumé is to inform the prospective employer of how qualified you are for to the position for which you are applying. (Refer to Procedure 21-1.)

A resumé has certain basic elements. At the top should be your name, address, phone number, and perhaps e-mail address. This information can be aligned left, centered, or run across the page. It should be emphasized somehow either by bolding or enlarging the print and perhaps drawing a line across the page to set it apart. If you are applying for a specific advertised position, you should list it by name at the top, aligned to the left, a couple of spaces below your personal information. This would identify the position for which you are applying, which might be important in case the employing facility has more than one position available. You could enter it as follows: Position Desired: Clinical medical assistant.

The next resumé sections include information about your education and your employment experiences. Listing your education begins with the most recent experience first. If you have completed a couple of educational programs, perhaps earning a degree, it probably is not appropriate to list your high school. Also, if listing the dates of completion might be a disadvantage age-wise, the dates can be omitted. The employment experience format will depend upon which resumé style is most appropriate for the position for which you are applying. Again, dates could be an item to consider if you have long gaps in employment, changed jobs frequently, or lack recent work experience. It is a good idea to identify your job titles, responsibilities, and key skills performed with each position, especially if you can demonstrate progress and increased responsibility. Select your employment listing style from the following information.

Resumé Styles

There are four major styles of resumés that are most frequently used, each with a particular focus: the **functional** style, the skills style, the **targeted** style and the **chronological** style. You can tailor your **qualifications** and experiences in the most appropriate style to best present yourself for the position **specifications**.

A *functional style* resumé works well for people who have had internships or cooperative work experience, such as a medical assistant externship. The style highlights previous work experience that provided you with experience for the job for which you are applying. When listing experience, you enter the job title first, showing the prospective employer your progress at work. If you have experience with a prestigious com-

PROCEDURE PROCEDURE PROCEDURE PROCEDURE PROCEDURE PROCEDURE PROCEDURE PROCEDURE

21-1  Prepare a Resumé

PURPOSE: To document information concerning education, experience, and abilities for employment consideration.

EQUIPMENT: High-quality paper, dictionary, thesaurus, telephone book, computer, and a quality printer.

PERFORMANCE OBJECTIVE: Provided with access to all equipment and supplies, prepare a resumé following the steps in the procedure. The document must be without errors, organized attractively on the page, and printed on appropriate paper.

1. Write your complete legal name, address, and phone number. This information may be arranged flush left or centered at the top of the page.
   (Refer to Figures 21-4A, B, and C for the particular style of resumé that is appropriate for you and your needs. Use reference materials listed above for accuracy, expression, and correct spelling in composing your resumé.)

2. List the position desired next to the heading of Job Objective, Job Target, or Postion Desired.

3. List your educational background, beginning with the most recent or present date.

4. List all pertinent employment experience, beginning with the most recent or present date or enter information in an alternative resumé style. **RATIONALE: Listing only the pertinent employment experience will allow you to provide necessary information and keep your resumé to the desired 1-page limit.**

5. List memberships/affiliations in professional organizations.

6. List community service, including volunteer programs and activities as may be appropriate.

7. State on the bottom of the resumé that references, transcripts, and certificates will be furnished on request.

8. Print the completed resumé on a sheet of bond paper.

9. Check the finished copy for errors.

10. Ask a reliable person to proofread your resumé.

11. Have a number of copies printed on quality paper for distribution.

---

pany, it may be to your advantage to list the company name first, then your job title. Either way is acceptable; however, be consistent and list all experiences in the same format. You can skip any positions that do not apply to the desired position, and they do not have to be listed in chronological order. It is most impressive if the listing is from most important to least, regardless of the dates of employment. As an example, if your work experience is limited prior to the medical assistant program, you might list your externship as the most applicable, followed by nurse assistant employment and self-employed child care. You can eliminate, for example, the fast-food restaurant and housekeeping jobs. Figure 21-4A is an example of a functional resumé of a recent medical assistant graduate.

The *skills style* resumé is best for highlighting experiences in a number of unrelated jobs and courses. It might also work well for individuals making a significant career field change. It emphasizes what you can do, not where you have been employed. You can list any applicable skills acquired through jobs, education, volunteer activities, and life experiences. For example, your summer receptionist job with an insurance company, a classified sales position at a small newspaper, and a volunteer position arranging meals on wheels deliveries

seem quite diverse, but the common elements of telephone skills and scheduling experience would be your areas of experience. The key is to **categorize** your experiences to match the skills required for the position. These skills would make you a good candidate for a receptionist in a medical facility.

The *targeted style* resumé will arrange information to focus on a specific job opportunity by highlighting the work experience and job skills that are requested by the employer. For example, if an opening indicated the position was for an administrative assistant with possible opportunity for office management, your resumé should reflect that opportunity. Usually this style will have a position statement such as Targeted Position, Professional Goal, or Career Objective. In this case it would be followed by a statement; for example, Career Objective: Administrative Medical Assistant position with the opportunity to advance to office manager. The work experiences listed should stress administrative competencies and any areas that could be considered as management skills. Remember that positions you hold with organizations could be applicable, such as a treasurer or a committee chairperson. Additional educational accomplishments such as computer training, an insurance seminar, or a time management workshop

Sarah Miller
510 State Street
Silverton, MO
(123) 456-7890

EDUCATION
20XX–20XX   Silverton Community College
                   AS Medical Assisting
20XX–20XX   Northern University
                   CPR for the Professional: January, 20XX
RELATED EXPERIENCE
20XX   **MEDICAL ASSISTING EXTERNSHIP**
                   (160 hours)
                   Primary Care Physicians, Silverton, MO
                   • Prepared patients for examination, took
                     vital signs, and charted chief complaint.
                   • Performed diagnostic tests, including
                     throat cultures, rapid strep test, EKGs
                   • Performed clerical duties, including
                     answering telephones, filing, writing
                     referrals, scheduling appointments.
                   • Data entry of patient information and
                     insurance payments.

19XX–20XX   **HEALTH CARE AIDE**
                   Manor Care Center, Silverton, MO
                   Performed personal care, took vital signs,
                   range-of-motion exercises
19XX–19XX   **SELF EMPLOYED CHILD CARE PROVIDER**
                   Responsible for child's care and safety.
SPECIAL SKILLS
                   Keyboarding 45 wpm
                   Microsoft Word, MediSoft, Practice
                   Management Software (PMS)
OTHER EXPERIENCE
1996–1997   **CASHIER**
                   Allen's Supermarket, Silverton, MO
                   Head checker

FIGURE 21-4A   Functional style resumé

Sharon R. Beach
4270 Hilldale Drive
Fernridge, CA 95061
(406) 555-1122

Job Target: Clinical Medical Assistant
Clinical Skills:
   • Assist with patient examination
   • CPR and first aid
   • Phlebotomy
   • Basic clinical laboratory skills
   • Electrocardiography
Achievements:
   • Certified Medical Assistant
   • Bachelor's degree in Nutrition
   • CPR certification
Employment Experience:
XXXX–Present   Fernridge Family Health Center
                   Clinical Medical Assistant
XXXX–XXXX   Brownsville General Hospital
                   Phlebotomist/ECG Technician
XXXX–XXXX   Ronald L. Botkin, D.O.—General Practice
                   Administrative and Clinical Medical Assistant
Professional Affiliations:
   • Member—American Association of Medical Assistants
Education:
XXXX   Baldwin Community College
XXXX   Brownsville University

FIGURE 21-4B   Targeted style resumé

after a few years of employment and additional education, your qualifications will change and you can make use of this information to improve your job status.

Other Resumé Entries

There are other areas of your life that would be appropriate to list on your resumé. These are primarily evidence of your success and personal involvement, such as the following.

Professional Affiliations

You should list your membership in a professional organization and identify any leadership position you have held. This shows your involvement in your profession and willingness to assume responsibility for its operation. You may list them alphabetically or in order of importance from most to least, as in Figure 21-4C.

Professional Achievements and Awards

List your certification status to indicate your commitment to a recognized professional credential. Also list any awards, scholarships, or recognitions you have been given; these show you have outstanding abilities.

Community Service

Willingness to give of one's time and energy in community service is an admirable

would be very desirable. Figure 21-4B is an example of a resumé targeted for a clinical position.

The *chronological style* resumé is the most common and the more traditional format. It lists education achievements followed by work experience, starting with the present or most recent job and progressing back in time. This style is most appropriate for people who have employment experiences that are closely related to their desired position. It works best when there are no long periods of unemployment between jobs, which can become obvious with this style. This format is probably the easiest to prepare and works well for most job applicants. If you have extensive work experience or have worked for several employers, it is appropriate that you focus on the last 10 to 15 years of employment. Figure 21-4C is an example of a chronological style format.

If you are young or have little work experience, this discussion may seem unrelated to you, but remember,

Sandy Lynn Beach, CMA
4030 Newbank Road
Wheelersburg, Ohio 45794
(614) 555-1212

Desired Position: Clinical Medical Assistant

EDUCATION:
XXXX to date: Attending evening courses in Nursing,
                             Southern Ohio Technical College
                             Lucasville, Ohio
XXXX–XX: Certificate, Ohio Valley Training Academy,
                             Wellston, Ohio. Major: Medical Assisting
XXXX: Diploma, Portsmouth East High School,
                             Portsmouth, Ohio. Major: General Business

EMPLOYMENT EXPERIENCE:
XXXX to date: Administrative Medical Assistant to Wilber
                             Roth, M.D., Rolling Hills, Ohio
XXXX–XX   Admissions Clerk, Green Meadows Com-
                             munity Hospital, Green Meadows, Ohio
XXXX–XX: Cashier, Garden Inn Restaurant, Hilldale, Ohio

ACHIEVEMENTS: AAMA National Certification 19XX

PROFESSIONAL ASSOCIATIONS:
    American Association of Medical Assistants
    Ohio State Society of Medical Assistants
    Scioto County Chapter of Medical Assistants

COMMUNITY SERVICE:
    Red Cross Volunteer
    Big Sisters Association Volunteer

References, transcripts, and certificates furnished upon request.

FIGURE 21-4C Chronological style resumé

trait and should be listed on the resumé. Employers recognize this quality and realize you have concern for others.

These additional pieces of information about you can set you apart from other candidates. Professional membership, achievements, and volunteer activities usually indicate a person who is living a full life—a happier, healthier, and productive person.

At the bottom of the resumé, be sure to make a statement that references, **transcripts**, and professional certificates will be furnished upon request. These documents verify your resumé entries and will be required if you interview for the position. You should prepare a list of three to four nonfamily persons who know you well and can recommend you to an employer. Be sure to ask these individuals if you may use them for a reference before you put them on your list.

A resumé that is basic but complete and properly arranged will attract an employer's attention. One that is flashy, too lengthy, or too wordy may well be discarded. A one-page resumé is a preferred length. It must be well organized and grammatically correct.

You should always have someone proofread your resumé, because often our own mistakes go unnoticed. Spelling must be accurate. There is no need for being **elaborate** in style. A resumé that is printed on a soft ivory or light gray high-quality paper will stand out and is easily retrieved in a pile of others.

Make sure that you refrain from dark colors that make print difficult to read. Dark shades and flashy fonts may be appropriate for graphic design or artistic positions, but not for the usually conservative medical job market. It is also recommended that you have your resumé printed at a print shop or that you use a high-quality laser printer to produce your copies. A poor-quality reproduction will not make the favorable impression you need to gain an interview.

Remember that as you gain work experience and acquire educational credentials, it will be necessary to update your resumé. Employment dates will change, and hopefully job responsibilities will show growth. Items of lesser importance should be deleted as more impressive accomplishments are achieved. Always try to maintain your resumé on a single page if at all possible; however, don't reduce the font size below 10 or reduce the margins trying to make it fit. If you do have enough quality items to list that you need to use the second page, be certain the most important information is on the first page.

THE COVER LETTER

After you have perfected your resumé, you should do the same to compose a cover letter to send with it. The letter must state *why* you should be hired for the desired position. The cover letter should be addressed to the person who decides who is interviewed and hired. Finding out the name of the office manager or supervisor may be done by making a simple phone call and asking (be sure to get the correct spelling). Personalizing the letter will gain more attention than will the standard form letter. Let the employer know that your skills and qualifications will be an asset. Make the letter simple and direct to convey what makes you the person for the job. Be sure to request an interview and make it clear when and how you can be reached. Figures 21-5A and B give sample cover letters. Remember that your resumé should provide a general overall description of your assets and qualifications. The cover letter should be specific and targeted toward a particular person or department. It should be sent in answer to an ad, in request for an interview, or at an individual's request.

Both cover letter and resumé must be error free. Employers eliminate numerous resumés by pitching those with spelling or grammatical errors, tears, or smudges, or those that are too wordy or unorganized. Faxing a resumé may produce a "muddy" look and is only recommended when requested by an employer.

Date

Karla Baker, CMA
Office Manager
Hilldale Medical Center
Hilldale, Ohio 45102

Dear Ms. Baker:
I have completed training in medical assisting at Ohio Valley
Training Academy. It has provided me with skills in both
administrative and clinical areas. I am very interested in securing
a position in your health care facility as a dual Medical Assistant. I
have Achieved National Certification as indicated an my resumé.

Please let me know if I may schedule an appointment for an
interview. I can be reached at home on Tuesday and Thursday
afternoons and every evening at 555-8131.

Thank you for your consideration.

Sincerely,

Sandy Lynn Beach, CMA

FIGURE 21-5A   Cover letter for a resumé

4270 Hilldale Drive
Fernridge, CA 95061
(406) 555-1122
Date

Ms. Doreen Castle
Office Manager
Hopkin's Medical Clinic
739 Mountainview Way
Great Valley, CA 95068

Dear Ms. Castle:
I read your ad in the local paper regarding the opening for a
full-time clinical medical assistant at Hopkin's Medical Clinic. I
feel that my training and experience makes me a worthy
candidate for this position. I am a Certified Medical Assistant
and have a bachelor's degree in Nutrition.

My experience in patient education regarding therapeutic diets
has helped me to sharpen my communication skills. I also have
excellent clinical skills and am currently enrolled in a CPR
certification class.

At your earliest convenience, I would like to meet with you for
an interview to discuss matching my qualifications to your
needs. Please call me at the number listed above to schedule
an appointment. I can be reached at home every evening and
on Wednesday afternoons.

Yours truly,

(Miss) Sharon R. Beach, CMA

FIGURE 21-5B   Cover letter for a resumé

APPT—Appointment	MED—Medical
ASST—Assistant	MGR—Manager
BGN or BEG—Beginning	MOS—Months
COL—College	NEC—Necessary
DEPT—Department	NEG—Negotiable
EDUC—Education	OFC—Office
EOE—Equal Opportunity	PD—Paid
Employer	POS—Position(s)
EXP—Experience	PT—Part Time
F—Female	REF—References
FB—Fringe Benefits	REQ—Required
FT—Full Time	SAL—Salary
GRAD—Graduate	SEC—Secretary
H—Handicapped	T—Temporary
HS—High School	TRANSP—Transportation
HR—Hour	WPM—Words Per Minute
HRS—Hours	WK—Week
IMMED—Immediate	WKENDS—Weekends
INT—Interview	W/—With
LIC—License	Yrs—Years
M—Male	

FIGURE 21-6   Some abbreviations used in the "Help Wanted" section of the newspaper

CLASSIFIED ADVERTISEMENTS

You may send your resumé to a prospective employer in response to a **classified** ad in the local newspaper. A classified ad is a request for qualified applicants to send information about themselves to a prospective employer. The employer may then request an interview with those who meet the requirements for the position instead of interviewing all persons who may wish to apply. This method of screening saves time for the employer and makes the resumé the most important means of communication. Figure 21-6 shows abbreviations commonly used in classified advertisements.

In responding to a classified ad, it is customary to write a cover letter to accompany your resumé. Begin the letter by stating that you read the ad in the paper, so the recipient knows how you learned about the position (See Figure 21-5B). This cover letter expresses your desire to be interviewed for the position and describes briefly who you are and what you have to offer.

PUBLIC EMPLOYMENT SERVICES

All states offer assistance in locating jobs through a state employment service. Local offices of this agency will have job openings on file, possibly including the one you are looking for. You simply walk in, fill out the general forms, wait your turn, and then have a conference with an employment counselor. If there are listings that call for your type of experience and training, you will have immediate leads to begin contacting. If no appropriate listings are currently on file, the employment counselor will place your name on file and notify you when listings do materialize. Because this agency is supported by tax dollars, there is no fee for the service.

PRIVATE EMPLOYMENT AGENCIES

Private employment agencies offer similar services. A cover letter and resumé should be sent to the agency explaining your area of expertise and desired employment. Many agencies specialize in the medical field and can give efficient service in locating openings in medical assisting. Many potential jobs are "fee paid," meaning that the employer pays the agency's fees. In general, you should avoid positions that require you to pay the fee. Fees for finding employment positions are generally based on a percentage of the first year's wages of an employee. Often, arrangements may be made for the fee to be paid in installments. The decision is obviously yours. You may be definitely interested in a particular position for which you will have to pay a fee. Carefully weighing the advantages and disadvantages will help you decide if the cost is worth it to you in the long run. A substantial pay increase is an obvious advantage. If you have been waiting for a certain position to open for a relatively long time, it may well be a wise choice to secure it by paying a fee.

OTHER CONTACTS

A resumé with a cover letter requesting an interview may be sent to many medical offices or health care facilities even if there is no position available. If you wish to be employed in a particular facility, making it known may spark an interest in you as a prospective employee should there be an opening. Introducing yourself through correspondence and specifying your interest in employment should a position become available can be very productive. Employers may keep your letter and resumé on file for as long as a year and respond as the need arises.

Additional information about job opportunities may be obtained at the public library. There are also many job opportunities you can check out by using the computer. Online information about jobs in every field is listed and updated regularly. Doing a job search is quick and easy. You can find opportunities without traveling miles and spending lots of time and money in the process. Taking advantage of one or all of the different ways to find employment should ensure you of a position in an area of your liking. But always check to be sure you know if any costs are involved before you sign any forms or complete any contracts. Even a seemingly small percentage can take a lot of money out of your pocket over a period of time. And be aware, getting information from the Internet is not usually free. You may need to provide a credit card number, on which charges will be made to obtain the information you want. If you seek the services of an employment agency or register with the employment placement center on your campus, be sure to check back with a specific person often to reaffirm your interest in becoming employed. Many services, periodicals, and books deal with occupational information, and library personnel can be very helpful.

Membership in professional associations is also quite helpful in the job search. Not only may an association's publications include classified ads, but personal contact with other members at meetings may provide invaluable information about job openings. Participation in community service groups can put you in touch with yet another network of persons who may have information about job openings.

Watch for industry-sponsored job fairs where employers will have a table or booth to meet prospective employees. This type of recruitment is usually reserved for large organizations, but many hospitals, clinics, and care facilities cooperate in health fairs. Finally, you should not overlook your friends and acquaintances; the job one of them happens to mention in conversation could turn out to be just the one you have been waiting for.

ACHIEVE UNIT OBJECTIVES

- Complete the Workbook activities to meet the learning objectives.
- Practice the procedures in this unit to meet the performance objectives.
- Apply your knowledge at the end of this chapter in completing the Critical Thinking Challenge and Activities, as well as the StudyWARE on your Student CD-ROM.

UNIT 3
CAREER ENTRY AND SUCCESS

OBJECTIVES

Upon completion of this unit, you will be able to achieve the following:

LEARNING Objectives

1. Spell and define, using the glossary at the back of the text, all of the Words to Know in this unit.

2. **Discuss how career entry has changed.**

3. **List five comments about the importance of appearance of your job application when applying for a job.**

4. **Identify six things to remember or prepare for on the day of your interview.**

5. **List personal grooming characteristics that might keep you from being hired.**

6. **List four areas of your personal life that could lead to arbitrary discrimination when being considered for a job.**

7. **Explain why you should send a follow-up letter after an interview.**

8. **List the qualities employers regard as most important in employees.**

9. **Define a job description.**

10. **Describe reasons for employment termination.**

11. **Describe ways to advance in employment.**

12. **List the most important qualities necessary for job advancement.**

PERFORMANCE Objectives

1. **Complete a job application.**

2. **Write an interview follow-up letter.**

WORDS TO KNOW

arbitrary	evaluation	negate
competent	fringe	obligation
contemporary	irreconcilable	transition
demeanor		

CERTIFICATION CONNECTION

CMA

Displaying professional
   attitude

Interviewing as a job
   candidate

Professional presentation

Now that you have completed your externship and prepared your resumé, you are ready to seek employment. Whether this will be your first full-time job or a change in your career, it is an exciting time. You have prepared yourself; now it is time to get that job and enter your new career.

CAREER ENTRY

According to recent statistics, there is an increasing need for qualified medical assistants across the nation. Employers in the health care field are recognizing the benefits of employing medical assistants who have had specific training in the field. Of course, this eliminates the need for extensive and expensive additional training on the job. Externship plans are very successful in educational programs because they provide the soon-to graduate medical assistant student 160 hours of experience in a medical office. The supervisor allows the instructor to periodically visit the facility and observe the student's performance. Other training programs, not accredited by CAHEEP or ABHES, require that students observe for a certain number of hours to fulfill the program's standards. In either case, the trend is welcomed following the past practice of hiring assistants without any training in the field for full- or part-time employment in physicians' offices or clinics.

The **transition** from student to medical assistant poses certain adjustment considerations to all concerned in the health care setting. Employers have an **obligation** to assist the new employee to feel accepted in the profession and to give helpful advice with patience. The new employee is obligated to strive to perform skills with both proficiency and efficiency. An effort to get along with others is required of each member of the health care team. A smooth transition with a new member of the team is possible if each employee recognizes the value of each person in each position to fulfill the health care needs of the patients.

APPLICATION FORMS

Filling out an application for employment may be your next step. These forms may range from the simple to the complex. Figure 21-7 shows an example of an application form that asks for a minimal amount of information. Much of the information is the same as what is contained on your resumé. Remember to take a copy of your resumé with you to help you fill out the job application. Be sure to transcribe dates and all other information correctly, completely, and accurately. When you are nervous or if you are hurried, mistakes are often made, such as transposing numbers, leaving a space blank, or even placing the wrong information in a space. Take adequate time to complete whatever forms are necessary in a neat and attractive manner. It is not considered proper to ask for a phone directory or any other reference when applying for a job. You are supposed to show that you are prepared. In filling out an application for employment, you must be accurate and honest. Being prepared with dates, names, addresses, phone numbers, and other detailed information will expedite completion of the form. Some appli-

EMPLOYMENT APPLICATION FORM

PERSONAL

NAME   DATE _____

(LAST)   (FIRST)   (MI)

ADDRESS—STREET   CITY   STATE   ZIP

PHONE NUMBER   SOCIAL SECURITY NUMBER

POSITION DESIRED:

EXPECTED SALARY OR HOURLY WAGE:

EDUCATION

NAME OF SCHOOL	ADDRESS	DATE(S)	DEGREE/CERTIFICATE
HIGH SCHOOL			
VOCATIONAL/TECHNICAL			
COLLEGE			
OTHER			

WORK EXPERIENCE—Give present position (or last position held first).

JOB TITLE:	EMPLOYER	ADDRESS	DATES
DUTIES PERFORMED:			
JOB TITLE:	EMPLOYER	ADDRESS	DATES
DUTIES PERFORMED:			

REFERENCES—LIST THREE PERSONS (OTHER THAN RELATIVES) WHO HAVE KNOWN YOU FOR AT LEAST 2 YEARS

NAME/TITLE	ADDRESS	TELEPHONE NUMBER

FIGURE 21-7 An example of an employment application form

cations are extremely lengthy (several pages). It may be best if this type is taken home to complete, because it may take a considerable amount of time.

Because the job application will probably reach the personnel manager's office before you do, it must speak well for you; it must make a good impression on the person who reads it. Applications must be complete, neat, and legible, or they will be discarded promptly. Reading and following the instructions on the form is of utmost importance. Take time to read the instructions and follow them precisely when completing an employment application form. If the printed instructions on the form say to print all information in black ink, you should do just that and not use cursive style or another color of ink. One of the functions served in having candidates complete the application form is to find out

how well they follow directions. The applicant in Figure 21-8 is carefully thinking before writing on the form to avoid making any errors. The application form will provide the employer not only with factual information about you but with many other insights as well.

Refer to Procedure 21-2 to practice completing an application.

If you take sufficient time and interest in completing the application, you will be more likely to be given a personal interview. Additionally, because of the Immigration Reform Act of 1986, employers are required by federal law to ask you for documents that show both your identity and eligibility to work in the United States. Employers will make copies of your documents and return them to you. Further, the Employment Eligibility Verification Form I-9 must be completed and

21-2  Complete a Job Application

PURPOSE: To accurately and neatly complete an application for employment.

EQUIPMENT: Job application, pen, copy of resumé, list of needed names, addresses and phone numbers, and copies of educational achievements.

PERFORMANCE OBJECTIVE: With access to all equipment, complete a job application, following all directions, and entering all information neatly and without error.

1. Assemble all necessary equipment and supporting documents.
2. Read the application, noting the instructions for completion.
3. Neatly enter your personal information.
4. Enter your educational information, referring to diplomas, certificates, and transcripts for accurate dates.
5. Enter work experience information, beginning with current or last position worked and proceeding backwards. **NOTE: Refer to prepared lists for accurate addresses.**
6. Enter any other information requested. **NOTE: Applications vary as to information requested.**
7. List the names and phone numbers of personal references. **NOTE: List only those from whom you have received approval.**
8. Review the application, checking for missed or incorrectly entered information.
9. Check for accuracy of spelling and general appearance.
10. Present or mail the application to the prospective employer.

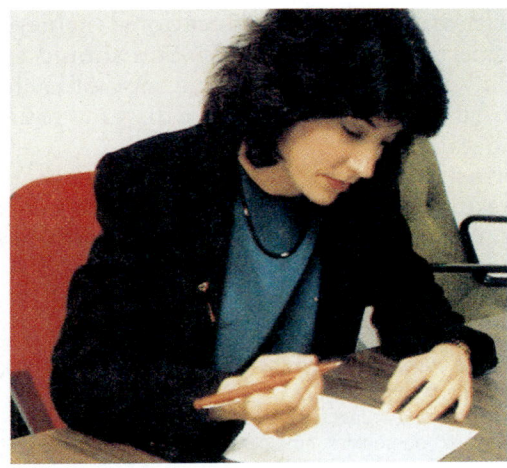

FIGURE 21-8 This applicant is carefully thinking over information before writing it on the application form to prevent making errors.

filed in the employee's record along with other important documents. Employers must verify that you are legally entitled to work in the United States. All applicants and employers must comply with this law. Refer to Chapter 10 for more details.

Because of the professional setting (medical field) for which you are seeking employment, many employers require that the background of prospective employees is checked. Among the areas of concern are the person's credit rating, police record, and chemical use/abuse. You may be asked to produce documents or give authorization for the employer to find out about your personal records before you may be considered for hiring.

THE INTERVIEW

An interview is a face-to-face meeting between you and your prospective employer. The day of the scheduled interview you should allow sufficient time to get ready. If you chew gum or smoke cigarettes, leave these at home for this trip. Neither has any place at a job interview.

When applying for a job, your appearance is extremely important. Even if you are merely picking up an application to take home to complete or returning it after you have completed it, your appearance, including your attitude, will certainly be noticed. You should dress for success any time a prospective employer may see you. Other employees will surely notice you and relay the information to the employer, especially if a negative impression is given. Appearance is an outward indication of who you are. Remember what you learned about nonverbal communication. If you are a sincere, **competent**, and dedicated person, then by all means attend to your appearance accordingly. Nonverbal messages, though silent, can speak loudly.

Most employers expect appropriate attire, and some require adherence to a very specific policy concerning type of dress and general appearance.

If you are interviewing for a clinical position, ask beforehand about what type of clothing to wear. Your inquiry will most likely be taken as showing genuine interest. Often, employers will want to see you dressed in what you perceive as a "uniform" to see how you will look on the job.

Women who prefer to wear business attire should dress conservatively in a navy, gray, tan, or brown tailored suit or pantsuit. Bright colors, jewelry, miniskirts, and frilly outfits are not considered professional attire. Men should also follow this advice and dress conservatively, avoiding outrageous ties, jewelry, and fad clothes. Remember that you want to make a positive impression with the interviewer concerning yourself and your qualifications, not your taste in fashions and accessories. A medical assistant who is more interested in meeting the requirements of the job than in being up with the latest fad is more appealing to a personnel manager.

All matters concerning personal cleanliness are vital. The following characteristics are sure to interfere with or **negate** the possibility of employment: bad breath, dirty or untrimmed fingernails, chipped nail polish, dirty or unkempt hair, overpowering aftershave or perfume, unclean teeth, unpleasant or offensive body odor, or untended complexion problems.

The point is this: no matter how well qualified or eager you are, you may not find anyone willing to pay for your services if you fail in certain matters of personal hygiene. Take nothing for granted. Make strict adherence to proper personal grooming a rigid daily rule.

Rushing usually detracts from your appearance and **demeanor**. If the address of the facility is not familiar to you, get directions and plan your time beforehand. (It is a good idea to go to the facility a day or two before the scheduled interview to check out the area to determine the approximate travel time, exact location, parking, bus route, and so on to avoid getting lost or being delayed.) You should arrive about 10 to 15 minutes before the appointment. (You may be instructed to arrive up to an hour or more before the interview to complete an application form or to take required preemployment tests.) Arriving too early will make you appear insecure. Being late for almost any reason will make you appear irresponsible and a poor candidate for the position. If you happen to find yourself in a situation beyond your control, a telephone call explaining the delay and a sincere apology are in order. Being on time is a sign of reliability, dependability, and conscientiousness.

You will be able to give your undivided attention to the interviewer if all of your responsibilities are in order before you enter the facility. If you have children, it is best to leave them with a child care provider. Taking children to an interview is inappropriate and quite distracting. If you are preoccupied with worry about personal problems, illness, a parking meter, or anything else, you will not be able to interview well. As soon as you know the date of the interview, make plans to allocate your time so that you can be stress free to get ready, travel to the site, interview, and return without rushing. An interview is an investment in yourself and your career. It is worth your giving sufficient time and effort for a successful outcome.

Introducing yourself with a handshake should initiate a friendly and pleasant conversation. Your manner should tell the interviewer you are happy to be there.

The interview ought to allow sufficient time for each of you to inquire about the other and to discuss the requirements of the position. Often, the interviewer will have reviewed your resume.

You should be prepared to answer questions concerning your career goals and objectives, how you feel about changes, why you decided on this career, your further educational plans, and so on (Figure 21-9). Look at the questions commonly asked by interviewers that are listed in the figure. Review these and draft answers for yourself. It is good to have thought-out answers before going in for the interview. Your answers should be brief, concise, and honest.

Remember to be prepared with the list of references and verification of your educational achievements and any certifications you hold. You should take the originals with you, but having a copy of each document to give to the interviewer will show your attention to details.

In terms of perspective and dimension, the section of the resumé that lists community services is an appealing area to many prospective employers. It is an in-

1. What are your qualifications for employment in our facility?
2. Do you have plans for continuing education? If yes, what are your plans?
3. What were your favorite subjects in school and why?
4. Why are you seeking employment with us?
5. What made you decide to enter the medical assisting field?
6. What is your most rewarding experience in life thus far?
7. What are your long-range career goals?
8. What motivates you to do your best?
9. What is the most difficult problem you ever had to deal with? And how did you handle it?
10. What does success mean to you?
11. What relationship should exist between supervisors and those under their supervision?
12. How would you describe yourself?
13. Do you work well under pressure?
14. What are your strengths and weaknesses?
15. What two things are most important to you in a job?

FIGURE 21-9 A list of commonly asked questions during employment interviews

dicator of your concern for others, your involvement, and your energy level and time management skills. Some employers may ask what prompted your interest in a particular service area. Be prepared to respond honestly.

Contemporary federal laws are designed to deal with arbitrary discrimination in hiring practices. Toward this end, you should not be asked questions concerning your age, cultural or ethnic background, marital status, or parenthood. Nevertheless, these issues may come up in the course of your interview. You are not required to provide this information if you choose not to. The purpose of the interview is to ascertain the relevance of your experience and character to the job at hand. Should any of these unrelated issues come up, be careful to analyze the context in which they arose (it could be from something you said). In any case, if you are honestly convinced that you have been denied a job because of **arbitrary** discrimination, be advised that this is illegal, and you have legal recourse.

At some point during the interview, the interviewer may give you a written job description of the position for which you are applying. You will probably be given time to look it over and then asked if you would feel confident about performing the job described. An honest answer is the best. Avoid hedging or bluffing about issues, because an experienced interviewer will pick up on your insecurities. Remember that body language tells the rest of the story. If there are one or two duties you have never performed before or one or two pieces of equipment that you know little about, say this but add that you are eager to learn. The employer will appreciate the initiative in your answer. If the job description sounds totally unfamiliar or if you feel it would be an impossible task, it is best to say so. The interviewer will appreciate your openness.

Some positions may have no job description, and the duties involved will be discussed during the interview. Knowing that there are probably as many duties not mentioned as mentioned will give you an idea of the amount of work the job requires.

By the time all of these matters have been dealt with, the interview will be starting to wind down. The interviewer beginning to reach closure will ask you if you have any further questions. If issues of salary, raises, and advancement have not been dealt with previously, this is an appropriate time to mention them. This is also the logical point for you to ask about any other matters you are uncertain about (Figure 21-10). However, do not drag out this time. Let the interview end smoothly. When it is over, rise and thank the interviewer for his time. Firmly shake hands if the interviewer extends a hand (Figure 21-11). Remember to smile and be pleasant and polite as you exit with confidence. See Figure 21-12 for the "dos and don'ts" of applying for a job.

1. To see a job description
2. About hours—work day schedule
3. Rate of pay (if not discussed by the close of the interview)
4. Chances for advancement or promotion
5. About continuing education—in-service programs (are expenses paid?)
6. **Fringe** benefits:
   a. Health insurance plan
   b. Dental insurance plan
   c. Eye care
   d. Vacation/time off
   e. Membership dues in AAMA/ARMA
   f. Profit sharing
   g. Retirement plan
   h. Tuition reimbursement
   i. Other
7. Frequency of job performance evaluations

FIGURE 21-10   A list of questions you, the applicant, might ask during the interview

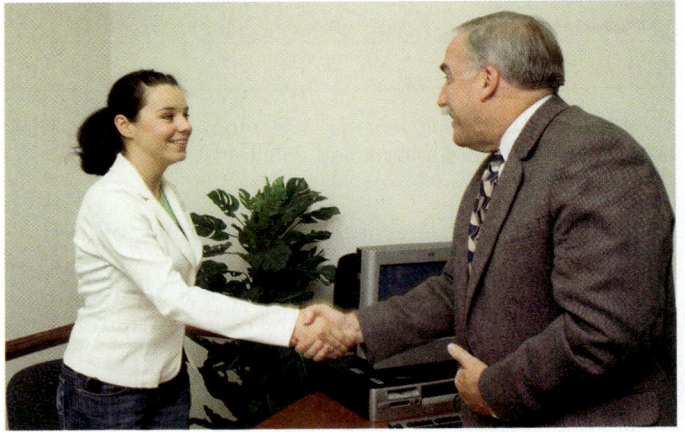

FIGURE 21-11   A firm handshake at the conclusion of the interview conveys courtesy and mutual respect.

WHEN INTERVIEWING OR APPLYING FOR A JOB:	
DO	**DON'T**
Arrive on time (10–15 minutes early)	Be late!
Show interest—enthusiasm!	Ask too many questions
Be immaculate in appearance	Make excuses
Display a positive attitude	Talk about personal problems
Use courtesy	Act over-confident
Act composed and poised	Drum fingers, swing leg, tap foot
Dress appropriately	Overdress
Keep good posture (sit still and straight)	Chew gum or smoke

FIGURE 21-12   Remember these tips when applying for a job or going for an employment interview.

INTERVIEW EVALUATION					
Subject	Excellent	Good	Satisfactory	Needs Improvement	Poor
Appearance					
Attitude					
Eye contact					
Self-control					
Voice					
Grammar					
Responses					
Manners					
Resumé					
Comments					
Date					
Employer		Title			
Address		Phone			
Applicant					

FIGURE 21-13 Employers may use a form such as this after an interview to record information about an applicant

The interviewer may talk to a number of people about a specific job opening in the office. To help the interviewer remember specific facts and traits about each individual, a form such as the one shown in Figure 21-13 may be filled out.

You may be one of many candidates interviewing for a particular job. Therefore, any decision may take some time. Out of courtesy and to enhance your image with the interviewer, take the time to compose a follow-up letter shortly after the interview has taken place. Figure 21-14 offers a sample letter. A typed thank you letter or a neatly hand-written note is an indication of your interest, persistence, and follow-through ability. Refer to Procedure 21-3 to write an interview follow-up letter.

WHAT EMPLOYERS WANT MOST IN EMPLOYEES

The personal investment that you have made in regard to your education and skills training, along with all of the effort you have put forth in producing a resumé and interviewing for employment, does not stop with being hired. After securing a position, you must continually strive to do your best. An employer will expect you to perform with increasing expertise in your position as you continue to gain experience.

Sandy Lynn Beach
4030 Newbank Road
Wheelersburg, OH 45794

January 10, 20XX

Karla Baker, CMA
Office Manager
Hilldale Medical Center
Hilldale, OH 45102

Dear Ms. Baker:

Thank you very much for granting me an interview for the clinical medical assistant's position on your staff. The interview was both challenging and stimulating; I found it to be an enjoyable and rewarding experience.

You outlined the duties and responsibilities that come with the position very specifically. This is the type of position for which I have been trained; I feel confident that if I am offered the position, I can handle the responsibilities and become an asset to your staff.

Again, thank you for considering me for this position. I would be very appreciative if you would inform me of your final decision at your earliest convenience (OR: I look forward to hearing from you soon).

Sincerely,

Sandy Lynn Beach, CMA

FIGURE 21-14 A sample follow-up letter

Desirable employee qualities that employers generally rank as most important are listed as follows:

1. Communication skills (oral and written)
2. Cooperation
3. Courteousness
4. Dependability
5. Enthusiasm
6. Initiative
7. Interest
8. Math skills
9. Punctuality
10. Reading skills
11. Reliability
12. Responsibility
13. Time management skills

These qualities are fast becoming increasingly more important in holding a job. Becoming proficient in grammar, including both the written and spoken word, is a must. Speaking in a well-educated manner is necessary to portray a professional image of not only yourself but of the facility where you are employed. You become a member of a team of medical personnel who

PROCEDURE PROCEDURE PROCEDURE PROCEDURE PROCEDURE PROCEDURE PROCEDURE PROCEDURE

21-3  Write an Interview Follow-up Letter

PURPOSE: To produce an error-free letter as an indication of interest and appreciation following an employment interview.

EQUIPMENT: Computer, high-quality paper, addressee's name and address, and dictionary.

PERFORMANCE OBJECTIVE: With access to all needed equipment and supplies, write an error-free interview follow-up letter. The letter must express appreciation for the interview, restate desire and capability for position, and request notification of decision.

1. Assemble the needed information and equipment.
2. Enter your name and address in a letterhead format.
3. Enter the date.
4. Enter the addressee information.
5. Enter a salutation.
6. Write the first paragraph, expressing appreciation for the interview.
7. Write the second paragraph, restating your preparation for and confidence in your ability to perform in the position.
8. Write a closing paragraph, again expressing appreciation and requesting notification of the decision. You may want to express a willingness to re-interview for further evaluation.
9. Enter the closing.
10 Enter your typed name four spaces below.
11. Sign the letter, make a copy, and place the original in an addressed envelope to be mailed.

---

reflect each other to the public you serve. Good communication skills include refraining from the use of slang and phrases that are not familiar or offensive to patients and coworkers. Getting together with friends to relax and enjoy leisure time is the appropriate way to let down and have fun. Even though your work day should be pleasant and enjoyable, you must respect and remember the professional code of conduct and follow it. Effective communication in a professional setting requires that employees speak in an educated manner. The person who speaks politely using good communication skills in proper English imparts confidence to coworkers and patients. Many evening classes, such as a business English course, offer a basic review in grammar. Taking the initiative to improve oneself is admirable. Employers recognize these efforts, and for those who demonstrate ambition, rewards will surely follow.

At Work and On Time

Attendance is most important because schedules must be changed and reassignments made when an employee is absent, especially when it is unexpected. An absent employee affects everyone because work must be divided among the other team members. Scheduling personal appointments should be done on your day off or after working hours. If there is an important engagement for which you need time off, you should ask for a meeting with your supervisor to discuss making

arrangements well in advance of the date. Remember that *only when it is absolutely necessary* should you call in sick. If you are not sure about the office policy regarding this issue, you should ask your employer. Employees have a responsibility to report a personal or serious illness to their supervisor as soon as possible. When an emergency involves an accident or acute medical problem, notification of the circumstance will be received with sympathy and concern. Generally, employers are most understanding about illness when the reason is genuine. If child care is a problem, and the reason for absence is caused by needing someone to care for children, the supervisor should be made aware of the situation. Often, supervisors may be helpful in assisting with information that could be a possible solution to the problem. However, repeated occurrences of calling in "sick" just to take a day off will become annoying and may lead to disciplinary action. Usually, offenders are more likely to take off on Mondays and Fridays for long weekends. These are days when schedules are full and all employees are needed. If one is placed on probation and warned about poor attendance practices and the warnings go unheeded, it could ultimately result in the employee's dismissal.

It is equally important to be on time daily. If you are scheduled to be at work at 8:00 AM, you should be at the work site and ready to begin at 8:00 AM and not just coming in the door at that time. Arriving a few minutes early is a wise practice, because it will allow time to put your personal belongings away and give you time to begin your day without being rushed. Being prompt is a valuable personal quality appreciated by both employers and patients. Leaving early is not advised unless absolutely necessary and with permission of the supervisor in advance. When one leaves before the scheduled time, it puts an added burden on other team members to finish your job. With each member of the health care team doing what is expected, the work will be shared, and the group's efficiency will be noticed by your employer. This makes for a harmonious working relationship among employees.

Take Care of Yourself

You have studied throughout this text about various patient education materials and guidelines for better health. You must have realized by now that you should be practicing what you are expected to teach patients. This can only help you to feel better about yourself, which will be evident to others with whom you come in contact. In good health, you will be more productive, be more energetic, and display better coping skills. All of the qualities important to employers should also be important to you. The secret to success is simple. Strive toward fulfilling the goals you set, and do everything in your power to reach them, which simply means to always do the best you can. Your personal satisfaction is surely one goal that will be realized if you follow this plan.

When you obtain employment, you must dedicate yourself to the task of keeping the job. This is where your work history begins, and it will follow you throughout your working life. If the health care field remains your chosen career area and if medical assisting is your point of entry, then you must be determined to become the very best medical assistant you can. Ultimately, your eventual advancement into a more responsible position and higher pay will depend largely upon your demonstrated capabilities in performing your administrative and clinical tasks. However, the aforementioned employee qualities will also become significant factors in paving the way for advancement.

Consider this scenario: A physician employs two medical assistants; both are the same age and possess relatively equal administrative and clinical skills. The only differences between the two come down to appearance and attitude. One maintains a considerably nicer appearance than the other, along with a more positive attitude. As the physician's volume of business expands and a promotion and salary increase for one of the positions becomes inevitable, which one will likely get the nod from the physician? You do not have to be a genius to figure this one out. In the end, it comes down to common sense.

THE JOB DESCRIPTION

The health care team is made up of many members who are delegated to perform specific functions. Each member should have a detailed outline of the duties required of their employment position. This detailed outline giving particular information about the duties and responsibilities of the position is called a job description. Because it can be helpful to both parties, this document may be referred to often during the interview process. The interviewer can show the applicant a detailed explanation of what would be expected on the job and observe the reaction to it. The applicant can be given a few minutes to read over the job description to get a better idea of what is involved in the job. Then, the applicant can ask specific questions and can see what steps are necessary to advance (if not already skilled in all procedures listed).

If there is no job description where you are applying for a job or you do not have one at your present job, it is wise to compose one. An example of a simple job description format is shown in Figure 21-15. This can be altered easily and used to document the duties and re-

Sample Job Description

Position: Clinical medical assistant

Job Summary: Prepare patients for exams, assist physician with examinations and treatments, provide patient education

Job Requirements: Responsibilities:
- Follow standard precautions, CLIA/OSHA regulations
- Perform patient education regarding exam preparation, treatments, and follow-up care
- Assist physician(s) with patient exams and treatments
- Document patient information accurately
- Assist as needed at the request of office manager
- Cleaning and stocking patient rooms as necessary

Responsible to: Physician(s) and Clinical Supervisor

Job Qualifications: Certified medical assistant, current CPR certification

_____   _____
Employee's signature   Date

_____   _____
Office Manager's signature   Date

FIGURE 21-15 An example of a job description

sponsibilities of your job. The job description should contain the following information:

- Title of the position
- Person(s) responsible to
- Summary of the position
- Primary duties of the job
- Expectations of the job (regarding job performance)
- Requirements of the position (education, certification, and so on)
- Qualifications of the job
- Additional criteria per facility

As you may have realized, the job description is helpful in setting guidelines, outlining educational requirements and qualifications, and establishing standards and goals of the facility. Knowing what is expected of you and having it in writing will safeguard misunderstandings and keep better communication links open. It also is important in protecting employees from being asked to perform duties and responsibilities for which they have little or no training and were not hired to perform.

Part of your job responsibilities will be to attend regularly scheduled office staff meetings. Most facilities hold regular weekly staff meetings where suggestions, problems, and other important information is discussed. Figure 21-16 shows the health care team gathered to discuss important in-house matters, decisions regarding patient care, in-service scheduling, and other topics at a staff meeting. This is not the time or place to discuss personal problems or requests. It is vital, however, to have private meetings to discuss personal goals, promotion opportunities, pay increase possibilities, educational pursuits, etc.

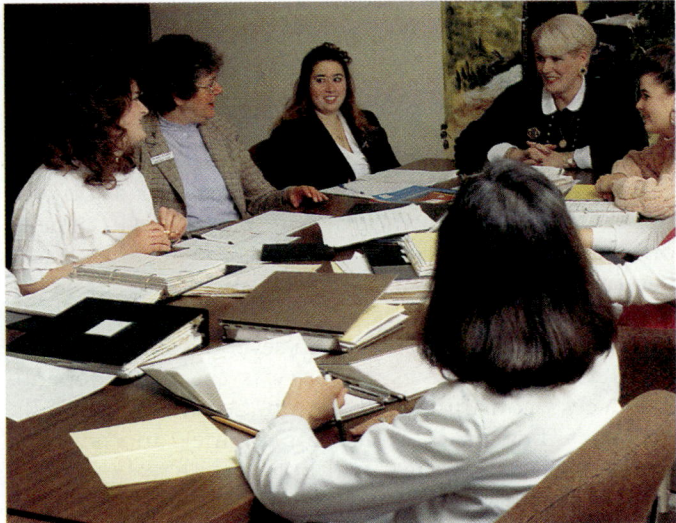

FIGURE 21-16 Attendance of scheduled staff meetings is a vital part of your job.

THE EMPLOYEE EVALUATION AND REVIEW

Most employers require that employees have regular, routine, or periodic reviews or **evaluations** regarding their work performance. The time schedule may vary from place to place, but usually the reviews are held initially every 3 months for the first year and then every 6 months thereafter. Some physicians/employers prefer to have annual reviews scheduled, unless there is a problem or the employee requests it more often. Evaluations should be regarded in a positive light. Some employers may provide you with an evaluation form for you to do your own evaluation. This gives you the opportunity to indicate how you perceive your performance. When you get together with the facility person who is responsible for doing evaluations, you can compare the two and discuss whether and where you have a difference of perception. It may sound easy, but it is very difficult to do a self-evaluation. If you feel you do well, you may hesitate to say so for fear it will be interpreted as bragging. If you realize a problem, you don't know whether to list it or not because it might not be as you perceive it.

Evaluations are generally conducted by the supervisor, the office manager of the facility, and sometimes by the physician-employer. Whoever holds this meeting with the employee offers insightful observations about the person. This is done to point out both positive and negative areas of which the employee may or may not be aware. The review, or evaluation as it is also referred to, is meant for both employer and employee to have just this opportunity. Your supervisor or evaluator may use a form similar to the one shown in Figure 21-17. Usually it will be completed and then offered to you to read. You should be asked to sign it at the bottom, indicating that you have read, discussed, and understood the rating on the form. You may request a copy if it is not offered. The original will remain in your employee record and be filed with all of the other documents pertaining to your employment. It is a good idea to study the form and note the rating scale. If you take the review seriously and with an open mind, you will most likely find out some good points and sometimes a couple of negative things about yourself that you may not have realized before. Try to improve on the negative things (e.g., poor attendance, poor grammar, appearance) before the next review. Showing improvement immediately and continuing on with the improvement will make good points on the next review. If you show a poor attitude, it will only make matters worse. Remember that the supervisor's job responsibilities require that this evaluation be performed. You should not take the suggestions or reprimands as personal insults, but as opportunities to improve.

Employee s name _____ Job title/position _____ Date hired _____

Supervisor _____ Title _____ Date of evaluation _____

Scheduled evaluation/review: ___Initial ___3 month ___6 month ___annual ___*other

*Explain _____

Previous review date _____ Rating _____

Comments _____

Total days/times: absent_____ Tardy_____ Left early_____

Rate the following areas of the employee appropriately using the scale from 1 to 10:
            1   2   3   4   5   6   7   8   9   10

Job knowledge: very little / limited / adequate / average / good / superior / outstanding ____

Quality of work: very poor / fair / good / acceptable / excellent / superior / outstanding ____

Quantity of work: inferior/ inadequate/ does just enough/ average/superior/outstanding ____

Speed: very slow / below average / average / above average / outstanding ____

Initiative: lacking / needs pushing / adequate / good / excellent / outstanding ____

Judgment: poor / unreliable / limited / reliable / superior / outstanding ____

Cooperation: very uncooperative / difficult / cooperative / excellent / outstanding ____

Adaptability: poor / slow / satisfactory / good / excellent / superior / outstanding ____

Appearance: poor/unprofessional/avg/reluctantly complies with dress code/outstanding____

Attendance: poor / average / good / excellent / superior / outstanding ____
                                                   Total ____

Since last evaluation the employee has:
____improved ____made no noticeable change ____regressed
Recommendation for pay raise: ____Yes ____No
Overall impression:
____unsatisfactory ____fair ____satisfactory ____excellent ____outstanding
Comments of employee's strengths and weaknesses:_____

Supervisor's signature_____
Employee's signature_____

FIGURE 21-17 An example of an employee evaluation form, which employers may use in documenting employment progress

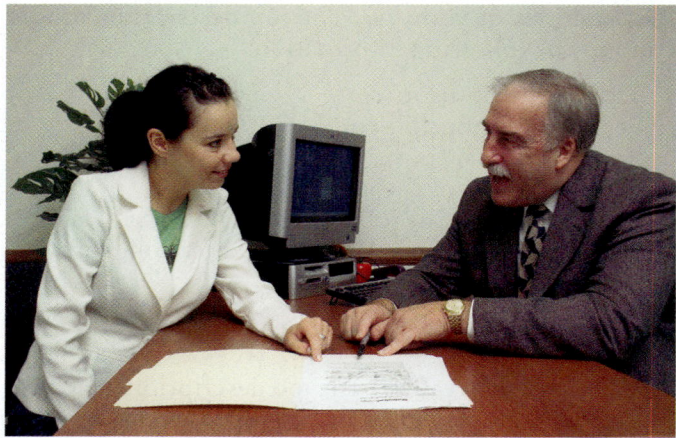

FIGURE 21-18 Employer discussing evaluation in an open communication manner

cusing and calm and discuss the problem. Chances are it may be a misunderstanding that can easily be talked out. Open dialogue and clear communication works wonders and leads to a better working relationship between you and your employer (Figure 21-18). Many positive results are achieved from reviews for both employee and employer.

ADVANCEMENT

Progressing in employment is up to you. The desire to advance in your field of choice is the first step to consider. Job satisfaction is also a major issue. If you enjoy your work and find your duties challenging and rewarding, you may want to stay in that position. If your salary meets your needs and you like what you do, staying with that job can be quite fulfilling. However, a motivating factor in moving up into a higher position or even changing jobs is most often for an increase in pay. Note: Cost-of-living raises (given to keep up with the economy) do not reflect one's job performance, but merit raises do. A merit raise is given to those employees who deserve recognition and praise for a job well done. Chances of advancement in your job will depend on several factors. Those employees who are offered better paying positions and positions with more responsibility are the ones who show the greatest interest. Interest can be displayed in several ways. Primarily, the person who shows initiative is the most dependable, seeks continuing education, acquires new skills, exhibits efficiency in a pleasant manner, and communicates well with others will be the first to be considered for a promotion. To move forward to a higher position in your place of employment means that you have been recognized by your employer or supervisor for your efforts, and you are being rewarded with either a raise in pay, a promotion, or both.

The expression "constructive criticism" usually elicits a note of negativity that, even though spoken with good intentions, keeps us from listening to or taking the responsibility for whatever someone is trying to tell us. Usually, weaknesses are brought up and explained as objectively as possible, and suggestions are given for how one could go about changing the behavior or improving the lacking skill. The challenge to improve may be motivated by a reward appropriate to the success of the task. You should use this meeting to your advantage. Let the employer/supervisor know your intentions regarding promotion goals. Ask questions tactfully about all concerns regarding policy, dress code, or whatever else you feel is important. You may ask about or schedule your vacation during this meeting.

Those who have an excellent work performance may be surprised or even insulted that a supervisor would bring up a trivial weakness. Supervisors who see potential in others are obligated to encourage professional growth and development. All of us tend to ask more of those who are good at what they do and further expect the best from them. Employers are no different. This is actually a compliment but is often viewed as demanding and unfair. Try to remain unac-

Continuing Education

Because the medical field in general is always changing and improving in health care technology, it is your responsibility to keep up with these changes. This is necessary if you want to reach peak performance at your job. To do this, you must take advantage of continuing education. This can be done in a variety of ways. Of course, the primary means of obtaining current information is to read. Physicians usually subscribe to several medical news publications that you can read on breaks or at lunch time. Keeping up with the latest in managed health care, new medications, and other newsworthy items is admirable and will be noticed by your employer. It will also help you perform your duties and give you a better appreciation for your role in patient care.

Other ways to better yourself and attain further education is to attend courses related to your area of interest in the medical field at a community college or university. Many night and weekend classes are offered for convenience to those who work during the day. You may want to take a refresher course in medical terminology or anatomy, for instance. Some find a favorite niche, such as medical records, transcription, or laboratory procedures, and realize that to advance in a particular area, additional education and credentialing is necessary. Discussing your goals with your supervisor is certainly advised so that reorganizing your work schedule to allow adequate time for classes can be arranged. The professional organizations AAMA and ARMA specifically address the needs of the medical assistant by offering continuing education programs at national, state, and local levels. Through these programs, there are continuing education units (CEUs) offered for keeping certification status current. There are also educational articles printed in the PMA (*The Professional Medical Assistant*) magazine that offer CEUs. AAMA will also consider CEU approval for educational programs offered by other professional organizations.

In addition, local hospitals offer educational seminars on a variety of topics for health care professionals. They welcome the attendance of those interested in learning more about patient care. You may ask to be put on the mailing list to keep you informed of future program offerings.

A perfect opportunity to inform your supervisor about your involvement in continuing education (if not already known) is during your scheduled evaluation. Employers are very receptive to and impressed by employees who take the initiative in self-improvement and involve themselves in professional organizations that offer continuing education to members. This conveys to the employer that you are interested in advancement and are willing to put forth the additional effort to move forward in your profession. Your involvement in leadership roles within the organization also gives the employer further insight into your appreciation of your career and its importance.

TERMINATING EMPLOYMENT

There are many reasons for a medical assistant to terminate employment—relocation, advancement to a more responsible position, a higher paying job, illness, educational pursuits, pregnancy, or a change in lifestyle. There is, however, a major responsibility that an employee has to an employer; that is giving at least 2 weeks' notice (Figure 21-19). This is done to give the employer time to fill the position that you will vacate. The notice, a letter of resignation, should be directed to your immediate supervisor, your physician-employer, or another appropriate member of the staff, with copies to whoever else is appropriate for your place of employment. The letter should include the date that will be your last working day. Employers appreciate this consideration because it allows for a smoother transition of personnel. There may be time for a new person to be hired to work with you so that you can help in the training and explain your job description in more detail. Often, however, this is not the case, and there is not sufficient time for the person who is leaving to train the new employee. If it is known that termination is evident because of a major move, or whatever the case may be, it is certainly considerate to inform your employer as far in advance as possible to assist in providing a smooth transition of your duties to another competent person. This is another reason to have a complete job description for every employee's position. Even without a former employee to point out duties and responsibilities, the job description should have enough detail to help the new employee perform the job with a minimum amount of difficulties.

Employment can also be terminated by the employer. This can be an unpleasant experience for both employer and employee. The usual cause for termination initiated by the employer is failure of an employee to satisfactorily perform job responsibilities. Deficiencies can include being tardy, high absenteeism, failure to get along with co-workers and patients, poor work habits, undependability, dishonesty, poor attitude, and uncooperativeness. Another reason that the employer may terminate one's employment could be from **irreconcilable** issues caused by personality conflicts. After legitimate efforts to resolve differences have failed, there is often no other recourse but to terminate the employment of the one who cannot, does not, or will not fit in with other staff members.

In some situations, through employer–employee communication, one may be able to ask if it is possible to change the situation from being fired to accepting a letter of resignation. This is mentioned because misunderstandings *do* happen from time to time. Having a

Date

Marlene Blackstone, CMA
Office Manager
Sports Medicine Center
7386 Canyon Road
Anywhere, U.S.A. 10000

Dear Ms. Blackstone:

It is with much regret that I submit this letter as my notice of resignation. My employment over the past five years in sports medicine has been an interesting experience for me. I have learned much in working with such a fine group of professionals. I am grateful for having had this opportunity.

My husband has taken a new position with his company; we are being transferred out of state. I will miss working with everyone at the center. I am giving my two week notice from the date of this letter. My last day will be (insert date).

My thanks to all of you for making my years of employment at the center something that I can look back on with fond memories.

Sincerely,

Patsy J. Keene, RMA

Date

Maxwell S. Mitchell, M.D.
472 Circle Drive
Anywhere, U.S.A. 10000

Dear Dr. Mitchell:

Please accept this as my letter of resignation. During my employment in your practice I have learned a great deal, and I have greatly enjoyed working for you. However, (at this point the writer may choose to add a sentence or two elaborating on the specific reason for leaving).

My X years of employment with you have been a valuable experience for me; thank you for the opportunity to work and learn.

In accordance with your personnel regulations, this letter is my two week notice; my last day in the office will be (at least two weeks hence).

Sincerely,

Your name and title or position with your signature

FIGURE 21-19 Sample letters of resignation

poor work record is something that could follow a person and make it difficult to get another job in the future.

It is much better to resign from a position than to be terminated. If your employer will accept a resignation, thank him or her sincerely and write your resignation effective for whatever date is decided—immediately or in 1 or 2 weeks.

EMPLOYEE RECORDS

When a new employee is hired, a file is established to keep all pertinent information regarding that person throughout their employment. It should be kept in strict confidence. The employee's record is kept private, just as a patient's record. The employment application form, resumé, reference letters, signed contract, tax forms, signed documents regarding compliance with OSHA/CLIA regulations and office policies, and any other relevant information must be placed in this file in case there is a reason for the employer or the employee to refer to any of the filed information in the future. Dates of an employee's vacation, regularly scheduled day off, evaluations, incident/accident reports, reprimands/warnings, and all other relevant information must be filed or recorded. Employees have the right to request a copy of any documents contained in their file.

A formal written request signed by the employee is advised to obtain quick reply. Employees also have the right to request a conference with the employer or supervisor as needed to discuss concerns. Again, it is best to put all requests in writing to make it a matter of record and obtain a faster response.

SUMMARY

Employers in medical practice have begun to realize the worth of trained medical assistants. Certified medical assistants (CMAs) or registered medical assistants (RMAs) are usually considered for employment over untrained applicants. In some managed care employment contracts, it may require that only CMAs or RMAs be hired. Currently, this is true in some states more than in others. Certification is becoming a requirement for employment in medical practice as regulations tighten. Keeping yourself up-to-date by attending continuing education programs, seminars, meetings, and other informative ways will make you a valued employee. By opting to become certified or registered, you will demonstrate that you are competent in basic entry-level skills. Further, you will demonstrate to a prospective employer that you have pride in the profession and in your professional skills.

A FINAL NOTE

Throughout this chapter, much emphasis has been directed toward securing and maintaining employment. Although it may seem to you that employers ask the impossible as you review their expectations, you must keep in mind that an employee is paid for work performed. Gainful employment is a mutually agreed to contract that is either written or implied. To assist you in gaining a better understanding of why employers have such expectations, you may find it interesting to know how and where they originated.

The concept of the "work ethic" originated from the 16th century's Protestant Ethic. During this period, work was considered a sacred task, and success in one's work was a sign of divine grace. One was looked down on by society in general if one was thought to have moral flaws, such as being lazy, having no ambition, or other undesirable characteristics. Essentially this ideal has not changed. The work ethics of today are basically the same as the original with some minor changes. The word *responsible* can be substituted for sacred. And being a success in one's work is a sign of *ambition, hard work, and perseverance*. These expectations are fair, realistic, and sensible. It simply means that one should give an honest day's work for an honest day's wage. Taking the responsibility of providing for oneself financially usually makes most people aware that it is necessary to keep a job. Being a part of the health care team means that health care workers also have to be team players!

Our best wishes for your successful and rewarding career in medical assisting!

ACHIEVE UNIT OBJECTIVES

- ■ **Complete the Workbook activities to meet the learning objectives.**
- ■ **Practice the procedures in this unit to meet the performance objectives.**
- ■ **Apply your knowledge at the end of this chapter in completing the Critical Thinking Challenge and Activities, as well as the StudyWARE on your Student CD-ROM.**

CRITICAL THINKING CHALLENGE

IMPACTING THE PATIENT, THE PRACTICE, AND YOUR CAREER

Steven was one of five applicants for a clinical position with Dr. Sells. He had just finished his training and an externship and was eager to get a job. The other applicants had some training and two had work experience, one as an administrative assistant and another as a phlebotomist. Steven had indicated on his resumé and in his interview that he had a lot of experience with drawing blood and doing ECGs as well as the usual clinical skills. He realized he needed to have something more than the others to get the position. In reality, his phlebotomy experience was limited to the training arm in the classroom and about five blood draws during his externship. He had done a few ECGs on classmates, but only two while at the clinic. He thought he knew enough to get by, and he needed the job so he could pay his bills.

QUESTIONS

1. How might Steven's less-than-honest assessment of his competencies affect a patient?
2. How might his statements affect the practice?
3. How could his actions affect his career?

ACTIVITIES

1. Go online and search for resumé samples. See if you can find a site that has information for health occupations.

2. After you and a partner have completed employment applications, role play conducting an interview for each other.

3. Make a performance evaluation for a partner and conduct a performance review.

4. Write an interview follow-up letter for a clinical assistant position.

StudyWARE™ CHALLENGE

- Study with the flash cards for Chapter 21 to review the key terms in this chapter.
- Solve the crossword puzzle for Chapter 21.
- Complete the true/false quiz in test mode for Chapter 21.

RESOURCES

Nolan, S. (2006, February). Resumes. *The Columbus Dispatch*, Classified Section.

Purdue University, Online Writing Lab. (2001). *Resume Styles*. Retrieved January 31, 2007, from http://owl.english.purdue.edu/handouts/pw/p_yrestyles.html.

University of Minnesota, Office of Human Resources. (n.d.). *Resume Tutor: Choosing a format*. Retrieved January 31, 2007, from www1.umn.edu/ohr/careerdev/resources/resume/format.html.

WEB LINKS

www.careerbuilder.com (CareerBuilder.com)
Job interview tips.

www.job-interview-helper.com (Job Interview Helper)
Job interview tips.

www.jobmedicalsupport.com (Job Science.com)
Provides information on searching for a medical assisting job through the Internet.

www.usawebpages.com (Mission of World Wide Webpages Corporation)
Maintains a world wide web directory that allows you to locate business webpages by geographic location and category.

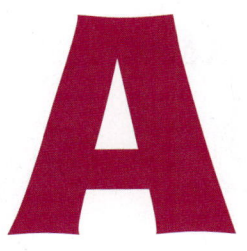

Medical Assistant Role Delineation Chart

ADMINISTRATIVE

ADMINISTRATIVE PROCEDURES

- Perform basic clerical functions
- Schedule, coordinate, and monitor appointments
- Schedule inpatient/outpatient admissions and procedures
- Understand and apply third-party guidelines
- Obtain reimbursement through accurate claims submission
- Monitor third-party reimbursement
- Perform medical transcription
- Understand and adhere to managed care policies and procedures
- *Negotiate managed care contracts (adv)*

PRACTICE FINANCES

- Perform procedural and diagnostic coding
- Apply bookkeeping principles
- Document and maintain accounting and banking records
- Manage accounts receivable
- Manage accounts payable
- Process payroll
- *Develop and maintain fee schedules (adv)*
- *Manage renewals of business and professional insurance policies (adv)*
- *Manage personnel benefits and maintain records (adv)*

CLINICAL

FUNDAMENTAL PRINCIPLES

- Apply principles of aseptic technique and infection control
- Comply with quality assurance practices
- Screen and follow up patient test results

DIAGNOSTIC ORDERS

- Collect and process specimens
- Perform diagnostic tests

PATIENT CARE

- Adhere to established triage procedures
- Obtain patient history and vital signs
- Prepare and maintain examination and treatment areas
- Prepare patient for examinations, procedures, and treatments
- Assist with examinations, procedures, and treatments
- Prepare and administer medications and immunizations
- Maintain medication and immunization records
- Recognize and respond to emergencies
- Coordinate patient care information with other health care providers

GENERAL (TRANSDISCIPLINARY)

PROFESSIONALISM

- Project a professional manner and image
- Adhere to ethical principles
- Demonstrate initiative and responsibility
- Work as a team member
- Manage time effectively
- Prioritize and perform multiple tasks
- Adapt to change
- Promote the CMA credential
- Enhance skills through continuing education

COMMUNICATION SKILLS

- Treat all patients with compassion and empathy
- Recognize and respect cultural diversity
- Adapt communications to individual's ability to understand
- Use professional telephone technique
- Use effective and correct verbal and written communications
- Recognize and respond to verbal and nonverbal communications
- Use medical terminology appropriately
- Receive, organize, prioritize, and transmit information
- Serve as liaison
- Promote the practice through positive public relations

LEGAL CONCEPTS

- Maintain confidentiality
- Practice within the scope of education, training, and personal capabilities
- Prepare and maintain medical records
- Document accurately
- Use appropriate guidelines when releasing information
- Follow employer's established policies dealing with the health care contract
- Follow federal, state, and local legal guidelines
- Maintain awareness of federal and state health care legislation and regulations
- Maintain and dispose of regulated substances in compliance with government guidelines
- Comply with established risk management and safety procedures
- Recognize professional credentialing criteria
- Participate in the development and maintenance of personnel, policy, and procedure manuals
- *Develop and maintain personnel, policy, and procedure manuals (adv)*

INSTRUCTION

- Instruct individuals according to their needs
- Explain office policies and procedures
- Teach methods of health promotion and disease prevention
- Locate community resources and disseminate information
- *Orient and train personnel (adv)*
- *Develop educational materials (adv)*
- *Conduct continuing education activities (adv)*

OPERATIONAL FUNCTIONS

- Maintain supply inventory
- Evaluate and recommend equipment and supplies
- Apply computer techniques to support office operations
- *Supervise personnel (adv)*
- *Interview and recommend job applicants (adv)*
- *Negotiate leases and prices for equipment and supply contracts (adv)*

*Denotes advanced skills.

Reprinted with permission of the American Association of Medical Assistants.

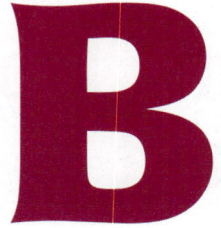

Certified Medical Assistant (CMA) Certification Examination Outline

I. A–F General
  A. Medical Terminology
    1. Word building and definitions
    2. Uses of terminology
  B. Anatomy and Physiology
    1. Body as a whole, including multiple systems
    2. Systems, including structure, function, related conditions, and diseases
  C. Psychology
    1. Basic principles
    2. Developmental stages of the life cycle
    3. Hereditary, cultural, and environmental influences on behavior
    4. Defense mechanisms
  D. Professionalism
    1. Displaying professional attitude
    2. Job readiness and seeking employment
    3. Performing within ethical boundaries
    4. Maintaining confidentiality
    5. Working as a team member to achieve goals
  E. Communication
    1. Adapting communication to an individual's ability to understand (e.g., patients with special needs)
    2. Recognizing and responding to verbal and nonverbal communication
    3. Patient instruction
    4. Professional communication and behavior
    5. Evaluating and understanding communication
    6. Interviewing techniques
    7. Receiving, organizing, prioritizing, and transmitting information
    8. Telephone techniques
    9. Fundamental writing skills
  F. Medicolegal Guidelines and Requirements
    1. Licenses and accreditation
    2. Legislation
    3. Documentation/reporting
    4. Releasing medical information
    5. Physician-patient relationship

II. G–Q Administrative
  G. Data Entry
    1. Keyboard fundamentals and functions
    2. Formats
    3. Proofreading
  H. Equipment
    1. Equipment operation
    2. Maintenance and repairs
  I. Computer Concepts
    1. Computer components
    2. Care and maintenance of computer
    3. Computer applications
    4. Internet services
  J. Records Management
    1. Needs, purposes, and terminology of filing systems
    2. Process for filing documents
    3. Organization of patient's medical record
    4. Filing guidelines
    5. Medical records
  K. Screening and Processing Mail
    1. U.S. Postal Service
    2. Private services
    3. Postal machine/meter
    4. Processing incoming mail
    5. Preparing outgoing mail
  L. Scheduling and Monitoring Appointments
    1. Utilizing appointment schedules/types
    2. Appointment guidelines
    3. Appointment protocol
  M. Resource Information and Community Services
    1. Services available
    2. Appropriate referrals
    3. Follow-up
    4. Patient advocate
  N. Managing Physician's Professional Schedule and Travel
    1. Arranging meetings (e.g., dates, facilities, accommodations)
    2. Scheduling travel

3. Integrating meetings and travel with office schedule

O. Managing the Office
   1. Maintaining the physical plant
   2. Equipment and supply inventory
   3. Maintaining liability coverage
   4. Time management

P. Office Policies and Procedures
   1. Patient information booklet
   2. Patient education
   3. Instructions for patients with special needs
   4. Personnel manual
   5. Policy and procedures manuals/protocols
   6. Compliance plan

Q. Managing Practice Finances
   1. Bookkeeping systems (e.g., single, double entry, pegboard, computer)
   2. Coding systems
   3. Third-party billing
   4. Accounting and banking procedures
   5. Employee payroll

III. R–Z Clinical

R. Principles of Infection Control
   1. Principles of asepsis
   2. Aseptic technique
   3. Disposal of biohazardous material
   4. Practice Standard Precautions

S. Treatment Area
   1. Equipment preparation and operation
   2. Principles of operation
   3. Restocking supplies
   4. Preparing/maintaining treatment areas
   5. Safety precautions

T. Patient Preparation and Assisting the Physician
   1. Performing telephone and in-person screening
   2. Vital signs
   3. Examinations
   4. Procedures
   5. Explanation and instructions
   6. Instruments, supplies, and equipment

U. Patient History Interview
   1. Components of patient history
   2. Documentation guidelines

V. Collecting and Processing Specimens; Diagnostic Testing
   1. Methods of collection
   2. Processing specimens
   3. Quality control
   4. Performing selected tests
   5. Vision testing
   6. Hearing testing
   7. Respiratory testing
   8. Medical imaging

W. Preparing and Administering Medications
   1. Pharmacology
   2. Preparing and administering oral and parenteral medications
   3. Prescriptions
   4. Maintaining medication and immunization records
   5. Medication disposal
   6. Principles of IV therapy

X. Emergencies
   1. Preplanned action
   2. Assessment and triage

Y. First Aid
   1. Establishing and maintaining an airway
   2. Identifying and responding to:
      a. Bleeding/pressure points
      b. Burns
      c. Cardiac and respiratory arrest/CPR
      d. Choking/Heimlich maneuver
      e. Diabetic coma/insulin shock
      f. Fractures
      g. Poisoning
      h. Seizures
      i. Shock
      j. Syncope
      k. Wounds
   3. Signs and symptoms
   4. Management

Z. Nutrition
   1. Basic principles
   2. Special needs

Reprinted courtesy of the American Association of Medical Assistants. For more information about the CMA exam, visit www.aama-ntl.org.

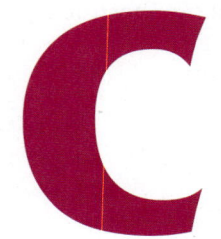

Registered Medical Assistant (RMA) Certification Examination Outline

I. General Medical Assisting Knowledge
   A. Anatomy and Physiology
      1. Body system structure and function
      2. Disorders and diseases
   B. Medical Terminology
      1. Word parts
      2. Definitions
      3. Common abbreviations and symbols
      4. Spelling
   C. Medical Law
      1. Medical law
      2. Licensure, certification, and registration
      3. Terminology
   D. Medical Ethics
      1. Principles of medical ethics
      2. Ethical conduct
   E. Human Relations
      1. Patient relations
      2. Interpersonal relations
   F. Patient Education
      1. Patient instruction
      2. Patient resource materials
      3. Documentation

II. Administrative Medical Assisting
   A. Insurance
      1. Terminology
      2. Plans
      3. Claims
      4. Coding
      5. Insurance finance applications
   B. Finance and Bookkeeping
      1. Terminology
      2. Patient billing
      3. Collections
      4. Fundamental medical office accounting procedures
      5. Banking procedures
      6. Employee payroll
      7. Financial mathematics
   C. Medical Receptionist/Secretarial/Clerical
      1. Terminology
      2. Reception
      3. Scheduling
      4. Oral and written communication
      5. Records and chart management
      6. Transcription and dictation
      7. Supplies and equipment management
      8. Computer applications
      9. Office safety

III. Clinical Medical Assisting
   A. Asepsis
      1. Terminology
      2. Bloodborne pathogens and Universal Precautions
      3. Medical asepsis
      4. Surgical asepsis
   B. Sterilization
      1. Terminology
      2. Sanitization
      3. Disinfection
      4. Sterilization
      5. Recordkeeping
   C. Instruments
      1. Identification
      2. Usage
      3. Care and handling
   D. Vital Signs and Mensurations
      1. Terminology
      2. Blood pressure
      3. Pulse
      4. Respiration
      5. Temperature
      6. Mensurations
   E. Physical Examinations
      1. Medical history
      2. Patient positioning
      3. Methods of examination
      4. Specialty examinations
      5. Visual acuity
      6. Allergy
      7. Terminology
   F. Clinical Pharmacology
      1. Terminology
      2. Parenteral medications

3. Prescriptions
4. Drugs

G. Minor Surgery
   1. Surgical supplies
   2. Surgical procedures

H. Therapeutic Modalities
   1. Modalities
   2. Alternative therapies

I. Laboratory Procedures
   1. Safety
   2. CLIA '88
   3. Quality control program
   4. Laboratory equipment

5. Laboratory testing
6. Terminology

J. Electrocardiography
   1. Standard, 12-lead ECG
   2. Mounting techniques
   3. Other ECG procedures

K. First Aid
   1. First aid procedures
   2. Legal responsibilities

Reprinted courtesy of the American Medical Technologists. For more information about the RMA exam, visit www.amt1.com.

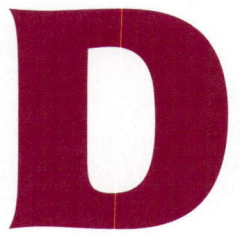

Certified Medical Administrative Specialist (CMAS) Certification Examination Outline

I. Medical Assisting Foundations
   A. Medical Terminology
   B. Anatomy and Physiology
   C. Legal and Ethical Considerations
   D. Professionalism
II. Basic Clinical Medical Office Assisting
   A. Basic Health History Interview
   B. Basic Charting
   C. Vital Signs and Measurements
   D. Asepsis in the Medical Office
   E. Examination Preparation
   F. Medical Office Emergencies
   G. Pharmacology
III. Medical Office Clerical Assisting
   A. Appointment Management and Scheduling
   B. Reception
   C. Communication
   D. Patient Information and Community Resources
IV. Medical Records Management
   A. Systems
   B. Procedures
   C. Confidentiality
V. Health Care Insurance Processing, Coding, and Billing
   A. Insurance Processing
   B. Coding
   C. Insurance Billing and Finances

VI. Medical Office Financial Management
   A. Fundamental Financial Management
   B. Patient Accounts
   C. Banking
   D. Payroll
VII. Medical Office Information Processing
   A. Fundamentals of Computing
   B. Medical Office Computer Applications
VIII. Medical Office Management*
   A. Office Communications*
   B. Business Organization Management*
   C. Human Resources*
   D. Safety
   E. Supplies and Equipment
   F. Physical Office Plant
   G. Risk Management and Quality Assurance

Note: Asterisked areas addressed by the Medical Office Management job function may or may not be performed by the Certified Medical Administrative Specialist at entry-level practice. Nevertheless, the competent Specialist should have sound knowledge of these management functions at certification level.

Reprinted courtesy of the American Medical Technologists. For more information about the CMAS exam, visit www.amt1.com.

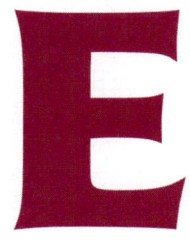

Measurements and Abbreviations

CONVERTING MEASUREMENTS

LENGTH	Centimeters	Inches	Feet
1 centimeter	1.000	0.394	0.0328
1 inch	2.54	1.000	0.0833
1 foot	30.48	12.000	1.000
1 yard	91.4	36.00	3.00
1 meter	100.00	39.40	3.28

Inches

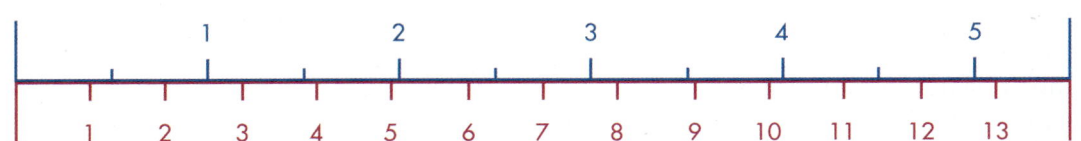

Centimeters

Comparison of Centimeters and Inches

VOLUMES	Cubic Centimeters	Fluid Drams	Fluid Ounces	Quarts	Liters
1 cubic centimeter	1.00	0.270	0.033	0.0010	0.0010
1 fluid dram	3.70	1.00	0.125	0.0039	0.0037
1 cubic inch	16.39	4.43	0.554	0.0173	0.0163
1 fluid ounce	29.6	8.00	1.000	0.0312	0.0296
1 quart	946.0	255.0	32.00	1.000	0.946
1 liter	1000.0	270.0	33.80	1.056	1.000

WEIGHTS	Grains	Grams	Apothecary Ounces	Pounds
1 grain (gr)	1.000	0.064	0.002	0.0001
1 gram (gm)	15.43	1.000	0.032	0.0022
1 apothecary ounce	480.00	31.1	1.000	0.0685
1 pound	7000.00	454.0	14.58	1.000
1 kilogram	15432.0	1000.00	32.15	2.205

RULES FOR CONVERTING ONE SYSTEM TO ANOTHER

Volumes

Grains to grams—divide by 15
Drams to cubic centimeters—multiply by 4
Ounces to cubic centimeters—multiply by 30
Minims to cubic millimeters—multiply by 63
Minims to cubic centimeters—multiply by 0.06
Cubic millimeters to minims—divide by 63
Cubic centimeters to minims—multiply by 16
Cubic centimeters to fluid ounces—divide by 30
Liters to pints—divide by 2.1

Weights

Milligrams to grains—multiply by 0.0154
Grams to grains—multiply by 15
Grams to drams—multiply by 0.257
Grams to ounces—multiply by 0.0311

Temperature

Multiply centigrade (Celsius) degrees by $\frac{9}{5}$ and add 32 to convert Fahrenheit to Celsius.
Subtract 32 from the Fahrenheit degrees and multiply by $\frac{5}{9}$ to convert Celsius to Fahrenheit.

COMMON HOUSEHOLD MEASURES AND WEIGHTS

1 teaspoon	= 4–5 cc. or 1 dram
3 teaspoons	= 1 tablespoon
1 dessert spoon	= 8 cc. or 2 drams
1 tablespoon	= 15 cc. or 3 drams
4 tablespoons	= 1 wine glass or ½ gill
16 tablespoons (liq)	= 1 cup
12 tablespoons (dry)	= 1 cup
1 cup	= 8 fluid ounces or ½ pint
1 tumbler or glass	= 8 fluid ounces or 240 cc.
1 wine glass	= 2 fluid ounces, 60 cc.
16 fluid ounces	= 1 pound
4 gills	= 1 pound
1 pint	= 1 pound

MEDICAL SYMBOLS

℥	ounce	′	foot, minute
O	pint	″	inch, second
#	pound, number	$\overline{aa}$	equal parts
℞	recipe, prescription	°	degree
		%	percent

♂	male	×	multiply
♀	female	÷	divide
$\overline{s}$	without	=	equals
$\overline{c}$	with	∞	infinity
—	minus, negative, alkaline reaction	↑	increase
		↓	decrease

ABBREVIATIONS

a, aa	of each
abd	abdomen
a.c.	before meals
ad lib	as desired
A & P	anterior and posterior
aq	aqueous, water
BE, ba.en.	barium enema
blf	black female
bib	drink
b.i.d., BID	twice a day
bm, BM	bowel movement
blm	black male
BP, B/P	blood pressure
BUN	blood urea nitrogen
$\overline{c}$	with
C	centrigrade
Ca	calcium
cap	capsule
CBC	complete blood count
CC	chief complaint
CCU	coronary care unit
CHF	congestive heart failure
cm^3	cubic centimeter
CNS	central nervous system
c/o	complains of
CO_2	carbon dioxide
comp	compound
COPD	chronic obstructive pulmonary disease
CPR	cardiopulmonary resuscitation
CSF	cerebrospinal fluid
CVA	cerebrovascular accident
cysto	cystoscopy
D & C	dilatation and curettage
Dil, dil	dilute
DOA	dead on arrival
DPT	diphtheria, pertussis, tetanus
dr.	dram
dx, Dx	diagnosis
ECG	electrocardiogram
EEG	electroencephalogram
EENT	eye, ear, nose, throat
EKG	electrocardiogram

elix	elixir	NB	newborn
ER	emergency room	NKA	no known allergies
et	and	no.	number
expl lap	exploratory laparotomy	noxt.	at night
ext.	extract	NPO	nothing by mouth
		N & V	nausea and vomiting
F	fahrenheit		
F	female	O	pint
FBS	fasting blood sugar	OB	obstetrics
FH	family history	OD	overdose
fl	fluid	OP	outpatient
fl. dr.	fluid dram	OR	operating room
fl. oz.	fluid ounce	os	mouth
Fx	fracture	oz	ounce
GB	gallbladder	Path	pathology
GI	gastrointestinal	PBI	protein bound iodine
Gm	gram	p.c.	after meals
GP	general practitioner	Peds	pediatrics
gr	grain	per	through, by
gtt, Gtt, gtts	drop, drops	PID	pelvic inflammatory disease
GU	genitourinary	PKU	phenylketonuria
GYN	gynecology	PO, p.o.	by mouth
		prn	as desired, needed
H, h	hour	pro time	prothrombin time
HCL	hydrochloric acid	Psych	psychiatry
Hgb	hemoglobin	pt	patient, pint
HPI	history present illness	pulv	powder
Hx	history	Px	physical examination
hypo	hypodermic, under		
		q	every
ICU	intensive care unit	q 4 h	every 4 hours
I & D	incision and drainage	qh	every hour
IM	intramuscular	q.i.d., QID	four times a day
inj	injection	qns	quantity not sufficient
I & O	intake and output	qs	quantity sufficient
IPPB	intermittent positive pressure breathing	qt	quart
IT	inhalation therapy		
IUD	intrauterine device	R	right
IV	intravenous	Ra	radium
IVP	intravenous pyelogram	RBC	red blood cells
		REM	rapid eye movement
k	potassium	rep	let it be repeated
KUB	kidney, ureter, and bladder	R/O	rule out
		ROM	range of motion
L, lb	pound	ROS	review of systems
lat	lateral	Rx	prescription, take
liq	liquid		
LLQ	left lower quadrant	s̄	without
LMP	last menstrual period	sig	instructions, directions
LUQ	left upper quadrant	SOB	short of breath
		sol	solution
m	minim	solv	dissolve
M	male	s.o.s.	distress signal
mm	millimeter	sp. gr.	specific gravity
MS	multiple sclerosis	stat	immediately
		syr.	syrup

T	temperature
T & A	tonsilectomy and adenoidectomy
tab	tablet
TIA	transient ischemic attack
t.i.d.	three times a day
tinct.	tincture
TPR	temperature, pulse, respiration
TUR	transurethral resection
UA	urinalysis
ung.	ointment
URI	upper respiratory infection
UTI	urinary tract infection
VD	venereal disease
vin	wine
VS	vital signs
WBC	white blood cells
WF	white female
WM	white male
WNL	within normal limits
wt., Wt.	weight

DO NOT USE ABBREVIATIONS

The use of some medical abbreviations has resulted in medication errors due to their ambiguous nature. In 2004 a "Do Not Use" list of abbreviations was issued by the Joint Commission on Accreditation of Healthcare Organizations as a national patient safety goal. The list contained abbreviations, symbols, and dose designations that had been frequently misinterpreted and involved harmful medication errors. It was determined these should *never* be used in medical communication. You can find this list by going to the Joint Commission's web site, www.jointcommission.org and searching for "do not use list."

In addition to the abbreviations identified by the Joint Commission, the Institute for Safe Medication Practices (ISMP) and the U.S. Food and Drug Administration (FDA) have started a campaign to eliminate additional abbreviations in order to prevent medication errors. The list was compiled from errors reported to the USP-ISMP Medication Error Reporting Program. You can find the list below by going to ISMP's web site, www.ismp.org, and searching for "error-prone abbreviations."

ISMP's List of *Error-Prone Abbreviations, Symbols,* and *Dose Designations*

The abbreviations, symbols, and dose designations found in this table have been reported to ISMP through the USP-ISMP Medication Error Reporting Program as being frequently misinterpreted and involved in harmful medication errors. They should NEVER be used when communicating medical information. This includes internal communications, telephone/verbal prescription, computer-generated labels, labels for drug storage bins, medication administration records, as well as pharmacy and prescriber computer order entry screens.

The Joint Commission on Accreditation of Healthcare Organizations (JCAHO) has established a National Patient Safety Goal that specifies that certain abbreviations must appear on an accredited organization's do-not-use list; we have highlighted these items with a double asterisk (**). However, we hope that you will consider others beyond the minimum JCAHO requirements. By using and promoting safe practices and by educating one another about hazards, we can better protect our patients.

Abbreviations	Intended Meaning	Misinterpretation	Correction
µg	Microgram	Mistaken as "mg"	Use "mcg"
AD, AS, AU	Right ear, left ear, each ear	Mistaken as OD, OS, OU (right eye, left eye, each eye)	Use "right ear," "left ear," or "each ear"
OD, OS, OU	Right eye, left eye, each eye	Mistaken as AD, AS, AU (right ear, left ear, each ear)	Use "right eye," "left eye," or "each eye"
BT	Bedtime	Mistaken as "BID" (twice daily)	Use "bedtime"
cc	Cubic centimeters	Mistaken as "u" (units)	Use "mL"
D/C	Discharge or discontinue	Premature discontinuation of medications if D/C (intended to mean "discharge") has been misinterpreted as "discontinued" when followed by a list of discharge medications	Use "discharge" and "discontinue"
IJ	Injection	Mistaken as "IV" or "intrajugular"	Use "injection"
IN	Intranasal	Mistaken as "IM" or "IV"	Use "intranasal" or "NAS"
HS	Half-strength	Mistaken as bedtime	Use "half-strength" or "bedtime"
hs	At bedtime, hours of sleep	Mistaken as half-strength	
IU**	International unit	Mistaken as IV (intravenous) or 10 (ten)	Use "units"
o.d. or OD	Once daily	Mistaken as "right eye" (OD-oculus dexter), leading to oral liquid medications administered in the eye	Use "daily"
OJ	Orange juice	Mistaken as OD or OS (right or left eye); drugs meant to be diluted in orange juice may be given in the eye	Use "orange juice"
Per os	By mouth, orally	The "os" can be mistaken as "left eye" (OS-oculus sinister)	Use "PO," "by mouth," or "orally"
q.d. or QD**	Every day	Mistaken as q.i.d., especially if the period after the "q" or the tail of the "q" is misunderstood as an "i"	Use "daily"
qhs	At bedtime	Mistaken as "qhr" or every hour	Use "at bedtime"
qn	Nightly	Mistaken as "qh" (every hour)	Use "nightly"
q.o.d. or QOD**	Every other day	Mistaken as "q.d." (daily) or "q.i.d. (four times daily) if the "o" is poorly written	Use "every other day"
q1d	Daily	Mistaken as q.i.d. (four times daily)	Use "daily"
q6PM, etc.	Every evening at 6 PM	Mistaken as every 6 hours	Use "6 PM nightly" or "6 PM daily"
SC, SQ, sub q	Subcutaneous	SC mistaken as SL (sublingual); SQ mistaken as "5 every;" the "q" in "sub q" has been mistaken as "every" (e.g., a heparin dose ordered "sub q 2 hours before surgery" misunderstood as every 2 hours before surgery)	Use "subcut" or "subcutaneously"
ss	Sliding scale (insulin) or ½ (apothecary)	Mistaken as "55"	Spell out "sliding scale;" use "one-half" or "½"
SSRI	Sliding scale regular insulin	Mistaken as selective-serotonin reuptake inhibitor	Spell out "sliding scale (insulin)"
SSI	Sliding scale insulin	Mistaken as Strong Solution of Iodine (Lugol's)	
1/d	One daily	Mistaken as "tid"	Use "1 daily"
TIW or tiw	3 times a week	Mistaken as "3 times a day" or "twice in a week"	Use "3 times weekly"
U or u**	Unit	Mistaken as the number 0 or 4, causing a 10-fold overdose or greater (e.g., 4U seen as "40" or 4u seen as "44"); mistaken as "cc" so dose given in volume instead of units (e.g., 4u seen as 4cc)	Use "unit"

Dose Designations and Other Information	Intended Meaning	Misinterpretation	Correction
Trailing zero after decimal point (e.g., 1.0 mg)**	1 mg	Mistaken as 10 mg if the decimal point is not seen	Do not use trailing zeros for doses expressed in whole numbers
No leading zero before a decimal dose (e.g., .5 mg)**	0.5 mg	Mistaken as 5 mg if the decimal point is not seen	Use zero before a decimal point when the dose is less than a whole unit

Courtesy of the Institute for Safe Medication Practices, www.ismp.org. Reprinted with permission.

Dose Designations and Other Information	Intended Meaning	Misinterpretation	Correction
Drug name and dose run together (especially problematic for drug names that end in "L" such as Inderal40 mg; Tegretol300 mg)	Inderal 40 mg Tegretol 300 mg	Mistaken as Inderal 140 mg Mistaken as Tegretol 1300 mg	Place adequate space between the drug name, dose, and unit of measure
Numerical dose and unit of measure run together (e.g., 10mg, 100mL)	10 mg 100 mL	The "m" is sometimes mistaken as a zero or two zeros, risking a 10- to 100-fold overdose	Place adequate space between the dose and unit of measure
Abbreviations such as mg. or mL. with a period following the abbreviation	mg mL	The period is unnecessary and could be mistaken as the number 1 if written poorly	Use mg, mL, etc. without a terminal period
Large doses without properly placed commas (e.g., 100000 units; 1000000 units)	100,000 units 1,000,000 units	100000 has been mistaken as 10,000 or 1,000,000; 1000000 has been mistaken as 100,000	Use commas for dosing units at or above 1,000, or use words such as 100 "thousand" or 1 "million" to improve readability

Drug Name Abbreviations	Intended Meaning	Misinterpretation	Correction
ARA A	vidarabine	Mistaken as cytarabine (ARA C)	Use complete drug name
AZT	zidovudine (Retrovir)	Mistaken as azathioprine or aztreonam	Use complete drug name
CPZ	Compazine (prochlorperazine)	Mistaken as chlorpromazine	Use complete drug name
DPT	Demerol-Phenergan-Thorazine	Mistaken as diphtheria-pertussis-tetanus (vaccine)	Use complete drug name
DTO	Diluted tincture of opium, or deodorized tincture of opium (Paregoric)	Mistaken as tincture of opium	Use complete drug name
HCl	hydrochloric acid or hydrochloride	Mistaken as potassium chloride (The "H" is misinterpreted as "K")	Use complete drug name unless expressed as a salt of a drug
HCT	hydrocortisone	Mistaken as hydrochlorothiazide	Use complete drug name
HCTZ	hydrochlorothiazide	Mistaken as hydrocortisone (seen as HCT250 mg)	Use complete drug name
MgSO4**	magnesium sulfate	Mistaken as morphine sulfate	Use complete drug name
MS, MSO4**	morphine sulfate	Mistaken as magnesium sulfate	Use complete drug name
MTX	methotrexate	Mistaken as mitoxantrone	Use complete drug name
PCA	procainamide	Mistaken as Patient Controlled Analgesia	Use complete drug name
PTU	propylthiouracil	Mistaken as mercaptopurine	Use complete drug name
T3	Tylenol with codeine No. 3	Mistaken as liothyronine	Use complete drug name
TAC	triamcinolone	Mistaken as tetracaine, Adrenalin, cocaine	Use complete drug name
TNK	TNKase	Mistaken as "TPA"	Use complete drug name
ZnSO4	zinc sulfate	Mistaken as morphine sulfate	Use complete drug name

Stemmed Drug Names	Intended Meaning	Misinterpretation	Correction
"Nitro" drip	nitroglycerin infusion	Mistaken as sodium nitroprusside infusion	Use complete drug name
"Norflox"	norfloxacin	Mistaken as Norflex	Use complete drug name
"IV Vanc"	intravenous vancomycin	Mistaken as Invanz	Use complete drug name

Symbols	Intended Meaning	Misinterpretation	Correction
℥	Dram	Symbol for dram mistaken as "3"	Use the metric system
♍	Minim	Symbol for minim mistaken as "mL"	
x3d	For three days	Mistaken as "3 doses"	Use "for three days"
> and <	Greater than and less than	Mistaken as opposite of intended; mistakenly use incorrect symbol; "< 10" mistaken as "40"	Use "greater than" or "less than"
/ (slash mark)	Separates two doses or indicates "per"	Mistaken as the number 1 (e.g., "25 units/10 units" misread as "25 units and 110" units)	Use "per" rather than a slash mark to separate doses
@	At	Mistaken as "2"	Use "at"
&	And	Mistaken as "2"	Use "and"
+	Plus or and	Mistaken as "4"	Use "and"
°	Hour	Mistaken as a zero (e.g., q2° seen as q 20)	Use "hr," "h," or "hour"

**These abbreviations are included on the JCAHO's "minimum list" of dangerous abbreviations, acronyms and symbols that must be included on an organization's "Do Not Use" list, effective January 1, 2004. Visit www.jcaho.org for more information about this JCAHO requirement.

GLOSSARY

ABHES—Accrediting Bureau of Health Education Schools.

abandonment—to desert, to give up entirely.

abbess—a mother superior; a woman who is the head of an abbey of nuns.

abbreviations—shortened form.

abdomen—the cavity in the body between the diaphragm and the pelvis.

abdominal—pertaining to the abdomen.

abdominopelvic—pertaining to the anterior body cavity below the diaphragm.

abduction—to move away from the midline.

ablation—a surgical procedure using a resectoscope inserted into the uterus through the cervix.

abortion—the termination of pregnancy; spontaneous or induced.

abrasion—an injury caused by rubbing or scraping off the skin.

abrupt—sudden; blunt, curt.

absolute—free as to condition, unlimited in power.

absorb—to suck or swallow up, to drink in.

abstinent—refraining from use; being away from.

absurd—contrary to sense or reason.

abuse—to maltreat; to use wrongly.

accelerator—increasing action or function.

accommodation—the process of the lens changing shape to permit close vision.

account history—the past financial record.

accountant—one who keeps, audits, and inspects the financial records of individuals or businesses.

accounts receivable (A/R)—money owed to the practice by patients.

accreditation—the assignment of credentials; approval given for meeting established standards.

accredited—certified as being of a specified quality; accepted as valid.

accumulated—to pile up; collect; gather.

accuracy—correctness, exactness.

accurate—correct, exact, without error.

accurate and precise testing (APT)—refers to a standard for performing laboratory procedures to ensure reliability of results.

acetylcholine—a hormone released at the parasympathetic and skeletal nerve endings.

Achilles' tendon—a tendon attaching the gastrocnemius muscle of the leg to the heel.

achromatic—a condition of total color blindness.

acidosis—a disturbance of the acid–base balance of the body.

acne valgaris—a skin condition characterized by inflammation of sebaceous glands and producing pimples.

acquaintance—the state of knowing a person or subject.

acquire—to gain by one's own efforts or actions; to get.

acquired immunodeficiency syndrome (AIDS)—a viral disease that renders the immune system ineffective.

acquisition—acquired by one's own efforts.

acromegaly—a chronic condition characterized by enlargement of bones of the extremities and some bones of the head; thickening of facial soft tissues.

acronym—a word formed from the initial letters of each major word in a term.

action potential—the temporary electrical charge within a cell.

activate—to make active or more active.

active listening—participation in the conversation with another by paraphrasing words and phrases or giving approving or disapproving nods.

acuity—refers to the sharpness or clearness of vision or hearing.

acupuncture—involves the insertion of needles at various points in the body to treat disease or relieve pain.

acute—sharp, severe; having a rapid onset, severe symptoms, and a short course; not chronic.

acute glomerulonephritis—the rapid onset of inflammation of the glomerulus of the kidney.

acute phase—a period of increased symptoms and severity of the disease.

acute renal failure—the sudden cessation of kidney function.

adapt—the act of or the result of adjusting to a new circumstance or change.

addiction—the state of being governed or controlled by a habit, as with alcohol or drugs.

additive—a substance deliberately added to a material to fulfill some specific purpose such as enhancing taste or color or prolonging shelf life.

adduction—to draw together toward the midline.

adenitis—inflammation of lymph nodes or a gland.

adequate—equal to the requirement or occasion, sufficient.

adhere—to stick fast, become firmly attached; to be devoted to.

adjective—a word added to (modifying) a noun to quantify or limit it.

adjustments—changes to fit or bring into harmony.

administer—to manage; to conduct, as in business.

administrative—duties that manage or direct activities; in medical assisting, refers to tasks other than clinical in nature; front office duties.

admissions clerk—a person who processes information and forms for a patient who will be entering the health facility.

adrenal—pertaining to the adrenal glands, which sit atop each kidney.

adrenaline—an internal secretion derived from the adrenal glands; can be commercially prepared from animal glands; acts as a stimulant.

adrenocorticotropic hormone (ACTH)—a hormone secreted by the anterior lobe of the pituitary gland.

advance directives—a living will; a document, written in advance, that states the patient's wishes regarding end-of-life care.

advantageous—beneficial, profitable.

adverb—a word added to (modifying) a verb, an adjective, or another adverb.

adverse—opposed to; unfavorable.

advocate—one who pleads for or defends a cause or a person.

aerobe—a microorganism that can live and grow only in the presence of oxygen.

afebrile—without fever.

affiliate—to unite, to join, or become connected.

agar—a dried mucilaginous substance, or gelatin, extracted from algae, used as a culture medium.

agent—one that acts or has the power or authority to act for another.

aggression—pushiness, assuming the offensive without cause; forcefulness.

aging of accounts—dividing accounts into categories according to the amount of time since the first billing date.

Al-Anon—a support group for family members of alcoholics.

Alateen—a support for teenagers with an alcoholic parent.

albino—a person who lacks pigment in the skin, hair, and eyes, either partial or total; a person with albinoism.

alcohol—a liquid generated by the fermentation of sugar and other carbohydrates.

alcoholic—an individual who uses alcohol to excess.

Alcoholics Anonymous—an organization formed to assist alcoholics to refrain from the use of alcohol.

alcoholism—a chronic, progressive, and potentially fatal disease characterized by tolerance and physical dependency on the ingestion of alcohol.

aldosterone—a mineralocorticoid hormone secreted by the adrenal cortex.

alignment—being in proper position.

alimentary canal—the intestinal tract, from the esophagus to the rectum, and accessory organs.

allege—to state positively but not under oath and without proof; to affirm.

allergens—any substance which causes an allergic reaction.

allergic rhinitis—inflammation of the nose caused by an allergy.

allergist—a physician specializing in the care of patients with allergies.

allergy—an altered or acquired state of sensitivity; abnormal reaction of the body to substances normally harmless.

allosteric protein—a protein found in erythrocytes that transports oxygen in the blood; hemoglobin.

alopecia—the loss of hair; baldness.

alpha-fetoprotein screening (AFP)—a blood test during pregnancy to detect birth defects.

alpha search—look by alphabetical order.

alternative—different from the usual or conventional.

alveoli—microscopic air sacs in the lung.

amber—orange/yellowish color.

amblyopia—lazy eye; a condition characterized by the inward turning of the affected eye.

ambulate—to walk, not be confined to bed.

ambulatory—refers to walking, being mobile.

amenity—pleasantness, pleasant ways, civilities.

amenorrhea—absence of menses; without menstruation

ammonia—strong-smelling inhalants used to revive a person who has fainted; also known as ammonia inhalants or spirits of ammonia.

amnesia—loss of memory.

amniocentesis—the use of a needle to withdraw amniotic fluid from the amniotic sac.

amniotic—pertaining to the amniotic fluid within the amniotic membrane surrounding the fetus.

amphetamine—a central nervous system stimulant, often referred to as an upper.

amplifier—a device on an electrocardiograph that enlarges the ECG impulses.

ampule—a small glass container that can be sealed and its contents sterilized.

amputate—to cut off, remove a part.

anaerobe—a microorganism having the ability to live without oxygen.

anal—pertaining to the anus or outer rectal opening.

analysis—the examination of anything to determine its makeup; a description of the process or the examination, point by point.

analytical—characterized by a method of analysis, a statement of point-by-point examination.

anaphylactic—a severe and rapid multisystem allergic reaction.

anaphylaxis—a hypersensitive reaction of the body to a foreign protein or a drug; the term implies symptoms severe enough to produce serious shock, even death.

anatomic—pertaining to the anatomy or structure of an organism.

anatomical position—the position with the human body upright, facing forward, with the palms facing toward the front of the body.

anatomy—the study of the physical structure of the body and its organs.

anchor—the attachment of a skeletal muscle; the wrapping at the start of a gauze or elastic bandage.

anemia—a deficiency of red blood cells, hemoglobin, or both.

aneroid—operating without a fluid; when used in reference to a sphygmomanometer, measuring by a dial instead of a mercury column.

anesthesia—without sensation, with or without loss of consciousness.

anesthesiologist—one who studies anesthiology.

anesthesiology—the study of anesthesia.

anesthetic—an agent that produces insensibility to pain or touch, either generally or locally.

anesthetize—to cause a loss of sensation, loss of consciousness.

aneurysm—a widening, external dilation caused by the pressure of blood on weakened arterial walls.

angina—pain and oppression radiating from the heart to the shoulder and left arm; a feeling of suffocation.

angiography—a radiologic study of an artery using a radiopaque medium.

angioplasty—an invasive procedure to alter the interior of a blood vessel.

angle—the inclination of two straight lines that meet in a point.

annotate—to provide with explanatory notes.

annotating—to provide critical or explanatory notes.

annuity—a sum of money to be received yearly, either in a lump sum or by installments.

anorexia (nervosa)—loss of appetite; with anorexia nervosa, loss of appetite for food not explainable by disease, which may be a part of psychosis.

anorexic—one suffering from anorexia.

antagonize—to annoy; to arouse opposition.

antecubital—the inner surface of the arm at the elbow.

anteflexed—abnormal bending forward.

anterior—before or in front of.

anteverted—a forward placement.

antibody—a protein substance carried by cells to counteract the effect of an antigen.

antibody-mediated—humoral immunity; when antibodies and complement work together to destroy antigens.

anticipation—expect, forsee.

anticoagulant—a substance that prohibits the coagulation of blood.

antigen—any immunizing agent that, when introduced into the body, may produce antibodies.

antihistamine—a class of drugs used to counteract allergic reactions or cold symptoms.

antiseptic—an agent that will prevent the growth or arrest the development of microorganisms.

antitoxin—a protein that defends the body against toxins.

anuria—the absence of urine.

anus—the external opening of the anal canal.

anxiety—a condition of mental uneasiness arising from fear or apprehension.

aorta—the main trunk of the arterial system of the body.

apex—the point, tip, or summit of anything; in reference to the heart, the point of maximum impulse of the heart against the chest wall.

Apgar—refers to a method for assessing the condition of newborns.

apical—referring to the apex.

apnea—the absence of breathing.

aponeurosis—extension of connective tissue beyond a muscle in round or flattened tendons; a means of insertion or origin of a flat muscle.

apostrophe—a punctuation mark showing the absence of a letter or letters or possession.

apothocary—one who dispenses drugs and medicines.

appearance—outward show.

appendectomy—the excision of the appendix.

appendicitis—inflammation of the appendix.

appendicular—pertaining to the limbs or things that append (attach) to other parts.

appointment—an engagement; a meeting at a particular time.

apprehension—anticipation of something feared, dread; a mental conception.

apprenticeship—a training or learning period; study under the guidance of a skilled, experienced worker.

apprise—to inform.

appropriate—correct, suitable.

aqueous humor—a watery, transparent liquid that circulates between the anterior and posterior chambers of the eye.

arachnoid—a delicate, lacelike membrane covering the central nervous system.

arbitrary—depending on will or whim, self-willed; depending on choice or discretion.

ardently—eagerly, passionately, intensely.

areola—a ringlike coloration about the nipple of the breast.

aromatherapy—the use of essential oils from plants for a therapeutic effect.

arrhythmia—without rhythm; irregularity.

arteriography—a radiologic study of an artery using a radiopaque medium.

arterioles—small blood vessels connecting arteries with capillaries.

arteriosclerosis—a degeneration and hardening of the walls of arteries.

artery—a blood vessel carrying blood away from the heart, usually filled with oxygenated blood.

arthritis—inflammation of a joint.

articulate—to join together, as in a joint.

artifact—something extraneous to what is being looked for. Activity that causes interference on EKGs.

artificial insemination—the mechanical placement of semen containing viable sperm into the vagina.

ascending—referring to that portion of the colon that ascends from the lower right quadrant to the upper right quadrant of the abdomen.

ascertain—to make certain.

ascites—an abnormal accumulation of fluid in the abdomen.

ASCLS—American Society for Clinical Laboratory Science.

asepsis—a condition free of organisms.

aseptic technique—means of performing tasks without contamination by organisms.

asphyxiation—suffocation, loss of consciousness as the result of too little oxygen and too much carbon dioxide.

aspiration—removal by suction.

assault—physical harm; a violent attack.

assess—to determine, to appraise the condition or state.

assets—anything owned that has exchange value, all the entries on a balance sheet that show the property or resources of a person or business.

associate's degree—a degree granted by a junior college at the end of a two-year course.

asthma—an allergic reaction to a substance resulting in wheezing, shortness of breath, and difficulty in breathing.

astigmatism—blurring of the vision caused by an abnormal curvature of the cornea.

asymmetry—lack of same size, shape, and position of parts or organs on opposite sides.

atelectasis—lack of air in the lungs caused by the collapse of the alveoli of the lungs.

atherosclerosis—fatty degeneration of the walls of the arteries.

atmosphere—any surrounding influence.

atria—the upper chambers of the heart.

atrial depolarization—the excitement and contraction caused by the SA node at the beginning of the cardiac cycle.

atrioventricular—see **AV node.**

atrium—cardiac auricle; the upper chamber of the heart.

atrophy—wasting away of a muscle.

attachment—the point at which something attaches or originates.

attenuated—diluted; to reduce virulence of a pathogenic organism.

at the time of service (ATOS)—when service is rendered; real time.

attitude—state of thought or feeling.

attribute—quality or characteristic; to give credit for.

atypical—deviated from normal.

audible—loud enough to be heard.

audiometer—a device to measure the degree of hearing ability.

audiometry—testing of the hearing sense.

audit—inspection.

auditory—pertaining to the sense of hearing; the external canal of the ear.

augmented—refers to leads 4, 5, and 6 of the standard 12-lead ECG tracing; these leads are of different voltage.

aural—the ear; temperature measurement using tympanic infrared scanner.

auscultate—to listen for sounds produced by the body.

auscultation—the process of listening for sounds within the body.

authorization—the giving of authority.

authorize—to give permission.

autoclave—a pressurized device designed to heat aqueous solutions above their boiling point to achieve sterilization. It was invented by Charles Chamberland in 1879.

autoimmune—a condition wherein the person's antibodies react against their own normal tissues.

autologous—given by oneself.

automation—behavior in an automatic or mechanical fashion.

autonomic—spontaneous; the part of the nervous system concerned with reflex control of bodily functions.

autonomous—self-governing.

autotrophs—microorganisms that feed on inorganic matter.

auxiliary—to provide aid.

AV node—atrioventricular node; the beginning of the bundle of His in the right atrium; nerve fibers responsible for the contraction of the ventricles.

axial—pertaining to the spinal column, skull, and rib cage of the skeleton.

axilla—the underarm area, armpit.

axillary—referring to the underarm area.

axon—an extension from a nerve cell.

ayurvedic—the traditional healing system of India that may be the oldest formal medical system in the world.

bacteria—unicellular microorganism concerned with the fermentation and putrefaction of matter; disease-causing agent.

balance—to bring into or keep in equilibrium; to have equal weight and power.

bandage—a piece of cloth used to hold a dressing in place, to support a body part; provide compression, or to protect from external contamination.

bankruptcy—the state of being bankrupt, being legally declared unable to pay debts.

barbiturate—a sedative or hypnotic drug, also known as a downer.

barrier—to prevent access; bar passage.

barter—to give one thing in exchange for another.

Bartholin's glands—two small mucous glands, situated one on each side of the vaginal opening at the base of the labia minora.

baseline—the initial information on which additional data is based.

basophil—a granulated white blood cell.

battery—any illegal beating of another person.

benefits—anything that promotes or enhances well-being.

benign—nonmalignant; not cancerous.

benign hypertrophy—nonmalignant enlargement.

bereavement—sadness as a result of death of a loved one.

bereavement time—time that an employee can take off when a family member or very close friend dies.

beriberi—a disease resulting from lack of vitamin B, thiamine.

biceps—the muscle of the upper arm that flexes the forearm.

biconvex—the curving out on both sides.

bicuspid—heart valve between the left atrium and left ventricle, also known as the mitral valve.

biennially—happening once in 2 years.

bile—a secretion of the liver; a greenish-yellow fluid with a bitter taste.

bilirubin—a yellow breakdown product of normal heme catabolism. Its levels are elevated in certain diseases, and it is responsible for the yellow color of bruises and the brown color of feces.

bimanual—two-handed; with both hands.

bimonthly—occurring once in 2 months.

binge—a spree; to overindulge, such as with alcohol or food.

binocular—pertaining to the use of both eyes; possessing two eyepieces as with a microscope.

biochemistry—a science concerned with the chemistry of plants and animals.

biofeedback—a method, usually with the help of electronic equipment, that enables a person to learn to control otherwise involuntary bodily functions.

biohazard—organism, or substance derived from an organism, that poses a threat to (primarily) human health.

biohazardous—any material that has been in contact with body fluid and is potentially capable of transmitting disease.

biopsy—excision of a small piece of tissue for microscopic examination.

birthday rule—a means to identify primary responsibility in insurance coverage.

bizarre—odd, unusual, strikingly out of the ordinary.

bladder—a membranous sac or receptacle for a secretion; the gallbladder, urinary bladder.

bleb—An elevation of the epidermis; a blister; in the lungs refers to a bubble-like structure from destroyed alveoli.

blood pressure—the amount of force exerted by the heart on the blood as it pumps the blood through the arteries.

body mechanics—the use of appropriate body positioning when moving and lifting objects to avoid injury.

body surface area (BSA)—refers to the total surface of the human body.

bolus—a mass of masticated food ready to be swallowed.

bonding—the attachment of two persons; the relationship between a parent and a baby.

bookkeeper—one who records the accounts and transactions of a business.

booster—a subsequent injection of immunizing substance to increase or renew immunity.

bowel—refers to intestines.

Bowman's capsule—part of the renal corpuscle; surrounds the glomerulus of the nephron.

brachial—refers to the brachial artery in the arm; the artery used in measuring blood pressure.

brachytherapy—a type of radiation therapy that places radioactive isotopes in or near the tumor.

bradycardia—slow heart rate.

braille—printing for the blind, using a system of raised dots.

brain scan—a diagnostic test using a scanner to measure radioisotopes within the brain.

breach—violation of a law, contract, or other agreement.

brochure—a small pamphlet or booklet of information.

bronchi—the primary divisions of the trachea.

bronchiole—small terminal branches of the bronchi that lack cartilage.

bronchitis—inflammation of the mucous membranes of the bronchial tree.

bruit—an adventitious sound of venous or arterial origin heard on auscultation; usually refers to the sound produced by the mixing of arterial and venous blood at dialysis shunts.

BSA—see **body surface area.**

buccal—the mouth; oral cavity.

bulbourethral glands—two small glands, one on each side of the prostate gland, terminating in the urethra by way of a duct.

bulimia nervosa—a condition characterized by alternating periods of overeating followed by forced vomiting and the use of laxatives to remove food from the body.

bundle—a number of things bound together.

bunion—a bursa with a callus formation.

bursa—a sac or pouch in connective tissue chiefly around joints.

business associate agreement (BAA)—an agreement with a company that ensures the company understands the person's expectations as to what the company will do with the privileged information they will have access to and the consequences of an inappropriate disclosure.

CAAHEP—Commission on Accreditation of Allied Health Education Programs.

caduceus—the wand of Hermes or Mercury; used as a symbol of the medical profession.

calculate—to compute.

calculator—an electronic or mechanical device for the performance of mathematical computations.

calculi—commonly called stones; usually composed of mineral salts.

calibration—a set of graduated markings to indicate values.

callus—in fractures, refers to the formation of new osseous material around the fracture site.

calorie—a unit for measuring the heat value of food.

calyces—two or more calyx.

calyx—the cuplike division of the kidney pelvis.

cancellation—to strike out by crossing with lines; marking a postage stamp or check or to delete an appointment or event.

cancellous—a latticework structure, as the spongy tissue of bone.

cancer—a malignant tumor or growth; specifically the hyperplasia of cells with infiltration and destruction of tissue.

cancerous—refers to a malignant growth.

cannula—a tube or sheath enclosing a trocar (triangular bore needle); after insertion, the trocar is removed.

capillary—a microscopic blood vessel connecting arterioles and venules.

capitation—a structure of payment based on the number served.

caption—heading, title, or subtitle.

carbohydrate—an organic combination of carbon, hydrogen, and oxygen as a sugar, a starch, or cellulose.

carbon dioxide—a gas found in the air, exhaled by all animals; the chemical formula is CO_2.

carbon monoxide—a colorless, odorless, poisonous gas caused by the incomplete combustion of carbon.

carboxyhemoglobin—combined carbon monoxide and hemoglobin in red blood cells.

carbuncle—a staphylococcal infection following furunculosis, characterized by a deep abscess of several follicles with multiple draining points.

carcinoembryonic antigen—a tumor marker that can be detected in the blood when tested.

carcinogen—cancer-causing agent.

carcinoma—a malignant tumor from epithelial tissue.

cardiac—pertaining to the heart.

cardiac sphincter—the muscle that encircles the esophagus where it enters the stomach.

cardinal signs—principal signs: temperature, pulse, respiration, and blood pressure.

cardiologist—a physician specializing in the care of patients with diseases of the heart.

cardiology—the study of the heart and its diseases.

cardiovascular—pertaining to the heart and blood vessels.

caregiver—the person responsible for another's care and well-being.

carotid—pertaining to the carotid artery.

carpal—bone of the wrist.

carpal tunnel syndrome (CTS)—the symptoms associated with the entrapment of the median nerve within the carpal bones and the transverse ligament at the wrist.

carrel—a small, partitioned space.

carrier—one who carries, transports; with insurance, it's the company who provides the policy.

cartilage—a strong, tough, elastic tissue forming part of the skeletal system; precalcified bone in infants and young children.

CAT scan—see **computerized transaxial tomography.**

cataract—an opacity of the lens of the eye resulting in blindness.

catarrhal—pertaining to inflammation of mucous membranes; causing severe spells of coughing with little or no expectoration.

catarrhal stage—inflammation of the mucous membranes.

catastrophic—of great consequence; disastrous.

categorize—to arrange by class or kind; to place like things together.

catheterization—to insert a catheter into a cavity (for example, urinary bladder to remove urine) to remove body fluid.

caudal—pertaining to any taillike structure.

caustic—capable of burning; an agent that will destroy living tissue.

cauterize—to burn with an electrical cautery or chemical substance.

cautery—an iron or caustic used to burn tissue.

cavities—a hollow space, such as within the body or organs.

cecum—the beginning of the ascending portion of the large intestine that forms a blind pouch at the junction with the small intestine.

celiac disease—dilation of the small and large intestines.

cell—structural and functional unit of all living organisms; sometimes called the building block of life.

cell-mediated—direct cellular response to antigens.

cell membrane—the structure that surrounds and encloses a cell.

central—situated at or related to a center.

centrifuge—a machine for the separation of heavier materials from lighter ones through the use of centrifugal force.

centriole—an organelle within the cell.

cerebellum—lower or back brain below the posterior portion of the cerebrum.

cerebral—pertaining to the cerebrum of the brain.

cerebrospinal—referring to the brain and spinal cord.

cerebrospinal fluid—the liquid that circulates within the meninges of the spinal cord and ventricles and meninges of the brain.

cerebrovascular accident—a stroke; hemorrhage in the brain.

cerebrum—the largest part of the brain. It is divided into two hemispheres with four lobes in each hemisphere.

certificate—a written declaration of some fact.

certificate of completion—a document awarded upon fulfillment of a program's criteria.

certificate of waiver—refers to a list of basic laboratory tests that may be performed in the physician's office by non-laboratory personnel.

certification—written declaration.

certified—holding a certificate; being certificated; guaranteed in writing.

certified ophthalmic technician (COT)—a person trained and certified in diagnostic testing procedures and limited examination of the eye.

cerumen—waxlike brown secretion found in the external auditory canal.

cervical—pertaining to the neck portion of the spinal column; also to the entrance into the uterus.

cervicitis—an inflammation of the cervix of the uterus.

cervix—the entrance into the uterus.

cesarean—surgical removal of an infant from the uterus.

cessation—ceasing or discontinuing.

chaos—a state of complete confusion; disorder.

charting—the recording of observations, subjective and objective findings, diagnostic procedures, treatments, and other pertinent data in the patient file.

chemical—a simple or compound substance used in chemical processes.

chemotherapy—the use of chemical agents in the treatment of disease, usually associated with cancer therapy.

Cheyne-Stokes—a breathing pattern characterized by alternating periods of apnea and hyperventilation.

chief complaint—the main reason for seeking medical care.

chiropractic—a system of healing based upon the theory that disease results from a lack of normal nerve function; treatment by scientific manipulation and specific adjustment of body structures, such as the spinal column.

chiropractor—a health care provider who uses chiropractic methods to treat patients.

chlamydia—a sexually transmitted disease caused by a bacteria that lives as an intracellular parasite.

chloroform—a liquid compound that yields a gas that dulls pain and causes unconsciousness.

cholecystectomy—surgical removal of the gallbladder.

cholecystolithiasis—an abnormal presence of stones in the gallbladder.

cholelithiasis—stones in the gallbladder.

cholenergic—nerve fibers capable of secreting acetylcholine.

cholera—an acute, specific, infectious disease characterized by diarrhea, painful cramps of muscles, and a tendency to collapse.

cholesterol—a sterol present in the tissues which contributes to heart disease when elevated; transported in the blood plasma of all animals.

chorionic gonadotropin—a hormone detectable in the urine of a pregnant female soon after conception.

choroid—the vascular coat of the eye between the sclera and the retina.

chromosome—structures within the cell's nucleus that store hereditary information.

chronic—continuing a long time, returning; not acute.

chronic glomerulonephritis—the slow, progressive destruction of the glomerulus of the kidney.

chronic leukemia—a form of leukemia characterized by insidious onset and slower progress.

chronic obstructive pulmonary disease (COPD)—a syndrome characterized by chronic bronchitis, asthma, and emphysema, or any combination of these conditions, resulting in dyspnea, frequent respiratory infections, and thoracic deformities from attempting to breathe.

chronic renal failure—the end result of the progressive loss of kidney function.

chronologic—the arrangement of events, dates, etc., in order of occurrence.

chyme—the mixture of partially digested food and digestive secretions found in the stomach and small intestines during digestion of a meal.

cilia—hairlike projections from epithelial cells, as in the bronchi.

circulatory—refers to the circulatory system; the process of blood flowing through the vessels to all the cells of the body.

circumcision—surgical removal of the foreskin of the penis.

circumference—the distance around a circle; with mensurations, the measurement of the head.

circumversion—rotation of an extremity in a circular motion.

cirrhosis—an interstitial inflammation with hardening of the tissues of an organ, especially the liver.

civil law—pertaining to the rights of private individuals; legal proceedings concerning rights that are not criminal.

clarity—clearness, absence of cloudiness.

classified—arranged in a group or classification according to some system.

clause—part of a sentence with a subject and a predicate.

claustrophobia—an abnormal fear of being in enclosed or confined places.

clavicle—the collar bone, articulating with the sternum and scapula.

CLIA—see **Clinical Laboratory Improvement Amendments.**

clinical—based on observation; in medical assisting, pertains to duties considered "back office"; not administrative in nature.

Clinical Laboratory Improvement Amendments (CLIA)—legislation dealing with the operation of a clinical laboratory.

clitoris—an erectile organ located at the anterior junction of the labia minora.

clonal—the duplicated copy; with immunity it is the cells produced to attack antigens.

clone—an exact copy.

coagulation—lessening of the fluidity of a liquid substance; clotting or curdling.

coccyx—the tailbone; the last four bones of the spine.

cochlea—the snail-shaped portion of the inner ear.

coercion—to force or compel; to restrain or constrain by force.

coitus—sexual intercourse between a man and a woman.

colitis—inflammation of the colon.

collaborate—to work together.

collateral—subordinate, secondary; property deposited as security for a loan.

colleague—an associate at work, usually one of similar status.

colon—the large intestine.

colorimeter—an instrument used for measuring the amount of pigments and determining the amount of hemoglobin in the blood.

colostomy—incision of the colon for the purpose of making a more or less permanent opening.

colposcopy—a diagnostic examination to visualize the cervix through a colposcope.

coma—an abnormal deep stupor from which a person cannot be aroused by external stimuli.

coma scale—refers to the Glascow Coma Scale used to determine level of consciousness.

combining forms—in medical terminology, the word root with a combining form vowel (usually an "o") that aids in making the word pronounceable, particularly when adding a suffix that begins with a consonant.

comminuted—a crushed bone fracture with many fragments.

commiserate—to feel or express sympathy or pity for.

common bile duct—a duct carrying bile from the hepatic and cystic ducts to the duodenum.

commonality—people in general; a body corporate or its membership.

communicable—capable of being transmitted from one person or species to another, also known as contagious.

communication—the act of communicating; information given; a means of giving information.

compatible—able to be mixed or taken together without destructive changes (as in blood typing and cross-matching); matching; not opposed to.

compensate—to make amends; be equivalent to.

compensation—anything given as an equivalent or to make amends; pay.

competency—demonstrated capability, being able; a task to achieve.

competent—fit, able, capable.

complement—a group of about 20 inactive enzyme proteins present in the blood.

complementary—something that will add to or make another thing complete or whole.

complete blood count—a test requested by a doctor or other medical professional that gives information about the cells in a patient's blood; also known as a CBC; amongst the most commonly performed blood tests in medicine.

complexity—the state of being complicated.

compliance—consent; conformity to formal or official requirements.

complicated—not simple, involved; having many parts; not easy to solve.

complimentary—express appreciation; given without charge.

compose—to form by putting together, creating.

compound—not simple, composed of two or more parts; with fractures, refers to bone fragments piercing the skin externally.

comprehensive—covering all areas; inclusive.

compression—to exert force against, press.

computed transaxial tomography (CAT)—computed axial tomography, a medical imaging method employing tomography in which digital geometry processing is used to generate a three-dimensional image of the internals of an object from a large series of two-dimensional x-ray images taken around a single axis of rotation.

computer—a mechanical, electric, or electronic device that stores numerical or other information and provides logical answers at high speed to questions bearing on that information.

computerized—to store in a computer; to put in a form a computer can use; to bring computers into use to control an operation.

computerized axial tomography (CAT)—a series of x-ray views of the body used to construct a three-dimensional picture.

conceal—to hide, to keep secret, to withhold, as information.

conceive—to become pregnant; the uniting of the sperm and ovum.

conception—the union of the sperm of a male and the egg of a female; fertilization.

conceptualize—to form a concept, thought, notion, or understanding.

concise—condensed, short.

condenser—part of a microscope substage that regulates the amount of light directed on a specimen.

confidential—revealed in confidence; secret information.

confidentiality—to be held in confidence; a secret.

confinement—restriction within certain limits.

confirmation—making firm or sure; convincing proof.

confirmed—verified or ratified.

conflict—a clash of opinions or interests; a fight or struggle; an inner moral struggle; to come into opposition.

confrontation—to stand face to face with.

congenital—existing at birth.

congestive heart failure—a complex condition of inadequate heart action with retention of tissue fluids; may be either right- or left-side failure, or both.

congratulations—to express pleasure; a recognition of accomplishment.

conjunction—meeting; a word that connects.

conjunctiva—a mucous membrane that lines the eyelids and covers the anterior sclera of the eyeball.

connective—that which connects or binds together; one of the five main tissues of the body.

connotations—something implied or suggested.

consciousness—awareness, full knowledge of what is in one's own mind.

consecutive—following in order, successive.

consecutively—a series of things that follow each other.

conserve—to keep from damage or loss; to maintain.

constipation—a sluggish action of the bowel; usually refers to an excessively firm, hard stool that is difficult to expel or lack of a bowel movement over a time.

constrict—to narrow; to become smaller because of contraction of a sphincter muscle.

contact dermatitis—inflammation and irritation of the skin caused by contact with an irritating substance.

contagious—catching; able to be transmitted by contact.

contaminate—to place in contact with microorganisms.

contemporary—happening or existing at the same time; a person living at the same time as another.

content—the matter dealt with in a field of study; matter contained.

context—the part of a written or spoken statement that surrounds a particular word or passage and can clarify its meaning.

contraception—against conception.

contract—to draw together, reduce in size, or shorten.

contraction—the muscle action of the uterus during labor; in spelling and punctuation, the shortening of a word by the omission of one or more letters, which are replaced with an apostrophe.

contracture—permanent shortening or contraction of a muscle.

contradiction—to deny; to assert to the contrary of.

contrast—to show difference; in radiology, refers to a radiopaque medium used to outline body organs.

contributory—giving a share; helping toward a result.

controversial—open to dispute; relating to discussion of opposing views.

conventional—growing out of custom; not spontaneous.

convey—to impart, as an idea; to transfer.

convulsion—attack of involuntary muscular contractions often accompanied by unconsciousness.

cooperate—to work together.

coordination—a state of harmonious adjustment or function.

coordination of benefits—when both spouses have health care insurance, the policy provision that limits benefits to 100% of the cost; also known as dual coverage.

coordinator—a person who works for harmonious functioning of parts or agents toward the production of a desired result.

COPD—see **chronic obstructive pulmonary disease.**

cornea—the transparent extension of the sclera that lies in front of the pupil of the eye.

coronal (plane)—a line drawn through the side of the body from head to toe, making a front and back section.

coronary—referring to the arteries surrounding the heart muscle; also refers to a "heart attack," which involves the coronary arteries.

coroner—an official who investigates a sudden, suspicious, or violent death to determine the cause. In some communities this position has been replaced by the medical examiner.

corpus luteum—the yellow body that develops in the ruptured graafian follicle after the ovum has been discharged.

correspondence—communication by the exchange of letters.

cortex—the outer portion of the kidney.

corticosteroids—hormones used to treat inflammation.

COT—see **certified ophthalmic technician.**

countershock—(in cardiology) a high-intensity, short-duration, electric shock applied to the area of the heart, resulting in total cardiac depolarization.

courteous—polite, considerate, and respectful in manner and action.

CPT—see **Current Procedural Terminology.**

cramp—a spasmodic, painful contraction of a muscle or muscles.

cranial—pertaining to the cranium or skull.

cranium—the skull; the eight bones of the head enclosing the brain; generally applied to the 28 bones of the head and face.

crenated—notched or scalloped, as the crenated condition of blood corpuscles.

cretinism—a congenital condition caused by the lack of the hormone thyroxin.

criminal law—of, involving, or having the nature of a crime.

crisis—the turning point of a disease; a very critical period; an emergency situation.

criterion—a standard of criticism or judgment (plural: criteria).

critique—a critical examination of a thing or situation, to determine its nature, worth, or conformity to standards.

Crohn's disease—an inflammation of the GI tract with debilitating symptoms.

cross-match—a blood test used to ensure compatibility of the donor to the recipient when transfusing blood.

crutches—staffs with a cross-piece at the top to place under the arms of a lame person.

cryosurgery—the use of a substance at subfreezing temperature to destroy or remove tissue.

cryptorchidism—failure of the testicles to descend into the scrotum.

CTD—see **cumulative trauma disorder.**

CTS—see **carpal tunnel syndrome.**

cultivate—to form and refine; to improve.

culture—a method of growing a microbial organism to determine what it is, its abundance in the sample being tested, or both. It is one of the primary diagnostic methods of microbiology.

cumulative trauma disorder (CTD)—an injury resulting from repetitive movement of a body part.

curette—an instrument to scrape material from a cavity.

currency—any form of money.

current—happening now; of the present time; the latest information.

Current Procedural Terminology (CPT)—a numerical listing of procedures performed in medical practice; a standardized identification of procedures. Published by the American Medical Association.

curriculum—a course of study at a school or university.

Cushing's syndrome—a disorder resulting from the hypersecretion of glucocorticoids from the adrenal cortex.

cusp—a sharp point or apex.

customarily—by custom, the usual course of action under similar circumstances.

cyanosis—a bluish discoloration of the skin caused by lack of oxygen.

cyst—a bladder; any sac containing fluid.

cystic—pertaining to a cyst; of disease, refers to a condition with multiple cysts.

cystic fibrosis—a disease condition of fibrous tumors that have undergone cystic degeneration, accumulating fluid in the interspaces; also known as fibrocystic disease.

cystitis—inflammation of the urinary bladder.

cystoscope—an instrument for examining the interior of the urinary bladder.

cytokine—a nonantibody protein of the immune system that regulates immune response.

cytologist—one who studies cells and interprets slides.

cytology—the study of cell life and cell formation.

cytoplasm—cellular matter, not including the nucleus of a cell.

cytotechnologist—a laboratory specialist who prepares and examines tissue cells to study cell formation.

cytotoxic—capable of destroying cells.

DACUM—an acronym for "design a curriculum."

daltonism—the inability to distinguish between red and green.

data—facts from which conclusions can be inferred.

date of birth (DOB)—the date a person is born, including the month, day, and year.

date of service (DOS)—the calendar date a service begins or is provided.

D & C—see **dilatation and curettage.**

DEA—see **Drug Enforcement Administration.**

debilitated—weakened; impaired the strength of.

debit—to deduct, to charge.

débridement—to clean up or remove, as is done with damaged tissue around a wound.

decibel—a unit of measure to express the degree of loudness of sound.

decline stage—becoming less intense, subsiding; a period of time when the symptoms of disease start to disappear.

dedicated—committed to; set apart for a special use.

deductible—an amount to be paid before insurance will pay.

deductions—to deduct or subtract; remove, take away.

defamation—to slander, or to attack the reputation of an individual or group.

defecate—to pass stool or move bowels.

defibrillation—to cause fibrillation to end; restore to normal action.

defibrillator—a device designed to deliver an electric shock to a patient, in an effort to stop pulseless ventricular fibrillation or ventricular tachycardia.

dehydration—withdrawal of water from the tissues naturally or artificially.

delegation—a person or group of persons officially elected or appointed to represent another or others; to entrust power

delete—to remove, erase.

delirium tremens—a psychic disorder involving hallucinations, both visual and auditory, found in habitual users of alcohol.

deltoid—the muscle of the shoulder.

demeanor—behavior; bearing.

demography—the study of population statistics concerning births, marriage, death, disease, and many other indicators.

dendrite—an extension from a nerve cell.

denial—a refusal to believe or accept; disowning.

denomination—a category or classification of currency.

denote—to indicate, to mean.

dental assistant—a health care worker employed by a dentist to perform management and clinical functions and provide chairside assistance.

dental hygienist—a licensed health care provider who is trained to x-ray and perform prophylactic treatments on teeth.

dentist (DDS)—a licensed health provider who cares for the teeth, repairing and replacing as needed.

deoxyribonucleic acid (DNA)—material within the chromosome that carries the genetic information.

dependable—that which may be relied upon.

dependence—that on which one depends; reliance.

depict—to represent by a picture; portray.

depleted—consumed, emptied, exhausted.

deposit—to entrust money to a bank or other institution.

deposition—testimony given under oath.

depressant—a drug that causes a slowing down of bodily function or nerve activity.

depressed—a state of depression, a period of low spirits; referring to a fracture, usually a fracture of the skull where bone fragments are driven (depressed) inward.

deprivation—to be deprived; without; having to do without or unable to use.

dermatitis—an inflammation of the skin, often the result of an irritant.

dermatologist—a physician who specializes in the diseases and disorders of the skin.

dermatology—the study of the skin and its diseases.

dermis—true skin.

descending—refers to the portion of the large intestine from the splenic flexure to the sigmoid.

description—a word picture.

desensitization—the process of making an individual less susceptible to allergens.

desensitizing—a process of exposing a patient to small levels of an allergen to gradually build up a nonallergic reaction.

design—working plan; layout; sketch.

designate—to point out; indicate; appoint.

detection—find out or discover.

detrimental—harmful, injurious.

deuteranopia—the difficulty in differentiating between the shades of green and bluish reds and some neutral shades.

devastate—to lay waste, plunder, destroy.

development—the advancement of abilities and knowledge.

dextrose—a simple sugar, also known as glucose.

diabetes mellitus—a metabolic disease caused by the body's inability to use carbohydrates.

diabetic—one afflicted with the condition diabetes.

diabetic coma—a diabetic emergency that can be fatal if not treated promptly and properly.

diagnostic—referring to measures that assist in the recognition of diseases and disorders of the body.

dialysis—removal of the products of urine from the blood by passage of the solutes through a membrane.

diaphanography—a type of transillumination used to examine the breast, using selected wavelengths of light and special imaging equipment.

diaphoresis—profuse sweating.

diaphragm—the muscle of breathing that separates the thorax from the abdomen.

diarrhea—frequent bowel movements, usually liquid or semisolid.

diarthrosis—a movable joint; another word for synovial.

diastole—the relaxation phase of the heartbeat; the period of least pressure.

dictation—spoken words; recorded voice communication.

dietician—one who is trained in dietetics, which includes nutrition, and in charge of the diet of an institution.

differential—refers to determining the number of each type of leukocyte in a cubic millimeter of blood.

diffuse—to scatter or spread.

diffusion—a process whereby gas, liquid, or solid molecules distribute themselves evenly through a medium.

digestion—the process by which food is broken down, mechanically and chemically, in the gastrointestinal tract and converted into absorbable forms.

digestive—pertaining to digestion.

digitally—pertaining to or resembling a finger or toe, as an examination using a finger or fingers.

dilate—to enlarge, expand in size; to increase the size of an opening.

dilation and curettage (D & C)—dilation of the cervix and scraping of the interior lining of the uterus.

dimpling—a condition characterized by indentations in the skin.

diphtheria—an acute infectious disease characterized by the formation of a false membrane on any mucous surface, usually in the air passages, interfering with breathing.

diplomate—an advanced status of medical practice.

direct payment—payment made directly to the physician by the insurance company.

disability—a legal incapacity.

disaster—an occurrence inflicting widespread destruction and distress.

disciplinary—designed to correct or punish breaches of conduct.

discipline—self-control, conduct, system of rules.

disclose—to uncover, reveal.

discoid—a type of lupus that is confined to the skin; also called cutaneous.

discreet—wisely cautious, prudent.

discrepancy—inconsistencies; variances.

discretion—the use of judgment, prudence.

disease—sickness, illness, ailment.

disinfection—the process of applying antimicrobial agents to non-living objects to destroy microorganisms.

dislocation—the displacement of a part; usually refers to a bone temporarily out of its normal position in a joint.

dispense—to distribute; to deal out in portions.

displacement—the transfer of emotions about one person or situation to another person or situation.

disposition—the act or manner of putting in a particular order; arrange.

dissect—to cut into parts for examination; to separate.

distal—farthest from the center, from the medial line, or from the trunk.

distend—to become inflated, to stretch out.

distinctive—unmistakable, different from anything else.

distort—to misrepresent; to twist out of usual shape.

diversion—the act of diverting or turning aside.

diverticulitis—inflammation of the diverticula.

diverticulum—a sac or pouch in the walls of a canal or organ, particularly the colon.

divulge—to make public; to make known; reveal.

DNA—see **deoxyribonucleic acid.**

doctorate—a postgraduate degree conferred following extensive course work, an individual research project, and the writing of a dissertation; a PhD.

doctrine—the principles of any branch of knowledge; a belief held or taught.

documentary—presenting facts without inserting fictional matter.

domestic—not foreign; private.

dominant—strongest; prevailing, the prime or main.

dominant gene—the prevailing gene.

dorsal—pertaining to the back.

dorsalis pedis—a pulse point palpable on the instep of the foot.

douche—an irrigation of the vagina.

dowel—a round piece of wood.

downtime—refers to being offline; computer failure; time when nothing is scheduled.

dribbling—uncontrolled leakage of urine from the bladder.

drill—disciplined repetitious exercises as a means of perfecting a skill or procedure.

droplet—a very small drop.

droplet infection—a disease that results from contamination with water-based microorganisms.

Drug Enforcement Administration (DEA)—a division of the federal government responsible for the enforcement of laws regulating the distribution and sale of drugs.

dual—referring to two; having two parts.

duodenum—the first segment of the small intestine.

dura mater—the outer membrane covering the brain and spinal cord.

duration—the amount of time a thing continues.

dwarfism—a condition caused by inadequate growth hormone during childhood.

dysmenorrhea—painful menstruation.

dysplasia—precancerous cells; with cervix are precursors to cervical cancer.

dyspnea—difficult or labored breathing.

dyspneic—difficulty in breathing.

dystrophy—progressive atrophy or weakening of a part, such as the muscles.

dysuria—painful urination; difficulty in urination.

ECG or EKG—see **electrocardiogram.**

echocardiography—ultrahigh-frequency sound waves directed toward the heart to evaluate function and structure of the organ.

echoes—reflections of sound.

ectopic—in an abnormal position; in pregnancy refers to the embryo or fetus being outside the uterus.

eczema—a noncontagious skin disease characterized by dry, red, itchy, and scaly skin.

edema—a condition of body tissues containing abnormal amounts of fluid, usually intercellular; may be local or general.

effacement—the thinning out of the cervix during labor.

efficiency—the ratio of energy expended to results produced.

ejaculation—the expulsion of seminal fluid from the male urethra.

ejaculatory duct—the duct from the seminal vesicle to the urethra.

elaborate—to improve by successive operations; to work out in detail.

elasticity—ability to return to shape after being stretched.

electrical—charged with electricity; run by electricity.

electrocardiogram (EKG, ECG)—a graphic record of the electric currents generated by the heart; a tracing of the heart action.

electrocardiogram technician (ECG tech)—a person trained in obtaining electrocardiograms, a record of cardiac impulses.

electrocardiograph—a machine for obtaining a graphic recording of the electrical activity of the heart.

electrocautery—an apparatus used to cauterize tissue with heat from a current of electricity.

electrocoagulation—coagulation of tissue by means of a high-frequency electric current.

electrode—an instrument with a point or a surface that transmits current to the patient's body.

electroencephalography (EEG)—recording of the electric currents generated by the brain; a tracing of brain waves.

electrolyte—a substance that, in solution, conducts an electric current.

electromagnet—a soft iron core that temporarily becomes a magnet when an electric current flows through a coil surrounding it.

electromagnetic—a specialized field of radiology that involves the use of both electrical and magnetic fields for diagnosis of disease processes.

electromagnetic radiation—rays produced by the collision of a beam of electrons with a metal target in an x-ray tube.

electromyography—the insertion of needles into selected skeletal muscles for the purpose of recording nerve conduction time in relation to muscle contraction.

electron—a minute particle of matter charged with the smallest known amount of negative electricity; opposite of proton.

electronic—operated by the use of electrons.

elements—substances in their simplest form; the basic building blocks of all matter.

elicit—to draw out, to derive by logical process.

elimination—to remove, get rid of, exclude; also to pass urine from the bladder or stool from the bowel.

elite—choice, superior, select.

ellipses—a mark or series of marks used in writing or printing to indicate an omission, especially of letters or words.

emaciation—to become abnormally thin; the loss of too much weight.

emancipated minor—no longer under the care, custody, or supervision of a parent or guardian.

embolism—the presence of an obstruction in a blood vessel.

embolus—a circulating mass in a blood vessel; foreign material that obstructs a blood vessel.

embryo—the first 8 weeks of development after fertilization.

emergency—an unexpected occurrence or situation demanding immediate action.

emergency medical technician (EMT)—an individual trained to respond in emergency situations and provide appropriate initial medical treatment.

emesis—to vomit.

emetic—medication that induces vomiting.

empathy—sympathetically trying to identify one's feelings with those of another.

emphysema—a chronic lung disease characterized by overdistention of the alveolar sacs and inability to exchange oxygen and carbon dioxide.

empirically—based on observations or experiment.

empyema—exudate (pus) within the pleural space of the chest cavity.

enact—to make into law.

encompass—to surround, enclose.

encounter—to meet, unexpectedly or by chance.

endocardium—the serous membrane lining of the heart.

endocervical—the lining of the canal of the cervix.

endocrine—a gland that secretes directly into the blood stream.

endocrinologist—a physician specializing in the diseases and disorders of the endocrine system.

endocrinology—the study of the endocrine or ductless glands of internal secretion.

endocytosis—a cellular process to bring large molecules of material into the cytoplasm of the cell.

endometrium—the mucous membrane lining of the uterus.

endoplasmic reticulum—an organelle within the cytoplasm of a cell.

endorse—to approve, recommend, or sponsor.

endorsement—the act of endorsing; approving.

endoscope—an instrument consisting of a tube and optical system for observing the inside of an organ or cavity.

enema—the instillation of fluid into the rectum and colon.

engorge—to fill with blood to the point of congestion; to devour or engulf.

enhance—to intensify, improve.

enthusiasm—intense interest; zeal; passion.

entity—a thing having reality.

enucleation—surgical excision of the eyeball.

enumerate—to count separately, name one by one.

enunciate—to speak or pronounce clearly.

envelope—to enclose completely with a cover; a paper container for a letter.

environment—surroundings.

enzyme—a complex chemical substance produced by the body, found primarily in the digestive juices, that acts upon food substances to break them down for absorption.

eosinophil—a white blood cell or cellular structure that stains readily with the acid stain eosin; specifically an eosinophilic leukocyte.

epidemic—affecting many persons at one time.

epidermis—the outer layer of the skin; literally *over the true skin*.

epididymis—a convoluted tube resting on the surface of the testicle that carries sperm from the testicle to the vas deferens.

epigastric—pertaining to the area of the abdomen over the stomach.

epiglottis—a cartilagenous lid that closes over the larynx when swallowing.

epilepsy—a chronic disease of the nervous system characterized by convulsions and often unconsciousness.

epinephrine—a hormone produced by the adrenal medulla.

epiphysis—a portion of bone not yet ossified; the cartilagenous ends of the long bones that allow for growth.

episiotomy—an incision in the perineum to avoid tearing during childbirth.

epistaxis—nosebleed; hemorrhage from the nose.

epithelial—pertaining to a type of cell or tissue that forms the skin and mucous membranes of the body.

equity—the value of property beyond the total amount owed on it.

equivalent—equal to in value, size, or effect.

erectile—refers to tissue that is capable of erection, usually caused by vasocongestion.

ergonomics—the applied science of being concerned with the nature and characteristics of people as they relate to design and activities with the intention of producing more effective results and greater safety.

erythema—diffuse redness over the skin because of capillary congestion and dilation of the superficial capillaries.

erythrocyte—a red blood cell (RBC).

erythropoiesis—the formation of red blood corpuscles.

eschar—slough, especially after a cauterization.

esophagus—a collapsible tube from the pharynx to the stomach, through which pass the food and water the body ingests.

essential—necessary; when referring to blood pressure, indicates an elevation without apparent cause.

esthetic—relating to the principles of beauty and taste.

estrogen—a female hormone produced by the ovaries.

ether—a colorless liquid used to produce unconsciousness and insensibility to pain.

ethical—right, according to the principles of ethics.

ethics—standards of conduct and moral judgement.

etiology—the study of the cause of disease.

etiquette—conventional rules for correct behavior.

euphoria—a feeling of well-being, elation.

eustachian tube—refers to the tube of the middle ear that connects to the pharynx.

evacuants—a medication that promotes emptying of the bowels.

evacuate—to empty, especially the bowels.

evacuation—withdrawal, to remove, to make empty.

evaluation—assessment; judgment concerning the worth, quality, significance, or value of a situation, person, or product.

eversion—the movement of the sole of the foot away from the median plane.

evoke—to call forth or up; summon; elicit.

excretion—the process of expelling material from the body.

exemplify—to show by example.

exempt—excluded; not liable; freedom from duty or service; privileged.

exemption—freed from or not liable for something to which others are subject.

exfoliate—to scale off dead tissue.

exhale—to breathe out.

exhaustion—extreme fatigue.

exocrine—a gland that secretes substances through a duct into the body.

exocytosis—a cellular process that moves materials within the cell to the outside.

exogenous—originating outside an organ or part.

exophthalmia—abnormal protrusion of the eyeball.

exorcism—the act of expelling an evil spirit.

expectorate—to spit, to expel mucus or phlegm from the throat or lungs.

expedient—suitable means for achieving or attaining a purpose or end; of immediate advantage, convenient.

expedite—to hasten.

expended—spent or used, as with money or energy.

experience—observation or practice resulting in knowledge; knowledge gained by seeing and doing.

expertise—special knowledge or skill.

expiration—the expulsion of air from the lungs in breathing.

explicit—clearly and definitely expressed; unambiguous; leaving no room for questions.

express—to utter; to make known in words or by action.

expressed—said in words or by action.

extend—movement of a joint to increase the angle of that joint.

extensive—having a wide range.

extensor—the muscle of a muscle team that extends a part, allowing the joint to straighten.

external—the outermost part of the body.

externship—a supervised employment experience in a qualified health care facility as part of the educational curriculum.

extinguish—to put out; put an end to.

extinguisher—a device for putting out fire.

extracellular—outside the cell.

extract—a substance distilled or drawn out of another substance.

extremities—the terminal parts of the body—the arms, legs.

exudate—pus; the collection of purulent material in a cavity.

exudative—pertaining to any fluid that filters from the circulatory system into lesions or areas of inflammation.

eyewash—a device using water to remove foreign material from the eyes, usually in emergency situations.

facility—a building; in medical situations, a building for the care and treatment of patients.

facsimile—an exact copy.

facultative—able to live under conditions of temperature or oxygen supply that vary; having the capability to adapt to more than one condition, as a facultative anerobe.

faith—belief in the doctrines of religion; a firm belief in something for which there is no proof.

fallopian tube—the ovaduct; the passageway for the ova from the ovary to the uterus.

familial—pertaining to the same family.

family practice—one which cares for patients of all ages and all conditions not requiring specialization.

fascia—a fibrous membrane covering, supporting, and separating muscles; may also unite the skin with underlying tissue.

fast—to abstain from food; without food or water.

fatal—causing death.

fax—a message that is transmitted over phone lines and printed by the recipient's equipment.

feasible—possible; practicable.

febrile—pertaining to a fever.

fecal—pertaining to feces.

feces—stool, bowel movement.

fee schedule—listing of allowable charge.

femoral—pertaining to the artery that lies adjacent to the femur.

femoral point—the pressure point on the femoral artery.

femur—the thigh bone of the leg.

fenestrated—having a window or opening.

fertilization—impregnation of the ovum by the sperm; conception.

fetal—pertaining to a fetus, pregnancy beyond the third month.

fetal alcohol syndrome—a group of birth defects in infants born to mothers who persisted to consume alcohol during gestation.

fetal monitor—a device to access fetal heart beat.

fetus—an embryo after 8 weeks of gestation.

fibrillation—the quivering of muscle fibers; ineffective, rapid but weak heart action.

fibroid—a tumor made up of fibrous and muscular tissue.

fibrosis—abnormal formation of fibrous tissue.

fibula—a long bone in the leg from the knee to the ankle.

filtration—the movement of solutes and water across a semipermeable membrane as a result of a force, such as gravity or blood pressure.

fiscal—of or pertaining to finances in general.

fissure—an ulcer, split, crack, or tear in the tissue.

fistula—an abnormal tubelike passage from a normal cavity or an abscess to a free surface.

flatulence—the existence of flatus or intestinal gas.

flatus—intestinal gas.

flex time—refers to the practice of permitting work hours within a range of time.

flexed—bent, as at a joint.

flexibility—easily bent, compliant, yielding to persuasion.

flexible—the ability to adapt to circumstances; ability to flex and bend; nonrigid.

flexor—the muscle of a muscle team that bends a part.

flora—plant life as distinguished from animal life; plant life occurring or adapted for living in a specific environment, as flora in the intestines.

flu—an abbreviation for the word influenza; a respiratory or intestinal infection.

fluoroscope—a device consisting of a fluorescent screen in conjunction with an x-ray tube to make visible shadows of objects interposed between the screen and the tube.

flushed—sudden reddish coloration of the skin.

follicle—a small excretory duct or sac or tubular gland; a hair follicle.

folliculitis—a staphylococcal infection of a hair follicle.

forceps—an instrument used to grasp tissue and to clamp blood vessels.

foreign (body)—anything that is not normally found in the location; usually refers to dirt, splinters, etc.

foreskin—loose skin covering the end of the penis.

forge—to imitate, especially to counterfeit, as a signature.

formaldehyde—a colorless, pungent gas used in its liquid form to harden tissue for pathologic study, or as a germicide, disinfectant, or preservative, according to the strength of the solution.

formalin—wood alcohol containing 40% formaldehyde.

fortitude—courageous endurance.

fovea centralis—a depression in the posterior surface of the retina that is the place of sharpest vision.

Fowler's—a full or partial sitting examination position.

fracture—the sudden breaking of a bone.

fraudulent—characterized by cheating and deceit; obtained by dishonest means.

frequency—the need to void urine often, though usually only a small amount at one time.

friction—resistance of one surface to the motion of another surface rubbing over it.

fringe (benefits)—benefits included in or added to the salary paid, such as health insurance, retirement fund, etc.

frontal—anterior; the forehead bone; refers to the plane drawn through the side of the body from the head to the foot.

functional—practical, working, useful.

fundus—that portion of an organ most remote from its opening; with uterus, the body of the uterus above the openings of the fallopian tubes.

fungus—a vegetable, cellular organism that subsists on organic matter, such as bacteria or mold; a disease condition that causes growth of fungal lesions on the surface of the skin.

furuncle—the medical term for a boil.

gait—manner of walking.

gallbladder—a small sac suspended beneath the liver that concentrates and stores bile.

galley proofs—printed matter in preliminary form, to be corrected.

galvanometer—an instrument that measures current by electromagnetic action.

gamete—a germ cell; any reproductive body.

ganglion—a mass of nerve tissue that receives and sends out nerve impulses.

gangrene—a form of necrosis; the putrefaction of soft tissue.

gastric—pertaining to the stomach.

gastrocnemius—the large muscle in the calf of the leg.

gastroenterologist—a physician specializing in the care of patients with diseases and disorders of the gastrointestinal tract.

gastroenterology—the study of the stomach and intestines and their diseases.

gastrointestinal (GI)—pertaining to the stomach and intestines.

gastrointestinal (GI) system—also called the digestive tract, alimentary canal, or gut, the system of organs within multicellular animals that takes in food, digests it to extract energy and nutrients, and expels the remaining waste.

gastroscopy—examination of the stomach with a gastroscope.

gatekeeper—one who regulates access to someone or something; in insurance, a primary care physician who coordinates the patient's referral to specialists and hospital admissions.

gauge—the size of a needle bore; the smaller the number the larger the needle bore.

gene—a substance within the chromosome that dictates heredity.

generate—to produce, as heat, ideas, power.

generic—general; characteristic of a genus or group.

genetic—pertaining to the genes.

genital herpes—fluid-filled lesions on the external genitalia, which are contagious upon direct contact.

genitalia—the external sexual organs.

genogram—a graph of family health history.

genucubital—pertaining to the elbows and knees; the knee-elbow position.

genupectoral—pertaining to the knees and chest; the knee-chest position.

geriatrics—the study and treatment of the diseases of old age.

gerontologist—a physician specializing in the care of the aged.

gestation—period of intrauterine fetal development.

gestational diabetes—form of diabetes found in pregnant women.

gigantism—a condition resulting from the overproduction of growth hormone during childhood.

glance—a quick look or view.

glaucoma—a disease of the eye characterized by increased intraocular pressure.

glomerulonephritis—inflammation of the glomerulus of the nephron of the kidney.

glomerulus—the microscopic cluster of capillaries within the Bowman's capsule of the nephron.

glucohemoglobin—sugar in the blood.

glucose—a colorless or yellow, thick, syrupy liquid obtained by the incomplete hydrolysis of starch; a simple sugar.

gluteus maximus—the large muscle of the buttocks.

glycohemoglobin—test that indicates the average blood sugar over the past 2 months.

glycosuria—sugar in the urine.

glycosylation—the process of adding sugars to proteins or lipids.

goiter—an enlargement of the thyroid gland.

Golgi apparatus—an organelle within the cytoplasm of a cell.

gonadotropic—related to stimulation of the gonads.

gonads—the sex glands, the ovaries in the female and the testicles in the male.

gonorrhea—a venereal disease of the reproductive organs, which is highly contagious upon direct contact.

gooseneck lamp—a light fixture with a flexible portion that allows adjustment.

graafian follicle—the vesicle in which ova are matured and which releases them when ripened.

graft—a constructed part.

Gram negative—bacteria that take on a pink color with Gram staining process.

Gram positive—bacteria that take on a purple color with Gram staining process.

greenstick—an incomplete fracture, occurring in children.

grillwork—a bar-like device, usually constructed of heavy metal; an open grating for a door or window.

groin—the depression between the thigh and the trunk of the body; the inguinal region.

gross—exclusive of deductions; total; entire.

gross anatomy—refers to the study of those features that can be observed with the naked eye by inspection and dissection.

guaiac—a solution used to test for the presence of occult blood in the stool.

guaiac test paper—a screening agent to test for hidden blood.

guarantee—assurance that something will be done as specified; a pledge.

guarantor—a person who makes or gives a guarantee or pledge, often to pay another's debt or obligation in the event of default.

guilds—associations of persons engaged in the same trade or calling for mutual protection.

GYN—see **gynecology.**

gynecologist—a physician specializing in the care of diseases and disorders of women, particularly the genital organs.

gynecology (GYN)—the study of diseases of the female, particularly of the organs of reproduction.

haemophilus—bacterial strains that grow best in hemoglobin.

hallucinogen—a substance that causes hallucinations.

hamstring—a group of muscles of the posterior thigh.

handicap—to hinder; those who are physically disabled or mentally retarded.

hangover—the malaise that follows ingestion of a considerable amount of alcohol.

harassment—continual annoyance; persecution.

harbor—place of protection; in health care, surfaces that allow microorganisms to hide and grow.

hard copy—information printed on a solid surface, such as paper, instead of displayed on a CRT screen or stored on a disk.

hardware—the visible parts of a computer system (keyboard, disk drive, monitor, and printers).

harmonious—having parts combined in a proportionate, orderly, or pleasing arrangement; being peaceable or friendly.

hazard—danger; risk.

HCFA—Health Care Financing Administration.

health—a state of complete physical and mental or social well-being.

health maintenance organization (HMO)—a type of managed care operation that is typically set up as a for-profit corporation with salaried employees.

health reimbursement arrangement (HRA)—an account with employer contributions used to pay for medical expenses.

health savings account (HSA)—a tax-sheltered savings account, with contributions from the employer and employee, which can be used to pay for medical expenses.

healthcheck—a federally mandated Medicaid program for health care of children up to 21 years of age.

heart block—a condition in which impulses from the SA node fail to carry over to the AV node, resulting in a slow heart rate and a different rate of contraction between the upper and lower heart chambers.

heart murmur—a sound produced by the leakage of blood through a heart valve.

heartburn—a burning sensation beneath the breastbone, usually associated with indigestion.

height—the vertical length of an object or person.

hematocrit—an expression of the volume of red blood cells per unit of circulating blood.

hematologist—a physician specializing in the care of patients with disorders and diseases of the blood and blood-forming organs.

hematology—the study of the blood and its diseases.

hematoma—a tumor or swelling that contains blood.

hematuria—blood in the urine.

hemodialysis—a process whereby blood is passed through a thin membrane and exposed to a dialysate solution to remove waste products.

hemoglobin—the combination of a protein and iron pigment in the red blood cells that attracts and carries oxygen in the body.

hemolysis—dissolution; the breaking down of red blood cells.

hemophilia—hereditary condition, transmitted through sex-linked chromosomes of female carriers; affects males only, causing inability to clot blood.

hemorrhage—abnormal discharge of blood either internally or externally from venous, arterial, or capillary vessels.

hemorrhoidectomy—surgical excision of hemorrhoidal tissue.

hemorrhoids—varicose veins of the anal canal.

hemostat—a type of forceps.

hemothorax—blood within the pleural space of the chest cavity.

heparin—a substance formed in the liver that inhibits the coagulation of blood.

hepatic—pertaining to the liver.

hepatitis—inflammation of the liver.

hepatitis B—acute infection of the liver transmitted through blood or body fluids.

herbal—pertaining to plants, particularly to their medicinal qualities.

hernia—a projection of a part from its normal location.

herniorrhaphy—the surgical repair of a hernia.

herpes simplex—the medical term for fever blister, an acute viral infection of the face, mouth, or nose.

herpes zoster—the medical term for shingles, an acute viral infection of the dorsal root ganglia.

hesitancy—difficulty in starting a urine stream.

heterosexual—sexual attraction toward the opposite sex.

heterotrophs—microorganisms that feed on organic matter.

HHS—U.S. Department of Health and Human Services.

hiatus—pertains to a herniation of the stomach through an opening or hiatus.

HIB/hib—*Hemophilus influenzae* type B.

hiccough—(also hiccup) a result of the spasmodic closing of the epiglottis and spasm of the diaphragm.

hiccup—see **hiccough.**

high-power field (hpf)—refers to microscope lens.

hilum—the recessed area of the kidney where the ureter and blood vessels enter.

hinge—a type of joint.

Hippocratic oath—refers to the oath taken by a doctor bonding him to observe the code of medical ethics contained in the oath by Hippocrates in the 4th century.

histamine—a substance normally present in the body.

histologist—(histotechnologist) a person engaged in the study of the microscopic structure of tissue.

histology—the study of cells.

histoplasmosis—a fungal infection caused by an organism found in bird and bat droppings.

histotechnologist—a laboratory specialist who prepares tissues for microscopic examination and diagnosis.

holistic—considering the whole or entire scope of a situation.

Holter monitor—a device that attaches electrodes to a patient's chest for the purpose of obtaining a 24-hour ECG tracing in an accessory tape recorder.

homeopathy—a system of medical practice that treats a disease by the administration of minute doses of a remedy that would in healthy persons produce symptoms similar to those of the disease.

homeostasis—maintenance of a constant or static condition of internal environment.

homosexual—sexual attraction toward the same sex as oneself.

honesty—the state of being truthful, trustworthy; genuine.

horizontal—not vertical; flat and even; level; parallel to the plane of the horizon.

hormone—a chemical substance secreted by an organ or gland.

hospice movement—an organization dedicated to providing care with dignity people who are terminally ill.

hostility—unfriendliness, enmity.

human chorionic gonadotropin (hCG)—a hormone produced in pregnancy that is made by the embryo soon after conception.

human immunodeficiency virus (HIV)—a retrovirus that causes acquired immunodeficiency syndrome (AIDS), a condition in humans in which the immune system begins to fail, leading to life-threatening opportunistic infections.

human organism—the collective higher individual resulting from the organization of cells, tissues, organs, and organ systems.

humble—modest, unassuming.

humerus—the long bone of the upper arm.

humor—something that is designed to be amusing or comical.

humoral—antibody-mediated immunity.

hyaline membrane disease—a condition resulting from incomplete development of the respiratory system in premature infants.

hydrocele—the accumulation of fluid in the scrotum.

hydrochloric acid—a digestive juice found in the stomach.

hygiene—the study of health and observance of health rules.

hygienist—one who provides health-related services, such as dental procedures.

hymen—a membranous fold partially or completely covering the vaginal opening.

hyperglycemia—increase of blood sugar, as in diabetes.

hyperopia—a defect of vision so that objects can only be seen when they are far away; farsightedness.

hypersensitive—oversensitive; abnormally sensitive to a stimulus of any kind.

hypertension—elevated blood pressure.

hyperthermia—higher than normal temperature.

hyperthyroidism—a condition caused by excessive secretion of the thyroid glands.

hypertonic—having a higher concentration of salt than found in a red blood cell.

hyperventilation—excessive deep and frequent breathing.

hyphen—a punctuation mark used to divide or create compound words.

hypnosis—a state that resembles sleep but is induced by suggestion.

hypoallergenic—unlikely to cause an allergic reaction.

hypochondriac—pertaining to the upper outer regions of the abdomen below the thorax; also someone with a morbid fear of disease, resulting in abnormal concern about one's health.

hypogastric—referring to an abdominal area in the middle lower third of the abdomen.

hypoglycemia—deficiency of sugar in the blood.

hypotension—abnormally low blood pressure.

hypothalamus—a structure of the brain between the cerebrum and the midbrain; lies below the thalamus.

hypothermia—below normal body temperature.

hypothyroidism—a condition caused by a marked deficiency of thyroid secretion.

hypotonic—having a lower concentration of salt than found in a red blood cell.

hypoxia—a lack of oxygen.

hysterectomy—surgical removal of the uterus.

hysteroscopy—a procedure using the hysteroscope to view the endometrium of the uterus.

ICD—see **International Classification of Diseases.**

I & D—see **incision and drainage.**

identification—anything by which a person or thing can be identified.

idiopathic—disease without recognizable cause.

idle—uninvolved; doing nothing.

ileocecal—the valve between the end of the small intestine and the cecum.

ileostomy—a surgical opening from the ileum onto the abdominal wall.

ileum—the last section of the small intestine.

iliac—the edge or crest of the pelvic bone.

ilium—the hip bone.

illegible—impossible to read.

illicit—improper; unlawful; not sanctioned by custom or law; illegal.

illuminating—enlightening; throwing light on.

imaging—a representation or visual impression produced by a lens, mirror, etc.

immobilize—to keep out of action or circulation; stationary.

immune—protected or exempt from a disease.

immunization—becoming immune or the process of rendering a patient immune.

immunoassays—a biochemical test that measures the level of a substance in a biologic liquid, typically serum or urine, using the reaction of an antibody or antibodies to its antigen.

immunodeficiency—lacking the components necessary to mount an immune response.

immunoglobulin—a large protein molecule that assists in the immune response.

immunologic—pertaining to immunology.

immunology—a broad branch of biomedical science that covers the study of all aspects of the immune system in all organisms.

immunosuppressed—a condition wherein the immune system has been overpowered and cannot function adequately.

impacted—refers to a fracture where the broken ends are jammed together.

impaction—a collection of hardened feces in the rectum that cannot be expelled.

impending—to be at hand or about to happen.

implant—something implanted into tissue; a graft; artificial part.

implement—a tool or instrument for doing something; to put into effect.

implementation—put into effect.

implication—involvement, bringing into connection.

implied—hinted, suggested.

impotence—inability of a male to obtain or maintain an erection.

impulse—a charge transmitted through certain tissues, especially nerve fibers and muscles, resulting in physiologic activity.

inappropriate—not appropriate, out of place.

incident report—a report giving detailed information about an emergency situation and how it was handled.

incineration—burn, setting afire.

incision—cut.

incision and drainage (I & D)—cutting into for the purpose of providing an exit for material, usually a collection of pus.

inclined—leaning or tending toward.

incompetent—not capable; not legally qualified; deficient.

incomprehensible—beyond belief, not to be grasped by the mind.

incongruous—lacking harmony or agreement.

incontinent—unable to control the bladder or bowel.

increments—becoming greater; amount of increase; gain.

incubation—the interval between exposure to infection and the appearance of the first symptom.

incus—the anvil, the middle bone of the three in the middle ear.

indemnity—to compensate for damage done or loss caused.

indigent—needy, poor, destitute.

indigestion—difficulty in digesting food.

induction—the process of causing or producing; to bring on.

inevitable—unavoidable, destined to occur.

infarction—infiltration of foreign particles; material in a vessel causing coagulation and interference with circulation.

infectious—capable of producing infection; denoting a disease in the body caused by the presence of germs; tending to spread to others.

infectious mononucleosis—a disease seen most commonly in adolescents and young adults, characterized by fever, sore throat, leg and muscle soreness and fatigue (symptoms of a common cold or allergies). Mononucleosis is caused by the Epstein-Barr virus (EBV).

inferior—below, under.

inferior vena cava—the large vein that carries deoxygenated blood from the lower half of the body into the heart.

infertility—inability to achieve conception.

infirmity—illness, disease.

inflict—to strike, to cause punishment.

influenza—an acute illness characterized by fever, pain, coughing, and general upper respiratory symptoms.

infrared—pertaining to those invisible rays just beyond the red end of the visible spectrum that have a penetrating heating effect.

infusion—to instill; introduction of a substance into a vein.

ingested—to eat.

inguinal—referring to the region where the thigh joins the trunk of the body; the groin.

inguinal canal—a passageway in the groin for the spermatic cord in the male.

inguinal hernia—the presence of small intestine in the inguinal canal.

inhale—to breathe in.

initial—the first; beginning; the first letter of each of a person's names.

initiate—to get something started, begin.

initiative—the action of taking the first step; ability to originate new ideas.

innate—inborn; inherent.

inoculating loop—a laboratory instrument used to transfer organisms from one source to another.

inorganic—not living; occurring in nature independently of living things.

inseminate—to impregnate with semen.

insertion—the place where a muscle is attached to the bone that it moves.

insidious—hidden, not apparent.

insignificant—unimportant; petty; of little or no value.

insomnia—abnormal inability to sleep.

inspect—to examine closely.

inspection—the first part of a physical examination; close observation.

inspiration—to breathe in, inhale.

instill—to slowly drop liquid onto a surface or into a cavity.

institute—to originate as a custom.

insufficient—not as much as needed.

insulin—a hormone secreted by the islets of Langerhans in the pancreas.

insulin shock—a condition of excess insulin or lack of blood sugar.

insurance—a contract to guarantee compensation for a specified situation.

intact—unbroken, undamaged.

intangible—that which cannot be touched, easily defined, or grasped.

integrity—soundness of character; honesty in particular.

integumentary—the skin; a covering.

integumentary system—the largest organ system by surface area, comprising skin, hair, nails, and sweat glands and their products (sweat and mucus). It distinguishes, separates, and protects. The name derives from the Latin *integumentum*, which means "a covering."

intellectualization—to employ reasoning to avoid confrontations or stressful situations.

intelligence—the ability to learn or understand.

interaction—to act upon one another.

intercede—to mediate, plead on behalf of another.

intercostal—between the ribs.

interference—confusion of desired signals caused by undesired signals, as in artifacts on an ECG.

interferon—a lymphokine that helps regulate the activities of macrophages and natural killer cells.

interjection—a part of speech; an exclamation.

interleukin—a substance that is a messenger between leukocytes.

intermediate—in the middle.

intermittent—stopping and starting again at intervals.

intermuscular—within the muscle.

internal—the innermost part(s) of the body.

Internal Revenue Service—the division of federal government charged with implementing tax laws and collecting taxes.

International Classification of Diseases (ICD)—a comprehensive listing of diseases and disorders of the human body.

interneurons—neurons connecting sensory to motor neurons.

internist—a physician specializing in the care of patients with internal diseases.

internship—a time following graduation wherein practice of the profession is performed.

interpersonal—between persons.

interpret—to explain, translate; to determine the meaning.

interpretive—computerized analysis of ECG tracings.

interval—time between events; space.

intervention—taking action to modify, hinder, or change an effect.

interventional hysterosalpingography—a diagnostic examination to evaluate the fallopian tubes.

intervertebral—between the vertebrae.

interview—a meeting between two people where one asks questions of the other.

intestine—the alimentary canal extending from the pylorus of the stomach to the anus.

intimidate—to make afraid, to frighten.

intimidation—to make afraid; to deter with threats.

intoxicated—a condition caused by the overindulgence in alcoholic beverages.

intracellular—within the cell.

intradermal—within the skin.

intramuscular (IM)—type of injection administered into a muscle.

intraocular—within the eyeball.

intrauterine device (IUD)—an object inserted into the uterus to prevent pregnancy.

intravenous—to insert into the vein.

intravenous pyelography (IVP)—the insertion of a radiopaque material into the vein for the purpose of x-raying the kidneys and ureters.

intricate—complicated, complex, elaborately interwoven.

intubation—insertion of a tube into the larynx for entrance of air.

intuition—the immediate knowing or learning of something without the conscious use of reasoning.

inunction—the process of administering drugs through the skin.

invasive (procedure)—diagnostic methods involving entry into living tissue.

inventory—an itemized list of goods in stock.

inversion—the movement of the sole of the foot toward the median plane.

in vivo—that which takes place inside an organism.

involuntary—independent of or even contrary to will or choice.

iodine—a nonmetallic element belonging to the halogen group.

ipecac—an emetic; causes vomiting.

iris—the colored, contractible tissue surrounding the pupil of the eye.

irrational—lacking the power to reason; senseless.

irreconcilable—cannot be brought into agreement.

irrelevant—not pertinent, not to the point.

irreparable—damaged beyond possibility of repair.

irrigate—to wash out with a liquid.

ischemia—temporary and localized anemia caused by obstruction of the circulation to a part.

ischium—posterior and inferior portion of the hip bone.

Ishihara—refers to an eye test to determine color vision.

islets of Langerhans—clusters of cells in the pancreas.

isotonic—having the same concentration of salt as found in a red blood cell.

issue—to send forth; to put into circulation.

IVP—see **intravenous pyelography.**

Jaeger—a system for measuring near vision acuity.

jaundice—a yellowish discoloration of the sclera and skin due to the presence of bile pigments in the blood.

jejunum—the middle segment of the small intestine, which measures approximately 8 feet in length.

jeopardize—to put at risk.

journal—a record of happenings; a diary.

journalizing—entries on the daily log.

judgment—a decision; ability to make the right decisions.

keloid—an overgrowth of new skin tissue; a scar.

ketone (acetone)—products of metabolism generated from carbohydrates, fatty acids, and amino acids in humans.

keying—pressing a lever or button, as on a typewriter, with the finger to operate the machine.

kidney—a bean-shaped organ that excretes urine and is located retroperitoneally, high in the back of the abdominal cavity.

KUB—kidneys, ureters, and bladder; refers to a radiologic study.

kyphosis—a convex curvature of the spine; humpback.

L & A—light and accommodation.

labia majora—the two large folds of adipose tissue lying on each side of the vulva of the female; external genitalia.

labia minora—the two mucocutaneous folds of membrane within the labia majora.

laboratory technician—a health care worker who performs specialized chemical, microscopic, and bacteriologic tests of blood, tissue, and body fluids.

laboratory—a room or building in which scientific tests or experiments are conducted.

laceration—a cut or tear.

lacrimal—pertaining to tears; the glands and ducts that secrete and convey tears.

Lamaze—a program or method of managing labor during birth.

laminectomy—the removal of a portion of the vertebral posterior arch.

lancet—a sharp, pointed instrument used to pierce the skin to obtain a capillary blood sample.

laryngeal—pertaining to the larynx.

laryngectomy—surgical removal of the larynx or voice box.

laryngitis—inflammation of the vocal cords.

larynx—the voice box.

lateral—pertaining to the side.

latissimus dorsi—the large muscle of the back.

lavage—the washing out of a cavity.

laxative—a substance that induces the bowels to empty.

ledgers—the principal account books of a business establishment, containing the credits and debits.

legible—easy to read, readable.

Legionnaires' disease—an acute bronchopneumonia.

leisure—spare or free time, away from the pressure and responsibilities of work.

lens—a part of the eye that bends or refracts images onto the retina.

lesion—an injury or wound; a circumscribed area of pathologically altered tissue.

lethal—deadly; capable of causing death.

lethargic—sluggishness, apathy.

leukemia—a disease characterized by a great excess of white blood cells; it exists in a lymphatic and myelogenous form; it is often fatal, especially in adults.

leukocyte—a white blood cell.

leukocyte esterase—a urine test for the presence of white blood cells and other abnormalities associated with infection.

liability—anything to which a person is liable, responsible, legally bound.

liaison—intercommunication between two entities.

license—a legal permit to engage in an activity.

licensed practical nurse (LPN)—an individual trained in basic nursing techniques, to provide direct patient care under the supervision of an RN or physician.

ligament—fibrous tissue that connects bone to bone.

ligation—to tie off; the process of binding or tying.

limbs—refers to the arms and legs.

limited—to restrict; to hold within fixed bounds.

limited check—a check that will be marked void if written for more than a certain amount. This type of check is often used for payroll or insurance payments.

listlessness—lack of desire, interest.

liter—a unit of measure; 1,000 mL or approximately 1 quart.

lithotomy—an examination position wherein the patient lies upon the back with thighs flexed upon the abdomen and legs flexed upon the thighs.

lithotripsy—destruction of stone; stonecrusher.

liver—the largest gland in the body, located in the upper right quadrant of the abdomen beneath the diaphragm.

living will—advance directive; a document, written in advance, that states the patient's wishes regarding end-of-life care.

LMP—last menstrual period.

longevity—a long duration of life; lasting a long time.

longitudinal fissure—the deep cleft between the two hemispheres of the cerebrum.

lordosis—abnormal anterior curvature of the lumbar spine.

low-power field (lpf)—refers to microscope lens.

lubb dupp—sounds made by the heart.

lumbar—pertaining to the back, specifically to the five vertebrae above the sacrum.

lumbar puncture—the insertion of a needle between the vertebrae in the lumbar area for the purpose of withdrawing spinal fluid.

lumen—the space within an artery, vein, or capillary; the space within a tube.

lung—the organ of respiration, located within the thoracic cavity.

lupus erythematosus—a chronic autoimmune disease that causes changes in the immune system.

luteinizing—a hormone effect that causes ovulation and progesterone in the female and sperm production and testosterone in the male.

Lyme disease—a disease caused by a spirochete that is carried by the deer tick.

lymph—a body fluid formed within the tissue spaces and circulated throughout the body.

lymphatic system—a network of transparent vessels carrying lymph fluid throughout the body.

lymphedema—excess lymph fluid in the tissues.

lymphocyte—a type of white blood cell.

lymphokine—a cytokine produced by a T-cell.

lysosomes—an organelle within the cytoplasm of the cell.

macrophage—a phagocytic cell that destroys antigens.

macule—a discolored spot or patch on the skin neither elevated nor depressed.

magnetic—having the properties of a magnet, able to attract.

magnetic resonance imaging (MRI)—a diagnostic test using magnetic waves to visualize internal body structures.

magnify—to make something look larger than it really is.

mailable—a standard for judging written correspondence as satisfactory for sending.

maintenance—to preserve; the act or work of keeping something in proper condition.

malaise—a feeling of discomfort or uneasiness.

malignant—a cancerous growth; tumor.

malinger—to pretend illness to escape dealing with a situation or obligation.

malleus—the largest of the three bones of the middle ear, also called the hammer.

malnutrition—lack of necessary or proper food substances in the body.

mammary glands—the breasts.

mammogram—an x-ray of the breast.

mammography—the process of using low-dose x-rays to examine the human breast. It is used to look for different types of tumors and cysts.

management—the act, manner, or practice of managing, handling, or controlling something.

mandate—an order of authorative command; instruction.

manifestation—act of disclosing; revelation; display.

manipulation—the passive movement of a joint to determine the range of flexion and extension.

manipulation therapy—any treatment or procedure involving the use of the hands; additional manual skills used by osteopathic physicians.

marginal—close to the lower limit of acceptability.

marrow—the soft tissue in the hollow of long bones.

massage—manipulation of tissues for therapeutic purposes by rubbing, kneading, or tapping with the hands.

masses—a multitude; a large number of people.

mastectomy—surgical removal of a breast.

matrix—a format for establishing a time schedule for appointments.

maturation index (MI)—a measurement of cellular maturity.

maturation—refers to a stage of cellular development.

maturity—a state of full development.

measles—a highly contagious disease characterized by the presence of maculopustular eruptions.

mechanical—pertaining to machinery.

medial—pertaining to the middle or midline.

Medicaid—a government health care program.

Medicare—a federal health program for paying certain medical expenses of the aged.

Medigap—refers to situations not covered by Medicare insurance.

medulla—the inner section of the kidney.

medulla oblongata—enlarged portion of the spinal cord; the lower portion of the brainstem.

melanin—a pigment that gives color to the skin, hair, and eyes.

melanocytes—cells that produce the pigment of the skin, melanin.

membrane—a thin, soft, pliable layer of tissue that lines a tube or cavity or covers an organ or structure.

menarche—the first menstrual period.

Meniere's disease—a disorder of the ear characterized by nausea, vomiting, tinnitus, and hearing loss.

meninges—the membranes covering the brain and spinal cord.

meningitis—inflammation of the meninges of the brain and/or spinal cord.

meniscus—a concave level of fluid in a tube or cylinder.

menopause—the permanent cessation of menstruation.

menorrhagia—excessive menstrual flow, hemorrhage.

menstruation—periodic discharge of bloody fluid from the uterus.

mensuration—the process of measuring.

mercury—a liquid metal used in measurement devices such as thermometers and sphygmomanometers; chemical symbol, Hg.

merit—to deserve reward or praise; excellence.

mesentery—a peritoneal fold connecting the intestine to the posterior abdominal wall.

metabolism—the successive transformations to which a substance is subjected from the time it enters the body to the time it or its decomposition products are excreted, and by which nutrition is accomplished and energy and living substance are provided.

metabolized—the successive transformation of a substance from the time it enters the body to the time it or its decomposition products are excreted, and by which nutrition is accomplished and energy and living substance are provided.

metacarpal—pertaining to the five bones of the hand between the wrist and the phalanges.

metastasis—movement of cancer cells from one part of the body to another.

metastasize—the process whereby malignant cells leave the primary lesion and migrate to another location.

metatarsal—the five bones of the feet between the instep and the phalanges.

methodical—systematic, following a plan or method.

MI—see **myocardial infarction.**

microbes—organisms that are microscopic (too small to be visible to the human eye).

microbial—related to microbes.

microfiche—a sheet of microfilm capable of accommodating and preserving a considerable number of book pages in reduced form.

microfilming—using a machine to put copies of written data such as a patient file into a smaller, storable format.

microhematocrit—packed cell volume (PCV) that measures the proportion of blood volume that is occupied by red blood cells.

microorganism—a microscopic living body not perceivable by the naked eye.

microscopic—visible only with a microscope.

microscopic anatomy—an area of study that deals with features that can be seen only with a microscope.

micturtion—the passing of urine.

midbrain—that portion of the brain connecting the pons and the cerebellum.

midline—the middle.

midsagittal—an imaginary vertical plane made by dividing the body down the middle, creating equal right and left sides; also known as the midline.

migraine—a severe headache with characteristic symptoms.

mineralocorticoid—a biologic principle of the adrenal cortex involved in regulating body fluid and electrolytes.

minute—a measurement of time equal to 60 seconds; very small, tiny.

misalignment—out of alignment; not straight.

misspelled—to spell incorrectly.

mitochondria—an organelle within the cytoplasm of the cell.

mitosis—the division of a cell.

mitral—the valve in the heart between the chambers of the left side, also known as the bicuspid.

mobility—quality of being mobile; easy to move.

modifier—changes; limits the meaning.

modifies—changes the form or quality of; alters slightly.

molten—melted.

monilia—a family of parasitic fungi or molds.

moniliasis—an infection of the mucous membranes by yeast-like fungi.

monitor—to oversee or observe.

monoclonal—a laboratory-produced hybrid cell that produces antibodies.

monocular—possessing a single eyepiece, as with a microscope.

monocyte—single nucleated cells that leave the blood and enter into tissues to become macrophages.

monogamous—an exclusive relationship between two people.

monokine—a cytokine produced by macrophages or monocytes.

monotone—a single, unvaried tone; having the same pitch; a tiresome sameness.

mons pubis—a pad of fatty tissue and coarse skin overlying the symphysis pubis in the female.

moral—a principle of right and wrong in conduct.

morality—right living; virtue.

mores—folkways that, through general observance, develop the force of a law.

morphology—a branch of biology dealing with the form and structure of organisms.

motor—refers to the nerves that permit the body to respond to stimuli.

mouth—the oral cavity; can also refer to the opening to organs.

MRI—see **magnetic resonance imaging.**

mucosa—pertaining to mucous membrane.

MUGA—see **multiple-gated acquisition scan.**

multi-skilled—having more than one skill area for employment.

multichannel—refers to the capability of ECG equipment of processing impulses from multiple leads.

multiple-gated acquisition scan (MUGA)—a diagnostic test to evaluate the condition of the myocardium of the heart.

mumps—an acute contagious disease characterized by inflammation of the parotid gland and other salivary glands.

murmur—a soft blowing or rasping sound heard on auscultation of the heart.

muscle team—a pair of skeletal muscles, one that flexes and one that extends the joint.

muscle tone—a state of muscle contraction in which a portion of the fibers are contracted while others are at rest.

muscle—a type of tissue composed of contractile cells or fibers that effect movement of the body.

muscular—pertaining to muscles.

musculoskeletal—pertaining to the muscular and skeletal systems.

mutation—a change in an inheritable characteristic; cellular change caused by an influence.

myelin—a fatlike substance forming the principal component of the myelin sheath of nerve fibers.

myelography—an x-ray examination of the spinal cord following an injection of a radiopaque material.

myocardial infarction (MI)—blockage of a coronary artery that interrupts the flow of blood to the heart muscle.

myocardium—the muscle layer of the heart.

myometrium—the muscular structure of the uterus.

myopia—a defect in vision so that objects can only be seen when very near; nearsightedness.

myxedema—a condition resulting from the hypofunction of the thyroid gland.

Nagel's rule—a method of predicting the anticipated date of delivery when pregnant.

narcolepsy—overwhelming attacks of sleep that the victim cannot inhibit; sleeping sickness.

narcotic—a drug capable of producing sleep and relieving pain or inducing unconsciousness and even death, depending upon the dosage.

nasal—pertaining to the nose.

nasal speculum—an instrument permitting visualization of the inside of the nasal cavity.

naturopathy—a multidisciplinary approach to health care based on the belief that the body has the power to heal itself.

nausea—an inclination to vomit.

needle holder—instrument used to hold a suture needle during the suturing process.

negate—to deny the existence or truth of.

neglect—to ignore or pay no attention to; to leave uncared for.

negligent—guilty of neglect; lacking in due care or concern; act of carelessness.

negotiable—capable of being discussed and terms arranged.

neoadjuvant—new attachment process; giving chemotherapy prior to surgery to shrink the tumor before removal.

neonate—a newborn infant.

neoplasm—a new growth.

neoplastic—new abnormal tissue formation; cancer-related.

nephrologist—a physician specializing in the diseases and disorders of the kidney.

nephrology—the study of the kidney and its diseases.

nephron—the structural and functional unit of the kidney.

nephrotic syndrome—term applied to renal disease of whatever cause characterized by massive edema, proteinuria, and usually elevation of serum cholesterol and lipids.

nerve—a group of nervous tissues bound together for the purpose of conducting nervous impulses.

nervosa—loss of appetite for food not connected with a disease; part of a psychosis.

net—remaining after all deductions have been made; to clear as profit.

neurilemma—a thin membranous sheath enveloping a nerve fiber.

neurologist—a physician specializing in the diseases and disorders of the nervous system.

neurology—the study of the nervous system and its diseases.

neuron—a nerve cell.

neurosurgery—surgical procedures performed on the nervous system.

neutrophil—a granulated white blood cell.

nicotine—a poisonous alkaloid extracted from tobacco leaves.

nit—the egg of a louse or other parasitic insect.

nitrite—a urine test that is positive in urinary tract infections from the presence of bacteria reducing nitrates to nitrite.

nocturia—having to void at night.

node—a knot, knob, protuberance, or swelling.

nomenclature—a system of technical or scientific names.

nominal—too small to be considered, or a very small amount.

nomogram—representation by graphs, diagrams, or charts of the relationship between numerical variables.

non compos mentis—general legal term for all forms of mental illness.

nonchalant—unconcerned, indifferent.

noninvasive procedurer—a diagnostic method not requiring entry into body tissue.

nonpathogen—an organism that does not produce a disease.

nonspecific urethritis—inflammation of the urethra in males and vaginitis or cervicitis in females caused by bacteria or an allergy to substances used by a sexual partner.

norepinephrine—a hormone secreted by adrenal medulla in response to sympathetic stimulation.

normal saline—a solution with the same salt content as that found within a red blood cell.

noun—the name of anything, such as a person, place, object, occurrence, or state.

NREM (non–rapid eye movement)—a stage of sleep in which the sleeper does not experience rapid eye movement. In a healthy young adult, NREM sleep usually accounts for 75%–90% of sleep time.

nuclear—pertaining to the nucleus of an atom.

nuclear medicine—the branch of medicine that uses radionuclides in the diagnosis and treatment of disease.

nuclear medicine technologist—an individual trained in the specialized field of operating cameras that detect and map the radioactive drug in a patient's body to create diagnostic images.

nucleolus—a structure found within the nucleus of the cell.

nucleus—the vital body in the protoplasm of a cell.

numeric—denoting a number or system of numbers.

nurse assistant (NA)—a person trained to assist nurses and attend to patients.

nurse midwife—a nurse trained in the delivery of babies.

nurse practitioner—an RN with advanced clinical experience and education in a special branch of practice.

nurture—to care for, train, or educate.

nutrition—refers to edible material, food, things that nourish.

nutritionist—a member of the health care team who studies and applies the principles and science of nutrition.

obese—weighing more than 30% of ideal body weight.

objective—the end toward which action is directed; of a disease symptom, perceptible to persons other than the one affected; on a microscope, a lens or series of lenses.

obligate—to bind legally or morally.

obligation—responsibility; a moral, social, or legal tie.

obliterate—to blot out; leave no trace; destroy.

observant—quick to notice, watchful.

obsolete—out of use, discarded, no longer useful.

obstetrician—a physician who specializes in the care and treatment of women during pregnancy and childbirth.

obstetrics—the branch of medicine dealing with women during pregnancy, childbirth, and postpartum.

obstructed—blocked.

obturator—anything that obstructs or closes a cavity or opening; refers to that internal portion of an examining instrument that facilitates the introduction of the instrument into the body and is then withdrawn, permitting visualization of the internal area.

occipital—pertaining to the back part of the head, the posterior lobe of the cerebrum.

occlude—to close up, obstruct.

occluder—a device to block viewing when conducting an eye examination.

occult—obscure; hidden.

occulta—obscure; hidden.

occupational medicine—diagnosing and treating disease or conditions arising from occupational circumstances.

Occupational Safety and Health Administration (OSHA)—an agency of the United States Department of Labor. It was created by Congress under the Occupational Safety and Health Act, signed by President Richard M. Nixon, on December 29, 1970. Its mission is to prevent work-related injuries, illnesses, and deaths by issuing and enforcing rules (called standards) for workplace safety and health.

occupational therapist (OT)—a health care worker involved in the use of purposeful activity with individuals who are limited by physical injury or illness, psychosocial dysfunction, developmental or learning diabilities, poverty and cultural differences, or the aging process to maximize independence, prevent disability, and maintain health.

occupational therapy assistant (OTA)—a person trained to assist an occupational therapist.

O.D.—oculus dexter, or right eye.

office manager—(business office manager) an individual responsible for the overall operation of the medical office.

ointment—a salve; a fatty, soft substance having antiseptic or healing properties.

olfactory—pertaining to the sense of smell.

oliguria—scanty production of urine.

oncogenes—a gene in a tumor cell.

oncologist—a doctor who has been specially trained in the study of tumors and cancer.

oncology—the branch of medicine dealing with tumors, usually malignant.

on-site—at the location.

ophthalmic—pertaining to the eye.

ophthalmic technician (OT)—an individual trained for assisting ophthalmologists with patients as well as procedures associated with the eyes.

ophthalmologist—a physician specializing in the diseases and disorders of the eye.

ophthalmology—the study of the eye and its diseases.

opportunistic—seizing the opportunity; taking advantage of the situation.

opposition—action against, resistance.

optic—pertaining to the eye or sight.

optic disc—the blind spot where the optic nerve exits from the retina of the eye.

optometrist—a person who measures the eye's refractive power and prescribes correction of visual defects when needed.

oral—pertaining to the mouth.

orbital—refers to the cavity within the skull where the eye is located.

organ—a part of the body constructed of many types of tissue to perform a function.

organ of Corti—terminal acoustic apparatus in the cochlea of the inner ear.

organelles—functional structures within the cytoplasm of a cell.

organic—pertaining to or derived from animal or vegetable forms of life.

origin—the beginning or source of anything; of muscles, the anchor.

orthopedics—the branch of medicine dealing with the structure and function of bones and muscles.

orthopedist—a physician who corrects deformities and treats diseases and disorders of the bones, joints, and spine.

orthopnea—respiratory condition in which breathing is possible only in an erect sitting or standing position.

orthostatic—standing; concerning an erect position.

O.S.—oculus sinister, or left eye.

os—pertains to a mouth or opening.

oscilloscope—an instrument that displays a visual representation of electric variations on the fluorescent screen of a cathode ray tube.

OSHA—U.S. Occupational Safety and Health Administration.

osmosis—the process of diffusion of water or another solvent through a selected permeable membrane.

osseous—bonelike, concerning bones.

osteopathy—any bone disease; also refers to a school of medicine based on the belief that the bony fragment of the body largely determines the structural relations of its tissues.

osteoporosis—a condition resulting from a decrease in the amount of calcium stored in the bone.

OTA—see **occupational therapy assistant.**

OTC—see **over the counter.**

otic—pertaining to the ear.

otitis—inflammation of the ear; can be referenced to the external, middle, or internal ear.

otorhinolaryngologist—a physician specializing in diseases and disorders of the ear, nose, and throat.

otorhinolaryngology—the study of the ear, nose, and larynx and their diseases.

otosclerosis—condition characterized by progressive deafness caused by the fixation of the stapes of the middle ear.

O.U.—oculus uterque, or each eye.

ovary—the female gonad, which produces hormones causing the secondary sex characteristics to develop and be maintained.

over-the-counter (OTC)—referring to accessible, nonprescription drugs.

overdraft—an amount beyond what is currently in the account.

ovulation—the periodic ripening and rupture of a mature graafian follicle and the discharge of the ovum.

ovum—an egg, the female gamete or reproductive cell.

oxalate—a salt of oxalic acid.

oxygen—a colorless, odorless, tasteless gas found in the air; chemical symbol, O_2.

oxygenate—combine or supply with oxygen.

pacemaker—the SA node of the heart; also refers to an artificial device that initiates heartbeat.

pallor—lack of color, paleness.

palpate—to feel; to examine by touch.

palpation—the technique of examination using the fingers or hands.

pancreas—an organ that secretes insulin and pancreatic digestive juice.

pancreatitis—inflammation of the pancreas.

pandemic—epidemic over a large region; epidemic in many regions.

panic value—an important indicator on a lab test that indicates immediate notification of the health care provider.

pantomime—motions or gestures used for expressive communication.

Papanicolaou (Pap) smear—a test to detect cancer cells in the mucus of an organ.

papillae—small protuberances or elevations, such as the taste buds of the tongue.

papillary muscles—muscular attachments to the undersides of the heart valves from the walls of the ventricles, which open the valves during the relaxation phase of the heartbeat.

papule—red, elevated area on the skin.

parabasal—beside, near, an accessory to the base or lower part.

paralytic ileus—paralysis of the intestinal wall with symptoms of acute obstruction.

paramedic—health care providers who provide emergency and supportive medical care; have additional training beyond EMT status.

parameter—quantity to which an arbitrary value may be given as a convenience in expressing performance or for use in calculations.

parasite—an organism that lives in or on another organism without rendering it any service in return.

parasympathetic—a division of the autonomic nervous system.

parathyroid—small endocrine glands located close to the thyroid gland.

parenteral—other than by mouth.

parietal—a central portion of the cerebrum located on each side of the brain.

paroxysmal—a sudden attack of a disease; fit of acute pain, passion, coughing, or laughter.

paroxysmal stage—occurring repeatedly; recurrent symptoms.

patella—the kneecap.

pathogen—any microorganism or substance capable of producing a disease.

pathologic—a condition caused by a disease.

pathologist—a physician specializing in the interpretation and diagnosis of changes caused by disease in tissues and body fluids.

pathology—the study of the nature and cause of disease.

pathophysiology—the study of mechanisms by which disease occurs, the responses of the body to the disease process, and the effects of both on normal function.

patience—calm in waiting, endurance without complaint.

patient care technician (PCT)—a health care worker who uses both nursing and medical assisting skills to provide patient care in a hospital setting.

patronize—to treat condescendingly.

payee—a person to whom money is paid.

PCT—see **patient care technician**.

PDR—*Physician's Desk Reference.*

pectoralis major—the principal muscle of the chest wall.

pediatrician—a physician specializing in the diseases and disorders of children.

pediatrics—the branch of medicine dealing with the care of children and their diseases.

pediculosis—the scientific name for lice.

peer—equal; usually refers to someone of similar standing or status.

peer review—assessment by other physicians or scientists in the same field.

pelvic—pertaining to the pelvis.

penis—the male external sex organ.

peptic—pertaining to digestion; can also refer to an ulcer of the upper digestive tract.

per capita—for each person.

perceive—to become aware of through the senses; to understand.

percentage—rate or proportion of each hundred.

percentile—any value in a series dividing the distribution of its members into 100 groups of equal frequency.

perception—awareness through the senses; the receipt of impressions; consciousness.

percussion—tapping the body lightly but sharply to determine the position, size, and consistency of an underlying structure.

percussion hammer—a hard, rubber-surfaced instrument used to test tendon reflex action.

performance—to execute an undertaking; an action; success in working.

perfusion—passing of a fluid through spaces; the act of pouring over or through.

pericarditis—inflammation of the pericardium, the covering of the heart.

pericardium—the membranous sac that covers the heart.

perineum—the region between the vagina and anus of the female and the scrotum and anus of the male.

periodic—occurring, appearing, or done again and again, at regular intervals.

periodical—appearing at regular intervals of time.

periosteum—the fibrous membrane covering the bone except at the articulating surfaces.

peripheral—pertaining to a portion of the nervous system; an item attached to a computer system.

peristalsis—a progressive, wavelike muscular movement that occurs involuntarily in the urinary and digestive system.

peritoneal—pertaining to the peritoneum.

peritoneum—the membrane that lines the abdominal cavity and covers the abdominal organs.

permeable—capable of being penetrated; allowing entrance.

pernicious anemia—a severe anemia characterized by progressive decrease in the production of red blood cells.

perplexing—troubling with doubt, puzzling.

PERRLA—an acronym meaning pupils equal, regular, react to light and accommodation.

persecute—treat badly; do harm to again and again; pursue to injure.

perserverance—the act of continuing steadfastly, especially in the face of discouragement.

personal protective equipment (PPE)—protective clothing, goggles, or gloves designed to protect the wearer's body or clothing from contamination by blood or other potentially infectious materials for job-related occupational safety and health purposes.

personality—the personal or individual qualities that make one person different from another.

perspective—a view of things, or facts, in which they are in the right relations.

pertinent—having to do with what is being considered; relevant or to the point.

pertussis—an acute infectious disease characterized by a paroxysmal cough, ending in a whooping inspiration.

petechiae—small, purplish, hemorrhagic spots on the skin.

petition—a written plea in which specific court action is sought.

petty—small, having little value, mean, narrow-minded.

pH—a measure of acidity or alkalinity.

phagocyte—a white blood cell that engulfs and destroys antigens.

phagocytosis—ingestion and digestion of bacteria and particles by phagocytes.

phalanges—bones of the fingers and toes.

phalanx—any one of the bones of the fingers or toes.

phantom limb—an illusion following amputation of a limb that the limb still exists.

pharmaceutical—concerning drugs or pharmacy.

pharmacist (RPH)—a licensed health care provider who prepares and dispenses drugs.

pharmacology—the study and practice of compounding and dispensing medical preparations.

pharmacy technician (PT)—an assistant to a pharmacist who prepares and in some situations administers medication.

pharynx—the throat; that portion of the alimentary canal between the mouth and the esophagus.

phenylalanine—an amino acid of a protein.

phenylketonuria (PKU)—a genetic disorder resulting from the body's failure to oxidize an amino acid, perhaps because of a defective enzyme.

phimosis—a narrowing of the opening of the foreskin of the penis.

phlebitis—inflammation of a vein.

phlebotomist—a health care worker who specializes in obtaining blood samples.

photocopy—a photographic reproduction of written matter made by a special device.

photophobia—sensitive to light; avoiding light.

physical—pertaining to the body; also used for the examination of the body.

physical medicine—the branch of medicine dealing with the treatment of disorders and diseases with mechanical devices, as in physical therapy.

physical therapist (PT)—one who is licensed to assist in the examination, testing, and treatment of physically disabled or handicapped people through the use of special exercise, application of heat or cold, use of sonar, and other techniques.

physician—a medical doctor; one skilled in the practice of medicine.

physician's assistant (PA)—a person trained in certain aspects of the practice of medicine to provide assistance to the physician.

Physicians' Desk Reference (PDR)—one of the reference books that lists information about medications.

physician's office laboratory (POL)—a designated room in the physician's office where laboratory procedures and tests are performed by qualified persons.

physiology—the study of the function of the cells, tissues, and organs of the body.

pia mater—innermost of the three meninges of the brain and spinal cord.

pigment—any coloring matter.

pineal body—a small endocrine gland attached to the posterior part of the third ventricle of the brain.

pinocytosis—the process whereby a cell engulfs large amounts of liquid.

pitch—the frequency of vibrations of sound that enable one to classify sound on a scale from high to low.

pitfall—trap or hidden danger.

pituitary—a small endocrine gland attached to the base of the brain; the "master" gland.

PKU—see **phenylketonuria.**

placebo—an inactive substance that is given as a medicine for its suggestive effect.

placenta—the structure through which the fetus obtains nourishment during pregnancy; the afterbirth.

plague—a deadly epidemic or pestilence.

planes—a flat or relatively smooth surface; points of reference by which positions or parts of the body are indicated.

plasma—the liquid part of the lymph and blood.

platelet—a type of cell found in the blood that is required for clotting.

pleura—a serous membrane that covers the lungs and lines the thoracic cavity.

pleurisy—inflammation of the pleura.

plexuses—a network of nerves.

plight—unfavorable situation or distressed condition.

plural—the form of a term that indicates more than one.

pneumoencephalography—an x-ray examination of ventricles and subarachnoid spaces of brain following withdrawal of cerebrospinal fluid and injection of air or gas via a lumbar puncture.

pneumonia—inflammation of the lung caused primarily by microbes, chemical irritants, vegetable dust, or allergy.

pneumonitis—an inflammation of the lungs, also known as pneumonia.

pneumoconiosis—a respiratory condition caused by inhalation of dust particles from mining or stone cutting.

pneumothorax—a collection of air or gas in the pleural cavity that displaces lung tissue.

podiatrist—(chiropodist) a person trained to diagnose and treat diseases and disorders of the feet.

podiatry—the branch of medicine dealing with disorders of the feet.

poison—a substance that, if taken internally or applied externally, is a threat to life.

POL—see **physician's office laboratory.**

policy—a high-level overall plan; general principles of an organization.

polio—(poliomyelitis) an acute, infectious, systemic disease that causes inflammation of the gray matter of the spinal cord.

polling—pertains to obtaining an unauthorized FAX transmission.

polycystic kidney disease—a condition of multiple cysts in the kidney.

polycythemia—an excess of red blood cells.

polyneuralgia—pain in many nerves.

polyp—a tumor with a pedicle, especially on mucous membranes, such as in the nose, rectum, or intestines.

polyuria—excessive secretion and discharge of urine.

pons—a portion of the brainstem connecting the medulla oblongata and cerebellum with upper portions of the brain.

popliteal—pertains to the area in back of the knee.

portal—pertaining to the portal circulation of blood from impaired internal organs to the liver for processing before entering the inferior vena cava.

positive—strongly affirmative.

positron emission tomography (PET scan)—a form of imaging permitting visualizing the physiologic function of the body.

post mortem—pertaining to or occurring during the period after death; common term for autopsy.

posted—to transfer charges from the day sheet to patient account records.

posterior—toward the rear or back or toward the caudal end.

postmark—a dated cancellation of a stamp by the post office that also identifies the place of posting.

postoperative (post-op)—after or following a surgical procedure.

postpartum—the period following delivery of a baby.

postscript (PS)—an addition to a letter written after the writer's name has been signed.

posture—the position and carriage of the body as a whole.

potential—possible; ability to develop into actuality.

power of attorney—a legal document authorizing a person to act as another's attorney, legal representative, or agent.

PPM—see **provider-performed microscopy.**

practice management system (PMS)—computer system used to keep and generate the records and reports of the practice.

practitioner—one who practices the profession of medicine.

preauthorization—prior approval of insurance coverage and necessity of procedure.

precancerous—a state just prior to the development of cancer.

precautions—care beforehand; a preventive measure.

precise—exact; definite; very accurate.

precision—exactness, accuracy.

precordial—pertaining to that area of the chest wall over the heart for the placement of ECG chest leads.

preferred provider organization (PPO)—an organization of physicians who network together to offer discounts to purchasers of health care insurance.

prefix—a word component added to the beginning of a word root or combining form that typically modifies the remaining part of the term.

pregnancy—the condition of being with child.

preliminary—coming before, leading up to.

premium—the amount paid or payable (for example, an insurance policy premium).

prenatal—the period before birth.

preoperative (preop)—the preparatory period preceding surgery.

preposition—a word that shows the relationship of an object to some other word in the sentence.

presbycusis—impairment of acute hearing in old age.

presbyopia—a defect of vision in advancing age involving loss of accommodation.

prescribe—to lay down as a rule or direction; to order or advise the use of.

prescription—a written direction for the preparation of a medicine.

prevention—the act of keeping something from coming to pass; to hinder.

preventive—tending to prevent or hinder; something used to prevent disease.

primary—occurring first in time, development, or sequence; earliest.

prioritize—to arrange in order of importance.

priority—preference; state of being first in time, place or mark.

pro tem—acting as (a temporary position); for the time being.

process—to treat or prepare by some method.

processor—performing a whole sequence of actions or operations.

proclivity—an inclination or predisposition toward something.

procrastination—intentionally delaying action of something that should be done; to postpone.

procrastinator—one who intentionally delays or postpones action.

proctology—the study of the rectum and anus and their diseases.

proctoscope—an instrument for the inspection of the rectum.

proctoscopy—instrumental inspection of the rectum.

procure—to get or obtain.

procurement—to obtain; acquire.

productivity—the amount of work accomplished in a period of time.

professional—conforming to the technical or ethical standards of a profession.

professionalism—professional status, methods, character, or standards.

proficiency testing (PT)—the measurement of acquired knowledge and skills; a means of assessing the competency of someone or of something.

proficient—well advanced in an art, occupation, skill, or branch of knowledge; unusually knowledgeable.

profit sharing—a system by which employees receive a share of the profits of a business enterprise.

progesterone—a hormone secreted by the graafian follicle following the expulsion of the ovum.

programmed—arranged; planned; a sequence of actions performed by a computer.

progress notes—record of the continuing progress and treatment of a patient.

progress report—an upgrading of current findings.

project—to produce and send forth with clarity and distinctness.

projection—a defense mechanism of trying to blame another for one's own inadequacies.

prolapse—dropping of an internal part of the body; usually refers to uterus or rectum.

prominent—conspicuous, outstanding.

promissory—containing a pledge to pay.

prompt—to urge to action, to inspire.

prone—a position, lying horizontal with the face down.

pronoun—a word used instead of a noun, to indicate without naming.

proofread—reading of printed proofs to discover and correct errors.

prophylactic—preventing disease.

proprietary—privately owned and managed and run as a profit-making organization.

proprietorship—the amount by which assets exceed liabilities.

prostaglandins—a group of chemical substances secreted by mast cells or basophils that constricts smooth muscles in some organs.

prostate—a gland of the male reproductive system that surrounds the proximal portion of the urethra.

prostatectomy—excision of part or all of the prostate gland.

prosthesis—an artificial replacement of a missing body part.

protanopia—a problem in which the perception of reds and sometimes yellow and green become confusing.

protected health information (PHI)—confidential health information that is protected under Health Insurance Portability and Accountability Act (HIPAA).

protein (albumin)—a normal substance found in serum but when found in urine means the presence of an excess of serum proteins excreted in the urine rather than reabsorbed by the renal tubules; a nutrient found in foods such as eggs, meat, fish, legumes, and soy products that provides energy to the body.

prothrombin—chemical substance existing in circulating blood which aids in the clotting process.

protocol—a plan of treatment, usually experimental, used to determine effectiveness of new treatments or medications.

protozoan—a single-cell animal.

provider-performed microscopy (PPM)—refers to microscopic procedures done in the physician's office laboratory.

provisions—the act of providing; something provided for the future; a stipulation.

proximal—nearest the point of attachment.

proxy—one who has authority to vote or act for another; a certificate of authorization to vote.

prudent—careful; wise in practical affairs.

pruritic—pertaining to an itching sensation.

pruritus—severe itching.

pruritus ani—itching around the anus.

PS—see **postscript.**

psoriasis—a chronic inflammatory disease characterized by scaly patches.

psychedelics—hallucinogenic drugs.

psychiatrist—a physician specializing in the diseases and disorders of the mind, including neuroses and psychoses.

psychiatry—the branch of medicine dealing with the diagnosis, treatment, and prevention of mental illness.

psychological—of the mind; mental.

psychologist—a person specializing in the study of the structure and function of the brain and related mental processes.

psychology—the study of mental processes, both normal and abnormal, and their effects upon behavior.

psychoneuroimmunology—a science studying the connection between the brain, behavior, and immunity.

psychopathic—concerning or characterized by a mental disorder.

psychosis—mental disturbance of such magnitude that there is personality disintegration and loss of contact with reality.

psychosomatic—pertaining to interrelationships between the mind or emotions and body.

psychotherapy—the treatment of disease by hypnosis, psychoanalysis, and similar means.

PT—see **pharmacy technician** or **proficiency testing**.

ptosis—a drooping or dropping of an organ or part, for example the eyelid or the kidney.

puberty—the period of life at which one becomes functionally capable of reproduction.

pubic—pertaining to the middle section of the lower third of the abdomen, also referred to as the hypogastric.

pulmonary—concerning or involving the lungs.

pulmonary edema—the presence of interstitial fluid in the lung tissue.

pulmonary embolis—a blockage in the pulmonary artery or one of its branches.

pulse deficit—the difference between the pulse rate measured radially and apically.

pulse pressure—difference between the systolic and diastolic measurements.

pulse—throbbing caused by the regular alternating contraction and expansion of an artery.

punctual—prompt; being on time.

punctuality—a desirable trait of being on time for appointments, work, etc.

punctuation—standardized marks in written matter to clarify meaning.

puncture—a hole made by something pointed.

pupil—the contractible opening in the center of the iris for the transmission of light.

purge—to empty; to cleanse of impurities; clear.

Purkinje—network of fibers found in the cardiac muscle that carries the electrical impulses resulting in the contraction of the ventricles.

pustular—pertaining to a collection of pus that has accumulated in a cavity formed by the tissue on the basis of an infectious process.

pustule—small elevation of the skin filled with lymph or pus.

pyelonephritis—inflammation of the kidney, pelvis, and nephrons.

pyloric—pertaining to the opening between the stomach and the duodenum.

pyrogen—capable of producing fever.

QNS—quantity not sufficient.

quackery—the pretense to knowledge or skill in medicine.

quad-base—refers to a cane with four "feet."

quadrant—one of four regions, as of the abdomen, divided for identification purposes.

quadriceps femoris—a large muscle on the anterior surface of the thigh that is composed of four separate muscles.

qualifications—a quality or attainment that fits a person for a place or position.

quality assurance (QA)—inclusive policies, procedures, and practices as standards for reliable laboratory results that includes documentation, calibration, and maintenance of all equipment, quality control, proficiency testing, and training.

quality control (QC)—inclusive laboratory procedures as standards to provide reliable performance of equipment, including test control samples, documentation, and analyzing statistics for diagnostic tests.

radial—referring to the radial artery or pulse taken in the radial artery.

radiation—the emission and diffusion of rays; a product of x-ray and radium.

radioactive—capable of emitting radiant energy.

radioactive agents—agents used to diagnose certain medical problems or treat certain diseases.

radiograph—a record produced on a photographic plate, film, or paper by the action of x-ray or radium.

radiologist—one who diagnoses and treats disease by the use of radiant energy.

radiology—the study of radiation and its uses.

radiology technician—an individual trained in the administration of x-rays.

radionuclides—a type of atom used in nuclear medicine for the diagnosis and treatment of disease.

radiopaque—impenetrable to the x-ray or other forms of radiation.

radius—a long bone of the forearm.

rales—an unusual sound heard in the bronchi on examination of respirations.

ramification—a subdivision or consequence.

random—by chance; without plan.

range of motion (ROM)—refers to the degree of movement of the body's joints and extremities.

rapport—relationship characterized by harmony and cooperation.

ratchet—locking mechanism of an instrument

rational—based on reasoning, sensible.

rationalization—to explain on rational grounds, to devise plausible explanations for one's acts.

RAST—short for radioallergosorbent test, a blood test used to determine what a person is allergic to. This is different from a skin allergy test, which determines allergy by the reaction of a person's skin to different substances.

Raynaud's phenomenon—a symptom of lupus characterized by fingers that turn white or blue in the cold.

reactivity—rate of nuclear disintegration in a reactor.

reagent—a substance involved in a chemical reaction.

realm—kingdom or empire, as used in text.

reason rule—refers to the purpose or reason for doing a test or procedure, an insurance company criteria for reimbursement.

receipt—a written acknowledgement that something has been received.

reception—the fact or manner of being received; a social gathering.

receptionist—one employed to greet telephone callers, visitors, patients, or clients.

receptor—peripheral nerve ending of a sensory nerve that responds to stimuli.

recessive gene—apparently suppressed in crossbred offspring in preference for a characteristic from the other parent.

recipient—one who receives.

reciprocity—mutual exchange, especially the exchange of special privilege.

reconcile—process to bring checkbook and bank statement into agreement.

rectal—referring to the rectum.

rectocele—the protrusion of the posterior vaginal wall and anterior wall of the rectum through the vagina.

rectum—the lower part of the large intestine between the sigmoid and the anal canal.

recumbent—lying down.

recurrent—returning at intervals.

reduce—to restore the ends of a fractured bone to their usual relationship.

redundant—extra, not needed, repetitive.

reference—a source of information or authority.

reflex—an involuntary response to a stimulus.

reflexology—massaging of the hands or feet based on the belief that pressure applied to specific points on these extremities benefits other parts of the body.

reflux—a return or backward flow.

refractive—the degree to which a transparent body deflects a ray of light from a straight path.

regimen—regulation of diet, sleep, exercise, and manner of living to improve or maintain health.

register—a formal or official recording of items, names, or actions; a record of money that has been spent.

registered—legally certified or authenticated.

registered nurse (RN)—an individual trained through formal training in the field of nursing.

registry—a list of persons qualified in a particular area of expertise.

regression—a defense mechanism of retreating to the thoughts and actions of an earlier, "safer," age.

regulate—control or direction.

Regulations in the POL—standards set for quality assurance and quality control in the physician's office laboratory to ensure reliable diagnostic tests.

regulatory—to control according to a rule; to adjust so as to make work accurately.

rehabilitate—to put back in good condition; to restore.

rehabilitation centers—facilities that assist in developing appropriate socialization skills, family and community reintegration, and increased independence.

rehabilitative therapy—treatment that offers the highest level of patient care and programs that will enhance the physical, psychological, and emotional health of the population served in most of these facilities.

reimbursement—to pay back or compensate for money spent, or losses or damages incurred.

reiterate—to say or do again.

rejuvenate—to make young again; to give youthful qualities to.

relapse—recurrence of a disease or symptoms; returning to a previous condition.

reliable—dependable, can be relied upon.

reluctant—marked by unwillingness.

rely—to depend on, to trust.

REM (rapid eye movement)—a stage of sleep in which the sleeper experiences rapid eye movement. In a healthy young adult, REM sleep accounts for 10%–25% of sleep time.

remedy—anything that relieves or cures a disease.

remission—a period that is disease- and symptom-free.

remote—from a distance; far removed in time and place; indirect.

renal—pertaining to the kidney.

renal failure—loss of function of the kidneys' nephrons.

renal threshold—the concentration at which a substance in the blood normally not excreted by the kidney begins to appear in the urine.

render—to present or to deliver, as a service or statement.

renovate—restore; to make new again.

repolarization—reestablishment of a polarized state in a muscle or nerve fiber following contraction or conduction of a nerve impulse.

repression—to force painful ideas or impulses into the subconscious.

reproductive—concerning reproduction.

reputable—having a good reputation; well thought of.

res ipsa loquitur—the thing speaks for itself.

residency—physician training period in a specialty field of medicine.

residual barium—barium remaining in the intestinal tract following evacuation at the completion of x-ray studies.

residual—pertaining to that which is left as a residue.

resistance—opposition, ability to oppose.

resonance—quality of the sound heard on percussion of the chest; the intensification and prolongation of a sound by reflection or by vibration of a nearby object.

resource—a source of support or supply.

respectful—showing respect; honoring; treat with consideration.

respiration—the taking in of oxygen and its use in the tissues and the giving off of carbon dioxide.

respiratory therapy technician—a person trained to perform procedures of treatment that maintain or improve the ventilatory function of the respiratory tract.

respiratory—pertaining to respiration.

respite—a temporary cessation of something that is painful or tiring; to delay, postpone.

respondeat superior—let the master answer.

restricted—limited; only for a certain group.

resumé—a summary, especially of work experiences.

resuscitation—an emergency first aid procedure for a victim of cardiac arrest. It is part of the chain of survival, which includes early access (to emergency medical services), early CPR, early defibrillation, and early advanced care. It is also performed as part of the choking protocol if all else has failed; revival from apparent or possible death.

retardation—slowing, delay, lag; slow in development, mental or physical.

retention—inability to void urine that is present in the bladder.

reticuloendothelial—pertaining to that group of cells that appear to aid in the making of new blood cells and the disintegration of old ones.

retina—the innermost layer of the eye that receives the image formed by the lens.

retinopathy—a degeneration of the retina caused by a decrease in blood supply.

retraction—a shortening; the act of drawing backward or state of being drawn back.

retractor—instrument used to hold back tissue, making the operative site easier to visualize.

retroflexed—refers to the body of the uterus being bent backward.

retrograde—refers to an x-ray procedure in which a radiopaque material is instilled by catheter into the bladder, ureters, and kidneys.

retroperitoneal—behind the peritoneum; posterior to the peritoneal lining of the abdominal cavity.

retroverted—refers to the entire uterus being tilted backward.

retrovirus—one with RNA (ribonucleic acid) genetic material.

revalidation—the renewing or reconfirmation of credentials.

revoke—to cancel, withdraw, take back.

Rh factor—an antigenic substance in human blood similar to the A and B factors that determine blood groups; apparently present only in red blood cells.

rhinitis—inflammation of the nasal mucosa.

rhinoplasty—plastic surgery of the nose.

rhythm—a measured time or movement; regularity of occurrence.

ribosome—an organelle within the cytoplasm of the cell.

rickets—a disease of the bones primarily due to the deficiency of vitamin D.

risk—chance; hazard; chance of loss or injury; degree of probability of loss.

R/O—rule out.

Roentgen—refers to x-rays.

Role Delineation Study—occupational analysis study conducted by AAMA and the National Board of Medical Examination in 1997 that identifies the most up-to-date entry-level areas of competence of the medical assisting profession.

ROM—see **range of motion.**

rotate—to move around; to turn on an axis.

rubella—(German measles) a mild contagious viral disease that may cause severe damage to an unborn child.

rubeola—(measles) an acute, highly contagious disease marked by a typical cutaneous eruption.

SA node—see **sinoatrial node.**

sacrilege—the crime of misappropriating what is consecrated to God or religion.

sacrum—five fused vertebrae that lie between the coccyx and the lumbar vertebrae of the spinal column.

safety—freedom from danger or loss.

sagittal—refers to a plane that is made by dividing the body down the center, creating a right and left side.

saliva—a digestive secretion of the salivary glands that empties into the stomach.

salivary glands—three pairs of glands that secrete the saliva that begins the digestion of food, primarily the breakdown of starch or complex carbohydrates.

salpingectomy—surgical removal of the fallopian tube or tubes.

salpingo-oophorectomy—surgical excision of the ovary and fallopian tube.

salve—an ointment.

sanitization—the process of applying antimicrobial agents to nonliving objects to destroy microorganisms.

sarcoma—malignant tumors of the connective, muscle, or bone tissue.

sartorius—a long narrow muscle of the thigh; the longest muscle of the body.

scan—to look over quickly but thoroughly.

scapula—the shoulder blade.

schedule—to arrange a timetable; to place in a list of things to be done.

sciatica—inflammation and pain along the sciatic nerve felt at the back of the thigh running down the inside of the leg.

scientific—based upon or using the principles and methods of science; systematic; exact.

sclera—the white or sclerotic outer coat of the eye.

scoliosis—lateral curvature of the spine.

screening—a preliminary or indicating procedure.

script—manuscript; type designed to look like handwriting.

scrotum—the double pouch containing the testes and part of the spermatic cord.

scrupulously—with great attention to detail; with great care.

scurvy—a disease caused by lack of fresh fruits, vegetables, and vitamin C in the diet.

sebaceous—an oily, fatty matter; glands secreting such matter.

sebum—oily secretion of the sebaceous glands of the skin.

secondary—one step removed from the first; not primary.

secretary—one employed to conduct correspondence; a person responsible for records and correspondence.

secretion—separation of certain materials from the blood by the activity of a gland.

sector—a section or division.

security—freedom from fear or anxiety.

sedate—to produce a state of calmness; process of allaying nervous excitement; using an agent to produce a tranquilizing effect.

sedentary—pertaining to sitting; inactivity.

sedimentation—formation or depositing of sediment; of blood, refers to the speed at which erythrocytes settle when an anticoagulant is added to blood.

segment—a part or section of an organ or a body.

seizures—a sudden attack of pain, disease, or certain symptoms.

self-control—control of ones emotions, desires.

semen—the mixture of secretions from the various glands and organs of the reproductive system of the male, which is expelled at orgasm.

semicircular canals—structures located in the inner ear.

semilunar—the valves of the heart located between the ventricles and the pulmonary artery and aorta.

senility—feebleness of body or mind caused by old age.

sensitivity—abnormal susceptibility to a substance.

sensorineural—refers to a sensory nerve.

sensorineural deafness—a loss of hearing caused by transmission failure of the nerves within the inner ear or the auditory nerve.

sensory—refers to the nerves that receive and transmit stimuli from the sense organs.

septum—a membranous wall dividing two cavities, as within the heart or the nose.

sequence—order of succession.

sequentially—arranged in sequence; in an order.

series—a group; a set of things in the same class coming one after another.

serrated—notched, toothed.

serrations—etchings located on the blades of an instrument to keep it from slipping.

serum—blood plasma in which clotting factors (such as fibrin) have been removed naturally by allowing the blood to clot prior to isolating the liquid component

sharps—any object that can cut, prick, stab, or scrape the skin.

sheath—a covering structure of connective tissue, such as the membrane covering a muscle.

shelf life—that length of time that sterile items are given before they are considered unsuitable as maintaining sterility.

shiatsu—a massage with the fingers applied to those specific areas of the body used in acupuncture.

shock—a condition in which the pulse becomes rapid and weak, the blood pressure drops, and the patient is pale and clammy.

sickle cell anemia—a blood disorder in which the red blood cells are shaped like sickles.

sigmoid—an S-shaped section of the large intestine between the descending colon and the rectum.

sigmoidoscopy—an inspection of the sigmoid with an instrument.

signature—a signing of one's own name.

simple—referring to a bone fracture, one without involvement of the skin surface.

Sims'—an examination position with the patient lying on the left side.

simultaneous—occurring at the same time.

singular—the form of a term that indicates the presence of only one.

sinoatrial (SA) node—the source of the nerve impulse that initiates the heartbeat; the pacemaker.

sinusitis—inflammation of the sinuses.

skeletal—pertaining to the skeleton or bony structure; also to the muscles attached to the skeleton to permit movement.

skip—a person who owes money but cannot be located.

skull x-ray—a radiologic examination of the skull.

sleep apnea—brief episodes of the cessation of breathing during sleep.

sling—a hanging support for an injured arm.

slough—to cast off, as dead tissue.

smooth—a type of involuntary muscle tissue found in internal organs.

snap locks—metal locking devices.

Snellen chart—the chart of alphabetic letters used to evaluate distant vision.

Social Security number (SSN)—unique nine-digit number assigned by the U.S. government.

software—computer programs necessary for directing the computer hardware to perform specific functions.

solace—an easing of grief, to comfort.

sole—only.

solicit—to ask for.

somatic—pertaining to the body as distinguished from the mind; physical.

sonar—a device that transmits high-frequency sound waves in water and registers the vibrations reflected back from an object.

sonogram—record obtained by ultrasound.

sophisticated—not simple or natural; very refined; highly complex or developed in form, technique, etc.

sound—that which is or can be heard; free from damage, safe, secure.

spasm—an involuntary sudden movement or convulsive muscular contraction.

spastic colon—spasmodic contractions of the large intestine.

specific gravity—the ratio of dissolved substances in a solvent as compared with the ratio of dissolved substances in distilled water, most commonly comparing the ratio of dissolved substances in a urine specimen when compared with distilled water.

specifications—any point or particular specified; mention in detail.

specificity—something specially suited for a given use or purpose; a remedy regarded as a certain cure for a particular disease.

specified—named particularly; mentioned in detail.

specimen—a sample; a representative piece of the whole.

speculum—an instrument that permits viewing inside a body cavity.

sperm—the male gamete or sex cell.

spermatozoan—a sperm cell.

sphincter—a circular muscle constricting an opening.

sphygmomanometer—a device that measures blood pressure; also called manometer.

spina bifida occulta—a disorder characterized by a defect in the spinal vertebrae with or without protrusion of the spinal cord and meninges.

spinal—pertaining to the spinal column, canal, or cord.

spinal fusion—the surgical implanting of a bone fragment between the processes of two or more spinal vertebrae to render them immobile.

spiral—having a circular fashion.

spirometer—an apparatus that measures the volume of inhaled and exhaled air.

spleen—an oval, vascular, ductless gland below the diaphragm in the upper left quadrant of the abdomen.

splinter—a thin sharp piece of wood.

spontaneous—involuntary; produced by itself; unforced.

spores—hard capsules formed by certain bacteria that allow them to resist prolonged exposure to heat.

sports medicine—the branch of medicine dealing with the care of athletes to prevent and treat sports-related injuries.

sprain—the forcible twisting of a joint with partial rupture or other injury of its attachments.

sputum—substance ejected from the mouth containing saliva and mucus; usually refers to material coughed up from the bronchi.

stability—the ability of a reagent to remain constant after being opened.

stabilize—to make steady; firmly fixed; constant.

staging—a method for determining the extent of the disease process with cancer.

standard—conforming to a custom or law.

standardization—process of bringing into conformity with a standard; pertaining to ECG, a mark made at the beginning of each lead to establish a standard of reference.

stapes—one of the three bones of the middle ear.

stasis ulcer—an open lesion caused by stagnant or inadequate blood supply to an area.

STAT (statim)—immediately.

stationery—writing materials, especially paper and envelopes.

stature—height.

statutory—legally enacted; deriving authority from law.

stenosis—narrowing or constriction of a passage or opening.

sterile—without any organisms.

sterile gauze square—a piece of dressing for a wound.

sterilization—the elimination of all transmissible agents (such as bacteria and viruses) from a surface, a piece of equipment, food, or biologic culture medium, including spores.

sternocleidomastoid—a muscle of the chest arising from the sternum and inner part of the clavicle.

sternum—the breastbone.

stethoscope—an instrument used in auscultation to convey to the ear the sounds produced by the body.

stimulant—a substance that temporarily increases activity.

stipulations—terms of an agreement.

stomach—a dilated, saclike, distensible portion of the alimentary canal below the esophagus and before the small intestine.

stool—bowel movement, feces.

strabismus—an eye disorder caused by imbalance of the ocular muscles.

strain—injury to muscles from tension caused by overuse or misuse.

stratagem—a trick or deception.

stress—to put pressure on; emphasize; urgency; tension, strained exertion. Topical; causing strain or injury to the skin.

striated—a type of muscle tissue marked with stripes or striae.

stricture—the narrowing of an opening, tube, or canal, such as the urethra or esophagus.

stylus—a pen; the ECG writer.

subarachnoid—the space between the pia mater and the arachnoid containing cerebrospinal fluid.

subcutaneous—beneath the skin.

subdural—beneath the dural mater; the space between the arachnoid and the dura mater.

subjective—relating to the person who is thinking, saying, or doing something; personal; of a disease symptom, felt by the individual but not perceptible to others.

sublimation—to express certain impulses, especially sexual, in constructive, socially acceptable forms.

sublingual—under the tongue.

subpoena duces tecum—court process initiated by a party in litigation, compelling production of specific documents and other items, and material in relevance to facts in issue in appending judicial proceedings.

subsequent—coming after, following.

substantial—considerable, large.

suction—withdrawal by pressure; a sucking action.

sudden infant death syndrome (SIDS)—the sudden, unexplainable death of an infant.

suffix—an addition to the end of a term that changes the grammatical function of the term.

superficial—on the surface.

superior vena cava—large but short vein that carries deoxygenated blood from the upper half of the body to the heart's right atrium.

superior—above or higher than.

supernatant—floating on the surface.

supervisor—one who oversees; has control; in charge.

supine—lying horizontally on the back.

supplement—something added; an additional or extra section.

support—to hold up; to bear part of the weight of.

suppository—a medicated conical- or cylindrical-shaped material that is inserted into the rectum or vagina.

suppression—the shutdown of kidney function; the absence of urine excretion; in psychology, it is the deliberate exclusion of an idea, desire, or feeling from consciousness.

suppressor—one that holds back or stops an action.

suprapubic—above the pubic arch.

surfactant—a fatty molecule on the respiratory membranes.

surgeon—a physician with advanced training in operative procedures.

surgery—the branch of medicine dealing with manual and operative procedures for correction of deformities and defects and repair of injuries.

surrogate—a substitute; in place of another.

surveillance—the process of watching or observing.

susceptible—having little resistance to a disease or foreign protein.

suspicion—mistrust, not believing statements.

suture—to unite parts by stitching them together.

symmetry—the state in which one part exactly corresponds to another in size, shape, and position.

sympathetic—a portion of the autonomic nervous system.

symphysis pubis—the junction of the pubic bones on the midline in front.

symptom—any perceptible change in the body or its functions that indicates disease or the phase of a disease.

synapse—the minute space between the axon of one neuron and the dendrite of another.

syncope—fainting; a transient form of unconsciousness.

syndrome—the combination of symptoms with a disease or disorder.

synergism—something stimulating the action of another so that the effect of both is greater than the sum of the individual effects.

synovial—a movable joint; also called diarthroses.

synthetic—not real or natural.

syphilis—a communicable venereal disease spread by sexual contact.

system—a group of organs working together to perform a function of the body.

systematically—by a system or plan.

systemic—pertaining to a whole system.

systole—the contraction phase of the heart; the greatest amount of blood pressure.

tachycardia—abnormal rapidity of heart action.

tact—delicate perception of the right things to say and do without offending.

tactile—relating to the sense of touch.

tar—a sticky, brown or black carcinogenic substance.

targeted—marked, the object of desire; aimed for.

tarry—a stool that has the appearance of tar.

tarsal—pertaining to the seven bones of the instep of the foot.

taut—tightly drawn; tense.

technical—relating to some particular art, science, or trade; also, requiring special skill or technique.

technologist—one skilled in technology; able to apply the technical methods in a particular field of industry or art.

technology—the practice of any or all of the applied sciences that have practical value and/or industrial use.

teleconference—a meeting held over phone lines incorporating video equipment.

temperature—degree of heat of a living body; degree of hotness or coldness of a substance; usually refers to an elevation of body heat.

temporal—relating to the temporal bone on the skull.

tendon—fibrous connective tissue serving to attach muscles to bones.

tendonitis—inflammation of the tendon.

tentative—experimental, provisional, temporary.

terminal—final, end; a terminal illness, refers to a condition that cannot be reversed.

termination—ending.

testes—the male gonads of the scrotum that produce sperm.

testosterone—a male hormone secreted by the testes that causes and maintains male secondary sex characteristics.

tetanus—an acute infectious disease caused by the toxins of the bacillus tetani.

tetany—intermittent tonic spasms resulting from inadequate parathyroid hormone.

thalamus—a portion of the brain lying between the cerebrum and the midbrain.

theories—beliefs not yet tested in practice; the general principles on which a science is based.

therapeutic—having medicinal or healing properties; pertaining to results obtained from treatment.

therapist—one who practices the curative and preventive treatment of disease or an abnormal condition.

thermal—characterized by heat; heat activated.

thermally—pertaining to heat activation.

thermography—a technique for sensing and recording on film hot and cold areas of the body by means of an infrared detector that reacts to blood flow.

thermometer—an instrument used to measure temperature.

thesaurus—a treasury of words, quotations, knowledge; a collection of words with their synonyms and antonyms.

ThinPrep—a method for preparing cytology specimens.

third-party reimbursement—payment made by a party other than the one providing or receiving the service, such as a physician or patient. Examples of whom you would receive third-party reimbursement from are an insurance company or an attorney.

thoracic—pertaining to the thorax or chest.

thorax—the chest; the body cavity enclosed by the ribs and containing the heart and lungs.

thready—term used to describe a weak pulse that may feel like a thread under the skin surface.

thrive—vigorous growth.

thrombophlebitis—inflammation of a vein associated with the formation of a blood clot.

thrombosis—the formation of a blood clot or thrombus.

thymus—an unpaired organ located in the mediastinal cavity anterior to and above the heart.

thyroid—an endocrine gland located anteriorly at the base of the neck.

thyroidectomy—the surgical removal of the thyroid gland.

tibia—a long bone in the leg from the knee to the ankle.

tibialis anterior—a muscle of the leg.

tinnitus—a ringing or tinkling sound in the ear that is heard only by the person affected.

tissue—a collection of similar cells and fibers forming a structure in the body.

tolerance—the difference between the maximum and minimum; the amount of variation allowed from a standard.

tongue—the muscular organ of the mouth that assists in the production of speech, contains the taste buds, and provides the ability to swallow.

tongue depressor—a flat wooden stick used to depress the tongue.

tonometer—instrument for measuring intraocular tension or pressure.

topical—pertaining to a specific area; local.

tort—any wrongful act, damage, or injury done willfully, negligently.

torticollis—stiff neck caused by spasmotic contraction of neck muscles drawing the head to one side with the chin pointing to the other; can be congenital or acquired.

total quality management (TQM)—refers to a management style that uses QA and QC to maintain quality of performance throughout the total process, not just to ensure the end result is satisfactory or corrected.

tourniquet—any constrictor used on an extremity to produce pressure on an artery and control bleeding; also used to distend veins for the withdrawal of blood or the insertion of a needle to instill intravenous injections.

toxin—poisonous substance or compound of vegetable, animal, or bacterial origin.

toxoid—a toxin treated so as to destroy its toxicity, but it is still capable of inducing formation of antibodies on injection.

TQM—see **total quality management.**

trace—the production of a sketch by means of a stylus passing over the paper, as in electrocardiography.

trachea—a cartilaginous tube between the larynx and the main bronchus of the respiratory tree.

tracheotomy—a surgically made opening in the trachea through which a person will breathe.

traction—the process of pulling; with fractures, traction is applied in a straight line to stretch the contracted muscles and permit realignment of the bone fragments.

trait—a feature; a distinguishing feature of character or mind.

transaction—dealing accomplished.

transcript—a copy made directly from an original record, especially an official copy of a student's educational record.

transcription—writing over from one book or medium into another; typing in full in ordinary letters.

transdermal—through the skin.

transducer—a device that transforms power from one system to another in the same or different form.

transfusion—injection of the blood of one person into the blood vessels of another.

transient ischemic attack (TIA)—temporary interruption of blood flow in the brain caused by small clots closing off blood vessels.

transillumination—inspection of a cavity or organ by passing a light through its walls.

transition—passing from one condition, place, or activity to another.

transmission—the process of sending from one place to another.

transmitted—sent from one person, thing, or place to another.

transpose—putting one in place of another, the accidental misplacing of words or letters.

transurethral—literally means through the urethra; refers to the removal of the prostate by going through the urethral wall.

transverse—lying across; the segment of large intestine that lies across the abdomen; a line drawn horizontally across the body or a structure.

trapezius—the large muscle of the back and neck.

trauma—any injury, physical or mental.

traumatic—caused by or relating to an injury.

traumatize—to cause trauma or injury.

treadmill—an apparatus with a movable platform that permits walking or running in place.

tremulousness—the process of involuntary shaking or trembling.

Trendelenburg—a position with the head lower than the feet.

trephining—cutting out a circular section.

triage—a system of sorting and identifying the severity of injuries.

trial balance—bookkeeping strategy to confirm accuracy in debits and credits in ledger.

triangular—having three angles and three sides.

triangular bandages—bandages having three angles and three sides.

triceps—the posterior muscles of the arm that work as a team with the biceps; the triceps straighten the elbow.

trichomoniasis—infestation with parasitic protozoa; usually refers to vaginal involvement.

tricuspid—a valve in the right side of the heart, between the chambers; literally means three cusps or leaflets.

triglycerides—a combination of glycerol and fatty acids in the blood.

trimester—divided into three sections; the third segment or period.

tritanopia—the inability to distinguish the color blue.

trivial—of little value, insignificant.

truncated—to cut the top or end off; to lop; with insurance.

tuberculosis—an infectious disease caused by the tubercle bacillus; pulmonary tuberculosis is a specific inflammatory disease of the lungs that destroys lung tissue.

tumor—a swelling or enlargement; a neoplasm; often used to indicate a malignant growth.

tuning fork—an instrument used to determine the sensation of hearing.

turbidity—flaky or granular particles suspended in a clear liquid giving it a cloudy appearance; usually refers to cloudy urine.

turgor—normal tension; with the skin means the resistance to being deformed and the length of time to return to normal.

tympanic membrane—the eardrum.

typhoid—an acute infectious disease acquired by ingesting contaminated food or water.

Tzanck smear—examination of tissue from the lower surface of a lesion in vesicular disease to determine the cell type.

ulcer—an open lesion on the skin or mucous membrane of the body characterized by loss of tissue and the formation of a secretion.

ulceration—suppuration of the skin or mucous membrane; an open lesion.

ulna—a long bone in the forearm from the elbow to the wrist.

ultimately—in the end, finally.

ultrasonic scanning—a process of scanning the body with sound waves to produce a picture on a screen of underlying internal structures.

ultrasound technologist—also known as diagnostic medical sonographers, these individuals are specially trained to use ultrasound equipment to direct high-frequency sound waves into specific areas of a patient's body to produce images of the shape, position, or movement of organs, fluid accumulations, masses, or fetuses.

umbilical—pertaining to the umbilicus or navel of the abdomen.

unemployment—the state of being without work; also, a limited federal program to provide some income for those who are without work.

unique—one of a kind, unmatched.

unit clerk—a secretarial position on the health care team of a patient care facility.

universal—relating to the universe; general or common to all.

universal emergency medical identification—worn by patients who have conditions that could have emergency episodes, such as heart conditions, diabetes, epilepsy, allergies, or a laryngectomy, to alert health workers of the patients' conditions when they cannot do so on their own.

universal precautions—steps taken by health care workers to prevent exposure to communicable diseases.

unobtrusive—not forced upon others; not thrusted forward or pushed out.

unproductive—not productive; no accomplishment.

unstructured—without specific arrangement.

unwittingly—not knowing, unaware; unintentional.

upper respiratory infection (URI)—inflammatory process involving the nose and throat, may include the sinuses; refers to symptoms associated with the common cold.

uremia—a condition in which products normally found in the urine are found in the blood.

ureter—a tube carrying urine from the kidney to the urinary bladder.

urethra—a membranous canal for the external discharge of urine from the bladder.

urgency—the sudden need to expel urine or stool.

urgent—requiring immediate attention.

URI—see **upper respiratory infection.**

urinalysis—an analysis of the urine; a test performed on urine to determine its characteristics.

urinary—pertaining to secreting and containing urine: the kidneys, ureters, bladder and urethra.

urinary meatus—the opening through which urine passes from the body.

urinary tract infection (UTI)—infection occurring within the kidneys, ureters, and/or urinary bladder.

urination—the act of urinating or voiding of urine.

urine—fluid secreted from the blood by the kidneys, stored in the bladder, and discharged from the body by voiding.

urobilinogen—the colorless product of bilirubin reduction formed in the intestines by bacterial action.

urologist—a doctor who has been specially trained in studies of the urinary system.

urology—the study of the urine and diseases of the urinogenital organs.

urticaria—an inflammatory condition characterized by the eruption of wheals that are associated with severe itching; commonly called hives.

uterus—a muscular, hollow, pear-shaped organ of the female reproductive tract in which a fertilized ovum develops into a baby.

UTI—see **urinary tract infection.**

utilization—to put to profitable use.

utilize—to use or make use of.

vaccination—inoculation with modified harmless viruses or other microorganisms to produce immunity, a preventive against diseases.

vaccine—any substance for prevention of a disease.

vagina—a musculomembranous tube that forms the passageway from the uterus to the exterior.

vaginal—pertaining to the tissues of the vagina.

vaginitis—inflammation of the vagina.

vagus—the 10th cranial nerve that has both motor and sensory function, affecting the heart, stomach, and other organs.

valve—any one of various structures for temporarily closing an opening or passageway or for allowing movement of fluid in one direction only.

varices—enlarged, twisted veins.

varicose—pertaining to varices; distended, swollen veins, most commonly found in the legs.

vas deferens—the excretory duct of the testes.

vasectomy—the cutting out of a portion of the vas deferens.

vein—a blood vessel carrying blood toward the heart after receiving it from a venule.

vena cava—one of two large veins that empty into the right atrium of the heart.

venereal—pertaining to or transmitted by sexual contact.

venipuncture—the puncture of a vein; the insertion of a needle into a vein for the purpose of obtaining a blood sample or instilling a substance.

venom—any of a variety of toxins used by several groups of animal species.

venous—pertaining to a vein.

ventilation—admission and circulation of fresh air; with the lungs, refers to a diagnostic test to determine air exchange and presence of an embolism.

ventilatory—that which ventilates, lets in fresh air.

ventral—pertaining to the anterior or front side of the body.

ventricle—one of the two lower chambers of the heart; also used in reference to cavities within the brain.

venule—a minute vein; a blood vessel that connects a capillary with a vein.

verb—the part of speech that expresses an action.

verify—to prove to be true; to support by facts.

veritable—actual, genuine.

vermiform appendix—the appendix; a small tube attached to the cecum.

verrucae—warts; small, circumscribed elevations of the skin formed by hypertrophy of the papillae.

vertebrae—the bones in the spinal column.

vertex—the top of the head, the crown.

vesicle—a small sac or bladder containing fluid; a small, blisterlike elevation on the skin containing serous fluid.

vested—settled; complete; absolute; continuous.

viable—capable of living.

vial—a small glass tube or bottle containing medication or a chemical.

video display terminal—the computer monitor.

vigilance—the act of watching for something to happen or watching for danger.

villi—tiny projections from a surface; the villi of the small intestine that absorb nutrients during the process of digestion.

villous adenoma—a type of polyp that is invasive and malignant.

viral shedding—that time when a virus is the most active and most contagious.

virulent—full of poison; deadly; malignant.

virus—a very simple, frequently pathogenic, microorganism capable of replicating within living cells.

viscera—internal organs.

visceral—pertaining to viscera, the internal organs, especially the abdomen.

visualization—the formation of mental visual images.

vital capacity—the total volume of air exchanged from forced inspiration and forced expiration.

vital—essential; pertaining to the preservation of life (the vital signs).

vitreous humor—the substance that fills the vitreous body of the eye behind the lens.

void—to pass urine from the urinary bladder; to make ineffective or invalid.

volatile—easily changed into a gas or tending to change into a vapor; usually considered potentially dangerous.

voltage—a measure of electromotive force.

volume—the amount of space occupied by an object as measured in cubic units.

voluntary—under one's control; done by one's own choice.

vomit—to expel the contents of the stomach through the mouth.

voucher—a document that serves as proof that terms of a transaction have been met.

vulnerable—liable to injury or hurt; capable of being wounded.

vulva—the female external genitalia, including the clitoris, the labia minora, and the labia majora.

waived—laboratory testing that is simple in nature and nonthreatening to the patient if performed or interpreted incorrectly.

waiver—to give up; forgo; waiving of a right or claim.

warrant—to justify, to give definite assurance as to the value of; to authorize.

warranted—justification for some act, belief.

wart—see **verrucae.**

watermark—a mark imprinted on paper that is visible when it is held to the light, usually a sign of quality.

weight—the amount of heaviness.

wheals—more or less round and evanescent elevations of the skin, white in center with a pale red edge, accompanied by itching.

wheelchair—a chair fitted with wheels by which a person can propel oneself.

whorl—a type of fingerprint in which the central papillary ridges turn through at least one complete circle.

wick—a small piece of cotton to absorb or provide moisture or medication.

withdrawal—a removal of something that has been deposited.

womb—nonmedical name for the uterus.

word processor—a system or machine that produces typewritten documents.

word root—a component of a medical term that does not have a combining form vowel attached.

work-in—to make time or space for.

writer—the person who writes; the author.

xiphoid—a process that forms the tip of the sternum.

x-linked—connected to the cell's sex chromosome; a characteristic of the sex chromosome.

x-ray technician—a person with specialized training in the techniques to prepare x-ray films to visualize the tissues and organs of the body.

year to date (YTD)—begins with the 1st date of the calendar year to present.

yoga—a system of exercises for attaining bodily or mental control and well-being.

Z-track (IM)—a method of injecting medication intramuscularly.

zygote—a cell produced by the union of an ovum and a sperm.

GLOSARIO

abadesa—madre superiora; una mujer que es la cabeza de una abadía de monjas.

abandono—desertar, dejar por completo.

abdomen—la cavidad en el cuerpo entre el diafragma y la pelvis.

abdominal—perteneciente al abdomen.

abdominopélvico—perteneciente a la cavidad anterior del cuerpo bajo el diafragma.

ABHES—por sus siglas en inglés, Oficina de Acreditación de las Escuelas de Educación en las Ciencias de la Salud.

ablación—procedimiento quirúrgico en que se usa un resectoscopio insertado en el útero por la cervix.

abogado—uno que alega o defiende una causa o a una persona.

aborto—la terminación del embarazo antes de la etapa de viabilidad; espontáneo o inducido.

abrasión—una lesión causada por el frote o raspadura de la piel.

abreviación—forma corta.

abrupto—súbito; brusco, seco.

absoluto—libre de condición, ilimitado en su poder.

absorber—chupar o tragar, tomar.

abstinente—Persona que renuncia a algo.

abstracto—resumen de las partes principales de una obra extensa.

absurdo—contrario al sentido o a la razón.

abusar—maltratar, lastimar una y otra vez.

accesible—capaz de ser alcanzado.

accidente cerebrovascular—embolia cerebral; hemorragia en el cerebro.

acción potencial—la carga eléctrica temporal en una célula.

acelerador—aumento de la acción o de la función.

acetilcolino—hormona liberada en las terminaciones nerviosas parasimpatéticas y las terminaciones nerviosas esqueléticas.

acidez—sensación de quemazón bajo el hueso del esternón, usualmente asociada con indigestión.

ácido clorhídrico—jugo digestivo encontrado en el estómago.

ácido desoxirribonucleico (ADN)—el material dentro del cromosoma que porta la información genética.

acidosis—disturbio del balance ácido-base del cuerpo.

acné—una condición de la piel caracterizada por la inflamación de las glándulas sebáceas y que produce barros.

acomodación—proceso por el cual el lente cambia de forma para permitir la visión cercana.

acoso—molestia continuada; persecución.

acreditación—la asignación de credenciales; aprobación otorgada por reunir los estándares establecidos.

acreditado—certificado; que cumple los estándares establecidos; aceptado como válido.

acromegalia—condición crónica caracterizada por el agrandamiento de los huesos de las extremidades y de algunos huesos de la cabeza; engrosamiento de los tejitos suaves faciales.

acrónimo—una palabra formada de las letras iniciales de cada palabra principal de un término.

actitud—estado de pensamiento o de sentimiento.

activar—hacer activo o más activo.

actual—que sucede ahora; del tiempo presente; la última información.

acumulado—amontonar; recoger; juntar.

acupuntura—involucra la inserción de agujas en varios puntos del cuerpo para tratar una enfermedad o aliviar el dolor.

adaptabilidad—el acto o el resultado de ajustarse a nuevas circunstancias o cambios.

adecuado—igual a lo requerido o a la ocasión, suficiente.

adenitis—inflamación de los ganglios linfáticos o de una glándula.

adherir—pegarse rápido, unirse de manera firme; ser devoto a.

adicción—el estado de estar gobernado o controlado por un hábito, como por alcohol o drogas.

adjetivo—una palabra añadida a (que modifica) un sustantivo para cuantificarlo o limitarlo.

administración—acción o práctica para manejar o controlar una situación.

administrador de consultorio—persona responsable por el funcionamiento del consultorio médico.

administrar—manejar; conducir-dirigir, como un negocio.

administrativo—deberes que manejan o dirigen actividades; en asistencia médica, se refiere a los deberes diferentes de aquellos por naturaleza clínica; deberes de oficina de recepción.

ADN—ver ácido desoxirribonucleico.

adquirir—obtener por esfuerzos o acciones propias; contraer.

adquisición—obtenido por esfuerzo personal.

adrenalina—una secreción interna derivada de las glándulas adrenales; se puede preparar comercialmente de glándulas animales; actúa como estimulante.

adrenal—relacionado con las glándulas adrenales que se sientan encima de cada riñon.

aducción—alejarse del eje del cuerpo.

aductar—acercar al eje del cuerpo.

adverbio—una palabra añadida (que modifica) un verbo, un adjetivo, u otro verbo.

adverso—opuesto, desfavorable.

aerobio—un microorganismo que sólo puede vivir y crecer en la presencia de oxígeno.

afebril—sin fiebre.

afiliarse—unirse, adherirse o conectarse.

agar—sustancia seca mucilaginosa, o gelatina, extraída de alga, usada como medio de cultivo.

agente—uno que actúa o tiene el poder o la autoridad de actuar por otro.

agotado—consumido, vacío, exhausto.

agravio—cualquier acto malintencionado, daño o lesión causada en forma intencional o por negligencia.

agresión—cualquier paliza ilegal a otra persona.

agresivo—insistente, que asume la ofensiva sin causa, vigoroso.

agudo—cortante, severo; tiene un comienzo rápido, síntomas severos y un curso corto; no crónico.

ajustes—cambios para que se acomode o poner en armonía.

Al-Anon—grupo de apoyo para familiares de alcohólicos.

Al-Ateen—apoyo para adolescentes de un padre o madre alcohólico.

albino—persona que carece de pigmentación en la piel, cabello u ojos, total o parcialmente; una persona con albinismo.

alcohol—líquido generado por la fermentación de azúcar y de otros carbohidratos.

alcohólico—individuo que usa alcohol en exceso.

Alcohólicos Anónimos—una organización formada para ayudar a que los alcohólicos se abstengan de usar alcohol.

aldosterona—hormona mineralocorticoide secretada por la corteza adrenal.

aleatorio—al azar; sin plan.

alegar—afirmar pero no bajo juramente y sin prueba; aducir.

alergia—estado alterado o adquirido de sensibilidad; reacción anormal del cuerpo a sustancias normalmente inofensivas.

alergista—médico especializado en el cuidado de pacientes con alergias.

alineamiento—estar en la posición adecuada.

alopecia—pérdida del cabello; calvicie.

alostérico—una proteína que se encuentra en los eritrocitos que transporta oxígeno en la sangre; hemoglobina.

alquitrán—sustancia carcinógena pegajosa, de color café o negro.

alquitranado—feces que tienen la apariencia del alquitrán.

alucinógeno—una sustancia que causa alucinaciones.

alvéolos—sacos microscópicos de aire en el pulmón.

ámbar—color anaranjado/amarilloso.

ambiente—lo que nos rodea.

ambliopía—ojo perezoso; condición del ojo caracterizada porque el ojo afectado se voltea hacia adentro.

amenidad—agradabilidad, amabilidades, cortesías.

amenorrea—ausencia de períodos menstruales; sin menstruación.

aminiocentesis—el uso de una aguja para extraer el fluido amniótico del saco amniótico.

amniótico—relacionado con el fluido amniótico adentro de la membrana amniótica que rodea al feto.

amplificador—un dispositivo en un electrocardiograma que amplía los impulsos del ECG.

ámpula—un pequeño contenedor de vidrio que puede ser cerrado y su contenido esterilizado.

amputar—cortar, remover una parte.

anaerobio—un microorganismo que tiene la habilidad de vivir sin oxígeno.

anafilaxis—una reacción hipersensitiva del cuerpo a una proteína o droga extraña; el término implica síntomas lo suficientemente severos para producir un shock serio, o aun la muerte.

análisis—el examen de cualquier cosa para determinar su composición; descripción del proceso o del examen, paso por paso.

analítico—caracterizado por un método de análisis, una declaración del examen paso por paso.

anal—relacionado con el ano o la apertura exterior del recto.

anatomía general—se refiere al estudio de aquellas características que pueden ser observadas a simple vista por inspección y disección.

anatomía microscópica—area que estudia las características que sólo son visibles a través del microscopio.

anatomía—el estudio de la estructura física del cuerpo y de sus órganos.

anatómico—relacionado con la anatomía o la estructura de un organismo.

ancla—la atadura de un músculo esquelético; la envoltura al principio de una gasa o de un vendaje elástico.

anemia drepanocítica—trastorno de la sangre en el cual los glóbulos rojos presentan la forma de la hoz.

anemia perniciosa—anemia severa caracterizada por la reducción progresiva en la producción de glóbulos rojos.

anemia—una deficiencia de células rojas de la sangre, hemoglobina, o de ambas.

aneroide—operando sin fluido; cuando se usa en referencia a un esfigmomanómetro, se mide por el marcador en vez de por la columna de mercurio.

anestesia—sin sensación, con o sin consciencia.

anestésico—un agente que produce insensibilidad al dolor o al toque, ya sea general o local.

anestesiología—el estudio de la anestesia.

aneurisma—ensanchamiento, dilación externa causada por la presión de la sangre en las paredes arteriales débilitadas.

anfetamina—estimulante del sistema nervioso central.

angina—dolor u opresión que irradia del corazón al hombro y al brazo izquierdo; sensación de asfixia.

angiografía—un estudio radiológico de una arteria usando un medio radiopaco.

ángulo—la inclinación de dos líneas derechas que se encuentran en un punto.

ano—la apertura externa del canal anal.

anorexia—pérdida de apetito; con anorexia nerviosa, pérdida del apetito por comida sin explicación por enfermedad, que puede ser parte de una psicosis.

anormalidad—persona, cosa o condición que no es normal.

anotación—entradas en un diario.

anotaciones del progreso—relación escrita del tratamiento y progreso de un paciente.

anotando—proveer notas críticas o de explicación.

anotar—proveer notas explicatorias.

ansiedad—la condición mental de desasosiego que surge del miedo o de la aprensión.

antagonizar—molestar; crear oposición.

antecubital—la superficie interior del brazo o del codo.

anteflexión—doblarse hacia delante de manera anormal.

anterior—antes o enfrente de.

anticipación—esperar, prever.

anticoagulante—una sustancia que prohibe la coagulación de la sangre.

anticonceptivo—contra la concepción.

anticuerpo—una sustancia proteínica cargada por las células para contrarrestar el efecto del antígeno.

antígeno carcinoembriónico—un marcador de tumor que puede ser detectado en la sangre cuando es examinada.

antígeno—cualquier agente inmunizante que cuando es introducido en el cuerpo, puede producir anticuerpos.

antihistamínico—una clase de drogas usada para contrarrestar reacciones alérgicas o síntomas del resfriado.

antiséptico—agente que va a prevenir el crecimiento o impedir el desarrollo de microorganismos.

antitoxina—una proteína que defiende al cuerpo de toxinas.

antógeno—dado por uno mismo.

anualidad—una suma de dinero que se recibe anualmente, ya sea en una sola suma o por cuotas.

anuria—la ausencia de orina.

aorta—el tronco principal del sistema arterial del cuerpo.

aparato de Golgi—un organelo dentro del citoplasma de una célula.

apariencia—representación exterior.

apendectomía—la extirpación del apéndice.

apéndice vermiforme—apéndice; tubo pequeño adherido al ceco.

apendicitis—la inflamación del apéndice.

apendicular—perteneciente a las extremidades o cosas que son apéndices (adheridas) a otras partes.

apical—en referencia al ápice.

ápice—el punto, la punta o la cumbre de cualquier cosa; en referencia al corazón, el punto de impulso máximo del corazón contra la pared del pecho.

aplicable—capaz de ser aplicado, adecuado.

apnea—la ausencia de respiración.

apoderado—persona que tiene la autoridad de votar o actuar por otra persona.

aponeurosis—extensión del tejido conectivo más allá del músculo en tendones redondos o aplanados; medio de inserción u origen de un músculo plano.

apóstrofe—un signo de puntuación que muestra la ausencia de una letra o letras; posesión.

aprehensión—anticipación de algo temido, tener miedo; una concepción mental.

apremio—situación desfavorable o condición desesperada.

aprendizaje—un entrenamiento o período de aprendizaje; estudio bajo la guía de un trabajador calificado o con experiencia.

apropiado—correcto, adecuado.

aracnoides—una membrana delicada como encaje que cubre el sistema nervioso central.

arbitrario—dependiente de un deseo o capricho, obstinado; que depende de elección o discreción.

ardientemente—ansiosamente, apasionadamente, intensamente.

área de superficie corporal (ASC)—se refiere a la superficie total del cuerpo humano.

aréola—coloración como anillo alrededor del pezón del seno.

armonioso—que tiene sus partes combinadas en un arreglo proporcionado, ordenado o placentero; el ser pacífico o amistoso.

arritmia—sin ritmo; irregularidad.

artefacto—algo ajeno a aquello que se está buscando. Actividad que causa interferencia en los ECG.

arteria—un vaso sanguíneo que lleva la sangre desde el corazón, usualmente lleno de sangre oxígenada.

arterioesclerosis—una degeneración y endurecimiento de las paredes de las arterias.

arteriolas—pequeños vasos sanguíneos que conectan las arterias con los capilares.

articular—unir, como en una articulación.

artritis—inflamación de una articulación.

artrografía—estudio radiológico de una arteria usando un medio radiopaco.

asalto—daño físico; un ataque violento.

ASC—área de superficie corporal.

ascendiente—se refiere a la porción del colon que asciende del cuadrante inferior derecho al cuadrante superior derecho del abdomen.

ASCLS—siglas que en inglés significan American Society for Clinical Laboratory Science, en español corresponden a la Sociedad Americana de la Ciencia del Laboratorio Clínico.

asepsis—una condición libre de organismos.

asfixia—sofocación, pérdida de conocimiento como resultado de poco oxígeno o de mucho dióxido de carbono.

asimetría—ausencia del mismo tamaño, forma y posición de partes u órganos en lados opuestos.

asistente del terapeuta ocupacional (OTA por sus siglas en inglés)—persona entrenada para asistir al terapeuta ocupacional.

asistente dental—trabajador de la salud empleado por un dentista para llevar a cabo funciones administrativas y clínicas y darle asistencia.

asma—reacción alérgica a una sustancia que produce respiración sibilante, falta de respiración y dificultad para respirar.

asociado—conectar en pensamiento; unirse como amigo o como socio; un grado otorgado por una universidad al finalizar un programa de dos años.

aspirar—remover por succión.

astigmatismo—visión borrosa causada por una curvatura anormal de la córnea.

astilla—pedazo de madera delgado y puntiagudo.

ataque—repentina ocurrencia de dolor, enfermedad o de ciertos síntomas.

atelectasis—falta de aire en los pulmones causada por el colapso de los alvéolos de los pulmones.

atenuado—diluido; reducir la virulencia de un organismo patógeno.

ateroesclerosis—degeneración adiposa de las paredes de las arterias.

atípico—desviado de lo normal.

atmósfera—cualquier influencia alrededor.

atributo—cualidad o característica; dar crédito.

atrio—aurícula cardíaca; cámara superior del corazón.

atrofia—mengua de un músculo.

audible—lo suficientemente alto para ser escuchado.

audiometría—prueba del sentido de audición.

auditorio—perteneciente al sentido de audición; canal externo del oído.

aumentado—se refiere a los conductores 4, 5 y 6 de los 12 conductores estándar del trazo del ECG; estos conductores son de diferente voltaje.

auricular—del oído; medida de temperatura usando un escáner timpánico infrarrojo.

auriculoventricular—ver AV.

auscultar—escuchar los sonidos producidos por el cuerpo.

autocontrol—dominio de los deseos y las emociones.

autoinmune—la condición por la cual los anticuerpos de una persona reaccionan en contra de sus propios tejidos normales.

automatización—comportamiento de modo automático o mecánico.

autónomo—autogobernado; espontáneo; parte del sistema nervioso relacionado con el control reflejo de las funciones corporales.

autorización—la concesión de autoridad.

autótrofo—microorganismos capaces de elaborar su propia materia orgánica a partir de materia inorgánica.

axial—perteneciente a la columna vertebral, cráneo, y la pared torácica.

axila—área debajo del brazo, sobaco.

axilar—referente al área debajo del brazo.

axón—una extensión de la célula nerviosa.

ayuno—abstenerse de comida; sin comida o agua.

bacteria—microorganismo unicelular relacionado con la fermentación y putrefacción de la materia; agente causante de enfermedades.

balance—poner o mantener en equilibrio; tener igual peso y poder.

bancarrota—el estado de estar quebrado, haber sido declarado legalmente incapaz de pagar deudas.

barbitúrico—un sedativo o droga hipnótica, también llamado tranquilizante.

bario residual—bario remanente en el tracto intestinal después de la evacuación al final de una sesión de exámenes de rayos X.

barrera—prevenir el acceso; prohibir el paso.

basófilo—célula blanca granulada de la sangre, que se tiñe fácilmente.

bazo—glándula ovalada, vascular y sin conductos localizada debajo del diafragma en el cuadrante posterior izquierdo del abdomen.

beneficio—cualquier cosa que promueve o aumenta el bienestar.

beneficios adicionales—beneficios incluidos en o agregados al salario pagado, como seguro de salud, pensión de retiro, etc.

benigno—no maligno; no canceroso.

beriberi—enfermedad como resultado de falta de vitamina B, tiamina.

bíceps—el músculo de la parte alta del brazo que flexiona el antebrazo.

biconvexo—la curvatura en ambos lados.

bicúspide—válvula del corazón entre el atrio izquierdo y el ventrículo izquierdo, también llamada válvula mitral.

bienal—que sucede una vez en 2 años.

bien—cualquier cosa que tiene valor de cambio, todas las entradas en una hoja de balance que muestran las posesiones o recursos de una persona o de un negocio.

bilis—una secreción del hígado; fluido verdoso-amarillento que tiene un sabor amargo.

bimanual—a dos manos; con las dos manos.

bimensual—que ocurre una vez en 2 meses.

binocular—perteneciente al uso de los dos ojos; que posee dos piezas para el ojo como en un microscopio.

biopsia—extracción de un pequeño pedazo de tejido para ser examinado bajo microscopio.

bioquímica—la ciencia relacionada con la química de las plantas y de los animales.

bisagra—un tipo de articulación.

bizarro—extraño, inusual, llamativamente fuera de lo ordinario.

bloqueo del corazón—una condición en la cual los impulsos del nódulo sinoatrial no traspasan al nódulo atrioventricular, causando un ritmo cardíaco lento y una rata diferente de contracción entre las cámaras alta y baja del corazón.

boca—cavidad bucal; también, relativo a la apertura de los organismos.

bolo—masa de comida masticada lista para ser tragada.

borradura—el adelgazamiento del cervix durante el parto.

borrar—remover, suprimir.

boticario—persona que dispensa drogas y medicinas.

bradicardia—ritmo cardíaco lento.

braille—impresión para los ciegos, usando un sistema de puntos en relieve.

braquial—se refiere a la arteria braquial del brazo; la arteria que se usa para medir la presión sanguínea.

broche de cerradura—mecanismo de metal para cerrar.

bronquíolo—pequeñas ramas terminales de los bronquios que carecen de cartílago.

bronquios—las divisiones primarias de la tráquea.

bronquitis—inflamación de las membranas mucosas del árbol bronquial.

bucal—de la boca; cavidad oral.

bulimia—una condición caracterizada por períodos alternos de comer en exceso seguidos de vómito forzado y del uso de laxativos para eliminar comida del cuerpo.

bulto—número de cosas ligadas.

bursa—saco o bolsillo con tejido conectivo principalmente alrededor de las coyunturas.

búsqueda alfa—buscar por orden alfabético.

búster—inyección subsecuente de sustancia inmunizante para aumentar o renovar la inmunidad.

CAAHEP—por sus siglas en inglés, Comisión de Acreditación de Programas de Educación en las Ciencias de la Salud.

cabestrillo—venda sujeta al hombro para sostener la mano o el brazo lastimado.

caduceo—la vara de Hermes o Mercurio; usada como símbolo de la profesión médica.

calambre—una contracción espásmica y dolorosa de un músculo o músculos.

calcitonina—hormona producida por la glándula tiroides esencial en el metabolismo del calcio en los huesos.

calcular—computar.

cálculos—comúnmente llamados piedras; compuestos usualmente de sales minerales.

calibraciones—juego de marcas graduadas para indicar valores.

calibre—el tamaño del ojo de la aguja; mientras más pequeño el número, más grande el ojo de la aguja.

cálices—dos o más cáliz.

calificaciones—cualidades o talentos de los que dispone una persona para ocupar ciertos cargos o ejecutar ciertas acciones.

cáliz—la división que se parece a una tasa de la pelvis del riñón.

callos—en las fracturas se refiere a la formación de nuevo material óseo alrededor del sitio de la fractura.

caloría—unidad para medir el valor calórico de la comida.

campo de baja potencia (LPF, low-power field, por sus siglas en inglés)—relativo al lente del microscopio.

canal alimenticio—el tracto intestinal, del esófago al recto y órganos accesorios.

canal inguinal—un pasaje en la ingle para el cordón espermático en el macho.

canales semicirculares—estructuras localizadas en el oído interno.

cancelación—tachar cruzando con líneas; marcar una estampilla o un cheque para borrar una cita o un evento.

cáncer—un tumor o crecimiento maligno; específicamente la hiperplasia de las células con infiltración y destrucción de tejido.

cánula—un tubo o envoltura que rodea un trocar (aguja triangular de perforación); después de la inserción, se remueve el trocar.

caos—estado de confusión completa: desorden.

capa—Estructura que recubre un tejido conectivo, como la membrana que cubre el músculo.

capacidad vital—Volumen total de aire intercambiado entre la inspiración forzada y la expiración forzada.

capción—encabezamiento, título o subtítulo.

capilar—un vaso sanguíneo microscópico que conecta las arteriolas y las vénulas.

capitación—una estructura de pago basado en el número servido.

cápsula de Bowman—parte del corpúsculo renal; rodea el glomérulo de la nefrona.

carbohidrato—una organización orgánica de carbón, hidrógeno y de oxígeno como en azúcar, un almidón o celulosa.

carboxihemoglobina—la combinación de monóxido de carbón y hemoglobina en las células rojas de la sangre.

carbúnculo—una infección de estafilococo que sigue a la forunculosis, caracterizada por abcesos profundos de varios folículos con múltiples puntos de drenaje.

carcinogenesis—la transformación maligna de una célula.

carcinogénico—agente causante de cáncer.

carcinoma—un tumor maligno de tejido epitelial.

cardíaco—perteneciente al corazón.

cardiología—el estudio del corazón y sus enfermedades.

cardiólogo—médico especializado en el cuidado de los pacientes con enfermedades del corazón.

cardiovascular—perteneciente al corazón y a los vasos sanguíneos.

carótida—perteneciente a la arteria carótida.

carpales—huesos de la muñeca.

cartílago—un tejido fuerte, duro, elástico, que forma parte del sistema esquelético; hueso precalcificado en bebés y niños pequeños.

CAT scan—ver tomografia axial computarizada.

catarata—una opacidad del lente del ojo que resulta en ceguera.

catarral—perteneciente a la inflamación de las membranas mucosas; causando ataques severos de tos con poca o ninguna expectoración.

catastrófico—de gran consecuencia; desastroso.

categorizar—organizar por clase o naturaleza; poner juntas las cosas que son similares.

cateterizar—insertar un catéter en una cavidad (por ejemplo, en la vejiga para remover orina) y para remover fluidos corporales.

caudal—perteneciente a caulquier estructura como la cola.

caústico—capaz de quemarse; un agente que destruirá tejido vivo.

cauterio—una plancha o un caústico usado para quemar tejido.

cauterizar—quemar con un cauterio eléctrico o con una sustancia química.

cavidades—espacio hueco como dentro del cuerpo o de los órganos.

central—situado o relacionado a un centro.

centrífuga—una máquina para la separación de materiales pesados de los más livianos a través del uso de la fuerza centrífuga.

centríolo—organelo dentro de la célula.

cerciorarse—asegurarse.

cerebelo—parte baja o trasera del cerebro bajo la parte posterior del encéfalo.

cerebral—que pertenece al encéfalo del cerebro.

cerebro medio—Porción del cerebro que conecta el pons y la corteza cerebral.

cerebroespinal—que se refiere al cerebro y a la columna vertebral.

certificación—una declaración escrita.

certificado de renuncia—se refiere a una lista de exámenes básicos de laboratorio que pueden ser realizados en la oficina de un médico por personal que no pertenece a un laboratorio.

certificado—en posesión de un certificado; estar certificado; una garantía por escrito; una declaración escrita de un hecho.

cerumen—la secreción café y serosa que se encuentra en el canal auditivo externo.

cervical—perteneciente a la porción del cuello de la columna vertebral; también a la entrada del útero.

cervix—la entrada al útero.

cesación—cesar o descontinuar.

cesárea—extracción quirúrgica de un bebé del útero.

Cheyne-Stokes—un patrón de respiración caracterizado por períodos alternos de apnea e hiperventilación

cianosis—una decoloración azulosa de la piel causada por falta de oxígeno.

ciática—Inflamación y dolor a lo largo del nervio ciático que corre desde la parte posterior del muslo hacia abajo por el interior de la pierna.

ciego—el comienzo de la porción ascendente del intestino grueso que forma una bolsa ciega en la unión con el intestino delgado.

científico—Basado en, o que utiliza los principios y métodos de la ciencia; sistemático, exacto.

CIE—ver Clasificación Internacional de las Enfermedades.

cifosis—Curvatura convexa de la espina; joroba.

cigoto—Célula producida por la unión de un óvulo y de una esperma.

cilia—proyecciones como cabellos de las células epiteliales como en los bronquios.

circulación portal—Relativo a la circulación de la sangre desde órganos internos hasta el hígado para procesamiento antes de entrar la vena cava inferior.

circulatorio—se refiere al sistema circulatorio; el proceso de fluido de la sangre a través de los vasos a todas las células del cuerpo.

circundar—rodear, cerrar.

circunscición—extirpación quirúrgica del prepucio del pene.

circunvolutivo—Tipo de huella dactilar en la cual los surcos centrales dan por lo menos una vuelta completa.

cirrosis—una inflamación intersticial con endurecimiento de los tejidos de un órgano, especialmente del hígado.

cirugía—Rama de la medicina que estudia los procedimientos manuales y operativos para la corrección de deformidades y defectos, y para reparar lesiones.

cirujano—Médico con entrenamiento avanzado en operaciones para la corrección de deformidades y defectos, y para reparar lesiones.

cistitis—inflamación de la vejiga urinaria.

cistoscopio—instrumento para examinar el interior de la vejiga urinaria.

cita—un compromiso; una reunión a una hora en particular.

citología—el estudio de la vida celular y de la formación celular.

citoplasma—materia celular sin incluir el núcleo de una célula.

citotecnólogo—un especialista de laboratorio quien prepara y examina el tejido de las células para estudiar su formación.

citotóxico—capaz de destruir células.

civil—perteneciente a los derechos de los individuos privados; procedimientos legales que conciernen derechos que no son criminales.

clamidia—bacteria que vive como un parásito intracelular y causa una enfermedad de transmisión sexual.

claridad—claro, ausencia de opacidad.

Clasificación Internacional de Enfermedades (CIE)—listado comprensivo de enfermedades y desórdenes del cuerpo humano.

clasificado—arreglado en un grupo o clasificación de acuerdo a algún sistema.

claustrofobia—temor anormal de estar en espacios cerrados o confinados.

cláusula—parte de una frase con sujeto y predicado.

clavícula—el hueso del cuello, que se articula con el esternón y la escápula.

CLIA—ver Enmienda al Mejoramiento del Labotarorio Clínico.

clínico—basado en observación; en asistencia médica, pertenece a los deberes considerados tras bambalinas; de naturaleza no administrativa.

clítoris—órgano eréctil localizado en la unión anterior de la labia menor.

clon—copia exacta.

cloroformo—un compuesto líquido que produce un gas que mitiga el dolor y causa inconsciencia.

coagular—disminuir la fluidez de una sustancia líquida; coágular o agrumar.

cocle—porción en forma de concha del oído interno.

coerción—forzar, imponer; restringir o constreñir a la fuerza.

coito—relación sexual entre hombre y mujer.

colaborar—trabajar juntos.

colateral—subordinado, secundario; propiedad depositada como garantía por un préstamo.

colecistomía—la extirpación quirúrgica de la vejiga.

colega—un asociado en el trabajo, usualmente uno de estatus similar.

colelitiasis—piedras en la vejiga.

cólera—una enfermedad aguda, específica e infecciosa caracterizada por diarrea, calambres dolorosos de los músculos y tendencia al colapso.

colinérgicas—fibras nerviosas capaces de secretar acetilcolina.

colirio—un objeto que usa agua para remover material extraño de los ojos, usualmente en situaciones de emergencia.

colitis—inflamación del colon.

colon—intestino grueso.

colon espástico—contracciones espasmódicas del intestino grueso.

colonoscopia—un examen diagnóstico para visualizar el colon por medio de un colonoscopio.

colorímetro—instrumento usado para medir la cantidad de pigmentos y determinar la cantidad de hemoglobina en la sangre.

colostomía—incisión en el colón con el propósito de hacer una apertura más o menos permanente.

coma—un letargo profundo y anormal del que una persona no puede ser despertada por un estímulo externo.

compatibilidad—relación caracterizada por la armonía y la cooperación.

compatible—capaz de ser mezclado o tomado en conjunto sin cambios destructivos (como en tipo de sangre y pruebas sanguíneas cruzadas); asemejar; no opuesto a.

compensación—cualquier cosa dada como un equivalente o para hacer enmiendas; pagar.

compensar—hacer enmiendas; ser equivalente.

competencia—habilidad demostrada.

competente—persona con los conocimientos necesarios y aptitudes avanzadas para la realización de una actividad artística o un trabajo determinado.

competente—apto, hábil, capaz.

complejidad—el estado de ser complicado.

complementario—expresar aprecio; dar sin cobrar.

complemento—un grupo de cerca de 20 proteínas enzimáticas inactivas presentes en la sangre.

complicado—no simple, involucrado; tener muchas partes; no fácil de resolver.

componer—formar juntando, creando.

comprensivo—que cubre todas las áreas; inclusivo.

compresión—ejercer fuerza contra, presionar.

compuesto—no simple, formado por dos o más partes; con fracturas, se refiere a los fragmentos de hueso que perforan la piel externamente.

computador—un aparato mecánico, eléctrico o electrónico que guarda información numérica o de otra clase y provee respuestas lógicas a alta velocidad a preguntas basadas en esa información.

computarizado—guardar en un computador; poner de forma que el computador pueda usar; poner los computadores en uso para controlar una operación.

comunal—gente en general; un cuerpo corporativo y su membresía.

comunicación—el acto de comunicar; información dada; forma de dar información.

concebir—quedar embarazada; la unión del esperma y del óvulo.

concepción—la unión del esperma del macho y del huevo de la hembra; fertilización.

conciso—condensado, corto.

condensador—parte debajo de la platina del microscopio que regula la cantidad de luz dirigida a un espécimen.

conducta—comportamiento, presencia.

conducto biliar común—un conducto que lleva la bilis de los conductos hepáticos y cístico al duodeno.

conducto eyaculatorio—el ducto de la vesícula seminal a la uretra.

conectivo—que conecta o une; uno de los cinco tejidos principales del cuerpo.

confiabilidad—seriedad, fiabilidad.

confiable—fiable, seguro.

confiable—sobre lo cual se puede contar.

confiar—fiar, tener fe en algo o alguien.

confidencialidad—ser tenido en confidencia; secreto.

confidencial—revelado en confidencia; información secreta.

confinamiento—restricción dentro de ciertos límites.

confirmación—hacer firme o seguro; prueba convincente.

confirmar—verificar o ratificar.

conflicto—colisión de opiniones e intereses; una pelea o lucha; una lucha interna moral; estar en oposición.

confrontar—encarar.

conjunción—reunión; una palabra que conecta.

conjuntiva—membrana mucosa que cubre los párpados y cubre la esclerótica anterior de la bola del ojo.

conminuto—una fractura del hueso con muchos fragmentos.

conmiseración—sentir o expresar simpatía o lástima.

connotación—algo implicado o sugerido.

conocido—el estado de conocer a una persona o sujeto.

consciencia—pleno conocimiento de lo que está en la propia mente.

consecutivamente—una serie de cosas que se siguen una a la otra.

consecutivo—que sigue en orden, sucesivo.

conservar—evitar daño o pérdida, mantener.

constipación—una acción indolente del intestino; usualmente se refiere a una deposición excesivamente firme y dura que es difícil de expeler o a la falta de movimiento del intestino por un período de tiempo.

constreñir—angostar; volverse más pequeño por contracción de un músculo del esfínter.

consuetudinario—por costumbre, la conducta habitual bajo circunstancias similares.

contable—persona que registra las cuentas y transacciones de un negocio.

contador—aquel que mantiene, verifica e inspecciona los registros financieros de individuos o negocios.

contagioso—pegadizo; capaz de ser transmitido por contacto.

contaminar—poner en contacto con microorganismos.

contemporáneo—que sucede o existe al mismo tiempo; una persona que vive al mismo tiempo que otra.

contenido—la materia que hace parte de un campo de estudio; materia contenida.

contexto—la parte de una declaración escrita o hablada que rodea una palabra o un pasaje en particular y que puede clarificar su significado.

contracciones—la acción del músculo uterino durante la labor del parto.

contrachoque—(en cardiología) un choque eléctrico y de corta duración, aplicado al área del corazón y que resulta en una despolarización total cardíaca.

contractura—acortamiento permanente o contracción de un músculo.

contradicción—el acto de contradecir; negar; afirmar lo contrario de.

contraer—juntar, reducir en tamaño o acortar.

contraste—mostrar diferencia; en radiología, se refiere al medio radiopaco que se usa para resaltar los órganos del cuerpo.

contributivo—dar una parte; ayudar hacia un resultado.

controvertido—abierto a la disputa; relativo a la discusión de puntos de vista opuestos.

convencional—dejar de estar de moda; no espontáneo.

convulsión—ataque de contracciones musculares involuntarias a menudo acompañadas de inconsciencia.

cooperar—trabajar juntos.

coordinación—un estado de ajuste o función armoniosa.

coordinador—persona que se encarga del funcionamiento armónico de las personas o agentes involucrados en una tarea o proyecto con el fin de obtener los resultados esperados.

copia dura—información impresa en una superficie sólida, como papel, en lugar de estar exhibida en una pantalla o guardada en un disco.

córnea—la extensión transparente de la esclerótica que yace enfrente de la pupila del ojo.

coroide—la envoltura vascular del ojo entre la esclerótica y la retina.

coronario—se refiere a las arterias que rodean el músculo del corazón; también se refiere a un "ataque al corazón", que involucra las arterias coronarias.

corregir pruebas—leer pruebas impresas con el objeto de corregir errores.

cortés—educado, considerado y respetuoso en manera y acciones.

cortex—la porción externa del riñón.

corticoesteroides—hormonas usadas para tratar la inflamación.

coto—un agrandamiento de la glándula tiroides.

coxis—el hueso de la cola; los últimos cuatro huesos de la columna vertebral.

craneal—perteneciente al cráneo o a la calavera.

cráneo—la calavera; los ocho huesos de la cabeza que contienen el cerebro; generalmente se aplica a los 28 huesos de la cabeza y la cara.

creación de imágenes—una representación o impresión visual producida por un lente, espejo, etc.

crenado—dentado u ondulado, como la condición dentada de los corpúsculos sanguíneos.

cretinismo—una condición congénita causada por la falta de la hormona tiroxina.

criminal—involucrar o tener la naturaleza de un crimen.

criocirugía—el uso de una sustancia a temperaturas bajo cero para destruir y/o extirpar tejido.

criptorquidismo—incapacidad de los testículos de descender al escroto.

crisis—el momento crucial de una enfermedad; un período muy crítico; una situación de emergencia.

criterio—un estándar de crítica o juicio.

crítica—un examen crítico de una cosa o situación, para determinar su naturaleza, valor o conformidad a estándares.

cromosoma—estructuras dentro del núcleo de la célula que almacenan la información hereditaria.

crónico—que continúa por un largo tiempo, que retorna; no agudo.

cronológico—la organización de eventos, fechas, etc., en orden de ocurrencia.

cuadrante—cuarta una de las cuatro partes del círculo. Este término se utiliza para identificar regiones en partes del cuerpo, como en el abdomen, por ejemplo.

cubículo—un espacio dividido, pequeño.

cubierta—cerrar completamente con algo que cubre; el contenedor de papel de una carta.

cúbito—hueso largo del antebrazo que se encuentra entre el codo y la muñeca.

cuerpo lúteo—el cuerpo amarillo que se desarrolla en la ruptura del folículo de De Graaf después de que el óvulo ha sido soltado.

cuerpo pineal—glándula endocrina pequeña adjunta a la parte posterior del tercer ventrículo del cerebro.

cultivar—formar y refinar; mejorar.

cumplimiento—consentimiento; conformidad con requerimientos formales u oficiales.

curandero—persona que pretende practicar medicina, pero que realmente no tiene mucho entrenamiento y usa métodos muy cuestionables.

cureta—un instrumento para raspar material de una cavidad.

currículo—un programa de estudio en un colegio o universidad.

D & C—ver dilatación y curetaje.

DACUM—un acrónimo en inglés que en español significa "diseño de currículo".

dar parte—informar

datos—hechos a partir de los cuales se infieren conclusiones.

deambular—caminar, no estar confinado a una cama.

DEA—ver Drug Enforcement Administration.

debilitado—endeble; menoscabar la fortaleza de.

débito—deducir, cobrar.

débridement—limpiar o remover, como se hace con el tejido dañado alrededor de una herida.

dedicado—comprometido a; apartar para uso especial.

deducciones—deducir o restar; remover, quitar.

deducible—una cantidad que debe pagarse antes de que el seguro pague.

deducir—inferir, derivar por proceso lógico.

defecar—expeler los excrementos o mover los intestinos.

defibrilación—causar la terminación de la fibrilación; restaurar la acción normal.

deficiencia renal—pérdida de función de los nefrones en el riñón.

déficit de pulso—diferencia entre el pulso radial y el pulso apical.

delegación—una persona o grupo de personas oficialmente elegidas o nombradas para representar a otro u otros; para empoderar.

delirium tremens—un desorden síquico que involucra alucinaciones, tanto visuales como auditivas, encontrado en usuarios habituales del alcohol.

deltoide—el músculo del hombro.

demografía—el estudio de las estadísticas de población que conciernen nacimientos, matrimonios, muertes, enfermedades y otros indicadores.

dendrita—una extensión de una célula nerviosa.

denominación—una categoría o una clasificación de dinero.

denotar—indicar, significar.

dentista—un proveedor de salud licenciado que se ocupa de los dientes, de repararlos y reemplazarlos en la medida de lo necesario.

deposición—testimonio dado bajo juramento.

depositar—confiar dinero en un banco o en otra institución.

deprimido—un estado de depresión, un período de desanimo; refiriéndose a una fractura, usualmente una fractura del cráneo donde los fragmentos de hueso son empujados (deprimidos) hacia dentro.

deprivación—estar deprivado; sin; tener que arreglárselas sin algo o incapaz de usar.

dermatitis por contacto—inflamación e irritación de la piel causada por contacto con una sustancia irritante.

dermatitis—una inflamación de la piel, a menudo el resultado de un irritante.

dermatología—el estudio de la piel y sus enfermedades.

dermatólogo—un médico que se especializa en las enfermedades y los desórdenes de la piel.

dermis—piel de verdad.

desalineamiento—no alineado, no derecho.

desastre—una ocurrencia que inflije destrucción y aflicción extendidas.

descendente—se refiere a una porción del intestino grueso del pliegue esplénico al sigmoide.

desconcertante—sorprendente, extraño, misterioso.

describir—representar con un dibujo; retratar.

descripción—un dibujo con palabras.

desempleado—estado de no tener trabajo.

desensibilización—el proceso de hacer a un individuo menos susceptible a los alérgenos.

deshidratación—privación de agua de los tejidos natural o artificialmente.

designar—senalar; indicar; nombrar.

desorden traumático acumulativo (DTA)—lesión como resultado de movimientos repetitivos de una parte del cuerpo.

desplazamiento—la transferencia de emociones acerca de una persona o situación a otra persona o situación.

despolarización atrial—la excitación y contracción causada por el SA node al principio del ciclo cardíaco.

detección—encontrar o descubrir.

detrimento—dañino, lesionante.

devastar—desperdiciar, saquear, destruir.

dextrosa—un azúcar simple, también conocida como glucosa.

diabetes mellitus—una enfermedad metabólica causada por la inhabilidad del cuerpo de usar carbohidratos.

diabético—alguien afectado con la condición de diabetes.

diafanografía—un tipo de transiluminación usado para examinar el seno, usando diferentes longitudes de onda luz y equipo especializado de creación de imágenes.

diaforesis—sudor profuso.

diafragma—el músculo de la respiración que separa al tórax del abdomen.

diagnóstico—se refiere a las medidas que asisten en el reconocimiento de las enfermedades y los desórdenes del cuerpo.

diálisis—remoción de los productos de la orina de la sangre por el paso de solutos a través de una membrana.

diario—un registro de acontecimientos; periódico.

diarrea—movimientos frecuentes de los intestinos, usualmente líquidos o semisólidos.

diartrosis—una articulación movible; otra palabra para sinovial.

diástole—la fase de relajación del latido cardíaco; el período de menor presión.

dictado—palabras habladas; comunicación de voz grabada.

dietista—el que es entrenado en dietética, que incluye nutrición, y a cargo de la dieta de una institución.

difamación—calumniar o atacar la reputación de un individuo o grupo.

diferencial—se refiere a la determinación del número de cada tipo de leucocitos en un milímetro cúbico de sangre.

difteria—una enfermedad aguda e infecciosa caracterizada por la formación de una falsa membrana en cualquier superficie mucosa, generalmente en los pasajes del aire, interfiriendo con la respiración.

difusión—un proceso por el cual gas, líquido o moléculas sólidas se distribuyen en forma uniforme a través de un medio.

difuso—regado o esparcido.

digestión—el proceso por el cual la comida es descompuesta mecánica y químicamente, en el tracto gastrointestinal y convertida en formas absorbibles.

digestivo—perteneciente a la digestión.

digital—perteneciente a o pareciéndose a un dedo de la mano o del pie, como a un examen usando uno o varios dedos.

dilatación y curetaje (D & C)—dilatación de la cervix y raspado del forro interior del útero.

dilatar—agrandar, expandir en tamaño; aumentar el tamaño de una apertura.

dióxido de carbón—un gas encontrado en el aire, exhalado por todos los animales; la fórmula química es CO_2.

diplomado—estatus avanzado de práctica médica.

directiva—plan general a alto nivel; principios de una organización.

disciplina—autocontrol, conducta, sistema de reglas.

disciplinario—diseñado para corregir o castigar faltas de conducta.

disco óptico—punto ciego donde el nervio óptico sale de la retina.

discoide—un tipo de lupus confinado a la piel; también llamado cutáneo.

discreción—el uso de juicio, prudencia.

discrepancia—inconsistencias; variaciones.

discreto—poco llamativo, que no molesta.

discreto—sabiamente cuidadoso, prudente.

disectar—cortar en partes para examinar; separar.

diseño—un plan de trabajo; esquema; trazado.

dislocar—el desplazamiento de una parte; usualmente se refiere a un hueso temporalmente fuera de su posición normal en una articulación.

dismenorrea—menstruación dolorosa.

disnea—respiración difícil o trabajosa.

dispensa—renuncia.

dispensar—distribuir; repartir en porciones.

disposición—el acto o la manera de poner en un orden particular; arreglar.

dispositivo intrauterino (DIU)—un objeto insertado en el útero para impedir embarazos.

distal—lo más alejado del centro, de la línea media o del tronco.

distender—inflarse, estrecharse.

distintivo—inconfundible, diferente de cualquier otra cosa.

distorsionar—tergiversar; cambiar de su forma usual.

distribución de ganancias—sistema a través del cual los empleados reciben una parte de las ganancias de la empresa.

distrofia—atrofia progresiva o debilitamiento de una parte, como de los músculos.

disuria—dolor al orinar; dificultad para orinar.

diversión—el acto de divertir o poner a un lado.

diverticulitis—inflamación de los divertículos.

divertículo—un saco o vejiga en las paredes o un canal u órgano, particularmente el colon.

divulgar—descubrir, revelar; hacer público; hacer conocido; revelar.

doctorado—un grado de posgrado conferido después de completar extensos cursos, un proyecto individual de investigación y escribir una disertación; un Ph.D.

doctrina—los principios de cualquiera rama del conocimiento; una creencia que se tiene o se enseña.

documental—la presentación de hechos sin incluir aspectos de ficción.

doméstico—no extranjero; privado.

dominante—el más fuerte; el que prevalece, el primero o principal.

dorsalis pedis—un punto de pulso palpable en el empeine del pie.

dorsal—perteneciente a la espalda.

Drug Enforcement Administration (DEA por sus siglas en inglés)—en español equivale a la Administración para el Cumplimiento de las Leyes Antidrogas; una división del gobierno federal responsable del cumplimiento de las leyes que regulan la distribución y venta de drogas.

DTA—ver desorden traumático acumulativo.

ducha—irrigación de la vagina.

duelo—tristeza como resultado de la muerte de una persona querida.

duodeno—el primer segmento del intestino delgado.

duración—la cantidad de tiempo por la que algo continúa.

duramadre—la membrana exterior que cubre el cerebro y la médula espinal.

ECG/EKG—ver electrocardiograma.

ecocardiografía—ondas de sonido de frecuencia ultra-alta dirigidas hacia el corazón para evaluar la función y la estructura del órgano.

ecos—reflejo de sonido.

ectópico—en posición anormal; en embarazo se refiere a cuando el embrión o feto está fuera del útero.

eczema—enfermedad no contagiosa de la piel caracterizada por piel seca, roja, con picazón y escamosa.

edema pulmonar—presencia de fluido intersticial en el tejido pulmonar.

edema—una condición de los tejidos del cuerpo que contienen cantidades anormales de fluido, usualmente intercelular; puede ser local o general.

eficiencia—la rata de energía utilizada para producir resultados.

ejemplificar—mostrar con ejemplo.

elasticidad—la habilidad de volver a la forma original después de haber sido estirado.

eléctrico—cargado con electricidad; que funciona con electricidad.

electrocardiógrafo—una máquina para obtener un registro gráfico de la actividad eléctrica del corazón.

electrocardiograma (ECG, EKG)—un registro gráfico de las corrientes eléctricas generadas por el corazón; un trazado de la actividad del corazón.

electrocauterio—un aparato usado para cauterizar el tejido con calor de una corriente de electricidad.

electrocoagulación—coagulación de tejido por medio de una corriente eléctrica de alta frecuencia.

electrodo—un instrumento con una punta o una superficie que transmite corriente al cuerpo del paciente.

electroencefalograma—registro gráfico de las corrientes eléctricas generadas por el cerebro; un trazado de las ondas cerebrales.

electroimán—un núcleo de hierro suave que se convierte en imán de manera temporal cuando una corriente eléctrica fluye a través de un alambre que lo rodea.

electrolito—una sustancia que, en solución, conduce una corriente eléctrica.

electromiografía—la inserción de agujas en músculos esqueléticos selectos con el propósito de registrar el tiempo de conducción de los nervios en relación con la contracción muscular.

electrónico—operado por el uso de electrones.

electrón—una partícula diminuuta de materia cargada con la cantidad más pequeña conocida de electricidad negativa; lo opuesto al protón.

elementos—sustancias en su forma más simple; los bloques básicos de construcción de toda materia.

eliminar—remover, descartar, excluir; también el paso de la orina desde la vejiga o las heces desde el intestino.

elipsis—una marca o serie de marcas usadas en la escritura o en la impresión para indicar una omisión, especialmente de letras o palabras.

elite—escogencia, superior, selecto.

emaciado—convertirse en delgado anormalmente; la pérdida de demasiado peso.

embarazo—período desde el momento de la concepción hasta el parto.

embolia pulmonar—obstrucción en la arteria pulmonar o en una de sus ramas.

émbolo—una masa que circula en un vaso sanguíneo; material extraño que obstruye un vaso sanguíneo.

embrión—las primeras 8 semanas de desarrollo después de la fertilización.

emergencia—un evento o situación inesperados que demandan acción inmediata.

emesis—vomitar.

emético—medicina que induce el vómito.

empatía—tratar de identificar los sentimientos propios con los de otra persona.

empiema—un exudado (pus) dentro del espacio pleural de la cavidad torácica.

enanismo—una condición causada por el crecimiento hormonal inadecuado durante la niñez.

encéfalo—la parte más grande del cerebro. Se divide en dos hemisferios con cuatro lóbulos en cada hemisferio.

encuentro—encontrarse, inesperadamente o por suerte.

endocardio—la membrana serosa que reviste el corazón.

endocervical—el revestimiento del canal del cervix.

endocitosis—un proceso celular para traer grandes moléculas de material al citoplasma de la célula.

endocrinología—el estudio de las glándulas endocrinas o sin ductos de secreción interna.

endocrinólogo—un médico que se especializa en las enfermedades y desórdenes del sistema endocrino.

endocrino—una glándula que secreta directamente en el torrente sanguíneo.

endometrio—la membrana mucosa que recubre el útero.

endosar—aprobar, recomendar, patrocinar.

endoscopio—un instrumento que consiste de un tubo y un sistema óptico para observar el interior de un órgano o cavidad.

endoso—el acto de endosar; aprobar.

enema—la instalación de fluido en el recto y colon.

enfermedad celíaca—dilatación de los intestinos grueso y delgado.

enfermedad de Crohn—una inflamación del tracto gastrointestinal con síntomas debilitantes.

enfermedad de Lyme—enfermedad que se transmite a través de la picadura de una garrapata que se encuentra en los venados.

enfermedad de membrana hialina—una condición que resulta del desarrollo incompleto del sistema respiratorio en bebés prematuros.

enfermedad del Legionario—bronconeumonía aguda.

enfermedad policística—condición caracterizada por muchos quistes.

enfermedad pulmonar crónica obstructiva (EPCO)—un síndrome caracterizado por bronquitis crónica, asma y enfisema, o cualquier combinación de estas condiciones, que resulta en disnea, infecciones respiratorias frecuentes y deformaciones torácicas como resultado de dificultad para respirar.

enfermedad—dolencia, achaque, indisposición.

enfermedad—dolencia, afección.

enfermera practicante—enfermera registrada (RN por sus siglas en inglés) con experiencia clínica avanzada y educación especializada en una rama particular de la medicina.

enfermera practicante licenciada (LPN por sus siglas en inglés)—persona entrenada en técnicas básicas de enfermería, con el objeto de proporcionar cuidado directo al paciente bajo la supervisión de una enfermera registrada (RN por sus siglas en inglés) o de un médico.

enfisema—una enfermedad crónica del pulmón caracterizada por la sobredistensión de los sacos alveolares y la inhabilidad para el intercambio de oxígeno y dióxido de carbono.

engullir—llenar con sangre hasta el punto de congestión; devorar o absorber.

Enmienda al Mejoramiento del Labotaorio Clínico (EMLC)—legislación relacionada con la operación de un laboratorio clínico.

enrejado—un artefacto como barra, usualmente construído de metal pesado; una rejilla abierta para una puerta o ventana.

entidad—una cosa que tiene realidad.

entusiasmo—interés intenso; celo; pasión.

enucleación—la extracción quirúrgica del ojo.

enumerar—contar separadamente, uno por uno.

enunciar—hablar o pronunciar claramente.

enzima—una sustancia química compleja producida por el cuerpo, que se encuentra principalmente en los jugos digestivos, que actúa sobre las sustancias alimenticias para descomponerlas para ser absorbidas.

eosinófilo—una célula blanca sanguínea o estructura celular que se mancha fácilmente con el ácido eosino; específicamente un leucocito eosinofílico.

EPCO—ver enfermedad pulmonar crónica obstructiva.

epidemia—que afecta a muchas personas al mismo tiempo.

epidermis—la capa superior de la piel; literalmente sobre *la verdadera piel*.

epidídimo—tubo enroscado que descansa en la superficie del testículo que lleva la esperma del testículo al vas deferens.

epífisis—una porción del hueso que todavía no se ha osificado; las terminaciones cartilaginosas de los huesos largos que permiten el crecimiento.

epigástrico—perteneciente al área del abdomen sobre el estómago.

epiglotis—tapa cartilaginosa que se cierra sobre la laringe al tragar.

epilepsia—una enfermedad crónica del sistema nervioso caracterizada por convulsiones y a menudo inconsciencia.

epinefrina—una hormona producida por la médula adrenal.

episiotomía—una incisión en el perineo para evitar rasgaduras durante el parto.

epistaxis—sangrado nasal; hemorragia de la nariz.

epitelial—perteneciente a un tipo de célula o tejido que forma la piel y las membranas mucosas del cuerpo.

equidad—el valor de la propiedad más allá de la suma total que se debe.

equipo muscular—par de músculos, uno flexiona mientras el otro extiende.

equivalente—igual a en valor, tamaño o efecto.

eréctil—se refiere al tejido que es capaz de erección, usualmente causado por vasocongestión.

ergonomía—la ciencia aplicada que se preocupa por la naturaleza y las características de la gente en cuanto se relaciona con el diseño y actividades, con la intención de producir resultados efectivos y mayor seguridad.

eritema—enrojecimiento disperso sobre la piel causado por una congestión capilar y por la dilatación de capilares superficiales.

eritrocito—una célula roja de la sangre (CRS)

eritropoyesis—la formación de corpúsculos de glóbulos rojos.

escanear—observar rápida pero cuidadosamente.

escáner del cerebro—prueba de diagnóstico en que se usa un escáner para medir los radioisótopos dentro del cerebro.

escaner ultrasónico—procedimiento de inspección del cuerpo a través de ondas sonoras que producen una imagen de las estructuras internas del cuerpo en una pantalla.

escápula—omóplato, paletilla.

escara—costra, especialmente después de una cauterización.

esclera—membrana de color blanco nacarado, gruesa, resistente y fibrosa, que constituye la capa externa del globo ocular.

escoliosis—curvatura lateral de la columna vertebral.

esconder—mantener secreto, retener, como información.

escorbuto—enfermedad causada por la falta de frutas frescas, vegetales y vitamina C en la dieta.

escroto—bolsa de piel que cubre los testículos y parte del tubo espermático.

esencial—necesario; cuando se refiere a presión arterial, indica una elevación sin causa aparente.

esfigmomanómetro—aparato que mide la presión sanguínea; también llamado manómetro.

esfínter cardíaco—el músculo que rodea el esófago donde entra al estómago.

esfínter—músculo circular que encoge una apertura.

esguince—torcedura contundente de una articulación con ruptura parcial, o lesión de sus ligamentos.

esófago—un tubo plegable de la faringe al estómago a través del cual pasa la comida y el agua que ingiere el cuerpo.

espasmo—movimiento repentino involuntario o contracción muscular convulsiva.

especificado—declarado en particular; mencionado en detalle.

específico—dícese de algo idóneo para un propósito o fin particular; medicamento que obra especialmente en una enfermedad.

espécimen—muestra; pedazo representativo del todo.

esperma—gameto masculino o célula sexual masculina.

espermatozoon—célula de la esperma.

espina bífida—trastorno caracterizado por un defecto en la espina vertebral con o sin protrusión de la columna vertebral y de las meninges.

espinal—relativo a la columna vertebral, al canal vertebral o a la espina dorsal.

espiral—curva abierta que se aleja cada vez más de su centro.

espirómetro—aparato que mide el volumen de aire inhalado y exhalado.

esponjoso—estructura enrejada, como el tejido esponjoso del hueso.

espontáneo—de propio movimiento; natural; no forzado.

espora—cápsula dura formada por ciertas bacterias que le permiten resistir una exposición prolongada al calor.

esputo—sustancia expectorada que contiene saliva y moco; usualmente se refiere al material que se escupe proveniente de los bronquios.

esqueletal—relativo al esqueleto o a la estructura ósea; relativo también a los músculos adjuntos al esqueleto para permitir el movimiento.

estabilizar—devolver a un estado constante; firme, seguro.

establecimiento—un edificio; en situaciones médicas, un edificio para el cuidado y tratamiento de pacientes.

estandarización—proceso a través del cual se logra la conformidad con unas normas establecidas; en un electrocardiograma, la marca de referencia establecida al comienzo de una curva.

estatura—altura de una persona medida desde los pies hasta la cabeza.

estatutorio—legalmente representado; promulgado.

estenosis—estrechamiento o restricción de un conducto o apertura.

estéril—sin organismos; que no produce.

esternocleidomastoideo—músculo del pecho que surge del esternón y la parte interior de la clavícula.

esternón—hueso plano del pecho con el cual se articulan las costillas.

estético—relativo a los principios de belleza y gusto.

estetoscopio—instrumento utilizado en auscultación para transmitir al oído los sonidos producidos por el cuerpo.

estilógrafo—instrumento de tinta para escribir; instrumento que escribe en el electrocardiograma.

estimulante—sustancia que aumenta la actividad en forma temporal.

estipulaciones—términos de un acuerdo.

estómago—órgano en forma de saco, dilatado y distensible, que forma parte del canal alimenticio y está localizado bajo el esófago y antes del intestino delgado.

estrabismo—trastorno del ojo causado por un desequilibrio de los músculos oculares.

estratagema—ardid, treta, engaño.

estresar—ejercer presión; enfatizar; tensionar; agotamiento. Tópico: causar lesión en la piel.

estriado—tipo de tejido muscular marcado por rayas o estrías.

estribo—uno de los tres huesos del oído medio.

estrictura—estrechamiento de una apertura, tubo o canal, como la uretra o el esófago.

estrógeno—hormona femenina producida por los ovarios.

etapa de declinación—volverse menos intenso, subsidir; período de tiempo en que los síntomas de la enfermedad empiezan a desaparecer.

éter—un líquido incoloro utilizado para producir inconsciencia e insensibilidad al dolor.

ética—estándares de conducta y juicio moral.

ético—correcto, de acuerdo a los principios de la ética.

etiología—el estudio de la causa de las enfermedades.

etiqueta—reglas convencionales para un comportamiento correcto.

euforia—sensación de bienestar, exaltación.

evacuación—separación, remover, vaciar.

evacuar—pasar orina desde la vejiga; vaciar, especialmente los intestinos.

evaluación—estimación; juicio concerniendo la importancia, calidad, significado, o valor de una situación, persona o producto.

evocar—provocar o llamar; invitar; sacar.

examen de conocimientos prácticos—medida de los conocimientos y las aptitudes de una persona para la realización de un trabajo determinado. Medida de evaluación de la competencia de alguien.

examen de Tzanck—inspección de tejido proveniente de la superficie inferior de una lesión para determinar el tipo de célula.

exceso—gasto extraordinario; demasiada indulgencia, como con el alcohol o la comida.

excreción—el proceso de expeler material del cuerpo.

exención—librado o no responsable por algo a que otros están sometidos.

exento—excluido, no responsable; exoneración del servicio o deber; privilegiado.

exfoliación viral—período durante el cual un virus presenta mayor actividad y es más contagioso.

exfoliar—desescamar tejido muerto.

exhalar—expirar.

exocitosis—un proceso celular que mueve materiales desde el interior de la célula hacia fuera.

exocrino—una glándula que secreta sustancias a través de un ducto al cuerpo.

exoftalmia—protrusión anormal del ojo.

exógeno—que se origina fuera de un órgano o parte.

exorcismo—el acto de expeler un espíritu maligno.

expectorar—escupir, expeler moco o flema de la garganta o pulmones.

expediente—una forma adecuada para lograr u obtener un propósito o un fin; de ventaja inmediata, conveniente.

expedir—apurar.

expedir—enviar; poner en circulación.

experiencia—conocimiento que resulta de la observación y la práctica.

expiración—la expulsión del aire de los pulmones al respirar.

explícito—claramente y definidamente expresado; no ambiguo; sin espacio para preguntas.

exploración—investigación preliminar o indicación de un procedimiento.

expresado—dicho en palabras o por acción.

expresar—decir; dar a saber por palabras o por acción.

extenso—que tiene una amplia gama.

extensor—el músculo de un grupo de músculos que extiende una parte, permitiendo que la articulación se enderezca.

externado—una experiencia de empleo supervisada en un establecimiento de salud calificado como parte del currículo educativo.

extinguidor—aparato para extinguir fuego.

extinguir—apagar; terminar.

extracelular—fuera de la célula.

extraer—una sustancia destilada u obtenida de otra sustancia.

extraño—cualquier cosa que no se encuentre normalmente en el sitio; usualmente se refiere a sucio, astillas, etc.

extremidad fantasma—ilusión de que la extremidad aún existe, después de ser amputada.

extremidad—se refiere a las partes terminales del cuerpo—los brazos, las piernas.

exudar—pus; la recolección de material purulento en una cavidad.

eyaculación—la expulsión de líquido seminal de la uretra masculina.

facsímil—una copia idéntica.

factible—posible; practicable.

factor Rh—sustancia antígena en la sangre similar a los factores A y B que determinan el grupo sanguíneo; aparentemente, el factor Rh sólo está presente en los glóbulos rojos.

facultativo—capaz de vivir bajo condiciones de temperatura o suministro de oxígeno variable; tener la capacidad de adaptarse a más de una condición, como una anerobia facultativa.

fagocito—glóbulo blanco que absorbe y destruye antígenos.

fagocitosis—ingestión y digestión de bacterias y otras partículas por parte de fagocitos.

falanges—huesos de las manos y los pies.

falsificar—imitar, especialmente falsear, como una firma.

familiar—perteneciente a la misma familia.

faringe—garganta; porción del canal alimentario entre la boca y el esófago.

farmaceuta—profesional licenciado que prepara y dispensa medicinas.

farmacéutico—relativo a las medicinas.

farmacología—el estudio y la práctica de preparar y dispensar medicinas.

fascia—una membrana fibrosa que cubre, sostiene y separa músculos; también puede unir la piel por debajo con tejido.

fatal—que causa muerte.

febril—perteneciente a una fiebre.

fecal—perteneciente a heces.

feces—desecho de los intestinos.

felicitaciones—expresar placer; reconocimiento de un logro.

femoral—pertenece a la arteria que yace adyacente al fémur.

fémur—el hueso del muslo de la pierna.

fenestrado—que tiene una ventana o apertura.

fenilalanina—aminoácido de una proteína.

fenilcetonuria (PKU por sus siglas en inglés)—trastorno genético que afecta el modo en que el cuerpo procesa las proteínas, probablemente debido al déficit de una encima. Se manifiesta por una deficiencia intelectual grave y trastornos neurológicos.

fenómeno de Raynaud—síntoma del lupus caracterizado por dedos que se vuelven azules o blancos a causa del frío.

fertilización—la impregnación del óvulo por el esperma; concepción.

fetal—perteneciente a un feto, embarazo después del tercer mes.

feto—un embrión después de la octava semana de gestación.

fibrilación—la vibración de fibras musculares; inefectiva, acción rápida pero débil del corazón.

fibroide—un tumor hecho de tejido fibroso y muscular.

fibrosis quística—una condición de una enfermedad de tumores fibrosos que ha sufrido degeneración quística, acumulando fluido en los intersticios; también conocida como enfermedad fibroquística.

fibrosis—formación anormal de tejido fibroso.

fiebre tifoidea—enfermedad infecciosa aguda adquirida tras la ingestión de comida o agua contaminada.

filigrana—marca transparente en el papel y los billetes de banco que sólo es visible cuando se ve en contraluz.

filo—cualquier objeto afilado que puede cortar, pinchar, punzar, apuñalar o rasguñar la piel.

filtración—el movimiento de solutes y agua a través de una membrana semipermeable como resultado de una fuerza, como la gravedad o la presión arterial.

fimosis—estrechez de la "boca" del prepucio, piel que recubre el glande.

firma—nombre de una persona en un papel.

fiscal—de o perteneciente a las finanzas en general.

fisiatría—rama de la medicina que estudia los trastornos y enfermedades de la mecánica del cuerpo, y sus formas de tratamiento. También conocida como Medicina Física y Rehabilitación.

físico—relativo al cuerpo.

fisiología—estudio de la función de las células, tejidos y órganos del cuerpo.

fisioterapista—persona licenciada para examinar y ofrecer tratamiento a pacientes con deficiencias fisiológicas o anatómicas a través de ejercicios especiales, aplicación de terapias de frío o calor, utilización del sonar y otras técnicas.

fístula—un pasaje anormal en forma de tubo de una cavidad normal o un absceso a una superficie libre.

fisura—una úlcera, división, apertura o rasgadura en el tejido.

fisura longitudinal—incisura profunda que divide los dos hemisferios del cerebro.

flato—gas intestinal.

flatulencia—la existencia de flato o gas intestinal.

flebitis—inflamación de una vena.

flebotomista—trabajador en el área de la salud con formación especial en la práctica de abrir venas para extraer muestra de sangre para ser analizadas en el laboratorio.

flexibilidad—fácilmente doblado, que acata, cediendo a la persuasión.

flexionado—doblado, como en una articulación.

flexor—el músculo de un grupo de músculos que dobla una parte.

flora—la vida de la planta en cuanto se distingue de la vida animal; la vida de las plantas que ocurre o se adapta para vivir en un entorno específico, como la flora de los intestinos.

fluido cerebroespinal—el líquido que circula dentro de las meninges de la columna vertebral y ventrículos y meninges del cerebro.

fluoroscopio—un aparato que consiste de una pantalla fluorescente junto con un tubo de rayos X que hace visibles las sombras de los objetos interpuestos entre la pantalla y el tubo.

foliculitis—una infección de estafilococo del folículo piloso.

folículo grafiano—el vesículo en el cual los huevos son madurados y que los libera cuando están maduro.

folículo—un pequeño conducto o saco excretor o glándula tubular; un folículo piloso.

folleto—un pequeño panfleto u opúsculo de información.

fondo—la porción de un órgano más remota de su apertura; en el útero, la porción del útero que se encuentra arriba de las aperturas de las trompas de falopio.

formaldehído—un gas incoloro y punzante, usado en su forma líquida para endurecer tejidos para estudios patológicos, o como germicida, desinfectante o preservativo, de acuerdo a la fortaleza de la solución.

formalina—alcohol de madera que contiene 40% de formaldehído.

fortaleza—resistencia valerosa.

forúnculo—el término médico para un nacido.

fotocopia—reproducción fotográfica de material escrito.

fotofobia—sensitividad hacia la luz.

fovea centralis—una depresión en la superficie posterior de la retina que es el lugar de la visión más aguda.

fractura—la ruptura repentina de un hueso.

fraudulento—caracterizado por hacer trampa y engaño; obtenido por medios deshonestos.

frecuencia—la necesidad de vaciar orina a menudo, aunque usualmente sólo en una pequeña cantidad cada vez.

fricción—la resistencia de una superficie al movimiento de otra superficie que frota sobre ella.

frontal—anterior; el hueso de la frente; se refiere al plano dibujado por el lado del cuerpo de la cabeza a los pies.

fuera de línea—se refiere a no estar en línea; falla de computador; tiempo en el que nada ha sido programado.

funcional—práctico; que funciona; útil.

fundido—derretido por el calor.

fusión espinal—implantación quirúrgica de un fragmento óseo entre los espacios de dos o tres vértebras espinales para inmovilizarlas.

galvanómetro—un instrumento que mide corriente por acción electromagnética.

gameto—una célula germen; cualquier cuerpo reproductivo.

ganglión—una masa de tejido nervioso que recibe y envía impulsos nerviosos.

gangrena—una forma de necrosis; la putrefacción de tejidos suaves.

garante—una persona que hace o da una garantía o promesa, a menudo pagar la deuda o la obligación del otro en el evento de incumplimiento.

garantía—seguridad de que algo será hecho como está especificado; una promesa.

garantizar—justificar; dar certeza definitiva del valor de algo; autorizar.

gastar—disponer o usar, como de dinero o energía.

gástrico—perteneciente al estómago.

gastrocnemio—el músculo grande en la pantorrilla.

gastroenterología—el estudio del estómago e intestinos y sus enfermedades.

gastroenterólogo—un médico especializado en el cuidado de pacientes con enfermedades y desórdenes del tracto gastrointestinal.

gastrointestinal (GI)—perteneciente al estómago y a los intestinos.

gastroscopia—examen del estómago con un gastroscopio.

generar—producir, como calor, ideas, poder.

genérico—general; características de un género o grupo.

genético—perteneciente a los genes.

genitales—órganos sexuales externos.

genograma—registro de la historia de la salud de la familia.

genucubital—perteneciente a los codos y rodillas; la posición rodilla-codo.

gen—una sustancia dentro del cromosoma que dicta la herencia.

genupectoral—perteneciente a las rodillas y al pecho; la posición rodilla-pecho.

geriatría—el estudio y tratamiento de las enfermedades de la vejez.

gerontólogo—un médico especializado en el cuidado de los ancianos.

gestación—período de desarrollo fetal intrauterino.

gigantismo—una condición que resulta de la sobreproducción de la hormona de crecimiento durante la niñez.

ginecología (GIN)—el estudio de las enfermedades de las mujeres, particularmente de los órganos de reproducción.

ginecólogo—un médico especializado en el cuidado de las enfermedades y desórdenes de las mujeres, particularmente de los órganos genitales.

GIN—ver ginecología.

glándula bulbouretral—dos pequeñas glándulas, una en cada lado de la glándula de la próstata, que terminan en la uretra por medio de un ducto.

glándulas de Bartholin—dos pequeñas glándulas mucosas, situadas una a cada lado de la apertura vaginal en la base de la labia minora.

glándulas mamarias—senos.

glándulas salivares—tres pares de glándulas que secretan la saliva, la cual inicia la digestión de la comida, y se encarga primordialmente de la descomposición de los almidones y los carbohidratos complejos.

glándulas sebáceas—órganos de la piel que secretan sebo.

glaucoma—una enfermedad del ojo caracterizada por aumento de presión intraocular.

glicosuria—azúcar en la orina.

glomerulonefritis—inflamación de los glomérulos del nefrón del riñón.

glomérulo—un racimo microscópico de capilares dentro de la cápsula de Bowman del nefrón.

glucohemoglobina—azúcar en la sangre.

glucosa—un líquido incoloro o amarillo, espeso y almibarado obtenido de la hidrólisis incompleta del almidón; un azúcar simple.

glúteo máximo—el músculo grande de los glúteos.

gónadas—las cláusulas del sexo, los ovarios en la hembra y los testículos en el macho.

gonadotrópico—relacionado con el estímulo de las gónadas.

gonadotropina coriónica—una hormona que se encuentra en la orina de una mujer embarazada poco después de la concepción.

gonorrea—una enfermedad venérea de los órganos reproductivos, que es altamente contagiosa por contacto directo.

goteo—filtración incontrolada de orina de la vejiga.

gotica—una gota muy pequeña.

graficar—registro de observaciones, hallazgos subjetivos y objetivos, procedimientos diagnósticos, tratamientos y otros datos pertinentes en la carpeta del paciente.

gram-negativo—bacteria que se tiñe de rosado con el proceso de teñido de Gram.

gram-positivo—bacteria que se tiñe de morado con el proceso de teñido de Gram.

gremios—asociaciones de personas interesadas en el mismo oficio o reunidas para protección mutua.

gripe—influenza; una infección respiratoria o intestinal.

guayaco—una solución usada para probar la presencia de sangre oculta en las heces.

guión—manuscrito.

HCFA—siglas en inglés para Health Care Financing Administration que en español significan Administración para la Financiación del Cuidado de la Salud.

heces—materia fecal, movimientos intestinales.

hematocrito—una expresión del volumen de las células rojas por unidad de sangre circulante.

hematología—el estudio de la sangre y de sus enfermedades.

hematólogo—un médico especializado en el cuidado de los pacientes con desórdenes y enfermedades de la sangre y de los órganos que la forman.

hematoma—un tumor o hinchazón que contiene sangre.

hematuria—sangre en la orina.

hemodiálisis—un proceso en el cual la sangre es pasada a través de una membrana delgada y expuesta a una solución dializada para remover productos de desecho.

hemofilia—condición hereditaria, trasmitida a través de cromosomas ligados al sexo de portadores femeninos; afecta a los hombres únicamente, causando inhabilidad de coagular la sangre.

hemófilo—cepa bacterial que crece mejor en la hemoglobina.

hemoglobina—la combinación de una proteína y un pigmento de hierro en los glóbulos rojos que atrae y lleva oxígeno en el cuerpo.

hemorragia—descarga anormal de sangre tanto interna como externamente de vasos venosos, arteriales o capilares.

hemorroidectomía—extirpación quirúrgica de tejido hemorroidal.

hemorroides—venas varicosas del canal anal.

hemotórax—sangre dentro del espacio pleural de la cavidad del pecho.

heparina—una sustancia formada en el hígado que inhibe la coagulación de la sangre.

hepático—perteneciente al hígado.

hepatitis—inflamación del hígado.

hernia inguinal—la presencia del intestino delgado en el canal inguinal.

hernia—una proyección de una parte de su localización normal.

herniografía—la reparación quirúrgica de una hernia.

herpes genital—lesiones llenas de fluido en los genitales externos, que son contagiosos al contacto directo.

herpes simple—el término médico para ampollas de fiebre, una aguda infección viral en la cara, la boca o la nariz.

herpes zóster—un término médico para culebrilla, una infección viral aguda de los ganglios dorsales.

heterosexual—atracción sexual hacia el sexo opuesto.

heterótrofo—microorganismos que se alimentan de materia orgánica.

HHS—siglas en inglés para Health and Human Services que en español significan Servicios Humanos y de Salud.

hiato—pertenece a la herniación del estómago a través de una apertura o hiato.

hidrocele—acumulación de fluido en el escroto.

hígado—la glándula más grande del cuerpo, localizada en el cuadrante superior derecho del abdomen debajo del diafragma.

higiene—el estudio de la salud y de la observancia de las reglas de la salud.

higienista—el que provee servicios relacionados con la salud, tales como procedimientos dentales.

higienista dental—proveedor de salud licenciado que está entrenado para tomar rayos X y efectuar tratamientos profilácticos en los dientes.

hilio—el área retirada del riñón donde entran la uretra y los vasos sanguíneos.

himen—un pliegue membranoso que cubre parcial o completamente la apertura vaginal.

hiperglicemia—un aumento del azúcar en la sangre, como en diabetes.

hiperopia—un defecto de la visión que hace que los objetos sólo puedan ser vistos cuando están muy lejos; hipermetropía.

hipersensitivo—muy sensible; anormalmente sensible a un estímulo de cualquier clase.

hipertensión—elevada presión arterial.

hipertermia—temperatura más alta de lo normal.

hipertiroidismo—una condición causada por excesiva secreción de las glándulas tiroides.

hipertónico—que tiene una concentración más alta de sal que las encontradas en los glóbulos rojos.

hipertrofia benigna—agrandamiento no maligno.

hiperventilación—respiración excesivamente profunda y frecuente.

hipo—el resultado del cierre espástico de la epiglotis y espasmo del diafragma.

hipoalergénico—poco probable que cause una reacción alérgica.

hipocondríaco—perteneciente a las regiones superiores y exteriores del abdomen bajo el tórax, también alguien con temor mórbido a la enfermedad, resultando en una preocupación anormal acerca de la propia salud.

hipocrático—se refiere al juramento tomado por un doctor que lo obliga a observar el código de ética médica contenido en el juramento hecho por Hipócrates en el siglo IV.

hipogástrico—se refiere a un área abdominal en el tercio medio bajo del abdomen.

hipoglicemia—deficiencia de azúcar en la sangre.

hipotálamo—una estructura del cerebro entre el cerebelo y el cerebro medio; yace bajo el tálamo.

hipotensión—presión arterial anormalmente baja.

hipotermia—temperatura corporal más baja de lo normal.

hipotiroidismo—una condición causada por una marcada deficiencia de secreción tiroidea.

hipotónico—que tiene una menor concentración de sal que la encontrada en un glóbulo rojo.

hipoxia—falta de oxígeno.

histamina—una sustancia presente normalmente en el cuerpo.

histerectomía—extirpación quirúrgica del útero.

histeroscopia—un procedimiento que usa el histeroscopio para ver el endometrio del útero.

histólogo—(histotecnólogo) una persona comprometida al estudio de las estructuras microscópicas de los tejidos.

histoplasmosis—una infección de hongos causada por un organismo que se encuentra en las heces de pájaros y murciélagos.

historia financiera—los registros financieros pasados.

hoja de vida—sumario de experiencia laboral.

holístico—considera la totalidad o el alcance completo de una situación.

homeostasis—el mantenimiento de una condición constante o estática de un entorno interno.

homólisis—disolución; descomposición de los glóbulos rojos.

homosexual—atracción sexual hacia el mismo sexo de uno mismo.

honestidad—el estado de ser verdadero, confiable; genuino.

hongo—un organismo vegetal y celular, que subsiste en materia orgánica, como bacteria o moho; la condición de una enfermedad que causa el crecimiento de lesiones de hongos en la superficie de la piel.

honrado—de buena reputación.

horizontal—no vertical; plano y parejo; nivelado; paralelo a la línea del horizonte.

hormona adrenocorticotrópica (HACT)—una hormona secretada por el lóbulo anterior de la glándula pituitaria.

hormona—una sustancia química secretada por un órgano o glándula.

hostilidad—animadversión, enemistad.

hoyuelos—una condición caracterizada por las hendiduras en la piel.

hpf—siglas en inglés que significan high-power field; en español significa campo de alto poder; se refiere al lente del microscopio.

húmero—el hueso largo del brazo.

humilde—modesto, no pretensioso.

humor acuoso—líquido aguado y transparente que circula entre la cámara anterior y posterior del ojo.

humor vítreo—sustancia que ocupa el cuerpo vítreo del ojo detrás del lente.

humoral—inmunidad mediada por anticuerpos.

I & D—ver incisión y drenaje.

ictericia—una descoloración amarillenta de la esclerótica y de la piel debida a la presencia de pigmento de bilis en la sangre.

identificación—cualquier cosa por la cual una persona o una cosa puede ser identificada.

idiopático—una enfermedad sin causa reconocible.

IHB/ihb—influenza hemófila tipo B.

ilegible—imposible de leer.

íleo paralítico—parálisis de la pared intestinal con síntomas de obstrucción aguda.

ileocecal—la válvula entre el final del intestino delgado y el ciego.

íleon—la última sección del intestino delgado.

ileostomía—una apertura quirúrgica del íleon encima de la pared abdominal.

ilíaco—el borde o la cresta del hueso pélvico.

ilícito—impropio, ilegal; no permitido por la costumbre o la ley; fuera de la ley.

ilion—el hueso de la cadera.

iluminar—aclarar, esclarecer.

impacción—una colección de heces endurecidas en el recto que no puede ser expulsada.

impactado—se refiere a una fractura cuando los extremos rotos están apretujados.

impedimento—obstaculizar; aquellos que están físicamente incapacitados o mentalmente retardados.

implante—algo implantado en un tejido; un injerto; parte artificial.

implementación—poner en práctica.

implemento—una herramienta o instrumento para hacer algo; poner en práctica.

implicación—envolvimiento, poner en contacto.

implicado—insinuado, sugerido.

impotencia—inhabilidad de un macho para obtener o mantener una erección.

improductivo—que no logra resultados.

impulso—una carga transmitida a través de ciertos tejidos, especialmente fibras nerviosas y músculos, que resultan en actividad fisiológica.

inapropiado—no apropiado, fuera de lugar.

incapacidad—una inhabilidad legal.

incas—el yunque, el hueso de la mitad de los tres en el oído medio.

incinerar—quemar, poner fuego.

incisión y drenaje (I & D)—cortar con el propósito de proveer una salida para un material, usualmente una colección de pus.

incisión—corte.

inclinado—recostado o propender a.

incompetente—no capaz; no calificado legalmente; deficiente.

incomprensible—increíble, sin que pueda ser entendido por la mente.

incongruo—falta de armonía o acuerdo.

inconscientemente—involuntariamente, sin tener conocimiento, sin intención.

incontinente—incapaz de controlar la vejiga o el intestino.

incrementos—agrandar; cantidad de aumento; ganancia.

incubación—el intervalo entre la exposición a la infección y la aparición del primer síntoma.

indemnización—compensar por daño hecho o pérdida causada.

indigente—necesitado, pobre, destituto.

indigestión—dificultad en digerir comida.

inducción—acción de causar o producir; generar.

inevitable—ineludible, destinado a ocurrir.

infarto—infiltración de partículas extrañas; en un vaso el material que causa coagulación e interferencia con la circulación.

infarto del miocardio (MI por sus siglas en inglés)—obstrucción de la arteria coronaria que interrumpe el flujo de sangre hacia el músculo del corazón.

infeccioso—capaz de producir infección; denota una enfermedad en el cuerpo causada por la presencia de gérmenes; tendencia a extenderse a otros.

inferior—abajo, debajo.

infertilidad—inhabilidad de lograr concepción.

infligir—asestar, causar castigo.

influenza—una enfermedad aguda caracterizada por fiebre, dolor, tos y síntomas generales del aparato respiratorio superior.

infrarojo—perteneciente a esos rayos invisibles que se encuentran más allá del final rojo del espectro visible que tienen el penetrante efecto de calentar.

infusión—infundir; introducción de una sustancia en una vena.

ingenio—inteligencia; facultad para discurrir o inventar.

ingerir—comer.

ingle—la depresión entre la cadera y el tronco del cuerpo; la región inguinal.

inguinal—se refiere a la región donde el muslo se une con el tronco del cuerpo; la ingle.

inhalar—respirar hacia adentro.

inicial—el primero; comienzo; la primera letra del nombre de cada persona.

iniciar—comenzar algo; empezar.

iniciativa—la acción de dar el primer paso; la habilidad de originar nuevas ideas.

injerto—una parte construída.

inminente—estar a la mano o a punto de suceder.

inmovilizar—mantener fuera de acción o circulación; estacionario.

inmune—protegido o exento de una enfermedad.

inmunización—volverse inmune o el proceso de hacer a un paciente inmune.

inmunodeficiencia—falta de los componentes necesarios para crear una respuesta inmune.

inmunoglobulina—una molécula de proteína grande que ayuda a la respuesta inmune.

inmunológico—perteneciente a la inmunología.

inmunosuprimido—una condición en la cual el sistema inmune ha sido vencido y no puede funcionar adecuadamente.

innato—congénito; inherente.

inorgánico—no viviente; ocurre en la naturaleza de forma independiente de las cosas vivas.

inseminar—impregnar con semen.

inserción—el lugar donde un músculo se une al hueso que mueve.

insidioso—oculto, no aparente.

insignificante—pequeño, de poco valor; mezquino.

insignificante—no importante; mezquino; de poco o ningún valor.

insomnio—incapacidad anormal de dormir.

inspeccionar—examinar de cerca.

inspección—la primera parte de un examen físico; observación cercana.

inspiración—respirar hacia adentro, inhalar.

instituir—originar como una costumbre.

insuficiencia cardíaca congestiva—una condición compleja de una acción cardíaca inadecuada con retención de líquidos de tejidos; puede ser una falla del lado derecho, izquierdo, o de ambos.

insuficiente—no tanto como se necesita.

insulina—una hormona secretada por las isletas de Langerhans en el páncreas.

intacto—no roto, no dañado.

intangible—lo que no puede ser tocado, fácilmente definido o captado.

integridad—solidez de carácter; honestidad en particular.

integumentario—la piel; una cubierta.

intelectualización—el empleo del racionamiento para evitar confrontaciones o situaciones de estrés.

inteligencia—la habilidad de aprender o entender.

interacción—actuar el uno con el otro.

interceder—mediar, rogar por otro.

intercostal—entre las costillas.

interferencia—confusión de las señales deseadas causada por señales indeseadas, como en artefactos en un ECG.

interferón—una lymphokina que ayuda a regular las actividades de los macrófagos y células destructoras naturales.

interjección—parte del habla; una exclamación.

interleukina—una sustancia mensajera entre leucocitos.

intermedio—en el medio.

intermitente—que para y arranca de nuevo a intervalos.

internado—etapa después de la graduación en que se practica la profesión.

internista—un médico especializado en el cuidado de pacientes con enfermedades internas.

interpersonal—entre personas.

interpretar—explicar, traducir; determinar el significado.

intervalo—tiempo entre eventos; espacio.

intervención—tomar acción para modificar, impedir o cambiar un efecto.

intervertebral—entre las vértebras.

intestinal—se refiere a los intestinos.

intestino—el canal alimentario que se extiende desde el píloro del estómago al ano.

intimidación—producir miedo; impedir con amenazas.

intimidar—producir miedo, asustar.

intoxicación—condición causada por la exageración en el consumo de bebidas alcohólicas.

intracelular—dentro de la célula.

intradermal—dentro de la piel.

intramuscular—dentro del músculo.

intraocular—dentro del ojo.

intravenoso—insertar en la vena.

intrincado—complicado, complejo, entretejido elaboradamente.

intubación—la inserción de un tubo en la laringe para la entrada de aire.

intuición—el conocimiento o aprendizaje inmediato de algo sin el uso consciente del razonamiento.

inunción—el proceso de administrar drogas a través de la piel.

invasivo—método de diagnóstico que involucra la entrada en el tejido vivo.

inventario—una lista pormenorizada de productos en existencia.

involuntario—independiente o aun en contra de la voluntad o escogencia.

iris—el tejido coloreado, contráctil que rodea la pupila del ojo.

irracional—sin el poder de la razón; sin sentido.

irreconciliable—situación en la que no se puede llegar a un acuerdo.

irrelevante—no pertinente.

irreparable—dañado más allá de la posibilidad de ser reparado.

ishahara—se refiere a una prueba del ojo para determinar visión de color.

isletas de Langerhans—ramos de células en el páncreas.

isotónico—que tiene la misma concentración de sal que se encuentra en un glóbulo rojo.

isquemia—anemia temporal y localizada causada por la obstrucción de la circulación de una parte.

isquión—porción posterior e inferior del hueso de la cadera.

Jaeger—un sistema para medir la agudeza de la visión cercana.

juanete—una bursa con formación callosa.

juicio—una decisión; la habilidad de tomar las decisiones correctas.

KUB (por sus siglas en inglés)—riñones, uréteres y vejiga. Relativo a un estudio radiológico.

L&A—luz y acomodación.

labia mayor—los dos pliegues grandes de tejido adiposo que se encuentran a cada lado de la vulva; genitales externos.

labia menor—los dos pliegues mucocutáneos de membrana dentro de la labia mayor.

laboratorio—espacio o edificio en el cual se conducen análisis o experimentos científicos.

laceración—cortadura o herida.

lagrimal (o lacrimal)—relativo a las lágrimas; las glándulas y ductos que secretan las lágrimas.

Lamaze—programa o método que prepara a la mujer embarazada para el momento del parto.

laminectomía—extirpación de una porción del arco posterior vertebral.

lanceta—instrumento afilado y punteado utilizado para perforar la piel con el objeto de obtener una muestra de sangre a nivel capilar.

laringe—caja vocal. Parte superior de la tráquea cuyos cartílagos sostienen las cuerdas vocales.

laríngeo—relativo a la laringe.

lateral—relativo al lado o costado.

lattissimus dorsi—el músculo grande de la espalda.

laxativo—sustancia que induce la evacuación de los intestinos.

legible—fácil de leer.

lengua—órgano muscular de la boca que ayuda en la producción de palabras, contiene las papilas gustativas y asiste en la acción de tragar.

lente—parte del ojo que refracta las imágenes en la retina.

lesión—herida; área circunscrita de tejido patológicamente alterado.

letal—mortal; capaz de causar la muerte.

letra script—fuente diseñada para parecer escrita a mano.

leucemia—enfermedad caracterizada por un exceso de glóbulos blancos; existe en forma linfática y mielógena; es a menudo fatal, especialmente en adultos.

leucocito—glóbulo blanco.

liaison—término francés que significa intercomunicación entre dos entidades.

libro de contabilidad—documento que contiene el registro de los créditos y débitos de una empresa.

licencia—permiso legal para ejecutar una actividad determinada.

liendre—huevo del piojo o de otro insecto parasítico.

ligado al cromosoma X—conectado al cromosoma sexual de la célula; una característica del cromosoma sexual.

ligadura—proceso a través del cual se amarra o se aprieta.

ligamento—tejido fibroso que conecta los huesos entre sí.

limitar—restringir, confinar, circunscribir.

línea de base—la información inicial en la que se basan datos adicionales.

linfa—fluido que se forma al interior de los espacios entre los tejidos y que circula a través del cuerpo.

linfocito—tipo de glóbulo blanco.

lisosoma—organelo que se encuentra al interior del citoplasma en la célula.

lista de honorarios—listado de cobros permitidos.

litotomía—posición para examinar al paciente en la cual el paciente se acuesta de espaldas con los muslos flexionados sobre el abdomen y las piernas flexionadas sobre los muslos.

litotripsia—destrucción de cálculos renales.

litro—medida de capacidad equivalente a 1,000 ml o aproximadamente un cuarto.

longevidad—larga duración de vida.

lordosis—curvatura anterior anormal de la espina lumbar.

lubb dupp—sonidos cardiacos normales.

lumbar—relativo a la espalda, específicamente a las cinco vértebras sobre el sacro.

lumen—espacio al interior de una arteria, una vena o un vaso capilar; espacio al interior de un tubo.

lupus eritomatoso—enfermedad autoinmune crónica que causa cambios en el sistema inmunológico.

luteinización—efecto hormonal que causa ovulación y progesterona en la mujer, y producción de esperma y testosterona en el hombre.

macrófago—célula fagocítica que destruye antígenos.

mácula—parche en la piel descolorado pero sin elevaciones o depresiones.

maduración—relativo a las fases de desarrollo celular.

madurez—fase de mayor desarrollo.

magnético—que tiene las propiedades de atracción del imán.

magnificar—hacer aparecer algo más grande de lo que es realmente.

malestar—sensación de incomodidad.

maligno—bulto o tumor canceroso.

malinger—fingir enfermedad para escapar una situación u obligación.

malleus—el más grande de los tres huesos del oído medio, también llamado "martillo".

mamografía—rayos X de los senos.

mandato—orden de mando; instrucción.

manifestación—acción de revelar o de exponer.

mantenimiento—actividad de preservar; acciones para conservar algo en condición apropiada.

marcapasos—nodo sinoatrial del corazón; también, aparato eléctrico que provoca en forma artificial la contracción del corazón cuando ésta no puede efectuarse normalmente.

marginal—cercano al límite más bajo de aceptación.

masa—multitud; grupo grande de personas.

mastectomía—operación quirúrgica para extirpar un seno.

matasellos—cancelación fechada de una estampilla por la oficina de correos; también identifica la dirección de la oficina de correos.

matriz—formato para establecer horarios para citas.

meato urinario—apertura a través de la cual la orina es evacuada del cuerpo.

mecánica corporal—el uso de posicionamiento adecuado del cuerpo cuando se mueve o cuando se levantan objetos para evitar lesiones.

mecánico—relativo a maquinaria.

mediado por anticuerpos—inmunidad humoral; cuando los anticuerpos y complementos trabajan juntos para destruir los antígenos.

medial—relativo al medio o a la línea central.

Medicaid—programa de salud del gobierno.

Medicaire—programa de salud a nivel federal destinado a pagar ciertos tratamientos de salud para pacientes de edad avanzada.

medicina deportiva—rama de la medicina que estudia la manera de prevenir y tratar lesiones causadas por la práctica del deporte.

medicina nuclear—rama de la medicina que utiliza radionúclidos en el diagnóstico y tratamiento de enfermedades.

medicina ocupacional—rama de la medicina que estudia el diagnóstico y tratamiento de enfermedades ocurridas en el trabajo.

médico—doctor entrenado en la práctica de la Medicina.

médico asistente—persona entrenada en ciertos aspectos de la práctica de la medicina con el objeto de proporcionar ayuda al médico.

médico de familia—el que cuida los paciente de todas las edades y todas las condiciones que no requieren especialización.

Medigap—relativo a situaciones no cubiertas por Medicare.

médula—tejido suave que se encuentra en el hueco de los huesos largos.

médula renal—sección interna del riñón.

medulla oblongata—porción alargada de la médula espinal; la porción más baja del tronco encefálico.

melanina—pigmento que da color a la piel, cabello y ojos.

melanocito—células que producen el pigmento de la piel, melanina.

membrana—capa de tejido muy delgada, suave y doblable que cubre un tubo, cavidad, órgano o estructura.

membrana celular—estructura que rodea y encierra la célula.

membrana timpánica—tímpano.

menarquía—primer período menstrual.

meninges—membranas que cubren el cerebro y la médula espinal.

meningitis—inflamación de las meninges.

menisco—concavidad que forma la superficie de un líquido contenido dentro de un tubo o cilindro.

menopausia—cesación permanente de la menstruación.

menor emancipado—que ya no está bajo el cuidado, la custodia o supervisión de un padre o guardián.

menorragia—flujo menstrual excesivo; hemorragia.

menstruar—descargar fluido sanguíneo del útero en forma periódica.

mensura—medida, medición.

mercurio—metal líquido utilizado en aparatos de medida tales como termómetros y esfigmomanómetros. Su símbolo químico es el Hg.

mérito—lo que hace digna de elogio o recompensa a una persona; excelencia.

mesenterio—doblez peritoneal que conecta al intestino con la pared abdominal posterior.

metabolismo—transformaciones sucesivas a las que se somete una sustancia desde el momento en que entra en el cuerpo hasta que dicha sustancia o sus desechos son excretados, y a través de las cuales el cuerpo se nutre y adquiere la energía para su subsistencia.

metacarpos—los cinco huesos de la mano que se encuentran entre la muñeca y las falanges.

metástasis—movimiento de células cancerosas de una parte del cuerpo a otra.

metatarsos—los cinco huesos de los pies que se encuentran entre el empeine y las falanges.

metódico—sistemático, que sigue un plan o método.

MI–índice de maduración (por sus siglas en inglés)—medida de maduración celular.

MI—infarto del miocardio (por sus siglas en inglés).

microbiano—relativo a los microbios.

microficha—hoja de microfilme con la capacidad de almacenar una cantidad considerable de información en forma reducida.

microorganismo—cuerpo viviente microscópico que no se puede percibir a simple vista.

microscópico—visible sólo a través de un microscopio.

micturación—acción de orinar.

mielina—sustancia grasosa que envuelva las fibras nerviosas.

mielografía—examen de la médula espinal a través de rayos X con inyección de un material radio-opaco.

miembros—relativo a los brazos y/o las piernas.

migraña—dolor de cabeza severo con síntomas característicos.

mineralocorticoide—hormona de la corteza adrenal que influye en el metabolismo del sodio y del potasio y regula el fluido del cuerpo y los electrolitos.

minuto—medida de tiempo equivalente a 60 segundos.

miocardio—capa muscular del corazón.

miometrio—estructura muscular del útero.

miopía—defecto de la vista que sólo permite ver los objetos próximos al ojo.

mitocondria—organelo que se encuentra en el citoplasma de la célula.

mitosis—división celular.

mitral—válvula en el corazón localizada entre las cámaras del lado izquierdo.

mixedema—condición que resulta de la hipofunción de la glándula tiroidea.

modificador—que cambia; que limita el significado.

modificar—cambiar la forma o cualidad de alguna cosa; alterar ligeramente.

moneda—cualquiera forma de dinero.

monilia—familia de hongos parásitos o mohos.

monitor fetal—un dispositivo para tener acceso al latido del corazón fetal.

monitor Holter—un aparato que adhiere electrodos al pecho de un paciente con el propósito de obtener el trazado de un electrocardiograma de 24 horas en una grabadora portátil.

monitorear—observar.

monocitos—células mononucleares que abandonan el sistema sanguíneo y entran en los tejidos para convertirse en macrófagos.

monoclonal—célula híbrida producida en laboratorio capaz de producir anticuerpos.

monocular—que posee un solo ojo, como el microscopio.

monograma—registro obtenido por ultrasonido.

monótono—tono único; invariable, aburrido, rutinario.

monóxido de carbón—un gas venenoso incoloro, inodoro, causado por la combustión incompleta del carbón.

mons pubis—relleno de tejido graso y piel gruesa que recubre el symphisis pubis en la mujer.

moralidad—virtud.

mores—acciones que, a través del acatamiento general, adquieren la fuerza de la ley.

morfología—rama de la biología que estudia la forma y estructura de los organismos.

motor—relativo a los nervios que permiten que el cuerpo responda a estímulos.

motricidad—cualidad del movimiento; de fácil movimiento.

MRI—resonancia magnética (por sus siglas en inglés). Examen de diagnóstico que utiliza ondas magnéticas para visualizar las estructuras internas del cuerpo.

mucosa—perteneciente a la membrana mucosa.

mudar—dejar una cosa como, por ejemplo, tejido muerto.

MUGA (multiple-gated acquisition scan)—por sus siglas en inglés, examen de diagnóstico para evaluar la condición del miocardio del corazón.

muleta—un bastón con una pieza atravesada en la parte superior para ponerlo bajo el brazo de la persona lisiada.

multicanal—relativo a la capacidad del equipo de ECG de procesar impulsos provenientes de múltiples procedencias.

murmuro—soplo suave o sonido áspero que se escucha durante la auscultación del corazón.

muscular—relativo a los músculos.

músculo—tipo de tejido compuesto de células contráctiles o fibras que generan el movimiento del cuerpo.

musculoesqueletal—relativo a los sistemas muscular y esquelético.

músculos papilares—grupos de músculos que van agarrados desde las paredes de los ventrículos del corazón hasta la parte inferior de las válvulas del corazón y cuya función es abrir las válvulas durante la fase de relajación del latido.

mutación—cambio en una característica heredada; cambio celular causado por una influencia.

narcolepsia—deseo irresistible e incontrolable de dormir a cualquier hora.

narcótico—droga capaz de producir el sueño y la relajación muscular, o capaz de inducir inconsciencia e incluso la muerte, dependiendo de la dosis.

nasal—relativo a la nariz.

náusea—ganas de vomitar.

nefrología—el estudio del riñón y de sus enfermedades.

nefrólogo—médico especializado en las enfermedades y los trastornos del riñón.

nefrón—unidad estructural y funcional del riñón.

negación—el rechazo a creer o a aceptar; desconocer.

negar—no admitir la existencia o veracidad de algo.

negligente—descuidado; que no pone todo el cuidado y aplicación que debiera.

negociable—asunto capaz de ser discutido y sus términos acordados.

neonato—infante recién nacido.

neoplástico—nueva formación de tejido anormal (cancerosa).

nervio—grupo de tejidos nerviosos que conducen la sensibilidad y el movimiento.

nervosa—pérdida de apetito sin conexión con una enfermedad; parte de una psicosis.

neto—valor restante después de deducir los gastos y descuentos; beneficios y ganancias; excluyente de deducciones; total; entero.

neumoconiosis—condición respiratoria causada por la inhalación de partículas de polvo provenientes de labores como la minería o el trabajo con piedra.

neumoencefalografía—examen por rayos X de los ventrículos y espacios subaracnoides del cerebro después de extraer fluido cerebroespinal e inyectar aire o gas a través de una puntura lumbar.

neumonía—inflamación del pulmón causada primordialmente por microbios, irritantes químicos, polvo vegetal o alergias.

neumotórax—colección de aire o gas en la cavidad pleural que desplaza el tejido pulmonar.

neurilema—capa membranosa delgada que recubre la fibra nerviosa.

neurocirugía—procedimientos quirúrgicos efectuados en el sistema nervioso.

neurología—estudio del sistema nervioso y de sus enfermedades.

neurólogo—médico especializado en las enfermedades y los trastornos del sistema nervioso.

neurona internuncial—neuronas que conectan las neuronas sensoriales a las motoras.

neurona—célula nerviosa.

neutrófilo—glóbulo blanco granulado.

nicotina—alcaloide venenoso extraído de las hojas de tabaco.

nicturia—necesidad de evacuar durante la noche.

no estructurado—sin orden.

no invasivo—método de diagnóstico que no requiere penetrar el tejido corporal.

no patógeno—organismo que no produce enfermedad.

nodo—nudo, protuberancia o inflamación.

nódulo AV—nódulo auriculoventricular; principio del nodo de His en la aurícula derecha/atrio; fibras nerviosas responsables de la contracción de los ventrículos.

nomenclatura—sistema de nombres científicos o técnicos.

nominal—demasiado pequeño para ser considerado, o cantidad muy pequeña.

nomograma—representación—a través de gráficos, diagramas, cuadros o tablas—de las relaciones entre variables numéricas.

non compos mentis—término legal general para todas las formas de enfermedad mental.

nonchalant—término francés que alude a una persona indiferente o despreocupada.

norepinefrina—hormona secretada por la médula adrenal en respuesta a una estimulación simpática.

norma de cumpleaños—manera de identificar la responsabilidad primaria en caso de cobertura de seguros.

nuclear—relativo al núcleo de un átomo.

núcleo—cuerpo vital en el protoplasma de la célula.

nucleolo—estructura que se encuentra en el interior del núcleo de la célula.

numérico—denota un número o sistema de números.

nutrición—relativo al material comestible, comida, cosas que nutren.

nutricionista—miembro del equipo de profesionales de la salud que estudia y aplica los principios de la ciencia de la nutrición.

nutrir—alimentar, cuidar.

O. D.—por sus siglas en latín (oculus dexter), u ojo derecho.

O. S.—por sus siglas en latín (oculus sinister), u ojo izquierdo; también, boca o apertura.

O. U.—por sus siglas en latín (oculus uterque), o cada ojo.

objetivo—fin hacia el cual se dirige la acción; del síntoma de una enfermedad, perceptible por personas diferentes de la afectada; en un microscopio, lente o serie de lentes.

obligar—atar legal o moralmente.

obliterar—borrar, no dejar trazo alguno; destruir.

observante—quien percibe rápidamente; agudo observador.

obsoleto—anticuado; caído en desuso.

obstetra—médico especializado en el cuidado y tratamiento de mujeres durante el embarazo y parto.

obstetricia—rama de la medicina que se encarga del cuidado y tratamiento de mujeres durante el embarazo y parto.

obturador—cualquier cosa que obstruye o cierra una cavidad o apertura; relativo a la porción interna de un instrumento de examen que facilita la introducción del instrumento dentro del cuerpo y es después retirada, permitiendo la visualización del área interna.

occipital—perteneciente a la parte posterior de la cabeza, el lóbulo posterior del cerebro.

ocluir—cerrar, obstruir.

oculto—oscuro, escondido.

oficinista de admisiones—una persona que procesa la información y los formularios para un paciente que va a ingresar al establecimiento de salud.

oftalmología—el estudio del ojo y de sus enfermedades y trastornos.

oftalmólogo—médico especializado en las enfermedades y trastornos del ojo.

ojeada—una mirada o visión rápida.

olfativo—perteneciente al sentido del olfato.

oliguria—producción escasa de orina.

oncogén—gene en la célula de un tumor.

oncología—rama de la medicina que estudia tumores, usualmente malignos.

oportunista—persona que aprovecha la oportunidad o toma ventaja de una situación.

oposición—actividad en contra de algo, resistencia.

óptico—relativo al ojo o a la visión.

optómetra—técnico que mide el poder refractivo del ojo y, de ser necesario, prescribe una fórmula correctiva de cualquier defecto visual.

oral—relativo a la boca.

orbital—relativo a la cavidad del cráneo donde está ubicado el ojo.

organelo—estructura funcional al interior del citoplasma de la célula.

orgánico—perteneciente a o derivado de formas de vida animal o vegetal.

órgano—parte del cuerpo construida a partir de diferentes tipos de tejidos para desempeñar una función necesaria para la vida.

órgano de Corti—aparato acústico terminal en la cóclea del oído interno.

origen—principio o procedencia de algo.

orina—fluido secretado de la sangre por los riñones, depositado en la vejiga, y evacuado del cuerpo a través de la orinación.

orinación—acto de orinar.

ortopedia—rama de la medicina que estudia la estructura y función de huesos y músculos.

ortopedista—médico que corrige las deformidades y trata enfermedades y trastornos de los huesos, las articulaciones y la columna vertebral.

ortopnea—condición respiratoria en la cual el paciente sólo puede respirar cuando está sentado o parado.

ortostático—relativo a la posición erecta; parado.

osciloscopio—instrumento de medida electrónico para la representación gráfica de variaciones eléctricas.

óseo—relativo a los huesos.

OSHA (Occupational Safety and Health Administration)—organización gubernamental encargada de la seguridad y la salud ocupacional.

osmosis—proceso de difusión de agua o de otro solvente a través de una membrana permeable.

osteopatía—cualquier enfermedad de los huesos; relativo a la escuela de medicina basada en la creencia según la cual el fragmento óseo del cuerpo determina en gran medida las relaciones estructurales de sus tejidos.

osteoporosis—condición causado por la reducción del calcio en los huesos.

OTC—por sus siglas en inglés "over the counter" se refiere a los medicamentos que se pueden adquirir sin prescripción médica.

otitis—inflamación del oído; puede referirse al oído externo, medio o interno.

otorrinolaringología—rama de la medicina que estudia las enfermedades y trastornos del oído, la nariz y la laringe.

otorrinolaringólogo—médico especializado en las enfermedades y trastornos del oído, la nariz y la garganta.

otosclerosis—condición caracterizada por la pérdida progresiva de la audición. El hueso esponjoso que rodea el laberinto del oído y los huesillos de éste van perdiendo progresivamente la facultad de conducir el sonido.

ovario—gónada femenina encargada de producir las hormonas que desarrollan y mantienen las características sexuales de la mujer.

"over the counter" (OTC, por sus siglas en inglés)—se refiere a los medicamentos que se pueden adquirir sin prescripción médica.

ovulación—proceso de formación y de su maduración de un folículo ovárico que culmina en la emisión de un óvulo.

ovum—huevo, el gameto o célula reproductora femenina.

oxalato—sal de ácido oxálico.

oxigenar—combinar con oxígeno o proveer oxígeno.

oxígeno—gas incoloro, inodoro y sin sabor que se encuentra en el aire. Su símbolo químico es O_2.

paciencia—esperar con tranquilidad, soportar con resignación.

pagaré—que contiene la promesa de pagar.

palidez—falta de color.

palpar—sentir, examinar con el tacto.

páncreas—órgano que secreta insulina y jugos digestivos.

pancreatitis—inflamación del páncreas.

pandémico—relativo a la extensión de una enfermedad contagiosa a muchas regiones o a una región extensa.

pantomima—expresarse por medio de gestos y movimientos.

Papanicolau (Pap por sus siglas en inglés)—examen que detecta células cancerosas en la mucosa de un órgano.

papelería—materiales para escribir, especialmente papel y sobres.

paperas—enfermedad contagiosa caracterizada por la inflamación de la glándula parótida y otras glándulas salivares.

papila—pequeñas protuberancias o elevaciones de la piel o de las membranas mucosas, tales como las papilas gustativas que se encuentran en la lengua.

pápula—área roja y elevada en la piel; elevación evanescente de la piel, más o menos redonda, blanca en el centro con un borde rojo pálido, acompañada de comezón.

par—igual. Usualmente se refiere a alguien con un status o una posición similar.

parabasal—al lado a cerca de la base o a la parte inferior.

paramédico—profesional de la salud que proporciona cuidado médico de emergencia y cuidado de apoyo.

parámetro—cantidad que se determina en forma arbitraria con el objeto de establecer comparaciones.

parasimpático—división del sistema nervioso autónomo.

parásito—organismo que vive en o sobre otro organismo, a expensas de ese otro organismo.

paratiroides—glándulas endocrinas situadas cerca de la glándula tiroides.

parenteral—que no se administra a través de la boca.

parietal—porción central de la corteza cerebral localizada a cada lado del cerebro.

paroxístico—ataque repentino de una enfermedad; ataque de dolor agudo, ataque de tos, ataque de risa, ataque de pasión.

paso—manera de caminar.

patela—rótula.

patofisiología—estudio de los mecanismos mediante los cuales ocurre una enfermedad, las respuestas del cuerpo al proceso de la enfermedad, y los efectos de ambos en una función normal.

patógeno—cualquier microorganismo o sustancia capaz de producir una enfermedad.

patología—estudio de la naturaleza y la causa de las enfermedades.

patológico—condición causada por una enfermedad.

patólogo—médico especializado en la interpretación y diagnóstico de cambios generados por una enfermedad determinada en tejidos y fluidos corporales.

pectoral mayor—el músculo principal de la pared del pecho.

pediatra—médico especializado en las enfermedades y los trastornos de la infancia.

pediatría—rama de la medicina que proporciona cuidad y tratamiento a los niños que sufren enfermedades.

pediculosis—enfermedad de la piel producida por el rascamiento motivado por la infestación de piojos.

peligro biológico—cualquier material que ha estado en contacto con un fluido corporal y que es potencialmente capaz de transmitir una enfermedad.

peligroso—arriesgado, de cuidado.

pélvico—relativo a la pelvis.

pene—órgano sexual externo masculino.

péptico—relativo a la digestión; también se refiere a una úlcera en el tracto digestivo superior.

per cápita—expresión latina que significa por cabeza. Se aplica a lo que corresponde por persona.

percentil—cualquier valor en una serie que divide la distribución de sus miembros en 100 grupos de igual frecuencia.

percepción—adquisición de consciencia o de conocimiento a través de los sentidos; recepción de impresiones.

percibir—adquirir consciencia de una sensación; comprender.

percusión—acción de golpear el cuerpo suave pero puntualmente para determinar la posición, el tamaño y la consistencia de una estructura subyacente.

perfusión—acción de verter o hacer correr un líquido.

pericardio—saco membranoso que recubre el corazón.

pericarditis—inflamación del pericardio, la cubierta del corazón.

pericia—un conocimiento especial o una habilidad.

periférico—relativo a una porción del sistema nervioso; aparato conectado a un computador.

perineo—región entre la vagina y el ano en la mujer, o la región entre el escroto y el ano en el hombre.

periódico—relativo a una acción que ocurre una y otra vez, a intervalos regulares.

periostio—membrana fibrosa que recubre la superficie del hueso excepto las las articulaciones que están cubiertas por cartílago.

peristalsis—serie de contracciones musculares normales, coordinadas y rítmicas que ocurren automáticamente para hacer pasar los alimentos a través del tracto digestivo, y para hacer pasar los líquidos por el sistema urinario.

peritoneal—relativo al peritoneo.

peritoneo—membrana serosa que forma la envoltura de la cavidad abdominal, y que rodea la mayor parte de los órganos abdominales.

permeable—capaz de ser penetrado; que permite la entrada.

peroné—un hueso largo en la pierna de la rodilla al tobillo.

perseverancia—cualidad de quien persiste sin flaquear.

personalidad—cualidades individuales que hacen a cada individuo diferente de los demás.

perspectiva—visión de cosas o hechos desde un punto determinado.

pertinente—perteneciente a una cosa. Relevante, relacionado con lo que está siendo considerado; que viene a propósito.

petechiae—manchas hemorrágicas pequeñas en la piel.

petición—súplica que se expresa por escrito a una autoridad con el fin de demandar acción legal.

pH—medida de acidez o alcalinidad.

piamadre—de las tres meninges del cerebro y la columna vertebral, es la que se encuentra más hacia el interior.

pielografía intravenosa (PIV)—la inserción de un material radiopaco en la vena con el propósito de tomarle radiografías a los riñones y uréteres.

pielonefritis—inflamación del riñón, pelvis y nefrones.

pigmento—todo material que genera color.

pilórico—relativo a la apertura entre el estómago y el duodeno.

pinocitosis—proceso a través del cual una célula absorbe grandes cantidades de líquido.

pirógeno—capaz de producir fiebre.

pituitaria—glándula endocrina adjunta a la base del cerebro; la glándula "maestra".

PIV—ver pielografía intravenosa.

placenta—estructura a través de la cual el feto se alimenta durante el embarazo.

plaga—epidemia o pestilencia que puede llegar a ser fatal.

plano coronal—una línea trazada de la cabeza a los pies, creando una sección delantera y trasera.

plano—superficie lisa; también, punto de referencia.

plasma—componente líquido de la linfa y la sangre.

plateleta—células de la sangre que evitan y detienen el sangrado.

pleura—membrana serosa que cubre los pulmones y reviste la cavidad torácica.

pleuresía—inflamación de la pleura.

plexo—red de filamentos nerviosos o vasculares.

poder—documento legal por el cual se autoriza a una persona a actuar en representación de otra.

podiatra—médico entrenado para diagnosticar y tratar enfermedades y trastornos de los pies.

podiatría—rama de la medicina que estudia las enfermedades y trastornos de los pies.

POL—laboratorio en consultorio médico (por sus siglas en inglés). Algunos consultorios han designado un espacio para establecer su propio laboratorio en el cual personas calificadas efectúan análisis y otros procedimientos de laboratorio comunes.

policitemia—trastorno en el cual hay un exceso de glóbulos rojos en la sangre.

polio (poliomielitis)—enfermedad sistémica aguda e infecciosa que causa inflamación de la materia gris de la espina dorsal.

pólipo—tumores o crecimientos exagerados de tejido que pueden estar adheridos por un pedículo. Generalmente, se encuentran en membranas mucosas como el útero, los intestinos, el recto y la nariz.

poliuria—secreción excesiva de orina.

"polling"—término inglés que significa obtener una transmisión de fax no autorizada.

pons—porción de la corteza cerebral que conecta la médula oblongada y el cerebelo con las porciones superiores del cerebro.

popliteo—perteneciente al área posterior de la rodilla.

porcentaje—tasa o proporción por cada cien.

posdata—lo que se añade a una carta después de la firma.

posparto—período siguiente al parto.

posterior—la parte de atrás.

postoperatorio—etapa siguiente a una operación quirúrgica.

postura—posición y manejo del cuerpo en su totalidad.

potencial—que tiene la posibilidad de suceder o existir.

PPMP (por sus siglas en inglés)—análisis microscópicos realizados en el laboratorio del consultorio médico.

práctica—ejercicios disciplinados y repetitivos como medio para perfeccionar una destreza o un procedimiento.

preautorización—decisión por parte de la compañía de seguros de establecer la necesidad de un procedimiento médico antes de efectuarse, y de cubrir los gastos por dicho procedimiento.

precanceroso—grado previo al desarrollo del cáncer.

precaución—cuidado previo; medida preventiva.

precisión—exactitud, certeza.

precisión—corrección, exactitud.

preciso—exacto, definido, certero, correcto.

precordial—perteneciente al área del pecho sobre el corazón donde se ubican los electrodos para realizar el electrocardiograma.

preliminar—antes de; que precede.

prenatal—período antes del nacimiento.

preoperatorio—período preparatorio que precede a la cirugía.

prepucio—la piel suelta que cubre el final del pene.

presbicusis—pérdida de la audición relacionada con la edad.

presbiopía—defecto de la visión que consiste en la dificultad para enfocar objetos que están cerca.

prescribir—señalar, determinar, dar dirección. Ordenar o aconsejar el uso de.

prescripción—orden escrita para la preparación y administración de una medicina.

presentar—pronunciar una declaración u ofrecer un servicio.

presión de pulso—diferencia entre la medida sistólica y la medida diastólica.

presión sanguínea—la cantidad de fuerza que ejerce el corazón en la sangre cuando bombea la sangre por las arterias.

prevención—acción de evitar que algo suceda; disposición que se toma para evitar algún peligro.

preventivo—que impide que algo suceda. Acción tomada para evitar una enfermedad.

prima—cantidad pagada o pagable (por ejemplo, la prima de una póliza de seguros).

primario—primero en orden o grado.

prioridad—preferencia; el primero.

priorizar—dar preferencia; ordenar en orden de importancia.

pro tem—posición temporal; por el momento.

procesador—ejecutar una secuencia de acciones u operaciones.

procesar—tratar o preparar información por medio de un método.

proclividad—inclinación o predisposición hacia algo.

procrastinación—diferir o aplazar una acción.

proctología—estudio del recto y el ano y de sus enfermedades.

proctoscopia—inspección instrumental del recto.

proctoscopio—instrumento para la inspección del recto.

procurar—hacer esfuerzos por conseguir una cosa. Ocasionar, originar.

productividad—cantidad de trabajo efectuado en un período de tiempo.

profesional—persona que se ciñe a las técnicas y normas de su trabajo.

profesionalismo—óptima realización de un trabajo.

progesterona—hormona secretada por el folículo graafiano después de la expulsión del óvulo.

programado—planeado, planificado. Secuencia de acciones ejecutadas por un computador.

programar—establecer un calendario; ingresar en la lista de actividades por realizar.

prolapsis—caída de una parte interna del cuerpo; usualmente se refiere al recto o al útero.

prominente—eminente, destacado, preponderante.

prono—acostado contra el vientre.

pronombre—palabra que hace las veces del nombre y toma el género y número de éste.

propiedad—dominio que se tiene sobre lo que se posee.

propietario—persona que posee un inmueble o finca raíz y que lo administra en forma privada con ánimo de lucro.

prostaglandinas—grupo de sustancias químicas secretadas por mastocitos o basófilos. Estas sustancias químicas encogen los músculos lisos en algunos órganos.

próstata—glándula del sistema reproductivo masculino que rodea la porción proximal de la uretra.

prostatectomía—intervención quirúrgica para extraer la totalidad o parte de la glándula prostática (próstata).

prótesis—extensión artificial que reemplaza una parte del cuerpo que falta.

protocolo—plan de tratamiento, a menudo experimental, utilizado para determinar la efectividad de nuevos tratamientos o medicinas.

protozoario—animal unicelular.

protrombina—sustancia química existente en la sangre que ayuda a la coagulación.

provechoso—beneficioso, lucrativo.

provisiones—conjunto de cosas necesarias; estipulación.

provocar—mover a alguien a hacer algo; inspirar.

proximal—punto más cercano al centro (tronco del cuerpo) o al punto de unión al cuerpo.

proyectar—disponer, preparar con intención y claridad.

prudente—cauteloso. Que actúa con juicio.

prueba de galera—material impreso en forma preeliminar, para ser corregido.

prueba precisa y cierta (PPC)—se refiere a un estándar para realizar procedimientos de laboratorio para asegurar la veracidad de los resultados.

pruebas sanguíneas cruzadas—prueba de sangre usada para asegurar la compatibilidad del donante con el receptor cuando hay transfusión de sangre.

prurito—picazón severo.

pruritus ani—picazón alrededor del ano.

psicodélicos—drogas alucinógenas.

psicología—estudio de los procesos mentales, tanto normales como anormales, y sus efectos sobre el comportamiento.

psicológico—relativo a la mente.

psicólogo—persona especializada en el estudio de la estructura y función del cerebro y sus procesos mentales.

psiconeuroinmunología—ciencia que estudia la conexión entre el cerebro, el comportamiento y la inmunología.

psicopático—relativo a un trastorno mental.

psicosis—disturbio mental de tal magnitud que se presenta una desintegración de la identidad y una pérdida del contacto con la realidad.

psicosomático—relativo a la interrelación entre las emociones y el cuerpo.

psicoterapia—tratamiento de enfermedades mentales a través de hipnosis, psicoanálisis y otras técnicas.

psiquiatra—médico especializado en las enfermedades y los trastornos de la mente, incluyendo neurosis y psicosis.

psiquiatría—rama de la medicina que se encarga del diagnóstico, tratamiento y prevención de las enfermedades mentales.

psoriasis—enfermedad inflamatoria crónica caracterizada por parches escamosos en la piel.

ptosis—caída de un órgano o parte, por ejemplo el párpado superior o el riñón.

pubertad—época de la vida en que se manifiesta la aptitud para la reproducción.

púbico—perteneciente a la sección media del tercio bajo del abdomen, también llamado hipogastro.

pulmón—órgano de la respiración localizado al interior de la cavidad torácica.

pulmonar—relativo a los pulmones.

pulso—palpitación causada por el proceso intermitente de contracción y expansión de una arteria.

punción—perforación realizada por un instrumento puntudo.

puntuación—conjunto de signos ortográficos que se emplean para puntuar y aclarar el significado de una frase.

puntual—pronto, diligente, exacto; a tiempo.

puntura lumbar—inserción de una aguja entre las vértebras en el área lumbar con el objeto de extraer fluido de la espina.

pupila—apertura del iris para la transmisión de luz.

purgar—evacuar, purificar.

Purkinje—red de fibras en el músculo cardiaco que transportan los impulsos eléctricos resultantes en la contracción de los ventrículos.

pústula—elevación pequeña de la piel llena de linfa o pus.

QA—certificación de calidad (por sus siglas en inglés). Conjunto de reglas, procedimientos y prácticas que se utilizan como estándares para obtener resultados de laboratorio confiables. La certificación de calidad se aplica a los diferentes procesos que incluyen la calibración y el mantenimiento del equipo, el control de calidad, los exámenes de competencia y entrenamiento para los técnicos del laboratorio.

QC—control de calidad (por sus siglas en inglés). El control de calidad determina estándares confiables para garantizar el óptimo desempeño del equipo de laboratorio.

QNS—cantidad no suficiente (por sus siglas en inglés).

quadriceps femoris—músculo grande en la superficie anterior del muslo que está compuesto de cuatro músculos.

queloide—engrosamiento de nuevo tejido de piel; una cicatriz.

químico—una sustancia simple o compuesta usada en procesos químicos.

quimo—la mezcla de comida parcialmente digerida y las secreciones digestivas que se encuentran en el estómago y el intestino delgado durante la digestión de una comida.

quimoterapia—el uso de agentes químicos en el tratamiento de la enfermedad, asociado usualmente con terapia de cáncer.

quiropráctica—un sistema de sanación basado en la teoría de que la enfermedad resulta de la falta de función normal de los nervios; el tratamiento por la manipulación científica ajuste específico de las estructuras del cuerpo, como la columna vertebral.

quiropráctico—proveedor de salud que usa los métodos quiroprácticos para tratar pacientes.

quiste—una vejiga; cualquier saco que contiene fluido.

quístico—perteneciente a un quiste; en enfermedad, se refiere a una condición con múltiples quistes.

R/O—descartar (por sus siglas en inglés).

racional—basado en la razón.

racionalización—explicar con la razón; concebir explicaciones plausibles por actos determinados.

radiación electromagnética—rayos producidos por la colisión de haz de electrones con un objetivo de metal en un tubo de rayos X.

radiación—emisión y difusión de rayos; producto de los rayos X y del radio.

radial—relativo a la arteria radial o al pulso que se ha tomado en la arteria radial.

radio—hueso largo del antebrazo.

radioactivo—capaz de emitir energía radiante.

radiografía—fotografía por rayos X o por efecto del radio que visualiza los tejidos y órganos del cuerpo.

radiología—estudio de la radiación y de sus usos y beneficios en el diagnóstico y tratamiento de enfermedades.

radiólogo—médico que diagnostica y trata enfermedades a partir del uso de energía radiante.

radionúclidos—tipo de átomo utilizado en medicina nuclear para el diagnóstico y tratamiento de enfermedades.

radio-opaco—impenetrable por los rayos X y otras formas de radiación.

rales—sonido inusual escuchado en los bronquios durante el examen de la respiración.

ramificación—subdivisión o consecuencia.

raquitismo—enfermedad de los huesos debida primordialmente a una deficiencia de vitamina D.

rasgo—característica.

RDS—examen de certificación (por sus siglas en inglés). RDS (Role Delineation Study) es un estudio de análisis ocupacional realizado en 1997 por la AAMA (Asociación Americana de Asistentes Médicos) y por NBME (Junta Nacional de Exámenes para Médicos) con el fin de identificar los conocimientos y aptitudes básicas necesarias para los profesionales de la salud entrenados en asistencia médica.

reactividad—tasa de desintegración nuclear de un reactor.

reagente—sustancia involucrada en una reacción química.

realzar—intensificar, mejorar.

reason rule—se refiere al propósito o razón para ejecutar un examen o procedimiento; criterio utilizado por una compañía de seguros para determinar la cobertura.

recepción—acción o efecto de recibir; reunión social.

recepcionista—persona encargada de recibir a los visitantes, pacientes o clientes, y de contestar llamadas.

receptor—terminación nerviosa periférica de un nervio sensorial que responde a estímulos.

recesivo—que tiende a la recesión; característica aparentemente suprimida durante la concepción para dar prioridad a una característica dominante; organismo que posee una o más características recesivas.

recibo—constancia escrita de que algo ha sido recibido.

recipiente—aquel que recibe.

reciprocidad—intercambio mutuo, especialmente el intercambio de privilegios especiales.

reconciliar—proceso a través del cual se comparan las cuentas llevadas en el talonario de cheques con el extracto de cuenta.

recreo—tiempo libre, alejado de las tensiones y responsabilidades del trabajo.

rectal—relativo al recto.

recto—parte inferior del intestino grueso entre el sigmoide y el canal anal.

rectocel—protrusión de la pared vaginal y de la pared anterior del recto a través de la vagina.

recurrente—que vuelve a suceder.

recurso—fuente de apoyo o de provisiones y suministros.

reducir—restaurar las terminaciones de un hueso fracturado a su relación normal.

redundante—repetitivo; reiterativo; superfluo.

reembolsar—pagar o recompensar por dinero que ya se ha gastado, o por pérdidas o daños en los que se ha incurrido.

referencia—fuente de información o autoridad.

reflejo—responsa involuntaria a un estímulo.

refracción—modificación en la dirección y velocidad de una onda al cambiar el medio en que se propaga. Se produce refracción de la luz cuando ésta pasa del medio aéreo al líquido.

refractivo—que produce refracción.

régimen—regulación de dieta, hábitos de sueño, ejercicio y estilo de vida para mantener una buena salud y/o mejorarla.

registrado—legalmente certificado o autenticado.

registro—documentación formal u oficial de ítems, nombres o acciones; relación de dinero que se ha gastado; listado de personas calificadas en un área particular.

regla de Nagel—método para predecir la fecha de nacimiento.

regulaciones en el POL—estándares establecidos para certificación de calidad (QA por sus siglas en inglés) y control de calidad (QC por sus siglas en inglés) en el laboratorio de un consultorio médico (POL por sus siglas en inglés) con el fin de garantizar resultados confiables.

regular—establecer control o dirección.

regulatorio—control basado en reglas establecidas; acción de adaptarse a ciertas reglas con el fin de alcanzar la mayor eficiencia y resultados precisos y confiables.

rehabilitar—devolver a su condición de funcionamiento normal; restaurar.

reincidencia—recurrencia de una enfermedad o de unos síntomas; vuelta a una condición previa.

reino—dominio, esfera.

reiterar—decir o hacer más de una vez.

rejuvenecer—renovar, otorgar cualidades juveniles.

reluctante—reacio, contrario a algo.

remedio—cualquier cosa que alivie o cure una enfermedad.

remisión—período durante el cual el paciente está libre de síntomas o de la enfermedad que lo aquejó.

remoto—a distancia; que sucedió hace mucho tiempo o en un lugar lejano.

renal—relativo al riñón.

renovar—restaurar, dar la apariencia de nuevo.

Rentas Internas—Internal Revenue en inglés; la división del gobierno federal encargada de implementar las leyes de impuestos y de la recolección de impuestos.

repolarización—reestablecimiento de un estado polarizado en una fibra nerviosa o muscular después de la contracción o conducción de un impulso nervioso.

represión—acción de contener o forzar ideas o impulsos dolorosos en el inconsciente.

reproductivo—relativo a la reproducción.

res ipsa loquitur—expresión latina que significa que la cosa habla por sí misma.

resaca—malestar que sigue a la ingestión de una cantidad considerable de alcohol.

residencia—período durante el cual el médico recibe entrenamiento y especialización en la rama de la medicina de su escogencia.

residual—relativo a lo que queda como residuo o remanente.

resistencia—oposición.

resonancia—cualidad del sonido escuchada en la percusión del pecho; intensificación y prolongación del sonido por reflexión o por la vibración de un objeto cercano.

respetuoso—considerado, honorable.

respiración—acción de tomar oxígeno para el funcionamiento del cuerpo y de soltar dióxido de carbono.

respiratorio—relativo a la respiración.

respiro—tregua, aplazamiento de algo que es doloroso o agotador.

respondeat superior—expresión latina que significa "dejar que el maestro responda".

responsabilidad—deber, obligación.

responsabilidad legal—cualquier cosa por la que una persona es responsable o por la que está legalmente atada u obligada.

restringido—limitado; exclusivo para cierto grupo.

retención—incapacidad de evacuar la orina que está en la vejiga.

retículo endoplásmico—un organelo dentro del citoplasma de una célula.

reticuloendotelial—relativo al grupo de células que parecen ayudar en la producción de glóbulos rojos y en la desintegración de los que ya han cumplido su función.

retina—capa más profunda del ojo que reciba la imagen formada por el lente.

retinopatía—degeneración de la retina causada por una reducción del suministro de sangre.

retiro—remoción de algo que ha sido depositado.

retracción—reducción o disminución en el volumen de los tejidos; acción de echarse para atrás.

retraso—acción de ir despacio, de llegar tarde o de posponer. Desarrollo físico o mental lento.

retroflexionado—relativo al útero cuando éste se voltea hacia atrás.

retrógrado—relativo a un procedimiento con rayos X para el cual un material radio-opaco se instila a través de un catéter en la vejiga, uréteres y riñones.

retroperitoneal—detrás del peritoneo; posterior a la cubierta peritoneal de la cavidad abdominal.

retrovertido—relativo al útero cuando el órgano se voltea hacia atrás en su totalidad.

retrovirus—partículas infecciosas que contienen sólo el material genético RNA.

revalidación—renovación o confirmación de credenciales.

revocar—cancelar, retirar, retractar.

ribosoma—organelo al interior del citoplasma de la célula.

riesgo—peligro. Probabilidad de pérdida, daño o lesión.

rinitis—inflamación de la mucosa nasal.

rinitis alérgica—inflamación de la nariz causada por una alergia.

riñon—un órgano en forma de frijol que excreta orina y está localizado retroperitonealmente, alto en la parte de atrás de la cavidad abdominal.

rinoplastia—cirugía plástica de la nariz.

ritmo—espacio de tiempo o movimiento medido; que ocurre en forma regular.

roentgen—relativo a los rayos X. Unidad de cantidad de radiación.

ROM—rango de movimiento (por sus siglas en inglés). Se refiere al grado de movimiento de articulaciones y extremidades.

rotar—mover(se) alrededor de un eje.

rubéola—enfermedad viral contagiosa leve pero que puede causar graves daños en el feto de la mujer embarazada que desarrolla la enfermedad.

rubor— repentina coloración rojiza de la piel.

ruptura—violación de la ley, de un contrato o de otro acuerdo.

sacrilegio—profanación de una cosa sagrada. Atentado contra una persona digna de veneración.

sacro—cinco vértebras fusionadas que se encuentran entre el cóccix y la vértebra lumbar de la columna vertebral.

sagital—relativo al plano resultante de la división del cuerpo por la mitad creando un lado derecho y un lado izquierdo.

saliva—secreción digestiva de las glándulas salivares.

salpingectomía—remoción quirúrgica de una o de las dos trompas de Falopio.

salpingo-ooforectomía—extirpación quirúrgica de uno o ambos ovarios y de una o las dos trompas de Falopio.

salud—estado de completo bienestar físico y mental o social.

sancionar—convertir en ley.

sarampión—enfermedad aguda altamente contagiosa caracterizada por la presencia de erupciones maculopustulares.

sarcoma—tumor maligno de los tejidos conectivos, músculos o huesos.

sartorio—músculo largo y delgado del muslo; el músculo más largo del cuerpo.

sebo—secreción grasa de la piel.

secreción—separación de ciertos materiales por actividad glandular.

secretaria—persona encargada de la correspondencia.

sector—sección y división.

secuencia—orden o sucesión.

secuencialmente—organizado en secuencia, en orden.

secundario—que viene en segundo lugar.

sedar—producir un estado de calma; utilizar un fármaco u otro agente para producir un efecto tranquilizante.

sedentario—que permanece sentado demasiado tiempo; inactividad.

sedimentación—formación o depósito de sedimento. En la sangre, se refiere a la velocidad en la que los eritrocitos se asientan cuando se agrega un anticoagulante a la sangre.

segmento—parte o sección de un órgano o del cuerpo.

seguridad—ausencia de miedo o ansiedad; ausencia de peligro o pérdida.

seguro—a salvo, libre de daño; un contrato que garantiza una compensación por una situación específica.

semen—mezcla de secreciones de varias glándulas y órganos del sistema reproductivo masculino, que se expele durante el orgasmo.

semilunar—válvulas del corazón localizadas entre los ventrículos y la arteria pulmonar y la aorta.

senilidad—debilidad del cuerpo y de la mente debida a la vejez.

sensibilidad—susceptibilidad anormal a una sustancia.

sensorial—relativo a los nervios que reciben y transmiten estímulos desde los órganos de los sentidos.

septo—pared membranosa que divide dos cavidades, como en el corazón o la nariz.

serie—grupo de cosas de la misma clase ordenadas una después de otra.

serrado—que tiene dientes como un serrucho.

SIDS—por sus siglas en inglés, fallecimiento repentino e inexplicable de un infante menor de un año.

sífilis—enfermedad venérea comunicable que se propaga por contacto sexual.

sigmoide—sección del intestino largo en forma de S localizada entre el colon descendiente y el recto.

sigmoidoscopia—inspección del sigmoide con un instrumento.

signos cardíacos—principales signos: temperatura, pulso, respiración y presión arterial.

simetría—estado en el cual una parte corresponde exactamente a la otra en tamaño, forma y posición.

simpático—porción del sistema nervioso autónomo.

simple—relativo a una fractura ósea sin implicación de la superficie de la piel.

simultáneo—que ocurre al mismo tiempo.

sinapsis—el espacio diminuto entre el axón de una neurona y la dendrita de otra.

síncope—colapso. Condición en la cual el pulso se vuelve rápido pero débil, la presión sanguínea disminuye, y el paciente se ve pálido y sudoroso.

síncope—desvanecimiento, desmayo; forma transciende de inconsciencia.

síndrome—combinación de síntomas con una enfermedad o trastorno.

síndrome de alcoholismo fetal—grupo de defectos en infantes nacidos de madres que consumieron alcohol durante el embarazo.

síndrome de Cushing—un desorden que resulta de la hipersecreción de los glucocorticoides de la corteza adrenal.

síndrome del tunel carpal (STC)—los síntomas asociados con el atrapamiento del nervio intermedio en los huesos carpales y en el ligamento transverso de la muñeca.

síndrome nefrótico—término aplicado a la enfermedad renal de cualquier causa caracterizada por edema masivo, proteinuria, y a menudo elevación de los niveles de colesterol y de lípidos.

sinergismo—una cosa que estimula la acción de otra que hace que el efecto de las dos es más grande que la suma de los efectos individuales.

sinovial—articulación móvil, también llamada diartrosis.

síntoma—cualquier cambio perceptible del cuerpo o de sus funciones que indica una enfermedad o la fase de una enfermedad.

sinusitis—inflamación de los senos nasales.

sistema—grupo de órganos que trabajan juntos con el fin de ejecutar una función del cuerpo.

sistema linfático—red de vasos transparentes que transportan el fluido linfático a través del cuerpo.

sistemático—que sigue un sistema o plan.

sístole—la fase de contracción del corazón; la cantidad de presión sanguínea máxima.

SN—nodo sinoatrial (por sus siglas en inglés). Fuente del impulso nervioso que origina el latido del corazón; marcapasos.

sobregiro—cantidad que excede de los créditos o fondos disponibles en una cuenta.

Sociedad Americana para la Ciencia del Laboratorio Clínico—American Society for Clinical Laboratory Science (ASCLS por sus siglas en inglés).

sofisticado—opuesto a lo simple o natural; muy refinado; altamente complejo o avanzado en forma, estilo, técnica, etc.

solaz—descanso, placer. Consuelo de una pena.

solicitar—pedir.

sólo—solamente.

solución normal salina—solución con el mismo contenido salino al que se encuentra en el interior de una célula sanguínea.

somático—físico. Relativo al cuerpo, a diferencia de la mente.

sonar—aparato que transmite ondas sonoras de alta frecuencia en agua y registra las vibraciones reflejadas desde un objeto.

sonido—lo que se puede oír.

soplo—sonido adventicio de origen venoso o arterial que se escucha en la auscultación; usualmente se refiere al sonido producido por la mezcla de la sangre arterial y venosa at dyalisis shunts.

soportar—sostener; aguantar parte del peso.

sordera sensorineural—pérdida de audición causada por una falla en la transmisión de los nervios al interior del oído interno del nervio auditivo.

STC—ver síndrome de tunel carpal.

suave—tipo de tejido muscular involuntario que se encuentra en órganos internos.

subaracnoide—espacio entre la piamadre y el aracnoide que contiene fluido cerebroespinal.

subcutáneo—debajo de la piel.

subdural—debajo de la dura-madre; espacio entre el aracnoide y la dura-madre.

subjetivo—relativo a la persona que está pensando, diciendo o haciendo algo; personal; relativo al síntoma de una enfermedad, sentido por el paciente pero no percibido por otros.

sublimación—expresión de ciertos impulsos, especialmente sexuales, en formas constructivas y socialmente aceptables.

sublingual—bajo la lengua.

subpoena duces tecum—expresión latina que se refiere a un proceso en la corte iniciado por una parte en litigio, producción contundente de documentos específicos y otros ítems, y material relevante a los hechos en cuestión en procedimientos judiciales adjuntos.

subsecuente—siguiente, que viene después.

substancial—considerable, importante, grande.

succión—aspiración por presión; acción de chupar o sorber.

superficial—en la superficie.

superior—sobre o más alto.

supernatante—que flota en la superficie.

supervisor—persona a cargo; que se asegura de que se cumplan las reglas y los procedimientos para lograr los resultados esperados.

supino—acostado boca arriba.

suplemento—algo agregado; sección adicional o extra.

supositorio—material medicado en forma de cono o de cilindro para insertar en el recto o vagina.

suprapúbico—sobre el arco púbico.

supresión—cesación del funcionamiento del riñón, ausencia de secreción de orina; en psicología, se refiere a la exclusión deliberada de una idea, deseo o sentimiento de la consciencia.

supresor—persona que calla o impide una acción.

surfactante—molécula grasa en las membranas respiratorias.

susceptible—que tiene poca resistencia a una enfermedad o a una proteína foránea.

sustituto—persona que reemplaza a otra persona.

sutura—costura de los bordes de una llaga o herida.

symphisis pubis—conexión de los huesos púbicos en la media línea al frente.

tabla de Snellen—tabla de letras del alfabeto utilizada para evaluar la visión a distancia.

tacto—sentimiento delicado de las conveniencias; destreza en la manera de decir las cosas sin ofender.

tálamo—porción del cerebro que descansa entre el cerebro y el mesencéfalo o cerebro medio.

tallo verde—una fractura incompleta que le ocurre a los niños.

taquicardia—rapidez anormal de la acción cardiaca.

tarsos—los siete huesos del empeine.

TCO—ver técnico certificado de oftalmología.

teclear—presionar una palanca o tecla, como en una máquina de escribir, operar la máquina con el dedo.

técnica aséptica—forma de realizar tareas sin contaminación de organismos.

técnico certificado de oftalmología—una persona entrenada y certificada en procedimientos de exámenes de diagnóstico y en el examen limitado del ojo.

técnico de emergencia médica (TEM)—un individuo entrenado para responder en situaciones de emergencia y proveer tratamiento médico inicial adecuado.

técnico de laboratorio—profesional especializado en el área de la salud que lleva a cabo análisis químicos, microscópicos y bacteriológicos en sangre, tejidos y fluidos corporales.

técnico en radiología—persona entrenada en las técnicas para preparar el filme y tomar la radiografía.

técnico farmaceuta (PT por sus siglas en inglés)—trabajador de la salud entrenado para asistir al farmaceuta en la preparación y la dispensación de medicinas.

técnico para el cuidado de pacientes (PCT por sus siglas en inglés)—trabajador de la salud entrenado tanto en enfermería como en asistencia médica para proporcionar ayuda a pacientes durante su permanencia en el hospital.

técnico—relativo a un arte, ciencia u oficio particular; que requiere un talento especial.

tecnología—la práctica de una ciencia o de todas las ciencias aplicadas que tienen un valor práctico o un uso industrial.

tecnólogo—persona entrenada en una tecnología particular; capaz de aplicar los métodos de la técnica necesaria en un área o arte particular.

tejido—colección de células similares y fibras que forman la estructura del cuerpo.

teleconferencia—reunión sostenida a través de líneas telefónicas con la incorporación de equipos de video.

temblor—movimiento involuntario.

temperatura—grado de calor de un cuerpo viviente; grado de calor o frío de una sustancia; usualmente se refiere a la elevación del calor corporal.

temporal—relativo al hueso temporal del cráneo.

tendinitis—inflamación de un tendón.

tendón de Aquiles—un tendón que une el músculo gastrocnemio de la pierna al talón.

tendón de la corva—un grupo de músculos del muslo posterior.

tendón—tejido conectivo fibroso cuya función es unir los músculos a los huesos.

tentativo—experimental; provisional, temporal.

teoría—creencia no comprobada en la práctica; principio general en el que se basa una ciencia.

terapeuta de la respiración—persona entrenada para efectuar procedimientos con el fin de mantener o mejorar la función ventilatoria del tracto respiratorio.

terapeuta ocupacional—trabajador de la salud encargado de diseñar y llevar a cabo actividades con pacientes que están limitados por enfermedad o lesión física, disfunción psicológica, retraso mental o problemas de aprendizaje, pobreza o diferencias culturales, o vejez, con el objeto de maximizar la independencia de estos pacientes, prevenir su invalidez y mejorar su salud.

terapeuta—persona que practica los tratamientos curativos y preventivos de una aenfermedad o de una condición anormal.

terapéutico—que tiene propiedades medicinales o curativas; relativo a los resultados obtenidos después de un tratamiento.

terapia de manipulación—tratamiento o procedimiento que implica el uso de las manos; movimiento de una coyuntura para determinar su rango de extensión y de flexión; técnicas manuales utilizadas por osteópatas.

tercera parte—en la industria de los seguros médicos, persona que no es el paciente, esposo o pariente responsable de pagar una porción o la totalidad de los costos médicos incurridos por el paciente.

térmico—relativo al calor; activado por el calor.

terminación—finalización.

terminal—final; enfermedad terminal, se refiere a una condición que no se puede revertir.

terminología procedimental actual (TPA)—listado numérico de procedimientos efectuados en una práctica médica; identificación estandarizada de procedimientos. Publicado por la Asociación Médica Americana.

termografía—técnica para detectar y registrar en filme áreas frías y áreas calientes del cuerpo por medio de un detector infrarrojo que reacciona al flujo sanguíneo.

termómetro—instrumento utilizado para medir la temperatura.

testículos—gónadas masculinas del escroto que producen la esperma.

testosterona—hormona masculina secretada por los testículos que causa y mantiene las características masculinas secundarias.

tetania—espasmos tónicos intermitentes causados por una inadecuada cantidad de hormona paratiroides.

tétano—enfermedad infecciosa aguda causada por las toxinas del bacilo tetani.

thesaurus—diccionario de sinónimos y antónimos.

thin prep—método para preparar especimenes para citología.

TIA—ataque isquémico transiente, por sus siglas en inglés. Interrupción temporal del flujo sanguíneo en el cerebro causado por pequeñas coagulaciones que obstruyen los vasos sanguíneos.

tibia—hueso largo de la pierna que se encuentra entre la rodilla y el tobillo.

tibialis anterior—músculo de la pierna.

tiempo flexible—se refiere a la práctica de permitir horas de trabajo dentro de un rango de tiempo.

timo—órgano localizado en la cavidad mediastinal anterior y sobre el corazón.

tinnitus—zumbido o tintineo en el oído que sólo lo oye la persona afectada.

tirante—tenso, ajustado.

tiroidectomía—extracción quirúrgica de la tiroides.

tiroides—glándula endocrina localizada en la base anterior del cuello.

tolerancia—diferencia entre lo máximo y lo mínimo; cantidad de variación permitida por un estándar.

tomografía axial computarizada (TAC)—una serie de imágenes de rayos X del cuerpo usadas para construir una imagen tridimensional.

tono muscular—estado de contracción muscular en el cual una porción de lasa fibras se contraen mientras las otras están en estado de relajación.

tono—frecuencia de vibraciones de sonido que permite clasificar el sonido en una escala de alto a bajo.

tonómetro—instrumento para medir la tensión o presión intraocular.

tópico—relativo a un área específica; local.

torácico—relativo al tórax o al pecho.

tórax—pecho; cavidad encerrada por las costillas y que contiene el corazón y los pulmones

torcedura—lesión de un músculo debido a la tensión causada por el uso incorrecto o el abuso.

torniquete—cualquier método utilizado para apretar una extremidad para producir presión en una arteria y controlar el sangrado; también se utiliza para dilatar una vena para la extracción de sangre o para la inserción de una aguja con el fin de instilar inyecciones intravenosas.

tortícolis—rigidez del cuello causada por la contracción de los músculos del cuello. Dichos músculos tiran la cabeza hacia un lado mientras tiran la barbilla hacia el otro lado. Este trastorno puede ser congénito o adquirido.

tosferina—enfermedad infecciosa aguda que afecta la parte superior de las vías respiratorias. Se caracteriza por vigorosos y repetidos ataques de tos. Típicamente, la persona tose de 5 a 10 veces sin poder tomar aliento. Cuando la tos finaliza, el aire es inhalado con tanta fuerza que suena al entrar en la tráquea.

toxina—sustancia venenosa o compuesto de vegetal, animal o bacterial.

toxoide—toxina tratada con el fin de destruir su toxicidad, pero sigue siendo capaz de inducir la formación de anticuerpos mediante su inyección.

TPA—ver terminología procedimental actual.

TQM—gestión de calidad total, por sus siglas en inglés. Se refiere a un estilo de gestión que utiliza QA (certificación de calidad) y QC (control de calidad) para mantener la más alta calidad de ejecución a través de la totalidad del proceso, y no sólo para asegurar que los resultados sean correctos o satisfactorios.

tracción—acción de tirar; en el caso de fracturas, se aplica tracción en línea recta para estirar los músculos contraídos y permitir el reajuste de los fragmentos óseos.

trampa—peligro escondido para engañar a alguien.

tranquilizante—droga que causa el retraso de la función corporal o de la actividad nerviosa.

transacción—acuerdo entre persona s o empresas.

transcribir—escribir en un libro o documento lo que está escrito en otro libro o documento.

transcripción—copia realizada directamente de un registro original, especialmente de una copia oficial de los registros educativos de un estudiante.

transdermal—que atraviesa la piel.

transductor—dispositivo que recibe la potencia de un sistema mecánico, electromagnético o acústico y la transmite a otro, generalmente en forma distinta.

transfusión—inyección de la sangre de una persona en las venas de otra persona.

transición—acción de pasar de una condición, lugar o actividad a otra.

transiluminación—colocación de una luz a través de una cavidad u órgano del cuerpo para inspeccionarlo.

transmitido—enviado de una persona, lugar o cosa a otra.

transmitir—impartir, como una idea; transferir.

transponer—poner una cosa en lugar de otra; trastocar letras o palabras.

transportador—el que carga, transporta: en seguros, es la compañía que provee la póliza.

transuretral—a través de la uretra; se refiere a la extirpación de la próstata a través de la pared uretral.

transverso—acostado a través; segmento del intestino grueso que reposa de un lado al otro del abdomen; línea horizontal dibujada de un lado al otro del cuerpo o de cualquier estructura.

trapecio—músculo grande de la espalda y cuello.

tráquea—tubo cartilaginoso entre la laringe y el bronquio principal del árbol respiratorio.

traqueotomía—apertura en la tráquea realizada quirúrgicamente para lograr que el paciente pueda respirar.

trastorno—condición patológica de la mente o del cuerpo.

traumático—causado por o relacionado con una lesión.

traumatizar—causar trauma o lesión.

trazo—en electrocardiografía, dibujo básico producido por el estilógrafo en una hoja de papel.

"treadmill", trotadora o cinta rodante—aparato con una plataforma móvil que permite caminar o correr en un mismo sitio.

trendelenburg—posición con la cabeza ubicada más abajo que los pies.

trepanar—cortar una sección circular.

trial balance—balance de comprobación, balance de sumas y saldos. Listado de los saldos de toda cuenta del libro mayor que se prepara al cierre del período contable. Incluye la sumatoria de todos los débitos y créditos en forma separada, debiendo ser iguales ambas columnas. Garantiza que el pase del libro diario al libro mayor ha sido realizado correctamente. Sirve de base para la preparación del balance general.

triangular—figura que tiene tres ángulos y tres lados.

tríceps—músculos posteriores del brazo que trabajan en conjunto con el bíceps; los tríceps enderezan el codo.

tricomoniasis—infestación de parásitos protozoarios; usualmente sucede en la vagina.

tricúspide—válvula al lado derecho del corazón, entre las cámaras. Literalmente significa tres cúspides.

trimestral—dividido en tres secciones; el tercer segmento o período.

trivial—insignificante, de poco valor.

trocar—dar una cosa a cambio de otra.

tromboflebitis—inflamación de una vena asociada con la formación de un coágulo sanguíneo.

trombosis—formación de un trombo o coágulo sanguíneo.

truncar—mutilar, disminuir.

tuberculosis—enfermedad infecciosa causada por el bacilo tubercle; la tuberculosis pulmonar es una enfermedad inflamatoria específica de los pulmones que destruye los tejidos pulmonares.

tubo de eustaquio—se refiere al tubo del oído medio que conecta con la faringe.

tubo de falopio—el ovaducto; el pasaje del ovario al útero.

tumor—inflamación o agrandamiento; neoplasma; a menudo se utiliza este término para indicar un crecimiento maligno.

turbidez—partículas escamosas o granulares suspendidas en un líquido transparente que le dan una apariencia turbia o nublada; este término se utiliza en referencia a la orina.

úlcera—lesión abierta en la piel o en las membranas mucosas del cuerpo, caracterizada por pérdida de tejido y la formación de una secreción.

úlcera stasis—lesión abierta causada por estagnación o por un inadecuado suministro de sangre a un área.

umbilical—relativo al ombligo.

umbral renal—concentración en la cual una sustancia en la sangre no excretada normalmente por el riñón empieza a aparecer en la orina.

ungüento—medicamento externo compuesto de resina y diversos cuerpos grasos; sustancia grasosa y suave con propiedades antisépticas o curativas.

único—que no tiene igual. Sólo hay uno en la especie.

universal—relativo al universo; general o común a todos.

UPM—ultimo período menstrual (LMP por sus siglas en inglés).

uremia—condición en la cual productos que normalmente sólo se encuentran en la orina se encuentran también en la sangre.

uréter—tubo que lleva la orina del riñón a la vejiga.

uretra—canal membranoso para la descarga externa de la orina desde la vejiga.

uretritis no específica—inflamación de la uretra en hombres, y vaginitis o cervicitis en mujeres, causada por bacteria o por una alergia a una sustancia utilizada por el compañero sexual.

urgencia—necesidad repentina de evacuar orina o feces.

URI—infección de las vías respiratorias superiores, por sus siglas en inglés. Proceso inflamatorio que involucra la nariz y la garganta, y puede incluir los senos nasales; se refiere a los síntomas asociados con la gripa común.

urianálisis—análisis de la orina para determinar sus características.

urología—rama de la medicina que estudia las enfermedades y trastornos de los órganos genitourinarios.

urticaria—condición inflamatoria caracterizada por la erupción de pápulas acompañadas de comezón severa.

útero—órgano muscular hueco en forma de pera que pertenece al sistema reproductivo femenino al interior del cual un óvulo fertilizado se desarrolla hasta convertirse en un bebé.

UTI—infección del tracto urinario, por sus siglas en inglés. Infección que ocurre al interior de los riñones, uréteres o vejiga.

utilizar—usar para algún beneficio.

vacilación—dificultad en comenzar un torrente de orina.

vacuna—sustancia que ayuda a prevenir una enfermedad.

vacunación—inoculación con virus inofensivos modificados o con otros microorganismos con el fin de producir inmunidad y prevenir enfermedades.

vagina—tubo musculomembranoso que forma el conducto que va desde el útero hasta el exterior del cuerpo de la mujer.

vaginitis—inflamación de la vagina.

vago—el décimo nervio craneal que tiene una función motora y una función sensorial y que afecta el corazón, el estómago y otros órganos.

vale—documento que sirve como prueba de que los términos de una transacción se han cumplido.

valorar—determinar, evaluar la condición o el estado.

válvula—una de las varias estructuras que cierran temporalmente una apertura o conducto, o que permiten el movimiento de fluido en una sola dirección.

várices—venas agrandadas y retorcidas.

varicoso—relativo a las várices; venas hinchadas y dilatadas, a menudo de las piernas.

vas deferens—tubo excretorio de los testículos.

vasectomía—corte de una porción del vas deferens.

vejiga—un saco membranoso o recipiente para una secreción; la vesícula biliar, la vejiga urinaria.

vena—vaso sanguíneo que conduce la sangre hacia el corazón después de recibirla de una vénula.

vena cava—una de las dos venas grandes que llevan la sangre al atrio derecho del corazón.

venipuntura—puntura de una vena; inserción de una aguja con el propósito de obtener una muestra de sangre o de instilar una sustancia.

venoso—relativo a la vena.

ventilatorio—que permite la circulación de aire fresco.

ventral—relativo a la parte anterior o frontal del cuerpo.

ventrículo—una de las dos cámaras inferiores del corazón; también se refiere a las cavidades al interior del cerebro.

vénula—vena diminuta; vaso sanguíneo que conecta un capilar con una vena.

veraz—genuino, real.

verbo—parte de la frase que expresa una acción.

verificar—comprobar la veracidad; certificar con hechos.

verruga—elevación pequeña de la piel formada por la hipertrofia de una papila.

vértebra—huesos en la espina dorsal.

vértice—corona, tope de la cabeza.

vértigo de Meniere—trastorno del oído caracterizado por náuseas, vomito, tinnitus y pérdida auditiva.

vesícula—vejiga o pequeño saco que contiene fluido; elevación de la piel parecida a una ampolla, que contiene fluido seroso.

vesícula biliar—un pequeño saco suspendido debajo del hígado que concentra y guarda la bilis.

viable—con posibilidad de vida.

vial—botella o tubo pequeño de vidrio en el que se guarda medicina o un químico.

vientre—nombre no médico del útero.

villi—vellosidades. Proyecciones pequeñas de una superficie; las vellosidades del intestino delgado absorben nutrientes durante el proceso de la digestión.

virulento—venenoso, letal, maligno.

virus—microorganismo simple, con frecuencia patógeno, capaz de reproducirse al interior de las células.

visceral—relativo a las vísceras, los órganos internos, especialmente el abdomen.

vital—esencial; relativo a la preservación de la vida.

volátil—sustancia que se convierte fácilmente en gas o en vapor; esta cualidad es a menudo altamente peligrosa.

voltaje—medida de fuerza electromotora.

volumen—cantidad de espacio ocupado por un objeto. Se mide en unidades cúbicas.

voluntario—bajo control propio.

vomitar—expeler los contenidos del estómago a través de la boca.

vulnerable—propenso a sufrir lesiones o accidentes.

vulva—genitales externos femenino, incluidos el clítoris, la labia menor y la labia mayor.

xifoide—proceso que forma la punta del esternón.

yacente—acostado.

yeyuno—el segmento medio del intestino delgado, que mide aproximadamente 8 pies de longitud.

yodo—un elemento no metálico que pertenece al grupo alógeno.

z-tract—método a través del cual se inyecta una medicina en forma intramuscular.

Page numbers followed by *f* reference figures. Page numbers followed by *t* reference tables.

Medical Assisting: Administrative and Clinical Competencies, 6th Ed. Student CD-ROM

Minimum System Requirements

Operating System: Microsoft Windows 98 SE, Windows 2000, or Windows XP
Processor: Pentium PC 500 MHz or higher (750 Mhz recommended)
Memory: 64 MB of RAM (128 MB recommended)
Free Disk Space: 650MB
Screen Resolution: 800 x 600 pixels
Color Depth: 16-bit color (thousands of colors)
Macromedia Flash Player 9. The Macromedia Flash Player is free, and can be downloaded from
   http://www.adobe.com/products/flashplayer

Installation Instructions

1. Insert disc into CD-ROM drive. The StudyWare™ installation program should start automatically. If it does not, go to step 2.
2. From My Computer, double-click the icon for the CD drive.
3. Double-click the *setup.exe* file to start the program.

Technical Support

Telephone: 1-800-477-3692, 8:30 A.M.-5:30 P.M. Eastern Time
Fax: 1-518-881-1247
E-mail: delmarhelp@thomson.com

StudyWare™ is a trademark used herein under license.

Microsoft® and Windows® are registered trademarks of the Microsoft Corporation.
Pentium® is a registered trademark of the Intel Corporation.

IMPORTANT! READ CAREFULLY: This End User License Agreement ("Agreement") sets forth the conditions by which Thomson Delmar Learning, a division of Thomson Learning Inc. ("Thomson") will make electronic access to the Thomson Delmar Learning-owned licensed content and associated media, software, documentation, printed materials, and electronic documentation contained in this package and/or made available to you via this product (the "Licensed Content"), available to you (the "End User"). BY CLICKING THE "I ACCEPT" BUTTON AND/OR OPENING THIS PACKAGE, YOU ACKNOWLEDGE THAT YOU HAVE READ ALL OF THE TERMS AND CONDITIONS, AND THAT YOU AGREE TO BE BOUND BY ITS TERMS, CONDITIONS, AND ALL APPLICABLE LAWS AND REGULATIONS GOVERNING THE USE OF THE LICENSED CONTENT.

1.0 SCOPE OF LICENSE

1.1 <u>Licensed Content</u>. The Licensed Content may contain portions of modifiable content ("Modifiable Content") and content which may not be modified or otherwise altered by the End User ("Non-Modifiable Content"). For purposes of this Agreement, Modifiable Content and Non-Modifiable Content may be collectively referred to herein as the "Licensed Content." All Licensed Content shall be considered Non-Modifiable Content, unless such Licensed Content is presented to the End User in a modifiable format and it is clearly indicated that modification of the Licensed Content is permitted.

1.2 Subject to the End User's compliance with the terms and conditions of this Agreement, Thomson Delmar Learning hereby grants the End User, a nontransferable, nonexclusive, limited right to access and view a single copy of the Licensed Content on a single personal computer system for noncommercial, internal, personal use only. The End User shall not (i) reproduce, copy, modify (except in the case of Modifiable Content), distribute, display, transfer, sublicense, prepare derivative work(s) based on, sell, exchange, barter or transfer, rent, lease, loan, resell, or in any other manner exploit the Licensed Content; (ii) remove, obscure, or alter any notice of Thomson Delmar Learning's intellectual property rights present on or in the Licensed Content, including, but not limited to, copyright, trademark, and/or patent notices; or (iii) disassemble, decompile, translate, reverse engineer, or otherwise reduce the Licensed Content.

2.0 TERMINATION

2.1 Thomson Delmar Learning may at any time (without prejudice to its other rights or remedies) immediately terminate this Agreement and/or suspend access to some or all of the Licensed Content, in the event that the End User does not comply with any of the terms and conditions of this Agreement. In the event of such termination by Thomson Delmar Learning, the End User shall immediately return any and all copies of the Licensed Content to Thomson Delmar Learning.

3.0 PROPRIETARY RIGHTS

3.1 The End User acknowledges that Thomson Delmar Learning owns all rights, title and interest, including, but not limited to all copyright rights therein, in and to the Licensed Content, and that the End User shall not take any action inconsistent with such ownership. The Licensed Content is protected by U.S., Canadian and other applicable copyright laws and by international treaties, including the Berne Convention and the Universal Copyright Convention. Nothing contained in this Agreement shall be construed as granting the End User any ownership rights in or to the Licensed Content.

3.2   Thomson Delmar Learning reserves the right at any time to withdraw from the Licensed Content any item or part of an item for which it no longer retains the right to publish, or which it has reasonable grounds to believe infringes copyright or is defamatory, unlawful, or otherwise objectionable.

4.0   PROTECTION AND SECURITY

4.1   The End User shall use its best efforts and take all reasonable steps to safeguard its copy of the Licensed Content to ensure that no unauthorized reproduction, publication, disclosure, modification, or distribution of the Licensed Content, in whole or in part, is made. To the extent that the End User becomes aware of any such unauthorized use of the Licensed Content, the End User shall immediately notify Thomson Delmar Learning. Notification of such violations may be made by sending an e-mail to delmarhelp@thomson.com.

5.0   MISUSE OF THE LICENSED PRODUCT

5.1   In the event that the End User uses the Licensed Content in violation of this Agreement, Thomson Delmar Learning shall have the option of electing liquidated damages, which shall include all profits generated by the End User's use of the Licensed Content plus interest computed at the maximum rate permitted by law and all legal fees and other expenses incurred by Thomson Delmar Learning in enforcing its rights, plus penalties.

6.0   FEDERAL GOVERNMENT CLIENTS

6.1   Except as expressly authorized by Thomson Delmar Learning, Federal Government clients obtain only the rights specified in this Agreement and no other rights. The Government acknowledges that (i) all software and related documentation incorporated in the Licensed Content is existing commercial computer software within the meaning of FAR 27.405(b)(2); and (2) all other data delivered in whatever form, is limited rights data within the meaning of FAR 27.401. The restrictions in this section are acceptable as consistent with the Government's need for software and other data under this Agreement.

7.0   DISCLAIMER OF WARRANTIES AND LIABILITIES

7.1   Although Thomson Delmar Learning believes the Licensed Content to be reliable, Thomson Delmar Learning does not guarantee or warrant (i) any information or materials contained in or produced by the Licensed Content, (ii) the accuracy, completeness or reliability of the Licensed Content, or (iii) that the Licensed Content is free from errors or other material defects. THE LICENSED PRODUCT IS PROVIDED "AS IS," WITHOUT ANY WARRANTY OF ANY KIND AND THOMSON DELMAR LEARNING DISCLAIMS ANY AND ALL WARRANTIES, EXPRESSED OR IMPLIED, INCLUDING, WITHOUT LIMITATION, WARRANTIES OF MERCHANTABILITY OR FITNESS FOR A PARTICULAR PURPOSE. IN NO EVENT SHALL THOMSON DELMAR LEARNING BE LIABLE FOR: INDIRECT, SPECIAL, PUNITIVE OR CONSEQUENTIAL DAMAGES INCLUDING FOR LOST PROFITS, LOST DATA, OR OTHERWISE. IN NO EVENT SHALL THOMSON DELMAR LEARNING'S AGGREGATE LIABILITY HEREUNDER, WHETHER ARISING IN CONTRACT, TORT, STRICT LIABILITY OR OTHERWISE, EXCEED THE AMOUNT OF FEES PAID BY THE END USER HEREUNDER FOR THE LICENSE OF THE LICENSED CONTENT.

8.0   GENERAL

8.1   <u>Entire Agreement</u>. This Agreement shall constitute the entire Agreement between the Parties and supercedes all prior Agreements and understandings oral or written relating to the subject matter hereof.

8.2   <u>Enhancements/Modifications of Licensed Content</u>. From time to time, and in Thomson Delmar Learning's sole discretion, Thomson Delmar Learning may advise the End User of updates, upgrades, enhancements and/or improvements to the Licensed Content, and may permit the End User to access and use, subject to the terms and conditions of this Agreement, such modifications, upon payment of prices as may be established by Thomson Delmar Learning.

8.3   <u>No Export</u>. The End User shall use the Licensed Content solely in the United States and shall not transfer or export, directly or indirectly, the Licensed Content outside the United States.

8.4   <u>Severability</u>. If any provision of this Agreement is invalid, illegal, or unenforceable under any applicable statute or rule of law, the provision shall be deemed omitted to the extent that it is invalid, illegal, or unenforceable. In such a case, the remainder of the Agreement shall be construed in a manner as to give greatest effect to the original intention of the parties hereto.

8.5   <u>Waiver</u>. The waiver of any right or failure of either party to exercise in any respect any right provided in this Agreement in any instance shall not be deemed to be a waiver of such right in the future or a waiver of any other right under this Agreement.

8.6   <u>Choice of Law/Venue</u>. This Agreement shall be interpreted, construed, and governed by and in accordance with the laws of the State of New York, applicable to contracts executed and to be wholly preformed therein, without regard to its principles governing conflicts of law. Each party agrees that any proceeding arising out of or relating to this Agreement or the breach or threatened breach of this Agreement may be commenced and prosecuted in a court in the State and County of New York. Each party consents and submits to the nonexclusive personal jurisdiction of any court in the State and County of New York in respect of any such proceeding.

8.7   <u>Acknowledgment</u>. By opening this package and/or by accessing the Licensed Content on this Web site, THE END USER ACKNOWLEDGES THAT IT HAS READ THIS AGREEMENT, UNDERSTANDS IT, AND AGREES TO BE BOUND BY ITS TERMS AND CONDITIONS. IF YOU DO NOT ACCEPT THESE TERMS AND CONDITIONS, YOU MUST NOT ACCESS THE LICENSED CONTENT AND RETURN THE LICENSED PRODUCT TO DELMAR LEARNING (WITHIN 30 CALENDAR DAYS OF THE END USER'S PURCHASE) WITH PROOF OF PAYMENT ACCEPTABLE TO THOMSON DELMAR LEARNING, FOR A CREDIT OR A REFUND. Should the End User have any questions/comments regarding this Agreement, please contact Thomson Delmar Learning at delmarhelp@thomson.com.